KU-511-689

Physical Activity, Fitness, and Health

International Proceedings and Consensus Statement

Claude Bouchard, PhD
Laval University
Roy J. Shephard, MD, PhD, DPE
University of Toronto
Thomas Stephens, PhD
Thomas Stephens & Associates, Manotick, Ontario

Editors

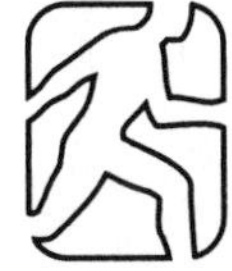

Human Kinetics Publishers

Library of Congress Cataloging-in-Publication Data

Physical activity, fitness, and health : international proceedings and consensus statement / [edited by] Claude Bouchard, Roy J. Shephard, Thomas Stephens & Associates.

p. cm.

Proceedings of the second International Conference on Physical Activity, Fitness, and Health, held in Toronto in May 1992.

Includes bibliographical references.

ISBN 0-87322-522-8

1. Exercise--Physiological aspects--Congresses. 2. Physical fitness--Congresses. 3. Health--Congresses. I. Bouchard, Claude. II. Shephard, Roy J. III. International Conference on Physical Activity, Fitness, and Health (2nd : 1992 : Toronto, Ont.)

QP301.P554 1994

613.7--dc20 93-38996

CIP

ISBN: 0-87322-522-8

The articles in this book were presented at the Second International Consensus Symposium on Physical Activity, Fitness, and Health, held May 5 to May 9, 1992, in Toronto, Canada.

Developmental Editor: Rodd Whelpley; **Managing Editor**: John Wentworth; **Assistant Editors**: Dawn Roselund, Valerie Hall, Anna Curry, and Jackie Blakley; **Copyeditors**: Dawn Barker, Jane Bowers, and Peggy Darragh; **Proofreaders**: Dawn Barker, Kathy Bennett, Karen Dorman, Pam Johnson, and Elizabeth Ragsdale; **Production Director**: Ernie Noa; **Typesetters**: Julie Overholt, Kathy Fuoss, Sandra Meier, Yvonne Winsor, Ruby Zimmerman, and Angie Snyder; **Text Designer**: Keith Blomberg; **Layout Artists**: Julie Overholt and Tara Welsch; **Cover Designer**: Jack Davis; **Photographer (cover)**: David R. Stocklein Photography; **Printer**: Braun-Brumfield

Printed in the United States of America 10 9 8 7 6 5 4 3 2

Human Kinetics

Web site: http://www.humankinetics.com/

United States: Human Kinetics, P.O. Box 5076, Champaign, IL 61825-5076
1-800-747-4457
e-mail: humank@hkusa.com

Canada: Human Kinetics, Box 24040, Windsor, ON N8Y 4Y9
1-800-465-7301 (in Canada only)
e-mail: humank@hkcanada.com

Europe: Human Kinetics, P.O. Box IW14, Leeds LS16 6TR, United Kingdom
(44) 1132 781708
e-mail: humank@hkeurope.com

Australia: Human Kinetics, 57A Price Avenue, Lower Mitcham, South Australia 5062
(08) 277 1555
e-mail: humank@hkaustralia.com

New Zealand: Human Kinetics, P.O. Box 105-231, Auckland 1
(09) 523 3462
e-mail: humank@hknewz.com

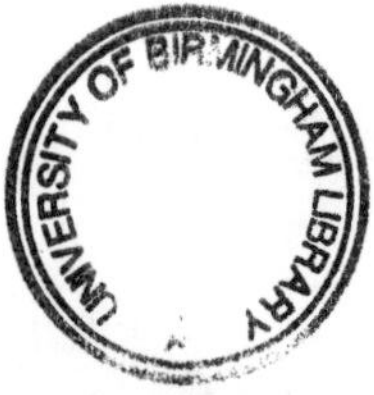

Contents

List of Participants and Contributors

Barbara AINSWORTH
Department of Physical Education
University of North Carolina
CB #8700, Fetzer Gymnasium
Chapel Hill, NC 27599-8700, USA

Per Olof ÅSTRAND
Department of Physiology III
Karolinska Institute
Box 5626
Stockholm S-114-86, Sweden

Richard L. ATKINSON
Department of Internal Medicine
Eastern Virginia Medical School
V.A. Medical Center
Hampton, VA 23667, USA

Mark A. BABCOCK
Department of Preventive Medicine
John Rankin Laboratory of Pulmonary Medicine
University of Wisconsin
504 N. Walnut Street
Madison, Wisconsin 53705, USA

R. James BARNARD
Department of Kinesiology
University of California at Los Angeles
1804 Life Science
Los Angeles, CA 90024, USA

Oded BAR-OR
Children's Exercise Nutrition Center
Chedoke Hospital
McMaster University
Hamilton, Ontario, Canada L8N 3Z5

Tom BENDIX
Department of Rheumatology
Copenhagen Back Center
national University Hospital
Tagensvej 20
DK-2200 Copenhagen, Denmark

Michael BERGER
Division of Metabolism and Nutrition
Heinrich Heine University
Düsseldorf, Germany

Fin BIERING-SØRENSEN
Fysiurgisk Hospital
Rigshospitalet
National University Hospital
25, Havnevej
DK-3100 Hornbæk, Denmark

Steven N. BLAIR
Department of Epidemiology
Institute for Aerobics Research
12330 Preston Road
Dallas, TX 75230, USA

Kari BØ
Norwegian University of Sport and Physical Education
P.O. Box 40
KRINGSJÅ 0807, Oslo 8, Norway

Claude BOUCHARD
Physical Activity Sciences Laboratory
Laval University
Ste-Foy, Québec, Canada GIK 7P4

Joanna L. BOWTELL
Department of Anatomy and Physiology
University of Dundee
Dundee DD1 4HN, Scotland

George A. BROOKS
Department of Physical Education
University of California at Berkeley
103 Harmon Gymnasium
Berkeley, CA 94720, USA

Gail E. BUTTERFIELD
Palo Alto VA Medical Center
3801 Miranda Avenue
Palo Alto, CA 94304, USA

Marshall W. CARPENTER
Women and Infants Hospital
101 Dudley Street
Providence, RI 02905, USA

Richard CASABURI
Division of Respiratory and Critical Care Physiology and Medicine
Harbour-UCLA Medical Center
1000 W. Carson St.
Torrance, California 90509, USA

Carl J. CASPERSEN
Cardiovascular Health Branch
Centers for Disease Control (K-47)
1600 Clifton Road
Atlanta, GA 30333, USA

Tom CHRISTENSEN
Department of Surgery F
Bispebjerg Hospital
Copenhagen, DK-2400, Denmark

Naama W. CONSTANTINI
Woman's Hospital
St-Luke's-Roosevelt Hosptial
Antenucci Building
428 W 59th Street
New York, New York 10019, USA

David C. CUMMING
Department of Obstetrics and Gynecology
University of Alberta
1D1 Walter Mackenzie Health Science Center
Edmonton, Alberta, Canada T6G 2R7

Caroline DAVIS
Bethune College
York University
Downsview, Ontario, Canada M3J 1P3

Michael D. DELP
Department of Medical Physiology
University of Missouri
W116-Veterinary Medical Building
Columbia, Missouri 65211, USA

Kenny DE MEIRLEIR
Sportgeneeskunde 2109
AZ Jette Polykliniek
NIV - 1 Laarbeekin 101
1090 Brüssel, Germany

Jerome A. DEMPSEY
Department of Preventive Medicine
University of Wisconsin
Madison, WI 53705, USA

Jean-Pierre DESPRÉS
Physical Activity Sciences Laboratory
Laval University
Ste-Foy, Québec, Canada GlK 7P4

Rod K. DISHMAN
Department of Exercise Science
University of Georgia
Athens, GA 30602, USA

Barbara DRINKWATER
Department of Medicine
Pacific Medical Center
Seattle, WA 98144, USA

Holly J. DROUGAS
Department of Surgery
Vanderbilt University
Nashville, TN 37232, USA

John V.G.A. DURNIN
Institute of Physiology
The University of Glasgow
Glasgow, G12 8QQ, United Kingdom

V. Reggie EDGERTON
Department of Kinesiology
University of California at Los Angeles
Los Angeles, CA 90024, USA

Randy E. EICHNER
Department of Medicine (EB-271)
University of Oklahoma Health Sciences Center
Oklahoma City, OK 73190, USA

Jenny ETNIER
Department of Exercise Science
Arizona State University
Tempe, Arizona 85287, USA

Robert FAGARD
Department of Medicine
University of Leuven K. U.L.
U.Z. Pellenberg, Weligerveld I
B-3212 Pellenberg, Belgium

Mary C. FAHRENBACH
The Division of Preventive Cardiology
The Miriam Hospital
Providence, Rhode Island 02906, USA

John A. FAULKNER
Department of Physiology
University of Michigan Medical School
7775 Medical Science II - Box 0622
Ann Arbor, MI 48109, USA

Ludwig-Emil FEINENDEGEN
German Nuclear Research Centre
Postfach 1913
5170 Jülich, Germany

Hans G. FISCHER
Institute for Cardiology and Sports Medicine
German University of Sport Sciences
Cologne, Germany

Victor FROELICHER
Cardiology Section
VA Medical Center
Stanford University School of Medicine
Palo Alto, CA 94304, USA

Lise GAUVIN
Department of Exercise Science
Concordia University
7141 Sherbrooke Street West
Montréal, Québec, Canada H4B 1R6

Adria GIACCA
Department of Physiology (Rm 3358)
Medical Science Building
University of Toronto
Toronto, Ontario, Canada M5S 1A8

Norman GLEDHILL
Bethune College, Room 343
York University
Downsview, Ontario, Canada M3J 1P3

Andrew P. GOLDBERG
Geriatrics Service (18)
Baltimore Veterans Administration Medical Center
10 North Greene Street
Baltimore, MD 21201, USA

Howard J. GREEN
Department of Kinesiology
University of Waterloo
Waterloo, Ontario, Canada N2L 3G1

Uwe GUDAT
Division of Metabolism and Nutrition
Heinrich Heine University
Düsseldorf, Germany

James M. HAGBERG
Division of Cardiology
Heart Institute
University of Pittsburgh
School of Medicine
Pittsburgh, PA 15213, USA

Lawrence E. HART
Department of Medicine and Clinical Epidemiology
McMaster University Chedoke-McMaster Hospital
Box 2000, Station "A"
Hamilton, Ontario, Canada L8N 3Z5

Herschel R. HARTER
LSU Medical Center, Shreveport
711 Wood Street
Monroe, Louisiana 71201, USA

William L. HASKELL
Stanford Center for Research in Disease Prevention
Stanford University School of Medicine
730 Welch Road, Suite B
Palo Alto, CA 94304-1583, USA

Wolf-Dieter HEISS
Max-Planck-Institute for Brain Research
Städtische Krankenanstalten
Ost-Merheimer Str. 200
5000 Köln-Merheim, Germany

Karl HERHOLZ
Max-Planck-Institute for Brain Research
Städtische Krankenanstalten
Ost-Merheimer Str. 200
5000 Köln-Merheim, Germany

Hans HERZOG
German Nuclear Research Research Centre
Postfach 1913
5170 Jülich, Germany

James O. HILL
University of Colorado Health Sciences Center
Center for Human Nutrition
Campus Box C225
4200 East Ninth Avenue
Denver, CO 80262, USA

Wildor HOLLMANN
Institut für Kreislaufforschung und Sportmedizin
Deutsche Sporthochschule
5000 Köln 41, Carl Diem Weg
Köln, Müngersdorf, Germany

Robert T. HYDE
Department of Health Research and Policy
Stanford University School of Medicine
HRP Building, Room 113
Stanford CA 94305, USA

Kurt JØRGENSEN
The August Krogh Institute
University of Copenhagen
13 Universitetsparken
DK-2100 Copenhagen, Denmark

Robert KAMAN
Departments of Physiology, Public Health and Preventive Medicine
Texas College of Osteopathic Medicine
Fort Worth, TX 76107, USA

James B. KAMPERT
Department of Health Research and Policy
Stanford University School of Medicine
HRP Building, Room 113
Stanford, CA 94305, USA

Harold W. KOHL
Institute for Aerobics Research
12330 Preston Road
Dallas, TX 75230, USA

Daniel M. LANDERS
Exercise and Sport Research Institute
Department of Health and Physical Education
Arizona State University
Tempe, AZ 85287, USA

M. Harold LAUGHLIN
Departments of Veterinary Biomedical Sciences and Medical Physiology
University of Missouri
W117-Veterinary Medical Building
Columbia, MO 65211, USA

I-Min LEE
Department of Epidemiology
School of Public Health
Harvard University
677 Huntington Avenue
Boston, MA 02115, USA

Pierre LEFÈBVRE
Département de Médecine
Centre Hospitalier Universitaire de Liège
Domaine Universitaire du Sart Tilman
Bloc central +2-B35
B-4000 Liège, Belgique

Arthur S. LEON
Division of Applied Physiology-Nutrition
Division of Epidemiology
School of Public Health
University of Minnesota
Minneapolis, MN 55455, USA

Anne B. LOUCKS
Department of Zoological and Biomedical Sciences
Ohio University
Athens, OH 45701-2979, USA

Duncan MacDOUGALL
Department of Physical Education
McMaster University
1280 Main Street West
Hamilton, Ontario, Canada L8S 4K1

Caroline A. MACERA
Department of Epidemiology and Biostatistics
School of Public Health
University of South Carolina
Columbia, NC 29208, USA

Robert M. MALINA
Department of Kinesiology and Health Education
University of Texas at Austin
Austin, TX 78712, USA

Claus MANNICHE
Department of Rheumatology
Hvidovre Hospital - University Hospital
kettegaards Allé 30
DK-2650 Hvidovre, Denmark

Errol B. MARLISS
Nutrition and Food Science Centre
McGill University 687 Pine Ave West
Montréal, Québec, Canada H3A 1A1

Richard McALLISTER
Departments of Veterinary Biomedical Sciences and Medical Physiology
University of Missouri
W116-Veterinary Medical Building
Columbia, Missouri 65211, USA

Edward McAULEY
Department of Kinesiology
University of Illinois at Urbana-Champaign
215 Freer Hall
Urbana, IL 61801, USA

Neil McCARTNEY
Department of Physical Education
McMaster University
Hamilton, Ontario, Canada L8S 4K1

John D. McKENZIE
Department of Radiology
Duke University Medical Center
Durham, NC 27706, USA

Barry McPHERSON
Faculty of Graduate Studies
Wilfrid Laurier University
75 University Street
Waterloo, Ontario, Canada N2L 3C5

Robert K. MERRITT
Cardiovascular Health Branch
Center for Chronic Disease Prevention and Health Promotion
Centers for Disease Control (K-47)
1600 Clifton Road
Atlanta, GA 30333, USA

David J. MILLWARD
Nutritional Research Unit
London School of Hygiene and Tropical Medicine
St. Pancras Hospital
4 St. Pancras Way
London NW1 2PE, England

Jere H. MITCHELL
UT Southwestern Medical Center
5323 Harry Hines Boulevard
Dallas, TX 75235, USA

Henry J. MONTOYE
Biodynamics Laboratory
University of Wisconsin-Madison
Madison, WI 53706, USA

Sean MOORE
Department of Pathology
McGill University
3775 University Street
Montréal, Québec, Canada H3A 2B4

William P. MORGAN
Sport Psychology Laboratory
University of Wisconsin-Madison
Madison, WI 53706, USA

Frank M. MOSES
Gastroenterology Service
Walter Reed Army Medical Center
6900 Georgia Avenue
Washington, DC 20307-5001, USA

Michelle MOTTOLA
Faculty of Kinesiology
The University of Western Ontario
Thames Hall
London, Ontario, Canada N6A 3K7

Eric A. NEWSHOLME
Department of Biochemistry
Merton College
University of Oxford
South Parks Road
Oxford OX1 3QU, United Kingdom

Henrik NIELSEN
Department of Rheumatology
Copenhagen County Hospital
University Hospital - Ndr. Ringvej
DK-2600 Glostrup, Denmark

David C. NIEMAN
Department of Health, Leisure and Exercise Sciences
Appalachian State University
Boone, NC 28608, USA

Tim D. NOAKES
Department of Physiology
University of Cape Town Medical School
Observatory 7925, South Africa

Pekka OJA
President Urho Kaleva Kekkonen Institute for Health Promotion Research
Kaupinpuistonkatu 1
SF-33500 Tampere 50, Finland

Neil OLDRIDGE
Department of Health Sciences
University of Wisconsin-Milwaukee
P.O. Box 413
Milwaukee, WI 53201, USA

Ralph PAFFENBARGER
Department of Health Research and Policy
Stanford University School of Medicine
Stanford, CA 94305-5092, USA

Richard S. PANUSH
Department of Medicine
New Jersey Medical School
Old Short Hills Road
Livingston, NJ 07039, USA

M. PARRY-BILLINGS
Cellular Nutrition Research Group
Department of Biochemistry
University of Oxford
South Parks Road
Oxford OX1 3QU, United Kingdom

Russell R. PATE
Department of Exercise Science
School of Public Health
University of South Carolina
Columbia, SC 29208, USA

Robert W. PATTON
Department of Health, Physical Education, Recreation and Kinesiology
University of North Texas
Fort Worth, TX 76107, USA

Louis PÉRUSSE
Physical Activity Sciences Laboratory
Laval University
Ste-Foy, Québec, Canada G1K 7P4

John C. PETERS
The Proctor & Gamble Company
Cincinnatti, OH 45230, USA

Steven J. PETRUZZELLO
Department of Health and Physical Education
Arizona State University
Tempe, Arizona 85287, USA

Michael J. PLYLEY
School of Physical and Health Education
University of Toronto
Toronto, Ontario, Canada M5S 1A1

Janet POLIVY
Department of Psychology
Erindale Campus
University of Toronto
Mississauga, Ontario, Canada L5L 1C6

Kenneth E. POWELL
Division of Injury Control
Centers for Disease Control
Mailstop F-36
1600 Clifton Road, N.E.
Atlanta, GA 30333, USA

Z. QING SHI
Department of PHysiology
Medical Sciences Building
University of Toronto
Toronto, Ontario, Canada M5S 1A8

Susan QUAGLIETTI
V.A. Medical Center
Stanford University School of Medicine
Palo Alto, CA 94304, USA

Art QUINNEY
Faculty of Physical Education and Sports Studies
University of Alberta
Edmonton, Alberta, Canada T6G 2H9

Rainer RAURAMAA
Kuopio Research Institute of Exercise Medicine
Puistokatu 20
70110 Kuopio, Finland

Peter RAVEN
Department of Physiology
Texas College Osteopathic Medicine
Fort Worth, TX 76107-2690, USA

Elizabeth READY
Faculty of Physical Education and Recreation Studies
University of Manitoba
Winnipeg, Manitoba, Canada R3T 2N2

W. Jack REJESKI
Department of Health and Sport Science
Wake Forest University
Winston-Salem, NC 27109, USA

Michael J. RENNIE
Department of Anatomy and Physiology
The University of Dundee
Dundee DD1 4HN, Scotland

Erik A. RICHTER
August Krogh Institute
University of Copenhagen
13 Universitetsparken
DK-2100 Copenhagen Õ, Denmark

Roland R. ROY
Brain Research Institute
University of California
1804 Life Sciences
Los Angeles, CA 90024, USA

Walter SALAZAR
Department of Exercise Science
Arizona State University
Tempe, Arizona 85287, USA

James F. SALLIS
Department of Psychology
San Diego State University
San Diego, CA 92182, USA

Art SALMON
ParticipACTION
P.O. Box 64
40 Dundas Street West
Toronto, Ontario, Canada M5G 2C2

Jukka T. SALONEN
Research Institute of Public Health
University of Kuopio
P.O.B. 1627
70211 Kuopio, Finland

Judy M. SEFTON
Alberta Centre for Well-Being
Edmonton, Alberta, Canada T6G 2H9

Mike SHARRATT
Faculty of Applied Health Sciences
University of Waterloo
Waterloo, Ontario, Canada N2L 3G1

Roy J. SHEPHARD
School of Physical and Health Education
University of Toronto
Toronto, Ontario, Canada M5S 1A1

James S. SKINNER
Exercise and Sport Research Institute
Arizona State University
Tempe, AZ 85287-0404, USA

Marcia L. STEFANICK
Stanford Center for Research in Disease Prevention
Stanford University School of Medicine
Palo Alto, CA 94304-1583, USA

George STELMACH
Exercise and Sport Science Institute
Arizona State University
Tempe, AZ 85287-0404, USA

Thomas STEPHENS
Thomas Stephens & Associates
Box 837, 1118 John Street
Manotick, Ontario, Canada K4M 1A7

John R. SUTTON
Cumberland College of Health Sciences
The University of Sydney, P.O. Box 170
Lidcombe, N.S.W., Australia 2141

Jerry R. THOMAS
Department of Exercise Science and Physical Education
Arizona State University
Tempe, AZ 85287-0701, USA

Paul D. THOMPSON
University of Pittsburgh Heart Institute
Montefiore University Hospital
5 South, 3459 Fifth Avenue
Pittsburgh, PA 15213, USA

Charles M. TIPTON
Department of Exercise and Sport Sciences
University of Arizona
Ina E. Gittings Building
Tucson, AZ 85721, USA

Angelo TREMBLAY
Physical Activity Sciences Laboratory
Laval University
Ste-Foy, Québec, Canada GlK 7P4

Arthur C. VAILAS
Biodynamics Laboratory
University of Wisconsin
2000 Observatory Drive
Madison, WI 53706, USA

James C. VAILAS
Manchester Sports Medicine Clinic
35 Kosciusko St.
Manchester, New Hampshire 03101, USA

Mladen VRANIC
Department of Physiology (Rm 3358)
Medical Science Building
University of Toronto
Toronto, Ontario, Canada M5S 1A8

Ilkka M. VUORI
President Urho Kekkonen Institute for Health Promotion Research
Kaupinpuistonkatu 1
SF-33500 Tampere 50, Finland

Janet WALBERG-RANKIN
Division of Health and Physical Education
College of Education
Virginia Polytechnic Institute and State University
Blacksburg, Virginia 24060, USA

Leonard M. WANKEL
Faculty of Physical Education and Recreation
University of Alberta
E-411 Physical Education Building
Edmonton, Alberta, Canada T6G 2H9

Michelle P. WARREN
Department of Obstetrics and Gynecology
St-Luck's-Roosevelt Hospital
Antenucci Building
New York, NY 10019, USA

Lindsay M. WEIGHT
Department of Physiology
Medical School Observatory 7925
University of Cape Town
Cape Town, South Africa

Garry D. WHEELER
Rick Hansen Centre
Department of Physical Education
University of Alberta
Edmonton, Alberta, Canada T6G 2R7

Brian J. WHIPP
Department of Physiology
St-George's Hospital Medical School
University of London
Cranmer Terrace, Tooting
London SW17 ORE, England

Dr. Timothy P. WHITE
Department of Human Biodynamics
University of California
Berkeley, CA 94720, USA

Melvin H. WILLIAMS
Human Performance Laboratory
Old Dominion University
Health and Physical Education Building
Norfolk, VA 23529-0196, USA

Jack H. WILMORE
Department of Kinesiology and Health Education
The University of Texas at Austin
Austin, TX 78712, USA

Alvin L. WING
Department of Health Research and Policy
Stanford University School of Medicine
HRP Building, Room 113
Stanford, CA 94305, USA

Peter D. WOOD
Stanford Center for Research in Disease Prevention
Stanford University School of Medicine
Palo Alto, CA 94304-1583, USA

Bernard ZINMAN
Department of Medicine
Medical Sciences Building
University of Toronto
Toronto, Ontario, Canada M5S 1A8

Preface

In May of 1992, the Second International Consensus Symposium on Physical Activity, Fitness, and Health was held in Toronto, Ontario, Canada. This book contains the text of the consensus achieved during the 4-day symposium, along with chapters of definitions and information about the organization and conduct of the event. The consensus also focuses on the relationships among physical activity, fitness, and health. The 70 chapters prepared by the invited experts detailing the evidence that forms the basis of the consensus are presented in extenso.

Acknowledgments

The editors of this book thank the members of the organizing committees of both the Consensus Symposium and the immediately following International Conference on the topic of physical activity, fitness, and health. The editors are particularly grateful to Dr. Barry McPherson, Wilfrid Laurier University; Dr. Norman Gledhill, York University; Dr. Art Quinney, University of Alberta; and Art Salmon, ParticipACTION, who contributed so much to the development and organization of these events.

The Consensus Symposium Organizing Committee and the Panel of International Advisors

The editors express their gratitude to their colleagues who served on the Consensus Symposium Organizing Committee over a 3-year period, as well as the members of the International Advisory Panel for their contributions to the development and conduct of the Consensus Symposium.

Other Guests and Support Personnel

The editors are greatly indebted to Ms. Dayle Levine, Executive Assistant, for her support throughout the planning, organization, and execution of the symposium. She played a key role in providing administrative support for the conduct of the meeting. Our thanks also go to Dr. Caroline Davis for organizing the registration and assisting during the consensus process. We are indebted to Dr. Davis's family for the hospitality extended to all participants during one evening of the symposium. Special thanks go to Ms. Veronica Jamnik for her organization of the hospitality and social events and assistance during the consensus meeting. We especially appreciate Mr. Stan Murray who coordinated on-site transportation.

Finally, we express our gratitude to all volunteers who helped us prepare and complete the meeting. These volunteers were Janet Bannister, Kelly Broadhurst, Debbie Childs, Michelle Dionne, Tony Doherty, Maria Gurevich, Brandon Hale, Marjorie Hammond, Lyse Jobin, Wendy Keeves, Jodi Liebsman, Denise Mercier, Patricia Murray, Helen Prlic, Marion Reeves, Joe Reischer, Sandra Sawatzky, Ann Marie Vandire, and Lori Wadge.

The Symposium and Conference Organizers gratefully acknowledge the support of the following sponsors and patrons:

Major Sponsors

Ontario Ministry of Tourism and Recreation

Government of Canada, Fitness and Amateur Sport

Additional Sponsors

Air Canada
Canada 125
Canadian Association of Sport Sciences
Canadian Bureau for Active Living
Conners Brewery
Health and Welfare Canada—National Health Research and Development Program
Heart and Stroke Foundation of Canada
Heart and Stroke Foundation of Ontario
Imperial Oil Limited
McDonald's Restaurants of Canada Limited
Medical Research Council of Canada
Merck Frosst Canada Inc.
Molson Breweries of Canada
Ontario Ministry of Citizenship—Office for Seniors' Issues
Ontario Ministry of Health
Ontario Physical and Health Education Association
ParticipACTION
Servier Canada Inc.
Toshiba—Portable Computers and Printers

Patron Universities

Université Laval, Ste-Foy, Québec
University of Alberta, Edmonton, Alberta
Wilfrid Laurier University, Waterloo, Ontario
York University, Downsview, Ontario

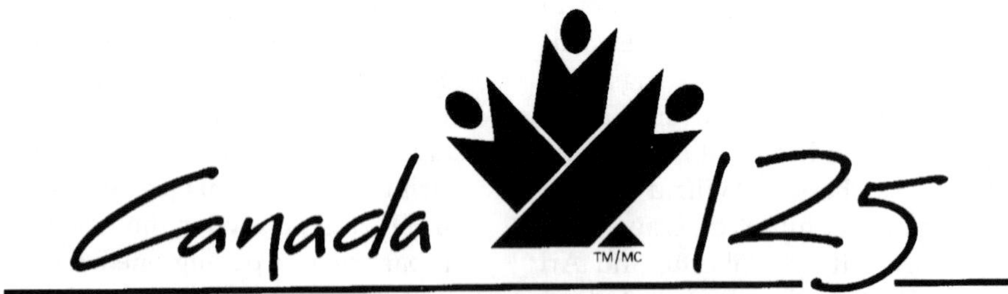

The International Consensus Symposium and The International Conference on Physical Activity, Fitness, and Health were held in conjunction with the celebration of Canada's 125 years of Confederation.

PART I

The Consensus Statement and Introductory Chapters

Chapter 1

Symposium Objectives and the Consensus Process

Canada, and particularly Toronto, has a longstanding tradition with regard to the organization of consensus meetings pertaining to the broad topics of exercise and health. An early initiative was the International Conference on Physical Activity and Cardiovascular Health convened by Roy Shephard in 1966. Toronto was also the site of the 1988 International Consensus Conference on Exercise, Fitness, and Health. In 1992, to coincide with Canada's 125th birthday, two further international meetings were convened in Toronto over a 10-day period. The first of the most recent meetings was the Second International Consensus Symposium on Physical Activity, Fitness, and Health. The full proceedings of the Consensus Symposium, including the consensus text and 70 chapters detailing the supportive evidence form the basis of this volume. The second meeting was a Conference on Physical Activity, Fitness, and Health (the Active Living Conference). The conference was open to all those interested in the areas of program and policy development as it pertains to physical activity, fitness, and health. The proceedings of that conference are presented in a separate publication also from Human Kinetics Publishers.

The objectives of the 1992 Second International Consensus Symposium on Physical Activity, Fitness, and Health were as follows:

- To revise and expand the 1988 Consensus Statement from the perspective of the biological, social and behavioral sciences.
- To achieve a better integration of the evidence regarding the respective and interactive contributions to health of regular physical activity and physical fitness.
- To review in greater depth the evidence linking the components in a general model.
- To provide a better description of the effects of growth, gender, aging and social environments upon the basic model.
- To provide a better quantification of the amount of habitual physical activity associated with each outcome (i.e., the dose–response issue).
- For each topic, to identify the type (experimental, epidemiological, clinical), the quality, and the extent of evidence supporting the conclusions.
- To identify in greater detail, and in a more systematic manner, areas of needed research and the most pressing questions to be addressed.
- To contribute to the knowledge base for the 1992 Conference on Active Living.

The Consensus Symposium Organizing Committee

A Consensus Symposium Organizing Committee took responsibility for the planning, the program development, the organization and the conduct of the event. The members of the Committee and their functions were as follows:

Dr. Claude BOUCHARD
Chairperson of the Consensus Symposium Organizing Committee
Université Laval
Ste-Foy, Québec

Dr. Norman GLEDHILL
Chair of Finance Committee
York University
Downsview, Ontario

Ms. Dayle LEVINE
Executive Assistant
York University
Downsview, Ontario

Dr. Barry McPHERSON
President of the Conference and Consensus Symposium Board
Wilfrid Laurier University
Waterloo, Ontario

Dr. Art QUINNEY
Chairperson of Active Living Conference Organizing Committee
University of Alberta
Edmonton, Alberta

Dr. Elizabeth READY
University of Manitoba
Winnipeg, Manitoba

Mr. Art SALMON
Chair of the Site Committee
ParticipACTION
Toronto, Ontario

Dr. Roy J. SHEPHARD
University of Toronto
Toronto, Ontario

Dr. Thomas STEPHENS
Consultant
Manotick, Ontario

The International Advisors

In addition, a panel of seven advisors from five countries assisted the Consensus Symposium Organizing Committee. The members of this International Advisory Panel were:

Dr. Per-Olof ÅSTRAND
Stockholm, Sweden

Dr. Steven N. BLAIR
Dallas, Texas, USA

Dr. Barbara L. DRINKWATER
Vashon, Washington, USA

Dr. Wildor HOLLMANN
Cologne, Germany

Dr. William P. MORGAN
Madison, Wisconsin, USA

Dr. Eric A. NEWSHOLME
Oxford, England

Dr. John SUTTON
Lidcombe, Australia

Planning of the Consensus Symposium

After 18 months and several meetings of the Consensus Symposium Organizing Committee, the preparation of numerous working documents, an extensive literature search, and frequent exchanges with the International Advisors, a total of 72 topics were selected for inclusion in the program.

A bank of names of individuals with expertise on each topic was created, based on the advice of members of the Consensus Symposium Organizing Committee and the International Advisory Panel. For each name on the list, a computer searched all papers published over the last five years, based on the Institute for Scientific Information literature banks. This list was compiled for each of about 600 scientists. The three to five most productive persons for each topic were retained, and a Science Citation Index or Social Science Citation Index study was carried out on each of them, using the services of the Institute for Scientific Information. The citation surveys were undertaken for about 350 scientists. The process yielded a first and second choice of experts for approximately 65 of the 72 topics. Further consultation was needed to identify the most active group of scientists for the remaining topics.

Invitations were issued to one or two experts per topic about 15 months prior to the Consensus Symposium. Each expert was given the following assignments:

- To prepare a two-page draft of the consensus text proposed for the topic at least three months before the meeting.
- To prepare a full paper documenting the research available on the topic, to be delivered before the symposium with the understanding that it would be revised before publication.
- To attend the 4-day Consensus Symposium in Toronto.
- To participate in the development of the final consensus text.

A document describing the model and the key concepts upon which the Consensus Symposium was based (see chapter 3 by Bouchard and Shephard) was distributed to all participants 6 months prior to the meeting. A series of criteria to be used in the evaluation of the available evidence was also distributed to all participants well ahead of the meeting.

The Consensus Development Process

Based on drafts of the 72 consensus proposals, a preliminary consensus text was prepared and revised by the three editors of this publication. After several rounds of corrections and amendments, the preliminary consensus document was made available to all invited participants about one month prior to the meeting. This text served as the basis for the discussion at the Consensus Symposium.

During the Consensus Symposium, the invited experts were divided into eight working groups. These working groups were constituted around clusters of topics determined by affinity of subject matter. In addition to attending plenary sessions, each working group met for 6 to 8 hours per day, reviewing the evidence and amending or rewriting the consensus statement for the topics that had been assigned to that group. A group leader organized the agenda and ensured that discussion proceeded in an orderly manner. In particular, leaders were encouraged to seek input from all participants, to avoid retreating to bland compromise, and to seek consensus but not necessarily unanimity. Administrative and secretarial support was provided to prepare and distribute revised drafts to members of each group. The major themes, the leaders, the invited participants, and the topics discussed by each group are listed here.

Group 1	Topics
ASSESSMENT, DETERMINANTS, AND ADJUVANTS	
Group Leader: Neil Oldridge, Milwaukee, USA	
Ainsworth, Barbara E.	
Butterfield, Gail E.	Physical activity and nutrition in the context of fitness and health (with A. Tremblay)
Caspersen, Carl J.	Measurement of health status and well being (with K.E. Powell)
Dishman, Rod K.	Determinants of participation in physical activity (with J.F. Sallis)
Gledhill, Norman	
Kaman, Robert	Costs and benefits of an active versus an inactive society (not reviewed by Group 1)
Leon, Arthur S.	Methods of assessing physical activity during leisure and work (with H.J. Montoye)
Montoye, Henry J.	Methods of assessing physical activity during leisure and work (with A.S. Leon)
Oja, Pekka	Laboratory and field tests for assessing health-related fitness (with J.S. Skinner)
Powell, Kenneth E.	Measurement of health status and well being (with C.J. Caspersen)
Sallis, James F.	Determinants of participation in physical activity (with R.K. Dishman)
Skinner, James S.	Laboratory and field tests for assessing health-related fitness (with P. Oja)
Tremblay, Angelo	Physical activity and nutrition in the context of fitness and health (with G.E. Butterfield)
Vuori, Ilkka	Adjuvants to physical activity (with J.H. Wilmore)
Wilmore, Jack H.	Adjuvants to physical activity (with I. Vuori)

Group 2	Topics
HEART AND VASCULAR	
Group Leader: Peter Raven, Fort Worth, USA	
Barnard, James R.	Physical activity, fitness, and claudication (peripheral vascular disease)
Blair, Steven N.	Physical activity, fitness, and coronary heart disease
Fagard, Robert	Physical activity, fitness, and hypertension (with C.M. Tipton)
Froelicher, Victor F.	Physical activity, fitness, and CHD rehabilitation
Haskell, William	Dose–response issues from a biological perspective (not reviewed by Group 2)
Kohl, Harold W.	Physical activity, fitness, and stroke
Laughlin, M. Harold	Physical activity and the microcirculation
Mitchell, Jere	Cardiovascular adaptation to physical activity (with P. Raven)
Moore, Sean	Physical activity, fitness, and atherosclerosis
Thompson, Paul D.	Risk of exercising: medical risks and sudden death
Tipton, Charles M.	Physical activity, fitness, and hypertension (with R. Fagard)
Rauramaa, Rainer	Physical activity, fibrinolysis, and platelet aggregability

Group 3	Topics
PULMONARY, DIGESTIVE, AND URINARY	
Group Leader: Michael J. Plyley, Toronto, Canada	
Bø, Kari	Physical activity, fitness, and bladder
Dempsey, Jerome A.	Pulmonary adaptation to physical activity
Eichner, Randy E.	Physical activity and free radicals
Goldberg, Andrew P.	Physical activity, fitness, and kidney diseases
Hart, Lawrence E.	Assessing the level and quality of evidence and identifying research needs (not reviewed by Group 3)
Moses, Frank M.	Physical activity and digestive processes
Noakes, Tim D.	Physical activity and iron metabolism
Quinney, Art	
Whipp, Brian J.	Physical activity, fitness, and chronic lung diseases

Group 4	Topics
METABOLISM	
Group Leader: Elizabeth Ready, Winnipeg, Canada	
Atkinson, Richard	Physical activity, fitness, and severe obesity
Brooks, George A.	Physical activity and carbohydrate metabolism
Després, Jean-Pierre	Physical activity and adipose tissue
Faulkner, John A.	Physical activity and skeletal muscle (with H.J. Green)
Giacca, Adria	Physical activity, fitness, and Type I diabetes (with M. Vranic)
Green, Howard J.	Physical activity and skeletal muscle (with J.A. Faulkner)
Hill, James O.	Physical activity, fitness, overweight, and moderate obesity
Lefebvre, Pierre	Physical activity, fitness, and Type II diabetes
Rennie, Michael J.	Physical activity and protein metabolism
Richter, Eric A.	Hormonal adaptation to physical activity (with J.R. Sutton)
Stefanic, Marcia L.	Physical activity, lipid metabolism, and lipid transport (with P.D. Wood)
Sutton, John R.	Hormonal adaptation to physical activity (with E.A. Richter)
Vranic, Mladen	Physical activity, fitness, and Type I diabetes (with A. Giacca)
Wood, Peter D.	Physical activity, lipid metabolism, and lipid transport (with M.L. Stefanic)

Group 5	Topics
INFECTION, TRAUMA, AND RISKS	
Group Leader: Mike Sharratt, Waterloo, Canada	
Biering-Sørensen, Fin	Physical activity, fitness, and back pain
Christensen, Tom	Physical activity, fitness, and recovery from surgery or trauma
Drinkwater, Barbara L.	Physical activity, fitness, and osteoporosis
Lee, I-Min	Physical activity, fitness, and cancer
Newsholme, Eric A.	Physical activity, fitness, immune function, and immune disorders
Nieman, David C.	Physical activity, fitness, and infection

Group 5 (Cont.)	Topics
Panush, Richard S.	Physical activity, fitness, and osteoarthritis
Pate, Russell R.	Risk of exercising: musculoskeletal injuries and recreational vehicle accidents
Shephard, Roy J.	Demography of health-related fitness level within and between populations (reviewed by Group 1)
Vailas, Arthur C.	Physical activity and bone and connective tissue

Group 6	Topics
SOCIAL AND PSYCHOLOGICAL ISSUES	
Group Leader: Lise Gauvin, Montréal, Canada	
Landers, Daniel M.	Physical activity, fitness, and anxiety
McAuley, Edward	Physical activity and psychosocial outcomes
McPherson, Barry	
Morgan, William P.	Physical activity, fitness, and depression
Polivy, Janet	Physical activity, fitness, and compulsive behaviors
Rejeski, Jack W.	Dose–response issues from a psychosocial perspective
Stephens, Thomas	Demography of participation in physical activity within and between populations (reviewed by Group 1)
Thomas, Jerry R.	Physical activity and intellectual performance
Wankel, Leonard M.	Physical activity and lifestyle behavior
Williams, Melvin H.	Physical activity, fitness, substance misuse and abuse

Group 7	Topics
BRAIN, NERVOUS SYSTEM, AND AGING	
Group Leader: Duncan MacDougall, Hamilton, Canada	
Åstrand, Per Olof	Physical activity and fitness: evolutionary perspective and trends for the future (not reviewed by Group 7)
Durnin, John	
Edgerton, Reggie V.	Physical activity and peripheral nervous system
Hagberg, James M.	Physical activity, fitness and health, and aging
Hollmann, Wildor	Physical activity and the brain
McCartney, Neil	Physical activity, fitness, and the physically disabled

Group 7 (Cont.)	Topics
Paffenbarger, Ralph	Physical activity, fitness, and quality-adjusted life expectancy (not reviewed by Group 7)
Stelmach, George	Physical activity and perceptual and sensory mechanisms

Group 8	Topics
REPRODUCTIVE HEALTH AND GROWTH	
Group Leader: Michelle Mottola, London, Canada	
Bar-Or, Oded	Childhood and adolescent physical activity and fitness and adult risk profile
Carpenter, Marshall W.	Physical activity, fitness, and health of the pregnant mother and fetus
Cumming, David C.	Physical activity, fitness, and reproductive health in men
Loucks, Anne B.	Physical activity, fitness, and menstrual cycles
Malina, Robert M.	Physical activity, fitness, and growth and development
Pérusse, Louis	Heredity, activity level, fitness, and health (with C. Bouchard) (not reviewed by Group 8)

The working groups were instructed to produce the most valid and complete consensus statement for each topic that had been assigned to them based on the available scientific evidence after taking into account the quality of that evidence. The consensus statement was to be prepared in terms of current status of knowledge and important research questions to be addressed. The consensus document is included in chapter 2.

It is important to recognize that each invited expert reviewed critically and approved the consensus text only for the topics that are indicated above as being on the agenda of his or her particular working group. However, the full consensus document was not reviewed and approved by all the experts taking part in the Consensus Symposium. The three editors assumed responsibility for the final text, paying attention to overall organization of text, redundancies, terminology, grammar, and spelling.

Although this consensus statement has not been reviewed in its entirety by all the symposium attendees, each section represents the collective views of several scientists who spent many hours reviewing and debating the evidence assembled by one of the working group members over the previous year. Thus, the editors feel confident that this statement represents the informed opinion of the most active scientists in each area concerning the relationships of physical activity, fitness and health.

Chapter 2

The Consensus Statement

Assessing the Level and Quality of Evidence

A meaningful consensus document should provide clinicians and researchers with guidance based on current scientific evidence, rather than merely outlining recommendations supported by available literature. Although it is plausible to assert that only the conclusions derived from methodologically defensible studies should be included in consensus documents, the reality of the scientific process demands otherwise. In many instances, consensus guidelines have to draw on somewhat imperfect or incomplete evidence. Defining minimally acceptable criteria for the validity and applicability of published data is therefore essential. To assist with this sort of endeavor, clinical methodologists have developed a comprehensive set of critical appraisal criteria that can be used to scrutinize both clinical and basic science literature.

Criteria have been generated to evaluate studies that deal with clinical measurement, diagnosis, the effectiveness of treatment, prognosis, disease, causation, quality of care, and health economics. Study designs are carefully weighted within each of these categories. Overviews (either meta-analyses or traditional review articles) can also be appraised according to defined criteria. Although randomized control trials are usually considered the benchmark of robust methodology, the findings from studies with other designs merit consideration in instances where randomized control trials are either inappropriate or unavailable.

One study that examined the choice of research methodology in various areas of the sports sciences demonstrated that cohort and cross-sectional designs were the most popular choices, accounting for 72% of all epidemiological studies published in an arbitrary sample of the sports science literature over a 12 month period. A case series approach was identified in 13% of the papers and case control studies constituted 7% of the total. Only 8% of the published papers were randomized control trials.

When applying critical appraisal criteria to this body of literature, the author of this particular review suggested that randomization had not been used, when perhaps it should have been, in approximately six out of every seven therapeutic studies and in two of every three studies on sports physiology or biomechanics. Furthermore, many of the sample sizes reported in the survey would have given inadequate statistical power to support the hypotheses that were advanced. A tendency to overlook the inherent limitations of numerator-based data was a further perceived inadequacy in the spectrum of 756 papers included in the review.

These findings suggest that a higher standard of sports science research will be possible once investigators appreciate the potential advantages of stronger research designs and receive the level of funding required for larger and more sophisticated investigations.

Assessment of Physical Activity, Fitness, and Health

Methods of Assessing Physical Activity During Leisure and Work

The various methods currently available to assess physical activity vary greatly in their applicability in epidemiologic research, intervention studies, clinical practice, and personal assessment. Many measurement problems stem from the fact that physical activity is a complex behavior which generally accounts for 15% to 40% of a person's total energy expenditure. This behavior encompasses physical activity on the job, self-care, household chores, home and yard maintenance, transportation, and discretionary leisure-time activities including fitness-promoting exercise and sports. Health-related dimensions include not only the contribution of physical activity to total energy expenditure, but intensity, duration, and frequency.

About 50 different individual assessment techniques are included under six general categories of physical activity assessment tools (see Table 2.1). Factors affecting selection of an appropriate measurement technique include: the nature of the problem under study; the dimension of physical activity related to health outcomes; the size and demographics of the study population; practicality in terms of cost; time to administer and process

Table 2.1 Physical Activity Assessment Procedures

1. Calorimetry:
   a) Direct heat exchange (in insulated chamber or "space-suit")
   b) Indirect (respirometry)
2. Physiologic markers:
   a) Heart rate monitoring
   b) Doubly isotopically labeled water
   c) Cardiorespiratory endurance ($\dot{V}O_2$max)
3. Mechanical and electronic motion detectors:
   a) Pedometer
   b) In-shoe step counters
   c) Electronic motion sensors
   d) Accelerometers
4. Behavioral observations
5. Dietary energy intake (food diary)
6. Occupational and leisure-time survey instruments:
   a) Job classification
   b) Global self-assessment
   c) Activity diaries or records
   d) Recall questionnaires
   e) Quantitative histories

the measurements; appropriateness and acceptability to study subjects; compatibility and nonreactivity with usual daily activities; and the reliability and validity of the instrument used.

Calorimetry and doubly labeled water can provide accurate measurements of average daily energy expenditure under controlled laboratory conditions. The precise measurement of energy intake under conditions of weight maintenance also provides a good estimate of daily energy expenditure. In addition, behavioral observation techniques and physical activity diaries or records yield information about specific activity patterns. Although these methods are not practical for use in large population studies, they are useful with small samples and for validation of physical activity survey questionnaires. Other less accurate validation techniques commonly employed for validating survey instruments include heart rate monitoring, electronic and mechanical motion detection, and various measurements of physical fitness, particularly $\dot{V}O_2$max, and associations with chronic diseases (e.g., coronary heart disease).

Questionnaire methods are currently the most popular and practical approaches for large population studies because of the volume and detail of information that they provide relative to cost and time invested. Assignment of levels of physical activity according to specific job categories or occupational titles also has been commonly employed in population studies because of its simplicity; however, the accuracy of this technique for physical activity classification is questionable. Global self-reports, which require individuals to respond to a limited number of simple questions about their usual physical activity habits, have good repeatability and fair validity. A wide variety of self- or interviewer-administered physical activity questionnaires of various lengths and complexities are currently available.

It is possible to select and/or score questionnaires to assess different physical activity dimensions. The length of the recall periods in these questionnaires generally varies from one week to a year, but some assess "usual" physical activity participation patterns, and the emphasis usually is on high intensity activities. The retrospective quantitative history (for example, the Minnesota Leisure-Time Physical Activity Questionnaire) is a more comprehensive form of survey procedure; it asks for the month-by-month frequency and duration of an extensive list of activities. The trade-off is greater cost, because increased time is required for administration and data processing.

IMPORTANT RESEARCH TOPICS

1. Standardized physical activity questionnaires are needed to identify and monitor secular trends over the entire spectrum of energy expenditure and dimensions of physical activity for representative samples of various populations and cultures in different areas of the world, including relevant subsets based on age and gender. Such questionnaires also can be useful for behavioral research to better define determinants of physical activity and exercise, and assess the effects of interventions.
2. The reliability and validity of existing and new physical activity questionnaires should be determined using existing and improved criteria standards.
3. Additional research is required to develop objective measures of physical activity (such as improved motion sensors) better suited to epidemiologic investigations, as well as for assessing clinical interventions and personal activity guidance.
4. There is a need to identify the most concise survey questions that reflect specific health-related dimensions of physical activity.
5. Basic research is also needed on how people encode, store, and recall specific information about physical activity.

Laboratory and Field Tests for Assessing Health-Related Fitness

In the assessment of physical and physiological fitness, it is important to identify whether the information relates to performance or health-related fitness. Most of the current methods for assessing fitness have evolved in the context of performance-related fitness. Their usefulness as measures of health-related fitness has not been systematically evaluated. It is important to distinguish between *performance-related norms* (e.g., below average, average, and above average) which are used to classify people in relation to their peers and *health-related criterion standards* (e.g., undesirable, minimal, acceptable, and desirable) which are used for screening, guidance, and encouragement. Most adults do not need to be tested. Instead, they need information about minimal and desirable levels of the various aspects of health-related fitness required for good health and independence. And they need to know about the amount and types of exercise needed to reach these levels. Unfortunately, little is known about the minimal levels of such factors as muscular strength or flexibility that are needed at different age groups and in different health states.

Morphological Fitness

For large scale practical assessment of body composition factors involved in health-related fitness, the body mass index, selected skinfolds from the limbs and trunk, and the waist to hip circumference ratio will provide reasonable estimates of (a) body fat content and (b) regional fat distribution (especially subcutaneous fat).

IMPORTANT RESEARCH TOPICS

6. More direct methods are needed to determine body composition. Simpler and more accurate indirect methods are also needed for field surveys. Further study is needed of the influence of such factors as age, gender, and disease upon population differences of body composition.
7. There is a need to modify techniques for the assessment of body composition, developing prediction equations and reference values that will allow the indirect assessment of body fatness, including regional fat distribution and the amount of abdominal visceral fat.

Bone Strength

In the context of health, bone strength is essentially synonymous with bone mineral density. The loss in bone mineral density with age is associated with a higher risk of osteoporosis and bone fractures. Exercise may lower the risk of fractures and osteoporosis by countering bone loss, by enhancing neuromuscular abilities that help to avert falls, and by reducing the impact if a fall occurs. Although there is evidence that exercise increases peak bone mass and attenuates the bone loss with age, the exact dose-response relationship between exercise and bone mineral density is not known. Densitometry is the best method to obtain useful, accurate information on bone mineral density, but will probably remain a research tool for some time to come. There are non-invasive methods to measure bone "stiffness," but too few studies have been carried out to evaluate their usefulness adequately.

IMPORTANT RESEARCH TOPICS

8. Simpler, inexpensive methods are needed to assess bone health.
9. Long-term prospective studies are needed to determine: (a) the health importance of bone "stiffness," (b) the sensitivity of densitometry and other indirect methods to measure the changes in bone mineral density and in bone stiffness that occur as a result of age or various interventions, and (c) the accuracy with which densitometric and other indirect methods can predict the risk of fractures in various populations.

Muscular Fitness

Although it is clear that strength and health are related, once strength falls below levels needed to accomplish the activities of daily living, the association among health, strength, and endurance of muscle groups other than the legs (e.g., those in the upper body) is poorly known. Research on health-related muscular fitness has focused on the possible role of a lack of trunk muscle strength and endurance in the development of back, neck, and shoulder problems. It is unclear what types and combinations of muscular fitness (isometric, isotonic, isokinetic power, strength, or endurance) are most important in this regard. The performance of specific muscle groups can be assessed in the laboratory, but this generally requires equipment be used under strictly controlled and standardized conditions. The practical health application of the data obtained remains questionable.

Traditional field tests of trunk-muscle fitness include repeat sit-ups and a variety of static or dynamic back extension tests. None of these procedures is fully satisfactory with respect to feasibility, safety, reliability, and validity when assessing large groups of individuals.

Flexibility

General flexibility is believed to be important for health, especially in terms of extending the period of independence in older adults. Trunk flexibility may also have health implications for back, neck, and shoulder problems. Several observational, cross-sectional studies have found that poor thoraco-lumbar and/or lumbar mobility may be related to an increased risk of back problems.

The static range of motion of specific joints can be assessed accurately in the laboratory, but there are problems of standardization and of equipment. Field assessment of trunk flexibility includes variations of the sit-and-reach and stand-and-reach tests. Maximal reach tests are affected by the relative length of upper and lower limbs, involve a significant tolerance component, and may be unsafe for some people. Interpretation of the results is difficult. Lateral spine bending is an unambiguous, simple, and safe test, but its health-related role is unknown.

IMPORTANT RESEARCH TOPICS

10. More studies are needed to establish firmly the relationship between musculoskeletal fitness and physical function or other aspects of health.
11. Criterion standards of trunk muscle strength and endurance and trunk mobility are needed in different populations, especially in older adults.
12. Standardized, feasible and safe field tests of muscle strength and endurance and flexibility are needed.
13. The validity, feasibility, safety and subject acceptability of most field tests of musculoskeletal fitness need to be studied in different populations.

Motor Fitness

Postural control can affect musculoskeletal health by decreasing the risk of falls which may lead to bone fractures. The assessment of postural control is a complex task and its complete determination may require several approaches using kinematic and biomechanical methods.

IMPORTANT RESEARCH TOPICS

14. More research is needed to establish the relationship between postural control and physical function as well as other aspects of health.
15. The scientific quality (validity, reliability, and feasibility) of the present tests of postural control needs to be assessed and new tests developed.

Cardiorespiratory Fitness

The two health-related components of cardiorespiratory fitness are maximal aerobic power and the ability to perform prolonged submaximal exercise (submaximal cardiorespiratory capacity). The traditional objective laboratory assessment of $\dot{V}O_2max$ usually requires a treadmill or a cycle ergometer, apparatus involving rhythmic, dynamic exercise with a large and standardized muscle mass capable of maximally stressing the systems for transporting and utilizing oxygen. For direct measurement of oxygen consumption, gas analysis equipment is needed.

It has been argued that cardiorespiratory capacity or efficiency during submaximal work may be important for reducing fatigue in heavy industry or, in an older person, extending the ability to undertake the activities of daily living. However, there is no direct evidence that the ability to perform prolonged submaximal exercise is related to health. While $\dot{V}O_2max$ is conceptually and methodologically unambiguous, the exact characteristics of submaximal cardiorespiratory capacity need to be defined, and appropriate assessment methods need to be developed. Measures of cardiovascular function during submaximal exercise may be useful in this regard.

There is little inherent reason to measure $\dot{V}O_2max$ for health-related purposes. If a submaximal procedure of adequate precision was available, a better approach might be to estimate maximal aerobic power from submaximal tests, so that large numbers of middle-aged and older adults could be evaluated with less risk. Indirect field tests of maximal aerobic power currently provide reliable and valid estimates of population averages.

IMPORTANT RESEARCH TOPICS

16. More research is needed to establish a firm relationship between cardiorespiratory fitness (maximal and submaximal factors) and various components of health.
17. Within the context of health-related fitness, more precise and valid tests of submaximal cardiorespiratory capacity are needed.

Metabolic Fitness

Metabolic fitness has been defined as resulting "from adequate hormonal actions, particularly for insulin, normal blood and tissue carbohydrate and lipid metabolism, and a favorable ratio of lipid to carbohydrate oxidized." It has been shown that various aspects of health are associated with glycemic status, lipid-lipoprotein profile, and the ratio of lipid to carbohydrate oxidation. It has also been shown that regular endurance training favorably affects these factors.

Although the concept of metabolic fitness makes intuitive sense, there is no consensus about a definition since this might include many other factors (e.g., other hormones and substrates). Nor do we know how all these factors should be measured and applied to health-related fitness. There are standardized procedures for measuring fasting blood glucose, glucose and insulin responses to a glucose load, and fasting blood lipid and lipoprotein profiles. However, there are no standardized tests that would evaluate the ratio of lipid to carbohydrate oxidation and allow its relevance to health to be studied.

IMPORTANT RESEARCH TOPICS

18. The conceptual definition of metabolic fitness should be clarified and extended.
19. Other physiological and biochemical factors which might be involved in metabolic fitness need to be explored.

Measurement of Health Status and Quality of Life

The careful study of physical activity and health requires precise measurement of both concepts. The measurement of health is complex, depending on the conceptual and pragmatic definition used. There are at least five facets of health, with potential for corresponding measures. A genetic facet governs basic health structure and influences the other four facets of health. Biochemical, physiologic, and morphologic conditions reflect a facet of health that determines disease, illness, organ impairment, disability, or handicap. A functional facet, closely related to this, includes the capacity to undertake the usual activities and requirements of daily life. Mental facets include mood and cognitive processes. The facet of health potential includes longevity, functional potential, and the extent of any disability. Measurement genres reflect these facets and include mortality, morbidity, risk factor prevalence, use of medical care, disability, physical function, mental function, functional activities, bodily well being, emotional well being, self-concept, global perceptions of health, and healthy life years. Physical activity impinges upon most of these facets and measures of health.

Measures of health status depend on the goals of the assessment and how one makes and uses the observations. The objective may be to evaluate or to predict health. Alternatively, there may be a wish to test the response to clinical interventions, health promotion efforts, or systems for the delivery of medical care. Such evaluations can stimulate economic, social, and political reform, but must consider changes in and vagaries of disease and health classification. Health status measures have to date tended to focus on disease events rather than individual health. However, individual measures, like health risk appraisals, can help to evaluate and encourage efforts at health promotion.

Traditional measures have focused on the absence of health. Mortality statistics take death as an end point and try to attribute specific causes of death. They can also project life expectancy at specified ages. Common measures of morbidity are disease incidence, case-fatality ratios, hospital admissions, bed-days, treatment costs, and lost days of work for specific causes. Morbidity and mortality statistics should separate disease events from measures of disease or illness burden like hospital days and treatment costs. However, combined morbidity and mortality measures like quality-adjusted life expectancy may be more useful in evaluating program effectiveness. Medical care cost indicators reflect the economic burden of mortality, morbidity and other direct and indirect costs associated with specific diseases. International and intercultural comparisons of these and other measures of health status may be impeded by differences in classification schema, data collection procedures, and geopolitical circumstances, which may also change over time.

Because of the high costs of collecting and compiling data, morbidity statistics usually come from smaller, less representative samples than the total population. Errors in recording, classifying, or processing data limit the utility of morbidity and mortality statistics, and inevitably they do not reflect positive health status.

Problems in conceptualizing constructs, especially positive health status, have hindered the measurement of health. Moreover, inadequate data sources and resources have restricted the development of measures even when appropriate measurement concepts exist. Nonetheless, progress continues in the development of measures that reflect well-being and functioning. Well-being includes concepts like bodily well-being, emotional well-being, self-concept, and global perceptions of health. Functioning includes physical and cognitive functioning, and the capacity to perform both the discretionary and the essential activities of daily living. Investigators have used such population-based measures as two-week disability days, disability-free life expectancy, and psychological well-being as measures of the quality of life. Global health measures include healthy life expectancy or disability-free life expectancy. Such measures of positive health may be useful in international and intercultural comparisons. The availability of data for many measures is limited by the validity of the existing instruments and the capacity to reflect a simple summary score.

Different measures of health are appropriate to different age groups and to each sex to the extent that their sociologic, behavioral, and health concerns and needs differ. Morbidity and mortality statistics are more useful in reflecting the health status of older adult populations who are affected by a variety of chronic diseases. Estimated years of potential life lost can help to emphasize diseases that kill younger populations, especially where chronic disease morbidity or mortality are very low. Quality of life measures have proven valuable in reflecting the health status of older adults where functional impairment, morbidity and disability are commonplace. These measures may also be useful in reflecting the positive health of younger age groups, even where morbidity, disability, and functional impairment are rare. However, quality of life measures suitable for younger populations are only starting to evolve.

IMPORTANT RESEARCH TOPICS

Because physical activity has an important influence on health, the following research recommendations apply to physical activity as it relates to the measurement of health. Each research recommendation reflects both generic as well as condition-specific health facets. They should focus on positive health. They should also represent the needs, interests, and special concerns of varying population subgroups, including children, women, older adults and the disadvantaged. Specifically, research efforts should include the following.

20. Develop reliable and valid measures that are sensitive to changes in individual and population health.
21. Develop outcome measures suitable for epidemiologic research, health promotion programs and preventive services, as well as composite measures for the assessment of functioning morbidity, mortality, and disability (e.g., quality adjusted life years).
22. Explore different methods of refining, weighing, and identifying the structure, utility, and preference of various health states in order to elucidate the meaning of composite health scores such as quality-adjusted life expectancy.

Physical Activity, Fitness, and Health: Status and Determinants

Demography of Leisure-Time Physical Activity

Recent questionnaire surveys in Australia, Canada, and the United States suggest that about 40% of adults are active enough in their leisure-time to obtain a variety of health benefits. That is, they exercise regularly at activities of at least moderate intensity. Ten percent of adults in these countries report exercising at least three times weekly for 20 or more minutes at an intensity considered sufficient to develop and/or sustain cardiorespiratory fitness. Depending on how "sedentary" is defined, at least one third to one half of adults in these countries fall into this category.

In Australia, Canada, Finland, the former German Democratic Republic, and the United States, there has been a modest increase in the self-reported prevalence of healthful levels of exercise over at least the past decade. This increase does not extend to heavy exercise for all these countries. In Australia, there is some hint of a recent levelling off while heavy exercise has recently become less common in Canada.

Although good data on non-leisure activity are scarce, Finnish surveys show steadily decreasing occupational activity, including bicycling to work. This is probably typical of countries where increased exercise has been reported, but it is not possible to make any statements about long-term trends in total energy expenditure.

There is considerable consistency among nations in the relationship of self-reported, leisure-time, physical activity levels to sex, age, and education. Sex differences are minimal when exercise intensity is moderate or light, that is, males and females report spending about the same amount of time exercising. Male-female differences are most pronounced when the definition of "active" involves high-intensity exercise (except when "high intensity" is defined relative to capacity in a sex-specific manner). Males are, on average, 50% more likely to report being vigorously active than females. Women appear to have increased their overall exercise levels more rapidly than men in the 1980s, but this is probably not true of vigorous exercise.

National surveys of physical activity consistently reveal that, by most definitions, including total active time or total energy expended per week, exercise prevalence declines steadily with age. When age-specific values for relative intensity are used as a means of defining vigorous activity, this trend disappears. The only population survey that included children and adolescents shows a precipitous drop in activity on leaving high school. Older adults increased their exercise levels more than younger ones during the 1980s.

Leisure-time physical activity is consistently more common among groups with more education. Recent surveys in Australia, Britain, Canada, and the United States all reveal that the most educated group is 50 to 200% more likely than the least educated group to undertake deliberate exercise. There is mixed evidence as to the fate of the education gap over the recent past. Canadian data show a modest narrowing of the gap from 1981 to 1988, whereas a slight widening was found in the United States for the period 1986 to 1990.

IMPORTANT RESEARCH TOPICS

23. Further monitoring of leisure-time activity in adult populations is needed to identify (a) whether the prevalence of exercise is still increasing, and (b) if women, older adults, and less educated groups are closing the gap by becoming more active more quickly than the rest of the population.
24. New studies are required to determine (a) if other countries, including less industrialized countries, have similar activity levels, and (b) if occupational demands and other sources of physical activity are diminishing as suspected.
25. Better data are needed on people with low levels of activity, children, and older adults and on forms of physical activity other than deliberate exercise (occupational activity, personal transportation, household chores). Customarily-used questionnaire methods will have to be adapted for these purposes.
26. Population surveys should provide sufficient detail on activity type, intensity, frequency, duration, seasonality, and social context to permit investigation of exercise stimuli and dosages relevant to all dimensions of health-related fitness. Guidelines are needed to develop the questionnaires for such surveys.
27. Definitions of exercise dose should be standardized with respect to intensity, frequency, and duration. When relative intensity is used, age- and sex-related adjustments should be consistently applied, and should be based on better data than are currently available.

Determinants of Participation in Physical Activity

As the health consequences of physical activity and inactivity become better documented, it becomes more important to understand the factors that influence participation in active leisure behavior (exercise). These influences, often termed "determinants," can be categorized as personal attributes, environmental characteristics, and features of the physical activity itself.

Though most studies prior to 1988 were conducted on non-representative samples, two-thirds of the more recent studies have employed community samples. Therefore, their findings should be more widely generalizable than earlier results, at least to "whites" from North America and Australia. Whereas earlier studies had focused on men, two thirds of the studies currently reviewed had women and men as subjects. Previous reviews had called for prospective studies, and half of the studies currently reviewed had follow-ups ranging from 7 weeks to 15 years. The continuing shortcomings are the emphasis on maintenance and dropout rather than adoption of exercise, and the restriction to vigorous exercise rather than including lower intensity activities.

Demographic variables continue to be among the most consistent and strongest correlates of vigorous exercise. In general, younger, male, well-educated, and, in North America, non-hispanic, "white" subgroups tend to be more active than others. Contrary to popular belief, there is little relationship between exercise patterns during youth, obesity, or smoking, and adult exercise habits. Self-efficacy, self-schemata, expectation of benefits, intention to exercise, and barriers are generally related to exercise participation, while attitudes and knowledge are not. In cross-sectional and prospective studies, social factors, especially specific social support for exercise, are usually significant correlates of exercise behavior. Few physical environment variables have been studied, but objectively measured access to facilities is related to participation in formal exercise programs. Both the intensity and the perceived effort of exercise are negatively correlated with participation. These findings suggest that most people prefer lower intensity activities.

Consistent associations were found in every category of determinants. These findings emphasize the importance of viewing exercise behavior as being influenced by many personal and environmental forces.

Twenty recent studies were reviewed. They represent methodological advances over the interventions reviewed for the 1988 consensus. Internal validity and generalizability have improved. Prior to 1988, most intervention studies used uncontrolled case and cohort designs. Since 1988, more than half the studies have used randomized or quasi-experimental designs, including large samples of males and females of various ages. A few studies of ethnic and minority groups have appeared, but such studies have largely been limited to the United States.

The existing literature permits the following conclusions regarding interventions designed to increase exercise participation.

1. Educational counseling and behavior modification or cognitive-behavior modification principles can be implemented with exercise programs. They are generally accompanied by an increased frequency of exercise or of the time spent in exercising at least for the limited periods of observation (typically 4 to 20 weeks).

2. With the exception of studies closely linked with onsite programs or periodic supervision (e.g., work site, clinics, or schools), the studies do not demonstrate that either exercise intensity or the total volume of daily physical activity has been increased enough to improve physical fitness, or to reduce the risk of future morbidity or mortality.

3. Most studies have used either indirect measures of exercise behavior (e.g., self-reports) or simple measures of physical fitness, based on heart rate or treadmill time. The absence of uniform outcome measures prevents a clear comparison of results across studies.

4. Most interventions have not been based on a broader theoretical model of behavioral change, such as stage theories, nor have they considered overall activity history or the companion literature on the determinants of exercise behavior.

Interventions, regardless of type, are usually associated with moderate increases in the frequency of exercising. An increase in adherence success from about 4 in 10 participants without intervention, to about 6 in 10 participants following intervention, is typical. The superiority of behavior change interventions versus a reduction in the intensity, duration, and frequency of the usual prescriptions used for increasing physical fitness merits direct testing.

Increases in physical activity or fitness associated with the interventions diminished as follow-up time increased. Few comparisons have used an attention-control condition. Therefore, generalizations about the effectiveness of specific components of the interventions for specific populations are not possible.

Although there have been too few studies since 1988 to permit meaningful clustering of effect sizes according to other important characteristics of the studies, it appears that the size of the intervention effects reported has been inversely related to the scientific quality of the studies.

IMPORTANT RESEARCH TOPICS

28. Research on determinants should focus on personal and environmental variables that can be manipulated and applied in interventions. When feasible, findings from observational studies need to be verified by experimental research. Genetic and biological factors influencing exercise behavior also need to be understood.
29. Determinants, and their relative importance, are likely to vary for different populations, population subgroups, and cultures. These differences need to be investigated. What are the similarities and differences in the determinants of

exercise behavior for men and women, and for peoples of different ages, ethnic groups, education, and geographic locations?

30. More and better studies of the determinants of various dimensions of exercise behavior, particularly different intensities and types, including sedentary behaviors, are needed.
31. More studies of the determinants of the adoption of regular exercise are needed. Continued study of adherence, long-term maintenance, and relapse is also recommended.
32. Studies should use valid measures of physical activity as well as valid measures of potential determinants that are comparable across studies. Objective measures of environmental determinants should be developed.
33. The primary need is for the development and evaluation of efficacious approaches that encourage the adoption and long-term maintenance of exercise behavior. Personal, environmental, and exercise characteristics reported as important in observational studies should be targeted in intervention research. Interventions probably require tailoring to specific populations, subpopulations, and cultures, but the means of tailoring are as yet not well developed. Face-to-face interventions, suited to clinically-based applications, should be compared with mediated interventions (e.g., television, telephone, and mail) suited for large-scale population-interventions to determine their relative effectiveness. Methods for documenting and improving the quality of intervention (e.g., program leadership) should be studied.
34. Interventions have disproportionately emphasized a change of personal attributes (e.g., attitudes, intentions, and self-efficacy) among exercise participants, but the efficacy of the interventions which have been used in attempts to change these psychological attributes has not been established. There is a need to evaluate interventions that target variables in the social and physical environments.
35. There is a need to develop valid measures for assessing the rewarding experiences and outcomes of exercise participation that can reinforce participation and minimize the likelihood of relapse to sedentary habits.
36. There is a need to determine the types, intensities, durations, locations, social settings and times of exercise that maximize the likelihood of its adoption and maintenance.
37. There is a need to standardize, or to reconcile, different measures of exercise behavior.

Assessing Population Levels of Health-Related Fitness: Methodological Concerns

Demographic studies within populations have yielded useful information on growth, aging, and sex-related differences of health-related fitness. Effects of socio-economic status and overall lifestyle have also been demonstrated, and associations between individual markers of fitness have been explored. However, the interpretation of demographic data is currently hampered. Key considerations include the following:

- Whether the samples of subjects tested are representative of the populations under discussion.
- The extent of allowance for specific factors that distort cross-sectional survey results.
- The ability to counter the problems that develop when longitudinal observations are collected over several decades.
- The severe technical constraints that are imposed by measurement techniques appropriate to large-scale surveys.
- The interactive impact of such surveys upon population fitness and health.

In terms of sampling, a large proportion of data has been obtained on convenience samples. Because of barriers such as geography and language, even entire communities may be representative only of themselves. In larger communities, data may be restricted to those born in a single year, with complications from cohort effects. Relatively few investigators have attempted to collect data on stratified random samples of national populations. Such information becomes heavily distorted because a high proportion of older individuals are excluded from the evaluation.

Even if large samples are recruited, the results of cross-sectional surveys are affected by climatic factors, selective migration, intercurrent pathologies, and differences in the life experience of various age cohorts. Seasonal factors, once recognized, are readily countered by spreading observations randomly over the entire year. The problem of chronic disease becomes widespread in older segments of most communities, complicating comparisons of data both within and between populations. Activity patterns, nutrition and lifestyle differ between age-cohorts in many communities, further limiting the potential for meaningful comparisons.

Longitudinal surveys do not resolve all technical difficulties. The constancy of methodology and of subjective responses to testing must be assured. The effects of aging tend to become confounded with secular trends in community behavior, and except in isolated communities, sample attrition is a major problem. Currently, the ideal approach is a mixed cross-sectional/longitudinal design.

International standardization of methodology has rarely been applied in interpopulation comparisons. Occasional surveys have applied high technology methodology to large populations, but usually the interpretation of data is complicated by the use of very simple test procedures that lack a strong relationship to health-related fitness.

Intrapopulation comparisons commonly examine effects of age, sex, socio-economic factors, activity patterns, and overall lifestyle. Sampling problems are less critical when making comparisons within a given population. However, whether comparing men to women, or children of various ages, there remains a critical need for agreement on methods of allowing for interindividual differences in body size. Gender-related differences also become confounded with cultural influences. Probably because of methodological problems, large-scale surveys show surprisingly little influence of reported activity upon estimates of fitness. Likewise, the observed relationship between fitness and other facets of lifestyle has been quite limited. On the other hand, there are substantial differences of activity patterns related to socio-economic status.

Interpopulation comparisons are currently severely limited by the lack of representative data. Body mass for height appears to be substantially lower in many of the economically poorer countries, and such regions generally show health advantages in terms of blood pressure and serum cholesterol. However, if aerobic power is expressed in ml/(kg × min), there are surprisingly few differences among different countries.

The challenges to future investigators are to adopt more appropriate sampling techniques, to devise methodology that remains valid within the context of a large survey, and to establish dose/response relationships that will enable a definition of clinically significant interpopulation differences in the variables under examination.

IMPORTANT RESEARCH TOPICS

38. Sampling techniques—there is a pressing need to develop better recruitment methods to reduce the response bias inherent in most current population studies, particularly the underrecruitment of older individuals and those from lower socio-economic strata.
39. Choice of criteria for population health—should we be concerned with the mean level of fitness reached by a given population or with the proportion of that population who fail to meet a certain minimum standard on selected variables?
40. Significant fitness levels—populations may score well on one criterion, but poorly on another. Thus, in assessing interpopulation differences, there is a need to identify which are the most important components of fitness from the viewpoint of health. It will be necessary to determine how these variables interact with each other, and to develop accurate and internationally standardized techniques for the assessment of such fitness on samples of population.
41. Significant covariates—in assessing the impact of fitness levels upon health, it is necessary to develop and to use simple, standardized techniques to assess important covariates such as cigarette smoking, nutrition and exposure to air pollutants.
42. There remains a need to carry out well-controlled interpopulation comparisons of health-related fitness, using standardized techniques.

Physical Activity, Nutrition, Fitness, and Health

Physical activity increases the utilization of many nutrients. The ability to perform vigorous exercise depends on the replacement of these nutrients through diet. Of particular concern are the nutrients used as fuel and water. Other nutrients are also of interest, such as the vitamins used during fuel oxidation, and the vitamins and minerals necessary for oxygen transport and protection against increased oxygen flux. However, much misinformation is currently purveyed to the public regarding the need for special ergogenic aids at all levels of exercise, and such misinformation should be countered.

Lipids and carbohydrates are normally the main sources of food energy. A small carbohydrate intake seems sufficient to allow a complete oxidation of lipids without detrimental ketone body production. Prolonged aerobic exercise induces an increase in carbohydrate utilization and a depletion of carbohydrate stores; the latter effect is associated with an increase in postexercise lipid oxidation. The enzymatic adaptations observed after exercise favor glycogen resynthesis, which is maximized by the ingestion of a high carbohydrate diet. Under high-fat diet conditions, the body still gives a priority to the restoration of carbohydrate reserves. The notion that glucose or sugar feeding during the hour before exercise induces an insulin hypoglycemia, and thus increases glycogen use at the beginning of exercise, remains controversial. Moreover, there is little support for the idea that such a practice impairs endurance capacity.

A minimal lipid intake is necessary to supply the body with essential fatty acids. Current dietary recommendations assure sufficient levels of essential fatty acids but avoid an excessive lipid intake, thus minimizing the risks of cardiovascular disease, cancer, and obesity. These recommendations apply to both inactive and exercising persons.

Research indicates that amino acids provide not more than 5 to 15% of the total energy expended during exercise. However, the magnitude of this increased utilization leads to only a slight increase in protein needs with strenuous physical activity. Given an adequate mixed diet, the slight increase has little consequence for fitness and health. Most people in most countries report consuming over twice the quantity of protein recommended daily for sedentary individuals, leaving more than adequate margin to cover any slight increase of needs with physical activity and tissue hypertrophy. Of concern may be the individual who combines a low energy intake with an increased protein requirement. Supplemental protein and individual amino acids, if they have any effect, act by adding energy to the system.

The increased energy output accompanying physical activity is important in controlling body mass. However, the ability of exercise to induce an energy deficit depends also on the adjustment of postexercise energy intake, and possible adaptive changes in resting metabolic rate.

Exercise increases body heat production. Heat is partly removed from the body by the evaporation of water, thus fluid replenishment is necessary if plasma volume and the ability to thermoregulate are to be maintained. Unfortunately, the thirst mechanism is usually inadequate to ensure *ad libitum* replacement of losses. Of particular concern are individuals exercising in the heat (where fluid losses may be great), and the elderly (in whom the thirst mechanism is diminished). Replenishment may be adequately accomplished with water under most circumstances.

Vitamins and minerals are essential to health. There is no clear evidence to suggest increased needs for the majority of these nutrients arise from physical activity. Zinc, copper, and chromium are of particular concern, however, because the intake of these nutrients by the general population is below present recommended dietary allowance. Cumulative losses in sweat, at least in the case of zinc and copper, can be significant. With the concern over increased free-radical production during exercise, there is a growing interest in the possible role of the antioxidants (e.g., vitamins C and E) in preserving fitness and health. However, there is insufficient research to draw conclusions at this time. Supplementation of iron and calcium may be of some benefit for some women. Interactions of trace minerals may result in a precipitation of deficiencies if intakes are imbalanced. A diet designed to promote overall health should be sufficient to cover needs of physical activity without supplementation, provided energy requirements are met.

IMPORTANT RESEARCH TOPICS

43. What are the mechanisms by which exercise can increase postexercise energy intake and expenditure, and what is the contribution of increases in postexercise energy intake and expenditure to the potential energy deficit induced by exercise?
44. Does exercise affect the minimal requirements of carbohydrate and lipids?
45. Does exercise have an effect on macronutrient preference (e.g., carbohydrate)?
46. Does exercise affect the need for micronutrients (e.g., chromium)?
47. What is the best way to replenish fluid during and after exercise—with water alone or in conjunction with carbohydrate and/or electrolytes?
48. Do nutrient needs with exercise change across various segments of the population at various ages?
49. Does the supplementation of protein to levels of ≥ 2.0 g/day per kg of body weight enhance the increase in fat-free mass associated with resistance training? If so, will the increase in fat-free mass be reflected by an increased resting metabolic rate which could facilitate fat loss?

50. Will the supplementation of calcium in combination with resistance and aerobic exercise training reduce bone mineral losses in young amenorrheic and postmenopausal women with aging?

Adjuvants to Physical Activity

Adjuvants to physical activity are defined as those measures or practices which, because of their potential physiological effects, are used in the hope of enhancing the benefits or reducing the potential detrimental effects of physical activity on fitness and health. Although there are many measures or practices that could be discussed, this statement focuses on electrical stimulation, massage, sauna, sudation garments, and questionable exercise devices.

Electrical Stimulation

Electrical stimulation increases isometric strength and isokinetic strength at both slow and fast contraction speeds. The magnitude of these effects is inversely related to the initial muscle strength of the individual. There seems to be no effect on muscular endurance. Contrary to ordinary strength training, electrical stimulation probably activates Type II better than Type I muscle fibers. In patients, these effects may translate to improved functional status. Electrical stimulation may alleviate postoperative pain, enabling the patient to conduct muscular training more effectively. Thus, electrical stimulation is a well-founded adjuvant to muscle training in the rehabilitation of injured (e.g., knee-operated) exercise participants and patients with neurological disorders, but it does not seem to give any extra benefit over equivalent voluntary training of healthy individuals.

Massage

Massage is widely and increasingly used with several intents, such as to enhance muscular relaxation and joint mobility prior to exercise; to prevent and alleviate muscular cramps, soreness, and pain; to hasten recovery after strenuous efforts; and to speed up the healing of soft tissue injuries, thereby restoring flexibility and joint mobility. These benefits are expected on the basis of the alleged physiological effects of massage.

A large proportion of exercise participants and patients receiving massage perceive its effects to be positive and useful, but this could be in part due to nonspecific placebo effects. However, massage has specific physiological effects, decreasing alpha motorneuron excitability, slightly increasing the range of motion in some joints, and slightly increasing the cutaneous and muscle blood flow. The practical significance of these effects remains to be proven. Recent studies have not shown massage to cause changes in serum beta-endorphins, muscle strength, circulatory responses to submaximal exercise, or short-term recovery from intense muscular activity. In conclusion, the physiological effects and preventive, therapeutic, and restorative efficacy of massage have been inadequately studied. Therefore, the use of massage as an adjuvant to exercise has to be considered at present as mainly "educated empiricism."

Sauna

Sauna has been suggested for numerous purposes including warming-up before training and competition, mental and physical relaxation before and after training and competition, facilitation of mental and physical recovery, weight reduction, prevention and treatment of musculoskeletal injuries, prevention of respiratory infections, training of the circulatory system and autonomous regulation, as well as acclimation to heat. Most of these proposed benefits are based more on perceived effects, reasoning, and indirect evidence than on well-conducted research.

On the basis of proven physiological effects, sauna has been used to reduce fluid loss and thus an acute weight reduction on certain types of athletes, for neuromuscular relaxation, and for heat acclimation. However, the temporary impairment of fluid and electrolyte balance, and of motivation for all-out effort that are caused by especially intensive bathing, as well as practical problems of environmental control, considerably limit the use of sauna. Favorable psychosomatic effects like stimulation-relaxation, facilitation of recovery from strenuous effort, and decreased postexercise musculoskeletal symptoms are commonly experienced among frequent sauna users. On the other hand, sauna bathing is not an efficient stimulus or substitute for circulatory training. Furthermore, intensive sauna bathing, or sauna followed by sudden cold exposure (e.g., a plunge into a cold lake or a shower), may increase the risk of cardiovascular complications and thermal injury. The risks are probably greater under certain conditions and in certain populations (e.g., infrequent use, pregnancy, cardiovascular disease, elderly).

Sudation (Sweat-Inducing) Garments

Sudation garments are used to create a temporary hot microclimate by preventing evaporative heat loss. Their intent is to enhance exercise-heat tolerance, and thus the person's performance capacity in hot climates. The few, but well-conducted studies specifically addressing this problem indicate that, at least in well-trained subjects, training in sudation garments does not offer significant advantages over training in ordinary exercise clothing. Neither increase exercise heat tolerance as much as training in warm conditions. This finding, and the extra physical and perceived demands of wearing sudation garments during training, do not support their use as a means to enhance exercise-heat tolerance.

Sudation garments are used to enhance the temporary weight loss induced by sweating. An increase of skin and deep body temperatures offers a strong stimulus for sweating. Skin and deep body temperature and sweating all increase more when the same exercise is performed in sudation garments rather than ordinary training clothing. Thus, exercise in a sudation garment enhances the acute weight reduction, or causes an equivalent weight reduction for less energy expenditure. From a practical point of view, the extra physical and perceived demands of using sudation garments, and the negative impact of fluid and electrolyte losses on physical performance capacity, limit the usefulness of sudation garments as a means of achieving an acute weight reduction. Hyperthermia, dehydration, and thermal injury can all result from the use of sudation garments.

Selected Exercise Devices

There are many exercise devices which have proven beneficial effects upon fitness and health (e.g., treadmills, cycle ergometers, resistance equipment). However, there are also many very questionable commercial exercise devices (e.g., bust developers and vibrating machines) that have no apparent scientific rationale. Most of these devices are associated with the multi-billion dollar weight-loss and figure-control industry. Some are passive devices that require no exertion or additional energy expenditure on the part of the user. Others include active movement, but the claims by each for spot reduction or figure enhancement are unfounded.

Unfortunately, few research studies have examined the efficacy of exercise devices that fall into the "questionable" category. In most cases, claims are made without supporting research data, and the scientific community expresses its skepticism on the basis of an evaluation of these claims against established scientific fact. Where actual scientific studies have been conducted, the resulting data generally do not support the manufacturer's claims. In some cases, manufacturers have been successfully prosecuted for fraudulent claims.

IMPORTANT RESEARCH TOPICS

51. What is the physiological basis for the muscle strengthening that is associated with neuromuscular electrical stimulation, for example, functional overload of Type I fibers (as in voluntary contraction), or preferential Type II fiber recruitment based on the specific characteristics of electrical stimulation?
52. What are the structural and functional effects in muscles, ligaments, and tendons of different types of massage after strenuous exercise and in post-injury rehabilitation?
53. The potential therapeutic and restorative benefits of sauna bathing for health and fitness should be further investigated.
54. Since many of the proposed adjuvants to physical activity are used for the purposes of inducing weight loss or reshaping the body figure, are there adjuvants that might work synergistically with physical activity to produce long-term changes in metabolic rate? Agents that increase sympathetic activity or body temperature would be likely candidates.

Human Adaptation to Acute and Chronic Physical Activity

Physical Activity and the Cardiovascular System

The acute response to muscular exercise provides the greatest challenge to the cardiovascular system, demanding a complex integration of the local regulation of blood flow to the active skeletal muscle and neural regulation of the hemodynamic response. In sustained dynamic exercise, the active muscle must receive a blood flow appropriate to its increased metabolic needs, and at the same time the brain and heart must receive an adequate blood flow to maintain their normal functions. In static exercise, the mechanical obstruction to skeletal muscle blood flow caused by increased intramuscular pressure opposes effects from the local dilation of the resistance vessels.

During intense dynamic exercise, there is a marked increase in oxygen delivery to the muscles;

this is accomplished by an increase in heart rate, stroke volume, and total body arterio-venous oxygen difference. However, there is only a small increase in mean arterial pressure, and peripheral vascular resistance is markedly decreased. Vasodilation in the resistance vessels of the active skeletal muscle can increase local blood flow to 250-300 ml/100g of muscle/minute, explaining the marked decrease in peripheral vascular resistance. The underlying mechanism is not known; however, many metabolic stimuli have been suggested. During dynamic exercise involving a large proportion of the skeletal muscle mass, the ability to increase cardiac output, and thereby maintain mean arterial blood pressure, is the factor limiting maximal oxygen uptake.

During "static" exercise with contractions of the skeletal muscle maintained at approximately 30 to 50% of the maximal voluntary force, there is little increase in oxygen consumption, a moderate increase in cardiac output and heart rate, and no change in stroke volume. Total peripheral vascular resistance remains relatively constant, with a marked increase in mean arterial blood pressure.

Both dynamic and static exercise lead to increased activity of the sympathetic nervous system and decreased activity of the parasympathetic nervous system. Two neural mechanisms are responsible: central neural mechanism ("central command") and a reflex mechanism ("exercise pressor reflex"). The exercise pressor reflex is mediated by Group III muscle afferents, which respond mainly to mechanical perturbations, and Group IV muscle afferents, which respond mainly to metabolic changes in the contracting skeletal muscle. The arterial baroreceptors, cardiopulmonary receptors, and the reflexes that they mediate also appear to be involved in the control of blood pressure during exercise.

Metabolites and other substances produced in active skeletal muscle have three major roles in orchestrating the cardiovascular response: (a) to act locally in causing vasodilation of the resistance vessels; (b) to activate sensory receptors in skeletal muscle which reflexly excite medullary cardiovascular control areas via Group IV afferent nerve fibers, thereby increasing sympathetic neuronal outflow to the heart and blood vessels; and (c) to modulate the sympathetic control of the resistance vessels in the active skeletal muscle.

The chronic adaptation of the cardiovascular system to repeated bouts of muscular exercise depends on the type and intensity of the activity that has been undertaken. Dynamic exercise training leads to an increase in maximal oxygen uptake, due to an enhanced ability to increase stroke volume and to widen the total body arterio-venous oxygen difference. The ability to deliver a greater peak stroke volume may reflect an eccentric hypertrophy of the left ventricle rather than an increase in the contractile state. Other results of dynamic exercise include increases in total blood volume, vascular capacitance, venous compliance, vascular reactivity to receptor agonists, and decreased afterloading. These changes affect cardiovascular regulation and may contribute to orthostatic intolerance.

With static exercise training, there is no appreciable increase in maximal oxygen uptake. However, eccentric hypertrophy of the left ventricle can again develop, increasing the ability to deliver the same stroke volume against a markedly increased mean arterial pressure (afterload).

IMPORTANT RESEARCH TOPICS

55. What is the local mechanism causing vasodilation in the resistance vessels of exercising skeletal muscle?
56. How is the metabolic demand in contracting skeletal muscle sensed and how does it affect the cardiovascular response?
57. Is there a change in sympathetic outflow to exercising skeletal muscle with training, and if so, what is its effect?
58. What is the relative importance of central command and the exercise pressor reflex in matching the cardiovascular response to the type and intensity of exercise, and how are the two mechanisms integrated?
59. What are the factors limiting maximal oxygen intake in different physiological and pathophysiological conditions?
60. What is the effect of gender and age on the acute cardiovascular response and adaptation to exercise?

Physical Activity and the Microcirculation of Cardiac and Skeletal Muscle

Exercise training increases the capacity of the cardiovascular system to transport nutrients to active skeletal muscle tissue. The increased vascular transport capacity makes possible an enhanced peak rate of oxidative metabolism in active muscles. Aerobic training increases the vascular transport capacity in both cardiac and skeletal muscle by augmenting both the peak blood flow and capillary exchange capacity. The increases in transport capacity result from both structural adaptations and altered control of vascular resistance. Structural vascular adaptations take at least two forms: increases in the cross-sectional area and length of the large and small arteries and veins (i.e., vascular growth) and increased numbers of capillaries (and other microvessels) per gram of muscle (i.e., angiogenesis).

Vascular adaptation induced by endurance exercise training develops relatively uniformly throughout the myocardium, whereas it seems less uniformly distributed in skeletal muscle. Increased capillary density and increased vascular transport capacity occur around muscle fibers that experience the largest increase in activity during exercise. However, vascular adaptation may not be heterogenous in the skeletal muscle of all species.

Angiogenesis has been demonstrated in the coronary circulation; endurance exercise training causes moderate cardiac hypertrophy, while maintaining or increasing the capillary density and increasing the arteriolar density. Changes in coronary vascular control induced by endurance exercise training include altered coronary responses to vasoactive substances, changes in endothelium-mediated vasoregulation, and alterations in the cellular-molecular control of intracellular free Ca^{2+} in both endothelial and vascular smooth muscle cells.

IMPORTANT RESEARCH TOPICS

61. There is a need for anatomical data, describing the effects of exercise training on small arteries, arterioles, venules, and small veins, in order to understand structural vascular adaptation and vascular remodeling.
62. The hypothesis that structural and functional vascular adaptations occur around muscle fibers that experience the greatest relative increase in activity during training bouts needs to be tested systematically in humans.
63. The hypothesis that exercise training induces changes in local control of microvascular resistance must be tested in both skeletal and cardiac muscles.
64. The interactions of microvascular adaptations induced by exercise training with disease states such as atherosclerosis, hypertension, and diabetes require elucidation.
65. The effects of weight training on skeletal muscle microvascular beds also require further investigation.
66. The signal or signals initiating structural and functional adaptive responses should be defined.

Physical Activity and the Pulmonary System

The responses to exercise in the young untrained healthy pulmonary system [$\dot{V}O_2max$ < 50-55 ml/(kg × min)] can be summarized as follows: the alveolar to arterial oxygen partial pressure difference widens two- to three-fold during maximal exercise, due primarily to an increased nonuniformity in distribution of alveolar ventilation relative to pulmonary capillary flow. Expiratory air flow is rarely limited significantly by airway collapse. The transpulmonary pressure developed by the inspiratory muscles reaches about 50% of their dynamic capacity. A significant compensatory but highly variable hyperventilatory response to heavy and maximum exercise occurs in all healthy untrained subjects (decrease in partial pressure of CO_2 in arterial blood 5 to 15 Torr). Based on voluntary mimicking of the exercise pleural pressure volume loop, the oxygen cost of hyperpnea is estimated to average 8-10% of $\dot{V}O_2max$ in subjects who require maximal ventilation in the range of 100 to 130 l/min. In long-term, heavy endurance exercise, breathing frequency and ventilatory output gradually rise. Dead space ventilation also rises, but alveolar ventilation remains adequate. At very heavy sustained work rates (> 85% $\dot{V}O_2max$) significant diaphragmatic fatigue occurs.

Adaptation of the healthy pulmonary system to the "training stimulus" may be summarized as follows: total lung capacity and its subdivisions do not change more than a few percent with prolonged, general physical training. Reported differences in some highly trained athletes, young or old, are most likely the result of pre-selection. Phylogenic differences in highly fit versus sedentary species show that the lung lacks adaptability compared to the highly adaptable structural capacities of muscle mitochondria, muscle capillaries, and heart muscle mitochondria. The diaphragm at all ages is adaptable to whole body physical training in terms of changes in aerobic capacity and perhaps even in fiber type.

Demand versus capacity in the highly fit, healthy pulmonary system may be described as follows. Diffusion limitation for oxygen at the alveolar capillary level becomes significant and arterial hypoxemia occurs as the increase in pulmonary blood flow exceeds the individual's ability to expand the pulmonary capillary blood volume. If the respiratory minute volume exceeds 150 to 160 l/min, the expiratory flow rate becomes limited by airway collapse, inspiratory muscles develop more than 90% of their maximal available pressure, and ventilation is mechanically limited. In such circumstances, the local oxygen consumption of the respiratory muscles will exceed 400 ml/min or 15% of $\dot{V}O_2max$. With endurance exercise in excess of 85% of $\dot{V}O_2max$, significant diaphragmatic fatigue occurs. The elastic recoil of the lung diminishes with normal aging, even in the non-smoking healthy human. Expiratory flow limitation is then reached even at moderate work rates, the functional residual capacity reaches resting levels or above, and the oxygen cost of exercise hyperpnea is increased relative to younger subjects.

The role of pulmonary system is a limiting factor to $\dot{V}O_2max$ and endurance exercise performance in the following fashion. In the young untrained or moderately trained human with a $\dot{V}O_2max \leq$ 55 ml/(kg × min) or a peak respiratory minute volume < 120 l/min, diffusion limitation does not occur and the oxygen cost of breathing is not high enough to influence the ventilatory response significantly. In such subjects $\dot{V}O_2max$ or endurance performance is not determined to any significant extent by limitations of the lung and chest wall. At $\dot{V}O_2max \geq$ 65 ml/(kg × min), an appreciable number of subjects will experience a significant limitation of $\dot{V}O_2max$ because of arterial oxyhemoglobin desaturation. The extent of this limitation is equivalent to at most 10 to 15% of $\dot{V}O_2max$. In highly fit humans with a peak respiratory minute volume in excess of 140 to 150 l/min, the oxygen cost of maximum ventilation will likely limit endurance performance significantly.

Several mechanisms responsible for the regulation of exercise hyperpnea have been identified in isolation. These include: (a) descending neural influences from higher locomotor areas of the central nervous system; (b) ascending neural signals from locomotor muscles initiated by mechanical and/or chemical changes in the locomotor muscles; and (c) humoral stimuli, including "CO_2 flow" to the lung.

The hyperventilatory response to heavy exercise is not yet accounted for. It remains correlated with increases in circulatory mediators from working muscle, including [H+], K+, norepinephrine and NH_3. Primary receptors and sensory pathways for transduction of the stimulus are controversial. Some of these same humoral stimuli change with duration of heavy exercise and have been implicated, along with body temperature, as potential mediators of the "tachypneic drift" during prolonged exercise. Regulation of upper airway calibre, respiratory muscle recruitment, and breathing pattern appear to optimize work of breathing during exercise.

IMPORTANT RESEARCH TOPICS

67. The relative contributions of basic neural and humoral control mechanisms to exercise hyperpnea and hyperventilation need quantification.
68. The contribution of the respiratory muscles of the chest wall and abdomen to exercise hyperpnea and the mechanisms which regulate the specific recruitment of these muscles need detailed study.
69. It is unclear whether there is an accumulation of extravascular lung fluid at high levels of exercise. New techniques are needed to measure pulmonary extravascular fluid.
70. What factors cause maldistribution of alveolar ventilation, pulmonary capillary flow, and the ratio of alveolar ventilation to pulmonary capillary flow during heavy exercise?
71. How do pulmonary and cardiovascular control systems interact during exercise to regulate efferent sympathetic nervous activity and peripheral vascular resistance?
72. Longitudinal studies are needed to examine the adaptability of the pulmonary system to physical training in humans. Important issues include: effects on the strength and endurance of the respiratory muscles, the importance of maturation and aging on any local training "effect," and the effects upon the morphology of the lungs and chest wall.

Physical Activity and Hormonal Adaptation

Exercise requires major metabolic and cardiovascular adjustments to increase the supply of oxygen and fuels to the working muscles, while maintaining homeostasis. Changes in autonomic nervous activity and in hormone secretion help to accomplish these adjustments. Although the endocrine glands are the main source of hormones, a sharp distinction between the nervous and endocrine systems is no longer appropriate, because substances previously considered hormones may be released from nerves (e.g., gastrin), and neurotransmitters may spillover into the blood and act as hormones (e.g., norepinephrine). Changes in effective plasma hormone concentrations may be due to changes in secretion, plasma volume, binding, and/or clearance.

A single bout of exercise increases plasma concentrations of a large variety of hormones and decreases concentrations of only a few hormones. Although only studied for some hormones, the general impression is that the large changes in plasma concentrations of amine and peptide hormones seen during exercise result mainly from changes in secretion rate rather than changes in the rate of clearance. However, the clearance of hormones degraded primarily in the liver (e.g., the steroid hormones) may be expected to decrease during exercise, as splanchnic blood flow decreases.

A key role in the neuro-endocrine response to exercise is an increase of sympatho-adrenal activity and a resultant suppression of insulin secretion. These responses have major effects on metabolism and circulatory regulation, facilitating fuel supply and utilization. Increased plasma concentrations of certain hormones also affect metabolism (glucagon, growth hormone, cortisol) and fluid balance (renin, angiotensin, aldosterone, atrial natriuretic factor, vasopression). The signals eliciting changes in secretion of these hormones seem to include both *feedforward* and *feedback* regulatory mechanisms.

Hormonal responses to exercise are changed by endurance training, and the resting concentrations of some hormones may also be changed. In general, the hormonal response to a given absolute work rate is lessened after endurance training. However, the hormonal response to exercise at a given relative submaximal load is unchanged. During high intensity or maximal exercise, the response of the glucoregulatory hormones may be unchanged or even accentuated in the trained individual.

Changes in plasma catecholamine concentrations may be one of the mechanisms whereby aerobic training decreases resting arterial blood pressure. Whether resting plasma concentrations of catecholamines change with training remains controversial.

In both cross-sectional and longitudinal studies, training is associated with a lower post-absorptive concentration of insulin than that seen in untrained subjects. Although effects of training on gonadal function are unknown, intense endurance training has been associated with a reduction in plasma gonadal steroid concentrations in both women and men, namely decreased levels of estradiol and progesterone in women and testosterone in men. These gonadal steroidal changes may be associated with an impairment in pituitary luteinising hormone pulsatility.

Training-related changes in neuro-endocrine activity are often accompanied by changes in target tissue sensitivity and/or responsiveness. For instance, the responsiveness of adipose tissue lipolysis to catecholamines is increased by training, and insulin sensitivity is increased in trained subjects compared with untrained individuals. These changes in target tissue sensitivity more or less offset any effect of lower hormone concentrations in submaximal exercise and offer the possibility of increased maximal responsiveness to a physiological challenge. The major part of these adaptations occurs and disappears within a few days to a few weeks of beginning and ending training, respectively.

Mechanisms behind the changes in hormone concentrations and target tissue sensitivity with training are still not known. In vitro studies demonstrate that muscle contractions alone can enhance hormone sensitivity of muscle but changes in non-muscle tissues (e.g., adipose tissue) also occur.

IMPORTANT RESEARCH TOPICS

73. There is a need to identify the signals and to determine the relative roles of feed-forward versus feedback in controlling hormone secretion during exercise. The effects of training on these variables should also be studied.
74. The mechanisms involved in the adaptation of target tissues to exercise training need elucidation.
75. Possible interactive effects of diet and training on changes in hormone secretion and target tissue adaptations should be explored.
76. The effects of environment, gender, and genetic variation on hormone secretion and target tissue adaptations should be examined.

Physical Activity and Skeletal Muscle

Contractions of skeletal muscles provide the basis for all physical activities. Force is developed during an isometric contraction, whereas when muscle fibers shorten or lengthen, power (force × velocity) is produced or absorbed, respectively. Disuse, trauma, or disease each impair the ability of skeletal muscles to develop and sustain force and power and therefore decrease physical and physiological fitness. Conversely, increases in physical activity may increase absolute or sustained force or power. Adequate levels of muscular power and endurance enable human beings to perform the activities of daily living throughout their varied life spans.

Within a motor unit, properties of fibers are more homogenous than throughout whole muscles. The fibers within a given motor unit may be classified as slow, fast fatigue resistant, or fast fatiguable. Muscle fibers may also be classified on the basis of myofibrillar ATPase activity (Type I, Type IIA, Type IIB, Type IIC) or the activities of both the myofibrillar ATPase and oxidative enzymes (slow-oxidative, fast-oxidative-glycolytic, and fast-glycolytic). The numbers and sizes of the different types of motor units in a given muscle determine functional capability. Recruitment of motor units occurs on the basis of size, from small, slow units for low intensity tasks, through the additional recruitment of fast fatigue resistant units for moderate intensity tasks, to fast fatiguable units for high intensity tasks. The interaction of the recruitment pattern and the habitual intensity of daily physical activity play a key role in motor unit adaptation and consequently the characteristics of the muscle fibers.

Physical activities involve various combinations of shortening, isometric, and lengthening contractions. Shortening contractions generate the power for movements of the organism or of external objects, and are energetically demanding. Measurements of work performed or power output provide the best estimates of the intensity of physical activity. The response can only be compared in terms of relative intensities of the maximum power during a single contraction.

Fatigue is defined as a loss in the development of force and/or velocity, that results from physical activity, and is reversible by rest. Fatigue is induced by accumulation of the products of ATP hydrolysis, including inorganic phosphate and hydrogen ions, which can potentially impair excitation-contraction coupling in the muscle. In long-term physical activity, a depletion of muscle glycogen stores may impair the ability of the muscle to develop force. Depending on the intensity and duration of the physical activity, full recovery occurs within minutes or hours. Decreases in force development that persist for more than 24 hours after physical activity are due to contraction-induced injury.

Training modifies the morphological, metabolic and molecular properties of muscle, altering the functional attributes of fibers in specific motor units. Adaptations for strength and endurance may occur independently, although training programs may produce increases in both attributes.

Bed-rest, immobilization, and weightlessness reduce recruitment and/or loading. Each model has differing effects. Immobilization and weightlessness result in a decrease in muscle mass and in the cross-sectional area of single fibers. Maintenance of a given level of physiological fitness requires a certain intensity, duration, and frequency of physical activity. Following a period of sustained increase or decrease in physical activity, adaptations may be reversed. During detraining, muscle fiber changes regress toward pretraining values, but some adaptations are sustained for considerable periods of time. The decrease in absolute force results from both the decrease in muscle cross-sectional area, and reduction in force developed per unit area.

During the early stages of strength training, maximum power can increase as a result of neurophysiological adaptations despite the absence of morphological or biochemical changes. Heavy-resistance strength training subsequently results in an increase in muscle cross-sectional area in all three fiber types. In addition, the proportion of Type IIA fiber subtypes is altered. Following ablation of synergistic muscles, the myosin isoform expression shifts from the fast toward slow-type. Peptide mapping suggests that a true transformation of myosin occurs in the hypertrophied fibers.

Endurance training increases the capacity of muscles to sustain force and power. The primary adaptations to prolonged physical activity are metabolic, hormonal, and cardiovascular changes that enhance the ability to oxidize all fuels including fatty acids during prolonged physical activity, to conserve carbohydrates (particularly muscle glycogen concentration), and to attenuate metabolic acidosis. If the intensity and duration of the endurance training program is sufficient, mitochondrial capacity increases in all fiber types. Although endurance training reduces blood flow during submaximal exercise, higher blood flows to the contracting muscles are observed during exercise at high intensities. Endurance training programs do not appear to induce any substantial changes in the major fiber types. For most individuals of all ages, increased physical activity and the associated improvements in strength, power, and endurance has the potential to improve the intensity and diversity of daily activities that can be performed without fatigue or the possibility of injury. This increase in capacity for the activities of daily living improves quality of life.

IMPORTANT RESEARCH TOPICS

77. To determine the mechanism responsible for fatigue during different intensities of physical activity.

78. To establish the interrelationships among the measurements made on skeletal muscle in vitro, in situ, and in vivo and the validity of extrapolating from observations on single permeabilized fibers to fibers in vivo.
79. To determine the relative role of the type of muscle progenitor cells and the subsequent environmental factors that ultimately result in diverse populations of muscle cells.
80. To determine the functional significance of the diversity of protein isoforms of muscle throughout the life span.
81. To establish the biomechanical behaviors of synergistic muscles during varied programs of exercise.
82. To establish the basis for age-related deficits that occur in skeletal muscles.
83. To determine the effects of training programs on the properties of skeletal muscle fibers.
84. To establish the significance of specific muscle adaptations in modifying hormonal, electrolyte, metabolic, and cardiovascular capacities.
85. To determine mechanisms underlying susceptibility to, and recovery from, the injury to skeletal muscle induced by various forms of exercise.
86. To develop programs of regular muscular activity that are affordable, safe, and acceptable to large numbers of sedentary people.

Physical Activity and Adipose Tissue

Adipose tissue is the most important organ for lipid storage. During prolonged exercise, the fuel mixture oxidized by the skeletal muscle varies, depending upon the intensity and the duration of exercise, but lipid mobilized from adipose tissue contributes significantly to the energy supply.

Endurance training can induce net lipid mobilization from adipose tissue, eventually leading to a reduction in adipose tissue mass if the increased mobilization is not fully compensated by mechanisms increasing lipid storage. To reduce adipose tissue mass, an exercise program without dietary restriction must generate a substantial energy expenditure, and the minimal prescription commonly recommended for improving cardiorespiratory fitness is often insufficient. Under these circumstances, dietary interventions generally produce a greater energy deficit, and thus, faster rates of decrease in body mass than exercise training alone. Weight loss induced by endurance training is, however, associated with a better preservation of fat free mass than hypocaloric diets. With endurance training, men generally show a greater reduction in body fat than women. Metabolic improvements associated with the reduction of adipose tissue mass include changes of carbohydrate and lipid metabolism that may reduce the risk of developing diabetes and cardiovascular disease.

The regulation of adipose tissue mass depends upon several metabolic processes, including lipolysis, and reesterification and storage through the hydrolysis of circulating triglycerides by the enzyme lipoprotein lipase. In lean subjects, endurance training increases the lipolytic response of adipose cells to catecholamines. Adipose tissue lipoprotein lipase is also increased, which contributes to the replenishment of adipose tissue lipid stores between exercise sessions. Much less information is available regarding obese subjects. Gender and site-specific differences in the response of adipose tissue lipolysis to catecholamines have been reported, this variation being partly attributed to alterations in the ratio of alpha (inhibitory) to beta (stimulatory) adrenergic receptors. The relative role of these factors in the response of adipose tissue lipolysis to exercise training has not been established. Gender differences in the acute response of abdominal and femoral adipose cell lipolysis to endurance exercise have been reported. Gluteal adipose cell lipolytic response to catecholamines is acutely increased following endurance exercise in men but not in women. These results may explain the apparently greater ability of men to lose gluteal fat in response to training. The response of adipose tissue lipoprotein lipase to insulin is increased in obese patients after weight loss. No information is currently available on the effects of endurance training on the regulation of adipose tissue lipoprotein lipase activity by insulin in humans.

Processes other than lipoprotein lipase activity must be involved in lipid accretion in adipose cells, as a normal adipose tissue mass has been reported in individuals with no lipoprotein lipase activity. Insulin-stimulated glucose transport is increased in adipose cells after training, which may contribute to the replenishment of adipose tissue lipids after exercise.

Plainly, human adipose tissue metabolism can adapt to endurance training. Endurance training that generates a large energy expenditure can reduce adipose tissue fat mass. Upper body fat is more readily mobilized than lower body fat during training. Endurance training may reduce the quantity of atherogenic visceral adipose tissue, especially when initial levels are high. Factors influencing the response of visceral adipose tissue to training include gender and age, as well as the initial stores of total body and abdominal visceral fat. The abdominal adipose depot appears to be more readily mobilized than peripheral depots. Reductions in adipose tissue mass are a consequence of decreases in average adipose cell size, but there is no change in fat cell number.

IMPORTANT RESEARCH TOPICS

87. Which mechanisms are responsible for the apparently greater loss of body fat in response to endurance training in men than in women?
88. What are the gender and site-specific differences in the effects of endurance training on adipose tissue metabolism?
89. What are the effects of endurance training on adipose tissue metabolism in various age groups and under various hormonal conditions (menopause, hormone replacement)?
90. Is there any relationship between the phase of the menstrual cycle, reproductive status, and the acute response of adipose tissue metabolism to exercise?
91. Are there differences between obese and lean individuals in the effects of endurance training on the metabolism of adipose cells obtained from various depots?
92. How does insulin regulate lipoprotein lipase activity in adipose tissue and its acute and chronic response to endurance exercise?
93. What are the mechanisms responsible for the genetic variation in the response of adipose tissue metabolism to endurance training?

Physical Activity and Connective Tissue

Connective tissue is the most abundant tissue type of the human body. Among the various forms of connective tissue, the dense fibrous elements (bone, ligament, tendon, and cartilage) have been the most studied under conditions of habitual exercise. However, increasing research interest has recently been directed toward exercise-induced adaptations of connective tissue in cardiac and skeletal muscle. The fibrillar collagen network in bones, ligaments, tendons and cartilage is more compact than the collagen domain in skeletal muscle. Composition, micro-architecture, cell type, and metabolism vary among the forms of connective tissue. It has been suggested that the adaptation of morphological, biochemical, and biomechanical properties to exercise is driven primarily by physical forces. The biomechanical aspects of locomotion (torsion, compression, and tension) translate into changes in mechanical stresses that present local elements of skeletal muscle, bone, ligament, cartilage, and tendon with a unique load history. This load history alters connective tissue metabolism and structure, leading to unique tissue adaptations. The biomechanical parameters of exercise characterize the types of activity that produce particular adaptations. Therefore, a specific characterization of the exercise undertaken is essential in determining the characteristics of connective tissue adaptation.

Unfortunately, there is a dearth of information characterizing and quantifying the in vivo load histories of the connective tissues in the various body segments. Few have been successful in measuring in vivo tissue loads and/or strains during exercise in human and animal models. Therefore, the approach of scientists has been focused primarily on tissue adaptations to exercise with the assumption that they are the result of physical challenges. This approach is partly valid, because connective tissue structural adaptation does not always follow Wolff's Law which asserts that change in connective tissue mass is directly proportional to the magnitude of the applied force. In addition, the level of tissue organization is a function of the direction of the applied force. However, the exercise stimulus involves not only biomechanical criteria, but also alterations of endocrine profile. Connective tissue anabolism and catabolism (turnover) are modified by exercise. Studies have documented exercise-induced endocrine changes which have the potential to alter connective tissue turnover and structure.

Exercise stimulates the metabolism of connective tissues. Nonetheless, not all studies support the hypothesis that exercise alone enhances connective tissue strength and organization. Other factors such as age, diet, endocrine status, and environment can enhance or reduce the effects of exercise.

Increases in the circulating metabolites of connective tissue structural proteins are seen in marathon runners, indicating an increase of tissue turnover. Biopsy data in both humans and animals verify that exercise increases the secretion and resorption of extracellular matrix proteins. The changes in concentration of these metabolites vary with time, indicating the temporal basis of connective tissue responses to exercise. Tissue studies support the hypothesis that exercise adaptation is multiphasic. For example, exercise "up-regulates" the synthesis and secretion of collagen, but there is a "down-regulation" in the formation of stable collagen crosslinks (a marker of maturation). However, at some point in time, a steady-state of adaptation is achieved and maturation is enhanced. Collagen has a long half-life in many of the dense fibrous connective tissues (110 days in tendon) and continues to be modified throughout the life of the protein. It is uncertain whether exercise alters the half-life of mature collagen.

Some preliminary evidence suggests that strenuous exercise increases the degradation of mature collagen. This would imply that an initial phase of connective tissue adaptation involves the resorption of mature collagen and its replacement by "younger" protein with fewer stable crosslinks. Other evidence shows that tissues of strenuously exercised rats have relatively more (percent of total) connective tissue mass, with fewer stable collagen crosslinks, resulting in a lower maximum stress and elastic modulus. However, the structural and material properties of connective tissues improve as the duration of training is increased. Most studies have reported results at a single point in time. This may partly account for the lack of consensus regarding connective tissue adaptations to exercise.

IMPORTANT RESEARCH TOPICS

94. The exercise dose-response should be evaluated for connective tissue structure and organization over various time periods.
95. Quantitative in vivo force-displacement data should be collected during locomotion.
96. An in-depth examination of connective tissue adaptations should be made in populations of differing age, sex, endocrine status, diet, and disease state in various environments.
97. Biomarkers of connective tissue metabolism in various body fluids should be validated to allow measurements during training.
98. Changes in such biomarkers should be correlated with the short- and long-term effects of exercise on the musculoskeletal system.
99. A non-invasive technology should be developed to assess connective tissue responses to exercise.
100. Studies should determine whether acute exercise causes degradation of mature collagen.

Physical Activity and Digestive Processes

Gastrointestinal symptoms are a common source of disability. The interaction between physical activity and the digestive processes is complex. We lack primary knowledge of much of the basic gastrointestinal physiology associated with exercise. Investigative techniques are hampered by artifacts from body motion, variations in study populations, and differing exercise test protocols. However, significant acute gastrointestinal problems such as nausea, vomiting, diarrhea, and gastrointestinal bleeding are associated with exercise. There are few studies of adaptations of the gastrointestinal system to chronic exercise, or the influence of exercise on gastrointestinal disease.

Surveys suggest that endurance runners have a relatively high frequency of digestive complaints, particularly nausea and diarrhea. Other symptoms include: a frequent urge to defecate or actual defecation with exercise, abdominal cramps, a loss of appetite, heartburn, chest pain, belching, and rarely, rectal bleeding. These complaints, while usually not severe, are troublesome and may impair exercise performance.

Studies examining the effects of exercise on gastroesophageal reflux show it to be potentiated by exercise, particularly when running postprandially. Acid exposure can be controlled by histamine receptor blockade. Esophageal motility changes with exercise. Low- and moderate-intensity exercise accelerates gastric emptying of liquid, while high intensity exercise delays it. Changes in the gastric emptying of solids appear similar, but data are more limited. Scanty data suggest only minor changes in gastric acid secretion with exercise. Changes in small intestinal motility and absorption with moderate exercise are also small, and of uncertain clinical significance. Colonic transit is unchanged or accelerated by both moderate exercise and aerobic training. The etiology of exercise-associated gastrointestinal motility changes may include alterations in visceral blood flow, neurohormonal axis, abdominal pressure and position, trauma, and medications.

The gastrointestinal hemorrhage that is associated with exercise may present as occult, asymptomatic bleeding, but less commonly and potentially more seriously, it may also manifest itself as acute bleeding from gastritis or colitis. Possible etiologies include ischemic damage, trauma, the effects of chronic medications including aspirin and non-steroidal anti-inflammatory drugs, and underlying pre-existent disease. Small randomized clinical trials suggest that cimetidine may be an effective therapy in selected cases of gastrointestinal bleeding.

Liver-associated enzyme activities may be abnormal transiently following strenuous exercise, but such changes rarely reflect significant hepatic disease or damage. Exercise acutely reduces hepatic blood flow. Aerobic training may enhance hepatic synthetic function as manifested by increased rates of aminopyrine and antipyrine metabolism.

IMPORTANT RESEARCH TOPICS

101. There is a pressing need to improve investigative techniques for evaluation of gastrointestinal physiology during exercise.
102. The etiology of exercise-induced gastrointestinal symptoms such as nausea, vomiting, diarrhea, and abdominal pain, and its relation to recognized gastrointestinal physiologic changes, needs to be established.
103. The physiological mechanisms responsible for exercise-related alterations in gastric emptying require clarification.
104. The pathophysiology and therapy of exercise-associated gastrointestinal hemorrhage remains unknown, and further work is required to elucidate it.
105. The interaction of exercise with diseases of the gastrointestinal system remains to be explored.
106. Liver, biliary system, and pancreatic function should be evaluated during exercise in both health and disease.

Physical Activity and Carbohydrate Metabolism

Many exergonic processes occur in skeletal muscle cells, but during contraction the hydrolysis of ATP becomes dominant. Whereas the phosphorylation of ADP is immediately accomplished by creatine phosphate and creatine phosphotransferase, sustained contractions require the participation of glycolysis and oxidative phosphorylation to maintain the mitochondrial-chemiosmotic gradient, and thus, the cellular ATP-ADP ratio. Muscle glycogenolysis and glycolysis provide the energy for short bursts of activity.

In sustained aerobic activity, carbohydrate utilization through glycolysis is again the main source of reducing equivalents for mitochondrial respiration during moderate- or high-intensity exercise. The availability of carbohydrates in the form of exogenous (blood) glucose is required for optimal cardiac function both in isolated working rabbit hearts, as well as in the intact beating human heart. The transition of rest to exercise is marked by increased utilization of most fuel sources, with the greatest relative gain in the utilization of muscle carbohydrate (glycogen). Muscle glycogen depletion is associated with fatigue. Thus, carbohydrate availability is required to support the energy needs of exercise of moderate or greater intensity.

Whereas the rate of mitochondrial respiration is tightly coupled to the energetics of muscle contraction, the coupling between glycolytic flux and mitochondrial requirements for oxidizable substrates is looser. Muscle contraction induces both increased glucose uptake and glycogenolysis. Additionally, epinephrine (Beta 2-adrenergic stimulation) can accelerate the rate of glycogenolysis in resting as well as contracting muscle. Thus, resting and contracting muscle both show a net release of lactate, especially at the onset of exercise or under the influence of epinephrine.

Lactate released from contracting skeletal muscle and other storage sites (e.g., inactive muscle, adipose, liver) may serve as a fuel source at cellular sites with a high rate of respiration (e.g., heart, lung, and red skeletal muscle). In post-absorptive human beings, exercising at approximately 50% of $\dot{V}O_2max$, the utilization of blood lactate approximates that of glucose. At higher relative power outputs, or with the imposition of added stress such as the hypobaric hypoxia of altitude, the utilization of blood lactate can even exceed that of glucose.

In the postprandial state, hepatic glucose production may be supported by glycogenolysis and gluconeogenesis. During prolonged exercise in the post-absorptive state, gluconeogenesis from lactate (i.e., the Cori Cycle) becomes essential for the maintenance of hepatic glucose production and thus blood glucose homeostasis. Under the latter circumstances, gluconeogenic or Beta 2-adrenergic blockade results in a fall of hepatic glucose production, hypoglycemia, and fatigue.

Resting muscle utilizes only a relatively small proportion of hepatic glucose production. During moderate- to high-intensity exercise, the significant increase in metabolic rate and overall carbohydrate utilization of the contracting muscle require a redistribution of glucose flux. However, the increase of hepatic glucose production during exercise still provides only a small fraction of the carbohydrate utilized by the contracting muscle at the onset of exercise or during moderate- to high-intensity exercise. The majority of the carbohydrates required by the contracting muscle is derived from intramuscular glycogen stores.

Synthesis accompanies the degradation of skeletal muscle glycogen during exercise. Studies utilizing infusion of ^{3}H-glucose and ^{14}C-lactate into laboratory animals demonstrate the incorporation of glucose into muscle and liver glycogen pools, including tissues where net glycogenolysis is occurring.

The increased lipid oxidation capacity of trained muscle spares glycogen during exercise, and the increased glucose uptake capacity may promote glycogen storage during recovery from exercise. A training-induced increased mass of mitochondrial reticulum allows a greater oxidation of both carbohydrate and lipid in high-intensity exercise; it also permits increased lipid utilization, and glycogen sparing during moderate-intensity exercise.

Endogenous carbohydrate fuel sources are of primary importance in sustaining physical activities ranging from short bursts to prolonged exercise. Complex cell-to-cell and tissue-to-tissue interactions are involved in the supply of glucose and lactate as energy sources for muscle contraction during exercise. Local contraction-induced events as well as the sympathetic-adrenal system appear extremely important in controlling the exchange of carbohydrate energy forms during exercise.

IMPORTANT RESEARCH TOPICS

107. What are the pathways of hexose disposal during rest, exercise, and recovery?
108. What are the regulating factors which allow whole-body muscle glycogen stores to be mobilized during sustained exercise?
109. How is the fuel selection of exercising muscle regulated?
110. Which healthful dietary habits can be encouraged to improve exercise tolerance in both the general population and athletes?
111. What are the mechanisms which allow substrates to interact to supply fuels during exercise? For instance, how effective is increased muscle glucose uptake and supporting glycogenolysis during exercise?

Physical Activity, Lipid and Lipoprotein Metabolism, and Lipid Transport

The class of compounds described as lipids is quite diverse. However, only free fatty acids which are stored in their ester form (triacylglycerols or triglycerides) are important as a metabolic fuel. To utilize lipids as fuel, the muscle must take up, activate, and translocate free fatty acids into mitochondria, supplying acetyl coenzyme A to the citric acid cycle. Sources of free fatty acids for oxidation include: (a) circulating free fatty acids, which are mobilized from adipose tissue following hydrolysis of stored triglycerides by hormone-sensitive lipase; (b) circulating lipoprotein triglycerides, which are hydrolyzed on the surface of the muscle capillary endothelium by lipoprotein lipase, the activity of which is relatively high in cardiac and oxidative skeletal muscle fibers; and (c) intramuscular triglycerides, which are more abundant in oxidative muscle fibers. Utilization of free fatty acids during exercise depends on the intensity of activity, the subject's state of training and the diet.

In acute response to physical activity, fat is oxidized in progressively increasing amounts as the total energy expenditure increases, so that lipids may cover up to 90% of oxidative metabolism in prolonged bouts of exercise (greater than one hour) at moderate-intensity (< 50% $\dot{V}O_2max$). As the intensity of exercise increases (> 70% $\dot{V}O_2max$), fat is used in decreasing amounts, and glycogen becomes the predominant energy source.

With the onset of exercise, an initial fall in plasma free fatty acids concentration, arising from an increased uptake by the working muscle, is followed by increased plasma free fatty acid levels. This is due to liberation of free fatty acids from adipose tissue as lipolysis is stimulated by hormone-sensitive lipase activity in response to increased sympathoadrenal activity and decreased insulin levels. A major fraction of the free fatty acids liberated is reesterified within the adipocyte. Free fatty acids, which are released into the blood stream, are bound to the protein albumin and are transported to the working muscle. For any given individual and exercise intensity, there is a close relationship between the arterial free fatty acid concentration and the amount of free fatty acids taken up and oxidized in muscles. However, several lines of evidence suggest that hydrolysis of circulating lipoprotein triglycerides and intramuscular triglycerides contribute to the provision of free fatty acids for exercising muscles. The latter sources may be of greater importance following endurance training or consumption of a high-fat diet.

Endurance training increases the capability for fat oxidation. The absolute mass of the skeletal muscle mitochondria increases with training, resulting in increased concentrations of enzymes for the citric acid cycle, fatty acid and ketone body oxidation, and the electron transfer system. There is a greater reliance on fat as a source of energy during submaximal exercise at the same absolute work rate in trained individuals. Endurance training results in an increased lipolytic responsiveness to Beta-adrenergic stimulation, concomitant with lower plasma catecholamine concentrations. Training increases the activity of both skeletal muscle and adipose tissue lipoprotein lipase, thereby facilitating the use of circulating triglycerides as a fuel source in trained muscles and promoting the clearance of circulating triglycerides even at rest.

Active men and women generally exhibit decreased plasma concentrations of triglycerides and increased levels of high-density lipoprotein cholesterol in comparison with sedentary individuals, suggesting that their risk of heart disease is reduced. Randomized, controlled clinical trials of at least 12 weeks duration show that sedentary men who adopt a program of regular aerobic exercise reduce plasma triglycerides and increase high-density lipoprotein cholesterol. There are fewer similar studies in women that have yielded less consistent results; however, these also generally show decreases in plasma triglycerides. Loss of body fat generally accompanies increases in aerobic exercise when the intake of food energy is unchanged or reduced, and is occasionally seen even if food intake is increased, if the training is long and hard enough. Fat loss may bring about changes in lipoproteins, even in the absence of exercise, but several lines of evidence suggest that exercise training affects lipoproteins independently of fat loss. Increased skeletal muscle lipoprotein lipase activity, for instance, contributes to lipoprotein metabolism. In single-leg training studies, lipoprotein triglycerides is lower and high-density lipoprotein cholesterol is higher in blood draining the trained leg compared to arterial blood, but no such differences are seen in the untrained leg. Exercise training can result in a reduction in total and abdominal fat which may contribute further to long-term improvements in lipoprotein metabolism. Additionally, changes in diet composition (relative quantity of fat and carbohydrate) can significantly modify the effects of training on lipoproteins. It remains to be determined whether sex differences are important in the effects of training on lipid and lipoprotein metabolism.

IMPORTANT RESEARCH TOPICS

112. How is fuel selection regulated during exercise?
113. What variables influence the sources of fatty acid, which are utilized as fuels, during exercise?
114. What is the best nutritional plan to optimize fat utilization during exercise without impairing performance?
115. Is there an optimal work intensity, frequency, and duration that maximizes fat utilization in most individuals bringing about the greatest benefits in weight regulation and weight-related problems, such as lipoprotein disorders and diabetes?
116. Which diet and exercise programs would increase the utilization of centrally-deposited fat?
117. Are there sex differences in the influence of exercise upon lipid and lipoprotein metabolism, and do these differ across the life cycle?

Physical Activity, Protein, and Amino Acid Metabolism

Exercise is associated with an increased catabolism of protein and amino acids. This is shown by an increased production of urea (with an increased nitrogen excretion in sweat and urine) and increased amino acid oxidation (as shown by production of labelled CO_2 from ^{13}C and ^{14}C carboxyl-labelled leucine and $^{15}NH_3$ from ^{15}N glycine). The net negative nitrogen balance may be masked, unless precautions are taken to account for losses in sweat, the delayed pattern of urinary nitrogen excretion, and the difficulty of observing small changes in the large body urea pool. However, the use of stable-isotope tracers to follow urea production rate and the transfer of label from amino acids to labelled urea suggests that urea production increases less than would be expected from other measures (e.g., leucine oxidation and the amount of amino acid delivered to the liver). The contradiction may be resolved if, as seems likely, exercise causes the liver to increase the production of acute phase proteins (such as fibrinogen or fibronectin). These substances are relatively branched-chain amino acid depleted compared to tissue protein, which is the likely source of the branched-chain amino acids oxidized in exercise.

The amount of amino acids in the free tissue and blood amino acid pool is increased during short-term exercise. This increase is almost certainly due to a fall in the ratio of whole body protein synthesis to breakdown. During high-intensity short-term exercise, ammonia production increases markedly, probably as a result of the action of adenosine deaminase at the expense of AMP, without replenishment of AMP from amino acids. Alanine production increases in this type of exercise to the extent that pyruvate is made available by glycolysis; this may help to limit acidosis. In longer-term exercise, some amino acid pools are diminished markedly. For example, muscle glutamate and blood branched-chain amino acids fall, probably due to an increased rate of transamination of branched-chain amino acids; whereas the production of alanine, aspartate, glutamine and ammonia rises. The exact source of carbon for the amino acids exported from muscle in this type of exercise remains unclear; muscle protein, glycogen and glucose are all possible precursors. The proportion of each is unknown, and may vary according to substrate availability.

During exercise, branched-chain amino acid oxidation is increased; this is due to an increased delivery (branched-chain amino acid transporters have a high capacity, but a low affinity), an increased net muscle breakdown, and an increase in the proportion of the branched chain ketoacid dehydrogenase that is in the active form. Activation of the dehydrogenase is closely correlated with metabolic state and probably also with the intensity and duration of exercise. It is inversely correlated with pre-existing glycogen stores, so that amino acid oxidation would be minimized under conditions of high glycogen availability.

Amino acid oxidation contributes a small fraction of energy needs compared with that derived from other fuels. It may nevertheless be important in sparing other sources of glucose and in providing a source of new carbon for gluconeogenesis. There is growing evidence that branched-chain amino acid oxidation is incomplete and branched-chain hydroxyacids are released from muscle to gluconeogenic tissues. The exercise-induced efflux of alanine and glutamine from muscle is taken up by the splanchnic bed, thus enabling the cycling of nitrogen from the periphery to the viscera with potential benefits for pH regulation and gluconeogenesis.

There is an acute decrease of protein synthesis in contracting muscle during exercise. Possible causes include a fall in ATP: ADP and in ribosome aggregation. There is conflicting evidence concerning muscle protein breakdown during exercise. Some workers claim that it is depressed and others that it is elevated. Part of the confusion may be due to the heterogeneity of the protein pool and the many proteolytic processes involved (e.g., ATP-dependent and independent processes would react differently). There may also be a time-dependent phenomenon, with muscle breakdown being depressed during exercise but elevated afterwards.

There is no doubt that muscle protein synthesis can rise markedly after exercise. The changes are so large they suggest that a remodeling-associated increase in breakdown must also occur, since the total protein mass increases relatively slowly. In young healthy men, there is no evidence that growth hormone supplements increase muscle protein accretion, although growth hormone may help rehabilitation after injury and in the maintenance of muscle mass in elderly men. Immobilization results in wasting because of a fall in muscle protein synthesis. This can be minimized by early remobilization or electrical stimulation.

The influence of large muscle exercise on dietary protein requirements is equivocal. During aerobic exercise, the increased utilization of some essential amino acids (e.g., the branched-chain amino acids) suggests that dietary protein requirements might be increased. This might be important for people living on a low protein diet (e.g., vegetarians or people of the developing world), or for any individual maintaining activity on an energy-reduced slimming diet. Nevertheless, there is no good evidence of any such change in requirements. Even if there were, because of the protein dense nature of the diet of most people in the developed world, satisfaction of energy requirements would inevitably satisfy protein needs for omnivores.

During an increase in training, individuals may show an adaptive increase in protein accretion. There is little evidence to suggest that once a plateau of fitness is reached, protein turnover (expressed per unit of lean body mass) is elevated by habitual exercise. Habitual exercise probably has a beneficial effect in maintaining muscle mass (and possibly protein turnover) in the elderly.

IMPORTANT RESEARCH TOPICS

118. Why is it so difficult to see the expected changes in urea turnover in relation to branched-chain amino acid oxidation? Can synthesis of acute phase proteins during or after exercise explain the "mopping up" of amino acids released from body protein?
119. Are the partial oxidation products of valine and isoleucine (their hydroxy acid

analogues) an important source of carbon for gluconeogenesis?

120. Do amino acid and protein metabolism have roles in acid-base homeostasis during and after exercise?
121. What changes in turnover of specific proteins occur in muscle during and after exercise and what are the mechanisms?
122. Does exercise increase protein requirements and is this important for people on low-protein diets?
123. What interplay exists between growth or aging and exercise-induced changes in protein and amino acid metabolism?
124. What influence does a manipulation of the carbohydrate and protein content of the diet have on protein metabolism during exercise and training?

Physical Activity, Fitness, Immune Function, and Glutamine

There is limited evidence that some forms of low-intensity exercise may be beneficial to the immune system, whereas high intensity and long duration exercise may be detrimental to the immune system. There is a nutritional link between muscle and the immune system, which might in part explain the effects of exercise on immune function.

Lymphocytes and macrophages play a quantitatively important role in the immune response, undergoing increased rates of production, recruitment, and activity. It has generally been thought that lymphocytes and macrophages obtain most of their energy by metabolism of glucose, and that resting lymphocytes, which have not been subjected to an immune response, are metabolically and nutritionally quiescent. This is not so. Glutamine is an extremely important fuel for both macrophages and lymphocytes: the rate of glutamine utilization is similar to or even greater than that of glucose. However, neutrophils do not appear to use glutamine at such a high rate. A high rate of glutamine utilization, but only partial oxidation, is characteristic of other cells (enterocytes, thymocytes, colonocytes, fibroblasts, and possibly endothelial cells). A hypothesis has been put forward which suggests that a high rate of glutamine utilization provides optimal conditions to regulate the use of the intermediates of the glutamine utilization pathway for synthesis of such compounds as purine and pyrimidine nucleotides for DNA and RNA synthesis essential for proliferation of cells. A decrease in the rate of glutamine utilization by lymphocytes would thus be expected to decrease the rate of cell proliferation. This has been shown to be the case in cultures of rat and human lymphocytes.

The importance of a high rate of glutamine utilization by these cells may be to permit a rapid immune response. The overall rate of glutamine utilization may be very high, since there are many lymphocytes in the body (approximately 1500 g in humans). This raises the important questions of the source and availability of this glutamine.

Glutamine is made available in the lumen of the intestine from the digestion of protein. However, the absorptive cells of the small intestine probably utilize almost all that is absorbed from a normal diet unsupplemented with glutamine. A major tissue involved in endogenous glutamine production is skeletal muscle: it contains a high concentration of glutamine, it has the enzymic capacity to synthesize glutamine, and it is known to release glutamine into the bloodstream at a varying rate.

The key process in the control of the rate of glutamine release by muscle is the glutamine transporter that carries glutamine across the plasma membrane. The rate of this process may be influenced by a number of hormones. Consequently, the process of glutamine synthesis may not be important to the acute control of glutamine release by muscle. Subsequently, this would impact on the plasma concentration of free glutamine.

Muscle can then be considered an important tissue source for providing substrate to the immune system. Failure of muscle to provide enough glutamine could result in impaired immune function. Therefore, an important question is what happens to the plasma glutamine levels after exercise?

Preliminary investigation in human subjects suggests that changes in the level of plasma glutamine during exercise varies with the nature of the exercise task. For example, the plasma glutamine concentration is decreased after a 42-km marathon but increased after sprints. Similarly, in the overtrained state, the plasma glutamine concentration is significantly lower in overtrained athletes compared with that in optimally trained athletes. The concentrations of alanine and branched-chain amino acids are similar in the plasma of trained and overtrained athletes. These changes are consistent with the hypothesis that a variation in the rate of glutamine release by muscle could influence the ability of the immune system to respond to an immune challenge.

IMPORTANT RESEARCH TOPICS

125. What happens to the plasma glutamine level when overtrained athletes engage in acute exercise?

126. What is the effect of different intensities and durations of exercise on arteriovenous differences in glutamine concentration for legs or arms in humans?
127. Do lymphocytes in vivo utilize glutamine at rates consistent with those predicted from in vitro experiments?
128. Will the provision of glutamine or glutamine-containing peptides during and/or after strenuous bouts of exercise decrease the risk of upper respiratory tract infections associated with such activity?
129. What is the effect of various training regimes on the plasma glutamine level?
130. Would previous exercise training facilitate glutamine release from muscle after undergoing surgery, thus improving the rate of recovery of the patient?

Physical Activity and Iron Metabolism

The belief that regular physical activity causes a specific anemia, the so-called "sports anemia," is entrenched in the scientific literature. However, the criteria for diagnosing such an anemia are inadequate. Thus, the incidence of the condition and its etiology are not clearly established.

The increased frequency of abnormalities in biochemical measures of iron status in the physically active individual, including low serum ferritin concentrations (8 to 22% in males; 9 to 82% in females), reduced hemoglobin concentrations (9 to 60%) and absence of stainable bone marrow stores, suggest that regular physical activity can impair whole-body iron metabolism. Factors that might explain these findings include: iron deficiency, increased rates of hemolysis, a dilutional effect, or activation of an acute phase response.

Conventional biochemical criteria for the diagnosis of iron-deficiency anemia include a blood hemoglobin concentration lower than 140 g/l in males and 120 g/l in females and one or both of the following: < 12 mg/l serum ferritin concentration, and < 18% transferrin saturation. When these stringent criteria are used to diagnose iron-deficiency anemia in the physically-active, the prevalence of iron deficiency ranges between 0 to 4% in both men and women. The prevalence in active women is not different from that of sedentary females but the prevalence in active males is higher than in the general population.

Factors that may explain changes in measures of iron status in the physically active include: a low intake of heme-iron, especially in vegetarian athletes; increased iron losses in sweat, urine, and feces (although these losses are typically small in normal subjects); impaired gastrointestinal iron absorption, and a disproportionate increase in blood volume relative to the increase in red cell mass causing a dilutional "pseudo anemia." These changes are not part of an acute phase response.

Iron therapy improves the exercise capacity of subjects with proven iron deficiency. A number of studies show that treatment of subjects with either low serum ferritin concentrations or reduced hemoglobin concentrations do not influence laboratory measures of maximal exercise performance.

IMPORTANT RESEARCH TOPICS

131. There is a need to establish adequate criteria for the assessment of hematological status in physically active individuals. The prevalence and etiology of iron deficiency and iron deficiency anemia need to be determined on the basis of these criteria.
132. There is a need to study the possibility that whole-body iron kinetics is substantially altered in the physically active person. In particular, there is a need to determine the cause of the low serum ferritin concentrations in the physically active.
133. There is a need to study whether iron therapy enhances prolonged submaximal exercise performance in individuals with low serum ferritin concentrations without anemia, or vice versa.

Physical Activity, Fibrinolysis, and Platelet Aggregability

Blood coagulation, fibrinolysis and platelet aggregation are intimately involved with early as well as advanced stages of atherosclerosis. The majority of published data relating physical activity with coagulation, fibrinolysis, and platelet function are restricted to young healthy subjects who have been exposed to a single bout of physical exercise. Measurements suggest that heavy exercise transiently increases in vitro blood coagulation, whereas moderate intensity effort is sufficient to activate fibrinolysis. Acute effects on platelet aggregability remain to be elucidated.

Available data suggest decreased plasma fibrinogen concentration, increased fibrinolytic and diminished antifibrinolytic activity after intensive exercise training in clinically healthy older men. In addition, limited data in middle-aged, overweight, mildly hypertensive men suggest that regular moderate-intensity exercise training inhibits platelet aggregability.

IMPORTANT RESEARCH TOPICS

134. Does physical activity have a dose–response related influence on blood coagulation, fibrinolysis, and platelet function?
135. What are the temporal relationships of any effects of physical activity on blood coagulation, fibrinolysis, and platelet function?
136. Do drugs, diet and physical activity have interactive effects on blood coagulation, fibrinolysis, and platelet aggregability?
137. Does physical activity influence the thrombotic mechanisms involved in atherosclerosis?

Physical Activity and Free Radicals

Oxygen-free radicals are essential in certain physiologic reactions, but can be potentially harmful, and contribute to several human diseases. If oxygen-free radicals accumulate unduly in cells, they can damage DNA, protein, and lipids. The body defends against oxygen-free radicals by means of scavenger enzymes, metal-binding proteins, and "antioxidants" such as vitamins E, C, and beta carotene.

Because oxygen-free radicals form during normal aerobic metabolism, they may be harmful to tissues, especially those with high rates of oxygen utilization or those subject to ischemia/reperfusion during exercise. Consequently, researchers are exploring the possible roles of oxygen-free radicals in physical activity, health, and disease.

Clinical research is hampered because assays for oxygen-free radicals are indirect and lack standardization. The most commonly used methods gauge either consumption of "antioxidants" (for instance, changes in blood concentrations of reduced glutathione) or the production of "oxidant damage," as measured by lipid peroxidation products in breath (pentane) or serum (thiobarbituric, acid-reactive substances).

The few studies of oxygen-free radicals in exercisers show these trends:

- Vigorous exercise tends to increase breath pentane production and serum thiobarbituric, acid-reactive substance concentration, and/or lower erythrocyte reduced glutathione concentration.
- Increments in serum concentrations of muscle enzymes (e.g., creatine kinase) tend to parallel increments in serum thiobarbituric, acid-reactive substances in exercisers with a known eccentric or tissue-damaging component.
- The muscle and red-cell content of scavenger enzymes may correlate with fitness.
- Exercise-induced changes in oxygen-free radicals are evanescent and do not accumulate after repeated days of exercise. There is no cogent evidence that supplements of antioxidant vitamins can mitigate exercise-induced free radical formation.

IMPORTANT RESEARCH TOPICS

138. Tools are needed to discriminate between oxidative stress and tissue damage from exercise.
139. These tools should be employed to determine whether physical activity increases free radical formation.
140. If physical activity is shown to increase free radical formation, the roles of free radicals in the etiology of exercise-induced pathology need to be examined.

Physical Activity and the Brain

Recent evidence indicates that regional brain blood flow increases during supine dynamic exercise and that this increase is influenced by exercise intensity. The increase in regional brain blood flow during exercise is not associated with an increased glucose turnover.

Physical exercise may increase the concentrations of certain circulating endorphins. The magnitude of these changes is related to both exercise intensity and duration. The effects of increases in concentrations of these peptides is unclear, but they are known to depress pain sensitivity and to elevate pain tolerance.

IMPORTANT RESEARCH TOPICS

141. How is blood flow distributed, modified, and regulated in specific regions of the brain during different forms of exercise?

142. Is there a relationship between changes in regional blood flow and glucose turnover in specific regions of the brain?
143. Does brain substrate utilization change during exercise?
144. What endogenous substances are involved in central nervous system fatigue?
145. What are the roles of specific neuromodulators and neurotransmitters (e.g., serotonin, dopamine, norepinephrine, and gama-amino-butyric acid) in the execution and modulation of exercise?
146. Can physical activity influence incidence and/or the progression of neuropathologies such as schizophrenia, migraine, and Alzheimer's disease?

Physical Activity and Perceptual and Sensory Mechanisms

There are few data on the effects of exercise on sensation and perception. In the broader context of cognitive-motor functioning, some data show that habitually physically active individuals have more rapid motor responses than sedentary individuals.

There are few reliable data from intervention studies to show any benefit of exercise on cognitive-motor functioning in young or middle-aged subjects. In contrast, there are some data that show an improved efficiency in the perception-action cycle (i.e., response speed) in the elderly. Unfortunately, none of these studies have used methodologies which permit localization of the improved efficiency.

There are few theories underlying research in this area and most studies have been conducted in a nonsystematic fashion. Data which suggest that exercise may benefit perception-action efficiency are confounded by design problems, failure of replications, and poorly assessed dependent variables. These studies also exhibit problems in describing exercise programs, assessing fitness levels, obtaining stable cognitive-motor measures, and accounting for changes in variance estimates.

A number of studies have shown that good health is associated with efficient cognitive-motor processes. For example, some individuals who are afflicted with coronary heart disease, cerebral vascular disease and atherosclerosis exhibit impaired cognitive-motor functioning (slowed response speed). Since such diseases covary with age, much of this work has attempted to disassociate primary aging processes from the secondary declines produced by pathological conditions.

Movement speed is usually faster in physically active than in sedentary adults. Moreover, some studies on older adults who exercise regularly show better scores on psychomotor and cognitive tests (WAIS, STROOP, and Memory tests). Despite these positive results, exercise interventions have failed to improve the cognitive-motor performance of sedentary older adults consistently.

As with the evidence in young and healthy subjects, cognitive-motor research in older individuals suffers from a nonsystematic approach, with little emphasis on hypothesis-driven experiments. Further, the interpretation of the cross-sectional evidence which purports to demonstrate a benefit for older adults who are physically active can be criticized. For example, stimuli to achieve high fitness levels are highly correlated with factors which optimize cognitive-motor function (motivation, instructional set, intelligence, educational level, and socioeconomic status).

IMPORTANT RESEARCH TOPICS

147. Does physical activity affect cognitive-motor processing in young and middle-aged individuals? What are the processes and mechanisms by which exercise influences the cognitive-motor functions?
148. Does physical activity slow the rate loss of cognitive-motor processing found among the elderly? If so, what types of exercise are most effective?
149. Can physical activity restore some of the typical declines in cognitive-motor processing that are found in the elderly? If so, what types of exercise are most effective?

Physical Activity, the Nervous System, and Neural Adaptation

Our current understanding of neural adaptation to physical activity involves many aspects of human behavior. Future work should address issues related to the higher levels of neural integration within the spinal cord, as well as by supraspinal centers that initiate or modulate movement. The mammalian spinal cord can execute complex motor tasks in the absence of supraspinal control, facilitating the study of neural and muscular plasticity in spinally impaired mammals, including humans. For example, the spinal cord can regain the ability to generate stepping after the removal of supraspinal control. Further, the ability of the spinal cord to generate stepping can be modified by training in specific motor tasks.

The most useful concept underlying the neurophysiological regulation of muscle force is the "size principle," that is, the order of recruitment of motor units is inversely related to parameters associated with the size of the motor unit. This concept forms the basis of the neurophysiological phenomena that are eventually integrated to form efferent signals within each motor pool. Because virtually all movements require the recruitment of components from two or more motor pools, generalized recruitment strategies, not only within but also across motor pools, need to be identified. To understand how force output of motor units is generated, the interactive dynamics among multiple motor units and between muscle units and connective tissue-tendon-bone interfaces must be defined more clearly. For example, muscle fibers of fast motor units gradually taper in cross-sectional area and often end midfascicularly, whereas the fibers of a slow unit appear to be more uniform in size throughout their length and to extend the fascicle boundaries.

Neurophysiological, morphological, and behavioral studies suggest that neural pathways involved in the control of movement are, in part, activity (impulse) dependent. For example, there are clear changes that occur in the spinal stretch reflex in reponse to short- and long-term exposure to microgravity. Moreover, postural deficiencies remain for hours to weeks following spaceflight. Other examples of neuroplasticity include: (a) evidence that monkeys can enhance or depress the monosynaptic reflexes, (b) decerebrated cats can learn to modify their stepping to avoid an obstacle, and (c) the cat spinal cord can be trained to either perform stepping or to stand without a supraspinal input. Activity dependency is a factor in the neonatal development of sensory as well as motor systems. This activity dependency is evident throughout life, although the potential for adaptation decreases with age. Changes vary from modulations of ionic transport properties in specific receptor channels to anatomical modifications of neural pathways. Significant progress is being made toward understanding long-term potentiation, memory, learning, and the role of excitatory amino acids in producing these functional modifications.

Although it has been shown that neuromuscular activity can affect some of the mechanical and metabolic properties of motor units, there is also considerable activity-independence of those properties. For example, a normal range of motor unit (and muscle fiber) types can persist even after six months of electrical silence. Some motor neurons and some muscle fibers can change from a slow to a fast type in response to experimental reductions of activity, whereas others are quite resistant to this adaptation.

Several studies suggest that the number of muscle fibers innervated is determined by the type of motoneuron, but this may not be activity dependent. The level of activity may be important in guiding the coordination of motor axons to a specific number and type of muscle fiber. In humans, beyond the seventh decade of life there is a progressive loss in the motoneurons innervating fast muscle fibers. It appears that orphaned muscle fibers may be reinnervated by slow motoneurons.

IMPORTANT RESEARCH TOPICS

150. Are the fundamental differences found in the architecture of fast and slow muscle units general phenomena?
151. How does the arrangement of muscle fibers affect the mechanical output of motor units?
152. To what extent are the properties of the muscle fibers activity dependent or genetically determined?
153. What are the respective roles of passive and active loading in maintaining the mechanical and metabolic properties of the muscle fiber, motor unit, and muscle?
154. What are the primary spinal cord neuromodulators and neurotransmitters associated with locomotion?
155. To what extent do the kinetics and kinematics of a movement reflect the properties of the neural pathways versus musculoskeletal design?
156. What are the morphological and neurochemical mechanisms that govern the ability of a neuronal network to learn, initiate, and control a specific motor task?
157. Is the development of coordinated motor skills in children influenced by increased physical activity?
158. Is the rate and level of recovery of coordinated motor skills in the motor-impaired affected by physical activity?

Physical Activity and Cognitive Function

Many aspects of intellectual performance have been correlated to physical activity, often with the suggestion that intellectual performance responds positively to increased levels of physical activity (chronic and/or acute). Included in the list of potential benefits are academic performance as well as intellectual functioning (e.g., memory and cognitive response). Among the wide-ranging and broad generalizations proposed, only the following conclusions seem warranted.

The beneficial effects of chronic exercise on cognitive function (i.e., memory, intelligence, reaction time) are small but consistent. Cross-sectional data comparing fit and unfit individuals indicate that fit individuals display faster reaction times. However, data regarding the beneficial impact of exercise on choice reaction time are equivocal for the elderly. Perceptual-motor training which consists of low levels of physical activity has no beneficial effect upon cognitive function.

IMPORTANT RESEARCH TOPICS

159. Are the effects of exercise upon cognitive function linear?
160. Are the effects of exercise on cognitive function general in nature or specific to certain types of cognitive activity?
161. Is exercise a practicable intervention for delaying the debilitating effects of aging on cognitive performance?
162. Do the beneficial effects of exercise on cognitive function disappear upon termination of the activity?
163. Do the effects of exercise on cognitive function generalize to children?
164. How are the effects of exercise on cognitive function best explained?

Physical Activity and Lifestyle Behavior

A "healthy lifestyle" is exemplified when an individual, within the context of his/her own individual biological restrictions and particular physical and social environment, lives a life which reflects a consistent pattern of healthy behavior. Of particular interest is the relationship of exercise to behaviors such as smoking, dietary practices including alcohol consumption, and various self-protective behaviors such as seat belt use. Although the general quality of the evidence pertaining to the relationship of physical activity and other leisure behavior is weak, certain conclusions seem warranted.

Correlational studies indicate a week inverse association of both smoking status (smoking versus nonsmoking) and smoking consumption (number of cigarettes per day), with the level of leisure-time physical activity. Retrospective and prospective observational studies of selected activity groups indicate that although active groups generally smoke less than do the inactive groups at baseline, these differences do not increase at follow-up. Although the inverse relationship of exercise and smoking has been consistently reported across both male and female populations, the reported relationship is somewhat stronger in males.

Metabolic ward research indicates that an increase of physical activity, at least to a moderate level (daily energy expenditure increased to 125% of base level), results in a corresponding increase in the food energy intake of non-obese individuals. Under similar, controlled conditions, obese individuals do not adjust their energy intake. More active individuals report better nutritional practices (e.g., lower percentage of saturated fat, more balanced diet, a good breakfast). No consistent relationship is evident between exercise and alcohol consumption.

IMPORTANT RESEARCH TOPICS

165. Randomized prospective intervention studies should be conducted to investigate the influence of physical activity on other lifestyle behaviors. Such studies require a clear theoretical framework, valid measures, and control for potential confounders, especially socioeconomic status.
166. Future research investigating the relationship of physical activity to other lifestyle behaviors should determine the motives underlying the pertinent behaviors, using in-depth qualitative studies, as appropriate.
167. There is a need for research that examines physical activity of various types and intensity, and takes into account the social conditions of the activity as these affect tobacco and alcohol use, in particular.
168. Research should investigate whether lifestyle change programs are more effective if they focus on specific target behaviors (e.g., physical activity) than on overall lifestyle.
169. Is the efficacy of different behavior change strategies specific to population

groups (e.g., age, sex, education level) or to differing motivations?

170. What role, if any, does health-related fitness play in the relationship of physical activity to other lifestyle behaviors?

Physical Activity and Psychosocial Outcomes

Definitive statements in the research literature are hampered by inconsistent operational definitions of physical activity, psychosocial outcomes, and psychological health. Psychosocial outcomes can be of a behavioral, perceptual, affective, physiological, or cognitive nature. The current literature has focused on the anxiolytic, stress-dampening, and anti-depressant effects of exercise and physical activity (which are dealt with later). A more modest segment of the literature deals with the effects of physical activity on self-perceptions of personal efficacy, self-esteem, and psychological well-being (positive affect). These conclusions are based on this latter literature.

There is a positive relationship between exercise habits and self-esteem for both adults and children. The consistency of this association is strengthened when esteem is measured at the level of specific domains rather than globally, and where exercise is valued by the individual.

There is a positive association between acute and chronic forms of exercise and psychological well-being. This relationship is stronger when measures of positive affect are employed. However, there is no evidence that the relationship between exercise and psychological well-being holds for individuals in an overtrained state.

There is a consistent positive association between exercise and self-efficacy. This relationship holds for both acute and chronic exercise, normal and clinical populations, and for adult males and females. Some evidence exists to suggest that aerobic fitness and self-efficacy are positively related, and that the effect of exercise on positive affect is mediated by self-efficacy.

IMPORTANT RESEARCH TOPICS

171. What are the relationships among the positive psychosocial outcomes of self-esteem, self-efficacy, and psychological well-being as a function of exercise participation?
172. Are changes in affect and esteem a function of underlying change in self-efficacy, or are other social, psychological, biological, or environmental factors implicated?
173. What role, if any, does physical fitness play in the enhancement of positive psychosocial outcomes?
174. Longitudinal studies employing randomized designs with adequate follow-up and conceptually and psychometrically-sound measures are required to extend and replicate an understanding of the effects of exercise on positive psychosocial outcomes.

Physical Activity and Fitness in Disease

Physical Activity, Fitness, and Atherosclerosis

Physical activity may influence the initiation, progression, regression, and the thrombo-embolic consequences of atherosclerosis by a variety of mechanisms. Effects on HDL provide one of several possible links between exercise and atherosclerosis.

Studies of the effects of exercise on various parameters of blood coagulation, insulin resistance and glucose intolerance, and lipoprotein metabolism are described in other sections of this statement, but there are no human studies of progression or regression of atherosclerosis as modified by exercise alone.

There are studies showing a reduction in the extent of lesion formation through exercise in experimental animals kept on atherogenic diets. There are no animal studies examining the effect of exercise on atherosclerosis induced by injury. Angiographically documented regression has been observed in studies which have included exercise as part of the therapeutic regimen.

IMPORTANT RESEARCH TOPICS

Several relevant research topics can also be found in the sections dealing with fibrinolysis, platelet aggregability, lipid metabolism, and Type II diabetes.

175. Randomized, clinical trials should be implemented to evaluate exercise alone

or exercise compared to other interventions in the treatment of established atherosclerotic lesions.

176. Exercise-induced modification of atherosclerosis caused by endothelial injury should be examined in experimental animals who are not receiving dietary lipid supplements.

Physical Activity, Fitness, and Coronary Heart Disease

Sedentary living is associated with a high incidence of coronary heart disease. This observation is supported by numerous prospective studies from Europe and North America based on groups of apparently healthy individuals who were followed for fatal and nonfatal coronary heart disease for up to 20 years. The majority of studies show an inverse relationship of coronary heart disease rates across physical activity levels. There is near unanimity that physical activity provides some protection against coronary heart disease in studies that have used good or excellent epidemiological methods, including valid and reliable assessment of physical activity and comprehensive surveillance of disease endpoints. There is an approximate doubling in risk of coronary heart disease when the least active individuals are compared with their most active peers. The association of inactivity to coronary heart disease is not due solely to the confounding influences of other favorable lifestyle behaviors.

Several recent studies have assessed physical fitness at baseline by either maximal or sub-maximal exercise testing. There is an inverse gradient of coronary heart disease death rates across fitness groups. The gradient across the distribution of exposure seems much steeper for the fitness-coronary heart disease studies than for activity-coronary heart disease studies. The relative risk for coronary heart disease in the least active compared to most active is approximately 2.0. When fitness is the exposure variable, relative risks as high as 8.0 are seen when comparing least fit with most fit individuals. Although the reasons for these differences in relative risk between activity and fitness studies are unclear, there may be less misclassification in the fitness studies, because habitual physical activity is difficult to assess reliably. Physical fitness is an excellent overall marker of physical activity and may provide precision for studies on the physical activity-coronary heart disease hypothesis.

Data on the relationship between activity and coronary heart disease in women are less convincing than the data from studies on men. However, the relationship between fitness and cardiovascular disease mortality show similar relative risks in men and women when individuals with low and high fitness levels are compared. Possibly, physical activity has not been assessed accurately in women because most activity assessment techniques have been developed for use with men.

There is a strong inverse gradient of coronary heart disease rates across activity or fitness levels. Low levels of activity or fitness precede the development of coronary heart disease in healthy individuals. Results are consistent within and across populations, and the epidemiological findings are plausible and coherent with the results from clinical and experimental investigations. The current literature thus strongly supports the concept that sedentary living habits increase the risk for coronary heart disease.

IMPORTANT RESEARCH TOPICS

177. What are the specific type, intensity, duration, frequency, and total amount of physical activity required to prevent coronary heart disease?
178. What is the role of physical activity in the prevention of coronary heart disease in women and minority groups?
179. What is the relative importance of lifetime and current patterns of physical activity with respect to the risk of coronary heart disease?
180. Is the risk of coronary heart disease reduced in sedentary, middle-aged, and older men and women if they convert to a more active way of life?
181. What are the independent and interactive contributions of physical activity and fitness to the risk of coronary heart disease?

Physical Activity, Fitness, and CHD Rehabilitation

Cardiac rehabilitation is defined by the World Health Organization as "the sum of activities required to ensure cardiac patients the best possible physical, mental, and social conditions so that they may, by their own efforts, resume as normal a place as possible in the life of the community . . . and that . . . rehabilitation cannot be regarded as an isolated form of therapy, but must be integrated into the whole treatment of which it constitutes only one facet."

As a general principle, low-level physical activity should begin within the first few days of infarction. Periodic exposure to gravitational stress during the early stages of convalescence decreases the complications of bed rest. Prescribed exercise should be gradually increased throughout the period of hospitalization, until it approximates the level of physical activity required for resumption of self-care at home. Such a plan prepares the patient for a predischarge exercise test, which can be used in addition to clinical features to stratify the risk of a recurrence. Early mobilization has no adverse effects on short- or long-term morbidity and mortality.

Among patients requiring supervised exercise, less than 30% require continuous electrocardiogram monitoring. In short-term (8 to 12 week) studies of supervised exercise programs, exercise capacity improved whether the patients were in a usual care or active intervention group. However, the exercise groups typically had a 20 to 25% greater exercise capacity than the usual care treatment groups. Low-risk survivors may not need a closely supervised cardiac rehabilitation program and may graduate directly to rehabilitation at home.

Limited data suggest that patients with anterior Q-wave myocardial infarctions might develop detrimental ventricular shape distortion after exercise training, but this has not been verified. In general, patients with ventricular dysfunction improve exercise capacity from exercise training. Older post-myocardial infaction patients seem to benefit from exercise training as much as younger ones.

Several meta-analyses of randomized trials of cardiac rehabilitation involving thousands of patients have demonstrated a 20% reduction of risk for total mortality, and a 25% reduction in the risk for fatal reinfarction. However, most of these studies have involved structured exercise programs continued for long periods post myocardial infarction. Current estimates are that the incidence of cardiac arrest is approximately one death per 100,000 patient-hours of exercise in supervised cardiac rehabilitation programs. Cardiac rehabilitation improves functional capacity and reduces symptoms in patients after surgery for coronary artery bypass and cardiac transplantation.

IMPORTANT RESEARCH TOPICS

182. Does exercise training improve the quality of life and survival in patients with heart failure?
183. Can exercise training in patients with coronary heart disease improve myocardial perfusion and function?
184. Does cardiac rehabilitation lower health care costs and improve psychosocial outcomes?

Physical Activity, Fitness, and Stroke

Stroke incidence and mortality are major public health problems in developed countries. Atherosclerosis is thought to be the underlying pathologic cause of most thromboembolic (ischemic) strokes, whereas hypertensive disease is the major pathologic determinant of hemorrhagic stroke. There is little direct evidence relating physical activity and/or physical fitness to the risk of thromboembolic or hemorrhagic stroke. Data from animal models are scarce.

Data relating physical activity to the risk of stroke are equivocal. Weaknesses of study design, including incomplete or non-existent control for potential confounding variables, often temporally incorrect and inadequate measures of physical activity, and potentially incomplete case definition and ascertainment, contribute to equivocal conclusions. No published studies have examined physical fitness and the risk of stroke.

Physical activity and fitness could be related to a lower risk of thromboembolic stroke either directly or indirectly (by influencing other factors thought to increase the risk of stroke). The potential mechanisms for any direct influence on atherosclerotic plaque or lesions in the arteries to the brain are unknown.

Physical activity or fitness may also alter the risk of hemorrhagic stroke. Such alteration may be based on blood pressure effects and the intensity of physical activity. Moderate exercise lowers resting blood pressure and may thus lower the risk of hemorrhagic stroke. High-intensity exercise could conceivably induce hemorrhagic stroke and such a tendency has been found in stroke-prone hypertensive rats.

IMPORTANT RESEARCH TOPICS

185. Is there an association between habitual physical activity and/or fitness and the risk of stroke?
186. Is there an increased risk of stroke during acute, intense physical activity, and

if so, is this risk influenced by the type of exercise?

187. What is the role that physical activity plays in atherosclerotic plaque formation and regression?
188. What is the role that physical activity plays in atherosclerotic plaque rupture?
189. What is the interaction of physical activity and/or fitness with other established risk factors for stroke?

Physical Activity, Fitness, and Peripheral Vascular Disease

More than 30 studies, almost all without any control group, have documented that regular exercise increases physical performance capacity in patients with peripheral vascular disease of the lower extremities. Both the walking distance before the onset of claudication and the maximum walking distance are increased. Gains in performance have ranged from less than 50% to more than 1,000%. The increase in performance is unrelated to the extent of disease or the duration of training. The extent of ischemic stimulus imposed during the training may be a critical factor.

The mechanism responsible for the improvement in performance is unknown. There is evidence to support the development of collateral vessels, an increase in maximum blood flow, a redistribution of flow within the ischemic leg and an increase in blood fluidity. Biochemical changes including an increase in aerobic enzymes have been reported, but these changes are unlikely to be major factors in the increase of performance because of the deficient oxygen supply.

IMPORTANT RESEARCH TOPICS

190. Does regular physical activity prevent the development or delay the presentation of peripheral vascular disease?
191. What are the stimuli and mechanisms responsible for adaptation to exercise training in patients with peripheral vascular disease?
192. What is the most effective exercise prescription for patients with peripheral vascular disease?
193. Does regular exercise have an effect on atherosclerosis and on related risk factors in patients with peripheral vascular disease?
194. How do the short- and long-term results of regular exercise compare with other hygienic, medical, and invasive interventions in patients with peripheral vascular disease?
195. What is the best exercise testing protocol for evaluating the severity of peripheral vascular disease?

Physical Activity, Fitness, and Blood Pressure

Hypertension is a risk factor for heart disease and stroke, and a major public health problem. At the present time, the primary risk factors for high blood pressure have been identified as genetic predisposition, advanced age, high body mass index, excessive sodium intake, increased consumption of alcohol, and lack of regular exercise. Blood pressure measurements during exercise have not proven to be good independent predictors of either future hypertension in normotensive populations or of the incidence of cardiovascular events in hypertensives.

Studies in humans and animals have repeatedly demonstrated that normotensive and hypertensive populations exhibit a postexercise decrease in resting blood pressure below preexercise levels. This may persist for several hours. The mechanism and the significance of such observations are not known.

Most cross-sectional epidemiological studies show an inverse relationship between resting blood pressure and fitness levels, habitual physical activity, or exercise. However, in the majority of studies, the difference between the most and least physically active or fit subjects was seldom more than 5 mmHg. In longitudinal studies, physical activity and fitness were inversely related to the development of hypertension.

When the effects of chronic endurance exercise were examined with experimental designs that included nonexercising subjects or control conditions, 48 groups of "healthy" normotensive and hypertensive subjects were identified, mostly men. These studies indicate that relative to controls, endurance training was associated with a mean reduction of systolic/diastolic blood pressure of 3/3 mmHg in the groups with a normal average pressure; of 6/7 mmHg in borderline hypertensives; and of 10/8 mmHg in hypertensives. In the genetic spontaneously hypertensive rat, endurance training studies have consistently demonstrated that trained rats will have resting systolic or mean arterial pressures that are 10 mmHg lower than their untrained controls. In adult hypertensive rats, the lower resting pressures of trained populations are because training prevents the increase in pressure that occurs with aging.

Endurance training in humans has not consistently reduced the blood pressure response during dynamic exercise. Monitoring of blood pressure during 24 hours showed that a training-induced decrease of blood pressure during the daytime was not observed during the night when the subjects were sleeping.

The hemodynamic mechanism underlying the hypotensive effect of endurance training remains controversial as the observed decrease in blood pressure could be due to a reduction of cardiac output and/or systemic vascular resistance. Reductions in circulating norepinephrine concentrations are associated with decreases in pressure.

Most studies indicate that strength-training does not lead to persistent changes in blood pressure; some have found limited decreases. However, any hypotensive effect seems smaller than the effect that can be achieved by dynamic aerobic training.

IMPORTANT RESEARCH TOPICS

196. What mechanisms are responsible for the acute reduction in resting blood pressure after exercise?
197. What is the optimal exercise prescription for the hypertensive patient?
198. What mechanisms are responsible for the reductions in resting and exercise blood pressures observed in endurance-trained hypertensive patients?
199. How does endurance training compare and interact with other nonpharmacological interventions and with pharmacological treatments of hypertensive patients?
200. What are the risks and benefits of weight-resistive exercises for hypertensive patients?
201. What is the role of physical activity in the prevention of hypertension and its sequelae?

Physical Activity, Fitness, and Type I Diabetes

There are few well-conducted, randomized controlled studies of habitual activity in Type I diabetes, but those available suggest that physical activity has both psychological and physiological benefits and that these apply to both diabetic and nondiabetic subjects. Exercise training increases insulin sensitivity, and may reduce insulin requirements in insulin-treated diabetics. Exercise may also have beneficial effects on the cardiovascular system and on lipoprotein profiles. However, no conclusive evidence exists that glycemic control is improved. Therefore, exercise is not recommended for the improvement of glycemia; rather, it should be recommended in the uncomplicated, well-controlled Type I diabetic, for the same reasons as for a nondiabetic individual.

Type I diabetics should not be discouraged from engaging in sport or recreational activities on the basis of their insulin dependency. However, patients should be instructed in self-monitoring, because their glycemic response to exercise is often abnormal, depending on the degree of insulinization achieved with their current insulin regimen.

In nondiabetic subjects, plasma glucose levels do not change during mild to moderate exercise; the exercise-induced increase in glucose uptake is matched by a corresponding increase in glucose production. In contrast to nondiabetic individuals, the subcutaneous absorption of insulin does not decrease and may even increase during physical activity in insulin-treated diabetics, particularly if the injected limb is physically active. Therefore, the increase in glucose uptake induced by physical activity may not be matched by a corresponding increase in glucose production, with a resulting acute hypoglycemia. Hypoglycemia can also occur in insulin-treated diabetic subjects several hours after physical activity, because of the exercise-induced increase in insulin sensitivity.

Underinsulinization also results in abnormalities of fuel homeostasis during physical activity. If the insulin deficiency is substantial, the exercise-induced increase in glucose uptake is attenuated and the increase in glucose production results in a worsening of hyperglycemia.

Intensive physical activity can be more deleterious to diabetic control than moderate activity of similar duration. The normal hyperglycemic response to exhausting exercise is exaggerated even in well-controlled Type I diabetics, who are unable to respond to hyperglycemia with increased insulin secretion.

With proper instructions and careful monitoring, most uncomplicated Type I diabetics can exercise safely. Blood glucose self-monitoring is mandatory before any unplanned, prolonged or vigorous physical activity. Exercising Type I diabetics should always have glucose reading strips, and a readily absorbed form of carbohydrate available. It is very important that they monitor their blood glucose concentrations prior to, during, and after exercise and adjust their carbohydrate intake accordingly. Metabolic control is more easily achieved and the risk of hypoglycemia is lessened if exercise is carefully planned.

Diabetics treated with conventional therapy (one or two daily injections with or without short-acting insulin) should not engage in physical activity at the peak of action of the injected insulin. Exercise is best carried out postprandially in these patients. The overall risk of hypoglycemia is greater with intensified insulin treatment (multiple injection regimens or Continuous Subcutaneous Insulin Infusion) than with conventional treatment. However, the risk of exercise-related hypoglycemic events can be lessened by reduction of premeal insulin boluses and basal insulin infusion. Patients treated with Continuous Subcutaneous Insulin Infusion or with a regimen of daily insulin boluses and bed-time intermediate insulin can safely exercise in both the postabsorptive and the postprandial state.

Clinical impressions and common sense suggest that caution should be used in recommending exercise to diabetic patients with the following:

- Proliferative retinopathy, because of the possibility of intraocular hemorrhages and retinal detachment during heavy exercise.
- Severe peripheral neuropathy or vascular disease (exercise can then traumatize the insensitive or ischemic foot).
- Autonomic neuropathy with postural hypotension (since heavy exercise might precipitate hypotensive episodes or cardiac arrhythmia). With less severe autonomic neuropathy, particular attention should be paid to the maintenance of proper hydration.
- Diabetic nephropathy with heavy proteinuria (for the possibility that exercise-induced dehydration and increase in proteinuria may precipitate acute renal failure).
- Coronary heart disease in the immediate post-infarct period (for the possibility that the elevated incidence of arrhythmia in diabetes may be further increased by exercise) and in patients with unstable angina or moderate to severe heart failure. In patients with stable coronary heart disease and in the later phases of postinfarct rehabilitation, exercise is recommended, but careful preexercise evaluation, and judicious and supervised training programs are indicated.
- Cerebrovascular disease with recurrent transient ischemic attacks (for the possibility that perfusion of the brain may be jeopardized by an exercise-induced lowering of systemic vascular resistance).

IMPORTANT RESEARCH TOPICS

202. What are the independent roles of insulin, glycemia, and the free fatty acid-glucose cycle in the exercise-induced rise in glucose uptake, clearance, oxidation, and storage? And, what is the status of glucose transporters?
203. What are the mechanisms of alteration in counter-regulatory responses observed during physical activity in Type I diabetics with and without autonomic neuropathy?
204. How do the metabolic effects of moderate and strenuous physical activity differ in Type I diabetes?
205. What is the antiatherogenic potential of the reduction in insulin dosage induced by exercise training in diabetic patients?
206. Long-term controlled studies in large populations are needed to evaluate the risks and benefits of acute and chronic exercise in diabetics.
207. There needs to be objective assessment of the risks of exercise in patients with diabetic complications, in particular, for those with proliferative retinopathy.

Physical Activity, Fitness, and Type II Diabetes

Type II diabetes or non-insulin-dependent diabetes mellitus comprises some 80% of diabetic patients. Its prevalence in most western countries is 2 to 3% and, in some epidemiological studies, one case is undiagnosed for every case that is known. In some populations like the Pima Indians in Arizona, the prevalence of Type II diabetes is over 30%. Non-insulin-dependent diabetes mellitus comprises a heterogeneous group of conditions, is more prevalent among obese persons, and is associated with an impairment of insulin secretion plus resistance to insulin. These two abnormalities seem linked in a vicious circle; chronic hyperglycemia impairs both insulin secretion and insulin sensitivity ("glucose toxicity"). The major site of insulin resistance appears to be in the skeletal muscle, particularly in the mechanisms leading to muscle glycogen accumulation. There is a strong hereditary component in Type II diabetes, but in contrast to Type I diabetes, there is no evidence that Type II diabetes mellitus is linked with the genes of the major histocompatibility region (such as Class II antigens of the HLA system).

Several studies in healthy volunteers have shown that physical activity and exercise training increase insulin sensitivity. Furthermore, in middle-aged individuals, regular exercise tends to improve tolerance to orally ingested glucose and to modify favorably several recognized risk factors for cardiovascular disease such as excess total and abdominal fat, adverse plasma lipoprotein levels, and mild-to-moderate arterial hypertension.

Numerous descriptive studies have shown that the prevalence of Type II diabetes mellitus is higher in inactive urban than in active rural populations. Furthermore, cross-sectional studies have shown that the prevalence of Type II diabetes (or abnormal glucose tolerance) is greater among sedentary individuals than among their active counterparts, independent of age and body mass index. Two epidemiological studies of large populations have shown that in both men and women the relative risk of developing Type II diabetes is lower in subjects who exercise regularly. This protective benefit of exercise is especially pronounced in persons with a high body mass index, a history of arterial hypertension, or a family history of diabetes. Thus, the concept has emerged that increased physical activity is associated with a reduced incidence of Type II diabetes. The prevalence of insulin resistance in non-diabetic sedentary individuals (~25% of adults) is such that an improvement in insulin sensitivity, produced by regular aerobic exercise training, may reduce the risk of non-insulin-dependent diabetes in a significant portion of the population.

Many studies have included physical activity as part of the treatment of Type II diabetes mellitus. Potential beneficial effects of physical training include lower blood glucose and glycosylated hemoglobin levels, lower fasting and postprandial plasma insulin levels, increased insulin sensitivity, favorable changes in plasma lipid profiles, increased cardiovascular fitness and physical work capacity, increased antithrombotic activity, and an improved self-esteem and sense of well being. However, exercise in Type II diabetic patients is not without risk or contraindications similar to those discussed for Type I diabetes. Practical considerations include: preexercise evaluation, the nature of the exercise prescription itself and appropriate precautions.

The literature indicates that exercise has a definite potential to improve glucose tolerance and reduce the insulin response in patients with impaired glucose tolerance or very early non-insulin-dependent diabetes mellitus. Evidence for exercise-induced improvement in metabolic control in more severe forms of non-insulin-dependent diabetes mellitus is scant. However, the exercise programs evaluated to date have generally involved low to moderate intensities of exercise, prescribed for only a few weeks. The amount of exercise required for improvements in blood glucose control is unknown and may be greater than the minimal amount needed to improve cardiovascular fitness. The feasibility of using exercise training in this population may also be lower than for the general population. Even when an exercise program is feasible in a given patient, compliance is not always achieved.

IMPORTANT RESEARCH TOPICS

208. Is there an optimal combination of exercise mode, intensity, duration, and frequency for preventing Type II diabetes or improving control in patients with manifest Type II diabetes?
209. To what extent are the effects of exercise independent of changes in body mass?
210. How does exercise improve insulin sensitivity in Type II diabetes?
211. What are the risks of an exercise program in Type II diabetes?
212. To what extent does the risk/benefit ratio of physical training programs differ between various subgroups of diabetic patients?
213. How long do the beneficial metabolic and/or cardiovascular effects of an exercise program persist after the cessation of physical activity, and how is this persistence modified by the state of training of the individual?
214. How can one improve the compliance of Type II diabetic patients to exercise programs?

Physical Activity, Fitness, and Moderate Obesity

Obesity, a condition characterized by an excessive percentage of body fat, results from an energy intake that exceeds the habitual energy expenditure. Physical activity is an important variable to consider in understanding and treating obesity since it is the principal discretionary component of energy expenditure and it can modify both energy intake and body composition.

It is likely that physical inactivity contributes to the development of obesity in some individuals and that activity helps prevent obesity in others. Studies in rodents have demonstrated that both inactivity and exercise cessation lead to an increased body fat content. Moreover, exercise can attenuate the increase in body fat that would otherwise occur when rodents are given high-fat diets.

The cause and effect relationship between inactivity and obesity is less clearly established for humans. Most data suggest that many obese persons engage in low levels of habitual physical activity relative to their non-obese counterparts. However, it is not possible to conclude that physical inactivity has caused the obesity. Prospective research using better techniques to quantify physical activity is needed to demonstrate a causal relationship between inactivity and obesity.

It may be erroneous to target physical inactivity as the sole cause of obesity. For example, even if an individual displays a reduced level of physical activity, obesity could only result if the energy intake was inappropriately high for the individual's overall level of energy expenditure. Thus, obesity would result not from inactivity alone but from a failure to match energy intake with energy expenditure.

When an obese person begins an exercise program, a condition of negative energy balance develops unless there is compensation (increased intake, decreased spontaneous activity) for the energy expended in exercise. Most data suggest moderately obese humans do not show complete energy compensation when they exercise. The negative energy balance thus produces a loss of body mass and/or a change in body composition, the extent of which is determined by the magnitude of the negative energy balance.

Exercise and exercise training may increase total daily energy expenditure in multiple ways. Initially, the increase is due largely to the increase of energy expenditure during the exercise bout. Any increase in postexercise energy expenditure is not likely to be significant with the moderate intensities of exercise usually used to treat obesity. With sustained and repeated bouts of exercise, there may be an increase in fat-free mass, which in turn, would increase resting energy expenditure. Neither an acute bout of exercise nor the level of aerobic fitness appears to alter the resting energy expenditure (after accounting for fat-free mass).

Exercise increases lipid oxidation and generally produces some reduction in body fat stores. The loss of body fat is greater the more exercise is undertaken and (for a given dose of exercise) the higher the body fat content of the person beginning exercise. Changes in body composition are somewhat dependent on the mode of exercise, but decreases in body fat occur with both aerobic exercise and resistance training.

Exercise alone is often dismissed as ineffective in treating obesity. A major reason is the small energy deficit produced by exercise in relation to the large energy deficit that can be induced by food restriction programs. The effectiveness of exercise as a treatment for obesity has not been adequately evaluated in studies using sustained exercise for long periods of time. It is difficult to maintain exercise compliance in obese subjects over very long periods of time. The weight loss produced by exercise alone does not produce the decline of resting energy expenditure seen with food restriction.

There is no reason to conclude from existing data that exercise is not at least additive to food restriction in terms of producing fat loss. Some of the confusion in the literature is due to inappropriate outcome expectations. Few studies have evaluated the extent of fat loss due to exercise in relation to the estimated energy deficit produced by exercise.

Regular exercise can alter fuel oxidation, and exercise has been suggested to modify the composition of the weight loss produced by food restriction alone. Much data suggest that exercise may increase fat loss and decrease the loss of fat-free mass. Many studies show a greater total fat loss with exercise and food restriction than with food restriction alone, despite similar changes of body weight. This benefit of exercise remains controversial, and may depend on the mode of exercise used and the duration of the exercise program.

Food restriction induces a decline in energy expenditure along with a decline in body mass. There is currently no indication that exercise prevents this decline. However, if exercise preserves fat-free mass, this could result in a higher resting energy expenditure following weight loss than would occur with food restriction alone.

Persons who are successful in achieving and maintaining a reduction in body weight are highly likely to be exercisers. It is not clear, however, if or how exercise provides an advantage in weight maintenance. It is possible that persons who exercise are also those who are most successful in making permanent lifestyle changes (e.g., modifying diet).

The risks of using exercise with a moderately obese population are small and consist primarily of musculoskeletal injuries due to beginning exercise at excessive intensities. Although the benefits of exercise in the treatment of obesity remain somewhat controversial, the potential benefits far outweigh the risks. It would seem prudent to include exercise in an obesity treatment program. Exercise increases the overall size of the energy deficit, increases lipid oxidation, and may increase relative fat loss. It also remains a good predictor of long-term success in weight reduction.

IMPORTANT RESEARCH TOPICS

215. Does physical inactivity cause obesity in human beings?
216. What are the mechanisms involved in matching energy intake and energy expenditure, and how are these affected by exercise and by exercise training?
217. How much energy compensation occurs when moderately obese humans begin an exercise program? Does this change over time?
218. What modes of exercise are most effective in reducing body fat content and increasing fat-free mass?
219. What are the mechanisms whereby exercise provides an advantage in the long-term maintenance of a reduced body weight?
220. Under what conditions does the combination of exercise and food restriction alter the composition of any weight that is lost?

Physical Activity, Fitness, and Severe Obesity

Severe obesity should be considered separately from moderate obesity, as adipocyte hyperplasia accompanies severe obesity. Adipocyte hyperplasia is associated with resistance to weight loss by lifestyle modification (diet, exercise, and behavioral modification). The 1991 National Institutes of Health Consensus Development Conference on Surgery for Severe Obesity defined severe obesity as a body mass index (BMI) of 40 or above, or a BMI of 35 or above if associated with complications. There are an extremely limited number of studies evaluating exercise in severe obesity as defined by these BMI values.

Conclusions from studies evaluating effects of exercise training on body mass and body composition in the severely obese are conflicting. Exercise training preferentially reduces body fat, while preserving fat-free mass. The degree of obesity and the type, intensity, frequency, and duration of exercise all affect weight loss. The limited ability of some severely obese individuals to exercise sufficiently may limit the effects of increased physical activity upon body mass, composition, or metabolic variables. Given the slow rate of weight loss with exercise and some degree of energy compensation by the subjects, the length of the studies was generally insufficient to expect major differences in body mass.

Most studies that have evaluated insulin levels and/or insulin sensitivity with exercise in the severely obese have shown improvements, although some have found no effect. Any effects on glucose tolerance are minimal, and several studies show no effect. Resting norepinephrine levels are often increased in severely obese individuals, and in general, such levels are decreased by weight loss because of exercise training or dieting. Lipoprotein profiles may improve with exercise training, even in the absence of weight loss.

Severely obese people have poor levels of health-related fitness. Strenuous exercise may be more uncomfortable for the very obese than for the general population, and this could contribute to the poor adherence to exercise programs reported in such populations. The occurrence of arthritis, venous statis lesions, thermal stress, and skin rashes in the severely obese also limit their exercise tolerance. Most available studies have shown modest increases in exercise endurance and maximum aerobic power in severely obese subjects after participation in an exercise training program.

IMPORTANT RESEARCH TOPICS

Additional studies comparing exercise training in the severely obese versus control, or moderately obese subjects should address the following questions.

221. Do the severely obese form a separate subgroup in terms of their response to an exercise training program?
222. Are there sex differences in the metabolic profiles and in the response to treatment of severely obese individuals?
223. How can compliance of the severely obese to an exercise regimen be improved?
224. What is the relative importance of the various components of the exercise prescription for the severely obese, including: type, intensity, duration, and frequency of effort?
225. Can exercise be used for long-term maintenance of weight loss in the severely obese? Is there a role for a combination of exercise and drugs in the

induction or maintenance of weight loss?

226. How do dietary energy and macronutrient content affect the ability of severely obese subjects to exercise, the outcome of weight-loss programs, and the complications of their obesity?
227. Does pre- or postsurgery exercise alter the outcome of obesity surgery in any way?

Physical Activity, Fitness, and Osteoarthritis

Osteoarthritis is the most common of over 100 types of arthritis, but it has a poorly understood multifactorial etiology. It leads to cartilaginous degeneration and is associated with clinical symptoms. Factors important in pathogenesis include genetic predisposition, trauma, inflammation, and biochemical characteristics. Immunologic events, occupational and environmental influences, and recreational patterns also have possible importance. The physical characteristics of the participant, biomechanical factors, age, sex, hormonal influences, state of nutrition, characteristics of the playing surface, unique features of particular sports, and the duration and intensity of effort can all influence the effects of exercise participation. A uniform view of the clinical, radiologic, and pathologic criteria that can be used to define osteoarthritis has not yet been reached. This has limited understanding of osteoarthritis and has created difficulties in analyzing the effects of exercise and sport-related activities on the risk of developing osteoarthritis.

There is currently little definitive information about the impact of physical activity on the development of osteoarthritis. Data on the relationship between exercise and osteoarthritis from animal studies have been inconsistent. In humans, numerous retrospective studies have alleged a possible relationship between sports participation and osteoarthritis. They include observations of osteoarthritis developing in joints subjected to sport-related stresses in wrestlers, boxers, baseball pitchers, cyclists, sports parachutists, cricketers, gymnasts, ballet dancers, soccer players, and American football players. Similarly, evidence that osteoarthritis follows repetitive occupational activities is inconsistent and inconclusive. Most of these data are difficult to evaluate because of methodological inadequacies.

Observations generally suggest that individuals who have run long distances for many years without clinical discomfort have not developed osteoarthritis at a rate that differs from nonrunner populations. Those individuals with underlying anatomic and/or biomechanical abnormalities appear to be at greater risk of subsequent development of osteoarthritis, and such observations seem valid for other sports activities as well. Limited data suggest that physical activity (carried out within the limits of comfort, putting joints through the normal range of motion, and without underlying joint abnormality) does not lead to joint injury, even if pursued over many years. Preliminary studies of therapeutic exercise programs for selected patients with rheumatoid arthritis and osteoarthritis have suggested clinical benefits.

IMPORTANT RESEARCH TOPICS

228. Further studies should define and quantify the physical stress imposed by various activities carefully. Future investigations of exercise and osteoarthritis require appropriate study and control populations. Observations should be of sufficient duration and sample size sufficient to provide definitive information. Studies are needed using standardized clinical and radiologic assessments of joint degeneration, with objective quantification of the patients' functional status, and an assessment of other risk factors. These are difficult studies to conduct, and unfortunately may never be done.

Physical Activity, Fitness, and Osteoporosis

Weight-bearing or resisted physical activity is essential for bone health. Without gravitational or mechanical loading on the axial and appendicular skeleton, there is a rapid and marked loss of bone density. Whether the generalized decrease in physical activity as one ages has a cumulative negative impact on bone mass is unknown. However, there is ample evidence that active individuals have a greater skeletal mass than those who are inactive. There are also data to support the concept that those who are sedentary can increase bone mass by becoming more physically active.

Exercise may be most effective in maximizing bone mass in young adults and maintaining bone mass during the mature adult years. On average, active people of all ages have a higher bone-mineral density than those who are sedentary. Data from cross-sectional studies indicate that active women and men less than 50 years of age average, respectively, 8% and 10% higher vertebral bone mineral density than their inactive peers. On the other hand, longitudinal data for the effect of exercise on lumbar bone mineral density in this age group are less numerous, and certainly less impressive, with changes ranging from −12 to 8%. This discrepancy may be due to the choice of physical activity and details of the exercise protocol rather than to the potential osteogenic effect that exercise might have on bone.

The positive effect of exercise on bone is also observed in postmenopausal women and older men. Cross-sectional studies show that active women have a higher bone mass than sedentary women (+7%). When sedentary older women participate in long-term physical activity programs (> 8 months) there is usually a slight increase in their lumbar bone mineral density, ranging from 1 to 8%, depending on the type of activity that is undertaken. However, the absolute level attained remains well below that of young normal women.

The most important question is whether the exercise-induced changes can decrease the risk of osteoporotic fractures by increasing bone density, by modifying bone microarchitectural, or by decreasing the likelihood of falls. Three epidemiologic studies report fewer hip fractures among men and women with a history of physical activity than in less active groups, but the studies were limited in their control of confounding factors. A conclusive assessment of the protective effect of exercise thus remains to be done.

Five general principles should be considered in planning or evaluating an exercise program to promote bone health:

- The Principle of Specificity: exercise provides a local osteogenic effect.
- The Principle of Overload: there must be a progressive increase in the intensity of the exercise for continued improvement.
- The Principle of Reversibility: the positive effect of exercise on bone would be lost if the exercise program were to be discontinued.
- The Principle of Initial Values: those who have the lowest bone mass have the greatest potential for improvement.
- The Principle of Diminishing Returns: as the biological ceiling of bone density is approached, more and more effort is required to obtain further gain.

In spite of its beneficial effect on bone, there is no evidence that exercise can substitute for hormone replacement therapy as a means of preventing bone loss in the early postmenopausal period. Experience with young hypoestrogenic athletes (usually with a negative energy balance) demonstrates that the positive effect of exercise on bone is greatly diminished if estrogen levels are subnormal despite rigorous activity. Physical activity can be an important adjunct to any hormone replacement therapy that is required and may help older individuals to improve coordination, balance, and muscle strength. These effects may decrease the likelihood of fracture independent of bone mass by preventing falls and/or minimizing the trauma of a fall.

IMPORTANT RESEARCH TOPICS

229. How do the general principles of training apply to the skeletal system? What is the magnitude, the frequency, and the distribution of an effective load; how are different parts of the skeleton affected; and what is the time course of the response?
230. How does exercise interact with endogenous hormones, and what biochemical markers reflect the effect of this interaction upon bone?
231. What is the appropriate exercise prescription for maintaining and increasing bone mass during childhood, adolescence, maturity, and the early and late postmenopausal years?
232. What are the interactive effects on bone mass of increased physical activity, nutrition, and pharmacologic interventions?
233. How does vertebral collapse affect other physiologic systems such as cardiovascular and respiratory function, and what is the potential of physical activity to prevent or ameliorate such adverse effects?
234. How might exercise affect structural factors other than bone mass which might decrease the risk of osteoporotic fractures?

Physical Activity, Fitness, and Back Pain

Back pain is a syndrome typically identified by individual self-report. Because of the subjective nature of back pain, interpretation of existing data is problematic. Methods for evaluation of "back fitness" are much less standardized than for cardiorespiratory function. The reproducibility is best for isometric trunk muscle tests.

A history of heavy physical work, forward bending, static work, torsion, and in particular, heavy lifting are strongly correlated with the incidence of low back pain. The causal role of sedentary occupations is less clear and often has not been addressed properly in epidemiological studies.

There is a lack of adequate data regarding the relationship between physical activity or sport participation and back pain in the general population. Various reports suggest that young athletes with low back pain have underlying structural problems. Anecdotal data suggest that back pain in sport is also caused by acute traumatic injury or effects of cumulative overuse.

Cadaver studies indicate that physical activity strengthens both the vertebrae and the intervertebral discs. Symmetric disc degeneration is associated with sedentary work, and vertebral osteophytosis is related to heavy work. Movement facilitates the nutrition of the intervertebral disc. However, other factors, like smoking, also influence disc degeneration.

A reduction of the amount of weight lifted and other ergonomic modifications of the work site can reduce the risk of certain types of occupational low back pain. The possible contributions of trunk muscular strength and endurance, trunk flexibility, and cardiovascular fitness are still questionable.

There is no unanimity as to the most appropriate treatment for existing low back pain. Trunk exercise rehabilitation programs seem beneficial in the treatment of both acute and chronic low back pain. The benefit apparently depends on the dosage rather than the use of dynamic versus isometric or extension versus flexion exercises. No randomized studies have demonstrated the superiority of the multidisciplinary treatment in comparison to exercise alone.

IMPORTANT RESEARCH TOPICS

235. A systematic approach is needed to address factors which potentially contribute to low back pain.
236. Randomized intervention studies are needed in which one or more aspects of lifting techniques are modified in one group of individuals to test the value of such changes in work site practice.
237. Interaction between physical fitness programs and other important factors, like psychosocial issues such as job responsibility and job satisfaction, should be investigated to avoid an overly-narrow focus on single-factor etiology.
238. The role of physical activity, muscular performance, and cardiovascular fitness in the prediction and prevention of back pain needs further elucidation.
239. Further research is needed in order to answer the question of intensity versus type of exercise in the treatment and prevention of back pain.
240. Standardization of dynamic trunk muscle function tests is required.

Physical Activity, Fitness, and Chronic Lung Disease

Patients with obstructive and restrictive lung disease have impaired pulmonary-mechanical function and inefficiencies of pulmonary gas exchange. This imposes increased ventilatory demands upon a system with limited response capabilities. Consequently, the tolerable range of work rates is constrained.

In obstructive pulmonary diseases, the increased flow-resistive work of breathing increases the oxygen consumption, CO_2 output and blood flow demands of the respiratory muscles, increasing the propensity to shortness of breath. Shortness of breath can be further exacerbated by hypoxemia. An increased dispersion of ventilation to perfusion ratios results in increased dead space to tidal volume ratio and arterial hypoxemia. The latter, in addition to provoking dyspnea, often results in hyperventilation with a decreased arterial CO_2 pressure. The consequence is an increased ventilatory demand for a given work rate.

The maximum attainable ventilation and the maximum achievable airflow are both reduced in obstructive lung disease. When the exercise ventilation approaches the maximal attainable ventilation, the exercise airflow encroaches upon (and may exceed) the outer limits of the patient's maximum expiratory flow-volume curve. This mechanical limitation is typically accompanied by a high rating of dyspnea, constraining further increases in work rate. Consequently, the peak O_2 intake, heart rate and blood lactate are all typically low during maximum exercise. When expiratory airflow is the dominant cause of functional impairment, the duration of inspiration can be shortened to prolong the time available for expiration. As a result, the mean inspiratory airflow and, consequently, inspiratory work increases. However, this strategy appears to be employed only by patients with severe expiratory air flow obstruction. End-expiratory lung volume increases during exercise in subjects with chronic obstructive pulmonary disease. This contrasts with normal subjects, in whom the end-expiratory lung volume decreases during exercise.

Exercise itself can provoke an increase of airway resistance in subjects with bronchial asthma. The exercise-induced bronchospasm is typically observed immediately postexercise. During the exercise session, an improvement in airflow is often seen. However, some subjects do develop bronchospasm during exercise. The postexercise bronchoconstriction reaches a peak during the first 15 minutes of recovery and then subsides slowly. Airway resistance may not return to preexercise levels for more than an hour. Respiratory heat and water loss appear to be the predominant mechanisms of the exercise-induced bronchospasm. The consequent hypoxemia is a result of an increased dispersion of ventilation to perfusion ratios in the lung.

Programs to improve exercise function in patients with obstructive lung disease should be designed to do the following:

- Reduce ventilatory demand, for example, administration of bronchodilators, supplemental oxygenation, pulmonary rehabilitation, and physical training.
- Improve respiratory performance, for example, bronchodilators (especially in patients who become bronchospastic during exercise), respiratory muscle training, and breathing pattern optimization.
- Reduce perception of breathing, for example, supplemental oxygen, pharmacologic, and psychogenic agents.

Patients with restrictive forms of pulmonary disease, such as diffuse interstitial fibrosis, have an increased elastic work of breathing, with a reduction of total lung capacity and its subcompartments. They respond to exercise with a rapid, shallow breathing pattern and report a high degree of dyspnea at maximum tolerable exercise. The combination of increased dispersion of ventilation to perfusion ratios and the low tidal volume leads to a high dead space to tidal volume ratio. Hyperventilation is commonly seen. Arterial hypoxemia results from both increased dispersion of ventilation to perfusion ratios and a diffusion impairment consequent to a reduced pulmonary capillary volume. These factors increase the ventilatory demand at a given work rate.

The inspiratory muscle load is abnormally high, and during exercise the ratio of tidal volume to inspiratory capacity closely approaches 1.0. The maximum exercise ventilation approaches the maximum attainable ventilation and breathing frequencies above 50 per min are quite typical. Oxygen supplementation can be used to reduce both the hypoxemia and a component of the dyspnea in restrictive lung disease, allowing an increased work capacity. However, neither the dyspnea nor the hyperventilation is abolished by this tactic.

IMPORTANT RESEARCH TOPICS

241. Establish the mechanisms of exertional dyspnea in patients with lung disease, with special reference to the interaction between pulmonary-mechanical and chemoreceptor mediation.
242. Develop improved methods of ameliorating exertional dyspnea.
243. Establish optimum training protocols to reduce the ventilatory demands of exercise and to increase the sustainable levels of ventilation.
244. Continue the search for the mechanism causing a mismatch of alveolar ventilation-to-perfusion ratios and also seek a means of reducing the mismatch.
245. Establish the contribution of deterioration of extrapulmonary systemic function (e.g., cardiovascular and muscular performance) to the impaired exercise tolerance and exertional dyspnea in patients with lung disease.
246. Determine the molecular mechanisms of exercise-induced bronchospasm and develop methods for effective prophylaxis.
247. Establish the genetic and environmental basis of obstructive and restrictive lung diseases, with the goal of preventing or alleviating the pulmonary disease.

Physical Activity, Fitness, and Kidney Diseases

The quality of life and long-term survival of patients with endstage renal disease (ESRD) are reduced, due to an accelerated development of atherosclerosis and eventual death from cardiovascular disease. The functional capacity of this population is poor. Fewer than half of the patients with endstage renal disease can increase their energy expenditure beyond the level required for walking, and most spend the majority of their time at rest. Chronic uremia, cardiovascular and musculoskeletal disease, anemia, and hypervolemia, along with poor motivation, depression, fatigue, and physical inactivity all reduce the exercise capacity of patients with chronic renal failure.

The high prevalence of hypertension, dyslipoproteinemia, reduced high density lipoprotein levels, glucose intolerance, and hyperinsulinemia accelerates atherosclerosis, causing substantial morbidity and premature mortality from cardiovascular disease in patients with endstage renal disease. This has led investigators to test the hypothesis that exercise training would improve cardiovascular function, reduce blood pressure, and improve lipid and glucose metabolism in this population.

Patients with endstage renal disease have a maximal aerobic power that is reduced on average by 50%, and a maximal heart rate that is decreased by 20 to 40 beats per minute, relative to healthy people of comparable age. Endurance training for as little as 10 weeks increased $\dot{V}O_2max$ by 15 to 20% in a selected group of dialysis patients. However, training for more than six months was needed to reduce hypertension, reduce plasma triglyceride and insulin levels, raise high-density lipoprotein cholesterol, and improve glucose tolerance. Exercise training also improved muscle strength, hematological function, and psychosocial status. These changes were associated with a reduction in antihypertensive medications, and a return to employment in some exercising patients.

Multisystem involvement, severity of disease, and differences in treatment warrant that patients with endstage renal disease undergo a complete medical examination and a graded exercise test prior to exercise training. Once a stable medication, dialysis, and dietary regimen is established, compliant dialysis patients will benefit from exercise training by improving cardiovascular function, reducing risk factors for atherosclerotic cardiovascular disease, and enhancing psychosocial status and quality of life. The high risk of cardiovascular complications, increased prevalence of multiple comorbidity, frequent psychological dysfunction, and poor compliance are major factors limiting the successful conduct of exercise programs in patients with endstage renal disease. Nevertheless, there is substantial need to improve the physical health of patients with chronic renal failure, to prevent the cardiovascular complications associated with endstage renal disease, and to reduce the stress of transplantation and immunosuppressive therapy.

IMPORTANT RESEARCH TOPICS

248. Can the accelerated atherosclerosis, loss of musculoskeletal function, chronic disease, fatigue, and depression be attenuated sufficiently by exercise training to reduce medical complications and improve the quality of life in patients with chronic renal failure?
249. What are the mechanisms by which exercise (a) improves cardiovascular, metabolic, and musculoskeletal function; (b) reduces risk factors for cardiovascular disease; and (c) enhances the psychological status of patients with endstage renal disease.
250. Can early physical rehabilitation delay the progression of renal disease in patients with declining renal function by reducing metabolic, cardiovascular, musculoskeletal, hematologic and immunologic complications?
251. Are there optimal exercise regimens for uremic patients that are safe, maximize adherence, and improve both physiological function and psychological status?
252. What are the effects of erythopoietin with and without exercise on the exercise capacity and the prevalence of cardiovascular risk factors in patients with endstage renal disease?
253. Is exercise training safe and effective in improving the health and functional capacity of older patients with endstage renal disease and comorbidity, including diabetes and cardiovascular disease?
254. Multicenter longitudinal studies are needed to determine if exercise training will reduce chronic morbidity and cardiovascular complications, improve quality of life and socioeconomic status, and prolong survival in patients with endstage renal disease.

Physical Activity, Fitness, and Bladder Control

Available data on the interrelationship between physical activity, fitness, and bladder control are sparse. Lack of bladder control during physical activity is primarily a female problem, and is often caused by stress urinary incontinence. Reported prevalence rates of female incontinence vary from 8 to 52%. The large variability of results may be explained by differences in study populations, response rates, definition of the condition, and the physical activity level of the respondents. A prevalence of 33% has been shown in a gynecological practice of exercising women, and a prevalence of 26% in female physical education students.

Continence requires a higher urethral than bladder pressure (a positive closure pressure). Factors which are necessary to maintain a positive closure pressure include: (a) normal function of the central nervous system and peripheral nerves innervating the bladder, urethra, and the pelvic floor muscles; (b) normal function of the pelvic floor muscles and the smooth and striated muscles of the urethral wall to close the urethra; and (c) possibly an adequate hormonal milieu to maintain submucosal and mucosal function.

A number of risk factors for stress urinary incontinence have been identified. These include pregnancy, parity, and age. However, high prevalence rates of stress urinary incontinence have also been demonstrated in young nulliparous women.

Incontinence leads to a reduction in the sense of well-being and the quality of life, with withdrawal from physical activities, especially activities that are performed in groups. High impact activities (running and jumping) may provoke leakage in those with stress urinary incontinence. Jumping with legs in alternating abduction and adduction (jumping jacks) is the activity most likely to cause symptoms. There are no data that reveal whether chronic physical activities could cause stress urinary incontinence. Longitudinal studies would be necessary to answer this question.

Stress urinary incontinence can be treated by surgery, pharmacological agents, electro-stimulation, strength training of the pelvic floor muscles, and bladder training. On the basis of current research, it is not possible to establish the most effective form of treatment. Common problems in the studies include: uncontrolled designs; the use of different, unreliable and invalid outcome variables; inadequate assessment of pelvic floor muscle function and strength; and variations in the duration of treatment and exercise regimens.

There is no evidence that general physical activity can either prevent or treat stress urinary incontinence. However, specific pelvic floor muscle strength training is effective in 60% of women, as demonstrated in a controlled randomized study. But over 30% of women are unable to contract the pelvic floor muscles correctly: The most common errors are the contraction of gluteal, hip adductor, or abdominal muscles or the performance of a Valsalva maneuver instead of pelvic floor muscle contractions. Most women are able to learn a correct contraction. Hence, to be effective the exercise has to be thoroughly taught. A controlled randomized study has shown that a combination of 8 to 12 maximal contractions, 3 times a day, and group exercise once a week are effective if performed for a period of at least 6 months. Pelvic floor muscle exercises should be the first choice of treatment because they are effective, noninvasive and complication-free.

IMPORTANT RESEARCH TOPICS

255. There is a need to develop reproducible and valid outcome measures of stress urinary incontinence, and methods to assess bladder and urethral function during exercise.
256. What is the normal function of the urethra and pelvic floor muscles during different forms of exercise?
257. What are the mechanisms of incontinence in nulliparous females?
258. Can strenuous exercise, such as weight lifting or marathon running, cause urinary incontinence?
259. What is the optimal mode of pelvic floor muscle exercise, the frequency of training and the duration of the exercise period when treating female stress urinary incontinence?
260. What is the mechanism through which pelvic floor muscle exercise acts to prevent and treat stress urinary incontinence?
261. Can urinary incontinence be prevented by early strength training of the pelvic floor muscles?

Physical Activity, Fitness, Immune Function, and Infection

Several infectious diseases affect highly active individuals. This may be because they perform in an environment in which certain pathogenic microorganisms are particularly widespread, or, in certain types of sport, because abrasions or other tissue injuries are likely. Highly active persons may also be at increased risk of various infections because of cross-infection from others with whom they make close contact, and from potential immunosuppression due to a combination of psychosocial stress and direct physiological effects linked to overtraining and/or participation in competitive athletic events.

Much attention has recently focused on physical and psychological stress, as potential factors modulating immune function, immune status, and upper respiratory tract infections. Because of the high incidence of upper respiratory tract infections in the general population, an understanding of the relationship between exercise and upper respiratory tract infections has potential public health implications.

The relationship between upper respiratory tract infections and exercise can apparently be modeled as a "J" curve. The risk of upper respiratory tract infections seems to decrease below that of a sedentary individual when one engages in moderate exercise training, but rises above average during periods of very heavy endurance exercise training and following exhausting endurance events.

Unusually heavy training and/or bouts of intense exercise lead to unfavorable changes in certain markers of immune function. Potential factors related to these changes may include the effects of cortisol, epinephrine, and the acute phase response to skeletal muscle damage. Several epidemiological studies have shown that risk of upper respiratory tract infections is increased in athletes following marathon-type events. Psychological stress, which alone has been shown to suppress immune function, may be a contributing factor. Regular moderate exercise training, on the other hand, may decrease the risk of acquiring an infection. Several of the immune system changes that occur during moderate exercise could improve host protection.

Various aspects of physical performance are reduced during an infectious episode. If an athlete experiences a sudden and unexplained deterioration in performance during training or competition, clinical evidence suggests that, among other possibilities, infection should be suspected. Several studies have demonstrated that exhausting exercise after contracting an infection may increase the risk of a corresponding final myocarditis. For this reason, clinicians recommend that intense exercise be restricted until full recovery.

Acquired immunodeficiency syndrome (AIDS) is a major public health problem. Questions have been raised regarding HIV transmission during sports that require close physical contact. The following recommendations regarding HIV infections in the athletic setting have taken into account earlier suggestions made by various sports medicine agencies:

- There is no evidence for HIV transmission during sports.
- Athletes infected with HIV should be allowed to participate in all sports.
- There is no justification for HIV screening prior to sports participation.
- There is a very low potential risk of transmitting HIV in some sports (e.g., boxing, wrestling).
- Each coach and trainer should receive training on the cleaning of equipment and the minimization of this risk.

Based on limited research, exercise programs for HIV-infected individuals do not appear to alter the course of disease, but may improve or preserve the individual's quality of life.

IMPORTANT RESEARCH TOPICS

262. More research is needed to improve our understanding of the threshold work rate below which exercise becomes protective and above which it is detrimental for upper respiratory tract infections.
263. Further research is warranted to elucidate the clinical significance of transient exercise-induced changes in immune status and function, and to determine which variables best predict potential changes in host protection.
264. There is also a need to examine the relation of upper respiratory tract infections in athletes and the involvement of the immune system in the tissue repair process that occurs following strenuous exercise. Could the active enmeshment of the immune system in the muscle tissue repair and inflammation process mean that protection from upper respiratory tract infections is compromised?
265. Larger, randomized, long-term, exercise training studies with HIV-infected individuals are needed to determine whether negative immune system changes can be attenuated.

Physical Activity, Fitness, and Cancer

The hypothesis that increased physical activity may be of benefit in preventing cancer development is not a new idea; the first study was reported in 1922. Early human studies (conducted up to the 1970s) yielded equivocal findings. The measurement of physical activity in these studies tended to be imprecise. Instead of measuring activity on an individual basis, investigators inferred the amount of activity from membership in a group (e.g., a specific occupation or participation in varsity sports teams). The investigators also did not consider potential confounding factors, such as body mass index and diet. Moreover, they studied only fatal cases, rather than the incidence or prevalence of the disease.

Studies of all-site cancers yielded inconsistent results. When investigators focused on site-specific cancers, the most consistent finding to emerge was an association between increased physical activity and a decreased risk of colon cancer. This observation has been consistent for both case-control and cohort study designs of varying strengths. Because cancer is a disease with a long induction period, randomized clinical trials are not feasible. Investigators studying populations from a number of developed countries have observed a protective relationship. There have been fewer studies of women than of men; nonetheless, current evidence suggests that the same relationship exists for women as for men. The protective effect of physical activity has also been documented in various ethnic groups. Although not consistently reported by all investigators, a dose-response relation appears to exist. That is, increasing amounts of physical activity appear to confer greater degrees of protection against colonic cancers. The lag time for a protective effect of physical activity remains unclear, but two studies in which physical activity during university was assessed, reported no association between such activity and the subsequent risk of colon cancer. We do not know whether different types and patterns of physical activity might offer varying degrees of protection against colon cancer. Whether certain subsites within the colon are more strongly protected by physical activity than other sites also remains unresolved. Body mass index and diet do not appear to confound, but may modify, the relationship between physical activity and the risk of developing colon cancer. A plausible mechanism for the protective relationship exists: physical activity appears to stimulate colonic peristalsis, but to decrease segmentation. This may reduce contact between the colonic mucosa and potential carcinogens in the fecal stream, both because of the shortened transit time and because of the decrease in mixing that occurs during segmentation.

Current evidence suggests that the risk of developing rectal cancer is not associated with the level of habitual physical activity. The absence of any relationship has been shown in studies conducted in several countries, and in studies of men as well as women. The situation may differ from that associated with colon cancer, because the rectum is only intermittently filled with feces, and increased peristalsis in the large bowel may not greatly affect the duration of contact between fecal material and the rectal mucosa.

A few studies have examined the influence of physical activity on the risk of developing prostatic cancer. A protective effect, no effect, and a harmful effect of physical activity have all been reported. The biological basis for a protective relationship is plausible: high levels of testosterone may be associated with an increased risk of this cancer, and some investigators have found strenuous physical activity to decrease resting testosterone levels.

The association between physical activity and the risk of breast cancer is another area of research yielding equivocal results; two studies have reported protection and two studies of weaker design have suggested no relationship. The first study noted that physical activity protected against cancers of the female reproductive system as well. Again, a plausible mechanism for a protective relationship exists; physical activity appears to alter the gonadal hormone milieu in women, and this altered profile may reduce the risk of cancers of the breast and the reproductive system. Data pertaining to the influence of physical activity on the risk of other site-specific cancers have been scarce.

There is a paucity of data on physical fitness as it relates to all-site cancer risk. The one study of this topic reported an inverse association between physical fitness, assessed by the endurance time of a maximal treadmill test, and all-site cancer mortality. To the extent that the resting heart rate can serve as a proxy for physical fitness, one other study of three populations has reported a direct relation between resting heart rate and all-site cancer mortality, colon cancer mortality, and colon cancer incidence.

IMPORTANT RESEARCH TOPICS

266. More data are needed pertaining to the effects of physical activity on the risks of cancer at sites other than the colorectum.
267. Once a relationship has been established for a specific cancer site, we need to address the following additional issues:
    - Does the observed relationship hold for both sexes, various ethnic groups, and populations with differing lifestyles?
    - At which periods of life should an individual be physically active in order to accrue any benefit?

- What types and patterns of physical activity are the most beneficial?
- Will an individual who changes from physically inactive to physically active behavior be protected against developing cancer? Conversely, will an individual who changes from an active to an inactive lifestyle lose this protection?
- Do body mass index and diet modify the relationship between physical activity and risk of the cancer?

268. Does physical activity confer uniform protection for all subsites within the colon? Or are certain subsites more strongly protected by physical activity than other sites?
269. What are the effects of physical activity in individuals who already have developed cancer?

Physical Activity, Fitness, and Recovery From Surgery or Trauma

Surgical trauma is followed by a convalescence period with decreased physical activity, decreased physical fitness, and increased feelings of fatigue extending to at least the first postoperative month. Daily physical activity (the average time spent standing and walking) is reduced in such patients during the first 6 weeks after both major and minor surgery. Those patients who are most active preoperatively also tend to be the most active in the postoperative period.

The voluntary muscle force of the elbow flexor muscles is decreased 10 to 20 days after major surgery. Measurements of handgrip force have also been made in many studies, but the results are variable. However, the response of adductor pollicis muscle to electrical stimulation is unchanged after major surgery. The oxygen uptake during standard submaximal exercise after major surgery is unchanged compared to preoperative findings. The pulse rate both at rest and during exercise is increased after surgical trauma. During identical intensities of exercise before and 20 days after surgery, the serum lactate concentration is significantly higher postoperatively. The decrease in physical activity and exercise tolerance after surgery are correlated with the postoperative decrease in body mass.

The increase in fatigue after surgery correlates with the degree of surgical trauma, the decrease in voluntary muscle force and endurance, the higher heart rate during standard submaximal bicycle exercise, and the decrease in body mass and average skinfold thickness. This increase in fatigue is independent of age and sex, preoperative anxiety, general anesthesia and duration of surgery, postoperative pain relief, and the extent of the increment in serum lactate during a standard submaximal exercise test.

Possible mechanisms to explain postoperative changes include an endocrine-metabolic response to the surgical trauma, immobilization, and decreased energy intake. A positive effect of exercise training is found after cardiac surgery, renal transplantation, and lower limb amputation. Inadequate enteral nutrition during 4 days (5 MJ/day) has no influence on either postoperative fatigue or the decrease in body mass. Intravenous nutrition during 10 days (13 MJ/day) has a positive effect on body mass and exercise tolerance postoperatively. It seems likely that the problem of recovery from surgery is multifactorial.

IMPORTANT RESEARCH TOPICS

270. What are the relative effects of epidural analgesia versus general anesthesia on physical activity and fitness after surgery?
271. What are the effects of pre- and early postoperative training on the recovery of function after surgery?
272. Does sufficient enteral nutrition influence the recovery of function?
273. Does the completeness of pain relief affect physical activity after surgery?
274. Are there interactions between analgesia or anesthesia, pre- and postsurgery exercise training, nutrition and pain relief affecting recovery?

Physical Activity, Fitness, and Neuromuscular Disorders

The debilitating and often progressive nature of many neuromuscular diseases limits the physical activity of the affected individuals sufficiently to cause further deconditioning, which in turn accelerates their loss of functional capacity.

Individuals with neuromuscular diseases can be broadly categorized into two groups, according to whether they have apparently normal or reduced muscle mass. A lower than normal muscle mass resulting from destructive or atrophic myopathies is associated with weakness and premature fatigue; the dystrophies best represent this class of disorders. Muscle mass is more normal in disorders of muscle activation, such as myasthenia gravis, and defects of energy metabolism, such as McArdle's disease. There has been little systematic research on physical activity, training, and performance in these disorders. Nor has there been adequate assessment of the effects of exercise interventions upon the ability to undertake the activities of daily living. Information is particularly limited in those with impaired muscle activation or relaxation, and individuals with multiple sclerosis.

The maximal oxygen intake of male patients with muscular dystrophy is low, ranging from less than 15 ml/(kg × min) in Duchenne patients up to approximately 30 ml/(kg × min) in those with slowly progressive dystrophies. Submaximal exercise responses, such as the tight coupling of increases in cardiac output to increases in $\dot{V}O_2$, appear to be normal. At peak exercise, there is often a lower than expected heart rate and arteriovenous O_2 difference, the greatest deficits being associated with the most severe forms of disease and the least muscle mass. The contribution of physical inactivity to the low exercise tolerance in dystrophy has not been established. Very limited observations suggest that training may improve $\dot{V}O_2max$ by 20 to 25% in some patients. However, one study reported concurrent increases in markers of muscle damage.

The muscle strength in dystrophy may range from almost nothing in end-stage Duchenne, to 70 to 80% of normal in more slowly progressive forms of dystrophy. There is often a direct relationship between strength and muscle mass, but incomplete motor unit activation can also contribute to weakness. Case reports of exercise-induced overwork weakness, in addition to little evidence of strength gains in Duchenne patients with minimal muscle mass, suggest little or no benefit is obtained from resistance training in these patients. The best controlled studies in other classes of dystrophy, however, demonstrate large gains in dynamic and isometric strength in response to resistance training in subjects who initially possess more than 10% of the anticipated normal strength for their age and sex.

There is considerable information on exercise responses in patients with phosphofructokinase deficiency and in McArdle's disease. Such individuals can perform mild exercise effectively, but heavy exercise is associated with pain, contractures, and extreme fatigue. The $\dot{V}O_2max$ of these patients is markedly reduced. In progressive exercise, the cardiac output increases much more than would be expected for a given rise in $\dot{V}O_2$.

The exercise responses of patients with disorders of lipid metabolism and of mitochondrial electron transport have also received some attention. The diverse nature of these disorders results in exercise responses that range from severely impaired to approximately normal. Data on exercise training as a potential therapeutic modality are almost nonexistent.

IMPORTANT RESEARCH TOPICS

Future research in this area of investigation must be more rigorously standardized, with larger sample sizes, most likely in multicenter trials.

275. Which patients with neuromuscular disease can benefit from endurance and resistance training in terms of their ability to undertake the activities of daily living?
276. Are conventional methods of exercise prescription appropriate for patients with neuromuscular disease?
277. What are the appropriate physiological and psychological tests to assess changes in the performance of daily activities?
278. What is the effect of endurance and resistance training on overwork weakness and muscle damage in the various forms of neuromuscular disease?
279. Can endurance or resistance training counter the deleterious effects associated with various progressive neuromuscular diseases?
280. What is the interaction among medications, exercise, and neuromuscular diseases?

Physical Activity, Fitness, and Depression

The efficacy of psychotherapy and pharmacological therapy in the treatment of depression is well documented, but it has been estimated that 21% of individuals who experience major depressive disorders are not seen in any service settings, and as many as 56% are seen by their physicians without receiving mental health services. There is also evidence that those individuals who receive treatment may not be well served. When one considers the cost and potential side-effects of antidepressant drugs, a search for nonpharmacological interventions is understandable. Psychotherapy can be particularly effective in the treatment of "non-biological" depression, and an effective adjunct when used in concert with biological interventions, but it requires a substantial investment of time and money. Finally, because of the pandemic nature of depression, neither drug therapy nor psychotherapy offers an acceptable solution. The best solution is prevention, not treatment. One potential strategy is exercise.

Exercise is associated with a decreased level of mild to moderate depression. The relationship between chronic physical activity and depression is equivocal in individuals who are not clinically depressed. However, there is limited research evidence suggesting that acute physical activity may reduce scores on depression inventories in nonclinically depressed individuals.

Excessive amounts of physical training (i.e., overtraining) increase depression scores in a dose–response manner in healthy young men and women. Severe depression requires professional treatment (e.g., medication, electroconvulsive therapy, and/or psychotherapy). The effects of exercise as an adjunct to treatment for severe depression are unclear at this time. Physically healthy people who require psychotropic medication may safely exercise if both the exercise prescription and medications are titrated under close medical supervision.

IMPORTANT RESEARCH TOPICS

281. Is the alleviation of depression observed in clinically depressed individuals following programs of chronic physical activity caused by physical activity? If so, what is responsible for the antidepressant effect?
282. If vigorous exercise reduces depression, what mode, intensity, duration, and frequency of activity maximize this effect?
283. Since excessive exercise (overtraining) causes an adverse disturbance of mood, what is responsible for these affective changes?
284. What role does exercise play in the prevention, onset, and treatment of depression within an overall therapeutic milieu?
285. What are the acute and chronic effects of exercise on brain histochemical, biochemical, and behavioral indicators of depression?

Physical Activity, Fitness, and Anxiety

Current estimates from the U.S. suggest that 12 percent of its citizens suffer from a disruption of their "normal" lifestyle due to anxiety and anxiety-related problems. Panic attack has become the most frequent type of psychopathology. Although most anxiety disorders continue to be treated with psychotropic drugs, an increasing number of primary care physicians are routinely prescribing exercise as a treatment for anxiety. The increasing clinical awareness of the role of exercise in reducing anxiety has prompted the U.S. National Institutes of Mental Health to identify this as a topic of immediate concern.

Due to the complexity of the construct of anxiety there has not been any consistency in its measurement. Anxiety is usually recognized as a moderate to high point along the physiological arousal continuum; the individual perceives a lack of control, which manifests itself in excessive worry, fear, and heightened sympathetic arousal. This perceived lack of control eventually leads to a disruption of normal behavior patterns, with such manifestations as erratic performance and an inappropriate attentional focus.

Since increased arousal is a necessary but not a sufficient condition for the diagnosis of an anxiety response, many investigators have used physiological measures to infer anxiety. Others have focused on psychological, paper and pencil measures of anxiety. These latter measures have either been "state" measures ("how I feel right now") or "trait measures" ("how I feel in general").

At least 26 published reviews support the anxiolytic (anxiety-reducing) nature of exercise, but most reviewers caution that early studies (a) were correlational or cross-sectional in type, (b) lacked appropriate control groups, and (c) suffered from many other methodological problems (e.g., inadequate sample size, or the use of inappropriate statistical tests), thus preventing a clear interpretation of findings. Better studies dealing with the exercise-anxiety relationship are now available. A literature search ending in June, 1991, identified 148 studies on this topic, from which several conclusions may be drawn.

There is a small to moderate relationship showing that physically fit people have less trait anxiety than those who are unfit. Research designs which maximize statistical power (within subject design or optimal sample size) and have randomized group assignment are associated with larger reductions in anxiety.

When compared to untreated control groups or baseline values, state anxiety is reduced following both an acute bout of aerobic exercise and an aerobic exercise training program. The anxiolytic effects of exercise on state anxiety begin within 5 minutes after acute exercise and continue for at least 2 hours.

Reductions in state and trait anxiety are associated with activites involving continuous, rhythmic (aerobic) exercise rather than resisted, intermittent exercise. Regardless of the intensity or duration of exercise, anxiety is reduced following acute or chronic exercise. The greatest reductions in trait anxiety occur in exercise programs that continue for more than 15 weeks.

In most of the state anxiety studies, exercise has not reduced anxiety any more or less than other known anxiety-reducing treatments (e.g., relaxation, meditation, and quiet rest). Reductions in anxiety following exercise are observed irrespective of whether physiological, behavioral, or self-report measures are employed. The relationship between reductions in anxiety and increases in physical fitness is equivocal, but individuals who initially have a low level of fitness or are very anxious achieve the greatest reductions in anxiety from an exercise training program.

IMPORTANT RESEARCH TOPICS

286. What are the key task elements (e.g., continuous versus resisted activities, social context) which cause various exercise modes to differ in their anxiolytic effects?
287. What is the time course of the reduction in anxiety following acute exercise, and how long is anxiety reduced following an exercise program?
288. Is there a significant correlation between fitness gains with prolonged aerobic training and changes in anxiety?
289. What explanations underlie the reduction in anxiety following exercise?

Physical Activity, Fitness, and Compulsive Behavior

There has been a variety of reports of a relationship between participation in a fitness program and some sort of compulsive quality to the activity. Case studies have documented the appearance of withdrawal symptoms, self-destructive exercising because the individual cannot go without an exercise "fix," and other evidence suggesting the development of an addiction or compulsion to exercise. This negative condition contrasts with the common view that regular exercise is a positive behavior with many beneficial effects. Some attempts have been made to quantify positive and negative types of exercise participation patterns through questionnaires and interviews. Another focus of research on compulsive fitness training has been the hyperactive behavior of many eating disorder patients, particularly those with anorexia nervosa. Such individuals frequently drive themselves to exercise in a compulsive manner, usually as a means of losing weight.

High levels of physical activity are frequently noted in patients with diagnosed eating disorders, particularly anorexia nervosa. This sign appears early in the syndrome but is slow to remit. Young females who are engaged in activities which emphasize high levels of physical activity, a thin body shape, and a high level of competitiveness have a greater risk of developing eating disorders than the rest of their peer group. Some competitive athletes (predominantly female) use unhealthy and dangerous weight-loss techniques in an attempt to achieve an unrealistically low body mass. They resemble eating disorder patients in this respect, though their motivation may be enhanced performance rather than appearance. Despite the widespread belief that high levels of physical activity are associated with the personality characteristics seen in patients with eating disorders, there is no evidence to support this view.

A small subset of regular exercisers develop an unhealthy compulsion to exercise even when such exercise is harmful to their physical and mental health, social functioning and job performance. Case reports suggest that compulsive behaviors associated with exercise develop in many of these individuals.

IMPORTANT RESEARCH TOPICS

290. Research is needed on the construct validity of compulsive physical activity as distinct from an eating disorder.
291. More correlational and experimental investigations are needed to identify the factors responsible for compulsive exercising to the point of injury, social disruption, or vocational interference. There is a need to understand the prevalence and etiology of such a disorder and to determine which individuals are particularly vulnerable.
292. Research should be conducted into treatment modalities that will help compulsive exercisers return to an appropriate level of physical activity.

Physical Activity, Fitness, and Substance Misuse and Abuse

Drug abuse is an international health problem. Governments spend billions of dollars in associated health care costs, and millions of individuals experience personal tragedies and wasted lives. Even elite athletes in their prime are not exempt from risk. Thus, reducing drug abuse is a major worldwide health objective. Efforts to curtail drug abuse have to date concentrated on tactics designed to reduce supply and demand, but although controlling the supply of drugs may be helpful, officials generally agree that such approaches cannot succeed if the demand remains high. A reduction of demand is critical to prevention.

In order to prevent drug abuse through appropriate interventions, the risk factors must be known, but the causes of drug abuse are complex. Research concentrating on children and adolescents has identified a number of possible risk factors predictive of drug abuse: antisocial behavior; adverse personality traits, personal attitudes, and beliefs; family-related factors such as interpersonal relationships, parental attitudes, and behaviors; school-related factors such as academic success; peer-related factors such as the social acceptance of drugs; and genetic factors. Although many questions remain unanswered concerning the most appropriate preventive approach, one strategy which may be effective involves social learning techniques, such as the development of general coping skills through enhancement of personal and social competence. Multiple behavioral techniques may be involved, and the best opportunity currently offered appears to involve comprehensive community planning.

Physical activity and exercise may confer significant benefits relative to the prevention of drug abuse and may be an important component of a comprehensive prevention program. Such exercise-related benefits as improved mood, enhanced self-concept, increased self-confidence, and reduced symptoms of both anxiety and mild-to-moderate depression suggest that physical activity and exercise may provide a useful adjunct in alcohol and other substance abuse prevention and treatment programs.

Unequivocal evidence indicates that misuse or abuse of alcohol, cigarettes, smokeless tobacco, marijuana, cocaine, or anabolic/androgenic steroids impair health with an adverse impact on various health-related risk factors. Among participants in certain exercise and sport activities, there is an increased prevalence of substance misuse and abuse (for instance, anabolic steroids by bodybuilders and smokeless tobacco use by professional baseball players). Despite theoretical rationale and popular beliefs that exercise training may mitigate some of the adverse health risks of substance abuse, there are few data to support such a prophylactic effect.

IMPORTANT RESEARCH TOPICS

293. Can exercise training mitigate some of the adverse health effects of alcohol abuse or cigarette smoking?
294. Can certain forms of physical activity help to prevent substance misuse or abuse?
295. In those activities in which there is a higher prevalence of substance misuse and abuse, what conditions (for example, social context or task demands) predispose individuals to such behavior?
296. How useful is exercise training as a therapeutic adjunct in substance abuse treatment programs?
297. If exercise training is useful in the prevention or treatment of substance misuse or abuse, what are the underlying explanations?

Physical Activity and Fitness Across the Life Cycle

The Relationship of Physical Activity to Growth, Maturation, and Fitness

Physical activity is popularly viewed as having a favorable influence on the growth, biological maturation, and physical fitness of children and youth. Inferences are based largely on comparisons of physically active and inactive individuals, and short-term experimental studies. Longitudinal studies that span childhood and adolescence and that control for physical activity are limited. Inferences about the effects of physical activity based on youngsters training regularly for specific sports have limited relevance to the general population of children and youth, since elite young athletes are a highly specialized group.

Regular physical activity has no apparent effect on statural growth and on commonly used indices of biological maturation (skeletal age, age at menarche, and age at peak height velocity). In well-nourished children and youth, these variables are primarily regulated by genetic factors. Data suggesting later menarche in female athletes are associational and retrospective, based on small samples, and do not control for other factors that influence the age at menarche.

In contrast, regular physical activity is an important factor in the regulation of body mass. Regular physical activity is often associated with a decrease in fatness in both sexes and occasionally with an increase in fat-free mass, at least in boys. Changes in fatness depend on continued activity (or restriction of energy intake) for their maintenance. Information about the possible influence of physical activity upon patterns of fat distribution in children and youth is lacking.

Regular physical activity is generally associated with greater skeletal mineralization, greater bone density, and increased bone mass. Findings are based largely on studies of experimental animals. The effects of activity on skeletal muscle are specific to the type of training program, for example, resistance or endurance training. Metabolic responses of muscle to training in growing individuals are similar to those observed in adults, but the magnitude of the response varies. There is a lack of information on the influence of physical activity on adipose tissue metabolism and cellularity in children and youth.

Active children generally show better responses to standardized motor, strength, and aerobic power tests than inactive children. Responses to short-term training programs are generally specific to the type of program or intervention. Regular instruction and practice of motor skills result in improved motor fitness, whereas strength training programs result in significant gains in muscular strength and endurance. Training-induced increments in strength are not accompanied by increases in muscle mass in prepubertal boys. Data on responses to strength training are generally unavailable for girls. There is apparently relatively little trainability of maximal aerobic power in children under 10 years of age. It is not certain whether this observation is the consequence of low trainability, initially high levels of activity, or inadequacies of training programs. During puberty, responses to aerobic training improve considerably.

Given the limitations of cross-sectional surveys, the short-term nature of most training programs, and the lack of adequate longitudinal data that span several years during both childhood and adolescence, it is difficult to partition training- or activity-related changes from those which accompany normal growth and maturation. Training-associated changes in body composition and fitness are in the same direction as those that accompany normal growth and maturation.

Interage correlations (tracking) of fitness indicators from childhood through late adolescence are generally moderate to low, and have limited predictive utility. Tracking of fitness from adolescence to adulthood is also only moderate.

IMPORTANT RESEARCH TOPICS

298. Can growth, maturation, and fitness be differentially influenced by regular physical activity prior to and during puberty? Prospective longitudinal studies that control for physical activity and that span both the prepubertal and the pubertal years are needed.
299. Is the fitness of children more responsive to regular physical activity at certain phases of growth and maturation than others?
300. What factors influence interindividual variability in trainability during childhood and youth?
301. Is physical activity per se or fitness a better predictor of a physically active lifestyle? Should more time and effort be devoted to the assessment and encouragement of a physically active lifestyle in children and youth rather than to the assessment and development of fitness per se?

Childhood and Adolescent Physical Activity, Fitness, and Adult Risk Profile

Little information is available about relationships among children's activity and/or fitness, and their present and future health status. Such paucity of information reflects the limited validity and precision of methods that assess free-living activity during childhood; a lack of knowledge as to what constitutes "health-related" fitness in children; and limited information on the tracking of activity patterns, fitness, and associated indices of health from childhood to adulthood. Most of the current evidence is limited to cross-sectional comparisons of risk factors between active and less active (or fit and less fit) children and to short-term intervention studies.

Among otherwise healthy children, a high resting arterial blood pressure has been associated with low aerobic fitness. Exercise intervention in healthy children does not induce a reduction in blood pressure. In some, but not all studies, adiposity is more prevalent in less active children. Short-term training programs induce a mild decrease in the percentage of body fat and, possibly, a mild increase in fat-free mass. The effect of training on the distribution of body fat is unknown. Physical activity and fitness seem to be associated with high serum high-density lipoprotein cholesterol and low serum triglyceride levels. Short-term training trials do not seem to modify the lipid or the lipoprotein profile of healthy children.

Children with chronic cardiorespiratory disease may benefit from training. This has been shown for those with asthma (exercise programs leading to a reduction in medication and possibly, a lessening of exercise-induced bronchoconstriction at a given intensity of submaximal exercise); cystic fibrosis (training programs yielding improved endurance of the respiratory muscles and an increased expulsion of mucus from the airways); and following surgery for congenital cardiac defects (where exercise tolerance and hemodynamic function are both improved by training). Short-term beneficial effects have also been shown for children with obesity (a reduction in the percentage of body fat and an improved lipoprotein profile), and for those with primary hypertension (a reduction in resting blood pressure). The long-term benefits of exercise have been studied only in children with obesity. In such individuals exercise as a single intervention has only a limited effect. Programs combining training, nutritional education, and behavioral modification may sustain weight control over several years.

The tracking of fatness, blood pressure, and lipoprotein profile from childhood to early adulthood is moderate to low, but is better from adolescence to early adulthood, particularly at the high risk limits of the distributions. Information on the tracking of physical activity patterns and attitudes toward physical activity from childhood to adulthood is inconclusive.

IMPORTANT RESEARCH TOPICS

Assuming that financial resources for pediatric exercise research are limited, preference should be given to longitudinal and interventional studies of children who already have adult risk factors for coronary artery disease, and those with family history of premature coronary artery disease.

302. What should be the "gold standard" for measuring the energy expenditure of children and youth under free-living conditions and for assessing behavioral aspects of physical activity?
303. Are there components of fitness that are related to health status during childhood and adolescence? Which of the components, if any, that are identified in childhood and adolescence can be related to health status in adulthood?
304. What factors underlie the decline in habitual physical activity during adolescence? What are the optimal educational and/or marketing strategies to increase physical activity among teenagers?
305. How well do patterns of, and attitudes toward, physical activity track from childhood through adolescence into adulthood?
306. Is there any ethnic or racial variation in physical activity, fitness, and risk factors during childhood and adolescence? If so, what are the underlying biological and cultural factors?
307. What is the optimal multidisciplinary program to promote the long-term control of juvenile obesity?

Physical Activity, Fitness, and Female Reproductive Function

Despite high levels of fitness, many physically active women have abnormal endocrinological reproductive function. Research does not support a specific etiological role for low fatness, low body mass, hyperandrogenism, or hyperprolactinemia in exercise-associated reproductive dysfunction. This statement concerns the effects upon female reproductive function of the "stress" of exercise, mediated by neurotransmitters and hormones of the hypothalamic-pituitary-adrenal axis, and energy availability, mediated by one or more yet to be identified metabolic signals.

Abruptly imposed, prolonged, strenuous exercise training induces anestrus, ovarian atrophy, and adrenal hypertrophy in animals of several species, but such a response is not observed with more moderate regimens. Reproductive hormonal disturbances accompanying abruptly imposed strenuous exercise training but not more moderate regimens have also been reported in women. The acute release of cortisol and other "stress" hormones during intense or prolonged exercise underlies the hypothesis that activation of the hypothalamic-pituitary-adrenal axis by physical activity disrupts the ovarian axis. It is unclear, however, whether the chronically elevated levels of cortisol observed in some amenorrheic athletes are related to strenuous exercise training.

Species differences exist, but many experiments in a wide range of species demonstrate that the activation of the hypothalamic-pituitary-adrenal axis is capable of disrupting reproductive function, and that it does so during exposure to some types of stress. The stresses most commonly employed in animal studies are electrical shock and immobilization. Although these studies tend to confirm the stress hypothesis, they also raise questions about whether the exercise effects on reproductive function may be confounded by the technique used to force the animals to exercise.

The "stress" of exercise has also been confounded with an exercise-induced energy deficit in many cross-sectional and longitudinal studies of animals and humans. In many experiments, exercise and energy availability were uncontrolled. Results of some animal studies have been confounded by using food rewards to motivate the animal to exercise. Since glucose administration prevents activation of the hypothalamic-pituitary-adrenal axis during prolonged exercise, the "stress" of prolonged exercise may reflect an acute reduction in the availability of glucose as an energy source. Similar endocrine abnormalities have been reported in physically active and sedentary amenorrheic women. Therefore, the etiology of amenorrhea in physically active women may not be uniquely associated with exercise.

Anestrus has been induced by food restriction, by the concurrent administration of pharmacological inhibitors of carbohydrate and fat metabolism, by insulin administration, and by cold exposure. This would suggest that the reproductive function of mammals depends upon fuel availability. The low dietary intake and higher prevalence of reproductive dysfunction in physically active women is consistent with the hypothesis that some physically active women self-impose a chronic energy deficit, resulting in a reduced basal metabolic rate.

There is evidence to implicate both the stress of exercise and energy availability as potential etiological factors of the reproductive endocrine dysfunction observed in some highly physically active women. Carefully controlled experiments with human subjects are needed to distinguish the independent contributions of stress and energy availability and to identify the mechanisms mediating these effects.

IMPORTANT RESEARCH TOPICS

308. What are the mechanisms of altered hormonal secretion in exercise-associated amenorrhea?
309. There is a need to characterize ovulatory dysfunction in menstruating, exercising women, including a determination of mechanisms, physiological significance, and clinical consequences.
310. Animal models should be used to study the effects of exercise and energy intake on the development, maturation, and subsequent function of the human female reproductive system.

Physical Activity, Fitness, and the Health of the Pregnant Mother and Fetus

The relationship of cardiac output to oxygen consumption and $\dot{V}O_2max$ appear to be unchanged by pregnancy, whereas the submaximal oxygen consumption and respiratory quotient at a given intensity of exercise are increased. Pregnancy-related changes in stroke volume during and after exercise have not been established. Pregnant women appear to thermoregulate adequately during brief exercise in thermoneutral environments, but thermoregulation has not been studied during prolonged exertion or in different environments. The effect of quantified exercise training on measures of exercise capacity during pregnancy has also not been examined in randomized, controlled trials.

The effects of exercise on catecholamine, insulin, glucagon, cortisol, and growth hormone concentrations have been incompletely examined in mother and fetus. Further studies of mother and fetus under varied and defined exertional conditions are required, as are similar studies in patients with Type I and II diabetes mellitus and disorders of maternal blood volume and pressure.

Fetoplacental homeostasis during maternal exertion has been investigated primarily in ungulate models. In these animals, the fetal oxygen uptake is maintained despite reduced uterine perfusion, even during very strenuous acute maternal exercise. Data on fetal heart rate changes and uterine activity during brief bouts of submaximal, human, maternal exertion suggest adequate fetal homeostasis. However, maximal exertion has been followed by fetal bradycardia in some instances. The implications of this finding to fetal homeostasis under conditions of very strenuous maternal exertion are unclear. Studies of the effects of prolonged maternal exertion on transplacental fuel kinetics are limited, as are controlled studies on the effects of maternal physical training, workplace exertion, and fitness on maternal and perinatal outcomes.

The interaction of chronic exertion with maternal conditions predisposing toward fetal growth retardation (for example, chronic hypertension, cardiac disease, or chronic cigarette smoking) may be important epidemiologically. Chronic exertion may improve glucose tolerance in gestational diabetes, and may have a therapeutic role in both this disorder and Type II diabetes. Neither the chronic nor the acute effects of exertion on insulin sensitivity, glucose kinetics and metabolic rate have been examined in pregnancy.

IMPORTANT RESEARCH TOPICS

311. Do women who are physically active have different perinatal outcomes in randomized, controlled studies where energy balance and expenditures have been adequately quantified in specific recreational and work environments?
312. What are the effects of pregnancy on the hormonal response to acute exercise?
313. What are the effects of prolonged bouts of maternal exertion and of present or prior physical training upon the cardiovascular, endocrinologic, and metabolic responses to exercise and upon perinatal outcomes?
314. What are the effects of exertion during pregnancy and the puerperium upon maternal cardiovascular and metabolic disease, and on fetoplacental disease —particularly disorders of fetal growth and development?
315. Do differences in maternal health-related fitness, attributable to racial or ethnic characteristics, alter the response to exertion during pregnancy and thereby affect the impact of exercise on maternal and fetal outcome?

Physical Activity, Fitness, and the Male Reproductive System

The male reproductive system consists anatomically of the hypothalamic-pituitary-testicular axis and the ejaculatory apparatus. The hypothalamic-pituitary-testicular axis is responsible for the manufacture and release of sex steroids, predominantly testosterone, and for the maturation and release of male gametes. Testicular function is controlled for the most part by luteinizing hormone and follicular stimulating hormone, both substances being released in a pulsatile fashion from the pituitary at 90-110 minute intervals, under gonadotrophin releasing hormone control. Gonadotrophin releasing hormone cannot satisfactorily be assessed in the systemic circulation, as it circulates predominantly in the pituitary portal system and has a half-life of less than 2 minutes. The pulsatile release of luteinizing hormone can be demonstrated because the luteinizing hormone half-life is 20 minutes; follicular stimulating hormone cannot usually be shown to be pulsatile, because its half-life exceeds 90 minutes. Luteinizing hormone is responsible for the manufacture of testosterone, whereas precursor availability is regulated to some degree by prolactin. Testosterone, in turn, inhibits both the production and the release of luteinizing hormone.

Testosterone is responsible for male differentiation in utero, development of secondary sexual characteristics at puberty and their maintenance during adult life. The hormone is also involved in the regulation of hepatic function, skeletal muscle growth, skeletal growth and maturation, gametogenesis in follicular stimulating hormone-primed tubules, and some behavioral aspects including sexuality. Animal data suggest that the speed of neuromuscular transmission is also affected by testosterone. Circulating testosterone is mainly bound to high-affinity, low-volume sex hormone binding globulin (~60%) and to low-affinity, high-volume albumin (~37%). The albumin-bound and free (~3%) testosterone are both biologically available.

Spermatogenesis is dependent upon testosterone and follicular stimulating hormone. The development of sperm takes up to 90 days from the initiation of gamete formation until its release into the epididymis. Full functional maturation of the sperm does not occur until after ejaculation. A peptide hormone, inhibin, is released from the testis during spermatogenesis, in turn, inhibiting both the production and the release of follicular stimulating hormone.

Short, intense bouts of exercise increase serum testosterone levels; there is debate as to what degree hemoconcentration, decreased clearance and/or increased synthesis are involved. The effects of short term exercise on serum luteinizing hormone and follicular stimulating hormone levels are unclear. It takes 20-40 minutes for a luteinizing hormone increment to induce a serum testosterone response. Because serum testosterone increments precede the time when luteinizing hormone is reported to have an effect, the testosterone increase does not involve gonadotropin stimulation of the testes.

There is a suppression of serum testosterone levels during and subsequent to more prolonged exercise and, to some extent, in the hours following intense short-term exercise. Again, the mechanisms are unclear; systems that might influence the decrease of testosterone synthesis include decreased gonadotropin, increased cortisol, changes in catecholamine or prolactin levels, and perhaps an accumulation of metabolic waste products.

Endurance training often induces a subclinical inhibition of serum testosterone levels. Changes in pulsatile luteinizing hormone release have been described, but they do not appear to be essential to the reduction of circulating testosterone levels. Clinical suppression of the hypothalamic-pituitary-testicular axis is unlikely in men. Anecdotal evidence suggests that a combination of dietary deficiencies with heavy exercise may result in decreased bone density and an increased risk of fractures. Semen quality is little affected by physical activity, with the exception of extremes of endurance training and associated weight loss. Thus, physical activity and training have measurable effects on the male reproductive system, but dietary alterations may be confounding factors. Such effects are generally physiological, and have no significant clinical consequence, except in extreme situations.

IMPORTANT RESEARCH TOPICS

316. What are the mechanisms of (a) testosterone increase with short-term exercise, (b) reduction of serum testosterone levels with acute exercise bouts of longer duration, and (c) the decrease in serum testosterone levels found with endurance training in some athletes?
317. Is there any long-term consequence of the reduced testosterone levels (both within the accepted physiological range and more profound reductions) which are observed in some athletes?
318. What is the impact of possible interactions between training and diet on testosterone responses?
319. What are the effects of exercise and training on male fertility and sexuality?

Physical Activity, Fitness, and Aging

Aging beyond the third decade is associated with a deterioration in most physiological systems. Lifestyle changes, including alterations in physical activity and diet, and disease processes also become manifest with aging, and may contribute to the functional deterioration that is evident in older individuals. Thus, many of the deteriorations of physiological function associated with aging may result from secondary aging processes, rather than primary biological aging.

Beneficial adaptations have been demonstrated cross-sectionally in older endurance-trained athletes and longitudinally in healthy sedentary individuals up to 80 years of age who have initiated endurance exercise training. These changes typically include a reduction of body fat, increases in maximal oxygen intake and maximal cardiovascular function, decreases of blood pressure in hypertensive individuals, and possibly an increase in bone density. Endurance training generally elicits the same adaptations, at least in relative terms, in older men and women as in young and middle-aged adults. Limited data indicate that low-intensity endurance exercise training may be as, or more, beneficial than higher intensity training in the elderly in terms of compliance, adherence, reductions in blood pressure in hypertensive individuals, and minimization of the risk of injuries.

It is unclear whether changes in glucose and lipid metabolism and cardiovascular disease risk factors resulting from endurance training are an effect of exercise per se, or are due to concurrent changes in body composition. Increases in habitual physical activity may convey nutritional benefits by increasing energy expenditure and energy intake, thus leading to a larger intake of essential nutrients—protein, minerals, and vitamins—with a correspondingly reduced likelihood of developing nutritional deficiencies.

Individuals up to ages in excess of 90 years can increase their muscular mass and strength of isolated muscle groups by specific resistive exercise training. This increase in muscular strength may yield significant functional benefits for the elderly. However, it is unclear whether older individuals can increase their total body fat-free mass significantly with resistive training.

Frail, older persons generally have greatly reduced muscle mass and strength and face a host of chronic diseases that predispose them to falls and impaired mobility. The reduced physical activity normally associated with institutionalization may further exacerbate their functional impairment. Increased levels of physical activity through walking and/or strengthening exercises may reverse many of the deleterious effects of a very sedentary lifestyle.

As a consequence of diminished exercise capacity, a large and increasing number of elderly persons will be living at or just above a level of physical ability for accomplishing the normal activities of daily living. Thus, a minor intercurrent illness may be enough to render them completely dependent. An increased level of habitual physical activity may maintain or improve physiological reserves, enhancing an older individual's ability to meet daily physical demands, and thus maintaining their independence. Increasing habitual physical activity levels and exercise training are valuable interventions for the elderly, having a favorable impact on numerous factors related to their heightened rates of mortality and disability.

IMPORTANT RESEARCH TOPICS

320. Can inevitable biological aging be differentiated from secondary aging processes?
321. What are the most appropriate training prescriptions for the various modes of exercise in order to promote health, fitness, and functional capacities in different populations of older men and women?
322. What factors predispose the elderly to falls, and to what extent can improvements in strength and flexibility decrease the incidence of falls?
323. Is it possible to decrease the rate of decline in fat-free mass in very old subjects?

Risks of Activity Versus Inactivity

Risk of Musculoskeletal Injuries

Among the greatest of the perceived risks of regular exercise is an increased risk in musculoskeletal injuries. Such injuries may be a deterrent to continued participation in exercise. Studies of patient groups treated in hospital emergency rooms and physician offices indicate that many persons experience musculoskeletal injury while they are engaged in either group or individual exercise and sporting activities. However, because such studies do not allow an estimation of the rates of injury in specified populations, they fail to provide information concerning the incidence of risk factors for musculoskeletal injuries during exercise participation or its absence. Such information is needed to evaluate this aspect of the cost-benefit ratio associated with being a regular exerciser.

The present statement is based on studies of adults, and because our interest is in the broad public health impact of exercise, special attention has been directed to the forms of exercise that are most prevalent in the adult population.

Some of the most commonly practiced activities in North America are, in order of decreasing prevalence, walking, gardening, running/jogging, aerobic dance, bicycling, weight lifting, and swimming. Our knowledge of the incidence of musculoskeletal injury is very limited for most of these activities. The one notable exception is distance running, for which the risk of musculoskeletal injury has been shown to be quite high (25 to 75% per year for the committed runner, depending on the manner in which injury is defined). In habitual runners the most common sites of injury are the knee and foot/ankle. Injury rates in running do not vary significantly with age or sex, but running distance and history of lower extremity injury are risk factors for injury.

Walking is generally thought to involve a minimal risk of musculoskeletal injury, but there are no studies of the incidence of injury in exercise walkers. Among competitive swimmers, shoulder injuries are relatively common, but the incidence of injuries in those who swim for exercise and physical fitness is unknown. Among aerobic dancers, the annual activity-related injury rate approximates 50%, and the risk of injury increases with the frequency of participation. Bicycling carries a significant risk of traumatic head injury and fatal bicycle accidents occur at a rate of approximately 3 to 4 per 100,000 population per year. However, little is known about the incidence of less severe musculoskeletal injuries in adults who bicycle for exercise. The risk of head trauma can be substantially reduced by wearing an effective helmet. With the other most common forms of exercise (such as weight lifting, aerobic dance, racquet sports, and softball), clinical studies have provided information on the most common types of injuries. Unfortunately, general population studies that would indicate the incidence of injury in relation to exposure are lacking for such pursuits.

IMPORTANT RESEARCH TOPICS

324. What is the incidence of musculoskeletal injury, and what are the risk factors predisposing to injury among regular participants in popular forms of exercise such as walking, aerobic dancing, gardening, and bicycling? What is the relationship between the dose of exercise and the incidence of injury? What is the effect of concurrent participation in two or more different types of physical activity on the incidence of injury?

325. Is the overall risk of musculoskeletal injury different in habitually active persons than in those who are inactive?
326. Which types and patterns of exercise optimize the ratio between the risk of musculoskeletal injury and risk of disease development?
327. What are the short- and long-term financial, behavioral, and health consequences of exercise-related injuries?
328. To what extent are "training errors" and participation in ancillary training activities like stretching and weight-training related to the risk of injury in habitual runners and participants in other activities?

Cardiovascular Risks

The cardiovascular complications of physical activity include cerebrovascular accidents, aortic dissection and rupture, cardiac arrhythmias, myocardial infarction, and sudden death. There are few data for the general population indicating the likelihood of nonfatal cardiovascular complications of exercise, and estimates of the cardiac risks of physical activity for asymptomatic persons are based largely on the likelihood of provoking sudden death. Most exercise-related sudden deaths in individuals over 30 years of age are associated with atherosclerotic coronary artery disease. However, a variety of cardiac abnormalities is associated with exercise-related deaths in young subjects.

The absolute incidence of deaths during vigorous exercise in healthy men who exercise regularly has been estimated at one death per 15,000 men per year (seven per 100,000). The hourly death rate during vigorous activity is significantly higher than that observed during less vigorous activity or when at rest. There are few studies of incidence for exercise-related sudden death in women. Available data suggest that the incidence of exercise deaths is much lower in women, undoubtedly because of the lower prevalence of coronary artery disease in middle-aged women as well as their lower participation in vigorous exercise.

There are few data on the incidence of exercise-related sudden death among young men. Available figures are often based on military personnel, who represent a selected population. For example, the exercise death rate among male U.S. Air Force recruits during basic training is approximately one per 170,000 men per year (0.6 deaths per 100,000). These results cannot be applied to the general population, because recruits are medically screened, and myocarditis appears to be more frequent in this population. The exercise-related cardiovascular death rate in Rhode Island for men under age 30 has been estimated at one per 280,000 per year (0.36 deaths per 100,000). However, the denominator for this estimate is all Rhode Island men of this age, and is not restricted to young men who exercise.

Estimates of the risk of exercise in patients with coronary artery disease are based on questionnaire data obtained from supervised cardiac rehabilitation programs. Recent results suggest that one cardiac arrest, myocardial infarction, or death occurs in every 112,000; 294,000; and 784,000 patient-hours of participation, respectively. An earlier study estimated one cardiac arrest, myocardial infarction and death per 35,000, 233,000, and 116,000 patient-hours, respectively. The lower event rates in the more recent study may be due to physicians referring healthier patients or to changes in coronary artery disease treatment.

Epidemiologic evidence continues to suggest that the cardiovascular benefits of physical activity outweigh cardiovascular risks. Such results are based on occupational and recreational exercise histories, but rarely include enough middle-aged and older subjects with extremely vigorous levels of physical exertion to calculate reliable incidence figures. Some intriguing epidemiologic results and the frequency of anecdotal reports of sudden death in vigorous exercise raise the question as to whether the risks of extremely vigorous exercise may outweigh its benefits.

Some recent reports of cardiac function following prolonged exertion suggest that the myocardium can suffer reversible dysfunction. Such studies rely exclusively on Echo Doppler-derived indices, which may be misleading. Nevertheless, they raise the question as to whether exercise induces cardiac dysfunction, whether this is deleterious, and whether this phenomenon has clinical implications in patients with ischemia or permanent left ventricular dysfunction.

IMPORTANT RESEARCH TOPICS

329. What is the pathology of, and what are the mechanisms responsible for, the possible coronary artery injuries (such as plaque rupture) associated with exercise?
330. What is the incidence of exercise-induced sudden death when determined in large populations including sufficient numbers of men, women, and

children? There is also a need to establish reliable figures.

331. What are risks versus benefits of extreme exertion in middle-aged persons?
332. Are there any serious long-term consequences of repetitive exercise-induced ischemia?
333. Is the exercise induced left ventricular dysfunction suggested by Echo Doppler studies a real phenomenon and of clinical significance to healthy individuals or to patients with myocardial disease?

Dose–Response Issues

Dose–Response Issues From a Biological Perspective

Any exercise that requires sustained or repeated contractions of a relatively large muscle mass activates many of the body's systems to support the process of muscle contraction. During and following exercise, local biochemical factors, along with activation of the central nervous system, stimulate the release of various hormones and affect enzymes that regulate many key metabolic functions. There are major shifts in cardiorespiratory performance, and if the activity is of sufficient intensity and duration, the renal, gastrointestinal and immune systems may become involved. Exercise also exerts physical forces on the bones, muscles, and connective tissue as a result of muscle contractions or in response to gravity. The improvement in structure, function, or health status produced by repeated bouts of exercise results from the body's immediate responses to the exercise, to the adaptations that occur over time in the body's attempt to increase its capacity or efficiency to respond to the exercise stress, or to some combination of these two responses.

The dose aspect of the dose–response relationship involves various characteristics of exercise, including type (for instance, dynamic versus static, or the amount of muscle mass used), intensity (absolute and relative to the individual's capacity), duration of session, frequency of sessions, total number of sessions, and length of time over which the sessions are performed. Other factors to be considered are baseline exercise and fitness levels, nutritional factors that might interact with exercise (for example, the intake of calcium or estrogen use may influence the effects of exercise on bone), and genetic determinants of the response. As the exercise dose that improves clinical or health status is likely to be very different from that required to improve competitive performance, it is important that the parameters of the dose–response relationship not be confined to those typically adopted when evaluating the dose–response required to improve athletic performance.

To understand the dose of exercise required to produce a specific health-related response, it would be helpful to have some idea of the nature of the mechanism of action. For example, if the response is a reduction in systemic arterial blood pressure, then to understand the dose of exercise required, it would be useful to know the mechanism by which this decrease in blood pressure is achieved. Is the lower blood pressure due to a decrease in cardiac output, a decrease in peripheral vascular resistance, or both? And what biologic changes are likely to lead to a reduction in each of these variables?

The traditional approach to the exercise dose–response issue has been to consider that the dose of exercise must produce a "training response" to be of benefit. A "training response" is a progressive change in function or structure that results from performing repeated bouts of exercise, lasts longer than hours and days, and is usually considered to be independent of a single bout of exercise. However, there is increasing evidence that some of the health-related biologic changes produced by exercise may be due more to acute biological responses during and for some time following each bout activity than to a training-induced adaptation. Examples of this type of effect include a decrease in the insulin response to a glucose challenge and an increase in lipoprotein lipase activity. If such acute changes prove to provide significant clinical benefits, then major changes may need to be made in exercise program guidelines in order to promote specific aspects of health, for example, increased frequency of activity or multiple exercise bouts per day.

Clinically significant health-related outcomes from exercise may be due to several biologic changes that have different dose–response profiles. If this is the case, then the health benefit may occur only if the characteristics of the exercise program meet the required dose (stimulus) for each of the biologic effects. A possible example of this multi-dose-response condition concerns the relationships of physical activity to decreasing the clinical manifestations of coronary heart disease. Exercise may exert its protection for heart disease through several different biological effects (changes in variables such as lipoproteins, insulin, cardiac work rate, blood pressure, and coronary artery status); each perhaps with a different dose-response profile.

Currently we know a substantial amount about the dose of exercise required to achieve many health-related physical or biological changes, but we still know very little about the optimal or minimal dose of exercise required to induce such effects in a given individual. Information on health-related biological and physical changes is still incomplete, but is adequate for the design and implementation of specific exercise program recommendations.

IMPORTANT RESEARCH TOPICS

334. What is the exercise stimulus (dose) required for a significant improvement in the various key biological changes associated with major health outcomes? How can the type, intensity, duration, frequency of exercise, and the time course of the response be defined?
335. What is the magnitude of the inter-individual variation in the dose–response relationship for the major health-related biological changes produced by exercise? Which components of the variation are due to heredity and which are due to various environmental factors? Can we identify responders and nonresponders?
336. What acute effects does exercise have upon biological outcomes that have potential health benefits? Study of this issue should consider a wide variety of exercise profiles, including prolonged low-intensity exercise as well as short bouts repeated frequently.
337. Can one discriminate between the dose-response relationship for the prevention of various pathological conditions and that needed for their treatment? For example, do the dose–response characteristics of exercise that is effective in preventing the age-related increase in arterial blood pressure differ from those lowering an already elevated blood pressure?

Dose–Response Issues From a Psychosocial Perspective

There is limited knowledge on the relationship between the dose of physical activity and the subsequent psychosocial response. Available research is frequently limited by

- the absence of a theoretical framework;
- preexperimental designs;
- weak operational definitions of the exercise dose; and
- poor external validity.

An additional problem is the meaning ascribed to the phrase "psychosocial outcomes." One can argue that these include

- overt behavior (for example, sleep and social activity);
- perception of effort (for example, the rating of perceived exertion);
- cognition (for instance, control beliefs and mental performance);
- affect (for example, anxiety and vigor); and
- the physiological outcomes of psychosocial stress.

It is erroneous to assume that the dose–response relationships will be similar for each of these different outcomes. Additionally, the concept of dose–response is in and of itself reductionistic.

The effect of a given dose of activity on any single psychosocial outcome is dependent upon subjective interpretations of the exercise stimulus (for example, the perceived intensity of exertion). Cross-sectional data suggest that the length of training influences the impact of exercise upon trait anxiety and depression. The largest effect sizes for trait anxiety are seen with programs that continue for 15 weeks or more, whereas for depression the threshold duration is 17 weeks.

Limited research suggests that reductions in blood pressure reactivity to psychosocial stress following acute bouts of aerobic exercise vary directly with exercise demands (that is, intensity and duration). In individuals with low to moderate levels of fitness, high-intensity exercise does not seem any more efficacious in influencing mood changes than low-intensity exercise.

IMPORTANT RESEARCH TOPICS

338. How does the physical and social setting of exercise influence the outcome of different doses of physical activity?
339. How are dose–response relationships influenced by subjective interpretations of the exercise stimulus and the physical and social setting of the activity program?
340. Future study of dose–response relationships should include a broad range of outcome measures, so that we might

better understand the clinical implications of different doses of activity.

341. What are the interactions between dose and mode of activity with respect to psychosocial outcomes? Are there differences of response between discontinuous and continuous activities of varying intensities and durations?
342. What baseline variables modulate dose–response relationships?

Other Considerations

Physical Activity, Fitness, and Quality-Adjusted Life Expectancy

Results from various epidemiological surveys suggest that adequate amounts of regular exercise will maintain or improve fitness, preserve good health, and enhance the quality of life relative to sedentary individuals. Hypertensive-metabolic-atherosclerotic disease will also be avoided or deferred, and in some studies of athletic populations, the length of life is increased. To the extent that physical activity is inadequate, physical fitness is reduced, the quality of life deteriorates, hypertensive-metabolic-atherosclerotic disease becomes more prevalent, and the risk of premature death is increased.

The important relationship between these sequences is that avoidance or correction of the undesirable activity pattern can reverse the downward path of adverse outcomes and result in a return to a more positive health status. An inactive individual may become physically more active, an unfit person may regain fitness, the risk of hypertensive-metabolic-atherosclerotic disease can be reduced, and life becomes longer, healthier, and more satisfying; all these follow if physical activity is adequate and maintained over the life span.

Factors other than physical activity such as inheritance, infection, nutrition, injury, environmental, and situational circumstances can all intervene and either promote or detract from the good quality, prolonged life to which the individual aspires. Yet, the past decade has seen wide acceptance of evidence that adequate levels of leisure-time physical activity promote health-related fitness and positively influence health status, quality of life, and longevity, even though the requirements for promoting these advantages in the individual and on a population are not fully defined.

One study of male United States university alumni aged 45 to 84 years, followed from 1977 to 1985, has indicated that lower all-cause death rates accompany an increase in the vigor and frequency of walking, stairclimbing, sportsplaying, and physical activity in general. The lower death rates are also accompanied by lower levels of cigarette smoking, and a lower body mass index, and by normotensive and euglycemic status, but show little association with a history of prolonged parental survival. Sedentary men (leisure energy expenditure <8 MJ/week), who contributed 58% of the man-years in this particular study, were at 19 to 66% (95% confidence intervals) greater risk of mortality during the nine-year follow-up period than more active men. Cigarette smokers showed 54 to 127% added risk over nonsmokers. Hypertensives had a 28 to 76% higher risk than normotensives. The more obese individuals were at 0 to 40% greater risk than men who were more lean. However, a background of early death in one or both parents added little to the risk of premature mortality (–9 to 20%).

Eleven to 15 years after the initial assessment, 23% of the men had remained active, 16% had converted from physically active to a sedentary status (leisure energy expenditure <8 MJ/week), 19% had converted from sedentary status to physically active, and 42% continued to be sedentary. Men who had increased their physical activity reduced their risk of death from 5 to 42% relative to those who now exercised less. Men who had decreased their physical activity level (often times because of chronic illness) increased their risk of death only slightly (–10 to 56%) versus those who had continued sedentary. Men who took up moderate sportsplay, versus those who continued to avoid it, reduced their risk between 14 and 43%. Other lifestyle factors were also associated with longevity. Men who quit smoking reduced their death risk by 8 to 43%. Long-term hypertensives were at greater risk of death than those more recently reported hypertensive. Maintenance of a lean body mass had survival advantages over continued obesity, becoming obese, or losing weight from a previously obese status.

These findings for males aged 45 to 84 years translate into estimates of extended survival when subjects are followed through to a maximum age of 85 (85 years being the approximate male lifespan). Changed lifestyles added years totalling: 0.24 to 1.30 years, for increasing physical activity to adequate level; 0.55 to 1.61 years, for taking up moderate sports; and 0.25 to 1.83 years, for quitting cigarettes. Even among the elderly, the combination of adding moderate sportsplay and stopping the smoking habit yielded a substantial gain in longevity (for example, 1.62 years for men aged 65 to 74 years, and 0.63 years for those aged 75 to 84 years).

The men who took up a more active lifestyle between the 1960s and 1977 not only increased longevity, but also reported improvements in health. They were more likely to report that they "felt younger than their years" and that they "felt fine and enjoyed life" than were those who had remained sedentary. The men who became more active were also less likely to develop cardiovascular and metabolic disorders during the nine-year follow-up.

IMPORTANT RESEARCH TOPICS

343. How much, what kinds, how intense, and for whom should physical activity be prescribed in order to improve and/or maintain health (physical, psychological, social, cultural, and spiritual well-being)?
344. How much short- and long-term physical activity is needed to induce an optimal level of physiological fitness, that is, a functional integration of all body systems?
345. How can longevity be extended to its optimum, that is, with preservation and enhancement of high quality living?
346. How can physical activity, health-related fitness, dietary and other lifestyle habits, environmental circumstances, and heredity best be integrated in our search for optimal health?

Costs and Benefits of an Active Versus an Inactive Society

Can corporate or national health care costs be reduced by increasing the prevalence of regular exercise? By extension, is the cost of achieving any improvement in health that results from greater exercise offset by a reduction in the costs of medical services? Because an increasing share of individual health care costs are borne by company-funded employee insurance programs in the United States, recent studies in that country have focused on the individual as a member of a work site employee group. In other industrialized countries, most of which have public health insurance, there is also concern about rising medical costs. Sometimes the work site has been adopted as the unit of analysis, and other studies have examined the impact of physical activity upon the population. In the private sector, a further motivation for offering exercise programs has been to enhance productivity.

Several investigators have sought to determine whether the physically active employee or member of the community is more productive, is less frequently absent from work, is injured less often, changes employment less frequently, and has a higher morale than a more sedentary person. A number of studies show potentially beneficial associations between physical activity and these variables. Correlations are generally statistically significant, but the strength of these relationships is generally low, leaving decision-makers with a good deal of uncertainty regarding the cost-benefit ratio for programs designed to enhance employee or community fitness.

A more global concern, of special importance to health economists, is the impact of improved health on longevity, and hence, on the burden that might be imposed upon company-sponsored and/or national medical and pension benefits by longer-living retirees. If improved worker health, as an outcome of increased physical activity, is translated into increased longevity (and total medical care costs for these retirees per year of life were to stay the same), such an outcome could be viewed as a liability to society and to the former employer. However, there is some suggestive evidence that active individuals will develop less chronic disease in their later years, and will die without incurring the costly extended final illness seen in many sedentary people. A longer lifespan not only has a potential impact upon medical costs, but also implies a longer total period of pension distribution, if the age of retirement also remains constant. Again, this potential cost would be offset if the retirement of a healthier person were delayed to a more advanced age. The current trend seems to be in the opposite direction, as improved pension and investment income programs support earlier retirement, although it is unclear how far accumulating medical problems influence an individual's decision to take premature retirement.

Unlike biological studies of the effects of enhanced physical activity, cost-benefit questions are frequently studied in the context of a quasi-experimental research design. In a recent evaluation of over 400 published reports of health promotion program outcomes, the vast majority were deemed insufficiently well controlled to draw firm conclusions, let alone to establish causal relationships. Given the paucity of firm, well-controlled research, some proponents of corporate and community fitness programs have prematurely advanced conclusions regarding the economic benefits of such programs. In fact, poorly supported claims detract from the probable positive outcomes that may ultimately be demonstrated. But, even if no positive return on investment is eventually concluded from more sophisticated research, good health as an outcome of increased physical activity may be its own inherent return. In other words, cost-effectiveness may be demonstrated even in the absence of a favorable cost-benefit ratio defined in strict monetary terms.

IMPORTANT RESEARCH TOPICS

347. The economic impact of exercise on the individual and on society remains unanswered, due principally to the difficulty of measuring change in a poorly controlled experimental environment. One approach has been to develop computer simulation projections of costs and benefits based on normative population data, with sensitivity analyses included as an essential part of such studies. However, such initiatives await stronger input data from well-controlled stronger input data from well-controlled randomized trials.
348. Another issue to be resolved is the lack of standardized program elements, definitions, and descriptions of outcomes. Standardization of these various terms must be achieved to allow comparisons between studies.
349. What elements comprise an acceptable corporate or community program? How is the outcome modified if other lifestyle modules such as smoking cessation are added? How should medical costs be defined: direct costs or total costs? What are the social costs and benefits of extended survival? How can productivity, absenteeism and turnover be measured accurately?
350. Since the quantification of psychological and behavioral outcomes (such as improved morale and greater productivity) are currently an uncertain science, should research focus on program cost-effectiveness rather than on cost-benefit analysis?
351. How does cost-effectiveness differ between the work site programs in manufacturing and insurance companies which have been most often studied to other industry and community settings; for instance from white salaried employee groups to minority and hourly-rate groups, and from large organizations to employees from smaller companies.
352. Would cost-effectiveness ratios differ for those who are currently inactive? What is the marginal return on such investment?
353. Most work site studies have concentrated on in-house employee programs with well-developed facilities. Many corporate programs, especially for smaller companies, have purchased memberships in commercial or community programs such as the YMCA. What are the cost-benefit ratios and the cost effectiveness for such arrangements?

Heredity, Activity Level, Fitness, and Health

Interindividual differences in the base sequence of DNA are the source of human genetic variation. Each human being has about one variable DNA base for every 100 to 300 bases, so that each one of us is genetically unique. Inherited differences are likely to be involved in determining the health status of a person as well as the interrelationships between individual components of the physical activity-fitness-health paradigm.

The contribution of genetic factors to interindividual differences in the level of habitual physical activity has not been extensively studied, but available data suggest that it accounts for about 30% of the phenotypic variation. The evidence that heredity is involved in determining interindividual variability in health-related fitness is more abundant, although the quality of the evidence varies according to the component considered and the methods that have been used to estimate heritability. Most of the data are from twin studies; heritability estimates derived exclusively from twin data are generally higher than those based on family data or relatives by adoption, and often vary quite widely from one study to another. Significant genetic effects have been reported for most factors associated with morphological fitness, with typical values ranging from about 25% for total body fat content to 30 to 50% for regional fat distribution phenotypes. Such effects are presumably polygenic, but major gene effects have also been reported to contribute to the variation in body mass index and some regional fat distribution phenotypes. Heritability estimates of various muscular and motor fitness phenotypes are largely derived from twin data and are generally well over 50%. The use of a wide range of tests to assess this component of fitness has contributed to the highly heterogeneous heritabilities reported in the literature.

Among the components of cardiorespiratory fitness, blood pressure is the variable that has been most studied by geneticists; heredity accounts for about 30% of interindividual differences in resting blood pressure. The contribution of heredity to submaximal exercise capacity and maximal aerobic power reaches about 20 to 30% of the phenotypic variance. More studies are needed to assess the genetic contribution to cardiac and pulmonary functions. Because of its association with common familial diseases like diabetes and cardiovascular disease, several components of metabolic fitness have been studied extensively; for instance, heritability levels reaching about 50% of the age- and sex-adjusted phenotypic variance for plasma triglycerides, total cholesterol, and the various lipoprotein fractions have been commonly reported.

The genetic factors responsible for interindividual differences in health-related fitness do not operate in a vacuum, but are constantly interacting with lifestyle and personal characteristics, as well as with the social and physical environment. Therefore, genetic factors may influence the response of phenotypes to environmental stimuli like regular physical activity. There is now good evidence that the extent of the response of health-related fitness factors to regular physical activity or dietary intervention is strongly determined by unknown genetic characteristics. Inherited differences appear to be more important in determining the adaptive response to regular physical activity than in determining the absolute initial level of the health-related phenotypes.

IMPORTANT RESEARCH TOPICS

354. We need to identify the genes that contribute to interindividual differences in each health-related fitness phenotype.
355. We need to determine the impact of allelic variation at relevant genes on (a) the level of health-related fitness phenotypes, (b) the response of these phenotypes to regular physical activity, and (c) the covariation between these health-related fitness phenotypes. An important question is whether the genes associated with individual differences in the response to regular exercise are the same for each health-related fitness component.

Physical Activity and Fitness: Evolutionary Perspectives and Trends for the Future

On our approximately 4.6 billion-year old planet, the first forms of life are estimated to have appeared some 3.5 billion years ago. Two billion years later, the unicellular living organism with a nucleus had evolved. The fundamental biological principles that sustain life were developed by a process of natural selection. If a comprehensive textbook of biochemistry had been written 1.5 billion years ago, it would no doubt be up-to-date in its treatment of cell function. Processes such as the breakdown and resynthesis of ATP, PCr, glycolysis, and aerobic energy production via the Krebs citric cycle and the respiratory chain were already well-developed. Evolution was now ready for its next major step, the emergence of larger animals, an era which began some 700 million years ago. Mammals are represented during the last 220 million years of the process, and the first primates entered the scene some 120 million years ago.

African fossils reveal the presence of a hominid *Australopithecus* about 4 million years ago. Several species of this genus survived for several million years, and one was the ancestor of the genus Homo, *Homo habilis*, about 2 million years ago. The species *Homo sapiens* (modern man) has probably existed for at least 40,000 years to date. The transition from the lifestyle of a roaming hunter and food gatherer to the less mobile farmer began some 10,000 years ago. Technological developments during the last 100 years have introduced a rate of change far exceeding all that occurred during the preceding 4 million years of hominid evolution.

A consequence of these changes in lifestyle is that humans have participated in gigantic experiments without any control groups. Our ancestors lived in small bands of perhaps 15-30 individuals as a cooperative society "in which individuals and environments continuously interrelate and affect each other." An individual's age was not measured in years, but rather in terms of accumulated experience. Education began when a child had matured enough to understand the messages of his or her teacher. Thus, the boys learned from the "retired" hunter, who had entered a new niche in society, carrying out a task that was still intellectually and physically demanding and of vital importance to the future of the group. There were no well-defined relationships between socio-occupational roles and a person's age in that era!

Many expressions of human behavior, which were very appropriate adaptations to life in small bands, would be close to "catastrophic" if adopted by large and modern societies. Despite the currently expressed desire of some indigenous populations, there seems no way that humans could revert to their historic "natural" way of life. But with adequate insight into our biological heritage, we may be able to modify our current, partly self-destructive lifestyle. The human body has adapted to the needs of regular, moderate physical activity, and a continuation of such activity is essential for its optimal functioning. This volume illustrates the many scientific efforts to study the value of restoring an active lifestyle as a tactic for the primary and secondary prevention of various disorders and diseases. In the future, the early study of DNA sequences may allow us to determine individuals who are at a particularly high risk of morbidity and mortality from specific diseases. It may then be possible to develop and implement preventive programs adapted to the needs of those individuals. Will it also be possible to predict a person's response to a given training program or to a change in diet from a review of blood lipids, blood pressure, maximal aerobic power, muscle strength, endurance, and the like? To take an extreme viewpoint: do those involved in health promotion have the right to "manipulate" the lifestyle of 100 persons in order to save three lives, particularly if the remaining 97 people neither enjoy nor need the exercise program but are also strongly encouraged or even "forced" to participate? At present, we are unable to predict which three individuals would benefit from a more active lifestyle. But what about in the future?

The United States Census Bureau has estimated that the proportion of Americans who are older than 65 years will double from 12% of the population in 1986 to 24% in 2020. Other developed and developing societies face similar challenges. Current gerontological research has emphasized the average age-related losses of function and has neglected to consider the substantial heterogeneity of older persons, which is in part a consequence of activity history and in part a consequence of genetic individuality. The functional effects of the inherent aging process have, in consequence, been exaggerated, and the modifying effects of diet, physical activity, personal habits, and psychological factors have all been underestimated. Within the category of normal aging, a distinction should be drawn between "usual aging," in which extrinsic factors heighten the inevitable, inherent effects of aging, and "successful aging," in which extrinsic factors play a neutral or a positive role. Aging is necessarily associated with some reduction of maximal aerobic power and muscle strength, but the functional ability of an active 65-year-old Canadian exceeds that of a sedentary young adult. Being overweight is an additional handicap at any age. In combination with the other changes seen in the frail elderly, it makes walking, climbing stairs, getting up from a bed or a chair, or entering a bus or a train more difficult, fatiguing, and eventually impossible. Aging persons thus lose their independence and autonomy. As a consequence of a progressive loss of functional capacity, large and increasing numbers of elderly persons live below, at, or just above the "thresholds" of physical ability needed for independence. A minor intercurrent illness is then sufficient to make them completely dependent.

In the United States, the life expectancy at birth has increased from an average of 47 years in 1900 to approximately 75 years in 1988, and in other countries the average expectancy is now substantially greater than this. What are the upper limits to average human longevity? It has been calculated that if ischemic heart disease were to be eliminated, the life expectancy at birth would increase by 3.0 years for females and 3.5 years for males. If all forms of cancer (22.5% of all deaths in 1985) were also eliminated, life expectancy would increase by 7.0 years for females and 8.1 years for males. In other words, elimination of these two major categories of disease would not lead to any dramatic increase in life expectancy. Technological advances in terminal medical treatment rather than a reduction in the prevalence of risk factors for chronic disease have allowed frail elderly persons who are suffering from fatal degenerative diseases to survive longer after the onset of disease than was the case in the past. Research efforts by the medical community have focused on prolonging the duration of life rather than on preserving its quality. The time has come to shift the emphasis of research toward preserving and ameliorating function in people with the nonfatal diseases of aging. One sad but important factor is ethical, including human and legal aspects of euthanasia in seemingly hopeless cases.

In this bizarre world, we notice overfeeding and the negative effects of a sedentary lifestyle in developed countries, but do little to help the millions of people who are living under marginal or very poor conditions in the "Third World." It is impossible to follow the advice to exercise and be active in societies where there is not enough food to cover even the energy demands of basal metabolism. This planet produces more food than its population needs, but it is poorly and inequitably distributed. Medical advances, including mass vaccinations, allow more and more children to survive in "Third World" countries, but what quality of life will they face as they become adults? Life has always been complicated: if we transform hominid history over a 4-million-year period into a 400 m race, it has become more complicated during the last meter (10,000 years) and particularly during the last 10 mm (100 years).

We must take a global view, and not "forget" the urgent health needs of the "Third World." However, priority one of the health scientist, from a realistic viewpoint, is to concentrate on health promotion in the developed countries. Open-air recreational activities are an effective source of physical activity that is well anchored in our biological heritage. Education in "fauna and flora" was once essential to survival. Similar education today is unfortunately neglected, but it could create an excellent lifelong, hobby interest. There are those who do not like walking just for the sake of walking, but if a hobby like bird-watching demands some walking, they will be prepared to walk. And family members, neighbors, or even business associates can also go out to "walk and talk." The message of enhanced physical activity will seem more practicable and realistic when we find such ways to incorporate regular exercise into our daily living.

Chapter 3

Physical Activity, Fitness, and Health: The Model and Key Concepts

Claude Bouchard
Roy J. Shephard

This document describes the basic model used at the Consensus Symposium to specify the relationships between physical activity, health-related fitness, and health.

An Overview of the Model

The subject matter has been approached on the assumption that the relationships between the levels of physical activity, health-related fitness, and health are complex (see Figure 3.1). The model specifies that habitual physical activity can influence fitness, which in turn may modify the level of habitual physical activity. For instance, with increasing fitness, people tend to become more active while the fittest individuals tend to be the most active. The model also specifies that fitness is related to health in a reciprocal manner. That is, fitness not only influences health, but health status also influences both habitual physical activity level and fitness level.

Other factors are associated with individual differences in health status. Likewise, the level of fitness is not determined entirely by an individual's level of habitual physical activity. Other lifestyle behaviors, physical and social environmental conditions, personal attributes, and genetic characteristics also affect the major components of the basic model and determine their interrelationships. The program content of the Consensus Symposium was planned to explore the relationships outlined in this figure.

Physical Activity

An active individual values physical activity as an important part of her or his total life experience and seeks to integrate such activity into daily routines and leisure pursuits throughout all aspect and stages of life. Physical activity comprises any body movement produced by the skeletal muscles that results in a substantial increase over the resting energy expenditure. Under this broad rubric, we consider active physical leisure, exercise, sport, occupational work and chores, together with other factors modifying the total daily energy expenditure. From the viewpoints of fitness and health, all determinants of human energy expenditure merit careful consideration.

Leisure-Time Physical Activity

In most developed societies, after completion of work, travelling, domestic chores and personal hygiene, the average person has 3-4 hours of "free," leisure, or discretionary time per day (32,68). However, there is wide inter-individual variation, depending in part upon such personal circumstances as the duration of paid work, the division of labor in the home (women often accepting more domestic duties than men), the need for self-sufficiency activities (greater in those with a limited income), daily travel time (significant for many people who live in large metropolitan areas), and the number and age of dependents.

Leisure-time physical activity is an activity undertaken in the individual's discretionary time that leads to any substantial increase in the total daily energy expenditure. The element of personal choice is inherent to the definition. Activity is selected on the basis of personal needs and interests. In some instances, the motivation will be an improvement of health and/or fitness, and the pattern of activity undertaken will be consonant with this objective. But there are many other possible motivations (21,40,61) including aesthetic (pursuit of a designed body type or an appreciation of the beauty of movement), ascetic (the setting of a personal physical challenge), thrill of fast movement and physical danger, chance and competition, social contacts,

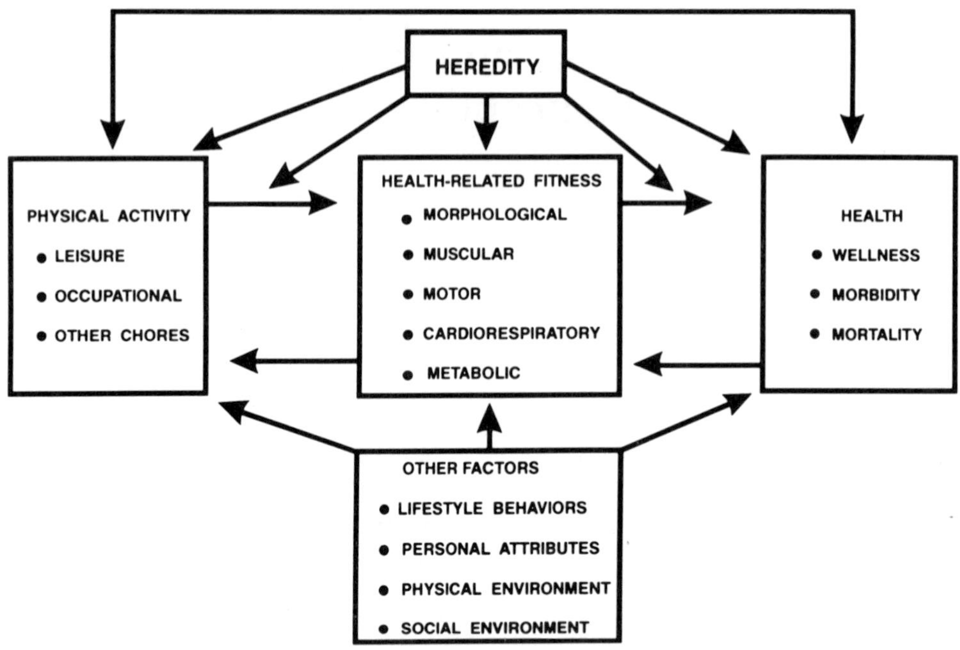

Figure 3.1 A model describing the relationships among habitual physical activity, health-related fitness, and health status.

fun, mental arousal, relaxation and detente, and even addiction to endogenous opioids.

Exercise

Exercise is a form of leisure-time physical activity that is usually performed on a repeated basis over an extended period of time (exercise training) with a specific external objective such as the improvement of fitness, physical performance, or health. When prescribed by a physician or exercise specialist, the optimum regimen advised typically covers the recommended mode, intensity, frequency, and duration of such activity (1).

Mode

The *mode* of exercise covers not only the type of activity to be performed (for instance, fast walking, jogging, or swimming), but also the *temporal pattern* of activity that is recommended (that is, continuous or intermittent activity), with a detailed specification of the duration of exercise and rest periods in the case of intermittent activity bouts. The issues of *intensity, frequency* and *duration* of exercise are therefore of considerable importance to prescription and activity assessment.

Intensity

The intensity of exercise can be expressed in either absolute or relative terms. The absolute intensity (for example, 20 kJ/min) is frequently used when classifying participants in occupational and epidemiological studies. Alternatively, absolute data may be expressed as a multiple of the individual's basal metabolic rate, thereby minimizing differences of energy expenditure between individuals due to differing body mass. Relative intensity is a percentage of the individual's maximal aerobic power output, maximal oxygen intake, or maximal heart rate. If due allowance is made for the influence of age on maximal aerobic power, the absolute and relative approaches can be reconciled (see Table 3.1).

Individual self-reports of activity participation can be categorized in terms of the intensity scales for occupation and leisure activity (see Table 3.2), taking account of both the pursuit and the frequency of its repetition. For instance, occasional swimming is likely to involve less intense activity than participation in a regular swimming program, and this in turn will involve less intense exercise than formal preparation for a major swimming competition.

Frequency

The frequency of leisure activity is normally reported as the number of sessions undertaken in a typical week, although occasional surveys have recorded less frequent participation, for example monthly. One important source of difficulty when reporting frequency is that many leisure activities

Table 3.1 A Characterization of the Intensity of Leisure Activity in Relation to the Subject's Age*

Categorization	Relative intensity (% $\dot{V}O_2max$)	Absolute intensity (METs)			
		Young	Middle-aged	Old	Very old
Rest	<10	1.0	1.0	1.0	1.0
Light	<35	<4.5	<3.5	<2.5	<1.5
Fairly light	<50	<6.5	<5.0	<3.5	<2.0
Moderate	<70	<9.0	<7.0	<5.0	<2.8
Heavy	>70	>9.0	>7.0	>5.0	>2.8
Maximal	100	13.0	10.0	7.0	4.0

*From reference 10. Note that currently there is a trend to prescribe fairly light and moderate intensity activities rather than heavier intensity activities.

are seasonal in nature. The epidemiologist thus finds it helpful to ask the frequency of participation during the past week or month and to overcome seasonal variations by questioning different individuals at different times during the year. Extending the reporting period to a full year is another approach but may suffer from recall problems.

Duration

The duration of an individual exercise session is usually reported in minutes or in hours. It is important that only the period of actual physical activity be considered, omitting travel, socializing, and preparations for participation (62). As with frequency, typical and usual duration is generally recorded although this may vary greatly.

Sport

In North America, sport implies a form of physical activity that involves competition. However, in Europe, the term sport may also embrace exercise and recreation (as in the UNESCO "Sport for All" movement, 51). There is some discussion as to whether required school programs and professional activities should be included in the category of sport because the important element of the participant's choice is then largely eliminated.

Table 3.2 Intensity of Occupational Work*

Intensity	Energy expenditure
Sedentary	<8.4 kJ/min
Light	8.4 - 14.7 kJ/min
Moderate	14.7 - 20.9 kJ/min
Heavy	20.9 - 31.4 kJ/min
Very heavy	>31.4 kJ/min

*Based on the categorization of reference 14.

Occupational Work

In the past, energy expenditures required by occupational work and the associated demands of transportation (on foot or on a bicycle) accounted for a major fraction of the total daily metabolism in a large segment of the labor force (24). This is still true in some developing societies (17), and even in the western world occasional occupational categories with a high energy demand can still be distinguished.

Heavy occupational demand has had considerable epidemiological interest (56) in the past, because it has typically been sustained for 30-40 hours per week over many years. However, in modern post-industrial societies there now tends to be an inverted gradient between "heavy" employment and daily energy expenditure, since leisure activities that are differentially accessible to the wealthy constitute the main fraction of the total daily energy expenditure (15). The standards defining a high or a very high intensity of occupational activity (Table 2; 14) differ from those applicable to "exercise." This is because in industry the duration of individual activity bouts is usually prolonged, often there are other adverse circumstances (such as a high environmental temperature, an awkward posture, or a heavy loading of small muscle groups), and normally the pace of working is set by such factors as a machine, a supervisor, or a union contract, rather than the individual.

Household and Other Chores

Automation has progressively reduced the energy demands associated with the operation of a household in developed societies, largely outdating the figures cited in the classical literature (24). While some individuals may deliberately seek out heavy activities such as sawing logs, most necessary domestic chores now fall into the "light" category of the industrial scale. The one possible exception is the care of dependents. Both playing with young children and the nursing of elderly relatives can involve quite heavy work.

Dose–Response

As with administration of a drug, there appears to be a relationship between the dose of physical activity—its mode, frequency, intensity, and duration—and the biological response in terms of improvement of fitness and health. The dose–response relationship is characterized by (a) a threshold below which little or no adaptation occurs, (b) a zone of increasing effect, and (c) a ceiling beyond which no further improvement is observed or signs of over-dosage may develop. As age increases, the margin between an effective and an excessive quantity of exercise narrows, with a corresponding requirement for a more careful prescription of physical activity. However, the dose–response issue is quite complex and needs to be considered in light of the diversity of the fitness components and health objectives.

The effects of a single dose of exercise may persist for several hours or days; thus, it is important to understand the interaction between the intensity, frequency, and duration of physical activity in determining the response.

Habitual Physical Activity

Physical activity is almost universally accepted as relevant to health, although the optimum pattern of activity (mode, intensity, frequency, and duration of individual bouts), interactions with nutritional status, and the cumulative impact of many years of participation, remain to be elucidated. It is desirable to combine the information on leisure physical activity, exercise, sports, occupational work, and other chores to assess the overall level of regular engagement in physical activity.

There is a need to integrate information on the intensity, frequency, and duration of physical activity to establish the pattern of activity over defined periods of time. One method of integration is to convert all data to an average weekly (leisure) energy expenditure (56). A second option is to compute an estimate of average 24-hour energy expenditure (28).

Energy Expenditure

The body conforms to the principle of the conservation of energy. Thus, long-term changes in an individual's body mass reflect the balance between their personal energy ingestion and energy expenditure. The liberation of heat energy by the body is expressed in joules, as an absolute value, as a ratio to estimated body surface area, per kilogram of body mass, or per kilogram of lean tissue mass. Important elements of overall daily energy expenditure in both sexes are the basal or resting metabolic rate, the energy cost of physical activity, and the thermic effect of food. In women, added demands are imposed by pregnancy and lactation.

In most circumstances, basal and resting metabolism account for the largest proportion of the individual's total daily energy expenditure. The rate of basal energy expenditure is relatively stable, although, if expressed per unit of body surface or body mass, it does show a small and progressive decrease with age. Small (about 10%) increases of resting metabolic rate are induced by ingesting a plethora of food (60), prolonged cold exposure (64), and possibly habitual activity or training (52); whereas restriction of food intake tends to reduce basal and resting metabolic rate.

Physical activity is clearly the most variable component of the total daily energy expenditure. Depending on the fitness of the individual, a five- to twenty-fold increase of metabolic rate can be sustained for a few minutes, and a healthy young adult can, if necessary, develop five to eight times the basal metabolic rate over an 8 hour working day. In a very sedentary elderly person, the total daily energy usage can be as low as 6 MJ, whereas in a highly active ultra-long distance athlete, expenditures can reach 30 to 40 MJ.

Basal and resting metabolism, the increase of metabolism following a meal, and the sustained increase of metabolism following exercise can all be assessed under the carefully controlled experimental conditions of a metabolic ward. Doubly-labelled water has been used to determine CO_2 production and thus to infer total energy expenditure over periods of 1 to 2 weeks (44), although such observations are relatively costly. If food intake can be assessed accurately for several weeks, and if body mass remains constant, then there is a 10 to 15% concordance between the individual's intake and expenditure of energy.

Health-Related Fitness

In general terms, fitness can be conceived as the matching of the individual to his or her physical and social environment. However, there is no universally agreed upon definition of fitness and of its components. The World Health Organization (75) defined fitness as "the ability to perform muscular work satisfactorily." In keeping with this definition, fitness implies that the individual has attained those characteristics that permit a good performance of a given physical task in a specified physical, social, and psychological environment. The components of fitness are numerous and are determined by several variables including the individual's pattern and level of habitual activity, diet, and heredity.

Fitness is operationalized in present day Western societies with a focus on two goals: performance and health. Performance-related fitness refers to those components of fitness that are necessary for optimal work or sport performance (10,29,57,58). It is defined in terms of the individual's ability in athletic competition, a performance test, or occupational work. Performance-related fitness depends heavily upon motor skills, cardiorespiratory power and capacity, muscular strength, power or endurance, body size, body composition, motivation, and nutritional status. In general, performance-related fitness shows a limited relationship to health (57).

Health-related fitness refers to those components of fitness that are affected favorably or unfavorably by habitual physical activity and relate to health status. It has been defined as a state characterized by (a) an ability to perform daily activities with vigor and (b) demonstration of traits and capacities that are associated with a low risk of premature development of hypokinetic diseases and conditions (58). Important components of health-related fitness include body mass for height, body composition, subcutaneous fat distribution, abdominal visceral fat, bone density, strength and endurance of the abdominal and dorso-lumbar musculature, heart and lung function, blood pressure, maximal aerobic power and capacity, glucose and insulin metabolism, blood lipid and lipoprotein profile, and the ratio of lipid to carbohydrate oxidized in a variety of situations. A favorable profile for these various factors presents a clear advantage in terms of health outcomes as assessed by morbidity and mortality statistics.

Fitness is best understood in terms of the components that should be taken into consideration for its assessment, and the context in which the concept is operationalized. There are various ways of defining the components of fitness and we are proposing an approach which, we believe, takes into consideration the most recent achievements in exercise and clinical sciences (see Table 3.3). They include morphological, muscular, motor, cardiorespiratory, and metabolic fitness components.

Table 3.3 The Components and Factors of Health-Related Fitness

Morphological component
Body mass for height
Body composition
Subcutaneous fat distribution
Abdominal visceral fat
Bone density
Flexibility
Muscular component
Power
Strength
Endurance
Motor component
Agility
Balance
Coordination
Speed of movement
Cardiorespiratory component
Submaximal exercise capacity
Maximal aerobic power
Heart functions
Lung functions
Blood pressure
Metabolic component
Glucose tolerance
Insulin sensitivity
Lipid and lipoprotein metabolism
Substrate oxidation characteristics

Morphological Component

The morphological component of physical and physiological fitness can be defined in terms of several factors that are associated with various morbid conditions and mortality rate.

The *weight for height* (or the *body mass for height*) relationship is often expressed as the body mass index (body mass in kg divided by height in m^2). High and very low body mass index values are both related to a higher all-cause mortality rate (72,73). Excessive weight for height is also associated with a greater likelihood of impaired glucose tolerance, hyperinsulinemia, hypertension, hypertriglyceridemia, and some dyslipoproteinemias (30,53,67). Body mass indices in the range of 20 to 25 are considered desirable among young adults (35). Desirable values tend to shift slightly upward with age (body mass indices of 26 and 27; 2).

It is commonly accepted that *body fat content* is the source of the risk of morbidity and mortality associated with a high body mass index. However, there is no epidemiological study that has assessed the relationship between total body fat content and health outcomes. Nonetheless, small-scale laboratory studies indicate that percentage of body fat and fat mass are significantly correlated with blood lipid, lipoprotein, insulin levels, and blood pressure (19,45,50). In most cases, body composition has not been assessed by one of the direct methods but has been inferred from some combinations of body weight, body mass index, and skinfolds. The results of these studies are, however, consistent with those in which body composition was determined from underwater weighing or other well-accepted methods.

Subcutaneous fat distribution is considered as an important indicator of enhanced risk for cardiovascular disease morbidity and mortality and of non-insulin dependent diabetes mellitus (8). A male profile of regional fat distribution (a preponderance of fat on the trunk) is associated with insulin resistance and elevated blood insulin level (25,38, 42), a more atherogenic plasma lipid and lipoprotein profile (18,41), and a higher blood pressure (19,38). A high proportion of fat over the upper-half of the body is also associated with a higher mortality rate in both sexes (46,47). Studies in which the amount of fat on the trunk has been assessed by skinfolds or by computerized tomography indicate that both the metabolic alterations and the increased cardiovascular mortality rates are associated with this profile of fat distribution (18,22,23,36).

In addition to the effects of an accumulation of trunco-abdominal subcutaneous fat on the risk profile, *abdominal visceral fat* also exerts a profound influence on insulin and lipoprotein metabolism (18,27,43). Within the abdominal visceral depot, it is thought that fat depots draining to the portal circulation are those that exert the largest adverse effects on hepatic glucose, lipid, and insulin metabolism (3). The amount of abdominal visceral fat can only be assessed by computerized tomography or other medical imaging techniques. In other words, it is useful to distinguish a minimum of three morphological factors and not only the total amount of body fat content but also the percent fat or fat mass, the trunco-abdominal subcutaneous fat, and the abdominal visceral fat (5). Lower body fat (the female pattern of fat deposition) apparently has only limited metabolic implications.

Bone mass is measured as local radiographic density or total body calcium. It is maximal in the third or fourth decade of life. There follows a progressive decrease of *bone density* which may progress to clinical osteoporosis and an increased susceptibility to bone fracture. Risk factors for osteoporosis include inherited susceptibility, a decrease in estrogen levels, a calcium deficient diet, and a low level of habitual physical activity (65). As osteoporosis reaches epidemic levels among the senior citizens of the developed countries of the western hemisphere, it is of great importance to understand the associations between habitual physical activity, fitness, and bone density. Currently available data support the notion that some types of physical activity may exert beneficial effects on bone mineral content and bone strength (54,65,69). In the context of bone health and overall skeletal strength, it is also useful to recognize that cartilage, ligaments, and tendons are favorably influenced by repeated muscular contractions (54,69).

Another factor of some importance in the morphological component of fitness is *flexibility*, generally defined as the range of motion at a joint. Flexibility is specific for a given joint and is determined by a variety of factors including the bony and cartilagenous surfaces and the soft tissues around the articulation. It can be improved by specific exercise designed to increase the range of motion at that particular joint. Although the issue is not yet entirely clear, it has been suggested that maintaining normal joint flexibility may help in preventing some of the manifestations of upper and lower back pain and osteoarthritis.

Muscular Component

Muscular fitness is universally recognized as an important component of physical and physiological fitness. Three factors are of particular interest: muscular power, muscular strength, and muscular endurance. *Muscular power* is strictly the maximum rate of working of a muscle, measured in a single effort such as a vertical jump. However, muscular power is sometimes taken as the peak power developed on an external device for as long as five seconds. *Muscular strength* can include the maximum force using an "isometric" dynamometer, an isokinetic dynamometer, or one repetition maximal isotonic lifting device. *Muscular endurance* is usually expressed as the decrease of peak force with a specified number of repetitions of an isokinetic or isotonic contraction. All three factors can be improved regardless of sex or age, given an appropriate regimen of exercise. Habitual activity does not appear to alter the slope of the aging curve, but the physically active person begins from a higher level of function and may thus experience less health impairment at a later age (63).

The progressive loss of lean tissue and muscular fitness with aging leads to a situation where desired activities such as lifting a load from the floor, carrying groceries, or lifting the body from a chair become impossible (63). Strong muscles also contribute to functional health by reducing the loading of joint surfaces, increasing the stability of articulations, and allowing a greater perfusion of the active fibers for any given absolute force of muscle contraction (16,39). A person with a reasonable level of muscular fitness should thus be less liable to local ischemia, with less fatigue, greater endurance, and a smaller rise in blood pressure as exercise continues.

It has been suggested that muscular fitness may be helpful in the prevention of upper and lower back pain that is so common in industrialized societies. Maintaining a reasonable level of muscular fitness through regular physical activity may also be important for normal hormonal and substrate metabolism, particularly for the insulin sensitivity of the active skeletal muscle tissue (26).

Motor Component

Motor fitness is of particular importance during growth, when the child explores his or her movement potential and develops basic motor skills. Agility, balance, speed of movement, and motor coordination are major facets of the motor component of fitness. *Agility* is usually described as a high score on a test that requires agile movements, such as a shuttle run. *Balance*, likewise, is described by scores on various tests of whole body equilibrium, or by measures of body sway. *Speed of movement* and *motor coordination* are characterized by fast responses to simple and complex choice reaction tasks. Motor fitness contributes only marginally to physical and physiological fitness as seen in a health perspective, with the possible exception of preventing falls and avoiding accidents, particularly in elderly people.

Cardiorespiratory Component

The cardiorespiratory component of physical and physiological fitness has traditionally been seen as the most important from a health point of view. Although this is still the case, important nuances are beginning to emerge (11). Cardiorespiratory fitness can be defined in terms of a large number of factors, the most relevant of which are listed in Table 3.3.

Submaximal exercise capacity or endurance performance can be defined as the tolerance to low intensity power output for prolonged periods of time. It is determined primarily by the oxygen delivery system, but is also affected by the peripheral utilization of oxygen to regenerate ATP, substrate mobilization and utilization, thermoregulatory mechanisms, and other physiological and metabolic factors. A person with a poor submaximal exercise capacity will experience fatigue sooner and may find problems in undertaking the normal activities of daily life.

Maximal aerobic power is assessed by measuring the maximal oxygen intake of the individual. Maximal oxygen intake decreases by about 10% per decade throughout adult life (63). The elderly individual becomes adversely affected by this decrease as some of the tasks of normal daily life require an increasingly large fraction of the maximal aerobic power. The initial maximal aerobic power is correlated with health outcomes (4), particularly with cardiovascular disease, and some (49) but not all authors (20,55) have also found an effect on non-insulin dependent diabetes mellitus risk factors.

Heart functions are assessed by a variety of indicators, including the cardiovascular response to exercise. The heart rate for a given power output (adjusted for body mass), the exercise stroke volume and cardiac output, the exercise electrocardiogram and vectocardiogram, and various imaging techniques that assess myocardium perfusion are among such indicators.

Lung functions may be assessed by measuring static and dynamic lung volumes. In most circumstances, the cardiorespiratory fitness of a healthy adult is limited by cardiac rather than by respiratory function. Nevertheless, it is ultimately better to have larger pulmonary volumes and higher flow rates for several reasons. One such reason is so a person can have a functional margin to accomodate the hazards of exposure to cigarette smoke, industrial dusts, other air pollutants, and respiratory pathogens.

Blood pressure is of particular importance, because hypertension is associated with an increased risk of death from ischemic heart disease, cardiac failure, cerebrovascular accident, rupture of other major blood vessels, and renal failure. There may also be some disadvantages to a very low systemic blood pressure, particularly a tendency to faint on standing suddenly after a period of recumbency. Regular physical activity and an improved fitness level may have positive influences on both hypotensive or hypertensive states (31,37). In addition to resting measurements of blood pressure, further information can be derived from the blood pressure response to exercise.

Metabolic Component

Metabolic fitness results from adequate hormonal actions, particularly for insulin, normal blood and tissue carbohydrate, and lipid metabolism. A high ratio of lipid to carbohydrate oxidized also seems to be a desirable trait.

Glucose tolerance is improved by regular physical activity; the response to training is generally better in those with an initially impaired glucose tolerance (26). Plasma insulin levels decrease (48,70) with hyperinsulinemic patients responding best to regular physical activity (26). Such changes are seen with programs of walking (48) and other low intensity, long duration, exercise sessions that do not necessarily cause an increase of maximal oxygen intake (12,55,70). It is not fully established whether the insulin-lowering effect of regular physical activity and the apparent improvement of an insulin-resistant state result from an acute or a short-term persistent increase in the *insulin sensitivity* of skeletal muscle and other peripheral tissues, because of a reduction in insulin secretion, an increased rate of hepatic removal of insulin, or a combination of these mechanisms.

Lipid metabolism is also an important dimension of metabolic fitness. Low plasma triglycerides, total cholesterol, low-density lipoprotein cholesterol, and high plasma high-density lipoprotein cholesterol are generally recognized as characteristics associated with a low risk of atherosclerotic diseases, particularly coronary heart disease. Regular physical activity is thought to alter lipid transport in the direction of this favorable profile (34,74). There are indications that the lipid profile may be favorably altered with exercise at a lower intensity than has generally been thought to be required (33,48,66,71).

Finally, *substrate oxidation characteristics* under standardized conditions at rest or during steady-state exercise are important indicators of metabolic efficiency. For instance, the respiratory quotient as measured over a 24-hour period in a metabolic chamber is significantly correlated with the amount of fat and weight gained over a period of about two years (76). Oxidizing more lipids than carbohydrates in a variety of conditions seems to be a desirable metabolic characteristic from a performance, fitness, and weight control point of view.

Health

Defining health remains a major challenge, despite the progress made in treating diseases and increasing the average life duration in Western societies. At the 1988 Consensus Conference (10), health was defined as a human condition with physical, social, and psychological dimensions, each characterized on a continuum with positive and negative poles. Positive health is associated with a capacity to enjoy life and to withstand challenges; it is not merely the absence of disease. Negative health is associated with morbidity and, in the extreme, with premature mortality.

Morbidity can be defined as any departure, subjective or objective, from a state of physical or psychological well-being, short of death. Morbidity is measured as (a) the number of persons who are ill per unit of population per year, (b) the incidence of specific conditions per unit of population per year, and (c) the average duration of these conditions. On the other hand, wellness is a holistic concept, describing a state of positive health in the individual, and comprising physical, social, and psychological well-being.

Traditional illness and mortality statistics do not provide a full assessment of health as conceived in the context of this paper. A more comprehensive approach would require that the risk profile of the individual be established in terms of common health endpoints, an assessment of health-related fitness status, information on temporary and chronic disabilities, absenteeism, overall productivity, and use of all forms of medical services, including prescribed and non-prescribed drugs. If the quality of life is less than optimal, life expectancy should be adjusted to reflect a quality-adjusted value. This reflects the individual's summated quality of life on each of a range of criteria at each point in their lifespan.

Other Factors Affecting Physical Activity, Fitness, and Health

Three types of influence are important: lifestyle factors other than physical activity level, physical environment, and social environment and personal attributes.

Lifestyle

Lifestyle comprises the aggregate of an individual's actions and behaviors of choice which can affect health-related fitness and health status. Habitual physical activity is one such behavior over which the individual has a large measure of voluntary control. In addition, we are particularly concerned by smoking, diet (energy intake and dietary composition), and alcohol consumption as they impact health-related fitness and health in general. The association between habitual physical activity and other favorable lifestyle behaviors is in the expected direction but is not very strong. However, the relationship is strengthened if emphasis is placed upon those facets of physical activity that are undertaken with the deliberate intention of promoting health.

An understanding of the role of lifestyle on fitness and health should also include an assessment of sleeping patterns, perceived stress, drug addiction, and the general avoidance of health risks, such as wearing a seat belt; observing traffic regulations; scheduling regular medical, dental, and self-examinations; and avoiding hazardous sexual behavior (13,15).

Social Environment and Personal Attributes

In the present context, the social environment may be defined as the combination of social, cultural, political, and economic conditions that affect participation in physical activity, health-related fitness, and health status. Social networks may have a positive influence on attitudes toward physical activity and other healthy behaviors. Friends, members of the family, other relatives, social clubs, church organizations, and other groups are all part of the social milieu that can affect both health and the sense of well-being of an individual. All these elements of the social network can provide support for active living, but can also exert powerful influences in the opposite direction. Thus, a healthy public policy strives to provide political, economic, and cultural conditions conducive to good health practices. Examples are encouragement of bicycle commuting, restrictions on smoking in public places, and a building design that encourages stair climbing.

Several personal attributes shape the lifestyle pattern of a person, including the attitude toward physical activity and other healthy habits. These attributes include age, gender, socioeconomic status, personality characteristics, and motivation.

Physical Environment

Participation in leisure time physical activity, fitness level, and health status are all influenced by environmental conditions. These include temperature, humidity, air quality, altitude and climatic changes. Such conditions influence not only the ability to exercise, but also the physiological response to the demands of exercise. Certain types of physical activity may be hazardous to health because of prevailing environmental conditions.

Heredity and Individual Differences

Health is the culmination of many interacting factors, including the genetic constitution. The genotype represents the characteristics of the individual at a given gene or set of genes. Humans are genetically quite diverse; current estimates are that each human being has about one variable DNA base for every 100 to 300 bases. Variations in DNA sequence constitute the molecular basis of genetic individuality and of human genetic variation. Given these circumstances, an equal state of health and of physical and mental well-being is unlikely to be achieved for all. Some will thrive better and will remain free from disabilities for a longer period of time than others.

Genetic differences do not operate in a vacuum. They interact constantly with existing cellular and tissue conditions to provide a biological response commensurate with environmental demands. In that sense, the genes are constantly interacting with everything in the physical and social environment, as well as with lifestyle characteristics of the individual, that translate into a signal capable of affecting the cells of the body. Thus, overfeeding, a high fat diet, smoking, and regular endurance exercise are all powerful stimuli that may elicit strong biological responses. However, because of inherited differences at specific genes, the amplitude of adaptive responses varies from one individual to the other. Inheritance is one of the important reasons why we are not equally prone to diabetes, hypertension, or heart attacks. It is also one major explanation for individual differences in the response to dietary intervention or exercise training.

Genetic individuality is important in the present context because it has an impact on the physical activity, fitness, and health paradigm. Thus, there are inherited differences in the level of habitual physical activity (59) and for many components of health-related fitness (6,9). There is now highly suggestive evidence that genetic variation accounts for a substantial fraction of the individual differences in the response to regular exercise of health-related fitness factors and the various risk factors for cardiovascular disease and non-insulin dependent diabetes mellitus (7,9,10).

A recognition of the critical role of DNA sequence variation in human response to a variety of challenges and environmental conditions seems essential to all those interested in the physical activity, fitness, and health paradigm. It will augment our understanding of human variation and make us more cautious in defining fitness and health benefits that may be anticipated from a physically active lifestyle. Incorporating biological individuality into our thinking can only increase the relevance of our observations to the true human situation.

References

1. American College of Sports Medicine. The recommended quantity and quality of exercise for developing and maintaining cardiorespiratory and muscular fitness in healthy adults. *Med. Sci. Sports Exerc.* 22: 265-274; 1990.
2. Andres, R. Mortality and Obesity: The rationale for age-specific height-weight tables. In: Andres, R.; Bierman, E.L.; Hazzard, W.R. eds. *Principles of geriatric medicine.* New York: McGraw-Hill; 1985: 311-318.
3. Björntorp, P. Portal adipose tissue as a generator of risk factors for cardiovascular disease and diabetes. *Arteriosclerosis.* 10: 493-496; 1990.
4. Blair, S.N.; Kohl, H.W. III; Paffenbarger, R.S. Jr.; Clark, D.G.; Cooper, K.H.; Gibbons, L.W. Physical fitness and all-causes mortality: A prospective study of healthy men and women. *JAMA* 262: 2395-2401; 1989.
5. Bouchard, C. Heredity and the path to overweight and obesity. *Med. Sci. Sports Exerc.* 23: 285-291; 1991.
6. Bouchard, C. Genetic determinants of endurance performance. In: Shephard, R.J., Astrand, P.O. eds. *Endurance in sports.* Oxford: Blackwell Scientific, Vol. II of the Encyclopedia of Sports Medicine an IOC Medical Commission Publication; 1992: 149-159.
7. Bouchard, C. Discussion: Heredity, fitness, and health. In: Bouchard, C.; Shephard, R.J.; Stephens, T.; Sutton, J.R.; McPherson, B.D.; eds. *Exercise, fitness, and health: A consensus of current knowledge.* Champaign, IL: Human Kinetics; 1990: 147-153.
8. Bouchard, C.; Bray, G.A.; Van Hubbard, V.S. Basic and clinical aspects of regional fat distribution. *Am. J. Clin. Nutr.* 52: 946-950; 1990.
9. Bouchard, C.; Dionne, F.T.; Simoneau, J.A.; Boulay, M.R. Genetics of aerobic and anaerobic performances. *Exerc. Sport Sci. Rev.* 1992, 20: 27-58.
10. Bouchard, C.; Shephard, R.J.; Stephens, T.; Sutton, J.R.; McPherson, B.D. *Exercise, fitness, and health: a consensus of current knowledge.* Champaign, IL: Human Kinetics; 1990.
11. Bouchard, C.; Shephard, R.J.; Stephens, T.; Sutton, J.R.; McPherson, B.D. Exercise, fitness and health: the consensus statement. In: Bouchard, C.; Shephard, R.J.; Stephens, T.; Sutton, J.R.; McPherson, B.D.; eds. *Exercise, fitness, and health: a consensus of current knowledge.* Champaign, IL: Human Kinetics; 1990: 3-28.
12. Bouchard, C.; Tremblay, A.; Nadeau, A.; Dussault, J.; Després, J.P.; Thériault, G.; Lupien, P.J.; Serresse, O.; Boulay, M.R.; Fournier, G. Long-term exercise training with constant energy intake. 1: Effect on body composition and selected metabolic variables. *Int. J. Obes.* 14: 57-73; 1990.
13. Breslow, L. Lifestyle, fitness, and health. In: Bouchard, C.; Shephard, R.J.; Stephens, T.; Sutton, J.R.; McPherson, B.D.; eds. *Exercise, fitness, and health: A consensus of current knowledge.* Champaign, IL: Human Kinetics; 1990: 155-163.
14. Brown, J.R.; Crowden, G.P. Energy expenditure ranges and muscular work grades. *Br. J. Industr. Med.* 20: 277-283; 1963.
15. Canada Fitness Survey. *Fitness and lifestyle in Canada.* Ottawa: Directorate of fitness and amateur sport; 1983.
16. Clausen, J.P. Muscle blood flow during exercise and its significance for maximal performance. In: Keul, J.; ed. *Limiting factors of physical performance.* Stuttgart: Thieme Verlag; 1973: 253-266.
17. Collins, K. Energy expenditure, productivity and endemic disease. In: Harrison, G.A., ed. *Energy and effort.* London: Taylor and Francis; 1982: 65-84.
18. Després, J.P.; Moorjani, S.; Lupien, P.J.; Tremblay, A.; Nadeau, A.; Bouchard, C. Regional fat distribution of body fat, plasma lipoproteins, and cardiovascular disease. *Arteriosclerosis* 10: 497-511; 1990.
19. Després, J.P.; Tremblay, A.; Thériault, G.; Pérusse, L.; Leblanc, C.; Bouchard, C. Relationships between body fatness, adipose tissue distribution, and blood pressure in men and women. *J. Clin. Epidemiol.* 41: 889-897; 1988.
20. Després, J.P.; Moorjani, S.; Tremblay, A.; Poehlman, E.T.; Lupien, P.J.; Nadeau, A.; Bouchard, C. Heredity and changes in plasma lipids and lipoproteins after short-term exercise training in men. *Arteriosclerosis.* 8: 402-409; 1988.
21. Dishman, R.K. Determinants of participation in physical activity. In: Bouchard, C.; Shephard, R.J.; Stephens, T.; Sutton, J.R.; McPherson, B.D.; eds. *Exercise, fitness, and health: a consensus of current knowledge.* Champaign, IL: Human Kinetics; 1990: 75-101.
22. Ducimetière, P.; Richard, J.L. The relationship between subsets of anthropometric upper versus lower body measurements and coronary heart disease risk in middle-aged men. The Paris prospective study. *Int. J. Obes.* 13: 111-112; 1989.
23. Ducimetière, P.; Richard, J.L.; Cambien, F. The pattern of subcutaneous fat distribution in middle-aged men and the risk of coronary heart disease. The Paris prospective study. *Int. J. Obes.* 10: 229-240; 1986.

24. Durnin, J.V.G.A; Passmore, R. *Energy, work and leisure*. London: Heinemann; 1967.
25. Evans, D.J.; Hoffman R.G.; Kalkhoff, R.K. Kissebah, A.H. Relationship of body fat topography to insulin sensitivity and metabolic profiles in premenopausal women. *Metabolism*. 33: 68-75; 1984.
26. Exercise and NIDDM. *Diabetes Care*. 13: 785-789; 1990.
27. Fujioka, S.; Matsuzawa, Y.; Tokunaga, K.; Tarui, S. Contribution of intra-abdominal fat accumulation to the impairment of glucose and lipid metabolism in human obesity. *Metabolism*. 36: 54-59; 1987.
28. Furrie, A.D.; Stephens, T. Energy expenditure patterns in the Canadian population. In: Landry, F., ed. *Health risk estimation, risk reduction and health promotion*. Ottawa: Canadian Public Health Association; 1983: 103-114.
29. Gledhill, N. Discussion: Assessment of Fitness. In: Bouchard, C.; Shephard, R.J.; Stephens, T.; Sutton, J.R.; McPherson, B.D.; eds. *Exercise, fitness, and health: a consensus of current knowledge*. Champaign, IL: Human Kinetics; 1990.
30. Glueck, C.J.; Taylor, H.L.; Jacobs, D.; Morrisson, J.A.; Beaglehole, R.; Williams, O.D. Plasma high-density lipoprotein cholesterol: Association with measurements of body mass. *The Lipid Research Clinics Prevalence Study*. Circulation 62 (suppl IV): 62-69; 1980.
31. Hagberg, J.M. Exercise, fitness, and hypertension. In: Bouchard, C.; Shephard, R.J.; Stephens, T.; Sutton, J.R.; McPherson, B.D.; eds. *Exercise, fitness, and health: A consensus of current knowledge*. Champaign, IL: Human Kinetics; 1990: 455-466.
32. Hanke, H. *Freizeit in der DDR*. Berlin: Dietz Verlag; 1979.
33. Hardman, A.E.; Hudson, A.; Jones, P.R.M.; Norgan, N.G. Brisk walking and plasma high density lipoprotein cholesterol concentration in previously sedentary women. *Br. Med. J.* 299: 1204-1205; 1989.
34. Haskell, W.L. The influence of exercise training on plasma lipids and lipoproteins in health and disease. *Acta. Med. Scand.* Suppl 711: 25-37; 1986.
35. Health and Welfare Canada. Canadian guidelines for healthy weights. Ottawa: Supplies and Services Canada; 1989.
36. Higgins, M.; Kannel, W.; Garrison, R.; Pinsky, J.; Stokes, J. Hazards of obesity—The Framingham experience. *Acta. Med. Scand. Suppl.* 723: 23-36; 1988.
37. Holmgren, A. Vaso-regulatory asthenia. *Can. Med. Assoc. J.* 96: 853; 1967.
38. Kalkhoff, R.K.; Hartz, A.H.; Rupley, D.; Kissebah, A.H.; Kelber, S. Relationship of body fat distribution to blood pressure, carbohydrate tolerance, and plasma lipids in healthy obese women. *J. Lab. Clin. Med.* 102: 621-627; 1983.
39. Kay, C.; Shephard, R.J. On muscle strength and the threshold of anaerobic work. *Int. Z. Angew. Physiol.* 27: 311-328; 1969.
40. Kenyon, G.S. Six scales for assessing attitudes towards physical activity. *Res. Quart.* 39: 566-574; 1968.
41. Kissebah, A.H.; Vydelingum, N.; Murray, R.; Evans, D.V.; Hartz, A.J.; Kalkhoff, R.K.; Adams, P.W. Relation of body fat distribution to metabolic complications of obesity. *J. Clin. Endocrinol. Metab.* 54: 254-260; 1982.
42. Kissebah, A.H.; Peiris, A.N. Biology of regional body fat distribution: Relationship to non-insulin dependent diabetes mellitus. *Diabetes Metab. Rev.* 5: 83-109; 1989.
43. Kissebah, A.H.; Freedman, D.S.; Peiris, A.N. Health risks of obesity. *Med. Clin. North Am.* 73: 111-138; 1989.
44. Klein, P.D.; James, W.P.; Wong, W.W.; Irving, C.S.; Murgatroyd, P.R.; Cabrera, M. Dalosso, H.M.; Klein, E.R.; Nichols, B.L. Calorimetric validation of the doubly labeled water method for estimation of energy expenditure in man. *Hum. Nutr. Clin. Nutr.* 38: 95-106; 1984.
45. Krotkiewski, M.; Björntorp, P.; Sjöstrom, L.; Smith, U. Impact of obesity on metabolism in men and women. Importance of regional adipose tissue distribution. *J. Clin. Invest.* 72: 1150-1162; 1983.
46. Lapidus, L.; Benftsson, C.; Larsson, B.; Pennert, K.; Rybo, E.; Sjöström, L. Distribution of adipose tissue and risk of cardiovascular disease and death: A 12-year follow-up of participants in the population study of women in Gothenburg, Sweden. *Br. Med. J.* 289: 1261-1263; 1984.
47. Larsson, B.; Svardsudd K.; Welin, L.; Wilhelmsen, L.; Björntorp, P.; Tibblin, G. Abdominal adipose tissue distribution, obesity and risk of cardiovascular disease and death 13 year follow-up of participants in the study of men born in 1913. *Br. Med. J.* 288: 1401-1404; 1984.
48. Leon, A.S.; Conrad, J.; Hunninghake, D.B.; Serfass, R. Effects of a vigorous walking program on body composition, carbohydrate and lipid metabolism of obese young men. *Am. J. Clin. Nutr.* 32: 1776-1787; 1979.
49. Leon, A.S.; Connett, J.; Jacobs, D.R. Jr.; Rauramaa, R. Leisure time physical activity levels and risk of heart disease and death: The Multiple Risk Factor Intervention Trial. *JAMA*, 258: 2388-2395; 1987.
50. Mauriège, P.; Després, J.P.; Marcotte, M.; Ferland, M.; Tremblay, A.; Nadeau, A.; Moor-

jani, S.; Lupien, P.J.; Thériault, G.; Bouchard, C. Abdominal fat cell lipolysis, body fat distribution, and metabolic variables in premenopausal women. *J. Clin. Endocrinol. Metab.* 71: 1028-1035; 1990.

51. McIntosh, P.C. *"Sport for All" programmes throughout the world.* Paris: UNESCO contract 207604; 1980.
52. Molé, P. Impact of energy intake and exercise on resting metabolic rate. *Sports Med.* 10: 72-87; 1990.
53. National Research Council. *Diet and health. Implications for reducing chronic disease risk.* Washington, DC: National Academy Press: 1989: 563-592.
54. Oakes, B.W.; Parker, A.W. Discussion: Bone and connective tissue adaptations to physical activity. In: Bouchard, C.; Shephard, R.J.; Stephens, T.; Sutton, J.R.; McPherson, B.D.; eds. *Exercise, fitness, and health: a consensus of current knowledge.* Champaign, IL: Human Kinetics; 1990: 345-361.
55. Oshida, Y.; Yamanonchi, K.; Hazamizu, S.; Sato, Y. Long-term mild jogging increases insulin action despite no influence on body mass index or $\dot{V}O_2$max. *J. Appl. Physiol.* 66: 2206-2210; 1989.
56. Paffenbarger, R.; Hyde, R.T.; Wing, A.L. Physical activity and physical fitness as determinants of health and longevity. In: Bouchard, C.; Shephard, R.J.; Stephens, T.; Sutton, J.R.; McPherson, B.D.; eds. *Exercise, fitness, and health: a consensus of current knowledge.* Champaign, IL: Human Kinetics; 1990: 33-48.
57. Pate, R.R.; Shephard, R.J. Characteristics of physical fitness in youth. In: Gisolfi, C.V.; Lamb, D.R., eds. *Perspectives in exercise science and sports medicine, vol 2, Youth, exercise and sport.* Indianapolis, IN: Benchmark Press; 1989: 1-45.
58. Pate, R.R. The evolving definition of fitness. *Quest.* 40: 174-179; 1988.
59. Pérusse, L.; Tremblay, A.; Leblanc, C.; Bouchard, C. Genetic and familial environmental influences on level of habitual physical activity. *Am. J. Epidemiol.* 129: 1012-1022; 1989.
60. Rothwell, N.J.; Stocks, M.J. Luxuskonsumption, diet-induced thermogenesis—the case in favour. *Clin. Sci.* 64: 19-23; 1983.
61. Sachs, M.L. Compliance and addiction to exercise. In: Cantu RC, ed. *The exercising adult.* Lexington, MA: DA Heath; 1982: 19-27.
62. Shephard, R.J. *Endurance fitness (2nd ed).* Toronto: University of Toronto Press; 1977.
63. Shephard, R.J. *Physical activity and aging (2nd ed).* London: Croom Holm; 1987.
64. Shephard, R.J. Adaptation to exercise in the cold. *Sports Med.* 2: 59-71; 1985.
65. Smith, E.L.; Smith, K.A.; Gilligan, C. Exercise, fitness, osteoarthritis, and osteoporosis. In: Bouchard, C.; Shephard, R.J.; Stephens, T.; Sutton, J.R.; McPherson, B.D.; eds. *Exercise, fitness, and health: a consensus of current knowledge.* Champaign, IL: Human Kinetics; 1990: 517-528.
66. Sopko, G.; Jacobs, D.R.; Jeffery, R.; Mittelmark, M.; Lenz, K.; Hedding, E.; Lipcjik, R.; Gerber, W. Effects on blood lipids and body weight in high risk men of a practical exercise program. *Atherosclerosis.* 49; 219-229; 1983.
67. Stamler, J. Overweight, hypertension, hypercholesterolemia and coronary heart disease. In: Mancini, M.; Lewis, B.; Contaldo, F., eds. *Medical complications of obesity.* London: Academic Press; 1979: 191-216.
68. Stundl, H. *Freizeit und Erholungsport in der DDR.* Schorndorf: Karl Hofmann Verlag; 1977.
69. Tipton, C.M.; Vailas, A.C. Bone and connective tissue adaptations to physical activity. In: Bouchard, C.; Shephard, R.J.; Stephens, T.; Sutton, J.R.; McPherson, B.D.; eds. *Exercise, fitness, and health: a consensus of current knowledge.* Champaign, IL: Human Kinetics; 1990: 331-344.
70. Tremblay, A.; Nadeau, A.; Després, J.P.; St-Jean, L.; Thériault, G.; Bouchard, C. Long-term exercise training with constant energy intake. 2: Effect on glucose metabolism and resting energy expenditure. *Int. J. Obes.* 14: 75-84; 1990.
71. Tucker, L.A.; Friedman, G.M. Walking and serum cholesterol in adults. *Am. J. Publ. Health.* 80: 1111-1113; 1990.
72. Van Itallie, T.B.; Abraham, S. Some hazards of obesity and its treatment. In: Hirsch, J.; Van Itallie, T.B., eds. *Recent advances in obesity research IV.* London: John Libbey; 1985: 1-19.
73. Waaler, H. Height, weight and mortality. The Norwegian experience. *Acta. Med. Scand.,* Suppl 679; 1983.
74. Wood, P.D.; Stefanick, M.L. Exercise, fitness, and atherosclerosis. In: Bouchard, C.; Shephard, R.J.; Stephens, T.; Sutton, J.R.; McPherson, B.D.; eds. *Exercise, fitness, and health: a consensus of current knowledge.* Champaign, IL: Human Kinetics; 1990: 409-423.
75. World Health Organization. Meeting of investigators on exercise tests in relation to cardiovascular function. *WHO Technical Report.* 388; 1968.
76. Zurlo, F.; Lilioja, S.; Esposito-Del Puente, A.; Nyomba, B.; Raz, I.; Saad, M.; Swinburn, B.; Knowler, W.; Bogardus, C.; Ravussin, E. Low ratio of fat to carbohydrate oxidation as predictor of weight gain. *Am. J. Physiol.* 259: E650-E657; 1990.

Chapter 4

The Role of Evidence in Promoting Consensus in the Research Literature on Physical Activity, Fitness, and Health

Lawrence E. Hart

Consensus methodology began to emerge in 1977 with efforts by the National Institutes of Health (NIH) to develop a program for promoting a more effective interface between health research and health care. During the past 15 years the NIH has sponsored more than 70 consensus conferences, and under its direction several guidelines have been developed on topic selection, panel selection, speaker selection, and the general conduct of consensus meetings (8,14).

Although the consensus program advocated by the NIH has become widely recognized for its intrinsic strengths (8,13,22,25,30), opponents of the process have identified some of its more evident weaknesses (1,11,15,21,23). The strengths of the NIH model include the potential to translate a large body of research evidence into practical clinical policy; the potential for bringing together apparently conflicting viewpoints, with evidence as the "common denominator"; the ability to draw attention to important clinical issues; and the potential to obtain frontline input on the feasibility of evidence-generated clinical policy.

In contrast, the following have been highlighted as the perceived weaknesses of the consensus process: too much focus on compromise between viewpoints, to the detriment of research evidence; ambiguous or overly general recommendations; dominance of proceedings by a vocal few; inadequate time for considered conclusions; and poor or nonexistent impact on actual practice (17).

The Role of Evidence in the Consensus Process

It has been argued that the consensus process, as promoted by NIH, relies too much on group process, public relations, and "back room politics" (18) and thereby tends to underemphasize the role of evidence from research studies. Based on this charge, Lomas and his group (18) were interested to see if a consensus panel would be guided primarily by the results of research studies when the process was structured to emphasize the role of such evidence while still retaining the public, political, and consultative characteristics of the NIH model. They addressed the following specific research question: Does the consensus process produce better consensus when good evidence exists and less consensus when there is conflicting, poor, or no evidence?

A consensus conference on cesarean birth provided the forum for this exercise. Ten participants were asked to evaluate 224 clinical scenarios on their appropriateness for a cesarean section. Ratings were obtained before and immediately after the conference, and the level of agreement (consensus) among panelists was assessed separately for scenarios with good research evidence (evidence scenarios) and those with conflicting, poor, or no evidence (nonevidence scenarios). For each scenario, consensus among participants was measured as total agreement, partial agreement, or disagreement on the appropriateness of a cesarean section.

Before the conference, total or partial agreement existed for a larger percentage of the evidence than nonevidence scenarios (85% vs. 30%), with an opposite pattern for disagreement (15% vs. 70%). After the conference, possible improvement in the level of consensus occurred for 71% of the evidence and only 24% of the nonevidence scenarios.

Thus, the consensus process, as structured in the Lomas study, demonstrated a sensitivity to the availability of good evidence and suggested that aspects of both expert and public processes can be successfully combined. However, it was agreed that even greater improvement was possible if final recommendations were graded according to the availability of rigorous research evidence.

The role of evidence in the consensus process has been further explored by Kanouse, Brook, and Winkler (16), who concluded that "the purposes of the [consensus] program are better served if the panel approaches its task by asking, 'what meaningful guidance can we give to clinicians based on the current scientific evidence?' rather than 'what definitive recommendations will the biomedical literature support?' " (16,19). Herein lies probably the single most contentious issue in the debates surrounding choices of consensus approach: Is the purpose of consensus recommendations to establish the best possible guidance for clinical care despite imperfect or incomplete evidence, or is the purpose to promulgate science based only on watertight conclusions derived from methodologically incontestable studies (16)? The latter approach places great reliance on the randomized controlled trial (RCT), which substantively limits the resources that might be used to generate consensus within several research domains.

Within the sports sciences, for example, a review of the choices and applications of research methodology demonstrated that only 8% of published papers (extracted from a sampling of the peer-reviewed literature over a 12-month period) were RCTs, and that of 55 papers identified as diagnosis or therapy studies, only six utilized an experimental design (31). Moreover, when judging this literature according to a predetermined set of critical appraisal criteria, randomization was not found in use (where perhaps it should have been) in approximately six of every seven therapeutic studies and in two of every three studies on sports physiology or biomechanics.

Based on these findings, it seems clear that total reliance on the RCT in the sports science literature, as in other subspecialty areas, would yield a very small segment of published research that might be amenable to the consensus process. It is evident, however, that for many conditions RCTs have never been (and arguably could never be) carried out, and the only information base for generating consensus recommendations would be derived from uncontrolled clinical observations (28). The incorporation of nonexperimental evidence into consensus statements therefore seems to be unavoidable, but when utilizing such evidence it is especially important to exercise the utmost circumspection (28).

Given the dilemmas that arise when purportedly "less than optimal" data are considered in consensus exercises, it becomes important to identify methodologic guidelines that help to define even minimal standards for the validity and applicability of published research. Various approaches to identify guidelines might be invoked. The following model is only one that has been used successfully in different segments of the clinical and basic science literatures and may be applied ideally to the general domains of physical activity, fitness, and health.

Assessing the Quality of Evidence in Published Studies

In a proposed step-by-step approach critical appraisal criteria are used to scrutinize the selected literature, levels of evidence are applied to order and prioritize the studies that qualify for inclusion in the consensus document, and based on these levels of evidence, grades of recommendations are assigned to the outcomes of interest.

A Framework for Critical Appraisal

In the literature on physical activity, fitness, and health, as in the general biomedical literature, most research concentrates on one of four areas: effectiveness of therapy, etiology or causation, clinical course and disease prognosis, and diagnostic testing. This review will therefore focus primarily on methodologic issues within these categories.

1. Effectiveness of Therapy

When considering therapeutic interventions, it is esssential to identify whether or not the ultimate objective is to achieve cure, palliation, or symptomatic relief. Only then should a specific treatment be prescribed (29). Once having decided that treatment of some sort is warranted, the next step is to select the specific drug, operation, splint, exercise, or conversation that will best achieve this goal. Three possible ways are proposed (29):

1. On the basis of retrospective analyses of uncontrolled clinical experience, or the extension of current concepts of mechanisms of disease, it is possible to arrive at the therapy that *seems to work*. This is the method termed *induction*.
2. On the basis of prospective analyses of formal RCTs designed to expose worthless or dangerous treatments, it is possible to select therapies that *successfully withstand formal attempts to demonstrate their worthlessness*. This is the method termed *deduction*.

3. On the basis of recommendations from teachers, consultants, colleagues, advertisements, or pharmaceutical representatives, treatments can be accepted *on faith*. This method has been referred to as *abdication* (28).

Sackett (28) contends that the nonexperimental method tends to overestimate efficacy, and he provides three compelling reasons to support his argument:

1. Favorable treatment responses are more likely to be recognized and remembered by clinicians when their patients comply with treatment and keep follow-up appointments. However, there are already five documented instances in which compliant patients in the placebo groups of RCTs exhibited far more favorable outcomes (including survival) than their noncompliant companions (2,3,10,12,26). Because high compliance is therefore a marker of better outcomes—even when treatment is useless—uncontrolled clinical experiences often prompt the conclusion that compliant patients have received efficacious therapy.
2. Unusual patterns of symptoms or signs and extreme laboratory test results, even when reassessed a short time later, tend toward the more usual result (29). Because of this universal tendency for regression towards the mean, any treatment (regardless of its efficacy) initiated in the interim will appear efficacious.
3. Routine clinical practice is never "blind"; both patients and their clinicians know when active treatment is under way. As a result, both the placebo effect and the desire of patients and clinicians for success can cause both parties to overestimate efficacy.

For these reasons approaches based on uncontrolled clinical experience would run the attendant risk of promoting the application of treatments that might be useless or even harmful.

Clearly, the deductive (or hypotheticodeductive) method for selecting specific treatments is preferred (29). The best information on treatment efficacy in patients with a given disorder is determined by an RCT in which patients with the given disorder are randomly selected for the given treatment or for a placebo (or conventional therapy) and then followed up to ascertain clinically relevant prognosis and treatment. However, the proper evaluation of therapy requires more than randomization. The following are some of the questions that should be addressed (7,29) when attempting to distinguish useful from useless or even harmful therapy:

Was the Assignment of Patients to Treatments Really Randomized? Only true methods of randomization, where each patient has known assignment probabilities, are acceptable. Studies with pseudorandom methods of assignment, or those in which the randomization process is not defined, should be avoided.

Were All Clinically Relevant Outcomes Reported? All outcome variables should be clearly documented and incorporate all of the clinically relevant events.

Were Both Clinical and Statistical Significance Considered? Studies with very large sample sizes usually yield statistically significant results, but with absolute differences in outcome that are so small they are clinically meaningless. In contrast, studies with very small sample sizes often show impressive differences that are not statistically significant, acting essentially as a chance event. Therefore, definitions of what constitutes both clinical and statistical significance should be articulated at the design stage of the study.

Is the Therapeutic Maneuver Feasible in Your Practice? Therapeutic interventions in studies of interest should be described in sufficient detail to permit their reproduction elsewhere. Also, issues of *contamination* (patients not receiving the therapy to which they were randomized) and *cointervention* (the use of additional therapies, possibly at different rates in the study comparison groups) should be addressed.

Were All the Patients Who Entered the Study Accounted for at Its Conclusion? Accountability ensures against bias resulting from selectively reporting on only some of the patients. Reporting nonrepresentative subsets of patients amounts to a type of selection bias at the analysis stage of a study.

2. *Etiology or Causation*

Austin Bradford Hill and several other recognized methodologists have proposed some "applied principles of common sense" to assess articles that claim to show causation (20). These commonsense principles, when applied to clinical articles (or other sources), can be expressed in the following way (Table 4.1) (6,29):

Is the Study Likely to Provide a Valid Answer to the Clinical Question? It is important to determine whether the strongest possible research design was utilized in the study under scrutiny. Although a true experiment (i.e., an RCT) is likely to

Table 4.1 Guidelines for Determining Etiology and Causation

1. Is the study likely to provide a valid answer to the clinical question?
   a. Was the *type of study* the strongest that could have been performed under the circumstances?
   b. Were the opportunities for, and the determination of, *exposure* free from bias?
   c. Was the determination of outcomes (in a cohort study) or the distinction between *cases and controls* (in a case control study) free from bias?
2. In reporting the *strength* of the association, were *both clinical and statistical significance* considered?
   a. If the relative risk/odds were statistically significantly greater than 1, was this increase clinically important?
   b. If the relative risk/odds were not statistically significantly greater than 1, was the study large enough to exclude a clinically important increased risk?
3. What happens when you apply rules of evidence for causation?
   a. Is the association consistent from study to study?
   b. Is the temporal sequence of exposure and outcome in the right direction?
   c. Is there a dose–response gradient?
   d. Does the association make sense?

Note. From Sackett, D.L., Haynes, R.B., Guyatt, G.H., Tugwell, P. (29). *Clinical epidemiology. A basic science for clinical medicine* (p. 285). Boston: Little, Brown and Company. Reprinted by permission.

provide the most accurate answer to a question on causation, it is often infeasible to invoke this methodology; other study designs therefore need to be considered.

The next most powerful method is the cohort study which identifies two groups (or cohorts) of patients, only one of which receives the treatment of interest. According to this design, the two cohorts are followed forward in time, counting the adverse events that occur in each (29). Though advantageous in many settings, the cohort study is subject to various biases and therefore needs to be viewed with some caution.

A second type of nonexperimental design is the case control study in which investigators gather cases of patients who already have suffered some adverse event and *controls* who have not. Both groups are then asked whether they received the treatment of interest. If those patients who had the adverse outcome were more likely to have undergone the treatment, this would constitute some evidence, though not very strong, that the treatment might cause, or at least precipitate, the adverse outcome. In this design, the direction of inquiry is backwards in time (9,29). By conducting case control studies "after the fact," investigators face a formidable series of potential biases (27). It is because of this greater liability to bias that the case control study is regarded as a relatively weak design.

One final type of nonexperimental study deserves mention. This is the case series in which a description of several cases is provided and no comparison or control group is identified (9,29). In general, case series are prone to overinterpretation, especially by their authors. Because of their methodologic weakness, case series are best used to stimulate other, more powerful, investigations. All too often, however, they provoke authoritarian (rather than authoritative) clinical advice about etiology, prevention, and therapy (29).

In Reporting the Strength of the Association, Were Both Clinical and Statistical Significance Considered? Strength here means the odds favoring the outcome of interest with, as opposed to without, exposure to the putative cause; the higher the odds, the greater the strength.

Different tactics for estimating the strength of association are used in different types of studies. In the RCT and cohort study, it is possible to calculate strength (relative risk) by comparing outcome rates in exposed and nonexposed persons. In contrast, in the case control study, strength (here called the *odds ratio*) can only be indirectly estimated.

What Happens When You Apply Rules of Evidence for Causation? Questions (listed in decreasing order of importance) that address specific rules of evidence for causation are as follows:

- *Is the association consistent from study to study?* The repetitive demonstration (by different investigators using different research designs in different settings) of an association between exposure to the putative cause and the outcome of interest constitutes consistency.
- *Is the temporal sequence of exposure and outcome in the right direction?* A consistent sequence of events of exposure to the putative cause, followed by the occurrence of the outcome of interest, is required for a positive test of temporality.

- *Is there a dose–response gradient?* The demonstration of an increasing risk of severity of the outcome in association with an increased dose or duration of exposure satisfies this rule.
- *Does the association make sense?* Four questions address this issue:
  1. Does the association make epidemiologic sense?
     This criterion is met when the article's results are seen to agree with current understanding of the distribution of causes and outcomes in humans.
  2. Does the association make biologic sense? This element of "sense" asks whether the results of the article are in harmony with our current understanding of the response of cells, tissues, organs, and organisms to stimuli.
  3. Are the article's results in agreement with our current understanding of the distributions of causes and outcomes in humans?
  4. Is the association specific? The limitation of the association to a single putative cause and a single effect satisfies this test.

3. *Prognosis*

When critically appraising articles on prognosis, the following guidelines might be applied (5,29):

An Inception Cohort of Subjects Should Be Identified. This facilitates study of a representative set of cases rather than a biased subset enrolled some time after the initial diagnosis.

The Referral Pattern Should Be Described. This allows one to relate the study results back to a reference population.

There Should Be Complete Follow-Up of All Patients. This avoids bias where the persons lost to follow-up have a different distribution of outcomes than those who are followed successfully.

Objective Outcome Criteria Should Be Developed and Used. This helps to remove the element of subjectivity that typically adds "noise" to the system, making the study less likely to produce significant results.

Blind Outcome Assessments Should Be Used. This reduces deliberate or subconscious bias. Ideally, both the subject and the person assessing clinical outcomes should be blinded to the treatment assignments.

Adjustment for Extraneous Prognostic Factors Should Be Carried Out. Unless this guideline is met, the possibility exists that causal roles may be assigned to variables that are merely markers for the real prognostic factors.

4. *Diagnostic Testing*

A comprehensive evaluation of a diagnostic test might address the following questions (4,29):

Was There an Independent, "Blind" Comparison With a "Gold Standard" of Diagnosis? The subjects shown (by application of an accepted gold standard of diagnosis) to have the condition of interest, plus a second group of patients shown (by application of the same gold standard) not to have this condition should have undergone the diagnostic test. The test should have been interpreted by assessors who didn't know (i.e., they were blind to) whether a given subject really had the condition. Afterwards, these diagnostic test results should be compared with the gold standard. In general, a gold standard refers to a definitive diagnosis attained by biopsy, surgery, autopsy, long-term follow-up or some other recognized benchmark (4,29).

Did the Patient Sample Include an Appropriate Spectrum of Mild and Severe, Treated and Untreated Disease, Plus Individuals With Different but Commonly Confused Disorders? Obvious disease usually poses much less of a diagnostic challenge than the same condition in an early or mild form. The real clinical value of a new diagnostic test often lies in its predictive value among equivocal cases.

Was the Setting for the Study, as Well as the Filter Through Which Study Subjects Passed, Adequately Described? Because a test's predictive value changes with the prevalence of the target disease, the data on a diagnostic test should contain sufficient information on the study site and patient selection filter to permit generalizability of the test's predictive value.

Was the Reproducibility of the Test Result (Precision) and Its Interpretation (Observer Variation) Determined? Validity of a diagnostic test demands both the absence of bias (i.e., systemic deviation from the truth) and the presence of precision (i.e., the same test applied to the same unchanged subject must produce the same result).

Was the Term "Normal" Defined Sensibly? When test results are reported as "normal," sensible frames of reference for such normality should be provided.

If the Test is Advocated as Part of a Cluster or Sequence of Tests, Was Its Contribution to the

Overall Validity of the Cluster or Sequence Determined? Any single component of a cluster of diagnostic tests should be evaluated in the context of its application.

Were the Tactics for Carrying Out the Tests Described in Sufficient Detail to Permit Their Exact Replication? If a diagnostic test is recommended for general use, a description of its application should cover patient issues as well as the mechanics of performing the test and interpreting its results.

Was the Utility of the Test Determined? The ultimate criterion for a diagnostic test or any other clinical maneuver is whether the patient benefits. Published studies describing such tests should therefore be scrutinized to assess whether, besides accuracy and precision, the long-term consequences of the use of the test have been explored.

Levels of Evidence

Although no guidelines currently exist for determining levels of evidence in studies on physical activity, fitness, and health, such methodology has been explored elsewhere in the biomedical literature. One model that has been developed and adopted by a group of investigators seeking consensus on the use of antithrombotic agents (28) seems ideally suited for other areas of research and is therefore presented as an example of what might be applicable to the fitness and exercise sciences.

When summarizing what was known about the causes, clinical course, and management of clinical entities, participants in the consensus exercise on antithrombotic agents specified levels of evidence according to the following classification (28):

Level I: Randomized trials with low false-positive (alpha) and low false-negative (beta) errors (high power).

A low false-positive (alpha) error refers to a *positive* trial that demonstrated a statistically significant benefit from experimental treatment. By contrast, a low false-negative (beta) error (high power) infers a *negative* trial that demonstrated no effective therapy, yet was large enough to exclude the possibility of a clinically important benefit (i.e., had very narrow 95% confidence limits that excluded any clinically important improvement from the test treatment).

Level II: Randomized trials with high false-positive (alpha) and/or high false-negative (beta) errors (low power).

A high false-positive (alpha) error is conferred by a trial with an interesting positive trend that is not statistically significant. A high false-negative (beta) error (low power) denotes a *negative* trial in which therapy was judged to be ineffective. Yet because of small numbers of patients the trial could not exclude the real possibility of a clinically important benefit (i.e., had very wide 95% confidence limits on the effect of experimental therapy).

Level III: Nonrandomized concurrent cohort comparisons between contemporaneous patients who did and did not receive the intervention of interest.

In this case, the outcomes of patients who received (and complied with) the therapeutic regimen would be compared with those of a contemporaneous group of patients who did not (through refusal, noncompliance, contraindications, local practice, oversight, etc.) receive these same interventions.

Level IV: Nonrandomized historical cohort comparisons between current patients who did receive the intervention of interest and former patients (from the same institution or from the literature) who did not.

For attribution of Level IV evidence, the outcomes of patients who received an intervention (as a result of local treatment policy) would be compared with those of patients treated in an earlier era or at another institution (when and where different treatment policies prevailed).

Level V: Case series without controls.

Such series may contain useful information about clinical course and prognosis but can only hint at efficacy.

Grading of Recommendations

Particularly in therapeutic studies, the step following determination of levels of evidence relates to grading of recommendations (see Table 4.2). Again, various groupings and models can be used, and the one provided here is merely one example (28).

Grade A: Supported by at least one, and preferably more, Level I randomized trials.

Grade B: Supported by at least one Level II randomized trial.

Grade C: Supported only by Level III, IV, or V evidence.

The Impact of Meta-Analysis on Determining Levels of Evidence

Guidelines for critically appraising overviews and meta-analyses are presented in Table 4.3 (24).

A meta-analysis refers to an overview that incorporates a specific statistical strategy for assembling

Table 4.2 The Relationship Between Levels of Evidence and Grades of Recommendations

	Level of evidence	Grade of recommendation
Level I:	Large randomized trials with clearcut results (and low risk of error)	Grade A
Level II:	Small randomized trials with uncertain results (and moderate to high risk of error)	Grade B
Level III:	Nonrandomized contemporaneous controls	Grade C
Level IV:	Nonrandomized, historical controls	Grade C
Level V:	No controls, case series only	Grade C

Note. From Sackett, D.L. (28). *Chest,* **95**, 3S. Reprinted by permission.

Table 4.3 Guidelines for Evaluating Overviews and Meta-Analyses

1. Were the questions and methods clearly stated?
2. Were the search methods used to locate relevant studies comprehensive?
3. Were explicit methods used to determine which articles to include in the review?
4. Was the methodologic quality of the primary studies assessed?
5. Were the selection and assessment of the primary studies reproducible and free from bias?
6. Were differences in individual study results adequately explained?
7. Were the results of the primary studies combined appropriately?
8. Were the reviewers' conclusions supported by the data cited?

Note. From Oxman, A.D., Guyatt, G. (24). *Canada Medical Association Journal,* **138**, p. 698. Reprinted by permission.

the results of several studies into a single estimate (29). Ideally, overviews begin with a clearly stated question followed by a description of the methods used to conduct the exercise. The validity of an overview is threatened when it fails to begin with a comprehensive, bias-free search for all potentially relevant articles on the topic of interest. Also, the methodologic quality of the primary studies contributing to the overview must be rigorously evaluated. Having recognized these basic requirements, the most compelling rationale for meta-analysis is its ability to generate more precise estimates (reflected in narrower confidence intervals) of the true treatment effect, such as a relative risk reduction, than can be provided by any individual trial.

A poorly conducted overview that incorporates low-quality studies may be misleading, while a rigorously conducted exercise using high-quality articles adds three important elements to the determination of levels of evidence. First, it generates narrower confidence intervals on estimates of the effectiveness of treatment (which can be related to the clinically significant differences that might promote clinical utility). Second, it provides a more comprehensive assessment of the methodologic quality of individual trials. Finally, it can detect and initiate the examination of heterogeneity in estimates of effectiveness among multiple trials of the same treatment (personal communication).

The use of meta-analyses can influence the classification of levels of evidence by generating a pooled estimate of treatment efficacy across a spectrum of selected high-quality trials. Meta-analyses have their most important impact in Level II studies where they might demonstrate that two or more high-quality, homogeneous but small (and therefore Level II) trials can really provide Level I evidence of treatment efficacy. In other words, when Level II studies are pooled, the lower limit of the confidence interval around the pooled estimate may then become greater than the minimal clinically important difference, thus elevating the aggregate of several Level II studies to Level I evidence.

Although Level III, IV and V data can be subjected to meta-analysis as well, the results would not likely shift such studies into another level; this additional analysis is therefore not generally encouraged.

Levels of Evidence and Grades of Recommendations When Dealing With Clinical Signs or Symptoms

In much the same way that levels of evidence and grades of recommendations have been proposed for studies dealing with the causes, clinical course, and management of given clinical entities, so, too, have attempts been made to adopt similar frameworks when dealing with clinical diagnosis. One example of this type of model is as follows (personal communications):

Level I evidence: independent, blind comparison of elicited signs or symptoms with a *gold standard* for anatomy, physiology, diagnosis, or prognosis among a *large* number of *consecutive* patients suspected of having the target condition. For optimal patient recruitment, a sufficient number should be recruited to ensure narrow confidence limits on the resulting sensitivity, specificity, or likelihood ratios.

Level II evidence: independent, blind comparison of elicited signs or symptoms with a gold standard among a *small* number of *consecutive* patients suspected of having the target condition. When referring to small numbers in this context, it is implied that there are insufficient numbers of patients to have narrow confidence limits on the resulting sensitivity, specificity, or likelihood ratios.

Level III evidence: independent, blind comparison of signs or symptoms with a gold standard among *nonconsecutive* patients suspected of having the target condition. At this level, a problem arises with restriction of the study sample to a subset of patients who underwent and generated definitive results on the sign or symptom and the application of the gold standard. Such results tend to overestimate accuracy.

Level IV evidence: nonindependent comparisons of signs or symptoms with a gold standard among *grab* samples of patients who obviously have the target condition plus, perhaps, normal individuals. In addition to the selection bias of Level III, these studies limit their samples to obviously clearcut presentations (sometimes selected on the basis of their gold standard result) that do not need a clinical examination (other than pattern recognition), and exclude the "shades of grey" that constitute the clinical spectrum of early and late, mild and severe, and other commonly confused conditions. Results of studies in this category greatly overestimate accuracy.

Level V evidence: nonindependent comparisons of signs and symptoms with a standard of uncertain validity (which may incorporate the sign and symptom results in its definition) among *grab* samples of patients plus, perhaps, normal individuals. In addition to the biases of Level IV, these studies often include the sign or symptom results as part of a *lead standard*, resulting in a self-fulfilling prophecy. These results extravagantly overestimate accuracy.

Using this format, Level I evidence would generate a Grade A recommendation, Level II evidence a Grade B recommendation, and Levels III, IV and V evidence would generate no more than a Grade C recommendation.

Summary

It has been determined that the availability of robust evidence promotes effective consensus in various domains of the biomedical sciences. A number of different methodologic models have been used in the evaluation of published research and the one outlined in this paper is but one example that seems ideally applicable to the literature on physical activity, fitness, and health. A framework is provided for the critical appraisal of research data and the allocation of levels of evidence and grades of recommendation for selected studies.

Acknowledgments

I would like to thank Dr. Deborah Cook and Dr. David Sackett, Departments of Clinical Epidemiology and Biostatistics and Medicine, McMaster University, for their helpful input during the planning phase of this chapter.

References

1. Ahrens, E.H., Jr. The diet-heart question in 1985: Has it really been settled? Lancet. 1:1087-1089; 1985.
2. Asher, W.L.; Harper, H.W. Effect of human chorionic gonadotropin on weight loss, hunger, and feeling of well-being. Am. J. Clin. Nutr. 26:211-218; 1973.
3. Coronary Drug Project Research Group. Influence of adherence to treatment and response of cholesterol on mortality in the coronary drug project. N. Engl. J. Med. 303:1038-1041; 1980.
4. Department of Clinical Epidemiology and Biostatistics, McMaster University, Hamilton, ON. How to read clinical journals: II. To learn about a diagnostic test. Can. Med. Assoc. J. 124:703-710; 1981.
5. Department of Clinical Epidemiology and Biostatistics, McMaster University, Hamilton,

ON. How to read clinical journals: III. To learn the clinical course and prognosis of disease. Can. Med. Assoc. J. 124:869-872; 1981.

6. Department of Clinical Epidemiology and Biostatistics, McMaster University, Hamilton, ON. How to read clinical journals: IV. To determine etiology or causation. Can. Med. Assoc. J. 124:985-990; 1981.
7. Department of Clinical Epidemiology and Biostatistics, McMaster University, Hamilton, ON. How to read clinical journals: V. To distinguish useful from useless or even harmful therapy. Can. Med. Assoc. J. 124:1156-1162; 1981.
8. Fink, A.; Kosecoff, J.; Chassin, M. Consensus methods: Characteristics and guidelines for use. Am. J. Public Health. 74(4):979-983; 1984.
9. Fowkes, F.G.R.; Fulton, P.M. Critical appraisal of published research: Introductory guidelines. Br. Med. J. 302:1136-1140; 1991.
10. Fuller, R.; Roth, H.; Long, S. Compliance with disulfram treatment of alcoholism. J. Chronic Dis. 36:161-170; 1983.
11. Gleicher, N. Cesarean section rates in the United States. The short-term failure of the national consensus development conference in 1980. JAMA. 252:3273-3276; 1984.
12. Hogarty, G.E.; Goldberg, A.P. Drug and sociotherapy in the aftercare of schizophrenic patients. Arch. Gen. Psychiatry. 28:54-64; 1973.
13. Jacoby, I. The consensus development program of the National Institutes of Health. Current practices and historical perspectives. Int. J. Tech. Assess. Health Care. 2:420-432; 1985.
14. Jacoby, I. Evidence and consensus. JAMA. 2599-3039; 1988.
15. Kahan, J.P.; Kanouse, D.E.; Winkler, J.D. Variations in the content and style of NIH consensus statements, 1973-1983. Publication no. N-2237. Santa Monica, CA: Rand Corp.; 1984
16. Kanouse, D.E.; Brook, R.H.; Winkler, J.D. Changing medical practice evaluation of the NIH consensus development program. Ann Arbor, MI: Health Adm. Press; 1989.
17. Lomas, J. The consensus process and evidence dissemination. Can. Med. Assoc. J. 134:1340-1341; 1986.
18. Lomas, J. Words without action? The production, dissemination, and impact of consensus recommendations. Annu. Rev. Public Health. 12:41-65; 1991.
19. Lomas, J.; Anderson, G.; Enkin, M. The role of evidence in the consensus process. Results from a Canadian consensus exercise. JAMA. 259:3001-3005; 1988.
20. Marmot, M.G. Epidemiology and the art of the soluble. Lancet. 897-900; 1986.
21. May, W.E. Consensus or coercion. JAMA. 254:1077; 1985.
22. Mullan, F.; Jacoby, I. The town meeting for technology. The maturation of consensus conferences. JAMA. 254:1068-1072; 1985.
23. Oliver, M.F. Consensus or nonconsensus conferences on coronary heart disease. Lancet. 1087-1089; 1985.
24. Oxman, A.D.; Guyatt, G. Guidelines for reading literature reviews. Can. Med. Assoc. J. 138:697-703; 1988.
25. Perry, S.; Kalberer, J. The NIH consensus development program and the assessment of health care technologies. N. Engl. J. Med. 303:160-172; 1980.
26. Pizzo, P.A.; Robichaud, K.J.; Edwards, B.K. Oral antibiotic prophylaxis patients with cancer: A double-blind randomized placebo-controlled trial. J. Pediatr. 102:125-133; 1983.
27. Sackett, D.L. Bias in analytic research. J. Chronic Dis. 32:51; 1979.
28. Sackett, D.L. Rules of evidence and clinical recommendations on the use of antithrombotic agents. Chest. 95:2S-4S; 1989.
29. Sackett, D.L.; Haynes, R.B.; Guyatt, G.H.; Tugwell, P. Clinical epidemiology. A basic science for clinical medicine. 2nd ed. Boston: Little, Brown; 1991.
30. Stocking, B. First consensus development conference in United Kingdom: On coronary artery bypass grafting. 1. Views of audience, panel, and speakers. Br. Med. J. 291:713-716; 1985.
31. Walter, S.D.; Hart, L.E. Application of epidemiologic methodology to sports science research. In: Pandolf, K.B., ed. Exercise and sports science reviews. Baltimore: Williams & Wilkins; 1990:47-49.

Chapter 5

Physical Activity and Fitness: Evolutionary Perspective and Trends for the Future

Per-Olof Åstrand

Our Biological Heritage

I will present a brief sketch of our evolutionary history to remind us that it has taken a long time to become the way we are.

According to the natural sciences, it is assumed that our solar system was created some 4,600 million years ago (see ref. 4). Evidently, the atmosphere surrounding our planet at that time did not contain oxygen. This was a prerequisite for the evolution of life from nonliving organic matter. Without atmospheric oxygen, the ultraviolet radiation from the sun, in the absence of high-altitude ozone, reached the surface of the earth. This radiation then provided the energy for the photosynthesis of organic compounds from such molecules as water, carbon dioxide, and ammonia. The process that enabled living organisms to capture solar energy for the synthesis of organic molecules (e.g., glucose) can be traced clearly in fossils that are about 3,500 million years old. Similarly, the familiar anaerobic fermentation (i.e., glycolysis) is probably the oldest energy-extracting pathway found in life on earth.

The ancient organisms split water by photosynthesis, gradually releasing free oxygen into the atmosphere. It may have taken some 2,000 million years to create an atmosphere in which one of every five molecules was oxygen. As oxygen became toxic for many of the original oxygen producers, new metabolic patterns were developed (i.e., aerobic energy yield) that utilized oxygen as a hydrogen acceptor.

A new milestone in biological evolution was reached some 1,500 million years ago when the unicellular organism with a nucleus, the eukaryote, was developed (14). The energy-absorbing and energy-yielding processes typical for our cell activities today are merely copies of events that occurred thousands of millions of years ago, such as the ATP-ADP system. Actually, ATP is the principal medium for the storage and exchange of energy in almost all living organisms. The store of ATP is, however, very limited because it is a heavy fuel. Within 24 hours, a person will spend energy equivalent to the energy stored in ATP weighing 50% to 100% more than his or her own body weight, depending on how physically active he or she is. A very rapid resynthesis of ATP is therefore necessary, and the *anaerobic* processes, which are several thousand million years old, are supplemented by the *aerobic* energy yield taking place inside the mitochondria.

Thus, over thousands of millions of years of evolution, a unicellular living organism was created. By some sort of trial and error, the fundamental biological principles for maintaining life were developed. They are still in efficient operation. Actually, a comprehensive textbook of biochemistry written some 1,500 million years ago would no doubt still be up to date in its treatment of the functions of the cell.

Evolution was now ready for the next major step, the creation of larger animals. That stage probably began 700 million years ago (12). In this evolution of larger animals, the individual cell retained its original size (i.e., the same size as the unicellular organism living more than 1,000 million years ago), but more cells were grouped together to increase the size of the organism.

As an inevitable consequence of grouping thousands of millions of some 200 different types of cells together in one organism (the human being), the individual cell lost its intimate contact with the external environment. This problem was solved by bathing each cell in water (i.e., the interstitial fluid). Like the amoeba, each cell in our body (with some exceptions) is surrounded by fluid, the composition of which is basically very similar to that of the ancient oceans. The organism brought the sea water with it, so to speak, in a bag made of skin.

In the course of the diversification of the multicellular organisms, which occurred over the last 700 million years, new types of organisms appeared and dispersions took place within already established groups. It should be noted that the history of mammals covers the last 220 million years, if not more. The first primates (the order including man) can be traced back some 60 to 70 million years to a period when dinosaurs were still dominant. With the extinction of the dinosaurs, there was a mammalian dispersion into vacant niches. In another evolutionary explosion a dispersion of flowering plants, birds, and mammals occurred.

What then are the mechanisms that underlie the origin of species and their evolutionary relationships (i.e., Darwinism)? Lewin (8) summarized the current views held by different researchers in this field. According to modern synthesis, evolution is a consequence of the gradual accumulation of genetic differences due to point mutations and rearrangements in the chromosomes. The direction of an evolutionary change is determined by natural selection, promoting the variants that are best fitted to their environment. The fact remains, however, that fossils, on the whole, do not document a smooth transition from old morphologies to new ones. This was also discussed by Darwin. For millions of years, species remain unchanged in the fossil record suddenly to be replaced by something that is substantially different but clearly related (8).

Because the accumulation of small genetic changes cannot exclusively explain the development of new species, a new theory called *punctuated equilibrium* has been advanced. According to this theory, individual species may remain virtually unchanged for long periods of time. They are then suddenly punctuated by abrupt events in the environment, and a new species arises from the original stock. It is conceivable, however, that future fossil records may fill many of the gaps and provide some of the missing links. It may have been only 5 or as many as 20 million years ago that the family tree of primates developed a branch, the hominids, which finally resulted in *Homo sapiens sapiens*, the only surviving hominid.

Not until about 4 million years ago do the African fossils reveal the presence of the hominid genus *Australopithecus*. The pelvis permitted an upright posture and bipedal gait with the arms free. There are archaeological records of tools, pebble choppers, and small stones that are probably more than 3 million years old (9). Toolmaking was thus established before there was a marked brain expansion in the hominid stock. Although a few varieties have been identified, the *Australopithecus* was a relatively homogeneous genus that survived for more than 2 million years.

The next well identified member of our family tree may have been the first true man. *Homo habilis* existed from 2.3 to 1.5 million years ago. This species was replaced by *Homo erectus*, who had a modern pelvis and moved with a striding gait. They lived as hunters and food gatherers and had a wide geographical range. The body height was probably 150 to 160 cm. They made use of fire, as evidenced by a hominid occupation site 1.4 million years old.

The general public is probably most familiar with the Neanderthal man (*Homo sapiens neanderthalensis*), who from archaeologic findings appears to have been well established some 200,000 years ago (11). These were skilled hunters of large and small game, forming bands similar to those of more recent hunting people, and were probably linked into tribal groupings, or at least groups with a common language. They formed a human population complex extending from Gibraltar across Europe into East Asia. The Neanderthal population was as homogeneous as the human population of today. On the average, the brain encased in the Neanderthal skull was slightly larger than the brain of modern man. Although the Neanderthals had the same postural abilities, manual dexterity, and range and character of movement as modern man, they had more massive limb bones and a larger muscular mass and power. The disappearance of the Neanderthals occurred some 35,000 years ago. When they vanished from the scene anatomically, modern man, *Homo sapiens sapiens*, was already in existence.

There are different opinions concerning "the latest phase in human origins—the emergence of people like you and me, our species Homo sapiens, with its widespread varieties of physique and color" (11). According to one hypothesis, modern humans evolved in Africa and then spread throughout the world, developing racial features in the process. Modern humans and Neanderthals could be distinct lines that diverged from a common ancestor more than 200,000 years ago in Africa and Europe respectively. At a later stage they spread and in some parts of the world they shared the environment.

An alternative hypothesis is a "gene-flow" model with a genetic contribution varying from region to region, the rate of intermixture gradually increasing as modern man evolved. Stringer (11) points out that in the gene-flow model racial features preceded the appearance of modern man whereas the African model reverses the order. He supports the African model showing dispersal of early modern humans from Africa within the past 100,000 years. The dating of our origin as modern man is, however, controversial.

Most likely, a human being living 50,000 years ago had the same potential for physical and intellectual performance, could play a piano or construct a computer like anyone living today. So, from all indications, *Homo sapiens sapiens* has remained biologically unchanged for at least 50,000 years. By 30,000 years ago, modern man had spread to nearly all parts of the world. It was not until some 10,000 years ago that the transition from a roaming hunter and food gatherer to a stationary farmer began.

To illustrate the evolutionary time scale, let us compare the 4,600 million years our planet has existed with a 460-km journey (see Figures 5.1 and 5.2). Life began after the first 100 km depicted on the graph. Another 200 km passed before the unicellular organism with a nucleus was born. Multicellular animals were living at the 400-km mark. An evolutionary radiation of the mammalian stock began somewhere around the 453-km mark. The first hominid appeared approximately 6 km later. The *Australopithecus*, however, joined the journey some 400 m from the "now," and the Neanderthals disappeared about 3.5 m from the finish line. The cultivation of land and keeping of livestock occurred 1 m from our present position. A 100-year-old person today has merely covered a distance of 0.01 m or 10 mm of the 460-km journey (see Figures 5.1 and 5.2). During the last century there has been a technological evolution that has surpassed the achievements of the entire 399.99 m-journey!

The purpose of this brief summary has been to present an outline of our genetic background. Many structures and functions are common to different species in the animal kingdom. For instance, there appear to be no fundamental differences in structure, chemistry, or function between the neurons and synapses in man and those of a squid, a snail, or a leech (7). Therefore, we can learn a great deal from studying different species. It is remarkable that all living organisms have a genetic code based on the same principle. Powerful research techniques of molecular biology have made it possible to isolate and characterize individual genes that mediate some of the development decisions involved in establishing the embryonic body plan. The key is a family of genes known as homeobox genes, which subdivides the early embryo into fields of cells with the potential to become specific tissues and organs. The order of homeobox genes is similar in vertebrates and invertebrates, and therefore the first homeobox complexes must have evolved eons ago in flatworms and/or other primitive organisms that were the common ancestors of both human beings and insects.

The amazing conservation of the complexes throughout evolution suggests that once an efficient way to control embryonic cell development was found, it was easier to produce new body shapes by modifying that system than to develop entirely new strategies (3). Data indicate that man and the chimpanzee share more than 99% of their genetic material (15). However, minimal genetic changes can affect major morphological modifications. Consequently, one should be careful when extrapolating findings from one species to another, because over millions of years many species undergo minor or major modifications in their physical and other characteristics. In general, however, evolution is a very conservative process. For instance, all vertebrates, including the hominids, have backbones which are complicated in design and are quite similar in all animals that have them. This supports the hypothesis that backbones have evolved only once, that is, all vertebrates share a common ancestor with a backbone.

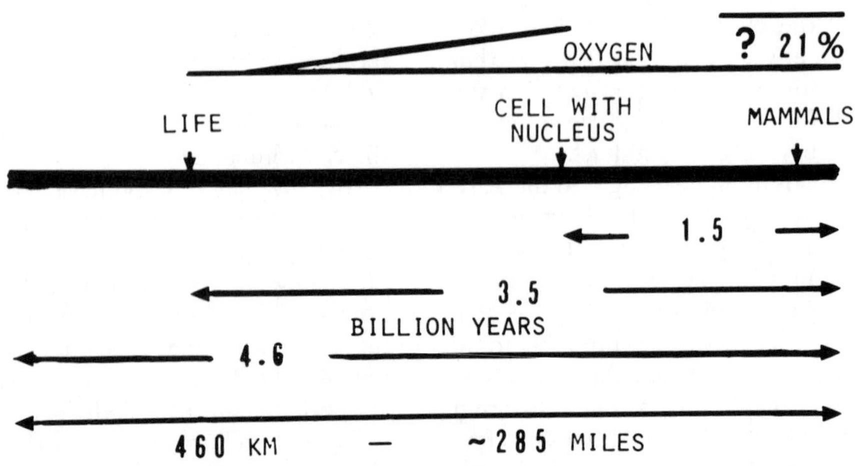

Figure 5.1 Our planet is probably some 4.6 billion years old. Let us translate those years to a 460-km journey. Biological evolution began some 1 billion years later. Cells with functioning nucleus thanks to the ATP-ADP cycling, glycolysis, Krebs citric cycle, and electron transport chain can be traced back 1.5 billion years—150 km from "now;" mammals appeared on the scene after almost another 130 km.

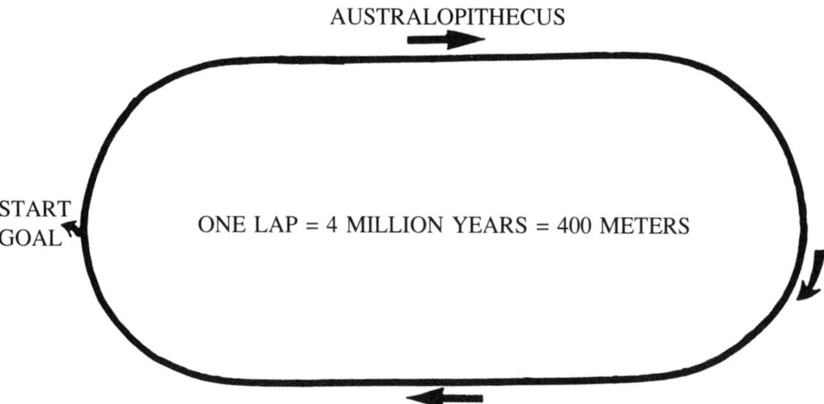

Figure 5.2 The hominid *Australopithecus* can be traced back approximately 4 million years. Let us symbolize those 4 million years by a 400-m track. He "gave up" after about 200 m. At this point, 2 million years ago, true *Homo* individuals appeared on the scene (*Homo habilis*, later on *Homo erectus*). After 399 m (10,000 years ago) farming and agriculture started, probably in the Middle East. This century equals the last 10 mm! *Homo sapiens neanderthalensis* became extinct approximately 35,000 years ago (3.5 m from "now"). Conclusion: During more than 99% of our existence we were hunters and food gatherers. Now we are exposed to an enormous experiment—without control groups. *From* Physical activity and fitness by P-O. Åstrand, © *The American Journal for Clinical Nutrition*, **55**(suppl.) 6:1231S-1236S, 1992. Reprinted by permission.

In general, vertebrate locomotion is genetically programmed. Fish can swim and birds can walk as soon as they hatch. Many species of mammals are well developed at birth. Thus, some are able to walk or run as soon as they are born, and some of them are able to attain a speed of 35 km $\times$ hour^{-1} when they are only a few days old. Evidently, survival may depend on their ability to get away. In the case of humans, who are utterly helpless at birth and entirely dependent on the parents' care, it may be to their advantage that they cannot remove themselves very far from their parents until they are mature enough to stand on their own feet.

The evolutionary process continues, and mammalian history has seen a wave of extinction, particularly severe for large mammals, including the hominids. Extinctions are a measure of the success of evolution in adapting organisms because particular adaptations provide entry into a relatively empty niche. In the balance between existence and extinction, the odds are not favorable. It has been estimated that 2,000 million species have appeared on earth during the last 700 million years, but that the number of multicellular species now living is only a few million (i.e., only 0.1% to 0.2% have survived).

The cortex of the human brain mirrors man's evolutionary success. Just as the proportions of the human hand, with its large opposable and muscular thumb, reflect successful adaptation for life in trees and later for the use of tools, so does the anatomy of the human brain reflect a successful adaptation for manual and intellectual skills. Where upright walking and toolmaking were the unique adaptations of the earlier phases of human evolution, the physiological capacity for speech provided the biological basis for the later stages. Indeed, it is by language that human social systems are mediated.

Speech is the form of behavior that differentiates man from other animals. The passing down of knowledge and experience by language from one generation to the next has enabled man, biologically unchanged for tens of thousands of years, to accelerate progress. In addition, it has enabled humans to apply their endowed intellectual resources in a technical revolution leading to entirely new and complex tools, weapons, shelters, boats, wheeled locomotion, and the ultimate exploratory voyage: space travel.

Nevertheless, in the midst of these splendid achievements, there are those who wonder whether the evolution of the human brain has gone too far. Although its ability to conceive, invent, create, and construct is astonishing, it remains to be seen whether or not it has retained or developed equally well its capacity for ethical conduct or responsible application of its endowed potential. When our ancestors roamed in small bands, the consequence of any destructive activity was quite limited. Because of social developments and technical innovations, however, basically the same brain is now capable of global destruction.

Like all higher animals, man is basically designed for mobility. Consequently, our locomotive apparatus and service organs constitute the largest part of our total body mass. The shape and dimensions of the human skeleton and musculature prevent the human body from competing with a gazelle in speed or an elephant in sturdiness, but it is indeed outstanding in diversity. The basic instrument of mobility is the muscle. It is a very old tissue. The earliest animal fossils were the burrowers living some 700 million years ago. By muscle force, these animals could dig into the seabed. They retained the metabolic pathways developed when the air had no oxygen (i.e., the anaerobic energy yield). Now, the pyruvic acid formed in our muscles under anaerobic conditions is removed by the formation of lactate. One alternative could have been the transformation of the pyruvate into ethyl alcohol. If the skeletal muscles had selected this alternative route, producing pyruvate by exercising to exhaustion or running uphill might have been a very popular endeavor!

The skeletal muscle is unique in its ability to vary its metabolic rate to a greater degree than any other tissue. In fact, active skeletal muscles may increase their oxidative processes to more than 50 times the resting level. Such an enormous variation in metabolic rate must necessarily create serious problems for the muscle cell, because although the consumption of fuel and oxygen increases 50-fold, the rate of removal of heat, carbon dioxide, water, and waste products must be similarly increased. To maintain the chemical and physical equilibrium of the cell, there must be a tremendous increase in the exchange of molecules between intracellular and extracellular fluid (i.e., fresh fluid must continuously flush the exercising cell). When muscles are thrown into vigorous activity, the ability to maintain the internal equilibriums necessary to continue the exercise is entirely dependent on those organs that service the muscle's demands. Food intake, digestion and handling of substrates, kidney function, and water balance are also very much affected by variation in metabolic rate.

Almost 100% of the biological existence of our species has been dominated by outdoor activity. Hunting and foraging for food and other necessities have been conditions of human life for millions of years. We are adapted to that style of life evidenced in our emotional, social, and intellectual skills. After a "brief" spell in an agrarian culture, we now live in an urbanized, highly technological society. There is obviously no way to revert to our natural way of life, which was not without its problems. With insight into our biological heritage, however, we may yet be able to modify our current lifestyle. Knowledge of the function of the body at rest, as well as during exercise under various conditions, is important as a basis for an optimization of our existence.

Children are spontaneously physically active. Unfortunately, in our modern society, we discourage them in this activity by furnishing houses and apartments to fit the parents' needs, keeping them indoors in schools and doing homework for many hours, creating heavily overpopulated "concrete deserts," and producing TV programs to capture their attention. The message is: Children should keep quiet and stay clean and neat! Vigorous physical activity is an asocial behavior in too many circumstances. From the time of puberty, human nature has an inclination toward physical laziness. No appetite center is developed for physical activity.

Some years ago I visited the bushmen in the Kalahari Desert, probably the last remaining Stone-Age people. They followed the lifestyle of the true hunters and food gatherers. Gathering sufficient food meant trudging long distances for the men in their hunting efforts and for the women and children in their collection of berries, melons, roots, and various plants. This walking, stopping, and squatting to dig, and walking again, is physically demanding. When the women gather enough and return home, they still have to collect and carry firewood for the cooking and the night fire. Most of the year, the game and food plants are not found in any abundance. To get enough to eat, the bushmen have to exercise for hours almost every day. The driving factor for the habitual physical activity is hunger and thirst, not a particular love for exercise. I never saw an adult bushman out jogging, but the walking was fast! The bushmen are well trained with emphasis on endurance.

In summation, close to 100% of the existence of the hominid/homo species has been dominated by outdoor activities. Hunting and foraging for food and other necessities in the wilds have been a condition of human life for millions of years. Evolutionary changes in the genetic code were promoted that made possible the survival of the hominids. We adapted to a lifestyle as hunter-gatherers, demonstrated in our emotional and social lives and our intellectual skills. Major adaptations for this survival were consonant; habitual physical activity, including endurance and peak effort alternated with rest and socialization. In relatively small bands individuals lived together.

Age was not measured in years. The old person was very important and respected in society because she or he was credited with experience essential for the well being and survival of the people. Therefore, the aging individual was still an important member of the group. I do not believe a person at that time had a well defined border between job and leisure time. More recently—but before our time—when an old man in a North

American Indian tribe did not fully qualify as a scout, a hunter, or a warrior, he became a teacher for boys in a "lecture hall" outdoors, giving lectures that were full of excitement. The old man entered a new niche in the society, still intellectually and physically demanding and of vital importance for the future of the tribe. Then one day he would say, "This is a good day to die!" (6).

Many expressions of human behavior that may not benefit large societies seem to work well within small bands. Archaeologists have shown, for example, that foraging can actually be more beneficial than herding and farming. Detailed analyses of skeletal remains reveal that in parts of North America a shift to agriculture was detrimental to nutrition, health, and longevity for certain groups. Similarly, in modern times it has become clear that when droughts strike southern Africa, groups that rely heavily on hunting and gathering tend to be affected less severely than groups that depend primarily on water-hungry herds and crops (16).

Daily physical activity involved the whole person—body, mind, and spirit—and was part of the total dynamic of a life in which individuals and environments continuously interrelated and affected each other.

Trends for the Future

There is virtually no way to revert to our "natural" way of life, but with insight into our biological heritage we may be able to modify the current, self-destructive elements of our modern lifestyle. For an optimal function of the human body, regular physical activity is essential. There are many scientific efforts that study effects of physical training and an active lifestyle in a broad sense in the field of primary and secondary prevention of specific diseases. In the future will it be possible by studies of the DNA sequence at a young age to determine who is at high risk of morbidity and mortality in specific diseases and to develop positive programs adapted to the individual?

Will it be possible to predict a person's response to a given training program, a change in diet, in blood lipids, blood pressure, maximal aerobic power, muscle strength, endurance, and so on? Will it be possible to reveal why some previously sedentary individuals improve their maximal aerobic power very dramatically when following a given training program while the response of others is almost negligible (2)? An extreme viewpoint asks what right we have to manipulate the lifestyle of 100 persons in a program if we save only three lives, where the remaining 97 did not like the program but were forced to participate. When a project starts, however, we are not able to predict who the three lucky ones will be.

The U.S. Bureau of Census has estimated that the percentage of Americans older than 65 will double from 12% in 1986 to 24% in 2020. Research in aging has emphasized average age-related health and fitness losses and neglected the substantial heterogeneity of older persons, again partly a consequence of genetic individuality. The effects of the aging process itself have, however, been exaggerated and the modifying effects of diet, exercise, personal habits, and psychological factors underestimated. Within the category of normal aging, a distinction can be made between "usual aging," in which extrinsic factors heighten the effects of aging alone, and "successful aging," in which extrinsic factors play a neutral or positive role. Research on the risks associated with usual aging and strategies to modify them should help elucidate how a transition from usual to successful aging can be facilitated.

Certainly, aging is obligatory and associated with reduced maximal aerobic power and reduced muscle strength, that is, with reduced fitness. Being overweight in addition to these handicaps is additionally unfortunate because these factors taken together make walking, climbing stairs, getting up from a bed or chair, or boarding a bus or train more difficult and fatiguing and eventually impossible. The aging person will lose her/his independence and autonomy. As a consequence of diminished exercise tolerance, a large and increasing number of elderly persons will be living below, at, or just above thresholds of physical ability, needing only a minor intercurrent illness to render them completely dependent.

A recent study reported a 2.5-fold post-training increase in maximal torque in the knee extensor muscles in subjects 87 to 96 years of age. The mid-thigh muscle area increased 9.0% ± 4.5% (5). Old people can also respond favorably to training of the oxygen transport system. Specificity training could take a high priority in order to develop optimal programs aiming at maintenance/improvement in functions of importance for successful aging. A person with an innate maximal oxygen uptake below average who follows recommended training programs and increases this maximum only some 5-10% may still be below average when evaluated in a treadmill test. Performance in laboratory tests is one thing, but it is more important to reduce or eliminate risk factors and to improve tolerance to demands of daily activities that have the potential to add life to years. It is a common opinion that ability to do quick, well-coordinated finger movements deteriorates at higher ages. It is, however, noteworthy that many musicians can perform perfectly at an advanced age. Arthur Rubinstein played very demanding Chopin compositions at the age of 88 years. Andrés Segovia, at 92 years of age, gave concerts on the classical guitar. However, hours of daily training are behind these achievements.

It is important to study the molecular mechanisms underlying reduced glucose tolerance, osteoporosis, factors triggering coronary heart disease, atherosclerosis, high blood pressure, and stroke—some diseases common in the elderly population. As pointed out by Verma (13) the idea of introducing genes to correct heritable and other disorders is nothing less than revolutionary. Perhaps that is one reason why the field has progressed somewhat more slowly than expected. As stated earlier, modern creatures are the product of millions of years of evolution. One cannot expect that the initial stabs at inserting genes into cells will yield normal, stable expression easily. However, promising experiments and observations are ongoing.

Gene therapy will never have the potential to correct all human diseases. Most human afflictions are not genetic. They are environmental, caused by extrinsic factors like microbial infections. Many of them spread because of poor sanitation, polluted drinking water, malnutrition, a sedentary lifestyle, smoking, alcohol, and other factors that are outside the scope of genetic engineering.

In the United States, life expectancy has increased from 47 years in 1900 to approximately 75 years in 1988. What are the upper limits to human longevity? It has been calculated that eliminating ischemic heart disease would only increase life expectancy at birth by 3.0 years for females and 3.5 years for males. Eliminating also all forms of cancer (22.5% of all deaths in 1985) would increase life expectancy by 7.0 years for females and 8.1 years for males (10). In other words, the effects of eliminating major diseases on life expectancy are not dramatic. Advances in medical treatment more than improvements in risk factors may be allowing elderly persons who are frail and who suffer from fatal degenerative diseases to survive longer after the onset of the disease than in the past. Current research efforts by the medical community are focused on prolonging life rather than preserving the quality of life. An obvious conclusion, therefore, is that the time has come to shift towards ameliorating the social function of people with nonfatal diseases of aging. Another sad but important factor in this discussion involves ethics, specifically the moral and legal aspects of euthanasia in hopeless cases.

In this world where we see overfeeding and negative effects of a sedentary lifestyle in developed countries, millions of people are starving and living under poor conditions. It is certainly impossible for them to follow our advice "Exercise! Be active!" when there is not enough food to cover the energy demand for basal metabolic rate. Through medical advances including mass vaccinations, more and more children survive, but in what life conditions? Since overpopulation is a real threat, effective birth control programs must have a very high priority in many developing countries.

How important is habitual physical activity during childhood and adolescence for optimal development, for prevention of various diseases during that period of time and for one's future? What sort of education is optimal to create a positive attitude and lifelong interest in sports? We know very little. One problem in physical education classes is the wide range in fitness and interest. The maturation age differs markedly. At chronological age 13 we can find a boy with weight 30 kg and height 130 cm; his classmate may weigh 80 kg and be 180 cm tall. Leg strength can be 150 and 850 N respectively. The *biological* age can vary from 9 (a boy) to 16 years of age (a girl), challenging a teacher.

In many industrial countries a current trend reduces or even abolishes compulsory time for physical education in schools and colleges. What will be the present and future effects of this ignorance? People are relatively well educated in the importance of a healthy lifestyle. In too many cases they do not apply that knowledge but postpone a change in lifestyle "until tomorrow," but there is always another tomorrow.

Recreational activities in the open air are well anchored in our biological heritage. The education in fauna and flora was in former times essential. A similar education today supplemented with serious discussion of our sensitive global ecology could create a lifelong interest, commitment, and promotion of excellent hobbies and activities. There are those who do not like walking just for the sake of walking unless enjoying a hobby like bird watching, which demands some walking. A suggestion for family members, neighbors, and business partners—why not go out and walk and talk?

Acknowledgment

This section is based in part on P.-O. Åstrand and R. Rodahl's *Textbook of Work Physiology*. See reference number 1.

References

1. Åstrand, P.-O.; Rodahl, R. Textbook of work physiology. New York: McGraw-Hill; 1986: chap. 1.

2. Bouchard, C.; Boulay, M.R.; Simoneau, J.-A.; Lartre, G.; Pérusse, L. Heredity and trainability of aerobic and anaerobic performances. Sports Med. 5:69-73; 1988.
3. De Roberties, E.M.; Oliver, G.; Wright, C.V.E. Homeobox genes and the vertebrate body plan. Sci. Am. 263(1):26-32; 1990.
4. Dickerson, R.E. Chemical evolution and the origin of life. Sci. Am. 239(3):62-78; 1978.
5. Fiatarone, M.A.; Marks, E.C.; Ryan, N.D.; Meredith, C.N.; Lipitz, L.A.; Evans, W.J. High-intensity strength training in nonagenarians. JAMA. 263:3029-3034; 1990.
6. Hill, R.B. Hanta yo. An American saga. New York: Warner Books; 1980.
7. Kandel, E.R. Small systems of neurons. Sci. Am. 241(3):66-76; 1979.
8. Lewin, R. Evolutionary theory under fire. Science. 210:883-887; 1980.
9. Lewin, R. Ethiopian stone tools are world's oldest. Science. 211:806-807; 1981.
10. Olshansky, S.J.; Carnes, B.A.; Cassel, C. In search of Methuselah: Estimating the upper limit to human longevity. Science. 250:634-640; 1990.
11. Stringer, C.B. The emergence of modern humans. Sci. Am. 264(6):68-74; 1990.
12. Valentine, J.W. The evolution of multicellular plants and animals. Sci. Am. 239(3):104-117; 1974.
13. Verma, I.M. Gene therapy. Sci. Am. 263(5):34-41; 1990.
14. Vidal, G. The oldest eukaryotic cells. Sci. Am. 250(2):32-41; 1984.
15. Washburn, S.L. The evolution of man. Sci. Am. 239(3):146-154; 1978.
16. Yellen, J.E. The transformation of the Kalahari!Kung. Sci. Am. 262(4):72-79; 1990.

Chapter 6

Heredity, Activity Level, Fitness, and Health

Claude Bouchard
Louis Pérusse

Geneticists estimate that each human being has about one variable DNA base for every 100 to 300 base pairs, which makes every one of us (with the exception of monozygotic twins) a genetically unique individual. This concept of genetic individuality is important to consider because, as we have learned from other areas of research, each genotype may be at a different risk for diseases associated with inactivity and a low level of health-related fitness. Figure 6.1 illustrates schematically how genes can influence physical activity, fitness, and health. Each component of the activity–fitness–health paradigm can be influenced by one or any number of combinations of the *n* genes involved, as illustrated in the figure. Moreover, as a result of genotype-environment interaction (G×E), genes can also determine how components of the model interact with each other. There is increasing evidence that the interaction between genes and environmental factors is an important component of the individual differences in health-related phenotypes. Gene–gene interactions (represented by double-headed arrows) can also have an impact on the phenotypes. After briefly reviewing the role of heredity in physical activity and in the various components of health-related fitness, we will provide some examples showing that the response of health-related fitness factors to regular physical activity or dietary intervention can be genotype-dependent.

Two Main Research Strategies

Two strategies are traditionally used by geneticists to study the role of genes in continuously distributed phenotypes in humans. As shown in Figure 6.2, they are referred to as the unmeasured genotype and the measured genotype approaches (39,40). The unmeasured genotype approach seeksto estimate the contribution of heredity to phenotypic variance and to find evidence for single genes with major effects on the phenotype. Because inference about the contribution of genes is made from the phenotype, this approach is also referred to as the top-down strategy. This approach uses various sampling designs (studying twins, nuclear families, families with adoptees, extended pedigrees, etc.) in combination with statistical tools like path analysis, variance component estimation, and complex segregation analysis.

The measured genotype approach, on the other hand, includes direct measurements of genetic variation at the protein or DNA levels and seeks to estimate the impact of allelic variation on the phenotypic variation. Since inference about the role of genes is made from DNA to the phenotype, this approach is referred to as the bottom-up strategy (40). Direct measures of genetic variation may be obtained either by protein polymorphism or DNA polymorphism (restricted fragment length polymorphism or RFLP, and Southern blotting, polymerase chain reaction [PCR] or PCR products, and other methods of assessing sequence variation). Recent advances in recombinant DNA technology have made possible the measure of genetic variation at the DNA level and provided the impetus necessary for the extensive use of the measured genotype approach in human genetics.

These two approaches can be used to provide evidence for the presence of G×E effects in humans. Using the unmeasured genotype approach, we recently proposed (10) that one way to test for the presence of a G×E effect in humans was to challenge several genotypes in a similar manner by submitting both members of monozygotic (MZ) twin pairs to a standardized treatment and compare the within- and the between-pair variances of the response to the treatment. The finding of a significantly higher variance in the response between pairs than that within pairs suggests that the changes induced by the treatment are more heterogeneous in genetically dissimilar individuals. In a series of experiments conducted on MZ

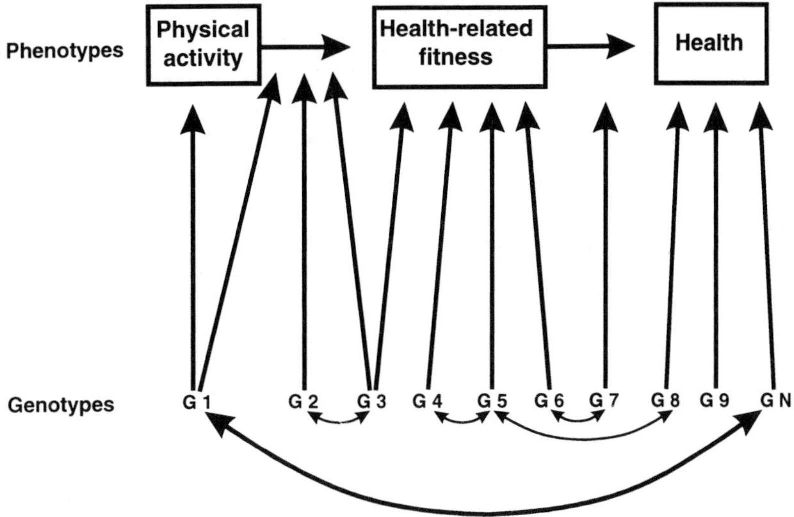

Figure 6.1 A simplified scheme to illustrate the various modes of influence of genes on the components of the activity-fitness-health paradigm.

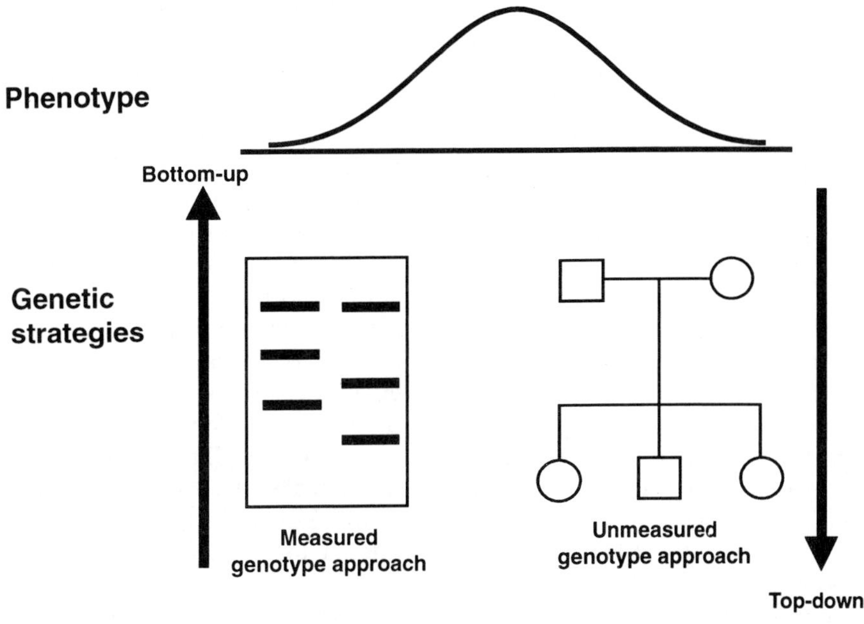

Figure 6.2 The two main strategies to study the role of genes in continuously distributed phenotypes (adapted from reference 39).

twins over the last 10 years in our laboratory, we used either exercise training or overfeeding as treatments to investigate G×E effects in health-related fitness phenotypes.

Three strategies can be used to provide evidence for G×E effect in humans with the measured genotype approach. In the first, the influence of a specific gene on a given phenotype is compared between populations with different ethnic and cultural backgrounds. In the second, the effect of a gene on the phenotype is studied between subgroups of individuals within the same population, but categorized on the basis of variables that can potentially affect the phenotype under study (e.g., sex, age, disease status, etc.). In the third strategy, the response to an environmental stimulus (exercise training, diet, or others) is investigated among individuals with different genotypes at a given gene. An important advantage of the measured genotype approach over the unmeasured genotype approach in the study of G×E is that it eventually makes possible the identification of the responsible genes, thereby providing a means for detecting individuals at a higher risk, say for a disease, because of differences in susceptibility to risk factors.

Genetic Effects on Activity Level

The contribution of genetic factors to the level of habitual physical activity or the amount of energy expended for daily physical activity has not been extensively studied. A review (9) of the available studies reveals the presence of familial resemblance for the level of habitual physical activity as assessed by various procedures. Using data from a stratified sample of the Canadian population obtained from a nationwide survey on physical fitness and physical activity habits (the 1981 Canada Fitness Survey), we studied the importance of familial resemblance in leisure-time energy expenditure (28). A total of 18,073 individuals living in 11,884 households across Canada completed a questionnaire on their physical activity habits. Detailed information on frequency, duration, and intensity of activities performed on a daily, weekly, monthly, and yearly basis was obtained and used to determine average daily energy expenditure (kJ/day/kg body weight). Familial correlations of 0.28, 0.12, and 0.21 were obtained in spouses (N= 1,024 pairs), parent-offspring (N=1,622 pairs), and siblings (N=1,036) respectively, suggesting a weak genetic contribution to interindividual differences in leisure-time energy expenditure (28). More recently, the familial resemblance in the level of habitual physical activity was investigated with the Caltrac accelerometer in 100 children, 4 to 7 years of age, 99 mothers and 92 fathers from the Framingham Children's Study (26). Data were obtained with the accelerometer for about 10 hours per day for an average of 9 days in children and 8 days in fathers and mothers over a period of one year. Active (accelerometer counts per h above the median) fathers or active mothers were more likely to have active children than inactive fathers or mothers, with an odds ratio of 3.5 and 2.0, respectively. When both parents were active, the children were 5.8 times more likely to be active than children of two inactive parents. These results suggest that unknown factors transmitted from parents to offsprings may predispose a child to be active or inactive.

Using data from the Quebec Family Study and the strategy of path analysis, we have studied the relative contribution of genetic and nongenetic factors to activity level (32). Two different indicators of physical activity were measured in 1,610 members of 375 families encompassing nine types of relatives by descent or adoption. Habitual physical activity and exercise participation were obtained from a 3-day activity record filled out by each individual during 2 weekdays and 1 weekend day. Each day of the activity record was divided into 96 periods of 15 min, and for each 15-min period, the individual had to note, on a scale from 1 to 9, the dominant activity of that period, each score representing a multiple of the resting metabolic rate. A score of 1 indicated that the individual was at rest, while a score of 9 indicated that the individual was engaged in an activity with an energy cost equivalent to about 9 times the resting metabolic rate. The scores 1 to 9 were summed over the 96 15-min periods of each day, and the average value for the 3 days was used as the indicator of habitual physical activity. The exercise participation indicator was computed as the average number of periods rated as 6, 7, 8, or 9 in each day. These categories were chosen because they correspond to activities thought to be of sufficient intensity to improve or maintain fitness. The results are summarized in Figure 6.3.

Most of the variation in these two indicators of physical activity level is accounted for by nontransmissible environmental factors with values of 71% for habitual physical activity and 88% for exercise participation. The transmission effect across generations was found to be significant but entirely accounted for by genetic factors for habitual physical activity with a value of 29%, while the transmission effect was entirely accounted for by cultural transmission (12%) for exercise participation with no genetic effect. Since habitual physical activity is the sum of scores 1 to 9 while exercise participation includes only sport activities, rated 6 to 9, activities rated 1 to 5 are likely to be those influenced by heredity. These results (32) were interpreted as an indication of inherited differences in the propensity to be spontaneously active.

Genetic Effects on Health-Related Fitness Phenotypes

Although the literature presents evidence for a role of genetic factors in most of the health-related fitness phenotypes, the quality of the evidence varies according to the phenotype considered. Because of their role in the etiology of many common diseases, some phenotypes like blood pressure, blood lipids and lipoproteins, and obesity have been more extensively studied by geneticists.

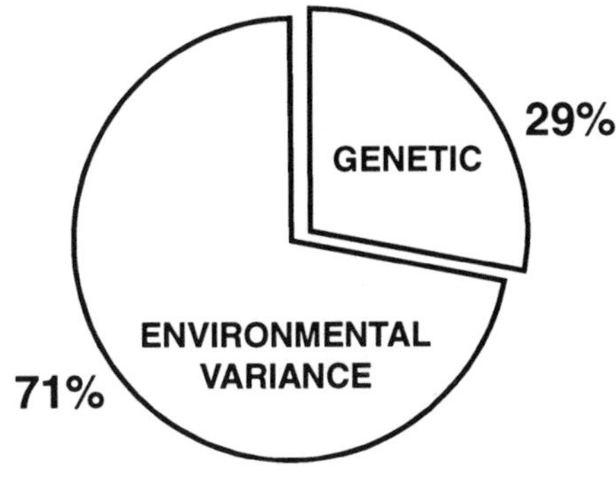

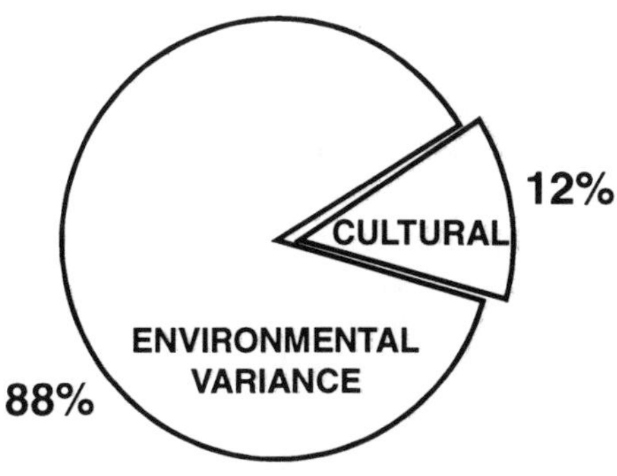

Figure 6.3 Components of phenotypic variance in habitual physical activity and exercise participation derived from a 3-day activity record and the BETA model of path analysis (adapted from reference 32).

Morphological Fitness

Obesity and regional fat distribution are the phenotypes of morphological fitness that have been most studied by geneticists. The genetics of obesity and regional fat distribution has been the object of a few reviews in recent years (4,5,8). Table 6.1 summarizes the trends emerging from these reviews regarding the contribution of genetic factors to obesity and regional fat distribution. The contributions of cultural inheritance, biological inheritance (heritability), and nontransmissible environmental factors to the age- and gender-adjusted phenotypic variance are presented along with the available evidence regarding the presence (yes) or the absence (no) of major gene effects. The body mass index (BMI), subcutaneous fat (sum of skinfold thicknesses), and percent body fat derived from underwater weighing are among the most commonly used phenotypes in genetic studies of obesity. They are characterized by a cultural transmission effect of about 30% and heritability levels ranging from 5% to 25%.

Results from a few studies suggest that BMI (25,33) and percent body fat (35) are influenced by major effects resulting from allelic variation possibly at a single gene. Evidence for commingling in the distribution of scores has been reported for subcutaneous fat (34), which is compatible with the presence of a major gene (indicated by a question mark), but not a proof of it. The phenotypes associated with regional fat distribution are generally characterized by slightly higher heritability levels with values reaching about 30% of the adjusted phenotypic variance. The trunk-to-extremity skinfolds ratio is the only regional fat distribution phenotype among those listed in Table 6.1 that has been found to be influenced by major effects associated with variation at a single gene.

Muscular Fitness

This fitness component is probably the one for which the evidence for a contribution of genetic factors is the least abundant. Heritabilities over 50% are generally observed for the various muscular fitness phenotypes (21). Most heritability estimates are derived from twin data and should therefore be interpreted with caution because of the limitations of the twin methodology. Two studies (29-30) used family data and the methodology of path analysis to study familial transmission of muscular fitness. In one study (29), we used the TAU model of path analysis to assess the contribution of transmissible factors in muscular endurance and muscular strength measurements obtained in 13,804 subjects who participated in the 1981 Canada Fitness Survey. The results showed that about 40% of the age- and sex-adjusted phenotypic variance in muscular endurance and muscular strength could be accounted for by factors transmitted from parents to offspring. In another study (30) we used the BETA model of path analysis that allows for partition of the transmissible variance into cultural and biological (genetic) components of inheritance, and found a genetic effect of 21% for muscular endurance and 30% for muscular strength. These results suggest that the heritability of muscular fitness does not exceed 30% of the phenotypic variance.

Cardiorespiratory Fitness

Cardiorespiratory fitness is a major component of health-related fitness and depends on a large number of phenotypes associated primarily with cardiac, vascular, and respiratory functions. Measurements of submaximal exercise capacity and maximal aerobic power are generally performed

Table 6.1 Summary of Current Evidence on the Genetics of Human Obesity and Regional Fat Distribution

Phenotype	Cultural inheritance	Biological inheritance	Nontransmissible factors	Major gene
BMI[a]	30%	5%	65%	Yes/No
Subcutaneous fat	30%	5%	65%	Unknown
Percent body fat	30%	25%	45%	Yes
Truncal abdominal fat	13%	28%	56%	No
Trunk/extremity skinfolds	30%	25%	45%	Yes
Subcutaneous fat/fat mass	10%	30%	60%	Unknown

[a]Two studies (25,33) support the hypothesis of a major gene for BMI, while another one (35) does not. Adapted from references 25, 33, 34, and 35.

to assess cardiorespiratory fitness. The contribution of genetic factors to these two phenotypes has been recently reviewed (7) and estimates of heritability were found to be lower for submaximal exercise capacity (less than 10%) than for maximal aerobic power (less than 25%). These inherited differences in cardiorespiratory fitness may be partly explained by interindividual differences in heart structures and functions, but relatively little is known about the role of heredity on these determinants despite evidence for significant familial aggregation (7).

Because of the high prevalence of hypertension in most developed countries and its association with an increased risk of death from myocardial infarction or stroke, the genetic and nongenetic determinants of blood pressure have been extensively studied in various populations. Overall, it is clearly established that blood pressure aggregates in families and heritability estimates reported from various populations are remarkably similar, accounting for about 30% of the interindividual differences (45). A recent study showed that systolic blood pressure measured in a population-based sample, in addition to being influenced by a polygenic effect accounting for 36% of the phenotypic variance, was influenced by allelic variation at a single gene whose effects were found to be both gender- and age-specific (31). The contribution of this major gene to systolic blood pressure variation was found to increase with age, accounting for about 1% and 6% of the variance at the age of 5 years and about 61% and 55% of the variance at the age of 50 years in males and females respectively (31).

Metabolic Fitness

There is increasing evidence for consideration of metabolic fitness in the relationship between physical activity and health. Metabolic fitness refers to normal blood and tissue carbohydrate, and lipid metabolisms and adequate hormonal actions, particularly insulin. A large number of studies on the genetics of metabolic fitness have been undertaken with blood lipids and lipoproteins as phenotypes because of their predominant role in the etiology of cardiovascular disease. As shown in Table 6.2, it is clearly established that genetic factors contribute to interindividual differences in blood lipids and lipoproteins. Heritability estimates generally account for about 25% to as much as 98% of the phenotypic variance, depending on the trait considered (19,40 for a review), with an average value of 50%. Table 6.2 also reveals that major gene effects have been reported for most of these phenotypes. Highly significant genetic effects have also been reported for fasting glucose and insulin values as well as for plasma fibrinogen, a protein involved in blood clotting. The glucose and insulin responses to a carbohydrate meal appear to be characterized by lower heritability estimates (less than 25%) than those for fasting values (13; results not shown).

The contribution of heredity to the various health-related fitness components thus ranges from low to moderate, and except for some phenotypes pertaining to muscular fitness and metabolic fitness, it rarely exceeds 50% of the phenotypic variance and is often below 25%. These low to moderate heritabilities should not be interpreted as an indication that genes are not important in the determination of these phenotypes. Moreover, these highly complex phenotypes are undoubtedly influenced by a variety of interactions between allelic variation at one or several genes and environmental factors. However, in most models used to estimate heritability, it is postulated that these gene–gene and gene–environment or lifestyle interactions are nonexistent. As illustrated in later sections of

Table 6.2 Summary of Heritability Estimates and Evidence for Major Gene Effects for Some Phenotypes of Interest[a]

Phenotype	Heritability %	Major gene
Triglycerides	25-47	No
Total cholesterol (CHOL)	49-64	Yes
LDL-CHOL	39-67	Yes
HDL-CHOL	28-56	Yes
APO AI	43	Yes
APO AII	30	No
APO B	50-70	Yes
LP (a)[b]	98	Yes
Fasting insulin	40-86	No
Fasting glucose	39-72	No
Plasma fibrinogen	51	No

[a]Adapted from references 19 and 40.
[b]From reference 24 (heritability derived from twin data).

the chapter, there is increasing evidence that interactions between genes and environmental factors or between various genes are common and contribute to interindividual differences in health-related fitness phenotypes. Consequently, they can no longer be ignored in the field of physical activity, fitness, and health.

Genetic Effects on Health Status

Improvements in sanitary conditions during the first half of this century have greatly contributed to the betterment of human health status in the Western world. These changes in living conditions allow for greater study of the contribution of genetic factors to human diseases and have increased the likelihood of detecting several forms of Mendelian diseases, as revealed by the rapid growth in the number of these diseases (23,38). For example, the incidence of some nutritional diseases (like rickets) showed a rapid decline when the nutrient involved (vitamin D) was identified and supplied to the population, but new cases continued to appear because of an inborn error of metabolism that is not fully compensated for by the nutritional supplementation (37). This example illustrates the changing heritability of human diseases as a consequence of changes in the environmental conditions and emphasizes the importance of genetic factors as determinants of diseases.

Despite their dramatic impact on an individual's health, chromosomal anomalies and single-gene Mendelian diseases have a relatively minor impact on the overall health status of the population because of their low prevalence. Common multifactorial diseases, however, are those having the greatest impact on the health of the community. It is important to note that there is increasing evidence that genetic factors are important determinants of these diseases. One example should suffice to demonstrate this point in the present context. In a recent study, the risks of premature death in adult adoptees with a biologic or adoptive parent who died of the same cause were compared to the risks of adoptees whose parents were both alive at that age (41). Relative risks were computed as the ratio of the cause-specific mortality rate among adoptees with at least one parent who died of the same cause to that among adoptees whose parents were both alive. As indicated in Table 6.3, the death of a biologic parent before the age of 50 resulted in relative risks of death in the adoptees of 2.0 for all natural causes and 4.5 for vascular causes compared to 1.0 and 3.0, respectively, for the death of an adoptive parent. These results suggest that genetic factors play an important role in the development of major diseases leading to premature death. Similar evidence can also be found for various morbid conditions.

Gene–Physical Activity Interactions

There is considerable evidence showing that there are interindividual differences in the response to training for many physical and physiological fitness phenotypes. To test the hypothesis that these differences were genetically determined, we performed several endurance and high-intensity intermittent training studies with pairs of MZ twins.

Table 6.3 Effect of the Death of a Biologic and Adoptive Parent Before Age 50 on the Rate of Adoptee Mortality from Concordant Causes

Cause of death	Biologic parent	Adoptive parent
Natural causes	2.0[a]	1.0
Vascular causes	4.5	3.0

[a]Values are relative risks derived from the ratio of the cause-specific mortality rate among adoptees with at least one parent who died of the same cause to that among adoptees whose parents were both alive. Adapted from reference 42.

We concluded from these studies (7) that the trainability of phenotypes governing aerobic and anaerobic performances is, to a large extent, determined by unknown genetic factors, that is, G×E effects are operating on these phenotypes. Table 6.4 summarizes the evidence for the contribution of a G×E effect for these phenotypes. There is about 2 to 12 times more variance between genotypes than within genotypes in their responses to exercise-training. This strongly suggests that unidentified genetic characteristics contribute to the variability in the response to training.

Few attempts have yet been made to identify genetic markers associated with this variable response to exercise-training. In one study (6), the training responses of maximal aerobic power and anaerobic performances were compared between carriers of enzyme variants for creatine kinase (CK) and adenylate kinase (AK1) and noncarriers (i.e., subjects having the common phenotype). No significant differences were observed between the two groups. We also considered associations between mitochondrial DNA polymorphisms and trainability and found a significantly lower $\dot{V}O_2$ max response to training in three subjects carrying an allele resulting from a base substitution in the subunit 5 of NADH dehydrogenase compared to noncarriers (16). In contrast, 3 subjects homozygous for the rare muscle CK-NcoI allele of 3.4 kb had a significantly higher $\dot{V}O_2$ max response to training than those carrying the two other CK-NcoI genotypes (Dionne et al., unpublished results). More research is needed to characterize the genetic basis of the interindividual differences in the response to exercise training. The search for associations, and subsequently linkage studies, with DNA sequence variation could lead to the identification of regions of the genome that could be involved in determining the response pattern.

Table 6.4 Evidence for Gene-Physical Activity Interactions in the Phenotypic Responses to Exercise-Training[a]

Phenotype	Approximate F ratio
Submaximal power output	2 to 4
Total work output in 90 min	10 to 12
$\dot{V}O_2$ max	6 to 9
Total work output in 10 s	2 to 3
Total work output in 90 s	8 to 10
Maximal O_2 pulse	6 to 10
Muscle fiber type composition	1 to 2
Muscle oxidative potential	2 to 5
Lipid substrate oxidation	2 to 5
Lipid mobilization	5 to 10

[a]The evidence is summarized by the ratio of between to within genotype variance. Summary based on several studies reported from our laboratory. See reference 7.

Gene–Diet Interactions

Using the unmeasured genotype approach, we studied the role of genotype in determining the response to diet by submitting both members of MZ twin pairs to short-term (12) and long-term (11) overfeeding experiments. Subjects had to eat a 4.2 MJ (1000 kcal) per day caloric surplus during periods of 22 days and 100 days in short-term and long-term overfeeding experiments, respectively. Both experiments resulted in significant changes for several morphological and metabolic fitness phenotypes, however, considerable interindividual differences in the adaptation to the extra calories were observed. An example of the results obtained for some morphological and metabolic fitness phenotypes is given in Table 6.5.

Long-term overfeeding resulted in significant increases in all morphological fitness phenotypes (results not shown). The F ratio of the between- to within-genotype variance indicates that there were two to six times more variance between pairs than within pairs in the response. These results suggest that the amount of fat stored in response to a caloric surplus is significantly influenced by the genotype of the individual. This genotype-overfeeding interaction effect appears to be more important for fat topography than for the amount of fat gained as indicated by higher F ratios for the amount of abdominal visceral fat gained. These findings suggest that genes determine not only gain in fat mass when subjected to a positive energy balance, but also the pattern of fat deposition among the various fat depots of the body. This has important implications for health because truncal-abdominal fat and, particularly, visceral fat are associated with greater risks of cardiovascular disease than total amount of body fat. The response of metabolic fitness phenotypes to short-term overfeeding (12) was also found to be genotype-dependent.

The results presented in Table 6.5 suggest that undetermined genetic characteristics specific to each individual are associated with the response to dietary changes. The use of the measured genotype approach could potentially contribute to the identification of some of the genes involved in determining this response. Genetic variation at the apolipoprotein gene loci could be helpful in this regard. The apolipoprotein E (apo E) gene is one of the most extensively studied genes of lipid metabolism, and its impact on plasma cholesterol levels

Table 6.5 Genotype-Overfeeding Interactions for Morphological and Metabolic Fitness Phenotypes[a]

Phenotype	F ratio
Body mass index	2.8*
Percent body fat	2.9*
Fat-free mass	2.3
Subcutaneous fat	2.8*
Abdominal visceral fat	3.6*
Abdominal visceral fat (adjusted for gains in fat mass)	6.1**

[a]The evidence is summarized by the F ratio of between to within genotype variance. Results are derived from a long-term overfeeding experiment with identical twins. Adapted from reference 11.
*$p < 0.05$; **$p < 0.01$

has been measured in several populations around the world. The gene for apo E is located on chromosome 19 and is polymorphic: Three common alleles designated ε_2, ε_3, and ε_4 code for three isoforms designated E_2, E_3, and E_4 that are associated with variation in plasma lipid levels (15). The comparison of the apo E effect on total cholesterol levels among various populations with different dietary habits provides indirect indication about the gene–diet interaction effect. Figure 6.4 presents the average effects of each apo E allele on total cholesterol in four populations (17).

The average effect of an allele, defined as the expected deviation of the mean of a group of individuals carrying that allele from the population mean, provides a measure of the influence of an allele on a given phenotype. For every population represented in the figure, the impact of the ε_2 allele is to lower, while the impact of the ε_4 allele is to raise cholesterol levels. Despite consistency in the direction of the effects across populations, the magnitude of the effects appears to vary. The cholesterol-raising effect of the ε_4 allele, for example, tends to be highest in populations like Tyrolea and Finland where a high-fat diet is eaten, and lowest in populations like Japan and Sudan who eat a low-fat diet. Results such as these have led to the proposal that the effect of this gene on plasma cholesterol was mediated by the diet (44).

Measured genetic variation at the apolipoprotein gene loci has also been used to study the role of genetic factors in the response to changes in the diet. Results of dietary intervention studies conducted on individuals from North Karelia, Finland, revealed that when subjects were switched from their habitual diet (high-fat low polyunsaturated to saturated fatty acid ratio or P/S) to a low-fat high P/S diet for 6 weeks and then switched back to their basal diet, considerable interindividual differences could be observed in the dietary response of serum lipids, lipoproteins, and apolipoproteins. When the results were analyzed, taking into account genetic polymorphism of apolipoproteins (42,43,47), significant gene-nutrient interactions were found. In the case of apo E polymorphism, results indicated that subjects homozygous for the ε_4 allele exhibited greater reductions in total cholesterol (CHOL) compared to subjects with other genotypes when switched to the low-fat high P/S diet and greater increases when brought back to the basal diet (42).

Sequence variation associated with the XbaI RFLP on the apo B gene was also associated with the response to dietary intervention. Subjects

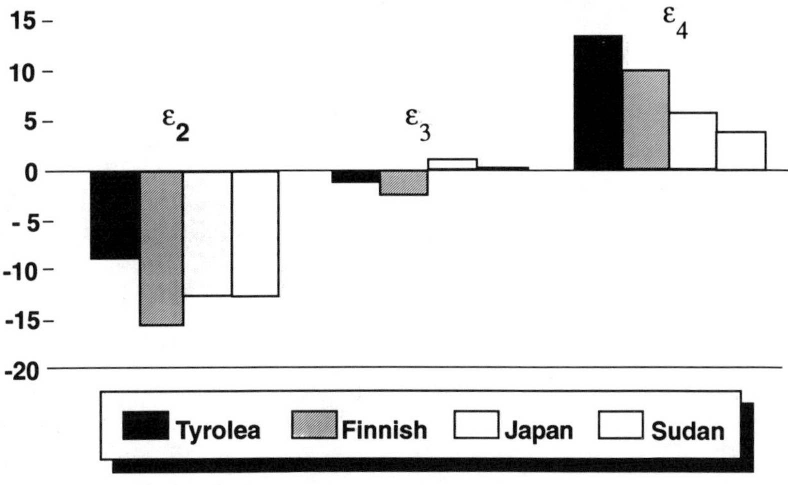

Figure 6.4 Average effects of the apo-E alleles on fasting plasma total cholesterol (mg/dl) in populations with different diets. See text for explanations (adapted from reference 17).

carrying the allele associated with the presence of the XbaI cutting site showed greater reductions in total CHOL, LDL-CHOL, HDL-CHOL, and apo B levels (43). The effects of genetic variation at the apo AII, apo AI-CIII-AIV gene cluster, apo B, apo E, and LDL-receptor genes on the response were further investigated on the same cohort (47). The major effect from the response to dietary changes was observed for the MspI-restricted fragment length polymorphism (RFLP) at the apo B gene locus, and it was found to account for 6.3% of the variation in changes of apo AI levels. Results of these studies as well as others summarized recently (1) are presented in Table 6.6. Despite some inconsistencies across studies, it appears that genetic variations at the apo B and apo E gene loci are involved in mediating plasma lipid response to dietary manipulations.

Most of these gene–nutrient interactions were documented on Finnish populations (of relatively few individuals) who are known to rank among those with the highest plasma cholesterol levels in the world and who differ from other ethnic groups in the relative frequencies of apo E alleles. Furthermore, the possibility that the response to diet depends on initial lipid values should not be excluded because most reported studies failed to adjust data for initial values. More definitive research is needed to identify genetic markers of the response to diet. However, available results strongly suggest that the concept of genetic individuality can no longer be ignored in studies designed to reduce risk of disease through dietary intervention. It is useful to recall that many animal studies are strongly supportive of the gene–nutrient interaction effect hypothesis.

Gene–Gene Interactions

Gender-specific influences of apolipoprotein polymorphisms on plasma lipids and lipoproteins provide another example of how interactions between genetic loci or between genes and environmental factors can influence health-related fitness phenotypes. The influence of apo E polymorphism on plasma lipids and lipoproteins was recently investigated in 374 men and 201 women specifically selected for their good health status (46). The ε_2 allele was found to be associated with lower plasma levels of total cholesterol, LDL-cholesterol, and apo B (LDL apo B) in both men and women, while the ε_4 allele was associated with higher levels of these traits, but in women only. As shown in Table 6.7, the contribution of apo E polymorphism to variation in total cholesterol, LDL-CHOL, HDL-CHOL, and apo B levels was found to be lower in males than in females.

Table 6.6 Genetic Variation in Apolipoproteins and the Response to Dietary Intervention

Population (REF)	Subjects	Type of diet	Gene loci	Association with response: Presence	Association with response: Lipid trait
North Karelia, Finland (42)	56 M; 54 F	Low fat, high P/S	Apo E	Yes	Chol, LDL-chol
North Karelia, Finland (43)	52 M; 51 F	Low fat, high P/S	Apo B	Yes	Chol, LDL-chol HDL-chol
North Karelia, Finland (47)	55 M; 52 F	Low fat, high P/S	Apo B	Yes	Apo A-I
			Apo E	No	
			Apo A-II	No	
			Apo AI-CIII-AIV	No	
			LDL receptor	No	
Oulu, Finland (36)	22 M; 22 F	High fat, high chol	Apo E	No	
Helsinki heart study (22)	117 dyslipidemic men	Low fat, high P/S	Apo E	Yes	Chol, LDL-chol
Adelaide, Australia (14)	38 hypercholesterolemic men	Low fat, high P/S	Apo E	Yes	Chol
Adelaide, Australia (2)	30 M; 21 F	Low fat, high P/S	Apo B	Yes	Chol
Texas, USA (3)	71 M	Low chol	Apo E	No	
			Apo B	No	

M, males; F, females; P/S, polyunsaturated to saturated fatty acids ratio.

Using the same population, Kessling et al. (20) studied associations between variability in apo B, apo AI-CIII-AIV and cholesterol ester transfer protein (CETP) gene region and blood lipids and lipoproteins in 229 male and 118 female subjects. Instead of using the traditional approach of searching for associations between a single (RFLP) and the phenotype, the authors used multiple RFLPs in each of the gene regions (4 for apo B; 6 for apo AI-CIII-AIV; 2 for CETP) to test whether genetic variability in any of the regions influences phenotypic variation in lipids and lipoproteins. The association patterns revealed striking differences between men and women: A total of 25 significant associations were observed in females compared to seven in men; and the contribution of genetic variability at these candidate genes to the phenotypic variation was found to be higher in women than in men. Among the significant associations reported, percentage of phenotypic variance accounted for by the genetic variation was found to range from 1.6% to 3.2% in men and from 1.8% to 13.0% in women. Examples of the influences of these polymorphisms on CHOL, LDL-CHOL, HDL-CHOL, and apo B levels are given in Table 6.7. The HincII apo B RFLP, for example, accounted for 1.6% and 2.5% of the variation in CHOL and LDL-CHOL, respectively, for men. The corresponding values for females reached 13.0% and 11.9%, respectively. The gender differences observed in these two studies (20,46) clearly show that pooling genders or adjusting data for gender effects should be avoided because it can dilute the estimated effect of genetic variation on the phenotype.

When the impact of a gene on a given phenotype is mediated by genetic variation at another gene locus, we are in the presence of a gene–gene interaction effect. For example, Pedersen and Berg (27) showed that variation in total CHOL and LDL-CHOL was influenced by an interaction between low-density lipoprotein receptor (LDLR) and apo E genes. They found that the cholesterol-raising and cholesterol-lowering effects of the ε_4 and ε_2 alleles, respectively, on total cholesterol levels were present only in individuals with a particular LDLR genotype. Another interesting example of gene–gene interaction has been reported by Hobbs et al. (18). These authors described a kindred with familial hypercholesterolemia in which one third of the individuals with a mutation at the LDL receptor gene, known to raise cholesterol levels, actually had plasma cholesterol values below the 25th percentile. They postulated that variation at another gene suppressed the cholesterol-raising effect of the LDL receptor mutation gene in these subjects (18). Through linkage analysis they were able to exclude the normal LDL receptor and its two ligands, apo B and apo E, as candidates for this suppressor gene. These examples of gene–gene and gene–environment interactions illustrate the complexity of gene actions and interactions and the relationships between genotype and phenotype.

Table 6.7 Percentage of Phenotypic Variance Accounted for by Genetic Variation in Apo AI-CIII-AIV, Apo B, Apo E, and CETP Genes

Phenotype and RFLP	Percentage of phenotypic variation ($R^2 \times 100$) Men	Women
Cholesterol		
apo AI-CIII-AIV XmnI	0.9	1.8
apo B HincII	1.6	13.0***
apo B PvuII	1.1	3.8*
apo E	1.9	15.6*
LDL-cholesterol		
apo B HincII	2.5	11.9***
apo B XbaI	1.4	3.8*
apo E	3.0	16.6***
HDL-cholesterol		
apo AI-CIII-AIV BamHI	1.5	5.0*
apo AI-CIII-AIV PvuII	1.3	3.1*
apo B XbaI	0.4	3.4*
CETP TaqI-2	0.3	10.1**
apo E	0.9	1.3
Apo B		
apo B Hinc II	1.7	11.7***
apo B PvuII	0.7	2.6*
apo E	3.4*	15.5*

Note. Adapted from references 20 and 46.
$^*p < 0.05$; $^{**}p < 0.005$; $^{***}p < 0.001$

Research Directions

Studies should be designed to incorporate both the measured and unmeasured genotype approaches and a variety of coherently related phenotypes permitting consideration in univariate or joint analysis. Special attention should be paid to gene–physical activity interactions and gene–gene interactions. To this end, physical activity intervention studies based on a panel of two-generation families with extensive phenotyping and intermediate phenotype assessment along with DNA banking would be particularly useful.

The greatest challenge at this time is to improve understanding of the potential of genetic and molecular medicine among the physical activity scientists, to train a new generation of these scientists to undertake these genetic studies, and to establish several competing centers of excellence where such investigations would be carried out routinely. Too few physical activity scientists and laboratories are involved in genetic and molecular biology research at the present time. Corrective measures and coordinated efforts are needed to explore the current revolution in the biological sciences, particularly in the DNA technology and the study of the human genome.

References

1. Abbey, M. The influence of apolipoprotein polymorphism on the response to dietary fat and cholesterol. Cur. Opin. Lipidol. 3:12-16; 1992.
2. Abbey, M.; Belling, B.; Clifton, P.; Nestel, P. Apolipoprotein B gene polymorphism associates with plasma cholesterol changes induced by dietary fat and cholesterol. Nutr. Metab. Cardiovasc. Dis. 1:10-12; 1991.
3. Boerwinkle, E.; Brown, S.A.; Rohrbach, K.; Gotto, A.M., Jr.; Patsch, W. Role of apolipoprotein E and B gene variation in determining response of lipid, lipoprotein, and apolipoprotein levels to increased dietary cholesterol. Am. J. Hum. Genet. 49:1145-1154; 1991.
4. Bouchard, C. Variation in human body fat: The contribution of the genotypes. In: Bray, G.A.; Ricquier, D.; Spiegelman, B., eds. Obesity: Towards a molecular approach. New York: Alan R. Liss, Inc.; 1990:17-28.
5. Bouchard, C. Etiology and pathogenesis: Genetic aspects of human obesities. In: Belfiore, F.; Jeanrenaud, B.; Papalia, D., eds. Obesity: Basic concepts and clinical aspects. Front diabetes. Basel, Karger; 1992:28-36.
6. Bouchard, C.; Chagnon, M.; Thibault, M.C.; Boulay, M.R.; Marcotte, M.; Côté, C.; Simoneau, J.A. Muscle genetic variants and relationship with performance and trainability. Med. Sci. Sports Exerc. 21:71-77; 1989.
7. Bouchard, C.; Dionne, F.T.; Simoneau, J.A.; Boulay, M.R. Genetics of aerobic and anaerobic performances. Exerc. Sport Sci. Rev. 20:27-58; 1992.
8. Bouchard, C.; Pérusse, L. Heredity and body fat. Annu. Rev. Nutr. 8:259-277; 1988.
9. Bouchard, C.; Pérusse, L.; Dériaz, O.; Després, J.P.; Tremblay, A. Genetic influences on energy expenditure in humans. In: Filer, L.J. ed. Child and adolescent obesity: What, how and who? Washington, DC: International Life Sciences Institute; [In press].
10. Bouchard, C.; Pérusse, L.; Leblanc, C. Using MZ twins in experimental research to test for the presence of a genotype-environment interaction effect. Acta Genet. Med. Gemellol. 39:85-89; 1990.
11. Bouchard, C.; Tremblay, A.; Després, J.P.; Nadeau, A.; Lupien, P.J.; Thériault, G.; Dussault, J.; Moorjani, S. The response to long-term overfeeding in identical twins. N. Engl. J. Med. 322:1477-1482; 1990.
12. Bouchard, C.; Tremblay, A.; Després, J.P.; Poehlman, E.T.; Thériault, G.; Nadeau, A.; Lupien, P.J.; Moorjani, S. Sensitivity to overfeeding: The Quebec experiment with identical twins. Prog. Food Nutr. Sci. 12:45-72; 1988.
13. Bouchard, C.; Tremblay, A.; Nadeau, A.; Després, J.P.; Thériault, G.; Boulay, M.R.; Lortie, G.; Leblanc, C.; Founier, G. Genetic effects in resting and exercise metabolic rates. Metabolism. 38:364-370; 1989.
14. Clifton, P.M.; Kestin, M.; Abbey, M.; Drysdale, M.; Nestel, P.J. Relationship between sensitivity to dietary fat and dietary cholesterol. Arteriosclerosis. 10:394-401; 1990.
15. Davignon, J.; Gregg, R.E.; Sing, C.F. Apolipoprotein E polymorphism and atherosclerosis. Arteriosclerosis 8:1-21; 1988.
16. Dionne, F.; Turcotte, L.; Thibault, M.C.; Boulay, M.R.; Skinner, J.S.; Bouchard, C. Mitochondrial DNA sequence-polymorphism, VO_2 max, and response to endurance training. Med. Sci. Sports Exerc. 23:177-185; 1991.
17. Hallman, D.M.; Boerwinkle, E.; Saha, N.; Sandholzer, C.; Menzel, H.J.; Csazar, A.; Utermann, G. The apolipoprotein E polymorphism: A comparison of allele frequencies and effects in nine populations. Am. J. Hum. Genet. 49:338-349; 1991.
18. Hobbs, H.H.; Leitersdorf, E.; Leffert, C.C.; Cryer, D.R.; Brown, M.S.; Goldstein, J.L. Evidence for a dominant gene that suppresses hypercholesterolemia in a family with defective low density lipoprotein receptors. J. Clin. Invest. 84:656-664; 1989.
19. Iselius, L. Genetic epidemiology of common diseases in humans. Weir, B.S.; Eisen, E.J.; Goodman, M.M.; Namkoong, G., eds. Proceedings of the 2nd international conference on quantitative genetics; May 31-June 5, 1987; Sunderland, MA: Sinauer Associates, Inc.; 1988:341-352.
20. Kessling, A.; Ouellette, S.; Bouffard, O.; Chamberland, A.; Bétard, C.; Selinger, E.; Xhignesse, M.; Lussier-Cacan, S.; Davignon, J. Patterns of association between genetic variability in apolipoprotein (Apo) B, Apo AI-CIII-AIV, and cholesterol ester transfer protein gene regions and

quantitative variation in lipid and lipoprotein traits: Influence of gender and exogenous hormones. Am. J. Hum. Genet. 50:92-106; 1991.

21. Malina, R.M.; Bouchard, C. Genetic considerations in physical fitness. In: Assessing physical fitness and physical activity in population-based surveys. DHHS publication no. 89-1253. Washington, DC: U.S. Dept. of Health and Human Services; 1989. Available from: U.S. Government Printing Office, Washington, DC.
22. Manttari, M.; Koskinen, P.; Ehnholm, C.; Huttunen, J.K.; Manninen, V. Apolipoprotein E polymorphism influence the serum cholesterol response to dietary intervention. Metabolism. 40:217-221; 1991.
23. McKusick, V.A. Mendelian inheritance in man. Catalogs of autosomal dominant, autosomal recessive, and X-linked phenotypes. 10th ed. Baltimore: Johns Hopkins University Press; 1992.
24. Hewitt, K.D.; Milner, J.; Breckenridge, C.; Maguire, G. Heritability of sinking pre-beta lipoprotein level: A twin study. Clin. Genet. 11:224; 1977.
25. Moll, P.P.; Burns, T.L.; Lauer, R.M. The genetic and environmental sources of body mass index variability: The Muscatine ponderosity family study. Am. J. Hum. Genet. 49:1243-1255; 1991.
26. Moore, L.L.; Lombardi, D.A.; White, M.J.; Campbell, J.L.; Oliveria, S.A.; Ellison, R.C. Influence of parents' physical activity levels on activity levels of young children. J. Pediatr. 118:215-219; 1991.
27. Pedersen, J.C.; Berg, K. Interaction between low density lipoprotein receptor (LDLR) and apolipoprotein E (apo E) alleles contributes to normal variation in lipid level. Clin. Genet. 35:331-337; 1989.
28. Pérusse, L.; Leblanc, C.; Bouchard, C. Familial resemblance in lifestyle components: Results from the Canada fitness survey. Can. J. Public Health. 79:201-205; 1988.
29. Pérusse, L.; Leblanc, C.; Bouchard, C. Intergeneration transmission of physical fitness in the Canadian population. Can. J. Sport Sci. 13:8-14; 1988.
30. Pérusse, L.; Lortie, G.; Leblanc, C.; Tremblay, A.; Thériault, G.; Bouchard, C. Genetic and environmental sources of variation in physical fitness. Ann. Hum. Biol. 14:425-434; 1987.
31. Pérusse, L.; Moll, P.P.; Sing, C.F. Evidence that a single gene with gender- and age-dependent effects influences systolic blood pressure determination in a population based-sample. Am. J. Hum. Genet. 49:94-105; 1991.
32. Pérusse, L.; Tremblay, A.; Leblanc, C.; Bouchard, C. Genetic and environmental influences on level of habitual physical activity and exercise participation. Am. J. Epidemiol. 129:1012-1022; 1989.
33. Price, R.A.; Ness, R.; Laskarzewski, P. Common major gene inheritance of extreme overweight. Hum. Biol. 62:747-765; 1990.
34. Rice, T.; Borecki, I.B.; Bouchard, C.; Rao, D.C. Commingling analysis of regional fat distribution measures: The Quebec family study. Int. J. Obes. 16:831-844; 1992.
35. Rice, T.; Borecki, I.B.; Bouchard, C.; Rao, D.C. Segregation of fat mass, measured using underwater weighing, and other body composition measures. Am. J. Hum. Genet. 52:967-973, 1993.
36. Savolainen, M.J.; Rantala, M.; Kervinen, K.; Jarvi, L.; Suvanto, K.; Rantala, T.; Kesaniemi, Y.A. Magnitude of dietary effects on plasma cholesterol concentration: Role of sex and apolipoprotein E phenotype. Atherosclerosis. 86:145-152; 1991.
37. Scriver, C.R. Changing heritability of nutritional disease: Another explanation for clustering. World Rev. Nutr. Diet. 63:60-71; 1989.
38. Scriver, C.R.; Beaudet, A.L.; Sly, W.S.; Valle, D. The metabolic basis of inherited disease. Vol. 1, 2. 6th ed. New York: McGraw-Hill Co.; 1989.
39. Sing, C.F.; Boerwinkle, E.A. Genetic architecture of inter-individual variability in apolipoprotein, lipoprotein and lipid phenotypes. In: Weatherall, D., ed. Molecular approaches to human polygenic disease. Chichester: Ciba Foundation Symposium 130; Wiley; 1987:99-127.
40. Sing, C.F.; Boerwinkle, E.A.; Moll, P.P.; Templeton, A.R. Characterization of genes affecting quantitative traits in humans. In: Weir, B.S.; Eisen, E.J.; Goodman, M.M.; Namkoong, G., eds. Proceedings of the 2nd international conference on quantitative genetics; Sunderland: Sinauer Associates; 1988:250-269.
41. Sorensen, T.I.A.; Nielsen, G.G.; Andersen, P.K.; Teasdale, T.W. Genetic and environmental influences on premature death in adult adoptees. N. Engl. J. Med. 318:727-732; 1988.
42. Tikkanen, M.J.; Huttunen, J.K.; Ehnholm, C.; Pietinen, P. Apolipoprotein E4 homozygosity predisposes to serum cholesterol elevation during high fat diet. Arteriosclerosis. 10:285-288; 1990.
43. Tikkanen, M.J.; Xu, C.F.; Hamalainen, T.; Talmud, P.; Sarna, S.; Huttenen, J.K.; Pietinen, P.; Humphries, S. XbaI polymorphism of the apolipoprotein B gene influences plasma lipid response to diet intervention. Clin. Genet. 37:327-334; 1990.

44. Utermann, G. Apolipoprotein E polymorphism in health and disease. Am. Heart J. 113:433-440; 1987.
45. Ward, R. Familial aggregation and genetic epidemiology of blood pressure. In: Laragh, J.H.; Brenner, B.M., eds. Hypertension: Pathophysiology, diagnosis and management. New York: Raven Press; 1990:81-99.
46. Xhignesse, M.; Lussier-Cacan, S.; Sing, C.F.; Kessling, A.M.; Davignon, J. Influences of common variants of apolipoprotein E on measures of lipid metabolism in a sample selected for health. Arterio. Thromb. 11:1100-1110; 1991.
47. Xu, C.F.; Boerwinkle, E.; Tikkanen, M.J.; Huttunen, J.K.; Humphries, S.E.; Talmud, P.J. Genetic variation at the apolipoprotein gene loci contribute to response of plasma lipids to dietary changes. Genet. Epidemiol. 7:261-275; 1990.

Chapter 7

Some Interrelations of Physical Activity, Physiological Fitness, Health, and Longevity

Ralph S. Paffenbarger, Jr.
Robert T. Hyde
Alvin L. Wing
I-Min Lee
James B. Kampert

We recognize trends and their importance even if we do not yet understand all the influences, mechanisms, and causal relations involved. This is why we find widespread recognition today of the importance of interrelated trends in physical activity, physiological fitness, health, quality of life, morbidity, mortality, and longevity, not to mention the prominent adjunctive area of interest, *diet*. We always hope to learn more. Because our main topic at present is physical activity, we will set aside dietary considerations, although in reality they are inseparable from any physical activity because life requires both energy intake and energy expenditure. Individuals in developed nations such as Canada and the USA are likely to find that their diet is more constant and plentiful than their physical exercise. Changes in diet might involve changes in nutrition, quantity, supplements, gustatory pleasure, or basic mealtime habits and perhaps clash with feedback and demand mechanisms of body systems. On the other hand, healthful improvements in physical activity patterns may be accomplished without adversely affecting appetite, diet, or energy intake. Both energy intake and energy output are determined primarily by individual behavior.

Modern society has tended to deprive people of physical activity rather than food. Trends of chronic disease now imply that adequate exercise is essential to preservation of good health, satisfying quality of life, and optimal longevity. Avoidance or postponement of morbidity is influenced by many variables capable of optimal adjustment, especially physical activity, either directly or through interactions. To the extent that physical exercise is a normal function of the body, it tends to promote optimal performance of all the body systems involved—musculoskeletal, cardiovascular-respiratory, hormonal-immunologic, hematologic, neurosensory, gastrointestinal, and so on (2).

The positive benefits of physical activity are best appreciated in contrast to the sluggishness or negative consequences associated with inactivity or sedentary living. This can be depicted in a pair of flow charts. The first sequence shows that where exercise is *adequate*, fitness is likely to be maintained or improved, good health is preserved, quality of life is favorable, systemic disease such as hypertensive-metabolic-atherosclerotic disease (HMAD) is avoided or deferred, and length of life is maximal: Physical activity → physiological fitness → high quality of life → low HMAD risk → long life. The second pattern shows the likely consequences of a downward trend of existence where lack of exercise reduces fitness to unfitness or debilitation, lifestyle and quality of life become unfavorable, health deteriorates toward HMAD, and risk increases of premature death or shortened life: Physical inactivity → physiological unfitness → low quality of life → high HMAD risk → short life.

One important relation between these two flow charts is that avoidance or correction of the problems inherent in the downward path of the second may result in an adherence or return to the beneficial status represented by the first. An inactive person may become more physically active, an unfit person may regain fitness, his or her lifestyle may become more favorable to avoidance of early HMAD, and he or she may expect to live a longer, healthier, and more satisfying life than if the habitual activity pattern had not been adjusted.

Current Status of Knowledge

The 1988 Toronto International Conference on Exercise, Fitness, and Health opened with a survey chapter entitled "Physical Activity and Physical Fitness as Determinants of Health and Longevity" (17), a topic similar to our present deliberations. In 1988 a good deal of time was devoted toward reaching a consensus on definitions of basic concepts such as physical activity, exercise, and fitness. Without denying the prominent role of cardiovascular-respiratory fitness, a broader concept of fitness was gained and appreciated under such terms as health fitness, whole body fitness, physiological or functional fitness, and functional capacity. These included attention to muscle strength, endurance, muscle power, agility, flexibility, reflexes, reaction time, metabolic efficiency, body composition, and other aspects of whole body fitness.

At the same time, physical activity variables were recognized as having relations to fitness and health outcomes. Type, duration, quantity, and intensity of physical exercise, for example, were discussed in terms of their relations to specific fitness variables and to assessed benefits and hazards for individuals of different age, health status, physique, and goals. The roles of these fitness and activity objectives in the planning and conduct of community health programs were also of great interest.

Both physical activity and physiological fitness are optional variables capable of favoring health and longevity. They have fundamentally different implications, however, because physical activity is a *process* and fitness is a *condition*. In this sense, physical activity is a dynamic, ongoing concept, and fitness a static or cross-sectional concept. Yet these are intertwined because fitness establishes bench marks and limitations for physical activity, and activity modifies fitness from one cross-sectional status to another.

None of these considerations have disappeared or diminished during the intervening years. We have accepted many of the findings of the 1988 Toronto Conference (5) and seek to refine, extend, and expand them here. For example, beneficial physical activity appears to fend off HMAD, and coronary heart disease (CHD) in particular (3,9,12,22,23), postponing mortality. Thus we now are asking how to promote such exercise and how to anticipate a longer and more active life, one of a higher quality that improved health makes possible. Optimum healthful longevity is the ultimate objective of all preventive medicine, the desired result that makes the entire program cost-effective (6,24,26). The achievement of good quality of life is of paramount importance today and in all the coming decades we can foresee. Although we now believe that exercise, fitness, and sound health are essential thereto, we are only beginning to examine the ways and means by which we can put our constructive efforts to best use.

Physical Activity and Health

A few recent or current studies have been looking at physical activity, fitness, and longevity. Professor Jeremy N. Morris of the London School of Hygiene and Tropical Medicine, who together with his colleagues pioneered studies of vigorous exercise and CHD (14,15), has extended those analyses to all-cause mortality or longevity among British civil servants (12,13). The first deck of Table 7.1 (A) is an excerpt of findings on rates and relative risks of CHD during a 9-year follow-up among 9,376 subjects, 45-65 years at entry in 1976, by patterns of sportsplaying characterized by intensity, duration, and frequency.

Vigorous sports (later referred to as "moderately vigorous") were defined as demanding 7.5 kilocalories (kcal) per minute or 6 METs or more, while less intense activity was considered *nonvigorous*. Duration was logged by totaling 5-minute increments, and frequency by ranking the number of episodes of sportsplay during the 4 weeks prior to study entry. Only 33% of the man-years represented any sportsplay, and 18% vigorous sportsplay; however, increasing frequency of the latter was associated with a gradient reduction in risk of CHD (p of trend <0.005). Cohort analysis for vigorous sportsplay showed that men 45-54 years required more energy expenditure to achieve beneficial levels of exertion than their elders, 55-64 years, who had lower functional capacity with advancing age. Nonvigorous sportsplay showed little benefit over none at all (p for trend > 0.05).

With regard to all-cause mortality and longevity in this study population, the 1990 report commented, "When non-coronary deaths were added to those from coronary heart disease, total death rates over the 9+ years of follow-up were lower in men with an exercise-related reduction in CHD, and their survival through middle age and into old age greater than in other men. Detailed analysis of mortality in general will have to be based on larger numbers and so a longer follow-up." In tendency at least, the British findings parallel results reported for Harvard alumni during the 1988 Toronto Conference except that the London study observed no benefit for levels of physical activity rated less than vigorous or moderate intensity (12).

Socioeconomic and other differences between the British and American study populations were

Table 7.1 Studies of Physical Activity and Longevity

A. Rates and relative risks of coronary heart disease (CHD)[a] among 9,376 British civil servants aged 45-64 at entry, in a 9+-year follow-up, 1976-1986, (87,563 man-years; 474 CHD cases), by patterns of sportsplaying (12).

Episodes of sportsplay in past 4 weeks	Vigorous sportsplay				Nonvigorous sportsplay			
	Man-years (%)	Number CHD cases	Cases per 1000 man-years	Relative risk of CHD[b]	Man-years (%)	Number CHD cases	Cases per 1000 man-years	Relative risk of CHD[c]
None	82	413	5.8	1.00	67	310	5.4	1.00
1-3	9	37	4.5	0.78	16	85	5.9	1.09
4-7	5	17	4.1	0.71	10	52	5.9	1.09
8-11	4	7	2.1	0.36	6	19	3.5	0.65
12+					1	8	6.8	1.26

[a]Age-adjusted; [b]p of trend <0.005; [c]p of trend >0.05.

B. All-cause mortality rates (deaths per 1,000 man-years) in a 26-year follow-up among 9,484 Seventh Day Adventist men, by attained age (50-99 yr, 10-year age groups) and physical activity status at entry (1960) (11).

Age (years)	Inactive	Moderately active	Highly active
50-59	4.0 (2.0,6.0)[a]	2.4	2.5
60-69	11.2 (9.2,13.2)	8.4	9.1 (7.1,11.1)
70-79	36.6 (32.7,40.5)	27.4 (25.4,29.4)	33.5 (27.6,39.4)
80-89	85.1 (75.3,94.9)	81.9 (78.0,85.8)	94.1 (80.4,108)
90-99	169.6 (154,185)	152.5 (143,162)	156.5 (125,188)

[a]95% confidence intervals in parentheses.

C. Relative risks (RR) of all-cause mortality[a] among the elderly in the Alameda County Health Study, 1965-1982, by age and physical activity status at entry (8).

Physical activity status	Age							
	38-49		50-59		60-69		70+	
	RR	(95% CI)	RR	(95% CI)	RR	(95% CI)	RR	(95% CI)
Low/high	1.48[b]	(1.08,2.02)	1.27[c]	(0.97,1.66)	1.38[b]	(1.09,1.75)	1.37[b]	(1.49,1.72)

[a]Adjusted for age, self-reported health status at baseline (entry), and six other risk factors (smoking, relative weight, alcohol use, sleep hours, breakfast habit, and snack habit). 95% confidence intervals in parentheses; [b]$0.001<p<0.01$; [c]$p<0.10$.

(continued)

Table 7.1 *(continued)*

D. Relative risks of coronary heart disease (CHD) and all-cause mortality[a] in a 17 to 20-year follow-up among 2,548 US railroad workers, 1957-1977, by leisure-time physical activity level at entry (27).

Leisure-time physical activity, kcal/wk	Relative risk of CHD mortality (95% CI)[b]	Relative risk of all-cause mortality (95% CI)
3,632	1.00	1.00
1,372	1.05 (1.00-1.11)	1.04 (1.01-1.08)
554	1.11 (1.00-1.23)	1.08 (1.01-1.15)
40	1.28 (0.99-1.63)	1.21 (1.03-1.42)

[a]Adjusted for age, systolic blood pressure, serum cholesterol, and smoking status; [b]95% confidence intervals in parentheses.

E. Relative risks of coronary heart disease (CHD) among 7,630 men aged 40-59 yr in an 8-year follow-up, in the British Regional Heart Study, by levels of physical activity index (25).

Physical activity	Number of men (%)	Relative risk of CHD[a]	
		Adjusted[b]	Further adjusted[c]
Inactive	686 (9.0)	1.0	1.0
Occasional	2,345 (30.7)	0.8 (0.5-1.2)	0.9 (0.5-1.3)
Light	1,761 (23.1)	0.8 (0.5-1.2)	0.9 (0.6-1.4)
Moderate	1,205 (15.8)	0.4 (0.2-0.8)	0.5 (0.2-0.8)
Moderately vigorous	1,120 (14.7)	0.4 (0.2-0.8)	0.5 (0.3-0.9)
Vigorous	513 (6.7)	0.8 (0.4-1.4)	0.9 (0.5-1.8)

[a]95% confidence intervals in parentheses; [b]adjusted for age, body mass index, social class, and smoking status; [c]also adjusted for systolic blood pressure, total cholesterol, HDL cholesterol, FEV1, breathlessness, and heart rate.

F. Rates and relative risks of stroke[a] among 7,630 men aged 45-59 yr in an 8.5-year follow-up in the British Regional Heart Study, by levels of physical activity index (29).

Physical activity	Number of men (%)	Number of stroke cases	Cases per 1000 per year	Relative risk of stroke
Inactive	686 (9.0)	21	3.1	1.0
Occasional	2,435 (30.7)	52	2.3	0.7
Light	1,761 (23.1)	29	1.7	0.5
Moderate	1,205 (15.8)	15	1.4	0.4
Moderately vigorous	1,120 (14.7)	9	1.0	0.3
Vigorous	513 (6.7)	2	0.5	0.2

[a]Age-adjusted.

considered among possible explanations for the varying outcomes described. Morris et al. had characterized their study population as more active than average Britons and perhaps more fit and active than the age-comparable Harvard alumni who might therefore show benefit from less exercise than the British to improve their health. Differing methods of activity assessment also might be involved, although the ratio of less active to more active individuals was about 2:1 in both populations. Relations of physical activity level and all-cause mortality will be explored further in this report, updating and extending the Harvard Alumni Health Study.

The second deck of Table 7.1 (B) presents findings from a 1991 report by Lindsted, Tonstad, and Kuzma on patterns of physical activity and mortality among 9,484 elderly Seventh Day Adventist men, during 1960-1985 (11). Baseline data were obtained from a self-administered lifestyle questionnaire completed in 1960. There were 4,000 deaths (42%) during follow-up, 12.5% at 91 years or older up to 105 years. The 5,803 men (61%) who reported moderate physical activity were older and had lower death rates than the 1,609 who were deemed highly active (17%) and the 2,022 who reported little or no physical activity (22%). The age-specific analysis was based on attained age, not on age at the time of the questionnaire in 1960. That is, 90-year-old survivors who had declared themselves highly active in 1960 were compared with 90-year-olds who had reported themselves inactive in 1960. Relative risks calculated from a univariate analysis of all-cause mortality among the three activity groups showed a significant difference in survival.

A multivariate analysis of all-cause mortality showed that interaction between activity level and age was significant for both moderate activity and high activity. At age 50 the respective relative risks were about equal, 0.61 to 0.66. Moderate activity continued protective beyond age 80 (relative risk = 0.85), but higher activity lost statistical significance at age 70 (relative risk = 0.89).

The analysis showed that crossover of risk for moderate activity occurred at 95.4 years (95% CI 81.7-109.4), and for higher activity at 78.2 years (95% CI 70.3-86.0). Crossover is the experience point at which the relative risk reaches 1.0 where inactivity and activity no longer influence survival. These findings reveal that moderate physical activity continues to be important well into old age; but at each age class, all-cause death rates were higher for the highly active than for the moderately active.

The study did not assess whether exercise habits of these men changed after 1960, but they were considered a stable and prudent population. They are likely to have followed the same trends as similar groups in whom influential lifestyle changes have been assessed during the same time period (12,18). In any event, this Loma Linda report is of high interest as a study of interrelations of physical activity, aging, and survival.

The third deck of Table 7.1 (C) presents physical activity status and mortality data on 4,174 adults at least 38 years of age in 1964, a cohort of the Alameda County [California] Study reported by Kaplan et al. in 1987 (8). In this age-specific analysis intended to focus on the elderly 60 years and older, two younger groups were included for comparison. The findings show that physical activity benefits continue into the later years of life beyond middle age.

Slattery, Jacobs, and Nichaman (27) studied leisure-time physical activity among male US railroad workers for relation to death from CHD and all causes in a 17- to 20-year follow-up period (Table 7.1, deck D). Some 2,500 men had been queried as to activity patterns and examined for other characteristics between 1957 and 1960, were reexamined from 1962 to 1964, and followed until 1977. The relative risk of CHD death was 1.28 for men who expended 40 kcal per week as compared with very active men who expended 3,632 kcal per week; the corresponding relative risk for all-cause mortality was 1.21. These risk estimates were adjusted for differences in age, cigarette smoking, blood pressure level, and serum cholesterol level. Leisure-time energy expenditure in light and moderate activities, as well as that of intense effort, showed independent relations to both CHD and all-cause mortality.

Professor A. Gerald Shaper and his colleague, Ms. Goya Wannamethee, from the Royal Free Hospital School of Medicine in London have been examining the relation between physical activity and risks of CHD and stroke in middle-aged men randomly chosen from general medical practices in 24 British towns, which are representative of the socioeconomic distribution of men in that country (25,29). Research nurses administered a standard questionnaire asking about physical activity, social habits, and a medical history. They made physical measurements and took electrocardiograms and blood samples, the latter for biochemical and hematological assessments.

The questions on leisure-time physical activities led to a complex classification system of 6 levels of energy expenditure that combine total effort and intensity of effort into six groups: inactive (9% of men), occasional (31%), light (23%), moderate (16%), moderately vigorous (15%), and vigorous (7%) (Table 7.1-E and F). All men, whether or not they showed evidence of CHD on initial examination, were followed for CHD morbidity and all-cause mortality, using established procedures in the British health care system. Men 45 to 59 years at entry were followed for CHD events over an 8-year period; men 40 to 59 years were followed for stroke events over an 8.5-year period.

With respect to CHD (Table 7.1-E), 488 men suffered at least one such major event. Risk of CHD decreased with increased physical activity; the groups reporting moderate or moderately vigorous activity experienced less than half the rate for inactive men; and vigorously active men experienced higher rates similar to those classified as occasionally or lightly active. Men who entered with *symptomatic* CHD experienced a lower rate of recurrence at occasional, light, and moderate levels of physical activity, but showed an increased rate at the moderately vigorous level. Men who entered with *asymptomatic* CHD experienced a higher rate of recurrence at light and moderate levels, declining again at moderately vigorous levels. Overall, men who reported sportsplaying (vigorous) activities of any weekly frequency had lower CHD rates than men reporting no sportsplaying. Excluding sportsplaying from the analysis, a significant inverse relation remained between physical activity and CHD incidence in the 8-year follow-up.

With respect to stroke (Table 7.1-F), 128 men suffered at least one such major event. Physical activity was inversely related to risk of stroke, both in men free of CHD and stroke at entry and in those with one or the other of these conditions. However, in *asymptomatic* men at entry, sportsplaying (i.e., vigorous activity) now was associated with an increased rate of CHD as compared with that for men engaged in moderate or moderately vigorous activity. In *symptomatic* men without CHD or stroke, those engaged in moderately vigorous or vigorous activity tended to experience a higher risk of CHD than inactive men.

These observations by Shaper and Wannamethee suggest that moderate physical activity (frequent walking or cycling, or very frequent recreational activities, or sportsplaying once a week) is associated with lower rates of CHD and stroke in men both with and without pre-existing CHD. They offer a cautionary note, however, suggesting there is no further lowering of rates from either disease among men engaging in the most vigorous activities. In fact, frequent sportsplay and recreational activities may be associated with higher risks than those for less vigorous, regular physical activities.

Physiological Fitness and Health

In 1988, we cited several reports on the influence of fitness on all-cause mortality (17). Since then a few additional reports have extended knowledge in this area. For example, Dr. Steven N. Blair and his colleagues of the Cooper Institute for Aerobics Research in Dallas, Texas, assessed fitness by treadmill performance in 10,244 men and 3,120 women aged 20-60+ years and followed them for 110,482 person-years, averaging 8+ years, for all-cause mortality (4). Mortality rates were lowest (18.6 per 10,000 person-years) among the most fit and highest (64.0) among the least fit men (Table 7.2, deck A), paralleling closely the results from studies of physical activity levels and mortality. Corresponding rates for the women were 8.5 and 39.5.

Since physical activity habits and fitness often are linked, these findings may imply that the beneficial effects of physical activity on health and survival are mediated via fitness status. Beneficial exercise is known to influence many body systems favorably, while systemic conditions may have roles in determining physiological fitness, for example, cardiovascular-respiratory fitness. The present conference has a major incentive to extend understanding of these matters found to be of great interest in the 1988 sessions. We do not have specific fitness data on the Harvard alumni, but their responses to questions about their physical activities and their degrees of satisfaction with their health status would seem to offer some clues to their general fitness status.

In a 7-year follow-up of a representative sample of the Canadian population, Arraiz, Wigle, and Mao used a home fitness test to distinguish the 807 subjects (37%) with a recommended level of fitness, 375 (17%) with minimally acceptable levels, and 992 (46%) with unacceptable levels (1). Compared with the most fit (Table 7.2, deck B), the relative risk of all-cause mortality was 1.6 (95% CI = 0.6-4.2) for subjects with minimally acceptable fitness levels and 2.7 (95% CI = 1.4-5.5) for those with unacceptable levels. Findings by fitness levels were similar for cardiovascular disease mortality but unrelated to risks of death from cancer of all sites.

Physical Activity and Mortality

Table 7.3 shows rates and relative risks of death, 1977-1985, among 11,864 Harvard alumni by patterns of physical activity assessed in 1977. These men had self-reported the absence of physician-diagnosed CHD on each of two mail questionnaires returned either in 1962 or 1966 and in 1977. Findings agree closely with earlier results among 16,936 alumni (including some of the same men) assessed in 1962 or 1966 and followed for all-cause mortality through 1978 (18,19). The impact of new, popular interest in physical activity and fitness appears evident among the alumni whose habitual participation in exercise such as walking and sportsplaying, as measured by prevalence or percentage of man-years, had increased appreciably by 1977 although 11 to 15 years had elapsed.

The most notable growth, 41% + 38% = 79% of man-years, was in moderate sportsplay defined as

Table 7.2 Studies of Physical Fitness and Longevity

A. Rates and relative risks of death[a] among Cooper Clinic men (10,244 middle-aged) and women (3,120 middle-aged) in an 8+ year follow-up, by gradients of physical fitness (4).

	Men			Women		
Quintiles of fitness by maximal treadmill test	Number deaths	Death per 10,000 man-years	Relative risk of death[b]	Number deaths	Death per 10,000 woman-years	Relative risk of death[b]
1 (low)	75	64.0	1.00	18	39.5	1.00
2	40	25.5	0.40	11	20.5	0.52
3	47	27.1	0.42	6	12.2	0.31
4	43	21.7	0.34	4	6.5	0.15
5 (high)	35	18.6	0.29	4	8.5	0.22

[a]Age-adjusted; [b]p of trend <0.05.

B. Relative risks (RR) of death among a representative sample of middle-aged Canadians (2,174 persons)[a] in a 7-year follow-up, by physical fitness tests (1).

Fitness levels	Number survivors	Number deaths	Crude RR of death	Adjusted RR of death[b]	(95% CI)
Recommended level	789	12	1.0	1.0	—
Minimum acceptable	363	7	1.3	1.6	(0.6,4.2)
Unacceptable	797	36	3.0	2.7	(1.4,5.5)

[a]Subjects aged 30-64 yr free of emphysema, heart disease, stroke, and diabetes; [b]adjusted for age, sex, body mass index, and smoking status.

at least 4.5 METs intensity, whereas stair-climbing prevalence was unchanged. The new exercise trend was echoed in the physical activity index compiled as total kcal per week from walking, stair-climbing, and sportsplay. In the 1960s, 62% of the alumni (by man-years experience) had an index below 2,000 kcal per week and 38% at or above that breakpoint. Corresponding percentages in 1977 were 58% and 42%, and comparative prevalences for successive 500-kcal increments of index were skewed likewise toward higher levels, revealing a consistent trend throughout the range up to 3,500 kcal per week.

There were 1,413 deaths during follow-up through 1977, and 730 more by 1985. Respective percentages of cause-specific deaths during the two follow-up intervals were: cardiovascular disease, 45% and 39%; cancer, 32% and 36%; other natural causes, 13% and 15%; and trauma, 10% and 10%.

Ages at entry ranged from 35-74 years in the first study and 45-84 years in the second. Because the entire study population had become older, higher death rates per 10,000 man-years would be expected in the second study than in the first; and they were. However, the increases were markedly greater among the less active men than among the more active, especially in relation to gradients of walking, physical activity index, and frequency and intensity of sportsplay. As stated earlier, Morris et al. noted similar patterns of mortality and survival among aging British civil servants classified by exercise status. Previous findings on CHD had shown that the vigorous Britons were less likely to develop CHD; their first attacks tended to be less severe, and to occur later in life; and they were more apt to survive than counterpart nonvigorous men. Vigorous job assignments conferred similar benefits on middle-aged San Francisco longshoremen and on London transit workers relative to sudden death (14,15,16).

Between 1962 and 1985 the large study population of Harvard alumni had ample time to be winnowed by deaths of many of its high-risk individuals, while survivors were proving their own hardiness and healthful habits. Table 7.3 appears to show just such an imbalance in death rates associated with levels of physical activity. Elements of sedentariness in terms of insufficient weekly physical activity were assessed as walking less than 5 km, stair-climbing fewer than 20 floors, and not engaging in any moderate sportsplay of at least 4.5 METs intensity. As will be seen, these findings may be translated into hypotheses and conclusions as to avoidance or postponement of morbidity, avoidance of premature death, preservation of desirable quality of life, and extension of longevity to an optimal healthy life span.

Table 7.4 shows the relative influence of selected types of physical activity on all-cause mortality among alumni during the 9-year follow-up period (1977-1985). It lists the age-adjusted death rates and relative risks of death associated with arbitrarily chosen levels and combinations of three types of physical activity assessed per week: walking 5+ km, stair-climbing 20+ floors, and actively playing sports requiring 4.5+ METs intensity.

Among men who did not engage in all three activities (4% of the man-years), there were 135.2 deaths per 10,000 man-years. When this rate was used as a standard for comparison, relative risks less than 1.00 were observed in the presence of any activity or combination of activities and were 0.63 for any single activity, 0.46 for any two, and 0.41 for all three.

In the 9-year follow-up interval, moderately vigorous sportsplay was the most influential in leading to decreased mortality, followed closely by walking and stair-climbing which were about equal in their strength of association with risk of death. Although intensity and persistence were neither measured nor considered in this analysis, moderate sportsplay certainly was more vigorous and sustained than were walking and climbing by these alumni.

Table 7.5 lists the prevalences of patterns of sedentary living as percentages of man-years of observation, the relative risks of death associated with the presence versus the absence of the adverse influences, and the population-attributable risks as estimated percentage reductions in death rates if the adverse influences had been shifted to favorable status. These relative risks and attributable risk estimates are derived from a multivariate analysis and proportional hazards models using Poisson regression methods. They contrast the effects of presence and absence of each of the four adverse patterns of

Table 7.3 Rates and Relative Risks of Death[a] Among Harvard Alumni, 1977-1985, by Patterns of Physical Activity

Physical activity (weekly)		Man-years (%)		Number deaths	Deaths per 10,000 man-years		Relative risk of death		p of trend
Walking (km)	<5	26		228	86.2		1.00		
	5-14	42		275	67.4		0.78		<0.001
	15+	32		194	57.7		0.67		
Stair-climbing (floors)	<20	37		341	80.0		1.00		
	20-54	48		293	62.9		0.79		0.001
	55+	15		80	59.6		0.75		
All sportsplay	None	12		156	88.9		1.00		
	Light only[b]	10		152	97.4		1.10		<0.001
	Light and moderate	36		208	59.7		0.67		
	Moderate only[c]	42		178	56.4		0.63		
Moderate sportsplay (h)	<1	30		308	92.9		1.00		
	1-2	41		126	58.2		0.63		<0.001
	3+	29		64	43.6		0.47		
Index (kcal)[d]	<500	12		197	110.3		1.00		
	500-999	18	58	135	69.1	78.9	0.63	1.00	
	1,000-1,499	15		111	68.9		0.62		
	1,500-1,999	13		73	61.4		0.56		<0.001
	2,000-2,499	10		51	52.4		0.48		
	2,500-2,999	8	42	44	64.6	55.4	0.59	0.70	
	3,000-3,499	6		36	74.7		0.68		
	3,500+	18		82	48.1		0.44		

[a]Age-adjusted; [b]<4.5 METs intensity; [c]4.5+ METs intensity; [d]sum of walking, stair-climbing, and all sportsplay.

Table 7.4 Rates and Relative Risks of Death[a] Among Harvard Alumni, 1977-1985, by Specific Combinations of Active Living

Walking ≥5 km/wk	Stair-climbing ≥20 floors/wk	Moderate sportsplay	Man-years (%)	Number deaths	Deaths per 10,000 man-years		Relative risk of death	
–	–	–	4	81	135.2		1.00	
–	–	+	8	53	69.2		0.51	
–	+	–	3	40	101.9	84.9[b]	0.75	0.63[b]
+	–	–	6	85	90.7		0.67	
–	+	+	11	54	62.5		0.46	
+	–	+	19	109	58.2	62.0[c]	0.43	0.46[c]
+	+	–	9	89	67.1		0.50	
+	+	+	40	178	55.1		0.41	

[a]Age-adjusted; [b]any one +; [c]any two +.

Table 7.5 Relative and Attributable Risks of Death[a] Among Harvard Alumni, 1977-1985, by Patterns of Sedentary Living

Sedentary living (weekly)	Man-years (%)	Relative risk of death	Individual attributable risk (%)	Population attributable risk (%)	p value
Walking <5 km	26	1.27 (1.08-1.50)	21.3	7.1 (1.9-12.0)	0.004
Stair-climbing <20 floors	37	1.22 (1.04-1.42)	17.7	8.5 (1.5-15.0)	0.013
No moderate sportsplay[b]	22	1.50 (1.27-1.77)	33.4	14.6 (8.3-20.4)	<0.001
Physical activity index <2,000 kcal[c]	58	1.40 (1.19-1.66)	28.8	20.4 (10.6-29.1)	0.001

[a]Adjusted for differences in age, other components of physical activity, cigarette smoking, hypertension, overweight-for-height, and parental mortality before age 65; [b]4.5+ METs intensity. 95% confidence intervals in parentheses; [c]in walking, stair-climbing, and sportsplay.

sedentary living—low levels of walking and stair-climbing, lack of moderate sportsplaying, and leisure-time physical activity totaling less than 2,000 kcal per week.

Each risk estimate is adjusted for difference in age, other components of physical activity, cigarette smoking, hypertension, overweight-for-height, and parental mortality before age 65. Over the 9-year follow-up period, alumni walking less than 5 km per week, or climbing fewer than 20 floors per week (about 400 steps), were respectively at 27% or 22% higher risk of death than men who walked or climbed further weekly. Men who did not play moderately vigorous sports were at 50% higher risk than men who did. The men with index below 2,000 kcal per week were at 40% higher risk of death than men physically more active. Thus, paucity of walking and stair-climbing and absence of recreational activities that require 4.5+ METs intensity of effort made independent contributions to higher risk of premature mortality.

As seen in the population-attributable risk estimates in the table, if weekly all 11,864 alumni had walked at least 5 km, or climbed 20+ floors, or played moderately intense games or sports, death rates accordingly might have been 7%, 8%, or 15% lower than were actually observed. In terms of physical activity index, the risk of death might have been reduced by 20% if every man had expended 2,000 or more kcal per week in walking, stair-climbing and recreational activities; and 146 of the 730 deaths during the 9-year follow-up might have been delayed.

Changes in Physical Activity and Mortality

Age-adjusted rates and relative risks of all-cause mortality are presented in Table 7.6 by continuities and changes in patterns of physical activity of the 11,864 alumni as determined from their questionnaires of 1962 or 1966 and again in 1977. These men had completed both a first and second questionnaire and were free of self-reported, physician-diagnosed CHD on both occasions. Moderate sportsplay and physical activity index are tabulated as being at favorable levels associated with reduced risk of death during the follow-up through 1985. Data are adjusted for differences in characteristics as in Table 7.5. Physical activity options (sportsplay and index) are categorized by four combinations of earlier and later participation status listed in order of presumed increasing benefit defined as lowered risk of death: (1) high-risk status unchanged, (2) low-risk status changed to high risk, (3) high risk changed to low, and (4) low-risk status continued.

As Table 7.6 shows, the findings for moderate sportsplay resemble those of the activity index pattern even though one is defined by metabolic equivalents (4.5+ METs) and the other in kilocalories per week. This might be expected because the index includes all sportsplay in hours per week equated to kcal. The few men who dropped moderate sportsplay (3% of man-years) were at 23% increased risk (not significant) over men who never had reported such recreation. When men with diagnosed cancer were excluded from the starting population, the added risk from discontinuing moderately intense activities was only 12%. These alumni had aged 11 to 15 years since answering the first questionnaire and were indeed in late middle age (58.2 ± 9.1 years). Yet remarkably, 38% of the man-years represented men who had taken up moderate sportsplay and 41% those who had continued it, so that three fourths of the group were alumni who participated in leisure-time activities of at least 4.5 METs intensity.

By index, 42% of the man-years represented alumni who had never reported enough activity to reach 2,000 or more kcal per week. Another 16% of man-years was contributed by men who by 1977 had dropped below the 2,000 kcal index level and showed a slightly higher (not significant) death rate during the follow-up through 1985 than men persistently sedentary. In contrast, men (prevalence 19% of man-years) who increased their index to favorable levels achieved a relative risk of 0.74, as low as the 0.79 ratio of their classmates who had been active at 2,000 or more kcal per week all along.

Figure 7.1 presents an age-specific analysis of the age-adjusted findings noted in Table 7.6. Although differences within the age classes are not significant, perhaps because of small numbers, the overall trends are of interest. Moderate sportsplay is again seen to be somewhat more influential than physical activity index, especially

Table 7.6 Rates and Relative Risks of Death[a] Among Harvard Alumni, 1977-1985, by Continuities and Changes in Patterns of Physical Activity Between 1962 or 1966 and 1977

Physical activity pattern	Status in 1962 or 1966	Status in 1977	Man-years (%)	Number deaths	Deaths per 10,000 man-years	Relative risk of death	*p* value
Moderate	No	No	18	234	84.1	1.00	—
sportsplaying	Yes	No	3	45	103.1	1.23 (0.88-1.63)	0.666
(4.5+ METs	No	Yes	38	184	59.6	0.71 (0.57-0.86)	0.007
intensity)	Yes	Yes	41	170	58.4	0.69 (0.58-0.90)	<0.001
Physical activity	No	No	42	346	72.9	1.00	—
index 2,000+ kcal/wk	Yes	No	16	147	87.6	1.20 (0.90-1.56)	0.077
(in walking, stair-	No	Yes	19	87	54.3	0.74 (0.58-0.95)	0.011
climbing, and	Yes	Yes	23	118	57.2	0.79 (0.63-0.98)	0.023
sportsplaying)							

[a]Adjusted for differences in age, other components of physical activity, cigarette smoking, hypertension, overweight-for-height, and parental mortality before age 65.

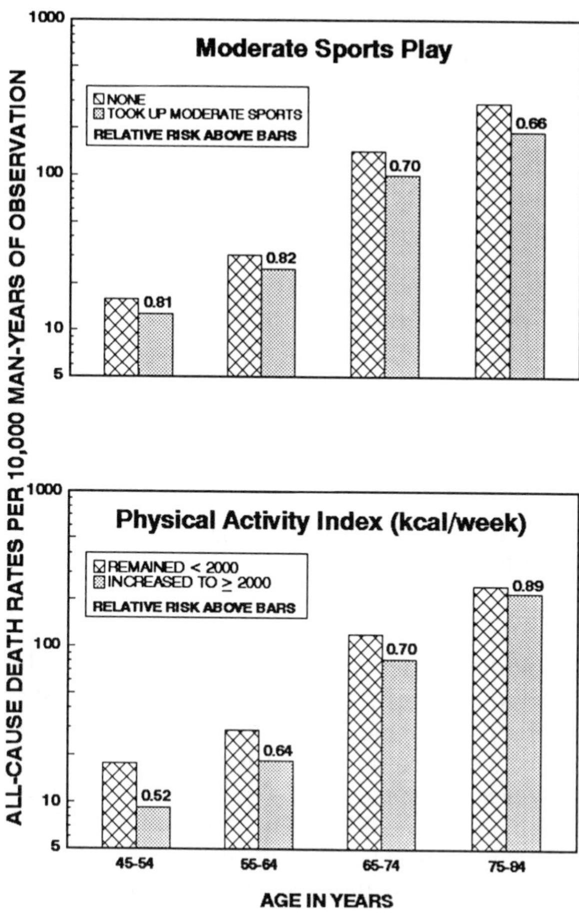

Figure 7.1. Age-specific rates and relative risks of death among Harvard alumni, 1977-1985, by continuities and changes in patterns of physical activity between 1962 or 1966 and 1977. These men had reported themselves free of physician-diagnosed coronary heart disease in 1977.

in the old-age bracket (75-84 years), though slightly less important in the lower age groups (45-64 years). This may imply that moderate sportsplay demanding at least 4.5 METs intensity tends to preserve fitness elements such as strength, endurance, and flexibility that otherwise would diminish with advancing age. The younger men have not had time to lose the important levels of physiological fitness that the older men must exert themselves to maintain. The fading advantage of mere physical activity index level in the upper age group, whose stair-climbing and walking may well have slowed down, appears to support this view. These observations also echo previous studies of these alumni, which showed that only continuing or current physical activity, not energy output earlier in life, protected middle-aged and elderly men against onset of morbidity and premature death (21,22).

Physical Activity and Longevity

If physical activity postpones death, one result should be increased longevity. Table 7.7 gives esti mated added years of life associated with maintaining or adopting adequate physical activity in terms of index of at least 2,000 kcal per week or moderate sportsplay demanding at least 4.5 METs intensity, versus life expectancy with less energy output. These estimates were derived from modified life-table analyses using the observed alumni mortality experience (1977-1985). Extrapolations to a younger age group (35-44 years) are included. The age-specific benefits decrease with advancing age, because the older men are nearer the natural life-span limit and have already passed through longevity brackets yet to be reached by the younger men. In each age group and overall, the time gained by moderate sportsplay is one fourth to one third more than that by physical activity index of at least 2,000 kcal per week, which might be anticipated from the death rate analyses described earlier.

Satisfaction with Living

Length of life or added longevity has meaning not only in calendar years or months but also in the quality of the life preserved or extended. Quality of life may be defined and assessed in various ways related to fitness, fulfillment, and satisfaction. Besides socioeconomic and health considerations, there are invaluable cultural and philosophical or spiritual aspects. Current reports reveal that much further study on the subject is needed (6,10,28). Results from questionnaire items designed to assess quality of life among the Harvard alumni are given in Table 7.8 contrasting active and sedentary groups adjusted for age and other lifestyle elements known to influence health, by percentages of those holding specified views on health and their prevalences of HMAD.

Predictably, active men were more likely to feel in control of their own well-being and efforts to achieve satisfactory health, and had lower prevalences of cardiovascular disease and non-insulin-dependent diabetes mellitus. A number of the differences were statistically significant, but none biologically spectacular. Perhaps the table reflects more clearly that the Harvard alumni were an elite, educated, accomplished, and affluent study population whose quality of life provided manifold opportunities for self-fulfillment and satisfaction plus optimum environmental security and personal

Table 7.7 Added Years of Life[a] to Age 85 from Continuities and Changes[b] in Patterns of Physical Activity as Estimated from the Mortality Experience of Harvard Alumni, 1977-1985

Age in 1977	Moderate sportsplay[c] vs. none	Physical activity[d] 2,000+ kcal/wk vs. less	Took up moderate sportsplay[c] vs. none	Physical activity[d] increased to 2,000+ from <2,000 vs. <2,000
[35-44][e]	[1.30]	[1.02]	[1.37]	[0.95]
45-54	1.25 (0.72-1.79)	0.99 (0.53-1.45)	1.31 (0.67-1.96)	0.91 (0.28-1.54)
55-64	1.07 (0.62-1.52)	0.85 (0.46-1.25)	1.13 (0.58-1.67)	0.79 (0.24-1.34)
65-74	0.73 (0.42-1.03)	0.58 (0.31-0.84)	0.74 (0.38-1.09)	0.52 (0.16-0.88)
75-84	0.28 (0.16-0.39)	0.21 (0.11-0.31)	0.26 (0.14-0.40)	0.20 (0.06-0.33)
45-84	1.06 (0.61-1.51)	0.84 (0.45-1.23)	1.08 (0.55-1.61)	0.77 (0.24-1.30)

[a]Adjusted for differences in age, other components of physical activity, cigarette smoking, hypertension, overweight-for-height, and parental mortality before age 65; [b]between 1962 or 1966 and 1977; [c]4.5+ METs intensity; [d]in walking, stair-climbing, and sportsplaying; [e]numbers in brackets are extrapolations.

health care. Regardless of importance, physical activity for fitness constituted only one sector of their outlook on life and would have to compete with all their other interests. Some of the latter might have almost as much or more influence on their levels of satisfaction, survival, and longevity.

Discussion

Evidence accumulates that risks of premature death as compared with its reciprocal, increased longevity, are related to physical activity expressed by participation or nonparticipation in moderately vigorous sportsplay and by high or low levels of weekly energy expenditure. Moreover, the findings among Harvard alumni from 1977 through 1985 corroborate closely the results obtained from similar investigations in this population between 1962 or 1966 and 1978 (18,19,21,22).

Patterns and trends of data in the present study appear to support further consideration of relations of physical activity, physiological fitness, and survival or longevity. As the population of alumni aged, death rates among the less active (and presumably less fit) were consistently greater than among the more active (and more fit) men of the same ages. As time passed, the original high-risk group tended to diminish or almost disappear by such attrition, while the original low-risk group was aging and probably tended to become less active and less fit. Therefore, in the latest decade of survival the physical activity and physiological fitness differences between the surviving risk groups have diminished while their death rates converged, especially in relation to physical activity index in kcal per week. It is likely also that the survivors of the original low-risk group may have been somewhat more active and fit than their classmates who died sooner. Even in the latest decade, however, the apparent saving influence of moderate sportsplay is still evident from the group differences in death rates and survival.

All of these patterns strongly support the hypothesis that adequately vigorous and continuing physical activity is conducive to maximal good health and longevity. Only further follow-up for at least another decade with questionnaires on lifestyles, quality of life, and health status might reveal how long the influences of physical activity on physiological fitness may continue to be important within the normal life span.

These observations are mindful of earlier findings (18,21,22) that former varsity athletes who dropped sportsplaying from their usual routines had higher death rates thereafter than college teammates who continued energetic exercise, and perhaps, higher death rates than classmates who have never engaged in organized sport effort. More importantly, the larger group of men who had avoided athletics in college but subsequently adopted a more active lifestyle experienced as low a death rate as alumni who had been physically active all along. The consistency of these associations of increased activity patterns with lower mortality rates—derived from thousands of man-years of alumni experience—is testimony to the importance of adopting an adequate exercise program. Similar observations among British civil servants extend and amplify this belief (12).

Individual attributable risk estimates of the projected benefits of favorable changes in physical activity (Table 7.5) had been computed from death

Table 7.8 Prevalences (Percentages) of Views on Health[a] and of Cardiovascular-Metabolic Disease[b] Among Harvard Alumni, 1988, by Patterns of Physical Activity

Item	Moderate sportsplay[c]			Physical activity 2,000+ kcal/wk[d]			Adopted moderate sportsplay[c]			Increased physical activity to 2,000+ kcal/wk from <2,000[d]		
	+	−	*p*	+	−	*p*	+	−	*p*	+	−	*p*
Attitudes and beliefs (frequency, %)												
I take adequate exercise for health.	52	42	<0.001	59	42	<0.001	45	38	<0.001	55	39	<0.001
One can adjust one's life-style for health.	73	60	<0.001	74	68	<0.001	70	58	<0.001	72	67	<0.001
I feel younger than my years.	86	80	<0.001	87	82	0.001	83	80	0.009	86	82	0.002
I feel fine and enjoy life.	94	91	0.002	94	92	0.019	92	91	0.131	92	92	0.670
I could do more for my health.	55	61	<0.001	52	60	<0.001	59	61	0.232	55	61	<0.001
Regular energetic exercise is important for health.	37	19	<0.001	41	27	<0.001	29	19	<0.001	36	25	<0.001
Cardiovascular disease or non-insulin-dependent diabetes mellitus (prevalence, %)	12	16	<0.001	12	14	0.024	14	17	0.074	12	15	0.025

[a]Age-adjusted; [b]adjusted for differences in age, cigarette smoking, hypertension, and overweight-for-height; [c]4.5+ METs intensity; [d]in walking, stair-climbing, and sportsplaying.

rates for the period 1977-1985. When real survival data were studied for alumni who actually had changed their exercise habits favorably between the 1960s and 1970s (Table 7.6), the percentages as benefits for each estimate were close: taking up moderate sportsplay, 33% estimated and 29% observed; avoiding sedentariness, 29% estimated and 26% observed. Thus, we may conclude that the adoption of an active lifestyle may reduce the risk of premature death and apparently (Table 7.8) enhance quality of life, or at least satisfaction with life, insofar as that can be measured.

Future Research

Many of the principal questions concerning influence of exercise on longevity remain unanswered, and the direction of future work might appropriately address some of the following: What kinds, how much, how intense, and for whom should physical activity be prescribed for optimal health (physical, psychological, social, cultural, and spiritual well-being)? What effects result from what kinds of *change* in physical activity patterns, and at what specific ages? How much physical activity (short-term and long-term) is needed to induce physiological fitness (a functional integration of all body systems), the zest for living, a reduced risk of HMAD, and an optimal longevity? What are the mechanisms by which physical activity may induce lower risk of HMAD and extend high quality living? What is the role of physical activity in the prevention or delay of recurrent or extended disease (secondary prevention)? How are physical activity, physiological fitness, dietary habits, other ways of living, environmental circumstances, and inherited tendencies (both lifestyles and diseases) *interactive* and *integrated* in man's search for his optimal health? No doubt answers to these questions will lead to another platform from which we may perceive a further range of new questions yet to be asked and answered.

Acknowledgments

This work was supported by U.S. Public Health Service research grants HL 34174 from the National

Heart, Lung and Blood Institute and CA 44854 from the National Cancer Institute. This is report No. L in a series on chronic disease in former college students.

References

1. Arraiz, G.A.; Wigle, D.T.; Mao, Y. Risk assessment of physical activity and physical fitness in the Canada health survey mortality follow-up study. J. Clin. Epidemiol. 45:419-428; 1992.
2. Astrand, P.-O.; Rodahl, K. Textbook of work physiology. 3rd ed. New York: McGraw-Hill; 1986.
3. Berlin, J.A.; Colditz, G.A. A meta-analysis of physical activity in the prevention of coronary heart disease. Am. J. Epidemiol. 132:612-628; 1990.
4. Blair, S.N.; Kohl, H.W., III; Paffenbarger, R.S., Jr.; Clark, D.G.; Cooper, K.H.; Gibbons, L.W. Physical fitness and all-cause mortality: A prospective study of healthy men and women. JAMA. 262:2395-2401; 1989.
5. Bouchard, C.; Shephard, R.J.; Stephens, T.; Sutton, J.R.; McPherson, B.D., editors. Exercise, fitness, and health. Champaign, IL: Human Kinetics; 1990.
6. Bunker, J.B.; Gomby, P.S.; Kehrer, B.H. Pathways to health: The role of social factors. Menlo Park, CA: Henry J. Kaiser Foundation; 1989.
7. Driver, B.L.; Brown, P.J.; Peterson, G.L., editors. Benefits of leisure. State College, PA: Venture Publishing, Inc.; 1990.
8. Kaplan, G.A.; Seeman, T.E.; Cohen, R.D.; Knudsen, L.P.; Guralnik, J. Mortality among the elderly in the Alameda County study: Behavioral and demographic risk factors. Am. J. Public Health. 77:307-312; 1987.
9. Kendrick, J.S.; Williamson, D.F.; Caspersen, C.J. Letter to the editor. Re: "A meta-analysis of physical activity in the prevention of coronary heart disease." Am. J. Epidemiol. 134:232-234; 1991.
10. King, A.C. Mini-series: Exercise and aging. Ann. Behav. Med. 13:87-90; 1991.
11. Linsted, K.D.; Tonstad, S.; Kuzma, J.W. Self-report of physical activity and patterns of mortality in Seventh-Day Adventist men. J. Clin. Epidemiol. 44:355-364; 1991.
12. Morris, J.N.; Clayton, D.G.; Everitt, M.G.; Semmence, A.M.; Burgess, E.H. Exercise in leisure-time, coronary attack and death rates. Br. Heart J. 63:325-334; 1990.
13. Morris, J.N.; Everitt, M.G.; Pollard, R.; Chave, S.P.W.; Semmence, A.M. Vigorous exercise in leisure-time: Protection against coronary heart disease. Lancet. 2:1207-1210; 1980.
14. Morris, J.N.; Heady, J.A.; Raffle, P.A.B.; Roberts, C.G.; Parks, J.W. Coronary heart disease and physical activity of work. Lancet. 2:1053-1057, 1111-1120; 1953.
15. Morris, J.N.; Kagan, A.; Pattison, D.C.; Gardner, M.; Raffle, P.A.B. Incidence and prediction of ischaemic heart disease in London busmen. Lancet. 2:552-559; 1966.
16. Paffenbarger, R.S., Jr.; Hale, W.E. Work activity and coronary heart mortality. N. Engl. J. Med. 292:545-550; 1975.
17. Paffenbarger, R.S., Jr.; Hyde, R.T.; Wing, A.L. Chronic disease in former college students: XXXVI. Physical activity and physical fitness as determinants of health and longevity. In: Bouchard, C.; Shephard, R.J.; Stephens, T.; Sutton, J.R.; McPherson, B.D., eds. Exercise, fitness, and health. Champaign, IL: Human Kinetics; 1990:33-48.
18. Paffenbarger, R.S., Jr.; Hyde, R.T.; Hsieh, C.; Wing, A.L. Chronic disease in former college students: XXX. Physical activity, all-cause mortality, and longevity of college alumni. N. Engl. J. Med. 314:605-613; 1986.
19. Paffenbarger, R.S., Jr.; Hyde, R.T.; Wing, A.L.; Hsieh, C.-c. Physical activity and longevity of college alumni. (Correspondence in reply to four letters.) N. Engl. J. Med. 315:399-401; 1986.
20. Paffenbarger, R.S., Jr.; Hyde, R.T.; Wing, A.L.; Lee, I.-M.; Jung, D.L.; Kampert, J.B. Chronic disease in former college students: XXXVII. The association of changes in physical-activity level and other lifestyle characteristics with mortality among men. N. Engl. J. Med. 328:538-545, 1993.
21. Paffenbarger, R.S., Jr.; Hyde, R.T.; Wing, A.L.; Steinmetz, C.H. Chronic disease in former college students: XXV. A natural history of athleticism and cardiovascular health. JAMA. 252:491-495; 1984.
22. Paffenbarger, R.S., Jr.; Wing, A.L.; Hyde, R.T. Chronic disease in former college students: XVI. Physical activity as an index of heart attack risk in college alumni. Am. J. Epidemiol. 108:161-175; 1978.
23. Powell, K.E.; Thompson, P.D.; Caspersen, C.J.; Kendrick, J.S. Physical activity and the incidence of coronary heart disease. Ann. Rev. Public Health. 8:253-287; 1987.
24. Russell, L.B. Is prevention better than cure? Washington, DC: Brookings Institute; 1986.
25. Shaper, A.G.; Wannamethee, G. Physical activity and ishaemic heart disease in middle-aged British men. Br. Heart J. 66:384-394; 1991.

26. Shephard, R.J. Costs and benefits of an exercising versus a nonexercising society. In: Bouchard, C.; Shephard, R.J.; Stephens, T.; Sutton, J.R.; McPherson, B.D., eds. Exercise, fitness, and health. Champaign, IL: Human Kinetics; 1990:49-60.
27. Slattery, M.L.; Jacobs, D.R., Jr.; Nichaman, M.Z. Leisure time physical activity and coronaryheart disease death: The U.S. railroad study. Circulation. 79:304-311; 1989.
28. Stewart, A.L.; King, A.C. Evaluating the efficacy of physical activity for influencing quality-of-life outcomes in older adults. Ann. Behav. Med. 13:108-116; 1991.
29. Wannamethee, G.; Shaper, A.G. Physical activity and stroke in British middle aged men. Br. Med. J. 304:597-601; 1992.

Chapter 8

Costs and Benefits of an Active Versus an Inactive Society

Robert L. Kaman
Robert W. Patton

Recently, the relationship between physical activity and health has been examined in the context of health care economics. Most observers agree that physical activity has a positive impact on the health of an individual (8). In fact, even light or moderate activity has been shown to contribute to significant health improvements (6). Simply stated, there appears to be a causal relationship between physical activity and improved health. By extension, if exercise does indeed improve the health of the individual, is the true cost of achieving that improvement in health offset by a reduction in the utilization of health care services? Is there a causal relationship between exercise and the reduction of health care utilization?

Because an increasing share of individual health care costs and the costs to society in general are borne by company-funded employee insurance programs, recent studies have focused on the individual as a member of a work site employee group. Work site fitness programs can be traced back to the early part of this century (12,16) and have evolved from simple gymnasiums in company basements to multimillion-dollar fitness centers and comprehensive health promotion programs addressing mental, spiritual, and emotional, as well as physical aspects of health. Studies have been initiated to determine if the cost of implementing such programs is offset by the benefit of reduced health care spending (11,14,18,23,25,27, 39,41,43,47,49,50,63).

In addition to a reduction in health care costs, researchers have expanded their analyses of program outcomes to determine whether the exercising (and thus healthier) employee is more productive, is absent less, is injured less often, leaves the company less frequently, and has a higher morale than the nonexercising, less healthy worker. Indeed, such conclusions have been drawn by several investigators. The strength of the correlations between exercise and program outcomes are generally statistically significant, but are at relatively low predictive levels, leaving the decision makers with a good deal of uncertainty regarding the determination of the cost–benefit of employee fitness programs (31,58).

Methodological Considerations in Applying a Cost–Benefit Analysis to Work Site Health Promotion Programs

Unlike the biological studies of the effects of enhanced physical activity, cost–benefit questions are best studied in the context of a quasi-experimental investigation. Within the quasi-experimental framework, a chain of logic is used to determine whether a specific program is related to a specific health outcome (38). The first question to ask when a difference between groups is observed is whether or not that difference is statistically significant. If a difference exists, the second question to ask is whether or not the affected subgroup has any characteristics other than exposure to the program studied that might influence this difference.

Even if a statistically significant difference has been measured between two groups, that difference may be the result of artifactual or indirect associations, rather than the result of the experimental treatment. Because of the inability to control treatments, most health promotion research findings have uncertain causality. A true test of the likelihood of a causal relationship between health promotion programs and some health outcomes include the following widely used criteria: (a) strength of the association, (b) dose–response relationship, (c) consistency of the association, (d) temporally correct association, (e) specificity of the association, and (f) coherence with existing information (outcome plausibility) (38).

Perhaps the single greatest barrier to effective program evaluation is that the researcher does not have access to all the necessary data. Issues of confidentiality or a lack of systematic data retrieval have prevented investigators from securing health care cost utilization and absentee records from personnel files. For example, health care utilization records for the employees of the federal government are not maintained by the work site personnel offices, but rather, can only be secured from the individual insurance carriers. To compound this particular problem, due to the particular nature of record keeping by the Health Maintenance Organizations (HMOs), utilization records of their clients simply are not released. Because HMOs typically serve 40 to 50% of a work force, this becomes a significant problem.

In an analysis of the economic implications of work site health promotion programs, Warner et al. (60) attempted to subject literature reports to a systematic analysis of outcomes. In fact, due to the lack of methodological rigor found throughout the 400 articles chosen for analysis, the authors ultimately relied on subjective judgments for their conclusions. Twenty-eight of the articles reviewed focused on exercise. The authors acknowledged the positive relationship between exercising workers and improvements in physiologic functioning, including measures such as blood pressure, pulse rate, and maximum oxygen uptake. They could not, however, find sufficient research knowledge satisfying the criteria for causality as defined above to economically justify such work site programs. Specifically, flaws in the economic analyses themselves, nonstandardization of definitions, limited participation, and self-selection were listed as problems with the research outcomes claimed. Table 8.1 from Warner et al. (60) summarizes those findings.

Studies continued to be published making positive claims for work site health promotion programs. The limitations of analysis remain, but work site programs continue to be promoted as economic solutions to rising health care costs. Whether this is so remains an uncertainty. On the other hand, the impact of work site health promotion programs, their fitness components in particular, and the impact of non–work site exercise may be defined in noneconomic terms (59). Perhaps those outcomes are the real benefit to society. It is instructive to assess all of the outcomes of exercise programs as documented in the literature. Those outcomes may be classified as reductions in absenteeism, increases in productivity, improvements in morale, and decreases in health care costs. Recently, Opatz et al. (42) have reviewed these outcomes, and have developed a consensus view of these measures. Table 8.2 summarizes those views (42).

Claims for those outcomes should be viewed within the context of the criteria for causality as detailed previously. In addition, outcomes should be related to program costs. In general, the five elements of cost, as defined by Grana (22), should be compared to the benefits claimed. Table 8.3 lists those elements (22).

It is fair to say that just as outcomes are not rigorously analyzed, most of the program costs are not included in the assessments. Without consideration of all the costs and all the benefits associated with such programs, it will remain difficult to render a final, subjective judgment on the economic and the noneconomic outcome (benefit) of them on society (7,57).

Current Findings Concerning Work Site Health Promotion Programs

Risk Reduction and Health Care Costs

Substantial evidence suggests that exercise program components within work site health promotion programs lower participants' health risks and therefore lower related health care costs. Numerous studies have been conducted on the relationship of risk reduction and health care costs (17,20,36,37,40,49,62). Anderson and Jose, in describing the design features of their program evaluation at Control Data (1,29), readily admitted an inability to establish the necessary controls for determining cause and effect. Entry of individuals into the program was noncontrolled, and implementation sites were not randomly selected resulting in a quasi-experimental design. Limited attempts at experimental control included matching program sites and evaluating treatments through pre- and posttime series and multiple time series.

Several conclusions were drawn from the StayWell program in general and from exercise programs specifically (and other individual components) that support an association between reduced risk (e.g., due to exercise) and reduced health care utilization. It is interesting to note that for the youngest age group studied, costs increased with exercise, while for the other age groups, costs decreased with increasing exercise. In addition, the lowest costs were associated with moderate rather than high levels of exercise. Both these observations, made in male groups only, may be attributable to the effects of exercise-related injuries. When female groups were observed, lack of exercise was related to higher claim levels; however, age was not a factor due to gynecological and obstetric costs in younger women.

Table 8.1 Research-Based Knowledge of the Health and Economic Effects of Workplace Health Promotion Programs

HP program	Articles reviewed	Epidemiology: prevalence and health impact	Health effects of behavior change	Cost information (types, measurements)	Cost-benefit or cost-effectiveness
Hypertension	38	✣	✣	✝	✛
Employee assistance programs (EAP)	33	✝	⊗	✛	⊕
Individual smoking cessation	48	✣	✝	✛	✛
Workplace smoking restriction policies	6	✝	⊕	⊗	❍
Nutrition and weight control	48	✝	✛	⊕	⊕
Exercise	28	✛	✛	⊗	⊕
Stress	35	✛	⊗	⊕	❍
Motor vehicle safety belts	13	✣	✣	✝	⊕
Back injury prevention	26	✛	✛	✛	❍
Health risk appraisals (HRA)	14	N/A	⊗	✣	⊕

Note. From Warner et al. (60). Symbols used are as follows: ✣—well understood, solid research base; ✝—generally understood, some good research but limited; ✛—some good information but more suggestive than definitive, category implies either a very few good studies or substantial number of scientifically weak studies; ⊗—very little research; ⊕—almost no research base, one or two relevant items. ❍—no research base; N/A—not available.

Table 8.2 Strength of Relationships

Area studies	Potential economic impact of health promotion		Benefit range per employee
	Short-Term	Long-Term	
Absenteeism	Moderate-strong	Inconclusive	1–2 days fewer absences
Employee health behavior	Moderate	Inconclusive	Not quantified
Health care costs	Moderate	Inconclusive	$51–$61 in lower medical costs
Productivity	Moderate-strong	Inconclusive	4–25% increased productivity
Computer simulation*	Promising	Inconclusive	N/A

*As an evaluation method.
Note. Data from Opatz et al. (42).

Another important observation made by the StayWell study was that health care claims were reduced proportionally with a reduction in all unhealthy behaviors. When all program costs, inflation, and turnover factors were analyzed, positive returns were projected for males and females across all age groups based on program participation and attendant reduced health risks.

The StayWell experience, supported in general in all of the program reports, suggests that the standardized health risk appraisal questionnaire, used as a universally-implemented, self-reported instrument of risk analysis, helps to identify those at high risk for illness. These individuals are also the subset of employees who are high users of health care resources. Targeting these individuals specifically for appropriate health promotion programming may be one of the most promising strategies for reducing health care costs.

Table 8.3 Program Costs Versus Program Benefits

Item of cost	Item of benefit
1. Personnel: staff, salaries, benefits, and consultant's fees	1. Decrease in disability (salary costs) for payment made during days off the job (including company contribution to workman's compensation)
2. Supplies, communication, travel	2. Decreased employee turnover
3. Space and overhead	3. Decreased absenteeism
4. Equipment	4. Increased productivity
5. Employee participation (hours away from work)	5. Decreased health care expenditures

Note. Data from Grana (22).

Several investigators have studied the impact of participation in work site fitness programs on the reduction in health care costs. In addition to the StayWell program, health care cost reduction outcomes from employee fitness programs have been reported earlier by investigators describing programs at the Prudential Insurance Company (9), Kimberly Clark (4), Blue Cross/Blue Shield of Indiana (20,40), Johnson and Johnson (61), Canada Life Insurance Company (46), and Mesa Petroleum (19).

Recently other studies have appeared suggesting an inverse relationship between participation in work site health promotion and health care costs. The Steelcase Incorporated health promotion program, evaluated by Yen et al. (64), resulted in average annual medical costs for 18 health-related measures which were $67 to $778 higher for high-risk employees than for low-risk employees. Risk was determined by responses to a health risk appraisal questionnaire, and surprisingly, exercise activity was not significantly related to reduced health care costs. Analysis of the data suggests that this observation may be related to the relatively low proportion (14%) of the total health care cost that cardiovascular disease, selected by this particular appraisal, represents in this work force.

Although exercise activity did correlate well with reduced risk for cardiovascular disease, the costs associated with this category of illness represented too small a fraction of the total health care bill to impact that total. This observation has not been documented extensively in the literature; however, when the authors of this chapter reviewed similar health care cost data from their own institution, cardiovascular disease-related costs were similarly low (an average of 10.78% of total costs over a 4-year study period) in that work force (Table 8.4). If this observation proves to have significant generalizability to other American employee groups, then despite the demonstrated cost of heart disease to society in general, the work site exercise programs' focus on cardiovascular exercise may need to be reexamined.

In addition, age and gender have been reported to have a large impact on exercise-related risk reduction and changes in health care costs. When the Steelcase data were reevaluated (64), controlling for the age/sex effects on costs, the relationship between costs and risk categories became significant for exercise as well as for cholesterol, relative body weight, and health risk age.

Injury as an element of health care costs has been evaluated earlier by Tsai et al. (56). In an urban, white-collar work force, no significant differences were noted in incidence or cost of injuries among participants and nonparticipants of an employee fitness program. That is, exercise did not impose a higher rate of injury among participants, although low utilizers (less than 1 or 1 time per week) had a slightly higher rate of injury than did nonparticipants and high utilizers (greater than 3 times per week).

Recently, incidence and cost of injury was reported by Whitmer (61) who studied Birmingham, Alabama's employee fitness program. The subgroup of fire fighters from within the entire city work force was evaluated. All fire fighters were given periodic performance tests and categorized as in excellent physical condition (16% of the total) or in very poor condition (8.3% of the total). During the 5-year term of the project, 14% of the excellent group experienced an injury, costing an average of $442 per injury. Sixty-eight percent of the very poor group had an injury with an average cost of $2,989. Apparently, being physically fit not only reduces work-related injuries in this work force, but when they do occur, they are less serious and much less expensive to treat. In addition, this study has reported no increase in employee health insurance costs during the past 5 years. Birmingham's average employee insurance cost has remained at $2,000 per year, while the average Alabama government employee health insurance cost has risen $1,000 during this same period.

The Birmingham program protocol included universal participation in an initial prescreening and Health Risk Analysis, and participants repeated these tests annually. Although not mandatory, this screen was made a *requirement* for enroll-

Table 8.4 Disease-Specific Health Care Costs

ICD-9 classification*	1988	1989	1990	1991	Avg.
Infectious disease	0.7**	0.4	0.4	0.4	0.48
Neoplasms (tumors)	5.8	6.4	5.5	4.3	5.50
Metabolic disease	1.5	1.2	2.3	1.9	1.73
Blood disorders	0.0	0.1	1.0	0.1	0.30
Nervous system disorders	1.8	3.8	4.2	4.4	3.55
Circulatory system	11.1	12.7	6.4	12.9	10.78
Respiratory system	8.1	4.4	3.4	3.6	4.90
Digestive system	12.6	13.5	9.1	7.8	10.75
Genitourinary system	8.9	10.5	9.5	9.8	9.68
Pregnancy & complications	1.0	2.4	3.4	10.4	4.30
Skin disorders	2.0	2.1	1.9	2.7	1.93
Musculoskeletal system	16.7	21.6	17.0	18.3	18.40
Congenital anomalies	1.0	0.4	2.3	0.3	1.00
Perinatal conditions	5.9	0.1	0.4	1.5	1.98
Ill defined conditions	6.6	6.5	7.7	4.7	6.38
Injury and poisonings	7.3	4.0	5.4	5.1	5.45
Miscellaneous	3.1	4.4	8.5	6.2	5.55
Total (dollars)	$475,796	$842,121	$886,737	$931,730	$784,096

*International Classification of Diseases—ninth edition.
**Percent of total yearly costs.

ment in the health insurance plan. Everyone participated in the screening. Fully 13% of all employees screened had heretofore undetected health problems that required medical attention.

Absenteeism

Shephard (46) reviewed 20 work site fitness programs and discovered that 14 of them reported an inverse relationship between exercise participation and absenteeism. While these studies consistently reported only one to two fewer absent days per year among participants, the collective economic impact of that reduction may become very significant in large work groups. In a recent 2-year study conducted at 41 intervention and 19 control sites within the DuPont Corporation, disability-related absenteeism was reduced an average of 0.4 days per employee per year for program participants compared to control group (nonparticipant) employees (5). Total savings reported amounted to over $3 million in 2 years.

Others have studied the relationship between measured fitness levels, rather than program participation, and absenteeism. Steinhardt et al. (52) reported significant inverse relationships between fitness and absenteeism among male, but not female, police officers in the Austin, TX, Police Department. For females, the relationship of absenteeism in the workplace to family issues (e.g., child care and pregnancy leave) obscured the fitness–absenteeism connection.

Tucker et al. (57) determined the extent to which measured cardiovascular fitness was associated with absenteeism due to illness in a large number of men and women (8,301) employed throughout the United States. Subjects in the poor fitness group had more than 2.5 times the rate of absenteeism compared to those in the excellent fitness category. The authors pointed out that if a causal relationship between cardiovascular fitness and absenteeism is assumed, employers could save substantial amounts of absenteeism costs by promoting fitness among employees. If the association is not causal, employers could still reduce absenteeism by simply recruiting physically fit employees. This observation agrees with the findings at the Tenneco Corporation reported earlier by Bernacki and Baun (2,3).

These authors observed that exercisers have fewer sick hours than nonexercisers, which was significant for females, but not males. In addition, females in both groups tended to have higher sickness-related absenteeism rates than males. Acknowledging that a high proportion of exercisers were active before the program was initiated, the authors agreed that the program appealed to a self-selected population of individuals whose high fitness levels correlated well with low absenteeism rates and high performance ratings. Thus, an argument in favor of an exercise facility at the workplace is that it will attract and retain individuals who are more likely to have low absenteeism rates and high levels of health and performance.

Finally, Jones et al. (28) compared absenteeism rates at different work sites with and without health promotion programs. Neither participation rates nor measured fitness levels were used in the analysis. Rather, employees at both control (no program) and experimental program sites who responded to health and lifestyle questionnaires at baseline and in the second year of the program were included. Although adjusted mean levels of absenteeism among wage earners in the program groups were found to decline over the study period and were significantly lower ($p<.01$) than the mean levels for nonprogram wage earners in the final year of the study, no differences were found for salaried personnel. In addition, the authors noted the great difficulty in securing reliable absenteeism data from employee records available. Interestingly, when the data was sorted to compare the effect of smoking on absenteeism within these groups, it seemed apparent that smokers had an average of 15 hr per year more sick leave than nonsmokers in both groups.

Despite the cumulative savings that may be realized in a large work force when absenteeism is reduced, the studies cited above as well as other program reports acknowledge low absenteeism rates even at work sites without health promotion intervention programs. Coupled with the difficulties of distinguishing sick leave days from personal leave, the relatively small margins for change, even in the best programs, suggest that absenteeism as a measure of the impact of work site health promotion programs may not be a reliable indicator.

Productivity

Some evidence exists that fitness related to participation in exercise programs has a positive impact on worker productivity (13,15,62). Measurement of productivity remains the confounding element of this issue. Only in very few cases may an objective measure of productivity be obtained, and a correlation between fitness and such a measure has not appeared in the literature. Rather, subjective measures of productivity have been used (3,44). The most common productivity ratings have been subjective supervisor evaluations and self-reported evaluations of attitudes and job-satisfaction (45). In some cases, productivity has been related simply to absenteeism: the fewer days absent, the higher the productivity outcome.

In an early study, Bernacki and Baun (3) noted the relationship between exercise adherence rates and subjective supervisor-conducted job performance ratings among 3,231 white-collar employees. They noted that a positive association did indeed exist between above-average job performance and exercise adherence, and that a negative association existed between poor job performance and exercise adherence. In all cases, no differences in performance were noted when prior performance was compared with current performance. The authors again concluded that although there appeared to be a positive relationship between exercise adherence in a corporate fitness program and above-average job performance, causality was not demonstrated.

In an interesting approach to this issue, Rudman (45) studied the impact of an on-site health and fitness center on worker productivity by assessing worker satisfaction as expressed in response to inquiries on a questionnaire. Job productivity was conceptualized in terms of: (a) job and company satisfaction and the carryover of job tasks outside the workplace, (b) perceived control over work conditions, and (c) beliefs about the effects of exercise on the completion of work tasks.

Results from the study seemed to suggest that implementation of an on-site health and fitness center had a positive effect on workers' attitudes extending beyond actual involvement in the center's programs. Although no direct measure of worker productivity was obtained, the indirect measures used in this study (e.g., job satisfaction, company loyalty, etc.) may be used to infer productivity outcomes. The assumption is that those who are satisfied at work are more likely to remain at the same company, care more about the quality of their work, and improve the work environment for others, and hence become more productive.

Finally, Golaszewski et al. (21) have taken a novel approach in estimating gains in productivity among workers engaged in a fitness program at the work site. Citing literature reports (10,42) that listed a 4% increase in productivity as the lowest gain noted in such programs, these authors simply multiplied the average salary of participants by this figure to arrive at an estimated increase in productivity. This multiplier, which the authors claim to be a conservative figure, nevertheless became the greatest financial benefit over time from the program.

In the absence of standardized, objective measures of productivity, this outcome may remain one with many hopeful claims, but with little substantive data to support them. Certainly, causality has not been demonstrated between participation in fitness programs and improved productivity. Nevertheless, there continues to be a thread of continuity between improved fitness and desirable work behaviors. Even if company support of fitness centers simply provides a convenient opportunity for already fit employees to exercise, such support may be justified as a strategy to recruit healthy and more productive individuals into the work force.

Turnover

A recurring theme encountered in the arguments by corporate managers who do not support employee fitness programs is that the ascribed benefit of improved health and fitness for a participant will not accrue to the providing company, but rather to some subsequent employer years hence. If the impact of increased physical activity is improved health and fitness for the individual, reduced health care costs and absenteeism may be measured on a long-term basis. The mobility of the American worker implies that he or she will remain at the current work site for only a limited time before moving on, taking his or her good health to the next employer (13,15,35,62). Despite the correlative notion that the original company has an equal chance of hiring similarly healthy employees from other companies, and the alternative argument that enhanced worker health may impose a greater burden on the pension system during an ensuing longer retirement, this issue has not been effectively examined.

In the single report published within the past 5 years (55) on the relationship of exercise adherence and turnover, there appeared to be a positive relationship between exercise and reduced job turnover among groups distinguished by gender and job classification. The strongest effect was seen among female clerical employees. Although no causality was demonstrated, the authors contend that the provision of an exercise program does play a role in retaining employees. Clearly, further studies on this issue seem in order.

Computer Simulation Analysis of Work Site Health Promotion Programs

Evaluation of work site health promotion programs continues to be hampered by "(1) the inability to employ true experimental designs and the resultant contamination of the subject selection/assignment procedure, (2) data availability constraints (and associated research design implications), (3) vulnerability to natural maturation processes, and (4) susceptibility to a Hawthorne Effect (51)." The Hawthorne Effect has been described as the improvement of the control population in the parameter measured in the absence of intervention. The incidental, heightened awareness by this group as a result of program publicity and baseline measurements has been suggested as a reason for this outcome (51). In addition, some companies have viewed completed program evaluation data as proprietary and have been unwilling to disclose evaluation results, while other programs have simply chosen to limit health promotion program funds to programming, assigning no resources to evaluation. Consequently, there remains a relatively small number of program evaluations in the literature.

In 1986 the President's Council on Physical Fitness and Sports estimated that of the 50,000 companies in the United States with 50 employees or more, 12,000 had some form of health promotion program (53). Of those, the Association for Fitness in Business estimated that 700 to 1,000 of these companies had facility-based programs. Of that group, only 10 such programs had published cost–benefit analyses by the end of 1988 (30). In a more recent review, Shephard constructed a similar table with additional cost–benefit analyses documented (48). Table 8.5, adapted from Kaman (30) and Shephard (48), summarizes those findings.

One strategy to overcome this problem is to develop valid computer simulation programs showing the costs, benefits, and effectiveness of work site health promotion programs. Basing projections on normative data (26,41) or on in-house data derived from sensitivity analyses, several studies have emerged as cost-effective models of evaluation. Terborg, in an unpublished but widely disseminated program report (54), utilized sensitivity analyses to project a positive annual benefit:cost ratio of \$1.24 to \$8.33 for participation in a work site fitness program. The analysis was strengthened by calculating actual program costs, participation rates, and actual reported data on health care utilization and sick leave. Productivity and turnover data were projected based on company data and on related assumptions of costs and benefit.

Murphy et al. (41) used normative data to project health care cost savings for work site intervention programs targeted to specific health care expenditures. Simple analysis of work force demographic data and subsequent projections of health risk formed the database for cost projections. Kaman et al. (32) showed that this approach may not be valid for all populations when compared to health risks measured by standardized health risk appraisal questionnaires.

Table 8.5 Cost:Benefit Ratios of Work Site Health Promotion Programs

Company	Benefit:Cost	Reference
1. Kennecott Copper (lifestyle)	$5.78	30*
2. Metropolitan Life (smoking cessation)	3.15	30*
3. Equitable Life (stress management)	5.52	30*
4. Blue Cross/Blue Shield of Indiana	2.51	30*
5. ALIEF ISD (Houston, TX)	2.15 (1985) 2.16 (1986)	30*
6. Mesa Petroleum Company	0.76 (1982) loss 1.07 (1983)	34
7. Prudential	1.91	30*
8. HEB ISD (TX)	1.41	30*
9. New York Telephone	1.95	30*
10. DuPont	2.05	48**
11. Pillsbury	3.63	48**
12. Coors Beer	3.75	60

*See Kaman (30) for details of references.
**See Shephard (48) for details of references.

Hatziandreu et al. (24) compared projected cost effectiveness of exercise to other health care interventions directed at cardiovascular disease. Exercise was more effective in costs-per-quality adjusted life years saved than treatment for either hypertension or angina, but surprisingly was less effective than bypass surgery for projected cases of heart disease among a nonexercising cohort population.

Keeler et al. (34) modeled an analysis on the lifetime costs incurred by individuals who exercise to varying degrees compared to those who do no exercise. Using data from the National Health Interview Survey and the RAND Health Insurance experiment, the lifetime subsidy from others who exercise to those with a sedentary lifestyle was calculated to be $1,900. The analysis included life expectancy projections for each group, a 5% annual discount rate, and the assumed effect of exercise on mortality. The authors concluded that these results provided a rationale for employer support of programs to increase employee exercise.

Comprehensive Analysis of Work Site Health Promotion Programs

Most program evaluations have reported only operating budgets as a measure of program cost, using fewer absentees and lower health care costs as measures of benefits. It is worthy to cite a comprehensive program evaluation, which has not yet appeared in a peer-reviewed journal but is available from the government printing office as a project report. Karch et al. (33) conducted a thorough cost–benefit and effectiveness analysis of the ARSTAF Corporate Fitness Project. This program, conducted over a 3-year period, included a self-selected population of 1,703 civilian and 1,646 military personnel working at the Pentagon. The evaluation outcome was relatively unremarkable in that the 3-year cost-benefit analysis achieved only a "break-even" result. Nevertheless, these investigators conducted a much more rigorous cost analysis, which included several elements of cost not usually found in most evaluations (e.g., start up, administrative overhead, office space, and utilities, etc.). Benefits were calculated (and projected) using rigorous conservative strategies as well.

This exercise-based program augmented with health education modules produced clear benefits in terms of lives saved and sick-leave reduction overall (female sick leave increased). Productivity measures produced a mixed result (self-reported measures decreased, while supervisor evaluations were positive) and did not contribute to the outcome. Finally, the original benefits calculated were reduced further when the outcome was discounted over the 3-year term of the project, resulting in the final break-even calculation.

Conclusions

The calculation of the economic impact of healthy lifestyles in general, and physical activity specifically, remains an inexact measure. Difficulties in obtaining precise measures of cost, sustaining randomly selected experimental and control populations, and obtaining reliable and standardized outcome data all contribute to the uncertainties of these analyses. Despite the difficulties, several notions appear to be correlatively if not causally linked to a positive relationship between improved fitness and reduced cost. Participants in work site fitness programs do seem to be at lower risk for ill health, utilize fewer health care services, are absent from the job less, may be more productive, and may stay with their companies longer than nonparticipants. The precise quantification of these apparent benefits and a causality link awaits continued progress in research design and data analysis. Further studies should address the following issues (42):

1. Generalizability: Manufacturing and insurance companies have been studied most often. Other industry programs should be evaluated as well.
2. Employee population issues: Most studies have focused on male-dominated, white-collar employee groups. Minority, blue-collar, and trade union workers should also be studied.
3. Company size: Most organizations studied have been large. The feasibility and the impact of these programs in small company settings must also be evaluated.
4. Cost–effectiveness: Emphasis should be redirected to studies of cost–effectiveness rather than cost–benefit until methodology is developed for obtaining accurate and comprehensive long-term dollar estimates of benefits (and costs).
5. Research design: Many work site evaluations use quasi-experimental designs which may allow selection bias, premeasurement sensitivity, multiple intervention interference, and other factors of uncertainty. Randomized selection and blindedness in design, if feasible, may help to minimize these limitations.
6. Standardization: There is a lack of standardized program elements and outcome definitions and descriptions. Standardization of these terms must be achieved before external validity may be claimed for individual study outcomes.

References

1. Anderson, D.R.; Jose, W.S. Employee lifestyle and the bottom line. Fitn. Bus. 2(3):86-91; 1987.
2. Bernacki, E.J. Can corporate fitness programs be justified? Fitn. Bus. 1(5):173-174; 1987.
3. Bernacki, E.J.; Baun, W.B. The relationship of job performance to exercise adherence in a corporate fitness program. J. Occup. Med. 26(7): 529-531; 1984.
4. Berry, C.A. An approach to good health for employees and reduced health care costs for industry. Health Insurance Association of America; 1981:9.
5. Bertera, R.L. The effects of workplace health promotion on absenteeism and employment costs in a large industrial population. Am. J. Public Health. 80(9):1101-1105; 1990.
6. Blair, S.N.; Kohl, H.W.; Paffenbarger, R.S.; Clarke, D.G.; Cooper, K.H.; Gibbons, L.W. Physical fitness and all cause mortality: A prospective study. JAMA. 262:2395-2401; 1989.
7. Blair, S.N.; Piserchia, P.V.; Wilbur, C.S.; Crowder, J.H. A public health intervention model for worksite health promotion. JAMA. 255(7):921-926; 1986.
8. Bouchard, C.; Shephard, R.J.; Stephens, T.; Sutton, J.R.; McPherson, B.D. Exercise, fitness, and health: The consensus statement. In: Bouchard, C.; Shephard, R.J.; Stephens, T.; Sutton, J.R.; McPherson, B.D., eds. Exercise, fitness, and health. Champaign, IL: Human Kinetics; 1990:3-27.
9. Brown, D.W.; Russell, M.L.; Morgan, J.L.; Optenberg, S.A.; Clarke, A.E. Reduced disability and health care costs in an industrial fitness program. J. Occup. Med. 26:809-815; 1984.
10. Carter, R.; Wanzel, R. Measuring recreation's effect on productivity. Recr. Manag. 18(6):42-47; 1975.
11. Chenoweth, D. Health promotion: Benefits versus costs. Occup. Health Saf. 37-41; 1983.
12. Conrad, C.C. A chronology of the development of corporate fitness in the United States. Fitn. Bus. 1(5):156-166; 1987.
13. Cox, M.; Shephard, R.J.; Corey, P. Influence of an employee fitness programme upon fitness, productivity, and absenteeism. Ergonomics. 24:795-806; 1981.
14. Demkovich, L.E. Business as a health care consumer, is paying heed to the bottom line. National Journal. 1980 April; 24:851-854.
15. Donoghue, S. The correlation between physical fitness, absenteeism, and work performance. Can. J. Public Health. 68:201-203; 1977.
16. Duggar, B.C.; Swengros, G.V. The design of physical activity programs for industry. J. Occup. Med. 11(6):322-329; 1989.
17. Durdeck, D.C.; Heinzelmann, F.; Schacter, J. The National Aeronautics and Space Administration—U.S. public health service health evaluation and enhancement program. Am. J. Cardiol. 30:784-790; 1972.

18. Elias, W.S.; Murphy, R.J. The case for health promotion programs containing health care costs: A review of the literature. Am. J. Occup. Ther. 40(11):759-763; 1986.
19. Gettman, L.R. Cost/benefit analysis of a corporate fitness program. Fitn. Bus. 1(1):11-17; 1986.
20. Gibbs, J.O.; Mulvaney, D.; Henes, C.; Reed, R.W. Worksite health promotion: Five year trend in employee health care costs. J. Occup. Med. 27:826-830; 1985.
21. Golaszewski, T.; Snow, D.; Lynch, W.; Yen, L.; Solomita, D. A benefit-to-cost analysis of a worksite health promotion program. J. Occup. Med. 34(12):1164-1172; 1992.
22. Grana, J. Weighing the costs and benefits of worksite health promotion. Corp. Cmnt. 6:18-19; 1985.
23. Gray, H.J. The role of business in health promotion: A brief overview. Prev. Med. 12:654-657; 1983.
24. Hatziandreu, E.I.; Kopland, J.P.; Weinstein, M.C.; Casperson, C.J.; Warner, K.E. A cost-effectiveness analysis of exercise as a health promotion activity. Am. J. Public Health. 78(11):1417-1421; 1988.
25. Herzlinger, R.E.; Calkins, D. How companies tackle health care costs. Part III. Harvard Bus. Rev. 3:70-80; 1986.
26. Huset, R. Tying your program to the bottom line. Health Action Managers. 1988; April 25:6-9.
27. Jones, L. Baker, M.R. The application of health economics to health promotion. Community Med. 8(3):224-229; 1986.
28. Jones, R.C.; Bly, J.L.; Richardson, J.E. A study of a work site health promotion program and absenteeism. J. Occup. Med. 32(2):95-99; 1990.
29. Jose, W.S.; Anderson, D.R. Control Data's staywell program: A health cost management strategy. In: Weiss, S.M.; Fielding, J.E.; Baum, A., eds., Health at work. Erlbaum; 1991:49-72.
30. Kaman, R.L. Costs and benefits of corporate health promotion. Fitn. Bus. 2(2):39-44; 1987.
31. Kaman, R.L.; Huckaby, J. Justification of employee fitness programs: Cost vs. benefit. Fitn. Bus. 3(3):90-95; 1988.
32. Kaman, R.L.; Licciardone, J.C.; Hoffmann, M.A. Comparison of health risk prevalence reported in a health risk appraisal and predicted through demographic analysis. Am. J. Health Promo. 5(5):378-383; 1991.
33. Karch, R.C.; Newton, D.L.; Schaeffer, M.A.; Zoltick, J.M.; Zajtchuk, R.; Rumbaugh, J.H. Cost-benefit and cost-effectiveness measures of health promotion in a military-civilian staff. The American University National Center for Health/Fitness ARSTAF Corporate Fitness Project Report, 1988 July. Available from: National Center for Health/Fitness, 4400 Massachusetts Ave., N.W. Washington, DC, 20016.
34. Keeler, E.B.; Manning, W.G.; Newhouse, J.P.; Sloss, E.M.; Wasserman, J. The external cost of a sedentary lifestyle. Am. J. Public Health. 79(8):975-981; 1989.
35. Kristein, M.M. The economics of health promotion at the worksite. Health Educ. Q. [Suppl.]. 9:27-36; 1982.
36. Lynch, W.D.; Teitelbaum, H.S.; Main, D.S. Comparing medical costs by analyzing high-cost cases. Am. J. Health Promo. 6(3):206-213; 1992.
37. Lynch, W.D.; Teitelbaum, H.S.; Main, D.S. The inadequacy of using means to compare medical costs of smokers and non-smokers. Am. J. Health Promo. 6(2):123-129; 1991.
38. Mausner, J.S.; Kramer, S. Analytical studies. In: Epidemiology—an introductory text. Philadelphia: Saunders; 1985:180-192.
39. McCoy, J. Wellness program can be a cost effective solution to soaring health care costs. Am. J. Compen. Bt. 278-284; 1988.
40. Mulvaney, D.E.; Gibbs, J.O.; Reed, W.R.; Grove, D.A.; Skinner, T.W. Staying alive and well at Blue Cross and Blue Shield of Indiana. In: Opatz, J.P., ed. Health promotion evaluation: Measuring the organizational impact. Stevens Point, WI: National Wellness Institute; 1987:131-141.
41. Murphy, R.J.; Elias, W.S.; Gasparatto, G.; Huset, R.A. Cost-benefit analysis in worksite health promotion evaluation. Fitn. Bus. 2(5):15-19; 1987.
42. Opatz, J.; Chenoweth, D.; Kaman, R. Economic impact of worksite health promotion programs. Northbrook, IL: Association for Fitness in Business Publications; 1991.
43. Ostwald, S.K. Cost benefit analysis: A framework for evaluating corporate health promotion programs. Am. Assoc. Occup. Health Nurses J. 34(8):377-382; 1986.
44. Pender, N.J.; Smith, L.C.; Vernoff, J.A. Building better workers. Am. Assoc. Occup. Health Nurses J. 35(9):386-390; 1987.
45. Rudman, W.J. Do onsite health and fitness programs affect worker productivity? Fitn. Bus. 2(1):2-8; 1987.
46. Shephard, R.J. Current perspectives on the economics of fitness and sport with particular reference to worksite programs. Sports Med. 7:286-389; 1989.
47. Shephard, R.J. The impact of exercise upon medical costs. Sports Med. 2:133-143; 1985.
48. Shephard, R.J. A critical analysis of work-site fitness programs and their postulated economic benefits. Med. Sci. Sports Exerc. 24(3):354-370; 1992.

49. Shephard, R.J.; Corey, P.; Cos, M.H. Health hazard appraisal—the influence of an employee fitness programme. Can. J. Public Health. 73:183-187; 1982.
50. Smith, K.J. A framework for appraising corporate wellness investments. Int. Auditor. 28-33, 1987.
51. Smith, K.; Everly, G. Problems in the evaluation of occupational health promotion programs: A case analysis. Am. J. Health Promo. 3(1):43-51; 1988.
52. Steinhardt, M.; Greenhow, L.; Stewart, J. The relationship of physical activity and cardiovascular fitness to absenteeism and medical care claims among law enforcement officers. Am. J. Health Promo. 5(6):455-460; 1991.
53. Survey. President's Council on Physical Fitness and Sports; 1986, Washington, DC.
54. Terborg, J.R. Cost benefit analysis of the Adolph Coors wellness program. Copyrighted, unpublished report. Available from: College of Business Administration, University of Oregon, Eugene, OR; 1988.
55. Tsai, S.P.; Baun, W.B.; Bernacki, E.J. Relationship of employee turnover to exercise adherence in a corporate fitness program. J. Occup. Med. 29(7):572-575; 1987.
56. Tsai, S.P.; Bernacki, E.J.; Baun, W.B. Injury prevalence and associated costs among participants of an employee fitness program. Prev. Med. 17:475-482; 1988.
57. Tucker, L.A.; Aldana, S.G.; Friedman, G.M. Cardiovascular fitness and absenteeism in 8,301 employed adults. Am. J. Health Promo. 5(2):140-145; 1990.
58. Walsh, D.C.; Egdahl, R.H. Corporate perspectives on worksite wellness programs: A report on the seventh Pew Fellows conference. J. Occup. Med. 31(6):551-556; 1989.
59. Warner, K.E. Selling health promotion to corporate America: Uses and abuses of the economic argument. Health Educ. Q. 14(1):39-55; 1987.
60. Warner, K.E.; Wickizer, T.M.; Wolfe, R.A.; Schildroth, J.E.; Samuelson, M.H. Economic implications of workplace health promotion programs: Review of the literature. J. Occup. Med. 30(2):106-112; 1988.
61. Whitmer, W. The city of Birmingham's wellness partnership contains medical costs. Bus. Health. 60-66; 1992.
62. Wilbur, C.S. The Johnson and Johnson program. Prev. Med. 12:672-681; 1983.
63. Wilson, D.M. Cost-effective fitness. Vancouver, BC: Hydro Health Services; 1982.
64. Yen, L.T.; Edington, E.W.; Witting, P. Associations between health risk appraisal scores and employee medical claims costs in a manufacturing company. Am. J. Health Promo. 6(1):46-54; 1991.

PART II

Assessment of Physical Activity, Fitness, and Health

Chapter 9

Methods of Assessing Physical Activity During Leisure and Work

Barbara E. Ainsworth
Henry J. Montoye
Arthur S. Leon

Most major contemporary chronic diseases and health problems (e.g., coronary heart disease, obesity, hypertension, non-insulin-dependent diabetes, osteoporosis, some types of cancer, and mental depression) appear to be associated with our modern habits of living, including low levels of physical activity (PA). Because of these associations, there has been a surge of interest during the last 30 to 40 years in the development of improved methods for assessing habitual PA and energy expenditure (EE) in free-living people. Assessment of PA was included previously as a topic in the 1988 Consensus Symposium on Physical Activity and Health (85). Many other reviews on techniques of assessing habitual physical activity have appeared during the past two decades (26,72,84,86, 87,89,127,136).

Our purposes here are to update these reviews, concentrating on ways of assessing habitual physical activity in free-living populations, and to suggest some future research directions in this field. PA measurement techniques are used in various settings to describe PA habits in populations, classify PA levels for intervention efforts, assess changes in PA over time, and to identify behavioral correlates of PA. Methods of estimating PA in both children and adults useful in observational epidemiologic studies are emphasized in this report. In addition, techniques are discussed which can be used to assess PA in clinical practice and in small intervention studies and to assess accuracy of field survey techniques.

The greatest obstacle to validating field methods of assessing habitual PA or total EE has been the lack of adequate criteria to assess accuracy of survey techniques. The practice of intercorrelating various field methods is of some value (concurrent validity), however, it is limited by inherent errors in all methods. For want of better criteria, work capacity or maximal oxygen uptake ($\dot{V}O_2max$) are commonly used for validation purposes (construct validity). However, measures of functional capacity and the ability to improve physical fitness with training have sizable hereditary components (22). Furthermore, functional capacity is significantly influenced by age, gender, and other habits besides PA (77), and leaves much to be desired as a validity criterion of habitual PA. Also, the type of exercise necessary to improve one's $\dot{V}O_2max$ may not be the only or even the essential type of PA related to disease prevention of specific medical conditions. Objective measures of physiological parameters associated with exercising, for example, heart rate and movement or acceleration of the body (also available as validation criteria) are discussed in the second half of this paper.

Comments in this manuscript about the validity, reliability, and feasibility of commonly used survey methods for estimating habitual PA are limited to those included under the following general categories: direct observations, PA records, survey questionnaires and interviews, objective mechanical and electronic devices for monitoring body movements, and physiological response to PA. Because of space limits we have omitted discussion of the use of direct and indirect calorimetry techniques for measuring EE (129) and the use of dietary records as a surrogate for EE (113). Regarding dietary records, in brief, there is a strong relationship between mean daily energy intake from 6 to 14 days of dietary records during weight maintenance and EE, especially if it is referenced against body weight (120).

Direct Observations

Direct observations provide a comprehensive and accurate PA assessment tool that allow characterization of habitual PA either directly or after review of film or videotapes. Direct observations have several advantages over survey techniques because they are not limited by recall or self-reporting biases of individuals. This technique can be used for either short or long periods of time, does not need equipment that may hinder movement of participants, and can be used in a variety of settings. However, direct observation is not practical for large-scale epidemiologic research because it is time-consuming, costly, intrusive, and may lead to alterations of typical behavior. Its usefulness is limited to small-scale studies, particularly involving younger children, and for validating survey questionnaires (64,66,94,100).

Physical Activity Records

Written or dictated PA records provide a detailed accounting of all or selected types of PA performed within a given time. PA records are useful in energy balance studies and can be used as a measure for validating PA survey questionnaires. Leisure-time and occupational PA are usually recorded with the quality and quantity of PA performed. However, PA records are not practical for large-scale epidemiological studies, because they call for much effort and time from study subjects and staff.

To improve accuracy in determining usual patterns of PA habits, PA records should include both weekdays and weekends for several days at a time, across all seasons of the year in order to minimize individual variability in daily PA. Physical activity records provide highly accurate indexes of mean daily EE for groups; however, individual variability in EE patterns may reduce the accuracy of PA records (36,60). Accuracy of PA records in estimating daily EE also depends on recorded details and the reference energy cost attributed to each activity used to develop the composite PA scores. PA records usually include general and specific descriptions of activities, their intensity or pace, duration in minutes, and whether or not they were done for leisure or occupational purposes. Various reference lists exist that identify energy costs for specific types of PA derived from indirect calorimetry assessments (74,83). EE in these lists is usually expressed in $kcal \cdot min^{-1}$ or $kcal \cdot kg^{-1} \cdot min^{-1}$ or METs. METs represent multiples of resting EE with 1 MET about equal to 3.5 ml of $O_2 \cdot kg^{-1} \cdot min^{-1}$. A Compendium of Physical Activities was recently developed from existing lists by the authors and their colleagues to reduce variability in scoring PA records and survey questionnaires (1).

A physical activity log (PA log) represents a modified form of PA records and provides a record of participation for specified types of PA. Activities are recorded in specific time periods or at the end of the day. PA logs have the advantage over PA records since only those activities of interest to the investigator are recorded. This increases ease and compliance in finishing, simplifies data processing, and improves the quality of the data obtained.

Survey Questionnaires and Interview Techniques

Survey instruments try to assess PA behaviors by self-reported responses or interviewer-completed assessments. Survey questionnaires or interviews provide a large volume of information on a variety of PA relative to their cost and time invested. Survey instruments are easy to administer, unobtrusive, nonreactive, and generally do not require much motivation or effort from the participant (12). For these reasons, they are the most popular types of PA assessment tools for epidemiologic research.

Survey instruments have been used to assess PA patterns for varying time frames, that is, 1 week, 1 month, 1 year, or a lifetime (18,69,122). There are many types of instruments with separate strengths and weaknesses. Most currently available questionnaires focus on participation in heavy intensity PA (Table 9.1).

The findings from validation studies show that heavy physical exertion and structured exercise or sports are easily recalled, while moderate-intensity activities, such as walking, gardening, and general household activities are less likely to be accurately recalled (56,63,101). One universal drawback of PA survey instruments is the difficulty in reliably assessing PA when an individual's PA habits often change. This helps explain the higher reliability coefficients observed for global surveys that assess general PA habits as compared to detailed recall instruments that assess PA over short periods of time.

Survey instruments also are used often to estimate the prevalence of PA in populations. Variability in the types of PA questionnaires used, activities surveyed, education level and gender of the respondents, reading level of the instruments, and the time frames sampled can lead to either an under- or an overestimation of PA habits in different populations (7,26,57). Hence, it is important to standardize the content and design of PA survey instruments used for population surveys. PA survey instruments that focus on organized sports and formal exercise participation appear to be more useful for accurately assessing habitual PA in men and young adults compared to women

Table 9.1 Physical Activity Survey Questionnaires and Interview Techniques

Method/ questionnaire[a]	Subject effort	Study expense	Type of activity[b]	Number of questions	Time frame	Mode of collection[c]	Summary index[d]	Reference
Global								
St. Louis Heart Health	Low	Low	EX	1	General	SAQ, MQ	2-point ordinal	Shapiro et al. (111)
NHIS	Low	Low	PA	1	General	PI	2-point ordinal	Slater et al. (117)
NSPHPC	Low	Low	PA	1	General	TI	6-point ordinal	Slater et al. (117)
Adventist Mortality	Low	Low	EX, JOB	1	General	SAQ	4-point ordinal	Lindsted et al. (79)
Parental Report	Low	Low	PA	1	General	PI	3-point ordinal	Murphy et al. (93)
Finnish	Low	Low	PA, JOB	2	Usual week	SAQ	4-point ordinal	Salonen et al. (105)
NHANES I	Low	Low	EX, PA	2	General	PI	3-point ordinal	Slater et al. (117)
Energy Balance	Low	Low	EX, PA	3	General	SAQ	Ordinal scale	Klesges et al. (63)
Lipid Research Clinics	Low	Low	EX, JOB	3	Usual day	SAQ, MQ	2- or 4-point ordinal	Ainsworth et al. (2)
Godin Leisure Time	Low	Low	EX	4	Usual week	SAQ, MQ	Unitless interval	Godin et al. (43,44)
MN Heart Health	Mod	Low	EX, JOB	6	Usual day	SAQ, PI	5-point ordinal	Jacobs et al. (56)
HIP-Job	Mod	Low	JOB, TRAN	6	General	SAQ, MQ	Unitless interval	Schechtman et al. (106)
NHIS/HPDP	Low	Low	PA, JOB	7	General	SAQ	kcal/kg/day; ordinal	Weiss et al. (130)
Stanford Usual	Low	Low	EX, PA	11	General	SAQ, MQ	6-point ordinal	Sallis et al. (103)
Recall								
Seven Day Recall	Mod	Low	PA	9	Past week	SAQ, PI	kcal/kg/day	Sallis et al. (104), Blair et al. (19)
CARDIA 7-Day Recall	Mod	Mod	PA, JOB	10	Past week	PI	kcal/kg/day	Sidney et al. (115)
College Alumnus	Mod	Low	EX, PA	7	Past week	SAQ, MQ	kcal/week	Paffenbarger et al. (95)
Baecke	Mod	Low	SP, PA, JOB	16	General	SAQ, MQ	Ordinal scale	Baecke et al. (8)
ARIC/Baecke	Mod/high	Low	SP, PA, JOB	39	Past year	SAQ, PI	Ordinal scale	Jacobs et al. (56)
Magnus	Mod	Mod	PA	—	Past year	PI	Ordinal scales	Magnus et al. (82)
ACLS 7-Day Recall	Mod	Low	EX, PA, SP	2	Past week	MQ	hr/week	Kohl et al. (67)
British Civil Servants	High	Mod	SP, PA	—	Past 48 hr	PI	Ordinal scale	Morris et al. (92)
Zutphen	Mod	Low	PA, JOB	15	Past month, week	SAQ	kcal/kg/day	Caspersen et al. (27)
Liverpool LTPA	Mod	Mod	EX, PA	—	Past 2 weeks	PI	kcal/day	Lamb et al. (70)
Behavioral Risk Factor	Mod	Mod	EX	3	Usual day	TI	kcal/kg/day	White et al. (133)

Quantitative History								
ACLS 3-Month Recall	Mod	Low	EX, PA, SP	8	Past 3 months	MQ	Unitless interval	Kohl et al. (67)
Tecumseh LTPA	High	Low/mod	EX, PA, JOB	100	Past year	PI	AMI/day	Montoye (87)
Tecumseh Occupation	Mod/high	Low/mod	JOB, TRAN	28	Past year	SAQ	kcal/day; kcal/week	Ainsworth et al. (3)
MN LTPA	High	Low/mod	EX, PA	64	Past year	PI	AMI/day; kcal/day	Taylor et al. (122)
MN LTPA Household	Mod	Low/mod	HH	10	Past year	PI	AMI/day; kcal/day	Jacobs et al. (56)
Four-Week History	Mod/high	Low/mod	EX, PA, HH	74	Past month	PI	AMI/day; kcal/day	Jacobs et al. (56)
3-Month Habitual	Mod/high	Low/mod	EX, TRAN, SP, PA	—	Past 3 months	PI	kJ/week	Verschuur et al. (123)
CARDIA	High	Low/mod	EX, SP, JOB	59	Past year	SAQ, PI	Exercise units	Jacobs et al. (58)
Life in New Zealand	High	Low/mod	EX, PA, HH, JOB	—	Past month	SAQ	PA units	Hopkins et al. (52)
Yale Elderly PA	Mod/high	Low/mod	EX, PA, HH	54	Past year	SAQ	kcal/week; hr/week	DiPietro et al. (35)
Elderly PAQ	Mod	Low/mod	PA, SP, HH	34	Past year	SAQ	PA units	Voorrips et al. (125)
Parker LTPA	High	Low/mod	PA, SP	47	Past year	SAQ	kcal/min	Parker et al. (96)
Historical PA	High	Low/mod	PA, SP	38	Lifetime	SAQ	kcal/week	Kriska et al. (69)
Diabetes PA	High	Low/mod	PA, JOB, EX, SP	>100	Life, past year, past week	PI	hr/week; kcal/kg/week	Kriska et al. (68)

[a]NHIS = National Health Interview Survey; NSPHPC = National Survey of Personal Health Practices & Consequences; NHANES I = National Health & Nutrition Examination Survey; MN Heart Health = Minnesota Heart Health; HIP-Job = Health Insurance of New York Study; NHIS/HPDP = National Health Informaton Survey/Health Promotion Disease Prevention; CARDIA 7-Day Recall = Coronary Artery Risk Development In Adolescents; ARIC/Baecke = Atherosclerosis Risk in Communities; ACLS 7-Day Recall = Aerobics Center Longitudinal Study; ACLS 3-Month Recall = Aerobics Center Longitudinal Study; Tecumseh LTPA = Tecumseh, Michigan Leisure Time Physical Activity; MN LTPA = Minnesota Leisure-Time Physical Activity; Yale Elderly PA = Physical Activity; Elderly PAQ = Physical Activity Questionnaire; Liverpool LTPA = Liverpool Leisure Time Physical Activity; Parker LTPA = One Year Leisure Time Physical Activity Survey; Diabetes PA = Assessment of Physical Activity in Pima Indians.

[b]Activity type: EX = exercise; PA = physical activity; JOB = occupational; TRAN = transportation to work; SP = sport; HH = household.

[c]Data collection mode: SAQ = self-administered questionnaire; MQ = mail questionnaire; PI = personal interview; TI = telephone interview.

[d]Summary index: kcal/kg/day = kilocalories · kilograms body weight^{-1} · day^{-1}; kcal/week = kilocalories · week^{-1}; hr/week = hours · week^{-1}; kcal/day = kilocalories · day^{-1}; AMI/day = activity metabolic units · day^{-1}; kJ/week = kilojoules · week^{-1}; PA units = physical activity units; kcal/min = kilocalories · minute^{-1}; kcal/kg/week = kilocalories · kilograms body weight^{-1} · week^{-1}.

and older people who in our society have been traditionally less likely to take part in such activities (35,51). Also, instruments that use terminology unfamiliar to participants may lead to incorrect information about PA habits. In the latter situation, interviewer-administered questionnaires provide more precise information than self-administered instruments because the interviewer can clarify questions and correct misinterpretations. A 4-week recall of PA once every 4 months appears to be the smallest time frame necessary to provide an accurate representative picture of one's year-round PA habit pattern because this approach accounts for seasonal variation in PA (56).

Little is known about the role of the memory processes (i.e., encoding, storing, and recalling of information) on the recall of PA habits (12). In a study of 44 adults, Klesges et al. (63) studied PA recall processes by comparing the accuracy of self-reports of voluntary PA performed during the past hour with simultaneous direct observation of the subject's PA. Results showed only moderate accuracy of recalled PA as compared to observed PA (r = .62). Also, sedentary activities were consistently underestimated while endurance activities were overestimated by over 300%.

Occupational Activity

Before 1970, most epidemiologic studies to evaluate the association between PA and health status focused on occupational PA. Assessment of occupational levels of energy expenditure in these studies was usually based solely on job titles under the misconception that all persons performing given job tasks expend similar amounts of energy. Because recent technological advances have led to a marked decline in heavy occupational PA and have changed the types of activities on the job, few job titles now accurately reflect the types of activities done and their true EE requirements. Furthermore, there is considerable variability in the types of activities within the same job classification, variability in estimated energy costs of job tasks, and seasonal changes in work requirements. Also, the PA gradient in many industries among jobs with different titles is so small that assessment tools may not be sensitive enough to differentiate between their energy costs.

Many occupational PA survey instruments focus primarily on heavy-intensity occupational PA and therefore are not applicable to most of the population who work in sedentary occupations. Hence, broader-scope occupational PA instruments that focus on the time spent in a wide range of activities of varying MET levels (including low intensity) are better suited to assess PA in most occupational settings. The recently developed Tecumseh Self-Administered Quantitative Occupational PA Questionnaire (3) and the CARDIA Seven Day Recall PA questionnaire (58,115) are two new instruments that measure time and EE of a wide spectrum of occupational activities of varying intensities. However, these two new instruments still show only moderate correlations with standard validation criteria.

Global Self-Assessment

Simple global PA assessment tools require only that a person respond to a few simple, direct questions about their usual PA habits. Global questionnaires now used in epidemiological research take less than 1 min to complete and have good repeatability and validity compared to physiologic validation parameters (2,43,56,106,130). Global self-report questionnaires do not provide detailed information about specific PA habits or total EE; rather, they only are concerned with whether or not individuals regularly perform high-intensity PA. However, they are useful to categorize an individual's cardiorespiratory fitness levels (43,106), or as independent variables in $\dot{V}O_2max$ prediction equations (4,55). Selected global PA instruments that have been used in epidemiological studies are listed in Table 9.1.

Recall Questionnaires

Most detailed self- or interviewer-administered recall PA questionnaires assess "usual" or actual PA participation during the previous 1 to 4 weeks. There are many such questionnaires which have been validated in recent years against measures of aerobic fitness, total and HDL-cholesterol levels, body composition, PA and food records, and motion detector readings (12,56,89). The principal advantages of recall questionnaires compared to the earlier discussed survey methods are that they provide information about specific types of PA performed, are easy to complete, and allow quantification of PA during the period assessed. For these reasons, recall questionnaires are the most commonly used types of assessment tools in epidemiological research. However, an important limitation is that PA recalled from a previous week or month may not accurately represent an individual's true year round activity pattern. Nevertheless, many such instruments have shown PA levels to be inversely associated with health status (99). Major recall questionnaires are listed in Table 9.1.

Quantitative Histories

Retrospective PA history instruments are designed to get detailed, qualitative, and quantitative information about PA during specified long-term time periods (usually 1 month or 1 year). Participants identify the type, frequency, and duration of specific activities from extensive lists of occupational and/or leisure-time activities. Such questionnaires are much longer and more detailed than other types of survey instruments and usually require trained interviewers for administration and scoring. Two other disadvantages of quantitative history questionnaires compared to other survey instruments are that they are more time-consuming for the participant to complete and require more time and effort by the study staff to accurately enter and analyze data. Therefore, quantitative PA history instruments generally are used only when detailed information about PA habits are needed and adequate funding and staffing is available. Examples of occupational and leisure-time quantitative PA instruments also are listed in Table 9.1.

The Minnesota Leisure Time Physical Activity (LTPA) Questionnaire is the most commonly used and most thoroughly evaluated quantitative history instrument (101,122). The LTPA questionnaire asks participants to indicate in which of 64 listed activities they participated during each month over the past 12-month period. The instrument yields duration and EE scores for total-, heavy-, moderate-, and light-intensity activities from estimates of the frequency and duration of PAs reported during each month of the past year. The instrument has been used in many studies to characterize PA habits in populations (32) and to test associations between PA and health outcomes (37,75,76,118,119). The 1-year test-retest reliability of this instrument is relatively high (r = .69) (38). The instrument also has been validated against measures of cardiorespiratory fitness, relative body weight and life habits (56,77,118), PA records (101), and dietary records (122). Also, a supplement to the LTPA questionnaire is available to assess household PA habits. A detailed description and validation data of the LTPA questionnaire and its household PA supplement were recently reported (101).

Objective Mechanical and Electronic Devices and Instruments

Pedometers

The pedometer is a simple mechanical movement counter which is clipped to a belt at the waist or worn on the ankle. Pedometers operate by counting steps in response to the vertical acceleration of the body during walking or running by causing a lever arm to move vertically and a ratchet to rotate. Pedometers tend to underestimate distances walked at slower speeds and overestimate distances during fast walking or running (16,126). Some brands of pedometers appear to be more accurate than others with the average error between instruments varying from +5% to +13% (42). Furthermore, the tension in the spring of each instrument may vary, so that readings among instruments of the same brand are not uniform (42). Irving and Patrick (54) observed that these instruments, despite their imprecision, could correctly differentiate gross differences in PA among five occupational groups. Further, Bassey, Blecher, Fentem, and Patrick (15) observed that the pedometer is useful in detecting the increased PA resulting from initiation of a walking program.

Other Motion Sensors

Electronic load transducers are available which can be inserted into the heels of shoes to monitor loads held, lifted, or carried, and walking activity (14,34). Such devices have not been used much in epidemiologic research, and little information is available on their accuracy in assessing habitual PA status and EE.

The Large-Scale Integrated Motor Activity Monitor (LSI) is a simple device that uses a mercury switch sensitive to a 3° tilt in a single axis. It is slightly larger than a wristwatch and can be worn on the trunk or limb. The LSI also can correctly distinguish between groups of adults who grossly differ in PA status (28,71). However, LSI readings do not correlate well with energy intake in children or with questionnaire assessment of LTPA in children, middle-aged men, or older women. Furthermore, the LSI readings correlate poorly with estimated $\dot{V}O_2$ levels during walking, running (91), and bicycle riding (53).

There are at least two advantages of the LSI as compared to pedometers. First, the standardization of the LSI is better because mechanical springs are not used, and second, the LSI operates on tilt rather than impact so that it can be used to assess a greater variety of activities than pedometers. However, some of the same limitations of pedometers also apply to the LSI. Also, the present cost of the LSI is prohibitive for use in large-scale field studies.

A motor sensor has been described which can be attached to the lateral thigh by an elastic band or tape and has six liquid mercury switches aligned on the faces of a cube (121). Berkowitz et al. (17) used this sensor to study the relationship of PA and body fat in 4- to 8-year-old children. Although they did not evaluate the validity of this instrument, three of these devices were very consistent in recording movement in over 20 trials of a subject walking on a treadmill at 2 mph and 3% grade.

Accelerometry

Motion results in acceleration of the limbs and body, which increases EE. However, even common activities such as walking, bending, and climbing stairs are quite complex and all their associated EE is *not* reflected in acceleration or deceleration of the mass of the body. Further, during activities such as bicycling and rowing, when an accelerometer is attached to the waist, little movement is recorded although the EE may be high.

On the other hand, in classifying individuals in a population by habitual PA status, we are dealing with a wide spectrum ranging from people who are extremely sedentary to those who routinely do considerable occupational and/or LTPA. In addition, in patient populations we often are concerned with documenting increased EE by intervention programs that add considerable PA to an otherwise sedentary lifestyle. For such applications, finer biomechanical considerations and problems assume less importance in terms of the development of movement instrumentation. Whereas a step-counting device is of limited value in studying EE related to complicated movements such as tennis, basketball, gardening, stair climbing, and housework, a more sophisticated instrument such as an accelerometer may be more useful.

One of us (Montoye) participated in the development of a small electronic single-plane accelerometer that has been useful for estimating habitual PA (53,91). The output of the accelerometer worn at the waist was almost identical to the vertical component of a force platform reached while subjects did bench stepping and knee bends (90). However, when the subject repeatedly bent over to touch the floor, agreement was poor. This probably resulted from the fact that the portable accelerometer was no longer maintained in a vertical position during this movement, which suggests the potential advantage of using a triaxial accelerometer. This portable accelerometer then underwent further modifications and was made commercially available under the trade name Caltrac (Hemokinetics; Madison, WI). In using the Caltrac, it should be stressed that it is vital that it fit tightly to the body in order to accurately measure accelerations and decelerations of the body mass (110).

The Caltrac has been used to estimate seasonal fluctuations in PA in older women (31), PA status in children (116), and daily EE in physical therapists (10). Intra- and interinstrument variability also has been studied. In laboratory tests with children walking or running on the treadmill, the correlation coefficient between instruments was about .8 to .9 (61,103). However, Gretebeck and Montoye (47) found that day-to-day Caltrac readings in 30 employed males correlated .72 (average rank order *r*) when expressed in kilocalories, but only .34 when expressed as METs. If only weekdays were considered, the rank orders were higher (.79 and .51, respectively). These differences in *r* values were probably not solely, or even primarily, a reflection of instrument variation, but more likely reflected true variability in PA on various days sampled.

In another validation study involving the Caltrac, Schutz, Froidevaux, and Jéquier (108) observed an *r* of .92 between EE measured by a whole body calorimeter and Caltrac readings in 29 women over a 24-hr period. However, the Caltrac underestimated EE by an average of 14%. In other laboratory investigations in which subjects walked or ran on a treadmill, *r*s of .80 to .94 were reported between $\dot{V}O_2$ levels and Caltrac readings (11,48,50).

Sallis et al. (103) recently reported *r* values of .54 and .42 between separate days of Caltrac recordings and monitored "activity heart rate" (daily HR minus resting HR) in children. In another study, the HR response of 20 high-school students during a basketball class was compared to Caltrac readings where a *r* of .92 was observed (9). In addition, a video camera was used to record the basketball class and MET values were assigned to observed activities at 15-s intervals. The estimates of EE by direct observations correlated .95 with the Caltrac readings.

On the other hand, Caltrac readings correlated poorly with PA questionnaire scores and an activity diary in a study including 45 adults (135). In another study involving 30 employed men, Caltracs were worn for 1 week and readings were compared with activity scores from five popular PA questionnaires (46). Correlation coefficients for estimated EE in kilocalories by the Caltrac were found to range from .28 to .87, and when the EE values were converted to METs, the *r* values varied from .40 to .69. In still another study, 222 children were directly observed in their homes in the evening for 1 hr and an activity rating derived for each child (64). When a parental estimate of habitual PA was compared with a 1-day activity recording by the Caltrac, the scores, surprisingly, were not significantly related.

Both the Caltrac and the LSI readings also were compared with directly observed PA in 50 adults during 1 hr of recreational activity (65). The relationships of the accelerometer and LSI readings with the overall mean rating of PA were found to be quite similar with measurements by the two instruments correlating well with each other. These same investigators (65) made similar comparisons among 30 school children in a day-care center. The correlations between PA as rated by an observer and the Caltrac or the LSI readings were found to be lower than the readings among adults. However, since errors in the measurements may be as great or greater than errors in the Caltrac readings, comparisons of this nature are of limited value.

Estimation of Energy Expenditure From Physiologic Data

Heart Rate Monitoring

Because of technical difficulties encountered in measuring EE by indirect calorimetry in the field, there is interest in finding simpler, less direct methods of recording physiologic data associated with EE. When work performance can be carefully controlled in the laboratory, for example on a treadmill or bicycle ergometer, $\dot{V}O_2$ and heart rate (HR) levels show a linear relationship over most of the range from resting to maximal levels. In using HR as a surrogate for PA, it is a common practice to bring the subject to the laboratory to establish an individualized HR-$\dot{V}O_2$ calibration curve, and then use this curve to convert HR recorded in the field into $\dot{V}O_2$ or EE values (24).

However, there are sources of error in this model. For example, high ambient temperature and humidity tend to raise the HR with little effect on $\dot{V}O_2$ requirements for the work task. In addition, exercise conditioning lowers the HR at which tasks at a given submaximal energy cost are performed. Women generally have a higher HR during similar levels of exercise as compared to men (88). Fatigue (20,81), state of hydration (81), body temperature, oxygen tension of the inspired air (altitude), and one's emotional state also significantly affect the HR-$\dot{V}O_2$ relationship. Certain kinds of activities (e.g., work limited to the arms even when the $\dot{V}O_2$ cost is the same as leg work) generally elicit a higher HR response than work done with the legs alone or the legs plus arms (29). Finally, static exercise increases the HR above that expected based on the work load (49).

Small portable recorders now are commercially available which record heart rates beat-by-beat. Among 13 such HR monitors evaluated, the Uniq Heart Watch was rated the best according to validity, stability, and functionality (73). Montoye has had experience using the Uniq Heart Watch under a variety of field conditions and generally found that it functioned exceedingly well in a study involving 30 employed men (47).

Ballor et al. (9), also using individual HR-$\dot{V}O_2$ calibration curves, reported a high correlation between HR estimates of EE and both Caltrac and videotaped estimates of PA during a basketball class. In two other studies in which individual HR-$\dot{V}O_2$ calibration curves were obtained, HR estimates of EE favorably compared with EE determined by doubly labeled water (DLW) measurements in free-living subjects (80,107). In one of these studies, Livingstone et al. (80) found that daily EE estimated from the HR was 2% higher than that obtained by DLW determinations. However, the range in percent differences varied from −22.2 to +52.1 (SD = 17.9%) among subjects. In the second of such investigations (107), involving six adults on 2 randomly selected days, the correlation coefficients between the DLW and HR estimates of EE varied from .53 to .73 depending on which prediction method for getting EE from HR was used.

The use of net HR (work HR minus resting HR) is a simple way to reduce subject-to-subject variation by adjusting for resting EE, individual HR characteristics, and state of training. It is much like using one point on an individual's HR-$\dot{V}O_2$ calibration curve with the assumption that the slopes of the curves are the same for various individuals. Washburn and Montoye (128) have shown that this method is much simpler, but is about as accurate as using a $\dot{V}O_2$-HR calibration curve on each subject.

The main problem with estimating EE from HR-$\dot{V}O_2$ calibration curves in individuals in industrialized countries is that average 24-hr EE level is low, and it is in this range where the greatest errors in prediction of EE from HR happen. This is illustrated by a careful validation study by Dauncey and James (33) using a whole body calorimeter. For most individuals, errors or variation at the lower end of the HR-$\dot{V}O_2$ curve led to large errors in predicting 24-hr EE.

Multiple Recorders

There are limits and problems with all types of mechanical and electronic devices proposed to estimate PA or total EE in free-living subjects. To improve these estimates, more complex recording systems have been developed. For example, Fouillot et al. (41) used a portable tape recorder to record the ECG in one channel, a 60-Hz timing pulse in another channel, and an event marker in the third channel. Taylor et al. (121) combined a movement sensor (six mercury switches mounted on the face of a cube) with HR recordings and 15-min activity logs kept by the subject. They tried to circumvent the problem of the effect of emotion on HR in this manner. Although PA recorded by a motion sensor agreed quite well with the subjects' PA logs, the subjects' assessment of anxiety showed poor agreement with elevated HRs during low levels of recorded PA, presumably because of anxiety.

Another multiple recording system has been described in which a two-channel portable tape recorder records both the ECG and footfall counts from a transducer under the heel (15). In addition, a portable, physiological monitoring system has recently been described that can record data from eight physiological sensors for a period of weeks (59). Still another system records ECG, and electromyogram readings from a thigh using a four-channel cassette recorder (5). It is encouraging that such multiple systems are being developed; however, none at the present time are practical for use in epidemiologic studies, and their validity in the field remains to be determined.

Doubly Labeled Water (DLW)

DLW is a relatively new approach for estimating EE in humans and is potentially applicable for use in both laboratory and field studies. The principle of this method is simple. A quantity of water with a known abundance of isotopes of hydrogen (deuterium or ^2H) and oxygen (^{18}O) is ingested by the study subject. In a matter of hours the isotopes distribute themselves in equilibrium with body water. The labeled hydrogen will gradually leave the body as part of water, mainly in the urine, sweat, and insensible water vapor loss. The ^{18}O leaves the body as part of both water and carbon dioxide molecules from energy metabolism. From the difference in elimination rates of these two isotopes, the production of $\dot{V}CO_2$ can be calculated. Then by knowing or estimating the respiratory exchange ratio ($\dot{V}CO_2/\dot{V}O_2$), O_2 uptake and thereby EE can be calculated for the time period under consideration.

However, while the cost of ^2H is minimal, the amount of ^{18}O needed for an EE determination now costs $300 to $500, which makes this method prohibitive in large-scale studies. When using this technique the dose of the two isotopes should be sufficient, so that following the observational period, the enrichment of body water provides isotope levels well above background levels. Probably a 2-week observation period in adults and 1 week in children provide maximum precision of this method. Since both isotopes are stable, there is no significant risk of radiation exposure to subjects.

Although the DLW method has never been validated in a field study (and it is probably infeasible), the validity of this method has been studied in human beings under controlled laboratory and metabolic ward conditions (102,109,131,132). Two criteria of EE have been used in such studies: (1) a calorimeter chamber in which direct and indirect (respiratory) measurements of EE were monitored, or (2) dietary balance studies in which energy intake and utilization were determined. The validity of the DLW technique for measurement of EE under such controlled conditions appears very satisfactory. However, the measurement error is conceivably much greater in field studies.

Conclusions

Promoting physical activity is a high-priority area for *Healthy People 2000 Objectives* because of the repeated demonstrations in epidemiologic studies of an association of sedentariness fostered by modern lifestyles and risk of coronary disease and other prevalent contemporary medical conditions. This has created a need for better techniques to assess PA in populations for further disease-specific epidemiologic research and to evaluate the effectiveness of public health strategies used to promote PA.

However, there are still problems with current instruments used to assess PA. There is no "gold standard" measurement technique. Furthermore, existing validation criteria, where various instruments account for different aspects of PA, only explain part of the variability in daily PA habits. Since questionnaires are used most often to characterize PA habits in epidemiological research, questions need to be identified that can measure various types of PA and will generalize to all socioeconomic, ethnic, gender, and age strata of the population.

References

1. Ainsworth, B.E.; Jacobs, D.R., Jr.; Leon, A.S.; Haskell, W.L.; Montoye, H.J.; Sallis, J.F.; Paffenbarger, R.S., Jr. Compendium of physical activities: Classification of energy costs of human physical activities. Med. Sci. Sports Exerc. 25:71-80; 1993.

2. Ainsworth, B.E.; Jacobs, D.R., Jr.; McNally, M.C.; Leon, A.S. Validity and reliability of self-reported physical activity status: The Lipid Research Clinics questionnaire. Med. Sci. Sports Exerc. 25:92-98; 1993.
3. Ainsworth, B.E.; Jacobs, D.R., Jr.; Leon, A.S.; Richardson, M.T.; Montoye, H.J. Assessment of the accuracy of physical activity occupational data. J. Occup. Med. [In press].
4. Ainsworth, B.E.; Richardson, M.T.; Jacobs, D.R., Jr.; Leon, A.S. Prediction of cardiorespiratory fitness using questionnaire data. Med. Exerc. Nutr. Health. 1:75-82; 1992.
5. Anastasides, P.; Johnston, D.W. A simple activity measure for use with ambulatory subjects. Psychophysiology. 27:87-93; 1990.
7. Arroll, B.; Beaglehole, R. Potential misclassification in studies of physical activity. Med. Sci. Sports Exerc. 23:1176-1178; 1991.
8. Baecke, H.A.H.; Burema, J.; Frijters, J.E.R. A short questionnaire for the measurement of habitual physical activity in epidemiological studies. Am. J. Clin. Nutr. 36:932-942; 1982.
9. Ballor, D.L.; Burke, L.M.; Knudson, D.V.; Olson, J.R.; Montoye, H.J. Comparison of three methods of estimating energy expenditure: Caltrac, heart rate, and video analysis. Res. Q. 60:362-368; 1989.
10. Balogun, J.A.; Farina, N.T.; Fay, E.; Rossmann, K.; Pozyc, L. Energy cost determination using a portable accelerometer. Phys. Ther. 66:1102-1109; 1986.
11. Balogun, J.A.; Martin, D.A.; Clendenin, M.A. Calorimetric validation of the Caltrac accelerometer during level walking. Phys. Ther. 69:501-509; 1989.
12. Baranowski, T. Validity and reliability of self-report measures of physical activity: An information-processing perspective. Res. Q. Exerc. Sports. 59:314-327; 1988.
14. Barber, C.; Evans, D.; Fentem, P.H.; Wilson, M.F. A simple load transducer suitable for long-term recording of activity patterns in human subjects. J. Physiol. (Lond.). 231:94-95; 1973.
15. Bassey, E.J.; Blecher, A.; Fentem, P.H.; Patrick, J.M. Daily physical activity monitored before, during and after a walking-programme in middle-aged subjects. In: Stott, F.; Raftery, E.B.; Clement, D.L.; Wright, S.L., eds. Proceedings of the 4th international symposium on ambulatory monitoring, and the second gent workshop on blood pressure variability. London: Academic Press; 1982:194-400.
16. Bassey, E.J.; Dallosso, H.M.; Fentem, P.H.; Irving, J.M.; Patrick, J.M. Validation of a simple mechanical accelerometer (pedometer) for the estimation of walking activity. Eur. J. Appl. Physiol. 56:323-330; 1987.
17. Berkowitz, R.I.; Agras, W.S.; Komer, A.F.; Kraemer, H.C.; Zeanah, C.H. Physical activity and adiposity: A longitudinal study from birth to childhood. J. Pediatr. 106:734-738; 1985.
18. Blair, S.N.; Dowda, M.; Pate, R.R.; Kronenfeld, J.; Hove, H.G., Jr.; Parker, G.; Blair, A.; Fridinger, F. Reliability of long-term recall of participation in physical activity by middle-aged men and women. Am. J. Epidemiol. 133:266-275; 1991.
19. Blair, S.N.; Haskell, W.L.; Ho, P.; Paffenbarger, R.S., Jr.; Vranizan, K.M.; Farquhar, J.W.; Wood, P.D. Assessment of habitual physical activity by a seven-day recall in a community survey and controlled experiments. Am. J. Epidemiol. 122:794-804; 1985.
20. Booyen, J.; Harvey, G.R. The pulse rate as a means of measuring metabolic rate in man. Can. J. Biomech. Physiol. 38:1301-1309; 1960.
22. Bouchard, C.; Boulay, M.R.; Simoneau, J.A.; Lortie, G.; Perusse, L. Heredity and trainability of aerobic and anaerobic performance: An update. Sports Med. 5:69-73; 1988.
24. Bradfield, R.B. A technique for determination of usual daily energy expenditure in the field. Am. J. Clin. Nutr. 37:461-467; 1983.
26. Caspersen, C.J. Physical activity epidemiology: Concepts, methods, and application to exercise science. In: Pandolf, K.B., ed. Exercise and sport sciences reviews, Vol. 17. Baltimore: Williams & Wilkins; 1989:423-473.
27. Caspersen, C.J.; Bloemberg, B.P.M.; Saris, W.H.M.; Merritt, R.K.; Kromhout, D. The prevalence of selected physical activities and their relation with coronary heart disease risk factors in elderly men: The Zutphen study, 1985. Am. J. Epidemiol. 133:1078-1092, 1991.
28. Cauley, J.A.; LaPorte, R.E.; Black-Sandler, R.; Schramm, M.M.; Kriska, A.M. Comparison of methods to measure physical activity in postmenopausal women. Am. J. Clin. Nutr. 45:14-22; 1987.
29. Cerretelli, P.; Prampero, P.E.D.; Sassi, G. The heart rate-$\dot{V}O_2$ relationship in different types of dynamic exercise. Arch. Fisiol. 65:358-365; 1967.
31. Cress, M.L.; Thomas, D.P.; Johnson, J.; Kasch, F.W.; Cassens, R.G.; Smith, E.L.; Agre, J.C. Effect of training on $\dot{V}O_2$max, thigh strength, and muscle morphology in septuagenarian women. Med. Sci. Sports Exerc. 23:752-758; 1991.
32. Dannenberg, A.L.; Keller, J.B.; Wilson, P.W.F.; Castelli, W.P. Leisure time physical activity

in the Framingham offspring study: Description, seasonal variation, and risk factor correlates. Am. J. Epidemiol. 129:76-88; 1989.

33. Dauncey, M.J.; James, W.P.T. Assessment of the heart rate method for determining energy expenditure in man, using a whole-body calorimeter. Br. J. Nutr. 42:1-13; 1979.
34. Dion, J.L.; Fouillot, J.P.; Leblanc, A. Ambulatory monitoring of walking using a thin capacitive force transducer. In: Stott, F.D.; Raftery, E.B.; Clement, D.L.; Wright, S.L., eds. Proceedings of the 4th international symposium on ambulatory monitoring, and the second gent workshop on blood pressure variability. London: Academic Press; 1982:420-425.
35. DiPietro, L.; Caspersen, C.; Ostfeld, A.; Nadel, E. A survey for assessing physical activity among older adults. Med. Sci. Sports Exerc. 25:628-642; 1993.
36. Durnin, J.V.G.A.; Namyslowski, L. Individual variations in the energy expenditure of standardized activities. J. Physiol. 143:573-578; 1958.
37. Folsom, A.R.; Caspersen, C.J.; Taylor, H.L.; Jacobs, D.R., Jr.; Luepker, R.V.; Gomez-Marin, O.; Gillum, R.F.; Blackburn, H. Leisure time physical activity and its relationship to coronary risk factors in a population-based sample: The Minnesota heart survey. Am. J. Epidemiol. 121:570-579; 1985.
38. Folsom, A.R.; Jacobs, D.R., Jr.; Caspersen, C.J.; Gomez-Marin, O.; Knudsen, J. Test-retest reliability of the Minnesota leisure time physical activity questionnaire. J. Chronic Dis. 39:505-511; 1986.
41. Fouillot, J.P.; Drospowski, T.; Tekaia, F.; Regnard, J.; Izou, M.-A.; Fourneron, T.; LeBlanc, A.; Rieu, M. Methodology of heart rate ambulatory monitoring recordings analysis, in relation to activity: Applications to sports training and workload studies. In: Stott, F.D.; Raftery, E.B.; Clement, D.L.; Wright, S.L., eds. Proceedings of the 4th international symposium on ambulatory monitoring, and the second gent workshop on blood pressure variability. London: Academic Press; 1982:377-383.
42. Gayle, R.; Montoye, H.J.; Philpot, J. Accuracy of pedometers for measuring distance walked. Res. Q. 48:632-636; 1977.
43. Godin, G.; Jobin, J.; Bouillon, J. Assessment of leisure time exercise behavior by self-report: A concurrent validity study. Can. J. Public Health. 77:359-361; 1986.
44. Godin, G.; Shephard, R.J. A simple method to assess exercise behavior in the community. Can. J. Appl. Sport Sci. 10:141-146; 1985.
46. Gretebeck, R.; Montoye, H.J. A comparison of six physical activity questionnaires with Caltrac accelerometer readings. Med. Sci. Sports Exerc. [Abstract]. 22:S79; 1990.
47. Gretebeck, R.J.; Montoye, H.J. Reproducibility of some measures of physical activity. Med. Sci. Sports Exerc. [In press].
48. Gutin, B.; Mukeshi, M. Validation of the Caltrac movement sensor using indirect calorimetry. Med. Sci. Sports Exerc. [Abstract]. 21:S112; 1989.
49. Hanson, O.E.; Maggio, M. Static work and heart rate. Int. Z. Angew. Physiol. 18:242-247; 1960.
50. Haymes, E.M.; Byrnes, W.C. Comparison of walking and running energy cost using the Caltrac and indirect calorimetry. Med. Sci. Sports Exerc. [Abstract]. 23:S60; 1991.
51. Henderson, K.A.; Bialeschki, M.D.; Shaw, S.M.; Freysinger, V.J. A leisure of one's own: A feminist perspective on women's leisure. State College, PA: Venture Publishing, Inc.; 1989.
52. Hopkins, W.G.; Wilson, N.C.; Russell, D.G. Validation of the physical activity instrument for the life in New Zealand national survey. Am. J. Epidemiol. 133:73-82; 1991.
53. Hunter, G.R.; Montoye, H.J.; Webster, J.G.; Demment, R.; Ji, L.L.; Ng, A. An investigation of the validity of a vertical accelerometer for estimation of energy expenditure in bicycle riding. J. Sports Med. Phys. Fitness. 29:218-222; 1984.
54. Irving, J.M.; Patrick, J.M. The use of mechanical pedometers in the measurement of physical activity. In: Stott, F.D.; Raftery, E.B.; Clement, D.L.; Wright, S.L., eds. Proceedings of the 4th international symposium on ambulatory monitoring, and the second gent workshop on blood pressure variability. London: Academic Press; 1982:369-376.
55. Jackson, A.S.; Blair, S.N.; Mahar, M.T.; Wier, L.T.; Ross, R.M.; Stuteville, J.E. Prediction of functional aerobic capacity without exercise testing. Med. Sci. Sports Exerc. 22:863-870; 1991.
56. Jacobs, D.R., Jr.; Ainsworth, B.E.; Hartman, T.J.; Leon, A.S. A simultaneous evaluation of ten commonly used physical activity questionnaires. Med. Sci. Sports Exerc. 25:81-91; 1993.
57. Jacobs, D.R., Jr.; Hahn, L.P.; Folsom, A.R.; Hannan, P.J.; Sprafka, J.M.; Burke, G.L. Time trends in leisure-time physical activity in the upper midwest 1957-1987: University of Minnesota studies. Epidemiology. 2:8-15; 1991.
58. Jacobs, D.R., Jr.; Hahn, L.P.; Haskell, W.L.; Pirie, P.; Sidney, S. Validity and reliability of

short physical activity history: Cardia and the Minnesota heart health program. J. Cardiopul. Rehabil. 9:448-459; 1989.

59. Jetté, M.; Landry, F.; Tiemann, B.; Blümchen, G. Ambulatory blood pressure and Holter monitoring during tennis play. Can. J. Sport Sci. 16:40-44; 1991.
60. Kalkwarf, H.J.; Haas, J.D.; Belko, A.Z.; Roach, R.C.; Roe, D.A. Accuracy of heart-rate monitoring and activity diaries for estimating energy expenditure. Am. J. Clin. Nutr. 49:37-43; 1989.
61. Kastango, K.B.; Freedson, P.S. Validation of a kilocalorie conversion of Caltrac activity counts. Med. Sci. Sports Exerc. [Abstract]. 23:S61; 1991.
63. Klesges, R.C.; Eck, L.H.; Mellon, M.W.; Fulliton, W.; Somes, G.W.; Hanson, C.L. The accuracy of self-reports of physical activity. Med. Sci. Sports Exerc. 22:690-697; 1990.
64. Klesges, R.C.; Haddock, C.K.; Eck, L.H. A multimethod approach to the measurement of childhood physical activity and its relation to blood pressure and body weight. J. Pediatr. 116:888-893; 1990.
65. Klesges, R.C.; Klesges, L.M.; Swenson, A.M.; Pheley, A.F. A validation of two motion sensors in the prediction of child and adult physical activity levels. Am. J. Epidemiol. 122:400-410; 1985.
66. Klesges, R.C.; Molderhauer, C.T. The FATS: An observational system for assessing physical activity in children and associated parent behavior. Behav. Assess. 6:333-345; 1984.
67. Kohl, H.W.; Blair, S.N.; Paffenbarger, R.S., Jr.; Macera, C.A.; Kronenfeld, J.J. A mail survey of physical activity habits as related to measured physical fitness. Am. J. Epidemiol. 127:1228-1239; 1988.
68. Kriska, A.M.; Knowler W.C.; LaPorte, R.E.; Drash, A.L.; Wing, R.R.; Blair, S.N.; Bennett, P.H.; Kuller, L.H. Development of a questionnaire to examine relationship of physical activity and diabetes in Pima Indians. Diabetes Care. 13:401-411; 1990.
69. Kriska, A.M.; Sandler, R.B.; Cauley, J.A.; LaPorte, R.E.; Hom, D.L.; Pambianco, G. The assessment of historical physical activity and its relation to adult bone parameters. Am. J. Epidemiol. 127:1053-1063; 1988.
70. Lamb, K.L.; Brodie, D.A. Leisure-time physical activity as an estimate of physical fitness: A validation study. J. Clin. Epidemiol. 44:4441-4452; 1991.
71. LaPorte, R.E.; Kuller, L.H.; Kupfer, D.J.; McPartland, R.J.; Matthews, G.; Caspersen, C. An objective measure of physical activity for epidemiologic research. Am. J. Epidemiol. 109:158-168; 1979.
72. LaPorte, R.E.; Montoye, H.J.; Caspersen, C.J. Assessment of physical activity in epidemiologic research: Problems and prospects. Public Health Rep. 100:131-146; 1985.
73. Leger, L.; Thivierge, M. Heart rate monitors: Validity, stability, and functionality. Phys. Sports Med. 16:143-151; 1988.
74. Leon, A.S. Approximate energy expenditures and fitness values of sports and recreational and household activities. In: Wilder, E.L., ed. The book of health and physical fitness. New York; Franklin Watts; 1981:283-341.
75. Leon, A.S.; Connett, J. Physical activity and 10.5 year mortality in the multiple risk factor intervention trial (MRFIT). Int. J. Epidemiol. 20:690-697; 1991.
76. Leon, A.S.; Connett, J.; Jacobs, D.R., Jr.; Rauramaa, R. Leisure-time physical activity levels and risk of coronary heart disease and death. JAMA. 258:2388-2395; 1987.
77. Leon, A.S.; Jacobs, D.R., Jr.; De Backer, G.; Taylor, H.L. Relationship of physical characteristics and life habits to treadmill exercise capacity. Am. J. Epidemiol. 113:653-660; 1985.
79. Lindsted, K.D.; Tonstad, S.; Kuzma, J.W. Self-report of physical activity and patterns of mortality in Seventh-Day Adventist men. J. Clin. Epidemiol. 44:355-364; 1991.
80. Livingstone, M.B.E.; Prentice, A.M.; Coward, W.A.; Ceesay, S.M.; Strain, J.J.; McKenna, P.G.; Nevin, G.B.; Barker, M.E.; Hickey, R.J. Simultaneous measurement of free-living energy expenditure by the doubly labeled water method and heart-rate monitoring. Am. J. Clin. Nutr. 52:59-65; 1990.
81. Lundgren, N.P.V. The physiological effects of time schedule work on lumber workers. Acta Physiol. Scand. [Suppl. 41]. 13:1-137; 1946.
82. Magnus, K.; Matroos, A.; Strackee, J. Walking, cycling, or gardening with or without seasonal interruption, in relation to acute events. Am. J. Epidemiol. 110:724-733; 1979.
83. McArdle, W.D.; Katch, F.I.; Katch, V.L. Exercise physiology: energy, nutrition, and human performance. 2nd ed. Philadelphia: Lea & Febiger; 1988:642-649.
84. Meijer, G.A.L.; Westerterp, K.R.; Verhoeven, F.M.H.; Koper, H.B.M.; Ten Hoor, F. Methods to assess physical activity with special reference to motion sensors and accelerometers. IEEE Trans. Biomed. Eng. 38:221-229; 1991.
85. Montoye, H.J. Discussion: Assessment of physical activity during leisure and work. In: Bouchard, C.; Shephard, R.J.; Stephens, T.; Sutton, J.R.; McPherson, B.D., eds. Exercise,

fitness, and health. Champaign, IL: Human Kinetics; 1990:71-74.

86. Montoye, H.J. Activity instrumentation. In: Webster, J.G., ed. Encyclopedia of medical devices and instrumentation, vol. 1. New York: Wiley; 1988:1-15.

87. Montoye, H.J. Estimation of habitual physical activity by questionnaire and interview. Am. J. Clin. Nutr. 24:1113-1118; 1971.

88. Åstrand, I. Aerobic work capacity in men and women with special reference to age. Acta. Physiol. Scand. 49(Suppl. 169):1-92; 1960.

89. Montoye, H.J.; Taylor H.L. Measurement of physical activity in populations studies. Hum. Biol. 56:195-216; 1984.

90. Montoye, H.J.; Servais, S.B.; Webster, J.G. Estimation of energy expenditure from a force platform and an accelerometer. In: Watkins, J.; Reilly, T.; Burwitz, L., eds. Sports science. London: Spon; 1986:375-380.

91. Montoye, H.J.; Washburn, R.; Servais, S.; Ertl, A.; Webster, J.G.; Nagle, F.J. Estimation of energy expenditure by a portable accelerometer. Med. Sci. Sports Exerc. 15:403-407; 1983.

92. Morris, J.N.; Chave, S.P.W.; Adam, C.; Sirey, C. Vigorous exercise in leisure time and incidence of coronary heart disease. Lancet. 1:333-339; 1973.

93. Murphy, J.K.; Alpert, B.S.; Christman, J.V.; Willey, E.S. Physical fitness in children: a survey method based on parental report. Am. J. Public Health. 78:708-710; 1988.

94. O'Hara, N.M.; Baranowski, T.; Simons-Morton, B.G.; Wilson, B.S.; Parcel, G.S. Validity of the observation of children's physical activity. Res. Q. Exerc. Sport. 60:4442-4447; 1989.

95. Paffenbarger, R.S., Jr.; Wing, A.L.; Hyde, R.T. Physical activity as an index of heart attack risk in college alumni. Am. J. Epidemiol. 108:161-175; 1978.

96. Parker, D.L.; Leaf, D.A.; McAfee, S.R. Validation of a new questionnaire for the assessment of leisure time physical activity. Ann. Sports Med. 4:72-81; 1988.

99. Powell, K.E.; Thompson, P.D.; Caspersen, C.J.; Kendrick, J.S. Physical activity and the incidence of coronary heart disease. Annu. Rev. Public Health. 8:253-287; 1987.

100. Puhl, J.; Hoyt, G.K.; Baranowski, T. Children's activity rating scale (CARS): Description and calibration. Res. Q. Exerc. Sport. 61:26-36; 1990.

101. Richardson, M.T. Evaluation of the Minnesota leisure time physical activity questionnaire. Minneapolis: University of Minnesota; 1991. Dissertation.

102. Roberts, S.B.; Coward, W.A.; Schlingenseipen, K.H.; Mohris, V.; Lucas, A. Comparison of the doubly labeled water ($^2H_2{}^{18}O$) method with indirect calorimetry and a nutrient-balance study for simultaneous determination of energy expenditure, water intake, and metabolizable energy intake in preterm infants. Am. J. Clin. Nutr. 44:315-322; 1986.

103. Sallis, J.F.; Buono, M.J.; Roby, J.A.; Carlson, D.; McClelland, C.; Morris, J.A. Reliability and validity of the Caltrac accelerometer as a physical activity monitor for children. Med. Sci. Sports Exerc. [Abstract]. 21:S112; 1989.

104. Sallis, J.F.; Haskell, W.L.; Wood, P.D.; Fortmann, S.P.; Rogers, T.; Blair, S.N.; Paffenbarger, R.S., Jr. Physical activity assessment methodology in the five-city project. Am. J. Epidemiol. 121:91-106; 1985.

105. Salonen, J.T.; Puska, P.; Tuomilheto, J. Physical activity and risk of myocardial impaired cerebral stroke, and death. Am. J. Epidemiol. 115:526-537; 1987.

106. Schectman, K.B.; Barzilai, B.; Rost, K.; Fisher, E.B., Jr. Measuring physical activity with a single question. Am. J. Public Health. 81:771-773; 1991.

107. Schulz, S.; Westerterp, K.R.; Brück, K. Comparison of energy expenditure by the doubly labeled water technique with energy intake, heart rate, and activity recording in man. Am. J. Clin. Nutr. 49:1146-1154; 1989.

108. Schutz, Y.; Froidevaux, F.; Jéquier, E. Estimation of 24 h energy expenditure by a portable accelerometer. Proc. Nutr. Soc. [Abstract]. 47: 23; 1988.

109. Seale, J.L.; Rumpler, W.V.; Conway, J.M.; Miles, C.W. Comparison of doubly labeled water, intake-balance and direct- and indirect-calorimetry methods for measuring energy expenditure in adult men. Am. J. Clin. Nutr. 52:66-71; 1990.

110. Servais, S.B.; Webster, J.G.; Montoye, H.J. Estimating human energy expenditure using an accelerometer device. J. Clin. Eng. 9:159-171; 1984.

111. Shapiro, S.; Weinblatt, E.; Frank, C.W.; Sager, R.V. The HIP study of incidence and prognosis of coronary heart disease. J. Chron. Dis. 18:527-558; 1965.

113. Shephard, R.J. Assessment of physical activity and energy needs. Am. J. Nutr. 50:1195-1200; 1990.

115. Sidney, S.; Jacobs, D.R., Jr.; Haskell, W.L.; Armstrong, M.A.; Dimicco, A.; Oberman, A.; Savage, P.J.; Slattery, M.L.; Sternfeld, B.; Van Horn, L. Comparison of two methods of assessing physical activity in the coronary

artery risk development in adolescents (CARDIA) study. Am. J. Epidemiol. 133:1231-1245; 1991.

116. Simons-Morton, B.G.; Huang, I.W. Heart rate monitor and Caltrac assessment of moderate-to-vigorous physical activity among preadolescent children. Med. Sci. Sports Exerc. [Abstract]. 23:S60; 1991.
117. Slater, C.H.; Green, L.W.; Vernon, S.W.; Keith, V.M. Problems in estimating the prevalence of physical activity from national surveys. Prev. Med. 16:107-118; 1987.
118. Slattery, M.L.; Jacobs, D.R., Jr. The inter-relationships of physical activity, physical fitness, and body measurements. Med. Sci. Sports Exerc. 19:564-569; 1987.
119. Slattery, M.L.; Jacobs, D.R., Jr.; Nichaman, M.Z. Leisure time physical activity and coronary heart disease death: The U.S. railroad study. Circulation. 79:304-311; 1989.
120. Sopko, G.; Jacobs, D.R., Jr., Taylor, H.L. Dietary measures of physical activity. Am. J. Epidemiol. 120:900-911; 1984.
121. Taylor, C.B.; Kraemer, H.C.; Bragg, D.A.; Miles, L.E.; Rule, R.; Savin, W.M.; DeBusk, R.F. A new system for long-term recording and processing of heart rate and physical activity in outpatients. Comput. Biomed. Res. 15:7-17; 1982.
122. Taylor, H.L.; Jacobs, D.R., Jr.; Schucker, B.; Knudsen, J.; Leon, A.S.; De Backer, G. A questionnaire for the assessment of leisure time physical activities. J. Chronic Dis. 31:741-755; 1978.
123. Verschuur, R.; Kemper, H. Habitual physical activity. Med. Sport Sci. 20:56-65; 1985.
125. Voorrips, L.E.; Ravelli, A.C.J.; Dongelmans, P.C.A.; Deurenberg, P.; Van Staveren, W.A. A physical activity questionnaire for the elderly. Med. Sci. Sports Exerc. 23:974-979; 1991.
126. Washburn, R.; Chin, M.K.; Montoye, H.J. Accuracy of pedometer in walking and running. Res. Q. Exerc. Sports. 51:695-702; 1980.
127. Washburn, R.A.; Montoye, H.J. The assessment of physical activity by questionnaire. Am. J. Epidemiol. 123:563-576; 1986.
128. Washburn, R.A.; Montoye, H.J. Validity of heart rate as a measure of mean daily energy expenditure. Exercise physiology, vol. 2. New York: AMS Press; 1986.
129. Webb, P.; Annis, J.F.; Troutman, S.J., Jr. Energy balance in man measured by direct and indirect calorimetry. Am. J. Clin. Nutr. 33:1287-1298; 1980.
130. Weiss, T.W.; Slater, C.H.; Green, L.W.; Kennedy, V.C.; Albright, D.L.; Wun, C.C. The validity of single-item self-assessment questions as measures of adult physical activity. J. Clin. Epidemiol. 43:1123-1129; 1990.
131. Welle, S. Two point vs. multipoint sample collection for the analysis of energy expenditure by use of the doubly labeled water method. Am. J. Clin. Nutr. 52:1134-1138; 1990.
132. Westerterp, K.R.; Brouns, F.; Saris, W.H.M.; Ten Hoor, F. Comparison of doubly labeled water with respirometry measurements at low- and high-activity levels. J. Appl. Physiol. 65:53-56; 1988.
133. White, C.C.; Powell, K.E.; Hogelin, G.C.; Gentry, E.M.; Forman, M.R. The behavioral risk factors survey: IV. The descriptive epidemiology of exercise. Am. J. Prev. Med. 3:304-310; 1987.
135. Williams, E.; Klesges, R.C.; Hanson, C.L.; Eck, L.H. A prospective study of the reliability and convergent validity of three physical activity measures in a field research study. J. Clin. Epidemiol. 42:1161-1170; 1989.
136. Wilson, P.W.F.; Paffenbarger, R.S.; Morris, J.N.; Havlik, R.J. Assessment methods for physical activity and physical fitness in population studies: A report of a NHLBI workshop. Am. Heart J. 111:1177-1192; 1986.

Chapter 10

Laboratory and Field Tests for Assessing Health-Related Fitness

James S. Skinner
Pekka Oja

When assessing physical fitness, it is important to identify whether the information obtained relates to performance or to health. The former refers to components that contribute to optimal job, sports, or daily performance, whereas the latter involves components related to health status. Table 10.1 contains the elements and components of health-related fitness discussed in this paper. The emphasis is on components shown by research to be related to health. As pointed out by Oja (77), health-related components are typically more universal and less activity-specific than those related to performance.

The relative importance of performance-related and health-related fitness varies with age and health status. For example, performance may be more important to healthy young men than to sedentary middle-aged persons or to those with diseases or disabilities that adversely affect their ability to exercise. Fitness for the elderly may be related to both performance and health. For example, adequate strength and balance are needed for independent living or for retention of function, as well as to avoid a higher risk of falling, which may have adverse effects on health.

Table 10.1 Components and Factors of Health-Related Fitness

Components	Factors
Morphological fitness	Body composition Bone strength
Musculoskeletal fitness	Muscular strength and endurance Flexibility
Motor fitness	Postural control
Cardiorespiratory fitness	Maximal aerobic power Submaximal cardiorespiratory capacity
Metabolic fitness	Carbohydrate metabolism Lipid metabolism

Pate (81) defines health-related fitness as a state characterized by (a) an ability to perform daily activities with vigor and (b) traits and capacities found in persons at low risk for prematurely developing diseases associated with inactivity. Within the conceptual framework of physical activity, fitness, and health, health-related fitness includes those components that have a positive effect on health, as well as those that can be improved by regular physical activity. For example, although the components listed in Table 10.1 can be influenced by genotype, age, and sex, they all adapt to physical activity and training in addition to being associated with health status. This paper will focus briefly on the evidence linking the various components with health, the types of laboratory and field tests that are used to assess each, and some research needs.

Discussion of health-related fitness and its assessment has been influenced by traditional negative concepts which define health as the absence of disease or disability. Given that there are no good definitions and few good indicators of "positive health," any discussion of health-related fitness assessment continues to be somewhat incomplete. For example, it can be argued that although muscle strength and endurance of the extremities do not directly affect health, the ability of the elderly to perform tasks requiring strength and endurance may be important for their independence and overall well-being.

Laboratory Versus Field Testing

While the administration of many health-related fitness tests may be similar in the field and in the laboratory, differences generally relate to cost, sophistication, and precision of control over extraneous factors which might affect results. For example, control of ambient temperature, humidity, and air movement can be important for laboratory tests, while field tests allow a larger variability in the environment as long as it does not significantly alter test performance or the body's physiologic responses.

Laboratory testing is generally conducted by professionally trained personnel. Because reliability and validity of the simplest self-test or group test may be questionable, specially trained personnel are also needed for field testing. A short, test-specific training course is often sufficient, however, as long as testing personnel have an adequate background.

Laboratory tests are usually done inside in space dedicated to testing, while field tests are often conducted in gymnasia, in large multipurpose rooms, and outside. Field tests usually are done with equipment available in ordinary communities and with methods accessible to and familiar to populations with an average level of education. Thus, cycle ergometers, dynamometers, and other types of equipment specially designed to measure, analyze, monitor, and record information are generally used only in the laboratory.

According to Sykes (106), the following criteria should be used to select field tests: (a) scientific quality (validity, reliability, and objectivity); (b) availability of reference values for each of the test items; (c) social acceptability and meaningfulness of the task; and (d) resource requirements. Although the same criteria are used in laboratory testing, field testing typically has more of a community or population orientation with a focus on creating interest in and awareness of exercise behavior by classifying and screening participants and by providing them with general exercise guidance.

Morphological Fitness

Body Composition

Health relationships. Most methods for assessing body composition use the two-component model of fat and fat-free tissue, with primary interest on the amount and percentage of body fat. Body fatness has health implications because of the significant association between fatness and increased risk for hyperlipidemia, hypertension, coronary heart disease (CHD), and diabetes (74). As an example, Després, Tremblay, Pérusse, Leblanc, and Bouchard (25) found a significant association between the amount of subcutaneous fat and serum HDL-cholesterol that was independent of overall obesity.

The simplest estimate of overall fatness is the body mass index (BMI) defined as the body mass in kilograms divided by (height in meters)^2. Both high and very low BMI values have been associated with a higher all-cause mortality (113). Buskirk (17) suggests that a BMI greater than 30 is associated with the point of upward deflection in the mortality curves prepared by Keys (51). Bray (9) has evaluated health risk using the BMI and other factors and found an increased health risk with a BMI greater than 25. The higher the proportion of truncal or abdominal fat, the greater was the risk. As expected, the presence of hyperlipidemia, diabetes, or hypertension further increased the risk of cardiovascular disease.

The pattern of fat distribution also has important health implications. Many studies have shown that regional body fat distribution may be a more important determinant of CHD and metabolic complications than total adiposity (24). As reviewed by Bouchard and Shephard (8), truncal-abdominal subcutaneous fat is associated with insulin resistance and high blood-insulin levels (52), more atherogenic plasma lipid and lipoprotein profiles (24), and higher blood pressure (26). Deep abdominal fat deposition is also associated with complications in lipoprotein, glucose, and insulin metabolism (24). Tremblay, Després, and Bouchard (110) showed that weight loss induced by exercise was associated with a greater mobilization of fat from the abdominal region in men. However, exercise alone had little effect on adiposity in women; this suggests gender differences in the health benefits of exercise training.

In agreement with Bouchard and Shephard (8), we feel that BMI, percent fat or fat mass, regional fat distribution (especially truncal-abdominal subcutaneous fat), and abdominal visceral fat should be measured or estimated when assessing health-related fitness.

Assessment methods. Many methods are available to assess body composition but Roche (89) concluded that none are completely accurate or valid and all need improvement. Direct assessment of body fatness is difficult without complicated analytical equipment. For example, while such laboratory techniques as neutron activation, nuclear magnetic resonance, computed tomography, whole-body ^{40}K, dual-energy absorptiometry, and isotope dilution are accurate, they are expensive and require complex instruments and highly trained technicians. Thus, while appropriate for research purposes, they are neither practical nor readily available for general fitness assessment.

Although hydrostatic weighing is less expensive, easier to perform, and considered by many the "gold standard" of indirect assessments of total body fatness, there are difficulties applying it to various groups (e.g., body fat tends to be overestimated in children and the elderly and underestimated in athletes). As well, the assumptions on which hydrostatic weighing is based may not always be valid. The reader is referred to the review by Skinner, Baldini, and Gardner (97) for more details.

More recent and practical methods for estimating total body fatness include bioelectric impedance and near-infrared (NIR) interactance. An excellent review by Baumgartner, Chumlea, and Roche (4) concluded the following about bioelectric impedance:

> The present whole-body and segment prediction equations are based on empirical and possibly fortuitous correlations. Nonetheless, these correlations have been demonstrated to be high across a range of samples with different sex, age, and ethnic compositions. Although the estimates obtained have been demonstrated generally to be accurate, this accuracy may be less for some types of individuals, especially patients with abnormal levels or distributions of body fluids. Thus, the present methods are most appropriate for epidemiologic and other field studies in which they will provide quick, easy, reliable and accurate estimates of body composition in normal individuals. (p. 218)

NIR interactance applies the principles of light absorption and reflection using NIR spectroscopy to estimate body composition. A portable, convenient, fast, noninvasive, and safe instrument called the Futrex (FTX) has made body composition assessment popular in hospitals, health clubs, and weight-loss clinics but there are questions about its validity. McLean and Skinner (66) compared skinfolds and FTX with estimates of total body fatness by hydrostatic weighing. Skinfolds correlated significantly better with hydrostatic weighing for 30 males and 31 females with a wide range of body fat. Only 52% were within 4% of their hydrostatic weighing values using the FTX, compared with 87% using skinfolds. This agrees with research findings that predictions based on skinfolds are usually within 3% to 5% of values estimated from hydrostatic weighing (62). The FTX overestimated body fat in lean subjects (less than 8% fat) and underestimated body fat in those with more than 30% fat. It was concluded that skinfolds give more information and more accurate estimates of body fat, especially at the extremes of the body fat continuum. Thus, while practical, NIR interactance is probably not accurate enough in its present form for assessing body fatness.

Although skinfold equations also have problems, skinfold thickness can be measured inexpensively and with reasonable accuracy and ease by adequately trained technicians using calipers. For an overview of some of the methodological problems, refer to the reviews by Skinner et al. (97) and by Brodie (12,13). Measuring skinfold thickness at a number of sites is the easiest way to obtain information on patterns of regional subcutaneous fat distribution. Values for each site should be compared to appropriate age and gender reference values for an adequate evaluation of their importance.

Computed axial tomography (CAT) is a reliable technique to measure the distribution and amount of subcutaneous and deep adipose tissue. Many investigators follow the general procedures described by Sjöström, Kvist, Cederblad, and Tylén (96). Because of irradiation and costs, however, CAT is not readily available. Although NIR interactance is somewhat expensive, it does not have the problem of radiation. More practical measures are needed which can give the same types of information without these inherent problems. Ferland et al. (29) used CAT to determine adipose tissue distribution and its association with body density and selected anthropometric measurements. They found a significant correlation between waist circumference and deep abdominal fat ($r = .76$). After correcting waist circumference for subcutaneous fat, however, this relationship was no longer significant, suggesting that subcutaneous and deep abdominal fat compartments expand independently. The amount of deep abdominal fat tended to level off in massively obese women, while subcutaneous fat increased at higher levels of obesity. Abdominal and subscapular skinfolds were most highly associated with deep abdominal fat. The ratio of waist girth to hip girth (WHR) was significantly correlated ($r = .49$) with deep abdominal fat but there was a large variation in deep fat at any given WHR, further suggesting an independent expansion of subcutaneous and deep abdominal fat compartments.

For practical assessment of factors involved in health-related fitness, a combination of the BMI, selected skinfolds from various regions of the body, and the WHR will provide reasonable estimates of (a) percent fat or fat mass, (b) regional fat distribution (especially truncal-abdominal subcutaneous fat), and (c) abdominal visceral fat.

Research needs. The future needs mentioned by Skinner et al. (97) in the earlier consensus can be restated, namely "more direct chemical data, simpler and more accurate indirect methods and further study of such factors as age, gender, disease and population differences are needed"(p. 112). Regarding health-related fitness, there is a need

1. to modify techniques and to develop equations and reference values for the indirect assessment of body fatness, regional fat distribution and abdominal fat.

2. to study population-specific differences in the response of total fatness, regional fat distribution and abdominal fat to such interventions as diet and exercise, as well as the impact of these interventions on health.

Bone Strength

Health relationships. In the context of health, bone strength is essentially synonymous with bone mineral density (BMD). There is a progressive loss of BMD with age. The rate of loss is higher in women (particularly after menopause) and starts at an earlier age. This loss may progress to the point of osteoporosis and a higher risk of bone fractures. There is a 12% to 20% higher mortality rate during the first 4 to 8 months after a hip fracture (73). Hip fractures are also associated with excess morbidity, because 20% of hip-fracture patients require full-time nursing care for more than 1 year (50) and only 25% regain full independence (112). Thus, osteoporosis and the associated risk of bone fractures are a major health problem in industrialized countries.

Risk factors for osteoporosis include being female, being of North European heritage, having a small or light body build, having a family history of osteoporosis, early menopause, and excessive use of alcohol and tobacco. Other factors include low estrogen levels (due to menopause, hard endurance training, or other factors), a diet deficient in calcium, and a low level of physical activity (100).

Given that there is no cure for osteoporosis and that fractures have such adverse health effects, it seems sensible to attempt to avoid the risk of fractures. Cross-sectional and prospective studies indicate that more active persons tend to have a lower risk of falls and fractures (20,57). Snow-Harter et al. (101) found a significant positive correlation between BMD and muscle strength in 59 women age 18 to 31 years. Muscle strength was an independent predictor of BMD and accounted for 15% to 20% of the total variance in BMD.

Exercise potentially lowers the risk of fractures and osteoporosis by countering bone loss, by enhancing neuromuscular abilities that help to avert falls, and by reducing the impact if a fall occurs. Although there is evidence that exercise increases peak bone mass and attenuates the loss with age, the exact dose–response relationship between exercise and BMD is not known.

Assessment methods. The most common methods to assess BMD are single-photon absorptiometry at the wrist and dual-energy absorptiometry (DPA) at the spine and hip. Dual-energy x-ray absorptiometry is more precise and produces less radiation than DPA. It can be used to accurately and reliably assess BMD of the spine, hip, extremities, and total body but is very expensive and not readily available. Quantitative computed tomography is currently limited to measures of the spine. The reader is referred to the review by Ostlere and Gold (79) for a more complete overview of these methods, as well as their advantages and disadvantages.

According to Ostlere and Gold (79), densitometry is unlikely to be a good procedure to screen for osteoporosis or to evaluate the effectiveness of its treatment. Although there is a high correlation between absolute BMD values and fractures of the hip and spine, it is not clear whether densitometry can predict the risk of future fractures. For example, almost all untreated women older than 75 years are at high risk for fractures. However, it is difficult to differentiate patients with fractures from those without fractures by measuring BMD (85). Patients with a recent hip fracture had the BMD of their contralateral hip measured using DPA. It was found that the BMD of the patients could not be distinguished from that of normal controls. One reason is the difficulty predicting BMD at one site from the BMD at another. Correlation coefficients of .4 to .7 have been reported for BMD in different bones and .8 for BMD at different sites on the same bone (36).

Given the cost of sophisticated, immobile equipment and the need for highly trained technicians to obtain useful, accurate information, densitometry will probably remain a research tool for some time to come. There are indirect, noninvasive methods to measure bone "stiffness" by low-frequency mechanical vibration (measuring resonance and impedance), ultrasonic wave propagation, and acoustic emission (22,102). While these methods are complementary to densitometry, they measure a different physical property of bone, and there have been too few studies to adequately evaluate their usefulness.

Research needs. Simpler, inexpensive methods are needed to assess bone health. Long-term prospective studies are needed to determine

1. the importance for health of bone "stiffness,"

2. the sensitivity of densitometry and the indirect methods to measure the changes in BMD and in stiffness that occur as a result of age or an intervention (e.g., exercise, hormonal replacement therapy, calcium supplements), and
3. the accuracy with which densitometric and indirect methods can predict the risk of fractures in various populations.

Musculoskeletal Fitness

Muscular Strength and Endurance

Health relationships. Although it is clear that strength and health are related, once strength falls below levels needed to accomplish daily activities, the association between strength/endurance of other muscle groups (e.g., those of the upper body) and health are poorly understood. Research on health-related muscular fitness has focused on the possible role of a lack of trunk muscle strength/endurance in the development of back, neck, and shoulder problems.

Weak trunk muscles are generally considered risk indicators of low-back pain (32,39,86). Several cross-sectional studies (49,67,75,99,104,108) have shown that patients with chronic back pain have less strength and endurance of trunk flexors and extensors during isometric and isokinetic contractions. However, these comparisons do not indicate whether the back pain is the cause or the consequence of poor muscle performance.

The predictive value of trunk muscular fitness for low-back problems has been evaluated in a few large-scale epidemiological studies. Biering-Sörensen (6) reported on a 1-year follow-up study of a representative community sample in Denmark. Isometric back endurance did predict first occurrence of low-back trouble among men but not women. In a 10-year follow-up study of metal factory employees, Leino, Aro, and Hasan (60) found that trunk extension and flexion performance at baseline explained a small but significant part of the variation in low-back status. Cady, Thomas, and Karwasky (19) showed that there were more thoracic and lumbar injuries and higher cost per injury among the least-fit fire fighters over a 10-year follow-up period. Unfortunately, strength was only one component of the measured fitness, and its independent effect cannot be assessed. Another drawback of the study was that it did not account for the notable age difference between the men with high and low levels of fitness. Battie et al. (2) studied musculoskeletal fitness and absenteeism over 4 years and found that workers with higher isometric lifting strength were actually at greater risk of future back problems than weaker workers.

A few attempts have been made to find out whether chronic back problems can be treated with muscular training. Mayer et al. (65) showed that intensive 3-week training of low-back patients greatly improved trunk strength and mobility and resulted in a better rate of return to work, less back surgery, and fewer patient visits than in a control group during a 2-year follow-up. Mellin, Hurri, Härkäpää, and Järvikoski (71,72) conducted a 3-week intensive multitreatment intervention, followed by a 3-month maintenance intervention for subjects with low-back pain. They found that the increase in lumbar and hip mobility correlated with the decrease in back pain in men and women; the increase in trunk strength showed the same correlation only in women. Similarly, the variance in back pain progress was explained more by mobility than by strength. Manniche, Benzen, Hesselsol, and Christensen (64) demonstrated in a 3-month randomized trial that (a) both modest and intensive back training improved back status, as assessed by a pain scale index during the treatment, and (b) the improvement that occurred with intensive training was retained during the 3-month follow-up.

Langrana and Lee (55) argue that low trunk-extension strength may be a better predictor of low-back trouble than low trunk-flexion strength because the psoas muscle adds 50% to the flexion strength of the back. Suzuki and Endo (104) suggest that the relative contribution of trunk-flexion strength excluding the psoas is not important for preventing low-back pain. Beimborn and Morrissey (5) use the ratio of trunk extension to flexion strength as the measure of trunk strength.

Repetitive loading of spinal tissue by lifting, bending, prolonged standing, or sitting fatigues spinal tissue and may predispose individuals to low-back pain. Thus, frequent overstress might be just as damaging to the back as occasional peak stresses (59). Deficient endurance of the trunk flexors (104) and extensors (6,49,59,86) has been associated with low-back trouble. Jörgensen and Nicolaisen (49) suggest that individuals with poor endurance of the back muscles are more exposed to postural stress, which may lead to incorrect spinal loading and consequently to low-back trouble.

Several mechanisms may be responsible for the possible health-protective effect of trunk strength and endurance. Due to a greater perfusion of the active fibers of strong muscles, there would be less local ischemia and fatigue for a given absolute force of muscle contraction (8). Another possible mechanism links the strength of the abdominal muscles to the strength of the erector spinae fascia (82). Because the abdominal oblique muscles insert into the fascia of the erector spinae, strong oblique muscles reinforce the erector spinae fascia and support the spinae, resulting in less strain on the back extensor muscles. Accordingly, Plowman (82) states that "the key abdominal muscles for low back health may be the internal and external obliques as opposed to the rectus abdominis itself" (p. 228) and speculates that fiber type composition of the back muscles may determine one's susceptibility to low-back pain. That is, an individual with predominantly slow-twitch fibers may be at risk of injury due to intense peak loads. Conversely, extended low-intensity work loads may be detrimental for those with a high percent of fast-twitch fibers.

In view of the available literature, strength and endurance of the trunk and supportive muscles may be associated with the development of low-back problems. However, the evidence is inconclusive and no unified view exists regarding the specific role of extensors versus flexors or strength versus endurance. Therefore, when assessing muscular fitness of the trunk, it seems prudent to measure both strength and endurance of the flexors and extensors.

Strength/endurance of the arms and legs also should be considered, because they may contribute to spinal health by facilitating normal function of the trunk muscles. Although there is no evidence of direct effects of strength and endurance of the extremities on health, it is obvious that decreased strength limits daily activity (18). There is evidence that both healthy and frail older adults preserve the trainability of skeletal muscle performance and thus have the potential to retain functional independence and well-being as they age (14).

Assessment methods. As summarized by Skinner et al. (97), laboratory assessment of muscle strength and endurance must consider the various types of contractions. Isometric strength is usually assessed by cable tensiometers for isolated muscle groups across a single joint or by dynamometers for large muscle groups. Maximal voluntary contraction (MVC) strength is often assessed isometrically because the forces are easy to measure. Modern dynamometers (e.g., Cybex, Orthotron, and Kin-Com) are computerized and can assess most major muscle groups.

Isotonic strength is assessed by the maximal weight lifted once by a muscle group (i.e., the one-repetition maximum or 1 RM). Because progressively heavier weights are lifted until the maximum is reached, the subjectivity in determining the number of trials needed may vary greatly and the ensuing fatigue may influence the outcome. Maximal isotonic contractions are limited by the lowest maximal force obtained at any joint angle throughout the range of movement. In contrast, isokinetic devices allow the maximal force to be exerted and measured throughout the range of motion under relatively constant velocity.

Muscular endurance may be expressed in absolute or relative terms. The assessment can be made with isometric, isokinetic, or isotonic contractions. The ability to hold an isometric contraction depends on the percent MVC applied. Over time, maximal tension drops and a characteristic fatigue curve is found. With isometric contractions above 60% MVC, there is occlusion of blood vessels to the muscle and the fatigue curve drops more steeply. Electromyography can be used to assess muscular fatigue by observing the increased muscle electrical activity during a constant isometric tension. One can also measure the recovery of force production at given percentages of maximal force following fatigue or the drop in isometric holding time after a given recovery period.

For a more complete review on the laboratory methods for assessing trunk muscle performance the reader is referred to the review of Beimborn and Morrissey (5).

Different curl-up protocols have been used to assess abdominal strength and endurance in the field. Subjects lie supine with knees bent at 90° to 140°, feet on the floor supported or unsupported, and the head in contact with the ground. Hands are free and directed towards the knees along the thighs or the ground (28) or interlocked behind the neck with the elbows contacting the thighs during the curl (84,92,115).

Dynamic endurance of abdominal muscles is usually assessed by the maximal number of curl-up repetitions, either with a time limit of 30 or 60 sec (1,46,115) or with a maximal limit of 100 to 120 repetitions (28,84). Isometric abdominal muscular endurance has been studied by holding the curl-up position for up to 240 sec, with time given every 30 sec (42).

The couch method (48,49) has been used to study isometric trunk extensor endurance. Subjects lie prone on a couch with their buttocks and legs fixed. The unsupported upper body is kept horizontal by the trunk extensors until exhaustion or until 240 sec. Viljanen, Viitasalo, and Kujala (115) measured dynamic short-term anaerobic strength production by repetition of trunk extensors from 50° of flexion to full extension.

Table 10.2 summarizes the studies on adults that have examined the validity, reliability, and other qualities of the trunk muscle field tests. Correlation coefficients of .92 (test-retest), .93 (intraobserver), and .90 (interobserver) have been reported for

Table 10.2 Assessment of Trunk Muscle Performance: Field Tests

Source	Subjects	Tests	Validity	Reliability	Other
Mälkiä (63)	1,110 M + W, 30–65 years; random sample of Finnish population	1. Abdominal dynamic endurance, 30 s, sit-up 2. Back dynamic endurance, 30 s, back extension		1-year test-retest; *r*: abdomen = .92, back = .82	
Jörgensen & Nicolaisen (48)	53 M, 27–60 years + 23 W, 22–61 years	1. Back isometric endurance, max 240 s, "the couch method" 2. Back isometric endurance at 60% MVC, "the pulling test"		2-week test-retest; *r*: couch = .89, pull = .82; coefficient of variation: couch = .19, pull = .24	Distribution: couch skewed, pull normal; omit 240 s limit in couch
Hyytiäinen et al. (42)	30 M, 35–44 years	1. Abdominal isometric endurance, max 240 s, curl-up 2. Back isometric endurance, max 240 s, "the couch method" 3. Abdominal dynamic strength, qualitative curl-up, 6 grades		1. Intraobserver reliability; *r*: Test 1 = .93, Test 2 = .74; Kappa = .57 for Test 3 2. Interobserver reliability; *r*: Test 1 = .90, Test 2 = .80; Kappa = .78 for Test 3 3. 1-week test-retest; means: no intraobserver differences, significant interobserver difference for back endurance	

Smidt et al. (98)	Normal 38 M, 25 years + 43 W, 25 years; back patients 21 M, 33 years	1. Qualitative sit-up, 4 grades 2. Qualitative double leg lowering, 5 grades 3. Qualitative prone trunk extension, 4 grades	Criterion measure—maximal trunk flexor and extensor torque by Kin-Com testing system: little differences in mean torques of grades for Tests 1 and 3; significant differences in mean torques of extreme grades for Test 2		
Faulkner et al. (28)	126 M + 136 W, 18–69 years	1. Curl-up, fingers reach patella 2. Curl-up, fingers slide 12 cm on mat (both 20 reps/min, max 120 reps)		2-3 day test-retest; consistency better for Test 1	Skewed distributions in both tests: 25% of young men do the max, majority of old can't do one; 10–20% had posttest pain

Note. M = men, W = women, MVC = maximal voluntary contraction.

different sit-up/curl-up protocols. Faulkner, Springings, and McQuarrie (28) found better test-retest consistency for fingers-to-patella than for fingers-on-mat curl-up; both tests had skewed distributions.

For the couch test of back muscles, studies have yielded test-retest correlation coefficients of .82 and .89, an intraobserver coefficient of .80, and an interobserver coefficient of .74. According to Jörgensen and Nicolaisen (48), the coefficient of variation (19%) for the couch method is modest. Hyytiäinen, Salminen, Suvitie, Wickström, and Pentti (42) found significant interobserver difference between test-retest means of the isometric endurance test.

Little attention has been given to the validity of the trunk muscle tests. Smidt, Blanpied, Anderson, and White (98) found little difference in criterion mean torques between qualitative grades of sit-up and couch test, whereas the extreme grades of the double leg-lowering test were significantly different. The authors concluded that these tests are poor discriminators of strength ability.

Posttest pain has been used to evaluate the appropriateness of curl-up tests (28). Subjects completing more curl-ups had a greater incidence of posttest pain. All subjects who experienced pain reported that it disappeared after a few days. The authors recommend (a) reducing the maximum from 240 sec to 120 sec to reduce the risk of post-exercise pain and (b) decreasing the reach distance for subjects older than 45 years because many older subjects could not complete a single curl-up.

Flexibility

Health realtionships. General flexibility is believed to be important for health, especially for independence in older adults. Trunk flexibility may have health implications for back, neck, and shoulder problems. Although flexibility has been defined more as a health-related fitness component than a performance-related one, it may be considered important for both components for most individuals (94).

Static flexibility refers to the degree to which a joint can be passively moved. Dynamic flexibility refers to the degree to which a joint can be moved as a result of muscular contraction and is the ability to move a joint quickly with little resistance (94). Flexibility is generally joint-specific and can be influenced by specific training (37,105).

Restricted spinal mobility is considered a risk factor for low-back disability (32,86), although relatively few studies have examined the role of thoracolumbar and lumbar mobility in the prevention of low-back disability. In a large 4-year longitudinal study, Battie et al. (2) studied aircraft manufacturing employee reports of back pain. Subjects were tested for lumbosacral, shoulder, and overall trunk flexion. While subjects of both genders with a history of back problems initially had slightly less mobility in all measurements (except for lumbar mobility in women), there was no association between flexibility and subsequent low-back pain. Burton, Tillotson, and Troup (15) cross-sectionally examined the relationship between low-back pain and lumbar mobility in persons aged 10 to 84 years. Results suggested that decreased lumbar mobility was not a prerequisite for low-back pain.

Other longitudinal and cross-sectional studies have found correlations between spinal mobility and low-back pain. For example, Biering-Sörensen (6) showed that diminished lumbar mobility in women, but not in men, was of some predictive value for the recurrence or persistence of low-back trouble. Mellin (70) studied thoracolumbar and lumbar mobility in low-back patients age 35 to 55 years. Thoracolumbar mobility correlated better with low-back pain than did lumbar mobility. Lateral flexion and rotation correlated more strongly with low-back pain than did measurements in the sagittal plane, with the exception of lateral rotation in women. Burton et al. (16) found in volunteers from 10 occupational groups that reduced lumbar extension was predictive of low-back trouble in men and that upper-lumbar flexibility was related to less chronicity of low-back pain in women.

In an intervention by Mellin (70), relations between spinal and lumbar mobility and low-back pain were examined among war veterans who suffered from chronic or recurrent low-back trouble. Treatment lasted 3 weeks and included heat and electrotherapy, massage, educational classes for low-back pain, as well as physical and back exercises. Although thoracolumbar lateral flexion and rotation, as well as lumbar flexion and extension mobility correlated significantly with low-back trouble, only thoracolumbar lateral flexion and rotation mobility correlated significantly with progress during treatment. In a later rehabilitation study by Mellin, Hurri, Härkäpää, and Järvikoski (71), the increase in lumbar and hip mobility was more important for subjective progress than the increase in trunk strength.

Several observational cross-sectional studies have found that poor thoracolumbar and/or lumbar mobility is related to an increased risk of back problems. A few observational follow-up studies have looked at the predictive role of spinal mobility in development of new back problems or in progress of existing problems. No firm conclusions about spinal mobility and spinal health can be made because of inconsistent results in the observational studies and nonexistence of randomized trials.

Assessment methods. Flexibility assessment has been reviewed in detail earlier (23,30,40,68). According to Skinner et al. (97), flexibility is easy to measure and requires a minimal amount of equipment (e.g., goniometers, fleximeters, anthropometers, tape measures, measuring sticks, and calipers). Electrogoniometers, photogoniometers, and radiogoniometers have also been used. For health-related assessment, simple methods that can be used in field conditions are often sufficient.

Spinal range-of-motion measurements are a standard part of clinical evaluations of patients with back pain and are extensively used to evaluate permanent impairment in individuals with long-standing back problems (3). The modified Schober test is the most widely used clinical test of spinal flexion. With the subject standing erect a mark is placed at the lumbosacral junction. After marks are placed 5 cm below and 10 cm above the lumbosacral junction, the subject bends forward as rapidly as possible. Lumbar flexion is expressed as the difference between this measurement and the initial distance of 15 cm (3). Side bending of the trunk, as measured with a tape measure, is a reproducible measure that is quick and easy to use and measures lateral mobility of the pelvis, lumbar and thoracic spine.

In the stand-and-reach test, fingertip-to-floor distance is measured while subjects maintain a fully flexed posture with heels on the floor, feet together or at shoulder width, and knees extended. Biering-Sörensen (6) found that fingertip-to-floor distance for both genders was significantly related to hamstring muscle length. Thus, this measure is a combined evaluation of hamstring tightness and spinal flexibility. The sit-and-reach test has traditionally been used in flexibility evaluations (1,46). With knees fully extended in a sitting position, subjects bend slowly forward with arms and fingers extended. Reach distance is then read, with zero being foot level. Similar to the stand-and-reach test, the sit-and-reach test is a measure of hamstring flexibility (44,45) and is therefore not an optimal measure of spinal mobility. The straight-leg raise is another flexibility test, which primarily measures hamstring flexibility (10).

Table 10.3 summarizes studies on the validity and reliability of trunk mobility tests. Forward-bending tests (stand-and-reach, sit-and-reach, modified Schober) yield high (.82 to .98) coefficients of test-retest, intertester, and intratester consistency. Coefficients of variation indicate low variability (1% to 5%) for the modified Schober but greater variability (14%) for the stand-and-reach test. On the other hand, Biering-Sörensen (6) found a statistically significant difference between test-retest means for the modified Schober test.

Based on reliability coefficients between .70 and .96, lateral bending is also a consistent test, although Rose (90) argues that the intratester least significant difference of 3 to 4 cm is unsatisfactory. According to Mellin (69), the segmental intercorrelation of tape and inclinometric assessments of lateral bending is best for the thoracolumbar segment.

The reliability coefficients for the straight-leg raise vary from .32 to .81. Shoulder mobility has been evaluated only by Battie, Bigos, Sheeky, and Wortley (3), who found that the test correlated better with sit-and-reach and side bending than with the modified Schober. Such mobility tests as trunk rotation and prone knee-bending have been studied by Frost, Stuckey, Smalley, and Dorman (31); reliability coefficients were low for the former and medium to high for the latter.

Because back function is central to health-related musculoskeletal fitness, a relevant test battery for the most important functional components is needed. Plowman (82) identified five critical areas of back function: (a) flexibility of the low back, (b) flexibility of the hamstrings, (c) flexibility of the hip flexors, (d) strength of the abdominal and lateral trunk muscles, and (e) strength and endurance of the trunk extensors. Her proposed test battery includes: graded sit-ups or partial curls, hip-flexor flexibility, lateral-trunk lift, trunk-extension endurance, and straight-leg raise or sit-and-reach.

Many computerized devices and protocols specific to muscle groups and contraction types can accurately and reliably assess strength and endurance of trunk flexors and extensors, as well as spinal mobility in the laboratory. For field assessment several curl-up protocols for trunk flexor strength and endurance, couch protocols for extensor strength and endurance, and trunk-bending protocols for mobility are reasonably reliable. However, the validity and feasibility of many of these tests have not been adequately studied.

Research needs.

1. More studies, especially well-controlled, randomized trials, are needed to firmly establish the relationship between musculoskeletal fitness and physical function or other aspects of health.
2. Criterion norms of trunk muscle strength and endurance and trunk mobility for different subpopulations are needed, especially in older adults.
3. Standardized, feasible, and safe field tests of back muscle strength/endurance and flexibility are needed.

Table 10.3 Assessment of Trunk Mobility: Field Tests

Source	Subjects	Tests	Validity	Reliability
Frost et al. (31)	12 M + 12 W, 20–55 years	1. Forward bending 2. Backward bending 3. Side bending 4. Rotation 5. Straight-leg raising 6. Prone knee-bending (3 testers, 3 measurements, 1-week test-retest)		r for day, tester, repetition, tester × day, tester × day × repetition: Test 1 = .98–.82, Test 2 = .79–.45, Test 3 = .91–.70, Test 4 = .13–.11, Test 5 = .68–.32, Test 6 = .82–.55
Biering-Sørensen (6)	127 M + W, 30–60 years; population sample	1. Modified Schober 2. Fingertip-to-floor 3. Length of hamstrings (6-month test-retest)	Intercorrelations: 1 vs. 2 = significant 1 vs. 3 = NS, 2 vs. 3 = significant	Coefficient of variation: Test 1 = 4.8% Difference of test-retest means: Test 1 = significant, Test 2 = NS, Test 3 = NS
Mellin (69)	39 healthy volunteers	1. Lateral bending, tape 2. Lateral bending, inclinometer (2 testers, 2-day test-retest)	Intercorrelations: pelvic = .40, thoracic = .30, lumbar = .48–.58, thoracolumbar = .58–.64	Test-retest r: intraobserver = .76–.96 interobserver = .85–.87
Battie et al. (3)	235 M + 670 W, 21–67 years; aircraft manufacturing employees	1. Shoulder flexibility 2. Modified Schober 3. Sit-and-reach 4. Side bending	Intercorrelations: 1 vs. 3 vs. 4 = .38–.44; 2 vs. 1 vs. 3 vs. 4 = .15–.24	
Gill et al. (35)	5 M + 5 W, 24–33 years	1. Fingertip-to-floor 2. Modified Schober 3. 2-inclinometer 4. Photometric (10-min test-retest)		Coefficient of variation: Test 1 = 14.1, Test 2 = 0.9–4.2, Test 3 = 1.7–33.9, Test 4 = 0.7–22.3
Gauvin et al. (33)	44 M + 26 W, 18–73 years; low-back patients	1. Fingertip-to-floor (2 testers, immediate test-retest)		Interclass correlation coefficient: intratester = .98, intertester = .95
Hyytiäinen et al. (42)	30 M, 35–44 years; shipyard employees	1. Fingertip-to-floor 2. Modified Schober 3. Straight-leg raising 4. Side bending (4 testers, 1-week test-retest)		Intratester r: Test 1 = .93, Test 2 = .88, Test 3 = .80–.81, Test 4 = .82–.87; intertester r: Test 1 = .96, Test 2 = .87, Test 3 = .52–.55, Test 4 = .84–.88
Rose (90)	3 M + 15 W, 19.5 years; physiotherapy students	1. Side bending (1 tester, 3-week test-retest)		Intertester r: .89–.78 Intratester least significant difference (LSD): 3.0–4.0 cm

Note. M = men, W = women, NS = not significant.

4. Validity, feasibility, safety, and subject acceptability of most field tests of musculoskeletal fitness should be studied in different populations.

Motor Fitness

Health relationships. Although the speed and agility components of motor fitness appear to have minor importance with respect to health, balance and coordination may have health consequences as determinants of postural control. Poor gait and balance are among the risk factors that predispose older individuals, particularly postmenopausal osteoporotic women, to falls that may lead to bone fractures (93).

Johansson (47) described postural control as a combination of balance and coordination, psychic control, and neuromuscular speed. Postural control is the manner in which the nervous system (a) activates muscles with optimal tension in different postures and movements and (b) maintains the center of body mass over its base of support against external perturbations. Johansson (47) suggests that postural control is diminished in patients with chronic back and neck pain when compared with healthy controls. Patients had a significantly shorter endurance time in certain posture tests. Accentuated equilibrium reactions and associated movements, as well as disturbances in coordination, were more common also among patients.

An eyes-open, unipedal balance index was found to be sensitive to fitness training (103) and to distinguish elderly nonfallers from fallers (34). Chandler, Duncan, and Studenski (21) confirmed findings that elderly fallers scored significantly lower on the postural stress test than young adults or nonfalling elderly persons. As there were no differences in balance strategy scores between young adults and healthy elderly subjects, poor performance cannot be attributed to age alone, but may be predictive of a pathological process that predisposes an individual to frequent falls.

Ring, Nayak, and Isaacs (88) administered the visual push test in elderly recent fallers, remote fallers, and nonfallers. They found that the mean amplitude of displacements was greater among fallers than nonfallers and that the mean sway path was greater in previous fallers than in recent fallers and nonfallers.

According to Oddsson (76), the high priority of postural control to the central nervous system has an implication for back injuries. Some injuries occur as a result of slips and falls which are apparently related to postural control. During fatigue, diminished control and coordination, along with reduced accuracy and speed of contraction, produce movement patterns that predispose an individual to back injury (80). Videman et al. (114) studied patient-handling skills, back injuries, and back pain in nurses and found that poor patient handling skill predisposed a nurse to back injury. Special training can improve these skills (111).

There is some evidence suggesting that the postural control component of motor fitness is related to musculoskeletal health by promoting spinal health and by decreasing the risk of falls which may lead to bone fractures. However, available results are at best sufficient for forming new hypotheses to study more exactly the possible relationships between motor fitness and health.

Assessment methods. Postural control is a complex phenomenon and cannot be evaluated with global measures of "balance." The integrity of the basic functional components (biomechanical, motor coordination, sensory organization) of the postural control system should be determined (41). The measurement of postural movement strategies ideally should include assessment of postural responses to external perturbations (expected and unexpected), voluntary center-of-body mass adjustments, and postural adjustments preceding voluntary limb movements (41).

Because of its complexity, assessment of postural control may require different approaches and methods. None of the present methods provides a sufficiently complete impression of the phenomenon. Laboratory analysis of gait and posture can be done using computerized kinematic or biomechanical force platform systems. These systems provide information on ground reaction forces and velocities, angular velocities, step characteristics, and so on. The utility of these types of analyses for assessing postural control has not been fully explored.

Clinically oriented tests of sway, balance, and gait appear useful for assessing postural control. In the original Rhomberg's test, subjects stand feet together with eyes open and then closed while the tester observes body sway. The Sharpened Rhomberg test and the one-legged stance test are later modifications. Wolfson, Whipple, Amerman, and Kleinerg (117) proposed a postural stress test to study activation of the balance reactions under varying environmental stimuli. In this test static balance is perturbed by gradually increasing destabilizing forces applied at the waist. Another version is the visual push-test (87) in which visual stimuli are varied while subjects stand on a force platform. Tinetti (109) designed a "performance-oriented evaluation of balance and gait" based on the performance of ordinary physical tasks requiring postural control.

Johansson (47) evaluated 16 field tests that assess postural control using patients with chronic back and neck pain. Qualitative observations of the total movement pattern and accentuated equilibrium reactions were determined. Four tests were best for assessing postural control in clinical situations: (a) "ski walking" (alternating long steps with reciprocal arm pendulum movements) 15 steps in a row (5 left, 5 right, 5 left), (b) the one-leg balance test in 20 sec, with the other foot positioned halfway up the calf of the supporting leg, (c) the one-leg balance test with slow neck rotation to the left and right, and (d) walking backwards 15 steps between two lines 20 cm apart. Most norm-referenced tests of balance measure the time subjects can maintain a particular equilibrium position. In these tests, visual inputs are reduced by eye closure (7,11,34,43,47,103). Somatosensory inputs are altered or reduced when subjects stand on one foot, stand on narrow rails, or stand with one foot in front of the other.

Bohannon, Larkin, Cook, Gear, and Singer (7) studied 184 people age 20 to 79 years. The one-leg balance was held longer with eyes open than with eyes closed. Similarly, more subjects failed to balance for 30 sec with eyes closed than with eyes open. The average balance time on one leg and the percentage of subjects balancing for 30 s diminished with age.

According to Stones and Kozma (103), the eyes-open test was more reliable ($r = .68$) than the eyes-closed test ($r = .32$). The eyes-open index had a higher age dependency and greater validity, evidenced by significantly higher relationships with respiratory functions and a significant improvement after subjects enrolled in a formal exercise program. Among noninstitutionalized elderly men, Iverson, Gossman, Shaddeau, and Turner (43) showed that the eyes-open balance test was activity dependent. Briggs, Gossman, Birch, Drews, and Shaddeau (11) demonstrated that foot dominance and wearing or not wearing shoes had no effect on balance time with the eyes open or closed.

The assessment of postural control is a complex task and its complete determination may require several approaches using kinematic and biomechanical methods. Nevertheless, relatively simple clinical tests of sway, balance, and gait are widely used to analyze postural control and may be useful when assessing health-related motor fitness.

Research needs.

1. More research is needed to establish the relationship between motor fitness and health in general and to identify the important health-related components of motor fitness.
2. The scientific quality (validity, reliability, and feasibility) of the present tests of postural control need to be assessed and new tests developed.

Cardiorespiratory Fitness

Health relationships. A key element of health-related fitness is cardiorespiratory fitness. It has been consistently shown that aerobic activity and cardiorespiratory fitness have important positive effects on cardiovascular health (61,83,116). Whether activity and fitness exert their effect in combination or independently remains an important challenge for more research (38). The role of endurance exercise and cardiorespiratory fitness in the prevention of hypertension, noninsulin dependent diabetes, and obesity is also gaining increasing support (8,116).

The two health-related factors of cardiorespiratory fitness are maximal aerobic power ($\dot{V}O_2max$) and the ability to perform prolonged submaximal exercise (submaximal cardiorespiratory capacity). $\dot{V}O_2max$ is the only objective measure of cardiorespiratory fitness and it, or a related measure, has been used almost exclusively in studies of exercise, fitness, and cardiovascular health. It has been argued that cardiovascular capacity or efficiency during submaximal work may also be important as a health-related component of cardiorespiratory fitness (8). It is possible that the positive effect of exercise on all or most of the mentioned disease states is mediated through a common metabolic adaptation to submaximal exercise (38).

For example, although there is no direct evidence that the ability to perform submaximal exercise is related to health, one has to do endurance exercise training to improve the ability to do maximal and submaximal exercise. As a result, this repeated endurance training may have a positive effect on various risk factors. Therefore, it is important to differentiate between maximal and submaximal components of cardiorespiratory fitness and to devise and select assessment methods for both. Although $\dot{V}O_2max$ is conceptually and methodologically unambiguous, the exact characteristics of submaximal cardiorespiratory capacity need to be defined and appropriate assessment methods need to be developed. It may be that the ability to perform prolonged submaximal exercise at a high intensity is an important ability in this regard (8,97).

Assessment methods. The traditional objective measurement of maximal cardiorespiratory fitness is $\dot{V}O_2max$. Laboratory assessment usually requires treadmills or cycle ergometers (i.e., apparatus involving rhythmic, dynamic exercise with a large muscle mass) that can be standardized for reproducible measurements and that are capable of maximally stressing the systems for transporting and utilizing oxygen. For the direct assessment of $\dot{V}O_2max$, gas analysis equipment is needed. The reader is referred to the review by Skinner et al. (97) for more details.

Various work protocols that consider individual differences in working capacity have been developed. Nevertheless, if the criteria for obtaining a maximal value have been met, there is little or no difference among protocols.

Except for research purposes, there is probably little reason to do maximal exercise tests with middle-aged and older adults. Thomas, Cunningham, Rechnitzer, Donner, and Howard (107) found test–retest reliability coefficients of .7 to .9 for three treadmill protocols with men aged 55 to 68 years. Although higher $\dot{V}O_2max$ values were found when tests were repeated, only one third of the men reached a plateau in $\dot{V}O_2max$; this raises more doubts about the value of and the need for maximal tests. A better approach might be to estimate maximal aerobic power from submaximal tests so that more people can be evaluated with less risk. As stated by Oja (77), maximal tests should be used primarily to evaluate athletic performance.

Two practical questions arise, however. Most submaximal tests determine heart rate (HR) at several levels of $\dot{V}O_2$ or power output (PO). By extrapolating the linear relationship between HR and either $\dot{V}O_2$ or PO to an individual's known or estimated maximal HR, the maximal $\dot{V}O_2$ or PO can be predicted. However, because of the large variation in maximal HR (95) and the concern about approaching or going to maximum, how does one select the correct maximal HR to which one should extrapolate? Similarly, if older persons are limited by muscular weakness and either cannot or will not push themselves to maximal levels of $\dot{V}O_2$, of what practical significance are these "maximal" values to their health, well-being, and independence?

There are tests to assess submaximal cardiorespiratory fitness but many are more closely associated with performance than with health. For example, there are tests which purport to measure the maximal amount of work than can be sustained for a prolonged period (97). Measures related to thresholds of anaerobic metabolism may be useful to evaluate the efficiency of the peripheral utilization of oxygen.

In the context of health, perhaps one should measure the cardiorespiratory responses to standard levels of work; these intensities should be at least moderate (50% to 70% $\dot{V}O_2max$), as defined by Bouchard and Shephard (8). Submaximal tests of progressively increasing intensity to some fixed end point (e.g., a known HR or onset of predetermined signs and symptoms) could provide useful information.

A variety of traditional and new laboratory techniques are available to assess cardiorespiratory fitness but the development of tools for field testing requires the reevaluation of old methods and the creation of new ones. Several valid and reliable indirect field tests of $\dot{V}O_2max$ are available. According to Oja, Laukkanen, Pasanen, Tyry, and Vuori (78), the correlation coefficient of measured and estimated $\dot{V}O_2max$ on the Canadian Home Fitness Test and the Cooper 12-min walk-run test was .91 and .90, respectively. The Åstrand-Ryhming nomogram had a standard deviation of less than 6.7% for men and 9.6% for women for two thirds of the original subjects. Recently, walking tests of 1 mile (53) and 2 km (78) have been developed to estimate $\dot{V}O_2max$ in the field. Both tests have good prediction validity (greater than 0.85) and test–retest reliability (greater than 0.90), as well as reasonably good cross-validity in different population groups. The feasibility of the latter test has also been evaluated and was acceptable for population assessment (56).

Research on the interrelationships between cardiorespiratory fitness and health has a long tradition. Although the evidence suggesting a protective effect of cardiorespiratory fitness on health is quite convincing, a well-controlled randomized trial providing a "definite" answer remains to be done. The importance of submaximal cardiorespiratory fitness is drawing increasing attention and may prove to be critical. Many valid and reliable traditional and new methods for the indirect assessment of $\dot{V}O_2max$ are available. New walking tests provide feasible tools for population assessment. The exact physiological characteristics of submaximal cardiorespiratory fitness need to be defined and specific assessment methods need to be developed.

Research needs.

1. Controlled, randomized trials are needed to firmly establish the relationships between cardiorespiratory fitness (maximal and submaximal components) and various components of health.
2. The conceptual and physiological meaning of these components and their possible health relationships need to be established.

3. There are no good tests of submaximal cardiorespiratory fitness within the context of health-related fitness and such tests need to be developed for both laboratory and field assessment.

Metabolic Fitness

Health relationships. According to Bouchard and Shephard (8), metabolic fitness "results from adequate hormonal actions, particularly for insulin, normal blood and tissue carbohydrate and lipid metabolism. A high ratio of lipid to carbohydrate oxidized also seems to be a desirable trait" (p. 18).

Recently, Kohl, Gordon, Villegas, and Blair (54) found that the risk of death increases with less favorable glycemic status and that cardiorespiratory fitness may attenuate the effects of impaired carbohydrate metabolism on mortality from all causes. Exercise programs of low intensity and long duration have been shown to improve the control of blood sugar, especially in those with poor control (27). Whether this is due to an acute or chronic effect of exercise is unclear. However, it is known that glucose levels, glucose metabolism, and insulin metabolism are improved with regular exercise, even though the exercise intensity may be too low to increase $\dot{V}O_2$max. Similarly, regular activity favorably affects lipid metabolism, resulting in lower levels of total cholesterol, LDL-cholesterol and triglycerides, and higher levels of HDL-cholesterol (118).

The ratio of lipid to carbohydrate oxidized (respiratory quotient or RQ) at rest and during submaximal exercise seems to be an indicator of metabolic efficiency. Zurlo et al. (119) found that the lower the RQ, the higher the metabolism of lipids. The RQ at rest was inversely related to the amount of fat and weight gained over many months. Leaf (58) suggests that the lower the RQ and the faster a person can lower the RQ during steady-state exercise below the anaerobic threshold, the better is that person's ability to perform prolonged submaximal exercise, and thus, the better his or her "fitness."

One reason why the RQ is lower during a standard submaximal exercise bout is that the same absolute power output represents a lower intensity relative to the higher $\dot{V}O_2$max in trained individuals. In addition, endurance athletes tend to work at higher relative intensities before they reach the threshold where the oxidation of carbohydrates begins to increase (91).

Assessment methods. While it is logical to assume that regular endurance exercise, a greater capacity to perform higher intensities of submaximal exercise, and possibly a high $\dot{V}O_2$max are closely interrelated and are components of metabolic fitness, there are no standardized exercise tests to measure this factor. Although the concept of metabolic fitness makes intuitive sense, there is no consensus about a definition that might include many other factors (e.g., other hormones or substrates) or how all these factors should be measured and applied to health-related fitness. While there are standardized procedures for measuring (a) fasting blood glucose, (b) glucose and insulin responses to a glucose load, (c) fasting blood lipid and lipoprotein profiles, and (d) RQ at rest and during exercise, there are no recognized exercise tests or protocols to evaluate these responses and levels so that their relevance to health could be studied.

Research needs.

1. The conceptual definition of metabolic fitness should be clarified and extended.
2. Protocols for standardized tests of metabolic fitness need to be developed so that cross-sectional and longitudinal studies can be carried out relative to glycemic control, lipid and lipoprotein profiles, and the ratio of lipid to carbohydrate oxidation.
3. Other physiological and biochemical factors which might be involved in metabolic fitness should be explored.

Conclusions

Most of the current methods for assessing fitness have evolved in the context of performance-related fitness. Their usefulness as measures of health-related fitness has not been systematically evaluated. With the exception of maximal cardiorespiratory fitness, the scientific bases of assessment methodology still need to be developed. Research in this area needs to address the technical aspects (e.g., repeatability, safety, feasibility, and cost-effectiveness of individual test items), as well as the validity and reliability of the concept of health-related fitness and its components.

Research is also needed to distinguish between performance-related *norms* (with such descriptors as below average, average, above average) which are used to classify people, and health-related *criterion standards* (with such descriptors as undesirable, minimal, acceptable, desirable) which are useful for screening, guidance, and encouragement. It should be remembered that most adults do not need to be tested. Instead, they need information about (a) minimal and desirable levels of the various aspects of health-related fitness required for good health and independence and (b) the amount and types of exercise needed to reach these levels. Unfortunately, little is known about the minimal levels of the different components that are needed for various populations, age groups, or health states.

Acknowledgments

We acknowledge the valuable contribution of Jaana Suni for compiling and organizing parts of the original material.

References

1. Balogun, J.A. Assessment of physical fitness of female physical therapy students. J. Orthop. Sports Phys. Ther. 8:525-532; 1987.
2. Battie, M.C.; Bigos, S.J.; Fisher, L.D.; Spengler, D.M.; Hansson, T.H.; Nachemson, A.L.; Wortley, M. The role of spinal flexibility in back pain complaints within industry. Spine. 15:768-773; 1990.
3. Battie, M.C.; Bigos, S.J.; Sheehy, A.; Wortley, M. Spinal flexibility and individual factors that influence it. Phys. Ther. 67:653-658; 1987.
4. Baumgartner, R.N.; Chumlea, W.C.; Roche, A.F. Bioelectric impedance for body composition. In Pandolf, K.; Holloszy, J.O., eds. Exercise and sport sciences reviews. Baltimore: Williams & Wilkins; 1990:193-224.
5. Beimborn, D.; Morrissey, M. A review of the literature related to trunk muscle performance. Spine. 13:655-660; 1988.
6. Biering-Sørensen, F. Physical measurements as risk indicators for low-back trouble over a one-year period. Spine. 9:106-119; 1984.
7. Bohannon, R.W.; Larkin, P.A.; Cook, A.C.; Gear, J.; Singer, J. Decrease in timed balance scores with aging. Phys. Ther. 64:1067-1070; 1984.
8. Bouchard, C.; Shephard, R.J. Physical activity, fitness and health: The model and key concepts. In Bouchard, C.; Shephard, R.J.; Stephens, T., eds. Physical activity, fitness, and health: Consensus statement. Champaign, IL: Human Kinetics; 1993:11-23.
9. Bray, G.A. Obesity. In: Brown, M.L., ed. Present knowledge in nutrition. Washington, DC: International Life Sciences Institute—Nutrition Foundation; 1990:23-38.
10. Breig, A.; Troup, J.D. Biomechanical considerations in the straight-leg raising test. Spine. 4:242-250; 1979.
11. Briggs, R.C.; Gossman, M.R.; Birch, R.; Drews, J.; Shaddeau, S. Balance performance among noninstitutionalized elderly women. Phys. Ther. 69:748-756; 1989.
12. Brodie, D.A. Techniques for measurement of body composition, part I. Sports Med. 5:11-40; 1988.
13. Brodie, D.A. Techniques for measurement of body composition, part II. Sports Med. 5:74-98; 1988.
14. Buchner, D.M.; Beresford, S.A.A.; Larson, E.B.; LaCroix, A.Z.; Wagner, E.H. Effects of physical activity on health status in older adults II: Intervention studies. Annu. Rev. Publ. Health. 13:469-488; 1992.
15. Burton, A.K.; Tillotson, K.M.; Troup, J.D.G. Variation in lumbar sagittal mobility with low-back trouble. Spine. 14:584-590; 1989.
16. Burton, A.K.; Tillotson, K.M.; Troup, J.D.G. Prediction of low-back trouble frequency in a working population. Spine. 14:939-946; 1989.
17. Buskirk, E.R. Obesity. In: Skinner, J.S., ed. Exercise testing and exercise prescription for special cases. Philadelphia: Lea & Febiger; 1987:149-174.
18. Buskirk, E.R.; Segal, S.S. The aging motor system: Skeletal muscle weakness. In: Spirduso, W.W.; Eckert, H.M., eds. Physical activity and aging. Champaign, IL: Human Kinetics; 1989:19-36.
19. Cady, L.D.; Thomas, P.C.; Karwasky, R.J. Program for increasing health and physical fitness of fire fighters. J. Occup. Med. 27:110-114; 1985.
20. Campbell, A.J.; Borrie, M.J.; Spears, G.F. Risk factors for falls in a community-based prospective study of people 70 years and older. J. Gerontol. 44:M112; 1989.
21. Chandler, J.M.; Duncan, P.W.; Studenski, S.A. Balance performance on the postural stress test: Comparisons of young adults, healthy elderly, and fallers. Phys. Ther. 70:410-415; 1990.
22. Christensen, A.B.; Ammitzboll, F.; Dyrbye, C.; Cornelissen, M.; Cornelissen, P.; van der Perre, G. Assessment of tibial stiffness by vibration testing in situ—I. Identification of mode shapes in different supporting conditions. J. Biomech. 19:53-60; 1986.
23. Corbin, C. Flexibility. Clin. Sports. Med. 3:101-117; 1984.

24. Després, J.P.; Moorjani, S.; Tremblay, A.; Nadeau, A.; Bouchard, C. Regional fat distribution of body fat, plasma lipoproteins, and cardiovascular disease. Arteriosclerosis. 10: 497-511; 1990.
25. Després, J.P.; Tremblay, A.; Pérusse, L.; Leblanc, C.; Bouchard, C. Abdominal adipose tissue and serum HDL-cholesterol: Association independent from obesity and serum triglyceride concentration. Int. J. Obes. 12:1-13; 1988.
26. Després, J.P.; Tremblay, A.; Thériault, G.; Pérusse, L.; Leblanc, C.; Bouchard, C. Relationships between body fatness, adipose tissue distribution, and blood pressure in men and women. J. Clin. Epidemiol. 41:889-897; 1988.
27. Exercise and NIDDM. Diabetes Care. 13:785-789; 1990.
28. Faulkner, R.A.; Sprigings, E.J.; McQuarrie, A.M. A partial curl-up protocol for adults based on an analysis of the procedures. Can. J. Sport Sci. 14:135-141; 1989.
29. Ferland, M.; Després, J.P.; Tremblay, A.; Pinault, S.; Nadeau, A.; Moorjani, S.; Lupien, P.J.; Thériault, G.; Bouchard, C. Assessment of adipose tissue distribution by computed axial tomography in obese women: Association with body density and anthropometric measurements. Br. J. Nutr. 61:139-148; 1989.
30. Fleischman, E. The structure and measurement of physical fitness. Englewood Cliffs, NJ: Prentice Hall; 1964.
31. Frost, M.; Stuckey, S.; Smalley, L.; Dorman, G. Reliability of measuring trunk motions in centimeters. Phys. Ther. 62:1431-1437; 1982.
32. Frymoyer, J.W.; Cats-Baril, W. Predictors of low-back pain disability. Clin. Orthop. 221: 89-98; 1987.
33. Gauvin, M.G.; Riddle, D.L.; Rothstein, J.M. Reliability of clinical measurements of forward bending using the modified fingertip-to-floor method. Phys. Ther. 70:443-447; 1990.
34. Gehlsen, B.M.; Whaley, M.H. Falls in the elderly: part II, balance, strength, and flexibility. Arch. Phys. Med. Rehabil. 71:739-741; 1990.
35. Gill, K.; Johnson, G.B.; Haugh, L.D.; Pope, M.H. Repeatability of four clinical methods for assessment of lumbar spinal motion. Spine. 13:50-53; 1988.
36. Guesens, P.; Dequeker, J.; Verstraeten, A.; Niis, J. Age, sex, and menopause-related changes of vertebral and peripheral bone: Population study with dual and single photon absorptiometry and radiogrammetry. J. Nucl. Med. 27:1540; 1987.
37. Harris, M.L. Flexibility: A review of the literature. Phys. Ther. 49:591-601; 1969.
38. Haskell, W.L. Dose-response relationship between physical activity and disease risk factors. In: Oja, P.; Telama, R., eds. Sport for all. Amsterdam: Elsevier Science; 1991:125-133.
39. Hildebrandt, V.H. A review of epidemiological research on risk factors of low back pain. In: Buckle, P.W., ed. Musculoskeletal disorders at work. London: Taylor & Francis; 1987:9-16.
40. Holland, G. The physiology of flexibility: A review of the literature. Kinesiol. Rev. 1:49-62; 1968.
41. Horak, F.B. Clinical measurement of postural control in adults. Phys. Ther. 67:1881-1885; 1987.
42. Hyytiäinen, K.; Salminen, J.; Suvitie, S.; Wickström, G.; Pentti, J. Reproducibility of nine tests to measure spinal mobility and trunk muscle strength. Scand. J. Rehabil. Med. 23:3-10; 1991.
43. Iverson, B.D.; Gossman, M.R.; Shaddeau, S.A.; Turner, M.E. Balance performance, force production, and activity levels in noninstitutionalized men 60 to 90 years of age. Phys. Ther. 70:348-355; 1990.
44. Jackson, A.W.; Baker, A.A. The relationship of the sit and reach test to criterion measures of hamstring and back flexibility in young females. Res. Q. Exerc. Sport. 57:183-186; 1986.
45. Jackson, A.W.; Langford, N.J. The criterion-related validity of the sit and reach test: Replication and extension of previous findings. Res. Q. Exerc. Sport. 60:384-387; 1989.
46. Jetté, M. The standardized test of fitness in occupational health: A pilot project. Can. J. Public Health. 69:431-437; 1978.
47. Johansson, C. Förändras postural kontroll vid kronisk smärta i rygg och nacke? Sjukgymnasten. 1:12-13; 1989.
48. Jörgensen, K.; Nicolaisen, T. Two methods for determining trunk muscle endurance: A comparative study. Eur. J. Appl. Physiol. 55:639-644; 1986.
49. Jörgensen, K.; Nicolaisen, T. Trunk muscle endurance: Determination and relation to low-back trouble. Ergonomics. 30:259-267; 1987.
50. Kelsey, J.; Hoffman, S. Risk factors for hip fracture. New Eng. J. Med. 316:404-416; 1987.
51. Keys, A. Overweight, obesity, coronary heart disease and mortality. Nutr. Rev. 38:297-307; 1980.
52. Kissebah, A.H.; Peiris, A.N. Biology of regional body fat distribution: Relationship to noninsulin dependent diabetes mellitus. Diabetes Metab. Rev. 5:83-109; 1989.

53. Kline, G.M.; Porcari, J.P.; Hintermeister, R. ; Freedson, P.S.; Ward, A.; McCarron, R.F.; Ross, J.; Rippe, J.M. Estimation of $\dot{V}O_2max$ from a one-mile track walk, gender, age and body weight. Med. Sci. Sports. Exerc. 19:253-259; 1987.
54. Kohl, H.W.; Gordon, N.F.; Villegas, J.A.; Blair, S.N. Cardiorespiratory fitness, glycemic status, and mortality risk in men. Diabetes Care. 15:184-192; 1992.
55. Langrana, N.; Lee, C. Isokinetic evaluation of trunk muscles. Spine. 9:171-175; 1984.
56. Laukkanen, R.; Oja, P.; Ojala, K.; Pasanen, M.; Vuori, I. Feasibility of a 2-km walking test for fitness assessment in a population study. Scan. J. Soc. Med. 20:119-126; 1992.
57. Law, M.R.; Wald, N.J.; Meade, T.W. Strategies for prevention of osteoporosis and hip fracture. Br. Med. J. 303:453-459; 1991.
58. Leaf, D.A. Fitness: A new look at an old term (measurements of human aerobic performance). Med. Hypotheses 18:33-46; 1985.
59. Lee, L.K.; Westers, B.; Mcinnis, S.; Ervin, L. Analyzing risk factors for preventive back education approaches: A review. Physiother. Can. 40:88-98; 1988.
60. Leino, P.; Aro, S.; Hasan, J. Trunk muscle function and low-back disorders: A ten-year follow-up study. J. Chronic. Dis. 40:289-296; 1987.
61. Leon, A.S. Physical activity and risk of ischemic heart disease—an update 1990. In: Oja, P.; Telama, R., eds. Sport for all. Amsterdam: Elsevier Science; 1991:251-264.
62. Lohman, T.G. Skinfolds and body density and their relation to body fatness: A review. Hum. Biol. 53:181-225; 1981.
63. Mälkiä, E. Muscular performance as a determinant of physical ability in Finnish adult population. Publications of the Social Insurance Institution 1983; AL:23. Turku: Social Insurance Institution; 1983.
64. Manniche, C.; Benzen, L.; Hesselsol, G.; Christensen, J. Clinical trial of intensive muscle training for chronic low-back pain. Lancet. 2:1473-1476; 1988.
65. Mayer, T.G.; Gatchel, R.J.; Kishino, N.; Keely, J.; Capra, P.; Mayer, H.; Barnett, J.; Mooney, V. Objective assessment of spine function following industrial injury: A prospective study with comparison group and one-year follow-up. Spine. 10:482-493; 1985.
66. McLean, K.P.; Skinner, J.S. Validity of Futrex-5000 for body composition determination. Med. Sci. Sports Exerc. 24:253-258; 1992.
67. McNeill, T.; Warwick, D.; Andersson, G.; Shulz, A. Trunk strength in attempted flexion, extension and lateral bending in healthy subjects and patients with low-back disorders. Spine. 5:52-58; 1980.
68. Mee, C. Staying flexible: Full range of motion. Alexandria, VA: Time-Life Books; 1987.
69. Mellin, G. Accuracy of measuring lateral flexion of the spine with a tape. Clin. Biomech. 1:85-89; 1986.
70. Mellin, G. Correlations of spinal mobility with degree of chronic low-back pain after correction for age and anthropometric factors. Spine. 12:464-468; 1987.
71. Mellin, G.; Hurri, H.; Härkäpää, K.; Järvikoski, A. A controlled study of the outcome of inpatient and outpatient treatment of low-back pain: part II. Effects on physical measurements three months after treatment. Scand. J. Rehabil. Med. 21:91-95; 1989.
72. Mellin, G.; Hurri, H.; Härkäpää, K.; Järvikoski, A. A controlled study of the outcome of inpatient and outpatient treatment of low-back pain: Part IV. Long-term effects on physical measurements. Scand. J. Rehabil. Med. 22:189-194; 1990.
73. Miller, C.W. Survival and ambulation following hip fracture. J. Bone Joint Surg. 60A:930; 1978.
74. National Research Council. Diet and health. Implications for reducing chronic disease risk. Washington, DC: National Academy Press; 1989:563-592.
75. Nummi, J.; Järvinen, T.; Stambej, U.; Wickström, G. Diminished dynamic performance capacity of back and abdominal muscles in concrete reinforcement workers. Scand. J. Work Environ. Health. 4(Suppl.1):39-46; 1978.
76. Oddsson, L.I. Control of voluntary trunk movements in man: Mechanism for postural equilibrium during standing. Acta. Physiol. Scand. 140:(Suppl.595); 1-11; 1990.
77. Oja, P. Elements and assessment of fitness in sport for all. In: Oja, P.; Telama, R., eds. Sport for all. Amsterdam: Elsevier Science; 1991: 103-110.
78. Oja, P.; Laukkanen, R.; Pasanen, M.; Tyry, T.; Vuori, I. A 2-km walking test for assessing the cardiorespiratory fitness of healthy adults. Int. J. Sports Med. 12:356-362; 1991.
79. Ostlere, S.J.; Gold, R.H. Osteoporosis and bone density measurement methods. Clin. Orthop. 271:149-163; 1991.
80. Parnianpour, M.; Nordin, M.; Kahanovitz, N.; Frankel, V. The triaxial coupling of torque generation of trunk muscles during isometric exertions and the effect of fatiguing isoinertial movements on the motor output and movement patterns. Spine. 9:982-992; 1988.

81. Pate, R.R. The evolving definition of physical fitness. Quest. 40:174-179; 1988.
82. Plowman, S.A. Physical activity, physical fitness, and low back pain. Exerc. Sport Sci. Rev. 20:221-242; 1992.
83. Powell, K.E.; Thompson, P.D.; Caspersen, C.J.; Kendrick, J.S. Physical activity and the incidence of coronary heart disease. Annu. Rev. Public Health. 8:253-287; 1987.
84. Quinney, H.A.; Smith, D.J.; Wenger, H.A. A field test for the assessment of abdominal muscular endurance in professional ice hockey players. J. Orthop. Sports Phys. Ther. 6:30-33; 1984.
85. Riggs, B.L.; Wahner, H.W.; Seeman, E.; Offord, K.P.; Dunn, W.L.; Mazess, R.B.; Johnson, K.A.; Melton, L.J. Changes in bone mineral density of the proximal femur and spine with aging. J. Clin. Invest. 70:716; 1982.
86. Riihimäki, H. Low-back pain, its origin and risk indicators. Scand. J. Work Environ. Health. 17:81-90; 1991.
87. Ring, C.; Matthews, R.; Nayak, U.S.L.; Isaacs, B. Visual push: A sensitive measure of dynamic balance in man. Arch. Phys. Med. Rehabil. 69:256-260; 1988.
88. Ring, C.; Nayak, U.S.L.; Isaacs, B. Balance function in elderly people who have and who have not fallen. Arch. Phys. Med. Rehabil. 69:261-264; 1988.
89. Roche, A. Body composition assessments in youth and adults. Columbus, OH: Ross Laboratories; 1985.
90. Rose, M.J. The statistical analysis of the intraobserver repeatability of four clinical measurement techniques. Physiotherapy. 77:89-91; 1991.
91. Sahlin, K. Discussion: Effects of exercise on aspects of carbohydrate, fat, and amino acid metabolism. In: Bouchard, C.; Shephard, R.J.; Stephens, T.; Sutton, J.R.; McPherson, B.D., eds. Exercise, fitness, and health. Champaign, IL: Human Kinetics; 1990:309-314.
92. Salminen, J. The adolescent back: A field survey of 370 Finnish schoolchildren. Acta Paediatr. Scand. Suppl.315:1-121; 1984.
93. Sattin, R.W. Falls among older persons: A public health perspective. Annu. Rev. Public Health. 13:489-508; 1992.
94. Shellock, F.G.; Prentice, W.E. Warming-up and stretching for improved physical performance and prevention of sports-related injuries. Sports Med. 2:267-278; 1985.
95. Sidney, K.; Shephard, R.J. Maximum and submaximum exercise tests in men and women in the seventh, eighth, and ninth decades of life. J. Appl. Physiol. 43:280; 1977.
96. Sjöström, L.; Kvist, H.; Cederblad, A.; Tylén, U. Determination of total adipose tissue and body fat in women by computed tomography, ^{40}K, and tritium. Am. J. Physiol. 250: E736-E745; 1986.
97. Skinner, J.S.; Baldini, F.D.; Gardner, A.W. Assessment of fitness. In: Bouchard, C.; Shephard, R.J.; Stephens, T.; Sutton, J.R.; McPherson, B.D., eds. Exercise, fitness, and health. Champaign, IL: Human Kinetics; 1990:109-120, 1990.
98. Smidt, G.; Blanpied, P.R.; Anderson, M.A.; White, R.W. Comparison of clinical and objective methods of assessing trunk muscle strength—An experimental approach. Spine. 12:1020-1024; 1987.
99. Smidt, G.; Herring, T.; Amundsen, L.; Rogers, M.; Russel, A.; Lehmann, T. Assessment of abdominal and back extensor function: A quantitative approach and results for chronic low-back patients. Spine. 8:211-219; 1983.
100. Smith, E.L.; Gilligan, K.A. Exercise, fitness, osteoarthritis, and osteoporosis. In: Bouchard, C.; Shephard, R.J.; Stephens, T.; Sutton, J.R.; McPherson, B.D., eds. Exercise, fitness, and health. Champaign, IL: Human Kinetics; 1990:517-528.
101. Snow-Harter, C.; Bouxsein, M.; Lewis, B.; Charette, S.; Weinstein, P.; Marcus, R. Muscle strength as a predictor of bone mineral density in young women. J. Bone Mineral Res. 5:589-595; 1990.
102. Steele, C.R.; Zhou, L.-J.; Guido, D.; Marcus, R.; Heinrichs, W.L.; Cheema, C. Noninvasive determination of ulnar stiffness from mechanical response—In vivo comparison of stiffness and bone mineral content in humans. J. Biomech. Eng. 110:87-96; 1988.
103. Stones, M.; Kozma, A. Balance and age in the sighted and blind. Arch. Phys. Med. Rehabil. 68:85-89; 1987.
104. Suzuki, N.; Endo, S. A quantitative study of trunk muscle strength and fatigability in the low-back pain syndrome. Spine. 8:69-74; 1983.
105. Swärd, L.; Eriksson, B.; Peterson, L. Anthropometric characteristics, passive hip flexion, and spinal mobility in reaction to back pain in athletes. Spine. 15:376-382; 1990.
106. Sykes, K. Measurement and evaluation of community physical fitness—concept and controversy. Health Educ. J. 48:190-197; 1989.
107. Thomas, S.; Cunningham, D.; Rechnitzer, P.; Donner, A.; Howard, J. Protocols and reliability of maximal oxygen uptake in the elderly. Can. J. Sport Sci. 12:144-151; 1987.
108. Thorstensson, A.; Arvidson, A. Trunk muscle strength and low-back pain. Scand. J. Rehabil. Med. 14:69-75; 1982.

109. Tinetti, M.E. Performance-oriented assessment of mobility problems in elderly patients. J. Am. Geriatr. Soc. 34:119-126; 1986.

110. Tremblay, A.; Després, J.P.; Bouchard, C. Alteration in body fat and fat distribution with exercise. In: Bouchard, C.; Johnston, F., eds. Fat distribution during growth and later health outcomes. New York: Alan R. Liss, Inc.; 1988:297-312.

111. Troup, D.; Rauhala, H. Ergonomics and training. Int. J. Nurs. Stud. 24:325-330; 1987.

112. U.S. Department of Health and Human Services. Public health service: Healthy people 2000—National health promotion and disease prevention objectives. Washington, DC: U.S. Government Printing Office; 1990.

113. Van Itallie, T.B.; Abraham, S. Some hazards of obesity and its treatment. In: Hirsch, J.; Van Itallie, T.B. eds. Recent advances in obesity research IV. London: John Libbey; 1985:1-19.

114. Videman, T., Rauhala, H.; Asp, S.; Lindström, K.; Cedercreutz, G.; Kämppi, M.; Tola, S.; Troup, J.D. Patient-handling skill, back injuries and back pain: An intervention study in nursing. Spine. 14:148-156; 1989.

115. Viljanen, T.; Viitasalo, J.T.; Kujala, U.M. Strength characteristics of a healthy urban adult population. Eur. J. Appl. Physiol. 63:43-47; 1991.

116. Vuori. I. Sport for all in health and disease. In: Oja, P.; Telama, R., eds. Sport for all. Amsterdam: Elsevier Science; 1991:33-43.

117. Wolfson, L.I.; Whipple, R.; Amerman, P.; Kleinerg, A. Stressing the postural response: A quantitative method for testing balance. J. Am. Geriatr. Soc. 34:845-850; 1986.

118. Wood, P.D.; Stefanick, M.L. Exercise, fitness, and atherosclerosis. In: Bouchard, C.; Shephard, R.J.; Stephens, T.; Sutton, J.R.; McPherson, B.D.; eds. Exercise, fitness, and health. Champaign, IL: Human Kinetics; 1990:409-423.

119. Zurlo, F.; Lilioja, S.; Esposito-Del Puente, A.; Nyomba, B.; Raz, I.; Saad, M.; Swinburn, B.; Knowler, W.; Bogardus, C.; Ravussin, E. Low ratio of fat to carbohydrate oxidation as a predictor of weight gain. Am. J. Physiol. 259: E650-E657; 1990.

Chapter 11

Measurement of Health Status and Well-Being

Carl J. Caspersen
Kenneth E. Powell
Robert K. Merritt

The measurement of health status and well-being as a reflection of the concept called health is a particularly complex endeavor (8). This chapter systematically reviews perspectives, characteristics, limitations, and other issues relevant to such measurement.

Any measurement of health status depends conceptually and pragmatically on the definition of health. More than 40 years ago the World Health Organization (WHO) issued the often-cited definition that health is "a state of complete physical, mental, and social well-being and not merely the absence of disease or infirmity" (86). This broad definition clearly calls attention to the fact that health encompasses more than not being physically ill. Terris (73) extended this concept by noting that health and disease may coexist. That is, disease presence does not necessarily reflect a loss of function and well-being. To that end he suggested replacing the word "disease" with "illness."

Last (43) elaborated and expanded the WHO definition, proposing that health encompasses several dimensions, including the following: (a) "freedom from the risk of disease and untimely death"; (b) "a state characterized by anatomical, physiological, and psychological integrity, ability to perform personally valued family, work and community roles"; (c) "ability to deal with physical, biological, psychological and social stress"; (d) "a feeling of well-being"; and (e) "a state of dynamic balance in which an individual or a group's capacity to cope with all the circumstances of living is at an optimum level." Each of these additional definitions has some benefits. For example, definitions (a), (b), and (c) fit in well with much of the anatomical, physiological, and psychological content of the consensus symposium. Definition (d) notes that how well one feels overall is as important as estimates of disease presence. Definition (e) adds an ambitious hope about optimal function. Definitions (c) and (e) extend the concept of health to both individuals and groups of people, thereby advancing a social perspective.

Bouchard and Shephard (9) for the consensus symposium have continued the effort to clarify the concept of health. They define health as "a human condition with physical, social, and psychological dimensions each characterized on a continuum with positive and negative poles. Positive health pertains to the capacity to enjoy life and to withstand challenges; it is not merely the absence of disease. Negative health pertains to morbidity and, in the extreme, with premature mortality." Thus, they too call attention to the various dimensions of health, noting that although these dimensions commonly move in concert, a positive and negative status for any one dimension may coexist with the opposing status of another dimension.

Beyond such conceptual definitions of health one must recognize that several facets influence health (4). A genetic facet governs basic health structure and even other facets of health status. Biochemical, physiologic, and anatomic conditions make up disease, disability, or handicap. Functional facets include usual activities of daily life. Mental facets include mood or feelings, as well as affective states, and are a reflection of well-being. Health potential is a facet that includes longevity, functional potential, and disability. Most of these facets can be operationally defined as a measurable construct pertaining to health.

We recognize that there is still argument about the number of measurable constructs pertaining to health status and well-being (52). Relying largely on those proposed by Stewart and King (71) we focused on eight constructs: mortality, morbidity, risk factor prevalence, use of medical care, disability, function (physical, mental, functional activities), well-being (bodily, emotional, self-concept, global perceptions of well being), and healthy life years. This total of 13 measurement categories (function consisting of three subconstructs, and well-being four) include many specific measures—69 of the most representative are considered herein.

The Review Process

We developed this paper by reviewing an array of literature and synthesizing it into a consensus among us. This consensus reflects our diverse educational backgrounds and undoubtedly also reflects a strong public health perspective derived from our status as employees at the Centers for Disease Control.

For each of the 13 distinctive—though not mutually exclusive—measurement categories of health status and well-being, we (a) elaborate upon several of them within the text, (b) evaluate some practical measurement characteristics (shown in detail for all 69 representative measures in Table 11.1), and (c) identify the potential use of measures in various settings (shown for all 69 measures, in Table 11.3). We arranged the data historically from the measurement category in longest use (mortality measures) to most recently developed (healthy life years).

To help the reader identify general trends or associations across the 13 measurement categories, we simplified and pictorially quantified the information from Tables 11.1 and 11.3. Table 11.2 thus summarizes the practical characteristics of the measures, and Table 11.4 summarizes the degree to which these measures are being or are likely to be used. As an additional aid, the glossary at the end of this chapter defines each of the 69 representative measures.

As the tables developed we found that they presented several different perspectives on the measurement of health status and well-being. We thus analyze the data through these consecutive viewpoints. From a historical perspective, we consider how long each measurement category has been in use. The utilitarian perspective examines the practical aspects of availability, costs, and so on, and considers how well the measures can be directly applied by various potential end-users. The age and developmental perspectives consider the different ways the measures apply to persons of varying chronologic, biologic, and psychologic levels. The context of this chapter necessitated (as did our own interests) an exercise science perspective sensitive to the role of physical activity measures in the 13 categories. Because health status measures can greatly influence health policy and programmatic responses to specific health problems, we also looked at the data from a public health perspective. The measurement issues pertaining to validity, simplicity, and the capacity to measure varying facets of health provided a methodological, statistical, and psychometric perspective. Finally, a futuristic perspective was imparted by the analyses' revealing current deficiencies in present data or usage and by their trying to anticipate future needs.

Historical Perspective

The sequence of measures in Table 11.1 are arranged roughly in a historical perspective. This ordering reflects the rich history behind the availability of and pattern of use for current measures of health status and well-being.

The more traditional health status measures have focused on the absence of health, sometimes called negative health. Because of the urgent social need to deal with death and serious illness, the most common—and generally most valid—health status measures are mortality and morbidity statistics (Tables 11.1 and 11.2). The widespread use of these data permit international comparisons.

Mortality statistics are measures that reflect the event of death as an end point and seek to attribute the specific cause(s) of death (53,87). Mortality measures can also project life expectancy at birth or as one achieves a given age (e.g., retirement age or age 65). Mortality measures are fruitfully used in epidemiologic studies to explore associations between physical activity and disease states (37,45,55,61).

Morbidity measures pertain to disease states and conditions that have not achieved a mortal end point. Common measures of morbidity are disease- or condition-specific incidence rates, hospital admissions, bed-days, treatment costs, and lost days of work for specific causes (32,53). Because of the high costs of gathering and compiling data, morbidity measures usually come from smaller, less representative samples than for the total population as in mortality measures (8,28).

Errors in recording, classifying, or processing data can limit the utility of morbidity and mortality statistics (8). Moreover, these two measurement categories do not reflect the more dynamic and positive aspects of health status.

The concept and measurement of risk factors is an established aspect of epidemiologic research, which seeks to know not only the distribution but the determinants of disease (43). A risk factor may be defined as "an aspect of personal behavior or lifestyle, an environmental exposure, or an inborn or inherited characteristic, which on the basis of

Table 11.1 Practical Characteristics of Measures for the Assessment of Health Status and Well-Being

Measures of health status	Data availability: By a basic source	Data availability: By age group[a]					Utility of data by age group					Chance that data are valid	Chance of low data cost to subject	Chance of low data costs for end-user to: gather	Chance of low data costs for end-user to: process	Measures positive health	Simple final measure	Can compare nations	Effects of physical activity on the measure
		I	C	Y	A	O	I	C	Y	A	O								
Mortality measures																			
Mortality rate[b]	####[c]	I	C	Y	A	O	I	C	Y	A	O	***[d]	***	***	*	*	***	***	**
Condition-specific mortality rate	####	I	C	Y	A	O	I	C	Y	A	O	***	***	***	*	*	***	***	***
Infant mortality	####	I	–	–	–	–	I	•	•	•	•	***	***	***	*	*	***	***	•
Maternal mortality	####	–	–	Y	A	–	•	•	Y	A	•	***	***	***	*	*	***	***	*
Condition-specific YPPL[e]	###	I	C	Y	A	O	I	C	Y	A	•	***	***	***	*	*	***	***	**
Life expectancy at birth or other ages	###	I	C	Y	A	O	I	C	Y	A	O	***	***	***	*	*	***	***	**
Morbidity measures																			
Condition-specific incidence	##	I	C	Y	A	O	I	C	Y	A	O	***	***	***	*	*	***	***	***
Condition-specific prevalence	##	I	C	Y	A	O	I	C	Y	A	O	***	***	***	*	*	***	***	***
Impairment prevalence	##	I	C	Y	A	O	•	•	Y	A	O	***	**	**	*	*	***	***	*
Days of restricted activity	##	I	C	Y	A	O	•	•	Y	A	O	***	**	**	*	*	***	***	***
Days of seeking medical attention	##	I	C	Y	A	O	•	C	Y	A	O	***	**	**	**	*	***	***	*
Days in a hospital	##	I	C	Y	A	O	I	C	Y	A	O	***	**	**	**	*	***	***	***
Active life expectancy	##	I	C	Y	A	O	•	•	•	A	O	**	**	**	**	*	**	**	***
Prevalence of risk factors																			
Smoking	###	–	C	Y	A	O	•	•	Y	A	O	***	**	**	*	**	***	***	*
Inactivity	###	–	C	Y	A	O	•	C	Y	A	O	**	**	**	*	**	**	**	•
Poor nutritional practices	###	I	C	Y	A	O	I	C	Y	A	O	**	**	**	*	**	**	**	**
High blood pressure	###	I	C	Y	A	O	I	C	Y	A	O	***	***	**	**	**	***	***	**
High blood cholesterol	###	I	C	Y	A	O	I	C	Y	A	O	***	**	**	**	**	***	***	**
Circumference ratios	###	–	C	Y	A	O	•	C	Y	A	O	***	**	**	**	**	***	***	***
Overweight, high body mass index	###	I	C	Y	A	O	I	C	Y	A	O	***	***	***	***	**	***	***	***
Use of medical care																			
Doctor visits per year	##	I	C	Y	A	O	I	C	•	A	O	***	**	**	*	*	***	**	**
Proportion not seeing a physician[f]	##	I	C	Y	A	O	I	C	Y	A	O	***	**	**	*	*	***	*	*
Interval since last doctor visit	##	I	C	Y	A	O	I	C	•	A	O	***	**	***	**	*	***	**	**
Short-stay hospital discharge rate	##	I	C	Y	A	O	•	•	•	A	O	***	**	**	*	*	***	**	**
Short-stay episodes per person per year	##	I	C	Y	A	O	•	•	•	A	O	**	**	***	*	*	***	**	**
Short-stay hospital days in a year	##	I	C	Y	A	O	•	•	•	A	O	**	***	***	*	*	***	**	**

Disability measures																			
Days of restricted activity[g]	##	–	C	Y	A	O	•	C	Y	A	O	***	**	**	*	*	***	**	***
Mobility limitation[h]	##	–	C	Y	A	O	•	C	Y	A	O	***	**	**	*	*	***	**	**
Activity limitation[i]	##	–	C	Y	A	O	•	C	Y	A	O	***	**	**	*	*	***	**	**
Activities of daily living (ADL)[j]	##	–	C	Y	A	O	•	C	Y	A	O	***	**	**	*	*	***	**	**
Function																			
Physical function																			
Overall mobility	##	–	–	Y	A	O	•	C	Y	A	O	**	**	**	**	**	***	**	***
Walking	##	–	–	Y	A	O	•	C	Y	A	O	**	**	**	**	**	***	**	***
Lifting	##	–	–	Y	A	O	•	C	Y	A	O	**	**	**	**	**	***	**	***
Reaching overhead	#	–	–	Y	A	O	•	C	Y	A	O	**	**	**	**	**	***	**	***
Going up and down stairs	##	–	–	Y	A	O	•	C	Y	A	O	**	**	**	**	**	***	**	***
Rising from or sitting down in a chair	#	–	–	Y	A	O	•	C	Y	A	O	**	**	**	**	**	***	**	***
Dexterity	#	–	C	Y	A	O	•	C	Y	A	O	**	*	**	*	**	***	***	**
Balancing	#	–	C	Y	A	O	•	C	Y	A	O	**	*	**	*	**	***	***	**
Flexibility	##	–	–	Y	–	–	•	•	Y	A	O	**	*	*	**	**	***	***	**
Strength	##	–	–	Y	–	–	•	•	Y	A	O	**	*	*	**	**	***	***	***
Mental function																			
Short-term memory	#	–	C	Y	A	O	•	•	•	A	O	***	**	*	**	**	***	***	*
Intelligible speech	#	–	C	Y	A	O	•	C	Y	A	O	***	**	*	**	**	***	***	•
Alertness	#	I	C	Y	A	O	•	C	Y	A	O	***	**	*	**	**	***	***	**
Orientation in time and space	#	–	C	Y	A	O	•	•	•	A	O	***	**	*	**	**	**	*	*
Visual and auditory perception	##	–	C	Y	A	O	I	C	Y	A	O	***	**	**	**	**	***	***	*
Confusion	#	–	C	Y	A	O	•	•	•	A	O	***	**	*	**	**	***	***	*
Attention	#	I	C	Y	A	O	•	C	Y	A	O	***	**	*	**	**	***	***	*
Comprehension	##	–	C	Y	A	O	•	C	Y	A	O	***	**	*	**	**	***	***	*
Problem solving	##	–	C	Y	–	–	•	C	Y	A	O	***	**	*	**	**	***	***	*
Literacy	###	–	C	Y	A	O	•	C	Y	A	O	***	**	*	**	**	***	***	•
Numeracy	###	–	C	Y	–	–	•	C	Y	•	•	***	**	*	**	**	***	***	•
Overall knowledge	#	–	C	Y	–	–	•	C	Y	•	•	***	**	*	**	**	***	***	•
Functional activities																			
Basic enabling activities																			
Personal care activities[k]	##	–	–	Y	A	O	•	C	Y	A	O	**	**	**	**	*	***	**	***
Skills of independence[l]	#	–	–	Y	A	O	•	C	Y	A	O	**	**	**	**	*	***	**	**
Productivity-oriented activities[m]	##	–	–	Y	A	O	•	•	•	A	O	**	**	**	**	**	*	**	***
Leisure/recreational activities	###	–	C	Y	A	O	•	•	•	A	O	**	**	**	**	**	*	***	***

(continued)

Table 11.1 *(Continued)*

Measures of health status	Data availability: By a basic source	By age group[a]: I	C	Y	A	O	Utility of data by age group: I	C	Y	A	O	Chance that data are valid	Chance of low data cost to subject	Chance of low data costs for end-user to: gather	process	Measures positive health	Simple final measure	Can compare nations	Effects of physical activity on the measure
Well-Being																			
Bodily well-being																			
Energy (see Glossary)	##	–	C	Y	A	O	•	C	Y	A	O	**	**	**	*	**	***	**	***
Pain	##	–	C	Y	A	O	•	•	•	A	O	**	**	**	*	**	**	**	**
Sleep	##	I	C	Y	A	O	I	C	Y	A	O	***	***	**	**	**	***	***	**
Emotional well-being																			
Positive affect	##	–	C	Y	A	O	•	C	Y	A	O	**	**	**	**	***	***	*	***
Anger/hostility/irritability	##	–	C	Y	A	O	•	C	Y	A	O	**	*	**	**	**	**	**	**
Anxiety	##	–	C	Y	A	O	•	C	Y	A	O	**	**	**	**	**	**	*	**
Depression	##	–	C	Y	A	O	•	C	Y	A	O	**	**	**	**	**	***	**	***
Self-concept																			
Self-esteem	##	–	C	Y	A	O	•	C	Y	A	O	**	**	**	**	***	**	*	***
Sense of mastery and control	#	–	C	Y	A	O	•	C	Y	A	O	**	**	***	**	***	**	*	**
Global perceptions of well-being																			
Health outlook	##	–	C	Y	A	O	•	•	•	A	O	**	**	**	***	***	***	***	***
Current health perceptions	##	–	C	Y	A	O	•	•	•	A	O	**	**	**	***	***	***	***	***
Life-satisfaction	##	–	C	Y	A	O	•	C	Y	A	O	**	**	**	***	***	***	***	**
Healthy life years	#	–	–	–	–	–	I	C	Y	A	O	*	**	*	**	***	**	*	**

[a]I = infant (under 1 year), C = child (ages 1–14), Y = youth (ages 15–24), A = adult (ages 25–64), O = older adult (ages 65 and older).

[b]Mortality rates are available in both crude and age-adjusted form.

[c]#### = data at the county level, ### = data to only the state level, ## = data to only the national level, # = data in smaller samples only.

[d]*** = high, ** = moderate, * = low, • = not applicable, – = not available..

[e]YPPL = years of potential life lost, usually before age 65 or some other selected age.

[f]The proportion not seeing a physician normally pertains to a time frame of the past year and is contingent on the patient's need to see a physician.

[g]Days of restricted activity includes being in bed, being off work/school, and having a reduced ability to perform usual activities.

[h]Mobility limitation pertains to being in bed or needing help getting around, in, or out of the house.

[i]Activity limitation pertains to being restricted in normal play, attending school but needing special classes, and being restricted in the workplace or in the home.

[j]Activities of daily living (ADL) include eating, dressing, bathing, toileting, preparing meals, and using the phone.

[k]Personal care activities include bathing, dressing, eating, and toileting.

[l]Skills of independence include household activities, self-direction, and task persistence.

[m]Productivity-oriented activities include tasks done at school or at the workplace.

Table 11.2 Summary of the Practical Characteristics of Measures for the Assessment of Health Status and Well-Being

<table>
<tr><th rowspan="2">Measurement category</th><th colspan="5">Practical characteristic of measure</th></tr>
<tr><th>Chance that data are valid</th><th>Chance of low subject cost</th><th>Measures positive health</th><th>Simple final measure</th><th>Can compare nations</th></tr>
<tr><td>Mortality measures</td><td>| | | | | | | | | |</td><td>| | | | | | | | | |</td><td>| | |</td><td>| | | | | | | | | |</td><td>| | | | | | | | | |</td></tr>
<tr><td>Morbidity measures</td><td>| | | | | | | | |</td><td>| | | | | | |</td><td>| | |</td><td>| | | | | | | | |</td><td>| | | | | | | | |</td></tr>
<tr><td>Prevalence of risk factors</td><td>| | | | | | | |</td><td>| | | | | | |</td><td>| | | | | |</td><td>| | | | | | | |</td><td>| | | | | | | |</td></tr>
<tr><td>Use of medical care</td><td>| | | | | | | |</td><td>| | | | | | |</td><td>| | |</td><td>| | | | | | | | | |</td><td>| | | | | |</td></tr>
<tr><td>Disability measures</td><td>| | | | | | | | | |</td><td>| | | | | |</td><td>| | |</td><td>| | | | | | | | | |</td><td>| | | | | |</td></tr>
<tr><td>Function</td><td></td><td></td><td></td><td></td><td></td></tr>
<tr><td>Physical function</td><td>| | | | | |</td><td>| | | | |</td><td>| | | | | |</td><td>| | | | | | | | | |</td><td>| | | | | | |</td></tr>
<tr><td>Mental function</td><td>| | | | | | | | | |</td><td>| | | | | |</td><td>| | | | | |</td><td>| | | | | | | | | |</td><td>| | | | | | | | |</td></tr>
<tr><td>Functional activities</td><td>| | | | | |</td><td>| | | | | |</td><td>| | | | |</td><td>| | | | | |</td><td>| | | | | | |</td></tr>
<tr><td>Well-Being</td><td></td><td></td><td></td><td></td><td></td></tr>
<tr><td>Bodily well-being</td><td>| | | | | | |</td><td>| | | | | | |</td><td>| | | | | |</td><td>| | | | | | | |</td><td>| | | | | | |</td></tr>
<tr><td>Emotional well-being</td><td>| | | | | |</td><td>| | | | |</td><td>| | | | | | |</td><td>| | | | | | | |</td><td>| | | | |</td></tr>
<tr><td>Self-concept</td><td>| | | | | |</td><td>| | | | | | |</td><td>| | | | | | | | | |</td><td>| | | | | |</td><td>| | |</td></tr>
<tr><td>Global perceptions of well-being</td><td>| | | | |</td><td>| | | | | | |</td><td>| | | | | | | | | |</td><td>| | | | | | | | | |</td><td>| | | | | | | | | |</td></tr>
<tr><td>Healthy life years</td><td>| | |</td><td>| | | | | | |</td><td>| | | | | | | | | |</td><td>| | | | | |</td><td>| | |</td></tr>
<tr><td>Numerical scale</td><td>0 3</td><td>0 3</td><td>0 3</td><td>0 3</td><td>0 3</td></tr>
</table>

Note. Each score is found by taking the arithmetic average of individual ratings across all measures within a category. The integer values of the numerical scale correspond to the following probabilities: 1 = low, 2 = moderate, 3 = high. Each symbol '|' is roughly equal to 0.33.

epidemiologic evidence is known to be associated with health-related condition(s) considered to be important to prevent" (43).

The risk factor concept is well evolved for coronary heart disease (CHD) (13). Among the more notable CHD risk factors are smoking, physical inactivity, poor nutritional practices (such as a high-fat, low-fiber, and high-sodium diet), high blood pressure, high serum cholesterol, high body mass index, and high proportion of total body fat (Table 11.1) (24). A compendium from the American Heart Association (1) provides methods for CHD risk factor measurement.

We did not compile a more extensive list of risk factors for diseases and conditions other than CHD owing to lack of space. For example, one might consider including measures of cardiorespiratory capacity (or aerobic power). However, we felt that a focus on physical inactivity would account for much of the nongenetic aspects of cardiorespiratory capacity. The interested reader should refer to Skinner and Oja (68) for further discussion and other potential measures. Further, other measures might include the assessment of blood-borne parameters (e.g., hemoglobin, ferritin, liver enzymes for alcohol intake, immune function, etc.) and additional measures taken as part of medical examinations (23,85) or employed as part of clinical services for the prevention of selected illnesses and conditions (78).

As Tables 11.3 and 11.4 show, measuring risk factor levels through establishing risk factor prevalence is a common way to assess health status. Unfortunately, this measurement often requires a somewhat arbitrary assessment of risk factor levels among variables (12). Moreover, like mortality and morbidity statistics, measures that identify the presence of a risk factor actually reflect negative states of health (Table 11.1). That is, although the absence of a risk factor can be thought of as healthy, it more aptly reflects the absence or reduced likelihood of disease (8).

Measures of the use of medical care can assess the individual and societal demands associated with seeking and receiving treatment for illness and disease. The most common measures for this category are usually found within administrative sources and correspond to visits to a primary care provider (e.g., physician) or to hospitals (see also Table 11.1) (40,53,63). The monetary aspects

Table 11.3 Likelihood of Using Measures for the Assessment of Health Status and Well-Being Within Selected Settings

	Policy-Related	Epidemiologic	Experimental	Clinical	Personal
Mortality measures					
Mortality rate (crude, age-adjusted)[a]	**[b]	**	•	•	•
Condition-specific mortality rates	***	***	•	•	•
Infant mortality	***	***	•	•	•
Maternal mortality	***	***	•	•	•
Condition-specific YPPL[c]	**	**	•	•	•
Life expectancy at birth or other ages	**	*	•	•	•
Morbidity measures					
Condition-specific incidence	***	***	*	•	•
Condition-specific prevalence	***	***	*	*	*
Impairment prevalence	***	***	**	*	*
Days of restricted activity[d]	***	***	*	*	*
Days of seeking medical attention	***	***	•	•	*
Days in a hospital	***	***	•	*	*
Active life expectancy	**	**	*	•	•
Prevalance of risk factors					
Smoking	***	***	***	***	***
Inactivity	***	***	***	***	**
Poor nutritional practices	***	***	***	***	**
High blood pressure	***	***	***	***	**
High blood cholesterol	***	***	***	***	**
Circumference ratios	**	***	**	*	*
Overweight, high body mass index	***	***	***	***	***
Use of medical care					
Doctor visits per year	***	***	*	***	**
Proportion not seeing a physician[e]	***	***	•	•	**
Interval since last doctor visit	**	**	*	***	*
Short-stay hospital discharge rate	***	***	*	•	•
Short-stay episodes per person per year	***	***	*	*	•
Short-stay hospital days in a year	***	***	*	*	*

Disability measures					
Days of restricted activity	***	***	**	**	***
Mobility limitation[f]	***	***	**	**	***
Activity limitation[g]	***	***	**	**	***
Activities of daily living (ADL)[h]	***	***	**	**	***
Function					
Physical function					
Overall mobility	***	***	***	***	***
Walking	***	***	***	**	***
Lifting	*	**	***	**	***
Reaching overhead	*	**	***	**	***
Going up and down stairs	***	***	***	***	***
Rising from or sitting down in a chair	**	***	***	***	***
Dexterity	**	**	***	**	**
Balancing	**	**	***	**	***
Flexibility	*	***	***	**	**
Strength	*	***	***	**	**
Mental function					
Short-term memory	•	***	***	***	*
Intelligible speech	*	*	**	***	**
Alertness	*	*	***	***	*
Orientation in time and space	**	**	**	***	•
Visual and auditory perception	***	**	**	***	***
Confusion	*	*	**	**	**
Attention	*	*	**	**	**
Comprehension	*	*	**	*	**
Problem solving	*	*	**	*	**
Literacy	***	***	**	•	***
Numeracy	***	***	**	•	***
Overall knowledge	*	**	**	•	***
Functional activities					
Basic enabling activities					
Personal care activities[i]	***	***	***	**	***
Skills of independence[j]	***	***	***	**	***
Productivity-oriented activities[k]	***	***	*	**	***
Leisure or recreational activities	***	***	**	*	***

(continued)

Table 11.3 ***(continued)***

	Policy-Related	Epidemiologic	Experimental	Clinical	Personal
Well-Being					
Bodily well-being					
Energy (see Glossary)	*	**	**	***	***
Pain	*	***	**	***	***
Sleep	*	**	**	***	***
Emotional well-being					
Positive affect	*	**	***	*	**
Anger/hostility/irritability	*	***	***	**	**
Anxiety	*	***	***	***	**
Depression	**	***	***	***	**
Self-concept					
Self-esteem	•	**	***	*	**
Sense of mastery and control	•	*	***	*	**
Global perceptions of well-being					
Current health perceptions	*	***	**	**	***
Health outlook	*	**	**	*	***
Life-satisfaction	*	**	**	*	***
Healthy life years	*	•	•	•	•

[a]Mortality rates are available in both crude and age-adjusted form.

[b]*** = high, ** = moderate, * = low, • = not applicable.

[c]YPPL = years of potential life lost, usually before age 65 or some other selected age.

[d]Days of restricted activity includes being in bed, being off work/school, and having a reduced ability to perform usual activities.

[e]The proportion not seeing a physician normally pertains to a time frame of the past year and is contingent on the patient's need to see a physician.

[f]Mobility limitation pertains to being in bed or needing help getting around, in, or out of the house.

[g]Activity limitation pertains to being restricted in normal play, attending school but needing special classes, and being restricted in the workplace or in the home.

[h]Activities of daily living (ADL) include eating, dressing, bathing, toileting, preparing meals, and using the phone.

[i]Personal care activities include bathing, dressing, eating, and toileting.

[j]Skills of independence include household activities, self-direction, and task persistence.

[k]Productivity-oriented activities include tasks done at school or at the workplace.

Table 11.4 Summary of the Likelihood of Using Measures for the Assessment of Health Status and Well-Being Within Selected Settings

<table>
<tr><th>Measurement category</th><th>Policy-Related</th><th>Epidemiologic</th><th>Experimental</th><th>Clinical</th><th>Personal</th></tr>
<tr><td>Mortality measures</td><td>| | | | | | | |</td><td>| | | | | | |</td><td>•</td><td>•</td><td>•</td></tr>
<tr><td>Morbidity measures</td><td>| | | | | | | | | |</td><td>| | | | | | | | | |</td><td>| | |</td><td>| |</td><td>| | |</td></tr>
<tr><td>Prevalence of risk factors</td><td>| | | | | | | | |</td><td>| | | | | | | | | |</td><td>| | | | | | | | |</td><td>| | | | | | | | |</td><td>| | | | | | | |</td></tr>
<tr><td>Use of medical care</td><td>| | | | | | | | |</td><td>| | | | | | | | |</td><td>| | |</td><td>| | | | |</td><td>| | | |</td></tr>
<tr><td>Disability measures</td><td>| | | | | | | | | |</td><td>| | | | | | | | | |</td><td>| | | | | | |</td><td>| | | | | |</td><td>| | | | | | | | | |</td></tr>
<tr><td>Function</td><td></td><td></td><td></td><td></td><td></td></tr>
<tr><td>Physical function</td><td>| | | | | |</td><td>| | | | | | | | |</td><td>| | | | | | | | | |</td><td>| | | | | | |</td><td>| | | | | | | | |</td></tr>
<tr><td>Mental function</td><td>| | | | |</td><td>| | | | | |</td><td>| | | | | | |</td><td>| | | | | | | |</td><td>| | | | | | |</td></tr>
<tr><td>Functional activities</td><td>| | | | | | | | | |</td><td>| | | | | | | | | |</td><td>| | | | | |</td><td>| | | | | |</td><td>| | | | | | | | | |</td></tr>
<tr><td>Well-Being</td><td></td><td></td><td></td><td></td><td></td></tr>
<tr><td>Bodily well-being</td><td>| | |</td><td>| | | | | | |</td><td>| | | | | | |</td><td>| | | | | | |</td><td>| | | | | | | | | |</td></tr>
<tr><td>Emotional well-being</td><td>| | | | | | |</td><td>| | | | | | | | |</td><td>| | | | | | | | | |</td><td>| | | | | | | |</td><td>| | | | | | |</td></tr>
<tr><td>Self-concept</td><td>•</td><td>| | | | |</td><td>| | | | | | | | | |</td><td>| | |</td><td>| | | | | | |</td></tr>
<tr><td>Global perceptions of well-being</td><td>| | | | | | |</td><td>| | | | | | | |</td><td>| | | | | | |</td><td>| | | |</td><td>| | | | | | | | | |</td></tr>
<tr><td>Healthy life years</td><td>| | | | | | |</td><td>| | | | | | |</td><td>•</td><td>•</td><td>•</td></tr>
<tr><td>Numerical scale</td><td>0 3</td><td>0 3</td><td>0 3</td><td>0 3</td><td>0 3</td></tr>
</table>

Note. Each score is found by taking the arithmetic average of individual ratings across all measures within a category. The integer values of the numerical scale correspond to the following probabilities: 1 = low, 2 = moderate, 3 = high. Each symbol '|' is roughly equal to 0.33. • = not applicable.

associated with these measures are health care cost indicators that reflect the economic burden of illnesses, diseases, and so on. In some instances, the inability to gain access to medical care where treatment is necessary can reflect unmet needs, which are especially common among disadvantaged groups (63).

A useful definition of disability is "limitations in physical or mental function, caused by one or more health conditions, in carrying out socially defined tasks and roles that individuals generally are expected to be able to do" (33). Hence, the effect on social tasks and roles is an important part of the definition. Disability measures include estimates of the number of days that individuals cannot perform normal levels of daily activity (e.g., days of restricted activity) and whether individuals require help performing basic functions of living (e.g., eating, dressing, or toileting) (22,33,50). Like mortality and morbidity measures, disability measures may be cause-specific to reflect the link to disease or injury. Many people use disability measures to rate the health of older adult populations; however, that rating reflects the more negative aspects of health.

Recently there has been a growing emphasis on characterizing and measuring more positive states of health and well-being. An important part of positive health is the concept of quality of life. Quality of life has been subjectively defined as "in a general sense, that which makes life worth living" (43). Two constructs related to quality of life are *function* and *well-being*. Function pertains to a person's ability to perform everyday tasks and activities (71). Function includes the subconstructs physical functioning, mental functioning, and the capacity to perform discretionary activities (e.g., social roles and recreation) and activities of daily living (71,80). Well-being pertains to more subjective internal states including how one feels both physically and emotionally and includes the subconstructs of psychological well-being, emotional well-being, self-concept, and global perceptions (71).

An extension of those two measurement categories is healthy life expectancy, sometimes called healthy life years (21,76). All three measurement categories reflect positive health facets and may also be useful in international and intercultural comparisons (8,64). Unfortunately, many measures of function and well-being rely on self-reported survey data or are not collected regularly (8). Nonetheless, there are many excellent sources on how to assess physical function (35,50,72,83), mental function (50,65), functional activities (50,72), bodily well-being (22,50), emotional well-being (22,50,65), self-concept (51,65), and global perceptions (10,50).

Quality of life is influenced by social components such as peace, justice, freedom, human dignity, income and employment, basic living necessities (e.g., food, housing, clothing), the environment, public safety, transportation, communication, and other factors like education, culture, and recreation. Such social components and factors will also influence other measures of health status and well-being (6,48). We thus expect that future research will encompass measures that traditionally pertain more to community health status than to the health of individuals in the community (17).

Utilitarian Perspective

The columns of Table 11.1 compare each row of measures with such practical criteria as the availability and utility of data, measurement validity, costs of data collection to the subject and end-user, the simplicity of the measure, and the capacity to compare nations. Other criteria could also be reviewed (5).

We considered data to be readily available in the United States when it existed uniformly at the county level. We also delineated availability at the state or national level, as well as at the level of isolated smaller samples, surveys, or studies. We recognized an apparent link between data availability and the costs for data gathering and data processing (see Table 11.1).

International comparisons of health status and well-being may be of interest to policy makers concerned with preventive and curative health care systems (8). The comparisons may influence the development of public health, economic, and social reforms. Mortality and morbidity measures are most likely to receive high ratings by us on the ability to compare countries (8). Other measures have also been compared internationally (64).

Measures of health status and well-being can be used in at least five different settings: policy-related, epidemiologic, experimental, clinical, and personal. Tables 11.3 and 11.4 show how likely persons from those five settings are to use or have interest in the measures. Where groups actually used the measures, we focused on what they currently used rather than what they should or could use. Policy makers and epidemiologists use measures based on past research or on what they can practically measure in large-scale, population-based studies. Experimenters are more likely to conduct smaller-scale studies than large, randomized controlled trials and to use measures appropriate for that scale. Clinicians choose measures that reveal what a patient can or cannot do, and what they in turn can do for those patients. An individual making personal decisions would be most concerned with the usefulness of the measure and with whether the measure was sensitive to change (as might result from behavior modification).

Measuring risk factors is useful to all five end-users (Tables 11.3 and 11.4). This wide application arises because risk factor change is presumed to beneficially influence health status. At the research level, risk factor prevalences are sensitive to short-term change. At the clinical level risk factor assessment has become a part of medical practice. At the individual level many are motivated to reduce the levels of their measured risk factors.

Most measurement categories have current—and similar—utility for the policy maker and epidemiologist, except perhaps for bodily well-being and self-concept (Tables 11.3 and 11.4). Those two measures are not commonly available in administrative data sources and are not currently useful to policy makers (59). Compared to policy makers, epidemiologists are more likely to use these measures (anger/hostility/irritability, anxiety, self-esteem, short-term memory). Perhaps policy makers do not use these measures because they do not translate into policy decisions. In contrast, condition-specific years of potential life lost, a useful measure for policy makers, is relatively uncommon in most epidemiologic work.

The row to row patterns of Table 11.4 for experimenters, clinicians, and individuals are very similar. Most similar is the lack of utility of mortality measures and healthy life years. Measures of mortal outcomes are of little use—or are understandably avoided—in these three settings comprising individuals or small groups. Although the concept of healthy life years may appear intrinsically motivating to subjects, patients, or individuals, the measure itself may have limited meaning in these settings.

Table 11.3, however, shows some salient differences among these three settings. On the whole, clinicians and individuals find greater utility in many of the measures of medical care use than experimenters. The latter tend neither to measure nor have much interest in productivity-oriented activities, perhaps owing to attendant measurement error in assessing physical activity (12,42). On the other hand, short-term memory, intelligible speech, and alertness (useful measures for clinicians and experimenters) would be of little use to an individual having limited means to modify those measures. Individuals also value not needing to see a physician, which makes such measures of little clinical concern. Moreover, clinicians would not use many measures (e.g., overall knowledge, leisure or recreational activities, sense of mastery and control, and life satisfaction) because these end-users (a) don't see the measures as part of clinical practice, (b) aren't convinced the measures influence patient outcome, (c) don't understand the numerical scores, and (d) have not been trained in using or have not been exposed to using those measures (18,52).

Age/Developmental Issues or Perspectives

Different health status measures can characterize populations of different age groups because these groups have distinct sociologic, behavioral, and health concerns (46). The second and third columns of Table 11.1 detail the availability and utility of measures for five age groups: infant (under 1 year), child (ages 1 to 14), youth (ages 15 to 24), adult (ages 25 to 64), and older adult (ages 65 and older).

Just as Table 11.2 summarized the practical characteristics detailed in Table 11.1, and as Table 11.4 summarized the likelihood of use by selected settings detailed in Table 11.3, Table 11.5 summarizes the availability and Table 11.6 the utility of the measures broken down by age group in Table 11.1.

The most striking feature of Table 11.5 is the limited number of measures available for assessing the health of infants. Only data on mortality, morbidity, and use of medical care are readily available for this age group. Two measures of mental function (alertness and attention) and bodily well-being (sleep) are somewhat available for infants (Table 11.1), as are certain risk factor measures (poor nutrition, high blood pressure, high cholesterol, and overweight). Table 11.6, however, reveals that many risk factor measures would, in fact, be less useful for infants than for older adults.

Table 11.5 shows that children's measures are generally available for most categories. The exceptions were physical function (none but flexibility and strength) and functional activities (only leisure and recreational activities) (Table 11.1).

Table 11.5 indicates that the measures were almost uniformly available for youth. For adults and older adults, data are similarly available and each had similar patterns across categories. For these two older age groups only two measures for physical function (flexibility and strength) and three measures of mental function (e.g., problem solving, numeracy, and overall knowledge) were generally lacking (Table 11.1).

In Table 11.6 mortality measures appear generally useful for all but older adults; specific measures varied in utility by age groups (Table 11.1). For example, maternal mortality measures seemed to add utility to the mortality category for youth and adults. Otherwise, mortality in those two groups is such a rare event that it did not seem to be very useful. An exception was the utility of estimated years of potential life lost (YPLL). YPLLs can help emphasize the importance of fatal diseases or injuries that kill younger populations (27).

Morbidity and mortality statistics seem to easily reflect the health status of older adult populations who have a variety of chronic diseases. At the same time, because death is an eventual outcome for older adults, measures like active life expectancy at age 65 are especially useful. Morbidity measures for infants and children, aside from condition-specific incidence and prevalence, days seeking medical attention, or days spent in a hospital, were not considered useful (Table 11.1).

Table 11.6 indicates that quality of life measures such as function and well-being are important measures for older adults among whom morbidity, disability, and functional impairment are common. Although potentially useful for children and youth, quality of life measures for these two age groups are only now beginning to evolve. Because younger persons are in generally good health, however, these measures may not discriminate health status among those age groups. We encourage epidemiologic and other research that will seek predictors of declining positive health in younger age groups.

Risk factor assessment may be the only hope of predicting the likelihood of chronic diseases with long latency like coronary heart disease among children and youth. However, we are uncertain whether risk factor assessment and modification (e.g., via physical activity) can fully predict future health status later in life (47).

Table 11.6 shows that measures of disability, physical and mental function, functional activities, emotional well-being, and self-concept were not very useful for infants. For children and youth we do not rate the following measures as being as useful as most of the other measurement categories: use of medical care, functional activities, and global perceptions of well-being. We list most of the measurement categories as being useful for adults and older adults. Although we found that measures of healthy life years would be useful for virtually all age groups, such measures were largely unavailable (Table 11.5).

While not listed in the tables, gender and race differences in health status and well-being are also known to prevail. For example, gender differences

Table 11.5 Summary of the Availability of Measures for the Assessment of Health Status and Well-Being for Five Age Groups

<table>
<tr><th>Measurement category</th><th>Infant</th><th>Child</th><th>Youth</th><th>Adult</th><th>Older adult</th></tr>
<tr><td>Mortality measures</td><td>| | | | | | | | | |</td><td>| | | | | | | | | |</td><td>| | | | | | | | | |</td><td>| | | | | | | | | |</td><td>| | | | | | | | | |</td></tr>
<tr><td>Morbidity measures</td><td>| | | | | | | | | |</td><td>| | | | | | | | | |</td><td>| | | | | | | | | |</td><td>| | | | | | | | | |</td><td>| | | | | | | | | |</td></tr>
<tr><td>Prevalence of risk factors</td><td>| | | | | |</td><td>| | | | | | | | | |</td><td>| | | | | | | | | |</td><td>| | | | | | | | | |</td><td>| | | | | | | | | |</td></tr>
<tr><td>Use of medical care</td><td>| | | | | | | | | |</td><td>| | | | | | | | | |</td><td>| | | | | | | | | |</td><td>| | | | | | | | | |</td><td>| | | | | | | | | |</td></tr>
<tr><td>Disability measures</td><td>•</td><td>| | | | | | | | | |</td><td>| | | | | | | | | |</td><td>| | | | | | | | | |</td><td>| | | | | | | | | |</td></tr>
<tr><td>Function</td><td></td><td></td><td></td><td></td><td></td></tr>
<tr><td>Physical function</td><td>•</td><td>| |</td><td>| | | | | | | | | |</td><td>| | | | | | | |</td><td>| | | | | | | |</td></tr>
<tr><td>Mental function</td><td>| |</td><td>| | | | | | | | | |</td><td>| | | | | | | | | |</td><td>| | | | | | | |</td><td>| | | | | | | |</td></tr>
<tr><td>Functional activities</td><td>•</td><td>| |</td><td>| | | | | | | | | |</td><td>| | | | | | | | | |</td><td>| | | | | | | | | |</td></tr>
<tr><td>Well-Being</td><td></td><td></td><td></td><td></td><td></td></tr>
<tr><td>Bodily well-being</td><td>| | |</td><td>| | | | | | | | | |</td><td>| | | | | | | | | |</td><td>| | | | | | | | | |</td><td>| | | | | | | | | |</td></tr>
<tr><td>Emotional well-being</td><td>•</td><td>| | | | | | | | | |</td><td>| | | | | | | | | |</td><td>| | | | | | | | | |</td><td>| | | | | | | | | |</td></tr>
<tr><td>Self-concept</td><td>•</td><td>| | | | | | | | | |</td><td>| | | | | | | | | |</td><td>| | | | | | | | | |</td><td>| | | | | | | | | |</td></tr>
<tr><td>Global perceptions of well-being</td><td>•</td><td>| | | | | | | | | |</td><td>| | | | | | | | | |</td><td>| | | | | | | | | |</td><td>| | | | | | | | | |</td></tr>
<tr><td>Healthy life years</td><td>•</td><td>•</td><td>•</td><td>•</td><td>•</td></tr>
<tr><td>Numerical scale</td><td>0 1</td><td>0 1</td><td>0 1</td><td>0 1</td><td>0 1</td></tr>
</table>

Note. Each score is found by taking the arithmetic average of individual ratings across all measures within a category. The integer values of the numerical scale correspond to the following ratings: 0 = not available, 1 = available. Each symbol '|' is roughly equal to 0.1. Infant = under 1 year, child = ages 1–14, youth = ages 15–24, adult = ages 25–64, older adult = ages 65 and older. • = data not available for age group.

in morbidity and mortality are primarily the result of differential risks acquired from social roles, stress, life-style, and preventive health practices (79). Race differences in morbidity and mortality may be accounted for more in terms of a social or social psychological etiology (e.g., social class, whether measured by level of education, income, or occupation) than a biological etiology (54).

Exercise Science Perspective

The last column of Table 11.1 shows the likelihood that physical activity affects the various measures of health status and well-being while Figure 11.1 summarizes the aggregate effect for each measurement category. For example, we judged the association between physical activity and certain morbidity and mortality measures to be quite high. We based this judgment on our understanding of the research linking physical activity to such outcomes as total and coronary heart disease mortality and risk factors (55,61,68,74). The influence of physical activity on physical and mental function seemed quite promising, especially among the older adults (11,20,71,82). Many of those associations with morbidity and mortality appear also to form the link between physical activity and medical care usage and costs (34,36). The evidence linking physical activity to physical fitness (68) seemed stronger than the evidence linking it with mental function. Physical activity may, however, have a pronounced effect on anxiety, self-esteem (41,49, 62), and well-being (70). On the other hand, physical activity may be more strongly linked to health outlook than to life satisfaction (a measure that may reflect many diverse components).

Although not the primary focus of our paper, ample data suggest that physical activity can enhance the quality of life for patients with certain diseases or conditions (25,26,39,56,57). That information is relevant to clinicians and to patients who may benefit from physical activity rehabilitation.

Public Health Perspective

Health status measures have been used to evaluate the health of general populations and to evaluate clinical interventions, health promotion efforts,

Table 11.6 Summary of the Utility of Measures for the Assessment of Health Status and Well-Being for Five Age Groups

<table>
<tr><th>Measurement category</th><th>Infant</th><th>Child</th><th>Youth</th><th>Adult</th><th>Older adult</th></tr>
<tr><td>Mortality measures</td><td>| | | | | | | |</td><td>| | | | | | |</td><td>| | | | | | | |</td><td>| | | | | | | |</td><td>| | | | |</td></tr>
<tr><td>Morbidity measures</td><td>| | | |</td><td>| | | | | |</td><td>| | | | | | | | |</td><td>| | | | | | | | | |</td><td>| | | | | | | | | |</td></tr>
<tr><td>Prevalence of risk factors</td><td>| | | | | |</td><td>| | | | | | | |</td><td>| | | | | | | | | |</td><td>| | | | | | | | | |</td><td>| | | | | | | | | |</td></tr>
<tr><td>Use of medical care</td><td>| | | | |</td><td>| | | | |</td><td>| | |</td><td>| | | | | | | | | |</td><td>| | | | | | | | | |</td></tr>
<tr><td>Disability measures</td><td>•</td><td>| | | | | | | | | |</td><td>| | | | | | | | | |</td><td>| | | | | | | | | |</td><td>| | | | | | | | | |</td></tr>
<tr><td>Function</td><td></td><td></td><td></td><td></td><td></td></tr>
<tr><td>Physical function</td><td>•</td><td>| | | | | | | |</td><td>| | | | | | | | | |</td><td>| | | | | | | | | |</td><td>| | | | | | | | | |</td></tr>
<tr><td>Mental function</td><td>|</td><td>| | | | | | | |</td><td>| | | | | | | |</td><td>| | | | | | | |</td><td>| | | | | | | |</td></tr>
<tr><td>Functional activities</td><td>•</td><td>| | | | |</td><td>| | | | |</td><td>| | | | | | | | | |</td><td>| | | | | | | | | |</td></tr>
<tr><td>Well-Being</td><td></td><td></td><td></td><td></td><td></td></tr>
<tr><td>Bodily well-being</td><td>| | |</td><td>| | | | | | |</td><td>| | | | | | |</td><td>| | | | | | | | | |</td><td>| | | | | | | | | |</td></tr>
<tr><td>Emotional well-being</td><td>•</td><td>| | | | | | | | | |</td><td>| | | | | | | | | |</td><td>| | | | | | | | | |</td><td>| | | | | | | | | |</td></tr>
<tr><td>Self-concept</td><td>•</td><td>| | | | | | | | | |</td><td>| | | | | | | | | |</td><td>| | | | | | | | | |</td><td>| | | | | | | | | |</td></tr>
<tr><td>Global perceptions of well-being</td><td>| | |</td><td>| | | | |</td><td>| | |</td><td>| | | | | | | | | |</td><td>| | | | | | | | | |</td></tr>
<tr><td>Healthy life years</td><td>•</td><td>•</td><td>•</td><td>•</td><td>•</td></tr>
<tr><td>Numerical scale</td><td>0 — 1</td><td>0 — 1</td><td>0 — 1</td><td>0 — 1</td><td>0 — 1</td></tr>
</table>

Note. Each score is found by taking the arithmetic average of individual ratings across all measures within a category. The integer values of the numerical scale correspond to the following ratings: 0 = not available, 1 = available. Each symbol '|' is roughly equal to 0.1. Infant = under 1 year, child = ages 1–14, youth = ages 15–24, adult = ages 25–64, older adult = ages 65 and older. • = data not available for age group.

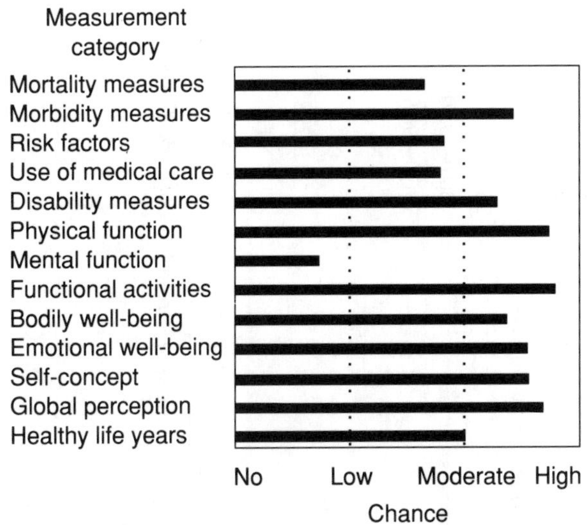

Figure 11.1 The chance that physical activity can affect 13 measurement categories for the assessment of health status and well-being.

and health care delivery systems (5). These evaluations have often resulted in improvements in public health. In some cases, similar measures have been used for each type of evaluation.

Health status measures usually come from administrative sources focusing on disease events rather than on individuals (8). Mortality measures are widely available from those sources and are used to reflect population health status. On the other hand, individual health status measures, like health risk appraisals, can help motivate and evaluate individual health promotion efforts.

Indicators of health care costs reflect the economic burden of mortality and morbidity as well as other direct and indirect costs associated with factors such as medical treatment, lost productivity, and absenteeism resulting from specific diseases (34,36). Although not included as a specific measure in our tables, such health cost indicators can help policy makers weigh the costs associated with a specific disease against those associated with risk reduction activities.

Table 11.7 offers some health status measures related specifically to several chronic diseases and conditions in the United States selected because of their established or potential link with physical inactivity (7,30,60). The data in Table 11.7 clearly suggest that reducing physical inactivity a small amount, even if it has but a modest association with each disease, could result in substantial

Table 11.7 Population-Based Health Status Indicators for Selected Chronic Diseases and Conditions in the United States

Disease/condition	ICD code(s)[a]	Death rate[b] (per 100,000)		Years of potential life lost[c]		Health care costs (billions)
		Crude	Age-adjusted	Total years lost	Years lost (per 100,000) before age 65	
All causes	All codes	882.0	535.5	12,276,000	5,698.2	$540[d]
Diseases of the heart	390.0–398.0, 402.0, 404.0–429.0	311.3	166.3	1,485,000	689.1	$ 95[d]
Ischemic heart disease	410.0–414.0	207.3	132.7	817,000	379.0	$ 65[d]
Malignant neoplasms (all sites)	140.0–208.0	197.3	12.6	1,826,000	847.6	$ 6.036[e]
Breast (women)	174.0–175.0	17.3	32.7	234,000	108.5	$ 1.265[e]
Colorectal	153.0–154.0	22.7	23.5	134,000	62.2	$ 1.301[e]
Lung	160.0–165.0	56.2	39.9	439,000	203.7	$ 1.598[e]
Prostate	185.0	15.2	12.3	18,000	8.4	$ .519[e]
Chronic obstructive pulmonary disease	490.0–496.0	33.7	19.4	133,000	61.9	$ 6.5[e]
Diabetes-related deaths	250.0	16.4	10.1	134,000	62.0	$ 13.8[e]
Cerebrovascular diseases	430.0–438.0	61.2	29.7	249,000	115.5	$ 20.4[d]
Depression	796.0–296.9	N/A	N/A	735,000	377.8	$ 4.2[f]
Obesity	N/A	N/A	N/A	N/A	N/A	N/A
Osteoarthritis	N/A	N/A	N/A	N/A	N/A	$ 2[f]
Osteoporosis	N/A	N/A	N/A	N/A	N/A	$ 3.8[f]
Low-back pain	N/A	N/A	N/A	N/A	N/A	$ 17.2[f]
Suicide	E950-E959	12.4	11.4	671,000	311.3	$ 0.3[e]

[a]Adapted from (53), p. 250; [b]Adapted from (53), pp. 85, 87, 89, 93, 99, 103; [c]Adapted from (53), p. 83; [d]From (19); [e]From (3); [f]From (75); N/A = not applicable.

reductions in mortality, morbidity, and related economic costs. However, this table does not present data on physical function or well-being because it is currently too difficult to attribute health care or other economic costs to them. Hence, policy makers likely will struggle to convince others of the societal costs associated with persons scoring poorly on measures representing those two categories. Also, this table does not include data on injuries, some of which are caused by physical activity (58).

Clearly, the measurement of health status and well-being can form the basis of economic, health care, and social reform. For example, monetary costs associated with various measures of health status focus attention on the burden of illness and disease and the reduction of health care costs. Measures of the use of medical care can focus attention on improvements in health care access. The combined use of these two and other measures can focus attention on improvements in public health.

In 1990 the Public Health Service of the U.S. Department of Health and Human Services released *Healthy People 2000* (76), which proposes 300 measurable objectives for the overall goal of improved quantity and quality of life. One all-encompassing objective called for improvements of healthy life years, focusing specifically on active life expectancy as a measurable goal. For example, the report recognized that in 1980 life expectancy (quantity of life) was 73.7 years at birth, of which 11.7 years were considered dysfunctional years. Active life expectancy—a simple reflection of quality of life—was 62 years. The Year 2000 target was a goal of 75 years for life expectancy and 65 years for active life expectancy. In that instance a complex, yet measurable, objective helps to focus on both the quantity and quality of American health.

Many of the measures we have presented have been used in drafting these national objectives. Health status objectives in *Healthy People 2000* represent health problems such as chronic disease (coronary heart disease, chronic lung cancer, diabetes, etc.), illnesses (pneumonia and influenza), intentional and unintentional injury, chronic back conditions, activity limitation, and HIV infection. The report's risk reduction objectives are often directly linked to health status objectives. They represented topics like behavioral patterns (physical activity, nutritional behaviors, alcohol use, smoking, sexual behaviors, seat belt use) and actions to reduce mental health disorders (e.g., depression, personal and emotional problems, stress, etc.) among others. Services and protection objectives focused on things such as clinical prevention services, access to medical care, and health promotion and disease prevention services offered through the school, work site, family, community, hospital, media, and public health agencies. The quantitative nature of the Year 2000 objectives demonstrate a commitment to create and track data over time. Surveillance of health status and well-being is thus critical.

One objective calls for the development of a set of health status indicators appropriate for federal, state and local agencies to establish and use (76). This would necessitate a data availability rating of "####" in Table 11.1. The current list of needed indicators (15) includes death rates (from all causes, motor vehicle crashes, breast and lung cancer, cardiovascular disease, homicide and suicide, and work-related injury), incidence rates (for AIDS, measles, primary and secondary syphilis, and tuberculosis), and indicators of risk factors (the prevalence of low birth weight, births to adolescents, prenatal care, childhood poverty, and the proportion of persons living in counties exceeding EPA standards for air quality).

The *Healthy People 2000* process and the objectives themselves recognize individual, group, and social roles in the promotion of health and the prevention of disease. The process has every potential to create both social and health care reforms in the United States, especially as communities become involved. Clearly the interest, availability, and meaning ascribed to health status and well-being measures will be one method of guiding and gauging the success of the *Healthy People 2000* process and its public health impact.

Psychometric/Statistical/ Methodological Perspective

Problems in conceptualizing constructs have hindered the measurement of health (8,52,80). Also, inadequate data sources and resources have restricted the development of measures when appropriate measurement concepts exist. Nonetheless, progress continues in the development of health status and quality of life measures that reflect the overall concepts of well-being and functioning (71).

Morbidity and mortality statistics should separate disease events from measures of burden like hospital days and treatment costs (8). However, combined morbidity and mortality measures such as quality-adjusted life expectancy may be useful in evaluating program effectiveness (38). Quality-adjusted life years (QALYs) have been used to analyze the cost-effectiveness of having physicians counsel their patients to exercise regularly to prevent coronary heart disease (31).

Short, yet feasible, valid, and reliable measures of health status should be incorporated in a variety of research efforts (52,59,71). Such measures are important to individuals and clinicians who have either limited means or limited wherewithal to make and interpret more complicated yet valid measures. Generic as well as disease-specific measures should also be further developed and refined (18,72).

Research efforts should develop suitable positive outcome measures for health promotion programs and preventive services besides combined measures for assessing morbidity, mortality, and disability (59), so that research may extend certain composite measures like healthy life years. To elucidate the meaning of composite health scores research must also explore different methods of refining, weighing, and identifying the structure of valuation and preference of various health states (21). For example, many experts disagree with the weighing factor that the QALYs use for selected health states (59).

Epidemiologic and other research will be needed to identify predictors of declining positive health as well as the dynamic, short-term changes that occur in health status in specific population groups (81).

Physical activity is a complex behavior having a variety of health-related dimensions that may relate differentially to specific health conditions and states (12,14,42). Hence, research should carefully establish the link between specific aspects of physical activity and well-considered measures of health states (e.g., well-being and function), disease outcomes, conditions, and perhaps composite health.

Summary, Conclusions, and Futuristic Perspective

This paper has systematically reviewed the literature on the measurement of health status and well-being focusing on a variety of perspectives, characteristics, limitations, and other issues.

Our review reveals a long-standing preference toward measures that largely reflect negative outcomes or diminished health states. This historical preference may also account for the greater availability, generally favorable validity, and international acceptance of the common measures of negative health states. In particular, mortality and morbidity measures have an array of users . . . such as policy makers, epidemiologists, and clinicians.

Interestingly, however, contemporary perspectives are focusing on the more positive measures of health status and well-being. The tables in this chapter demonstrate that the newer measures of positive health already are useful. Given time and serious effort, many of these measures should become more widely available, more valid, and even more useful. This development is likely to produce important public health and social reform. In the short run we expect to see an even greater profusion of constructs striving to measure our new understanding of positive health.

The different categories characterized in this review are not mutually exclusive. Some of the overlap occurs because the categories that better capture the essence of the constructs are not yet apparent. The overlap also occurs because of the multidimensionality of health status and well-being. Clearly, multiple measures of health will be needed. Although certain composite measures may be helpful in selected circumstances, a composite will be based on the relative merits of different components, each of which has its own utility and needs accurate measurement.

We have indicated our impression that physical activity can have important effects on a variety of measures of health status and well-being. The growing list of diseases for which regular physical activity has a preventive or ameliorative effect will be joined by a similarly impressive list of positive health measures abetted by physical activity. The categories for disability, function, and well-being provide rich areas of research for physical activity scientists. Meaningful associations, however, will depend on the development and refinement of measures for these categories and physical activity itself. To make measurement tools useful to the many different types of measurement settings this research should attend to various practical criteria. Ideally, this chapter will help focus such efforts.

Glossary of Health Status and Well-Being Measures

(Definitions are presented in the order they occur in Tables 11.1 and 11.3)

Mortality Measures

Mortality rate—total number of deaths during a given time interval, divided by the number in the population.

Condition-specific mortality rate—mortality rate for a specific cause.

Infant mortality rate—number of deaths of live-born children under 1 year of age during a given time interval, divided by the number of live births.

Maternal mortality—number of deaths during a given time interval assigned to causes related to pregnancy or the puerperium, divided by the number of live births during the same interval.

Condition-specific years of potential life lost—years of potential life lost before age 65 due to a specific cause.

Life expectancy (at birth or at other ages)—average number of years of life remaining to a person at a particular age based on a given set of age-specific death rates.

Morbidity Measures

Condition-specific incidence rate—number of new cases of a specified condition during a given period of time, divided by the population size.

Condition-specific prevalence rate—number of current cases, new and old, of a specified condition at a specific point in time, divided by the population size.

Impairment prevalence—number of people with a loss or an abnormal function of an organ.

Days of restricted activity—number of days on which a person cuts down on usual activities for more than one-half day because of an illness or an injury.

Days of seeking medical attention—number of days on which an examination, diagnosis, treatment, or advice is sought from a health care professional or provider.

Days in a hospital—number of nights an inpatient spends in a hospital.

Active life expectancy—age to which a person is expected to live free of disabling diseases or conditions.

Prevalence of Risk Factors

Smoking—smoking at least 100 cigarettes in a lifetime and currently smoking cigarettes on a regular (usually daily) basis.

Inactivity—generally having no leisure-time or occupational physical activity.

Nutritional practices—dietary choices concerning the specific type and amount of foods and nutrients ingested.

High blood pressure (adults)—systolic pressure greater than or equal to 140 mmHg and/or diastolic pressure greater than or equal to 90 mmHg.

Blood cholesterol—the concentration of cholesterol in plasma or serum.

Circumference ratios—indicators of body fat distribution. For example, a waist-hip ratio is determined by the waist circumference (at the umbilicus) in centimeters divided by hip circumference (at the largest circumference of the hips and buttocks) in centimeters.

Overweight, high body mass index—approximation of excess body weight for height or excess fat and/or muscle relative to a specific standard. One such standard, body mass index, is defined as body weight in kilograms divided by height in meters squared. Females with body mass index greater than or equal to 27.3 and males with body mass index greater than or equal to 27.8 are considered overweight.

Use of Medical Care

Doctor visits per year—number of visits per year to a doctor of medicine or doctor of osteopathy for examination, diagnosis, treatment, or advice.

Proportion not seeing a physician—number of people not seeking care from a physician within a specific time period, divided by the total number in the population.

Interval since last doctor visit—number of calendar days since last visiting a doctor.

Short-stay hospital discharge rate—number of formal releases from a hospital for any reason (e.g., discharge, transfer, death) during a given time interval (less than 30 days).

Short-stay episodes/person/year—number of short (less than 30 days) hospital stays per person per year.

Short-stay hospital days in a year—average number of nights per person spent in a hospital during a year considering only hospitalizations of less than 30 days.

Disability Measures

Days of restricted activity—number of days in which a person cuts down on usual activities for more than half a day because of an impairment or disability.

Mobility limitation—extent to which a person's physical abilities to move about within a house or community to accomplish routine tasks are limited.

Activity limitation—extent to which a person's usual or major activities are limited (e.g., reduced recreational or household activity, absence from school or place of employment).

Activities of daily living—physical functioning and independence in performing basic daily activities such as bathing, dressing, toileting, transferring from bed to chair, continence, and feeding.

Function (physical function)

Overall mobility—physical ability to move about within a house or community to accomplish routine tasks.

Walking—to go or travel on foot at a pace slower than a run.

Lifting—raising an object from a lower to a higher position.

Reaching overhead—raising both arms to a level higher than the head in order to manipulate objects.

Going up and down stairs—climbing and descending a reasonable number of stairs (1-3 flights) with ease.

Rising from and sitting down in a chair—sitting down on and getting up from a chair with ease.

Dexterity—skill in the use of the hands or body; adroitness.

Balance—skill-related component of physical fitness that relates to the maintenance of equilibrium while stationary or moving.

Flexibility—health-related component of physical fitness that relates to the range of motion available at a joint.

Strength—health-related component of physical fitness that relates to the amount of force that a muscle can exert against an external resistance.

Function (mental function)

Short-term memory—ability to recall and describe recent events, particularly those within the past day or two.

Intelligible speech—ability to communicate orally.

Alertness—attentiveness; a condition of preparedness or watchfulness.

Orientation in time and space—ability to know and express the current date and time on the clock, and to know and express one's geographic location in both the global (e.g., national) and local (e.g., building, street) sense.

Visual and auditory perception (sensory perception)—ability to receive, process, and understand visual and auditory stimuli.

Confusion—disturbed, emotional, and unclear thinking.

Attention—process of preferentially responding to a stimulus or range of stimuli.

Comprehension—understanding, mentally grasping; the process of reacting intelligently in a problem situation.

Problem solving—process involved in discovering the correct sequence of alternatives leading to a goal or to an ideational solution.

Literacy—ability to read and write.

Numeracy—ability to understand and perform numerical calculations.

Overall knowledge—all that has been perceived, grasped, and retained by the mind; learning; enlightenment.

Function (functional activities)

Personal care activities—basic daily activities such as bathing, dressing, toileting, transferring from bed to chair, continence, and feeding.

Skills of independence—ability to select appropriate tasks by oneself and to concentrate and persist in the effort to accomplish the task.

Productivity-oriented activities—job, school, household, or other tasks that contribute to the overall productivity of society.

Leisure/recreational activities—optional, refreshing, and enjoyable pursuits during time uncommitted to productivity-oriented activities.

Well-Being (bodily well-being)

Energy—capacity for action or accomplishment; resistance to fatigue.

Pain—unpleasant physical sensation due to damaged tissue or the stimulation of the free nerve ending receptors for pain on or in the tissue.

Sleep—ability to fall asleep promptly, stay asleep during the night, and arise feeling rested and energetic in the morning.

Well-Being (emotional well-being)

Positive affect—feelings of excitement, interest, pride, and pleasure with the way things are going.

Anger/hostility/irritability—tendency to be easily or persistently angry toward others or about one's life.

Anxiety—state of apprehension, tension, and worry.

Depression—mood disorder characterized by sadness and dejection, decreased motivation and interest in life, negative thoughts, and such physical symptoms as sleep disturbances, loss of appetite, and fatigue.

Well-Being (self-concept)

Self-esteem—positive or negative evaluation of oneself.

Sense of mastery and control—feeling that current and future events, including health events, are positively influenced by an individual's actions and decisions.

Well-Being (global perceptions of well-being)

Health outlook—individual's expectation for his or her future health status.

Current health perceptions—individual's rating of his or her present health status.

Life-satisfaction—general feeling of well-being indicated by taking pleasure in daily activities, finding life meaningful, having a feeling of success in achieving major goals, and having a positive self-image and optimism.

Healthy Life Year

Healthy life year—year free from chronic, disabling diseases and conditions, from preventable infections, and from serious injury; a year with the full range of functional capacity enabling one to enter into satisfying relationships with others, to work, and to play.

Sources

To create most of the definitions compiled in this glossary, we used published dictionaries, lists, glossaries, and other sources (1,14,16,17,29,43,44, 50,51,53,66,67,69,75,76,84).

Acknowledgments

The authors would like to gratefully acknowledge the comments of Professor Jeremy N. Morris of the London School of Hygiene and Tropical Medicine and the editorial suggestions and written contributions of Dr. Rick Hull. Their invaluable assistance has helped to improve the quality of this manuscript.

References

1. American Heart Association. Annotated bibliography of epidemiological methods of cardiovascular research. Dallas: American Heart Association; 1989.
2. American Heart Association. 1992 heart and stroke facts. Dallas: American Heart Association; 1991.
3. Amler, R.W.; Dull, H.B. Closing the gap: The burden of unnecessary illness. New York: Oxford University Press; 1987.
4. Bergner, M. Measurement of health status. Med. Care. 23:696-704; 1985.
5. Bergner, M.; Rothman, M.L. Health status measures: An overview and guide for selection. Annu. Rev. Public Health. 8:191-210; 1987.
6. Berkman, L.F. Social networks, support, and health: Taking the next step forward. Am. J. Epidemiol. 123:559-562; 1986.
7. Biering-Sørensen, F.; Bendix, T.; Jørgensen, K.; Manniche, C.; Nielsen, H. Physical activity, fitness and back pain. In: Bouchard, C.; Shephard, R.J.; Stephens, T., eds. Physical activity, fitness, and health. Champaign, IL: Human Kinetics; 1994:737-748 (this volume).
8. Blanchet, M. Assessment of health status. In: Bouchard, C.; Shephard, R.J.; Stephens, T.; Sutton, J.R.; McPherson, B.D., eds. Exercise, fitness, and health: A consensus of current knowledge. Champaign, IL: Human Kinetics; 1990:127-131.
9. Bouchard, C.; Shephard, R.J. Physical activity and fitness as determinants of health: The general model and basic concepts. In: Bouchard, C.; Shephard, R.J.; Stephens, T., eds. Physical activity, fitness, and health. Champaign, IL: Human Kinetics; 1994:77-88 (this volume).
10. Bowling, A. Measuring health: A review of quality of life measurement scales. Philadelphia: Open University Press; 1991.
11. Buchner, D.M.; Beresford, S.A.; Larson, E.B.; LaCroix, A.Z.; Wagner, E.H. Effects of physical activity on health status in older adults II: Intervention studies. Annu. Rev. Public Health. 13:469-488; 1992.
12. Caspersen, C.J. Physical activity epidemiology: Concepts, methods, and applications to exercise science. Exerc. Sport Sci. Rev. 17:423-473; 1989.
13. Caspersen, C.J.; Heath, G.W. The risk factor concept of coronary heart disease. In: Guidelines for graded exercise testing and prescription: A resource manual. Philadelphia: Lea & Febiger; 1988:111-125.
14. Caspersen, C.J.; Powell, K.E.; Christenson, G.M. Physical activity, exercise and physical

fitness: Definitions and distinctions for health-related research. Public Health Rep. 100:126-130; 1985.

15. Centers for Disease Control. Consensus set of health status indicators for the general assessment of community health status. MMWR. 40:449-451; 1991.
16. Definitions Workgroup, PHS Task Force on Improving Medical Criteria for Disability Determination. Unpublished manuscript. 1991.
17. Dever, G.E.A. Community health analysis: Global awareness at the local level. 2nd ed. Gaithersburg, MD: Aspen; 1991.
18. Deyo, R.A.; Patrick, D.L. Barriers to the use of health status measures in clinical investigation, patient care, and policy research. Med. Care. [Suppl. 3]. 27:S254-S268; 1989.
19. Elixhauser, A.; Weschler, J.M. The cost effectiveness of the primary prevention of cardiovascular disease: A review of the literature. Washington: Battelle, Human Affairs Research Centers; 1990.
20. Emery, C.F.; Blumenthal, J.A. Effects of physical exercise on psychological and cognitive functioning of older adults. Ann. Behav. Med. 13:99-107; 1991.
21. Erickson, P.; Kendall, E.A.; Anderson, J.P.; Kaplan, R.M. Using composite health status measures to assess the nation's health. Med. Care. [Suppl. 3]. 27:S66-S76; 1989.
22. Falvo, D.R. Medical and psychosocial aspects of chronic illness and disability. Gaithersberg, MD: Aspen; 1991.
23. Fischbach, F.T. A manual of laboratory & diagnostic tests. 4th ed. Philadelphia: Lippincott; 1992.
24. Fraser, G.E. Preventive cardiology. New York: Oxford University Press; 1986.
25. Friedman, R.; Tappen, R.M. The effect of planned walking on communication in Alzheimer's disease. J. Am. Geriatr. Soc. 39:650-654; 1991.
26. Froelicher, V.R.; Quaglietti, S. Physical activity and cardiac rehabilitation for patients with coronary heart disease. In: Bouchard, C.; Shephard, R.J.; Stephens, T., eds. Physical activity, fitness, and health. Champaign, IL: Human Kinetics; 1994:591-608 (this volume).
27. Gardner, J.W.; Sanborn, J.S. Years of potential life lost (YPPL)—what does it measure? Epidemiology. 1:322-329; 1990.
28. Gillum, R.F.; Blackburn, H.; Feinleib, M. Current strategies for explaining the decline in ischemic heart disease mortality. J. Chronic Dis. 35:467-474; 1982.
29. Hamilton, E.M.N.; Whitney, E.N.; Sizer, F.S. Nutrition: Concepts and controversies. New York: West; 1988.
30. Harris, S.S.; Caspersen, C.J.; DeFriese, G.H.; Estes, E.H. Physical activity counseling for healthy adults as a primary preventive intervention in the clinical setting. JAMA 261:3588-3598; 1989.
31. Hatziandreu, E.I.; Koplan, J.P.; Weinstein, M.C.; Caspersen, C.J.; Warner, K.E. A cost-effectiveness analysis of exercise as a health promotion activity. Am. J. Public Health. 78:1417-1421; 1988.
32. Health Care Financing Administration. The international classification of diseases, 9th revision, clinical modification (ICD-9-CM). 4th ed. DHHS publication no. (PHS) 91-1260. Washington, DC: Public Health Service; 1991. Available from: U.S. Government Printing Office, Washington, DC.
33. Institute of Medicine. Disability in America. Washington: National Academy Press; 1991.
34. Kaman, R.; Patton, R.W. Costs and benefits of an active versus an inactive society. In: Bouchard, C.; Shephard, R.J.; Stephens, T., eds. Physical activity, fitness, and health. Champaign, IL: Human Kinetics; 1994:134-144 (this volume).
35. Kane, R.A.; Kane, R.L. Assessing the elderly: A practical guide to measurement. Lexington, MA: Lexington Books; 1981.
36. Keeler, E.B.; Manning, W.B.; Newhouse, J.P.; Sloss, E.M.; Wasserman, J. The external costs of a sedentary life-style. Am. J. Public Health. 79:975-981; 1989.
37. Kohl, H.W.; McKenzie, J.D. Physical activity, fitness and stroke. In: Bouchard, C.; Shephard, R.J.; Stephens, eds. Physical activity, fitness, and health. Champaign, IL: Human Kinetics; 1994:609-621 (this volume).
38. Koplan, J.P. Health promotion, quality of life, and QALYS: A useful interaction. In: Published proceedings of the 1989 public health conference on records and statistics: Challenges for public health statistics in the 1990's. DHHS publication no. (PHS) 90-1214. 1989 July 17-19; Washington, DC: U.S. Dept. of Health and Human Services; 1989:294-296.
39. Kottke, T.E.; Caspersen, C.J.; Hill, C. Exercise in the management and rehabilitation of selected chronic diseases. Prev. Med. 13:47-65; 1984.
40. Kovner, A.R.; Jonas, S., editors. Health care delivery in the United States. 4th ed. New York: Springer; 1990.
41. Landers, D.M.; Petruzzello, S. Physical activity, fitness, and anxiety. In: Bouchard, C.; Shephard, R.J.; Stephens, T., eds. Physical activity, fitness, and health. Champaign, IL: Human Kinetics; 1994:868-882 (this volume).

42. LaPorte, R.E.; Montoye, H.J.; Caspersen, C.J. Assessment of physical activity in epidemiologic research: Problems and prospects. Public Health Rep. 100:131-146; 1985.
43. Last, J.M. A dictionary of epidemiology. 2nd ed. New York: Oxford University Press; 1988.
44. Last, J.M.; Wallace, R.B., eds. Maxcy-Rosenau-Last public health and preventive medicine. 13th ed. Norwalk, CT: Appleton and Lange; 1992.
45. Lee, I.-M. Physical activity, fitness, and cancer. In: Bouchard, C.; Shephard, R.J.; Stephens, T., eds. Physical activity, fitness, and health. Champaign, IL: Human Kinetics; 1994: chp. 55.
46. Lewis, C.C.; Pantell, R.H.; Kieckhefer, G.M. Assessment of children's health status. Field test of new approaches. Med. Care. [Suppl. 3]. 27:S54-S65; 1989.
47. Malina, R.M. Growth, exercise, fitness, and later outcomes. In: Bouchard, C.; Shephard, R.J.; Stephens, T.; Sutton, J.R.; McPherson, B.D., eds. Exercise, fitness, and health: A consensus of current knowledge. Champaign, IL: Human Kinetics; 1990:637-653.
48. Marmot, M.G. Psychosocial factors and cardiovascular disease: Epidemiological approaches. Eur. Heart J. 9:690-697; 1988.
49. McAuley, E. Physical activity and psychosocial outcomes. In: Bouchard, C.; Shephard, R.J.; Stephens, T., eds. Physical activity, fitness, and health. Champaign, IL: Human Kinetics; 1994:551-568 (this volume).
50. McDowell, I.; Newell, C. Measuring health: A guide to rating scales and questionnaires. New York: Oxford University Press; 1987.
51. Miller, D.C. Handbook of research design and social measurement. 5th ed. Newbury Park, CA: Sage Publications; 1991.
52. Mosteller, F.; Ware, J.E., Jr.; Levine, S. Finale panel: Comments on the conference on advances in health status assessment. Med. Care. [Suppl. 3]. 27:S282-S293; 1989.
53. National Center for Health Statistics. Health United States 1990. Hyattsville, MD: Public Health Service; 1991.
54. Navarro, V. Race or class or race and class: Growing mortality differentials in the United States. Int. J. Health Serv. 21:229-235; 1991.
55. Paffenbarger, R.S. Some interrelations of physical activity, physiological fitness, health, and longevity. In: Bouchard, C.; Shephard, R.J.; Stephens, T., eds. Physical activity, fitness, and health. Champaign, IL: Human Kinetics; 1994: 119-133 (this volume).
56. Painter, P.; Blackburn, G. Exercise for patients with chronic disease. Postgrad. Med. 83:185-187, 190-196; 1988.
57. Panush, R.S. Physical activity, fitness, and osteoarthritis. In: Bouchard, C.; Shephard, R.J.; Stephens, T., eds. Physical activity, fitness, and health. Champaign, IL: Human Kinetics; 1994:712-723 (this volume).
58. Pate, R.R.; Macera, C. Risk of exercising: Musculo-skeletal injuries and recreational vehicle accidents. In: Bouchard, C.; Shephard, R.J.; Stephens, T., eds. Physical activity, fitness, and health. Champaign, IL: Human Kinetics; 1994:1008-1018 (this volume).
59. Patrick, D.L.; Bergner, M. Measurement of health status in the 1990s. Annu. Rev. Public Health. 11:165-183; 1990.
60. Powell, K.E.; Caspersen, C.J.; Koplan, J.P.; Ford, E.S. Physical activity and chronic diseases. Am. J. Clin. Nutr. 49:999-1006; 1989.
61. Powell, K.E.; Thompson, P.D.; Caspersen, C.J.; Kendrick, J.S. Physical activity and the incidence of coronary heart disease. Annu. Rev. Public Health. 8:253-287; 1987.
62. Raglin, J.S. Exercise and mental health: Beneficial and detrimental effects. Sports Med. 9:323-329; 1990.
63. Robert Wood Johnson Foundation. Challenges in health care: A chartbook perspective 1991. Princeton, NJ: The Robert Wood Johnson Foundation; 1991.
64. Robine, J.M.; Brounard, N.; Colvez, A. The disability free life expectancy (DFLE) indexes: Comprehensive indexes of population health status. Rev. Epidemiol. Sante Publique. 35:206-224; 1987.
65. Robinson, J.P.; Shaver, P.R.; Wrightsman, L.S., editors. Measures of personality and social psychological attitudes. New York: Academic Press, Inc.; 1991.
66. Sarafino, E.P. Health psychology: Biopsychosocial interactions. New York: Wiley; 1990.
67. Sharkey, B.J. Physiological fitness & weight control. Missoula, MT: Mountain Press Publishing Co.; 1974.
68. Skinner, J.S.; Oja, P. Laboratory and field tests for assessing health-related fitness. In: Bouchard, C.; Shephard, R.J.; Stephens, T., eds. Physical activity, fitness, and health. Champaign, IL: Human Kinetics; 1994:160-179 (this volume).
69. Stedman, T.L. Stedman's medical dictionary. 25th ed. Baltimore: Williams & Wilkins; 1990.
70. Stephens, T. Exercise and mental health in the United States and Canada: Evidence from four population surveys. Prev. Med. 17:35-47; 1988.
71. Stewart, A.L.; King, A.C. Evaluating the efficacy of physical activity for influencing quality-of-life outcomes in older adults. Ann. Behav. Med. 13:108-116; 1991.

72. Stewart, A.L.; Ware, J.E., editors. Measuring functioning and well-being: The medical outcomes study approach. Durham, NC: Duke University Press; 1992.
73. Terris, M. Approaches to an epidemiology of health. Am. J. Public Health. 65:1037-1045; 1975.
74. Tipton, C.M.; Fagard, R. Physical activity, fitness and hypertension. In: Bouchard, C.; Shephard, R.J.; Stephens, T., eds. Physical activity, fitness, and health. Champaign, IL: Human Kinetics; 1994:633-655 (this volume).
75. U.S. Department of Health and Human Services. Disease prevention/health promotion: The facts. Palo Alto, CA: Bull Publishing; 1988.
76. U.S. Department of Health and Human Services. Healthy People 2000: National health promotion and disease prevention objectives—full report, with commentary. DHHS publication no. (PHS) 91-50212. Washington, DC: Public Health Service; 1991. Available from: U.S. Government Printing Office, Washington, DC.
77. U.S. House of Representatives. A discursive dictionary of health care. Washington, DC: U.S. Government Printing Office; 1976.
78. U.S. Preventive Services Task Force. Guide to clinical preventive services: An assessment of the effectiveness of 169 interventions. Baltimore: Williams & Wilkins; 1989.
79. Verbrugge, L.M. Gender and health: An update on hypotheses and evidence. J. Health Soc. Behav. 26:156-182; 1985.
80. Verbrugge, L.M. Recent, present, and future health of American adults. Annu. Rev. Public Health. 10:333-361; 1989.
81. Verbrugge, L.M.; Balaban, D.J. Patterns of change in disability and well-being. Med. Care. [Suppl. 3]. 27:S128-S147; 1989.
82. Wagner, E.H.; LaCroix, A.Z.; Buchner, D.M.; Larson, E.B. Effects of physical activity on health status in older adults I: Observational studies. Annu. Rev. Public Health. 13:451-468; 1992.
83. Wallace, R.B.; Woolson, R.F., editors. The epidemiologic study of the elderly. New York: Oxford University Press; 1992.
84. Webster's new world dictionary, third college edition. New York: Simon & Schuster; 1988.
85. Wilson, J.D.; Braunwald, E.; Isselbacher, K.J.; Petersdorf, R.G.; Martin, J.B.; Fauci, A.S.; Root, R.K., editors. Harrison's principles of internal medicine. 12th ed. New York: McGraw-Hill; 1991.
86. World Health Organization. Constitution of the World Health Organization. In: Basic documents. Geneva: World Health Organization; 1948.
87. World Health Organization. International classification of disease, 9th revision (ICD-9). Geneva: World Health Organization; 1975.

PART III

Physical Activity, Fitness, and Health: Status and Determinants

Chapter 12

The Demography of Physical Activity

Thomas Stephens
Carl J. Caspersen

National-level data on leisure-time physical activity from representative population surveys using reasonably comparable methods are now available for several countries, and data on trends over 10 or more years are available for most of these. It is thus possible to make some generalizations about the exercise behavior of adult populations in advanced industrial societies and about how this behavior has changed in the past decade. This paper offers such generalizations, compares the exercise practices of selected population subgroups, and identifies major outstanding issues of a conceptual and methodological nature. The focus is on leisure-time activity, because this is the subject of most of the surveys, although some data on occupational activity are available.

For data on current prevalence, the evidence presented here is generally restricted to national-level population estimates from well-documented reports and is taken from the most recent surveys known to the authors (see Table 12.1). Surveys of subnational areas have not been included if national-level data are available for the same country, although many of these are high quality. Some data are occasionally used to illustrate patterns in countries other than those in Table 12.1, even though their documentation is less than complete, in the hope of encouraging fuller reporting by survey officials in the future.

Population surveys of physical activity have been concentrated in Australia, Canada, Finland, and the United States, where several major studies have been carried out since at least the mid-1980s. Data are presented from multiple sources within these countries because different surveys often employ different methods and definitions, thus providing some evidence of validity and reliability. Where trend data are described, they are restricted to time series in which key definitions are internally consistent. Most are also consistent with respect to the time of data collection and design of the sample. The notable exception is Australia where the most recent data (8) were collected in Adelaide only from August 1990 to February 1991 while data collected variously in January and July from 1984 to 1987 (2) represent the national adult population; in this review, a published, pooled value (2) is used to represent Australian activity levels as of 1986.

Current Prevalence of Activity in Adult Populations

Recent surveys in Australia, Canada, England, and the United States indicate that only about 10% of the adult population of each country might be called "aerobically active," that is, engaging in vigorous activities during their leisure time on an average of at least three occasions weekly for 20 to 30 min or more per occasion. These results pertain to definitions that tend to incorporate a minimum threshold of intensity, although the height of this threshold varies: 7 METs (8), 50%+ of age-specific capacity (23), 60%+ of age- and sex-specific capacity (6,11), 7.5 kcal/min (1), 10 kcal/min (20), or perceived exertion of hard breathing and puffing (18). The definitions also specify frequency and duration of activity (or total time) (12) which equates to an average of at least three sessions per week for 20 min per session (see Table 12.2).

Results from Finland are apparently consistent with these findings (16); however, because less detail is available on the methods of this particular survey, its features do not appear in Table 12.1 nor the results in Table 12.2. In Finland, 15% of persons age 30 to 59 years were classified highly active.

One third of the American, Australian, Canadian, and English populations engage in leisure-time activities that are less vigorous or less frequent than is generally assumed to be needed for cardiorespiratory fitness, although they are usually active on a fairly regular basis and may well achieve weight control, cardiovascular, and other health benefits. In Finland (17), half the adult population is at least moderately active. These results

Table 12.1 Features of Recent National Surveys of Physical Activity

Country	Year	Agency	Age	Sample size	Method
Australia (18)	1989	National Heart Foundation	20–69	9,328	Questionnaire
Australia (8) (Adelaide)	1990-1991	Department of the Arts, Sport, Environment, Tourism, and Territories (DASETT)	18–78	3,384	Personal interview
Canada (23) (CFS)	1988	Canadian Fitness & Lifestyle Research Institute	10+	3,068	Questionnaire
Canada (12) (GSS)	1991	Statistics Canada (General Social Survey)	15+	11,924	Telephone interview
England (1)	1990	Sports Council & Health Education Authority	16+	4,316	Personal interview
Finland (17)	1991	National Public Health Institute	15–64	5,000	Postal questionnaire
USA (15) (NHIS)	1990	National Center for Health Statistics (National Health Interview Survey)	18+	41,104	Personal interview
USA (6,11) (BRFSS)	1990	CDC (Behavioral Risk Factor Surveillance System)	18+	48,745	Telephone interview

Table 12.2 Percentage of National Populations That Are "Aerobically Active" in Their Leisure Time (Various Definitions), by Sex

Country, Year	Definition	Total	Male	Female
Australia, 1989 (18)	Vigorous PA (hard breathing, puffing, panting) for 20+ min, 3+ times/week	5	6	4
Australia, 1990-1991 (8)	Greater than 3250 MET over 2 weeks (~1,600 kcal/week) and 6+ 20-min occasions of activities at 7+ MET	15	16	14
Canada, 1988 (23)	PA 50% or more of age-specific capacity, for 30+ min, 3+ times/week	11	14	8
Canada, 1991 (12)	Vigorous PA (10+ kcal/min) for a weekly total of at least 1 hr (600+ kcal/week)	15	20	10
England, 1990 (1)	12+ occasions over 4 weeks of vigorous PA (7.5+ kcal/min) *including occupational activity* for 20+ min (450+ kcal/week)	9	14	4
USA, 1990 (BRFSS) (6,11)	PA of 20+ min/occasion, 3+ times/week, at 60%+ of age- and sex-specific maximum cardiorespiratory capacity involving rhythmic contractions of large muscle groups	9	9	9

Note. PA = physical activity, MET = multiple of the resting metabolic rate.

(see Table 12.3) reflect a variety of definitions of "active" based on total time (or frequency and duration of activity) at levels of intensity which are either moderate or unspecified. If a minimum intensity threshold is specified, the requirement is for less demanding activity (e.g., 5.0-7.5 kcal/min[1]) than that reflected in Table 12.2.

Some surveys categorize physical activity into four categories (6,8,11,23), some use three (12,15,24), while the English survey (1) reports six levels. These variations complicate comparisons of the size of populations which are less than moderately active. However, the surveys in Table 12.4 all report the proportion of the population which

Table 12.3 Percent of National Populations That Are Moderately Active in Their Leisure Time (Various Definitions), by Sex

Country, Year	Definition	Total	Male	Female
Australia, 1989 (18)	Less vigorous PA (no puffing or panting)	31	33	29
Australia, 1990–1991 (8)	1500–3250 MET over 2 weeks (~735–1,600 kcal/week)	29	32	26
Canada, 1988 (23)	Low-intensity PA (less than 50% of age-specific capacity) for 30+ min, 3+ times/week	38	37	38
Canada, 1988 (24)	Daily average of 3 kcal·kg^{-1}, any intensity (~1,250 kcal/week)	33	42	25
Canada, 1991 (12)	2,000+ kcal/week, any intensity	32	39	26
England, 1990 (1)	12 or more 20-min occasions in 4 weeks of at least moderate activity (5–7.5 kcal/min) *including occupational* activity (300–450 kcal/week)	36	35	37
Finland, 1991 (17)	1/2 hr or more of activity to produce light sweating 2+ times/week	51	50	51
USA, 1990 (NHIS) (15)	Daily average of 3 kcal·kg^{-1}, any intensity (~1,250 kcal/week)	29	37	23
USA, 1990 (NHIS) (15)	Exercise or play sports regularly	41	44	38
USA, 1990 (BRFSS) (6,11)	PA of 20+ min/occasion, 3+ times/week, either not reaching 60% of age- and sex-specific capacity or not rhythmic contractions of large muscle groups, or both	32	32	32

Note. PA = physical activity, MET = multiple of the resting metabolic rate.

Table 12.4 Percent of National Populations That Are Sedentary in Their Leisure Time (Various Definitions), by Sex

Country, Year	Definition	Total	Male	Female
Australia, 1989 (18)	No exercise of any kind	27	27	27
Australia, 1990–1991 (8)	Less than 100 MET total over 2 weeks (~50 kcal/week)	23	22	24
Canada, 1988 (23)	0 - 1.4 kcal·kg^{-1}·day (~600 kcal/week)	43	36	49
Canada, 1991 (12)	<500 kcal/week	22	19	25
England, 1990 (1)	No 20-min occasions in 4 weeks of even moderate activity (5 kcal/min) *including occupational*	16	17	16
Finland, 1991 (17)	PA to produce light sweating a few times a year or less	15	17	14
USA, 1990 (BRFSS) (6,11)	No PA reported for the last month	31	29	32

Note. PA = physical activity, MET = multiple of the resting metabolic rate.

is inactive or sedentary, although even these definitions vary in their rigor. The prevalence of sedentarism generally ranges between one quarter and one third of adults except in Finland and England where it is much lower. However, the English figures include occupational activity.

With the exception of England, these findings on the prevalence of activity pertain to leisure-time activity only. However, it seems reasonable to include the English data because occupational activity typically does not add much to total energy expenditure. In Canada, where only 20% of the workforce in 1988 described their job as physically demanding and 51% as involving mostly sitting, there was no relationship between occupational and leisure-time activity (23). Office workers and manual laborers were about equally likely to exercise in their spare time, apparently disproving the contention that blue-collar workers are sedentary off the job because they are active on the job.

The Finnish surveys are the only ones to specify walking or cycling to work as forms of physical activity (18). In 1991 an impressive 37% of women and 27% of men working away from home spent 15+ min daily in physically active commuting.

Temporal Trends in Leisure-Time Activity

Compared to the mid-1980s (21), there are now several time series available which allow for the examination of trends in leisure-time activity in national populations. With some exceptions in vigorous activity, these point to recent increases in the prevalence of exercise.

For vigorous physical activity, the United States (6,11) shows a slight increase from the mid-1980s to 1990 (see Figure 12.1). There was no change in Australia during this period, while a decline was experienced in Canada between 1981 and 1988. This is consistent with other Canadian data suggesting that activity preferences are shifting toward less vigorous forms. For example, jogging was the only exercise activity among the top-ranked 18 to lose popularity in Canada between 1981 and 1988. Gardening, social dancing, and bowling—relatively low-level activities—all made notable gains during this period, while the popularity of bicycling, tennis, home exercise, and cross-country skiing—relatively demanding activities—all held steady (23).

Data from other countries, although not as well documented as the primary sources in this review, are consistent with the evidence for increased activity. Eastern Finland and the former German Democratic Republic reported distinct increases in vigorous activity from the 1970s through the mid-1980s (16). Unfortunately, these time series do not continue into the 1990s, while the Australian, Canadian, and United States series began relatively recently. This makes it difficult to draw firm conclusions about the nature of longer term trends in vigorous leisure-time activity, although the European data strengthen the general impression of increases in physical activity over the recent past.

For moderate levels of physical activity the evidence for recent increases is consistent (see Figure 12.2). In Canada (12,20,23,24), Finland (17), and the United States (5,6,11,15,19), moderate levels of exercise, by several definitions, became more common during the 1980s. Similar trends have been reported from telephone surveys in two major cities in Scotland for the period 1987 to 1991 (26).

Data from many of these same countries show declines in the prevalence of sedentarism (see Figure 12.3). Definitions vary, as they do with other categories of activity, yet the trends are the same: In Australia, Canada, Finland, and the United States, the sedentary population shrank during the 1980s. This is consistent with trends reported for Scotland for the period 1987 to 1991 (26).

Good trend data on occupational activity are even more scarce than for leisure-time activity. While automation and a reduced work week have undoubtedly resulted in an overall decrease in energy expenditure on the job (10), precise data are lacking for all countries but Finland. Surveys in that country (17) reveal that adults reporting heavy occupational work declined from 50% to 38% of the work force between 1972 and 1987, while there were also substantial declines in physically active

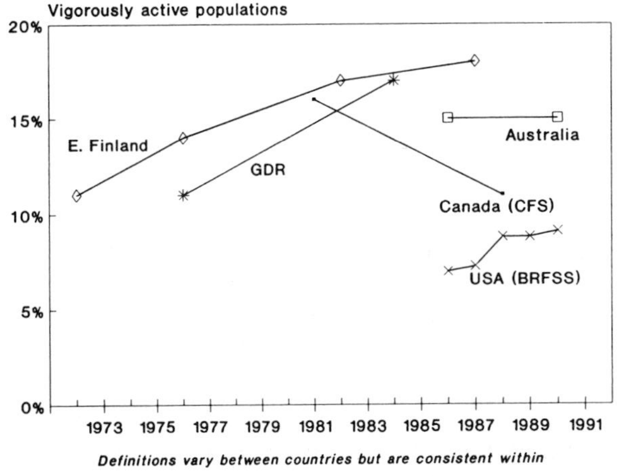

Figure 12.1 Temporal trends in vigorous leisure-time activity.

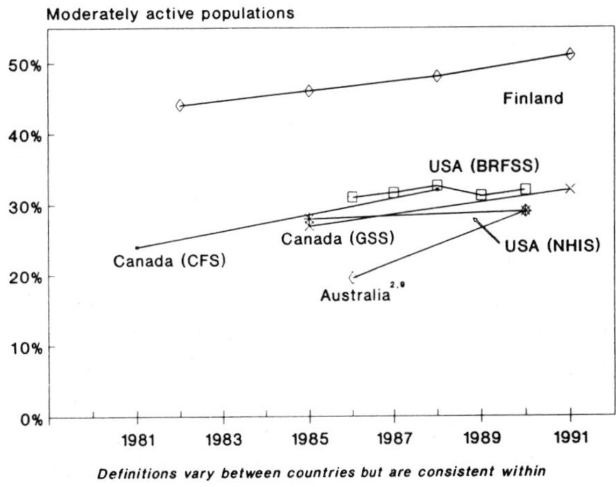

Figure 12.2 Temporal trends in moderate leisure-time activity.

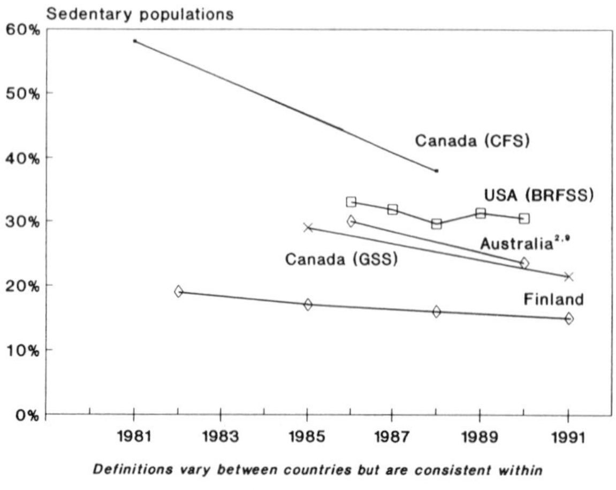

Figure 12.3 Temporal trends in sedentary leisure-time activity.

commuting to work. From 1982 to 1991, the proportion of men working away from home who spent more than 15 min walking or bicycling to work decreased from 41% to 27%; the equivalent proportion of women declined from 60% to 37%.

In summary, it is clear that there has been an increase in leisure-time physical activity in many industrialized countries in at least the past decade, and it appears that this development consists mainly of sedentary individuals becoming moderately active rather than there being any meaningful increase in the vigorously active population. This is supported by Canadian longitudinal data: Over the period 1981 to 1988, 26% of Canadians changed from being sedentary to moderately active, while only 5% increased their exercise level from moderately active to more highly active, and 6% decreased from highly to moderately active (23).

Seasonal Differences

Few surveys have published data on changes in physical activity *during* a given year, although many studies tacitly recognize this phenomenon by designing data collection to counteract such patterns. In the temperate climate of Australia, for example, only swimming has been found to vary substantially with the seasons, while other forms of physical recreation are remarkably stable—varying by less than 2% between winter and summer surveys (8).

In contrast, Canadian and Scottish data reveal wide seasonal swings in activity. Figure 12.4 shows the seasonal variations in Canada for those types of activity which consistently figure in the 10 most popular internationally (22). The peak–trough values differ by a factor of 2. However, these data do not include such popular winter sports as skating (ranked 7th overall in Canada in 1988), alpine skiing (ranked 8th), and cross-country skiing (ranked 13th) (23). Survey data collected from more than 13,000 adults in Glasgow and Edinburgh from January 1987 through June 1991 show considerable variation in both outdoor and indoor activities (26). In a fashion similar to the Canadian data, these surveys show that activity peaks in early summer and reaches a nadir in early winter.

While data on seasonality are rare, they indicate that, in these three countries at least, leisure-time activity levels correspond to seasonal changes in weather and length of day. Data from other countries covering a wider range of activities would be helpful in establishing the nature of and explanation behind these behavioral variations.

Demographic Correlates of Activity

Sex

The male/female ratio of active populations ranges widely depending on the definitions and the country. For aerobically active populations, the sex ratios range from 1.0 (USA) to 3.5 (England), with an average value around 1.8 (see Table 12.5, column 2). In other words, males in these countries are, on average, 80% more likely to be vigorously active than females. The major exception to this pattern occurs when high-intensity activities are scored on a sex-specific basis, as in the US Behavioral Risk Factor Surveillance System (6,11), although the Australian data (8) show equality of the sexes without such an adjustment.

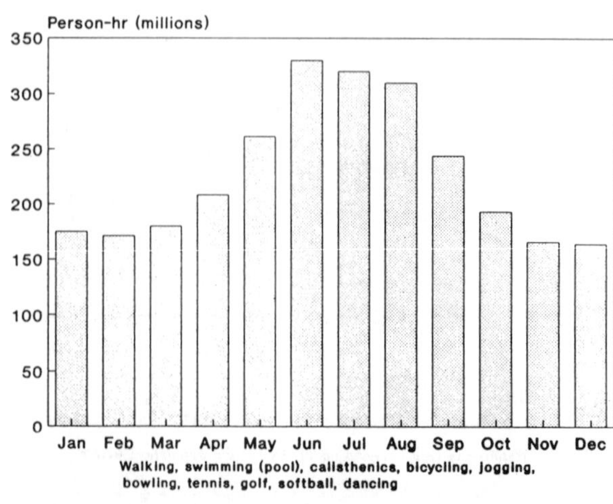

Figure 12.4 Seasonal trends in leisure-time activity.

Table 12.5 Differences Between the Sexes in Active, Moderate, and Sedentary Populations in Various National Surveys

Country, Year	M/F ratio		
	Aerobically active	Moderately active	Sedentary
Australia, 1989 (18)	1.5	1.1	.9
Australia, 1990–1991 (8)	1.1	1.2	.9
Canada, 1988 (23)	1.8	1.0	.7
Canada, 1991 (12)	2.0	1.5	.8
England, 1990 (1)	3.5	0.9	1.1
Finland, 1991 (17)	—	1.0	1.2
USA, 1990 (BRFSS) (6,11)	1.0	1.0	.9

Sex differences for moderate levels of activity are smaller than for vigorous activity (from 0.9-1.5), and are relatively trivial when intensity does not form part of the definition of active. When different definitions of "moderately active" exist for the same populations (see Table 12.3), those based on *frequency and duration* of activity have M:F ratios close to 1.0, while those that incorporate *intensity* tend to result in larger sex differences. For example, the M:F ratio for frequent low-intensity activity of 30+ min per occasion is 1.0 in Canada; for the same population, the ratio is 1.7 when the definition is based on total energy expenditure, thus giving a premium to activities of high absolute intensity (23).

An earlier review (21) concluded that women increased their exercise levels more rapidly than men in the early 1980s, but this may not be true of every country. Like much in this review, it depends on the definition. For example, the proportion of Canadians in the active category grew more quickly for men from 1981 to 1988 (23) and 1985 to 1991 in Canada (12,20) than it did for women. But when the definition of active is based strictly on time and does not account for intensity, the 7-year increases are the same for both sexes (23). Moreover, when sex-specific values are used in the United States for defining vigorous activity, women were found to be more likely than men to make gains in regular vigorous activity during the period 1986 to 1990 (6,11). In Finland the increases during the period 1982 to 1991 were equal for men and women.

Male-female differences in occupational activity are more rarely reported and appear to be even less consistent than those for leisure-time activity. In Canada (23) very similar proportions of men and women rate their work as heavy (21% and 18%, respectively), while in Finland the respective percentages are 44% and 32% (16). Although the definitions in these surveys are clearly different and international comparisons are thus compromised, it is not clear why there is a large sex difference in one country and not the other, or why these differences are opposite to those noted earlier for leisure-time activity.

Age

National cross-sectional surveys of physical activity are fairly consistent in reporting that exercise prevalence among adults declines with age (see Figure 12.5), as reported before (21,25), at least until age 65. Compared to younger adults, older adults exercise less often and choose activities that are lower in their absolute energy demands. However, there are important exceptions to this generalization. In Canada and Finland there is an increase in activity reported for the *oldest* age group compared to the next youngest. Also, if intensity of activity is defined *relative to age* as in the USA-BRFSS series, the expected decline in exercise prevalence plotted by age disappears and there is evidence of increased activity at age 65, or even younger, depending on the definition.

Although most surveys are confined to the adult population, those that include children show a precipitous drop in activity that coincides with the end of high school. For example, Canadians age 20 to 24 years are twice as likely to be sedentary as 10 to 14 year-olds and only 60% as likely to be in the active category (23).

Trend data for age groups show that older Americans increased their exercise levels more than younger ones during the early 1980s (21), and more recent figures indicate that this trend is continuing. Longitudinal data from Canada (23)

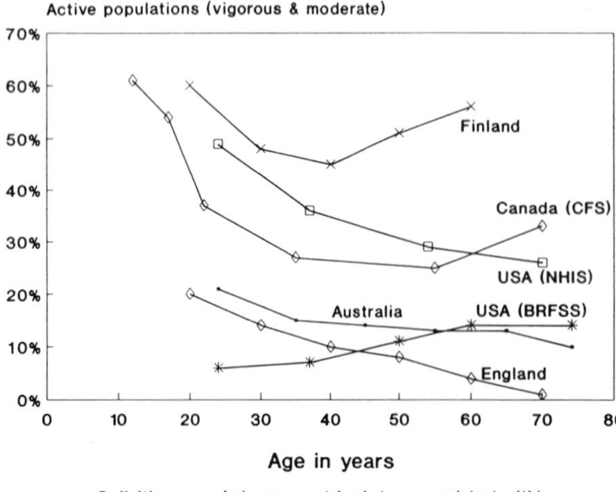

Figure 12.5 Age trends in leisure-time activity.

reveal that persons age 20 to 24 were the only age group that did not increase their leisure-time physical activity over the period 1981 to 1988, while a 1986 to 1991 series shows that the age group 15 to 24 had the smallest increase of all age groups in Canada (12,20). Similarly, in the United States, men and women age 18 to 29 and 30 to 44 were the only persons who did not increase their leisure-time physical activity from 1986 to 1990 (6,11).

Education

Leisure-time physical activity is consistently more common among groups with more education. Data from recent surveys in Australia, Canada, and the United States reveal that the most educated group is 1.5 to 3.1 times more likely to be active as the least educated group and only 30 to 60% as likely to be sedentary (see Table 12.6). (Unfortunately, none of these data are age-standardized.) Data for England (1) that are age-stratified are consistent with this pattern: Among both men and women, the least educated group in each of three age strata is twice as likely to be sedentary as the most educated group. Among the set of countries in this review, the education-level differences are most pronounced in the United States (most/least educated ratios of 2.8 and 3.1 in 1986 and 1990 BRFSS series). This steep education gradient in the United States has been noted in previous international comparisons of other health habits such as smoking and alcohol use (13).

There is little evidence to suggest this education gap is closing over time despite the efforts of public policy-makers. The 1981 to 1988 Canadian data (23) show a modest narrowing of this gap, but no such evidence was found in a review of United States sources covering most of the period 1971 to 1985 (21), while some widening of the gap was evident in the United States for the period 1986 to 1990 (6,11).

Summary

Recent surveys in Australia, Canada, Finland, and the United States indicate that only about 10% of adults engage in genuinely vigorous activities at least three times weekly for 20+ min at a time. Another third are active at a lower level—practicing leisure-time activities that are less vigorous or less frequent—while one quarter to one third are sedentary in their leisure time. The balance is defined as low-active.

In Australia, Canada, Finland, and the United States, there is clear evidence for an increased prevalence of exercise over at least the past decade, although the increase is generally of modest proportions and is most clearly seen for moderate levels of activity. In Australia and Canada there is some suggestion of a leveling off or even decline in the size of the vigorously active group; however, in all these countries and others there are signs that the sedentary population has shrunk.

There is considerable consistency among nations in the patterns of exercise levels related to sex, age, and education. Male-female differences are most pronounced for high-intensity leisure-time activity (except when "high-intensity" is defined in a sex-specific manner), and are smaller or nonexistent for other measures of activity.

Exercise prevalence generally declines steadily with age, although this trend may be obscured when the definition of "active" is based on age-specific cutpoints to classify the intensity of activities. Canada and Finland may provide important exceptions, because seniors in these two countries are more active than the next youngest group—even without the advantage of accounting for age in the definition of "active."

Leisure-time physical activity is consistently more common among groups with more education. This is particularly true in the United States but does not hold in Finland. From the perspective of international comparisons, Finland is the interesting exception to patterns generally seen in Australia, Canada, England, and the United States: There is equality of the sexes and education groups and little age-related decline in physical activity.

Table 12.6 Differences Between Education Groups in Active and Sedentary Populations in Various National Surveys

	% Active			% Sedentary		
Country, Year	High education	Low education	Ratio High:Low	High education	Low education	Ratio High:Low
Australia, 1990–1991 (8)	23	11	2.0	11	28	.4
Canada, 1988 (23)	41	27	1.5	33	52	.6
Finland, 1991 (17)	51	53	1.0	—	—	—
USA, 1990 (NHIS) (15)	37	20	1.9	—	—	—
USA, 1990 (BRFSS) (6,11)	14	5	3.1	18	52	.3

Outstanding Issues

Methodological Issues

A wide variety of methods is available to measure physical activity (4), but few other than questionnaires are suitable for population surveys. Simple measures including single-item questions show some promise as proxy measures of physical activity (28,29) and can prove useful for classifying activity into high/medium/low categories. Further work is needed to establish a simple but good interval-level variable, just as it is to establish the validity and reliability of more elaborate questionnaire techniques. Recent efforts in New Zealand (9) to establish validity and in the United States (3) to determine reliability of long-term recall are encouraging developments. The report of the recent Australian survey (8) is commendable for the detail provided on reliabilities of questionnaire items; their validity remains moot, however.

Inconsistencies of recall period and timing of data collection in various questionnaires can complicate comparisons between surveys. The 2-week period which is typical in many surveys may not be suitable for populations with large seasonal variations in activity such as in Canada, Scotland and the northern United States. Even when seasonal variations are small, as in Australia, basing temporal trends on data from surveys in January and July (2) may not be entirely straightforward. Further methodological work is needed to establish whether a recall period of 1, 2, or 4 weeks is the optimum for accurate and reliable reporting of physical activity.

Conceptual and Substantive Issues

There has been some convergence in the measurement and definition of the active population since earlier reviews on this topic, although some notable differences remain. Most large population surveys now collect sufficient detail on activity type, frequency, and average duration, making it possible to calculate summaries of energy expenditure expressed in total kilocalories (Canada) (12) or METs over the reporting period (Australia) (8) or average daily kilocalories per kilogram of body weight (Canada [23], United States [15]). While the cutpoints used with these energy expenditure indexes (e.g., 3 $kcal \cdot kg^{-1} \cdot day$ [15,23], 3250 MET/2 weeks [8]) are approximately equal to the total energy expenditure from the exercise dose recommended for cardiovascular benefit, these definitions, unlike the prescription itself, impose no requirements of vigorous intensity, minimum frequency, or minimum duration per occasion.

For this reason, a more rigorous definition of vigorous activity has developed, inspired by the United States health promotion objectives for the years 1990 and 2000 (14,27). This approach requires evidence of each of the elements of the prescription, namely vigorous activity, adequate duration, and sufficient frequency (7). This approach is reflected in the definitions of aerobic activity used in Australia, Canada, England, and the United States (BRFSS) (see Table 12.2).

There remains an unresolved definitional issue, however: Should vigorous activities be identified according to absolute or relative capacity, and if relative, should this take into account both age and sex? At this time, the American and Canadian approaches account for age, although the recent Canadian survey used a value of 50% of capacity compared to the American figure of 60%. Sex-specific values are used only in the United States. The impact of this is shown in Table 12.5 where the American male:female ratio for the prevalence of vigorous activity was 1.0 in 1990, compared to 2.0 in Canada and 3.5 in England. Settling this issue would facilitate international comparisons. Since it is clear that maximum cardiorespiratory capacity does indeed vary with age and sex (7), the issue is not *whether* to make age- and sex-specific adjustments, but *how* and what values to use.

Definitions vary in other details, although the general approaches have converged in recent surveys. For example, the operational definitions used to distinguish vigorous activities vary from a lower limit of 7.5 kcal/min (England [1]) to 10 kcal/min (Canada–GSS [20]). Similarly, definitions of "sedentary" based on energy expenditure range from less than 50 kcal/week (Australia [8]) to less than 600 kcal/wk (Canada [12]).

Once definitions have been agreed upon (or more likely, while definitions continue to evolve), further monitoring of leisure-time activity in adult populations is needed to identify whether: (a) the prevalence of activity is increasing or has reached a plateau, (b) women, older adults, and less educated groups are closing the gap by becoming more active more quickly than the rest of the population, (c) less industrialized countries than those in this review have similar activity levels, (d) occupational demands are diminishing as suspected, and (e) seasonal fluctuations in activity correspond to annual variations in weather and length of day.

References

1. Activity and Health Research. Allied Dunbar National Fitness Survey: Main findings. London: The Sports Council and the Health Education Authority; 1992.
2. Bauman, A.; Owen, N.; Rushworth, R.L. Recent trends and sociodemographic determinants of exercise participation in Australia. Community Health Stud. 14(1):19-26; 1990.
3. Blair, S.N.; Dowda, M.; Pate, R.R.; Kronenfield, J.; Howe, H.G., Jr.; Parker, G.; Blair, A.; Freidenger, F. Reliability of long-term recall of participation in physical activity by middle-aged men and women. Am. J. Epidemiol. 133(3):266-275; 1991.
4. Caspersen, C.J. Physical activity epidemiology: Concepts, methods, and applications to exercise science. Exerc. Sport Sci. Rev. 17:423-473; 1989.
5. Caspersen, C.J.; Christensen, G.M.; Pollard, R.A. Status of the 1990 physical fitness and exercise objectives—evidence from NHIS 1985. Public Health Rep. 101(6):587-592; 1986.
6. Caspersen, C.J.; Merritt, R.K. Trends in physical activity patterns among older adults: The behavioral risk factor surveillance system, 1986-1990. Med. Sci. Sports Exerc. 24(4):526; 1992.
7. Caspersen, C.J.; Pollard, R.A.; Pratt, S.O. Scoring physical activity data with special consideration for elderly populations. Proceedings of the 21st national meeting of the public health conference on records and statistics: Data for an aging population. 1987 July; Washington, DC.
8. Department of the Arts, Sport, the Environment, Tourism and Territories (DASETT). Pilot survey of the fitness of Australians. Canberra: Australia Government Publishing Service; 1992.
9. Hopkins, W.G.; Wilson, N.C.; Russell, D.G. Validation of a physical activity instrument for the life in New Zealand national survey. Am. J. Epidemiol. 133(1):73-82; 1991.
10. Koplan, J.P.; Powell, K.E. Physicians and the Olympics. JAMA. 252:529-530; 1984.
11. Merritt, R.K.; Caspersen, C.J. Trends in physical activity patterns among young adults: The behavioral risk factor surveillance system, 1986-1990. Med. Sci. Sports Exerc. 24(4):526; 1992.
12. Millar, W.J. Report on the 1991 General Social Survey. Ottawa: Statistics Canada; March 1992 (and custom tabulations).
13. National Center for Health Statistics; Stephens, T.; Schoenborn, C. Adult health practices in the United States and Canada. Vital and health statistics. Series 5, No.3. DHHS pub. no. (PHS) 88-1479. Washington, DC: Public Health Service; 1988. Available from: U.S. Government Printing Office, Washington, DC.
14. Office of Disease Prevention and Health Promotion. The 1990 health objectives for the nation: A midcourse review. Washington, DC: U.S. Department of Health and Human Services; 1986.
15. Piani, A.; Schoenborn, C.A. Health promotion and disease prevention: United States, 1990. Vital and health statistics. Series 10, No. X. DHHS pub. no. (PHS) 93-1513. Washington, DC: Public Health Service; 1992; [In preparation]. Available from: U.S. Government Printing Office, Washington, DC.
16. Powell, K.E.; Stephens, T.; Marti, B.; Heinemann, L.; Kreuter, M. Progress and problems in the promotion of physical activity. In: Oja, P.; Telama, R., eds. Sport for all. Amsterdam: Elsevier Science; 1991:55-73.
17. Puska, P.; Berg, M-A.; Peltoniemi, J. Health behaviour among Finnish adult population. Helsinki: National Public Health Institute, Department of Epidemiology and Health Promotion; 1992.
18. Risk Factor Prevalence Study Management Committee. Risk Factor Prevalence Study: Sur-

vey no. 3 1989. Canberra: National Heart Foundation of Australia and Australian Institute of Health; 1990.

19. Schoenborn, C.A. Health habits of U.S. adults, 1985: The "Alameda 7" revisited. Public Health Rep. 101:571-580; 1986.
20. Statistics Canada, Housing, Family and Social Statistics Division. Health and social support, 1985. General Social Survey, analysis series. Statistics Canada Catalogue no. 11-5612, no. 1. Ottawa: Minister of Supply and Services; 1987.
21. Stephens, T. Secular trends in adult physical activity: Exercise boom or bust? Res. Q. Exerc. Sport. 58(2):94-105; 1987.
22. Stephens, T.; Craig, C.L. Fitness and activity measurement in the 1981 Canada Fitness Survey. In: National Center for Health Statistics, Drury, T., ed. Assessing physical fitness and physical activity in population-based surveys. DHHS pub. no. (PHS) 89-1253. Hyattsville, MD: Public Health Service; 1989.
23. Stephens, T.; Craig, C.L. The well-being of Canadians: Highlights of the 1988 Campbell's Survey. Ottawa: Canadian Fitness and Lifestyle Research Institute; 1990.
24. Stephens, T.; Craig, C.L.; Ferris, B.F. Adult physical activity in Canada: Findings from the Canada Fitness Survey I. Can. J. Public Health. 77:285-290; 1986.
25. Stephens, T.; Jacobs, D.R.; White, C.C. A descriptive epidemiology of leisure-time physical activity. Public Health Rep. 100:147-158; 1985.
26. Uitenbroek, D.G.; McQueen, D.V. Leisure-time physical activity in Scotland: Trends 1987-1991 and the effect of question wording. Soz Praventivmed. 36; 1992.
27. U.S. Department of Health and Human Services. Healthy People 2000: National health promotion and disease prevention objectives—full report, with commentary. DHHS publ. no. (PHS) 91-50212. Washington, DC: Public Health Service; 1991. Available from: U.S. Government Printing Office, Washington, DC.
28. Washburn, R.A.; Goldfield, S.R.W.; Smith, K.W.; McKinlay, J.B. The validity of self-reported exercise-induced sweating as a measure of physical activity. Am. J. Epidemiol. 132(1):107-113; 1990.
29. Weiss, T.W.; Slater, C.H.; Green, L.W.; Kennedy, V.C.; Albright, D.L.; Wun, C.C. The validity of single-item, self-assessment questions as measures of adult physical activity. J. Clin. Epidemiol. 43(11):1123-1129; 1990.

Chapter 13

Determinants and Interventions for Physical Activity and Exercise

Rod K. Dishman
James F. Sallis

Understanding the knowledge, attitudes, and behavioral and social skills associated with adopting and maintaining a regular exercise program is a research need identified by the U.S. Public Health Service in the Year 2000 Objectives for the Nation (17). Similar policies for understanding and increasing physical activity have been issued in other industrialized nations (34,73,111).

In this chapter we examine the recent English language literature on the determinants of physical activity and exercise and on behavior change interventions for increasing and maintaining physical activity and exercise. Our purpose is to provide a view of what is, and what is not, known that updates the review of this topic that was prepared for the 1988 International Conference on Exercise, Fitness, and Health (22). Thus, we have focused on studies published from 1988 through January 1992. The review is also limited to studies of exercise or physical activities consistent with definitions conventionally used in public health (11). Single session and case studies (e.g., 35), though important, are not included. We have drawn from previous reviews (22,25,27,55,56,78,90,99) to describe the extant literature on the topic.

The known determinants of physical activity can be categorized as past and present personal attributes, past and present environments, and aspects of physical activity itself. Because few controlled studies have been conducted to experimentally manipulate variables presumed to operate as determinants and no population trials have been completed, we use the term *determinant* to denote a reproducible association or predictive relationship, rather than to imply cause-and-effect. For clarity, physical activity is distinguished from exercise that occurs in a supervised setting where time, place, activity, and type of participant may be restricted relative to spontaneous or free-living activity in a population base. Planning for participation, initial adoption of physical activity, continued participation or maintenance, and overall periodicity of participation can be distinguished from each other. Too few studies are available on children, the elderly, the disabled, ethnic and minority groups, or gender comparisons to permit conclusions about how determinants in these cases may differ from general observations.

In the following sections we describe the current scientific knowledge regarding the descriptive and predictive determinants of physical activity and the effectiveness of interventions designed to increase and maintain physical activity and exercise participation. Also, we provide an evaluation of the progress made in understanding the determinants during the past several years when judged against earlier scientific consensus (6). Finally, we discuss selected methodological issues as they bear on our recommendations for future research and application.

Determinants

The purpose of this section is to update the review of physical activity determinants in the previous volume (22) that was based on literature published in 1987 and before. Table 13.1 summarizes studies published from 1988 to 1991, with a few references from 1992. Articles were found through a combination of computer and manual searches. Unpublished studies were not reviewed. Papers primarily devoted to presenting a new measure related to physical activity determinants are described in a separate section in the text, as are studies primarily testing or comparing theories. A few studies with small sample sizes, very short follow-ups, an exclusive focus on sports participation, or analog studies were excluded from consideration. The studies reviewed consist of community or clinical samples, use a variety of physical activity measures reflecting a range of intensities, and include both cross-sectional and prospective designs.

Table 13.1 presents selected study characteristics and a simplified tabulation of results. Some studies had multiple dependent measures or reported multiple subgroups of subjects. In these cases, general trends were noted, the summary measure of physical activity was chosen, or specific findings were stated. The following list summarizes the information provided in each column.

Reference. Author and reference list number.

Sample. Number of males (M) and females (F), age range, ethnicity, other special characteristics. The source of the sample is noted (e.g., community sample or exercise class members).

Design. Cross-sectional, prospective, retrospective. Length of follow-up (time from baseline to last measurement).

Dependent Variable. The type of physical activity measure is noted, though fitness is accepted as a substitute for physical activity in a few cases. The following categories are used to note quality of the measure: (1) self-report of poor or unknown reliability/validity; (2) self-report with acceptable reliability/validity or poor objective measure; (3) well-validated self-report or acceptable objective measure.

Independent Variable, Related. This is a list of independent variables that were significantly associated with each physical activity. The direction of the association is summarized with a "+" or "–." No attempt was made to indicate the strength of the relationship.

Independent Variable, Not Related. This is a list of independent variables that were not significantly associated with physical activity.

Review of Recent Studies: General Findings

The 33 recent studies reviewed in Table 13.1 represent several major conceptual and methodological advances over the literature reviewed in past years (24,27). Many of the changes called for in previous reviews have been made in the recently published studies.

One of the shortcomings of the earlier studies was the reliance on clinical or other selected samples of questionable generalizability to the broader population. In Table 13.1, 24 of 33 studies are community samples not selected from exercise programs. The community samples included representative national samples from Australia (4,81) and Canada (114). Samples ranged from high school age to the elderly, and poor and minority populations were included in some samples. Physical activity determinants research in children has been reviewed elsewhere (106). The applicability of the findings to the entire population has been improved because 26 studies included both men and women.

Though cross-sectional studies can be useful, there are numerous advantages to prospective designs, and almost half of the studies reviewed (15 of 33) were prospective. Follow-ups ranged from 7 weeks to 15 years. Long-term follow-ups are important because the health benefits of physical activity accrue to those who are active regularly over a period of years. Thus, it is critical to understand what facilitates long-term participation. Long-term studies of children have particular promise for studying factors related to lifelong participation (50).

One distinct improvement in recent determinants studies is in the application of multidimensional models, theories, and assessment batteries. This recognition of multiple influences allows comparisons between different types of determinants. A continuing shortcoming of the determinants research is that virtually all studies focus on the maintenance/dropout phase or do not discriminate between maintenance and adoption. A very small number of studies addressed the problem of adoption (52,100,114). Because of the substantial numbers of sedentary adults in the population, it is essential to understand the determinants of physical activity adoption.

Development of Theory for Physical Activity Determinants Research

Numerous theories have been applied to the study of physical activity determinants. At least nine relevant theories were identified in 1988 (22,110). Since that time additional theories have been developed or applied to this topic. Self-schemata (51,52), the stages of change model (68), and personal investment theory (116) are three psychological theories that have recently been applied to the study of exercise behavior and have received some support. The social ecology framework (115) can be used to guide the investigation of social and physical environment influences on physical activity.

As strong determinants are confirmed by multiple studies, the next step is to explore influences on those determinants. Correlates of self-efficacy (45), exercise barriers (82,122), and exercise intentions (41) have been studied to date.

One very promising recent trend in physical activity determinants research has been the publication of studies comparing different theoretical formulations. All three studies involved comparisons with Ajzen and Fishbein's (2) social psychological

Table 13.1 Characteristics and Results of Studies on the Determinants of Physical Activity Published 1988 to Early 1992

Reference	Sample	Design	Dependent variable	Independent variable—related	Independent variable—not related
Bauman et al. (4)	8,202M; 8,851 F; random survey in Australia; age 14 and above	Cross-sectional	2-week recall (1)	Male (+), age (–), education (+), income (+), live in cities (+), childless (+)	Season
Brill et al. (7)	420 adult males; for athletes and nonathletes	Prospective; 56-month follow-up	Questionnaire (2)		Prior athlete status
Carron et al. (9)	47 exercise classes with 5 to 46 members; program on university campus	Prospective data from archives; 10-week follow-up	Attendance (3)	Class size (attendance highest in smallest and largest classes)	
Carron et al. (9) (study 1)	289 adults; 122 completed fitness class of elite sports; 67 dropped out	Cross-sectional	Attendance (2)	Group cohesion	
Cauley et al. (12)	368 M; 549 F; random samples of high and low income areas (white)	Cross-sectional	College Alumni Survey (3)	Age (–), male (+), socioeconomic status: + for sports; – for walking (in females)	
Dennison et al. (16)	453 men; 23 to 25 years old; took fitness tests while 10 to 18 years old	Prospective (fitness) and retrospective (adult survey); 5- to 15-year follow-up	7-day recall interview (3)	Aerobic fitness (+), sit-ups (+), sprint (+), sports after high school (+), spouse encouragement (+), education (+)	Pull-ups, broad jump, sports during high school, obesity as adult, parent encouragement, smoking history, health status
Dishman (21)	265 M; white men in exercise program	Cross-sectional and prospective; 6-month follow-up	7-day recall (3); attendance (3)		Prior athlete status

Dishman & Steinhardt (28)	158 M & F members of college physical activity course	Cross-sectional	7-day recall (3); 7-day diary (3)	Self-motivation (+)	
Dishman & Steinhardt (29)	43 M; 41 F; members of college physical activity course	Prospective; 9 weeks	7-day recall (3); attendance (3)	Internal health locus of control (+), exercise outcomes (benefits) (+), exercise barriers (–)	Internal exercise locus of control
Folsom et al. (36)	574 M; 685 F; random sample of blacks and whites age 25 to 75 years	Cross-sectional	Leisure-time activity survey (3)	Age (–), education (+), mean activity lower in blacks than whites	
Garcia & King (40)	42 M; 32 F; community sample age 50 to 64, randomized to intervention	Prospective; 12-month follow-up	Monthly adherence reports (1) or attendance (3)	Self-efficacy (+)	Self-motivation, perceived exertion, enjoyment, and convenience of exercise
Hovell et al. (46) (not included in Table 13.2; it is only study of walking)	1,080 M & F; community sample of adults who do not do vigorous exercise	Cross-sectional	Walking for exercise (1)	Self-efficacy (+), age (+), healthy diet (+), family support (+)	Modeling, friend support, barriers to exercise, benefits, knowledge, normative beliefs, sports media, home equipment, gender, education, smoking, alcohol, body mass index, exercise history, modeling history, injury history
Kaplan et al. (49)	3,158 M; 3,770 F; community sample age 16 to 94 years	Prospective; 9-year follow-up	Interview (2)	Education (+), black race (–), income (+), occupation status (+), married (+), group memberships (+), social isolation (–), depression (–), life satisfaction (+), perceived health (+)	
Kendzierski (52)	95 university students, sedentary at baseline	Prospective; 12-week follow-up	Reported adoption of exercise (1)	Exercise self-schemata	

(continued)

Table 13.1 *(continued)*

Reference	Sample	Design	Dependent variable	Independent variable—related	Independent variable—not related
King et al. (61)	80 M; 319 F; randomly selected employees	Cross-sectional	Active/not active categories (2)	Age (–), perceived health (+), safety concerns (–), exercise myths (–), physical discomfort (–), social support (+)	Relative weight, smoking, knowledge
Klesges et al. (62)	215 M; white men; 175 nonsmokers, 40 smokers	Cross-sectional	Multiple questionnaires (3)	Socioeconomic status (+), smoking (–)	
Krick & Sobal (64)	1,029 M; 1,362 F; probability sample	Cross-sectional	Numerous items (1)	Age (–), education (+), income (+)	Gender, drinking, sedative use, smoking, employment
Marcus et al. (68)	358 M; 420 F; recruited from worksites	Cross-sectional	Exercise stages of change (2)	"Pros" (+) and "cons" (–) of exercise	
McAuley & Jacobson (70)	58 F; exercise class members	Prospective; 4-month follow-up	Attendance, class, follow-up interview (2)	Total participation: self-efficacy (+)	Body fat, self-motivation, influence of instructor
McPhillips et al. (71)	508 M; 632 F; community sample age 50 years and older	Cross-sectional	2-week recall survey (2)	Age (– for moderate and heavy, + for light exercise), chronic disease history (–), obesity (–), smoking (–), physical and mental functioning (+)	
Myers et al. (72)	179 M; 203 F; convenience sample	Cross-sectional	Numerous items (1)	Barriers (–), positive physical education (+), lack of time (–)	Physical education history
Oldridge & Streiner (79)	120 M; cardiac rehabilitation patients	Prospective; 6-month follow-up	Dropout from program (2)	Age (–), smoking (–), white collar (+), severity of illness (+), cues to action (–, unexpected)	Health locus of control, other health beliefs (motivation, susceptibility, barriers)

Owen & Bauman (82)	8,202 M; 8,851 F; random sample in Australia	Cross-sectional	2-week recall (1)	Age (–), education (+), income (+)	Gender, location
Perusse et al. (85)	3,570 M; 3,466 F; representative sample in Canada	Cross-sectional	Survey (1)	Male (+), physical activity of family members (+)	
Reynolds et al. (92)	388 M; 355 F; 10th-grade students	Prospective; 16-month follow-up	Questionnaire (2)	Behavioral intention (+), self-efficacy (+, females), body mass index (–, females)	Stress, social influence
Sallis et al. (103)	2,053 M and F; community residents	Cross-sectional	Vigorous exercise item (2)	Proximity of exercise facilities	
Sallis et al. (104) (not included in Table 13.2; Sallis et al. (100) is prospective analysis of this sample)	1,021 M; 768 F; community sample age 18 to 90 years	Cross-sectional	Vigorous exercise item (2)	Self-efficacy (+), modeling (+), friend support (+), barriers (–), benefits (+), home equipment (+), age (–), education (+), smoking (–), healthy diet (+), coordination (+)	Family support, exercise knowledge, normative beliefs, sports media, gender, alcohol, body mass index, exercise history, modeling history, injury history, neighborhood environment, convenience of facilities
Sallis et al. (100)	1,739 M and F; community residents age 18 to 90 years	Prospective; 2-year follow-up	Vigorous exercise item (2)	Baseline physical activity (after adjustment for baseline and demographics): barriers (–), self-efficacy (+), neighborhood environment (–), injury as adult (+), friend support (+), family support (+)	Modeling, exercise knowledge, normative beliefs, sports media, home equipment, smoking, alcohol, healthy diet, body mass index, exercise history, modeling history, injury as child, coordination, convenience of facilities
Shea et al. (107)	1,532 M; 2,072 F; random sample of whites, blacks, and Hispanics age 20 to 64 years	Cross-sectional	Centers for Disease Control phone survey (2)	Education (+, Hispanic women only), Hispanic background (–), male gender (+, whites only)	Black race

(continued)

Table 13.1 *(continued)*

Reference	Sample	Design	Dependent variable	Independent variable—related	Independent variable—not related
Siegel et al. (108)	186 F; exercise or sport class members	Prospective; 7-week follow-up	Attendance (2)	Desire to develop skills (+), desire to use mind in activity (+), social reasons (+), health and fitness (−)	Desire for relaxation, change in routine
Steinhardt and Young (113)	423 M; 223 F employees	Prospective; 6-month follow-up	Worksite attendance categories	Attitudinal commitment (+), self-motivation (+), perceived physical competence (−), attraction to physical activity (+), age (−)	
Stephens & Craig (114)	1,977 M; 2,192 F; age 10 years and above; representative sample of Canada	Prospective; 7-year follow-up	Survey (2)	Baseline physical activity: age (−, except walking +), male gender (+), education (+), rated health status (+), obesity (−), social support (+), activity history (+), programs at work (+), perceived control over exercise (+), health benefits (+), intention to exercise (+)	
Treiber et al. (117)	89 M; 141 F; public school teachers; 119 M; 119 F; community sample, black and white	Cross-sectional	Baecke questionnaire (2)	Male gender (+), black race (−, on some measures), friend social support (+), family social support (+)	

Note. M = male; F = female; + = significant positive association; − = significant negative association. See text for explanation of numbers in parentheses in *Dependent variable* column.

theory. In one comparison, a similar model that included past exercise was slightly more effective at predicting exercise than the Ajzen and Fishbein theory (118). Two short-term studies indicated that social cognitive theory, including self-efficacy ratings, was significantly more effective in predicting exercise than the Ajzen and Fishbein theory (31,32). More studies that compete theories against one another are needed, and it might be most useful to choose very distinct theories.

Advances in the Measurement of Determinants

Most determinants studies have used either unvalidated measures of potential determinants or general purpose measures borrowed from other domains. In recent years investigators have begun to develop specific measures of potential determinants and evaluate their reliability and validity. Measures of the following constructs have been reported: physical self-perception (38), physical activity enjoyment (53), expected outcomes and barriers for physical activity (68,112), locus of control for physical fitness behaviors (121), social support (93,97), and self-efficacy (105). This trend should facilitate progress in the field, and more psychometric studies are encouraged.

The proliferation of measures of psychological variables may create some difficulties. Constructs and measures tend to be overlapping, therefore differentiation of measures is needed. Different measures of the same construct are used. This practice may lead to failure to replicate, hence use of well-evaluated measures across different studies is recommended. However, this is not meant to restrain the improvement of measures of psychological variables.

Determinants of Moderate Versus Vigorous Physical Activity

The growing body of evidence supporting the health benefits of moderate intensity physical activity led the U.S. Public Health Service (17) and the American College of Sports Medicine (3) to add recommendations for the public to engage in regular moderate intensity activity. However, few studies have examined differences in patterns and determinants of moderate and vigorous physical activity. Walking is consistently found to be the most commonly reported form of moderate intensity activity (114), but the absence of validated self-report measures of walking hinders research in this area.

The available studies strongly indicate that moderate and vigorous physical activities are controlled by different factors. The strong decline in total and vigorous activity with age is not seen with moderate activities. Studies reporting separate analyses for moderate intensity activities have consistently noted increased levels with age (46,71,114). While men are found to have higher levels of total and vigorous activity, in at least two studies women reported more walking (46,114). Walking and other forms of moderate activity appear to have important health benefits, and they may be more acceptable to older adults and to women.

Correlates of walking were examined in one sample which did not do vigorous exercise (46). Psychological and social variables that were significant in relation to walking tended to have the same associations as with vigorous exercise (104). However, the same determinants accounted for much less of the variance in walking. This may be due to error in measuring walking, or it could indicate that other variables not included in the study are important influences on walking. Research on determinants of moderate intensity physical activity is a high priority.

Determinants of Adoption Versus Maintenance of Physical Activity

Previous reviews (29,99) have emphasized the need to distinguish adoption, maintenance, and resumption of physical activity. Most studies have examined the issue of maintenance or dropout, and that trend continues. Only one study specifically assessed influences on resumption of exercise after dropout (102) and suggested that multiple episodes of dropout and resumption are common. Recent research also has focused on predicting inactivity rather than participation (82).

Some progress has been made in the last few years regarding research on adoption of physical activity. Over 20% of Canadian adults reported adopting regular physical activity between 1981 and 1988 (114), and factors that would motivate sedentary people to do so were identified (61). Sedentary students who perceived themselves as exercisers (self-schemata) were likely to adopt exercise in the near future (52). Adoption of vigorous exercise by a community sample of sedentary men during a 2-year period was predicted by self-efficacy, age (negative), and neighborhood environment. Adoption by women was predicted by education, self-efficacy, and friend and family support for exercise (100). In the same study, maintenance of vigorous exercise was predicted by some of the same variables. While some variables predicted both adoption and maintenance, it is interesting that the model was more successful in predicting adoption. These studies suggest that adoption can be predicted, but they have not adequately addressed the question of differences in determinants of adoption versus maintenance of physical activity.

Injury as a Determinant of Physical Activity

There is a well documented dose-response relationship between physical activity and orthopedic injuries (66). Injury rates may be as high as 50% per year in those who regularly engage in high intensity exercise like running (67,87). It is important to examine injury and participants' subjective responses to injury as a potential influence on the probability of adopting or maintaining physical activity.

In one study, subjects reported the reason for their last relapse from exercise (102). Injury was by far the most common reason given. Though subjects reporting temporary injuries were less likely than healthy individuals to report vigorous exercise, the injured reported significantly more walking for exercise (44). This is consistent with previous findings that intensity of exercise is related to injury risk and suggests that many injured people can still engage in regular walking. Because injury appears to be a strong influence on maintenance or drop-out from regular physical activity, intervention programs should teach participants to reduce risk of injury.

Genetic and Biologic Influences on Physical Activity

Though not usually subject to direct intervention, it is important to understand the role of genetic and biologic influences on physical activity. These factors may interact with or modify the actions of other influences. Recent Canadian data suggest an important heritable component of physical activity (85,86). In a study of family aggregation in a sample of over 1,300 persons, approximately 20% of the variation in daily physical activity was attributable to genetically transmissible variation (86).

Summary of Physical Activity Determinants Literature

Table 13.2 presents a summary of the physical activity determinants literature published since 1987. The format used in the Dishman review (22) was adapted to allow comparisons with pre-1988 studies. Results from subjects in supervised programs versus samples free-living in the community are reported separately. The small number of post-1987 studies with supervised samples reduces confidence in interpretations made from that column.

Demographic variables continue to have strong associations with physical activity (37), however some of these could be considered selection biases rather than causal determinants. Education, income, male gender, and age (negative) are consistent and powerful correlates of physical activity habits. Non-Hispanic whites appear to be more active than other ethnic groups, but it is difficult or impossible to disentangle the effects of ethnicity and socioeconomic status.

Pre-1988 studies found that the obese were generally less active than those with normal weight. However, the more recent studies were relatively consistent in finding no association between obesity and physical activity. This important question deserves more focused investigation.

Eighteen variables are included in the cognitive category. Self-efficacy receives the most support as a cognitive determinant in both types of studies. However, the lack of prospective studies that control for physical activity habit (101) limits our confidence over how much of the observed relationship between self-efficacy and activity is causal and how much reflects a selection effect; that is, active individuals report high self-efficacy due to past success. Self-schemata, expectation of benefits, and intention to exercise seem to be associated with physical activity, at least in community samples. Perceived barriers to exercise, including lack of time, are negatively associated in several recent community studies. Self-motivation has continued to receive generally consistent support. Those with mood disturbances appear less likely to be active, but attitudes and knowledge are not found to be related to activity. Small numbers of studies preclude interpretations of other psychological variables.

Although past physical activity during adulthood (usually measured at the study baseline) is consistently related to activity measured at follow-up, there continues to be little evidence that activity patterns in childhood or early adulthood are predictive of later physical activity. Likewise, other health-related behaviors, including smoking (48), are usually not found to be related to physical activity.

When social influences are studied, they are usually found to be associated with physical activity. Social support from family and friends is consistently related to physical activity in cross-sectional

Table 13.2 Summary of Physical Activity Determinants Literature for Studies Conducted in Supervised Settings and With Free-Living Samples During Two Time Periods

Determinant	Supervised: pre-1988 results	Supervised: 1988–1991 results	Free-Living: pre-1988 results	Free-Living: 1988–1991 results
Personal attributes:				
Demographics				
Age	00	~	~	—
Blue-collar occupation	—	~	~	
Childless				+
Education	+		++	++
Gender (male)			++	++
High risk for heart disease	~	~	~	
Income/socioeconomic status			++	++
Injury history				+
Overweight/obesity	~	0	~	00
Race (nonwhite)			~	—
Cognitive variables				
Attitudes	0	+	0	
Barriers to exercise		~		—
Control over exercise				0
Enjoyment of exercise	+		+	0
Expect health and other benefits	0	+	+	+
Health locus of control	+	0		
Intention to exercise	0		+	++
Knowledge of health and exercise	0		0	0
Lack of time	—		~	~
Mood disturbance	~		~	—
Normative beliefs	0			0
Perceived health or fitness	++		~	++
Self-efficacy for exercise	+	+	+	++
Self-motivation	+	++	++	+
Self-schemata for activity			+	+
Stress				0
Susceptibility to illness				0
Value exercise outcomes	0		0	

(continued)

Table 13.2 *(Continued)*

Determinant	Supervised: pre-1988 results	Supervised: 1988–1991 results	Free-Living: pre-1988 results	Free-Living: 1988–1991 results
Behaviors				
Alcohol				0
Contemporary program activity			0	
Diet	00		+	0
Past free-living activity during childhood			0	0
Past free-living activity during adulthood	+		+	++
Past program participation	++	+	+	
School sports	0		0	00
Smoking	—	~	0	0
Sports media use				0
Type A behavior pattern	~		+	
Environmental factors: Social environment		+		
Class size				
Exercise models				0
Group cohesion		+		
Physician influence			+	
Social isolation				~
Past family influences			+	0
Social support; friends/peers			+	++
Social support; spouse/family	++		+	++
Social support; staff/instructor	+	0		
Physical environment				
Climate/season	~		~	0
Cost	0		0	
Disruptions in routine	~			
Access to facilities: actual	+			+
Access to facilities: perceived	+		0	0
Home equipment				0
Physical activity characteristics				
Intensity	~		~	
Perceived effort	—		~	~

Note. ++ = repeatedly documented positive association with physical activity; + = weak or mixed evidence of positive association with physical activity; 00 = repeatedly documented lack of association with physical activity; 0 = weak or mixed evidence of no association with physical activity; — = repeatedly documented negative association with physical activity; ~ = weak or mixed evidence of negative association with physical activity. Blank spaces indicate no data available.

and prospective studies. Group factors may be important in exercise programs. This is a promising area for future research.

There is a wide variety of environmental variables that could be studied in relation to physical activity, but of those studied, most have not been found to have strong associations. However, there may be a problem with assessing environmental variables by self-report questionnaires. Objectively measured access to facilities was related to physical activity, while perceived access was usually not related. Measurement of physical environment variables poses a substantial challenge to investigators.

Both intensity and perceived effort of physical activity appear to be negatively associated with participation in physical activity. This is an important finding and should be taken into consideration in the design of physical activity interventions.

Consistent associations were found in every category of variables in Table 13.2. These findings reemphasize the importance of viewing physical activity as being influenced by many forces both inside and outside the person. The influences on physical activity cannot be understood unless characteristics of the person, the environment, and the activity itself are assessed.

Recommendations for Future Research on Physical Activity Determinants

The research to date has convincingly demonstrated the multidimensional nature of physical activity determinants and has identified some variables in each category that appear to be influences as well as those that are not supported. However, because of limitations of measurement methods, differences in sample characteristics, and limited numbers of studies that have used the same variables, it is not possible to attach effect sizes to specific variables with confidence. The results to date can still be useful in designing intervention programs. Programs should target long-term changes in key cognitive, social, and physical environment variables to maximize the probability of long-term behavior change.

Recommendations for improving the quality and public health utility of physical activity determinants research are as follows:

1. The relevance of determinants research for intervention design should be considered when designing studies. Determinants that are subject to change through educational programs and policy initiatives should be emphasized. However, it is still useful to understand the biologic and genetic context within which these other personal and environmental factors operate.
2. The interaction of demographic variables with modifiable determinants should be assessed. The physical activity of different population subgroups is likely to be influenced by different determinants. For example, how do determinants differ for people with different incomes, levels of education, at different ages, and from various ethnic groups? Answers to these types of questions can assist intervention planners to develop intervention strategies that are appropriate for key population subgroups.
3. The studies to date indicate that different processes underlie participation in moderate and vigorous physical activities. These differences have direct implications for public health policy and need to be further explored.
4. More studies of the determinants of the adoption of regular physical activity are needed.
5. Most of the theories that have been applied to the investigation of physical activity determinants are primarily or wholly psychological in nature. The data clearly indicate that psychological models alone are inadequate to explain participation in physical activity. Broader models are needed that incorporate psychological, environmental, and physical activity variables.
6. Virtually every study has relied on self-reports of physical activity and/or unvalidated self-report measures of determinants. Discrepant conclusions over the predictive validity of determinants can occur when objective measures of physical activity are contrasted with self-reported activity (26). It is critical that both dependent and independent measures be carefully developed and validated. Objective measures of physical activity are available (65) and should be applied to this area. Investigators must be more creative in developing measures of social and physical environment variables that do not rely on self-report.

Interventions

The purpose of this section is to update and expand the brief section on behavior change interventions included in the review prepared for the 1988 International Conference on Exercise, Fitness, and

Health (22) and two recent review articles (24,55). We have reviewed studies located through our personal retrieval systems and a Medline computer search of publications in the English language. Table 13.3 summarizes studies published from 1988 to 1991, including 1 study from 1992. Unpublished thesis and dissertation research is not included.

Table 13.3 presents selected characteristics of the studies and a tabulation of results. A format similar to Table 13.1 on determinants was employed, however we have added the type of physical activity and setting along with the type of intervention used. Interventions are coded as health education (HE), behavior modification (BM), and cognitive-behavior modification (CBM), or they are otherwise described in the table. The strength of scientific inference over the causal influence of an intervention depends on the research design used. Hence, we also have distinguished the quality of designs from high (A, fully randomized), to moderate (B, matched or nonequivalent control group), to low (C, cohort study without a control group).

Because sample sizes varied greatly among the studies and because statistical significance is dependent on sample size, an important consideration in comparing the results of the studies is the size of the effect observed for each intervention. For this purpose we have transformed all results to a correlation coefficient (r) according to procedures outlined by Friedman (39) and Rosenthal (95). Consistent with Cohen (15), we regard population values of r approximating .01, .26, and .37 as small, moderate and large, respectively. Because it is useful to view the results of interventions in terms of success rates, we also present binomial effect sizes (BES) according to Rosenthal and Rubin (96). The BES can be interpreted as the change in the proportion of exercise adherents in the experimental group compared with a control group. The .50 binomial probability of adherence in the absence of an intervention effect is consistent with naturalistic observations of exercise programs.

Review of Recent Studies: General Findings

The 20 recent studies reviewed in Table 13.3 represent a few methodological advances over the interventions reviewed for the 1988 Consensus (22). Prior to 1988 most intervention studies used uncontrolled case and cohort designs (24). Since 1988 most studies have used randomized or quasi-experimental designs with large samples of males and females of varying ages offering more internal validity and generalizability. A few studies of ethnic and minority groups have appeared.

It is generally accepted that recommendations to exercise regularly are not followed by the majority of people (10,13,14). Therefore, specific efforts to promote physical activity are needed. There are numerous theories that promote different approaches to behavior change that can be applied to physical activity behaviors. Educational interventions and reinforcement control and stimulus control strategies based on the traditions of behavior modification or cognitive-behavior modification have been successfully implemented with exercise. Behavioral approaches, including written agreements or contracts (e.g., 74,94), and reinforcement (e.g., 58,75) have been used successfully in experimental studies. Cognitive-behavioral approaches have included self-monitoring, goal setting, and feedback fashioned after the relapse prevention model of Marlatt and Gordon (e.g., 58,60) and educational modeling approaches consistent with social-cognitive theory (83,109). Health education approaches have relied on health risk appraisals, fitness testing, and counseling (1,8,33, 63,80,83,120).

In our view, the existing literature permits the following conclusions:

- Studies typically support that health education and behavior modification or cognitive-behavior modification principles can be implemented with exercise programs and are accompanied by increased frequency of activity or time spent in activity for limited periods of time (e.g., 4 to 20 weeks).
- With the exception of studies closely linked with onsite programs or periodic supervision (e.g., worksite, clinic, or school) the studies do not demonstrate that exercise intensity or total activity has been increased enough to reliably increase physical fitness or to reduce risk for future morbidity or mortality.
- The quasi-experimental nature of about one half of the literature limits confident conclusions about the cause-and-effect nature of the increased physical activity that has accompanied the interventions.
- Most studies have used indirect measures of physical activity (e.g., self-report) or indirect estimates of physical fitness based on heart rate or treadmill time; thus, their validity is uncertain. Only a few studies have attempted to verify self-reports of activity.
- The effect size for increased fitness when $\dot{V}O_{2peak}$ was measured is typically small, even when the effects for self-reported activity are large.
- Most interventions have not been based on a broader theoretical model of behavior change

Table 13.3 Characteristics and Results of Studies on Interventions to Increase Exercise and Physical Activity Published Since 1988

Study	Sample	Design	Activity/ Setting	Intervention length	Intervention type	Dependent variable	Follow-up	Outcome & effect size
Acquista et al. (1)	437 healthy adults	C—cohort, no control group	Leisure/ home-based	2 hr phone follow-up at 1–3 weeks & at 1 month; mail follow-up at 6 weeks	HE & counseling	Self-reported activity (walk, run, lift, carry; greater than 3 ×/week)	12 months	r = .20, BES = .40 to .60; Moderate
Bush et al. (8)	692 African-American children (10.5 years old)	B—random assignment of schools	Leisure/ school	3 years	Health screening and education with CBM	Fitness; exercise recovery pulse (adjusted for baseline, age, sex, and SES)	Yearly	Year 2 r = .02, BES = .49 to .51; Year 3 r = .06, BES = .47 to .53; Year 4 r = .04, BES = .48 to .52; Year 5 r = .02, BES = .49 to .51; Small
Farquhar et al. (33)	2,503 healthy adults	B—random assignment of communities	Leisure/ community free-living	5 years	HE	Resting HR (adjusted for age, sex, and education)	3 years	Year 1 r = .07, BES = .47 to .53; Year 2 r = .12, BES = .44 to .56; Year 3 r = .05, BES = .48 to .52; Small
Killen et al. (54)	1,130 healthy adolescents (14–16 years old)	A—randomized factorial	Leisure/ community free-living	7 weeks	HE/BM/CBM	Self-report; resting HR; BMI	2 months	r = .09, BES = .45 to .54; r = .14, BES = .43 to .58; r = .06, BES = .47 to .53; Small

(continued)

Table 13.3 *(continued)*

Study	Sample	Design	Activity/ Setting	Intervention length	Intervention type	Dependent variable	Follow-up	Outcome & effect size
King et al. (57)	38 healthy male adults	C—cohort, no control group	Parcourse/ worksite and aerobics/free-living	16 weeks	BM	Self-report frequency; recovery HR; weight		r = .52, BES = .24 to .76; r = .63, BES = .18 to .82; r = .32, BES = .34 to .66; Large
King et al. (58)	36 obese male adults	A—randomized factorial	Walk/jog/ supervised and home-based	1 year	BM/CBM	7-day recall interview (very hard; hard; moderate)		r = −.14, BES = .53 to .47; r = −.11, BES = .53 to .47; r = .05, BES = .53 to .57; Small
King et al. (59)	300 healthy adults	A—randomized factorial	Aerobic/ community home-based or supervised	1 year	Exercise intensity; home vs. group	Self-report (diary) $\dot{V}O_{2max}$; treadmill time		Intensity: r = −.05, BES = .52 to .48; Home-based: r = .23, BES = .38 to .62; r = .16, BES = .42 to .58; r = .21, BES = .40 to .60; Small to moderate
King et al. (60) (Adoption study)	48 healthy adults	A—randomized factorial	Aerobic/ home-based	1 year	BM/CBM	Self-report (frequency, duration) $\dot{V}O_{2peak}$		r = .18, BES = .41 to .59; r = .03, BES = .49 to .51; r = .08, BES = .46 to .54; Small to moderate
King et al. (60) (Maintenance study)	47 healthy adults	A—randomized factorial	Aerobic/ home-based	1 year	BM	Self-report (days/month); $\dot{V}O_{2peak}$		r = .31, BES = .34 to .65; r = .00, BES = .50; None to moderate

Knutsen & Knutsen (63)	1,060 men at risk for CHD and 809 wives	A—randomized control group	Leisure/ community free-living	2 home visits 1–2 years after screening	HE (physician counseling)	Self-report; BMI	7 years	Males $r = -.03$, BES = .51 to .49; $r = .03$, BES = .48 to .52; Females $r = .08$, BES = .46 to .54; $r = .00$, BES = .50; Small
Neale et al. (74)	96 medical clinic patients and employees	C—cohort, no control group	Leisure/ community free-living	12 weeks	BM	HR at 6.4 METs	6 months	$r = .17$, BES = .41 to .59; Moderate
Noland (75)	75 healthy adults	A—randomized factorial	Aerobic/ community free-living	18 weeks	BM	Recall questionnaire (frequency, duration, & intensity for adoption and maintenance groups)		Adopt $r = .40$, BES = .30 to .70; $r = .23$, BES = .39 to .61; $r = .24$, BES = .38 to .62; Maintain $r = .08$, BES = .46 to .54; $r = .12$, BES = .44 to .56; $r = .27$, BES = .36 to .64; Small to moderate
Ostwald (80)	39 healthy adults	C—no control group; random assignment to HE and fitness testing or HE, fitness testing, and group exercise	Aerobic/ worksite	12 weeks	HE/HE plus group exercise	Resting HR; treadmill time	1–2 months	HE: $r = .38$, BES = .31 to .69; $r = .62$, BES = .19 to .81; HE & group exercise: $r = .53$, BES = .23 to .77; $r = .30$, BES = .35 to .65; Moderate to large

(continued)

Table 13.3 *(continued)*

Study	Sample	Design	Activity/ Setting	Intervention length	Intervention type	Dependent variable	Follow-up	Outcome & effect size
Parcel et al. (83)	372 healthy children (9 years old)	B—randomized control group; assignment of schools	Aerobic/ school & community free-living	Two 6–8 week units	HE/curriculum change	Self-report	2 years	Year 1 $r = -.09$, BES = .54 to .46; Year 2 $r = -.10$, BES = .55 to .45; Small
Patterson et al. (84)	166 healthy families (Mexican-American and Anglo-American)	A—randomized factorial	Leisure/ physical activity at the San Diego Zoo	1 year	BM/CBM	Observation (meters traveled, % active, not using escalator)	5 months	Mexican-American $r = .82$, BES = .09 to .91; $r = .37$, BES = .31 to .69; $r = .49$, BES = .25 to .75; Large Anglo-American $r = -.02$, BES = .51 to .49; $r = -.33$, BES = .67 to .33; $r = .53$, BES = .23 to .77; Small to large
Pollock (88)	36 to 425 healthy men (21–71 years old)	A—randomized control group	Jogging, walking, cycling, circuit training/supervised program	16–24 weeks	Exercise intensity; duration; frequency	Attendance		$r = .19$, BES = .40 to .60; $r = .17$, BES = .42 to .58; $r = .07$, BES = .46 to .54; Small to moderate

Robison et al. (94)	94 healthy adults	B—random assignment of groups. Nonequivalent control group	Aerobic/ worksite	6 months	BM	Self-report (witnessed); resting HR; $\dot{V}O_{2max}$, treadmill time		r = .61, BES = .19 to .81; r = .11, BES = .45 to .55; r = .15, BES = .57 to .43; r = .06, BES = .47 to .53; Small to large
Simons-Morton et al. (109)	340 healthy children (8–9 years old)	B—randomized control group, assignment of schools	Aerobic/ school	Five 6–8 week units	HE/ curriculum change	Observation of school P.E. class activity (moderate to vigorous, HR ~ 170 bpm)	2 years	3rd grade r = .76, BES = .12 to .88; 4th grade r = .71, BES = .14 to .86; Large
Weber & Werthelm (119)	55 women (17–56 years old)	A—randomized control group	Not reported/ health club	12 weeks	CBM	Attendance (number of sessions, proportion of dropouts)		r = .34, BES = .33 to .67; r = .33, BES = .34 to .66; Moderate
Weir, Jackson, & Pinkerton (120)	206 adults	B—cohort with nonequivalent control group	Aerobics/ worksite	12 weeks	HE/fitness testing	Self-report (r = .56 with $\dot{V}O_{2max}$)	2–3 years	r = .43, BES = .29 to .71; Large

Note. A = high quality of design, B = moderate quality of design, C = low quality of design, HE = health education, BES = binomial effect size, CBM = cognitive-behavior modification, SES = socioeconomic status, HR = heart rate, BM = behavior modification, BMI = body mass index, CHD = coronary heart disease, MET = multiples of resting metabolic rate, P.E. = physical education, bpm = beats per minute. Effect sizes are in the order of the dependent variables.

such as stage theories (18,91) and have not considered activity history and the companion literature on the determinants of physical activity.

These conclusions indicate that education and behavior modification and cognitive-behavior modification interventions have shown potential *efficacy* for increasing exercise and physical activity, but their *effectiveness* for increasing exercise, physical activity, fitness, or health in the population remains unclear. Interventions, regardless of tradition or content, usually are associated with effect sizes for frequency of physical activity that are moderate, where binomial effect sizes suggest increases in success probabilities from about .40 to .60. The impact on changes in intensity and duration of physical activity is less clear. Since these effects are comparable to those found for lowered intensity, duration, and frequency of exercise prescriptions in fitness training studies for white males (84), the superiority of behavior change interventions over modifications in traditional fitness programming (e.g., 3) merits direct testing. Uncontrolled case and quasi-experimental multiple baseline studies published prior to 1988 have commonly reported increases of 50% to 200% (24). However, the absolute levels of the increased activity typically fall below the frequency, duration, and intensity required to increase physical fitness (3) and may not reach the level required to optimally decrease risk for disease morbidity or all-cause mortality (5).

Only about one half of the studies reported a follow-up to the intervention, and they typically showed that increases in physical activity or fitness associated with the interventions were diminished as follow-up time increased. Minimally effective intervention conditions for control comparisons have been rare. Therefore, generalizations are not possible about specific components of the interventions that are effective for specific populations. Many types of interventions have been associated with increased physical activity; however, the superiority of these interventions has not been directly compared. For this reason and because the few studies prior to 1988 employing attention, placebo, or minimally effective comparison conditions showed similar changes in physical activity when compared to the intervention condition, it is not clear that the components of the interventions employed exert a practically meaningful influence on physical activity beyond that exerted by social support and reinforcement. The superiority of behavior change interventions over increased attention from attending professionals still has not been convincingly shown.

Although there are too few studies since 1988 to permit meaningful clustering of effect sizes according to important characteristics of the studies, it appears that studies with the best experimental control report small-to-moderate effects compared to moderate-to-large effects of less controlled studies. Also, effects for self-reported physical activity seem to be larger than effects for changes in $\dot{V}O_{2peak}$. In general, we believe that the size of effects is inversely related to internal and external validity of the results. An illustration of this is the large effect typical of the several interventions based on health education and fitness testing. The methods of these studies are representative of prior studies for which it has been concluded by narrative review that little impact on physical activity occurred (23).

Future Directions

As part of the implementation plans to attain the U.S. Public Health Service physical fitness and exercise goals for 1990, The Workshop on Epidemiologic and Public Health Aspects of Physical Activity and Exercise was sponsored by the U.S. Department of Health and Human Services and held September 24 through 25, 1984, at the Centers for Disease Control in Atlanta, Georgia (89). After review and discussion by a panel of experts from the fields of public health and exercise science, the important recommendations and study questions for the determinants of physical activity were agreed upon for public health. Specific recommendations were made under each of the three categories that follow. The progress and current priority of these recommendations, based on research and events since the recommendations, was recently evaluated (19,20). An updating of those conclusions follows.

1. "First, there remains a need to conceptualize and, in a general way, rank determinants according to priority. Our knowledge will continue to benefit from replication, extension, and direct comparison of factors implicated by previous studies" (27, p. 168).

Though this recommendation has not been achieved, there has been progress in identifying some strong and consistent correlates of physical activity. The demographic variables of age, education, gender, and socioeconomic status continue to be supported. Cognitive variables have been extensively studied, but only perceived barriers, intention to exercise, mood disturbance, perceived health or fitness, and self-efficacy have been consistently related to physical activity. The only behavioral variable predictive of current physical activity is activity level in the recent past. Social support from family and peers has been found to be strong correlates and predictors of physical activity. Too few data on physical environmental influences have been reported to allow the priority of these variables to be reliably estimated. Amount of perceived effort or the intensity of exercise is usually inversely related to physical activity participation. The research to date has taught that some aspects of personal attributes, social and physical environments, and characteristics of the activities themselves are likely to exert an influence on physical activity. Many variables remain to be explored, and the need still exists for comparisons of variables within and between categories.

Little or no progress has been made in identifying and ranking the interactions of personal attributes and environments as they influence physical activity. This remains a priority for advancing theory and for selecting effective interventions for different population segments and physical activity settings, but it cannot occur until available theories are competitively contrasted or remodeled based on analyses of data from large population-based studies or large-sample clinical studies.

Progress has been made in identifying cognitive factors and interventions that influence the planning and adoption of physical activity (43) and in clarifying the effectiveness of behavioral and cognitive-behavioral interventions designed to increase and maintain physical activity (24). However, the most effective components of these interventions have yet to be identified. The relative importance, additivity, or interaction of population-based promotions of physical activity that are based on social-cognitive and educational models, versus clinical interventions, based on principles of behavior modification or cognitive-behavior modification, require study.

2. "Second, as our general knowledge grows, it will also be necessary to specify major activity determinants for certain populations and settings" (27, p. 169).

Little or no progress has been made in understanding how determinants differ according to age, race, gender, ethnicity, socioeconomic level, health status, and fitness level, or who is most likely to benefit from different intervention approaches. However, research has increased in these areas and remains a priority. An increase in intervention research in different nations is a favorable trend (77).

Progress has been made in clarifying differences and similarities between determinants of moderate leisure physical activity and vigorous exercise related to fitness in supervised and free-living settings (46,98). Progress has also been made toward establishing that sport history (21) and age (89) are probably selection biases, not true causes of contemporary inactivity. Family and peer influences, socioeconomic status, and education level may be selection bias effects, yet they have potential as true determinants. Their study remains a high priority.

Physical activity has not correlated consistently with other health behaviors. Although there may be correlations between physical activity and other health behaviors when variability within an individual is considered, it does not appear that variations between individuals in most health behaviors can be explained by variation in physical activity (76). This suggests that generalized health behavior theories or interventions will not be useful for exercise applications when they are focused on a population over a short period of time. Experimental or prospective studies are a high priority for deciding whether general or physical activity–specific theories and interventions are most effective for studying and increasing physical activity.

3. "Third, advancing age and elapsed time after initial adoption of an activity are among the most reliable predictors of inactivity. Thus, it seems likely that past activity environments and experiences are strong influences on present and future participation. Yet, little is known in these areas" (27, p. 169).

Little or no progress has been made in understanding how perceptions and preferences for types and intensities are formed and if they influence participation. This understanding remains a high priority for undertaking free-living physical activity and for its adoption in supervised leisure settings. Activity preferences may be less important for supervised exercise adherence when activities are varied and intensity is based on initial fitness level. Nevertheless actual intensity is still likely to be important.

Little or no progress has been made in understanding if determinants and dispositions for physical activity differ or change at a definable age within lifespan stages. It does now appear, however, that inactivity associated with age can be reversed with appropriate interventions (59). This priority has increased in importance due to increases in elderly populations and lack of evidence that schools have increased children's leisure physical activity (47).

Progress has been made in showing that stages in physical activity include planning, adoption, maintenance, and periodicity and that determinants can differ for each stage. Decision-based theories and interventions appear helpful for increasing planning and adoption. Integrating decision theories with social marketing strategies offers an important direction for future research and applications (30). In addition, social support, self-motivation, self-regulatory skills, and interventions like relapse prevention seem necessary to maintain or resume a physical activity pattern. The origin and time course for intrinsic reinforcement of physical activity remains unknown. Understanding the process of personal motivation for physical activity, however, remains a high priority for facilitating the success of public health promotion. More studies using qualitative methods are encouraged in this area (e.g., 42). Interfacing the fields of education, medicine, exercise science, behavioral science, public health, and public policy must be accelerated. Biologically-oriented theories of reinforcement should receive more research attention, and more needs to be known about genetically transmissable dispositions toward physical activity and inactivity.

In addition, future studies must consider unique cultural and economic-political differences between developed and developing or restructuring nations and between westernized and unwesternized nations. Theoretical models evolving from ideologies that place responsibility on the self to effect behavior change (e.g., most of the decision theories studied in exercise settings) will have less potential to explain or predict physical activity when social and environmental factors do not facilitate personal decision-making or direct personal control of behaviors like exercise due to cultural or economic restraints. These concerns also apply to disadvantaged segments of the population in generally affluent societies.

Acknowledgments

Thanks to Marlee Stewart Mikel, Donna Smith, Melinda Brewer, and Kecia Carrasco for their help in preparing this manuscript.

References

1. Acquista, V.W.; Wachtel, T.J.; Gomes, C.I.; Salzillo, M.; Stockman, M. Home-based health risk appraisal and screening program. J. Community Health. 13(1):43-52; 1988.
2. Ajzen, I; Fishbein, M. Understanding attitudes and predicting social behavior. Englewood Cliffs, NJ: Prentice Hall; 1980.
3. American College of Sports Medicine. Position statement on the recommended quality and quantity of exercise for developing and maintaining fitness in healthy adults. Med. Sci. Sports Exerc. 22:265-274; 1990.
4. Bauman, A.; Owen, N.; Rushworth, R.L. Recent trends and socio-demographic determinants of exercise participation in Australia. Community Health Stud. 14:19-26; 1990.
5. Blair, S.M.; Kohl, H.W.; Paffenbarger, R.S.; Clark, D.G.; Cooper, K.H.; Gibbons, L.W. Physical fitness and all-cause mortality: A prospective study of healthy men and women. JAMA. 262:2395-2401; 1989.
6. Bouchard, C.; Shephard, R.J.; Stephens, T.; Sutton, J.R.; McPherson, B.D., editors. Exercise, fitness, and health: A consensus of current knowledge. Champaign, IL: Human Kinetics; 1990.
7. Brill, P.A.; Burkhalter, H.E.; Kohl, H.W.; Blair, S.N.; Goodyear, N.N. The impact of previous athleticism on exercise habits, physical fitness, and coronary heart disease risk factors in middle-aged men. Res. Q. Exerc. Sport. 60:209-215; 1989.
8. Bush, P.J.; Zuckerman, A.E.; Taggart, V.S.; Theiss, P.K.; Peleg, E.O.; Smith, S.A. Cardiovascular risk factor prevention in black school children: The "know your body" evaluation project. Health Educ. Q., 16:215-227; 1989.
9. Carron, A.V.; Widmeyer, W.N.; Brawley, L.R. Group cohesion and individual adherence to physical activity. J. Sport Exerc. Psychol. 10:127-138; 1988.
10. Caspersen, C.J.; Christenson, G.M.; Pollard, R.A. Status of the 1990 physical fitness and exercise objectives—evidence from NHIS 1985. Public Health Rep. 101:587-592; 1985.
11. Caspersen, C.J.; Powell, K.E.; Christenson, G.M. Physical activity, exercise, and physical fitness: Definitions, and distinctions for health-related research. Public Health Rep. 101:126-146; 1985.
12. Cauley, J.A.; Donfield, S.M.; LaPorte, R.E.; Warhaftig, N.E. Physical activity by socioeconomic status in two population based cohorts. Med. Sci. Sports Exerc. 23:343-352; 1991.
13. Centers for Disease Control. Sex-, age-, and region-specific prevalence for sedentary lifestyle in selected states in 1985—the behavioral risk factor surveillance system. MMWR. 36:195-198, 203; 1987.
14. Centers for Disease Control. CDC surveillance summaries, June. MMWR. 39(No. SS-2):8; 1990.
15. Cohen, J. Statistical power analysis for the behavioral sciences. New York: Academic Press; 1977.
16. Dennison, B.A.; Straus, J.H.; Mellits, E.D.; Charney, E. Childhood physical fitness tests:

Predictor of adult physical activity levels? Pediatrics. 82:324-330; 1988.
17. Department of Health and Human Services. Healthy people 2000: National health promotion and disease prevention objectives. DHHS (PHS) 91-50212. Washington, DC: Public Health Service; 1991: p. 107. Available from: U.S. Government Printing Office, Washington, DC.
18. Dishman, R.K. Compliance/adherence in health-related exercise. Health Psychol. 1:237-267; 1982.
19. Dishman, R.K., editor. Exercise adherence: Its impact on public health. Champaign, IL: Human Kinetics; 1988.
20. Dishman, R.K. Exercise adherence research: Future directions. Am. J. Health Promo. 3:52-56; 1988.
21. Dishman, R.K. Supervised and free-living physical activity: No differences in former athletes and nonathletes. Am. J. Prev. Med. 4:153-160; 1988.
22. Dishman, R.K. Determinants of participation in physical activity. In: Bouchard, C.; Shephard, R.J.; Stephens, T.; Sutton, J.R.; McPherson, B.D., eds. Exercise, fitness, and health: A consensus of current knowledge. Champaign, IL: Human Kinetics; 1990:75-102.
23. Dishman, R.K. Physical activity in medical care. In: Torg, J.S.; Welsh, R.P.; Shephard, R.J., eds. Current therapy in sports medicine—2. Philadelphia: B.C. Decker, Inc; 1990:122-129.
24. Dishman, R.K. Increasing and maintaining exercise and physical activity. Behav. Ther. 22:345-378; 1991.
25. Dishman, R.K., ed. Exercise adherence volume II. Champaign, IL: Human Kinetics; [In press].
26. Dishman, R.K.; Darracott, C.R.; Lambert, L.T. Failure to generalize determinants of self-reported physical activity to a motion sensor. Med. Sci. Sports Exerc. 24:904-910; 1992.
27. Dishman, R.K.; Sallis, J.F.; Orenstein, D. The determinants of physical activity and exercise. Public Health Rep., 100:158-171; 1985.
28. Dishman, R.K.; Steinhardt, M. Reliability and concurrent validity for a seven-day recall of physical activity in college students. Med. Sci. Sports Exerc. 20:14-25; 1988.
29. Dishman, R.K.; Steinhardt, M. Internal health locus of control predicts free-living, but not supervised, physical activity: A test of exercise-specific control and outcome-expectancy hypotheses. Res. Q. Exerc. Sport. 61:383-394; 1990.
30. Donovan, R.J.; Owen, N. Social marketing and population-level intervention. In: Dishman, R.K., ed. Exercise adherence volume II. Champaign, IL: Human Kinetics; [In press].
31. Dzewaltowski, D.A. Toward a model of exercise motivation. J. Sport. Exerc. Psychol. 11:251-269; 1989.
32. Dzewaltowski, D.A.; Noble, J.M.; Shaw, J.M. Physical activity participation: Social cognitive theory versus the theories of reasoned action and planned behavior. J. Sport. Exerc. Psychol. 12:388-405; 1990.
33. Farquhar, J.W.; Fortmann, S.P.; Flora, J.A.; Taylor, C.B.; Haskell, W.L.; Williams, P.T.; Maccoby, N.; Wood, P.D. Effects of communitywide education on cardiovascular disease risk factors: The Stanford five-city project. JAMA. 264(3):359-365; 1990.
34. Fitness Canada. Active living: A conceptual overview. Toronto: Fitness Canada; 1991.
35. Fitterling, J.M.; Martin, J.E.; Gramling, S.; Cole, P.; Milan, M.A. Behavioral management of exercise training in vascular headache patients: An investigation of exercise adherence and headache activity. J. Appl. Behav. Anal. 21:9-19; 1988.
36. Folsom, A.R.; Cook, T.C.; Sprafka, J.M.; Burke, G.L.; Norsted, S.W.; Jacobs, D.R. Differences in leisure-time physical activity levels between blacks and whites in population-based samples: The Minnesota heart survey. J. Behav. Med. 14:1-9; 1991.
37. Ford, E.S.; Merritt, R.K.; Heath, G.W.; Powell, K.E.; Washburn, R.A.; Kriska, A.; Haile, G. Physical activity behaviors in lower and higher socioeconomic status populations. Am. J. Epidemiol. 133:1246-1256; 1991.
38. Fox, K.R.; Corbin, C.B. The physical self-perception profile: Development and preliminary validation. J. Sport. Exerc. Psychol. 11:408-430; 1989.
39. Friedman, H. Magnitude of experimental effect and a test for its rapid estimation. Psychol. Bull. 70:245-251; 1968.
40. Garcia, A.W.; King, A.C. Predicting long-term adherence to aerobic exercise: A comparison of two models. J. Sport. Exerc. Psychol. 13:394-410; 1991.
41. Gatch, C.L.; Kendzierski, D. Predicting exercise intentions: The theory of planned behavior. Res. Q. Exerc. Sport. 61:100-102; 1990.
42. Gauvin, L. An experiential perspective on the motivational features of exercise and lifestyle. Can. J. Sport Sci. 15(1):51-58; 1991.
43. Godin, G.; Shephard, R.J. Use of attitude-behavior models in exercise promotion. Sports Med. 10(2):103-121; 1990.
44. Hofstetter, C.R.; Hovell, M.F.; Macera, C.; Sallis, J.F.; Spry, V.; Barrington, E.; Callender,

C. Illness, injury, and correlates of aerobic exercise and walking: A community study. Res. Q. Exerc. Sport. 62:1-9; 1991.

45. Hofstetter, C.R.; Hovell, M.F.; Sallis, J.F. Social learning correlates of exercise self-efficacy: Early experiences with physical activity. Soc. Sci. Med. 31:1169-1176; 1990.
46. Hovell, M.F.; Sallis, J.F.; Hofstetter, C.R.; Spry, V.M.; Elder, J.P.; Faucher, P.; Caspersen, C.J. Identifying correlates of walking for exercise: An epidemiologic prerequisite for physical activity promotion. Prev. Med. 18:856-866; 1989.
47. Iverson, D.C.; Fielding, J.E.; Crow, R.S.; Christenson, G.M. The promotion of physical activity in the United States population: The status of programs in medical, worksite, community, and school settings. Public Health Rep. 100:212-224; 1985.
48. Johansson, G.; Johnson, J.V.; Hall, E.M. Smoking and sedentary behavior as related to work organization. Soc. Sci. Med. 32:837-846; 1991.
49. Kaplan, G.A.; Cohen, R.D.; Lazarus, N.B.; Leu, D.J. Psychosocial factors in the natural history of physical activity. Am. J. Prev. Med. 7:12-17; 1991.
50. Kemper, H.C.G. The natural history of physical activity and aerobic fitness in teenagers: The Amsterdam growth and health study. In: Dishman, R.K., ed. Exercise adherence volume II. Champaign, IL: Human Kinetics; [In press].
51. Kendzierski, D. Self-schemata and exercise. Basic Appl. Soc. Psychol. 9:45-61; 1988.
52. Kendzierski, D. Exercise self-schemata: Cognitive and behavioral correlates. Health Psychol. 9:69-82; 1990.
53. Kendzierski, D.; DeCarlo, K.J. Physical activity enjoyment scale: Two validation studies. J. Sport. Exerc. Psychol. 13:50-64; 1991.
54. Killen, J.D.; Telch, M.J.; Robinson, T.N.; Maccoby, N.; Taylor, C.B.; Farquhar, J.W. Cardiovascular disease risk reduction for tenth graders: A multiple-factor school-based approach. JAMA. 260(12):1728-1733; 1988.
55. King, A.C. Community intervention for promotion of physical activity and fitness. Exerc. Sport Sci. Rev. 19:211-260; 1991.
56. King, A.C.; Blair, S.N.; Bild, D.; Dishman, R.K.; Dubbert, P.M.; Marcus, B.H.; Oldridge, M.; Paffenbarger, R.S.; Powell, K.E.; Yeager, K. Determinants of physical activity and interventions in adults. Med. Sci. Sports Exerc. 24:S221-S236; 1992.
57. King, A.C.; Carl, F.; Birkel, L.; Haskell, W.L. Increasing exercise among blue-collar employees: The tailoring of worksite programs to meet specific needs. Prev. Med. 17:357-365; 1988.
58. King, A.C.; Frey-Hewitt, B.; Dreon, D.M.; Wood, P.D. Diet vs exercise in weight maintenance. Arch. Intern. Med. 149:2741-2746; 1989.
59. King, A.C.; Haskell, W.L.; Taylor, C.B.; Kraemer, H.C.; DeBusk, R.F. Group- vs. home-based exercise training in healthy older men and women. JAMA. 266:1535-1542; 1991.
60. King, A.C.; Taylor, C.B.; Haskell, W.L.; DeBusk, R.F. Strategies for increasing early adherence to and long-term maintenance of home-based exercise training in healthy middle-aged men and women. Am. J. Cardiol. 61:628-632; 1988.
61. King, A.C.; Taylor, C.B.; Haskell, W.L.; DeBusk, R.F. Identifying strategies for increasing employee physical activity levels: Findings from the Stanford/Lockheed exercise survey. Health Educ. Q. 17:269-285; 1990.
62. Klesges, R.B.; Eck, L.H.; Isbell, T.R.; Fulliton, W.; Hanson, C.L. Smoking status: Effects on the dietary intake, physical activity, and body fat of adult men. Am. J. Clin. Nutr. 51:784-789; 1990.
63. Knutsen, S.F.; Knutsen, R. The Tromso survey: The family intervention study—the effect of intervention on some coronary risk factors and dietary habits, a 6-year follow-up. Prev. Med., 20:197-212; 1991.
64. Krick, J.P.; Sobal, J. Relationships between health protective behaviors. J. Community Health. 15:19-34; 1990.
65. LaPorte, R.E.; Montoye, H.J.; Caspersen, C.J. Assessment of physical activity in epidemiologic research: Problems and prospects. Public Health Rep. 100:131-146; 1985.
66. Macera, C.A.; Jackson, K.L.; Hagenmaier, G.W.; Kronenfeld, J.J.; Kohl, H.W.; Blair, S.N. Age, physical activity, physical fitness, body composition, and incidence of orthopedic problems. Res. Q. Exerc. Sport. 60:225-233; 1989.
67. Macera, C.A.; Pate, R.R.; Powell, K.E.; Jackson, K.L.; Kendrick, J.S.; Craven, T.E. Predicting lower-extremity injuries among habitual runners. Arch. Intern. Med. 149:2565-2568; 1989.
68. Marcus, B.H.; Selby, V.C.; Niaura, R.S.; Rossi, J.S. Self-efficacy and the stages of exercise behavior change. Res. Q. Exerc. Sport. 63(1):60-66; 1992.
69. Marlatt, G.A.; Gordon, J. Relapse prevention. New York: Guilford Press; 1985.
70. McAuley, E.; Jacobson, L. Self-efficacy and exercise participation in sedentary adult females. Am. J. Health Promo. 5:185-191; 1991.

71. McPhillips, J.B.; Pellettera, K.M.; Barrett-Connor, E.; Wingard, D.L.; Criqui, M.H. Exercise patterns in a population of older adults. Am. J. Prev. Med. 5:65-72; 1989.
72. Myers, A.M.; Weigel, C.; Holliday, P.J. Sex- and age-linked determinants of physical activity in adulthood. Can. J. Public Health. 80:256-260; 1989.
73. National Heart Foundation of Australia. Risk factor prevalence study: No. 2-1983. Canberra: National Heart Foundation of Australia; 1985.
74. Neale, A.V.; Singleton, S.P.; Dupuis, M.H.; Hess, J.W. The use of behavioral contracting to increase exercise activity. Am. J. Health Promo. 4:441-447; 1990.
75. Noland, M.P. The effects of self-monitoring and reinforcement on exercise adherence. Res. Q. Exerc. Sport. 60(3):216-224; 1989.
76. Norman, R.M.G. The nature and correlates of health behavior. Health promotion studies series no. 2. Ottawa: Health and Welfare, Canada; 1986.
77. Oldenburg, B.; Bauman, A.; Booth, M.; Owen, N. Increasing levels of physical activity in the Australian community. Health Promo. J. Aust. 1:15-18; 1991.
78. Oldridge, N.B. Compliance and exercise in primary and secondary prevention of coronary heart disease: A review. Prev. Med. 11:56-70; 1982.
79. Oldridge, N.B.; Streiner, D.L. The health belief model: Predicting compliance and dropout in cardiac rehabilitation. Med. Sci. Sports Exerc. 22:678-683; 1990.
80. Ostwald, S.K. Changing employees' dietary and exercise practices: An experimental study in a small company. J. Occup. Med. 31(2):90-97; 1989.
81. Owen, N.; Bauman, A. The descriptive epidemiology of physical inactivity in adult Australians. Int. J. Epidemiol. 21:305-310; 1992.
82. Owen, N.; Bauman, A. Determinants of physical inactivity and of reasons for inactivity. Int. J. Epidemiol.; [In press].
83. Parcel, G.S.; Simons-Morton, B.; O'Hara, N.M.; Baranowski, T.; Wilson, B. School promotion of healthful diet and physical activity: Impact on learning outcomes and self-reported behavior. Health Educ. Q. 16(2):181-199; 1989.
84. Patterson, T.L.; Sallis, J.F.; Nader, P.R.; Rupp, J.W.; McKenzie, T.L.; Roppe, B.; Bartok, P.W. Direct observation of physical activity and dietary behaviors in a structured environment: Effects of a family-based health promotion program. J. Behav. Med. 11(5):447-458; 1988.
85. Perusse, L.; Leblanc, C.; Bouchard, C. Familial resemblance in lifestyle components: Results from the Canada fitness survey. Can. J. Public Health. 79:201-205; 1988.
86. Perusse, L.; Tremblay, A.; Leblanc, C.; Bouchard, C. Genetic and familial environmental influences on level of habitual physical activity. Am. J. Epidemiol. 129:1012-1022; 1989.
87. Pollock, J.L.; Carroll, J.F.; Graves, J.E.; Leggett, S.H.; Braith, R.W.; Limacher, M.; Hagberg, J.M. Injuries and adherence to walk/jog and resistance programs in the elderly. Med. Sci. Sports Exerc. 23:1194-1200; 1991.
88. Pollock, M.L. Prescribing exercise for fitness and adherence. In: Dishman, R.K., ed. Exercise adherence: Its impact on public health. Champaign, IL: Human Kinetics; 1988:259-277.
89. Powell, K.E.; Paffenbarger, R.S., Jr. Workshop on epidemiologic and public health aspects of physical activity and exercise: A summary. Public Health Rep. 100:118-126; 1985.
90. Powell, K.E.; Stephens, T.; Marti, B.; Heinemann, L.; Kreuter, M. Progress and problems in the promotion of physical activity. J. Public Health Policy. [In press].
91. Prochaska, J.O.; Marcus, B.H. The transtheoretical model: The applications to exercise. In: Dishman, R.K., ed. Exercise adherence volume II. Champaign, IL: Human Kinetics; [In press].
92. Reynolds, K.D.; Killen, J.D.; Bryson, S.W.; Maron, D.J.; Taylor, C.B.; Maccoby, N.; Farquhar, J.W. Psychosocial predictors of physical activity in adolescents. Prev. Med. 19:541-551; 1990.
93. Robbins, S.R.; Slavin, L.A. A measure of social support for health-related behavior change. Health Educ. 19:36-39; 1988.
94. Robison, J.I.; Rogers, M.A.; Carlson, J.J.; Mavis, B.E.; Stachnik, T.; Stoffelmayr, B.; Sprague, H.A.; McGrew, C.R.; Van Huss, W.D. Effects of a 6-month incentive-based exercise program on adherence and work capacity. Med. Sci. Sports Exerc. 24(1):85-93; 1992.
95. Rosenthal, R. Meta-analytic procedures for social research. Beverly Hills, CA: Sage Publications; 1984:1-149.
96. Rosenthal, R.; Rubin, D.B. A simple, general purpose display of magnitude of experimental effect. J. Educ. Psychol. 74:166-169; 1982.
97. Sallis, J.F.; Grossman, R.M.; Pinski, R.B.; Patterson, T.L.; Nader, P.R. The development of scales to measure social support for diet and exercise behaviors. Prev. Med. 16:825-836; 1987.

98. Sallis, J.F.; Haskell, W.L.; Fortmann, S.P.; Vranizan, K.M.; Taylor, C.B.; Solomon, D.S. Predictors of adoption and maintenance of physical activity in a community sample. Prev. Med. 15:331-346; 1986.
99. Sallis, J.F.; Hovell, M.F. Determinants of exercise behavior. Exerc. Sport Sci. Rev. 18:307-330; 1990.
100. Sallis, J.F.; Hovell, M.F.; Hofstetter, C.R. Predictors of adoption and maintenance of vigorous physical activity in men and women. Prev. Med. 21:237-251; 1992.
101. Sallis, J.F.; Hovell, M.F.; Hofstetter, C.R.; Barrington, E. Explanation of vigorous physical activity during two years using social learning variables. Soc. Sci. Med. 34:25-32; 1992.
102. Sallis, J.F.; Hovell, M.F.; Hofstetter, C.R.; Elder, J.P.; Faucher, P.; Spry, V.M.; Barrington, E.; Hackley, M. Lifetime history of relapse from exercise. Addic. Behav. 15:573-579; 1990.
103. Sallis, J.F.; Hovell, M.F.; Hofstetter, C.R.; Elder, J.P.; Hackley, M.; Caspersen, C.J.; Powell, K.E. Distance between homes and exercise facilities related to frequency of exercise among San Diego residents. Public Health Rep. 105:179-185; 1990.
104. Sallis, J.F.; Hovell, M.F.; Hofstetter, C.R.; Faucher, P.; Elder, J.P.; Blanchard, J.; Caspersen, C.J.; Powell, K.E.; Christenson, G.M. A multivariate study of determinants of vigorous exercise in a community sample. Prev. Med. 18:20-34; 1989.
105. Sallis, J.F.; Pinski, R.B.; Grossman, R.M.; Patterson, T.L.; Nader, P.R. The development of self-efficacy scales for health-related diet and exercise behaviors. Health Educ. Res. 3:283-292; 1988.
106. Sallis, J.F.; Simons-Morton, B.G.; Stone, E.J.; Corbin, C.B.; Epstein, L.H.; Faucette, N.; Iannotti, R.J.; Killen, J.D.; Klesges, R.C.; Petray, C.K.; Rowland, T.W.; Taylor, W.C. Determinants of physical activity and interventions in youth. Med. Sci. Sports Exerc. 24:S248-S257; 1992.
107. Shea, S.; Stein, A.D.; Basch, C.E.; Lantigua, R.; Maylahn, C.; Strogatz, D.S.; Novick, L. Independent associations of educational attainment and ethnicity with behavioral risk factors for cardiovascular disease. Am. J. Epidemiol. 134:567-582; 1991.
108. Siegel, D.; Johnson, J.; Newhof, C. Adherence to exercise and sports classes by college women. J. Sports Med. Phys. Fitness. 28:181-188; 1988.
109. Simons-Morton, B.G.; Parcel, G.S.; Baranowski, T.; Forthofer, R.; O'Hara, N.M. Promoting physical activity and a healthful diet among children: Results of a school-based intervention study. Am. J. Public Health. 81(8):986-991; 1991.
110. Sonstroem, R.J. Psychological models. In: Dishman, R.K., ed. Exercise adherence: Its impact on public health. Champaign, IL: Human Kinetics; 1988:125-154.
111. Sports Council of Great Britain. Sport, health, psychology, and exercise symposium. London: Sports Council of Great Britain; 1990.
112. Steinhardt, M.A.; Dishman, R.K. Reliability and validity of expected outcomes and barriers for habitual physical activity. J. Occup. Med. 31:536-546; 1989.
113. Steinhardt, M.A.; Young, D.R. Psychological attributes of participants and nonparticipants in a worksite health and fitness center. Behav. Med. 18(1):40-46; 1992.
114. Stephens, T.; Craig, C.L. The well-being of Canadians: Highlights of the 1988 Campbell's survey. Ottawa: Canadian Fitness and Lifestyle Research Institute; 1990.
115. Stokols, D. Establishing and maintaining healthy environments: Toward a social ecology of health promotion. Am. Psychol. 47:6-22; 1992.
116. Tappe, M.K.; Duda, J.A.; Menges-Ehrnwald, P. Personal investment predictors of adolescent motivational orientation toward exercise. Can. J. Sport Sci. 15:185-192; 1990.
117. Treiber, F.A.; Baranowski, T.; Braden, D.S.; Strong, W.B.; Levy, M.; Knox, W. Social support for exercise: Relationship to physical activity in young adults. Prev. Med. 20:737-750; 1991.
118. Valois, P.; Desharnais, R.; Godin, G. A comparison of the Fishbein and Ajzen and the Triandis attitudinal models for the prediction of exercise intention and behavior. J. Behav. Med. 11:459-472; 1988.
119. Weber, J.; Wertheim, H. Relationships of self-monitoring, special attention, body fat percent, and self-motivation to attendance at a community gymnasium. J. Sport Exer. Psychol. 11:105-114; 1989.
120. Weir, L.T.; Jackson, A.S.; Pinkerton, M.B. Evaluation of the NASA/JSC health related fitness program. Avia. Space Environ. Med. 60:438-444; 1989.
121. Whitehead, J.R.; Corbin, C.B. Multidimensional scales for the measurement of locus of control of reinforcements for physical fitness behaviors. Res. Q. Exerc. Sport. 59:103-117; 1988.
122. Yoshida, K.K.; Allison, K.R.; Osborn, R.W. Social factors influencing perceived barriers to physical exercise among women. Can. J. Public Health. 79:104-108; 1988.

Chapter 14

Demography of Health-Related Fitness Levels Within and Between Populations

Roy J. Shephard

Although implicit in the basic model of exercise, fitness, and health adopted for the 1988 consensus conference (12), no systematic attempt was made to synthesize information on the demography of health-related fitness at that meeting. Key questions include (a) whether samples are representative of the populations that have been tested, (b) what are the specific factors distorting cross-sectional survey results, (c) what problems arise when collecting longitudinal observations over several decades, (d) what constraints are imposed by measurement techniques appropriate to large-scale surveys, (e) what impact do such surveys have on health-related fitness, (f) where have clear population differences of health-related fitness been established within or between populations, and (g) what priorities are there for future research? Further discussion of the techniques adopted in individual surveys, the reported results (commonly biased), and the issues that arise when making comparisons within and between populations will be found in Drury (26), Shephard (82,86-88), and Shephard and Parizkova (98).

Population Sampling

The Fallacy of Convenience Sampling

Exercise scientists have often been content to report the results of careful measurements made on convenience samples of 4 to 6 healthy young men. Subjects have been drawn from laboratory staff or university students, the latter commonly being enrolled in physical education courses or attending programs in a Department of Athletics. It has usually been inferred that the findings from such studies were relevant to either all North Americans or Europeans, or at least to a substantial fraction of such populations (e.g., "white" males). Such an assumption is dangerous in any area of human biology, but is particularly suspect when the data refer to patterns of exercise and health-related fitness due to selective recruitment of the "worried well" (19). Moreover, both habitual physical activity and a healthy lifestyle are particularly prevalent in well-educated, single young men of above-average socioeconomic status (16,29,31,40) (Tables 14.1 and 14.2).

Indigenous Populations

Fitness enthusiasts with an anthropological bent have hypothesized that low levels of health-related fitness are endemic in "developed" nations because such societies have abandoned the physically demanding lifestyle of the neolithic hunter-gatherer cultures, a lifestyle to which the human body has adapted over many centuries of evolution (39,114,120).

Unfortunately, many of those interested in indigenous populations have studied very small and non-representative samples (82). In consequence, erroneous impressions have been formed. For example, an earlier generation of Canadian scientists believed that the Inuit had a very poor respiratory function (10,42) and a relatively low level of aerobic fitness (3).

The manual of methodology developed for the International Biological Programme (IBP) (115,116) stressed the number of subjects needed to demonstrate a statistically significant difference between groups, but gave no guidance on population sampling other than to suggest this be "random." One of the larger IBP studies examined the Canadian Inuit community of Igloolik. Here, for the first time, exercise scientists were able to secure informed consent and test participation by some 72% of a substantial indigenous settlement. Biological calibration assured the equivalence of both apparatus and techniques between medical observers and exercise scientists. Nevertheless, reported population averages for such measures of health-related

Table 14.1 Direction of Potential Biases When Health-Related Fitness Is Measured on a Small Sample of the Population

Characteristic	High age of sample	High socioeconomic status	High education level
Aerobic fitness	Positive	Negative	Positive
Skinfold thickness	Negative	Negative	Negative

Table 14.2 Influence of Level of Education on Percentage of Population Showing Selected Measures of Physical Activity

	Years education (29)					Level of education			
Pursuit	8	10	14	16		Less than high school	High school	Greater than high school	University
Walking	28%	42%	49%	51%	Canada Fitness Survey (31)				
Swimming	13	35	46	51	Active	41	56	58	63
Gymnastics	9	22	26	27	Moderate	31	34	33	31
Nordic skiing	3	7	13	14	Sedentary	25	8	7	5
Tennis	3	14	15	25	CFLRI (16)				
Golf	3	12	18	22	Active	27	32	34	41
Skating	13	19	23	24	Moderate	21	25	24	27
Ice-hockey	4	10	13	10	Sedentary	52	43	42	33

Note. Subjects older than 14 years who are physically active at least once in year (29); subjects older than 10 years, active more or less than 3 hr/week, 9 months/year (31); subjects older than 10 years, energy expenditure 3 kcal/kg/day (16).

fitness as the forced vital capacity and the 1 s forced expiratory volume differed substantially between the two teams of investigators. The reason was that the 28% of residents not tested by the exercise scientists tended to be the sick members of the population; these individuals were recruited selectively by the medical investigators, but some of the fittest members of the settlement were not interested in evaluation by the physicians.

Age-Related Biases

Both in Igloolik (82) and in various nationwide surveys (11,87) a substantial fraction of older potential subjects either refuse to participate or are excluded from testing on medical grounds (Table 14.3). The residual sample reporting for measurements of health-related fitness includes an excessive proportion of those who are fit and have adopted a healthy lifestyle (106) (Table 14.4).

Future surveys of health-related fitness will require preliminary paramedical screening procedures of greater specificity. Such tools should be simple to apply and of sufficient sensitivity to assure test safety, yet precise enough to exclude a much smaller proportion of older test volunteers. The recent revision of the Physical Activity Readiness Questionnaire (PAR-Q) (108) goes some way towards meeting these objectives. It excludes only about two thirds of test candidates who would have been rejected by the original PAR-Q instrument. Nevertheless, substantial numbers of older people will continue to be excluded from exercise testing, even with the best type of screening devices. There is thus a need to devise methods for a *post-hoc* adjustment of mean scores for missing subjects and for comparing participants and nonparticipants in terms of such readily ascertained noninvasive measures as age, body mass index, smoking habits, and habitual activity patterns.

Sampling by Community

Whether dealing with an indigenous population or a "developed" society, one of the more satisfactory

Table 14.3 Recruitment of Older Men to Studies of Health-Related Fitness

Study	Age range (years)	Response rate (%)	Author
Minnesota businessmen	45–55	92	Keys et al. (1963)*
Framingham residents	40–60+	66	Dawber et al. (1963)*
L.A. civil servants	40–59	75	Chapman (1964)*
Albany civil servants	40–59	89	Doyle et al. (1957)*
Chicago (W. Electric employees)	40–59	67	Paul et al. (1963)*
(People's Gas employees)	40–59	92	Stamler (1973)*
Tecumseh residents	40–59	83–88	Montoye (61)
California corporate employees	40–59	66	Rosenmann et al. (1975)*
Evans County, GA residents	45–64	92	McDonough et al. (1965)*
Men born 1913 in Göteborg, Sweden	50	88	Tibblin et al. (1975)*
Industrial health survey	40–67	84	Höglund & Gustafson (43)
Israeli civil servants	40–59	86	Medalie et al. (1968)*
Yugoslavia residents	35–62	93	Kozarevic et al. (1976)*
Puerto Rico residents	45–59	81	Gordon et al. (1974)*
Honolulu Japanese	45–59	81	Gordon et al. (1974)*
Lipid research clinics	20–69	85	Rifkind & Segal (70)
(Canadian clinics)	20–69	73	Hewitt et al. (41)
NHANES	25–74	70	Blair et al. (11)
Canada Fitness Survey	40–59	44	Stephens (106)

Note. *See Keys (53) for details on references.

Table 14.4 An Estimate of the Response Bias in the Canada Fitness Survey

Age (years)	Body mass index (kg/m²) M	F	Resting heart rate (beats/min) M	F	Blood pressure (mmHg) M	F
7–19	100.0	99.5	99.3	99.5	99.8/100.0	99.8/99.7
20–39	100.0	98.7	99.3	99.3	99.3/99.5	99.6/99.6
40–54	98.9	97.2	98.2	98.6	97.3/97.6	97.3/97.5
54–69	98.1	96.2	97.7	98.0	94.4/95.8	93.4/94.8

Note. Based on data reported by Stephens (106). Data for participants in active fitness tests, expressed as a percentage of average values for sample participating in simple physical measurements.

approaches to sampling is to test all willing individuals who meet minimal selection criteria. Examples of this approach include the Igloolik Inuit survey (82),the Framingham (22,51) and Tecumseh (60,61) studies in the United States, and the "Men Born in 1913" study from Göteborg, Sweden (118). Publicity regarding such surveys has its greatest impact in a small community where there is a corresponding increase of response. For instance, the overall response was 83% in the city of Tecumseh, Michigan (60,61). Nevertheless, there remains a steep age gradient for physically demanding components of the test battery; thus, only 50% of those age 50 to 69 years completed a simple step test in the Tecumseh study.

Even if sampling is very complete, doubt sometimes remains about the generality of results that are based upon a single community. The problem is most obvious in isolated settlements. For example, the Inuit from different circumpolar communities differ widely in their nutritional status and the extent of their acculturation to "white" society (82,84). Indeed, some groups are sufficiently separated to allow at least a theoretical potential for genetic drift. Thus a comparison of young adult male Inuit from three regions (82,84) suggested substantial intercommunity differences of aerobic power and average skinfold thicknesses (Igloolik, Northwest Territories: 53.5 ml/[kg·min], 6.5 mm; Upernavik, Greenland: 40.7 ml/[kg·min]; Wainwright, Alaska, 45.5 ml/([kg·min], 11.0 mm). But even in developed areas of Canada and the United States, small cities sometimes attract particular ethnic groups, and the labor force may be concentrated in a few specific industries with a preponderance of particular socioeconomic categories.

In larger cities, a project may become unmanageable unless the study is restricted to those born in specific years. However, the experience of the cohort that is examined may then differ from that of preceding or succeeding groups with respect to such factors as nutrition, habitual activity, health education, and exposure to the stresses of global warfare.

Representative Stratified Sampling

An alternative tactic is to recruit a representative or a stratified representative sample of a city or a nation. We attempted this in the medium-sized prairie city of Saskatoon (metropolitan population 150,000). We invited those whose names were drawn in a specified sequence from the local telephone directory to attend the university for a free fitness assessment (9). We recognized that in so doing we immediately excluded certain categories of people including those living in various types of institutions, those too poor to own a telephone, and those who had unlisted telephone numbers. But a much greater problem arose from subsequent attrition of the sample. Of 2,648 respondents, 118 were unsuitable for testing (for example, too old), 982 refused the test directly, and a further 649 were unable to agree upon a convenient time for testing. An additional 49 failed to keep their appointment, and another 72 were excluded by the physician supervising the tests, so that only 29.4% of the initial respondents were evaluated. Likewise, in Quebec, Landry et al. (55) were only able to persuade 23.6% of 1,000 randomly selected subjects to visit their laboratory for fitness testing.

The Canadian Association for Health, Physical Education, and Recreation adopted representative testing in their studies of health-related fitness in schoolchildren. Measurements were made on the *nth* pupil in classes from each of a representative list of schools provided by Statistics Canada (33,45). Where a refusal was encountered, they proceeded to test the *nth* + 1 pupil in the same class. Unfortunately, no information was provided on a possible bias introduced by the selection of classes where physical education was taught, nor did the report specify the number of students who refused to participate in the survey.

The Canada Fitness Survey undertook the ambitious task of recruiting a nationally representative sample of some 20,000 individuals for home-based assessments of activity patterns and health-related fitness (31). In order to facilitate data collection across a wide geographical area, and to obtain valid information that could be applied to subgroups of the Canadian population, the sample was cluster-stratified by province and type of community. The numbers tested were proportional to the square root of the population of a given province, and included those resident in rural areas, medium-sized towns, and large cities. The major constraint was that those to be interviewed and tested must live within one and a half hours drive of one of the 80 teams conducting the tests. Similar efforts to recruit representative national samples have been made in the Canada Health Survey (15), the U. S. National Health and Nutrition Examination Surveys (11,56) and the National Health Interview Survey (65). Other surveys of this type are planned in England and in New Zealand (44,77).

Cross-Sectional Biases

Because of high costs and logistic difficulties in tracing populations with a high annual turnover rate, the majority of studies of health-related fitness have been cross-sectional in type. Sometimes (as in the repeated AAHPERD studies of field performance [1] and in the analogous CAHPER studies [14], closely similar cross-sectional data have been collected after the lapse of 5 to 15 years. Attempts are commonly made to infer rates of growth and aging, as well as to make interpopulation comparisons from such cross-sectional data, but findings can be distorted by seasonal/climatic factors, selective migration, intercurrent pathologies, and cohort effects.

Seasonal and Climatic Factors

Seasonal and climatic factors may explain a substantial part of regional differences in health-related fitness across Canada (57). Studies from several countries have shown seasonal variations in the fitness of schoolchildren. In Québec, physical condition was poor in the summer and peaked in the late fall at the zenith of the hockey season (96). Likewise, Scandinavian children lost physical condition during the summer months when they were not participating in organized physical activity programs (7,54). In the Inuit community of Igloolik, the health-related fitness of adults was marginally lower during the winter than in the summer months; this was presumed due to the restriction of physical activity imposed by the harsh arctic climate (72).

Selective Migration

Miall, Ashcroft, Lovell, and Moore (58) noted a selective migration of tall individuals out of mining communities. This exaggerated the normal decrement of height with age in certain valleys of South Wales, with obvious consequences for the body mass index in these populations. In Canada, successive waves of immigration are well recognized. In any given year of cross-sectional testing, one decade of the population may include a predominance of those of British ancestry, another will be biased by United States draft-dodgers, and another by Vietnamese boat people, Tamils, or those fleeing from Hong Kong.

Intercurrent Pathologies

When dealing with older subjects a substantial proportion of a cross-sectional sample is affected by some form of chronic disease. In many such individuals, the disease process reduces some measure of health-related fitness such as maximal oxygen intake. Thus, Brown and Shephard (13) noted chronic disease in about 50% of female department store employees age 40 to 70 years. In some 25% of their sample the disease was judged to limit cardiorespiratory function. For affected individuals aged 40 to 49 years, aerobic power was only 90% of normal, and in those aged 50 to 59 years it was only 86% of normal.

In younger individuals chronic disease is less commonly a concern. Nevertheless, survey results have been distorted in some indigenous populations with a high prevalence of infections such as tuberculosis (82,84).

Cohort Effects

Cohort effects that have influenced health-related fitness include (a) wartime dietary shortages that influenced the growth of children (39) and the risk of atherosclerosis in adults (79), (b) a secular trend to a reduced consumption of saturated animal fats (32,49,111), (c) replacement of active recreation by passive entertainment such as television watching (2,97,101,109), (d) replacement of self-propulsion by the use of motorized vehicles (85), (e) the mechanization and subsequent automation of heavy industrial work (27), and (f) an increase followed by a decline of cigarette consumption (50,75,85,110). Indigenous populations commonly have had imposed upon them a process of acculturation to the lifestyle of "developed" societies (99).

Longitudinal Surveys

Examples of longitudinal studies include the ongoing study of the Igloolik community (71,73), the Framingham study (22), various studies of children in Holland, Belgium, and Québec (86), and the Canada Fitness Survey (in which, unfortunately, it was necessary to eliminate physiological measurements and to reduce the sample size when evaluation was repeated)(16). Longitudinal surveys are widely assumed to give values of irreproachable validity for such aspects of health-related fitness as growth and aging. However, in practice results can be beset with major technical problems, including inconsistencies of methodology, secular trends, sample attenuation, and statistical artifacts.

Methodological Concerns

If a longitudinal study is to be successful, the interest of the investigator, of supporting staff, and of funding agencies must be sustained over an extended period. Methodology must be held as constant as possible throughout, and because of observer aging, the traditional approach of biological calibration will need reinforcement by physical methods of standardizing equipment and procedures (48). Some measurements of health-related fitness, such as skinfold thicknesses, are particularly prone to interobserver variation (28,68,92, 119). If observers change over the course of a prolonged study, it is thus vital that the readings obtained by one observer be calibrated against his or her replacement.

One adverse corollary of a constant methodology is that new technologies cannot be exploited (11). The procedures used may thus seem very dated by the time a final report is prepared.

Secular Trends

Most communities have seen systematic secular trends in habitual physical activity, nutrition, and other aspects of personal lifestyle over the past 40 to 50 years (85,110,111). The effects of growth and aging upon an individual's health-related fitness are commonly confounded by variations in habitual physical activity (89,105) and exposure to cigarette smoke (110).

Systematic changes of lifestyle have been particularly rapid in many indigenous communities, as these populations have become acculturated to the lifestyle of "white," developed societies (38,73,99). In such communities the transition from a "primitive" culture to the lifestyle of a "developed" society has been accompanied by dramatic changes in various indices of health-related fitness such as maximal oxygen intake, skinfold thicknesses, and muscle strength (71,73,99). In the urban culture of North America, on the other hand, there has recently been a fitness boom, followed by a plateauing of interest in physical activity (89,105).

Sample Attenuation

A further problem arises from progressive sample attenuation as individuals lose interest in a study or change their place of residence. A geographically or linguistically isolated settlement may show moderate stability. For instance, the annual loss of schoolchildren from a study conducted in the largely unilingual francophone community of Trois Rivières was held to only 4% (86). On the other hand, the rate of population turnover in many North American cities is 20% per year or higher. Even if the sample is drawn on a nationwide basis, it becomes progressively harder to trace specific study participants as the period of observation is extended.

The loss of subjects is unfortunately not a random process. In general, it is the upwardly mobile, health-oriented individuals who tend to migrate. This is well illustrated by comparing the early mortality from arteriosclerotic and degenerative heart disease in those migrating from Italy to Australia and in those remaining in their homeland (74). Aging curves for a given community are further modified by a selective death of individuals with an adverse lifestyle, and (presumably) a poor level of health-related fitness (62,66).

Statistical Artifacts

The error of measurement of health-related variables is usually sufficiently large that it is desirable to report population averages rather than individual results. However, problems may then arise from a smoothing of the data. This is particularly true at the time of peak pubertal growth. Averaged data underestimate peak growth rates for such characteristics as body mass and maximal oxygen intake unless the results are first aligned in terms of the peak height velocity of the individual (59,69,107).

Mixed Cross-Sectional and Longitudinal Designs

Some studies, for example those conducted on the Igloolik community, have retested the entire population periodically. It is then possible to compare the impact of secular trends upon both cross-sectional and longitudinal data (Figure 14.1).

Techniques of Large-Scale Surveys

There is often substantial disagreement on an appropriate choice of measuring techniques when health-related fitness is to be measured in a well-equipped laboratory. Such disagreement may be further magnified when the procedures are simplified to allow large-scale demographic surveys. Specific issues include the interlaboratory standardization of methodology and the choice between a high- or low-technology approach to subject testing.

Interlaboratory Standardization

In the early 1960s (17), scientists began to appreciate that, while the results of a procedure such as respiratory gas analysis might be highly reproducible within a given laboratory, there were often

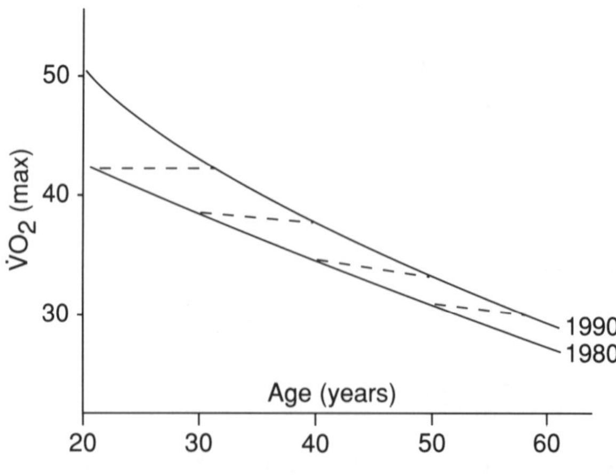

Figure 14.1 Diagram to illustrate the differing estimates of aging of the maximal oxygen intake ($\dot{V}O_2$max) obtained from cross-sectional (solid lines) and longitudinal (interrupted lines) studies. It is assumed that there has been an increase of habitual activity and thus of maximal oxygen intake over the decade of observation from 1980 to 1990.

large systematic differences in results from one laboratory to another. The first step in a meaningful demographic comparison is thus interlaboratory agreement upon standard procedures (114, 115), with ongoing physicochemical and/or biological calibration of all techniques from one laboratory to another (48).

One important key to success is an adequate budget for preliminary orientation sessions where a multiplicity of observers can learn common techniques, cross-validating these not only against each another, but also relative to some external standard. Given such preliminary training, the results of simple measurements such as blood pressure, height, body mass, skinfold thicknesses, and the sit-and-reach test of flexibility may be accepted with reasonable confidence, even if their interpretation remains open to some discussion.

Unfortunately, more than two decades after conclusion of the International Biological Programme, we are still far from standardizing procedures for the measurement of health-related fitness, largely because of personal pride and the vested interests that various laboratories have in conserving their existing methodology.

High-Technology Approach

If a whole community is to be evaluated, it is possible to airlift electric generators, voltage stabilizers, and all the equipment of a modern laboratory into quite remote locations (82,84). Unfortunately the high costs of air transportation and a requirement to duplicate key apparatus makes a high-technology survey very expensive. Further, if maximum effort tests are contemplated, it is necessary for a physician to remain on site throughout the survey.

Some investigators, particularly in the United States (26), have recommended adoption of a high-technology approach in national surveys of health-related fitness. The necessary test equipment can be built into large air-conditioned trailers and driven from one city to another, although a national survey then becomes a slow process, with potential difficulties in allowing for seasonal effects when comparing one community with another.

Low-Technology Approach

Other investigators have attempted to develop simple field measures of health-related fitness that use a minimum of equipment and do not require the presence of a supervising physician (30,87,88).

The biggest controversy has surrounded low-technology approaches to the estimation of aerobic fitness. Some field surveys have used the cycle ergometer to determine a directly measured or closely interpolated PWC_{170} (33,45). This test is reasonably effective in children, although the level of cardiorespiratory fitness can be underestimated if the resting heart rate is increased by either anxiety or a hot and humid environment (93). In adults, further complications arise from a variable decline in maximal heart rate with age. The Åstrand (6) prediction of maximal oxygen intake may be criticized on similar grounds, although the final version of this procedure did incorporate an *average* correction for the age-related decline in maximal heart rate.

In Canada, extensive use has been made of the Canadian Home Fitness Test (CHFT; 9,100). This was originally designed as a simple, self-administered motivational tool, but there have been subsequent attempts to develop multiple regression equations that would allow a prediction of maximal oxygen intake from the subject's body mass, the peak rate of stepping, the corresponding heart rate, and age (18,47,100). Provided that the heart rate is measured accurately (for instance, by electrocardiogram), the required stepping rhythm is accurately maintained, and subjects lift their center of mass the full height of the staircase at each cycle, the procedure seems no better and no worse than other submaximal procedures for the estimation of aerobic power (83,100).

Predictions have a coefficient of variation of 10% to 15% relative to the corresponding direct measurements of maximal oxygen intake, so little can be said about individual fitness from such an evaluation. On the other hand, the systematic error relative to direct measurements is fairly small, so that averaged data provide a useful measure of the cardiorespiratory status of a large population. The equation introduced by Jetté, Campbell, Mongeon, and Routhier (47) was based upon quite a small sample of subjects, and the proposed method of assessment gave a very low weighting to the immediate postexercise pulse rate. This method has the advantage that any effects of anxiety and habituation are minimized; however, it seems likely to reduce the impact of interindividual differences in fitness upon the test score. The structure of the equation also imposes a "ceiling" of performance upon those with a high level of aerobic fitness.

Currently, efforts are being made to develop more reliable equations for the prediction of aerobic power from the CHFT, based upon larger samples of healthy individuals and using additional test stages to accommodate very fit individuals

(100). However, such efforts seem doomed to failure unless an electronic device is available to monitor the heart rate accurately.

Those involved in the mass evaluation of schoolchildren have commonly used a battery of physical performance tests such as the time to run 50 meters and 1500 m, push-ups, pull-ups, sit-ups, a shuttle-run, and a standing broad jump or a vertical jump (1,14,76). The results of such assessments depend heavily upon environmental conditions, recent practice of the required gymnastic skills, motivation, body size, and physical aptitude rather than health-related fitness (20,21,24,25). Some authors have thus distinguished the concept of "performance-related fitness" (the primary factor examined by such tests) from health-related fitness (64).

Impact of Measurement

Data collection can in itself influence the results of fitness tests in several ways. If subject cooperation is involved, learning and habituation may at first improve test scores, but loss of interest can later lead to a deterioration of test performance (80). The phenomena of learning and habituation are well-recognized, but it is less certain how many measurements are needed to reach a plateau of performance with any given type of test, or how rapidly learning and habituation are dissipated between the individual test sessions of a longitudinal survey.

Test participation could theoretically have a positive influence upon the subsequent lifestyle of those evaluated (35,36). For example, discovery of an abnormal exercise electrocardiogram during a simple step test might encourage smoking cessation, or the onset of severe shortness of breath might encourage the adoption of a regular exercise program. If a high proportion of a community is evaluated, both the physical environment and the social norms of the community may also be altered in a manner favoring the adoption of a healthy lifestyle. Thus, one unexpected consequence of the Trois Rivières longitudinal study was the construction of an indoor swimming pool at the local primary school (86). However, in practice, the effects of a single fitness testing session are usually quite weak (35,36).

Results of Surveys

Intrapopulation Differences

Intrapopulation comparisons may relate to the effects of age, sex, activity patterns, lifestyle, socioeconomic gradients, and secular trends. As with interpopulation comparisons, the analysis of secular trends is often complicated by an unsuspected change of technique from one evaluation to another.

Age and Sex

Age comparisons must allow for an increase of stature during the period of growth and a decrease in both stature and the proportion of lean mass with aging. Unfortunately, there is no agreed-upon method to adjust data for changes of body size. Surveys of maximal oxygen intake thus show a sharp decline over the latter part of childhood if data are expressed per kilogram of body mass (8), an approach that reflects the approximate energy cost of displacing body mass. However, there is relatively little pubertal change of aerobic power if results are expressed relative to height squared (an approach that some have argued is dimensionally "correct," 112).

In elderly subjects, the decrease of stature, the loss of mineral from the bones and the resultant decrease in the density of lean tissue all have implications for the determination of optimum body mass (103). From an actuarial point of view, the optimal body mass increases steadily as a person ages (4). The resting blood pressure also apparently increases with age (117), but because this change is not shown by some indigenous populations with a "simpler" lifestyle (e.g., Solomon Islanders [63] and Navajo Indians [23]), it is unclear whether the increment reflects intrinsic aging or incipient pathological changes such as arteriosclerosis. Cross-sectional surveys such as the Canada Fitness Survey (31) show the anticipated loss of muscle strength and flexibility with aging, but again it is unclear how far intercohort differences of environment and age-related decreases of habitual physical activity have contributed to the observed gradients of function.

When making comparisons between men and women, the method of expressing data is again controversial. Strength and aerobic power are commonly standardized per unit of body mass, but the composition of the body mass that is used to "normalize" the data differs between the two sexes; breast tissue increases the proportion of body fat and a lighter bone structure reduces the density of lean tissue in the female. Men have 10% to 20% higher scores for most health-related fitness tests except flexibility (where women have a substantial advantage). It remains unclear how far sex effects reflect culturally-related differences of lifestyle, and how far they are genetically imposed.

Activity Patterns

From our underlying model we might anticipate a within-population gradient of health-related fitness with the level of habitual physical activity. We saw a substantial difference of aerobic power between continuing hunters and sedentary members of the Igloolik community (84). In urban samples, any relationship between reported activity and measures of health-related fitness seems relatively weak (34,35), but this may reflect difficulty in measuring physical activity patterns accurately and/or the fact that few people are active in North American society (87). Montoye (60) compared the most and the least active people in Tecumseh, finding only small differences of blood pressure (137/78 vs. 140/81 mmHg) and average skinfold thickness (20.9 vs. 23.1 mm) between the two groups. When the Canada Fitness Survey data were classified in terms of daily energy expenditure per kilogram of body mass (87,91), there was no gradient of fitness between sedentary, moderately active, and active individuals, and a classification depending upon spending a certain intensity of activity for 3 hr/week also showed only marginal intergroup differences in most indices of fitness.

Lifestyle

Correlations have been sought between the level of habitual physical activity and other facets of lifestyle, using such techniques as principal component analysis (78,90). In general, physical activity has shown little relationship to other types of health behavior, although many surveys have failed to distinguish health-related physical activity from sports with other appeals such as excitement, competition, or social interaction (87).

Urban/rural comparisons now favor urban areas (57,82,86,87), because of associated socioeconomic gradients, poorer exercise facilities in rural areas, and (in the case of children) because the rural students spend much of their leisure time sitting in school buses. Physical activity patterns also show a positive gradient from eastern to western Canada (57), in part because of climatic factors, and in part because of economic gradients.

Socioeconomic Differences

Participation in formal leisure activity programs shows a substantial social gradient (16,31) (see Table 14.1), but perhaps because of the physical demands of occupation, the gradient of health-related fitness with social class is less clearly established.

Secular Trends

Because of differences in sampling and measurement techniques, there is little data that can be used to assess secular trends in fitness. The surveys of Pett and Ogilvie (67) and the Canada Fitness Survey (31) allow a comparison of changes in body mass index (BMI) for representative samples of Canadians over a 27-year period (Table 14.5). Men showed little change of relative body mass over this period; however, older women were substantially lighter in 1981 than in 1954, reflecting the female trend to thinness. It is less clear if the women achieved the reduced BMI through a reduction of body fat or a loss of lean tissue. Howell and MacNab (45) and Gauthier, Massicotte, Hermiston, and MacNab (33) tested the PWC_{170} on comparable samples of Canadian children in 1966 and in 1981 using identical techniques. Over this period older girls showed a substantial gain in physical working capacity and thus in predicted maximal oxygen intake (Table 14.5).

Surveys of performance-related fitness have been repeated several times in both the United States and in Canada (1,14). Scores have apparently improved for some items, yet it is unclear how far this reflects the fact that students now have greater experience of the required test procedures. Longitudinal data for the settlement of Igloolik show a deterioration in most measures of health-related fitness (73,99), apparently in association with acculturation to an urban type of society.

Interpopulation Differences

Interpopulation fitness comparisons are severely limited by a lack of representative samples. Even when surveys have been coordinated by a single observer (e.g., the Seven Countries Study), a casual inspection of the data shows substantial intersample differences related to methodology rather than to phenotype (53).

The majority of population data refer to young adults, although there have also been some comparisons of growth patterns between developed and less industrialized countries (98). Where nutrition has been less plentiful, there has generally been a stunting of growth, and with extreme malnutrition the size of children has also been small in relation to height (113). Comparisons around the time of puberty have been complicated by the later maturation of those from less developed societies (82,86). In terms of aging, the 1971 survey of Igloolik suggested that the deterioration of aerobic power had a more convex form than in a developed society (71,82). It was reasoned that this reflected a

Table 14.5 Canadian Secular Trends of Body Mass Index (kg/m²) and Predicted Maximal Oxygen Intake [ml/(kg·min), estimated from PWC_{170}]

	Body mass index					Predicted aerobic power			
	Men		Women			Boys		Girls	
Age (years)	1954	1981	1954	1981	Age (years)	1966	1981	1966	1981
20–29	23.8	24.0	22.3	21.9	7–9	38.4	41.3	33.8	36.8
30–39	25.5	25.1	23.6	23.5	10–12	40.2	41.8	33.4	37.5
40–49	25.8	26.0	25.5	24.5	13–14	42.3	53.3	30.0	35.9
50–59	25.9	26.0	26.9	25.7	15–19	40.9	43.7	29.0	36.8
60+	25.7	26.5	27.0	25.8					

Note. Based on the data of Pett and Ogilvie (67), the Canada Fitness Survey (31), Howell and MacNab (45), and Gauthier et al. (33).

steep decline of physical activity when the younger generation were able to assume the responsibilities of hunting. Some support for this hypothesis was found from a change towards the more commonly seen pattern of aging as the overall level of physical activity declined among the younger members of the community (73,99).

Body Composition

Body mass data for the less industrialized countries in most instances show a substantial deficit relative to actuarial norms (82). In contrast, data for Canada, the United States, and many other leading industrial nations show a substantial proportion of the population exceeding actuarial recommendations (Tables 14.6 and 14.7).

Aerobic Power

The aerobic power of people in some of the less developed countries is apparently quite low (see Table 14.6), in part because of difficulties in determining maximal performance in such societies, in part because of difficulties in making an appropriate allowance for their smaller body size, and in part because of malnutrition. However, a number of groups including the Canadian Inuit, Chilean Indians, Israeli Yemenites, Tarahumara runners, New Guinea Kauls, active Nigerian Yoruba, active Tanzanians, and Venezuelan Warao show higher average figures than would be expected in young North American adults. This reflects a more active lifestyle, a much lower burden of body fat, and in some groups the necessity of traversing mountainous terrain (82).

Blood Pressure and Serum Cholesterol

A substantial volume of data on blood pressure and serum cholesterol levels is now available, in part as a result of the Seven Countries study (Table 14.7). The two variables seem generally related in middle-aged adults, although the highest values have been observed in regions such as Eastern Finland—which traditionally has consumed a high fat diet—with low values in regions where the consumption of fat has been restricted by poverty and/or tradition (e.g., Japan and parts of Yugoslavia). Recently, changes in typical national diets have substantially modified these regional differences.

Priorities for Future Research

Before embarking upon any massive international comparisons of fitness, further research should be directed to issues of sampling and the standardization of methodology. It will also be necessary to agree upon the magnitude of differences in health-related fitness that have clinical significance.

Issues of Sampling

Intergroup comparisons cannot be based upon convenience samples. Repeated large and representative surveys encompassing regions and/or countries with a variety of physical and sociocultural environments are needed before strong conclusions can be drawn about possible relationships between demographic differences of health-related fitness and corresponding differences in community health.

Table 14.6 Skinfold Thicknesses, Estimated Percentage of Body Fat, and Aerobic Power of Young Male Populations from Less Industrialized Societies

	XS mass skinfold				
Group	Mass (kg)	(mm)	(fat%)	Aerobic power [ml/(kg·min)]	Author
Arabs (Chaamba)		6.2			Wyndham (1966)
Australia (Aborigenes)		6.6			Wyndham (1966)
Canada (Inuit)		5.6		56.4	Shephard (1974)
Chile (Indians)				49.1	Donoso et al. (1974)
East Africa (Dorobo)				46.0	diPrampero (1969)
Easter Island	0.0			42.0	Ekblom & Gjessing (1968)
Ethiopia	−10.7			37.3	Areskog (1969)
	−13.0	6.0		39.9	Andersen (1971)
Israel					
Kurds	−0.4			48.4	Samueloff et al. (1973)
Yemenites	+2.5			52.4	Samueloff et al. (1973)
Jamaica	−5.3			47.0	Miller et al. (1972)
Malaya (Temiars)				53.2	Chan et al. (1974)
Mexico (Tarahumara)					
runners			11.1	63.0	Aghemo et al. (1971)
nonrunners			17.9	38.9	Aghemo et al. (1971)
New Guinea					
Tukisenta-Lagaip	5.0			45.1	Sinnett & Solomon (1968)
Kauls				53.2	Patrick & Cotes (1971)
Highland Lufas				67.0	Patrick & Cotes (1971)
Nigeria (Yoruba)					
active	−3.7			55.5	Davies et al. (1972)
inactive	−4.0			45.9	Davies et al. (1972)
Peru (Quechua)		6.3		49.3	Buskirk (1974)
Russia (Kirghiz)				33.9	Mirrakhimov (1972)
South Africa					
Bantu	−4.7	5.6		47.9	Wyndham (1966)
Kalahari		4.6		47.1	Wyndham (1966)
Tanzania					
active	−1.2			57.2	Davies (1973)
inactive	−4.1			47.2	Davies (1973)
Trinidad					
Negroes	−1.3	7.9		38.3	Edwards et al. (1972)
East Indians	−3.4	10.6		39.4	Edwards et al. (1972)
United States (Navajho)				44.0	Gardner (1971)
Venezuela (Warao)		5.9		51.2	Gardner (1971)
Zaire					
Hoto	−6.7			42.7	Ghesquiere (1971)
Twa	−7.7			47.5	Ghesquiere (1971)

Note. See Shephard (82) for details on references.

Some progress has been made in developing methods of population sampling, but there remains a need for appropriate methods of adjusting population data to allow for incomplete sampling of older age groups. Large biases are currently introduced into population averages by the selective omission of the diseased, lower socioeconomic groups, and those with an adverse lifestyle.

Standardization of Methodology

Even minor differences of experimental protocol can lead to large intersurvey differences of fitness scores. There thus remains an urgent need for international standardization of methodology applicable to high-technology and low-technology surveys. Before interpopulation comparisons can be made with confidence, procedures must be agreed

Table 14.7 Data on Health-Related Fitness for Subjects Age 40 to 45 Years Living in Various Countries

Group	Relative mass (%)	Skinfold (mm)	Blood pressure (mmHg)	Serum cholesterol (mmol/L)	Author
Canada					
(M/F/F—no contraceptive hormones)				5.48/5.50/5.24	Hewitt et al. (41)
(M/F)	111.2/111.7	13.6/20.3			Jetté (46)
Finland					
East	94	13	141/87	6.87	Keys (53)
West	98	16	133/80	6.43	Keys (53)
Finns (M/F)				7.21/7.00	Aromaa et al. (5)
Lapps (M/F)				7.29/6.95	Aromaa et al. (5)
Greece					
Corfu	94	16	130/81	5.00	Keys (53)
Crete	94	14	131/80	5.13	Keys (53)
Israel					
Civil servants				5.30	Goldbort et al. (37)
European (M/F)				5.43/5.15	Kark et al. (52)
Asiatic (M/F)				5.27/5.30	Kark et al. (52)
N. African (M/F)				5.09/4.95	Kark et al. (52)
Italy					
Crevalcore	105	23	136/84	5.03	Keys (53)
Montegiorgino	99	15	128/78	4.98	Keys (53)
Roma	108	26	135/86	5.37	Keys (53)
Japan					
Tanushinaru	89	15	120/68	4.33	Keys (53)
Ushibuka	91	15	126/75	4.20	Keys (53)
(M/F)			130/80 130/79		Lovell (1967)*
Kenya		11	113/72		Shaper (1967)*
Netherlands	99	24	140/90	6.04	Keys (53)
Norway					
(Bergen) (M/F)			141/? 140/?		Kantor, Winkelstein, et al. (51a)
Poland					
Plock (M/F)			143/85 148/85		Aleksandrow (1967)*
Krakow (M/F)			138/85 138/85		Aleksandrow (1967)*
South Seas					
Palau (M/F)			113/70 113/75		Lovell (1967)*
Saipan (M/F)			126/78 125/78		Lovell (1967)*
United Kingdom (M)			132/84	6.00	Mann et al. (55a)
(F)			130/81	5.60	Mann et al. (55a)
London (M/F)				6.03/5.89	Slack et al. (102)
United States					
U.S. Railroad	104	33	130/83	6.07	Keys (53)
Lipid Research Clinics				5.31/5.31	Hewitt et al. (1977)
Yugoslavia					
Dalmatia	94	15	136/85	4.72	Keys (53)
Slavonia	95	15	130/79	5.08	Keys (53)
VelikaKrsna	89	13	124/78	3.99	Keys (53)
Zrenjanin	103	23	126/80	4.40	Keys (53)

Note. See Stamler, Stamler, and Pullmann (104) for details on references. Subjects are men unless otherwise indicated.

upon between investigators, and it must be demonstrated that different observers can reach the same results when testing a common pool of subjects.

In high-technology surveys, there is a need to adopt uniform sites and procedures for skinfold measurement. Preferably, data should be reported as skinfold readings, because there is a bewildering array of equations to predict the percentage of body fat and interpopulation differences in the density of lean tissue preclude the development of an acceptable uniform equation (92). Twenty five years after the International Biological Programme Working Party (81,82), there remains a need for a common laboratory protocol for the determination of aerobic power. This should cover such issues as apparatus (use of treadmill, cycle ergometer, or step test), an appropriate duration of initial warm-up, a suitable ramp function for the increase of exercise intensity, and clear criteria for the attainment of maximal effort.

For the measurement of muscle strength and endurance, likewise, agreement is required for both apparatus and technique. Flexibility is thought to be an important component of health-related fitness in older individuals, but there is little agreement on which movements are critical to continued health, on the communality of scores between the widely used sit-and-reach test and function at other joints (94), or on an appropriate warm-up period prior to testing.

Many surveys of blood pressure still lack careful standardization for posture, preliminary rest periods, site and dimensions of the measuring cuff, rate of cuff deflation, choice of signal (phase four or phase five), and above all, familiarity with the observer (95,121). Equally, determining of blood glucose and lipid profiles require a standardized technique from one laboratory to another (41).

Low-technology, performance-type tests seem simple to perform, but again there is a pressing need for surveys that use absolutely identical techniques under closely matched environmental conditions. Finally, whether or not a high- or a low-technology approach is adopted, it is important that there be a much better standardization of tools and techniques for measuring covariates such as habitual activity patterns, smoking habits, and exposure to air pollutants from one population to another.

Clinical Significance of Differences

There is general agreement that an increase of body fat, a reduction of maximal oxygen intake, or an increase of systemic blood pressure are adverse changes in health-related fitness. However, there is a need to establish clearer dose–response relationships between community health and changes in each of these variables. For example, if we find a 1% difference of body fat between two populations, is this of clinical importance, or should we be concerned only if there is a 10% interpopulation difference in body fat? Furthermore, should estimates of community health be based upon population means for the various determinants of health-related fitness, or should we examine the proportions of various populations that exceed some arbitrary ceiling? Decisions on such questions seem an important prelude to future demographic comparisons. Only then can we determine an appropriate sample size, the necessary sensitivity of techniques, and an appropriate method of data analysis.

References

1. AAHPERD. Health related fitness test. Washington, DC: American Alliance for Health, Physical Education, Recreation and Dance; 1980.
2. Alderson, J.; Crutchley, D. Physical education and the national curriculum. In: Armstrong, N., ed. New directions in physical education vol. I. Leeds, UK: Human Kinetics; 1990: 37-62.
3. Andersen, K.L.; Hart, J.S. Aerobic work capacity of Eskimos. J. Appl. Physiol. 18:764-768; 1963.
4. Andres, R. The rationale for age-specific height-weight tables. In: Andres, R.; Bierman, E.L.; Hazzard, W.R. Principles of geriatric medicine. New York: McGraw-Hill; 1985: 311-318.
5. Aromaa, A.; Björksten, F.; Eriksson, A.W.; Maatela, J.; Kirjarinta, M.; Fellman, J.; Tamminen, M. Serum cholesterol and triglyceride concentrations of Finns and Finnish Lapps. Acta Med. Scand. 198:13-22; 1975.
6. Åstrand, I. Aerobic work capacity in men and women with special reference to age. Acta Physiol. Scand. [Suppl.]. 49:169:1-91; 1960.
7. Åstrand, P.O. Fysiologiska synpunkter på skolungdomens fysika fostran; preliminär rapport till Folksam. (Physiological aspects of growth: Preliminary report to till Folksam.) Stockholm: Central Gymnastic Institute; 1961.
8. Bailey, D.A. Exercise, fitness and physical education for the growing child. In: Orban, W.A.R., ed. Proceedings of the national conference on fitness and health. Ottawa: Health and Welfare Canada; 1974:13-22.

9. Bailey, D.A.; Shephard, R.J.; Mirwald, R.L. Validation of a self-administered home test of cardio-respiratory fitness. Can. J. Appl. Sport Sci. 1:67-78; 1976.
10. Beaudry, P.H. Pulmonary function of the Canadian Eastern Arctic Eskimo. Arch. Environ. Health. 17:524-528; 1968.
11. Blair, D.; Habicht, J.-P.; Alekel, L. Assessments of body composition, dietary patterns, and nutritional status in the national health examination surveys and national health and nutrition examination surveys. In: Drury, T., ed. Assessing physical fitness and physical activity in population-based surveys. Hyattsville, MD: U.S. Dept. of Health and Human Services; 1990:79-104.
12. Bouchard, C.; Shephard, R.J.; Stephens, T.; Sutton, J.R.; McPherson, B.D., eds. Exercise, fitness, and health: A consensus of current knowledge. Champaign, IL: Human Kinetics; 1990.
13. Brown, J.R.; Shephard, R.J. Some measurements of fitness in older female employees of a Toronto department store. Can. Med. Assoc. J. 97:1208-1213; 1967.
14. CAHPER. Fitness performance II. Test manual. Ottawa: Canadian Association for Health, Physical Education and Recreation; 1980.
15. Canada Health Survey. Ottawa: Health and Welfare Canada; 1982.
16. CFLRI. The well-being of Canadians: Highlights of the 1988 Campbell's survey. Ottawa: Canadian Fitness and Lifestyle Research Institute; 1990.
17. Cotes, J.E.; Woolmer, R.F. A comparison between twenty seven laboratories of the results of analysis of an expired gas sample. J. Physiol. 163:36P-37P; 1962.
18. Cox, M.H.; Thomas, S.G.; Weller, I.M.R.; Corey, P. Reliability and validity of a fitness assessment for epidemiological studies. Can. J. Sport Sci. 17:49-55; 1992.
19. Criqui, M. The problem of response bias. In: Kaplan, R.M.; Criqui, M.H., eds. Behavioral epidemiology and disease prevention. New York: Plenum Press; 1985.
20. Cumming, G.R. Body size and the assessment of physical performance. In: Shephard, R.J.; Lavallée, H., eds. Physical fitness assessment. Principles, practice and applications. Springfield, IL: C.C. Thomas; 1978:18-31.
21. Cumming, G.R.; Keynes, R. A fitness performance test for schoolchildren and its correlation with physical working capacity and maximal oxygen uptake. Can. Med. Assoc. J. 96:1262-1269; 1967.
22. Dawber, T.R. The Framingham Study: The epidemiology of atherosclerotic disease. Cambridge, MA: Harvard University Press; 1980.
23. DeStephano, F.; Coulehan, J.; Kennethewiant, M. Blood pressure survey on the Navajo Indian reservation. Am. J. Epidemiol. 109:335-345; 1979.
24. Drake, V.; Jones, G.; Brown, J.R.; Shephard, R.J. Fitness performance tests and their relationship to the maximal oxygen uptake of adults. Can. Med. Assoc. J. 99:844-848; 1968.
25. Drake, V.; White, D.; Shephard, R.J. The fitness performance of Canadian working men. With some comments on the adaptation of performance tests to a small gymnasium. J. Sports Med. Phys. Fitness. 9:152-161; 1969.
26. Drury, T. Assessing physical fitness and physical activity in population-based surveys. Hyattsville, MD: U.S. Dept. of Health and Human Services; 1989.
27. Edholm, O. The changing pattern of human activity. Ergonomics. 13:625-643; 1970.
28. Edwards, D.A.W.; Hammond, W.H.; Healy, M.J.R.; Tanner, J.M.; Whitehouse, R.H. Design and accuracy of calipers for measuring subcutaneous tissue thickness. Br. J. Nutr. 2:133-143; 1955.
29. Ferland, Y. Schooling and lesiure activities. Can. Stat. Rev. (November):vi-ix; 1980.
30. Fitness Canada. Canadian standardized test of fitness. Operations manual. 2nd ed. Ottawa: Fitness Canada; 1981.
31. Fitness Canada. Fitness and lifestyle in Canada. Ottawa: Fitness Canada; 1983.
32. Florey, Du V.C.; Melia, R.J.W.; Darby, S.C. Changing mortality from ischaemic heart disease in Great Britain 1966-76. Br. Med. J. (i):635-637; 1978.
33. Gauthier, R.; Massicotte, D.; Hermiston, R.; MacNab, R. Comparaison entre 1968 et 1983 de la capacité physique de travail des jeunes Canadiens agés de 7 à 17 ans. (Comparison of the physical working capacity of young Canadians aged 7 to 17 years between 1968 and 1983.) CAHPER J. 50(Sept/Oct.):2-7; 1983.
34. Godin, G.; Cox, M.; Shephard, R.J. The impact of physical fitness evaluation on the behavioral intentions towards regular exercise. Can. J. Appl. Sport Sci. 8:240-245; 1983.
35. Godin, G.; Desharnais, R.; Jobin, J.; Cook, J. The impact of physical fitness and health age appraisal upon exercise intentions and behavior. J. Behav. Med. 10:241-250; 1987.
36. Godin, G.; Shephard, R.J. A simple method to assess exercise behavior in the community. Can. J. Appl. Sport Sci. 10:141-146; 1985.

37. Goldbourt, U.; Holtzman, E.; Neufold, H.N. Total and high density lipoprotein cholesterol in the serum and the risk of mortality: Evidence of a threshold. Br. Med. J. 290:1239-1243; 1985.
38. Greksa, L.P.; Baker, P.T. Aerobic capacity of modernizing Samoan man. Hum. Biol. 54:777-799; 1982.
39. Harrison, G.A. Population structure and human variation. London: Cambridge University Press; 1979.
40. Health and Welfare, Canada. Canada's health promotion survey. Ottawa: Health and Welfare Canada; 1988.
41. Hewitt, D.; Jones, G.J.L.; Godin, G.J.; McComb, K.; Breckenridge, W.C.; Little, J.A.; Steiner, G.; Mishkel, M.A.; Baillie, J.H.; Martin, R.H.; Gibson, E.S.; Prendergast, W.F.; Parliament, W.J. Normative standards of plasma cholesterol and triglyceride concentrations in Canadians of working age. Can. Med. Assoc. J. 117:1020-1024; 1977.
42. Hildes, J.A.; Schaefer, O.; Sayed, J.E.; Fitzgerald, E.J.; Koch, E.A. Chronic pulmonary disease and associated cardiovascular disease in Igloolimiuts. In: Shephard, R.J.; Itoh, S., eds. Circumpolar health. Toronto: University of Toronto Press; 1976:327-331.
43. Höglund, D.; Gustafson, A. Prospective study among male employees in industry. Acta Med. Scand. 198:5-11; 1975.
44. Hopkins, W.G.; Walker, N.P.; Hulme-Moir, F.M. Physical activity in New Zealand—a pilot study. N.Z. J.H.P.E.R. 20:11-18; 1987.
45. Howell, M.L.; MacNab, R. The physical work capacity of Canadian children 7-17 years. Ottawa: Canadian Association for Health, Physical Education and Recreation; 1968.
46. Jetté, M. Anthropometric characteristics of the Canadian population. Nutrition Canada Survey, 1970-72. Ottawa: University of Ottawa; 1983.
47. Jetté, M.; Campbell, J.; Mongeon, J.; Routhier, R. The Canadian Home Fitness Test as a predictor of aerobic capacity. Can. Med. Assoc. J. 114:680-682; 1976.
48. Jones, N.; Kane, M. Inter-laboratory standardization of methodology. Med. Sci. Sports. 11:368-372; 1979.
49. Joossens, J.V.; Brems-Heyns, E.; Claes, J.H.; Graffar, M.; Kornitzer, M.; Pannier, R.; Van Houte, O.; Vuylsteek, K.; Carlier, J.; De Backer, G.; Kesteloot, H.; Lequime, J.; Raes, A.; Vastesaeger, M.; Verdonk, G. The pattern of food and mortality in Belgium. Lancet. (i):1069-1072; 1977.
50. Jossa, D. Smoking Behaviour of Canadians 1983. Ottawa: Minister of Supply and Services (Cat. # H39-66/1985E); 1985.
51. Kannel, W.B.; Sorlie, P.; McNamara, P. The relationship of physical activity to risk of coronary heart disease. The Framingham study. In: Larsen, O.A.; Malmborg, R.O., eds. Coronary heart disease and physical fitness. Baltimore, MD: University Park Press; 1971:256-260.
51a. Kantor, S.; Winkelstein, W.; Sackett, D.L. A method for classifying blood pressure: An empirical approach to the reduction of misclassification due to response instability. Am. J. Epidemiol. 84:510-523; 1967.
52. Kark, J.D.; Friedlander, Y.; Kaufmann, N.A.; Stein, Y. Coffee, tea, and plasma cholesterol. The Jerusalem lipid research clinic prevalence study. Br. Med. J. 291:699-704; 1985.
53. Keys, A. Seven countries. A multivariate analysis of death and coronary heart disease. Cambridge: Harvard University Press; 1980.
54. Knuttgen, H.G.; Steendahl, K. Fitness of Danish school children during the course of one academic year. Res. Q. 34:34-40; 1963.
55. Landry, F.; Carrière, S.; Poirier, L.; LeBlanc, C.; Gaudreau, J.; Moisau, A.; Carrier, R.; Potvin, R. Observations sur la condition physique des Québecois. (Observations on the physical condition of Québecois.) Union Méd. 109:1-6; 1980.
55a. Mann, J.L.; Lewis, B.; Shephard, J.; Winder, A.F.; Fenster, S.; Rose, L.; Morgan, B. Blood lipid concentrations and other cardiovascular risk factors: Distribution, prevalence, and detection in Britain. Br. Med. J. 296:1702-1706.
56. McDowell, A.J. Cardiovascular endurance, strength and lung function tests in the national health and nutrition examination surveys. In: Drury, T., ed. Assessing physical fitness and physical activity in population-based surveys. Hyattsville, MD: U.S. Dept. of Health and Human Services; 1989:21-77.
57. McPherson, B.D.; Curtis, J.E. Regional and community type differences in the physical activity patterns of Canadian adults. Ottawa: Canadian Fitness and Lifestyle Research Institute; 1986.
58. Miall, W.E.; Ashcroft, M.T.; Lovell, H.G.; Moore, F. A longitudinal study of the decline of adult height with age in two Welsh communities. Hum. Biol. 39:445-454; 1967.
58a. Mirrakhimov, M.M. Ovsyokogorhoi patologii cheloveka v Kirgizskoi, S.S. Klin. Med. (Moscow) 50:104-109; 1972.
59. Mirwald, R.L.; Bailey, D.A. Maximal aerobic power. London, ON: Sports Dynamics; 1986:1-80.

60. Montoye, H.J. Physical activity and health. An epidemiologic study of an entire community. Englewood Cliffs, NJ: Prentice Hall; 1975.
61. Montoye, H.J. Lessons from Tecumseh on the assessment of physical activity and fitness. In: Drury, T., ed. Assessing physical fitness and physical activity in population-based surveys. Hyattsville, MD: U.S. Dept. of Health and Human Services; 1989:349-376.
62. Paffenbarger, R. Contributions of epidemiology to exercise science and cardiovascular health. Med. Sci. Sports Exerc. 20:426-438; 1988.
63. Page, L.B.; Damon, A.; Moelleriag, R.C. Antecedents of cardiovascular disease in six Solomon Island societies. Circulation. 49:1132-1146; 1974.
64. Pate, R.; Shephard, R.J. Characteristics of physical fitness in youth. In: Gisolfi, C.V.; Lamb, D., eds. Perspectives in exercise science and sports medicine. Vol. 2. Youth, exercise and sport. Indianapolis: Benchmark Press; 1989:1-45.
65. Pearce, N.D. General population surveys—an overview. In: Drury, T., ed. Assessing physical fitness and physical activity. Hyattsville, MD: U.S. Dept. of Health and Human Services; 1989.
66. Pekkanen, J.; Marti, B.; Nissinen, A.; Tuomilheto, J.; Punsar, S.; Karvonen, M.J. Reduction of premature mortality by high physical activity: A twenty year follow-up of middle-aged Finnish men. Lancet. (i):1473-1477; 1987.
67. Pett, L.B.; Ogilvie, G.F. The report on Canadian average weights, heights and skinfolds. Hum. Biol. 28:177-188; 1956.
68. Prahl-Andersen, B.; Kowalski, C.J.; Heyendael, P. A mixed longitudinal interdisciplinary study of growth and development. London: Academic Press; 1979.
69. Preece, M.A.; Baines, M.J. A new family of mathematical models describing the human growth curve. Ann. Hum. Biol. 5:1-24; 1978.
70. Rifkind, B.M.; Segal, P. Lipid research clinics program reference values for hyperlipidemia and hypolipidemia. JAMA. 250:1869-1879; 1983.
71. Rode, A.; Shephard, R.J. Cardio-respiratory fitness of an arctic community. J. Appl. Physiol. 31:519-526; 1971.
72. Rode, A.; Shephard, R.J. Fitness of the Canadian Eskimo: The influence of season. Med. Sci. Sports. 5:170-173; 1973.
73. Rode, A.; Shephard, R.J. Fitness and health of an Inuit community: 20 years of cultural change. Ottawa: Circumpolar and Scientific Affairs; 1992.
74. Rose, G. Current developments in Europe. In: Jones, R.J., ed. Atherosclerosis II. Berlin: Springer-Verlag; 1970:310-314.
75. Rosenbaum, P.D.; Bursten, J. Canada's health promotion survey. Special study on labour force groups. Ottawa: Ministry of Supply and Services; 1988.
76. Ross, J.C. Evaluating fitness and activity assessments from the national children and youth fitness studies I and II. In: Drury, T., ed. Assessing physical fitness and physical activity in population-based surveys. Hyattsville, MD: U.S. Dept. of Health and Human Services; 1989:229-259.
77. Russell, D.; Wilson, N.; Worsky, T.; Hopkins, W. Life in New Zealand. A lifestyle survey of New Zealanders. In: Russell, D.G.; Buisson, D.H., eds. Lifestyle report. Dunedin: Human Performance Associates; 1989.
78. Santa Barbara, J. The relationship between physical activity and other health-related lifestyle behaviours. Ontario: Ministry of Culture and Recreation; 1982.
79. Schettler, G. Atherosclerosis, the main problem of industrialized societies. In: Schettler, G.; Goto, Y.; Hata, Y.; Klose, G., eds. Atherosclerosis IV. Berlin: Springer-Verlag; 1977.
80. Shephard, R.J. Learning, habituation and training. Int. Z. Angew. Physiol. 28:38-48; 1968.
81. Shephard, R.J. Endurance fitness. 2nd ed. Toronto: University of Toronto Press; 1977.
82. Shephard, R.J. Human physiological work capacity. London: Cambridge University Press; 1978.
83. Shephard, R.J. Current status of the Canadian home fitness test. Br. J. Sports Med. 14:114-125; 1980.
84. Shephard, R.J. Work physiology and activity patterns. In: Milan, F.A., ed. The human biology of circumpolar populations. London: Cambridge University Press; 1980:305-338.
85. Shephard, R.J. Ischemic heart disease and exercise. London: Croom Helm; 1981.
86. Shephard, R.J. Physical activity and growth. Chicago: Year Book Medical; 1982.
87. Shephard, R.J. Fitness of a nation. Lessons from the Canada Fitness Survey. Basel: Karger; 1986.
88. Shephard, R.J. Work capacity: Methodology in a tropical environment. In: Collins, K.J.; Roberts, D.F., eds. Capacity for work in the tropics. London: Cambridge University Press, 1988:1-30.
89. Shephard, R.J. Fitness boom or bust—the Canadian perspective. Res. Q. 59:265-269; 1988.
90. Shephard, R.J. Exercise and lifestyle change. Br. J. Sports Med. 23:11-22; 1989.

91. Shephard, R.J. An international perspective on critical issues in fitness testing of U.S. adults. In: Drury, T., ed. Assessing physical fitness and physical activity in population-based surveys. Hyattsville, MD: U.S. Dept. of Health and Human Services; 1989:433-450.
92. Shephard, R.J. Body composition in biological anthropology. London: Cambridge University Press; 1990.
93. Shephard, R.J.; Allen, C.; Bar-Or, O.; Davis, C.T.M.; Degré, S.; Hedman, R.; Ishii, K.; Kaneko, M.; LaCour, R.; diPrampero, P.E.; Seliger, V. The working capacity of Toronto schoolchildren. Can. Med. Assoc. J. 100:560-566, 705-714; 1968.
94. Shephard, R.J.; Berridge, M.; Montelpare, W. On the generality of the "sit and reach" test. Res. Q. 61:326-330; 1990.
95. Shephard, R.J.; Cox, M.; Simper, K. An analysis of PAR-Q responses in an office population. Can. J. Public Health. 72:37-40; 1981.
96. Shephard, R.J.; Lavallée, H.; Jéquier, J-C.; LaBarre, R.; Rajic, M.; Beaucage, C. Seasonal differences in aerobic power. In: Shephard, R.J.; Lavallée, H., eds. Physical activity assessment: Principles, practice and applications. Springfield, IL: C.C. Thomas; 1978:194-210.
97. Shephard, R.J.; Lavallée, H.; LaRivière, G.; Rajic, M.; Brisson, G.R.; Beaucage, C.; Jéquier, J-C.; LaBarre, R. La capacité physique des enfants Canadiens: Une comparaison entre les enfants Canadiens français, Canadiens anglais et Esquimaux. III. Psychologie et sociologie des enfants Canadiens français. (The physical capacity of Canadian children: A comparison between French Canadian children, English Candians and Eskimos. III. Psychology and sociology of French Canadian children.) Union Méd. Can. 104:1131-1136; 1975.
98. Shephard, R.J.; Parizkova, J. Human growth, physical fitness and nutrition. Basel: Karger; 1991.
99. Shephard, R.J.; Rode, A. Acculturation and the biology of aging. In: Fortuine, R., ed. Circumpolar health '84. Seattle: University of Washington Press; 1985:45-48.
100. Shephard, R.J.; Thomas, S.; Weller, I. The Canadian Home Fitness Test—An update. Sports Med. 11:358-366.
101. Sherif, C.W.; Rattray, G.D. Psychological development and activity in middle-childhood (5-12 years). In: Albinson, J.G.; Andrew, G.M., eds. Child in sport and physical activity. Baltimore: University Park Press; 1976:97-132.
102. Slack, J.; Noble, N.; Meade, T.W.; North, W.R.S. Lipid and lipoprotein concentrations in 1604 men and women in working populations in north-west London. Br. Med. J. (2):353-356; 1977.
103. Smith, E.L.; Gilligan, C. Health-related fitness of the older adult. In: Drury, T., ed. Assessing physical fitness and physical activity. Hyattsville, MD: U.S. Dept. of Health and Human Services; 1989:293-345.
104. Stamler, J.; Stamler, R.; Pullmann, T. The epidemiology of hypertension. New York: Grune & Stratton; 1967.
105. Stephens, T. Secular trends in adult physical activity. Exercise boom or bust? Res. Q. 58:94-105; 1987.
106. Stephens, T. Fitness and activity measurements in the 1989 Canada Fitness Survey. In: Drury, T., ed. Assessing physical fitness and physical activity. Hyattsville, MD: U.S. Dept. of Health and Human Services; 1989:401-432.
107. Tanner, J.M. Growth at adolescence. 2nd ed. Oxford: Blackwell Scientific Publications; 1962.
108. Thomas, S.; Reading, J.; Shephard, R.J. Revision of the physical activity readiness (PAR-Q) questionnaire. Can. J. Sport Sci. 17:338-345; 1992.
109. Tucker, L.A. The relationship of television viewing to physical fitness and obesity. Adolescence. 21:797-806; 1986.
110. U.S. Dept. of Health and Human Services. The health consequences of involuntary smoking. DHSS Publication CDC 87-8398. Rockville, MD: DHSS; 1986.
111. U.S. Dept. of Health and Human Services. Year 2000 objectives for the nation. Draft report. Rockville, MD: DHSS; 1990.
112. Von Döbeln, W. Kroppstorlek, energieomsättning och Kondition. (Body size, energy consumption and fitness.) In: Luthman, G.; Aberg, U.; Lundgren, N., eds. Handbok i ergonomi. (Handbook of ergonomics.) Stockholm: Almqvist & Wiksell; 1966.
113. Waterlow, J.C. Global nutritional status. Bull. WHO. 64:929-941; 1986.
114. Weiner, J.S. Proposals for international research. Human Adaptability Project, Document 5. London: Royal Anthropological Institute; 1964.
115. Weiner, J.S.; Lourie, J.A. Human biology: A guide to field methods. Oxford: Blackwell Scientific; 1969.
116. Weiner, J.S.; Lourie, J.A. Practical human biology. London: Academic Press; 1981.
117. Whelton, P.K. Hypertension in the elderly. In: Andres, R.A.; Bierman, E.L.; Hazzard, W.R., eds. Principles of geriatric medicine. New York: McGraw-Hill; 1985:536-551.

118. Wilhelmsen, L.; Tibblin, G.; Werkö, L. A primary preventive study in Göteborg, Sweden. Prev. Med. 1:153-160; 1972.
119. Womersley, J.; Durnin, J.V.G.A. An experimental study of the variability of measurements of skinfold thicknesses in young adults. Hum. Biol. 45:281-292; 1973.
120. Worthington, E.B. The evolution of IBP. London: Cambridge University Press; 1978.
121. Young, M.A.; Rowlands, D.B.; Stallard, T.J.; Watson, D.A.; Littler, W.A. Effect of environment on blood pressure: Home versus hospital. Br. Med. J. 286:1235-1236; 1983.

Chapter 15

Physical Activity and Nutrition in the Context of Fitness and Health

Gail E. Butterfield
Angelo Tremblay

Diet and exercise are considered two elements in a strong program for health and fitness, yet physical activity increases the utilization of many nutrients, and the long-term success of any program may depend on the replacement of the nutrients used through appropriate food choices. However, much misinformation is purveyed to the public regarding the "special" nutrient needs of active individuals. In reality, the major nutrients of concern are those used as fuel (carbohydrate, fat, and protein) and water. More mythology surrounds vitamins and minerals used for fuel oxidation and oxygen transport, and future research may focus in this area.

Carbohydrate

Carbohydrates are a class of molecules of different sizes and complexities whose main nutritional function is to store potential energy for the resynthesis of adenosine triphosphate (ATP). In the body, carbohydrate and lipid are the principal substrates for energy metabolism at rest and during exercise. In a sedentary individual the estimated carbohydrate intake which allows a complete lipid oxidation without significant ketone body production, has been found to be less than 100 g (60). Despite the apparently low minimal carbohydrate needs of inactive individuals, recommending bodies (National Research Council, Health and Welfare Canada) generally propose that carbohydrate contribute at least 50% of daily energy intake for optimal health.

Effects of Exercise on Carbohydrate Oxidation and Stores

The contribution of carbohydrate to energy metabolism is increased during exercise (15), despite the low body stores (i.e., 400–800 g) (40). This apparent paradox is not clearly understood but the high energy potential of carbohydrate per liter of oxygen consumed, which is explained by the additional production of ATP without oxygen through the glycolytic pathway (15), may justify its primary utilization when the energy expenditure is increased. Endurance capacity (time to exhaustion at a given work load) depends on glycogen stores (10); and dietary approaches favoring an increase in carbohydrate stores before prolonged exercise have been found effective in prolonging endurance.

When carbohydrate utilization and intake are discussed in the context of programs aimed at improving fitness and health in the general population, there is a lower acuity in comparison to endurance athletes. Nevertheless, even under these conditions, some factors can significantly modify carbohydrate utilization and postexercise metabolic regulation.

Intensity and duration of exercise have opposite effects on carbohydrate utilization. The fraction of the energy cost of exercise that is covered by carbohydrate metabolism increases with the intensity of exercise, whereas that fraction is progressively reduced when exercise is prolonged (15). The training status can also influence the composition of the fuel mix oxidized. Indeed, the proportion of carbohydrate in the substrate mix is lower in exercise-trained than in untrained individuals at rest (87) and during exercise (51).

Individual variations have been reported in the respiratory exchange ratio (RER) during exercise of similar intensity, even among a population of sedentary individuals. Moreover, recent data suggest that these variations are at least partly explained by genetically determined factors (13).

Diet composition can also significantly affect the composition of the fuel mix oxidized during exercise. The most established effect is the increase in carbohydrate oxidation induced by a high carbohydrate diet, or simply by the administration of a carbohydrate load before exercise. The resulting effect of all these factors is that carbohydrate utilization during and after a given exercise session varies substantially between individuals. Despite these variations, an exercise bout of moderate intensity and duration necessarily reduces the carbohydrate stores of the body and initiates postexercise adaptations with important nutritional implications.

Postexercise Carbohydrate Metabolism

Postexercise metabolic adaptations favor the resynthesis of glycogen stores which rapidly return to preexercise values under high-carbohydrate diet conditions (Table 15.1). The priority that is given to glycogen resynthesis is also observed under fasting conditions (62) but the rate of glycogen resynthesis is necessarily reduced.

The decrease in carbohydrate stores that occurs in response to prolonged exercise is accompanied by an increase in lipid oxidation in the postexercise resting state (11,87). Consequently, the increased carbohydrate utilization induced by exercise can be partly compensated for by a sparing effect of carbohydrate in the postexercise state. From a nutritional standpoint it is thus difficult to evaluate the net impact of a given exercise session on carbohydrate oxidation and balance.

Nutritional Implications

A high-carbohydrate diet is generally considered a necessary approach to rapidly restock carbohydrate stores. Kirwan et al. (54) recently demonstrated that a carbohydrate intake greater than 8 g/kg body weight/day may be necessary to prevent chronic glycogen depletion in individuals regularly performing a large amount of exercise. Such an intake of carbohydrate probably corresponds to 60% to 70% of total daily energy intake. A relatively high proportion (at least 50%) of energy from carbohydrate is recommended to the overall population (71), and 55% to 60% of energy from carbohydrate is more realistic for active persons. Even if a greater, ideal proportion might be recommended, the changes in food habits required by the majority of people would be so drastic that there is little chance of following such a guideline.

Table 15.1 Postexercise Adaptation in Carbohydrate Metabolism

Adaptation in carbohydrate metabolism	Reference
Increased glycogen synthase activity	48,56,79
Increased muscle glycogen synthesis	56,83
Return to preexercise glycogen levels in 24 hr	33,61

Fifteen years ago, Costill et al. (28) suggested that preexercise glucose intake could be associated with hypoglycemia and increased muscle glycogen utilization during exercise. As recently reviewed by Coyle (29), the two studies (28,41) which proposed this mechanism have not been repeated. Moreover, the preexercise sugar intake has been rarely associated with a reduction in endurance capacity (29). When these observations are applied in the context of fitness programs, there seems to be no convincing evidence to justify the recommendation to abstain from sugar intake before exercise.

The type of carbohydrate is another nutritional factor considered as potentially affecting carbohydrate metabolism. Basically, carbohydrates have been subdivided into simple and complex molecules. However, the observation that, within these categories, metabolic reactions may vary significantly has required the adoption of another classification. During the last decade the classification system which probably received the most attention is the glycemic index of food. This variable represents the ratio of the area under the blood glucose curve resulting from the ingestion of a given quantity of carbohydrate food and the area under the glucose curve resulting from the ingestion of the same quantity of white bread (50). The most obvious application of the glycemic index of food is the adaptation of the dietary regimen of diabetics. In these individuals, slow release carbohydrate, that is, carbohydrate foods with a low glycemic index, may form a useful part of the diet because their ingestion attenuates the burden imposed on a pancreas which cannot produce enough insulin to ensure normal glucose disposal (49,50).

The preoccupations of healthy individuals regularly practicing prolonged exercise are not the same and are rather oriented towards an efficient postexercise glycogen resynthesis. It has been suggested that a person ingest foods with moderate to high glycemic index after exhaustive exercise (i.e., foods whose glucose content becomes more rapidly available for glycogen restoration) (29). However, there is no objective evidence demonstrating that persons involved in moderate exercise programs aimed at the improvement of fitness and health status can really benefit from this recommendation. The advantage of complex carbohydrate, with its high fiber content, is of more consequence to the overall health of this group (71). However, the issue of the optimal carbohydrate composition in the postexercise state remains an important issue and should be the object of further investigation.

Lipid

The majority of molecules which are classified as dietary lipid are triacylglycerols. This form also makes up the lipid stored in adipose tissue. As is true for carbohydrate, the primary function of lipid in the body is to serve as energy substrate. Moreover, as several essential fatty acids cannot be synthesized by the body, an exogenous supply of these fatty acids is necessary even if body fat stores are substantial. In general, an intake of essential fatty acids corresponding to 3% of total energy intake is considered adequate to satisfy the needs of the body (44). However, if one considers that even the best food sources of these fatty acids contain a significant amount of other lipid molecules, it is difficult to follow this recommendation with a lipid intake lower than 10% of total energy intake, and even under these conditions a relatively strict lipid selection is necessary. A dietary fat intake close to the 30% recommended for the general population (71) would provide sufficient essential fatty acids without undue attention to lipid selection.

Exercise and Lipid Utilization

As discussed earlier, the increased contribution of carbohydrate to energy metabolism during exercise results in a reduction of the proportion of energy derived from lipid. Expressed in absolute terms, however, the amount of lipid oxidized during exercise may actually be increased.

In the postexercise state, the absolute as well as the relative contribution of lipid to energy metabolism has been shown to be increased (11,87). It is, however, noteworthy that this adaptation is more likely to occur after prolonged aerobic exercise than following an exercise of short duration, which may suggest that glycogen depletion is involved in the events leading to increased lipid metabolism after exercise. The quantification of this effect requires an indirect calorimetry metabolic chamber in which a subject can mimic a usual pattern of activities while gas collection is performed to determine substrate oxidation. The study of Bielinski, Schutz, and Jéquier (11) is, to our knowledge, the only investigation which has measured postexercise increase in lipid oxidation under standardized conditions. These authors observed an increase in lipid oxidation of 27 g during 17 hr following a prolonged vigorous exercise when compared to a control session not preceded by exercise. When these observations are taken together it is clear that exercise has the potential to significantly increase lipid oxidation. From a nutritional standpoint, the question that must be addressed is the extent to which this increase in lipid expenditure must be compensated by a corresponding lipid intake.

Nutritional Implications

For the great majority of individuals, the lipid compartment is by far the main energy reservoir of the body. Theoretically then, body fat should be the macronutrient compartment whose homeostasis is the least disturbed by the acute energy deficit associated with exercise. This idea is consistent with the data showing that lipid oxidation is increased in the postexercise state, presumably to favor the resynthesis of glycogen stores. Moreover, that individuals regularly practicing exercise tend to be leaner than sedentary individuals may also reflect that body fat stores can accomodate a certain reduction in their content without eliciting stimuli which would force a restoration of lipid balance.

Recent investigations, however, suggest that the ability of adipose tissue to serve as a buffer to negative energy balance is not unlimited. For instance, in ex-obese long distance runners whose training program included a running distance of about 100 km per week, the expected increase in adipose tissue lipolytic capacity was not observed after they had achieved a mean body weight loss of 39.5 kg (85). In obese women subjected to a dietary restriction, it has been found that a 10 kg fat loss has the potential to induce a mean reduction in resting lipid oxidation of 20 g/day (78).

The conceptual integration of these observations is depicted in Figure 15.1. In agreement with the numerous studies that have shown exercise-training to induce body weight and fat losses (14,86,91), energy and lipid deficits will be spontaneously tolerated by the body. However, when fat loss becomes substantial, the body reduces its lipid oxidation so that the excess lipid oxidation induced by exercise is completely compensated. When this threshold is reached, it is likely that the role of lipostatic factors (52) in the long-term control of energy intake is very significant. These factors may exert a strong enhancing effect on energy intake and contribute to protecting the remaining body lipid stores.

In summary, the acute increase in lipid oxidation resulting from exercise does not deserve a short-term compensation in lipid intake. However, it is

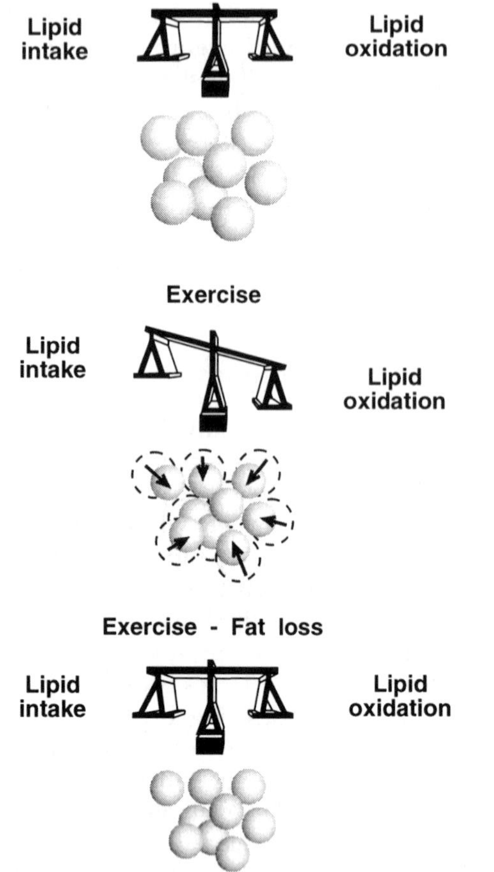

Figure 15.1 Short-term effect of exercise and long-term effect of exercise with substantial fat loss on lipid balance.

likely that a long-term cumulative lipid deficit can initiate adaptations in energy intake to prevent further fat loss.

Control of Energy Intake

The impact of exercise and exercise-training on energy balance is obviously associated with the energy cost of exercise and the increase in post-exercise resting metabolic rate (7,88) which may be observed in some individuals. However, the net effect of exercise on energy balance ultimately depends on the adaptations in energy intake occurring after exercise.

Many theories have been proposed to understand how food intake is regulated in humans. Most of them suggest that a specific metabolic process plays a key role in the regulation of energy intake and balance. Besides these metabolic hypotheses, behavioral factors also exert a significant effect on food intake in humans, which complicates nutritional investigations.

Despite these potential limitations in the study of the effect of exercise on energy intake, the available literature suggests two categories of variables, those relating to glucose and those to lipid, which contribute significantly in this context.

Mayer proposed that first the level of blood glucose (65), and then the rate of entry of glucose into cells or its availability for energy metabolism (66), could elicit signals affecting short-term feeding behavior (glucostatic theory). More recently, glycogen stores (32) and preprandial glycemia (23) have also been shown to represent important glucostatic factors.

Kennedy (52) suggested that factors related to adipose tissue morphology or metabolism affect long-term food intake (lipostatic theory). For instance, Björntorp et al. (12) showed that resistance to loss of body weight in response to a restrictive dietary regimen coincided with the incapacity to reduce fat cell size below a certain threshold. In ex-obese long distance runners, fat cell lipolysis appeared to be the critical factor associated with their inability to further lose body fat (85). Recent investigations have demonstrated a highly significant association between lipid oxidation and energy balance (77) and have emphasized the importance of this variable in the long-term control of energy intake and balance (78).

These observations suggest that diet composition and the ability to utilize lipid as an alternative fuel can affect the impact of exercise on energy intake. Indeed, an integration of the comments presented earlier on the priority given to postexercise glycogen resynthesis and on the role for glucostatic factors in the control of food intake necessarily lead to the conclusion that a high carbohydrate diet is essential to restore preexercise carbohydrate stores with a minimal energy intake. This issue has been the object of a recent study which showed that when a high-fat diet is consumed following a prolonged vigorous exercise, the postexercise increase in energy intake may largely exceed the increase in energy expended during exercise (89).

As indicated previously, both a high capacity to oxidize fat and the level of fat stores seem to be important determinants of variations in post-exercise energy intake. Indeed, recent data have shown that there is a significant correlation between the postexercise change in energy intake and the change in lipid oxidation (89). From a practical standpoint, this means that individuals displaying an increased relative lipid oxidation in response to a given exercise stimulus spare carbohydrate and are thus less prone to overeat after exercise.

These factors are particularly relevant when exercise is used as a mode of treatment of obesity. Fat oxidation is reduced in response to fat loss, due to the loss of body substance as well as a shift favoring an increased contribution of carbohydrate to energy metabolism (78). As depicted in Figure 15.1, this effect has the long-term consequence of completely eliminating the lipid deficit induced by exercise. Thus, a weight-reducing program including exercise will likely be tolerated for a time without any marked increase in energy intake due to the availability of substantial fat stores, whereas such a situation would be less likely in lean individuals. Accordingly, metabolic ward studies showed that a moderate fat loss induced by training in obese women was accomodated without a significant increase in energy intake (92), whereas lean individuals compensated by an increase in energy intake (93). These results are also concordant with a stronger impact of exercise training on weight loss in obese women than in leaner women (6).

Protein

Proteins are a group of structural and regulatory molecules each made up of a specific combination of 20 different nitrogen-containing building blocks called amino acids. Eight of these amino acids cannot be synthesized in the body and must be supplied by the diet if body proteins are to be synthesized. Although the magnitude of the requirement for each of these indispensible amino acids is presently in question (95), the dietary intake generally exceeds even the higher values proposed (17), and it is the requirement for total amino groups which drives the need for dietary protein.

Because protein, and especially the branched chain amino acid leucine (97), is used as a metabolic fuel during exercise, much controversy surrounds the need for protein in exercising individuals (17,57). There is now sufficient data in the literature to suggest that protein requirements do vary with the type and intensity of exercise performed and the total energy consumed.

The primary method used for determination of protein utilization with exercise has been the classic nitrogen balance technique. Because this measure is affected markedly by time on the diet (19,45), amount and quality of protein consumed (22), energy intake (22), and completeness of collections (21), a great deal of data presented in the literature is inappropriately collected and incorrectly interpreted.

Protein Needs With Endurance (Aerobic) Exercise

Early work (35,94) illustrated a fall in nitrogen balance in response to initiation of a moderate endurance exercise program, suggesting an increased need for protein under such circumstances. However, this decline corrected itself within 2 weeks of the start of exercise without dietary manipulation (36). Butterfield and Calloway (19) confirmed the transient nature of this decline in nitrogen balance with initiation of an exercise program such as that proposed in programs to improve fitness and health (45%–55% of maximum oxygen capacity [$\dot{V}O_2max$]). They found that nitrogen balance was more positive after the adaptation than before, suggesting that the protein intake required for nitrogen equilibrium in individuals performing moderate endurance exercise may actually be lower than that of the sedentary population, provided energy intake is adequate.

More recent work suggests that individuals who exercise at a higher intensity have protein needs that are elevated above those proposed for individuals performing low or moderately intense exercise (68,81). Meredith, Zachin, Frontera, and Evans (68), conducting a classic nitrogen balance regression assessment of trained male runners exercising daily at 75% of their $\dot{V}O_2max$, have estimated protein requirement in this group to be 0.94 g/kg body weight/day.

Protein need in exercise is also dependent on energy intake. Butterfield (16) has shown that feeding as much as 2 g protein/kg body weight/day to men running 5 or 10 miles per day at 65% to 75% of their $\dot{V}O_2max$ is insufficient to maintain nitrogen balance when energy intake is inadequate by as little as 100 kcal/day. Further evidence of the critical nature of energy intake in determination of protein need comes from the same laboratory (20) investigating protein requirements in women running 3 to 5 miles/day at about 65% of $\dot{V}O_2max$. Protein requirements were estimated at about 1.1 g/kg body weight/day in these women who consumed only 35 kcal/kg body weight/day to maintain body weight, a value considerably lower than would have been expected from the activity level of the runners. A high protein requirement under circumstances of low energy intake is not unexpected (22).

Protein Needs for Resistance Exercise

In the area of resistance exercise, where an increase in body mass is the main goal, the mythology of increased protein need is rampant. Weight lifters consume anywhere from 1.2 to 3.4 g protein/kg body weight/day (38,55), and in some cases, do so in the form of protein supplements. The basis for this practice is word of mouth and old reports which have been inappropriately interpreted. The often-quoted work of Celejowa and Homa (24) states that protein needs for maintenance of body mass in Olympic weight lifters is greater than 2 to 2.2 g/kg body weight/day. This conclusion is based on the observation that 5 of 10 subjects were in negative nitrogen balance over 11 days on a mean protein intake of 1.85 g/kg body weight/day. However, when measurement of nitrogen balance is attempted with protein intakes that vary from day to day, as was done in this study, it is difficult to interpret the data (96).

Since resistance exercise protein requirements were last reviewed (17,57), sufficient data have accumulated to allow division of the study into two areas: the need for maintenance (minimum protein required to accomplish nitrogen equilibrium), and the need for increasing lean tissue (maintaining a positive nitrogen balance).

Tarnopolsky, MacDougall, and Atkinson (81) showed that experienced body builders could maintain nitrogen equilibrium on intakes similar to those required by sedentary controls. However, the high protein intakes used to generate their regression lines may have resulted in overestimation of protein requirements (45). Recently, Butterfield, Cady, and Moynihan (18) and Meredith, O'Reilly, and Evans (67) have found protein requirement for maintenance in recreational weight lifters and body builders to be 0.78 and 0.52 g/kg body weight/day, respectively, provided energy intake was adequate but not excessive.

Requirement for maintenance of nitrogen balance under circumstances of initiation of a resistance exercise program may depend on the intensity of the exercise performed. Tarnopolsky, Lemon, MacDougall, and Atkinson (82) have estimated protein requirements in young novice male body builders exercising 6 days a week for 1.5 hr/day to be 1.5 g/kg body weight/day. Energy intake is not reported in this work. Hickson, Wolinshky, and Pivarnik (46) found no change in nitrogen excretion with the initiation of a program of 30 min of lifting 3 times per week at an intensity of about 50% of maximum capacity when subjects were consuming 0.8 g/kg body weight/day, the RDA for protein (72).

The data on the protein requirements for the accretion of tissue are not satisfying. Celejowa and Homa (24) found no increase in lean issue on 1.85 g protein/kg body weight/day; however, energy intake balanced energy output within 100 kcal/day. Other studies (9,63) suggest that energy surfeit may be required for increase in lean tissue and that there is a maximum rate of nitrogen accumulation of about 0.4 to 0.5 mg/added kJ (16).

Recently, Butterfield, Cady, and Moynihan (18) have attempted to establish the relevance of added protein in the accretion of lean tissue in recreational weight lifters. They found that when energy intake exceeded need by 400 kcal, increasing nitrogen intake from requirement (mean = 10 g N/day) to 1.5 times requirement (mean = 15 g N/day) had no significant effect on nitrogen retention. Any improvement in nitrogen balance seen with increased energy and protein intake could be explained by the energy contribution of the protein.

Nutritional Implications

Protein requirements may be slightly elevated by the initiation of an exercise program, be it endurance or resistance exercise. The magnitude of the elevation will depend on the intensity of the program and the overall energy balance attained. With programs of moderate intensity, such as those to improve overall health and fitness, increases in need would be minimal. However, to maximize the utilization of the protein ingested, sufficient energy to cover the increased energy output should be consumed. Under circumstances where a negative energy balance is desired to accomplish weight loss, additional protein may be required, although the work of Todd, Butterfield, and Calloway (84) suggests that a moderate exercise program may actually protect protein stores under circumstances of energy deficit if the protein intake is at least equal to the recommended dietary allowance (RDA).

If protein need for exercise is slightly elevated above that for sedentary individuals the usual protein intake of the population will more than meet these needs. Reports of food intake in athletes and nonathletes consistently indicate that protein represents from 12% to 20% of total energy intake (38), or 1.2 to 2 g/kg body weight/day in a 70 kg man consuming 2,800 kcal. The exception to this rule will be the small active women who may consume a low energy intake (64,69) in conjunction with an activity program. These women may consume close to the RDA for protein. If the data of Butterfield, Gates, Holloway, and Cherry (20) are correct, this value in conjunction with the low energy intake may be inadequate to maintain lean mass.

Diets having more protein than needed are to be avoided. As pointed out by the National Research Council (NRC) (71), protein foods are often also high in fat; consumption of excess protein creates difficulty in maintaining a low-fat diet. In addition, the hypercalciuric effect of high-protein diets is still considered by some a significant factor in calcium balance (53), and until the controversy is settled (80), a conservative approach is advised.

Water

Water is a nutrient essential to thermoregulation. It is lost from the body through evaporation at the rate of 1 L/580 kcal expended. During exercise sweat is secreted to provide the fluid for this evaporation, and body fluid compartments are altered. Sweat contains solutes, primarily urea and sodium, the loss of which further alters body compartments. Continued thermoregulation requires replenishment of both water and solutes, or physical performance will suffer and life may be threatened (76). Unfortunately, the thirst mechanism, normally thought responsible for maintenance of body fluids, is insufficient to insure complete rehydration after strenuous exercise (39).

Replenishing Body Fluid

The most effective means of rehydration of body fluids is a topic of controversy. Factors which determine effectiveness include rate of emptying from the stomach (27), absorption across the gut lining (34), and maintenance of the thirst mechanism (70). Sodium and carbohydrate-containing liquids have been shown to promote fluid absorption in the gut by acting as cofactors of a transport protein which shuttles both components across the cell wall. The osmotic gradient thus created promotes the movement of water (34). However, cool temperature and moderate osmotic pressure of the liquid consumed are of importance in initial exit from the stomach, a step which must be accomplished before the water can enter the interstitial compartment (27).

Nose, Mack, Shi, and Nadel (73) have shown that fluid consumption in conjunction with sodium consumption results in a more complete replenishment of fluid and solute losses than with water alone. These investigators propose that the consumption of solute with solvent maintains elevated plasma osmolality, which in turn prolongs both the volume-dependent drive and osmotic drive to drink and promotes continued fluid consumption.

However, other investigators have found water as effective as carbohydrate-electrolyte solutions in maintaining plasma volume and performance under conditions of extreme heat and prolonged exercise (8,58). These studies do not, however, address the question of rehydration after these arduous exercise periods, or the maintenance of the thirst mechanism necessary to accomplish that rehydration.

Nutritional Implications

Most individuals performing a program of exercise designed to maintain fitness and health will not lose sufficient fluid or solute while exercising to warrant consumption of specially formulated fluids for the purpose of replacing those losses. The rate of sodium loss in sweat will determine the rate of extracellular sodium depletion (70). In circumstances where sodium loss in sweat is significant, such as in untrained individuals or in the elderly, losses may require replacement. The elderly may also have a diminished thirst mechanism due to changes in anti-diuretic hormone (ADH) secretion. These factors taken together may put the elderly more at risk than other groups. Under these circumstances, ingestion of a fluid containing 20 to 30 mEq/L sodium and 5% to 10% carbohydrate may serve to better replenish losses than would water alone (34). An additional advantage of these fluids that should not be overlooked is palatability. Improved taste may enhance consumption, which in itself is a significant factor in rehydration.

Vitamins and Minerals

Vitamins and minerals are food components which serve as coenzymes in the reactions which release energy, transport and consume oxygen, and maintain cell integrity. Because of these important functions, their use as ergogenic aids has been rampant, although with little documented effect. The need for these food components in exercise has been reviewed recently (25,43), with the consensus that unless an individual is deficient in a given nutrient, supplementation with that nutrient does not have a major effect on performance. Nutrients at risk in the diets of active populations are similar to those of concern for the general population, including folate, vitamin B-6, calcium, and zinc. Because many women who exercise are also vegetarians, iron and perhaps vitamin B-12 may be of specific concern to this subgroup. Nutrients already at risk and lost in sweat in significant amounts will be further addressed.

Controversial Nutrients at Risk or Lost in Sweat and Urine

Recent reports suggest that significant amounts of some trace minerals may be lost in sweat (copper, zinc) or in urine (chromium) with exercise. Concern for the intake of these nutrients in active individuals arises in that these same nutrients are also of low nutrient density (g/1,000 kcal) in the food supply and are considered "at risk" in the general population. Thus, the fear arises that nutrient needs with increased activity will not be met by normal dietary intakes.

Chromium

Chromium is necessary for the action of insulin in increasing cellular uptake of glucose and amino acids. Consequently, it is very important for both cellular energy metabolism and protein synthesis. Chromium supplementation has been shown to improve glucose tolerance in some individuals with initial intolerance (1). Dietary chromium intake in the general population is reported to be lower than the safe and adequate levels recommended by the NRC (4,72), but inadequate data on chromium content of foods cannot be ruled out. Highly processed foods and foods high in simple carbohydrate—foods promoted for and consumed by athletes—are known to be low in chromium.

Anderson and colleagues (5) have shown that chromium is lost in the urine in response to exercise, possibly consequent to mobilization to optimize carbohydrate metabolism (Table 15.2). However, they have also found that basal urinary chromium losses in trained individuals are significantly lower than those found in untrained individuals on a constant chromium intake, suggesting that training increases the efficiency of vitamin storage (2). This idea is supported by the work of Vallerand, Cuerrier, Shapcott, Vallerand, and Gardiner (90) in which it was shown that exercising animals had higher levels of chromium in heart and kidney as compared to nonexercising animals on a similar chromium intake. Chromium levels in sweat have not been accurately measured at this time due to problems of contamination.

Recommendations have been made that athletes consume chromium supplements to insure adequate supplies, given urinary losses and usual dietary intakes (26), but no documentation of a positive effect of such supplementation has been found. One report of chromium supplementation increasing lean body mass in college weight lifters and football players (30) is flawed by lack of data on dietary intakes of protein and energy or prior chromium status. A more recent report by Hasten, Rome, and Franks (42) could not reproduce the effect in men, although women showed a slight increase in lean body mass in response to chromium supplementation. Here, too, neither the prior chromium status of the subjects nor their dietary intake were documented.

Copper

Copper is necessary for red blood cell formation (ceruloplasmin acts to bring iron out of stores) and for protection against free radicals (as enzymatic site in supraoxide dismutase), both functions related to physical activity. Reported intakes of copper are low in comparison to the safe and adequate levels recommended by the NRC (72). Supplementation with other nutrients, such as vitamin C (31), zinc (37), or fructose (74), has been shown to affect copper status.

The effect of exercise on copper status is questionable, however. Resina et al. (75) found decreased serum copper in runners when compared to controls, but included no data on dietary intake of the nutrient. Lukaski, Hoverson, Gallagher, and Bolonchuk (59) showed no adverse effect of physical activity on copper status in swimmers consuming adequate copper (Table 15.3). Urinary copper levels appear to be unchanged by exercise (5), but sweat losses of copper are high (58–500 μg/L) under any circumstances (47). Given high sweat losses and low dietary intakes, copper status with physical activity may be of concern. However, no reliable studies have been done to evaluate the possible benefit of copper supplementation to performance.

Zinc

Zinc is essential to the action of 70 to 100 key metabolic enzymes in the body. Of particular concern to physical activity is lactate dehydrogenase, however zinc is also involved in carbohydrate,

Table 15.2 Exercise and Training Effects on Urinary Chromium Excretion in Men Fed a Constant Chromium Intake

Subject	24-hr excretion, μg	
	Basal	Exercise
Trained	0.09 ± 0.01	0.12 ± 0.02
Untrained	0.21 ± 0.03	0.21 ± 0.02

Note. Adapted from Anderson et al. (2).

Table 15.3 Copper Nutriture in Swimmers

Measure	Sex	Preseason	Postseason
Intake	M	1.6±0.1	1.9±0.1
(mg/day)	F	1.3±0.1	1.4±0.1
Plasma levels	M	13.2±0.4	13.8±0.4
(μM/L)	F	15.7±1.4	15.9±1.3
Ceruloplasmin	M	425±19	446±17
(mg/L)	F	487±40	494±32

Note. Adapted from Lukaski et al (59).

lipid, and protein metabolism. Dietary intakes of the population are marginal (72), and there are many reports of intakes below the recommended dietary allowance in athletes.

Serum zinc levels, often used as a measure of status, are markedly affected by exercise. A single bout of exercise will transiently increase serum zinc, but the increase is followed 2 hr later by a drop below baseline (3). These swings have been attributed to redistribution of zinc stores and increased urinary losses. Sweat zinc is high (416–825 µg/L) (47), and losses with exercise may result in increased requirements (1), although Lukaski et al. (59) have shown no effect of training on measures of zinc status in male and female swimmers consuming a diet adequate in zinc (Table 15.4). Plasma zinc has been shown to decrease with training in some studies, but others find no difference in plasma zinc between athletes and control subjects (see ref. 1 for review). Dietary zinc intake has not been controlled in most reports.

Nutritional Implications

There are no data to suggest that supplementation of individual vitamins and minerals is of benefit to an individual performing moderate physical activity, provided overall nutrient needs are met by diet. Supplementation with trace minerals should be undertaken with caution as interactions between minerals are well documented and imbalanced intakes may precipitate a deficiency of one nutrient while "curing" the deficiency of another (72).

Summary

In summary, there is a relatively good consensus in the literature to suggest that a high-carbohydrate diet represents the optimal dietary regimen to restore preexercise substrate homeostasis with a minimal increase in energy intake. However, when this notion is considered in the context of obesity treatment, it must be taken into account that a substantial fat loss can alter significantly the composition of the fuel mix oxidized. When such a fat loss is achieved, the contribution of carbohydrate to energy metabolism is likely increased and the postexercise carbohydrate and energy intake must necessarily be increased to restore preexercise glycogen stores. The latter mechanism might be involved in the occurrence of resistance to further loss of fat which is generally observed in obese individuals after they reach substantial body weight and fat losses, even if their morphological status is not normalized.

Regarding protein, vitamins, and minerals, there is no evidence in the literature to suggest that increased levels of any of these nutrients would be required in individuals undertaking a moderate physical activity program for health and fitness. However, as some nutrients are normally at risk in the population (zinc, chromium, copper) and may be lost in significant amounts in sweat, special attention should be made to consume foods rich in these nutrients, such as meats or beans, and fruits and vegetables. Attention should be paid to replacing fluid losses, possibly with electrolyte and carbohydrate fluids.

Table 15.4 Zinc Nutriture in Swimmers

Measure	Sex	Preseason	Postseason
Intake	M	15.6±0.8	17.9±1.0
(mg/day)	F	10.4±0.8	10.4±0.9
Plasma levels	M	13.7±0.5	14.3±0.5
(µm/L)	F	12.7±0.5	12.6±0.5

Note. Adapted from Lukaski et al. (59).

References

1. Anderson, R.A. New insights on the trace elements, chromium, copper and zinc and exercise. Med. Sport Sci. 32:38-58; 1991.
2. Anderson, R.A.; Bryden, N.A.; Polansky, M.M.; Deuster, P.A. Exercise effects on chromium excretion of trained and untrained men consuming a constant diet. J. Appl. Physiol. 64:249-252; 1988.
3. Anderson, R.A.; Bryden, N.A.; Polansky, M.M.; Deuster, P.A. Exercise effects on urinary losses and serum concentrations of chromium, copper, iron, and zinc of trained and untrained runners. FASEB J. 3:1294; 1989.
4. Anderson, R.A.; Kozlovsky, A.S. Chromium intake, absorption and excretion of subjects consuming self-selected diets. Am. J. Clin. Nutr. 41:1177-1183; 1985.
5. Anderson, R.A.; Polansky, M.M.; Bryden, N.A. Strenuous running: Acute effects on chromium, copper, zinc, and selected clinical variables in urine and serum of male runners. Biol. Trace Element Res. 6:327-336; 1984.
6. Andersson, B.; Xu, X.; Rebuffé-Scrive, M.; Terning, K.; Krotkiewski, M.; Bjorntorp, P. The

effects of exercise-training on body composition and metabolism in men and women. Int. J. Obes. 15:75-81; 1991.

7. Bahr, R.; Ingnes I.; Vaage, O.; Sejersted, O.M.; Newsholme, E.A. Effect of duration of exercise on excess postexercise O_2 consumption. J. Appl. Physiol. 62:485-490; 1987.
8. Barr, S.I.; Costill, D.L.; Fink, W.J. Fluid replacement during prolonged exercise: Effects of water, saline, or no fluid. Med. Sci. Sports Exerc. 23:811-817; 1991.
9. Bartels, R.L.; Lamb, D.R.; Vivian, V.M.; Snook, J.T.; Rinehart, K.F.; Delaney, J.P.; Wheeler, K.B. Effects of chronically increased consumption of energy and carbohydrate on anabolic adaptations to strenuous weight training. In: Grandjean, A.C.; Storlie, J., eds. The theory and practice of athletic nutrition: Bridging the gaps. Report of the Ross Symposium. Columbus, OH: Ross Laboratories; 1989:70-80.
10. Bergstrom, J.; Hermansen, L.; Hultman, E.; Saltin, B. Diet, muscle glycogen and physical performance. Acta Physiol. Scand. 71:140-150; 1967.
11. Bielinski, R.; Schutz, Y.; Jéquier, E. Energy expenditure during the postexercise recovery in man. Am. J. Clin. Nutr. 42:69-82; 1985.
12. Björntorp, P.; Carlgren, G.; Isaksson, B.; Krotkiewski, M.; Larsson, B.; Sjostrom, L. Effect of an energy reduced dietary regimen in relation to adipose tissue cellularity in obese women. Am. J. Clin. Nutr. 28:445-452; 1975.
13. Bouchard, C.; Tremblay, A.; Nadeau, A.; Després, J.-P.; Thériault, G.; Boulay, M.R.; Leblanc, C.; Lortie, G.; Fournier, G. Genetic effect in resting and exercise metabolic rates. Metabolism. 38:364-370; 1989.
14. Bray, G.; Gray, D. Treatment of obesity: An overview. Diabetes Metab. Rev. 4:653-659; 1988.
15. Brooks, G.A.; Fahey, T.D. Exercise physiology: Human bioenergetics and its applications. New York: Wiley; 1984.
16. Butterfield, G.E. Whole body protein utilization in humans. Med. Sci. Sports Exerc. 19:S157-S165; 1987.
17. Butterfield, G.E. Amino acids and high protein diets. In: Lamb, D.R.; Williams, M.H., eds. Perspectives in exercise science and sports medicine, vol 4: Ergogenics—enhancement of performance in exercise and sport. Ann Arbor, MI: Brown and Benchmark; 1991:87-122.
18. Butterfield, G.E.; Cady, C.; Moynihan, S. Effect of increasing protein intake on nitrogen balance in recreational weight lifters. Med. Sci. Sports Exerc. 24:S71; 1992.
19. Butterfield, G.E.; Calloway, D.H. Physical activity improves protein utilization in young men. Brit. J. Nutr. 51:171-184; 1984.
20. Butterfield, G.E.; Gates, J.; Holloway, L.; Cherry, D. Energy and protein utilization in female runners. J. Appl. Physiol. [Submitted 1992].
21. Calloway, D.H.; O'Dell, A.C.F.; Margen, S. Sweat and miscellaneous losses in human balance studies. J. Nutr. 101:775-786; 1971.
22. Calloway, D.H.; Spector, H. Nitrogen balance as related to caloric and protein intake in active young men. Am. J. Clin. Nutr. 2:405-411; 1954.
23. Campfield, L.A.; Smith, F.J. Transient declines in blood glucose signal meal initiation. Int. J. Obes. 14(Suppl. 3):15-33; 1990.
24. Celejowa, I.; Homa, M. Food intake, nitrogen and energy balance in Polish weight lifters during a training camp. Nutr. Metab. 12:259-274; 1970.
25. Clarkson, P.M. Vitamins and trace minerals. In: Lamb, D.R.; Williams, M.H., eds. Perspectives in exercise science and sports medicine, vol 4: Ergogenics—enhancement of performance in exercise and sport. Ann Arbor, MI: Brown and Benchmark; 1991:123-182.
26. Clarkson, P.M. Nutritional ergogenic aids: Chromium, exercise and muscle mass. Int. J. Sports Nutr. 1:289-293; 1991.
27. Costill, D.L. Gastric emptying of fluids during exercise. In: Gisolfi, C.V.; Lamb, D.R. Perspectives in exercise science and sports medicine. vol 3: Fluid homeostasis during exercise. Carmel, IN: Benchmark Press; 1990:97-128.
28. Costill, D.L.; Coyle, E.; Dalsky, G.; Evans, W.; Fink, W.; Hoopes, D. Effects of elevated plasma FFA and insulin on muscle glycogen usage during exercise. J. Appl. Physiol. 43:695-699; 1977.
29. Coyle, E.F. Timing and method of increased carbohydrate intake to cope with heavy training, competition and recovery. J. Sports Sci. 9:29-52; 1991.
30. Evans, G.W. The effect of chromium picolinate on insulin controlled parameters in humans. Int. J. Biosoc. Med. Res. 11:163-180; 1989.
31. Finley, E.B.; Cerklewski, F.L. Influence of ascorbic acid supplementation on copper status in young adult men. Am. J. Clin. Nutr. 37:553-556; 1983.
32. Flatt, J.-P. Dietary fat, carbohydrate balance, and weight maintenance: Effects of exercise. Am. J. Clin. Nutr. 45:296-306; 1987.
33. Gaesser, G.A.; Brooks, G.A. Glycogen repletion following continuous and intermittent exercise to exhaustion. J. Appl. Physiol. 49:722-728; 1980.

34. Gisolfi, C.V.; Summers, R.; Schedl, H. Intestinal absorption of fluids during rest and exercise. In: Gisolfi, C.V.; Lamb, D.R. Perspectives in exercise science and sports medicine. vol 3: Fluid homeostasis during exercise. Carmel, IN: Benchmark Press; 1990:129-180.
35. Gontzea, I.; Sutzesco, P.; Dumitrache, S. The influence of muscular activity on nitrogen balance and on the need of man for protein. Nutr. Rep. Int. 10:35-43; 1974.
36. Gontzea, I.; Sutzesco, P.; Dumitrache, S. The influence of adaptation to physical effort on nitrogen balance in man. Nutr. Rep. Int. 11:231-236; 1975.
37. Goodwin, J.S.; Hunt, W.C.; Hooper, P.; Garry, P.J. Relationship between zinc intake, physical activity and blood levels of high-density lipoprotein cholesterol in a healthy elderly population. Metabolism. 34:519-523; 1985.
38. Grandjean, A.C. Macronutrient intake of U.S. athletes compared with the general population and recommendations made for athletes. Am. J. Clin. Nutr. 49:1070-1076; 1989.
39. Greenleaf, J.E.; Brock, P.J.; Keil, L.C.; Morse, J.T. Drinking and water balance during exercise and heat acclimation. J. Appl. Physiol. 54:414-419; 1983.
40. Hargreaves, M. Carbohydrates and exercise. J. Sports Sci. 9:17-28; 1991.
41. Hargreaves, M.; Costill, D.L.; Katz, A.; Fink, W.J. Effect of fructose ingestion on muscle glycogen usage during exercise. Med. Sci. Sports Exerc. 17:360-363; 1985.
42. Hasten, D.L.; Rome, E.P.; Franks, B.D. Anabolic effects of chromium picolinate on beginning weight training students. (Conference abstract.) Southeast Regional Chapter, American College of Sports Medicine; 1991.
43. Haymes, E.M. Vitamin and mineral supplementation to athletes. Int. J. Sports Med. 1:146-169; 1991.
44. Health and Welfare Canada. Recommendations on nutrition. Ottawa: Health and Welfare Canada; 1990.
45. Hegsted, D.M. Balance studies. J. Nutr. 101:307-311; 1975.
46. Hickson, J.F.; Wolinshky, I.; Pivarnik, J.M. Repeated days of body building exercise do not enhance urinary nitrogen excretions from untrained young adult males. Nutr. Res. 10:723-730; 1990.
47. Jacob, P.A.; Sandstead, H.H.; Munoz, J. M.; Klevay, L.M.; Milne, D.B. Whole body surface loss of trace metals in normal males. Am. J. Clin. Nutr. 34:1379-1383; 1981.
48. Jeffress, R.N.; Peter, J.B. Effects of exercise on glycogen synthetase in red and white skeletal muscle. Life Sci. 7:957-960; 1968.
49. Jenkins, D.J.A.; Wolever, T.M.S.; Taylor, R.H.; Griffiths, C.; Krzeminska, K.; Lawrie, J.A.; Bennett, C.M.; Goff, D.V.; Sarson, D.L.; Bloom, S.R. Slow release dietary carbohydrate improves second meal tolerance. Am. J. Clin. Nutr. 35:1339-1347; 1982.
50. Jenkins, D.J.A.; Wolever, T.M.S.; Thorne, M.J.; Jenkins, A.L.; Wong, G.S.; Josse, R.G.; Csima, A. The relationship between glycemic response, digestibility and factors influencing the dietary habits of diabetics. Am. J. Clin. Nutr. 40:1175-1192; 1984.
51. Karlsson, J.; Nordesjo, L.O.; Saltin, B. Muscle glycogen utilization during exercise after physical training. Acta Physiol. Scand. 90:210-217; 1974.
52. Kennedy, G.C. The role of depot fat in the hypothalamic control of food intake in the rat. Proc. R. Soc. Lond. [Biol.]. 140B:578-582; 1953.
53. Kerstetter, J.E.; Allen, L.H. Dietary protein increases urinary calcium. J. Nutr. 120:134-136; 1990.
54. Kirwan, J.P.; Costill, D.L.; Mitchell, J.B.; Houmard, J.A.; Flynn, M.G.; Fink, W.J.; Beltz, J.D. Carbohydrate balance in competitive runners during successive days of intense training. J. Appl. Physiol. 65:2601-2606; 1988.
55. Kleiner, S.M.; Bazarre, T.L.; Litchford, M.D. Metabolic profiles, diet and health practices of championship male and female body builders. J. Am. Diet. Assoc. 90:962-967; 1990.
56. Kochan, R.G.; Lamb, D.R.; Lutz, S.A.; Perrill, C.V.; Reimann, E.M.; Schlender, K.K. Glycogen synthase activation in human skeletal muscle: Effects of diet and exercise. Am. J. Physiol. 236:E660-E666; 1979.
57. Lemon, P.W.R. Protein and amino acid needs of the strength athlete. Int. J. Sports Nutr. 1:127-145; 1991.
58. Levine, L.; Rose, M.S.; Francesconi, R.P.; Neufer, P.D.; Sawka, M.N. Fluid replacement during sustained activity in the heat: Nutrient solution vs. water. Aviat. Space Environ. Med. 62:559-564; 1991.
59. Lukaski, H.C.; Hoverson, B.S.; Gallagher, S.K.; Bolonchuk, W.W. Physical training and copper, iron and zinc status of swimmers. Am. J. Clin. Nutr. 51:1093-1099; 1990.
60. MacDonald, I. Metabolic requirements for dietary carbohydrate. Am. J. Clin. Nutr. 45:1193-1196; 1987.
61. MacDougall, J.D.; Ward, G.R.; Sale, D.G.; Sutton, J.R. Muscle glycogen repletion after high-intensity intermittent exercise. J. Appl. Physiol. 42:129-132; 1977.
62. Maehlum, S.; Hermansen, L. Muscle glycogen concentration during recovery after prolonged

severe exercise in fasting subjects. Scand. J. Clin. Lab. Invest. 38:557-560; 1978.

63. Marable, N.L.; Hickson, J.F.; Korslund, M.K.; Herbert, W.G.; Desjardins, R.F.; Thye, F.W. Urinary nitrogen excretion as influenced by a muscle-building exercise program and protein intake variation. Nutr. Rep. Int. 19:795-805; 1979.
64. Marable, N.L.; Kehrberk, N.L.; Judd, J.T.; Prather, E.S.; Bodwell, C.E. Caloric and selected nutrient intakes and estimated energy expenditures for adult women: Identification of non-sedentary women with low energy intakes. J. Am. Diet. Assoc. 88:687-693; 1988.
65. Mayer, J. Glucostatic mechanism of regulation of food intake. N. Engl. J. Med. 249:13-16; 1953.
66. Mayer, J.; Thomas, D.W. Regulation of food intake and obesity. Science. 156:328-337; 1967.
67. Meredith, C.N.; O'Reilly, K.P.; Evans, W.J. Protein and energy requirements of strength trained men. Med. Sci. Sports Exerc. 24:S71; 1992.
68. Meredith, C.N.; Zachin, M.J.; Frontera, W.R.; Evans, W.J. Dietary protein requirements and body protein metabolism in endurance trained men. J. Appl. Physiol. 66:2850-2856; 1989.
69. Mulligan, K.; Butterfield, G.E. Discrepancies between energy intake and expenditure in physically active women. Brit. J. Nutr. 64:23-36; 1990.
70. Nadel, E.R.; Mack, G.W.; Nose, H. Influences of fluid replacement beverages on body fluid homeostasis during exercise and recovery. In: Gisolfi, C.V.; Lamb, D.R. Perspectives in exercise science and sports medicine. vol 3: Fluid homeostasis during exercise. Carmel, IN: Benchmark Press; 1990:181-206.
71. National Research Council, Committee on Diet and Health, Food and Nutrition Board. Diet and health: Implications for reducing chronic disease risk. Washington, DC: National Academy Press; 1989.
72. National Research Council, Food and Nutrition Board. Recommended dietary allowances. 10th ed. Washington, DC: National Academy Press; 1989.
73. Nose, H.; Mack, G.W.; Shi, X.; Nadel, E.R. Role of osmolality and plasma volume during rehydration in humans. J. Appl. Physiol. 65:325-331; 1988.
74. Reiser, S.; Smith, J.C.; Mertz, W., et al. Indices of copper status in humans consuming typical American diet containing either fructose or starch. Am. J. Clin. Nutr. 42:242-251; 1985.
75. Resina, A.; Fedi, S.; Gatteschi, L.; Rubenni, M.G.; Giamberardino, M.A.; Trabassi, E.; Imreh, F. Comparison of some serum copper parameters in trained runners and control subjects. Int. J. Sports Med. 11:58-60; 1990.
76. Sawka, M.N.; Pandolf, K.B. Effects of body water loss on physiological function and exercise performance. In: Gisolfi, C.V.; Lamb, D.R. Perspectives in exercise science and sports medicine. vol. 3: Fluid homeostasis during exercise. Carmel, IN: Benchmark Press; 1990:1-38.
77. Schutz, Y.; Flatt, J.P.; Jéquier, E. Failure of dietary fat intake to promote fat oxidation: A factor favoring the development of obesity. Am. J. Clin. Nutr. 50:307-314; 1989.
78. Schutz, Y.; Tremblay, A.; Weinsier, R.L.; Nelson, K.M. Role of fat oxidation in the long-term stabilization of body weight in obese women. Am. J. Clin. Nutr. 55:670-674; 1992.
79. Sherman, W.M.; Costill, D.L.; Fink, W.J.; Hagerman, F.C.; Armstrong, L.E.; Murray, T.F. Effect of a 42.2-km footrace and subsequent rest or exercise on muscle glycogen and enzymes. J. Appl. Physiol. 55:1219-1224; 1983.
80. Spencer, H.; Kramer, L. Does dietary protein increase urinary calcium? J. Nutr. 121:151; 1991.
81. Tarnopolsky, M.A.; MacDougall, J.D.; Atkinson, S.A. Influence of protein intake and training status on nitrogen balance and lean body mass. J. Appl. Physiol. 64:187-193; 1988.
82. Tarnopolsky, M.A.; Lemon, P.W.R.; MacDougall, J.D.; Atkinson, S.A. Effect of body building exercise on protein requirements. Can. J. Sport Sci. 15:225; 1990.
83. Terjung, R.L.; Baldwin, K.M.; Winder, W.W.; Holloszy, J.O. Glycogen repletion in different types of muscle and in liver after exercise. Am. J. Physiol. 226:1387-1391; 1974.
84. Todd, K.S.; Butterfield, G.E.; Calloway, D.H. Nitrogen balance in men with adequate and deficient energy intake at three levels of work. J. Nutr. 114:2107-2118; 1984.
85. Tremblay, A.; Després, J.-P.; Bouchard, C. Adipose tissue characteristics of ex-obese long distance runners. Int. J. Obes. 8:641-648; 1984.
86. Tremblay, A.; Després, J.-P.; Bouchard, C. The effects of exercise-training on energy balance and adipose tissue morphology and metabolism. Sports Med. 2:223-233; 1985.
87. Tremblay, A.; Fontaine, E.; Nadeau, A. Contribution of post-exercise increment in glucose storage to variations in glucose-induced thermogenesis in endurance athletes. Can. J. Physiol. Pharmacol. 63:1165-1169; 1985.
88. Tremblay, A.; Fontaine, E.; Poehlman, E.T.; Mitchell, D.; Perron, L.; Bouchard, C. The effect of exercise-training on resting metabolic rate in lean and moderately obese individuals. Int. J. Obes. 10:511-517; 1986.

89. Tremblay, A.; Plourde, G.; Després, J.-P.; Bouchard, C. Impact of dietary fat content and fat oxidation on energy intake in humans. Am. J. Clin. Nutr. 49:799-805; 1989.
90. Vallerand, A.L.; Cuerrier, J.P.; Shapcott, D.; Vallerand, R.J.; Gardiner, P.F. Influence of exercise training on tissue chromium concentrations in the rat. Am. J. Clin. Nutr. 39:402-409; 1984.
91. Wilmore, J.H. Body composition in sport and exercise: Directions for future research. Med. Sci. Sports Exerc. 15:21-31; 1983.
92. Woo, R.; Garrow, J.S.; Pi-Sunyer, F.X. Voluntary food intake during prolonged exercise in obese women. Am. J. Clin. Nutr. 36:478-484; 1982.
93. Woo, R.; Pi-Sunyer, F.X. Effect of increased physical activity on voluntary intake in lean women. Metabolism. 34:836-841; 1985.
94. Yoshimura, H. Adult protein requirements. Fed. Proc. 20:103-110; 1961.
95. Young, V.R.; Bier, D.M.; Pallet, P.L. A theoretical basis for increasing current estimates of the amino acid requirements in adult man with experimental support. Am. J. Clin. Nutr. 50:80-92; 1989.
96. Young, V.R.; Marchini, J.S. Mechanisms and nutritional significance of metabolic responses to altered intakes of protein and amino acids, with reference to nutritional adaptations in humans. Am. J. Clin. Nutr. 51:270-289; 1990.
97. Young, V.R.; Torun, B. Physical activity: Impact on protein and amino acid metabolism and implications for nutritional requirements. In: Nutrition in health and disease and international development: Symposium from XIIth international congress on nutrition. New York: Alan R. Liss, Inc.; 1981:57-85.

Chapter 16

Adjuvants to Physical Activity: Do They Help in Any Way?

Ilkka Vuori
Jack H. Wilmore

Many individual and environmental factors, in addition to physical activity, can affect fitness and health. Adjuvants to physical activity are defined as those measures or practices which, because of their potential physiological effects, are used to enhance the benefits or reduce the potential detrimental effects of physical activity on fitness and health. Measures or practices used as a substitute for physical activity or to improve performance capacity as an ergogenic aid are not included in this chapter.

Several of the more popular adjuvants to physical activity are reviewed in this chapter. Each will be discussed with respect to the rationale for its use, including the intended purpose and potential physiological justification, the actual physiological changes associated with its use, and the efficacy of its use with respect to potential benefits for fitness and health. With several adjuvants there is a major body of research to support or reject their use. This evidence is summarized, key studies are cited, and conclusions are drawn. With other adjuvants, however, there is inadequate research to make scientifically based conclusions. For these adjuvants, the conclusions drawn are based on the limited data available and on understanding of the basic physiological principles.

Current Status of Knowledge

Among the many measures or practices that could be considered as adjuvants to physical activity, this consensus statement will focus on electrical stimulation, massage, sauna, sudation garments, questionable exercise devices and spot reduction, and nutritional supplements.

Electrical Stimulation

Some studies in the 1960s suggested that muscle strength (69,89) and endurance (68) can be increased by electrical stimulation. This area of research received a strong impulse when Kots of the Soviet Union (75) presented an application of stimulation-producing vigorous muscular contractions while minimizing the pain and discomfort of the treatment. Detailed accounts on the rather extensive research on the effects and modes of application of percutaneous neuromuscular electrical stimulation (NMES) in sport and exercise are found in recent, thorough reviews by Currier in 1991 and Lake in 1992 (28,83).

NMES in Sport Rehabilitation

The effects on various muscle and performance characteristics NMES has as an adjuvant to voluntary muscle contractions have been investigated in several well-conducted studies especially on knee-operated patients, the quadriceps muscle group having been the primary focus. Most studies suggest that NMES significantly augments the effects of muscle training in terms of isometric (126) and isokinetic strength (115) especially at high contraction speeds (128), muscle mass (126), oxidative (45,126) and glycolytic muscle enzyme capacity (126), clinically assessed muscle function (45), and gait pattern (115). One study failed to show additional isometric strength gain when NMES stimulation was combined with voluntary muscle training (113).

The notion of NMES as a valuable adjuvant to voluntary training is supported by the findings of several well-conducted studies indicating that NMES was superior in preventing disuse muscle atrophy in knee-operated patients when compared to isometric exercise alone (50,53) and to cocontraction of quadriceps and hamstrings muscle groups (36). NMES, exercise, and their combination may be useful in different phases of rehabilitation because Grove-Lainey, Walmsley, and Andrew (54) found that isometric exercise alone was superior to NMES to maintain strength during the first 2 postoperative weeks, but during the next 4 weeks NMES was more beneficial. In addition, NMES seems to be useful in selective muscle strengthening and "muscle re-education" as well as in reducing traumatic edema (see 83 for details).

Use of NMES in Healthy Subjects

Most studies show that NMES increases the isometric strength of the most studied muscle group, quadriceps femoris, to the same degree as voluntary isometric exercise (29,30,56,78,80,84,91). However, Mohr, Carlson, Sulentic, and Landry (93) failed to find any effect on quadriceps' strength of NMES. Eriksson, Häggmark, Kiessling, and Karlsson (46) found significant increases, but there were no differences in isokinetic quadriceps' strength gains in groups receiving either NMES or performing isokinetic training. Kahanovitz et al. (73) came to a similar conclusion when comparing the effects of NMES and dynamic trunk muscle exercises on the isokinetic back muscle strength.

When NMES was combined with isometric (28,59) or dynamic (99,131) quadriceps training, no significant difference was seen in isometric (28) or dynamic muscle strength gain or in other muscle performance characteristics (59,99,131). However, when abdominal muscles of sedentary subjects were trained by combined NMES and static exercise or static exercise alone, the isometric strength of the abdominal muscles increased significantly more with NMES plus static exercise than with static exercise alone (5).

The effects of NMES on muscular endurance are unresolved at present. Some studies show increased endurance in abdominal (5) or back muscles (73), while other studies find no increase in the endurance of quadriceps femoris muscles (42,46).

Factors Affecting the Effectivity of NMES: Initial Muscle Status and Stimulus Characteristics

The results of different studies on the effects of NMES show large variation. Some of the most important factors causing this variation are the differences in the initial training status and in the electrical stimulation and exercise training programs. NMES is particularly effective in retaining and restoring the strength of weakened muscles, but its effects on normal muscle are much less clear. The preliminary observations suggesting remarkable effects of NMES combined with strength training in athletes (35) need to be verified in controlled studies.

There is now agreement on the characteristics of electrical stimulation for various applications suggesting that burst-modulated alternating current and biphasic pulsed current stimulators are the most versatile for sport rehabilitation. Because no single waveform suits all subjects, the stimulators should allow large selection of electrical current characteristics (for review see refs. 28,83).

Mechanism of Muscle Strength Increase Using NMES

Although the efficacy of NMES in the augmentation of muscle strength is well-substantiated, its mode of action is not completely understood. Delitto and Snyder-Mackler (37) have proposed two theories: physiological overload (as in voluntary muscle training), and reversal of voluntary recruitment order of different muscle fiber types causing preferential Type II fiber contraction. The prevailing assumption and basis for study design as well as for practical applications has been the overload principle. Although the overload principle does not fit with all observations, the reverse recruitment theory could partly explain the discrepancies. In this theory, the electrical current of NMES applied to skin recruits more lower resistance than higher resistance nerve fibers, leading to Type II muscle fiber recruitment instead of Type I fiber recruitment such as that in voluntary muscle contraction. Histological (19) and histochemical findings (37,126) support the reversed recruitment theory. This mode of action of NMES would support its use especially in the strengthening of weakened muscles and in the postoperative and other painful states when high-intensity voluntary contractions are not advisable or possible to perform.

In conclusion, NMES is shown to be an effective and useful adjuvant to sport rehabilitation either alone or combined with voluntary muscle training. It augments isometric strength and isokinetic strength at both slow and fast contraction speeds. These effects are inversely related to the initial muscle strength. NMES may also improve the functional status and may be useful in selective muscle strengthening and "re-education," in reducing posttraumatic edema, and in alleviating pain. The effect of NMES on muscle endurance is unresolved at the present time. NMES may somewhat augment the strength of even normal muscle, but its efficacy as an adjuvant to ordinary athletic training is questionable.

Massage

Massage is a group of manual techniques for the systematic manipulation of the soft tissues for preventive, therapeutic, and restorative purposes. "Swedish" massage, the most commonly used technique in the Western countries, consists of stroking, gliding, kneading, rolling, wringing, pulling, percussing, and vibrating activities performed by the massage therapist. The pressure, combined with heat or cold, can also be exerted by water jet. This water massage in various applications has gained popularity in sport. Massage encompasses a variety of techniques such as shiatsu, acupressure, and reflexology. The techniques of massage are described in great detail in numerous handbooks and manuals (10,65,76,133).

Massage is widely and increasingly used in sports for many purposes, for example, to enhance tissue elasticity, muscular relaxation, and joint mobility prior to performance; to prevent and alleviate muscular cramps, soreness, and pain; to hasten physical and mental recovery after strenuous efforts; and to speed up healing of soft tissue injuries and to restore flexibility and joint mobility in rehabilitation.

The benefits of massage are expected on the basis of its claimed physiological effects, including the following: (a) reflex relaxation of muscles caused by excitation of skin and deep tissue receptors; (b) stretching of individual muscles, tendons, and ligaments both longitudinally and transversely; (c) increasing blood and tissue fluid circulation and tissue permeability, thus enhancing waste product disposal and attainment of physiological equilibrium in the muscles; (d) liberation of neurotransmitter-like endorphins alleviating pain; (e) prevention and breakdown of fibrous adhesions; and (f) balancing the autonomic nervous system.

Despite the very long tradition from antiquity and wide use of massage, its physiological effects and preventive, therapeutic, and restorative efficacy have been inadequately studied (for review see ref. 20). It is obvious that a large proportion of athletes and patients receiving massage perceive its effects as positive and useful. However, this could be in part due to nonspecific placebo effects caused by the human touch and empathy.

Physiological Effects of Massage

One of the aims of massage in sports is to increase tissue extensibility in order to increase performance and to prevent injuries. Wiktorson-Möller, Öberg, Ekstrand, and Gillquist (127) found that in healthy subjects kneading massage increased significantly only ankle dorsiflexion of the six tested ranges of motion, and it significantly decreased isokinetic strength of the hamstrings and isometric strength of the quadriceps muscles. Stretching combined with general warming-up increased significantly all six ranges of motion, but did not affect muscle strength. Crosman, Chateauvert, and Weisberg (26) obtained more positive results, finding that in young, healthy women massage involving stroking, kneading, and friction to the posterior aspect of one randomly assigned lower extremity increased the range of passive motion significantly compared to the contralateral limb. The effect mostly disappeared in one week.

Massage has been claimed to increase muscle extensibility on the basis of direct mechanical and neurological effects (70). Beneficial effects of massage on both healthy and injured soft tissues are likely but scientifically unproven. Massage is used to stretch muscles, tendons, ligaments, and fascia, and this can be done very selectively regardless of joint range (133). Cyriax's deep friction massage is used to break down soft tissue scars and adhesions (23). Intensive massage also may cause temporary untoward effects evidenced by increased serum enzyme activities and decreased physical performance (2,15).

The claims of a neurological basis for the increased soft tissue extensibility caused by massage are supported by the finding that deep massage (petrissage) (94,116) reduces the level of motoneuron excitability, and consequently of muscle reflex activity. The effect is specific to the muscles being massaged, and it is probably caused by activation of cutaneous and especially deep muscle receptors (116). This mechanism may be important especially to reduce tension in fatigued or injured muscles, which are sensitive to reflex contractions. This view is also supported by the finding that mechanically-induced vibratory massage decreases electrical activity of resting muscle (110).

Massage is assumed to increase blood and lymph circulation and tissue permeability, and thus to enhance the disposal of harmful waste products and to decrease edema after strenuous exercise. Earlier studies (124,132) have shown that massage increases local blood flow. Part of this is due to increased skin circulation as evidenced by flushing. Hansen and Kristensen (57) using the ^{133}Xe disappearance rate method found that centripetal stroking massage caused a slight increase in muscular blood flow. No changes were seen in subcutaneous blood flow. Hovind and Nielsen (67) using the same method observed that petrissage including kneading, squeezing, and friction caused no changes in blood flow in healthy, young subjects, but *tapotement*, that is, percussion movements including hacking and bunching, increased muscle blood flow by 35% during the maneuver and for some minutes after it. Similar increases in blood flow are caused by very light exercise. Massage also increases skin blood flow (67) and lymph flow to a substantial degree (96) thus aiding in the reduction of edema.

Studies on the effects of massage on physical performance capacity and factors affecting it show variable results. Müller and Schulte am Esch (97) observed that calf massage between repeated bouts of strenuous exercise increased substantially dynamic exercise tolerance without influencing muscle oxygen supply. Balke, Anthony, and Wyatt (8) observed a small increase in treadmill working capacity and a 20% increase in muscular endurance associated with massage with an electromechanical device. Ask, Oxelbeck, Lundeberg, and Tesch (7) found that maximal muscle power output during leg extension was increased by 11% following massage. On the other hand, massage was found to have no effect on maximal stride frequency during simulated sprinting exercise (58), even causing a slight decrease in maximal voluntary contraction force (127). In treadmill tests at 80% intensity with and without a prior massage no differences were found in oxygen consumption, oxygen transport, or lactic acid concentration (13). Similarly, percussive vibratory massage did not cause sufficient circulatory or other effects to augment short-term recovery from intense muscular activity (21).

Most people find many forms of massage a pleasant experience, but only a few studies have addressed the psychological effects of massage. Weinberg, Jackson, and Kolodny (125) studied the relationship between exercise, massage, and positive mood enhancement by using a checklist method. Running and a 30-min massage consistently produced positive mood enhancement; however, none of several other sport activities significantly influenced the mood variables. The role of endorphins in mediating the mood effects of massage is obscure because in some studies endorphin serum concentration was not affected by massage (34,104) while in one study there was a slight increase (72). With respect to the autonomic nervous system, massage primarily seems to increase sympathetic activity (9).

In conclusion, the effects of massage and their practical significance have not been thoroughly studied. Massage causes a blend of specific and unspecific effects, which many people perceive to be positive for performance, fitness, and wellbeing. The structural-functional rationale of the use of massage is partly sound, suggesting considerable potential to enhance fitness and health. However, it may also cause undue discomfort and performance deterioration, and especially among athletes it may lead to unwarranted reliance and even a dependency on its availability. For these reasons, the real significance and proper uses of massage should be thoroughly studied.

Sauna

Sauna is a mild to severe heat stress causing a variety of physiological responses (for review see 60,61,123). In connection with exercise and sports, sauna has been suggested for numerous purposes including warming-up, mental and physical relaxation, facilitation of mental and physical recovery, weight reduction, prevention and treatment of musculoskeletal symptoms, prevention of respiratory infections, training of the circulatory system, and for effecting autonomic regulations and acclimation to heat. Many of these proposed benefits are based more on perceived effects, reasoning, and indirect evidence than well-conducted research. Finnish athletes use sauna regularly—primarily for hygienic and mental reasons, and rarely before training and competition except for required weight reduction in some sports (105,121).

Performance-Related Responses

Sauna causes elevation of body temperature, increase of sweating, increase and redistribution of cardiac output and blood flow, increase of ventilation and mild broncholysis, and numerous hormonal responses. The extent of these responses depends on habituation and the intensity and duration of exposure. Repeated exposures increase tolerance to sauna (see 81,122). The consequences of these effects on the determinants of physical performance capacity include temporarily decreased extra- and intracellular fluid volume (1,77), loss of electrolytes (1), decrease of ventilatory reserve but also decrease of ventilatory resistance (82), decreased muscle blood flow (40,107) and circulatory reserve (122), decreased maximal oxygen uptake (22,25,108), decreased aerobic endurance capacity (22,108), decreased peak blood lactate concentration at decreased muscle tension (38), decreased muscle strength (16,63,66,114,119), decreased rate of isometric force development (119), decreased muscle endurance (117), increased flexibility (85), and increased tolerance to heat (107).

Sauna does not affect glycogen or fat stores or increase metabolic rate in any practically significant amount. Sauna seems to decrease aggressiveness (95) and enhance sleep (103). Relaxation, tranquilization, improved mood, and enhanced readiness for interpersonal contacts are commonly perceived effects among athletes (121), and plasma β-endorphin level may be increased in sauna (71,118).

Use of Sauna in Exercise and Sports

Based on research evidence sauna could be used for acute weight reduction, for neuromuscular relaxation, for heat acclimation, to enhance recovery after strenuous effort, and as heat therapy after musculoskeletal injuries. However, the temporary impairment of several physiological functions seriously limit the use of sauna for acute weight reduction. At least part of it should be attained by physical exercise in order to prevent performance deterioration (22). However, the recommendation to prohibit the use of sauna to "make weight" (6) is unduly strong.

For heat acclimation sauna is impractical and rather inefficient without simultaneous exercise training (60,61,107); and for circulatory training sauna is inefficient (44,60,61,107). The findings that suggest regular sauna may decrease the incidence of the common cold (43,47,79) need verification by controlled studies.

Despite the very common use and widely perceived positive effects of sauna (especially among the Finns) to facilitate recovery after strenuous effort and to prevent and decrease postexercise musculoskeletal symptoms, there is a lack of firm scientific evidence to support this practice. However, heat is shown to have numerous positive musculoskeletal and psychological effects, and sauna is one way to apply heat.

Because sauna is a heat stress, there are also contraindications for its use. Many of them are based on practical knowledge and are not completely scientifically validated. Sauna is not advisable during acute, especially febrile, infections and inflammations, during the first days after traumatic or overuse injuries, and during the acute phase of prolapsed intervertebral disc and sciatica. Other contraindications are fatigue, severe dehydration, and hypoglycemia before their partial correction, disorders related to heat such as cramps and exhaustion, and cold disorders such as numbness, frostbite, freezing, and hypothermia. Persons having contagious or exudative skin diseases should not take sauna for hygienic reasons. On the other hand, mild to moderate sauna is well-tolerated even by young children, old people, and patients with various diseases. The risk of cardiovascular complications is increased by intensive and prolonged heat and especially by the sudden great change in temperature caused by plunging in cold water (for review, see 123).

In conclusion, sauna can serve as a valuable adjuvant to sports and physical activity, especially via its psychosomatic effects. Its physiological and psychological effects depend strongly on the duration and intensity of the sauna bath as well as on habituation.

Sudation Garments

The rationale for use of sudation garments in exercise and sport is to create a temporary, hot microclimate by preventing evaporative heat loss. This way of training has been proposed to increase exercise-heat tolerance more than similar training in ordinary exercise clothing in a cool environment, and could help athletes to train effectively for performances in a hot climate. Another use of sudation garments could be acute weight reduction based on increased sweating.

Training for Exercise-Heat Tolerance

Earlier uncontrolled studies on the effects of sudation garments have suggested either no additional benefit for (3,4,27) or significant improvement in (49,87,112) heat tolerance. Recent research by Dawson and co-workers has generated reliable data allowing firm conclusions and sound recommendations (31,32,33).

Dawson and Pyke (31) showed that training in lightweight nylon sweat clothing provided a significant challenge to the thermoregulatory system and appeared not to restrict running training. In a subsequent study Dawson and Pyke (see 31) had elite hockey players train either in ordinary or in sweat clothing in cool conditions. After 2 weeks of field training on self-paced intensity testing in interval running in hot, humid conditions only limited improvements were revealed in exercise-heat tolerance in the group using sweat suits, and the same adaptations also were largely seen in the control subjects. Next, Dawson, Pyke, and Morton (33) compared the effects of training in a sweat suit in cool conditions (20 °C, 50% relative humidity [RH]), and in normal clothing in the heat (34 °C, 60% RH). Testing for exercise-heat tolerance after 7-day interval treadmill running revealed changes typical of heat acclimation. However, the improvements were practically the same in both groups, indicating that sweat clothing was as effective as artificial heat exposure in stimulating improvements in exercise-heat tolerance in well-trained subjects.

The fourth study of Dawson, Pyke, and Morton (32) was designed to examine the effectiveness of training in sweat clothing in cool conditions to improve exercise-heat tolerance. Interval running tests in hot conditions after 10 carefully planned field training sessions revealed significant improvements in the group using sweat clothing. Most of these changes, however, were matched by the group training in normal clothing in the same temperature with the exceptions of a smaller rectal temperature change and greater sweating sensitivity during exercise in the subjects training in sweat suits.

Thus, at least in trained subjects, training in sudation garments does not improve exercise-heat tolerance more than training in ordinary clothing, but sweat clothing causes additional physical and psychological demands.

Sudation Garment Use in "Making Weight"

Increased internal body temperature is a strong stimulus for sweating (98), and they both increase more when the same exercise is performed in sweat clothing compared to ordinary training clothing (31,32). Thus, exercise in a sweat suit enhances acute weight reduction or causes the same weight loss with less effort. This may be an advantage in terms of less fatigue and sparing of muscle and liver glycogen. The advantage of a higher sweating rate may be lost if the sweat suit is too impermeable restricting the evaporation of the sweat from skin. This may suppress the local sweating rate (98,109). The practical difficulties, the extra physical and psychological demands (32), and the risk of significant disturbances in fluid, electrolyte, and thermal balance decrease the usefulness of sudation garments as a means for acute weight reduction in sports.

Spot Reduction and Questionable Exercise Devices

A number of exercise devices have been introduced on the consumer market over many years that have made numerous claims regarding the health and fitness benefits associated with their use. While several of these devices do provide benefits as an adjuvant to a physical activity program, many have been found to have no valid scientific basis for their claims. Most of those devices that have been found to have little or no benefit are associated with the multibillion dollar per year weight loss and slimming, or figure control, industry. Some of these are passive devices that require no exertion or energy expenditure on the part of the user, while others do include active movement. The claims, however, for spot reduction or figure enhancement are generally not supported by scientific research (48).

Unfortunately, few research studies have been conducted concerning the efficacy of exercise devices that would fall into the "questionable" category. In most cases, claims are made by the manufacturer without supporting research data, and the scientific community expresses its skepticism on the basis of an evaluation of these claims against established scientific fact. Where actual scientific studies have been conducted the resulting data generally do not support the manufacturer's claims. Questionable exercise devices include passive exercise devices, those designed for spot reduction, mechanical vibrators, and bust developers. Because most of these devices claim to have a specific influence on one segment or area of the body, the general area of spot reduction will be reviewed first.

Spot Reduction

For years it has been proposed that by exercising one specific area of the body it is possible to exert major changes on the fat content of that area. This concept has been referred to as spot reduction. What is the evidence for spot reduction? Mohr (92) reported significant decreases in waist and abdominal skinfold thicknesses following a 4-week program of six isometric abdominal contractions held for 6-s each, an exercise program she claimed could be considered a form of spot reduction. Unfortunately, there was no control group, or general (i.e., nonspecific) exercise group, to confirm that these changes were, in fact, the result of spot reduction, and not simply the result of a generalized reduction in subcutaneous fat throughout the body. To date, only one research study using an appropriate experimental design has supported the concept of spot reduction.

Using single-arm biceps curls and triceps extensions, Olson and Edelstein (101) reported a significant reduction in the triceps skinfold fat measurement on the arm that exercised compared to the control arm that did not exercise. Conversely, using a similar study design, Roby (106) found decreases in triceps skinfold fat measurements in both the trained (–1.0 mm) and untrained (–1.5 mm) arms following a 10-week program of forearm extension weight training exercise.

Noland and Kearney (100) conducted a 10-week study of 56 women randomly assigned to either a general or specific (spot-reduction) exercise group. While there were significant decreases pre- to post-training in skinfold thickness and girth measurements for both groups, there were no differences between the groups. Gwinup, Chelvam, and Steinberg (55) took a unique approach in their study of spot reduction. Using professional tennis players, they found substantially greater muscular development in the dominant arm, which was attributed to the difference in activity levels between the two arms. However, no differences were found between the arms in localized fat stores as assessed by multiple skinfold determinations.

Finally, Katch, Clarkson, Kroll, McBride, and Wilcox (74) observed the effects of a 27-day sit-up training program on adipose cell size and adiposity. Fat biopsies were obtained from the abdominal, subscapular, and gluteal regions both before and after this extensive training regimen (5,004 sit-ups total). Weight, total body fat, skinfold thicknesses, and girths did not change. While the fat cell diameters were reduced, there was no evidence to indicate a selective or preferential use of fat from the abdominal region compared with the subscapular and gluteal regions.

From the above, it is concluded that the overwhelming evidence does not support the concept of spot reduction. This is an important conclusion, as most of the questionable exercise devices to be discussed in the next section base many of their claims on the theory of spot reduction.

Questionable Exercise Devices

Hernlund and Steinhaus (64) conducted one of the first studies of what would be considered a questionable exercise device. They investigated the weight-reducing claims made for a mechanical vibrating machine which was commonly used in health clubs at that time for spot reduction and weight loss. After their subjects underwent 15 min of continuous mechanical vibration they found no evidence of changes in blood fat levels, and the small increases in oxygen uptake over the passive vibration and recovery sessions amounted to a total of only 11.4 kcal above seated resting energy expenditure levels for the same time period.

Wilmore et al. (129) investigated the claims of two exercise devices that were sold through the mail. The Astro-Trimmer is a rubber-surfaced belt which is placed directly against the skin around the waist and is connected to an elastic cord. The elastic cord attaches to a doorknob. The individual is to walk or jog in place 10 to 15 min leaning slightly forward, placing tension on the cord and belt. The Slim-Skins device is a pair of plastic pants that covers the body from midwaist to midthigh and has a plastic tube embedded in the pants that attaches to a vacuum cleaner hose. The pants are connected to the vacuum cleaner and the vacuum cleaner is operational during the 8- to 10-min exercise period, as well as during the 15-min period of seated recovery. The exercise period includes toe touches, jogging in place, bench squats without weights, seated toe touches, and a final set of jogging in place. The manufacturer claimed an average loss of 20.45 in. from the waist, abdomen, hips, and thighs over a 3-day period.

Subjects were divided into experimental or control groups for each of the two exercise devices, and body composition, skinfold fat, and girth measurements were obtained both before and after the 3-day (Slim-Skins) and the 5-day (Astro-Trimmer) programs. The programs for these two devices were followed exactly as specified in the manufacturer's instruction booklets. The test results were unable to confirm the manufacturer's claims for either of these two devices. While several of the measurements demonstrated significant alterations across trials, the changes were small, variable, or inconsistent with the expected results.

In a second study, Wilmore et al. (130) investigated the claims made for a bust-developer device that suggested that the bustline could be increased by 2 to 3 in. within 3 to 5 days. The exercise program consisted of a series of six upper body exercises performed with the exercise device, which consisted of two slightly curved pieces of plastic hinged in the center and joined by a spring at one end. The exercises were performed exactly as outlined by the manufacturer. Subjects were randomly assigned to either control or experimental groups. Anthropometric measures, measures taken from a series of breast photographs, breast volume, and body composition were assessed both before and after the 21-day program. These measures and the breast photography measures were unable to support the manufacturer's claims.

Martin and Kauwell (88) evaluated the efficacy of a continuous assistive–passive exercise device (CAPE) in sedentary women. The CAPE program utilized six tables which provided a combination of passive, continuously assisted, and light resistive exercise to the trunk and extremities. Sedentary, postmenopausal women were randomly assigned to one of three groups: CAPE program, moderate cycle ergometry, and control. Training consisted of one 10-min bout on each of the six CAPE tables twice per week, or one 30-min bout on the cycle ergometer at 70% to 85% of maximum heart rate twice per week for 12 weeks. The cycle group lost 1.1 kg of weight and increased maximal oxygen uptake ($\dot{V}O_2max$) by 9.2%, while the CAPE group significantly decreased their $\dot{V}O_2max$ and had no change in body weight, caloric intake, or skinfold thicknesses.

One final study should be mentioned as it provides interesting insight into the physiologic responses to a popular form of activity for children, adolescents, and young adults. While not making claims as passive exercise devices, video games have captured the attention of the public and have potentially reduced the amount of time the individual would normally spend in the pursuit of physical activity. Segal and Dietz (111) quantified the physiologic responses of playing a video game in 20 men and 12 women, age 16 to 25 years. Playing the arcade version of the video game "Ms. Pac-Man" while standing resulted in significant increases in heart rate, systolic and diastolic blood pressure, and oxygen consumption. Energy expenditure while playing the video game was increased by ≈80% over resting standing values. The authors concluded that the increase in metabolic rate and cardiovascular stimulation was similar in magnitude to mild-intensity exercise. Thus, video games, long considered a passive activity, do have a mild exercise component.

From the preceding, it is concluded that there is little or no evidence to support manufacturers' claims for questionable exercise devices. This is not unexpected considering that most of these devices base their claims on the theory of spot reduction. This conclusion pertains only to those devices that are either passive or that require little in the way of energy expenditure.

Nutritional Supplements

There have been a multitude of claims made as to the efficacy of various nutritional supplements as adjuvants to physical activity programs. This consensus statement will deal only with the supplement of protein, vitamins, and minerals.

Protein

For many years it was thought that protein had to be supplemented in rather large quantities in physically active people. This belief resulted from a theory prevalent in the mid-1800s that the muscle consumed itself as fuel to provide the energy substrate for its own contractions. It is now widely recognized that protein is used sparingly as a fuel for physical activity. Therefore, is there any advantage to increasing the intake of protein or specific amino acids relative to enhancing strength, muscle mass, or performance? There are two possible pathways by which increased protein intake could influence performance: more efficient use of protein as a major substrate for muscle contraction, or more effective replacement of that which was utilized during exercise; and enhanced synthesis of protein in response to resistance-type exercise training to increase muscle mass.

This first pathway involves primarily endurance-type rather than resistance-type exercise. Muscle glycogen, plasma glucose, plasma-free fatty acids, and plasma and muscle triglycerides have long been recognized as the major energy sources for endurance activity. With respect to protein, it is now recognized that during an acute bout of exercise there is a reduction in the rate of muscle protein synthesis and a possible increase in muscle proteolysis, thus increasing the pool of available free amino acids (39,52,120). However, amino acids provide not more than 5% to 15% of the total energy expended during exercise, depending on the type of exercise, its duration and intensity, and the composition of the diet for several days prior to exercise (17,52,120). The main use of free amino acids is through the oxidation of the branched-chain amino acids (leucine, isoleucine, and valine) and the use of alanine in gluconeogenesis to maintain blood glucose concentrations (120).

Thus, protein does appear to be a relatively small yet important energy source during endurance exercise. Does this mean that it is necessary to increase protein intake in those individuals who participate in endurance-type activity? Lemon and Proctor (86) estimate that regular endurance exercise may increase protein needs by 50% to 100%. The protein requirements may be as high as 1.6 g of protein/kg body weight/day for some endurance athletes, a value which is twice the American recommended daily allowance (RDA) of 0.8 g/kg/day. For most individuals, however, intakes of 1.2 to 1.4 g/kg/day should be adequate (86). Most active individuals who are consuming a balanced diet, with 12% to 15% of the caloric intake from protein, would normally be consuming between 1.2 to 2.0 g/kg/day from their diet alone and would not need to supplement protein. Recent interest has focused on branched-chain amino acid supplements and their potential for increasing performance. At least one study has demonstrated possible improvements in both mental and physical performance in subjects competing in either a 30-km cross-country race or a 42.2 km marathon (12).

The second pathway by which protein supplementation might benefit performance is through the potential enhancement of protein synthesis. Resistance-type training is used not only to increase muscle strength but also muscle mass. An increased muscle mass would be important to the performance of many athletes, but would also be important for those who have lost muscle mass through a combination of physical inactivity and aging. The key to increasing muscle mass is to increase protein synthesis and reduce protein degradation. Booth, Nicholson, and Watson (14) have concluded that increased protein synthesis is more important than reduced degradation for increasing muscle protein with training. Goldberg, Etlinger, Goldspink, and Jablecki (51), however, proposed that both an increased rate of synthesis and a decreased rate of degradation are responsible for the increase in muscle mass consequent to resistance training.

For maintenance of muscle mass, there appears to be no need to supplement protein in individuals performing resistance-type exercise, provided that total caloric intake is meeting the individual's energy needs and that protein constitutes 12% to 15% of the calories ingested (18). The role of protein supplementation in enhancing the protein synthesis with resistance-type exercise training has not been clearly established (18). It is clear that total caloric intake must be increased in order to achieve increases in muscle mass, but the need to specifically increase protein intake has not been established.

In summary, protein supplementation is generally considered unnecessary if individuals are in energy balance and are consuming 10% to 15% of their energy intake from protein (102). For those interested in increasing their fat-free mass through physical activity, it may be of some benefit to increase protein intake, although this has not been scientifically documented.

Vitamins

It has been clearly established that supplementation of vitamins and minerals is important and beneficial for those who have inadequate intake or insufficient body stores. In the absence of vitamin or mineral deficiencies, will supplementation above the RDA be an adjuvant to physical activity? Of the 13 substances classified as vitamins, only the B-complex vitamins and vitamins C and E have been extensively investigated relative to their role in and the possible need for supplementation with physical activity.

B-complex vitamins are involved with coenzyme activity in the metabolism of fats and carbohydrates and in the formation of erythrocytes (62). With respect to exercise, B-complex vitamins could potentially enhance endurance performance (24). When a B-complex vitamin deficiency is produced in individuals who have previously had adequate intake and body stores, endurance performance is decreased. B-complex vitamin supplementation of these deficient individuals will restore their endurance performance. While several studies have shown that the supplementation of one or a combination of the B-complex vitamins facilitates performance, the overwhelming majority of studies have found that supplementation is of no measurable value providing there is no preexisting deficiency.

Vitamin C has an important role in the formation of collagen, a critical protein in connective tissue, and serves to facilitate the absorption of iron. It also is involved in the metabolic reactions of amino acids, in the synthesis of catecholamines and the anti-inflammatory corticoids of the adrenal gland, and serves as an antioxidant. With respect to exercise, vitamin C could help reduce tissue damage associated with exercise and facilitate the repair of any resulting damage. While several studies have demonstrated small improvements in performance with vitamin C supplementation, it is the consensus of several recent reviews on this topic that even with the increased requirements for vitamin C with exercise, supplementation of vitamin C in the absence of deficiency has no ergogenic properties (11,24,62).

Vitamin E has received a great deal of attention over the years, as there have been numerous claims made regarding the health and medical benefits associated with its supplementation. Vitamin E is a fat-soluble vitamin that derives most of its activity from alpha-tocopherol, and has important antioxidant properties. It is postulated to be important during exercise due to its relationship with oxygen use and energy supply. Again, the results of studies concerning the value of supplementing vitamin E for improved exercise performance are mixed. However, the general consensus of recent reviews on vitamin E and exercise performance is that supplementation is of little or no value (24,62).

To summarize, a number of studies have shown that exercise can increase the need for some vitamins. However, for those individuals in energy balance who are consuming a nutritionally well-balanced diet, there is little evidence to support the use of vitamin supplements for fitness or health benefits. With the increasing concern over free-radical production during exercise, there is a growing interest in the role of the antioxidants (vitamins C and E) in preserving fitness and health (24). However, there is insufficient research to draw any conclusions at this time.

Minerals

Minerals are much less likely to be supplemented, possibly because fewer ergogenic properties have been ascribed to specific minerals in comparison to vitamins. Of the body's minerals, the major electrolytes in muscle, plasma, and sweat (sodium, chloride, potassium, calcium, and magnesium), and iron and calcium have been studied the most. Calcium is critical in the formation and maintenance of healthy bone. Reduced intake can lead to decreased mineralization of bone. Decreased mineralization of bone is also associated with reduced levels of estrogen, and is very common in female athletes who have become amenorrheic (41). It is unclear at this time as to the potential benefits of calcium supplementation in those who are meeting the RDA with their normal daily intake. For those who have normal menstrual function and estrogen levels, supplementation will most likely have little benefit. However, for those who are amenorrheic with low estrogen levels, calcium intakes of 1,500 mg/day can have a positive effect on cortical bone (41).

Iron plays a major role in the oxygen transport system, and substantial decreases in endurance performance will follow iron deficiency anemia.

There is no consensus as to the prevalence of iron deficiency. This is possibly due to the lack of a standardized criteria for iron deficiency. Clarkson (24) provides a three-stage approach for determining iron status. A reduction in serum ferritin levels indicative of *iron depletion* constitutes the first stage. Serum ferritin levels provide a good index of bone marrow iron stores. Continued iron deficiency resulting in an impairment in erythrocyte formation constitutes the second stage and is termed *iron-deficient erythropoiesis*. With the continued inability to form erythocytes, hemoglobin levels begin to fall, and this constitutes the third and final stage termed *iron deficiency anemia*.

While iron depletion is relatively common in athletes, the prevalence among athletes is no different than among nonathletes (24). Iron-deficient erythropoiesis and iron deficiency anemia are not considered prevalent in the athletic population. However, when iron deficiency anemia is present, endurance performance is impaired. Performance can be restored with iron supplementation in those with iron deficiency anemia; however, supplementation has little or no effect when individuals are iron depleted or have iron-deficient erythropoiesis (24).

With respect to the major electrolytes in muscle, plasma, and sweat, there are rather substantial alterations in their concentrations with exercise. With the loss of large volumes of sweat, there will be a loss of electrolytes from the body. The total loss of electrolytes is relatively small compared to the magnitude of the body stores, thus many investigators have concluded that the replacement of electrolytes during the activity is not necessary. However, it is important to replace the water that is lost in sweat, as this loss will lead to decreases in plasma volume, and water uptake in the small intestine is facilitated by a fluid that contains both sugar and sodium (90).

To summarize, the supplementation of iron or calcium may be of benefit for some, but only those with iron deficiency anemia or low estrogen levels, respectively. Further, there is possibly some benefit to supplementing electrolytes, primarily sodium, when using fluid replacement during exercise in order to facilitate the uptake of water in the small intestine.

References

1. Ahonen, E.; Nousiainen, U. The sauna and body fluid balance. Ann. Clin. Res. 20:257-261; 1988.
2. Ahonen, J.; Salorinne, Y.; Weber, T. Effect of various types of massage on muscular performance and release of muscle enzymes in athletes. Valmennus ja kuntoilu. 1:60-61; 1985.
3. Allan, J.R.; Crowdy, J.P.; Haisman, M.F. The use of a vapour barrier suit for the practical induction of artificial acclimatization to heat. I. Winter experiment. Army Personn. Res. Estab. Rep. 4:65; 1965.
4. Allan, J.R.; Haisman, M.F. Modification of the physiological responses to heat stress by physical training with and without extra clothing. Army Operat. Res. Estab. Rep. 11:64; 1964.
5. Alon, G.; McCombe, S.A.; Koutsantonis, S.; Stumhauzer, L.J.; Burgwin, K.C.; Parent, M. M.; Bosworth, R.A. Comparison of the effects of electrical stimulation and exercise on abdominal musculature. J. Orthop. Sports Phys. Ther. 8:567-573; 1987.
6. American College of Sports Medicine. Position stand on weight loss in wrestlers. Med. Sci. Sports 8:2; 1976.
7. Ask, N.; Oxelbeck, U.; Lundeberg, T.; Tesch, P.A. The influence of massage on quadriceps function after exhaustive exercise. Abstract. Med. Sci. Sports Exerc. 19:53; 1987.
8. Balke, B.; Anthony, J.; Wyatt, F. The effects of massage treatment on exercise fatigue. Clin. Sports Med. 1:189-196; 1989.
9. Barr, J.S.; Taslitz, N. The influence of back massage on autonomic functions. Phys. Ther. 50:1679-1691; 1970.
10. Basmajian, J.V., editor. Manipulation, traction and massage. Baltimore: Williams & Wilkins; 1985.
11. Belko, A.Z. Vitamins and exercise—an update. Med. Sci. Sports Exerc. 19:S191-S196; 1987.
12. Blomstrand, E.; Hassmén, P.; Ekblom, B.; Newsholme, E.A. Administration of branched-chain amino acids during sustained exercise—effects on performance and on plasma concentration of some amino acids. Eur. J. Appl. Physiol. 63:83-88; 1991.
13. Boone, T.; Cooper, R.; Thompson, W.R. A physiologic evaluation of the sports massage. Athletic training. JNATA. 26:51-54; 1991.
14. Booth, F.W.; Nicholson, W.F.; Watson, P.A. Influence of muscle use on protein synthesis and degradation. Exerc. Sport Sci. Rev. 10:27-48; 1982.
15. Bork, K.; Korting, G.W.; Faust, G. Das Verhalten einiger Serumenzyme nach Ganzkörper-Muskelmassage. Ein Beitrag zur Frage der physikalischen Behandlung bei Dermatomyositis. Arch. Derm. Fortschr. 240:342-348; 1971.

16. Bosco, J.S.; Terjung, R.L.; Greenleaf, J.E. Effects of progressive hypohydration on maximal isometric muscular strength. J. Sport Med. 8:81-86; 1968.
17. Brooks, G.A. Amino acid and protein metabolism during exercise and recovery. Med. Sci. Sports Exerc. 19:S150-S156; 1987.
18. Butterfield, G. Amino acids and high protein diets. In: Lamb, D.R.; Williams, M.H., eds. Ergogenics: Enhancement of performance in exercise and sport. Dubuque, IA: Brown & Benchmark; 1991:87-117.
19. Cabric, M.; Appell, H.-J.; Resic, A. Fine structural changes in electrostimulated human skeletal muscle. Evidence for predominant effects on fast muscle fibres. Eur. J. Appl. Physiol. 57:1-5; 1988.
20. Cafarelli, E.; Flint, F. The role of massage in preparation for and recovery from exercise. Sports Med. 14:1-9; 1992.
21. Cafarelli, E.; Sim, J.; Carolan, B.; Liebesman, J. Vibratory massage and short-term recovery from muscular fatigue. Int. J. Sports Med. 11:474-478; 1990.
22. Caldwell, J.E.; Ahonen, E.; Nousiainen, U. Differential effects of sauna-, diuretic-, and exercise-induced hypohydration. J. Appl. Physiol. 57:1018-1023; 1984.
23. Chamberlain, G.J. Cyriax's friction massage: A review. J. Orthop. Sports Phys. Ther. 4:16-22; 1982.
24. Clarkson, P.M. Vitamins and trace minerals. In: Lamb, D.R.; Williams, M.H., eds. Ergogenics: Enhancement of performance in exercise and sport. Dubuque, IA: Brown & Benchmark; 1991:123-176.
25. Craig, F.N.; Gummings, E.G. Dehydration and muscular work. J. Appl. Physiol. 21:670-674; 1966.
26. Crosman, L.J.; Chateavert, S.R.; Weisberg, J. The effects of massage to the hamstring muscle group on range of motion. J. Orthop. Sports Phys. Ther. 6:168-172; 1984.
27. Crowdy, J.P.; Haisman, M.F. The use of a vapour-barrier suit for the practical induction of artificial acclimatization to heat. II. Summer experiment. Army Personn. Res. Estab. Rep. 4:65; 1965.
28. Currier, D.P. Neuromuscular electrical stimulation for improving strength and blood flow, and influencing changes. In: Nelson, R.M.; Currier D.P., eds. Clinical electrotherapy. Norwalk, CT: Appleton & Lange; 1991:35-103.
29. Currier, D.P.; Lehman J.; Lightfoot, P. Electrical stimulation in exercise of the quadriceps femoris muscle. Phys. Ther. 59:1508-1512; 1979.
30. Currier, D.P.; Mann, R. Muscular strength development by electrical stimulation in normal subjects. Phys. Ther. 63:915-921; 1983.
31. Dawson, B.; Pyke, F.S. Artificially induced heat acclimation of team game players with sweat clothing: I. Responses to wearing sweat clothing during exercise in cool conditions. J. Hum. Movement Stud. 15:171-183; 1988.
32. Dawson, B.; Pyke, F.S.; Morton, A.R. Effects on exercise-heat tolerance of training in cool conditions in sweat clothing. Aust. J. Sci. Med. Sports. 20:3-10; 1988.
33. Dawson, B.; Pyke, F.S.; Morton, A.R. Improvements in heat tolerance induced by interval running training in the heat and in sweat clothing in cool conditions. J. Sports Sci. 7:189-203; 1989.
34. Day, J.A.; Mason, R.R.; Chesrown, S.E. Effect of massage on serum level of β-endorphin and β-lipotropin in healthy adults. Phys. Ther. 67:926-930; 1987.
35. Delitto, A.; Brown, M.; Sturbe, J.M.; Rose, S.J.; Lehman, R.C. Electrical stimulation of quadriceps femoris in an elite weight lifter: A single subject experiment. Int. J. Sports Med. 10:187-191; 1989.
36. Delitto, A.; Rose, S.J.; McKowen, J.M.; Lehman, R.C.; Thomas, J.A.; Shively, R.A. Electrical stimulation versus voluntary exercise in strengthening thigh musculature after anterior cruciate ligament surgery. Phys. Ther. 68:660-663; 1988.
37. Delitto, A.; Snyder-Mackler, L. Two theories of muscle strength augmentation using percutaneous electrical stimulation. Phys. Ther. 70:158-164; 1990.
38. DeVries, H.A.; Beckmann, P.; Huber, H.; Dieckmeir, L. Electromyographic evaluation of the effects of sauna on the neuromuscular system. J. Sports Med. Phys. Fitness. 8:61-69; 1968.
39. Dohm, G.L.; Tapscott, E.B.; Kasperek, G.J. Protein degradation during endurance exercise and recovery. Med. Sci. Sports Exerc. 19:S166-S171; 1987.
40. Drettner, B. The effect of the sauna bath on the peripheral blood flow. In: Acta societatis medicorum upsaliensis (Vol. LXIX). Uppsala, Sweden: Almqvist & Wiksell; 1964:279-290.
41. Drinkwater, B.L. Amenorrhea, body weight, and osteoporosis. In: Brownell, K.D.; Rodin, J.; Wilmore, J.H. Eating, body weight and performance in athletes: Disorders of modern society. Philadelphia: Lea & Febiger; 1992:235-247.
42. Duchateau, F.; Hainaut, K. Training effects of submaximal electrostimulation in a human

skeletal muscle. Med. Sci. Sports Exerc. 20:99-104; 1988.

43. Einenkel, D. Verbesserung des gesundheitszustandes von kindergartenkindern im kreis annaberg durch den regelmässigen besuch einer betriebsauna. Z. Arztl. Fortbild. 71:1069-1071; 1977.
44. Eisalo, A. Effects of the Finnish sauna on circulation. Studies on healthy and hypertensive subjects. Ann. Med. Exp. Biol. Fenn. [Suppl. 4]. 34; 1956.
45. Eriksson, E.; Häggmark, T. Comparison of isometric muscle training and electrical stimulation supplementing isometric muscle training in the recovery after major knee ligament surgery. Am. J. Sports Med. 7:169-171; 1979.
46. Eriksson, E.; Häggmark, T.; Kiessling, K.H.; Karlsson, J. Effects of electrical stimulation on human skeletal muscle. Int. J. Sports Med. 2:18-22; 1981.
47. Ernst, E.; Pecho, E.; Wirz, P.; Saradeth, T. Regular sauna bathing and the incidence of common colds. Ann. Med. 22:225-227; 1990.
48. Franklin, B.A. Myths and misconceptions in exercise for weight control. In: Storlie, J.; Jordan, H.A., eds. Nutrition and exercise in obesity management. New York: Medical & Scientific Books; 1984:53-92.
49. Gisolfi, C.V.; Wilson, N.C.; Claxton, B. Work-heat tolerance of distance runners. In: Milvy, P., ed. Marathon: Physiological, medical, epidemiological and psychological studies. New York: Annals of New York Academy of Sciences (Vol. 301); 1977:139-150.
50. Godfrey, C.M.; Jayawardena, H.; Quance, T.A.; Welch, P. Comparison of electro-stimulation and isometric exercise in strengthening the quadriceps muscle. Physiother. Can. 31:265-267; 1979.
51. Goldberg, A.L.; Etlinger, J.D.; Goldspink, D.F.; Jablecki, C. Mechanism of work-induced hypertrophy of skeletal muscle. Med. Sci. Sports. 7:185-198; 1975.
52. Goodman, M.N.; Ruderman, N.B. Influence of muscle use on amino acid metabolism. Exerc. Sport Sci. Rev. 10:1-26; 1982.
53. Gould, N.; Donnermeyer, D.; Gammon, G.G.; Pope, M.; Ashikaga, T. Transcutaneous muscle stimulation to retard disuse atrophy after open menisectomy. Clin. Orthop. 178:190-197; 1983.
54. Grove-Lainey, C.; Walmsley, R.P.; Andrew, G.M. Effectiveness of exercise alone versus exercise plus electrical stimulation in strengthening the quadriceps muscle. Physiother. Can. 35:5-11; 1983.
55. Gwinup, G.; Chelvam, R.; Steinberg, T. Thickness of subcutaneous fat and activity of underlying muscles. Ann. Intern. Med. 74:408-411; 1971.
56. Halbach, J.W.; Straus, D. Comparison of electro-myostimulation to isokinetic power of the knee extensor mechanism. J. Orthop. Sports Phys. Ther. 2:20-24; 1980.
57. Hansen, T.I.; Kristensen, J.H. Effect of massage, shortwave diathermy and ultrasound upon ^{133}Xe disappearance rate from muscle and subcutaneous tissue in the human calf. Scand. J. Rehabil. Med. 5:179-182; 1973.
58. Harmer, P.A. The effect of pre-performance massage on stride frequency in sprinters. Athl. Train. 26:55-59; 1991.
59. Hartsell, H.D. Electrical muscle stimulation and isometric exercise effects on selected quadriceps parameters. J. Orthop. Sports Phys. Ther. 8:203-209; 1986.
60. Hasan, J.; Karvonen, M.J.; Piironen, P. Physiological effects of extreme heat as studied in the Finnish "sauna" bath. Part I. Am. J. Phys. Med. 45:296-314; 1966.
61. Hasan, J.; Karvonen, M.J.; Piironen, P. Physiological effects of extreme heat as studied in the Finnish "sauna" bath. Part II. Am. J. Phys. Med. 46:1226-1246; 1967.
62. Haymes, E.M. Proteins, vitamins, and iron. In: Williams, M.H., ed. Ergogenic aids in sport. Champaign, IL: Human Kinetics; 1983:27-55.
63. Herbert, W.G.; Ribisl, P.M. Effects of dehydration upon physical working capacity of wrestlers under competitive conditions. Res. Q. Am. Assoc. Health Phys. Educ. 43:416-422; 1972.
64. Hernlund, V.; Steinhaus, A.H. Do mechanical vibrators take off or redistribute fat? J. Assoc. Phys. Ment. Rehabil. 11:96; 1957.
65. Hollis, M. Massage for therapists. Oxford: Blackwell Scientific; 1987.
66. Houston, M.E.; Marrin, D.A.; Green, H.J.; Thompson, J.A. The effect of rapid weight loss on physiological functions in wrestlers. Phys. Sportsmed. 9:73-78; 1981.
67. Hovind, H.; Nielsen, S.L. Effect of massage on blood flow in skeletal muscle. Scand. J. Rehabil. Med. 6:74-77; 1974.
68. Ikai, M.; Yabe, K. Training effect of muscular endurance by means of voluntary and electrical stimulation. Int. Z. Angew. Physiol. 28:55-60; 1969.
69. Ikai, M.; Yabe, K.; Ischii, K. Muskelkraft und muskulare ermunding bei willkurlicher anpassung und elektrischer reizung des muskles. Sportz. Sportmed. 5:197-204; 1967.

70. Jacobs, M. Massage for the relief of pain: Anatomy and physiological considerations. Phys. Ther. Rev. 40:93-98; 1960.
71. Jezova, D.; Vigas, M.; Tator, P.; Jurcovicova, J.; Palat, M. Rise in plasma β-endorphin and ACTH in response to hyperthermia in sauna. Horm. Metab. Res. 17:693-694; 1985.
72. Kaada, B.; Torsteinbo, O. Increase of plasma β-endorphins in connective tissue massage. Gen. Pharmacol. 20:487-489; 1989.
73. Kahanovitz, N.; Nordin, M.; Verderame, R.; Yabut, S.; Parnianpour, M.; Viola, K.; Mulvihill, M. Normal trunk muscle strength and endurance in women and the effect of exercises and electrical stimulation. Part 2: Comparative analysis of electrical stimulation and exercises to increase trunk muscle strength and endurance. Spine. 12:112-118; 1987.
74. Katch, F.I.; Clarkson, P.M.; Kroll, W.; McBride, T.; Wilcox, A. Effects of sit-up exercise training on adipose cell size and adiposity. Res. Q. Exerc. Sport. 55:242-247; 1984.
75. Kots, Y. Electro-stimulation. Moscow: State Central Institute of Physical Culture; 1977.
76. Kottke, F. 17 Massage. In: Knapp, M., ed. Krujsen's handbook of physical medicine and rehabilitation. Philadelphia: Saunders; 1982.
77. Kozlowski, S.; Saltin, B. Effect of sweat loss on body fluids. J. Appl. Physiol. 19:119-124; 1964.
78. Kramer, J.F.; Semple, J.E. Comparison of selected strengthening techniques for normal quadriceps. Physiother. Can. 35:300-340; 1983.
79. Krauss, H.; Diener, H.; Ernst, R.; Kanig, F. Methods and results of systematic physiotherapeutic measures in respiratory tract diseases in childhood. Kinderarztl. Prax. 49:485-492; 1981.
80. Kubiak, R.J.; Whitman, K.M.; Johnston, R.M. Changes in quadriceps femoris muscle strength using isometric exercise versus electrical stimulation. J. Orthop. Sports Phys. Ther. 8:537-541; 1987.
81. Kukkonen-Harjula, K.; Kauppinen, K. How the sauna affects the endocrine system. Ann. Clin. Res. 20:262-266; 1988.
82. Laitinen, A.; Lindqvist, A.; Heino, M. Lungs and ventilation in the sauna. Ann. Clin. Res. 20:244-248; 1988.
83. Lake, D.A. Neuromuscular electrical stimulation. An overview and its application in the treatment of sports injuries. Sports Med. 13:320-336; 1992.
84. Laughman, R.K.; Youdas, J.W.; Carrett, T.R.; Chao, E.Y.S. Strength changes in the normal quadriceps femoris muscle as a result of electrical stimulation. Phys. Ther. 63:494-499; 1983.
85. Lehman, J.F.; deLateur, B.J. Diathermy and superficial heat and cold therapy. In: Kottke, F.J.; Stillwell, G.K.; Lehman, J.F., eds. Krusen's handbook of physical medicine and rehabilitation. London: Saunders; 1982.
86. Lemon, P.W.R.; Proctor, D.N. Protein intake and athletic performance. Sports Med. 12:313-325; 1991.
87. Marcus, P. Heat acclimatization by exercise-induced elevation of body temperature. J. Appl. Physiol. 33:283-288; 1972.
88. Martin, D.; Kauwell, G.P.A. Continuous assistive-passive exercise and cycle ergometer training in sedentary women. Med. Sci. Sports Exerc. 22:523-527; 1990.
89. Massey, B.H.; Nelson, R.S.; Sharkey, B.C.; Comden, T.; Otott, G.C. Effects of high frequency electrical stimulation on the size and strength of skeletal muscle. J. Sports Med. Phys. Fitness. 5:136-144; 1965.
90. Maughan, R. Carbohydrate-electrolyte solutions during prolonged exercise. In: Lamb, D.R.; Williams, M.H., eds. Ergogenics: Enhancement of performance in exercise and sport. Dubuque, IA: Brown & Benchmark; 1991:35-76.
91. McMiken, D.F.; Todd-Smith, M.; Thompson, C. Strengthening of human quadriceps muscles by cutaneous electrical stimulation. Scand. J. Rehabil. Med. 15:25-28; 1983.
92. Mohr, D.R. Changes in waistline and abdominal girth and subcutaneous fat following isometric exercises. Res. Q. 36:168-173; 1965.
93. Mohr, T.M.; Carlson, B.; Sulentic, C.; Landry, R. Comparison of isometric exercise and high volt galvanic stimulation on quadriceps femoris muscle strength. Phys. Ther. 65:606-612; 1985.
94. Morelli, M.; Seaborne, D.E.; Sullivan, S.J. Changes in H-reflex amplitude during massage of triceps surae in healthy subjects. J. Orthop. Sports Phys. Ther. 14:55-59; 1990.
95. Morgan, W.P. Psychological effect of weight reduction in the college wrestler. Med. Sci. Sports. 2:24-27; 1970.
96. Mortimer, P.S.; Simmonds, R.; Rezvani, M.; Robbins, M.; Hopewell, J.W.; Ryan, T.J. The measurement of skin lymph flow by isotope clearance-reliability, reproducibility, injection dynamics, and effects of massage. J. Invest. Dermatol. 95:677-682; 1990.
97. Müller, E.A.; Schulte am esch, J. Die wirkung der massage auf die leistungsfähigkeit von muskeln. Int. Z. Angew. Physiol. Eincsl. Arbeistphysiol. 22:240-257; 1966.
98. Nadel, E.R. Control of sweating rate while exercising in the heat. Med. Sci. Sports. 11:31-35; 1979.

99. Nobbs, L.A.; Rhodes, E.C. The effect of electrical stimulation and isokinetic exercise on muscular power of the quadriceps femoris. J. Orthop. Sports Phys. Ther. 8:260-268; 1986.
100. Noland, M.; Kearney, J.T. Anthropometric and densitometric responses of women to specific and general exercise. Res. Q. 49:322-328; 1978.
101. Olson, A.L.; Edelstein, E. Spot reduction of subcutaneous adipose tissue. Res. Q. 39:647-652; 1968.
102. Paul, G.L. Dietary protein requirements of physically active individuals. Sports Med. 8:154-176; 1989.
103. Putkonen, P.T.S.; Elomaa, E. Sauna and physiological sleep: Increase slow-wave sleep after heat exposure. In: Teir, H.; Collan, Y.; Valtakari, P., eds. Sauna studies. Helsinki; 1976: 270-279.
104. Puustjärvi, K.; Hänninen, O.; Leppäluoto, J. Effect of massage on endorphin levels and some physiological parameters. [Abstract]. Acta Physiol. Hung. 68:243; 1986.
105. Rehunen, S. The sauna and sports. Ann. Clin. Res. 20:292-294; 1988.
106. Roby, F.B. Effect of exercise on regional subcutaneous fat accumulations. Res. Q. 33:273-278; 1962.
107. Rowell, L.B. Cardiovascular adjustments to thermal stress. In: Shephard, J.T.; Abbound, F.M., eds. Handbook of physiology. Section 2. The cardiovascular system. Vol. 3. Peripheral circulation and organ blood flow. Part 2. Bethesda, MD: American Physiological Society MD; 1983:967-1023.
108. Saltin, B. Aerobic work capacity and circulation at exercise in man with special reference to the effect of prolonged exercise and/or heat exposure. Acta Physiol. Scand. [Suppl]. 230:1-52; 1964.
109. Sargent, F. Depression of sweating in man: So-called "sweat gland fatigue." In: Ellis, R.A.; Silver, A.F., eds. Advances in biology of skin. Vol. 3. London: Pergamon Press; 1962.
110. Schmidt, K. Das verhalten der elektrischen muskelaktivität nach maschineller vibrationsmassage. Dtsch. Med. Wochenschr. 93:114-116; 1968.
111. Segal, K.R.; Dietz, W.H. Physiologic responses to playing a video game. Am. J. Dis. Child. 145:1034-1036; 1991.
112. Shvartz, E.; Saar, E.; Meyerstein, N.; Benor, D. Heat acclimatization while wearing vapour-barrier clothing. Aerospace Med. 44:609-612; 1973.
113. Sisk, T.D.; Stralka, S.W.; Deering, M.B.; Griffin, J.W. Effect of electrical stimulation on quadriceps strength after reconstructive surgery of the anterior cruciate ligament. Am. J. Sports Med. 15:215-220; 1987.
114. S'Jongers, J.J.; Vogelaere, P.; Caremans, J.; Poortmans, J.; van Fraechem, J.; Ego, S. Evolution de diverses variables physiologiques au cours du sauna, dans une population de jounes sujets masculins, myoennement entraines. Schweiz. Z. Sportmed. 25:101-118; 1977.
115. Snyder-Mackler, L.; Ladin, Z.; Schepsis, A.A.; Young, J.C.; Massachusetts, B. Electrical stimulation of the thigh muscles after reconstruction of the anterior cruciate ligament. J. Bone Joint Surg. 73-A:1025-1036; 1991.
116. Sullivan, S.J.; Williams, L.R.T.; Seaborne, D.E.; Morelli, M. Effects of massage on alpha motoneuron excitability. Phys. Ther. 71:555-560; 1991.
117. Torranin, C.; Smith, D.P.; Byrd, R.J. The effect of acute thermal dehydration and rapid rehydration on isometric and isotonic endurance. J. Sports Med. Phys. Fitness. 19:1-9; 1979.
118. Vescovi, P.P.; Gerra, G.; Pioli, G.; Pedrazzoni, M.; Maninetti, L.; Passeri, M. Circulating opioid peptides during thermal stress. Horm. Metab. Res. 22:44-46; 1990.
119. Viitasalo, J.T.; Kyröläinen, H.; Bosco, C.; Alen, M. Effects of rapid weight reduction on force production and vertical jumping height. Int. J. Sports Med. 8:281-285; 1987.
120. Viru, A. Mobilisation of structural proteins during exercise. Sports Med. 4:95-128; 1987.
121. Vuori, I. Use of sauna by Finnish athletes. In: Their, H.; Collan, Y.; Valtakari, P., eds. Sauna studies. Helsinki; 1976:141-149.
122. Vuori, I. Sauna bather's circulation. Ann. Clin. Res. 20:249-256; 1988.
123. Vuori, I.; Vapaatalo, H., editors. Special issue on sauna. Ann. Clin. Res. 20; 1988.
124. Wakim, K.G; Martin, G.M.; Terrier, J.C.; Elins, E.C.; Krusen, F.H. The effects of massage on the circulation in normal and paralysed extremities. Arch. Phys. Med. 30:135; 1949.
125. Weinberg, R.; Jackson, A.; Kolodny, K. The relationship of massage and exercise to mood enhancement. Sports Physiol. 2:202-211; 1988.
126. Wigerstad-Lossing, I.; Grimby, G.; Jonsson, T.; Morelli, B.; Peterson, L.; Renström, P. Effects of electrical muscle stimulation combined with voluntary contractions after knee ligament surgery. Med. Sci. Sports Exerc. 20:93-98; 1988.
127. Wiktorson-Möller, M.; Öberg, B.; Ekstrand, J.; Gillquist, J. Effects of warming up, massage, and stretching on range of motion and muscle strength in the lower extremity. Am. J. Sports Med. 11:249-252; 1983.

128. Williams, R.A.; Morrissey, M.C.; Brewster, C.E. The effect of electrical stimulation on quadriceps strength and thigh circumference in meniscectomy patients. J. Orthop. Sports Phys. Ther. 8:143-146; 1986.
129. Wilmore, J.H.; Atwater, A.E.; Maxwell, B.D.; Wilmore, D.L.; Constable, S.H.; Buono, M.J. Alterations in body size and composition consequent to Astro-Trimmer and Slim-Skins training programs. Res. Q. Exerc. Sport. 56:90-92; 1985.
130. Wilmore, J.H.; Atwater, A.E.; Maxwell, B.D.; Wilmore, D.L.; Constable, S.H.; Buono, M.J. Alterations in breast morphology consequent to a 21-day bust developer program. Med. Sci. Sports Exerc. 17:106-112; 1985.
131. Wolf, S.L.; Ariel, G.B.; Saar, D.; Penny, A.; Railey, P. The effect of muscle stimulation during resistive training on performance parameters. Am. J. Sports Med. 14:18-23; 1986.
132. Wolfson, H. Studies on effect of physical therapeutic procedures on function and structure. JAMA. 90:2019; 1931.
133. Ylinen, J.; Cash M. Sports massage. London: Stanley Paul; 1988.

PART IV

Human Adaptation to Acute and Chronic Physical Activity

Chapter 17

Cardiovascular Adaptation to Physical Activity

Jere H. Mitchell
Peter B. Raven

Cardiovascular Response to Exercise

Dynamic Exercise

The acute response to dynamic muscular exercise provides the greatest challenge to the cardiovascular system, which is met by a complex integration of the local regulation of blood flow to the active skeletal muscles and the neural regulation of the hemodynamic response. In dynamic exercise, the active muscle must receive a blood supply appropriate to its increased metabolic needs, while the brain, heart, and other organs receive an adequate blood flow to maintain function. During intense dynamic exercise there is a marked increase in oxygen consumption, which is accomplished by an increase in heart rate, stroke volume, and total body arteriovenous oxygen difference. Also, there is a moderate increase in mean arterial pressure and a marked increase in peripheral vascular conductance.

The marked vasodilation of the resistance vessels in the active skeletal muscles, which can increase blood flow 250 to 300 ml/100 g/min, is responsible for the marked increase in peripheral vascular conductance. The mechanism for this marked vasodilation is not known; however, many metabolic products have been proposed (i.e., increased K^+, increased H^+, adenosine, etc.). It appears that during dynamic exercise involving a large proportion of the skeletal muscle mass, the ability to increase cardiac output, and thereby maintain mean arterial blood pressure, is the limiting factor in determining maximal oxygen uptake. However, in some pathological conditions, the ability to take up oxygen by the skeletal muscle may become a limiting factor.

The circulatory response to dynamic exercise is directly related to the intensity of the work load (1) and is demonstrated by the linear increase in oxygen consumption to a progressive increase in the intensity of exercise until maximal oxygen uptake is reached as depicted in Figure 17.1 (2). Maximal oxygen uptake ($\dot{V}O_{2max}$) objectively measures the maximal oxygen delivery capacity of the circulatory system (2,3) and can be expressed by rearrangement of the Fick principle as follows:

$$\dot{V}O_{2max} = \dot{Q}_{max} \times \text{A-VO}_2\text{diff.}_{max}$$

where $\dot{Q}_{max}$ = maximal cardiac output and A-VO_2diff.$_{max}$ = the maximal extraction of oxygen measured as the difference between the arterial and mixed venous oxygen contents.

Oxygen uptake ($\dot{V}O_2$) at rest approximates 0.25 L/min while the $\dot{V}O_{2max}$ of a sedentary 70 kg man averages 3.0 L/min (or 43 ml O_2/kg/min). However, $\dot{V}O_{2max}$ can be substantially increased by endurance exercise training up to an individual's genetic optimum (4) and may range from 3.0 L/min to 6.0 L/min $\dot{V}O_{2max}$ for the general population. However, the absolute value (L/min) is dependent upon the individual's body size and when comparing values across gender a normalization for body weight (ml/kg) is required (5).

In young, healthy individuals performing upright exercise the increase in cardiac output approximates 5 L/min for each 1 L/min of oxygen uptake (Figure 17.2). The increase in cardiac output occurs as a result of a linear increase in heart rate from resting values of 60 to 70 beats/min to the individual's maximal heart rate of 180 to 190 beats/min and an initial increase in stroke volume from rest to its maximal level at approximately 40% $\dot{V}O_{2max}$ (Figure 17.2). During a progressive increase in work load, arterial hemoglobin saturation and arterial oxygen content remain relatively constant at 97% and 200 ml/L of blood, respectively. However, as the intensity of exercise progresses to $\dot{V}O_{2max}$ the venous oxygen content decreases substantially to a minimal level, ($\dot{V}O_{2max}$ of 30 ml/L of blood), due to the increased extraction of oxygen in the exercising muscles and the redistribution of blood away from resting muscles and visceral organs. This results in a maximal

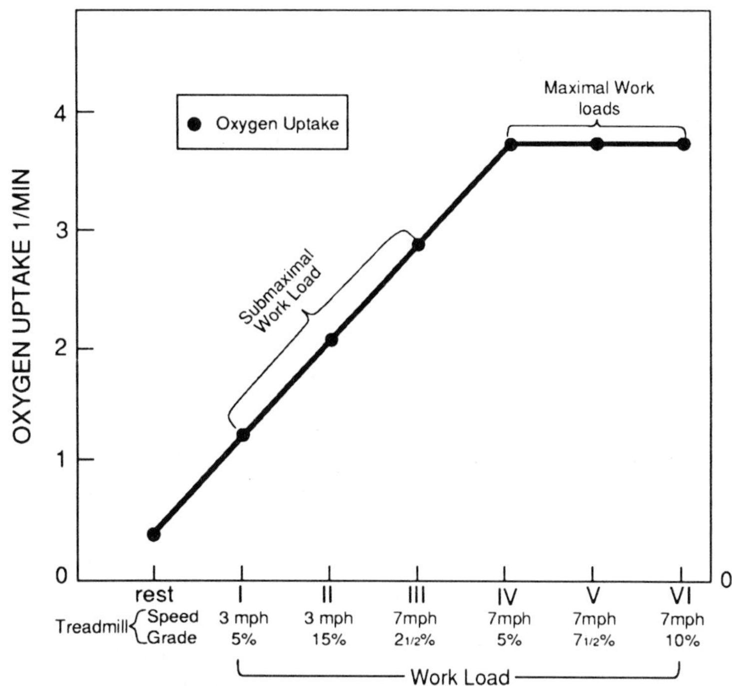

Figure 17.1 A schematic representation of oxygen uptake measured during a progressively increasing work load on a treadmill. Note the plateau of oxygen uptake at maximal work levels—the point of plateau is the accepted objective determination of maximal oxygen uptake of $\dot{V}O_2$max.
Note. From "Maximal Oxygen Uptake" by J.H. Mitchell and C.G. Blomqvist, 1971, *New England Journal of Medicine*, 284, p. 1018. Reprinted by permission of The New England Journal of Medicine.

arteriovenous oxygen difference (A-VO_{2diff}) of about 170 ml O_2/L of blood.

Resting systolic and diastolic blood pressures approximate 120 mmHg and 75 mmHg respectively with a calculated mean arterial pressure of 90 mmHg. As the intensity of exercise increases, systolic blood pressure increases markedly to around 240 mmHg at $\dot{V}O_{2max}$ while diastolic blood pressure decreases to approximately 60 mmHg at $\dot{V}O_{2max}$, resulting in a moderate increase in mean arterial pressure (Figure 17.2). This moderate increase (33%) in mean arterial pressure occurs despite a large (500%–600%) increase in cardiac output which is distributed to the working muscles.

As the intensity of exercise increases, the need for an increase in blood flow to the muscles is enhanced by large increases in skeletal muscle vascular conductance and a redistribution of the cardiac output via regional vasoconstriction in the nonexercising muscles and in the visceral organs. However, maximal vasodilation of the skeletal muscle can increase blood flow to above 250 ml/100 g/min, and if the entire muscle mass of the body was involved in the exercise, the flow demand would exceed the pumping capacity of the heart (6).

As work intensity increases and more and more muscle mass becomes maximally dilated, the maintenance of an adequate perfusion pressure appears to rely on active sympathetic vasoconstriction reducing blood flow to the working muscles (7). However, the neural control mechanisms responsible for the increased muscle sympathetic nerve activity are not entirely clear. In fact, major questions concerning the cardiovascular response to dynamic exercise focus on the neural control mechanisms that are involved in ensuring adequate perfusion to the exercising muscles.

Static Exercise

During sustained static or isometric contractions (e.g., weight lifting), perfusion of the exercising muscle is reduced in direct proportion to the intensity of the muscle contraction, expressed as a percentage of the individual's maximal voluntary contraction (% MVC) of the muscle (8). The static contraction causes a reduction in muscle blood flow which results in increased sympathetic neural activity and mean arterial pressure in an attempt to restore blood flow to the compromised muscle tissue (Figure 17.2). The magnitude of the cardiovascular response is related to both the intensity of muscle contraction (% MVC) and to the amount

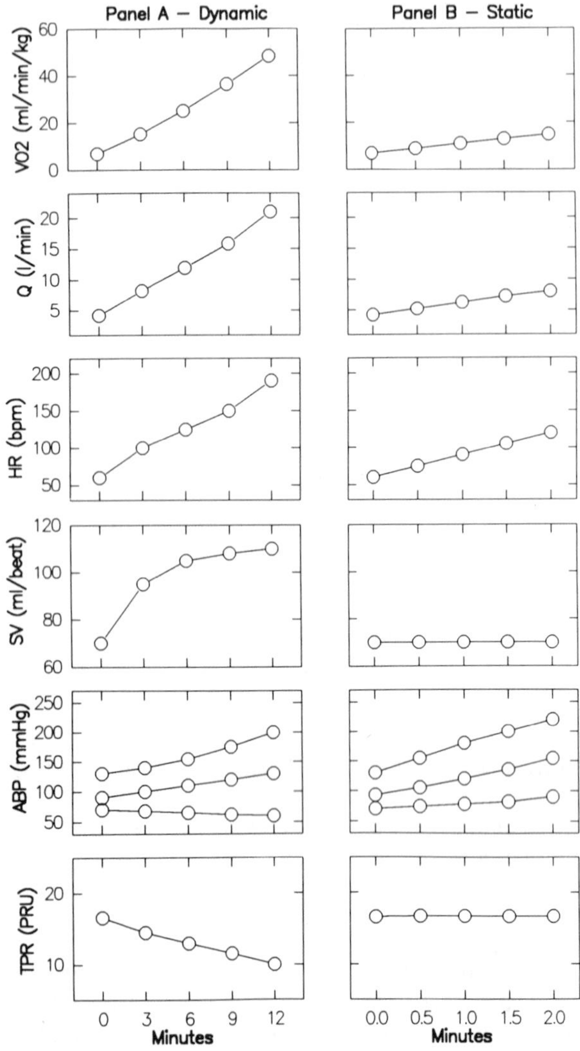

Figure 17.2 Panel A: A representative description of the cardiovascular responses to a progressively increasing work load to $\dot{V}O_2max$: $\dot{Q}$ = cardiac output; SV = stroke volume; HR = heart rate; ABP = systolic (top line), mean (middle line), and diastolic (bottom line) arterial blood pressure; TPR = total peripheral resistance.
Panel B: A representative description of the cardiovascular responses to a sustained isometric contraction (30% MVC): $\dot{Q}$ = cardiac output; SV = stroke volume; HR = heart rate; ABP = systolic (top line), mean (middle line), and diastolic (bottom line) arterial blood pressure; TPR = total peripheral resistance.

of skeletal muscle mass involved in the contraction (9). The increase in cardiac output is a result of an increased heart rate with no apparent increase in stroke volume (Figure 17.2). Surprisingly, the static, exercise-induced increase in mean arterial pressure appears to be a direct result of the increased cardiac output with little or no change in systemic vascular resistance (10).

Neural Control During Exercise

Two neural mechanisms play important roles in regulating the cardiovascular system during exercise (Figure 17.3). In one, which has been termed *central command*, the neural activity responsible for the recruitment of motor units activates in parallel the cardiovascular control area in the ventrolateral medulla, and in turn, determines the immediate changes in the level of efferent activity of the sympathetic and parasympathetic autonomic nervous system to the heart and blood vessels (11). In the other, which has been termed the *exercise pressor reflex*, stimulation of mechanoreceptors and chemosensitive metaboreceptors in the contracting skeletal muscle also determines the changes in autonomic nerve activity to the cardiovascular system. Neural impulses related to the mechanical activity within the skeletal muscle are thought to be transmitted primarily by Group III muscle afferent nerves which travel predominantly through the dorsal roots into the spinal cord (11-13). Subsequently, the afferent nerve traffic reaches the cardiovascular control areas in the ventrolateral medulla almost simultaneously with neural impulses from central command. Both central command and a reflex mechanism signaling mechanical activity provide information concerning the type and intensity of the muscle contraction and the mass of skeletal muscle involved in the physical activity.

Neural impulses related to the metabolic activity of the skeletal muscle are thought to be transmitted primarily by Group IV muscle afferents (13) and also pass predominantly through the dorsal roots into the spinal cord (11-13) and reach the same cardiovascular control area. Because Group IV afferent activity depends on an increase in the concentration of metabolites that are by-products of the increased activity in the contracting muscle, these neural signals occur later in the exercise than those emanating from the mechanoreceptors within the muscle (14,15).

The relative importance of these two neural mechanisms (central command vs. exercise pressor reflex) in determining the cardiovascular response to exercise is dependent upon the type of exercise (static or dynamic), the intensity of the exercise, the time after the onset of exercise, and the effectiveness of blood flow to meet the increased metabolic needs of the contracting muscle (11). However, the manner of integration of these two mechanisms in determining the cardiovascular response to exercise remains unknown; but it appears that they are somewhat redundant, rather than additive, and neural occlusion is operative. Further, the cardiovascular responses during exercise are importantly influenced by arterial

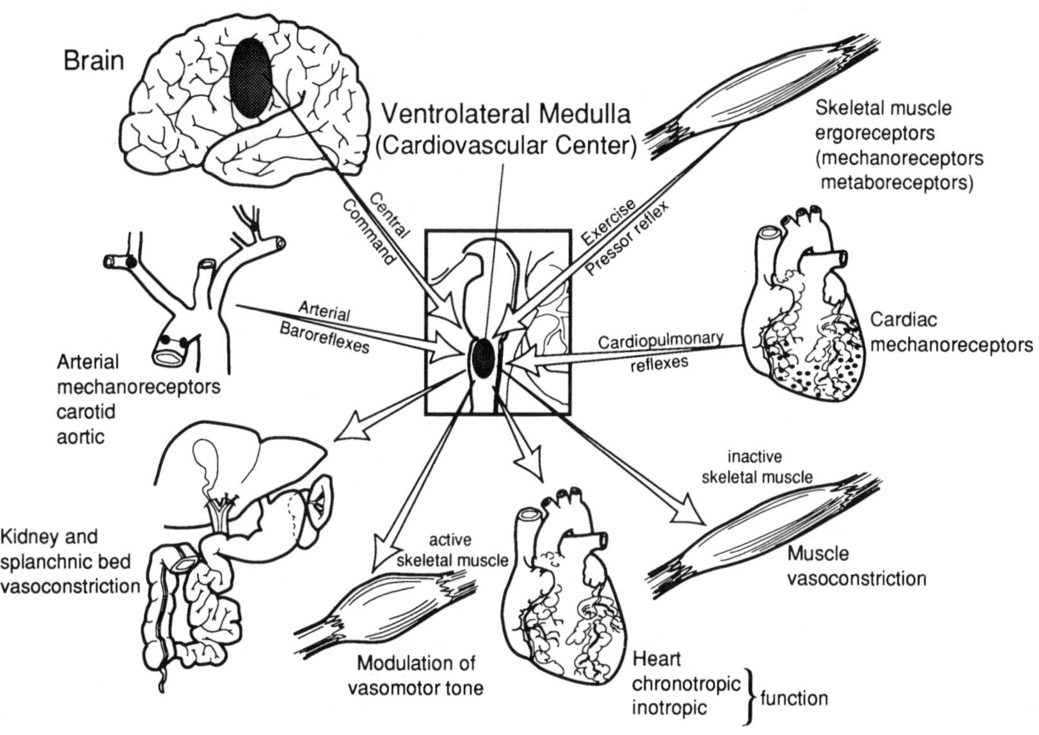

Figure 17.3 A schematic representation of the neural regulation of the cardiovascular system during exercise.

baroreflexes and cardiopulmonary mechanoreceptors.

Central Command

Neuromuscular blockade has been utilized to study the role of central command in determining the cardiovascular response to dynamic and static exercise (16,17). In these experiments the central effort required to perform physical activity is increased.

Studies utilizing this model have shown little effect of enhanced central command on the cardiovascular responses during dynamic exercise (16) (Figure 17.4). A graded exercise test was performed on a cycle ergometer until maximal oxygen uptake was achieved. This caused a progressive increase in heart rate, mean arterial pressure, and rate of perceived exertion. After neuromuscular blockade, the subjects performed their maximal effort on the cycle ergometer as the blockade subsided. During a high level of blockade, despite maximal effort as indicated by a high rating of perceived exertion, heart rate and blood pressure were related to the exercise intensity as measured by the oxygen uptake (not the central effort). As the blockade weakened and maximal effort continued, heart rate and blood pressure increased normally with oxygen uptake. Thus, the cardiovascular responses appeared to be determined by the actual work performed and not by the exerted neural effort or central command (16).

During static exercise, however, the cardiovascular responses are enhanced by neuromuscular blockade (17) (see Figure 17.5). Subjects performed static leg extension at the same absolute force and at the same relative force before and after a 50% reduction in muscle strength by the administration of curare. At the same absolute force the heart rate and blood pressure responses were greater during neuromuscular blockade, when central command was enhanced, than during the control study. However, at the same relative force, the cardiovascular responses were the same during neuromuscular blockade, when central command was the same, as during the control study. This study demonstrates that central command can be important in determining the cardiovascular responses to static exercise (17).

Microneurographic recordings of sympathetic nerve activity to resting muscle and to skin have

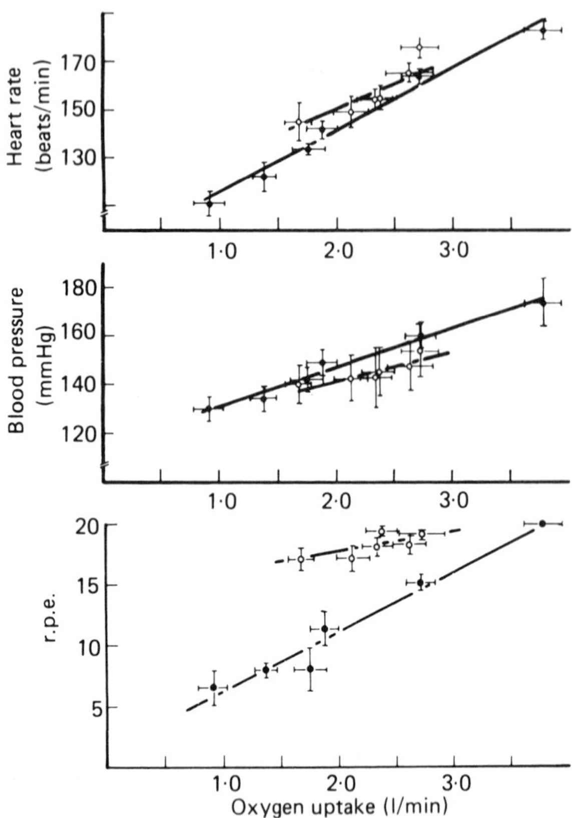

Figure 17.4 Effect of neuromuscular blockade on the cardiovascular responses and rate of perceived exertion (r.p.e.—units on a scale of 0-20) during submaximal and maximal exercise in 10 subjects. Exercise was performed during control (•) and during maximal effort as the blockade subsided (o). Values are means +/− SEM.
Note. From "Cardiovascular, Ventilatory and Catecholamine Responses to Maximal Dynamic Exercise in Partially Curarized Man" by H. Galbo, M. Kjaer, and N.H. Secher, 1987, *Journal of Physiology*, 389, p. 557. Reprinted by permission.

been used to study response to exercise in humans (18–21). With this technique it has been shown that central command is an important determinant of the increased sympathetic nerve activity (SNA) to the skin during static handgrip (21) (Figure 17.6). Static exercise was performed at 30% of maximal voluntary contraction for 2 min followed by postexercise ischemia for an additional 2 min. There was an immediate increase in skin SNA followed by a progressive increase during the 2 min of static contractions. During postexercise vascular occlusion, the skin SNA returned to normal. Thus, the predominant mechanism that increases skin SNA during static exercise is central command; and further, the muscle metaboreceptors have little if any effect (21).

It has also been shown with microneurographic recordings that the muscle metaboreceptors are important determinants of SNA to resting muscle during static exercise (19,21). Muscle SNA during static handgrip followed by postexercise ischemia was studied by Vissing et al. (21) (results are shown in Figure 17.6). There is no increase in muscle SNA during the first minute of static exercise; then a progressive increase occurs during the last minute. During postexercise vascular occlusion, muscle SNA remained elevated until the occlusion was released. Thus, the predominant mechanism that increases muscle SNA during static exercise is related to the activation of muscle metaboreceptors.

Exercise Pressor Reflex

Epidural anesthesia has been utilized to study the role of the exercise pressor reflex in determining the cardiovascular response to dynamic and static exercise (22,23). In these experiments the input from Group III and IV muscle afferents is partially blocked.

During dynamic exercise the normal increase in blood pressure is markedly attenuated by epidural anesthesia (22) (results are shown in Figure 17.7). Normal subjects performed a progressive exercise test on a cycle ergometer to exhaustion. During the controlled study there was a linear increase in heart rate with increased oxygen uptake and a progressive increase in mean arterial pressure. After epidural anesthesia the heart rate response during exercise was normal; however, there was a marked attenuation of the increase in blood pressure. Thus, the afferent neural activity from the working muscle (exercise pressor reflex) is important for blood pressure regulation during dynamic exercise in man but may not be necessary for eliciting the normal heart rate response.

Also during static exercise after epidural anesthesia, the increased central command required to develop force due to the concomitant muscular weakness does not cause enhanced cardiovascular responses (23) (Figure 17.5). Subjects performed static leg extension at the same absolute force and at the same relative force before and after epidural anesthesia, which not only reduced muscle strength by 50% (motoneuron blockade) but also inhibited the afferent feedback from the contracting muscles. At the same absolute force the heart rate and blood pressure responses were the same during epidural anesthesia when central command was blocked as during the control study. However, at the same relative force, the cardiovascular responses were less during epidural anesthesia, when central command was the same, as during the control study. In these studies the cardiovascular responses were not determined by

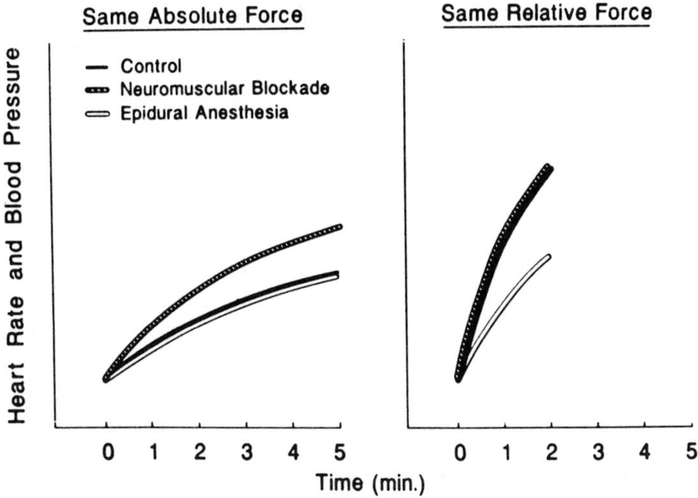

Figure 17.5 Effect of neuromuscular blockade and of epidural anesthesia on the cardiovascular responses to static exercise. In the left panel the effect of each intervention is compared to control at the same absolute force and in the right panel at the same relative force.
Note. From "Epidural Anesthesia and Cardiovascular Responses to Static Exercise in Man" by J.H. Mitchell, D.R. Reeves, Jr., H.B. Rogers, and N.H. Secher, 1989, *Journal of Physiology*, 417, p. 13. Reprinted by permission.

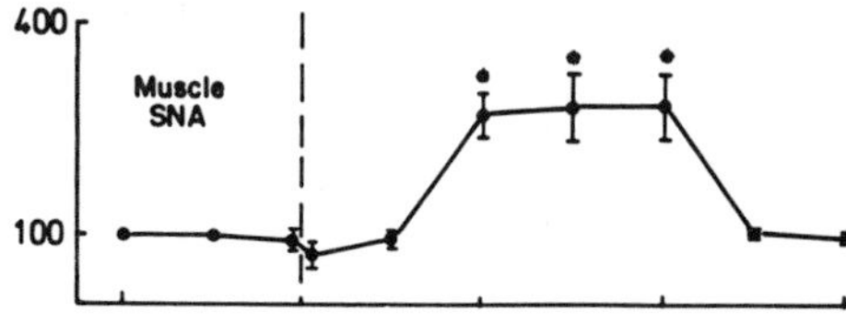

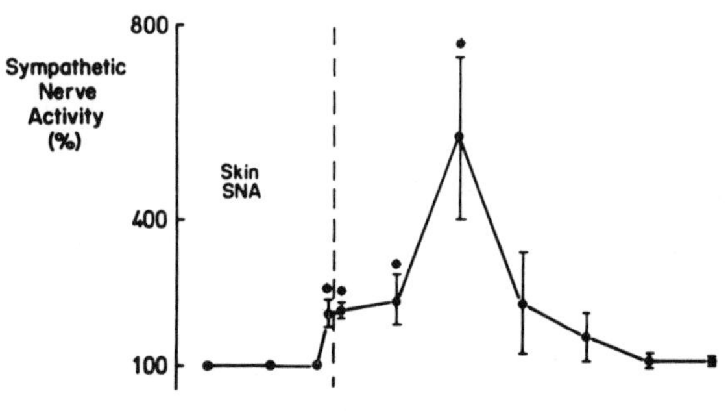

Figure 17.6 Response of muscle sympathetic nerve activity (SNA) and skin SNA to static handgrip and to postexercise ischemia.
Note. From "Stimulation of Skin Sympathetic Nerve Discharge by Central Command" by S.F. Vissing, U. Scherrer, and R.G. Victor, 1991, *Circulation Research*, 69, p. 228. Reprinted by permission.

the level of central command when the afferent feedback for the controlling muscles was inhibited by epidural anesthesia.

Further insight into the role of central command and the exercise pressor reflex during static exercise can be gained by comparing the results of the study by Leonard et al. (17) and Mitchell et al. (23), as shown in Figure 17.5. Central command is important in determining the cardiovascular responses to static exercise when the afferent feedback from the contracting muscles is not affected (neuromuscular blockade). However, central command does not appear to be important in determining the cardiovascular responses to static exercise when the afferent feedback from the working muscle is inhibited (epidural anesthesia). Thus the results of these two studies are complementary and support the concept that central command and the exercise pressor reflex both can be important in determining the cardiovascular response to static exercise in humans.

Arterial and Cardiopulmonary Mechanoreceptors

Recent work (11,24) has significantly advanced our knowledge of the role of central command and the exercise pressor reflex in the neural control of circulation during both static and dynamic exercise; however, the role of the arterial and cardiopulmonary mechanoreceptors during exercise remains to be determined (Figure 17.3). The arterial baroreceptors in the carotid sinus and aortic arch tonically inhibit the cardiovascular center and regulate the arterial blood pressure on a beat-to-beat basis. In the absence of these reflexes the blood pressure is much more labile. From animal model experiments it appears that

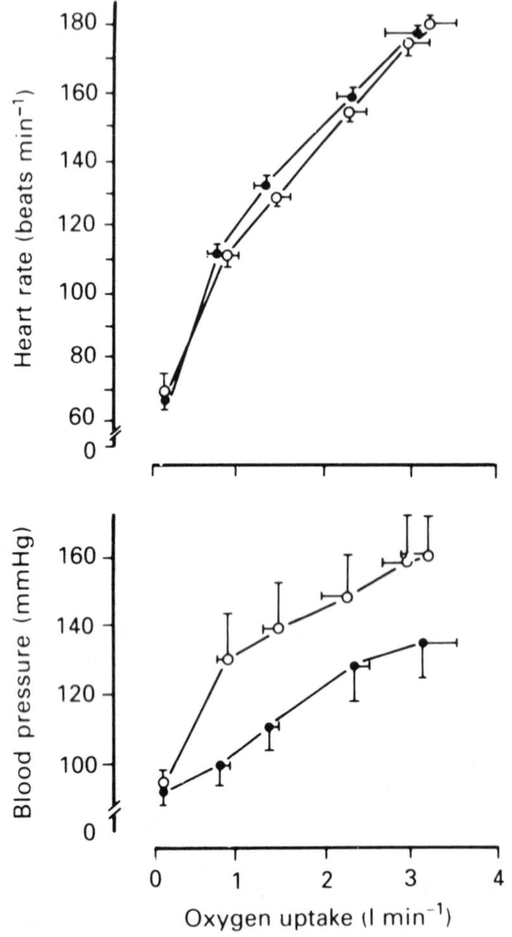

Figure 17.7 Effect of epidural anesthesia on the cardiovascular responses during a progressive exercise test to exhaustion in six subjects. Exercise was performed during control (o) and during epidural anesthesia (•). Values are means +/− SEM.
Note. From "Cardiovascular and Ventilatory Responses to Dynamic Exercise During Epidural Anesthesia in Man" by A. Fernandes, H. Galbo, M. Kjaer, J.H. Mitchell, N.H. Secher, and S.N. Thomas, 1990, *Journal of Physiology*, 420, p. 281. Reprinted by permission.

at the onset of exercise, whether dynamic or static, the arterial baroreflex is reset rapidly (25). The shape of the stimulus-response curve is unchanged, but the operating point or set point appears to be elevated progressively as the severity of the exercise increases (26). This upward shift of the stimulus-response curve, which only recently has been demonstrated in humans to be a parallel upward shift (27), permits the arterial blood pressure to reach higher levels during exercise without a change in the gain (Figure 17.8). This allows acute changes in pressure to be buffered as effectively during exercise as observed during rest (28).

Furthermore, the arterial mechanoreceptors appear to set a limit to the blood pressure increase occurring during exercise and are thought to be providing a buffer to the exercise pressor reflex (24). In studies in dogs during graded exercise in which the aortic arch mechanoreceptors were chronically denervated and the carotid sinuses were isolated from the circulation (29), there were large increases in arterial blood pressure as the intensity of work increased. Importantly, the cardiac output and heart-rate responses to the exercise were unaltered by the absence of the arterial baroreflexes. It appears, therefore, that the function of the arterial baroreflexes during exercise is to modulate cardiac output and total systemic vascular resistance to insure adequate perfusion pressure of the active skeletal muscle.

Another population of mechanoreceptors, the cardiopulmonary receptors located in the left ventricle, right atrium, and great veins are known to maintain a tonic inhibitory outflow via vagal

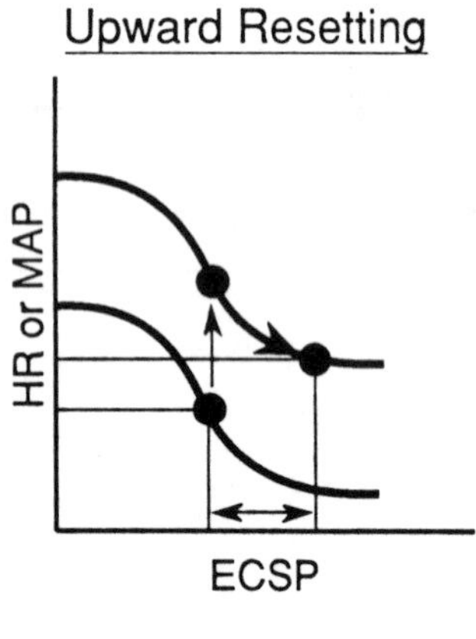

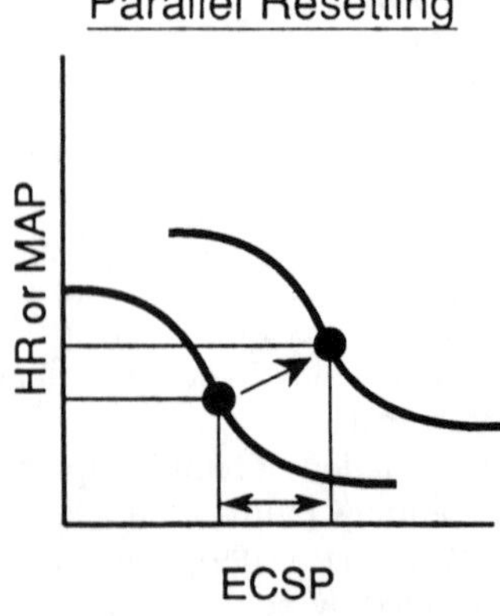

Figure 17.8 A conceptual illustration of two proposed mechanisms of carotid baroreceptor resetting during a steady-state rise in arterial pressure during dynamic exercise. The panel on the top illustrates an "upward resetting," while the panel on the bottom illustrates a "parallel resetting." The bottom panel appears to be the mechanism of resetting in humans.

afferents to the cardiovascular center (Figure 17.3). During upright standing the decreased inhibition allows for an increase in sympathetic outflow in response to prolonged reductions in central blood volume (30); unfortunately, their role during dynamic exercise is unknown. In the presence of normally functioning arterial baroreflexes, the sympathoinhibitory cardiopulmonary reflexes seem to be unnecessary for a normal response to isometric exercise (31); that is, they do not appear to modulate the muscle sympathetic nerve responses. By contrast, the arterial baroreflexes exert an inhibitory influence on the sympathetic activity to the skeletal muscles (32).

Gender

It appears that the qualitative cardiovascular response to static and dynamic exercise of women is similar to that of men. However, differences in development of women, attributed to differences between the sexes in reproductive and anabolic steroid hormone concentrations, raise questions as to whether the differences in anatomical structure and physiological functions result in altered quantitative cardiovascular responses to exercise (5).

Women have smaller blood volumes, heart size, and oxygen-carrying capacity because of lower hemoglobin concentrations and oxygen content of the blood (33,34). Consequently, the objective measure of oxygen delivery capacity ($\dot{V}O_{2max}$) is less in women than in men, even when normalized for body size. Because of women's apparent lower arterial oxygen content at rest and during exercise, the ratio of cardiac output to oxygen uptake ($\dot{Q}/\dot{V}O_2$) during submaximal work is higher in women than in men (33,34). This difference in the $\dot{Q}/\dot{V}O_2$ ratio reflects a hyperkinetic circulation in response to the reduced oxygen delivery. However, as noted for the differences in $\dot{V}O_{2max}$ when comparisons between the sexes are made, adjustments for surface area-to-mass ratio differences on cardiovascular variables need to be made before assuming differences due to gender. Other findings such as lower circulating blood volume resulting in a lower stroke volume and therefore a higher heart rate at the same $\dot{V}O_2$ need to be normalized for differences in body size (5,33–35).

The epidemiologic findings show that clinically relevant autonomic dysfunction diseases such as migraine (36), mitral valve prolapse (37,38), Reynaud's disease (36), multiple sclerosis, and postmenopausal hypertension (39) are more prevalent in women than in men. This suggests that the neural control of circulation during exercise (11) may be qualitatively and quantitatively different in the two genders. However, little or no information exists regarding this question. We are in need of data concerning the physiological function of the autonomic nervous system in women during exercise. Furthermore, the preceding ideas describing the interaction of central command, the exercise pressor reflex, and baroreflex function in the neural control of circulation during exercise have been based on findings that only use men as experimental subjects (11). Hence, whether the autonomic nervous system's function in women is different from men at rest and during exercise needs to be evaluated.

Age

During the developmental years the $\dot{Q}/\dot{V}O_2$ ratio is high compared to the adult years and reflects a hyperkinetic circulation to compensate for a reduced oxygen-carrying capacity resulting from lesser hemoglobin content and smaller blood volumes. As a person's age increases above 65 years, depending on lifetime activity history, structural and functional changes within the cardiovascular system result.

Maximal attainable heart rate (HR_{max}) progressively declines (a population average decline in HR_{max} can be expressed as $220 - Age = HR_{max}$.) Left ventricular function is impaired in that the heart (a) becomes less compliant as it becomes more rigid, (b) has a reduced intrinsic contractile function; (c) responds less to catecholamines, and (d) works against an increasing afterload because of increased impedance of the arterial tree and a reduced vasodilatory capacity in the peripheral arterioles (40). As aging occurs, the $\dot{Q}/\dot{V}O_2$ ratio is reduced and reflects a hypokinetic circulation which is compensated for by an increased oxygen extraction at the working tissues during submaximal exercise. Clearly, cardiac output and arteriovenous oxygen differences are maximized at lower work loads resulting in a reduced maximal oxygen-carrying capacity (41).

Average isometric strength is greater in men than in women and is probably related to man's greater mass of lean tissue (42). Isometric strength increases to a maximum through ages 30 to 40 years but then declines progressively as age advances. However, when one incorporates a strength-training program, or one's lifetime employment requires strength maneuvers throughout the working day, the age-related decline in isometric strength is reduced or absent. There is little information regarding the aging effect on the cardiovascular response to isometric exercise (42,43). However, animal studies indicate that regulatory mechanisms react differently to increases in blood pressure similar to those observed in static exercise in the elderly compared to the young adult. Baroreflex responsiveness appears attenuated in the elderly. In addition, there is a reduction in parasympathetic control of heart rate with increasing age (43,44).

Cardiovascular Adaptation to Exercise Training

Dynamic Exercise Training

Dynamic exercise or aerobic training results in several cardiovascular adaptations evident both at rest and during exercise (Table 17.1, Figure 17.9). Resting cardiac output is relatively unchanged by exercise training, whereas maximal cardiac output can be twice as high in a well-trained endurance athlete compared to an untrained subject of the same body size. The individual's genetic propensity for response to exercise training (4) and the length of time spent training are important factors in inducing an increase in maximal cardiac output (45).

Maximal cardiac output is the product of maximal heart rate and maximal stroke volume. Maximal heart rate is not affected by endurance training, hence the higher maximal cardiac outputs are a result of the heart's ability to eject a larger maximal stroke volume (Table 17.1 and Figure 17.9). Several factors are responsible for an increased maximal stroke volume. First, resting cardiac dimensions are increased; left ventricular chamber size is greater in endurance-trained subjects, indicated by greater end-diastolic volumes at rest and during exercise.

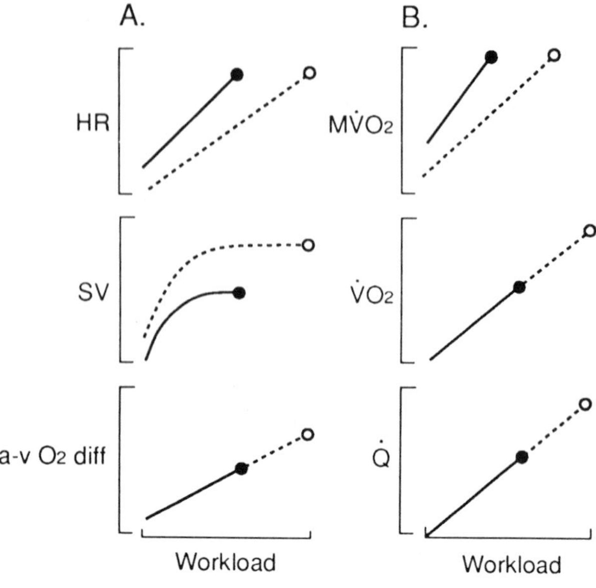

Figure 17.9 Cardiovascular responses to increasing work loads to a maximum. • = untrained subject; o = endurance trained subject; solid line = submaximal responses in untrained subject; dashed line = submaximal responses in trained subject; $\dot{Q}$ = cardiac output; HR = heart rate; SV = stroke volume; A-$\dot{V}O_2$ = total body oxygen consumption; $M\dot{V}O_2$ = myocardial oxygen consumption.
Note. From "Cardiorespiratory Adaptations to Training" by M.L. Smith and J.H. Mitchell. In *Resource Manual for Guidelines for Exercise Testing and Prescription* (pp. 62-65) by American College of Sports Medicine (Ed.), 1988, Philadelphia: Lea & Febiger. Reprinted by permission.

Endurance-trained athletes have a larger absolute left ventricular mass (eccentric hypertrophy) and left ventricular mass normalized to lean body mass than sedentary subjects (46,47) regardless of gender (Figure 17.10). The increased left ventricular mass and increased chamber size that develops

Table 17.1 Endurance Training–Induced Changes in Some Cardiovascular Variables

Variables	Resting	Submaximal exercise	Maximal exercise
Oxygen consumption	No change	No change	Increase
Heart rate	Decrease	Decrease	No change
Stroke volume	Increase	Increase	Increase
Cardiac output	No change	No change	Increase
Cardiac contractility	??	??	??
Muscle blood flow	No change	No change	Increase
Splanchnic blood flow	No change	No change	Decrease
Oxygen extraction	No change	No change	Increase

with endurance training occurs gradually over months or years of training. Also the increased left ventricular mass in endurance athletes correlates with the maximal oxygen uptake as shown in Figure 17.11. The increased maximal stroke volume is directly related to the increased chamber size and an increased preload. Evidence exists to suggest that the preload increase after endurance training is related to an increase in total blood volume consequent to an increased plasma volume (48). Also, effective left ventricular diastolic compliance (or the ability of the chamber to accept blood) appears to be increased after endurance training, a factor that enhances submaximal or maximal preload. The question as to whether cardiac contractility during rest or submaximal or maximal exercise is increased after training remains unanswered.

Cardiac output and the $\dot{Q}/\dot{V}O_2$ at submaximal work loads are not changed by endurance training. Hence, stroke volume is elevated at all levels of submaximal work in the trained state and heart rates are decreased. The result is an increased "efficiency" of the heart at submaximal work loads and results in a decreased double product (heart rate × arterial pressure) at submaximal work loads. As myocardial oxygen consumption is strongly correlated with the double product (HR × MAP), an important benefit of endurance training is the reduced work of the heart at any submaximal work load (49).

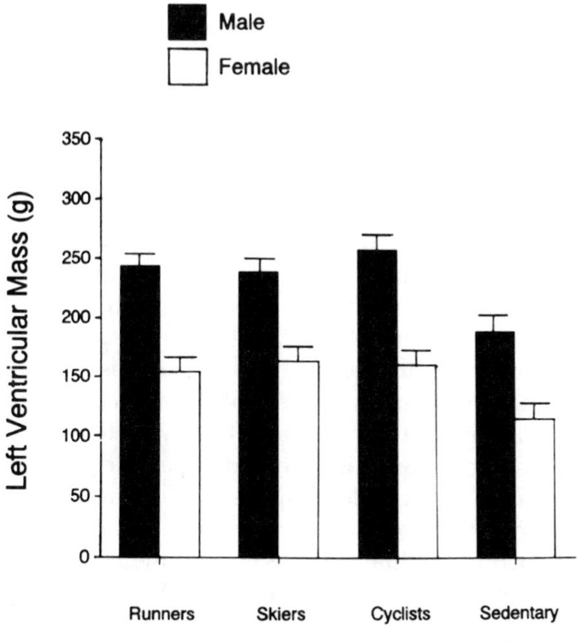

Figure 17.10 Ratios of left ventricular (LV) mass to lean body mass of endurance exercise trained competitive subjects compared to sedentary control subjects using magnetic resonance imaging.
Note. From "Left Ventricular Mass as Determined by Magnetic Resonance Imaging in Male Endurance Athletes" by M.C. Milliken, J. Stray-Gundersen, M. Peshock, J. Katz, and J.H. Mitchell, 1988, *American Journal of Cardiology*, 62, p. 301. Also from "Left Ventricular Dimensions and Mass Using Magnetic Resonance Imaging in Female Endurance Athletes" by M. Riley-Hagan, R.M. Peschock, J. Stray-Gundersen, J. Katz, R.W. Ryschon, and J.H. Mitchell, 1992, *American Journal of Cardiology*, 69, pp. 1067-1074.

Endurance training is associated with an increased maximal vascular conductance (45) and is affected by reduced peripheral resistance during submaximal and maximal exercise. This reduction in peripheral resistance enables the endurance athlete to achieve much higher maximal exercise cardiac outputs than that of a sedentary subject at similar arterial pressures. Although the mechanisms responsible for the augmented vascular conductance are not fully understood, an important factor is certainly the increase in vascularity associated with endurance training (50,51). The increased vascular space augments the fall in peripheral resistance as maximal vasodilation in skeletal muscle is approached during maximal exercise. Alterations in metabolic function at maximal work levels also may affect the maximal level of vasodilation that is achieved. Together these training effects reduce peripheral resistance at maximal work loads, thereby augmenting maximal cardiac output.

The ability to vasodilate (and increase blood flow) in the active tissue does not reach a maximum, however, even at maximal work loads. For example, when the pericardium was removed in untrained dogs, a greater rise in cardiac output and a greater fall in peripheral vascular resistance occurred at maximal exercise (52). In fact, the vasculature of the contracting skeletal muscle appears to maintain some degree of tonic vasoconstriction which has been shown to be increased when the active muscle mass was increased (7). Saltin (6) has proposed that if most of the skeletal muscle of the body was engaged in maximal dynamic exercise, a cardiac output of more than 60 L/min would be required to prevent a measurable fall in blood pressure. These findings strongly support the hypothesis that the pump capacity of the heart is the primary limitation to $\dot{V}O_{2max}$ in humans and remains the primary limitation in the trained human. However, Dempsey et al. (53) have noted significant arterial desaturation during maximal aerobic exercise of the highly trained endurance athlete. These data suggest that the lungs may also present some limitation to the achievement of maximal oxygen uptake in the well-trained endurance athlete.

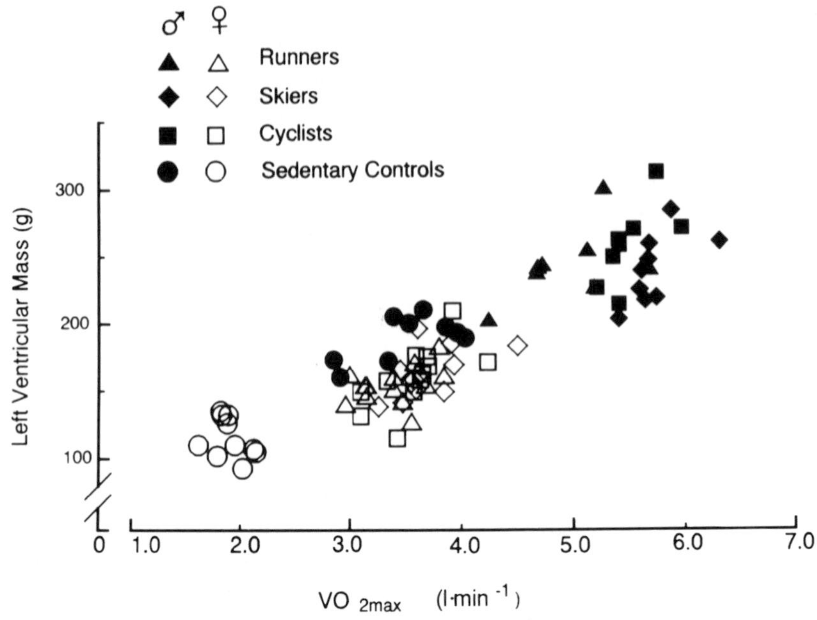

Figure 17.11 Left ventricular mass in grams (g) compared to maximal oxygen uptake ($\dot{V}O_2max$) in L/min (l·min^{-1}) in male and female sedentary subjects and endurance athletes.
Note. From "Left Ventricular Mass as Determined by Magnetic Resonance Imaging in Male Endurance Athletes" by M.C. Milliken, J. Stray-Gundersen, M. Peshock, J. Katz, and J.H. Mitchell, 1988, *American Journal of Cardiology*, 62, p. 301. Also from "Left Ventricular Dimensions and Mass Using Magnetic Resonance Imaging in Female Endurance Athletes" by M. Riley-Hagan, R.M. Peschock, J. Stray-Gundersen, J. Katz, R.W. Ryschon, and J.H. Mitchell, 1992, *American Journal of Cardiology*, 69, p. 1967.

Maximal total body oxygen extraction (the arteriovenous oxygen difference) increases after endurance training. This effect is brought about in part by an increase in the diffusion gradient for oxygen between the capillaries and the active skeletal muscle cells. The total myoglobin (the oxygen-carrying protein complex in skeletal muscle) content of trained muscle also increases and these changes will enhance the diffusion capacity of oxygen within the working muscle (54,55). Also, tissue oxygen extraction is increased by the increased capillary density that occurs with endurance training, and the total number and density (total number per gram of tissue) of capillaries increases (50,51). The increased capillary density results in an increased capillary diffusion surface area that is advantageous for nutrient and metabolic by-product exchange. Furthermore, Musch, Haidet, Ordway, Longhurst, and Mitchell (56) have demonstrated that endurance training increases the degree of shunting of blood away from the splanchnic and renal circulations at maximal exercise and will increase blood flow to the active skeletal muscle. This improved redistribution of blood flow during exercise acts in concert with the increased tissue oxygen extraction to augment total body arteriovenous oxygen difference. Hence, several training-induced adaptations within the skeletal muscle contribute to an augmented maximal arteriovenous oxygen difference.

Static Exercise Training

Training for weight lifting using progressive resistance concentric exercise or isometric (static) exercise increases lean muscle mass primarily by muscle fiber hypertrophy (57,58) and hyperplasia (of 5%–15%) via stem cell activation (59). This increase in lean body mass is associated with concentric cardiac hypertrophy of the left ventricle (60). Relatively little change is observed in aerobic capacity or the cardiovascular responses to dynamic exercise or lower body negative pressure in the weight-trained individual (61). Because of the increase in maximal voluntary contraction (MVC) capability of the weight-trained individual, the heart rate and blood pressure response to a given absolute force of contraction will be less following static exercise training. However, similar to the dynamic exercise response to training when expressed as the same relative force (same % MVC), the heart rate and blood pressure response will be the same at pre- and poststatic exercise training.

Effect of Exercise Training on Neural Control

Endurance-trained individuals often have a reduced heart rate at rest and at any level of submaximal exercise (45,59). The resting bradycardia has been attributed to a shift of autonomic balance in favor of the parasympathetic nervous system, a possible decrease in intrinsic heart rate (the rate obtained with complete ablation of the autonomic nervous system) and the increased central blood volume. However, the classic experimental models of cardiovascular regulation using isometric exercise and dynamic exercise (11) have not been carried out prior to and following exercise training, and only a few investigations have reported cross-sectional differences in the reflex control of blood pressure in endurance-trained men.

The primary findings of these cross-sectional investigations suggest reduced vasoconstriction and attenuated arterial and cardiopulmonary baroreflex responsiveness during lower body negative pressure–induced orthostatic hypotension (62–64). These findings have recently been confirmed in one longitudinal investigation prior to and following 8 months of aerobic training (65). Consistently, aerobic training produces increases in blood volume (48), decreases in resting heart rate, and increases in resting sinus bradycardia, an index of an increased vagal tone (66). Mechanistically the findings of reduced reflex control of blood pressure during orthostasis can be related to altered (a) sensory organ functions, (b) effector end-organ functions, and (c) central integration of afferent nerve traffic resulting in different efferent nerve traffic. All of these factors are components of the autonomic nervous system's control of circulation (11). Whether dynamic or static exercise training alters the autonomic nervous system's control of circulation, the neuropeptide regulation of baroreflexes or blood volume distribution during exercise is unknown.

Gender

The qualitative response to dynamic exercise training is relatively the same for men and women (5,33–35,67). Some investigations suggest that men increase their $\dot{V}O_{2max}$ by increasing stroke volume as a result of the increased blood volume and oxygen extraction A-VO_2diff.$_{max}$ while women only increase their stroke volume capacity (34). The cyclical effects of the hormones in postpubescent women and the subsequent retention and diuresis of body fluids result in cyclic variations in blood volume. Therefore, one questions whether the adaptive response to the dynamic exercise training of an increased blood volume and an increased oxygen content of the blood is similar in both men and women. However, in a review of 20 endurance-training studies, only 4 investigations used women as subjects and found qualitatively similar increases in blood volume (48). However, because of differences in training duration, age of the subjects, and lack of hormonal information it was impossible to establish important comparative differences (5,41,47,48,68,69).

Similar concerns regarding training duration, age of subjects, and lack of hormonal information make it difficult to compare the gender-related differences to resistance exercise training. It is well known that the absolute mass of skeletal muscle is different between postpubescent women and men; yet when strength is normalized for cross-sectional area the differences in strength were accounted for (42).

The mechanism(s) underlying the greater skeletal muscle hypertrophy in men is unknown. Skeletal muscle and cardiac muscle possess receptors for both androgens and estrogens (70–72). Because the role of androgens in stimulating protein synthesis is well known, the higher circulating androgens may account for the greater skeletal muscle hypertrophy in men compared with women. However, whether the concentric hypertrophy of the cardiac muscle due to resistance training in men and women is the same is unknown. Importantly, the higher circulating estrogens in women may be important in regulating energy metabolism rather than protein synthesis in muscle and requires further investigation. Also gender differences in smooth muscle structure and function are unknown.

The cardiovascular responses associated with isometric exercise include an increase in blood pressure. The increase in blood pressure is marked during fatiguing contractions and involves modest increases in heart rate and cardiac output with no change in vascular resistance (10,11). However, despite the apparent increased incidence of clinical manifestations of autonomic dysfunction in women compared with men, there are relatively few documented investigations comparing the cardiovascular responses of men and women to static exercise training.

Age

Earlier studies suggested that elderly individuals (65+ years) had a reduced capability to adapt to dynamic exercise training (41). However, a significantly greater number of investigations have reported marked improvement in physical performance and maximal oxygen uptake following a period of exercise training (73). Indeed, when moderate activity is maintained throughout life it appears that life expectancy and quality of life are increased (74). The central and peripheral cardiovascular adaptations associated with endurance

Table 17.2 The Effect of Aging on the Adaptations of the Cardiovascular System to Dynamic Exercise Training

Measurement	Young	Old
$\dot{V}O_{2max}$	++	+
$\dot{Q}_{max}$	++	+
HR_{max}	0 or –	?
Stroke $volume_{max}$	++	+
Left ventricular contractility	?	?
TPR_{max}	—	?
Exercise muscle blood $flow_{max}$	++	?
HR_{rest}	—	?
Blood pressure	—	?
End diastolic volume	++	?
End systolic volume	0	?
Vasomotor response	++	?
Parasympathetic control	++	?
Sympathetic control	?	?

+ = increase, ++ = large increase, 0 = no effect, – = decrease, — = large decrease, ? = questionable or unknown.

exercise training in the young appear manifest in the elderly (73). However, because the total amount of work involved in training is not equalized in comparisons of how the young and old train, the functional improvements due to training are usually less in the old than in the young.

One consistent finding with highly active elderly individuals and with individuals that have trained throughout life is that age-related decline in maximal heart rate is present (41). It appears, therefore, that neural control of circulation may decline with age regardless of activity history throughout life. Whether this implied loss of neural control of circulation has some role in the increasing incidence of the cardiovascular pathophysiology of the aged needs to be investigated. Furthermore, relatively little information is available concerning the effects of age on the adaptation of the cardiovascular system to dynamic or static exercise training. A summary of the findings of our current knowledge is shown in Table 17.2.

References

1. Taylor, H.L.; Buskirk, E.R.; Henschel, H.A. Maximal oxygen uptake as an objective measure of cardiopulmonary performance. J. Appl. Physiol. 8:73-80; 1955.
2. Mitchell, J.H.; Blomqvist, G.B. Maximal oxygen uptake. N. Engl. J. Med. 284:1018-1022; 1971.
3. Mitchell, J.H.; Sproule, B.J.; Chapman, C.B. The physiological meaning of the maximal oxygen intake test. J. Clin. Invest. 37:538-547; 1958.
4. Dionne, F.T.; Turlotte, L.; Thiboult, M.C.; Boulay, M.R.; Skinner, J.S.; Bouchard, C. Mitochondrial DNA sequence polymorphism, $\dot{V}O_{2max}$, and response to endurance exercise training. Med. Sci. Sports Exerc. 23:177-185; 1991.
5. Mitchell, J.H.; Tate, C.; Raven, P.B. Acute response and chronic adaptation to exercise in women. Med. Sci. Sports Exerc. [Suppl.]. 24:S258-S265; 1992.
6. Saltin, B. Physiological adaptation to physical conditioning: Old problems revisited. Acta Med. Scand. [Suppl]. 711:11-24; 1986.
7. Secher, N.H.; Clausen, J.P.; Klausen, K.; Noer, I.; Trap-Jensen, J. Central and regional circulatory effects of adding arm exercise to leg exercise. Acta Physiol. Scand. 100:288-297; 1977.
8. Asmussen, E. Similarities and dissimilarities between static and dynamic exercise. Circ. Res. 48:I3-I10; 1981.
9. Mitchell, J.H.; Schibye, B.; Payne, F.C., III; Saltin, B. Response of arterial blood pressure to static exercise in relation to muscle mass, force development, and electromyographic activity. Circ. Res. 48:I70-I75; 1981.

10. Friedman, D.B.; Peel, C.; Mitchell, J.H. Cardiovascular responses to voluntary and non-voluntary static exercise in humans. J. Appl. Physiol. 73:1982-1985; 1992.
11. Mitchell, J.H. Neural control of the circulation during exercise. Med. Sci. Sports Exerc. 22:141-158; 1990.
12. Longhurst, J.C.; Mitchell, J.H.; Moore, M.B. The spinal cord ventral root: An afferent pathway of the hind-limb pressor reflex in the cats. J. Physiol. 301:467-476; 1980.
13. Kaufman, M.P.; Longhurst, J.C.; Rybicki, K.J.; Wallach, J.H.; Mitchell, J.H. Effects of static muscular contraction on impulse activity of Groups III and IV afferents in cats. J. Appl. Physiol. 55:105-112; 1983.
14. Rybicki, K.J.; Kaufman, M.P.; Kenyon, J.L.; Mitchell, J.H. Arterial pressor responses to increasing interstitial potassium in hindlimb muscles of dogs. Am. J. Physiol. 247:R717-R721; 1984.
15. Rotto, D.M.; Stebbins, C.L.; Kaufman, M.P. Reflex cardiovascular and ventilatory responses to increasing H^+ activity in cat hindlimb muscle. J. Appl. Physiol. 67:256-263; 1989.
16. Galbo, H.; Kjaer, M.; Secher, N.H. Cardiovascular, ventilatory and catecholamine responses to maximal dynamic exercise in partially curarized man. J. Physiol. (Lond.). 389:557-568; 1987.
17. Leonard, B.; Mitchell, J.H.; Mizuno, M.; Rube, N.; Saltin, B.; Secher, N.H. Partial neuromuscular blockade and cardiovascular responses to static exercise in man. J. Physiol. (Lond.). 359:365-379; 1985.
18. Valbo, A.B.; Hagbarth K-E.; Torebjörk, H.E.; Wallin, B.G. Somatosensory proprioceptive and sympathetic activity in human peripheral nerves. Physiol. Rev. 59:919-957; 1979.
19. Mark, A.L.; Victor, R.G.; Nerhed, C.; Wallin, B.G. Microneurographic studies of the mechanisms of sympathetic nerve responses to static exercise in humans. Circ. Res. 57:461-469; 1985.
20. Victor, R.G.; Seals, D.R.; Mark, A.L. Differential control of heart rate and sympathetic nerve activity during dynamic exercise: Insight from intraneural recordings in humans. J. Clin. Invest. 79:508-516; 1987.
21. Vissing, S.F.; Scherrer, U.; Victor, R.G. Stimulation of skin sympathetic nerve discharge by central command. Circ. Res. 69:228-238; 1991.
22. Fernandes, A.; Galbo, H.; Kjaer, M.; Mitchell, J.H.; Secher, N.H.; Thomas, S.N. Cardiovascular and ventilatory responses to dynamic exercise during epidural anaesthesia in man. J. Physiol. 420:281-293; 1990.
23. Mitchell, J.H.; Reeves, D.R., Jr.; Rogers, H.B.; Secher, N.H. Epidural anesthesia and cardiovascular responses to static exercise in man. J. Physiol. (Lond.). 417:13-24; 1989.
24. Rowell, B.; O'Leary, D.S. Reflex control of the circulation during exercise: Chemoreflexes and mechanoreceptors. J. Appl. Physiol. 69:407-418; 1990.
25. DiCarlo, S.E.; Bishop, V.S. Onset of exercise shifts operating point of arterial baroreflex to higher pressures. Am. J. Physiol. 262:H303-H307; 1992.
26. Melcher, A.; Donald, D.E. Maintained ability of carotid baroreflex to regulate arterial pressure during exercise. Am. J. Physiol. (Heart Circ. Physiol., 10). 241:H838-H849; 1991.
27. Potts, J.T.; Shi, X.R.; Raven, P.B. Carotid baroreflex responsiveness I: Modulation of heart rate and blood pressure during dynamic exercise in man. Am. J. Physiol. [Submitted 1992].
28. Joyner, M.J.; Shepherd, J.T. Arterial baroreceptor function and exercise. In: Persson, P.B.; Kirchheim, H.R., eds. Baroreceptor reflexes. Berlin, Heidelberg: Springer-Verlag; 1991:237-255.
29. Walgenbach, S.C.; Donald, D.E. Inhibition by carotid baroreflex of exercise-induced increases in arterial pressure. Clin. Res. 52:253-262; 1983.
30. Joyner, M.J.; Shepherd, J.T.; Seals, D.R. Sustained increases in sympathetic outflow during prolonged lower body negative pressure in humans. J. Appl. Physiol. 68:1004-1009; 1990.
31. Seals, D.R. Cardiopulmonary baroreflexes do not modulate exercise-induced sympathoexcitation. J. Appl. Physiol. 64:2197-2203; 1987.
32. Seals, D.R.; Victor, R.G. Regulation of muscle sympathetic nerve activity during exercise in humans. In: Holloszy, J.O., ed. Exercise and sport sciences reviews. Vol. 19. Baltimore: Williams & Wilkins; 1991:313-349.
33. Åstrand, P.-O.; Rodahl, K. Textbook of work physiology. Physiological basis of exercise. 3rd ed. New York: McGraw-Hill; 1986:1-756.
34. Drinkwater, B.L. Women and exercise: Physiological aspects. Exerc. Sport Sci. Rev. 12:21-51; 1984.
35. Drinkwater, B.L. Physiological responses of women to exercise. Exerc. Sport Sci. Rev. 1:126-154; 1973.
36. Cooke, J.P.; Creager, M.A.; Osmundson, P.J.; Shepherd, J.T. Sex differences in control of cutaneous blood flow. Circulation. 82:1607-1615; 1990.
37. Gaffney, F.A.; Bastian, B.C.; Lane, I.B. Abnormal cardiovascular regulation in the mitral valve prolapse syndrome. Am. J. Cardiol. 52:316-320; 1983.

38. Gaffney, F.A.; Campbell, W.G.; Karlsson, E.S.; Blomqvist, C.G. Sex differences in response to orthostatic stress induced by lower body negative pressure. [Abstract]. Clin. Res. 6:232; 1978.
39. Anastos, K.; Charney, P.; Charon, R.A. Hypertension in women: What is really known? Ann. Intern. Med. 115:287-293; 1991.
40. Weisfeldt, M.L. Left ventricular function. In: Weisfeldt, M.L., ed. Aging. Vol. 12. New York: Raven Press; 1980:297-316.
41. Raven, P.B.; Mitchell, J.H. Effect of aging on the cardiovascular response to dynamic and static exercise in the aging heart: Its function and response to stress. In: Weisfeldt, M.L., ed. Aging. Vol. 12. New York: Raven Press; 1980:269-296.
42. Petrofsky, J.S.; Phillips, C.A. The physiology of static exercise. In: Pandolf, K.B., ed. Exercise sport sciences reviews. Vol. 14. New York: Macmillan; 1986:1-44.
43. Shock, N.W. Physiological aspects of aging in man. Annu. Rev. Physiol. 23:97-123; 1961.
44. Kenny, W.L. Parasympathetic control of resting heart rate: Relationship to aerobic power. Med. Sci. Sports Exerc. 17:451-455; 1985.
45. Blomqvist, C.G.; Saltin, B. Cardiovascular adaptations to physical training. Annu. Rev. Physiol. 45:169-190; 1983.
46. Milliken, M.C.; Stray-Gundersen, J.; Peshock, M.; Katz, J.; Mitchell, J.H. Left ventricular mass as determined by magnetic resonance imaging in male endurance athletes. Am. J. Cardiol. 62:301-305; 1988.
47. Riley-Hagan, M.; Peshock, R.M.; Stray-Gundersen, J.; Katz, J.; Ryschon, R.W.; Mitchell, J.H. Left ventricular dimensions and mass using magnetic resonance imaging in female endurance athletes. Am. J. Cardiol. 69:1067-1074; 1992.
48. Convertino, V.A. Blood volume: Its adaptation to endurance training. Med. Sci. Sports Exerc. 23:1338-1348; 1991.
49. Smith, M.L.; Mitchell, J.H. Cardiorespiratory adaptations to training. In: American College of Sports Medicine, ed. Resource manual for guidelines for exercise testing and prescription. Philadelphia: Lea & Febiger; 1988:62-65.
50. Hudlicka, O. Growth of capillaries in skeletal and cardiac muscle. Circ. Res. 50:451; 1982.
51. Ingjer, J.; Brodal, P. Capillary supply of skeletal muscle fibers in untrained and endurance-trained women. Eur. J. Appl. Physiol. 38:291; 1978.
52. Stray-Gundersen, J.; Musch, T.I.; Haidet, G.C.; Ordway, G.A.; Mitchell, J.H. The effect of pericardiectomy on maximal oxygen consumption and maximal cardiac output in untrained dogs. Circ. Res. 58:523-530; 1986.
53. Dempsey, J.A. Is the lung built for exercise? Med. Sci. Sports Exerc. 18:143-155; 1986.
54. Holloszy, J.O. Adaptation of skeletal muscle to endurance exercise. Med. Sci. Sports Exerc. 7:155; 1975.
55. Meldon, J.H. Theoretical role of myoglobin in steady-state oxygen transport to tissue and its impact upon cardiac output requirements. Acta. Physiol. Scand. 440:S93; 1976.
56. Musch, T.I.; Haidet, G.C.; Ordway, G.A.; Longhurst, J.C.; Mitchell, J.H. Training effects on regional blood flow response to maximal exercise in foxhounds. J. Appl. Physiol. 62:1724-1734; 1987.
57. Gollnick, P.D.; Tunson, B.F.; Moore, R.L.; Reidy, M. Muscular enlargement and number of fibers in skeletal muscles of rats. J. Appl. Physiol. 50:936-943; 1981.
58. Gollnick, P.D.; Parsons, D.; Reidy, M.; Moore, R.L. An evaluation of mechanisms modulating muscle size in response to varying perturbations. In: Borer, R.T.; Edington, D.W.; White, T.P., eds. Frontiers of exercise biology. Champaign, IL: Human Kinetics; 1983:27-50.
59. Mikesky, A.E.; Giddings, C.J.; Matthews, W.; Gonyea, W.J. Changes in muscle fiber size and composition in response to heavy-resistance exercise. Med. Sci. Sports Exerc. 23:1042-1049; 1991.
60. Longhurst, J.C.; Kelly, A.R.; Gonyea, W.J.; Mitchell, J.H. Echocardiographic left ventricular masses in distance runners and weight lifters. J. Appl. Physiol. 48:154-162; 1980.
61. Smith, M.L.; Raven, P.B. Cardiovascular responses to lower body negative pressure in endurance and static exercise trained men. Med. Sci. Sports Exerc. 18:545-550; 1986.
62. Smith, M.L.; Graitzer, H.M.; Hudson, D.L.; Raven, P.B. Baroreflex function in endurance and static exercise trained men. J. Appl. Physiol. 64:585-591; 1988.
63. Smith, M.L.; Graitzer, H.M.; Hudson, D.L.; Raven, P.B. Effect of changes in cardiac autonomic balance on blood pressure regulation in men. J. Auton. Nerv. Syst. 22:107-114; 1988.
64. Smith, M.L.; Hudson, D.L.; Graitzer, H.M.; Raven, P.B. Blood pressure regulation during cardiac autonomic blockade: Effect of fitness. J. Appl. Physiol. 65:1789-1795; 1988.
65. Stevens, G.H.J.; Foresman, B.H.; Raven, P.B. Reduction in LBNP tolerance following prolonged endurance exercise training. Med. Sci. Sports Exerc. 24:1235-1244; 1992.
66. Smith, M.L.; Hudson, D.L.; Graitzer, H.M.; Raven, P.B. Exercise training bradycardia: The role of autonomic balance. Med. Sci. Sports Exerc. 21:40-44; 1989.

67. Martin, D.; Ranwell, G.P.H. Continuous assistive-passive exercise and cycle ergometry training in sedentary women. Med. Sci. Sports Exerc. 22:523-527; 1990.
68. Cress, M.E.; Thomas, D.P.; Johnson, J. Effect of training on $\dot{V}O_{2max}$ thigh strength, and muscle morphology in septuagenarian women. Med. Sci. Sports Exerc. 23:752-758; 1991.
69. Cononie, C.C.; Graves, J.E.; Pollock, M.L.; Phillips, M.I.; Sumners, C.; Hagberg, J.M. Effect of exercise training on blood pressure in 70-79 yr. old men and women. Med. Sci. Sports Exerc. 23:505-511; 1991.
70. Dubé, J.Y.; Lesage, R.; Tremblay, R.R. Androgen and estrogen binding in rat skeletal and perineal muscles. Can. J. Biochem. 54:50-55; 1976.
71. Krieg, M.; Smith, K.; Bartsch, W. Demonstration of a specific androgen receptor in rat heart muscle: Relationship between binding, metabolism and tissue levels of androgens. Endocrinology. 103:1686-1694; 1978.
72. Stumpf, W.E.; Aumuller, G. The heart: A target organ for estradiol. Science. 196:319-321; 1977.
73. Seals, D.R.; Hagberg, J.M.; Hurley, B.F.; Ehsoni, A.A.; Holloszy, J.O. Endurance training in older men and women I. Cardiovascular response to exercise. J. Appl. Physiol. Respir. Environ. Exerc. Physiol. 57:1024-1029; 1984.
74. Paffenbarger, R.S.; Hyde, R.T.; Wing, A.L.; Hsieh, C.-C. Physical activity all cause mortality and longevity of college alumni. N. Engl. J. Med. 314:605-613; 1986.

Chapter 18

Physical Activity and the Microcirculation in Cardiac and Skeletal Muscle

M. Harold Laughlin
Richard M. McAllister
Michael D. Delp

Exercise training (ET) has several well-known effects on the cardiovascular system that may promote the transport of nutrients to active striated muscle tissue. The primary function of vascular beds in cardiac and skeletal muscle is to supply muscle cells with nutrients and remove metabolic products. This transport is accomplished by at least two steps or processes: convective transport of blood to and through the capillaries (blood flow capacity), and transcapillary exchange between blood and tissue (capillary exchange capacity) (54,59,61,63). Current information indicates that ET of mammalian species induces adaptive changes in coronary and skeletal muscle vascular beds that improve the ability of these vascular beds to transport nutrients and metabolites.

Mechanisms for vascular adaptation induced by chronic increases in metabolic rate in striated muscle tissue can be grouped into two major categories: *structural adaptations* and *adaptations in the control of vascular resistance*. Structural vascular adaptation occurs in response to ET in at least two forms: *vascular remodeling and growth* (i.e., growth of vessels such as increased length and/or cross-sectional area of the existing large and small arteries and veins), and *angiogenesis* (i.e., increased numbers of capillaries and other microvessels per gram of muscle). Adaptive changes in the control of vascular resistance can be the result of altered neurohumoral control of the vascular bed, altered local control via changes in metabolic control systems, altered myogenic responses to mechanical stimuli, intrinsic changes in vascular smooth muscle cells and/or endothelial cells, or the effects of structural changes on the distribution of resistance throughout the microcirculation.

The approach of this review is to consider effects of ET on blood flow capacity (BFC), capillary diffusion capacity (CDC), and the contributions of structural vascular adaptation and alterations in control of vascular resistance to changes in transport capabilities in cardiac and skeletal muscle vascular beds. In addition, we examine and evaluate models of ET and methods used in the various studies to provide an assessment of the scientific quality of each study.

Assessment of Quality

Models of Exercise Training

The cardiorespiratory effects of ET can be influenced by species differences, adequacy of and type of ET program investigated, and age of the animal. In this review, a subject is considered to be in an endurance-trained state if repeated bouts of dynamic exercise have resulted in one or more of the following adaptations: increased skeletal muscle oxidative capacity and/or whole body maximal oxygen consumption, increased exercise tolerance, training bradycardia, cardiac hypertrophy, increased maximal cardiac output, and/or improved cardiac function. It is well known that many adaptations induced by ET are specific to the type of contractile activity involved in ET bouts (11). This is especially true of adaptations within skeletal muscle tissue (11). Similarly, the cardiovascular adaptations induced by rhythmic exercise (walking, running, swimming, or cycling) are different from those induced by resistance training.

It is important to determine if animal studies included in our deliberations have used models of ET which closely mimic known adaptations induced by endurance ET in humans. For example, the model of swim training rats does not mimic many human training responses (11). Also, weight training does not induce cardiovascular adaptations comparable to those seen with endurance ET (37,45). Even the treadmill-trained rat model does not mimic many of the cardiac adaptations seen in humans and large mammals (58,100).

Table 18.1 presents 21 studies of the effects of ET on coronary BFC. It can be seen that no independent estimate of the efficacy of the ET program was measured in one third of these studies. Many studies report heart weight:body weight ratios as evidence of a training effect. Heart weight:body weight data must be interpreted carefully since ET has effects on body weight in many models of ET (100). Even fewer of the studies presented in Table 18.2 present independent evidence of training efficacy. It is surprising that this is such a common weakness among studies of the effects of ET on skeletal muscle vascular beds and the coronary circulation.

It is well established that coronary structural vascular adaptation in rats is blunted in mature animals. Thus, some vascular adaptations induced by exercise in immature rodents may not reflect the type of vascular adaptation induced in mature humans and other large mammals.

Measurement of Blood Flow Capacity

Procedures utilized to estimate BFC should include control of key hemodynamic parameters to ensure that measurements are made under comparable conditions in trained and control animals so that vascular resistance is the major determinant of blood flow. In quality measurements of coronary BFC, factors that determine heart work and myocardial metabolic rate (arterial pressure, sympathetic tone to the heart, venous return, circulating catecholamines, arterial oxygen content, coronary perfusion pressures, and heart rate) must be controlled. The phrase "maximal blood flow" should be used to refer to a specific blood flow value measured during maximal vasodilation at a defined, physiologic perfusion pressure (90-120 mmHg). If maximal blood flow is to be estimated, it is essential to control perfusion pressure, because once maximal vasodilation has been produced, both blood flow and resistance are related to arterial pressure (61,63). BFC can best be estimated by measuring blood flow as a function of perfusion pressure during maximal vasodilation. The mathematical expression describing the relationship between blood flow and perfusion pressure can then be compared between control and trained groups. Maximal vasodilation correctly refers to the maximal response—that which is seen at (and beyond) the plateau in a dose response curve (61,63,65,98).

Effects of Training on the Coronary Microcirculation

Coronary Blood Flow Capacity

A summary of investigations of the effects of ET on coronary BFC is presented in Table 18.1. In forming this table animal models used, programs employed in ET, and methods used to measure coronary BFC were critically evaluated. The quality of each study was assessed by evaluating the quality of training and adequacy of coronary BFC measurements. Among studies reporting an unchanged coronary BFC in trained subjects (Table 18.1 A), only the study of Cohen (22) avoided complications of changes in myocardial oxygen consumption and extravascular resistance effects by using intracoronary infusion of vasodilator drugs. Cohen (22) also clearly demonstrated maximal adenosine vasodilation in mongrel dogs and greyhounds, but found no difference in coronary BFC. However, as pointed out by Cohen (22), the cardiac hypertrophy of greyhounds is partially determined by genetic factors and partially related to the animals' level of physical activity. As a result, it is a tenuous conclusion that these observations may correspond to what may happen with ET in other mammals. Thus, examination of these studies reporting no change in coronary BFC in ET animals reveals that all are flawed according to one or more of the stated quality assessment criteria.

It has been reported that during submaximal exercise, coronary blood flow is less in ET dogs than in untrained dogs and that during exercise at maximal intensities coronary blood flow is greater than or equal to that seen in untrained dogs (6,7,67,114). Similarly, Breisch, White, Nimmo, McKirnan, and Bloor (14) reported that transmural coronary blood flow during exercise at intensities producing maximal heart rates was not significantly different in trained and untrained pigs, and that transmural coronary blood flows were similar in trained and control pigs during systemic infusion of adenosine during exercise at this intensity. It is difficult to definitively interpret the results of these conscious animal experiments because critical hemodynamic factors could not be adequately controlled. As a result, coronary blood flows may have been influenced, at least in part, by factors other than coronary vascular resistance (61,63,65, 90,99).

Laughlin and colleagues have reported that ET dogs (55,65) and miniature swine (61) have an increased coronary BFC. In these studies (55,61,65), the determinants of myocardial oxygen demand, diastolic time, and extravascular resistance were

Table 18.1 Investigations of Effects of Exercise Training on Coronary Blood Flow Capacity (CBFC)

References	Species	Type of training	†Training program	**Efficacy of program	‡Hypertrophy	*$Quality assessment: Training model	*$Quality assessment: CBFC measurement
A. Studies reporting unchanged blood flow capacity in trained animals							
Bove et al. (13)	Dog	Run	8 mph, 4%; 75 min/d, 5 d/wk; 8 wk	HR, SM$\dot{V}O_2$	Y	E	G
Stone (114)	Dog	Run	?; 75 min/d, 5 d/wk; 8 wk	HR	Y	G	G
Barnard et al. (6)	Dog	Run	?; 2 hr/d, 5 d/wk; 12–18 wk	SM$\dot{V}O_2$, HR, $\dot{V}O_2$max	Y	E	G
Yipintsoi et al. (130)	Rat	Swim	?; 150 min/d, 5 d/wk; 10 wk	NM	Y	U	U
Carey et al. (16)	Dog	Run	8 mph, 10%; 50 min/d, 5 d/wk; 8 wk	HR	N	G	U
Liang et al. (67)	Dog	Run	?; 90 min/day, 5 d/wk; 12 wk	HR	N	G	U
Breisch et al. (14)	Pig	Run	70–80% max; 60 min/d, 5 d/wk; 12 wk	$\dot{V}O_2$max, HR	Y	E	U
Cohen (22)	Dog	Run	Greyhound compared to mongrels	NM	Y	U	E
B. Studies reporting increased blood flow capacity in trained animals							
Penpargkul & Scheuer (86)	Rat	Swim	?; 150 min/d, 5 d/wk; 10 wk	Cardiac function	Y	G	G
Spear et al. (110)	Rat	Run	26.8 m/min, 15%; 60 min/d, 5 d/wk; 18 wk	NM	Y	G	U
Laughlin et al. (57)	Dog	Run	10–20 km/hr, 10–20%; 75 min/d, 5 d/wk; 10 wk	SM$\dot{V}O_2$	Y	E	G
Schaible & Scheuer (97)	Rat	Swim	?; 150 min/d, 5 d/wk; 8 wk	HR, cardiac function	Y	G	E
	Rat	Run	20 m/min, 10%; 150 min/d, 5 d/wk; 8 wk	HR, cardiac function	Y	E	E

Scheel et al. (98)	Dog	Run	3.6 mph, 25%; 45 min/d, 5 d/wk; 6 wk	NM	N	U	G
Liang & Stone (68)	Dog	Run	?; 60 min/d, 5 d/wk; 4 wk	NM	N	U	U
Laughlin (55)	Dog	Run	6 mph, 10–20%; 75 min/d, 5 d/wk; 12–20 wk	$SM\dot{V}O_2$	N	G	E
Buttrick et al. (15)	Rat	Swim	?; 150 min/d, 5 d/wk; 8–10 wk	Cardiac function	Y	G	E
Laughlin & Tomanek (65)	Dog	Run	6 mph, 10–20%; 75 min/d, 5 d/wk; 12–20 wk	$SM\dot{V}O_2$	N	G	E
Laughlin et al. (61)	Pig	Run	4–6 mph, 0%; 85 min/d, 5 d/wk; 16–20 wk	$SM\dot{V}O_2$, HR	Y	E	E
DiCarlo et al. (26)	Dog	Run	?; 5 d/wk; 4 wk	NM	N	U	E
Baur et al. (8)	Rat	Run	27 m/min, 10%; 60 min/d, 5 d/wk; 16 wk	NM	N	U	G

†Training programs are described as: intensity (run = speed and grade), duration of training sessions, frequency of training sessions, and duration of training in weeks. **Efficacy of training programs as reported in the publications: HR = training bradycardia, $SM\dot{V}O_2$ = skeletal muscle oxidative capacity, $\dot{V}O_2max$ = whole body maximal oxygen consumption, NM = training efficacy was not measured in the study, cardiac function = improved cardiac function was measured in trained groups. ‡Hypertrophy refers to presence of cardiac hypertrophy: Y = hypertrophy present, N = no hypertrophy. *$Quality assessment: E = excellent, G = good, U = unsatisfactory. *Training model*: The quality of the training model was assessed with the following four criteria: (1) adequacy of the exercise stimulus, (2) similarity of the training program to human aerobic training, (3) quantifiable measures to demonstrate efficacy of training, and (4) does the model of training appear to have cardiorespiratory adaptations similar to those known to occur in humans? *Coronary blood flow capacity measurement* was assessed with the following three criteria: (1) Was maximal vasodilation rigorously defined? (2) Were hemodynamic parameters controlled (and/or comparable) in trained and sedentary animals during the measurement? (3) Was coronary blood flow capacity directly measured?

comparable in ET and sedentary animals. The estimates made by DiCarlo, Blair, Bishop, and Stone of coronary BFC are excellent because complications of changes in myocardial oxygen consumption, extravascular resistance effects, and mean arterial pressure, were avoided by using intracoronary infusion of vasodilator drugs in conscious dogs (26). DiCarlo et al. (26) used dose-response curves to establish maximal vasodilator effects with adenosine and beta-adrenergic agonists and found that both produced greater vasodilation in dogs following 4 weeks of training. These results suggest that coronary BFC was increased by ET. Among other studies finding increased coronary BFC, the studies of Buttrick, Schaible, and Scheuer (15) and Scheel et al. (98) also clearly established maximal vasodilation and conducted the measurements under comparable conditions in control and trained subjects. As a result, it is likely that the greater blood flow measured in ET coronary vascular beds as compared to controls was the result of lower minimal coronary vascular resistance.

In conclusion, studies of the effects of training on coronary BFC were judged based upon the following characteristics: (a) Adequate training programs were employed and ET was established by independent measures of training effectiveness, (b) maximal vasodilation was clearly established, and (c) direct measurements of BFC were made with adequate control of hemodynamic factors under comparable conditions in sedentary control and ET animals. Studies with good to excellent assessment of training and excellent assessment of coronary BFC estimates report that ET induces an increase in coronary BFC (15,55,61,65). Our review of available data indicates that the results of the more rigorously controlled studies of ET have consistently found greater coronary BFC in exercise trained subjects.

Coronary Capillary Diffusion Capacity

Capillary permeability–surface area product for EDTA, a functional index of coronary capillary diffusion capacity (CDC), has been found to be increased in ET dogs (55,65) and miniature swine (61). An increase in CDC could result from an increase in capillary permeability and/or increased capillary surface area available for exchange. An increase in capillary surface area available for exchange could be the result of capillary proliferation, that is, angiogenesis (discussed later) and/or from alterations in control of the microvascular bed so that the distribution of blood flow through the perfused exchange vessels is more closely matched to each capillary's exchange capacity (65). Because CDC increases as a function of flow in a maximally vasodilated coronary bed (65), it is possible that ET alters the distribution of resistance in the coronary vascular bed so that at any given coronary perfusion pressure the microvascular pressure is higher, resulting in more capillary exchange area exposed to blood. Indeed, current information indicates that the most reasonable explanation for the increased CDC in the trained heart is a change in distribution of blood flow in the capillary bed (i.e., altered microvascular control of blood flow and its distribution) (65).

Structural Coronary Vascular Adaptation

Tepperman and Pearlman were among the first to advocate the concept that ET results in increases in coronary vessel size and/or numbers (118). Several subsequent studies of ET (summarized in Table 18.2) with rats and other rodent models report similar results.

Small Coronary Arteries and Arterioles

Although most coronary vascular resistance is considered to reside in the small arteries and arterioles of the microcirculation, there have been few studies of the effects of ET on the size and/or number of these vessels. Breisch et al. (14) and White et al. (123) have reported that ET in miniature swine and domestic pigs causes increases in morphometrically determined arteriolar numerical densities. Coronary arterioles were defined as vessels with at least three layers of vascular smooth muscle and with diameters greater than 35 μm and less than 75 μm. Both arteriolar number density and arteriolar length density were found to be increased approximately 40% (14). These data indicate that ET may induce remodeling and/or growth of vascular control vessels of the coronary microcirculation. These and similar changes in other microvascular control vessels could have important functional significance on control of coronary blood flow and capillary exchange.

Coronary Capillary (and/or Microvascular Exchange) Vessels

There are many reports in the literature presenting capillary density (number of capillaries per square millimeter of tissue) and other morphometric indexes of myocardial capillarization in ET animals that indicate that ET either results in increases in capillarization or maintenance of normal levels of capillarization (5,39,99,120). Although it is clear

Table 18.2 Investigations of Exercise Training-Induced Structural Microvascular Adaptations in the Coronary Circulation

Reference	Species	Type of training	Frequency (d/wk)	Session duration & intensity	Training duration	**Efficacy of training	‡Cardiac hypertrophy	Technique	*Capillaries
Tepperman & Pearlman (118)	Rat	Run	Activity cages	0.5–1.5 miles/d	5 wk	NM	Y	Cast	No change relative to heart wt
	Rat	Swim	5–6	60 min/d	11 wk	NM	Y	Cast	Increase in total cast wt/heart wt
Stevenson et al. (113)	Rat	Run	2	10.5 m/min, 1.3 km/d	4 wk	NM	N	Cast	Increase in cast wt/heart wt
		Run	5	10.5 m/min, 1.3 km/d	2–4 wk	NM	N	Cast	No change
		Swim	5	60 min	4 wk	NM	N	Cast	Increase in cast wt/heart wt
		Swim	2	60 min	4 wk	NM	N	Cast	Increase in cast wt/heart wt
		Swim	4	120 min × 2/d	4 wk	NM	Y	Cast	Increase in cast wt/heart wt
Leon & Bloor (66)	Rat	Swim	5	60 min/d	10 wk	NM	Y	Perfusion fixation	↑C/F
		Swim	2	60 min/d	10 wk	NM	N	Perfusion fixation	↑C/F
Tomanek (121)	Rat	Run	6	1.0–1.5 mph, 40–50 min/d, 8% grade	12 wk	HR	N	Ink perfusion	↑C/F, ↔CND
Wyatt & Mitchell (129)	Dog	Run	5	4–8 mph, 1 hr/d, 10% grade	12 wk	NM	N	Fixation	↔CND
Carlsson et al. (17)	Rat	Swim	6	1 hr/d	2 wk	NM	N	^{3}H-thymidine	↑labeling
Wachtlova et al. (122)	Rabbit	Run	Spontaneous	Wild vs. caged	N/A	N/A	Y	PAS stain	↑C/F, ↑CND
Ho et al. (37)	Rat	Run	7	60 min, 36 m/min	16 wk	NM	N	Cast	Increase in cast wt/heart wt
	Rat	Weight train	7	—	16 wk	NM	N	Cast	No change in cast wt/heart wt

(continued)

Table 18.2 *(Continued)*

Reference	Species	Type of training	Frequency (d/wk)	Session duration & intensity	Training duration	**Efficacy of training	‡Cardiac hypertrophy	Technique	*Capillaries
Tharp & Wagner (119)	Rat	Run	3–5	18.8–26.8 m/min	8 wk	NM	Y	Ink perfusion (pelikan ink)	↓CND ↓C/F
Laughlin & Tomanek (65)	Dog	Run	5	10–20 km/min, 75 min, 10–20% grade	18 wk	$SM\dot{V}O_2$, performance, HR	N	Perfusion fixation	↔CND ↔C/F
Breisch et al. (14)	Pig	Run	5	60 min, 70–85% max	12 wk	↑$\dot{V}O_2$max, HR	Y	Perfusion fixation	↔CND ↔C/F
Anversa et al. (5)	Rat	Run	5	60 min/d, 13.4 m/min, 7.5% grade	7 wk	NM	N ↑RVW	Perfusion fixation	↑CND
		Run	5	90 m/d, 26.8 m/min, 15% grade	7 wk	NM	Y	Perfusion fixation	↑CND

**Efficacy of training programs as reported in the publications: NM = training efficacy was not measured in the study, HR = training bradycardia, N/A = not applicable, $SM\dot{V}O_2$ = skeletal muscle oxidative capacity, $\dot{V}O_2$max = whole body maximal oxygen consumption. ‡Cardiac hypertrophy: Y = hypertrophy present, N = no hypertrophy. *Capillaries: wt = weight, C/F = capillary to fiber ratio, CND = capillary numerical density, RVW = right ventricular weight.

that ET can produce increases in myocardial capillarization, it appears that this phenomenon can be best demonstrated in young animals. Two studies that compared the effects of treadmill ET on coronary capillary density in young (prepubescent) and old (postpubescent) rats found that capillary density only increased significantly when training commenced at an early age (47,121). Most investigators have failed to find increased capillarization in the heart with ET when training was commenced with adult animals (14,65,123,129). Since ET often produces moderate levels of cardiac hypertrophy, these results suggest that, even in adults, training results in angiogenesis of new capillaries but at a rate matched to cardiac hypertrophy. If not, capillarization would decrease in proportion to cardiac hypertrophy (5,65).

Small Coronary Veins and Venules

There appears to be no information on the effects of ET on these coronary vessels.

Adaptations of Coronary Vascular Control

There are many more publications available concerning exercise training-induced structural vascular adaptation than altered coronary vascular control mechanisms. This suggests that most investigators in this field have favored structural vascular adaptation as the primary mechanism in exercise training-induced increases in coronary transport capacity. However, support for the notion that ET induces alterations in coronary vascular control exists in at least three forms. First, there is considerable evidence that systemic cardiovascular control systems are altered by ET. Space does not allow a detailed review of the effects of endurance ET on systemic cardiovascular regulatory systems (for review see 9,25,91,93,100,107, and chapter 17). Training-induced alterations of coronary vascular control mechanisms may be one component of alterations in cardiovascular control mechanisms. Second, a number of investigations have directly examined vascular control mechanisms in the coronary circulation of ET animals. Finally, there are a number of studies that have applied a variety of in vitro techniques to examine vascular control mechanisms in the coronary circulation.

Neurohumoral Control of the Coronary Circulation

Gwirtz and Stone (35) and Liang and Stone (68) reported that ET alters neural control of the coronary circulation. Also, Bove and Dewey (12) reported diminished phenylephrine-induced vasoconstrictor responses of proximal coronary arteries in intact, anesthetized ET dogs. The vasodilator response of the intact coronary circulation of anesthetized ET dogs to alpha-adrenergic blockade with prazosin was reported to be enhanced as compared to control dogs (55). DiCarlo et al. (26) reported that ET for 4 weeks resulted in enhanced coronary resistance vessel sensitivity to both alpha- and beta-adrenergic agents and to adenosine. Finally, Laughlin et al. (65) reported that blockade of alpha-adrenergic receptors produced a larger increase in coronary plasma flow in ET pigs than in controls, and that adenosine produced greater coronary vasodilation in ET pigs.

Local Coronary Vascular Control

Local vascular control phenomena are regulatory responses that can be demonstrated in isolated perfused tissues removed from neural or humoral influences. Because local vascular control is the primary control system in the coronary circulation (30), it is likely that any training-induced change in control of the coronary circulation will include alterations in local control.

The metabolic theory of blood flow control holds that an increase in metabolic rate will release more vasoactive metabolites causing vasodilation and increased blood flow, while decreases in metabolic rate will release less metabolites, resulting in vasoconstriction and decreased blood flow. The hypothesis that metabolic control is altered in the coronary circulation by training has not been systematically investigated. However, there is evidence that metabolic control of the coronary vascular bed is altered by ET: (a) The relationship between heart rate (during atrial pacing) and coronary blood flow is shifted to the left (higher flow) in ET dogs (114), (b) diastolic coronary resistance is lower at any given heart rate in ET dogs (68), (c) reactive hyperemic responses produced by a 10-s coronary occlusion are augmented in ET dogs (57), (d) the coronary vascular bed is more sensitive to vasodilator effects of adenosine in ET dogs (26,55,65) and pigs (61), and (e) coronary vascular smooth muscle from ET pigs is more sensitive to the effects of adenosine (84). Training-induced alterations in metabolic vascular control could result from a shift in the relationship between metabolic rate and the release of vasoactive metabolites or from altered responses of coronary resistance vessels to vasoactive metabolites. Metabolic control may not be the only local control mechanism altered by ET since a recent preliminary report by Muller, Myers, Tanner and Laughlin indicates that training alters myogenic control of the coronary circulation—myogenic responses are enhanced in coronary arterioles isolated from ET pigs (81).

Contractile Behavior of Isolated Coronary Arteries

Training-induced changes in control of proximal coronary arteries include altered coronary responses in vasoactive substances (12,84,92), changes in endothelium-mediated vasoregulation (62,80,92), and alterations in the cellular–molecular control of intracellular free Ca^{2+} in both endothelial and vascular smooth muscle cells isolated from coronary arteries of ET animals (111,112).

Changes in Endothelial Function

The revelation of the importance of the endothelium in vascular control has produced a dramatic change in our understanding of blood flow control processes (24,27). It is now known that the endothelium can mediate vasodilator responses, vasoconstrictor responses, and vascular growth (proliferation) in response to several stimuli. The endothelium appears to be able to sense physical forces (shear stress and vessel stretch) imparted to and the chemical environment of the blood vessels, and release substances that modulate vascular tone and/or blood vessel structure to maintain homeostasis (24,27,38,44,51,52,88,94). This is a relatively new area of vascular biology which is rapidly expanding. Very little is known about potential effects of ET on vascular endothelium and endothelium-dependent vasoregulation. Muller et al. (80) reported that bradykinin-induced, endothelium-dependent vasodilation is enhanced in arterioles isolated from the hearts of ET pigs. It is clear that more research is needed to determine the importance of training-induced changes in endothelium-mediated vascular control.

Effects of Training on Skeletal Muscle Vascular Beds

Blood Flow Capacity of Skeletal Muscle

The increased maximal oxygen consumption characteristic of trained individuals has been attributed to increases in both maximal cardiac output and maximal arteriovenous oxygen difference (10, 20,93,100). The fact that the increased maximal cardiac output is believed to be directed to working skeletal muscle during exercise suggests that skeletal muscle BFC is also increased by ET. Both cross-sectional (73,104,108) and longitudinal (72,106) studies have obtained results suggestive of greater limb muscle BFC in trained individuals. In these studies, BFC was estimated with venous occlusion plethysmography by measuring reactive hyperemic responses to ischemia or ischemic exercise to fatigue. Evidence for training-induced increases in skeletal muscle BFC has also been provided in experiments using the ^{133}Xe washout technique to measure blood flow (21,49). Finally, Musch, Haidet, Ordway, Longhurst, and Mitchell (83) used radiolabelled microspheres to measure regional blood flow responses to maximal treadmill exercise in dogs before and after training. Their results indicated that 80% of the training-induced increase in maximal cardiac output was directed to active skeletal muscle (83).

BFC has also been shown to be increased in skeletal muscle of trained rats when maximal vasodilation was induced by metabolically demanding muscle contractions (70) and by infusion of papaverine (59,63,102). Regional blood flows measured with radiolabelled microspheres suggested that training-induced increases in BFC are localized in and around muscle fibers that have the greatest relative increases in activity during ET bouts (56, 59,63,70,102).

Skeletal Muscle CDC

Studies of the effects of ET on skeletal muscle CDC have found increases (63,102) or no change in CDC (29,63). One source of conflicting results is lack of maximal vasodilation during capillary exchange measurements (29,102). Also, techniques available for measuring CDC only reflect average capacity for relatively large masses of skeletal muscle. If CDC is increased in only a small percentage of muscle tissue, these averaging techniques may not be able to resolve such adaptations (29,63). In experiments in which the model of training is expected to induce adaptations in a large portion of the skeletal muscle tissue, results indicate that training increases CDC of skeletal muscle (63,102).

In conclusion, effective ET appears to be associated with increases in vascular transport capacity of skeletal muscle vasculature. Both BFC and CDC are increased. In skeletal muscle vascular beds of rats, training-induced adaptations are not homogeneously distributed throughout the tissue. Fiber type composition and fiber recruitment patterns during exercise-training bouts have important consequences for the distribution of training-induced adaptations in skeletal muscle (56,59,63,70,102). Increases in BFC and CDC of skeletal muscle vasculature could be due to structural adaptations or alterations in the control of blood flow and its distribution in the microvasculature.

Structural Vascular Adaptation

Small Arteries and Arterioles

There is limited information concerning the effects of ET on the size and/or number of small arteries and arterioles in skeletal muscle vascular beds. Lash and Bohlen (53) recently reported that arteriolar density was increased in spinotrapezius muscle but unchanged in gracilis muscle of rats following treadmill training. The fact that precapillary vascular resistance is decreased in hindquarters isolated from trained rats suggests that training induces changes in precapillary resistance vessels (29,102). There is a need for studies of exercise training-induced functional and structural adaptations in various skeletal muscle vascular beds.

Capillary (and/or Microvascular Exchange) Vessels

The effects of ET on the structure of skeletal muscle capillary beds has been extensively investigated. Numerous studies in humans, both cross-sectional and longitudinal in nature, have consistently demonstrated increased capillarization in response to training (96). Among animal studies there is evidence that training causes increases in skeletal muscle capillarization (2,3,18,71,89) as well as reports of no change (69,82,85). Causes for this controversy include models of training and lack of rigorous documentation of a trained state, choice of muscle tissue to examine, and failure to appreciate potential differences among capillary beds in different types of skeletal muscle.

Consideration of training regimen in various studies is necessary in critical interpretation of available literature concerning effects of ET on skeletal muscle capillarization. It is also important to evaluate the choice of muscle tissue for examination. For example, Ljungqvist and Unge (69) used swim training and assessed skeletal muscle capillarization in soleus muscle. It has been shown that blood flow is decreased in soleus of rats during swimming, suggesting that the muscle is not recruited extensively during swimming (60). Therefore, vascular adaptation would not be expected to occur in this rat skeletal muscle as a result of swim training. Similarly, Parizkova et al. (85) trained rats on a treadmill at 20 m/min and found no change in capillarization. This may have been an insufficient exercise intensity to promote increased capillary growth.

In our review of the literature we find that few studies have documented training efficacy with an independent measure of training-induced adaptation (69,82,89). The studies of Muller (82) and Ljungqvist and Unge (69) documented training efficacy by measuring heart weight:body weight ratios. This approach is not as rigorous as measuring skeletal muscle citrate synthase activity as done in an excellent study by Poole et al. (89). Their rats were trained with a moderate treadmill training program. Capillarization was examined in soleus muscle and efficacy of training was tested with skeletal muscle citrate synthase activity (35% increase). Their results indicated that training resulted in a 30% increase in capillary to fiber ratio (89).

Differences appear to exist in the effects of training on capillary beds within and among whole muscles. It is well established that skeletal muscle fibers are heterogeneous in both biochemical and physiological characteristics; however, fibers can be classified into three relatively homogeneous types: slow-twitch oxidative (SO), fast-twitch oxidative glycolytic (FOG), and fast-twitch glycolytic (FG) (96).

Although blood flows to inactive muscles of various fiber type composition are similar, locomotory activity results in heterogeneity of flow both among and within muscles, as demonstrated by *in situ* and *in vivo* studies (56). Postural activity causes increases in blood flow to SO fibers. In fact, blood flow in muscle during postural maintenance is directly related to percent SO fiber composition (56). With exercise, increases in blood flow in extensor muscles of the hip, knee, and ankle joints are related to percent FOG fiber composition, although FG fibers receive increases in blood flow during high-intensity exercise (56). These patterns of blood flow distribution are related to patterns of muscle fiber recruitment during exercise (56).

BFC has been found to be greatest in rat FOG fibers, followed in order by SO and FG fibers. Capillarization of muscle has a similar ordering in other rodents (18, 71). In humans, differences between SO and FOG fiber capillarization are less pronounced (96). ET has been reported to modulate relationships among fiber type composition and capillarization. Mai et al. reported that capillarization was increased by ET in muscles composed of FOG fibers but was not changed in SO or FG muscle tissue of guinea pigs following moderate intensity ET (71). This intensity of exercise would be expected to result in increased recruitment of FOG fibers and increased blood flow to FOG fibers during training bouts (56,103). More recently, a systematic series of investigations of capillary adaptations to three ET programs of differing intensities has shown that increases in capillarization occur in the areas of muscle with the greatest relative increase in fiber activity during training bouts (33,59,63,102).

These studies support the hypothesis that increases in capillarization are localized in the areas of muscle expected to have the greatest relative increase in fiber activity during training bouts. In contrast, training studies with human subjects indicate that capillarization is increased in muscle composed of all three types of fibers (4,46,48). This is surprising, for continuous, submaximal (70%-80% max) ET was utilized in these studies. Thus, during training bouts, little FG fiber recruitment would be expected. Another study that does not support the hypothesis of heterogeneous vascular adaptation is that of Lash and Bohlen, which reported aerobic, ET-induced increases in vascular density in rat skeletal muscle even if oxidative capacity of the muscle was not increased (53). Vascularization may have been increased to a greater extent in limb muscles showing increased oxidative capacity in the trained rats of Lash and Bohlen (53). However, this possibility cannot be evaluated since Lash and Bohlen only evaluated vascular density in spinotrapezius and gracilis muscle.

Small Veins and Venules

There appears to be no information in the literature concerning the effect of ET on these skeletal muscle microvessels. However, the fact that postcapillary vascular resistance is decreased in hindquarters from ET rats (29,102) is consistent with the hypothesis that ET alters the venous circulation of skeletal muscle.

Adaptations of Vascular Control

Neurohumoral Control

Alterations in sympathetic nerve activity (SNA) to skeletal muscle at rest and during exercise may be one component of an overall training-induced adaptation of sympathetic neural control of vascular resistance (36,50,75,76,95,115,116,124,125,128). Training-induced alterations in SNA have been investigated with measures of (a) plasma norepinephrine concentration, (b) skeletal and/or total vascular resistance, and (c) direct microneurographic recordings of SNA. Although plasma concentrations of catecholamines in resting subjects are not altered by ET (23,87,126), training attenuates the increase in plasma catecholamines associated with exercise at a given absolute intensity (23,87,126,127). However, plasma catecholamine concentrations are normal in trained subjects during exercise when equal relative exercise intensities are compared (23,87,127) and are reportedly greater during maximal exercise after training (126). Although measures of plasma catecholamine concentrations only provide an indirect estimate of SNA (19,32), these results suggest that SNA to skeletal muscle is attenuated after ET.

Two longitudinal studies, using microneurographic techniques to measure skeletal muscle SNA during static handgrip exercise, indicate that SNA is decreased by ET (105,109), although resting muscle SNA is not altered (101,117). However, a cross-sectional study was unable to detect an effect of aerobic fitness on SNA during static handgrip exercise (101). There is no information concerning the effects of ET on SNA in the skeletal muscle microcirculation. Thus, although there is clear evidence that cardiovascular control mechanisms are modified by ET (9,10,25,45,108,125), and that ET attenuates SNA to skeletal muscle during exercise, the impact of these changes on skeletal muscle microcirculation remains to be explored.

Local Vascular Control in Skeletal Muscle

Lash and Bohlen (53) reported that spinotrapezius muscle arterioles of ET rats exhibited greater vasodilation during skeletal muscle contractions than those from sedentary control rats. These results suggest that ET alters the exercise hyperemic response in the skeletal muscle microcirculation. It is not possible at this time to determine if this represents altered metabolic control or alterations in other local control mechanisms such as myogenic control or flow-induced vasodilation in skeletal muscle microvascular beds.

The effects of ET on peripheral vascular smooth muscle has also been investigated. Edwards, Tipton, and Matthes (28) reported that training did not appear to alter norepinephrine dose–response relationships in helical strips of aorta, femoral artery, or renal artery of rat. Gute, Muller, McAllister, and Laughlin (34) similarly reported that segments of femoral arteries isolated from sedentary and trained miniature swine demonstrated similar sensitivity and responsiveness to norepinephrine and KCl. Further, no training-induced alterations were found in vasodilator responses induced by sodium nitroprusside or adenosine (34). In conclusion, it appears that training does not alter vascular smooth muscle of femoral arteries. However, there is evidence that exercise training may alter local control mechanisms at the arteriolar level in skeletal muscle microcirculatory beds.

Changes in Endothelial Function

We are aware of only one study that investigated training-induced alterations in endothelium-dependent vascular control in the peripheral circulation (64). The results of this study revealed that the vasodilator effects of the endothelium-dependent vasodilator, acetylcholine, were enhanced in aortas of trained rats. Chronic increases in blood flow produced by femoral arteriovenous fistulas in dogs have also been shown to produce enhancement of endothelium-dependent vasodilation (77,78). Endothelium-mediated vasodilation was found to be enhanced in arterial rings isolated from the femoral artery proximal to the fistula (77). This effect was subsequently found to be the result of alterations in the release of EDRF (endothelium-derived relaxing factor) as evidenced by the finding that there was no change in sensitivity of the vascular smooth muscle to EDRF (78). There is currently no information concerning the effects of training on endothelium-mediated vascular control in the microcirculation of skeletal muscle.

Mechanisms for Training-Induced Vascular Adaptation

There is relatively little information available that directly addresses the question of how ET induces structural vascular adaptation in the coronary circulation and skeletal muscle vascular beds. This relative lack of information may be partially because vascular growth, remodeling, and angiogenesis in normal growth and development, in wound healing, and in pathology are also poorly understood, though currently under intense investigation. Structural vascular adaptation is the result of increased production of the components of blood vessels. Thus, some signal is produced by exercise training that stimulates vascular smooth muscle cells, endothelial cells, and fibroblasts to assemble more and/or larger blood vessels. This signal appears to be related to increased blood flow and/or increased metabolic activity of the muscle tissue as well as to muscle mass (1,39–43). A large number of angiogenic factors have been identified (31). However, the role of these factors in exercise training-induced vascular adaptation remains to be established.

Hudlická has proposed that microvascular angiogenesis, induced by increased activity in striated muscle tissues, is signaled by increased blood flow (40,43). This is an attractive hypothesis that is supported by as much experimental evidence as any current hypothesis for training-induced angiogenesis in cardiac and/or skeletal muscle. As reviewed by Hudlická (39,40,41), growth of vessels in normal development, in female reproductive tissues, and in exercise training-induced structural vascular adaptation in skeletal and cardiac muscle is consistently associated with increases in blood flow. In an important series of experiments, Hudlická and colleagues have demonstrated that several stimuli known to induce angiogenesis only did so when blood flow to the tissue is allowed to increase (39–43). Recent work from this group demonstrated that the increase in capillarization usually induced by chronic electrical stimulation of tibialis anterior and EDL muscles could be eliminated by ligation of the common iliac artery (42). These results reinforce the notion that increased blood flow is essential for angiogenesis in skeletal muscle.

Recently, Morrow, Kraus, Moore, Williams, and Swain (79) reported that continuous electrical stimulation of rabbit skeletal muscle resulted in increased concentrations of fibroblast growth factor (FGF), which is known to induce capillary angiogenesis (31). The signal for FGF release could be mechanical, metabolic, or increased blood flow. These results suggest the possibility that FGF is one angiogenic factor that is involved in training-induced structural vascular adaptation in skeletal muscle. Since training-induced vascular adaptation appears to be similar in cardiac and skeletal muscle, it is possible that FGF is important in vascular adaptation in both types of muscle tissue.

Another popular hypothesis for training-induced angiogenesis and structural vascular adaptation is the metabolic hypothesis (1), proposing that increases in metabolic demand and/or tissue hypoxia result in the release of a variety of signals stimulating growth and/or angiogenesis of the appropriate blood vessels. Differentiating the role of metabolic signals from signals related to increased flow is difficult due to the fact that hypoxia (and most of the metabolites of interest as metabolic signals for vascular growth) also stimulates increased blood flow. Adair et al. (1) proposed a feedback control model for blood vessel growth that emphasized the metabolic hypothesis. More research is required to define quantitative contributions of various factors in exercise training-induced structural vascular adaptation in skeletal muscle vascular beds and the coronary circulation.

Conclusions

Aerobic exercise training induces an increase in vascular transport capacity in both cardiac and skeletal muscle. This increased transport capacity is the result of increases in both BFC and CDC. These functional changes are the result of two major types of adaptive responses: structural vascular adaptation, and altered control of vascular resistance. Training-induced vascular adaptation is generally uniform throughout the myocardium. Vascular adaptation in rat skeletal muscle tissue is not uniformly distributed throughout the tissue. The most evident structural (increases in capillary density) and functional (increased vascular transport capacity) adaptations appear to occur in the skeletal muscle tissue with the greatest relative increase in activity during training bouts (i.e., around muscle fibers that experience the largest increase in activity during physical activity). A common weakness of investigations of the effects of training on striated muscle vasculature is that investigators have not consistently obtained independent measures of a training effect. As a result, if no changes were found in striated muscle vasculature, it is not possible to determine if training failed to induce vascular adaptation or if the subjects were not trained.

One bout of exercise induces a complex array of factors that may be involved in initiating training-induced adaptations. During exercise blood flow is increased in active skeletal muscle and the heart. Vasodilation and increased blood flow in cardiac muscle and active skeletal muscle are always associated with exercise. Vasodilation produces one of the likely "signals" for vascular adaptation: an alteration in mechanical forces in the vessel wall. The other major effect of vasodilation is increased blood flow, which will produce a second potential signal for vascular adaptation: increased shear stress in the blood vessels. Repetitive exposure to these two mechanical stimuli (stretch and shear stress) and/or metabolic signals during exercise training bouts may initiate both structural vascular adaptation and altered control of vascular resistance. Changes in concentrations of various hormones, peptides, and/or changes in neurohumoral stimuli during exercise may also act as signals or modifiers for vascular adaptation.

Structural vascular adaptation in the form of angiogenesis occurs in both cardiac and skeletal muscle. Changes in vascular control in the coronary circulation appear to include altered responses to some vasoactive substances, changes in endothelium-mediated vasoregulation, and alterations in the cellular-molecular control of intracellular free Ca^{2+} in both endothelial and vascular smooth muscle cells. Similar changes may occur in skeletal muscle vascular beds. An attractive, unifying hypothesis is that the adaptive strategy entails maintenance of normal shear stress in coronary and skeletal muscle arterial vessels. Thus, as a result of training-induced vascular growth and alterations in vascular control, shear stress during a bout of exercise is maintained in the normal range.

Acknowledgments

Work in the authors' laboratory is supported by NIH grant # HL-36531 and # HL-36088. M.H. Laughlin is the recipient of NIH Research Career Development Award # HL-01774, and R.M. McAllister is the recipient of a Fellowship from the Missouri affiliate of the American Heart Association.

References

1. Adair, T.H.; Gay, W.J.; Montani, J. Growth regulation of the vascular system: Evidence for a metabolic hypothesis. Am. J. Physiol. 259:R393-R404; 1990.
2. Adolfsson, J. The time dependence of training-induced increase in skeletal muscle capillarization and the spatial capillary to fibre relationship in normal and neovascularized skeletal muscle of rats. Acta Physiol. Scand. 128:259-266; 1986.
3. Adolfsson, J.; Ljungqvist, A.; Tornling, G.; Unge, G. Capillary increase in the skeletal muscle of trained young and adult rats. J. Physiol. 310:529-532; 1981.
4. Andersen, P.; Henriksson, J. Capillary supply of the quadriceps femoris muscle of man: Adaptive response to exercise. J. Physiol. 270:670-690; 1977.
5. Anversa, P.; Ricci, R.; Olivetti, G. Effects of exercise on the capillary vasculature of the rat heart. Circulation. [Suppl. I]. 75:I12-I18; 1987.
6. Barnard, R.J.; Duncan, H.W.; Baldwin, K.M.; Grimditch, G.; Buckberg, G.D. Effects of intensive exercise training on myocardial performance and coronary blood flow. J. Appl. Physiol. 49:444-449; 1980.
7. Barnard, R.J.; MacAlpin, R.; Kattus, A.A.; Buckberg, G.D. Effect of training on myocardial oxygen supply/demand balance. Circulation. 56:289-292; 1977.
8. Baur, T.S.; Brodowicz, G.R.; Lamb, D.R. Indomethacin suppresses the coronary flow response to hypoxia in exercise trained and sedentary rats. Cardiovasc. Res. 24:733-736; 1990.
9. Bedford, T.G.; Tipton, C.M. Exercise training and the arterial baroreflex. J. Appl. Physiol. 63:1926-1932; 1987.
10. Blomqvist, C.; Saltin, B. Cardiovascular adaptations to physical training. Annu. Rev. Physiol. 45:169-189; 1983.
11. Booth, F.W.; Thomason, D.B. Molecular and cellular adaptation of muscle in response to

exercise: Perspectives of various models. Physiol. Rev. 71:541-586; 1991.

12. Bove, A.A.; Dewey, J.D. Proximal coronary vasomotor reactivity after exercise training in dogs. Circulation. 71:620-625; 1985.
13. Bove, A.A.; Hultgren, P.B.; Ritzer, T.F.; Carey, R.A. Myocardial blood flow and hemodynamic responses to exercise training in dogs. J. Appl. Physiol. 46:571-578; 1979.
14. Breisch, E.A.; White, F.C.; Nimmo, L.E.; McKirnan, M.D.; Bloor, C.M. Exercise-induced cardiac hypertrophy: A correlation of blood flow and microvasculature. J. Appl. Physiol. 60: 1259-1267; 1986.
15. Buttrick, P.M.; Schaible, T.F.; Scheuer, J. Combined effects of hypertension and conditioning on coronary vascular reserve in rats. J. Appl. Physiol. 60:275-279; 1985.
16. Carey, R.A.; Santamore, W.P.; Michelle, J.J.; Bove, A.A. Effects of endurance training on coronary resistance in dogs. Med. Sci. Sports Exerc. 15:355-359; 1983.
17. Carlsson, S.; Ljungqvist, A.; Tornling, G.; Unge, G. The myocardial vasculature in repeated physical exercise. Acta Pathol. Microbiol. Immunol. Scand. [A]. 86:117-119; 1978.
18. Carrow, R.; Brown, R.; Van Huss, W. Fiber sizes and capillary to fiber ratios in skeletal muscle of exercised rats. Anat. Rec. 159:33-40; 1967.
19. Chang, P.C.; Kreik, E.; van der Krogt, J.; van Brummelen, P. Does regional norepinephrine spillover represent local sympathetic activity? Hypertension. 18:56-66; 1991.
20. Clausen, J. Circulatory adjustments to dynamic exercise and effect of physical training in normal subjects and in patients with coronary artery disease. Prog. Cardiovasc. Dis. 18:459-495; 1976.
21. Clausen, J.; Larsen, O.; Trap-Jensen, J. Physical training in the management of coronary artery disease. Circulation. 40:143-154; 1969.
22. Cohen, M.V. Coronary vascular reserve in the greyhound with left ventricular hypertrophy. Cardiovasc. Res. 20:182-194; 1986.
23. Cousineau, D.; Ferguson, R.J.; de Champlain, J.; Gauthier, P.; Côté, P.; Bourassa, M. Catecholamines in coronary sinus during exercise in man before and after training. J. Appl. Physiol. 43:801-806; 1977.
24. Daniel, T.O., Ives, H.E. Endothelial control of vascular function. NIPS. 4:139-142; 1989.
25. DiCarlo, S.E.; Bishop, V.S. Regional vascular resistance during exercise: Role of cardiac afferents and exercise training. Am. J. Physiol. 258:H842-H847; 1990.
26. DiCarlo, S.E.; Blair, R.W.; Bishop, V.S.; Stone, H.L. Daily exercise enhances coronary resistance vessel sensitivity to pharmacological activation. J. Appl. Physiol. 66:421-428; 1989.
27. Dzau, V.J.; Gibbons, G.H. The role of the endothelium in vascular remodeling. In: Rubanyi, G.M., ed. Cardiovascular significance of endothelium-derived vasoactive factors. Mount Kisco, NY: Futura Publishing Co. Inc.; 1991:281-291.
28. Edwards, J.G.; Tipton, C.M.; Matthes, R.D. Influence of exercise training on reactivity and contractility of arterial strips from hypertensive rats. J. Appl. Physiol. 58:1683-1688; 1985.
29. Edwards, M.T.; Diana, J.N. Effect of exercise on pre- and postcapillary resistance in the spontaneously hypertensive rat. Am. J. Physiol. 234:H439-H446; 1978.
30. Feigl, E.O. Coronary physiology. Physiol. Rev. 63:1-205; 1983.
31. Folkman, J.; Klagsbrun, M. Angiogenic factors. Science. 235:442-447; 1987.
32. Grossman, E.; Chang, P.C.; Hoffman, A.; Tamrat, M.; Kopin, I.J.; Goldstein, D.S. Tracer norepinephrine kinetics: Dependence on regional blood flow and the site of infusion. Am. J. Physiol. 260:R946-R952; 1991.
33. Gute, D.C.; Amann, J.F.; Laughlin, M.H. Effects of different exercise training protocols on skeletal muscle capillary density in the rat. Anat. Histol. Embryol. 19:83-84; 1990.
34. Gute, D.C.; Muller, J.; McAllister, R.; Laughlin, M.H. Effects of exercise training on femoral arterial smooth muscle in miniature swine. Med. Sci. Sports Exerc. 23:S88; 1991.
35. Gwirtz, P.A.; Stone, H.L. Coronary vascular response to adrenergic stimulation in exercise-conditioned dogs. J. Appl. Physiol. 243: 315-320; 1984.
36. Harri, M.N.E. Physical training under the influence of beta-blockade in rats. II. Effects on vascular reactivity. Eur. J. Appl. Physiol. 42: 151-157; 1979.
37. Ho, K.W.; Roy, R.R.; Taylor, R.; Heusner, W.W.; Van Huss, W.D. Differential effects of running and weight-lifting on the rat coronary arterial tree. Med. Sci. Sports Exerc. 15:472-477; 1983.
38. Holtz, J.; Giesler, M.; Bassenge, E. Two dilatory mechanisms of anti-anginal drugs on epicardial coronary arteries in vivo: Indirect, flow-dependent, endothelium-mediated dilation and direct smooth muscle relaxation. Z. Kardiol. 72 [Suppl. 3]:98-106; 1983.
39. Hudlická, O. Growth of capillaries in skeletal and cardiac muscle. Cir. Res. 50:451-461; 1982.

40. Hudlická, O. Capillary growth: Role of mechanical factors. NIPS. 3:117-120; 1988.
41. Hudlická, O. What makes blood vessels grow? J. Physiol. 444:1-24; 1991.
42. Hudlická, O.; Price, S. The role of blood flow and/or muscle hypoxia in capillary growth in chronically stimulated fast muscles. Pflugers Arch. 417:67-72; 1990.
43. Hudlická, O.; Tyler, K.R. Angiogenesis. New York: Academic Press; 1986.
44. Hull, S.S., Jr.; Kaiser, L.; Jaffe, M.D.; Sparks, H.V. Endothelium-dependent flow induced dilation of canine femoral and saphenous arteries. Blood Vessels. 23:183-198; 1986.
45. Hurley, B.F.; Seals, D.R.; Ehsani, A.A.; Cartier, L.-J.; Dalsky, D.P.; Hagberg, J.M.; Holloszy, J.O. Effects of high-intensity strength training on cardiovascular function. Med. Sci. Sports Exerc. 16:483-488; 1984.
46. Ingjer, F. Effects of endurance training on muscle fiber ATPase activity, capillary supply and mitochondrial content in man. J. Physiol. 294:419-432; 1979.
47. Jacobs, T.B.; Bell, R.O.; McClements, J.D. Exercise, age and the development of the myocardial vasculature. Growth. 48:148-157; 1984.
48. Klausen, K.; Andersen, L.; Pelle, I. Adaptive changes in work capacity, skeletal muscle capillarization and enzyme levels during training and detraining. Acta Physiol. Scand. 113:9-16; 1981.
49. Klausen, K.; Secher, N.; Clausen, J.; Hartling, O.; Trap-Jensen, J. Central and regional circulatory adaptations to one-leg training. J. Appl. Physiol. 52:976-983; 1982.
50. Kowalchuk, J.M.; Klein, C.S.; Hughson, R.L. The effect of beta-adrenergic blockade on leg blood flow with repeated maximal contractions of the triceps surae muscle group in man. Eur. J. Appl. Physiol. 60:360-364; 1990.
51. Kuo, L.; Davis, M.J.; Chilian, W.M. Endothelium-dependent, flow-induced dilation of isolated coronary arterioles. Am. J. Physiol. 259:H1063-H1070; 1990.
52. Lamping, K.G.; Dole, W.P. Flow-mediated dilation attenuates constriction of large coronary arteries to serotonin. Am. J. Physiol. 255:H1317-H1324; 1988.
53. Lash, J.; Bohlen, H.G. Functional adaptations of rat skeletal muscle arterioles to aerobic exercise training. J. Appl. Physiol. 72:2052-2062; 1992.
54. Laughlin, M.H. Coronary transport reserve in normal dogs. J. Appl. Physiol. 57:551-561; 1984.
55. Laughlin, M.H. Effects of exercise training on coronary transport capacity. J. Appl. Physiol. 58:468-476; 1985.
56. Laughlin, M.H.; Armstrong, R.B. Muscle blood flow during locomotory exercise. Exerc. Sport Sci. Rev. 13:95-136; 1985.
57. Laughlin, M.H.; Diana, J.N.; Tipton, C.M. Effects of chronic exercise training on coronary reactive hyperemia and coronary blood flow in the dog. J. Appl. Physiol. 45:604-610; 1978.
58. Laughlin, M.H.; Hale, C.C.; Novela, L.; Gute, D.; Hamilton, N.; Ianuzzo, C.D. Biochemical characterization of exercise-trained porcine myocardium. J. Appl. Physiol. 71:229-235; 1991.
59. Laughlin, M.H.; Korthuis, R.J.; Sexton, W.L.; Armstrong, R.B. Regional muscle blood flow capacity and exercise hyperemia in high-intensity trained rats. J. Appl. Physiol. 64: 2420-2427; 1988.
60. Laughlin, M.H.; Mohrman, S.J.; Armstrong, R.B. Muscular blood flow distribution patterns in the hindlimb of swimming rats. Am. J. Physiol. 246:H398-H403; 1984.
61. Laughlin, M.H.; Overholser, K.A.; Bhatte, M. Exercise training increases coronary transport reserve in miniature swine. J. Appl. Physiol. 67:1140-1149; 1989.
62. Laughlin, M.H.; Parker, J.L. Coronary vascular smooth muscle function in exercise-trained rats. FASEB J. 5:A662; 1991.
63. Laughlin, M.H.; Ripperger, J. Vascular transport capacity of hindlimb muscles of exercise-trained rats. J. Appl. Physiol. 62:438-443; 1987.
64. Laughlin, M.H.; Thorne, P.; Gute, D. Exercise training enhances endothelium-mediated vasodilator responses in rat. Med. Sci. Sports Exerc. 24:5116; 1992.
65. Laughlin, M.H.; Tomanek, R.J. Myocardial capillarity and maximal capillary diffusion capacity in exercise-trained dogs. J. Appl. Physiol. 63:1481-1486; 1987.
66. Leon, A.S.; Bloor, C.M. Effects of exercise and its cessation on the heart and its blood supply. J. Appl. Physiol. 24:485-490; 1968.
67. Liang, I.Y.S.; Hamara, M.; Stone, H.L. Maximum coronary blood flow and minimum coronary resistance in exercise trained dogs. J. Appl. Physiol. 56:641-647; 1984.
68. Liang, I.Y.S.; Stone, H.L. Effect of exercise conditioning on coronary resistance. J. Appl. Physiol. 53:631-636; 1982.
69. Ljungqvist, A.; Unge, G. Capillary proliferative activity in myocardium and skeletal muscle of exercised rats. J. Appl. Physiol. 43:306-307; 1977.
70. Mackie, B.; Terjung, R. Influence of training on blood flow to different skeletal muscle fiber types. J. Appl. Physiol. 55:1072-1078; 1983.

71. Mai, J.; Edgerton, V.; Barnard, R. Capillarity of red, white, and intermediate muscle fibers in trained and untrained guinea-pigs. Experientia. 26:1222-1223; 1970.
72. Martin, W.H.; Kohrt, W.M.; Malley, M.T.; Korte, E.; Stoltz, S. Exercise training enhances leg vasodilatory capacity of 65-yr-old men and women. J. Appl. Physiol. 69:1804-1809; 1990.
73. Martin, W.H.; Ogawa, T.; Kohrt, W.M.; Malley, W.T.; Korte, E.; Kieffer, P.S.; Schechtmann, K.B. Effects of aging, gender, and physical training on peripheral vascular function. Circulation. 84:654-664; 1991.
74. Martin, W.H.; Spina, R.J.; Korte, E.; Ogawa, T. Effects of chronic and acute exercise on cardiovascular β-adrenergic responses. J. Appl. Physiol. 71:1523-1528; 1991.
75. McAllister, R.M.; Lee, S.J.K. The effects of exercise training in patients with coronary artery disease taking beta-blockers. J. Cardiopulm. Rehabil. 6:245-250; 1986.
76. McLeod, A.A.; Kraus, W.E.; Williams, R.S. Effects of $beta_1$-selective and nonselective beta-adrenoceptor blockade during exercise conditioning in healthy adults. Am. J. Physiol. 53:1656-1661; 1984.
77. Miller, V.M.; Aarhus, L.A.; Vanhoutte, P.M. Modulation of endothelium-dependent responses by chronic alterations of blood flow. Am. J. Physiol. 251:H520-H527; 1986.
78. Miller, V.M.; Vanhoutte, P.M. Enhanced release of endothelium-derived factors by chronic increases in blood flow. Am. J. Physiol. 255:H446-H451; 1988.
79. Morrow, N.G.; Kraus, W.E.; Moore, J.W.; Williams, R.S.; Swain, J.L. Increased expression of fibroblast growth factors in a rabbit skeletal muscle model of exercise conditioning. J. Clin. Invest. 85:1816-1820; 1990.
80. Muller, J.M.; Myers, P.R.; Tanner, M.A.; Laughlin, M.H. The effect of exercise training on sensitivity of porcine coronary resistance arterioles to bradykinin. FASEB J. 5:A658; 1991.
81. Muller, J.M.; Myers, P.R.; Tanner, M.A.; Laughlin, M.H. Myogenic responses of coronary arterioles from exercise trained pigs. FASEB J. 6:A2080; 1992.
82. Muller, W. Subsarcolemmal mitochondrial and capillarization of soleus muscle fibers in young rats subjected to endurance training. Cell Tissue Res. 174:367-389; 1976.
83. Musch, T.I.; Haidet, G.C.; Ordway, G.A.; Longhurst, J.C.; Mitchell, J.H. Training effects on regional blood flow response to maximal exercise in foxhounds. J. Appl. Physiol. 62: 1724-1732; 1987.
84. Oltman, C.L.; Parker, J.L.; Adams, H.R.; Laughlin, M.H. Effects of exercise training on vasomotor reactivity of porcine coronary arteries. Am. J. Physiol. 263:H372-H382; 1992.
85. Parizkova, J.; Wachtlova, M.; Soukupova, M. The impact of different motor activity on body composition, density of capillaries and fibers in the heart and soleus muscles, and cell's migration in vitro in male rats. Int. Z. Angew. Physiol. 30:207-216; 1972.
86. Penpargkul, S.; Scheuer, J. The effects of physical training upon the mechanical and metabolic performance of the rat heart. J. Clin. Invest. 49:1859-1868; 1970.
87. Peronnét, F.; Cléroux, J.; Perrault, H.; Cousineau, D.; De Champlain, J.; Nadeau, R. Plasma norepinephrine response to exercise before and after training in humans. J. Appl. Physiol. 51:812-815; 1981.
88. Pohl, U.; Holtz, J.; Busse, R.; Bassenge, E. Crucial role of endothelium in the vasodilation response to increased flow in vivo. Hypertension. 8:37-44; 1986.
89. Poole, D.C.; Mathieu-Costello, O.; West, J.B. Capillary tortuosity in rat soleus muscle is not affected by endurance training. Am. J. Physiol. 256:H1110-H1116; 1989.
90. Raff, W.F.; Kosche, F.; Lochner, W. Extravascular coronary resistance and its relation to the microcirculation. Am. J. Cardiol. 29:598-603; 1972.
91. Raven, P.B.; Rohm-Young, D.; Blomqvist, C.G. Physical fitness and cardiovascular response to lower body negative pressure. J. Appl. Physiol. 56:138-144; 1984.
92. Rogers, P.J.; Miller, T.D.; Bauer, B.A.; Brum, M.M.; Bove, A.A.; Vanhoutte, P.M. Exercise training and responsiveness of isolated coronary arteries. J. Appl. Physiol. 71:2346-2351; 1991.
93. Rowell, L.B. Cardiovascular adaptations to chronic physical activity and inactivity. In: Human Circulation. New York: Oxford University Press; 1986:257-286.
94. Rubanyi, G.M.; Romero, J.C.; Vanhoutte, P.M. Flow-induced release of endothelium-derived relaxing factor. Am. J. Physiol. 250: H1145-H1149; 1986.
95. Sabel, D.L.; Brammell, H.L.; Sheehan, M.W.; Nies, A.S.; Gerber, J.; Horwitz, L.D. Attenuation of exercise conditioning by beta-adrenergic blockade. Circulation. 65:679-684; 1982.
96. Saltin, B.; Gollnick, P.D. Skeletal muscle adaptability: Significance for metabolism and performance. Handbook of physiology. Skel-

etal muscle. Bethesda, MD: American Physiological Society; 1983:555-631.

97. Schaible, T.F.; Scheuer, J. Effects of physical training by running or swimming on ventricular performance of rat hearts. J. Appl. Physiol. 46:854-860; 1979.
98. Scheel, K.W.; Ingram, L.A.; Wilson, J.L. Effects of exercise on the coronary and collateral vasculature of beagles with and without coronary occlusion. Circ. Res. 48:523-530; 1981.
99. Scheuer, J. Effects of physical training on myocardial vascularity and perfusion. Circulation. 66:491-495; 1982.
100. Scheuer, J.; Tipton, C.M. Cardiovascular adaptations to physical training. Annu. Rev. Physiol. 39:221-251; 1977.
101. Seals, D.R. Sympathetic neural adjustments to stress in physically trained and untrained humans. Hypertension. 17:36-43; 1991.
102. Sexton, W.L.; Korthuis, R.J.; Laughlin, M.H. High-intensity exercise training increases vascular transport capacity of rat hindquarters. Am. J. Physiol. 254:H274-H278; 1988.
103. Shepherd, R.; Gollnick, P. Oxygen uptake of rats at different work intensities. Pflugers Arch. 362:219-222; 1976.
104. Sinoway, L.I.; Musch, T.I.; Minotti, J.R.; Zelis, R. Enhanced maximal metabolic vasodilation in the dominant forearms of tennis players. J. Appl. Physiol. 61:673-678; 1986.
105. Sinoway, L.; Rea, R.; Smith, M.; Mark, A. Physical training induces desensitization of the muscle metaboreflex. Circulation. [Abstract]. 80:II-290; 1989.
106. Sinoway, L.I.; Shenberger, J.; Wilson, J.; McLaughlin, D.; Musch, T.; Zelis, R. A 30 day forearm work protocol increases maximal forearm blood flow. J. Appl. Physiol. 62:1063-1067; 1987.
107. Smith, M.L.; Raven, P.B. Cardiovascular responses to lower body negative pressure in endurance and static exercise-trained men. Med. Sci. Sports Exerc. 18:545-550; 1986.
108. Snell, P.G.; Martin, W.H.; Buckey, J.C.; Blomqvist, C.G. Maximal vascular leg conductance in trained and untrained men. J. Appl. Physiol. 62:606-610; 1987.
109. Somers, V.K.; Leo, K.C.; Green, M.P.; Mark, A.L. Forearm training attenuates the sympathetic nerve response to isometric handgrip. Circulation. [Abstract]. 78:II-177; 1988.
110. Spear, K.L.; Koerner, J.E.; Terjung, R.L. Coronary blood flow in physically trained rats. Cardiovasc. Res. 12:135-143; 1978.
111. Steno-Bittel, L.; Laughlin, M.H.; Sturek, M. Exercise training alters Ca^{2+} release from coronary smooth muscle sarcoplasmic reticulum. Am. J. Physiol. 259:H643-H647; 1990.
112. Steno-Bittel, L.; Laughlin, M.H.; Sturek, M. Exercise training depletes sarcoplasmic reticulum Ca^{2+} in coronary smooth muscle. J. Appl. Physiol. 71:1764-1773; 1991.
113. Stevenson, J.A.; Feleki, V.; Rechnitzer, P. Effect of exercise on coronary tree size in the rat. Cir. Res. 15:265-269; 1964.
114. Stone, H.L. Coronary flow, myocardial oxygen consumption and exercise training in dogs. J. Appl. Physiol. 49:759-768; 1980.
115. Svedenhag, J. The sympatho-adrenal system in physical conditioning. Acta Physiol. Scand. [Suppl.]. 543:1-73; 1985.
116. Svedenhag, J.; Martinsson, A.; Ekblom, B.; Hjemdahl, P. Altered cardiovascular responsiveness to adrenoceptor agonists in endurance-trained men. J. Appl. Physiol. 70:531-538; 1991.
117. Svedenhag, J.; Wallin, B.G.; Sundlöf, G.; Henriksson, J. Skeletal muscle sympathetic activity at rest in trained and untrained subjects. Acta Physiol. Scand. 120:499-504; 1984.
118. Tepperman, J.; Pearlman, D. Effects of exercise and anemia on coronary arteries in small animals as revealed by the corrosion-cast technique. Cir. Res. 9:576-584; 1961.
119. Tharp, G.D.; Wagner, C.T. Chronic exercise and cardiac vascularization. Eur. J. Appl. Physiol. 48:97-104; 1982.
120. Thomas, D.P. Effects of acute and chronic exercise on myocardial ultrastructure. Med. Sci. Sports Exerc. 17:546-553; 1985.
121. Tomanek, R.J. Effects of age and exercise on the extent of the myocardial capillary bed. Anat. Rec. 167:55-62; 1970.
122. Wachtlova, M.; Rakusan, K.; Poupa, O. The coronary terminal vascular bed in the heart of the hare and the rabbit. Physiol. Biochem. 14:328-331; 1965.
123. White, F.C.; McKirnan, M.D.; Breisch, E.A.; Guth, B.D.; Liu, Y.; Bloor, C.M. Adaptation of the left ventricle to exercise-induced hypertrophy. J. Appl. Physiol. 62:1097-1110; 1987.
124. Wiegman, D.L.; Harris, P.D.; Joshua, I.G.; Miller, F.N. Decreased vascular sensitivity to norepinephrine following exercise training. J. Appl. Physiol. 51:282-287, 1981.
125. Williams, R.S. Role of receptor mechanisms in the adaptive response to habitual exercise. Am. J. Cardiol. 55:68D-73D; 1985.
126. Winder, W.W.; Hagberg, J.M.; Hickson, R.C.; Ehsani, A.A.; McLane, J.A. Time course of sympathoadrenal adaptation to endurance exercise training in man. J. Appl. Physiol. 45:370-374; 1978.

127. Winder, W.W.; Hickson, R.C.; Hagberg, J.M.; Ehsani, A.A.; McLane, J.A. Training-induced changes in hormonal and metabolic responses to submaximal exercise. J. Appl. Physiol. 46:766-771; 1979.
128. Wolfel, E.E.; Hiatt, W.R.; Brammel, H.L.; Travis, V.H.; Horwitz, L.D. Plasma catecholamine responses to exercise after training with beta-adrenergic blockade. J. Appl. Physiol. 68:586-593; 1990.
129. Wyatt, H.L.; Mitchell, J. Influences of physical conditioning and deconditioning on coronary vasculature of dogs. J. Appl. Physiol. 45:619-625; 1978.
130. Yipintsoi, T.; Rosenkrantz, J.; Codini, M.A.; Scheuer, J. Myocardial blood flow responses to acute hypoxia and volume loading in physically trained rats. Cardiovasc. Res. 14:50-57; 1980.

Chapter 19

Pulmonary System Adaptations: Limitations to Exercise

Mark A. Babcock
Jerome A. Dempsey

This review of the respiratory response to exercise will examine the plasticity of the healthy lung and chest wall exposed to exercise and exercise training. A major point to be made is that this organ system, in comparison to the cardiovascular and neuromuscular systems, undergoes relatively little adaptation to chronic physical training. We also consider the implications this low level of plasticity may have on the balance (or imbalance) struck between demand versus capacity in the respiratory system during heavy short-term and endurance exercise. No attempt is made here to deal in depth with all aspects of limitations and we devote no discussion at all to the problem of regulatory mechanisms in the pulmonary system during exercise. Please consult recent reviews (12,13).

Summary of Key Responses to Maximum Exercise in the Young, Untrained Healthy Pulmonary System ($\dot{V}O_2$max less than or equal to 50–55 ml·kg^{-1}·min^{-1})

The pulmonary system of the young untrained adult responds to the exercise stimulus by a precise neuromechanical regulation of matching alveolar ventilation to metabolic demand (13), as well as through changes designed to optimize transfer of oxygen from alveolar gas to arterial blood such as maintenance of alveolar capillary diffusion distance, adequate red blood cell transit time through pulmonary capillary beds and ventilation to perfusion ratios that are high ($\dot{V}_A$:$\dot{Q}_C$~3–5) and fairly uniformly distributed at maximal exercise.

Several key mechanical responses occur during the progression from mild to maximum exercise:

1. Airway resistance remains unchanged because the upper airway is maximally dilated due to phasic activation of the airway abductor muscles. Intrathoracic bronchiolar smooth muscle also undergoes near maximum relaxation, and bronchodilation occurs.
2. End-expiratory lung volume (EELV) decreases because of expiratory muscle recruitment. Thus elastic energy stored in the chest wall during expiration is released, leading to a "passive assist" of inspiration upon initiation of next breath. In addition the increased intra-abdominal pressure lengthens the diaphragm, placing it in a more advantageous position on its length:tension relationship.
3. Tidal volume (V_T) is increased by encroaching on both inspiratory and expiratory reserve volumes so that less compliant areas of the pressure:volume (p:v) relationship of the respiratory system are avoided during exercise. Dynamic compliance is reduced slightly at maximum exercise.
4. Maximum flow rates achieved during tidal breathing do not reach the maximum available flow rate. The pleural pressure developed during expiration only reaches flow limiting pressures at low lung volumes near EELV at maximum exercise. Therefore expiratory pleural pressure does not reach a level where dynamic compression of airways would occur and limit expiratory airflow.
5. During tidal inspiration at peak pressure the inspiratory muscles generate only 40% to 60% of their capacity for dynamic pressure generation—as estimated under resting conditions for the volumes (muscle length) and flow rates (velocity of shortening) achieved during exercise (1,26).

What are the consequences of these ventilatory responses? First, the inspiratory and expiratory muscles appear to be operating within their capacity for pressure generation and at a level that would not be expected to cause fatigue (24,28).

Secondly, the oxygen cost of the exercise hyperpnea does not seem to be excessive (1). The typical, untrained young adult shown in Figure 19.1 who at $\dot{V}O_2max$ did not reach significant expiratory flow limitation and whose inspiratory muscles generated pressures of only 40% to 60% of their dynamic capacity, required a respiratory muscle $\dot{V}O_2$ of about 8% to 11% of their whole body $\dot{V}O_2max$ (1). Thirdly, the maximum expired gas flow ($\dot{V}_E$) required in these young, untrained subjects (~120L/m) is just beginning to reach the level where the effects of mechanical constraint on ventilatory output are becoming significant. This was shown by the reduced ventilatory response to superimposed carbon dioxide (CO_2) inhalation which was first evident at exercise intensities requiring these levels of $\dot{V}_E$ (9).

In long-term endurance exercise at a level greater than 65% of $\dot{V}O_2max$, breathing frequency and ventilatory output will gradually rise; thus the alveolar ventilation ($\dot{V}_A$) remains adequate but loses efficiency because of increasing dead space ventilation. This hyperventilation serves as a means to minimize [H^+] changes in both arterial and femoral venous blood (45). Only at very heavy, sustained work loads (greater than 85% $\dot{V}O_2max$) is the ventilatory work apparently sufficient to precipitate diaphragmatic fatigue in man (24,28).

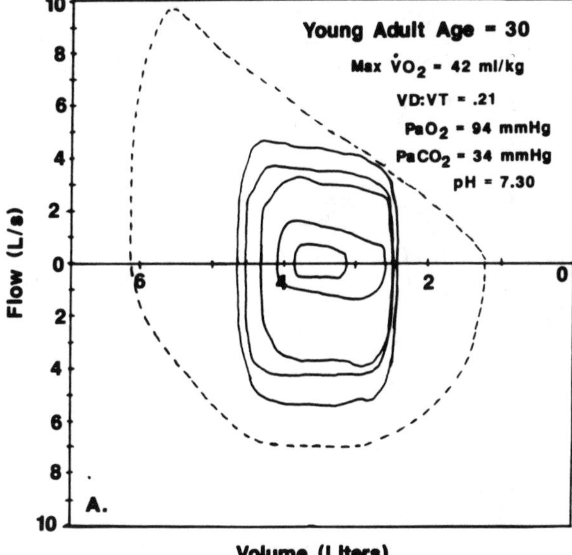

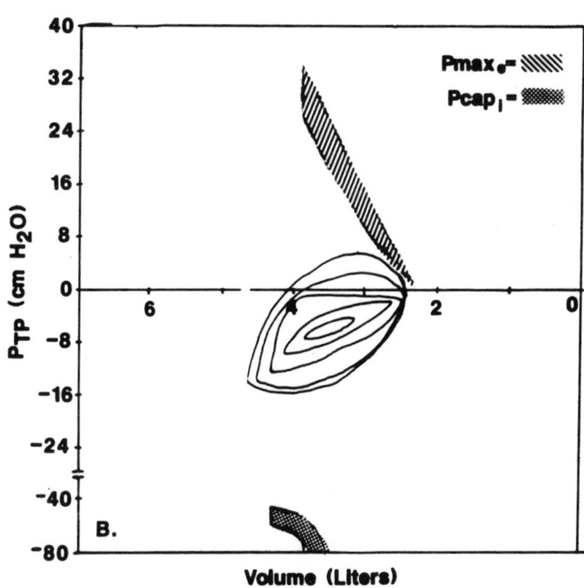

Figure 19.1 A typical ventilatory response to progressive exercise in an untrained young adult. The solid line represents the flow:volume (top) and pressure:volume (bottom) responses at rest and during progressively heavier work loads. Each loop represents the ensemble average of 20 breaths. The flow:volume loops are contained inside the maximal volitional flow:volume loop (broken line). No flow limitation is evident on the f:v loop and the inspiratory, and expiratory muscles are well short of their maximal pressure generation capacity during exercise.

Aging Effects on the Healthy (Nonsmoking) Pulmonary System

Figure 19.2 shows the flow:volume relation of an older adult at rest and during progressive exercise. Note that in comparison to the younger adult (Fig. 19.1), expiratory flow rates are lower at each lung volume and vital capacity is reduced. The functional residual capacity (FRC) and the lung volume at which airways close are increased compared to the young. These changes result from a loss of elastic recoil in the aging lung, leading to a dynamic narrowing or closure of airways at lower lung volumes during expiration compared to young adults.

The respiratory muscles in the older subject appear to be minimally affected by aging. The ability of the inspiratory muscles to generate pleural pressure across a range of lung volumes (lengths) or flow rates (velocity of shortening) was not different between young and older subjects (25). Animal studies also show that age-related changes in the diaphragm are minimal. For example, Type II muscle fiber size or distribution does not appear to change with aging (19). Negligible changes have been reported in capillary density (19), myosin heavy and light chains, and neuromuscular coupling of the aging diaphragm (42,43).

Gas exchange during exercise could be affected by aging because of six major changes. These are: (a) loss of elastic recoil of the lung (47), (b) decreased surface area of the lung (46), (c) decreased

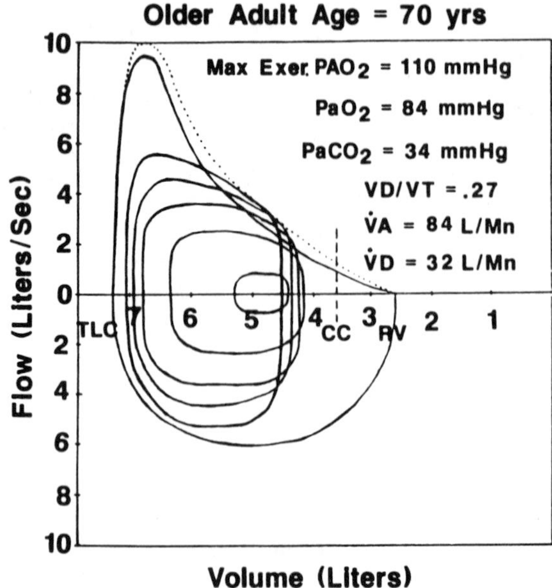

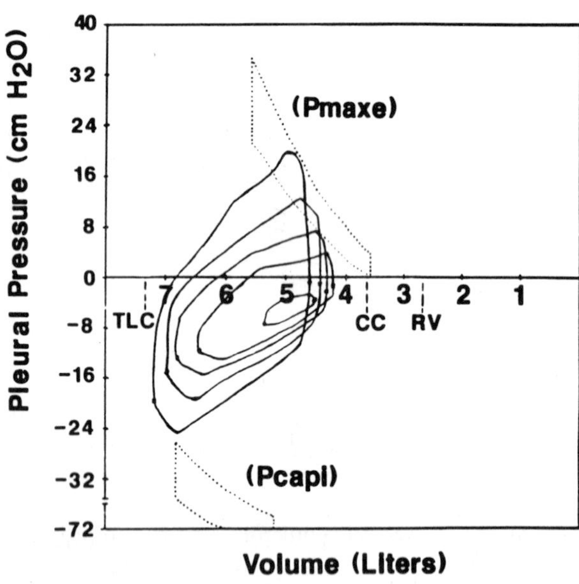

Figure 19.2 The group mean (n = 12) flow:volume (top) and pressure:volume (bottom) responses of older adults to progressive exercise. These individuals reach flow limitation during expiration at moderate work loads and an increasing proportion of expiration is flow limited. This is also evident from the pressure:volume loop, because the expiratory muscles reach their maximal effective expiratory pressure, thereby causing dynamic compression of the airways. Note the reduction in EELV in mild exercise and its increase back to resting levels at maximum exercise. Peak pressure generated by the inspiratory muscles reaches approximately 80% of the maximum available dynamic peak pressure (P_{capl}). TLC = total lung capacity; CC = closing capacity; RV = residual volume.

pulmonary capillary blood volume (14), (d) increased dead space ventilation (6), (e) decreased distensibility of the pulmonary arterial vasculature (36), and (f) reduced rib cage compliance. The effects of these changes with age will depend on the relative magnitudes of aging effects on the structural capacities of the pulmonary system on the one hand, versus the effects on maximum metabolic demand as determined by aging effects on cardiovascular and skeletal muscle capacities.

How Adaptable Is the Healthy Pulmonary System to the Training Stimulus?

In general whole-body exercise training results in relatively small changes in total lung capacity and its subdivisions (8). Longitudinal studies in animals are nearly unanimous in showing that diffusion surface area of the lung is not altered with physical training (2,4,5,39). A larger diffusion capacity in champion swimmers has been reported but the data do not indicate if this higher capacity was a result of training or had been present since childhood (31); further, there were several studies showing no alteration in diffusion capacity in the highly trained (37). There are some exceptions such as young, highly trained swimmers who show larger lung volumes (3,8) and older endurance athletes who show less aging effects on the lung elastic recoil and diffusion surface (25). The differences in highly trained athletes, young and old, could be due to preselection, as these characteristics of the pulmonary system are necessary for success in the sport.

Finally, two extreme examples underscore the relative absence of plasticity in the lung—at least in response to the stimulus offered by physical training. First, daily exercise training has recently been shown to be without effect on the morphologic dimensions of pulmonary diffusion surface, even in the maturing lung of the newborn animal (39). Secondly, when athletic versus nonathletic species of similar body mass but differing in $\dot{V}O_2$max two- to threefold (e.g., horse vs. cow) corresponding differences in pulmonary diffusion surface were less than 50% in contrast to the threefold greater locomotor muscle mitochondrial volume (22,27). These effects of training or athleticism contrast sharply with the well-documented adaptability of the lung diffusion surface to chronic hypoxia. Humans native to or long-term travelers at high altitude—regardless of fitness level—show 30% to 50% greater pulmonary diffusion capacity than do short-term travelers (7).

In contrast to the lung the respiratory muscles appear to be more susceptible to alterations by a training stimulus. Exercise training increases the strength and endurance of the muscles as indicated by the ability to generate, using volitional tests, a larger maximum pressure and to sustain a given level of pressure over a longer time period (8,38). Whether these changes coincide with biochemical or histochemical changes in the inspiratory muscles in humans is unknown; indeed, that only volitional tests have been used leaves us with no objective evidence that whole-body physical training actually induces significant changes in the end-organ.

Animal studies are conflicting but do favor a significant adaptation of at least some fiber types in at least some portions of the diaphragm in response to whole-body physical training. For example, the activity of succinate dehydrogenase (SDH), a marker enzyme for oxidative capacity, has been reported to increase (23,34), or not to change (20,30) in the diaphragm after whole-body endurance training. However, aerobic capacity in the costal portion of the diaphragm is clearly changed by exercise training (33,34). The abdominal expiratory muscles, in contrast, showed no increase in oxidative enzyme activity after training (48).

Thus, the diaphragm at all ages seems adaptable to whole-body exercise in terms of changes in aerobic capacity and perhaps even fiber type, although these changes are consistently much smaller than in limb locomotor muscle of similar fiber type. Furthermore, the functional significance of these changes to the prevention of fatigue or regulation of breathing during exercise, remains untested.

Demand Versus Capacity in the Trained, Healthy Pulmonary System

Because there is a relative lack of adaptability in structures of the lung diffusion surface and in the airways and lung parenchyma and a limited adaptability in the chest wall respiratory musculature in response to a physical-training stimulus compared to the cardiovascular system and skeletal muscle, the pulmonary system may lag behind. Thus, it would seem reasonable to postulate that the lung and chest wall will increase in importance as contributors to exercise limitation, the greater the exercise capacity (10). Current evidence, summarized following, supports this hypothesis, but also emphasizes that redundancy in different structures within the pulmonary system varies widely.

Pulmonary Gas Exchange

When many, but not all, highly trained, young human subjects exercised near or at the level of their $\dot{V}O_2max$ (greater than 65 $ml{\cdot}kg^{-1}{\cdot}min^{-1}$) the alveolar to arterial partial pressure of oxygen (A-a DO_2) difference widens to greater than 30 to 35 mmHg, and the oxygen saturation of arterial blood (SaO_2) declines below 90% and the arterial partial pressure of oxygen (PaO_2) falls below 75 mmHg (11,12,21,26,50). This decrease in O_2 saturation may be due to (a) significant amounts of ventilation to perfusion ($\dot{V}_A{:}\dot{Q}_C$) nonhomogeneity, (b) postpulmonary veno-arterial shunt or, (c) failure of alveolar to end-pulmonary capillary equilibrium (11). Certainly, as mixed venous oxyhemoglobin (HbO_2) saturation falls with exercise the $\dot{V}_A{:}\dot{Q}_C$ nonuniformity (*within* lung regions) and the small anatomic shunt contribute significantly and progressively to a normally widening A-a DO_2. But at exactly what level of exercise $\dot{V}O_2$, if any, alveolar to end-pulmonary capillary disequilibrium occurs remains unspecified (because of our inability to definitively separate all three potential contributors). We would speculate that the excessive widening of the A-a DO_2 in many of the athletes who had $\dot{V}O_2max$ greater than 65 to 70 $ml{\cdot}kg^{-1}{\cdot}min^{-1}$ is due to diffusion limitation.

In turn, why might this proposed diffusion disequilibrium occur? Much has been made recently of the potential fragility of the blood-gas barrier placed under the stress of a rising pulmonary capillary pressure at high flow rates leading to an accumulation of extravascular lung water, that is, pulmonary edema, at heavy exercise (16,40). Unfortunately, methods do not permit a direct testing of this hypothesis (17). In our highly trained athletes who experience exercise-induced arterial hypoxemia (11) all but one (of 30 tested thus far) showed an immediate return of arterial PO_2 and a narrowing of A-a DO_2 back to preexercising resting levels within 1 to 3 min—and usually within 30 s—following maximum exercise. These data provide very indirect evidence against the notion that extra-vascular lung water has accumulated at the alveolar-capillary interface, at least to an extent that would cause diffusion limitation during exercise.

On the other hand there is some evidence that left ventricular dysfunction may occur at the termination of very heavy exercise (40,41) and that relatively mild nonuniformities in $\dot{V}_A{:}\dot{Q}_C$ distribution during exercise may sometimes persist in recovery (40). In addition, elegant studies in the isolated dog lung lobe show extravascular fluid accumulation when blood flow rate increases sufficiently to cause pulmonary wedge pressure to exceed 25 mmHg (i.e., levels that would approximate those observed in some elite athletes), and this edema formation was enhanced via increased V_T and transpulmonary pressure (51).

So, there are inconclusive data on both sides of this question of exercise-induced pulmonary edema. We favor the speculation that any diffusion limitation in very heavy exercise in the highly fit occurs secondary to an inadequate red cell transit time in the pulmonary capillary secondary to an extraordinary maximum pulmonary blood flow through a normal size pulmonary capillary vascular volume (11). These exciting controversial questions need to be addressed in depth.

An equally intriguing flip side to this question is why *only* less than about one half of the human athletes tested to date actually experienced significant arterial hypoxemia at these high work loads? One answer may be the critical importance under these extreme conditions of high metabolic rate and markedly reduced mixed venous O_2 content of even very small interindividual differences in certain critical matchups of demand versus capacity due to:

- size of pulmonary capillary blood volume versus blood flow (11),
- variations in the distribution of red blood cell transit times throughout the lung,
- small maldistribution of the mechanical time constants among the smaller airways leading to propensities toward slightly lower regional $\dot{V}_A$:$\dot{Q}_C$ (underventilated) areas in some subjects than others, and
- individual differences in the degree of the hyperventilatory response, a factor in causing hypoxemia in at least a minority of cases (11,26).

In turn, these differences in ventilatory response are determined by the magnitude of *mechanical limitation* to flow and volume in maximum exercise on the one hand and the subject's *responsiveness* (of respiratory motor output) to the combination of mechanical constraints and increasing neurochemical stimuli on the other (26). It has been proposed that endurance athletes show a sluggish ventilatory response to chemical stimuli. However, this is clearly not the case during heavy and maximum exercise where some fit subjects show a marked hyperventilation that helps maintain a high PaO_2, and yet drives them to their mechanical limits for flow, volume, and pressure; whereas others show little or no hyperventilatory response (despite progressive arterial hypoxemia and acidosis) and remain well within their mechanical reserves for ventilatory output (25,26).

It is also important to note that the equine athlete shows very little heterogeneity in terms of pulmonary gas exchange during exercise, because virtually all thoroughbred horses demonstrate marked widening of A-a DO_2 and arterial hypoxemia that begins at 60% to 70% of their $\dot{V}O_2$max and worsens progressively with further exercise. CO_2 retention commonly occurs at slightly higher work loads. This "threshold" work rate for hypoxemia corresponds to about 80 to 100 ml·kg^{-1}·min^{-1} in these animals. Perhaps these data predict that if human athletes also eventually achieve maximum aerobic capacities of this magnitude, they too will uniformly experience frank failure of pulmonary O_2 transport.

The older human athlete presents yet an additional example of demand exceeding capacity—again to highly variable extents. Excessive A-a DO_2 and significant hypoxemia were observed in some older endurance athletes at $\dot{V}O_2$max, but at a prevalence rate (about 20%) that was even slightly less than that in the younger athletes. The interesting feature of these older healthy athletes was that the hypoxemia occurred at $\dot{V}O_2$max in the 45 to 55-ml·kg^{-1}·min^{-1} range, a level of maximum metabolic demand at which younger, healthy subjects never experience exercise-induced arterial hypoxemia. Apparently then, in some healthy subjects—especially those who continue heavy training schedules—the aging effect on reducing the magnitude of the alveolar capillary diffusion surface (capacity) exceeded the age-related decline in $\dot{V}O_2$max (demand). We emphasize that the norm is for the age-related decline in diffusion capacity to lag slightly behind that in $\dot{V}O_2$max, thus exercise-induced hypoxemia was a rare occurrence in the elderly athlete.

Lung and Chest Wall Mechanics

Demand also exceeds capacity among healthy subjects in terms of airway mechanics. Figure 19.3 shows the f:v and p:v relationships for young, highly trained subjects described previously. Not only did these subjects experience hypoxemia but the f:v loops show flow limitation over most of expiration at maximum exercise. During this flow limitation at the maximal work rate (the largest f:v and p:v loop) the subjects in general met or slightly exceeded the effective maximal expiratory pressure (P_{max}e) over a significant portion of the expiration. The P_{max}e is the level of pressure generation where maximum flow rate occurs at a given lung volume; producing more pressure will only cause compression of the airways. Therefore the flow rate will decrease and the subject does more work than necessary and essentially wastes energy.

This process is even more dramatic in the aging athlete (Fig. 19.4). In older (vs. young) subjects less pressure generation is needed to reach $P_{max}e$, which is consistent with the age-dependent loss of elastic recoil of the lung (25,26). When expiratory flow and inspiratory pressure development are very high the $\dot{V}O_2$ of respiratory muscles will exceed 400 ml·min^{-1} and approach 15% of whole-body $\dot{V}O_2max$ (1). At these work levels the respiratory muscles may compromise blood flow distribution and therefore O_2 delivery to working locomotor skeletal muscle.

When the work rate requires 85% $\dot{V}O_2max$ or more and exercise duration exceeds 10 min, significant diaphragm fatigue may also occur. The more intense the exercise the greater will be the metabolic and ventilatory requirements; this in turn leads to greater respiratory muscle fatigue (24).

In summary, more fit individuals are more likely to experience several manifestations of demand exceeding capacity:

- Arterial hypoxemia during maximal exercise
- Flow limitation during expiration when $\dot{V}_E$ exceeds 120 L/min
- Pressure development by inspiratory muscles during tidal breaths that reaches its dynamic (available) capacity for pressure generation
- High O_2 cost of breathing greater than or equal to 15% of $\dot{V}O_2max$
- Diaphragm fatigue during endurance exercise when work intensity exceeds 85% $\dot{V}O_2max$

In fit elderly subjects dynamic compression of airways occurs more readily during expiration as elastic recoil of the lung diminishes with age. This means that expiratory flow limitation occurs even at moderate work loads and EELV increases back to and above resting levels. A major consequence of this limitation in the fit elderly subject is an increased oxygen cost of ventilation.

Relative Susceptibilities to Failure Within the Pulmonary System

The types of data outlined herein show that demand can indeed exceed capacity in the healthy pulmonary system; they also suggest that not all elements of the pulmonary system have the same structural "reserve."

The normal pulmonary diffusion capacity (which is nearly equal in the trained and untrained human subject) appears to be the component with the greatest reserve. This evaluation

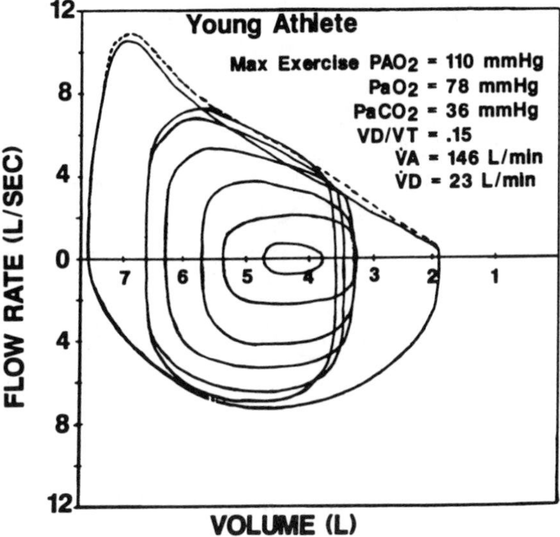

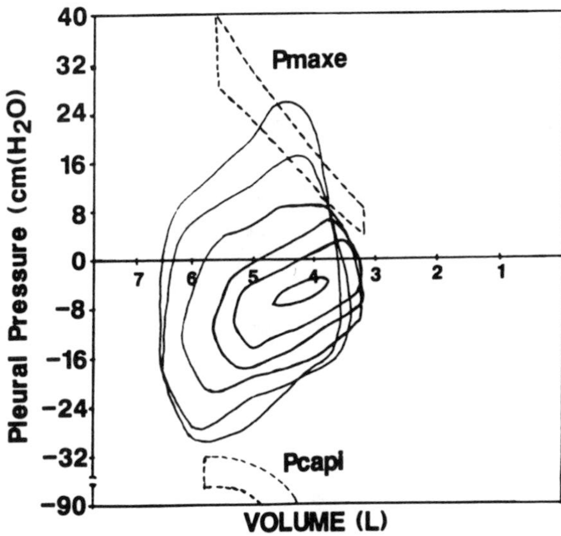

Figure 19.3 Mean ventilatory response to progressive exercise in young endurance athletes (n = 8). Tidal flow (top) and pressure (bottom) volume loops (solid lines) are plotted from rest through maximal exercise. The tidal flow:volume loops are plotted within the pre-(solid) and postexercise (dashed) maximal volitional flow:volume loops, and are positioned according to their measured end-expiratory lung volume. The tidal pressure:volume loops are plotted relative to the maximal effective pressure on expiration and the capacity for inspiratory muscle pressure generation on inspiration. At maximum exercise the highly trained athlete achieves expiratory flow limitation over most (55% to 65%) of their VT, and their inspiratory muscles generate peak pressures which approximate 90% to 100% of the available maximum P_{capi}.

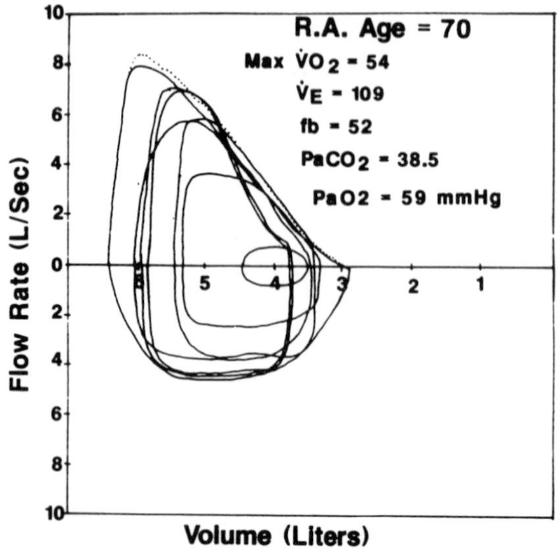

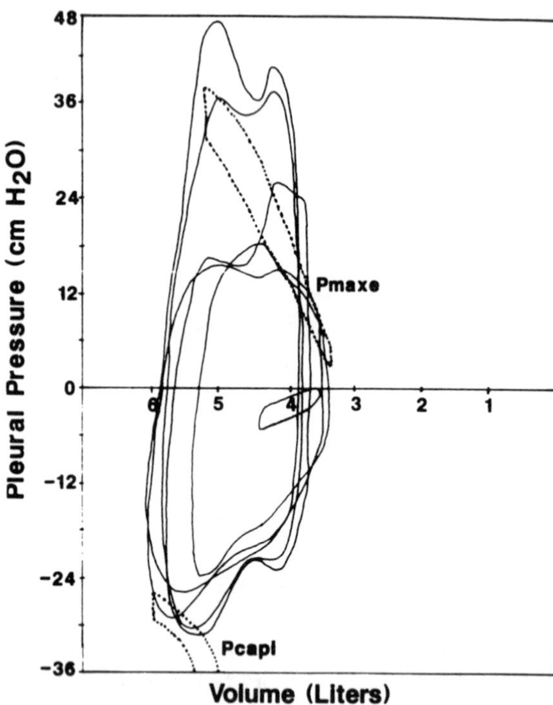

Figure 19.4 The ventilatory response to progressive exercise in a very fit older adult. The flow:volume (top) and pressure:volume (bottom) (solid lines) from rest to maximal exercise are plotted. The flow:volume loops are plotted within the pre- (solid) and post-exercise (dashed) maximal volitional flow volume loops relative to the measured EELV. The pressure: volume loops are plotted relative to the inspiratory capacity for pressure generation and the maximal effective pressure on expiration. Note that this subject reaches significant expiratory flow limitation at every work load above rest, that EELV initially fell and then rose above resting FRC, and that at both top two work rates the subject exceeds maximal effective capacity for pressure generation on expiration, achieving the available capacity for pressure generation by inspiratory muscles. fb = breathing frequency.

is based on the observation that significant exercise-induced arterial hypoxemia does not begin to develop until the demand for pulmonary oxygen transport ($\dot{V}O_2$max) exceeds normal by more than 150% to 160%; it is not even universally present probably until $\dot{V}O_2$max is greater than 200% of normal (i.e., extrapolating data in the human to the thoroughbred horse). Given the substantial effect of chronic hypoxia (as opposed to physical training) on pulmonary diffusion capacity, we would speculate that the athletic natives of high altitudes would experience the least chance of incurring diffusion limitation and exercise-induced arterial hypoxemia during heavy exercise at sea level.

Expiratory flow limitation, that is, dynamic airway compression, at the level of the intralobar airways appears to have considerably less reserve than does diffusion, judging from the findings that significant expiratory flow limitation (i.e., greater than 60% of V_T achieves expiratory flow limitation), begins to occur at ventilatory requirements accompanying a $\dot{V}O_2$max that is only 130% to 150% of the normal, untrained $\dot{V}O_2$max. We judge that this amount of flow limitation may represent a significant ventilatory limitation because it causes a reduction in the gain of ventilatory response, forces EELV to rise, and occurs coincidentally with a marked increase in the oxygen cost per liter $\dot{V}_E$ (a reduced mechanical efficiency of breathing).

The endurance capacity of the diaphragm may be the weakest link with the least reserve in view of the finding that significant diaphragmatic fatigue occurs as a result of heavy endurance exercise, even in the normally fit, untrained subject. We need to clarify, however, that these are very special circumstances that cause this diaphragmatic fatigue. Only 60% to 70% of the maximum dynamic capacity of the diaphragm for pressure generation is reached during tidal breathing under these heavy endurance conditions. (Indeed, to reach the dynamic capacity for inspiratory muscle pressure generation during exercise requires a $\dot{V}O_2$max in the 70- to 80-ml·kg^{-1}·min^{-1} range—which was only reached at maximum exercise loads sustained for a 2 to 3 min period.) Further, even maintaining this magnitude of pressure generation by the inspiratory muscles (or the diaphragm) is probably not sufficient by itself to cause diaphragmatic fatigue, even when maintained for periods of time equal to or greater than the duration of the whole-body endurance exercise itself (1).

We would postulate that it is not the capacity for pressure generation that is severely taxed during whole-body endurance exercise. Rather, it seems as though the background or internal milieu of metabolic acidosis—both within the diaphragm muscle and in the plasma (15)—and high levels of circulating catecholamines are required in combination with the high pressures repeatedly generated by the muscle to cause the working diaphragm to fatigue. These influences may work via an enhanced glycogen depletion and by preventing diffusion of hydrogen ions out of the working muscle cell, thereby intensifying intracellular acidosis in the diaphragm. To date these hypotheses have only been tested in part.

In summary, for the first two of these instances of demand exceeding capacity (i.e., pulmonary diffusion and expiratory flow limitation) we would speculate, based on our original hypothesis, that substantial redundancy or reserve exists in these functions at the $\dot{V}O_2$max achieved in the untrained state. These reserves are then eroded as training (or greater fitness) increases the maximum metabolic requirement together with the need for greater pulmonary O_2 transfer and expiratory flow rate, without concomitant adjustments in the structural capacities of the alveolar capillary surface for diffusion or the intrathoracic airways for accepting high expiratory flow rates.

With regard to the inspiratory muscles and the diaphragm of the trained or untrained subject, we believe their capacity for maximum pressure generation and for sustained endurance performance at high pressures exceeds by a comfortable margin that required for the ventilatory output demanded by whole-body, prolonged exercise. The exercise-induced diaphragmatic fatigue occurs because of the internal milieu created by the end products from exercising limb locomotor muscles.

We would further speculate that while intense physical training might increase the aerobic capacity of the diaphragm to some extent, the protection afforded by this adaptation against diaphragmatic fatigue during whole-body endurance exercise at a given relative intensity of $\dot{V}O_2$max is lost because the requirement for ventilation and therefore diaphragmatic pressure generation will be markedly increased in the subject with the higher $\dot{V}O_2$max. Thus, the trained subjects experience similar levels of diaphragmatic fatigue during exercise, although they are "protected" to some extent because their diaphragm sustains much greater absolute work loads (24).

In all components of the pulmonary system, adaptation to the chronic stimulus of training, or even genetic endowment afforded the highly fit athlete, is insufficient to prevent demand from exceeding structural capacity as fitness increases in the healthy human subject.

Role of Pulmonary System as a Limiting Factor in $\dot{V}O_2$max and in Endurance Exercise Performance

It is important to clarify that because the *limits* to airflow, respiratory muscle function, or diffusion may be met or surpassed during exercise does not automatically translate into the conclusion that these factors will necessarily be *limiting to* exercise performance. We now address this latter question.

First, what are the consequences of the arterial O_2 desaturation (84%–92% SaO_2) observed in the highly trained during short-term maximum or near maximum exercise? To address this question, trained and untrained subjects were provided a mildly hyperoxic gas mixture to breathe during an incremental exercise test that was just sufficient to maintain SaO_2 at resting levels. The results showed that the highly trained subjects who had reduced their air breathing SaO_2 to less than 92% increased their $\dot{V}O_2$max (75 vs. 70 $ml \cdot kg^{-1} \cdot min^{-1}$) when their exercise-induced hypoxemia was prevented. On the other hand, the moderately trained group's $\dot{V}O_2$max remained unchanged at 57 $ml \cdot kg^{-1} \cdot min^{-1}$ (35).

The extent of the influence of this "limiting factor" is probably at most 10% to 15% of the $\dot{V}O_2$max. That is, $\dot{V}O_2$max would increase about 15% when the maximum observed arterial desaturation (about 84%) is prevented with supplemental O_2. Thus, even at its peak influence, the effects of exercise-induced arterial hypoxemia are probably less than those imposed by limitations in maximum cardiac output. These data also support the notion of the critical importance of systemic O_2 transport in the determination of $\dot{V}O_2$max because the working locomotor muscles—even in the very highly trained—are apparently capable of extracting and metabolizing more O_2 when it is provided.

The pulmonary system may also limit exercise capacity when the ventilatory requirement is such that severe expiratory flow limitation is incurred. At this level of ventilatory work the oxygen cost of breathing may exceed 15% of $\dot{V}O_2$tot, sufficient to limit work output because the respiratory muscles may "steal" blood flow originally intended for locomotor muscles. The perception of the effort of ventilating at these high levels may also contribute to endurance exercise limitation. Attempts to test these hypotheses have focused on the effects of "unloading" using a proportional assist mechanical ventilator (18). In short- or long-term exercise, when the ventilatory response was in the 110- to 130-$L \cdot min^{-1}$ range, unloading produced little effect on the ventilatory response, on the $\dot{V}O_2$, or on the performance time. However, we have also observed when the highly fit performed endurance exercise at intensities in excess of 85% $\dot{V}O_2max$ ($\dot{V}_E$ greater than 130 $L \cdot min^{-1}$) unloading via $He:O_2$, inhalation significantly prolonged performance time, reduced dyspneic sensations, and increased the ventilatory response.

These results are consistent with the concept that significant pulmonary limitations to exercise are most likely to occur under very high demand conditions—whether via arterial hypoxemia or the generation of excessive ventilatory work. The examples discussed previously in the elderly athlete also remind us, however, that both of these limiting factors—exercise-induced arterial hypoxemia (rarely) and excessive respiratory muscle work—may occur in the healthy subject at work rates that require only 50 $ml \cdot kg^{-1} \cdot min^{-1}$ $\dot{V}O_2max$ if the pulmonary diffusion capacity or mechanical limits to flow rate are diminished, which commonly occurs with the normal aging process.

The third type of pulmonary system limitation identified earlier was that of diaphragmatic fatigue incurred during heavy endurance exercise. The biological significance of this fatigue has not been determined. It certainly does not prevent the occurrence of significant time-dependent hyperventilation during prolonged exercise. Clearly, unloading studies are needed to determine the effect of diaphragmatic fatigue on respiratory muscle recruitment and breathing pattern.

Biological limitations to oxygen transport and to exercise performance are rarely, if ever, confined to a single organ system; clearly, strong interactions occur among the organ systems to contribute in total to exercise limitation. These interactions have received little attention to date. For example, we have emphasized that excessive ventilatory work may contribute to exercise limitation via a high oxygen cost of breathing and therefore steal blood flow from limb locomotor muscles. This view is too narrow!

Extremely high intrathoracic pressures (± 30–35 cm H_2O Δ pleural pressure) are also generated by the respiratory muscles because of the high ventilatory requirement and flow limitations, and these changes might affect cardiac output. Natural quiet breathing at rest was associated with phasic changes in femoral venous blood flow (49). The increase in abdominal pressure during contraction of the diaphragm has also been shown to increase the venous return from the splanchnic area (44). Increases in pleural pressure may also affect the afterload on the left ventricle (decrease it) and the preload on the right atrium by increasing right ventricle wall stiffness (this would decrease preload by restricting the filling of the right ventricle) (32). Might these wildly swinging pressures—both intrathoracic and transdiaphragmatic—have a significant effect on venous return, cardiac filling and cardiac output, and perhaps even diaphragmatic blood flow, and therefore markedly limit $\dot{V}O_2$ or performance? This hypothesis needs testing across the broad continuum of demand versus capacity, perhaps by use of unloading experiments.

Another example of potentially strong interactive effects on the limitation to exercise performance is the observed fatigue of the diaphragm during exercise. As mentioned earlier, diaphragmatic fatigue did not occur in isolation. In addition to the high muscular work generated, this fatigue probably required anaerobic metabolism by the limb locomotor muscles that presented the diaphragm with the "opportunity" to experience lactate uptake and intracellular metabolic acidosis.

We urge adoption of a broader, interactive cause–effect view of biological limitations to exercise.

Acknowledgments

This work is supported by NHLBI. Mark Babcock is an American Lung Association Postdoctoral Fellow. We are indebted to Dana Van Hoesen for her excellent preparation of the manuscript and to Jeffrey Regnis for his helpful criticisms of the manuscript.

References

1. Aaron, E.A.; Johnson, B.E.; Seow, C.K.; Dempsey, J.A. Oxygen cost of exercise hyperpnea: Implications for performance. J. Appl. Physiol. 75(5):1818-1825; 1992.
2. Andrew, G.M.; Becklake, M.R.; Guleria, J.S.; Bates, D.V. Heart and lung functions in swimmers and non-athletes during growth. J. Appl. Physiol. 32(2):245-251; 1972.
3. Astrand, P.O.; Engstrom, L.; Eriksson, B.O.; Karlberg, P.; Nylander, I.; Saltin, B.; Thoren, C. Girl swimmers: With special reference to respiratory and circulatory adaptation and gynecological and psychiatric aspects. Acta. Paediatr. Suppl. 147: 5-71; 1963.
4. Bartlett, D. Postnatal growth of the mammalian lung: Influence of exercise and thyroid activity. Respir. Physiol. 9:50-57; 1970.
5. Bartlett, D.; Areson, J.G. Quantitative lung morphology in Japanese waltzing mice. J. Appl. Physiol. 4:446-449; 1978.

6. Brischetto, M.S.; Millman, R.P.; Peterson, D.D.; Silage, D.A.; Pack, A.I. Effect of aging on ventilatory response to exercise and CO_2. J. Appl. Physiol. 56:1143-1150; 1984.
7. Cerny, F.C.; Dempsey, J.A.; Reddan, W.G. Pulmonary gas exchange in non-native residents of high altitude. J. Clin. Invest. 52:2993-2999; 1973.
8. Clanton, T.L.; Dixon, G.F.; Drake, J.; Gadek, J.E. Effects of swim training on lung volumes and inspiratory muscle conditioning. J. Appl. Physiol. 62(1):39-46; 1987.
9. Clark, J.M.; Sinclair, R.E.; Lenox, J.B. Chemical and nonchemical components of ventilation during hypercapnic exercise in man. J. Appl. Physiol. 48:1065-1076; 1980.
10. Dempsey, J.A. Is the lung built for exercise? Med. Sci. Sports. 18:143-155; 1986.
11. Dempsey, J.A.; Hanson, P.G.; Henderson, K. Exercise-induced arterial hypoxemia in healthy humans at sea level. J. Physiol. (Lond.). 355:161-175; 1984.
12. Dempsey, J.A.; Powers, S.; Gledhill, N. Cardiovascular and pulmonary adaptation to physiological activity: Discussion. In: Bouchard, C.; Exercise, fitness, and health. Champaign, IL: Human Kinetics; 1990:205-216.
13. Dempsey, J.A.; Vidruk, E.H.; Mitchell, G. Pulmonary control systems in exercise: Update. Symposium on biological regulation during exercise at FASEB national meeting; 1984 April; St. Louis. Fed. Proc. 44:2260-2270; 1985.
14. Emirgil, C.; Sobol, B.J.; Campodonico, S.; Herbert, W.M.; Mechkati, R. Pulmonary circulation in the aged. J. Appl. Physiol. 23:631-640; 1967.
15. Fregosi, R.; Dempsey, J.A. The effects of exercise in normoxia and acute hypoxia on respiratory muscle metabolites. J. Appl. Physiol. 60:1274-1283; 1986.
16. Fu, Z.; Costello, M.L.; Tsukimoto, K.; Prediletto, R.; Elliott, A.R.; Mathieu-Costello, O.; West, J.B. High lung volume increases stress failure in pulmonary capillaries. J. Appl. Physiol. 74(1):123-133; 1992.
17. Gallagher, C.G.; Huda, W.; Rigby, M.; Greenberg, D.; Younes, M. Lack of radio graphic evidence of interstitial pulmonary edema after maximal exercise in normal subjects. Am. Rev. Respir. Dis. 137:474-476; 1988.
18. Gallagher, C.G.; Younes, M. Effect of pressure assist on ventilation and respiratory mechanics in heavy exercise. J. Appl. Physiol. 66:1824-1837; 1989.
19. Gosselin, L.E.; Betlach, M.; Vailas, A.C.; Thomas, D.P. Training-induced alterations in young and senscent rat diaphragm muscle. J. Appl. Physiol. 72(4):1506-1511; 1992.
20. Green, H.J.; Plyley, M.J.; Smith, D.M.; Kile, J.G. Extreme endurance training and fiber type adaptation in rat diaphragm. J. Appl. Physiol. 66(4):1914-1920; 1989.
21. Hopkins, S.R.; McKenzie, D.C. Hypoxic ventilatory response and arterial desaturation during heavy work. J. Appl. Physiol. 67(3):1119-1124; 1989.
22. Hoppeler, H.; Kayar, S.R.; Claassen, H.; Uhlmann, E.; Karas, R.H. Adaptive variation in the mammalian respiratory system in relation to energetic demand: III. Skeletal muscles: Setting the demand for oxygen. Respir. Physiol. 69:27-46; 1987.
23. Ianuzzo, C.D.; Noble, E.G.; Hamilton, N.; Dabrowski, B. Effects of streptozotocin diabetes; insulin treatment, and training on the diaphragm. J. Appl. Physiol. 52(6):1471-1475; 1982.
24. Johnson, B.D.; Babcock, M.A.; Suman, O.E.; Dempsey, J.A. Exercise induced diaphragmatic fatigue in healthy humans. J. Physiol. (Lond.). 460:385-405; 1993.
25. Johnson, B.D.; Reddan, W.G.; Seow, K.C.; Dempsey, J.A. Mechanical constraints on exercise hyperpnea in an aging population. Am. Rev. Respir. Dis. 143:968-977; 1991.
26. Johnson, B.D.; Saupe, K.W.; Dempsey, J.A. Mechanical constraints on exercise hyperpnea in endurance athletes. J. Appl. Physiol. 73:874-886; 1992.
27. Kayar, S.R.; Hoppeler, H.; Lindstedt, S.L.; Claassen, H.; Jones, J.H.; Essen-Gustavsson, B.; Taylor, C.R. Total muscle mitochondrial volume in relation to aerobic capacity of horses and steers. Pflugers Arch. 413:343-347; 1989.
28. Levine, S.; Henson, D. Low-frequency diaphragmatic fatigue in spontaneously breathing humans. J. Appl. Physiol. 64:672-680; 1988.
29. McCool, F.D.; Tzelepis, G.T.; Leith, D.E.; Hoppin, F.G. Oxygen cost of breathing during fatiguing inspiratory resistive loads. J. Appl. Physiol. 66:2045-2055; 1989.
30. Metzger, J.M.; Fitts, R.H. Contractile and biochemical properties of diaphragm: Effects of exercise training and fatigue. J. Appl. Physiol. 60(5):1752-1758; 1986.
31. Mostyn, E.M.; Helle, S.; Gee, J.B.L.; Bentivoglio, L.G.; Bates, D.V. Pulmonary diffusing capacity of athletes. J. Appl. Physiol. 18(4):687-695; 1963.
32. Permutt, S.; Wise, R.A.; Sylvester, J.T. Interaction between the circulatory and ventilatory pumps. In: Roussos, C.T.; Macklem, P.T., eds. The thorax. New York: Marcel Dekker; 1985:701-735.

33. Powers, S.; Criswell, D.; Lieu, F.-K.; Dodd, S.; Silverman, H. Diaphragmatic fiber type specific adaptation to endurance exercise. Respir. Physiol. 89:195-207; 1992.
34. Powers, S.K.; Lawler, J.; Criswell, D.; Dodd, S.; Grinton, S.; Bagby, G.; Silverman, H. Endurance-training-induced cellular adaptations in respiratory muscles. J. Appl. Physiol. 68(5): 2114-2118; 1990.
35. Powers, S.K.; Lawler, J.; Dempsey, J.A.; Dodd, S.; Landry, G.E. Effects of incomplete pulmonary gas exchange on $\dot{V}O_2$max. J. Appl. Physiol. 66(6):2491-2495; 1989.
36. Reeves, J.T.; Dempsey, J.A.; Grover, R.F. Pulmonary circulation during exercise. In: Weir, E.K.; Reeves, J.T., eds. Pulmonary vascular physiology and pathophysiology. New York: Marcel Dekker; 1989:107-133.
37. Reuschlein, P.L.; Reddan, W.G.; Burpee, J.F.; Gee, J.B.L.; Rankin, J. The effect of physical training on the pulmonary diffusing capacity during submaximal work. J. Appl. Physiol. 24:152-158; 1968.
38. Robinson, E.P.; Kjeldgaard, J.M. Improvement in ventilatory muscle function with running. J. Appl. Physiol. 52(6):1400-1406; 1982.
39. Ross, K.A.; Thurlbeck, W.M. Lung growth in newborn guinea pigs: Effects of endurance exercise. Respir. Physiol. 89:353-364; 1992.
40. Schaffartzik, W.; Poole, D.C.; Derion, T.; Tsukimoto, J.; Hogan, M.C.; Arcos, J.P.; Bebout, D.E.; Wagner, P.D. $\dot{V}_A/\dot{Q}$ distribution during heavy exercise and recovery in humans: Implications for pulmonary edema. J. Appl. Physiol. 72(5):1657-1667; 1992.
41. Seals, D.R.; Rogers, M.A.; Hagberg, J.M.; Yamamoto, C.; Cryer, P.E.; Ehsani, A.A. Left ventricular dysfunction after prolonged strenuous exercise in healthy subjects. Am. J. Cardiol. 61:875-879; 1988.
42. Smith, D.O. Physiological and structural changes at the neuromuscular junction during aging. In: Giacobini, E.; Filogamo, G.; Giacogini, G.; Vernadakis, A., eds. The aging brain: Cellular and molecular mechanisms in the nervous system. New York: Raven Press; 1982: 123-137.
43. Smith, D.O.; Rosenheimer, J.L. Aging at the neuromuscular junction. In: Johnson, J.E., Jr., ed. Aging and cell structure. New York: Plenum Press; 1984:111-137.
44. Takata, M.; Robotham, J.L. Effects of inspiratory diaphragm descent on inferior vena caval venous return. J. Appl. Physiol. 72:597-607; 1992.
45. Thompson, J.M.; Dempsey, J.A.; Chosy, L.W.; Shahidi, N.T.; Reddan, W.G. Oxygen transport and oxyhemoglobin dissociation during prolonged muscular work. J. Appl. Physiol. 37(5):658-664; 1974.
46. Thurlbeck, W.M. The effect of age on the lung. In: Dietz, A.A., ed. Aging—Its chemistry. Washington, DC: Association for Clinical Chemistry; 1980:88-109.
47. Turner, J.M.; Mead, J.; Wohl, M.E. Elasticity of human lungs in relation to age. J. Appl. Physiol. 25:664-671; 1968.
48. Uribe, J.M.; Stump, C.S.; Tipton, C.M.; Fregosi, R.F. Influence of exercise training on the oxidative capacity of rat abdominal muscles. Respir. Physiol. 88:171-180; 1992.
49. Willeput, R.; Rondeux, C.; deTroyer, A. Breathing affects venous return from legs in humans. J. Appl. Physiol. 57:971-976; 1984.
50. Williams, J.H.; Powers, S.K.; Stuart, M.K. Hemoglobin desaturation in highly trained athletes during heavy exercise. Med. Sci. Sports Exerc. 18(2):168-173; 1988.
51. Younes, M.; Bshouty, Z.; Ali, J. Longitudinal distribution of pulmonary vascular resistance with very high pulmonary blood flow. J. Appl. Physiol. 62:344-358; 1987.

Chapter 20

Hormonal Adaptation to Physical Activity

Erik A. Richter
John R. Sutton

Exercise is the most powerful physiologic perturbation experienced by healthy man. It requires major metabolic and cardiovascular adjustments to increase the supply of oxygen and fuels to the working muscles while at the same time maintaining internal homeostasis. To accomplish this task, changes in autonomic nervous activity as well as changes in hormone secretion occur during exercise. The rather sharp distinction between the nervous system and the hormonal system that was customary previously is no longer reasonable because substances earlier considered genuine hormones may be released from nerves (e.g., gastrin), and neurotransmitters may spill over into the blood and act as hormones (e.g., norepinephrine). Intracellular and extracellular fuel sources for muscle during exercise are illustrated in Figure 20.1. Fat and carbohydrates are present both inside and outside of the muscle cell. Protein and amino acids contribute about 2% to 10% of fuel sources depending upon availability of other fuels—for the most part carbohydrates.

A single bout of exercise is characterized by increased plasma concentrations of a large variety of hormones, and decreased concentrations of only a few hormones. Although only studied for some hormones, large changes in plasma hormone concentrations during exercise are generally the result of changes in secretion rate rather than changes in rate of clearance of the hormone. This is certainly the case for amine and peptide hormones. However, clearance for the many hormones that are degraded primarily in the liver may be expected to decrease during exercise as splanchnic blood flow decreases. This holds true for the steroid hormones, among others. Exercise-induced decrease in plasma volume will tend to increase plasma concentrations of all hormones.

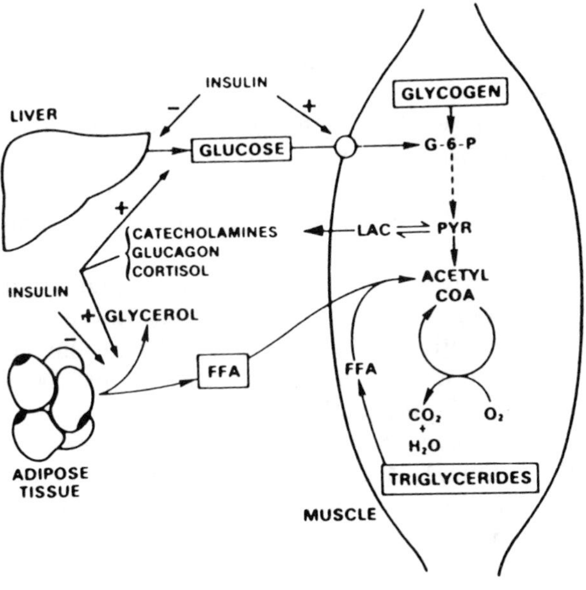

Figure 20.1 Intra- and extracellular fuel sources during exercise.

Hormonal Responses to a Single Bout of Exercise

Catecholamines

During exercise the concentration of epinephrine as well as of norepinephrine increases in proportion to the intensity and duration of exercise (Figure 20.2) (12,13). However, the epinephrine response (but much less so than that of norepinephrine) is also strongly influenced by the plasma glucose concentration (12,13). Therefore, if the pre-exercise diet has been carbohydrate-poor, the resulting early decline in plasma glucose concentration during prolonged exercise causes a marked increase in the plasma epinephrine concentration (14). The catecholamine response to exercise is also influenced by temperature, such that during hyperthermia, the norepinephrine response is exaggerated (63). In women, the response to exercise is higher in the follicular phase compared with the luteal phase (72).

The catecholamines have a variety of metabolic effects. Epinephrine primarily acts as a stimulator of glycogen breakdown in liver and muscle and of lipolysis in adipose and muscular tissue during exercise (1,5,24,81,83). While norepinephrine is only a weak stimulator of muscle glycogenolysis, its role in enhancing hepatic glycogenolysis is unclear (for review see [83]). Norepinephrine is a powerful stimulator of lipolysis in adipose tissue (81,91) but probably less so of muscle lipolysis (5).

Insulin, Glucagon

The plasma concentration of insulin decreases during exercise at an intensity above approximately 50% of $\dot{V}O_2$max (12,13). The decrease is most likely due to alpha-adrenergic inhibition of insulin secretion (12,13) rather than an increase in insulin clearance. In contrast, adrenergic mechanisms apparently play a minor role in the regulation of glucagon secretion in man. Thus, plasma glucagon concentrations are not influenced by alpha- and beta-adrenergic blockade when accompanying changes in glucose concentrations are compensated for (12,13). The main stimulus for glucagon secretion during exercise in man seems to be a decrease in plasma glucose concentration (12,13).

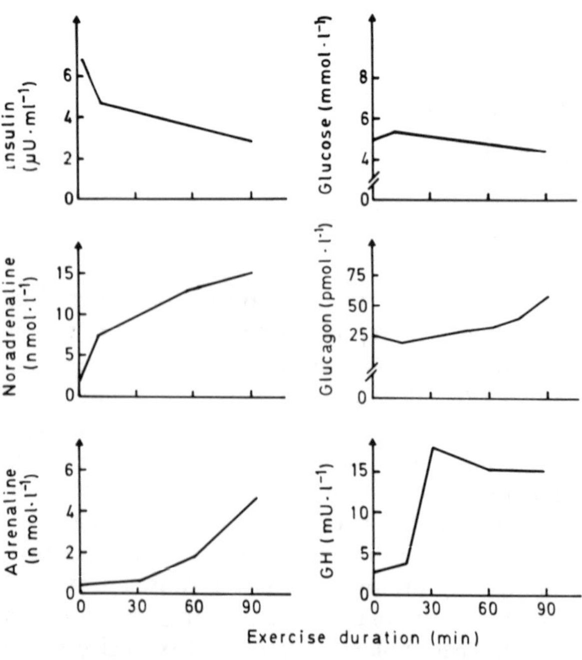

Figure 20.2 Typical changes in circulating levels of plasma glucose, insulin, glucagon, growth hormone and the catecholamines during exercise at 60% to 70% of $\dot{V}O_2$max in the postabsorbtive state.

Therefore, marked increases in glucagon concentrations only occur during prolonged exercise accompanied by a decrease in plasma glucose concentrations (Figure 20.2). The menstrual cycle apparently plays only a minor role in the insulin response to exercise (72). The decrease in plasma insulin concentration during exercise is of importance for increasing lipolysis (82) and probably also for allowing hepatic glucose production to increase (83). Furthermore, since insulin and contractions have additive effects on glucose transport in muscle (55), the decrease in plasma insulin concentration may be of importance for limiting muscle glucose uptake and thereby delaying exhaustion of hepatic glycogen stores.

Glucagon plays an important role in increasing hepatic glucose production in exercising dogs (83) but its role in humans is less clear. The primary argument against a role for glucagon in humans is the fact that plasma concentrations of glucagon usually only increase late in exercise (12,13) and even may decrease during short-term intense exercise (35) when hepatic glucose output is high. Recent experiments in man using the islet clamp technique indicate that rather large (3× above resting concentrations) increases in plasma glucagon concentration can increase hepatic glucose production during exercise (12).

ACTH, Cortisol, Growth Hormone, and Endorphins

Adrenocorticotropin (ACTH), growth hormone, and beta endorphin are released in a pulsatile manner from the anterior pituitary gland where ACTH is synthesized as part of a large precursor molecule that also contains beta endorphin. Cortisol will be released from the adrenal cortex and under the influence of ACTH, however, there is a time lag between the elevation of plasma ACTH and cortisol.

The early studies (73) demonstrated significant increases in growth hormone and cortisol concentrations with maximal exercise, which are similar in magnitude in both fit and unfit people when exercising to exhaustion. By contrast, at the same absolute level of work the response is greater in the unfit (67). Much more experimental work has been conducted to quantify and determine the various factors that regulate the anterior pituitary gland's responsiveness to exercise; in recent times that of the autonomic neuroendocrine activity has been highlighted (37). A number of seminal studies (37,38) demonstrate the role of central command in hormonal regulation (Figure 20.3).

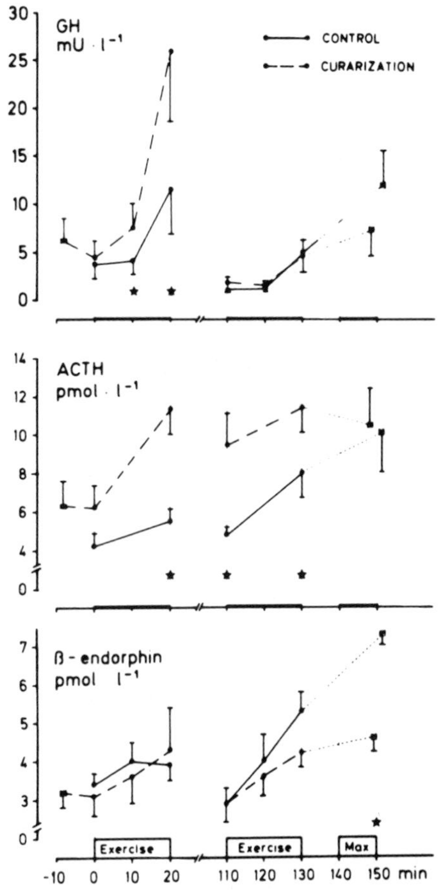

Figure 20.3 Concentrations of pituitary hormones (GH, ACTH, and [beta]-endorphin) in plasma at rest and during three exercise periods. Subjects were studied with and without partial neuromuscular blockade with tubocurarine. Values are means +/–SE of seven to eight observations. * denoted significant ($p < 0.05$) difference betwteen curare and control experiments. (Reproduced from reference 37 with permission.)

Using tubocurarine (37) to produce partial neuromuscular paralysis, these workers were able to demonstrate significant elevations in growth hormone and ACTH during submaximal exercise that was greater after blockade but at the same absolute oxygen uptake. In this study the catecholamine increases were also greater following tubocurarine. Surprisingly there was no difference in the beta endorphin responses with and without neuromuscular block at low levels of work. When the subjects worked at the same relative intensity during blockade the growth-hormone response was identical on both occasions. However, the response remained high with ACTH and slightly lower for beta endorphin. Subjects then went to maximal exercise, and growth hormone now was higher at exhaustion under control conditions, as was beta endorphin. However, ACTH was similar in both conditions.

This indicated that, although the relevant motor centers were probably activated maximally, the afferent neural traffic may well have been greater in experiments with the motor blockade. To follow up this possibility of enhanced, afferent neural traffic from working muscles affecting hormonal secretion, these same workers used epidural anesthesia and were able to demonstrate a decreased responsiveness of ACTH and beta endorphin during submaximal exercise. However, this was not the case with growth hormone (38).

The importance of psychological factors and emotional stress in stimulating hypothalamic-pituitary hormonal release has long been considered; and the anticipatory response of cortisol and presumably ACTH has resulted in doubling of the normal basal plasma concentrations of these hormones immediately prior to a race (69). In awake humans psychological factors are always present and may well be a confounding variable when attempting to dissect various control mechanisms. Such factors were eliminated in a study (79) demonstrating that direct electrical stimulation of subthalamic motor centers in paralyzed, decorticated cats will result in many of the endocrine responses seen during exercise, thus confirming that direct neural mechanisms definitely exist to elicit pituitary hormonal stimulation.

Some highly trained runners have been described as being in a chronic state of hypercortisolism (45,77). When a corticotropin-releasing hormone was injected into sedentary, moderately trained and highly trained athletes a reduced integrated response of both ACTH and cortisol was found in the highly trained group (45). The authors suggested highly trained athletes may exhibit chronically increased ACTH secretion. Beta endorphin appears to require a slightly greater intensity of exercise for its stimulation compared to ACTH or growth hormone. The effect of training appears to augment the beta endorphin response to exercise (4,11), but the much publicized role of beta endorphins in the determination of mood in "runners high" has not been realized by properly conducted placebo-controlled exercise studies with naloxone (18,68).

Renin, Aldosterone, Angiotensin, ANF, and Endothelin

Fluid balance is markedly altered by exercise. Thus, plasma volume is acutely diminished by 7% to 10% during exercise, due initially to fluid shifts but later also due to evaporation and sweating. Thus, the concentration of vasopressin, renin, angiotensin, and aldosterone in plasma increases in response to a single bout of exercise (15). Beta-adrenergic blockade can blunt the secretion of renin and hence of angiotensin and aldosterone (42). Another factor influencing the rate of aldosterone secretion could be the hyperkalemia that accompanies moderate to high intensity exercise (48). Atrial natriuretic factor (ANF) also increases during exercise, probably due to increased atrial filling pressure (16). In accordance with this assumption, alpha-1 and beta-1 adrenergic blockade decreased and increased, respectively, the concentration of ANF both at rest and during exercise (29,76). At either time the plasma renin activity and the angiotensin and aldosterone concentrations are higher in the luteal than the follicular phase (27).

Repeated bouts of exercise lead to an increase in plasma volume, which is accompanied by a more or less matched increase in red cell mass. The latter may be the result of increased concentrations of erythropoietin in plasma in response to each exercise session (80). However, the increase in red cell mass is often less than the increase in plasma volume, leading to hemoglobin concentrations that are in the low end of the normal range.

Endothelin is a recently discovered polypeptide produced in and released from the endothelial cells (90). It has marked vasoconstrictor effects (53,90); however, whether it has any metabolic effects is at present unclear. It was recently shown that the plasma response of endothelin-1 during prolonged submaximal exercise is biphasic: an initial decrease in its plasma concentration was followed by an increase (57) (Figure 20.4).

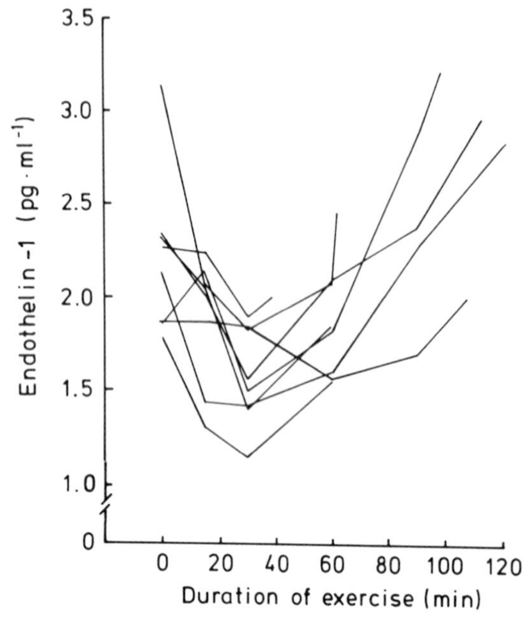

Figure 20.4 Plasma concentration of endothelin-1 in eight healthy subjects at rest and during bicycle exercise at 67% of $\dot{V}O_2max$ to exhaustion. Individual values are shown.

Reproductive Hormones

The ovarian and testicular hormones are under direct pituitary gonadotropic control, which in turn is under the pulsatile secretory regulation of the gonadotropin-releasing hormone (GNRH) from the hypothalamus. With exercise there is no change in gonadotropin concentration with fit or unfit subjects, male or female, with one exception. That is, FSH appears to increase during exercise in the follicular but not the luteal phase (26).

Exercise increases the plasma concentration of both estradiol and progesterone (26). These increases are independent of gonadotropin changes. The increases in the plasma concentration of the ovarian steroids were subsequently shown to be the result of a decreased metabolic clearance of estradiol, rather than increased secretion (28). In males major increases in testosterone have been demonstrated during exercise (40,70) (Figure 20.5). As with estradiol the increases in testosterone during exercise are shown to be the result of a decreased metabolic clearance of the hormone and not an increase in production (71) (Figure 20.6). Although it is beyond the scope of this chapter, chronic training appears to have a depressive effect on reproductive hormone functions resulting in hypothalamic hypogonadism in both females (8) and males (46). Although a decrease in plasma testosterone has been demonstrated in trained subjects, LH pulsatility remains intact (84).

Regulation of Hormonal Secretion During Exercise

Many changes in hormone secretion occur early in exercise at a time when blood-borne stimuli cannot account for the change in secretion. This has led to the hypothesis of feed-forward control of hormone secretion at the onset of exercise: Impulses from motor centers and afferent impulses from the working muscles elicit a work load dependent increase in sympathoadrenal activity and some pituitary hormones such as growth hormone (GH), ACTH, prolactin, and endorphins. The increase in sympathoadrenal activity depresses insulin secretion due to alpha-adrenergic stimulation of the pancreatic beta cell (13), and the increased secretion of the pituitary hormones increases the secretion of subordinate glands. This initial endocrine response is then modified throughout exercise by feedback mechanisms due to developing

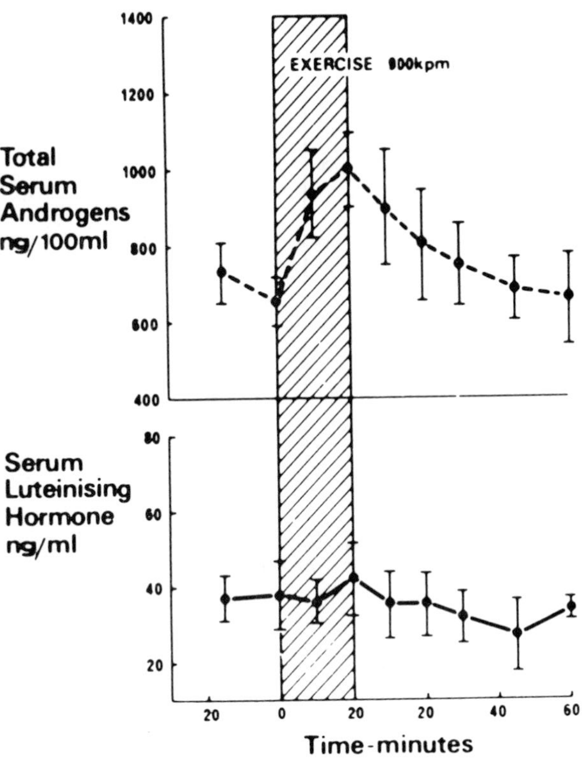

Figure 20.5 Concentration in serum of total androgens and luteinizing hormone (LH) before, during, and after exercise. (Reproduced from reference 71 with permission.)

metabolic error signals of which a decrease in plasma glucose concentration is the most powerful (12,13).

Modification of Hormonal Secretion by Training/Inactivity

Hormonal Changes at Rest

Norepinephrine. Conflicting results exist regarding whether endurance training decreases the activity in the sympathetic nervous system at rest. When endurance-trained athletes were compared with untrained subjects no difference in resting plasma norepinephrine concentrations were found (34–36,41,74), and peripheral sympathetic nervous activity measured directly by nerve recording was unrelated to training status (75). In two longitudinal studies of previously untrained subjects 4 to 5 months of endurance training, which increased $\dot{V}O_2max$ by 18% and 27%, respectively, did not significantly decrease resting plasma norepinephrine concentrations (54,74). Similar findings in short-term training studies in which comparable increases in $\dot{V}O_2max$ were obtained have been described by others (20,39,88).

However, a decrease in resting plasma norepinephrine concentrations as well as in sympathetic nervous activity (as reflected by whole-body norepinephrine spillover, which is the average rate at which norepinephrine released from sympathetic nerves enters plasma), was found in 10 out of 12 subjects after 4 weeks of hard endurance training (25). Furthermore, in that study, resting mean blood pressure decreased due to a decrease in total peripheral resistance in all 12 subjects. A training-induced decrease in plasma norepinephrine at rest was also found by Hespel et al. (21).

Epinephrine. Longitudinal training studies have shown that there is no effect of endurance training on the plasma concentration of epinephrine at rest (20,25,39,41,74,88). However, in athletes who have been training for years, it has been found that plasma concentration of epinephrine at rest is increased compared with controls (35,36). Thus, it may be that years of training induces adaptations in the adrenal gland that are not found in longitudinal studies over only a few months.

Other Hormones. Plasma concentrations of other hormones may be changed by training. For instance, the plasma concentration of insulin is lower in well-trained than in untrained subjects (35,89). Furthermore, in highly trained male runners, the resting (evening) plasma concentration of ACTH and cortisol was elevated compared to less-trained and untrained subjects, and the response to ovine corticotropin-releasing hormone was also diminished in the well-trained subjects, suggesting impairment of the hypothalamic-pituitary-adrenal axis (45). A difference in plasma cortisol concentration at rest (in the morning) between athletes and untrained subjects was however not found by others (19,35).

In male endurance-trained athletes testosterone and free testosterone were lower and LH higher than in sedentary controls (19); whereas a 6-month endurance training program decreased total and free testosterone without a change in LH levels or LH pulsatility (84). Thus, it is unclear to what reason the decrease in testosterone found with endurance training can be ascribed. The finding of changed hormonal status in athletes who endurance trained for years, but an absence of development of such changes in untrained subjects undergoing only months of training, suggest that long-term endocrine adaptations to years of endurance training take place. Another possibility is, of course, that the athletes are differently genetically equipped than the untrained controls.

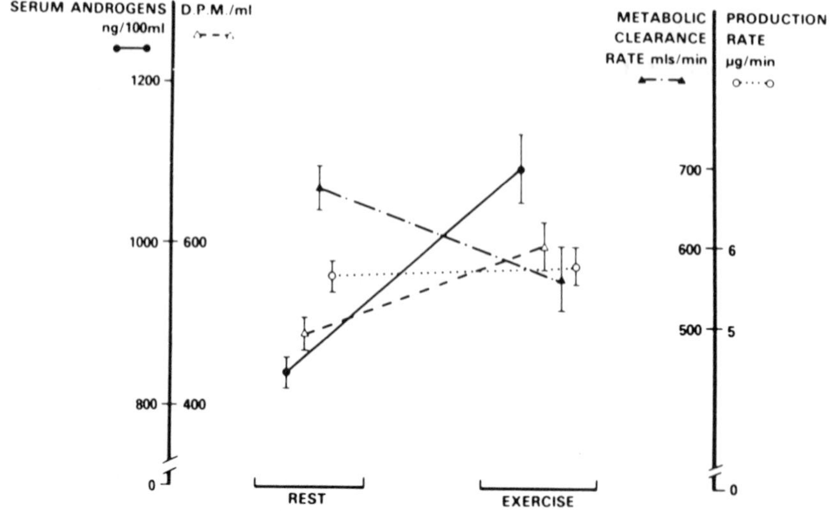

Figure 20.6 Concentrations in serum of total adrogens and metabolic clearance and production rate of testosterone at rest and during exercise. (Reproduced from reference 71 with permission.)

Functional Significance. The possible effect of exercise training on sympathetic nervous activity has attracted considerable interest as a possible means of treatment of mild hypertension and also as a means to lower blood pressure in normotensive individuals. Several studies in mild to moderate hypertensive patients have found a decrease in mean arterial blood pressure of 5 to 10 mmHg after training, yet many studies have methodological problems that weaken the conclusions. A recent review, however, concludes that physical endurance training in normotensive subjects causes a decrease in both systolic and diastolic blood pressure of on the average 4 mmHg (10). In hypertensive subjects the decrease averages 11/6 mmHg systolic/diastolic. Interestingly, the decrease in blood pressure is found only during the day and not during sleeping (10).

The functional significance of changes in plasma concentrations of epinephrine, testosterone, LH, and in some studies of ACTH at rest is not readily apparent—and there may be none, or if any it may be more of a deleterious than beneficial nature. It should, however, be realized that the observed hormonal changes between endurance-trained athletes and untrained controls represent differences obtained in highly selected subgroups of the population. However, the findings do raise the question as to whether or not the described hormonal changes seen in athletes (compared to untrained controls) mean that many years of hard endurance training imposes considerable stress on the body that for some body functions may be more harmful than beneficial.

Hormonal Changes During Exercise

The plasma concentration of the catecholamines increases during exercise depending on the relative exercise intensity (12,13). Endurance training makes the same absolute work load a relatively lesser work load; hence it follows that the plasma concentration of the catecholamines during exercise at a fixed work load decreases after training (20,54,74,88). It has even been described that during prolonged, low-intensity exercise at the same relative work load, the plasma concentration of the catecholamines was decreased after 6 weeks of endurance training (39). Surprisingly, a partial adaptation can be found after only a few days of training (17) and seems to be essentially complete after only 3 weeks (Figure 20.7) (87). The rapidity and magnitude of adaptation is probably dependent upon the intensity and frequency of training. It is interesting, however, that the hormonal adaptation occurs much more rapidly than the increase in $\dot{V}O_2max$. Thus, the early adaptation cannot be elicited by changes in relative work load. Possibly the rapid increase in plasma volume plays a role (17).

In contrast to these findings obtained before and after a rather short training period, cross-sectional studies have provided data that suggest that many years of hard endurance training may result in adaptations different than those found after only a few months of training. Thus, at the same absolute submaximal work load the epinephrine concentration in plasma was similar in athletes and in controls in spite of markedly lower norepinephrine concentrations in the former (35). Furthermore, it

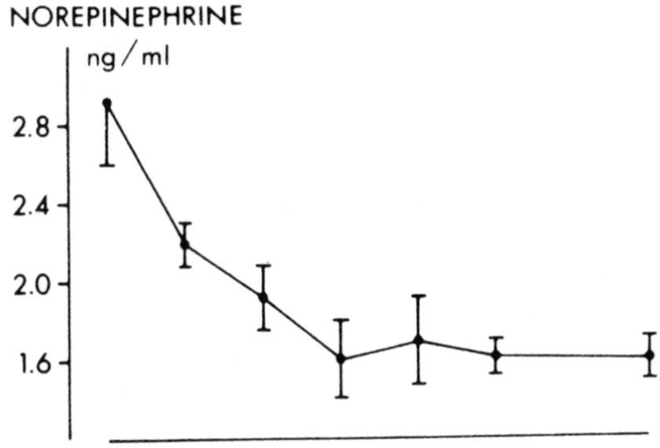

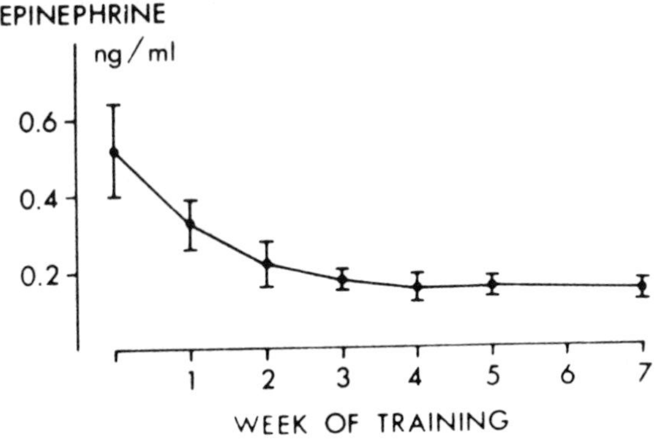

Figure 20.7 Plasma catecholamines after 5 min of exercise at the same absolute work load before and after training for 1 to 7 weeks. (Reproduced from reference 87 with permission.)

has been reported that during maximal and "supramaximal" exercise the epinephrine response but not the norepinephrine response was significantly larger in athletes than in sedentary controls (35). These findings may reflect that endurance-trained athletes may develop a higher maximum epinephrine secretion rate. Further support for this concept has been published (36), and is also supported by the finding of adrenal medullary hypertrophy in trained rats (65). Thus, although it may be that athletes are genetically predisposed to have a large capacity to secrete epinephrine, the rat study implies that neuroendocrine tissue, like muscle, may adapt to frequent use.

Following training, other hormones are also found in lower concentrations in plasma during exercise at a given absolute work load, for instance ACTH (3), glucagon (39), and GH (33).

Functional Significance. The functional significance of the training-induced decrease in plasma concentrations of the catecholamines and glucagon found during submaximal exercise is readily apparent when one views the hormonal response to exercise as a mechanism promoting fuel delivery to the working muscles while at the same time maintaining internal homeostasis, primarily plasma glucose. Thus, following training, when glycogen stores are increased and the muscles are able to rely more on fat combustion than before training, the need for hormonal response is less. This trend is further strengthened when sensitivity of target tissues is increased by training. It is in line with this thinking that the epinephrine and glucagon response to exercise is determined to a large extent by the plasma glucose concentration; thus secretion of these hormones is exaggerated when the plasma glucose concentration falls (12,13).

Changes in Hormone Sensitivity of Target Tissues

Sensitivity to Catecholamines

Hormonal adaptations to exercise training also relates to possible training-induced changes in hormone sensitivity of target tissues. For instance, the action of epinephrine is enhanced in adipocytes from trained subjects and rats (7,85). Although an increase in beta-adrenergic receptors in muscle following training has been reported in rats (86), 12 weeks of endurance training did not alter muscle beta-adrenergic density in humans (47). However, stimulation of oxygen consumption by epinephrine (probably primarily an alpha-adrenergic response [61]) was enhanced in perfused hind limbs from trained compared with untrained rats (56).

Sensitivity to Insulin

Exercise training has been shown to diminish the increase in plasma insulin concentration in response to a glucose load in both man (44,62) and rat (2). Nevertheless, glucose tolerance is unchanged or improved (2,44,62). These findings indicate that insulin action is enhanced in the trained state. This assumption has been directly confirmed using the euglycemic insulin clamp procedure (23,62). The tissues involved include adipose tissue (6,23,62,78), possibly liver (62), and probably more importantly skeletal muscle (23,52,62). Interestingly, the endocrine pancreas apparently adapts to the increased peripheral insulin sensitivity by being less responsive to hyperglycemia. Thus, during similar levels of sustained hyperglycemia insulin secretion in trained subjects is markedly lower than in untrained subjects (32,51). Also during stimulation with arginine, trained subjects secrete less insulin than untrained subjects (9a), indicating that the pancreatic adaptation to endurance training is not selective towards stimulation by glucose.

Conversely, decreased levels of activity impair insulin action in muscle. Thus, when normal volunteers had the knee joint of one leg immobilized by a splint for only 7 days, insulin action on thigh glucose uptake during euglycemic hyperinsulinemia was decreased compared to the nonimmobilized leg (Figure 20.8) (59). Similarly, muscle insulin sensitivity is decreased after 7 days of bed rest (50). In rodents limb immobilization also causes rapidly developing insulin resistance of muscle (64).

The mechanism behind the training-induced increased insulin sensitivity of muscle is not clear. Part of the effect is related to the effect of the last exercise bout, because a single exercise session causes an increase in insulin sensitivity of muscle (58,60) that lasts for at least 48 hr (49). However, in the trained state insulin sensitivity is increased beyond what can be accounted for by the effect of the last training session. It has recently been demonstrated that muscle of endurance-trained, middle-aged subjects contains twice as much of the insulin-regulatable glucose transporter GLUT 4 than muscle from untrained controls (22). This might in part explain the increased insulin action in trained muscle (22).

Increased insulin sensitivity might also be related to the increased capillarization of endurance-trained muscle (43). Accompanying the increased capillarization of muscle with training is an increase in muscle lipoprotein lipase activity (30), which has recently been shown to correlate closely with muscle insulin sensitivity (Figure 20.9) (31). Whereas this correlation may only reflect that both lipoprotein lipase activity and insulin sensitivity are related to muscle capillarization, the correlation may also reflect that the regulatory regions of the gene controlling lipoprotein lipase expression are very similar to those controlling GLUT 4 expression (personal communication).

The decreased plasma insulin concentration in the fasting state might be considered beneficial, as hyperinsulinemia has been suggested as an independent risk factor for development of arteriosclerosis (66). Thus, training diminishes or abolishes this risk factor. However, since trained subjects habitually consume much larger quantities of carbohydrates than sedentary subjects, the increased insulin sensitivity is offset by the increased intake of carbohydrates, and during the day, plasma insulin concentrations are no different in trained compared with untrained subjects (9).

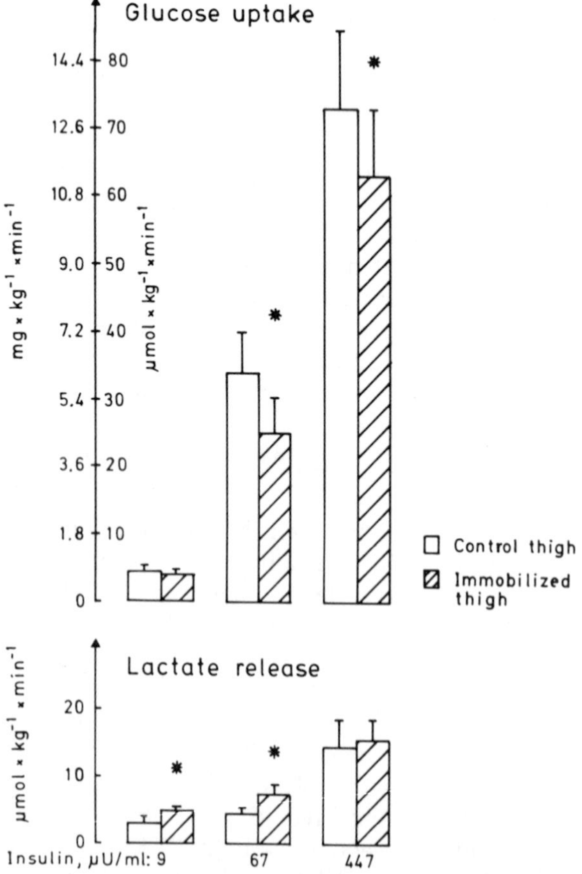

Figure 20.8 Dose–response relation for glucose uptake (top) and lactate release (bottom) in immobilized and control thighs. * $p < 0.05$ compared with control thigh. (Reproduced from reference 59 with permission.)

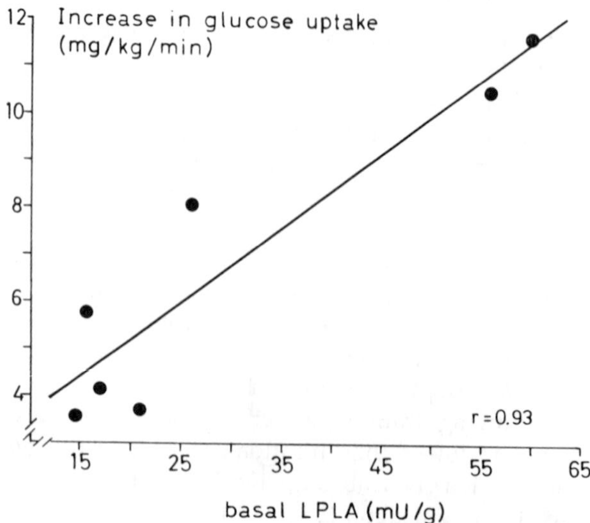

Figure 20.9 Relationship between insulin-stimulated thigh glucose uptake and muscle lipoprotein lipase activity. (Reproduced from reference 31 with permission.)

Major Unanswered Research Questions

Although major advances have been made toward the understanding of the mechanisms regulating hormone secretion during exercise, the precise role of and signals for feed-forward versus feedback control of hormone secretion remains to be defined. Furthermore, the relative role of the various neuroendocrine responses to exercise in regulating substrate utilization still remains somewhat elusive. In this regard, the adaptation of target tissues to training also plays a role, because different adaptations of hormone sensitivity in different organs may shift the relative role of various hormones in regulation of substrate utilization. It is of note that target tissue adaptation takes place in the muscles but also in organs not directly involved in exercise. Unraveling the mechanisms behind training-induced adaptations in target tissues is a major challenge for future research.

Finally, it is well known that acute changes in diet may cause marked changes in neuroendocrine activity during exercise. However, virtually nothing is known about the role of dietary composition for the adaptations that occur with endurance training. Thus, training on a fat-rich diet, for example, may cause very different adaptations than training on a carbohydrate-rich diet.

Acknowledgments

Authors were supported by grants from the Danish Medical (grant 12-9535) and Natural Sciences (11-7766) Research Council, Novo-Nordisk Research Fund, and the Medical Research Council of Australia.

References

1. Arner, P.; Kriegholm, E.; Engfeldt, P.; Bolinder, J. Andrenergic regulation of lipolysis in situ at rest and during exercise. J. Clin. Invest. 85:893-898; 1990.
2. Berger, M.; Kemmer, F.; Herberg, L.; Schwenen, M.; Gjinavci, A.; Berchtold, P. Effect of physical training on glucose tolerance and on glucose metabolism of skeletal muscle in anaesthetized normal rats. Diabetologia. 16:179-184; 1979.
3. Buono, M.; Yeager, J.; Sucec, A. Effect of aerobic training on the plasma ACTH response to exercise. J. Appl. Physiol. 63:2499-2501; 1987.
4. Carr, D.B.; Bullen, B.A.; Skrinar, G.S.; Arnold, M.S.; Rosenblatt, M.; Beitins, I.Z.; Martin, J.B.; McArthur, J.W. Physical conditioning facilitates the exercise-induced secretion of beta-endorphin and betalipotropin in women. N. Engl. J. Med. 305:560-563; 1981.
5. Cleroux, J.; vanNguyen, P.; Taylor, A.; Leenen, F.H. Effects of β1-vs. β1 + β2-blockade on exercise endurance and muscle metabolism in humans. J. Appl. Physiol. 66:548-554; 1989.
6. Craig, B.; Hammons, G.; Garthwaite, S.; Jarett, L.; Holloszy, J. Adaptation of fat cells to exercise: Response of glucose uptake and oxidation to insulin. J. Appl. Physiol. 51:1500-1506; 1981.
7. Crampes, F.; Beauville, M.; Riviere, D.; Garrigues, M. Effect of physical training in humans on the response of isolated fat cells to epinephrine. J. Appl. Physiol. 61:25-29; 1986.
8. Cumming, D.C.; Vickovic, M.M.; Wall, S.R.; Fluker, M.R. Defects in pulsatile LH release in normally menstruating runners. J. Clin. Endocrinol. Metab. 60:810-812; 1985.
9. Dela, F.; Mikines, K.J.; von Linstow, M.; Galbo, H. Twenty-four hour profile of plasma glucose and glucoregulatory hormones during normal living conditions in trained and untrained men. J. Clin. Endocrinal. Metab. 73:982-989; 1991.
9a. Dela, F.; Mikines, K.J.; Tronier, B.; Galbo, H. Diminished arginine-stimulated insulin secretion in trained men. J. Appl. Physiol. 69:261-267; 1990.
10. Fagard, R.; Bielen, E.; Hespel, P. Physical exercise in hypertension. In: Laragh, J.H.; Brenner, B.M., eds. Hypertension: Pathophysiology, diagnosis and management. Vol. 2. New York: Raven Press; 1990:1985-1998.
11. Farrell, P.A.; Kjaer, M.; Bach, F.W.; Galbo, H. Beta endorphin and adrenocorticotrophin response to supramaximal treadmill exercise in trained and untrained males. Acta Physiol. Scand. 130:619-625; 1987.
12. Galbo, H. Hormonal and metabolic adaptation to exercise. New York: Georg Thieme; 1983:1-116.
13. Galbo, H. Exercise physiology: Humoral function. Sport Sci. Rev. 1:65-93; 1992.
14. Galbo, H.; Holst, J.; Christensen, N.J. The effect of different diets and of insulin on the hormonal response to prolonged exercise. Acta Physiol. Scand. 107:19-32; 1979.
15. Geyssant, A.; Geelen, G.; Denis, C.; Allevard, A.; Vincent, M. Plasma vasopressin, renin activity and aldosterone: Effect of exercise and training. Eur. J. Appl. Physiol. 46:21-30; 1981.
16. Goetz, K. Physiology and pathophysiology of atrial peptides. Am. J. Physiol. 254:E1-E15; 1988.

17. Green, H.; Jones, L.; Houston, M.; Ball-Burnett, M; Farrance, B. Muscle energetics during prolonged cycling after exercise hypervolemia. J. Appl. Physiol. 66:622-631; 1989.
18. Grossman, A.; Bouloux, P.; Price, P.; Drury, P.L.; Lam, K.S.L.; Turner, T.; Thomas, J.; Besser, G.M.; Sutton, J. The role of opioid peptides in the hormonal responses to acute exercise in man. Clin. Sci. 67:483-491; 1984.
19. Hackney, A.; Sinning, W.; Bruot, B. Reproductive hormonal profiles of endurance-trained and untrained males. Med. Sci. Sports Exerc. 20:60-65; 1988.
20. Hartley, L.; Mason, J.; Hogan, R.; Jones, L.; Kotchen, T. Multiple hormonal responses to prolonged exercise in relation to physical training. J. Appl. Physiol. 33:607-610; 1972.
21. Hespel, P.; Lijnen, P.; VanHoof, R.; Fagard, R.; Goossens, W.; Lissens, W.; Moerman, E.; Amery, A. Effects of physical endurance training on the plasma renin-angiotensin-aldosterone system in normal man. J. Endocrinol. 116:443-449; 1988.
22. Houmard, J.A.; Egan, P.C.; Neufer, P.D.; Friedman, J.E.; Wheeler, W.S.; Israel, R.G.; Dohm, G.L. Elevated skeletal muscle glucose transporter levels in exercise-trained middle-aged men. Am. J. Physiol. 261:E437-E443; 1991.
23. James, D.; Kraegen, E.; Chisholm, D. Effects of exercise training on in vivo insulin action in individual tissues of the rat. J. Clin. Invest. 76:657-666; 1985.
24. Jansson, E.; Kaijser, L. Substrate utilization and enzymes in skeletal muscle of extremely endurance-trained men. J. Appl. Physiol. 62:999-1005; 1987.
25. Jennings, G.; Nelson, L.; Nestel, P.; Esler, M.; Korner, P. The effects of changes in physical activity on major cardiovascular risk factors, hemodynamics, sympathetic function and glucose utilization in man: A controlled study of four levels of activity. Circulation. 73:30-40; 1986.
26. Jurkowski, J.; Younglai, E.; Walker, C.; Jones, N.L.; Sutton, J.R. Ovarian hormone response to exercise. J. Appl. Physiol. 44:109-114; 1978.
27. Jurkowski, J.E.; Sutton, J.R.; Keane, P.M.; Viol, G.W. Plasma renin activity and plasma aldosterone during exercise in relation to the menstrual cycle. Med. Sci. Sports. 10:41; 1978.
28. Keizer, H.A.; Poortmans, J.; Bunniks, J. Influence of physical exercise on sex hormone metabolism. J. Appl. Physiol. 50:545-551; 1981.
29. Keller, N.; Møller, T.; Sykulski, R.; Storm, T.L.; Thamsborg, G. Effect of alpha-1 adrenoceptor blockade on plasma levels of atrial natriuretic peptide during dynamic exercise in normal man. Horm. Metab. Res. 19:344; 1987.
30. Kiens, B.; Lithell, H. Lipoprotein metabolism influenced by training-induced changes in human skeletal muscle. J. Clin. Invest. 83:558-564; 1989.
31. Kiens, B.; Lithell, H.; Mikines, K.J.; Richter, E.A. Effects of insulin and exercise on muscle lipoprotein lipase activity in man and its relation to insulin action. J. Clin. Invest. 84:1124-1129; 1989.
32. King, D.; Staten, M.; Kohrt, W.; Dalsky, G.; Elahi, D.; Holloszy, J. Insulin secretory capacity in endurance-trained and untrained young men. Am. J. Physiol. 259:E155-E161; 1990.
33. Kjaer, M.; Bangsbo, J.; Lortie, G.; Galbo, H. Hormonal response to exercise in humans: Influence of hypoxia and physical training. Am. J. Physiol. 254:R197-R203; 1988.
34. Kjaer, M.; Christensen, N.J.; Sonne, B.; Richter, E.A.; Galbo, H. Effect of exercise on epinephrine turnover in trained and untrained male subjects. J. Appl. Physiol. 59:1061-1067; 1985.
35. Kjaer, M.; Farrell, P.; Christensen, N.; Galbo, H. Increased epinephrine response and inaccurate glucoregulation in exercising athletes. J. Appl. Physiol. 61:1693-1700; 1986.
36. Kjaer, M.; Galbo, H. Effect of physical training on the capacity to secrete epinephrine. J. Appl. Physiol. 64:11-16; 1988.
37. Kjaer, M.; Secher, N.H.; Bach, F.W.; Galbo, H. Role of motor centre activity for hormonal changes and substrate mobilization in humans. Am. J. Physiol. 253:R687-R695; 1987.
38. Kjaer, M.; Secher, N.H.; Bach, F.W.; Sheikh, S.; Galbo, H. Hormonal and metabolic responses to exercise in humans: Effect of sensory nervous blockade. Am. J. Physiol. 257:E95-E101; 1989.
39. Koivisto, V.; Hendler, R.; Nadel, E.; Felig, P. Influence of physical training on the fuel-hormone response to prolonged low intensity exercise. Metabolism. 31:192-197; 1982.
40. Kuoppasalmi, K.; Naveri, H.; Harkonen, M.; Adlercreutz, H. Plasma cortisol, androstenedione, testosterone and luteinizing hormone in running exercise of different intensities. Scand. J. Clin. Lab. Invest. 40:403-409; 1980.
41. Lehmann, M.; Dickhuth, H.H.; Schmid, P.; Porzig, H.; Keul, J. Plasma catecholamines, beta-adrenergic receptors, and isoproterenol sensitivity in endurance trained and non-endurance trained volunteers. Eur. J. Appl. Physiol. 52:362-369; 1984.
42. Lijnen, P.J.; Amery, A.K.; Fagard, R.H.; Reybrouck, T.M.; Moerman, E.J.; De Schaepdryver, A.F. The effects of β-adrenergic receptor blockade on renin, angiotensin, aldosterone and catecholamines at rest and during exercise. Br. J. Clin. Pharmacol. 7:175-181; 1979.

43. Lillioja, S.; Young, A.; Culter, C.; Ivy, J.; Abbott, W.G.; Zawadzki, J.K.; Yki-Järvinen, H.; Christin, L.; Secomb, T.W.; Bogardus, C. Skeletal muscle capillary density and fiber type are possible determinants of in vivo insulin resistance in man. J. Clin. Invest. 80:415-424; 1987.
44. Lohmann, D.; Liebold, F.; Heilmann, W.; Senger, H.; Pohl, A. Diminished insulin response in highly trained athletes. Metabolism. 27:521-524; 1978.
45. Luger, A.; Deuster, P.; Kyle, S.; Gallucci, W.; Montgomery, L.; Gold, P.W.; Loriaux, D.L.; Chrousos, G.P. Acute hypothalamic-pituitary-adrenal responses to the stress of treadmill exercise. N. Engl. J. Med. 316:1309-1315; 1987.
46. MacConnie, S.E.; Barkan, A.; Lampman, R.M.; Schork, M.A.; Beitins, I.Z. Decreased hypothalamic gonadotropin releasing hormone secretion in male marathon runners. N. Engl. J. Med. 315:411-417; 1986.
47. Martin, W., III; Coggan, A.; Spina, R.; Saffitz, J. Effects of fiber type and training on β-adrenoceptor density in human skeletal muscle. Am. J. Physiol. 257:E736-E742; 1989.
48. Medbø, J.; Sejersted, O. Plasma potassium changes with high intensity exercise. J. Physiol. 421:105-122; 1990.
49. Mikines, K.; Sonne, B.; Farrell, P.; Tronier, B.; Galbo, H. Effect of physical exercise on sensitivity and responsiveness to insulin in humans. Am. J. Physiol. 254:E248-E259; 1988.
50. Mikines, K.J.; Richter, E.A.; Dela, F.; Galbo, H. Seven days of bed rest decrease insulin action on glucose uptake in leg and whole body. J. Appl. Physiol. 70:1245-1254; 1991.
51. Mikines, K.J.; Sonne, B.; Tronier, B.; Galbo, H. Effects of training and detraining on dose-response relationship between glucose and insulin secretion. Am. J. Physiol. 256:E588-E596; 1989.
52. Mondon, C.E.; Dolkas, C.B.; Reaven, G.M. Site of enhanced insulin sensitivity in exercise-trained rats. Am. J. Physiol. 239:E169-E177; 1980.
53. Pernow, J.; Hemsen, A.; Lundberg, J.M.; Nowak, J.; Kaijser, L. Potent vasoconstrictor effects and clearance of endothelin in the human forearm. Acta Physiol. Scand. 141:319-324; 1991.
54. Peronnet, F.; Cleroux, J.; Perrault, H.; Cousineau, D.; Champlain de, J.; Nadeau, R. Plasma norepinephrine response to exercise before and after training in humans. J. Appl. Physiol. 51(4):812-815; 1992.
55. Ploug, T.; Galbo, H.; Vinten, J.; Jørgensen, M.; Richter, E.A. Kinetics of glucose transport in rat muscle: Effects of insulin and contractions. Am. J. Physiol. 253:E12-E20; 1987.
56. Richter, E.A.; Christensen, N.J.; Ploug, T.; Galbo, H. Endurance training augments the stimulatory effect of epinephrine on oxygen consumption in perfused skeletal muscle. Acta Physiol. Scand. 120:613-615; 1984.
57. Richter, E.A.; Emmeluth, C.; Bie, P.; Helge, J.; Kiens, B. Biphasic response of plasma endothelin-1 concentration to exhausting submaximal exercise in man. Unpublished manuscript.
58. Richter, E.A.; Garetto, L.P.; Goodman, M.N.; Ruderman, N.B. Muscle glucose metabolism following exercise in the rat. J. Clin. Invest. 69:785-793; 1982.
59. Richter, E.A.; Kiens, B.; Mizuno, M.; Strange, S. Insulin action in human thighs after one-legged immobilization. J. Appl. Physiol. 67:19-23; 1989.
60. Richter, E.A.; Mikines, K.J.; Galbo, H.; Kiens, B. Effect of exercise on insulin action in human skeletal muscle. J. Appl. Physiol. 66:876-885; 1989.
61. Richter, E.A.; Ruderman, N.B.; Galbo, H. Alpha and beta adrenergic effects on metabolism in contracting, perfused muscle. Acta Physiol. Scand. 116:215-222; 1982.
62. Rodnick, K.; Haskell, W.; Swislocki, A.L.; Foley, J.; Reaven, G. Improved insulin action in muscle, liver and adipose tissue in physically trained human subjects. Am. J. Physiol. 253:E489-E495; 1987.
63. Rowell, L.B.; Brengelmann, G.L.; Freund, P.R. Unaltered norepinephrine-heart rate relationship in exercise with exogenous heat. J. Appl. Physiol. 62:646-650; 1987.
64. Seider, M.; Nicholson, W.; Booth, F. Insulin resistance for glucose metabolism in disused soleus muscle of mice. Am. J. Physiol. 242:E12-E18; 1982.
65. Stallknecht, B.; Kjaer, M.; Mikines, K.J.; Maroun, L.; Ploug, T.; Ohkuwa, T.; Vinten, J.; Galbo, H. Diminished epinephrine response to hypoglycemia despite enlarged adrenal medulla in trained rats. Am. J. Physiol. 259:R998-R1003; 1990.
66. Stern, M.; Haffner, S. Body fat distribution and hyperinsulinemia as risk factors for diabetes and cardiovascular disease. Arteriosclerosis. 6:123-130; 1986.
67. Sutton, J.R. Hormonal and metabolic responses to exercise in subjects of high and low work capacities. Med. Sci. Sports. 10:1-6; 1978.
68. Sutton, J.R.; Brown, G.M.; Keane, P.; Walker, W.H.C.; Jones, N.L.; Rosenbloom, D.; Besser, G.M. The role of endorphins in the hormonal and psychological responses to exercise. Int. J. Sports Med. 3:19; 1982.

69. Sutton, J.R.; Casey, J.H. The adrenocortical response to competitive athletics in veteran athletes. J. Clin. Endocrinol. Metab. 40:135-138; 1975.

70. Sutton, J.R.; Coleman, M.J.; Casey, J.; Lazarus, L. Androgen responses during physical exercise. Br. Med. J. 1:520-522; 1973.

71. Sutton, J.R.; Coleman, M.J.; Casey, J.H. Testosterone production rate during exercise. In: Landry, F.; Orban, W.A.R., eds. 3rd international symposium on biochemistry of exercise. Miami, FL: Symposia Specialists Inc.; 1978:227-234.

72. Sutton, J.R.; Jurkowski, J.E.; Keane, P.; Walker, W.H.C.; Jones, N.L.; Toews, C.J. Plasma catecholamine, insulin, glucose and lactate responses to exercise in relation to the menstrual cycle. Med. Sci. Sports Exerc. 12:83-84; 1980.

73. Sutton, J.R.; Young, J.D.; Lazarus, L.; Hickie, J.B.; Maksvytis, J. The hormonal response to physical exercise. Aust. Ann. Med. 18:84-90; 1969.

74. Svedenhag, J. The sympatho-adrenal system in physical conditioning. Acta Physiol. Scand. [Suppl. 543]. 125:1-73; 1985.

75. Svedenhag, J.; Wallin, B.; Sundlöf, G.; Henriksson, J. Skeletal muscle sympathetic activity at rest in trained and untrained subjects. Acta Physiol. Scand. 120:499-504; 1984.

76. Thamsborg, G.; Sykulski, R.; Larsen, J.; Storm, T.; Keller, N. Effect of beta 1-adrenoceptor blockade on plasma levels of atrial natriuretic peptide during exercise in normal man. Clin. Physiol. 7:313-318; 1987.

77. Villanueva, A.L.; Schlosser, C.; Hopper, B.; Liu, J.H.; Hoffman, D.I.; Rebar, R.W. Increased cortisol production in women runners. J. Clin. Endocrinol. Metab. 63:133-136; 1986.

78. Vinten, J.; Galbo, H. Effect of physical training on transport and metabolism of glucose in adipocytes. Am. J. Physiol. 244:E129-E134; 1983.

79. Vissing, J.; Iwamoto, G.; Rybicki, K.; Galbo, H.; Mitchell, J. Mobilization of glucoregulatory hormones and glucose by hypothalamic locomotor centers. Am. J. Physiol. 257:E722-E728; 1989.

80. Vitali, E.D.P.; Guegliemini, C.; Casoni, I.; Vedovato, M.; Gilli, P.; Farinelli, A.; Salvatorelli, G.; Conconi, F. Serum erythropoietin in cross-country skiers. Int. J. Sports Med. 9:99-101; 1988.

81. Wahrenberg, H.; Engfeldt, P.; Bolinder, J.; Arner, P. Acute adaption in adrenergic control of lipolysis during physical exercise in humans. Am. J. Physiol. 253:E383-E390; 1987.

82. Wasserman, D.; Lacy, D.; Goldstein, R.; Williams, P.; Cherrington, A. Exercise-induced fall in insulin and increase in fat metabolism during prolonged muscular work. Diabetes. 38:484-490; 1989.

83. Wasserman, D.H.; Cherrington, A.D. Hepatic fuel metabolism during muscular work: Role and regulation. Am. J. Physiol. 260:E811-E824; 1991.

84. Wheeler, G.D.; Singh, M.; Pierce, W.D.; Epling, W.F.; Cumming, D.C. Endurance training decreases serum testosterone levels in men without change in luteinizing hormone pulsatile release. J. Clin. Endocrinol. Metab. 72:422-425; 1991.

85. Williams, R.; Bishop, T. Enhanced receptor-cyclase coupling and augmented catecholamine-stimulated lipolysis in exercising rats. Am. J. Physiol. 243:E345-E351; 1982.

86. Williams, R.; Caron, M.; Daniel, K. Skeletal muscle beta-adrenergic receptors: Variations due to fiber type and training. Am. J. Physiol. 246:E160-E167; 1984.

87. Winder, W.; Hagberg, J.; Hickson, R.; Ehsani, A.; McLane, J. Time course of sympathoadrenal adaption to endurance exercise training in man. J. Appl. Physiol. 45:370-374; 1978.

88. Winder, W.; Hickson, R.; Hagberg, J.; Ehsani, A.; McLane, J. Training-induced changes in hormonal and metabolic responses to submaximal exercise. J. Appl. Physiol. 46:766-771; 1979.

89. Wirth, A.; Diehm, C.; Mayer, H.; Mörl, H.; Vogel, I. Plasma C-peptide and insulin in trained and untrained subjects. J. Appl. Physiol. 50:71-77; 1981.

90. Yanagisawa, M.; Kurihara, H.; Kimura, S.; Tomobe, Y.; Kobayashi, M.; Mitsui, Y.; Yazaki, Y.; Goto, K.; Masaki, T. A novel potent vasoconstrictor peptide produced by vascular endothelial cells. Nature. 332:411-415; 1988.

91. Yeaman, S. Hormone-sensitive lipase-a multipurpose enzyme in lipid metabolism. Biochim. Biophys. Acta. 1052:128-132; 1990.

Chapter 21

Response and Adaptation of Skeletal Muscle to Changes in Physical Activity

John A. Faulkner
Howard J. Green
Timothy P. White

Skeletal muscle constitutes approximately 40% of the mass of the human body. For a 70-kg person, the 28 kg of muscle mass consists of 660 skeletal muscles with specific properties that reflect genetic inheritance (see chapter 6) and habitual patterns of recruitment and loading (20). The voluntary contractions of skeletal muscles provide the basis for all physical activities. Physical and physiological fitness are indexes of the quality and quantity of the physical activity provided by skeletal muscles. Physical fitness is measured by gross whole-body activities of throwing, running, jumping, and dodging (see chapter 3), whereas physiological fitness is measured by specific tests of the absolute and sustained force and power of a given muscle, or muscle group (9, 20).

Indirectly and directly, physical and physiological fitness provide measures of the strength, power, and endurance of skeletal muscles. Disuse, trauma, or disease may jointly or in concert impair the ability of skeletal muscles to develop and sustain force and power and therefore decrease physical and physiological fitness (see chapter 3). Conversely, increases in habitual levels of physical activity may be precisely designed to increase absolute or sustained aspects of force or power and as a consequence improve performance on specific tests of physical fitness. Adequate levels of muscular power and endurance enable human beings to perform the activities of daily living throughout their life span (see chapter 9). Such levels increase the potential for a higher quality of life, however no definitive evidence currently supports any direct effect on longevity (see chapter 7).

Regardless of the mammalian species, the determinants of strength, power, and endurance are qualitatively similar. Furthermore, the response to single bouts and the adaptive changes to repeated bouts of physical activity are qualitatively, and in many circumstances, quantitatively similar in skeletal muscles of most, if not all, mammalian species. This review describes the continuum of physical activity; the determinants and measures of force, power, and endurance; the properties of motor units; the acute response of mammalian skeletal muscles to physical activity; and the adaptations resulting from chronic exposures to reductions and increases in physical activity. The primary focus is on studies of human beings; however, data on muscle preparations of small mammals studied in situ and in vitro and data on adaptations resulting from animal models of unweighting of limbs, ablation of synergistic muscles, and chronic electrical stimulation will be presented when these investigations provide insights into the physiological mechanisms involved.

Continuum of Physical Activity

The continuum of physical activity ranges from the almost complete absence of activity associated with bedrest or immobilization to high levels of activity associated with the training regimes of world-class power and endurance performers (Figure 21.1). During a given day, a total organism is in an inactive state, or minimally active state, more than a highly active state. Therefore, except for the diaphragm and postural muscles, the habitual state for skeletal muscles is one of relative inactivity. The lack of a significant range of physical inactivity limits studies of the response to changes in this condition. Conversely, the low baseline position of habitual daily physical activity for most people allows a wide range of responses to increases (Figure 21.1).

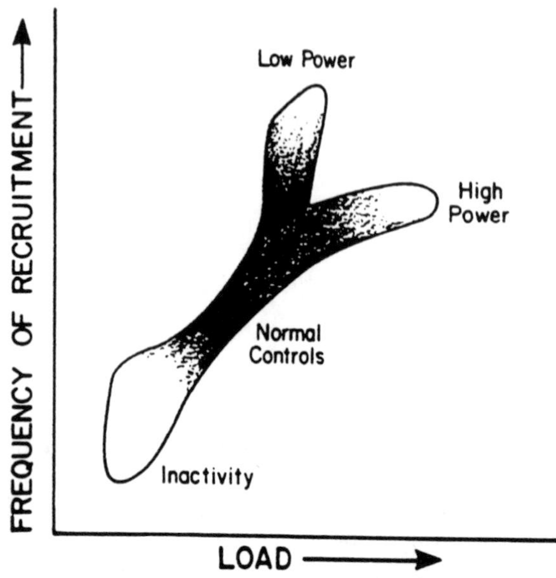

Figure 21.1 Physical activity is determined by the frequency of recruitment for contractions (ordinate) and the load on the muscle during the contraction (abscissa). Physical activity constitutes a continuum from the almost complete absence of activity associated with bed-rest or immobilization, through the nominal activity levels of sedentary subjects to high levels observed in physically active subjects. Toward the high end of the continuum, a dichotomy arises as endurance performers increase the frequency of recruitment cycles without increasing load significantly, whereas strength and power performers increase the load significantly without much of an increase in frequency.

Adaptations result from habitual changes in the intensity, duration, and frequency of physical activity achieved by variations in the recruitment, contraction, and subsequent loading of skeletal muscles. A muscle contraction is defined as activation of the force-generating capacity of the actomyosin complex within fibers with a tendency for the fibers in the muscle to shorten. Whether fibers shorten, remain at the same length (isometric), or lengthen depends on the external load applied relative to the force developed by the muscle. With activation, cross-bridges execute complete cycles from unbound, to weakly bound, to strongly bound, through the driving stroke, to strongly bound, and then back to the unbound, or possibly the weakly bound state (23). Only cross-bridges in the driving stroke will develop force during a shortening or isometric contraction, whereas cross-bridges in any bound state may contribute to the force that opposes the lengthening of a muscle (38).

Force, Power, and Endurance

For human beings the strength of muscle groups may be determined by maximum volitional contractions, or by the development of maximum isometric tetanic force with electrical stimulation of the motor nerve, or by direct muscle stimulation (53). In contrast, maximum force of muscles of small mammals can only be obtained by direct or indirect electrical stimulation (9). Assuming optimum fiber length and current flow, the maximum force of muscles is obtained by increasing the stimulation frequency until force plateaus (9). With supramaximum stimulation frequency, the isometric force developed by muscles is a function of the total cross-sectional area of the contracting fibers and the position of the fibers on the length–force relationship. Under these circumstances, all fiber types of all mammalian species develop a maximum force of about 280 kN/m^2 (20).

Gradations in the force developed by whole muscles in vivo will be influenced by the number and size of motor units recruited and the frequency of the stimulation. The product of the force and velocity at which muscle shortens or lengthens determines the power output, or power absorption, respectively. The velocity of unloaded shortening is determined by the myosin ATPase activity (5) and the length of the muscle fibers. When muscles are loaded, the velocity attained is also influenced by the magnitude of the load (77). Attenuations in force and power also occur due to the angles of fiber pinnation in relation to the overall longitudinal axis of the muscle and other architectural complexities (22).

Fatigue may occur during repeated contractions (46,76). Fatigue is defined as a loss in the development of force, velocity, or both, which results from muscle activity under load and is reversible by rest (19). Potential biochemical modulators of fatigue, which could act on any of the excitation–contraction sites, include concentrations of ATP, ADP, AMP, and IMP. Different ionic species of potassium, sodium, and magnesium have also been implicated in the development of fatigue (47). In single permeabilized muscle fibers, inorganic phosphate (23), and hydrogen ions (54) decrease force development. In single intact fibers, calcium (46) and possibly a change in calcium sensitivity have been associated with fatigue (43). Fatigue is an inevitable consequence of sustained, high-intensity physical activity (78), and an understanding of the underlying mechanisms of fatigue is of both physiological and practical significance. It is generally felt that in many physical activities potentially limited by fatigue participants select a strategy that permits the completion of a task or a distance with minimum fatigue. In contrast to the concept of fatigue, endurance is the duration a given force or power may be sustained, and physiological fitness of skeletal muscle is the maximum force or power that can be sustained for a given time (19).

Properties of Motor Unit

Within the neuromuscular system, fibers are organized functionally into motor units that consist of the cell body, the motor nerve and its branches, and the skeletal muscle fibers innervated by the branches (11). Burke, Levine, Zajac, Tsairis, and Engel (11) classified the motor units in cat skeletal muscles as slow (S), fast fatigue resistant (FR), and fast fatigable (FF) based on contraction time, a "sag" in the force record during unfused tetanus, and a fatigue test. Histochemical techniques for the classification of fibers in mammalian motor units are based on the activities of oxidative enzymes (58) and the differential sensitivity of myofibrillar ATPase activity to altered pH (59). Markers of glycolytic capacity are ambiguous and have not been found to be particularly useful in fiber classification schemes (58).

Classification of fibers within motor units by different histochemical techniques provides similar results, but the similarity is not sufficient to allow unambiguous interchange among the different classification schemes (20). For control limb muscles (11), a reasonable correlation has been established between the motor units classified by either of the two major histochemical techniques: Type I, IIA, IIB (8), or slow (S), fast-oxidative-glycolytic (FOG), and fast-glycolytic (FG) (58) and those classified by contractile properties (S, FR, FF) (11). In each scheme of fiber classification, the primary determinants of the classification (i.e., the myosin isoform and the oxidative enzymes) constitute a continuum (20). Therefore, classification of fibers into discreet types based on qualitative determination of "low" and "high" activity for these two characteristics is of limited value.

Response to Acute Exposure to Physical Activity

Physical activities involve various combinations of shortening, isometric, and lengthening contractions of the motor units that are recruited (19,48). In spite of the diversity of the types of contractions, shortening contractions generate the power necessary for movements of organisms or of external objects. In addition, shortening is the most demanding type of contraction metabolically (33). During most physical activities, energy will be expended for isometric contractions to provide a stable basis for the generation of power, and antagonistic muscles will co-contract, brake the velocity of the limb movement, or return the limb to its original position during repetitive movements as in cycling (19,48). Furthermore, the energy expended to perform the isometric and lengthening contractions is not expressed as external work.

The more complex the movement the greater the discrepancy between caloric expenditures and the amount of external work performed. Consequently, the examples of physical activity described will be single or repeated isovelocity shortening contractions of a fully activated single muscle, rather than the more complex volitional activities of walking or running. Unlike volitional activities, the electrically stimulated contractions of a single muscle do not involve selective recruitments of motor units, but rather all muscle fibers are recruited concurrently.

The metabolic changes that occur with muscle contraction are rapid and dramatic. Since a skeletal muscle contraction occurs within 10 ms of an action potential, a metabolic response must also occur within this time frame. The small decrease in ATP and increase in ADP and inorganic phosphate results in an acceleration in the hydrolysis of creatine phosphate to rephosphorylate ADP to ATP (38). Changes in the byproducts of ATP hydrolysis in conjunction with other activators lead to a cascade of enzymatic events that activate the glycolytic and oxidative phosphorylation pathways. With contractions of muscles, autoregulatory mechanisms increase muscle blood flow and increase the delivery of oxygen and metabolic substrates (2,45).

The immediate response to a series of muscle contractions is influenced by factors intrinsic and extrinsic to the muscle fibers (Figure 21.2). Intrinsic factors include the types of fibers, and the substrates, particularly ATP and glycogen, and metabolite concentrations in fibers. The extrinsic factors involve the delivery of oxygen, removal of metabolites, and regulation of muscle temperature and pH. The optimum temperature for sustained force is between 28 °C and 32 °C (18). Short-term power is enhanced by higher temperatures because of the direct effect of temperature on velocity of shortening up to at least 44 °C (65). In contrast, optimization of sustained power constitutes a complex interaction between mechanical and metabolic effects of temperature.

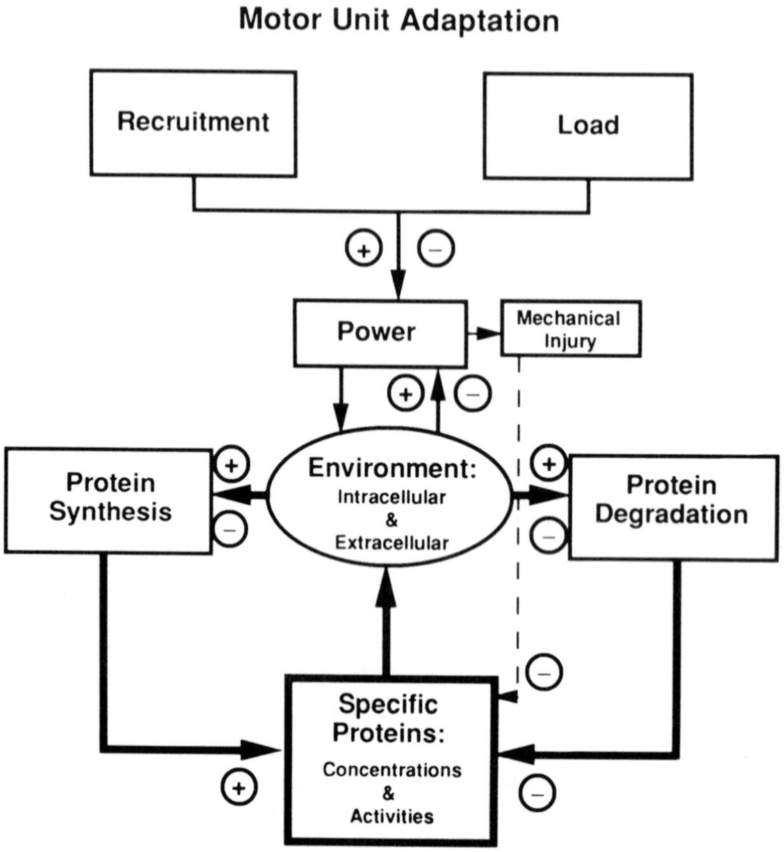

Motor Unit Adaptation

Figure 21.2 During changes in the level of physical activity the total power developed by a motor unit results from the recruitment of the fibers in motor units and the load against which the fibers contract. If the fibers shorten power will be developed (+), and if the fibers are lengthened power will be absorbed (−). Presumably, reduced power, sustained power, or high power result in acute changes in the cellular environment that then lead to an augmentation or inhibition of gene expression and/or specific proteases. If sustained, this will lead to altered rates of protein synthesis and degradation, respectively. This in turn will lead to changes in the concentrations or activities of specific proteins and thus chronically, but not permanently, alter the cellular environment. These adaptations may increase or decrease the capability of fibers in a motor unit to develop and maintain power. The adaptive responses to some physical activities are known, but the receptors, integrating centers, second messengers, and effectors involved have not been fully identified. Under certain circumstances muscle fibers are injured during acute contractions and the concentration of myofibrillar proteins is decreased directly.

The intensity with which a physical activity is performed is determined by the power (watts or W) developed by the muscles involved. The power is the amount of work done (joules) per unit time. During repeated isovelocity shortening contractions, the product of the number of contractions per second and the duration of each contraction in seconds gives the fraction of the total time during which the muscle is working, or the duty cycle (9). With the shortening velocity optimum for the development of power, the average force during repeated contractions holds constant only at the lowest duty cycles (9). At most duty cycles, during the first minute of repeated contractions the average force decreases and then plateaus at a steady-state value which will remain constant for up to 40 min.

The duty cycle is a critical determinant of the average force the muscle is able to develop during each of a series of shortening, isometric, or lengthening contractions. The average force during each contraction is a curvilinear function of the duty cycle (9). Eventually, a duty cycle is achieved at which the average force declines continuously. The sustained power, a product of the average force and velocity of shortening, has a parabolic relationship with the duty cycle (9). Similar to the single muscle, maximum power cycling has a parabolic relationship with pedaling rate expressed in revolutions per minute (67).

During a single contraction, fast fibers produce about three times the maximum power of slow fibers, and their ability to sustain power is about 15% higher (9). Consequently, the steady-state value for sustained power (W/kg) is a function of the fiber type and the duty cycle. In single permeabilized fibers, inorganic phosphate appears to modulate the development of force (23). The decrease in force is associated with an increase in inorganic phosphate possibly through a reversal of the reaction A·M·ADP·Pi → A·M·ADP+Pi. Reversal of this reaction would reduce force development by decreasing the number of cross-bridges in the force-producing portion of the cross-bridge cycle.

Wilkie (77) estimated a maximum power of 225 W/kg for the elbow flexor muscles of human beings. The value is close to that of 221 W/kg reported for EDL muscles of mice (10). With the assumptions of 28 kg of muscle in a 70-kg person, and equal muscle masses associated with the upper and lower limbs and with agonist and antagonist functions, a maximum value of active wet muscle mass of 7 kg is estimated (78). The product of 7 kg × 225 W/kg = 1,575 W which is in reasonable agreement with maximum peak performance for a single contraction (78).

Compared with the maximum power during a single contraction, sustained power during repetitive contractions is reduced (Figure 21.3). The magnitude of the reduction depends on the duty cycle and the decrease in the average force developed due to fatigue (9,19). From the maximum power developed during a single contraction to that developed during 10 s of peak physical activity, the power is already halved (78). During lengthening contractions a decrease in power due to injury is also a possibility (50,69). Depending on the intensity and duration of the physical activity, full recovery of force development after a bout of physical activity occurs usually within minutes or hours. Changes that persist for more than 24 hr after physical activity are likely due to injury (50,69) rather than to a failure to recover from the response to the physical activity.

For an individual, the power that can be sustained for a given time is dependent on the maximum capacity to develop power and on the degree to which the individual is trained for endurance activities (Figure 21.3). To clarify these relationships, the response to light (5%), moderate (about 10%), high (about 15%), and exhaustive (greater than 15%) intensities of physical activity will be described (Figure 21.3). The percentages are of the maximum power developed during a single contraction. For a moderately active adult subject, light, moderate, and high intensities are equivalent to walking, easy jogging, and hard running, respectively. During high-intensity physical activity, energy demand is greater than aerobic energy

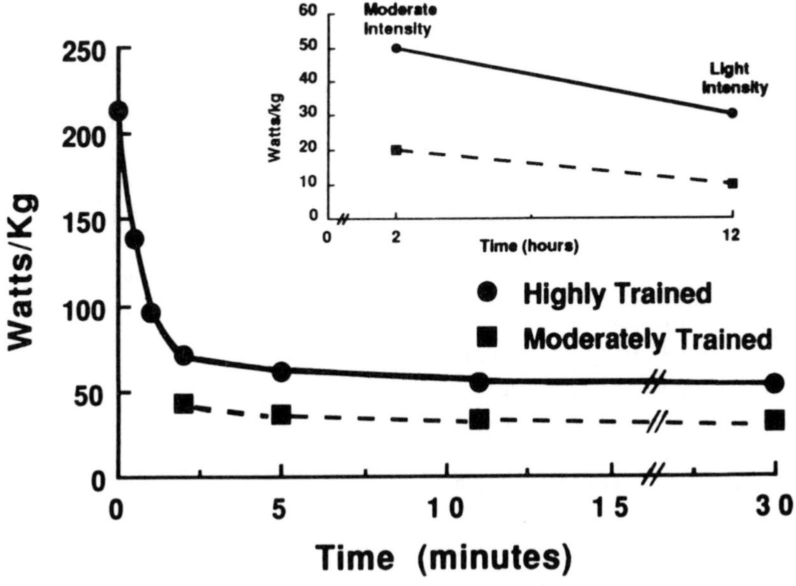

Figure 21.3 The relationship of normalized power output with the duration of the physical activity in minutes and in the inset in hours. The power is for cycling on a stationary cycle ergometer. The power is normalized per kg of active muscle on the assumption that 7 kg of muscle is active in each leg (see text). The data were modified from the data of Wilkie (78) with permission. The designations light, moderate, high, and exhaustive are for 12 hr, 2 hr, 5 min, and < 5 min. The data are in reasonable agreement with actual measurements of power of whole muscles during single (10) and repeated (9) contractions in situ. Note the significant difference in the effect of time on the relative power developed by highly trained endurance athletes and moderately trained adults.

supply. Consequently, high-intensity physical activity can elicit 100% of the subject's maximum oxygen consumption.

Response to Physical Activity of Light Intensity

Light activity, performed at 5% of maximum power produced during a single contraction, is about 10 W/kg of active muscle and equivalent to about 70 W on a bicycle ergometer. During general physical activities this intensity requires an aerobic energy expenditure of 16 ml/O_2/kg body weight per minute, or 4.5 MET (see chapter 3). The physiologic adjustment to physical activity of light intensity is rapid and complete. The transition from the delivery of energy by the hydrolysis of creatine phosphate and by glycolysis to almost complete dependence on oxidative phosphorylation occurs within the first minute. The average force per contraction remains near that of a single contraction with little evidence of fatigue (11).

Modestly trained young and adult subjects meet the force requirement of an activity of this intensity through recruitment of Type I and IIA motor units. Recruitment of Type IIB fiber motor units would be required by only the most poorly trained subjects. For poorly trained subjects, Type IIB fibers, when recruited, would lose average force rapidly (11), and endurance time (assuming a large percentage of Type IIB fibers) would be a matter of minutes. For most subjects light-intensity physical activity can be sustained without evidence of fatigue throughout an 8- to 12-hr period, and a minimal recovery period is required.

Response to Physical Activity of Moderate Intensity

At 10% of maximum power (equivalent to about 20 W/kg of active muscle and about 140 W on a bicycle ergometer), the metabolic requirement is about 9.0 MET. Compared with the average force developed during a single contraction, during activity of moderate intensity some loss of average force occurs during each of the repeated contractions. Throughout moderate physical activity, ATP concentration is maintained relatively constant by high energy phosphate reactions such as the creatine phosphokinase reaction. During a transition period of several minutes duration, energy output is constant, yet the contribution of the different metabolic pathways vary. After the transition period, oxygen consumption plateaus and oxidative phosphorylation is the predominant pathway throughout the remainder of the activity.

The magnitude of the power sustained during moderate activity is controlled by the balance between energy output and energy input. The concentrations of inorganic phosphate (23), hydrogen ions (54), and calcium (46) have each been implicated and may cause a reduction in the force or velocity either acting separately or in concert. Although a pseudo-steady state of metabolism is achieved, this intensity of activity can only be performed by most moderately trained subjects for a few hours. If this intensity of physical activity is carried on to the point of fatigue, blood glucose and muscle glycogen concentrations would be nearly exhausted (13).

Response to Physical Activity of High Intensity

Physical activity at an intensity 15% of maximum power achieved during a single contraction results in a value of about 30 W/kg of active muscle, about 210 W on a bicycle ergometer, or 13.5 MET. If physical activity is initiated at a high intensity, fatigue will occur within the first few minutes and maximum values of oxidative metabolism will not be reached. In the event the high-intensity physical activity is preceded by the muscle or muscle groups performing moderate intensity contractions for about 10 min or more, then the high-intensity activity can be sustained for minutes or even hours in the case of trained athletes.

In moderately trained subjects who may achieve maximum oxygen uptake cycling at this intensity, the exercise duration to fatigue typically will not exceed 5 to 10 min. In contrast, the highly trained person will perform high-intensity activities at 80% to 90% of maximum oxygen uptake and continue the activity for several hours. Critical substrates, primarily muscle glycogen, are metabolized and a degree of metabolic acidosis is produced. The increased inorganic phosphate, hydrogen ions, and impaired excitation contraction coupling all potentially contribute to a decreased power output. Depending on training state, glycogen depletion and metabolic acidosis appear to be key limitations at this intensity of effort (13).

Response to Physical Activity of Exhaustive Intensity

Unlike physical activity of high intensity that is enhanced by prior activity of light to moderate intensity, any prior activity decreases power during short-term exhaustive activities (66). Activity of an exhaustive intensity is not improved by prior activity because maximum force or power can only be sustained for a matter of seconds, and oxidative metabolism is not involved significantly. Energy flux is primarily through hydrolysis of creatine phosphate and glycolysis (66).

For skeletal muscles to contract at an exhaustive intensity requires high-frequency stimulation of most if not all of the motor units in the muscle or muscle groups. Whether the limbs are considered as a single muscle group of 7-kg mass, or alternatively contracting groups of 3.5 kg each, the transition from a single contraction to repeated contractions reduces the power to about 40% because the maximum duty cycle is about 0.4 (9) at 120 cycles/min (67). The velocity is at least optimum for the development of power and perhaps higher depending on the task desired. After even a few isovelocity shortening contractions at this frequency, the average force during each contraction declines (9). The exact mechanism of the decline remains controversial, but appears to be closely associated with a feedback regulation of cross-bridge mechanics (9). Depending on the task performed or the training effect desired, exhaustive intensities of contractions may be achieved by high loads, or high-duty cycles, or some combination of the two.

Isometric contractions with development of forces greater than 50% of the maximum voluntary force produce complete occlusion of blood flow. Consequently, delivery of oxygen and substrates and removal of metabolites is dependent on reactive hyperemia. The magnitude of the reactive hyperemia is aided by the ejection of much of the blood in the vascular bed of the muscle by the force of the contraction. The short duration of the contraction and the likelihood of complete occlusion of blood flow results in a reliance on the hydrolysis of creatine phosphate and by glycolysis for the maintenance of the ATP stores. With repeated high-force or power contractions at high-duty cycles, fatigue occurs rapidly resulting from mechanisms similar to those for high-intensity physical activity. Impaired transmission of action potentials and aspects of high-frequency fatigue, however, are of greater potential significance (76).

As with other intensities of physical activity, the precise mechanisms that limit the development of force and power are not known during exhaustive activities when the energy demand may be as much as sixfold greater than what can be supplied aerobically. The ability of a muscle to sustain force or power may be a function of the balance between the energy use during the contraction and the energy delivery and metabolite clearance during recovery. Conversely, in spite of the high-power outputs, factors other than energy imbalance may be implicated (12). Performance of high-power contractions can be enhanced by low-duty cycles, with seconds or even minutes in between contractions.

Adaptations to Chronic Changes in Physical Activity

The adaptations that occur in response to chronic reductions or increases in physical activity are characterized by modifications of morphological, biochemical, and molecular properties that alter functional attributes of fibers in specific motor units (Figure 21.2). Adaptations range from a diminished capacity to generate or maintain power in response to reduced physical activity, to a higher capacity to develop maximum power following strength training or to an enhanced capacity to maintain power for longer periods of time following endurance training. Adaptations for strength and endurance may occur independently, although training programs may produce increases in both attributes (37). The addition of heavy resistance training to endurance-training programs has no detrimental effect and enhances endurance performance under some circumstances (34). In addition to the high or low loading during contractions and the short or long duration of the periods of activity, training variables include the frequency of the training sessions per week and the total duration of the training sessions in months or years.

The combination of these factors and variables characterizes an habitual level of physical activity and provides a potential for training stimuli of varying intensities, durations, and frequencies (Figure 21.1). A training stimulus occurs when a change in the habitual level of physical activity is of sufficient magnitude and duration to produce a measurable adaptive response (Figure 21.3). Skeletal muscle adaptation to a chronic exposure to complete immobilization of limbs or to bed rest occurs within days, whereas the effects of detraining may take weeks or even months to be significant depending on the magnitude of the decrease (71). With increased physical activity, some metabolic adaptations may be observed within days (29). In contrast, most improvements in biochemical (3,17,29,37) and contractile properties (40) require weeks or months.

Maximum power can increase with no adaptive changes in morphological or biochemical properties of skeletal muscles. This type of neurophysiological adaptation is observed as a large improvement in strength and power during the early stages of a strength-training program, which presumably reflects the optimization of motor unit recruitment (63). Most adaptations that occur beyond the early training sessions are characterized by measurable morphological, biochemical, and molecular changes that influence directly the contractile and metabolic properties of skeletal muscle fibers (37). These adaptations may be either in the muscle group directly involved in the movement, in antagonistic muscles, or in fixator muscles that provide the force platform for the movement. Later improvements in a highly coordinated task may reflect optimization of motor unit recruitment between and amongst these different muscle groups.

The criterion for an adaptive response is a qualitative or quantitative alteration in one or more specific muscle proteins: contractile, regulatory, structural, metabolic, or transport (Figure 21.2). Adaptations occur in response to a specific training stimulus, and the adaptive response is regulated at multiple sites each controlled by negative feedback (Figure 21.2). Fibers within a motor unit are relatively homogeneous as to the concentrations and activities of metabolic, regulatory, and contractile proteins and consequently the contractile properties of fibers are similar (20,57,60). Conversely, the concentrations and activities of proteins in fibers of different motor units and the resultant contractile properties may show as much as a threefold difference (35).

The high degree of adaptive specificity results in unique modifications of specific morphological, biochemical, and molecular properties of skeletal muscle fibers in response to a given training stimulus (3). Fibers within motor units recruited during training are the fibers primarily affected. Furthermore within the recruited fibers, only elements that are stimulated beyond a threshold will undergo an adaptive change. The assumption is that the properties of fibers within a motor unit that adapt to a training stimulus do so in unison. Adaptations of muscle fibers in vitro appear to be mediated predominantly by the frequency and duration of stimulation and by the external load (20) with trophic factors playing at most a minor role. Mechanical forces generated in embryonic muscle cells growing in vitro appear to enhance muscle growth by soluble growth factors (74), but the role of growth factors in vivo has not been determined. The specificity of adaptations may result in improved performance in one physical activity with no change or even an impairment in another activity (52). The degree to which improved performance transfers from one physical activity to another depends on the amount of overlap in the physiological requirements of the two activities.

Adaptations to Chronic Reductions in Physical Activity

The concept of a chronic exposure to reduced physical activity assumes a baseline level with some modicum of physical activity (Figure 21.1). Consequently, models of reduced physical activity of specific skeletal muscles are achieved by further decreases in the neural input, biomechanical loading, or both. In human beings, studies have principally included bed rest, limb immobilization, unilateral leg suspension, or space flight. A reduction of physical activity by limb immobilization in human beings leads to a decrease in muscle fiber area and in the metabolic proteins that support endurance performance (51). Similar changes were observed following unloading of a lower limb of human beings for 4 weeks by suspension (7). The unweighting of the limb produced an 8% decrease in muscle cross-sectional area and a 20% decrease in muscle strength during both shortening and lengthening contractions.

Spaceflight or ground-based hind limb suspension has been employed to produce microgravity conditions for muscles (55,62,73). When exposures are of equally short duration, the magnitude of changes observed in muscles after hind limb suspension are not significantly different from those produced by space flight. The lack of a difference in results supports the validity of the ground-based model (55,62). In muscle unweighting by hind limb suspension of rats, contractile protein content decreases within the first few days, with the decrease more pronounced in slow soleus muscle than in fast muscles (73). The greatest rate of decrease in muscle mass and fiber cross-sectional area occurs in the first 7 days. In spite of continued unweighting, the rate slows and then plateaus at about 14 days (41). When chronic muscle unweighting by hind limb suspension is interspersed with minimal periods of weight bearing, the amount of muscle atrophy is decreased (28). After 28 days of suspension, the capacity of soleus muscles to generate maximum force decreases to a greater extent than the decrease in protein mass would predict (16).

For soleus muscles, the decrease in the development of force is twofold greater than that of the plantaris muscle. Slow soleus and fast plantaris muscles also differ as to the effect of unweighting on the maximum velocity of shortening (16). The maximum velocity of shortening of the soleus muscles increased, whereas that of the plantaris muscle did not change. The differences observed in the two muscles reflect either the habitual differences in the recruitment and loading of the two muscles, or an intrinsic difference in sensitivity to reduction in specific components of daily weight bearing.

During hind limb suspension of rats, the EMG activity is reduced initially in the plantar flexor muscles, but returns to close to control values after 7 days (1). In contrast, the EMG activity of the dorsiflexor tibialis anterior muscle remains increased throughout the period of hind limb suspension, yet the mass and contractile properties of this muscle are unaffected by the procedure of suspension (1). During hind limb suspension, unlike the unloaded plantar flexor muscles, the dorsiflexor muscles are loaded by the mass of the foot. These experiments emphasize the significant interactions among recruitment, the external load, and the force developed by the muscle group in the determination of the adaptive response.

Following a period of endurance training or strength training a decrease in the intensity of the daily activity usually results in a gradual regression back toward the pretraining values (15,24,44). The conclusion is that the maintenance of muscle adaptations requires a sustained increase or decrease in physical activity, and when the stimulus for adaptation is diminished or eliminated adaptations are reversible (15,44). The stability of adaptations to chronic physical activity appear to be a function of both the type and the duration of the training stimulus. In spite of the tendency for adaptation to regress, some adaptations are sustained for considerable periods of time in the absence of continued training (71).

Adaptation to Strength Activity

For humans, 12 weeks of heavy-resistance strength training leads to a 5% increase in quadriceps muscle cross-sectional area as measured by computerized tomography (40). Since muscle length is not likely to change, the circumference values provide an estimate of the gain in muscle mass. The increase in muscle mass following power lifting results from comparable increases in the cross-sectional area of Type I and Type II muscle fibers (51). Some investigators have reported a preferential Type II hypertrophy in the muscles of power lifters (20). Hypertrophy of single skeletal muscle fibers results from the increase in the number of myofibrils within the fiber (24). Vandenburgh et al. (74,75) demonstrated that when increased constant tension is applied to embryonic skeletal muscle, fibers differentiate in tissue culture via many of the same processes associated with fiber hypertrophy in vivo. These processes include sodium-dependent amino acid transport, sodium--potassium–ATPase activity, protein synthesis, and total protein and myosin heavy-chain accumulation. In addition, the myofibers responded to insulin and IGF-1 with a significant degree of hypertrophy.

Strength and power training has been shown to decrease mitochondrial protein concentration of muscles (51). Although strength training alone tends to reduce endurance, hypertrophied muscle does respond to an endurance training stimulus (61). Consequently, a decreased endurance capacity with strength training is not inevitable.

In muscles in which fibers are parallel to the long axis of the muscle, the number of fibers present may be determined from histochemical sections. Counts of the fibers in the cross section of parallel-fibered muscles with pennation may underestimate the number of fibers in the muscle due to some fibers not appearing in the cross section (49). If the fiber length (L_f):muscle length (L_m) ratio is less than 0.5, the relative number of fibers appearing in a cross section through the belly of the muscle depends on the L_f:L_m ratio. Therefore, the number of fibers in pennate muscles is best obtained by actual counts following nitric acid digestion (27). Following increased loading of the soleus muscle by ablation of synergistic muscles, no difference in fiber number was found between the muscles overloaded by removal of the synergistic muscles and the control muscles (27). The nascent muscle fibers observed in hypertrophied chicken anterior latissimus dorsi muscle (42) likely represent fibers regenerating following contraction-induced injury (50). The predominant mechanism for the hypertrophy of muscle in adult animals is hypertrophy of individual fibers.

In studies of strength training, the gains in force development of 30% to 40% invariably exceed the increase in cross-sectional area of the muscle. This increase is due in part to the optimization of recruitment patterns (63). A change in the orientation of individual fibers within a muscle might increase the angle of fibers relative to the long axis of the muscle. Under these circumstances the effective muscle fiber cross-sectional area would increase more than is indicated by computerized tomography (22).

In addition to the compensatory increase in muscle mass following ablation of synergistic muscles, the myosin isoform expression shifts from the fast toward the slow isozymes (4). Myosin isozymes were separated electrophoretically from the plantaris and soleus muscles of rats 11 weeks following ablation of the gastrocnemius muscle (32). Few adaptations occurred in the soleus muscle, but a threefold increase in the proportion of slow myosin (SM) was observed in the plantaris muscle, and fast myosin (FM2) decreased proportionately. Peptide mapping suggested that a true transformation of myosin had occurred in hypertrophied fibers of plantaris muscle (31).

Adaptations to Endurance Activities

Endurance training results in a significant increase in the capacity of muscles to sustain force and power. The primary adaptations to endurance training are metabolic and cardiovascular changes leading to an enhanced ability to oxidize fatty acids, conserve carbohydrates, and delay metabolic acidosis during prolonged physical activity (13,14,20,26,31,36,37). With endurance training, an approximate twofold increase in the oxidative activity of whole-muscle homogenates or of markers of mitochondrial protein concentration have been reported (3,17,36,37). Although the oxidative capacity of whole-muscle homogenates increases two-fold, this does not represent a two-fold increase in the maximum oxygen uptake of the total organism because of limitations in fiber recruitment and in the blood flow to fibers when a large muscle mass is activated (20). Other metabolic adaptations to physical activity, such as altered mobilization, storage, transport, and endogenous production of carbohydrates, lipids, and amino acids are developed in chapter 25.

Following endurance training, muscle blood flow at a given submaximal level of exercise may decrease or remain unchanged (2). In contrast, endurance training results in higher blood flows to the active muscles during exercise at $\dot{V}O_2$max (56). Armstrong, Laughlin, and Ripperger (2,45) have demonstrated increased blood flow to the oxidative portions of skeletal muscles with lower flows to the glycolytic portions both in anticipation of exercise and during exercise. Thus, a major adaptive response to endurance training is the redistribution of blood flow from the glycolytic fibers to the oxidative fibers within the active muscles.

Volitional endurance-training programs of 8 to 12 weeks increase the capillary:fiber ratio of human skeletal muscles by 5% to 10% (39). Small increases in the capillary density are not likely to affect maximum blood flow significantly when compared with the changes that can be produced by recruitment of the existing capillaries by vasodilation upstream, or recruitment by cell-to-cell communication (68). Increases in capillary density with endurance training may play a role in increasing the capillary transit time for red blood cells and thereby facilitate nutrient and gas exchange (see chapter 19).

Fibers in the soleus, medial gastrocnemius, and red portion of the vastus lateralis muscles of rats adapt to continuous running at submaximum velocities with increased concentrations of cytochrome *c*. In contrast, muscle fibers in the white portion of the vastus lateralis muscles require interval training at high velocities of running for large adaptive responses to occur (17). During running at different velocities, the responses of the three fiber types differ and may reflect altered recruitment of and power output by individual motor units. Alternatively, the different velocities of running may provide stimuli of varying intensities for adaptation of a given variable, such as cytochrome *c* concentration (17). This experiment (17) was not designed to provide an interpretation as to whether different fiber types have inherent differences in the threshold or capacity for adaptation.

A causal relationship exists between the training stimulus and the adaptive response, but the relationship is complex and not necessarily stoichiometric. The lack of stoichiometry results from the diversity of responses elicited in skeletal muscles by a given intensity of exercise performed by a total organism. Within an individual the diversity may arise from variations in the training stimulus or in the response. Subtle changes in recruitment and loading patterns may arise from day to day variations in hydration, nutrition, and fatigue, and such uncontrolled environmental factors as temperature, wind, and terrain. Among individuals, major differences in recruitment and loading patterns may arise from the differences in the fiber types present in the contracting muscles (25).

In quadriceps muscle, major differences in the proportions of fiber types exist even among such a homogeneous group as world-class marathon runners (20). Consequently, heterogeneity is to be expected between physically inactive and highly trained subjects. Because of the great variability in the functional properties of fibers among different individuals, a single training stimulus has the potential of eliciting a multitude of different adaptive responses due to variations in patterns of recruitment and loading as well as variations in the metabolic status of the skeletal muscle fibers recruited. In addition, physical activity is highly complex. Physical activity, or the power required to perform a task, may be altered by changes in a single variable or in a number of variables. The lack of a stoichiometric relationship between the training stimulus and the adaptive response constitutes a serious difficulty in investigating the relationship between a training stimulus and the adaptive response in a definitive or mechanistic manner.

Considerable interest has focused on the question: Does volitional endurance training provide a sufficient stimulus for the conversion of fibers from one type to another type? The concept of a conversion of fibers from Type II to Type I arose initially from cross-sectional studies of different groups of athletes. Compared to the 50% Type I (low myofibrillar ATPase) fibers normally observed in the muscles of control subjects, significantly greater percentages of Type I fibers (e.g., 70% to 80%), have been reported in the muscles of elite endurance athletes while sprinters and power lifters have approximately 80% Type II fibers (25,72). Furthermore, the difference exists only in the muscles involved in the sport (25,72). A strong genetic influence on the proportions of fiber types is observed in studies of twins (see chapters 3 and 6). None of the cross-sectional studies of elite athletes exclude the possibility that athletes who already have high percentages of certain fiber types select and subsequently excel in specific activities.

Although the oxidative capacity constitutes a continuum and a given fiber may not necessarily express a single myosin isozyme profile, the two independent characteristics have been blended into a variety of schemes for the classification of fibers (8,11,58). A prerequisite for meaningful interpretations of adaptations using a given classification scheme is that the fibers must be classified on the basis of variables actually measured. Endurance training increases the oxidative capacity of each of the three fiber types (4). If the intensity and duration of the endurance-training program is great enough, a percentage of the FG or IIB fibers may increase their oxidative capacity sufficient to change their fiber classification to FOG or IIA, however such a change in the percentages of fiber types is equivocal because oxidative capacity is a continuum (20).

An almost complete change from fast to slow or slow to fast fiber types has been shown with cross-innervation experiments (64). In addition, muscles exposed to chronic low-frequency stimulation demonstrate an increase in the percentage of Type I fibers and a decrease in the percentage of Type II. These experiments have established that the expression of myosin isozymes can be changed from fast to slow and vice versa (70). A number of experiments on rats and humans have been designed to determine if volitional recruitment can modify the type of myosin isozymes expressed in skeletal muscle fibers (20).

Gregory, Low, and Stirewalt (32) trained young rats for 10 weeks reaching a distance of 15 km/day, which is fourfold further than typical endurance-running protocols. Myosin isozymes, reported under nondenaturing conditions, showed a significant conversion from slow (SM) to fast (FM1, FM2, and FM3). Nevertheless, the possibility of selective hypertrophy of existing Type I and IIA fibers rather than a true conversion of fiber type could not be ruled out. Green and co-workers (30) studied 15 weeks of treadmill running at a final daily distance of 5.7 km. Of four muscles studied by the histochemical demonstration of myofibrillar ATPase, only the deep portion of the vastus lateralis muscle showed a significant increase in Type I fibers and decrease in Type II fibers.

The effect of 8 weeks of endurance training on myosin isozymes of histochemically typed fibers in human vastus lateralis muscle was evaluated by Baumann, Jaggi, Soland, Howald, and Schaub (6). The training induced a significant decrease in Type IIB fibers from 13% to 8%, which was not balanced by a significant increase in Type I or Type IIA fibers. Fragments of single fibers, which had been typed histochemically, were electrophoresed under denaturing conditions. Following training, biopsies from three of four subjects showed an increase in slow light chains and heavy chains in fibers classified Type IIA histochemically. The conclusion that the adaptations mark the beginning of a transition from Type II toward Type I fibers is not warranted. The gels were not quantified, and the differences observed were within the normal sampling variability for needle biopsies of human leg muscles. Modifications in isomyosin distribution in whole muscles of rodents have been reported in response to endurance training (21). These modifications, which to some degree are dependent on the type of muscle, consist of increases in intermediate myosins (i.e., fast myosins with a mixture of light chains).

Purified myosin fractions showed parallel changes in myosin light chains determined under denaturing conditions. Reiser, Moss, Giulian, and Greaser (60) have demonstrated in rabbit soleus muscle that fast and slow myosin frequently coexist in a single fiber. In these "mixed" fibers, the ratios of total fast to total slow light chains may be different from the ratio of fast to slow heavy chains. Under these circumstances, maximum unloaded shortening velocities of single fibers correlate highly with the proportion of fast heavy chain. Similarly, the proportion of fast myosin heavy chain is the primary determinant of the histochemical assay for myosin ATPase. Consequently, among individual muscle fibers many gradations of shortening velocity and staining intensities for myosin ATPase are possible. Partial conversion of "mixed" fibers is undoubtedly possible. Therefore, the demonstration of a change in the proportion of fast heavy chain is equivocal and cannot be taken as evidence of a complete conversion from fast to slow fiber type. None of the investigations resolves the issue of complete conversion from fast to slow myosin heavy chain, or vice versa, in individual fibers. The question whether or not volitional recruitment can provide the stimulus necessary to modify the expression of myosin isozymes remains unresolved and controversial.

Approaches and Areas of Needed Research

The promising avenues of research on the response and adaptation of skeletal muscle to physical activity will test hypotheses and will involve the utilization of the techniques developed primarily in biochemistry, bioengineering, cell and molecular biology, kinesiology, and physiology. The approaches will include the use of mono- and polyclonal antibodies, gene transfer and transgenic technology, quantitative gel electrophoresis, tissue culture, radiology, radioactive isotope tracers, and mechanics of muscles, motor units, and single fibers. These techniques coupled to animal model experiments or to the procedure of obtaining needle biopsies of human muscle tissue before and after well-designed training programs constitute a powerful investigative approach.

The substantive issues that require attention with respect to acute physical activity include: the causes of fatigue in different types of endurance, strength, and precision activities; the interrelationships among the measurements made on skeletal muscle in vitro, in situ, and in vivo and the related question of the validity of extrapolating from observations on single permeabilized fibers at 15 °C to fibers in vivo at 35 °C; the relative role of the type of muscle progenitor cells and the subsequent environmental factors that ultimately result in a diverse population of muscle cells poised for acute exercise; the functional significance of the diversity of myosin isoforms in adult muscles; the biomechanical behavior of functionally synergistic muscles composed of different fiber types and with fibers arranged at varying angles of pinnation; and the basis for age-related deficits that occur in skeletal muscles.

Equally important questions regarding the adaptive response to chronic changes in physical activity include: the identification of the mechanistic linkages and involved factors in plasma, sarcolemma, sarcoplasm, and nucleus between altered levels of recruitment and/or load and adaptive changes; the relative contribution of different and perhaps competing factors (hormone, mechanical, satellite cell, etc.) to the final steady state; the functional significance of the increased number of capillaries that can occur with endurance training; the effect of differences in the initial physiological status ranging from rudimentary to elite on the adaptive response to different types of training; the role of injury and subsequent degeneration and regeneration in the adaptation to training; and the basis for decreases in specific force capacity with atrophy, hypertrophy, and regeneration. Many gaps exist in the understanding of molecular mechanisms responsible for adaptations. For example, the role of satellite cells in muscle adaptation has been implicated but not adequately resolved (42). Areas of applied interest include: (a) the specific dose–response relationship between the adaptive response of specific proteins and the parameters of the physical activity training; (b) alterations in this relationship for people of different ages from early to late life; (c) alterations for persons with specific diseases or disabilities where physical activity might be useful in a therapeutic sense; and (d) countermeasures in environments of prolonged muscle unweighting such as during space flight.

Conclusions

The changes that occur in skeletal muscle with single bouts of physical activity and the adaptations that occur with decreases and increases in chronic exposures to physical activity constitute a significant and challenging field of study. The adaptive responses to altered levels of physical activity are highly complex. Research has focused primarily on the adaptive responses of whole muscles, or portions of muscles homogeneous as to fiber type. Currently, sufficient data are available to describe the adaptive response to stimuli of reduced activity, endurance training, and strength training. Even for these interventions, the relationship between stimulus and adaptive response has not been described adequately with regard to the threshold for activation of the response or the dose–response relationship. A wide variety of important problems remains to be investigated. Most important will be an understanding of the mechanical, biochemical, and molecular linkages between altered activity levels and adaptive responses. The design of definitive experiments and the utilization of a multitude of contemporary and traditional techniques could result in significant progress in this field of research that has such important implications for physical and physiological fitness and for the quality of life.

Acknowledgments

We acknowledge the valuable contributions of our colleagues whose names appear on joint publications. Gabriele Wienert typed the manuscript with skill and considerable tolerance for changes. Portions of this manuscript are based on "Adaptations of Skeletal Muscle to Physical Activity," by J.A. Faulkner and T.P. White. In *Exercise, Fitness, and Health,* (pp. 265-279) by C. Bouchard, R.J. Shephard, T. Stephens, J.R. Sutton, and B.D. McPherson (Eds.), 1990, Champaign, IL: Human Kinetics. The manuscript was written with partial grant support from National Institute of Dental Research Program Project DE-07687.

References

1. Alford, E.; Roy, R.R.; Hodgson, J.A.; Edgerton, V.R. Electromyography of rat soleus, gastrocnemius, and tibialis anterior during hind limb suspension. Exp. Neurol. 96:635-649; 1987.
2. Armstrong, R.B.; Laughlin, M.H. Exercise blood flow patterns within and among rat muscles after training. Am. J. Physiol. 246:H59-H68; 1984.
3. Baldwin, K.M.; Klinkerfuss, G.H.; Terjung, R.L.; Mole, P.A.; Holloszy, J.O. Respiratory capacity of white, red and intermediate muscle, adaptive response to exercise. Am. J. Physiol. 222:373-378; 1972.
4. Baldwin, K.M.; Valdez, V.; Herrick, R.E.; MacIntosch, A.M.; Roy, R.R. Biochemical properties of overloaded fast-twitch skeletal muscle. J. Appl. Physiol. 52:467-472; 1982.
5. Barany, M. ATPase activity of myosin correlated with speed of muscle shortening. J. Gen. Physiol. 50:197-218; 1967.
6. Baumann, H.; Jaggi, M.; Soland, F.; Howald, H.; Schaub, M.C. Exercise training induces transitions of myosin isoform subunits within histochemically typed human muscle fibres. Pflugers Arch. 409:349-360; 1987.
7. Berg, H.E.; Dudley, G.A.; Häggmark, T.; Ohlsén, H.; Tesch, P.A. Effects of lower limb unloading on skeletal muscle mass and function in humans. J. Appl. Physiol. 70:1882-1885; 1991.
8. Brooke, M.H.; Kaiser, K.K. Three "myosin adenosine triphosphatase" systems: The nature of their pH and sulfhydryl dependence. J. Histochem. Cytochem. 18:670-672; 1970.
9. Brooks, S.V.; Faulkner, J.A. Forces and powers of slow and fast skeletal muscles in mice during repeated contractions. J. Physiol. (Lond.). 436:701-710; 1991.
10. Brooks, S.V.; Faulkner, J.A.; McCubbrey, D.A. Power outputs of slow and fast skeletal muscles of mice. J. Appl. Physiol. 68:1282-1285; 1990.
11. Burke, R.E.; Levine, D.N.; Zajac, F.E., III; Tsairis, P.; Engel, W.K. Physiological types and histochemical profiles in motor units of the cat gastrocnemius. J. Physiol. (Lond.). 234:723-748; 1973.
12. Clausen, T. Significance at the Na^+ $-K^+$ pump regulation in skeletal muscle. News Physiol. 5:148-151; 1990.
13. Conlee, R.K. Muscle glycogen and exercise endurance: A twenty-year perspective. In: Pandolf, K.B., ed. Exercise sport science reviews. Vol. 15. New York: Macmillan; 1987:1-28.
14. Constable, S.H.; Favier, R.J.; McLane, J.A.; Fell, R.D.; Chen, M.; Holloszy, J.O. Energy metabolism in contracting rat skeletal muscle: Adaptation to exercise training. Am. J. Physiol. 253:C316-C322; 1987.
15. Coyle, E.F.; Martin, W.M., III; Sinacore, D.R.; Joyner, M.J.; Hagberg, J.M.; Holloszy, J.O. Time course of loss of adaptations after stopping prolonged intense endurance training. J. Appl. Physiol. 57:1857-1864; 1984.
16. Diffee, G.M.; Ciaozzo, V.J.; Herrick, R.E.; Baldwin, K.M. Contractile and biochemical properties of rat soleus and plantaris after hindlimb suspension. Am. J. Physiol. 260:C528-C534; 1991.
17. Dudley, G.A.; Abraham, W.A.; Terjung, R.L. Influence of exercise intensity and duration on biochemical adaptations in skeletal muscle. J. Appl. Physiol. 53:844-850; 1982.
18. Edwards, R.H.T.; Harris, R.C.; Hultman, E.; Kaijser, L.; Nordesjo, L.-O. Effect of temperature on muscle energy metabolism and endurance during successive isometric contractions, sustained to fatigue, of the quadriceps muscle in man. J. Physiol. (Lond.). 220:335-352; 1972.
19. Faulkner, J.A.; Brooks, S.V. Fatigability of mouse muscles during constant length, shortening, and lengthening contractions: Interactions between fiber types and duty cycles. In: Sargeant, T.; Kernell, D., eds. Neuromuscular fatigue. Amsterdam, Netherlands: Elsevier Science; 1993:116-123.
20. Faulkner, J.A.; White, T.P. Adaptations of skeletal muscle to physical activity. In: Bouchard, C.; Shephard, R.J.; Stephens, J.R.; McPherson, B.D., eds. Exercise, fitness, and health. Champaign, IL; Human Kinetics; 1990:265-278.
21. Fitzsimons, D.P.; Diffee, G.M.; Herrick, R.E.; Baldwin, K.M. Effects of endurance exercise on isomyosin patterns in fast- and slow-twitch skeletal muscles. J. Appl. Physiol. 68:1950-1955; 1990.
22. Gans, C. Fiber architecture and muscle function. In: Terjung, R.L., ed. Exercise sport science reviews. Vol. 10. Philadelphia: Franklin Institute; 1982:160-207.

23. Goldman, Y.E. Special topic: Molecular mechanism of muscle contraction. Annu. Rev. Physiol. 49:629-636; 1987.
24. Goldspink, G. Alterations in myofibril size and structure during growth, exercise and changes in environmental temperature. In: Peachey, L.D.; Adrian, R.H.; Geiger, S.R., eds. Handbook of physiology. Baltimore: Waverly Press; 1983:539-554.
25. Gollnick, P.D.; Armstrong, R.B.; Saubert, C.W., IV; Piehl, K.; Saltin, B. Enzyme activity and fiber composition in skeletal muscle of untrained and trained men. J. Appl. Physiol. 33:312-319; 1972.
26. Gollnick, P.D.; Bertorci, L.A.; Kelso, T.B.; Witt, E.H.; Hodgson, D.R. The effect of high intensity exercise on the respiratory capacity of skeletal muscle. Pflugers Arch. 415:405-413; 1990.
27. Gollnick, P.D.; Timson, B.F.; Moore, R.L.; Riedy, M. Muscular enlargement and number of fibers in skeletal muscles of rats. J. Appl. Physiol. 50:936-943; 1981.
28. Graham, S.C.; Roy, R.R.; Hauschka, E.O.; Edgerton, V.R. Effects of periodic weight support on medial gastrocnemius fibers of suspended rats. J. Appl. Physiol. 67:945-953; 1989.
29. Green, H.J.; Helyar, R.; Ball-Burnett, M.; Kowalchuk, N.; Symon, S.; Farrance, B. Metabolic adaptations to training precede changes in muscle mitochondrial capacity. J. Appl. Physiol. 72:484-491; 1992.
30. Green, H.J.; Klug, G.A.; Reichmann, H.; Seedorf, U.; Wiehrer, W.; Pette, D. Exercise-induced fibre type transition with regard to myosin and sarcoplasmic reticulum in muscles of the rat. Pflugers Arch. 400:432-438; 1984.
31. Green, H.J.; Reichmann, H.; Pette, D. Fibre type specific transformations in the enzyme activity pattern of rat vastus lateralis muscle by prolonged endurance training. Pflugers Arch. 399:216-222; 1983.
32. Gregory, P.; Low, R.B.; Stirewalt, W.S. Changes in skeletal muscle myosin isoenzymes with hypertrophy and exercise. Biochemistry. 238:55-63; 1986.
33. Hesser, C.M.; Linnarsson, D.; Bjurstedt, H. Cardiorespiratory and metabolic responses to positive, negative and minimum-load dynamic leg exercise. Respir. Physiol. 30:51-67; 1977.
34. Hickson, R.C.; Dvorak, B.A.; Gorostiaga, E.M.; Kurowski, T.T.; Foster, C. Potential for strength and endurance training to amplify endurance performance. J. Appl. Physiol. 65:2285-2290; 1988.
35. Hintz, C.S.; Lowry, C.V.; Kaiser, K.K.; McKee, D.; Lowry, O.H. Enzyme levels in individual rat fibers. Am. J. Physiol. 239:C58-C65; 1980.
36. Holloszy, J.O. Biochemical adaptations in muscle. Effects of exercise on mitochondrial oxygen uptake and respiratory enzyme activity in skeletal muscle. J. Biol. Chem. 242:2278-2282; 1967.
37. Holloszy, J.O.; Booth, F.W. Biochemical adaptations to endurance exercise in muscle. Annu. Rev. Physiol. 38:273-291; 1976.
38. Huxley, A. Reflections on muscle. Liverpool: Liverpool University Press; 1980.
39. Ingjer, F. Capillary supply and mitochondrial content of different skeletal muscle fiber types in untrained and endurance trained men: A histochemical and ultrastructual study. Eur. J. Appl. Physiol. 40:197-209; 1979.
40. Jones, D.A.; Rutherford, O.M. Human muscle strength training: The effects of three different regimes and the nature of the resultant changes. J. Physiol. 391:1-11; 1987.
41. Kasper, C.E.; White, T.P.; Maxwell, L.C. Running during recovery from hindlimb suspension induces transient muscle injury. J. Appl. Physiol. 68:533-539; 1990.
42. Kennedy, J.M.; Eisenberg, B.R.; Reid, S.K.; Sweeney, L.J.; Zak, R. Nascent muscle fiber appearance in overloaded chicken slow-tonic muscle. Am. J. Anat. 81:203-215; 1988.
43. Lamb, G.D.; Recupero, E.; Stephenson, D.G. Effect of myoplasmic pH on excitation-contraction coupling in skeletal muscle fibres of the toad. J. Physiol. (Lond.). 448:211-224; 1992.
44. Larsson, L. Effects of long-term physical training and detraining on enzyme histochemical and functional skeletal muscle characteristics in man. Muscle Nerve. 8:714-722; 1985.
45. Laughlin, M.H.; Ripperger, J. Vascular transport capacity of hindlimb muscles of exercise-trained rats. J. Appl. Physiol. 62:438-443; 1987.
46. Lee, J.A.; Westerblad, H.; Allen, D.G. Changes in tetanic and resting $[Ca^{2+}]_i$ during fatigue and recovery of single muscle fibers from xenopus laevis. J. Physiol. (Lond.). 433:307-326; 1991.
47. Lindinger, M.I.; Sjogaard, G. Potassium regulation during exercise and recovery. Sports Med. 11:382-401; 1991.
48. Luhtanen, P.; Komi, P.V. Force-, power-, and elasticity-velocity relationships in walking, running, and jumping. Eur. J. Appl. Physiol. 44:279-289; 1980.
49. Maxwell, L.C.; Faulkner, J.A.; Hyatt, G.J. Estimation of number of fibers in guinea pig skeletal muscles. J. Appl. Physiol. 37:259-264; 1974.
50. McCully, K.K.; Faulkner, J.A. Injury to skeletal muscle fibers of mice following lengthening contractions. J. Appl. Physiol. 59:119-126; 1985.
51. McDougall, J.D.; Elder, G.C.B.; Sale, D.G.; Moroz, J.R.; Sutton, J.R. Effects of strength

training and immobilization on human muscle fibers. Eur. J. Appl. Physiol. 43:25-34; 1980.
52. McDougall, M.J.N.; Davies, C.T.M. Adaptive response of mammalian skeletal muscle to exercise with high loads. Eur. J. Appl. Physiol. 52:139-155; 1984.
53. Merton, P.A. Voluntary strength and fatigue. J. Physiol. (Lond.). 123:553-564; 1954.
54. Metzger, J.M.; Moss, R.L. Greater hydrogen ion-induced depression of tension and velocity in skinned single fibres of rat fast than slow muscles. J. Physiol. (Lond.). 393:727-742; 1987.
55. Musacchia, X.J.; Steffen, R.D.; Fell, R.D.; Dombrowski, M.J. Skeletal muscle response to spaceflight, whole body suspension, and recovery in rats. J. Appl. Physiol. 69:2248-2253; 1990.
56. Musch, T.I.; Haidet, G.C.; Ordway, G.A.; Longhurst, J.C.; Mitchell, J.H. Training effects on regional blood flow response to maximal exercise in fox hounds. J. Appl. Physiol. 62:1724-1732; 1987.
57. Nemeth, P.; Pette, D.; Vrbova, G. Malate dehydrogenase homogeneity of single fibers of the motor unit. In: Pette, D., ed. Plasticity of muscle. New York: de Gruyter; 1980:45-54.
58. Peter, J.B.; Barnard, R.J.; Edgerton, V.R.; Gillespie, C.A.; Stemple, K.E. Metabolic profiles of three fiber types of skeletal muscle in guinea pigs and rabbits. Biochemistry. 14:2627-2633; 1972.
59. Pette, D.; Staron, R.S. Cellular and molecular diversities of mammalian skeletal muscle fibers. Rev. Physiol. Biochem. Pharmacol. 116:1-75; 1990.
60. Reiser, P.J.; Moss, R.L.; Giulian, G.G.; Greaser, M.L. Shortening velocity in single fibers from adult rabbit soleus muscles is correlated with myosin heavy chain composition. J. Biol. Chem. 260:9077-9080; 1985.
61. Riedy, M.; Moore, R.L.; Gollnick, P.D. Adaptive response of hypertrophied skeletal muscle to endurance training. J. Appl. Physiol. 59:127-131; 1985.
62. Roy, R.R.; Baldwin, K.M.; Edgerton, V.R. The plasticity of skeletal muscle: Effects of neuromuscular activity. In: Holloszy, J.O., ed. Exercise and sport sciences reviews. Vol. 19. Baltimore: Williams & Wilkins; 1991:269-312.
63. Sale, D.G. Neural adaptation to resistance training. Med. Sci. Sports Exerc. 20:S135-S145; 1988.
64. Salmons, S.; Hendrickson, J. The adaptive response of skeletal muscle to increased use. Muscle Nerve. 4:94-105; 1981.
65. Sargeant, A.J. Effect of muscle temperature on leg extension force and short-term power output in humans. Eur. J. Appl. Physiol. 56:693-698; 1987.
66. Sargeant, A.J.; Dolan, P. Effect of prior exercise on maximal short-term power output in humans. J. Appl. Physiol. 63:1475-1480; 1987.
67. Sargeant, A.J.; Hoinville, E.; Young, A. Maximum leg force and power output during short-term dynamic exercise. J. Appl. Physiol. (Respir. Environ. Exerc. Physiol.). 51:1175-1182; 1981.
68. Segal, S.S. Microvascular recruitment in hamster striated muscle: Role for conducted vasodilation. Am. J. Physiol. 261:H181-H189; 1991.
69. Sjoström, M.; Friden, J.; Ekblom, B. Endurance—what is it? Muscle morphology after an extremely long distance run. Acta Physiol. Scand. 130:513-520; 1987.
70. Sreter, F.A.; Pinter, K.; Jolesz, F.; Mabuchi, K. Fast to slow transformation of fast muscles in response to long-term phasic stimulation. Exp. Neurol. 75:95-102; 1982.
71. Staron, R.S.; Leonardi, M.J.; Karapondo, D.L.; Malicky, E.S.; Falkel, J.E.; Hagerman, F.C.; Hikida, R.S. Strength and skeletal muscle adaptations in heavy-resistance-trained women after detraining and retraining. J. Appl. Physiol. 70:631-640; 1991.
72. Tesch, P.A. Skeletal muscle adaptations consequent to long-term heavy resistance exercise. Med. Sci. Sports Exerc. 20:S132-S134; 1988.
73. Thomason, D.B.; Booth, F.W. Atrophy of the soleus muscle by hindlimb unweighting. J. Appl. Physiol. 68:1-12; 1990.
74. Vandenburgh, H.H.; Karlisch, P.; Shansky, J.; Feldstein, R. Insulin and IGF-I induce pronounced hypertrophy of skeletal myofibers in tissue culture. Am. J. Physiol. 260:C475-C484; 1991.
75. Vandenburgh, H.H.; Swasdison, S.; Karlisch, P. Computer-aided mechanogenesis of skeletal muscle organs from single cells in vitro. FASEB J. 5:2860-2867; 1991.
76. Westerblad, H.; Lee, J.A.; Lannergren, J.; Allen, D.G. Cellular mechanisms of fatigue in skeletal muscle. Am. J. Physiol. 261:C195-C209; 1991.
77. Wilkie, D.R. The relation between force and velocity in human muscle. J. Physiol. (Lond.). 110:249-280; 1950.
78. Wilkie, D.R. Man as a source of mechanical power. Ergonomics. 3:1-8; 1960.

Chapter 22

Physical Activity and Adipose Tissue

Jean-Pierre Després

Adipose tissue is the most important organ for lipid storage. During prolonged exercise the fuel mixture oxidized by the skeletal muscle varies depending upon the intensity and the duration of exercise. It is well accepted, however, that lipid mobilization from adipose tissue contributes significantly to the energy supply (5), although the exact contribution of adipose cells' fatty acids in the overall free fatty acid (FFA) supply to the muscle mitochondria remains uncertain and may vary among individuals. The simplest and most obvious example that adipose tissue lipids are utilized during endurance exercise is provided by the low levels of body fat measured in individuals who can achieve high levels of energy expenditure due to competitive endurance training (e.g., marathon runners) (20,35,79). However, as endurance athletes' low levels of body fat may also reflect a selection process, it is also important to investigate the effects of endurance exercise on adipose tissue morphology and metabolism in initially sedentary individuals.

Effects of Endurance Exercise Training on Adipose Tissue Mass

Review papers on the effects of exercise training on body fatness and published meta-analysis articles have indicated that total body weight and adipose mass losses induced by training, although often significant, are generally small when no dietary restriction is applied (6–11,26,27,34,36,37,42,44,70, 73,77,93,95,97,112).

Therefore, an exercise program aimed at weight loss must generate a large energy expenditure, and the minimal prescription recommended for improving cardiorespiratory fitness (1) may not be sufficient to substantially reduce adipose tissue mass (7,34,36,97). As an example, it has been previously calculated that a 40 min endurance exercise session, performed 4 to 5 times a week at about 75% of $\dot{V}O_2$ max could generate a net energy expenditure of approximately 200 kcal/day in men and a little more than 100 kcal/day in women (34,99). In this regard, Epstein and Wing (42) have reviewed 16 studies with five or more subjects in which individuals (mostly men) were exercise-trained from 8 to 26 weeks and the mean weight change was a loss of 0.20 lb/week. Wilmore (112) reviewed 16 and 37 exercise-training studies in women and men respectively and reported average weight losses of 0.15 lb/week in women and 0.16 lb/week in men.

It is therefore clear that dietary restriction can potentially induce faster rates of weight loss than exercise training alone. Weight loss induced by endurance exercise training is, however, associated with a better preservation of fat-free mass than hypocaloric diets (6,17,28–30,32,33,97). Indeed, in all exercise-training experiments that have been performed at the Physical Activity Sciences Laboratory over the years, there has not been a single study where a significant reduction in fat-free mass was found (17,28–30,32,33,38,98,99,101).

Thus, there is a higher proportion of fat in the body mass lost in response to endurance exercise training in comparison with hypocaloric diets.

Després et al. (30,36,38) as well as Tremblay, Després, and Bouchard (97) have reported, in concordance with previous observations (53,54), that there are gender differences in the sensitivity to lose weight in response to endurance exercise training, men generally responding better than women (30,36,38,97). A meta-analysis recently published has confirmed these studies in supporting the existence of a sex dimorphism in adipose tissue sensitivity to exercise training (6).

Such differences may be due to a compensatory increase in food intake in women and to gender differences in adipose tissue metabolism (36). In this regard, it has been previously estimated that 20 weeks of endurance exercise training performed 4 to 5 times a week, 40 min/day, at about 75% of the maximal aerobic power was associated with a net energy expenditure of 26,007 and 15,572 kcal in men and women respectively. This training should have generated weight losses of 4.3 kg and 2.6 kg (assuming a caloric equivalent of weight loss of 6,000 kcal/

kg) in men and women respectively, had no compensation in energy intake occurred (99).

In this previous experiment, a body weight loss of only 1.7 kg was observed in men whereas no significant change was noted in women (99). It is therefore very likely that a caloric compensation had occurred and that it was greater in women than in men. These results are consistent with those of Woo and Pi-Sunyer (113) who reported an increase in energy intake following exercise training in lean women but no increase in obese women. In obese women, several studies have indicated that the magnitude of weight loss that can be achieved by exercise training alone is small (26,33,55) and sometimes not significant (38,53, 54,56,59).

The gender difference in adipose tissue sensitivity to endurance exercise training will require further investigation but this phenomenon is consistent with results from animal studies. Indeed, body weight growth curves of exercise-trained male rats have often been found to be lower than sedentary male rats (25,71,73,85). Exercise-trained female rats, however, generally show normal body weight gain curves when compared to sedentary controls (72,73). When the energy expenditure produced by exercise training is further increased, or in situations where the energy intake is controlled, exercise-trained female rats have shown reductions in body fat content (93,108,109).

Mechanisms responsible for this apparent gender difference in adipose tissue sensitivity to exercise training are poorly understood and additional research in this area is clearly warranted. Thus, although a substantial reduction in caloric intake should not be recommended for the long-term regulation of adipose tissue mass, some control over food intake, especially over the lipid content of the diet, is important to optimize adipose tissue mobilization in response to exercise, especially in women. Although the loss of body fat induced by exercise training in initially sedentary individuals will be generally small, metabolic improvements associated with such a moderate reduction in adipose tissue mass will include improved carbohydrate metabolism and plasma lipid transport (7-13,26,32–34,36–38,53-56,101), which contribute to reduce the risk of developing diabetes and cardiovascular disease.

Effects of Endurance Exercise Training on Regional Adipose Tissue Distribution

It has been hypothesized, however, that the well-documented gender difference in adipose tissue distribution and in sex steroid levels may be involved in the sex dimorphism observed in the sensitivity of adipose tissue to exercise training (30,36). It is well known that men tend to accumulate fat in the upper part of the body, especially in the abdominal area, whereas women generally show a preferential accumulation of body fat in gluteal and femoral areas (102,103). The peripheral adipose tissue of women has been reported to have an impaired lipolytic response to catecholamines (58,76,92) and a high activity of lipoprotein lipase in comparison with abdominal fat depots (83). It is therefore possible that the greater prevalence of gluteal-femoral fat in women may be partly responsible for their lower sensitivity to lose weight in response to an exercise-training program.

On the other hand, men have been reported to have a greater proportion of abdominal adipose tissue and a higher accumulation of deep abdominal (visceral) fat than women (41). Visceral adipose tissue has a lively lipolysis (76,81,82) that responds poorly to insulin (14). Therefore, although the presence of high levels of abdominal visceral adipose tissue is associated with impairments in carbohydrate and lipid metabolism, this adipose depot can be readily mobilized during weight loss, especially if high levels are initially present (33,46,81,90).

These observations on the regional properties of adipose tissue in men and women are consistent with the preferential mobilization of upper body fat that has been observed in exercise-training studies reported by Després et al. (26,29,33,36,38) and Tremblay et al. (98,100). Indeed, a greater mobilization of trunk than extremity fat during weight loss produced by endurance exercise training has been reported in men (26,98), whereas a small loss of trunk fat was noted in women (26). In both sexes, however, a preferential mobilization of abdominal fat in comparison with femoral fat was consistently observed. Such preferential mobilization of abdominal adipose tissue has been confirmed by computed tomography studies (33,90).

A significant loss of visceral fat in response to endurance exercise training and a large energy deficit have also been observed in young adult men (Bouchard et al., unpublished observations). These results are concordant with those of another study in which healthy young and older men were exercised for a period of 6 months (90). In both groups, significant losses of visceral fat were noted but the reduction was more marked in older men.

It must be recognized, however, that the preferential loss of upper body fat during weight loss is not a unanimous finding. However, in addition to gender, several factors may influence the magnitude of abdominal adipose tissue loss such as the initial level of fatness, the initial level of abdominal adipose tissue, the subject's age, the intensity of exercise, and the energy deficit generated by the exercise-training program. In this regard, Tremblay et al. (100) have shown, in a large cohort of men and women studied for the 1981 Canada Fitness Survey, that subjects regularly involved in vigorous aerobic activities had lower levels of upper body fat than subjects participating in activities of lower intensity generating similar estimated levels of total energy expenditure. These results are concordant with the notion of a preferential loss of abdominal or upper body fat in response to endurance exercise training.

One must also consider that the pattern of adipose tissue distribution is strongly inherited (16) and that individual variation in the sensitivity of the various adipose depots to exercise training will likely be observed. In summary, it appears that the greater proportion of upper body and visceral adipose tissue in men may be partly responsible for their generally greater sensitivity to lose weight in comparison with women in response to an aerobic exercise program.

Effects of Endurance Exercise Training on Fat Cell Size and Number

The size of a given adipose depot is determined by the number and the size of the constituting adipose cells (49). Weight loss produced by endurance exercise training appears to reduce body fat mass solely through a reduction in adipose cell size (11,13,29,30,96,99). The low levels of body fat of ex-obese long distance runners, who had lost almost 40 kg of body weight by training for the marathon, could be entirely accounted for by a reduction in adipose cell size, as these subjects had apparently more adipose cells than control runners who had never been obese in the past (96). It therefore appears that endurance exercise training may, without any caloric restriction, generate a small but significant loss of body fat, especially in men, and that this reduction in the adipose tissue mass can be solely explained by changes in adipose cell size.

Effects of Endurance Exercise Training on Adipose Tissue Metabolism

The regulation of adipose tissue mass depends on several metabolic processes, the two most important being lipid mobilization through lipolysis and storage through the hydrolysis of circulating triglycerides by the enzyme lipoprotein lipase (LPL). An insulin-sensitive glucose transport can also be measured in human adipose cells, but whether human adipocytes have the ability to synthesize substantial quantities of lipids from this substrate remains a controversial issue (62). In the next sections, the acute and chronic responses of human adipose tissue metabolism to prolonged exercise will be reviewed.

Adipose Tissue Lipolysis

Free fatty acids (FFA) represent the major fuel oxidized during prolonged aerobic exercise. In addition to endogenous triglyceride stores and those of lipoprotein-triglycerides, adipose tissue represents the most important source of exogenous FFA for the working muscle (74). Through the hydrolysis of adipose tissue triglycerides, mainly under the control of catecholamines and insulin, free fatty acids can be released into the circulation, which may contribute to the energy supply to the working muscle. It has been shown that an increased availability of FFA increased their oxidation (66,78), potentially contributed to spare glycogen utilization (21,48,84), and reduced glucose uptake (47). Although additional studies are needed to understand further the effect of increased FFA availability on the balance between carbohydrate and lipid metabolism in the skeletal muscle, the adaptation of adipose tissue lipolysis to endurance training may have important implications for the regulation of energy supply and utilization of energy by the skeletal muscle.

Chronic Response of Adipose Cell Lipolysis to Endurance Exercise Training

An abundant literature is available on the chronic effects of prolonged exercise in rats (74,91). However, as there are differences between rats and humans regarding the adrenergic regulation of lipolysis (57), it has been important to study the adaptation of adipose tissue lipolysis in humans. However, such studies have been limited by the difficulty in obtaining large amounts of adipose tissue from biopsies. Therefore, it has not been possible to conduct several incubations from a single piece of adipose tissue. New techniques for the assay of very small concentrations of glycerol (by bioluminescence) (51) and for the in situ measurement of lipolysis (2,52) should allow a better characterization of the acute and chronic adaptive responses of adipose tissue lipolysis to aerobic exercise.

In 1983, Després, Savard, Tremblay, and Bouchard (35) reported that suprailiac adipose cells of highly trained marathon runners had higher epinephrine-stimulated lipolysis than sedentary controls. As such difference may have resulted from a selection bias, sedentary men and women were exercise-trained and higher epinephrine-stimulated lipolysis was observed after training (28,30,31). Other groups have since confirmed the significant adaptation of adipose tissue lipolysis to chronic endurance exercise (22,24,86).

Therefore, in lean subjects endurance exercise training has been reported to increase the lipolytic response of adipose cells to catecholamines in both men and women (22,24,28,30,31,75,86). The mechanism underlying the increased lipolytic response to catecholamines in trained subjects is not fully understood. It appears certain, however, that the reduction in fat cell size is not a major factor, as Després et al. (28,30,31) have reported an increased lipolytic response in the presence or absence of concomitant changes in adipose cell size following training. It has been previously speculated that the balance between $alpha_2$- and $beta_1$-adrenergic receptors may be involved (30); this ratio is critical in determining whether catecholamines will have a lipolytic or an antilipolytic effect (43). In men, it has been suggested that the greater lipolytic response noted after training could be due to an increased $beta_1$-adrenergic response (22). In women, alterations in both the $alpha_2$- (decreased efficiency) and in the $beta_1$- (increased efficiency) adrenergic pathways may be involved, the increase in the $beta_1$-adrenergic component being greater in women than in men (24).

No information is available, however, on the potential adaptation of adipose tissue lipolysis to exercise training in obese subjects. Regional differences in adipose tissue lipolysis response to catecholamines have been reported in obese men and women, this variation being partly attributed to alterations in the ratio of alpha- (inhibitory) to $beta_1$- (stimulatory) adrenergic receptors (57,58,60, 64,65). Further research on this topic is clearly warranted in both lean and obese subjects as the potential regional variation in the chronic adaptation of adipose tissue lipolysis to endurance exercise has received little attention so far.

Acute Response of Adipose Cell Lipolysis to Prolonged Endurance Exercise

Adipose tissue lipolysis can also acutely respond to a single bout of endurance exercise. Indeed, in nonobese subjects, 30 min of submaximal aerobic exercise resulted in an increase in the lipolytic responsiveness of gluteal adipocytes to catecholamines, which was unrelated to changes in $beta_1$- or $alpha_2$-adrenergic receptors (106,107). Gender differences were observed in the acute adaptation of lipolysis, male gluteal fat being more responsive than female gluteal adipose cells after exercise (106,107).

These results on the acute effects of prolonged exercise on adipose tissue lipolysis are consistent with those of Crampes, Beauville, Rivière, Garrigues, and Lafontan (23) who reported that desensitization of human fat cell $beta_1$- and $alpha_2$-adrenergic responses did not occur after a period of intense exercise in both trained and sedentary women. As the higher lipolytic responsiveness of adipocytes in endurance-trained women was still evident after a short period of exercise, the difference between trained and sedentary women probably reflected functional variations in the lipolytic cascade at some postreceptor levels and not a residual effect of the last exercise session in trained women. In addition, a single endurance exercise session of 90 min in moderately active men has also been associated with an increase in subcutaneous abdominal fat cells' lipolytic response to epinephrine (89).

More recently, Arner, Kriegholm, Engfeldt, and Bolinder (3), using a microdialysis probe, have suggested the presence of a differential adrenergic regulation of lipolysis in situ. Lipolysis was measured at rest to be under $alpha_2$-adrenergic control, whereas the beta-adrenergic component appeared to regulate adipose tissue lipolysis during exercise in nonobese subjects (3). Lipolytic activity was significantly higher in subcutaneous abdominal than in gluteal adipose tissue, and this regional variation was more apparent in women than in men. The acute adipose cell lipolytic response to catecholamines is therefore depot- and gender-dependent. Gluteal fat cells seemed to be more responsive to exercise in men than in women. In addition, gluteal adipose cells of men were also more responsive than abdominal subcutaneous adipose cells from both sexes (106). These results may help to explain the resistance of gluteal-femoral fat to exercise training in comparison with abdominal adipose tissue in women.

In summary, although the evidence available in humans is limited, it can be safely concluded that the lipolytic response to catecholamines is increased by endurance exercise training. Further work is clearly warranted, however, in both lean and obese men and women in order to identify the mechanisms involved in the acute and chronic adaptations of adipose tissue lipolysis to exercise training. Several studies that have been conducted in animals (74,91) have suggested that most of the adaptations could occur at postreceptor events, although different results may be obtained in humans as their adipocytes show both alpha- and beta-adrenergic responses to catecholamines (43,57,60)—whereas rat adipocytes are characterized mostly by a beta-adrenergic lipolytic response (57). The increased lipolytic response of exercise-trained adipose cells may contribute to increase or at least maintain the supply of exogenous FFA to the skeletal muscle despite the low levels of body fat and the reduced concentrations of plasma catecholamines during prolonged exercise observed in the endurance-trained individual.

Adipose Tissue Lipoprotein Lipase (LPL)

The enzyme lipoprotein lipase (LPL) plays a major role in the regulation of triglyceride stores in the adipose cell. Indeed, the main function of LPL is the hydrolysis of triglycerides transported by lipoproteins, a process that allows the uptake of FFA by the various tissues. Adipose tissue LPL is synthesized by the parenchymal cells of the adipose tissue (15). After glycosylation of the protein, the enzyme is then transported to the Golgi apparatus and secreted in vesicles. After exocytosis, LPL remains associated with capillary endothelial cells, where it binds to glycosaminoglycans (39). The enzyme hydrolyzes triglyceride in chylomicrons and very low density lipoproteins (VLDL) allowing the uptake, esterification, and storage as triglycerides (TG) by the adipose cells. LPL can be released by heparin but the origin of LPL activity measurable in the postheparin plasma is heterogeneous, as both the cardiac and skeletal muscles are also important sources of LPL (15). It is therefore important to specifically assess LPL in adipose tissue to derive valid information on the adaptation of this enzyme in this specific tissue, because the acute and chronic responses of muscle and adipose tissue LPL to endurance exercise have been reported to differ (67).

Chronic Response of Adipose Tissue LPL to Aerobic Exercise Training

Adipose tissue lipoprotein lipase has been reported to be increased in lean, endurance-trained subjects, an adaptation which may contribute to the replenishment of adipose tissue lipid stores between exercise sessions (63,67,68,87). Most lipoprotein lipase measurements have, however, been performed in the fasting state. In addition, we have no information on the mechanisms responsible for the increased LPL activity measured in the adipose tissue of endurance-trained subjects. The activity of adipose tissue LPL can be altered at various steps that include transcription, translation, glycosylation, and secretion (39). This enzyme has also been shown to respond to insulin (39,40). The increase in LPL activity produced by insulin appears to result from an increased proportion of active LPL available at the surface of the cell through modification of posttranslational mechanisms (69). The importance of posttranslational regulation of LPL activity is also supported by a recent study by Arner, Lithell, Wahrenberg, and Brönnegard (4) who reported no correlation between LPL messenger (mRNA) levels and adipose tissue LPL activity measured in abdominal and femoral depots.

The response of adipose tissue LPL to insulin is reportedly increased in obese patients after weight loss (40). However, no information is available on the effect of endurance exercise training on the regulation of adipose tissue LPL activity by insulin in humans. In addition, results are lacking on the effects of aerobic exercise training on adipose tissue LPL activity in obese men and women, with control over potential regional differences. Indeed, gender and regional differences in adipose tissue LPL activity have been reported (45,80,83), but no information is available on the interaction of these factors with exercise training.

Acute Response of Adipose Tissue LPL to Endurance Exercise

The acute response of adipose tissue LPL to prolonged exercise is also a complex phenomenon. One should expect a decrease in adipose tissue LPL in response to acute exercise, because increased plasma catecholamines and reduced insulin levels theoretically lead to a reduction in LPL activity (67). However, a 90 min endurance exercise session has been reported to increase adipose tissue LPL activity in nonobese men (89). These results are concordant with those of Lithell et al. (61) and Taskinen, Nikkila, Rehunen, and Gordin (94) who reported increased adipose tissue LPL activity after a single session of exercise. The physiological function of this acute adaptation remains unclear.

Because adipose tissue LPL is already high and its responsiveness to insulin is low in obese patients, it would also be relevant to study its acute response to exercise in obese men and women. Potential regional variation in adipose tissue LPL response to exercise should also be studied. Additional work is clearly needed regarding the effects of exercise on the regulation of adipose tissue LPL activity in obese subjects with various body fat distribution phenotypes.

Therefore, although we can conclude from the results available that human adipose tissue LPL acutely and chronically responds to prolonged exercise, studies on this topic are limited and several unanswered questions remain: Is there a potential regional variation in the adipose tissue LPL response to prolonged exercise and exercise training? What is the response of adipose tissue LPL in obese patients? What are the mechanisms responsible for the changes observed? Finally, it is not known whether exercise will acutely or chronically modify the adipose tissue LPL response to insulin in lean and obese men and women.

Glucose Transport and Lipogenesis

Processes other than LPL must be involved in lipid accretion in adipose cells, as a normal adipose tissue mass has been reported in individuals with no LPL activity (18). Although the contribution of adipose tissue to whole body lipogenesis appears to be small (62), an increase in the insulin-stimulated glucose conversion into lipids has been reported in adipose cells from endurance-trained athletes in comparison with sedentary controls (87). Such an adaptation may also contribute to the replenishment of adipose tissue lipids after exercise. In this study, it was not possible, however, to verify whether the ^{14}C-labeled lipids recovered were derived from the esterification of intracellular FFA with labeled glycerophosphate or were resulting from true *de novo* lipogenesis from labeled acetate.

Using the same methodology, Savard, Després, Marcotte, and Bouchard (88) have shown that 20 weeks of endurance training induced a significant increase in the conversion of ^{14}C-glucose into lipids. There is, however, little information on the chronic effects of endurance exercise on adipose tissue basal- and insulin-stimulated glucose uptake and lipogenesis in humans, although several studies have shown that these processes are increased in trained animals (50,104,105,111). The conversion of glucose into lipids has been reported to be significantly reduced by 90 min of aerobic exercise (89). The high plasma catecholamine concentrations and the reduction in plasma insulin levels observed during prolonged exercise, combined with an increase in intracellular FFA levels, may have contributed to the reduction of glucose conversion in lipids observed in this study (89).

In addition to LPL and lipogenesis, there is another important process by which lipids can accumulate in the human adipose tissue. An acylation-stimulating protein (ASP) has been identified as a potent stimulator of FFA uptake and esterification in various tissues (19,110). Uptake and esterification of FFA into TG by human adipose tissue is stimulated to a substantial extent by ASP (110). No information is available on the acute and chronic effects of endurance exercise on ASP levels and response in adipose cells. Further research in this area is clearly warranted as ASP may represent a very important regulator of adipose tissue TG stores under various physiological conditions.

Conclusion

There is evidence that human adipose tissue morphology and metabolism adapt to endurance exercise training. Endurance exercise training generating a large energy expenditure can potentially reduce adipose tissue stores via a reduction in adipose cell size. In this regard, the abdominal adipose depot appears to be more readily mobilized during exercise training-induced weight loss than peripheral depots. Endurance exercise may, in some instances, induce a preferential mobilization of central fat and a loss of visceral adipose tissue. The regional variation in the response of adipose tissue lipolysis to exercise training is to some extent consistent with the morphological changes observed. This reduction in adipose tissue mass is solely the consequence of a decrease in adipose cell size, as there is no evidence for a change in fat cell number. Adipose cell lipolytic response and LPL activity clearly adapt to endurance exercise training in humans, but further work is needed on: (a) gender differences, (b) regional variation in adipose tissue metabolic response to exercise training, (c) the LPL response to exercise training in various fat depots and its regulation by insulin, and (d) the adaptation of other metabolic pathways involved in lipid accretion in adipose tissue.

References

1. American College of Sports Medicine. The recommended quantity and quality of exercise for developing and maintaining cardiorespiratory and muscular fitness in healthy adults. Med. Sci. Sports Exerc. 22:265-274; 1990.
2. Arner, P.; Bolinder, J.; Eliasson, A.; Lundin, A.; Ungerstedt, U. Microdialysis of adipose tissue and blood for in vivo lipolysis studies. Am. J. Physiol. (Endocrinol. Metab.). 255: E737-E742; 1988.

3. Arner, P.; Kriegholm, E.; Engfeldt, P.; Bolinder, J. Adrenergic regulation of lipolysis in situ at rest and during exercise. J. Clin. Invest. 85:893-898; 1990.
4. Arner, P.; Lithell, H.; Wahrenberg, H.; Brönnegard, M. Expression of lipoprotein lipase in different human subcutaneous adipose tissue regions. J. Lipid Res. 32:423-429; 1991.
5. Askew, E.W. Role of fat metabolism in exercise. Clin. Sports Med. 3:605-621; 1984.
6. Ballor, D.L.; Keesey, R.E. A meta-analysis of the factors affecting exercise-induced changes in body mass, fat mass and fat-free mass in males and females. Int. J. Obes. 15:717-726; 1991.
7. Björntorp, P. Effects of exercise conditioning in obesity. In: Bray, G., ed. Obesity in perspective. Bethesda, MD: Department of Health, Education, and Welfare; 1975:397-406.
8. Björntorp, P. Exercise in the treatment of obesity. Clin. Endocrinol. Metab. 5:431-453; 1976.
9. Björntorp, P. Physical training in the treatment of obesity. Int. J. Obes. 2:149-156; 1978.
10. Björntorp, P. Physiological and clinical aspects of exercise in obese persons. Exerc. Sport Sci. Rev. 11:159-180; 1983.
11. Björntorp, P. Adipose tissue adaptation to exercise. In: Bouchard, C.; Shephard, R.J.; Stephens, T.; Sutton, J.R.; McPherson, B.D., eds. Exercise, fitness, and health: A consensus of current knowledge. Champaign, IL: Human Kinetics; 1990:315-323.
12. Björntorp, P.; Fahlen, M.; Grimby, G.; Gustafson, A.; Holm, J.; Renström, P.; Schersten, T. Carbohydrate and lipid metabolism in middle-aged, physically well-trained men. Metabolism. 21:1037-1044; 1972.
13. Björntorp, P.; Grimby, G.; Sanne, H.; Sjöström, L.; Tibblin, G.; Wilhemsen, L. Adipose tissue fat cell size in relation to metabolism in weight-stable physically active men. Horm. Metab. Res. 4:182-186; 1972.
14. Bolinder, J.; Kager, L.; Ostman, J.; Arner, P. Differences at the receptor and postreceptor levels between human omental and subcutaneous adipose tissue in the action of insulin on lipolysis. Diabetes. 32:117-123; 1983.
15. Borensztajn, J. Adipose tissue lipoprotein lipase. Chicago: Evener; 1987:79-132.
16. Bouchard, C.; Tremblay, A.; Després, J.P.; Nadeau, A.; Lupien, P.J.; Thériault, G.; Dussault, J.; Moorjani, S.; Pinault, S.; Fournier, G. The response to long-term overfeeding in identical twins. N. Engl. J. Med. 322:1477-1482; 1990.
17. Bouchard, C.; Tremblay, A.; Nadeau, A.; Dussault, J.; Després, J.P.; Thériault, G.; Lupien, P.J.; Serresse, O.; Boulay, M.R. Long-term exercise-training with constant energy intake. 1: Effect on body composition and selected metabolic variables. Int. J. Obes. 14:57-73; 1990.
18. Brun, L.D.; Gagné, C.; Julien, P.; Tremblay, A.; Moorjani, S.; Bouchard, C.; Lupien, P.J. Familial lipoprotein lipase-activity deficiency: Study of total body fatness and subcutaneous fat tissue distribution. Metabolism. 38:1005-1009; 1989.
19. Cianflone, K.; Sniderman, A.D.; Walsh, M.J.; Vu, H.; Gagnon, J.; Rodriguez, M.A. Purification and characterization of acylation stimulating protein. J. Biol. Chem. 263:426-430; 1989.
20. Costill, D.L.; Bowers, R.; Kammer, W.F. Skinfold estimates of body fat among marathon runners. Med. Sci. Sports. 2:93-95; 1970.
21. Costill, D.L.; Coyle, E.; Dalsky, G.; Evans, W.; Fink, W.; Hopes, D. Effects of elevated plasma FFA and insulin on muscle glycogen usage during exercise. J. Appl. Physiol. 43:695-699; 1977.
22. Crampes, F.; Beauville, M.; Rivière, D.; Garrigues, M. Effect of physical training in humans on the response of isolated fat cells to epinephrine. J. Appl. Physiol. 61:25-29; 1986.
23. Crampes, F.; Beauville, M.; Rivière, D.; Garrigues, M.; Lafontan, M. Lack of desensitization of catecholamine-induced lipolysis in fat cells from trained and sedentary women after physical exercise. J. Clin. Endocrinol. Metab. 67:1011-1017; 1988.
24. Crampes, F.; Rivière, D.; Beauville, M.; Garrigues, M. Lipolytic response of adipocytes to epinephrine in sedentary and exercise-trained subjects: Sex-related differences. Eur. J. Appl. Physiol. 59:249-255; 1989.
25. Crews, E.L., III; Fuge, K.W.; Oscai, L.B.; Holloszy, J.O.; Shank, R.E. Weight, food intake, and body composition: Effects of exercise and protein deficiency. Am. J. Physiol. 216:359-363; 1969.
26. Després, J.P. Obesity, regional adipose tissue distribution and metabolism: Effect of exercise. In: Romsos, D.R.; Himms-Hagen, J.; Suzuki, M., eds. Obesity: Dietary factors and control. Tokyo: Japan Scientific Societies Press; 1991:251-259.
27. Després, J.P.; Bouchard, C. Effects of aerobic training and heredity on body fatness and adipocyte lipolysis in humans. J. Ob. Weight Regul. 3:219-235; 1984.
28. Després, J.P.; Bouchard, C.; Savard, R.; Prud'homme, D.; Bukowiecki, L.; Thériault, G.

Adaptive changes to training in adipose tissue lipolysis are genotype dependent. Int. J. Obes. 8:87-95; 1984.

29. Després, J.P.; Bouchard, C.; Tremblay, A.; Savard, R.; Marcotte, M. Effects of aerobic training on fat distribution in male subjects. Med. Sci. Sports Exerc. 17:113-118; 1985.
30. Després, J.P.; Bouchard, C.; Savard, R.; Tremblay, A.; Marcotte, M.; Thériault, G. Effect of a 20 week endurance training program on adipose tissue morphology and lipolysis in men and women. Metabolism. 33:235-239; 1984.
31. Després, J.P.; Bouchard, C.; Savard, R.; Tremblay, A.; Marcotte, M.; Thériault, G. Level of physical fitness and adipocyte lipolysis in humans. J. Appl. Physiol. 56:1157-1161; 1984.
32. Després, J.P.; Moorjani, S.; Tremblay, A.; Poehlman, E.T.; Lupien, P.J.; Nadeau, A.; Bouchard, C. Heredity and changes in plasma lipids and lipoproteins after short-term exercise training in men. Arteriosclerosis. 8:402-409; 1988.
33. Després, J.P.; Pouliot, M.C.; Moorjani, S.; Nadeau, A.; Tremblay, A.; Lupien, P.J.; Thériault, G.; Bouchard, C. Loss of abdominal fat and metabolic response to exercise training in obese women. Am. J. Physiol. (Endocrinol. Metab.). 261:E159-E167; 1991.
34. Després, J.P.; Prud'homme, D.; Tremblay, A.; Bouchard, C. Contribution of low intensity exercise training to the treatment of abdominal obesity: Importance of "metabolic fitness." In: Guy-Grand, B.; Ricquier, D.; Lafontan, M.; Ailhaud, G., eds. Obesity in Europe 91. London: John Libbey; 1992:177-181.
35. Després, J.P.; Savard, R.; Tremblay, A.; Bouchard, C. Adipocyte diameter and lipolytic activity in marathon runners: Relationship with body fatness. Eur. J. Appl. Physiol. 51:223-230; 1983.
36. Després, J.P.; Tremblay, A.; Bouchard, C. Sex differences in the regulation of body fat mass with exercise-training. In: Björntorp, P.; Rossner, S., eds. Obesity in Europe I. London: John Libbey; 1989:297-304.
37. Després, J.P.; Tremblay, A.; Moorjani, S.; Nadeau, A.; Lupien, P.J.; Bouchard, C. Obésité abdominale et lipoprotéines: Effets de l'exercice. Sci. Sport. 6:265-273; 1991.
38. Després, J.P.; Tremblay, A.; Nadeau, A.; Bouchard, C. Physical training and changes in regional adipose tissue distribution. Acta Med. Scand. 723:205-212; 1988.
39. Eckel, R.H. Lipoprotein lipase. A multifunctional enzyme relevant to common metabolic diseases. N. Engl. J. Med. 320:1060-1068; 1989.
40. Eckel, R.H.; Yost, T.J. Weight reduction increases adipose tissue lipoprotein lipase responsiveness in obese women. J. Clin. Invest. 80:992-997; 1987.
41. Enzi, G.; Gasparo, M.; Biondetti, P.R.; Fiore, D.; Semisa, M.; Zurlo, F. Subcutaneous and visceral fat distribution according to sex, age, and overweight, evaluated by computed tomography. Am. J. Clin. Nutr. 44:739-746; 1986.
42. Epstein, L.H.; Wing, R.R. Aerobic exercise and weight. Addict. Behav. 5:371-388; 1980.
43. Fain, J.N.; Garcia-Sainz, J.A. Adrenergic regulation of adipocyte metabolism. J. Lipid Res. 24:945-986; 1983.
44. Forbes, G.B. Body composition as affected by physical activity and nutrition. Fed. Proc. 44:343-347; 1985.
45. Fried, S.K.; Kral, J.G. Sex differences in regional distribution of fat cell size and lipoprotein lipase activity in morbidly obese patients. Int. J. Obes. 11:129-140; 1987.
46. Fujioka, S.; Matsuzawa, Y.; Tokunaga, K.; Keno, Y.; Kobatake, T.; Tarui, S. Treatment of visceral fat obesity. Int. J. Obes. 15:59-65; 1991.
47. Hargreaves, M.; Kiens, B.; Richter, E.A. Effect of increased plasma free fatty acid concentrations on muscle metabolism in exercising men. J. Appl. Physiol. 70:194-201; 1991.
48. Hickson, R.C.; Rennie, M.J.; Conlee, R.K.; Winder, W.W.; Holloszy, J.O. Effects of increased plasma free fatty acids on glycogen utilization and endurance. J. Appl. Physiol. 43:829-833; 1977.
49. Hirsch, J.; Knittle, J. Cellularity of obese and nonobese human adipose tissue. Fed. Proc. 29:1516-1521; 1970.
50. Hirshman, M.F.; Wardzala, L.J.; Goodyear, L.J.; Fuller, S.P.; Horton, E.D.; Horton, E.S. Exercise training increases the number of glucose transporters in rats adipose cells. Am. J. Physiol. (Endocrinol. Metab.). 257:E520-E530; 1989.
51. Kather, H.; Schroder, F.; Simon, B. Microdetermination of glycerol using bacterial NADH-linked luciferase. Clin. Chim. Acta. 120:295-300; 1982.
52. Jansson, P.A.; Smith, U.; Lönroth, P. Interstitial glycerol concentration measured by microdialysis in two subcutaneous regions in humans. Am. J. Physiol. (Endocrinol. Metab.). 258:E918-E922; 1990.
53. Krotkiewski, M. Physical training in the prophylaxis and treatment of obesity, hypertension and diabetes. Scand. J. Rehabil. Med. [Suppl.]. 9:55-70; 1983.

54. Krotkiewski, M. Physical training in obesity with varying degree of glucose intolerance. J. Ob. Weight Regul. 4:179-209; 1985.
55. Krotkiewski, M.; Björntorp, P. Muscle tissue in obesity with different distribution of adipose tissue. Effects of physical training. Int. J. Obes. 10:331-341; 1986.
56. Krotkiewski, M.; Mandroukas, K.; Sjöström, L.; Sullivan, L.; Wetterqvist, H.; Björntorp, P. Effects of long-term physical training on body fat, metabolism, and blood pressure in obesity. Metabolism. 28:650-658; 1979.
57. Lafontan, M. Physiologie et pharmacologie de la mobilisation des lipides: Aspects actuels et futurs. Cah. Nutr. Diét. 21:19-46; 1986.
58. Lafontan, M.; Dang-Tran, L.; Berlan, M. Alpha-adrenergic antilipolytic effect of adrenaline in human fat cells of the thigh: Comparison with adrenaline responsiveness of different fat deposits. Eur. J. Clin. Invest. 9:261-266; 1979.
59. Lamarche, B.; Després, J.P.; Pouliot, M.C.; Moorjani, S.; Lupien, P.J.; Thériault, G.; Tremblay, A.; Nadeau, A.; Bouchard, C. Is body fat loss a determinant factor in the improvement of carbohydrate and lipid metabolism following aerobic exercise training in obese women. Metabolism. 41:1249-1256; 1992.
60. Leibel, R.; Edens, N.K.; Fried, S.K. Physiological basis for the control of body fat distribution in humans. Annu. Rev. Nutr. 9:417-443; 1989.
61. Lithell, H.; Hellsing, K.; Lunsqvist, G.; Malmberg, P. Lipoprotein lipase activity on human skeletal-muscle and adipose tissue after intense physical exercise. Acta Physiol. Scand. 105:312-315; 1979.
62. Marin, P.; Rebuffé-Scrive, M.; Smith, U.; Björntorp, P. Glucose uptake in human adipose tissue. Metabolism. 36:1154-1160; 1987.
63. Marniemi, J.; Peltonen, P.; Vuori, I.; Hietanen, E. Lipoprotein lipase of human postheparin plasma and adipose tissue in relation to physical training. Acta Physiol. Scand. 110:131-135; 1980.
64. Mauriège, P.; Després, J.P.; Prud'homme, D.; Pouliot, M.C.; Marcotte, M.; Tremblay, A.; Bouchard, C. Regional adipose tissue lipolysis in lean and obese men. J. Lipid Res. 32:1625-1633; 1991.
65. Mauriège, P.; Galitzky, J.; Berlan, M.; Lafontan, M. Heterogeneous distribution of beta and alpha-2 adrenoceptor binding sites in human fat cells for various deposits: Functional consequences. Eur. J. Clin. Invest. 17:156-165; 1987.
66. Molé, P.A.; Oscai, L.B.; Holloszy, J.O. Adaptation of muscle to exercise: Increase in level of palmityl CoA synthetase, carnitine palmityltransferase, and palmitylCoA dehydrogenase, and in the capacity to oxidize fatty acids. J. Clin. Invest. 50:2323-2330; 1971.
67. Nikkilä, E.A. Role of lipoprotein lipase in metabolic adaptation to exercise and training. In: Borensztajn, J., ed. Lipoprotein lipase. Chicago: Evener; 1987:187-199.
68. Nikkilä, E.A.; Taskinen, M.R.; Rehunen, S.; Harkonen, M. Lipoprotein lipase activity in adipose tissue and skeletal muscle of runners: Relation to serum lipoproteins. Metabolism. 27:1661-1671; 1970.
69. Ong, J.M.; Kern, P.A. Effect of feeding and obesity on lipoprotein lipase activity, immunoreactive protein, and messenger RNA levels in human adipose tissue. J. Clin. Invest. 84:305-311; 1989.
70. Oscai, L.B. The role of exercise in weight control. Exerc. Sport Sci. Rev. 1:103-123; 1973.
71. Oscai, L.B.; Holloszy, J.O. Effects of weight changes produced by exercise, food restriction, or overeating on body composition. J. Clin. Invest. 48:2124-2128; 1969.
72. Oscai, L.B.; Molé, P.A.; Holloszy, J.O. Effects of exercise on cardiac weight and mitochondria in male and female rats. Am. J. Physiol. 220:1944-1948; 1971.
73. Oscai, L.B.; Molé, P.A.; Krusack, L.M.; Holloszy, J.O. Detailed body composition analysis on female rats subjected to a program of swimming. J. Nutr. 103:412-418; 1973.
74. Oscai, L.B.; Palmer, W.K. Cellular control of triacylglycerol metabolism. Exerc. Sport Sci. Rev. 11:1-23; 1983.
75. Oscai, L.B.; Palmer, W.K. Discussion: Adipose tissue adaptation to exercise. In: Bouchard, C.; Shephard, R.J.; Stephens, T.; Sutton, J.R.; McPherson, B.D., eds. Exercise, fitness, and health: A consensus of current knowledge. Champaign, IL: Human Kinetics; 1990:325-330.
76. Ostman, J.; Arner, P.; Engfeldt, P.; Kager, L. Regional differences in the control of lipolysis in human adipose tissue. Metabolism. 28: 1198-1205; 1979.
77. Pacy, P.J.; Webster, J.; Garrow, J. Exercise and obesity. Sports Med. 3:89-113; 1986.
78. Paul, P.; Issekutz, B. Role of extramuscular energy sources in the metabolism of the exercising dog. J. Appl. Physiol. 22:615-622; 1967.
79. Pollock, M.L.; Miller, H.S.; Wilmore, J. Physiological characteristics of champion American track athletes 40 to 75 years of age. J. Gerontol. 29:645-649; 1974.
80. Pouliot, M.C.; Després, J.P.; Moorjani, S.; Lupien, P.J.; Tremblay, A.; Nadeau, A.; Bouchard, C. Regional variation in adipose tissue

lipoprotein lipase activity: Association with plasma high density lipoprotein levels. Eur. J. Clin. Invest. 21:398-405; 1991.

81. Rebuffé-Scrive, M.; Andersson, B.; Olbe, L.; Björntorp, P. Metabolism of adipose tissue in intraabdominal depots of nonobese men and women. Metabolism. 38:453-458; 1989.
82. Rebuffé-Scrive, M.; Andersson, B.; Olbe, L.; Björntorp, P. Metabolism of adipose tissue in intraabdominal depots in severely obese men and women. Metabolism. 39:1021-1025; 1990.
83. Rebuffé-Scrive, M.; Enk, L.; Crona, N.; Lönnroth, P.; Abrahamsson, L.; Smith, U.; Björntorp, P. Fat cell metabolism in different regions in women. Effect of menstrual cycle, pregnancy, and lactation. J. Clin. Invest. 75:1973-1976; 1985.
84. Rennie, M.J.; Winder, W.W.; Holloszy, J.O. A sparing effect of increased plasma fatty acids on muscle and liver glycogen content in exercising rat. Biochem. J. 156:647-655; 1976.
85. Richard, D.; Arnold, J.; Leblanc, J. Energy balance in exercise-trained rats acclimated at two environmental temperatures. J. Appl. Physiol. 60:1054-1059; 1986.
86. Rivière, D.; Crampes, F.; Beauville, M.; Garrigues, M. Lipolytic response of fat cells to catecholamines in sedentary and exercise-trained women. J. Appl. Physiol. 66:330-335; 1989.
87. Savard, R.; Després, J.P.; Deshaies, Y.; Marcotte, M.; Bouchard, C. Adipose tissue lipid accumulation pathways in marathon runners. Int. J. Sports Med. 6:287-291; 1985.
88. Savard, R.; Després, J.P.; Marcotte, M.; Bouchard, C. Endurance training and glucose conversion into triglycerides in human fat cells. J. Appl. Physiol. 58:230-235; 1985.
89. Savard, R.; Després, J.P.; Marcotte, M.; Thériault, G.; Tremblay, A.; Bouchard, C. Acute effects of endurance exercise on human adipose tissue metabolism. Metabolism. 36:480-485; 1987.
90. Schwartz, R.S.; Shuman, W.P.; Larson, V.; Cain, K.C.; Fellingham, G.W.; Beard, J.C.; Kahn, S.E.; Stratton, J.R.; Cerqueira, M.D.; Abrass, I.B. The effect of intensive endurance exercise training on body fat distribution in young and older men. Metabolism. 40:545-551; 1991.
91. Shepherd, R.E.; Bah, M.D. Cyclic AMP regulation of fuel metabolism during exercise: Regulation of adipose tissue lipolysis during exercise. Med. Sci. Sports Exerc. 20:531-538; 1988.
92. Smith, U.; Hammersten, J.; Björntorp, P.; Kral, J.G. Regional differences and effect of weight reduction on human fat cell metabolism. Eur. J. Clin. Invest. 9:327-332; 1979.
93. Stern, J.S.; Titchenal, C.A.; Johnson, P.R. Obesity: Does exercise make a difference? In: Berry, E.M.; Blondheim, S.H.; Eliahou, H.E.; Shafrir, E., eds. Recent advances in obesity research. London: John Libbey & Co., Ltd; 1986:352-364.
94. Taskinen, M.R.; Nikkilä, E.A.; Rehunen, S.; Gordin, A. Effect of acute vigorous exercise on lipoprotein lipase activity of adipose tissue and skeletal muscle in physically active men. Artery. 6:471-483; 1980.
95. Thompson, J.K.; Jarvie, G.J.; Lahey, B.B. Exercise and obesity: Etiology physiology and intervention. Psychol. Bull. 91:55-79; 1982.
96. Tremblay, A.; Després, J.P.; Bouchard, C. Adipose tissue characteristics of ex-obese long-distance runners. Int. J. Obes. 8:641-648; 1984.
97. Tremblay, A.; Després, J.P.; Bouchard, C. The effects of exercise-training on energy balance and adipose tissue morphology and metabolism. Sports Med. 2:223-233; 1985.
98. Tremblay, A.; Després, J.P.; Bouchard, C. Alteration in body fat and fat distribution with exercise. In: Bouchard, C.; Johnston, F.E., eds. Fat distribution during growth and later health outcomes. New York: Alan R. Liss, Inc.; 1988:297-312.
99. Tremblay, A.; Després, J.P.; Leblanc, C.; Bouchard, C. Sex dimorphism in fat loss in response to exercise-training. J. Ob. Weight Regul. 3:193-203; 1984.
100. Tremblay, A.; Després, J.P.; Leblanc, C.; Craig, C.L.; Ferris, B.; Stephens, T.; Bouchard, C. Effect of intensity of physical activity on body fatness and fat distribution. Am. J. Clin. Nutr. 51:153-157; 1990.
101. Tremblay, A.; Després, J.P.; Maheux, J.; Pouliot, M.C.; Nadeau, A.; Moorjani, S.; Lupien, P.J.; Bouchard, C. Normalization of the metabolic profile in obese women by exercise and a low fat diet. Med. Sci. Sports Exerc. 23:1326-1331; 1991.
102. Vague, J. La différenciation sexuelle, facteur déterminant des formes de l'obésité. Presse Med. 30:339-340; 1947.
103. Vague, J. The degree of masculine differentiation of obesities: A factor determining predisposition to diabetes, atherosclerosis, gout, and uric calculous disease. Am. J. Clin. Nutr. 4:20-34; 1956.
104. Vinten, J.; Galbo, H. Effect of physical training on transport and metabolism of glucose in adipocytes. Am. J. Physiol. (Endocrinol. Metab.). 244:E129-E134; 1983.
105. Vinten, J.; Petersen, L.N.; Sonne, B.; Galbo, H. Effect of physical training on glucose transporters in fat cell fractions. Biochim. Biophys. Acta. 841:223-227; 1985.

106. Wahrenberg, H.; Bolinder, J.; Arner, P. Adrenergic regulation of lipolysis in human fat cells during exercise. Eur. J. Clin. Invest. 21:534-541; 1991.

107. Wahrenberg, H.; Engfeldt, P.; Bolinder, J.; Arner, P. Acute adaptation in adrenergic control of lipolysis during physical exercise in humans. Am. J. Physiol. 253:E383-E390; 1987.

108. Walberg, J.L.; Molé, P.A.; Stern, J.S. Effect of swim training on the development of obesity in the genetically obese rat. Am. J. Physiol. 242:R204-R211; 1982.

109. Walberg, J.L.; Upton, D.; Stern, J.S. Exercise training improves insulin sensitivity in the obese Zucker rat. Metabolism. 33:1075-1079; 1984.

110. Walsh, M.J.; Sniderman, A.D.; Cianflone, K.; Vu, H.; Rodriguez, M.A.; Forse, R.A. The effect of ASP on the adipocyte of the morbidly obese. J. Surg. Res. 46:470-473; 1989.

111. Wardzala, L.J.; Crettaz, M.; Horton, E.D.; JeanRenaud, B.; Horton, E.S. Physical training of lean and genetically obese Zucker rats: Effect on fat cell metabolism. Am. J. Physiol. (Endocrinol. Metab.). 243:E418-E426; 1982.

112. Wilmore, J.H. Body composition in sport and exercise: Directions for future research. Med. Sci. Sports Exerc. 15:21-31; 1983.

113. Woo, R.; Pi-Sunyer, F.X. Effect of increased physical activity on voluntary intake in lean women. Metabolism. 34:836-841; 1985.

Chapter 23

Physical Activity and Connective Tissue

Arthur C. Vailas
James C. Vailas

The connective tissue system has a unique physiology that involves the interaction between physical and chemical stresses upon various types of connective tissue cells. There are many types of connective tissues; however, most of the discussion in this chapter will be focused on the different dense fibrous types such as cartilage, bone, skin, tendon, and ligament. Also, some discussion will include connective tissue adaptation in skeletal muscle.

Dense fibrous connective tissues are highly specialized tissues that are involved with the in vivo translation of mechanical stresses. Also, these tissues maintain the integrity and stability of joints during dynamic loading. Essentially, these tissues are constantly challenged in the living organism. The stimulus of exercise provides connective tissues with a rhythmical pattern of mechanical and chemical challenges. Therefore, various types of physical activity affect the pattern of physical and chemical stimuli and thus induce different tissue adaptations. Scientists are developing and revising theoretical models that characterize the relationships between mechanical stress history and tissue structure. This means that over some finite period of time, exercise causes connective tissue adaptations that result in changes of tissue structure and organization. These exercise-induced structural modifications have impacted on tissue biochemical and physical properties. Therefore, exercise alters the physical and chemical environment of connective tissues and creates a new set of biological parameters that are associated with homeostasis.

Connective tissue adaptations resulting from exercise can be modified further by environmental and organismic factors such as gravity, temperature, oxygen tension, barometric pressure, nutrition, age, and hormones. For example, hormone-receptor interactions can sometimes act synergistically or antagonistically to adaptations driven by mechanical stresses. Therefore, connective tissue responsiveness to physical stimuli can be modified by biological aging, endocrine changes, and other systemic factors.

A significant challenge to exercise physiologists is to develop noninvasive markers of connective tissue metabolism and other unique technologies that would monitor the connective tissue responses and adaptations to various exercise programs. These technologies would then be used to determine the efficacy of exercise prescription and provide a scientific data base for designing exercise programs. Also, these exercise programs have the potential of reducing the probability of musculoskeletal injury by enhancing tissue structure and organization. Exercise prescription can impact on the progression of musculoskeletal disorders such as osteoporosis and arthritis.

A Cellular Basis of Connective Tissue Adaptation

In the late 1800s Wolff advanced two important concepts that were fundamental to the understanding of connective tissue adaptation to mechanical stresses. These concepts are known as Wolff's law and characterize the relationships between load history and connective tissue adaptation. The first aspect of Wolff's law states a relationship between tissue size and the magnitude of force application. The second aspect relates to the direction of force application and its effect on tissue organization (123). More recently, others have demonstrated that altered dynamic load patterns induced unique changes in tissue macrostructure and regional orientation (104,124).

Exercise can potentially challenge connective tissue cells by physical and chemical pathways. There are a variety of possible cellular stimuli such as electrical (piezoelectric), mechanical (cyclic strain of cell membranes, streaming potentials, or shear stress), and/or hormones (Figure 23.1). For example, others

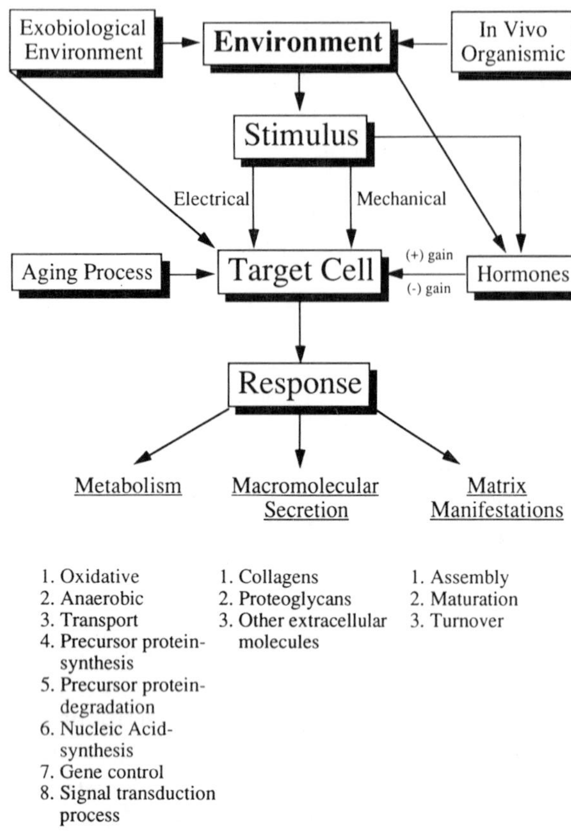

Figure 23.1 A schematic that illustrates cellular levels of regulation associated with connective tissue responses and adaptations.

have demonstrated that electric fields evoked changes in DNA synthesis, cell mitosis, collagen secretion (82), and bone remodeling (89). Because connective tissues are equilibrated in an electrolytic fluid, loading induces changes (*streaming potentials*) in tissue fluid flow, which causes movement of ions across cell surfaces and/or presents the cell with shear stresses that are proportional to the fluid flow rate (32,33). Therefore, exercise could potentially cause cyclic patterns of shear stresses, streaming potentials, or changes in tissue piezoelectric properties. Subsequently, these patterns of physiological stimuli could evoke changes in cell metabolism of second messengers (prostagland I_2 and cyclic AMP) which would affect protein turnover. There is a plethora of published data that show exercise alters connective tissue metabolism.

Some investigators believe that mechanical stresses cause a distortion of the cell membrane, thus altering cell shape (19,66,80). Distortions of the membrane would affect the flow of calcium and other cations and induce the secretion of proteinases. This would be another potential mechanism by which exercise can modulate protein turnover.

In general, exercise is known to alter the homeostasis of the endocrine system and thus change the secretion patterns of many hormones (anabolic and catabolic). Essentially, exercise is a complex stimulus that impacts on the homeostasis of connective tissues via multiple pathways of regulation (physical stress and/or chemical control). Therefore, connective tissue mass and organization are constantly being affected by exercise.

Muscle Connective Tissue Adaptations

Skeletal muscle with its tendons includes both loose connective tissue (in the intramuscular form) and dense connective tissue (in the form of its tendons). An important function of the intramuscular connective tissue is to bind the muscle cells together and ensure proper alignment (22). Also, skeletal muscle connective tissue is the structural scaffold for muscle force translation to tendon (53). An additional function of the intramuscular connective tissue network is to provide the needed lubrication between muscle fiber and muscle fiber bundle surfaces that enable the fibers to change shape (67). The extracellular matrix (ECM) is a large component of connective tissue and consists of a ground substance containing numerous proteins. One of the most important proteins in the ECM is collagen, because it provides strength and structure to the ECM.

The translation of muscular forces is facilitated by collagen (67). Collagen makes up 1% to 9% of the fat-free, dry mass of skeletal muscle (17,59). At present, there are 13 genetically different types of collagen that have been identified (16,17,64). The different collagen types are based on their supramolecular structure and can be classified as *fibrillar* and *nonfibrillar* collagens (17). Four types of collagen have been located in skeletal muscle connective tissue. Fibroblasts are the cells primarily responsible for secretion of this connective tissue protein, but myoblasts have been shown to be capable of synthesizing Types I, III, IV, and V collagen in vitro (18,87).

The intramuscular skeletal muscle connective tissue network is divided into three categories. The first is the *epimysium*, which surrounds the entire muscle and contains as its major constituent Type I collagen and Type III collagen as its minor constituent. Second is the *perimysium*, which circumscribes a bundle of muscle fibers called a *fascicle*. It also has Type I collagen as its primary component, Type III collagen as its secondary component, and Type V collagen in trace amounts. The perimysium is the structure that contains blood vessels, lymphatics, and nerves. The third is the *endomysium,* which encapsulates each individual muscle fiber. Its main collagen types are I and III, but the endomysium is also made up of Type IV (found in the basement membrane) and Type V collagens. The endomysium is the layer of connective tissue that includes the capillary supply and fibroblasts (67). Borg and Caufield (22) have shown that the endomysium is composed of myocyte-myocyte connections, myocyte-capillary connections, and a weave network linked with the basal laminae of myocytes.

Slow and fast skeletal muscles are structurally dissimilar because they have different amounts of collagen. In animal experiments with male rats aged 1 to 24 months it has been shown that "slow twitch" muscles contain a higher collagen concentration than "fast twitch" muscles (51-57). In rats, the soleus muscle contains the highest concentration of hydroxyproline (52). Slow twitch muscles have thicker perimysiums than fast twitch muscles (22,65). It has also been found that the total quantity of collagen in skeletal muscle increases with age (14,51,57). At present, there is a lack of consensus on whether collagen changes occurring with age are due to just growing old or to the decline in activity (51).

A sufficient exercise modality is required in order to produce changes in the collagen content of skeletal muscle. Endurance training on a treadmill for 3 to 7 weeks did not bring about alterations in skeletal muscle hydroxyproline concentration for 3-month-old male rats or in 1- to 6-month-old male mice (54,55,97). Also, a 3-week swimming study on adult male rats did not yield changes in the concentration of hydroxyproline in skeletal muscle (41). The work of Kovanen and colleagues (51, 54,55) has shown that 9 to 23 months of endurance training caused significant increases in the concentration of skeletal muscle hydroxyproline in 10- to 24-month-old male rats as compared to sedentary controls. Also, 45 days of treadmill endurance training did not produce any changes in hydroxyproline skeletal muscle concentration (75).

There have been few animal studies that have investigated connective tissue adaptations during skeletal muscle hypertrophy and most reported significant increases in collagen (62,63,65,92, 106,122). Tenotomy studies showed hypertrophy in 12-week-old male rats (106,122). Another study used adult fowl with a stretch-induced model of hypertrophy (65). These studies confirmed increases in collagen because of thicker perimysiums and endomysiums in the overloaded muscle as compared to the sham-operated or nonweighted muscle (65,106,122).

The regulation of procollagen (intracellular collagen) is dependent upon its synthesis and degradation. Procollagen's rate of turnover has been observed to be amplified during disease, tissue growth, and atrophy. This is independent of whether the overall collagen level increases or decreases (63,65). Both the synthesis and degradation of procollagen may be up- or down-regulated in response to exercise without a notable change in the extracellular collagen (tropocollagen). In skeletal muscle, prolylhydroxylase (PH), and galactosylhydroxylysylglucosyltransferase (GGT), intracellular biosynthetic enzymes of precursor collagen (procollagen) have their highest activity in 1-month-old male rats (52,98). PH activity in skeletal muscle has the capacity to increase with age (56,98).

It has been shown with adult male rats that 1 to 23 months of treadmill endurance training and 3 weeks of swimming endurance training can increase the activity of PH and GGT in skeletal muscle (46,47,52). With exercise-induced muscle damage seen in 4- to 6-month-old male mice after one bout of treadmill running for 9 hr, Myllyla, Salminen, Peltonen, Takala, and Vikko (75) reported that both the endurance-trained and untrained animals had an increase in PH activity of skeletal muscle. During stretch-induced hypertrophy of skeletal muscle in adult chickens there is approximately a five- to sevenfold increase in the synthesis of procollagen, a 60% decrease in the degradation of newly formed procollagen, approximately a fourfold rise in the degradation of mature tropocollagen, and an enhanced activity of PH (63,64,65). The subsequent collagen synthesis is presumably stimulated by the activation of fibroblasts (65). The tenotomy model for hypertrophy that was used with male rats also exhibited an increase in PH activity of skeletal muscle compared to the sham-operated limb (106).

At this time, few studies have examined the effect of physical training on collagen in human skeletal muscle. An aging study used 69-year-old men and women trained by walking/jogging, swimming, gymnastics, and ball games for 8 weeks. These elderly subjects showed significant improvements in $\dot{V}O_2max$ (determined indirectly by submaximal testing) from pre- to posttraining of 11% to 12%. Only the women exhibited a significant increase in their skeletal muscle PH activity from pre- to posttraining (96). A cross-sectional study of runners, cross-country skiers, and age-matched sedentary controls reported that significant increases in PH activity in the skeletal muscle of endurance athletes was 50% higher than that of sedentary controls (94–97).

The soleus muscle in rats has a higher concentration of collagen-stable cross-links than any other skeletal muscle that was measured (52). There is an increase in the cross-linking of collagen with age, and this is also true of the collagen present in skeletal muscle (52,67,121). Aging is also associated with an increase in the strength and stiffness of skeletal muscle (53). Collagen cross-linking can also be affected by exercise. It has been suggested by Kruggel and Field (58) that active muscles in cows have fewer cross-links and a higher percentage of tropocollagen than the less active muscles.

Conventional, standardized, strength training is achieved by emphasizing a small, repetitive number of maximal or near maximal contractions and attempting to overload skeletal muscle. Characteristically, the end result is an increase in both the synthesis of myofibrillar protein and the size of individual muscle fibers. An expansion of the muscle cross-sectional area is evidence of the effectiveness of the training regimen (133). It has been found by Fritz and Stauber (34) that force-induced lengthening of the soleus muscle in male rats had significant changes in the ECM as well as the myofibers. The strength training of skeletal muscle would seem to require a remodeling of the ECM in order to allow for skeletal muscle growth. In addition, this hypertrophy of skeletal muscle seems to have the ability to alter the content or the maturity of collagen (cross-linking) within the ECM surrounding muscle fibers.

In contrast, endurance training is attained by performing a large number of repetitive, moderate- to low-intensity contractions. Increases in mitochondrial volume density, oxidative enzyme activity, and capillary density are noted (42). Adaptations associated with endurance training may also include modifications in collagen content and maturity within the ECM. Since the ECM contains both the vasculature that supplies skeletal muscle as well as the collagen continuum that provides strength and structure, it would seem the intramuscular connective tissue is a site where changes could occur.

Studying the effects of strength and endurance training on skeletal muscle collagen might provide valuable insight into the mechanism of skeletal muscle hypertrophy. This information could in turn prove extremely useful when trying to minimize the atrophy of skeletal muscle, which is significantly associated with disuse of muscle (21) and with exposure to an antigravity environment such as space (70). Skeletal muscle is one of the main tissues that provides force for movement, and the knowledge gained from studying different training regimens and the plasticity of connective tissue will be important for determining whether the matrix has impacted upon muscle function and structure. There is also a definite lack of information regarding collagen changes in the skeletal muscle of humans.

Ligament and Tendon Adaptations

Ligaments and tendons have been shown to be metabolically active structures. They function like all other collagen-base structures of the body in that they respond to external stimuli. Roux hypothesized that mechanical tension stimulated proliferation of connective tissue (83). This theory was not confirmed until 1940 with animal models (93). More recent work by Vailas, Tipton, and Laughlin (109) provided more evidence that ligaments and tendons were not metabolically inert structures. They demonstrated oxygen consumption and enzymatic (cytochrome oxidase) changes to mechanical stimuli in animal models (109).

Similar to skin, bone, and muscle, ligaments and tendons are affected by many biological factors that can cause structural and chemical changes within them. In the human, movement is essential for maintaining a proper homeostasis of all connective tissue types. Many studies have shown that ligaments and tendons are altered structurally and chemically by activity, and even more so by inactivity (1,2–7,9–13,100–104,107–110,125–130, 134). The current research challenge is to quantify the tissue response at the cellular and structural level to a mechanical stress (exercise) so that a dose–response relationship can be established. The essential variables appear to be exercise history, age, and hormone interaction.

A primary focus is on collagen metabolism, because it is the basic protein for the stabilization of the musculoskeletal system. It constitutes 65% to 80% of the mass by dry weight of the tissue (10). Ligaments and tendons differ from other tissues because of the collagen type. These tissues primarily have Type I collagen, although ligaments are composed of some (9%–12%) Type III collagen. The microstructure of the collagen network, other macromolecules of the ground substance, and the cellular density of the fibroblasts are different between ligaments and tendons. Ligaments have more cells per mass than tendons (9,132).

The procollagen molecule is secreted out of the cell where peptidases convert it to tropocollagen. The molecules then configure themselves in a quarter-staggered packing arrangement and are covalently bonded by cross-links intramolecularly between the alpha chains and intermolecularly between adjacent tropocollagens (16,105). Cross-links are important to the collagen tensile strength characteristics and resistance to proteases. These cross-links result from enzyme-mediated reactions involving primarily lysine and hyroxylysine. The key enzyme in this process is lysyl oxidase, which is the rate-limiting step for collagen cross-linking. The most prevalent intermolecular cross-links in native insoluble collagen are the hydroxylysine-containing cross-links. There are different types of cross-links, reducible and nonreducible. The latter, found in mature collagen, accounts for stiffer, stronger, more stable collagen. Three types of reducible cross-links have been studied. The relative concentrations vary for different ligamentous and tendinous tissues and are usually expressed as a ratio. The conversion to a nonreducible cross-link appears to be a spontaneous, age-related process, but other factors like mechanical stress and hormones may have an effect (16,18). The amino acid residue identified with the nonreducible cross-links is *pyridinoline* (30,31,35). The concentration of cross-links and the ratio of the two types vary from species to species and tissue to tissue. For example, the rabbit anterior cruciate ligament (ACL) has 3 to 5 times more nonreducible cross-links than the patellar tendon (31).

The assembled triple helical tropocollagen molecules are known as a *collagen microfibril*. Several fibrils make a bundle, and bundles make the ligament or tendon. The ground substance and water provide the lubrication and spacing of the fibrils. These characteristics are essential for gliding and cross-tissue interactions (16,18,80). Water is 60% to 80% of total wet weight of tendon or ligament. Proteoglycans and glycoproteins that constitute the ground substance account for less than 1% of the total dry weight of the tendon and slightly more in the ligament (9,68). These proteins function to maintain the water within the tissues and are involved with intermolecular and cellular interactions (80).

The current research associated with structural and chemical adaptations to exercise was prompted by findings from immobilization studies on tendons and ligaments. Pioneering work by Akeson (2) noted a decrease in water content and ground substance with immobilization. Also, there was a significant turnover of collagen with synthesis and degradation occurring. In 1985 Akeson's most remarkable finding was the increase of the reducible collagen cross-links. Several other studies noted similar changes in the biomechanical properties. Immobilization caused a decrease in junctional strength of the tissue, small reduction in tissue mass, reduction in cross-sectional area, less organization of the collagen, and less stiffness and reduction of the gliding properties (2–6,9,60,69,76,77, 101,103,127). Another form of reduced activity, hind-limb unloading, has also induced changes in collagen structure and ground substance (107).

These structural and chemical changes from inactivity are reversible with mobilization; however, the time period is usually as long, if not longer, especially if the immobilization period is prolonged. In general, 6 weeks of immobilization will require 20 weeks or more to recover the junctional strength of the tissue that is the most affected by immobilization (103). A rabbit study by Woo and colleagues (126,127,129) showed that 1 year was required to recover the functional properties from 12 weeks of immobilization. These studies gave credance to the clinical practice of mobilizing long bone fractures after adequate internal fixation. Also, clinical emphasis is placed on immediate fixation of these fractures, because it is shown to provide quicker restoration of the soft tissue functions.

The positive effects of physical activity following immobilization prompted investigators to study the same functions in the normal tendon and ligament under exercise stress. Many studies provided the general impression that exercise did induce structural and chemical changes in ligaments and tendons. However, the pattern of changes do not mirror the changes observed with immobilization with more specific regards to onset, duration, and degree of change. Closer inspection of the data reveals conflicting findings. Some studies found an increase in strength, collagen density, and cross-sectional area (1,101,103,134). More recent studies involving nonhuman primate ligaments and swine tendons did not see significant changes in structural and mechanical properties (102,125). Close comparison of these studies indicated that some variables were different: animal species and age, tissue types and anatomy, exercise history, preexisting tissue injury, and mechanical and biochemical testing techniques (103). Most of the recent and current research focus on these variables either individually or in combination.

To illustrate the importance of tissue type and location, a study by Vailas, Zernicke, and Matsuda (111) on rat menisci showed differences in structural and chemical response of the posterior region. He noted 10% thicker menisci and higher concentrations of proteoglycans and collagen. Another study by Tipton (102) on nonhuman primates showed no change in the medial collateral ligament (MCL) with exercise, but he later states that it is probably because the animals do not stress their MCLs as much as the patellar tendon during locomotion (103). This illustrates the importance of exercise specificity and proper tissue analysis.

Research on the effects of aging and the load history of exercise includes studies involving hormonal changes. This is quite relevant because of the hormonal differences between the mature and immature animal model and the known changes of circulating hormones with exercise. Exercise intensity can cause variations in hormones, which can alter cellular metabolism of matrix substances (38). In hypophysectomized and thyroidectomized male rats, training increased the junctional strength of ligaments, but this was not seen in normal and sterilized female rats (101,103). A similar study by Vailas, Tipton, and Laughlin (109) showed a 60% reduction in enzymatic activity of a hypophysectomized rat tendon and ligament. He states that the lack of the training effect on the structural changes may be from inadequate loading of the tissues. This theory of inadequate loading was also noted in a later study by Vailas, Pedrini, and Pedrini-Mille (108). Despite the findings of increased collagen concentration with exercise (21,101), this study could not demonstrate any significant change in collagen concentration in the rat patellar tendon. Varying load history was the explanation. However, they did find an exercise effect on the glycoaminoglycans that was limited to an increase in galactosamine. This exercise effect on proteoglycans was noted in an early study with cyclic loading of fibrocytes (66).

With ongoing research the load history of exercise is becoming more relevant to the extent of the structural and biochemical adaptations to exercise. Two years of endurance training of male rats maintains and possibly slightly elevates ligament junctional strength; however, it is theorized that running on a grade intermittently or sprinting would cause further increases (103). Some studies showed that exercise caused an increase in procollagen turnover with minimal effects (39) on tropocollagen secretion. It appears that longer periods of training may be necessary, especially in the aging animal (94). Short-term, high-intensity load has minimal effects on adaptation. A recent study reported no change in enzymatic activity within a rat's Achilles tendon after a high-intensity, 3-hr bout of exercise (46). A closer look at the microstructure showed that training formed fewer cross-links (120). Prolonging the duration and increasing the intensity may lessen this effect, but this has yet to be demonstrated.

These exercise effects on the biochemical and structural elements of tendons and ligaments are of a lesser degree in the aging animal. With aging and without exercise load the properties of connective tissue will change (12,119). Amiel, Kuiper, and Wallace (12) analyzed the MCL and ACL of immature, young rabbits and mature rabbits. With age the water content and collagen concentration decreased. The young ligament had more reducible cross-links, whereas the older had an increase in the number of nonreducible cross-links. Other studies have shown that the mechanical properties of ligaments decrease in the aging animal (76,112). An explanation of this conflicting data is that the collagen bundle fragmentation as noted by Amiel et al. (12) and the alteration of the ground substance proteins with aging as noted by Vailas et al. (108) decreased the failure energy despite the ratio of nonreducible:reducible cross-links. Clinical studies have suggested that tendons are weaker in the older human, as indicated by the increased incidence of spontaneous ruptures of large tendons with age (15,43–45,50).

A recent study involving biopsies of intact tendons from fresh cadaveric individuals of different ages demonstrated an increased incidence of pathologic changes within the microstructure of the tendons. For example, the Achilles tendons of younger individuals with a mean age of 38 years had a 30% incidence of abnormal fibrils. Within older individuals with a mean age of 66 years there was a 50% incidence (45). The types of pathological changes noted included collagen fibril fragility, reduced periodicity of the fibers, vacuoules in the matrix, and tenocytes, lipid deposits, and accumulations of proteoglycans between fibrils. Amiel et al. (12) noted similar findings of lipid and "dense body" deposition and vacuole formation in the aging rabbit.

Exercise appears to have a beneficial effect on the properties of the aging tendon or ligament. A study on rats showed that exercise slowed the decline of galactosamine proteoglycans with age, however, the 28-month-old runner was similar to the 9-month-old sedentary rat (108). Furthermore, a positive response to increasing the intensity of exercise as suggested by Tipton, Vailas, and Matthes (103) showed that an increase in the grade of the running surface or intermittent sprinting will likely increase the junctional strength of male rat ligaments. A clinical study proposed that progression of pathological changes in the aging tendon may be slowed with exercise especially in the sedentary individuals (43,44). One possible cause for these changes is a decrease in arterial blood flow to the tendon rendering it relatively hypoxic. The hypoxic degeneration of tendon structure is the most common cause of spontaneous ruptures in human tendons (45).

Some concern is being raised about the effects of exercise on the immature tendon and ligament. Already in a relatively hypermetabolic state, immature connective tissue exposed to exercise seemed to cause further collagen turnover and a more disorganized collagen with more inferior mechanical properties. When the Achilles tendon of immature chickens were exposed to 8 weeks of endurance training 5 days/week, the new collagen deposition was 46% higher than matched sedentary controls (27). The mature cross-links also were reduced and the total number of reducible cross-links were decreased. Similar findings were noted in the menisci of immature chickens after 5 weeks of exercise with a change in the proteoglycan content (79). Vidiik's (116–120) findings of tissue strength correlated with the number of cross-links, suggesting that exercise-induced changes in immature tendons and ligaments may weaken the tissue and predispose it to injury. The proposed mechanisms for these changes most likely involve endocrine and mechanical stress factors during the early phase of adaptation. In the rabbit ligament model, longitudinal growth would increase with tension in the immature animal, but this could not be reproduced in the adult ligament even if growth hormone was administered (28).

These studies are limited; hence the issue of specifying load history for an immature animal and observing other, more beneficial changes has not been tested. As in clinical science, the musculoskeletal physiology of the growing athlete needs to be addressed differently than the adult. An example and a growing concern is the use of anabolic steroids in the growing athlete. These athletes have two potentially detrimental factors (anabolic steroids and excessive exercise) that can negatively affect tendon properties. Exercise and anabolic steroids have been shown to cause collagen dysplasia in the fibrils of mice (71,72) and change the crimp pattern in rat tendons (131). These factors compounded with the stress of growing are more likely to cause gross tendon dysfunction, or possibly failure, which is being observed more frequently among anabolic steroid users.

Cartilage Responses and Adaptations

Although there are many different cartilage types, most cartilages are designed to dissipate load during normal activity. In joints, load translation throughout cartilage affects chondrocyte metabolism during exercise (24,25,29,31,40,48,73,74,84,85, 113–115). For example, the rabbit studies of Saamanen, Tammi, Kiviranta, Jurvelin, and Helminen (84) showed an increase in keratan-rich proteoglycan (PG) content. Vailas and co-workers (111) also showed increases in the concentration of proteoglycans of rat menisci after 12 weeks of treadmill running. Also, they hypothesized that exercise-induced enhancement of collagen and PG concentration of menisci would lead to an increase in cartilage strength and stiffness.

Augmentation of cartilage strength and stiffness is a function of fluid flow within a large matrix of hydrophilic-aggregated macromolecules known as the *proteoglycans*, which are contained by the hydrophobic network of collagen during dynamic loading (74). The water content of articular cartilage ranges from 60% to 80% of the total tissue weight. Remaining constituents of cartilage are collagen and proteoglycans (PG). In comparison to other dense fibrous connective tissues, cartilage contains a higher concentration of PG. Loss of these large molecules by active proteases would reduce tissue stiffness (74).

Net loss of proteoglycans occurs with osteoarthritis (OA) (78). Also, cartilage undergoes degeneration during prolonged immobilization and may lead to osteoarthritis (24,78). The remobilization studies of Palmoski and Brandt (78) demonstrated that immobilization caused a significant decrease in PG synthesis and aggregation. Normal weight bearing restores the PG profile to *normal* in immobilized dogs. However, dogs that were subjected to high levels of exercise during the early stages of remobilization had a thinning of the cartilage layer with increases in degradation of newly aggregated PG (78). Therefore, exercise intensity and duration have the potential of either enhancing cartilage anabolism or resorption. Salter and Field (85,86) demonstrated that continuous passive motion of immobilized rabbit knees caused a slight repair of cartilage. He hypothesized that activity enhances the nutrient delivery to chondrocytes and stimulates the synthesis of structural macromolecules.

During growth and development PG aggregation of the meniscus is essential for structural stability (40). Therefore, the greater the level of PG aggregation with increasing collagen the more strong and stiff the cartilage (74). Pedrini-Mille, Pedrini, and Maynard (79) published results that demonstrated early aggregation of PG of *avian meniscus* in endurance-trained chickens. These studies supported the hypothesis that exercise of nominal intensity and duration augments the synthesis of matrix macromolecules and aggregation of PG. Exercise could be of clinical importance by minimizing the degeneration of cartilage in patients that have osteoarthritis.

Proteoglycans are more easily extracted from OA specimens (88). The smaller PG molecules in OA tissue are not confined within the collagen network and diffuse into the synovial fluid during dynamic loading (88). This rationale would argue against the prescription of exercise in OA patients. However, other clinical studies such as those of Minor, Hewett, Webel, and Anderson (73) show that aquatic and aerobic walking reduce the level of joint pain and increase range of motion. Minor and colleagues' findings would support a prescription of exercise for OA patients. This area of research needs further study in order to determine whether exercise is positively efficacious for individuals suffering from osteoarthritis.

Cartilage in the joint capsule receives nourishment from a limited blood supply and synovial fluid (91). Simkin, Huang, and Benedict (90,91) reported increases in blood flow of the menisci of exercised adult dogs using a standard microsphere technique. Increases in blood flow by exercise would stimulate the cartilage repair process. Subsequently exercise would improve nutrient delivery and ensure a greater metabolic turnover.

Connective Tissue Biomarkers

The half-life of many ECM proteins is long in comparison to proteins of other tissues. For example, the estimated half-life of collagen in tendons is approximately 110 days. Also, many of these large ECM proteins have precursor forms that are compartmentalized within the cell. Subsequently, synthesis and degradation processes are confined within the intracellular domain. These precursor macromolecules are transported to the cell membrane and undergo further posttranslational modification prior to secretion. Therefore, extracellular turnover of ECM proteins is regulated by processes associated with resorption and secretion (64).

Collagen, the most abundant ECM protein in the body, is synthesized as procollagen and degraded inside the cell by specific proteases. However, some of the procollagen is exocytosed with some modifications such as cleavage by N-terminal and C-terminal peptidases, and accumulation in the ECM as tropocollagen. This highly specialized protein continues to be modified throughout its life span by altering its intra- and intermolecular cross-links. Among many functions collagen cross-linking provides strength and chemical stability (30,31). Essentially, the intracellular turnover of precursor ECM proteins is different from the extracellular turnover rate, which is often slow.

Little is known about the coregulation of (intracellular vs. extracellular) ECM proteins. However, exercise has been documented to affect the turnover of all forms of ECM proteins (29,59,99,111, 113–115). These ECM proteins have unique chemical characteristics, and scientists have been interested in identifying ECM metabolites and correlating the concentration changes with some alteration of connective tissue metabolism (26,81,99). More recently, exercise physiologists have used unique ECM metabolites in urine and plasma and correlated these changes with exercise duration and intensity (88,98).

There are few noninvasive technologies available for exercise scientists to study connective tissue responses and adaptations in man. Every noninvasive diagnostic has limitations associated with use criteria and interpretation. However, more research is needed to validate and establish applications of these technologies. Takala, Vuori, and Anttinen (98) studied ultramarathon runners and showed dramatic increases in the concentration of Type III procollagen aminopropeptide in human plasma. They also correlated these increases to an elevation in GGT in skeletal muscle of postexercise athletes. This enzyme is specific to the glycosylation of procollagen. This acute response to exercise can only be applied to the up-regulation of the precursor form.

The most promising marker for studying collagen metabolism in man is the discovery of a collagen cross-link residue in urine (81), where Robins and Duncan have isolated a compound known as *hydroxylysylpyridinoline* (HP), which is specific to Type I and II mature collagen sources. Also, the urinary HP is not a substrate of any organ system (81). The urinary excretion of HP increases with various bone diseases and in ovarianectomized rats (81). Preliminary studies from our laboratory have discovered the presence of HP in human plasma. The plasma resting levels of HP increased after 9 weeks of heavy exercise training (Figure 23.2). More studies are needed to determine the optimal conditions for measuring HP in exercising humans.

Specific noninvasive markers of connective tissue metabolism are useful in characterizing responses and adaptations to exercise. One can also use noninvasive tissue analyses by enhancing the resolution of quantitative computerized tomography (QCT), magnetic resonance imaging (MRI), dual photon absorption (DPA), and other devices of imaging connective tissue. The combination of biomarkers and imaging may provide exercise physiologists the opportunity of studying mechanisms of connective tissue adaptations in exercising humans.

Clinical Relevance of Exercise Prescription

A better understanding of the microstructural and cellular adaptations of connective tissue to exercise will help the clinician formulate better exercise programs that are more specific for the individual

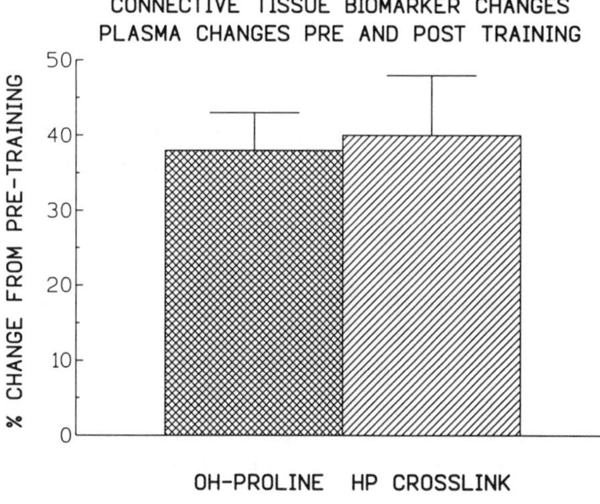

Figure 23.2 Summarized data obtained from a 9-week exercise training study of male subjects (n=10, age range 20-35 yrs.) that were subjected to an endurance exercise program of moderate to high intensity work sessions (65-75% VO_2 maximum for 20-30 minutes in duration/5 days per week). Plasma samples were taken from each subject for hydroxyproline and HP content pre- and posttraining (48 hours from the last bout of exercise). Values represent mean and standard deviations percent change from pretraining.

and the type of activity. Major considerations are age and skeletal maturity. The goal is to enhance activity performance without causing injury to the tissues (e.g., rupture), or more commonly, microstructural failure in tendons or ligaments as seen in overuse syndromes. Another goal of a proper exercise regimen is to prevent or slow the normal degenerative processes of aging such as tendon ruptures or bone osteoporosis; and in the presence of injury to the tissues, an exercise program can enhance tissue repair.

The key elements of an exercise program are the duration of the exercise and the intensity. The clinician should be cognizant of the possibility of weakening tissues by overexercising or accelerating exercise intensity, especially in the young athlete. Otherwise this may predispose the athlete to injury. Occurrence of positive adaptations of the tissues will usually require several weeks of exercise; and this period is more likely to be longer in the older individual. In order to obtain further changes beyond initial adaptations to a steady-state exercise regimen, the level of intensity should be increased gradually. However, this should not occur until the tissues have adjusted to the previous level of exercise.

To accurately determine the time to make adjustments to connective tissues may require the use of clinical markers like plasma biomarkers. If that becomes the case, then clinical studies will be needed to measure biomarker changes for different age groups and sexes to establish reference data. Eventually, with enough reproducible data, guidelines can be established to help set parameters for exercising in specific age groups and sexes without having to obtain plasma samples. The use of biomarkers, or indicators, may offer a better method of assessing adaptation or injury. Nevertheless, by the time a ligament or tendon injury manifests itself clinically, enough structural damage has probably occurred to require a significant rest period. Typically, for a partial tear of a large tendon or ligament 6 to 9 weeks of protected activities are necessary to provide good recovery. That is a substantial amount of time for an athlete, especially during an active sport season. Premorbid indicators like plasma biomarkers may be correlated to microstructural injury, which may be easier to evaluate and thus expedite injury treatment.

Magnetic resonance imaging may prove helpful, but presently it is used to confirm clinical diagnoses of more significant injuries. There is not enough clinical MRI data to quantify MRI signal changes of ligaments or tendons with actual structural damage. It will be interesting to determine whether or not the preclinical MRI changes already noted in menisci, ligaments, and tendons of the aging and athletically active population correlate with alterations of urine and plasma marker levels. Therefore, guidelines must be established for the type of sport recommended for an individual in addition to age and sex classifications.

Acknowledgments

I would like to express my gratitude for the contributions made by the following individuals; Drs. James Hodgdon and Hal Goforth, Naval Health Research Center; Dr. Judith Bautch, University of Wisconsin School of Nursing; Nancy Swan and Laura Liedtke, R.N., M.S. Work effort and publication costs were supported by Navy and NASA grants N66001-88-C0276, NAG-2568, and NCC 2-619.

References

1. Adams, A. Effect of exercise on ligament strength. Res. Q. 37:163-167; 1966.
2. Akeson, W.H. An experimental study of joint stiffness. J. Bone Joint Surg. 43A:1022-1034; 1961.

3. Akeson, W.H.; Amiel, D.; Abel, M.F. Effects of immobilization on joints. Clin. Orthop. 219:28-37; 1987.
4. Akeson, W.H.; Amiel, D.; Mechanic, G.L. Collagen cross-linking alterations in joint contractures: Changes in the reducible cross-links in periarticular connective tissue collagen after nine weeks of immobilization. Connect. Tissue Res. 5:15-19; 1977.
5. Akeson, W.H.; Frank, C.B.; Amiel, D. Ligament biology and biomechanics. In: Finnerman, G., ed. AAOS symposium on sports medicine. St. Louis: Mosby; 1985:11-15.
6. Akeson, W.H.; Woo, S.L.-Y.; Amiel, D. The connective tissue response to immobility: Biochemical changes in periarticular connective tissue of the immobilized rabbit knee. Clin. Orthop. 93:356-362; 1973.
7. Amiel, D.; Akeson, W.H.; Harwood, F.L. The effect of immobilization on the types of collagen synthesized in periarticular connective tissue. Connect. Tissue Res. 8:27-32; 1980.
8. Amiel, D.; Akeson, W.H.; Harwood, F. Stress deprivation effect on metabolic turnover of the medial collateral ligament. Clin. Orthop. Rel. Res. 172:265-270; 1982.
9. Amiel, D.; Billings, E.; Akeson, W.H. Ligament structure, chemistry, and physiology. In: Daniel, D., ed. Knee ligaments: Structure, function, injury, and repair. New York: Raven Press; 1990.
10. Amiel, D.; Billings, E.; Harwood, F.L. Collagenase activity in anterior cruciate ligament: Protective role of the synovial sheath. J. Appl. Physiol. 69:902-906; 1990.
11. Amiel, D.; Frank, C.B.; Harwood, F.L. Tendons and ligaments: A morphological and biochemical comparison. J. Orthop. Res. 1:257; 1984.
12. Amiel, D.; Kuiper, S.D.; Wallace, C.D. Age-related properties of medial collateral ligament and anterior cruciate ligament: A morphologic and collagen maturation study in the rabbit. J. Gerontol. 46:159-165; 1991.
13. Amiel, D.; Woo, S.L.-Y.; Harwood, F.L. The effect of immobilization on the collagen turnover in connective tissue: A biochemical-biomechanical correlation. Acta Orthop. Scand. 53:325-332; 1982.
14. Analaqueeb, M.; Alzaid, N.; Goldspink, G. Connective tissue changes and physical properties of developing and skeletal muscle. J. Anat. 139:677-689; 1984.
15. Arner, O.; Lindholm, A.; Orell, S.R. Histologic changes in subcutaneous rupture of the Achilles tendon. A study of 74 cases. Acta Chir. Scand. 116:484-490; 1958-1959.
16. Bailey, A.J.; Robins, S.P.; Balian, G. Biological significance of the intermolecular cross-links of collagen. Nature. 251:105; 1974.
17. Bailey, A.J.; Simms, T.J. Meat tenderness: Distribution of molecular species of collagen in bovine muscles. J. Sci. Food Agric. 28:565-570; 1977.
18. Berg, R.; Prockop, D. The thermal transition of a non-hydroxylated form of collagen: Evidence for a role for hydroxyproline in stabilizing the triple helix of collagen. Biochem. Biophys. Res. Commun. 52:115-120; 1973.
19. Binderman, I.; Shimshoni, Z.; Somjen, D. Biomechanical pathways involved in the translation of physical stimulus into biochemical message. Calcif. Tissue Int. 36:S82-S85; 1984.
20. Booth, F.; Gould, E. Effects of training and disease on connective tissue. Exerc. Sport Sci. Rev. 83:112; 1975.
21. Booth, F.W.; Gould, E.W. Effects of training and disuse on connective tissue. Exerc. Sport Sci. Rev. 3:83-107; 1975.
22. Borg, T.; Caufield, J. Morphology of connective tissue in skeletal muscle. Tissue Cell Res. 12:197-207; 1980.
23. Butler, D.L.; Grood, E.S.; Noyes, F.R. Biomechanics of ligaments and tendons. Exerc. Sport Sci. Rev. 6:125-182; 1978.
24. Caterson, B.; Lowther, D.A. Changes in the metabolism of the proteoglycans from sheep articular cartilage in response to mechanical stress. Biochem. Biophys. Acta. 540:412-422; 1978.
25. Comper, W.D.; Laurent, T.C. Physiological function of connective tissue polysaccharides. Physiol. Rev. 58:255-315; 1978.
26. Cundy, T.; Bartlett, M.; Bishop, M. Plasma hydroxyproline in uremia: Relationships with histologic and biochemical indices of bone turnover. Metab. Bone Dis. Rel. Res. 46:297-303; 1983.
27. Curwin, S.L.; Vailas, A.C.; Wood, J. Immature tendon adaptation to strenuous exercise. J. Appl. Physiol. 65:2297-2301; 1988.
28. Dahners, L.E.; Sykes, K.E.; Muller, P.R. A study of the mechanisms influencing ligament growth. J. Orthop. Rel. Res. 12:1569-1572; 1989.
29. Engstrom, A.; Hallgreen, R. Circulating hyaluronic acid varies with physical activity in health and rheumatoid arthritis. Arthritis Rheum. 30:1333-1338; 1987.
30. Eyre, D.R.; Koob, T.J.; Van Ness, K.P. Quantitation of hydroxypyridinium crosslinks in collagen by high-performance liquid chromatography. Anal. Biochem. 137:380-384; 1984.

31. Eyre, D.R.; Oguchi, H. Collagens their measurement, properties and a proposed pathway of formation. Biochem. Biophys. Res. Commun. 92:403-407; 1980.
32. Frangos, J.A.; Eskin, S.G.; McIntire, I.V. Flow effects on prostacyclin production by human endothelial cells. Science. 227:1477-1479; 1985.
33. Frangos, J.A.; McIntire, L.V.; Eskin, S.G. Shear stress induced stimulation of mammalian cell metabolism. Biotech. and Bioeng. 32:1053-1060; 1988.
34. Fritz, V.; Stauber, W. Characterization of muscles injured by forced lengthening. Med. Sci. Sports Exerc. 20:354-361; 1988.
35. Fujimoto, D.; Moriguchi, T. Pyridinoline, a non-reducible crosslink of collagen. J. Biochem. 83:863-868; 1978.
36. Gosh, P.; Southerland, J.; Bellenger, C. The influence of weight bearing exercise on articular cartilage of meniscetomized joints. J. Orthop. Rel. Res. 252:101-113; 1990.
37. Harper, J.; Amiel, D.; Harper, E. Collagenase production by rabbit ligaments and tendon. Connect. Tissue Res. 17:253-259; 1988.
38. Harvey, S.; Klandorf, H.; Foltzer, C. Endocrine responses of ducks (Anas platyrhynchos) to treadmill exercise. Gen. Comp. Endocrinol. 48:415-420; 1982.
39. Heikkinen, E.; Vuori, I. Effect of physical activity on the metabolism of collagen in aged mice. Acta Physiol. Scand. 84:543-549; 1972.
40. Heinegard, D.; Inerot, S.; Olsson, S.E.; Saxne, T. Cartilage proteoglycans in degenerative joint disease. J. Rheumatol. 14:110-112; 1987.
41. Hitchcock, T.F.; Light, T.R.; Bunch, W.H. The effect of immediate constrained digital motion on the strength of flexor tendon repairs in chickens. J. Hand Surg. 12A:590-595; 1987.
42. Holloszy, J.O. Adaptation of skeletal muscle to endurance training. Med. Sci. Sports Exerc. 7:155-164; 1975.
43. Jozsa, L.; Kvist, M.; Balint, J.B. The role of recreational sport activity in Achilles tendon rupture. A clinical pathoanatomical and sociological study of 292 cases. Am. J. Sports Med. 17:338-343; 1989.
44. Jozsa, L.; Reffy, A.; Balint, J.B. The pathogenesis of tendolipomatosis: An electron microscopical study. Int. Orthop. 7:251-255; 1984.
45. Kannus, P., Jozsa, L. Histopathological changes preceding spontaneous rupture of a tendon. J. Bone Joint Surg. 73:1507-1525; 1991.
46. Karpakka, J.; Vaananen, K.; Orava, S.; Takala, T. The effects of pre-immobilization, training and immobilization on collagen synthesis in rat skeletal muscle. Int. J. Sports Med. 11:484-488; 1990.
47. Karpakka, J.; Vaananen, K.; Virtanen, P. The effects of remobilization and exercise on collagen biosynthesis in rat tendon. Acta Physiol. Scand. 139:139-145; 1990.
48. Kiviranta, I.; Tammi, M.; Jurvelin, J.; Saamanen, A.; Helminen, H.J. Moderate running exercise augments glycosaminoglycan and thickness of articular cartilage in the knee joint of young beagle dogs. J. Orthop. Res. 6:188-195; 1988.
49. Klein, L.; Dawson, M.H.; Heiple, K. Turnover of collagen in the adult rat after denervation. J. Bone Joint Surg. 59A:1065-1067; 1977.
50. Konn, G.; Everth, H.J. Morphologie der spontanen sehnenzerreissungen. Hefte Unfall. 91:255-262; 1967.
51. Kovanen, V. Effects of aging and physical training on rat skeletal muscle. Acta Physiol. Scand. S577:1-56; 1989.
52. Kovanen, V.; Palokangas, H.; Suominen, H. Hydroxypridinium crosslinks and prolyl-4 hydroxylase in eight different skeletal muscles of 26-30 month-old wistar rats. Med. Sci. Sports Exerc. 23:S122; 1991.
53. Kovanen, V.; Suominen, H. Effects of age and life long endurance training on the passive mechanical properties of rat skeletal muscle. Compr. Gerontol. A. 2:18-23; 1988.
54. Kovanen, V.; Suominen, H. Age and training-related changes in the metabolism of rat skeletal muscle. Eur. J. Appl. Physiol. 58:765-771; 1989.
55. Kovanen, V.; Suominen, H.; Heikkinen, E. Mechanical properties of fast and slow muscle in rats: Effects of endurance training. Acta Physiol. Scand. 108:173-180; 1980.
56. Kovanen, V.; Suominen, H.; Heikkinen, E. Collagen of slow twitch and fast twitch muscle fibers in different types of rat-skeletal muscle. Eur. J. Appl. Physiol. 52:235-242; 1984.
57. Kovanen, V.; Suominen, H.; Peltonen, L. Effects of aging and life long physical training on collagen in slow and fast skeletal muscle in rats. Cell Tissue Res. 248:247-255; 1987.
58. Kruggel, W.; Field, R. Crosslinking of collagen in active and quiescent bovine muscle. Growth. 38:495-499; 1974.
59. Larizza, D.; Lorini, R.; Franchini, M. Urinary hydroxylysine and hydroxylysyl glycosides excretion in patients with Turner's syndrome. Horm. Metab. Res. 17:432-433; 1985.
60. Laros, G.S.; Tipton, C.M.; Cooper, R.R. Influence of physical activity on ligament insertions. J. Bone Joint Surg. 53A:275-286; 1971.
61. Laseter, J.T.; Russell, J.A. Anabolic steroid-induced tendon pathology: A review of the literature. Med. Sci. Sports Exerc. 23:1-3; 1991.

62. Laurent, G. Rates of collagen synthesis in lung, skin, and muscle obtained in cows by a simplified method using 3H-proline. Biochem. J. 206:535-544; 1982.
63. Laurent, G. Dynamic state of collagen: Pathways of collagen degradation in cows and their possible role in regulation of collagen mass. Am. J. Physiol. 252:C1-C9; 1987.
64. Laurent, G.; McNulty, R.; Gibson, J. Changes in collagen synthesis and degradation during skeletal muscle growth. Am. J. Physiol. 249:C352-C355; 1985.
65. Laurent, G.; Sparrow, M.; Bates, P. Collagen content and turnover in heart and skeletal muscles of the adult fowl and the changes during stretch-induced growth. Biochem. J. 176:419-427; 1978.
66. Leung, D.Y.; Glagon, S.; Mathews, M.B. Cyclic stretching stimulates synthesis of matrix components by arterial smooth muscle in vitro. Science. 191:475-477; 1975.
67. Light, N.; Champion, A. Characterization of muscle epimysium, perimysium and endomysium collagens. Biochem. J. 219:1017-1026; 1984.
68. Lindahl, U.; Hook, M. Glycosaminoglycan and their binding to biological macromolecules. Annu. Rev. Biochem. 47:385-417; 1978.
69. Loitz, B.J.; Zernicke, R.F.; Vailas, A.C. Effects of short-term immobilization versus continuous passive motion on the biomechanical and biochemical properties of the rabbit tendon. Clin. Orthop. Rel. Res. 244:265-271; 1989.
70. Martin, T. Protein and collagen content of rat muscle following space flight. Cell Tissue Res. 254:251-253; 1988.
71. Michna, H. Organization of collagen fibrils in tendon: Changes induced by an anabolic steroid. II. A morphometric and stereologic analysis. Virchows Arch. [B] 52:87-89; 1986.
72. Michna, H. Tendon injuries induced by exercise and anabolic steroids in experimental mice. Int. Orthop. 11:157-162; 1987.
73. Minor, M.A.; Hewett, J.E.; Webel, R.R.; Anderson, S.K. Efficacy of physical conditioning exercise in patients with rheumatoid arthritis and osteoarthritis. Arthritis Rheum. 32:1396-1405; 1989.
74. Mow, V.C.; Holmes, M.H.; Lai, W.M. Fluid transport and mechanical properties of articular cartilage: A review. J. Biomed. 17:377-394; 1984.
75. Myllya, R.; Salminen, A.; Peltonen, L.; Takala, T.; Vihko, V. Collagen metabolism of mouse skeletal muscle during repair of exercise injuries. Pflugers Arch. 407:64-70; 1986.
76. Noyes, F.R.; Grood, E.S. The strength of the anterior cruciate ligament in humans and Rhesus monkeys. J. Bone Joint Surg. 58A: 1074-1082; 1976.
77. Noyes, F.R.; Torvik, P.J.; Hyde, W.B. Biomechanics of ligament failure. J. Bone Joint Surg. 56A:1406-1418; 1974.
78. Palmoski, M.J.; Brandt, K.D. Running inhibits the reversal of atrophic changes in canine knee cartilage after removal of a leg cast. Arthritis Rheum. 24:1329-1337; 1981.
79. Pedrini-Mille, A.; Pedrini, V.A.; Maynard, J.A. Response of immature chicken meniscus to strenuous exercise: Biochemical studies. J. Orthop. Res. 6:196-204; 1988.
80. Pitaru, S.; Aubin, J.E.; Bhargava, U. Immunoelectron microscopic studies on the distributions of fibronectin and actin in a cellular dense connective tissue: The periodontal ligament of the rat. J. Periodont. Res. 22:64-74; 1987.
81. Robins, S.P.; Duncan, A. Pyridinium crosslinks of bone collagen and their locating in peptides isolated from rat femur. Biochem. Biophys. Acta. 914:233-239; 1987.
82. Rodan, G.A.; Bourreet, L.A.; Norton, L.A. DNA synthesis in cartilage cells is stimulated by oscillating electric fields. Science. 199:690-692; 1978.
83. Roux, W. Gesammelte abhandlunger uber entwicklungsmechanik der organism. Leipzig: Engelmann; 1:458-460; 1985.
84. Saamanen, A.; Tammi, M.; Kiviranta, I.; Jurvelin, J.; Helminen, H. Levels of chondroitin-6-sulphate and non-aggregating proteoglycans at articular cartilage contact sites in the knees of young dogs subjected to moderate running exercise. Arthritis Rheum. 32:1282-1292; 1989.
85. Salter, R.B. The biologic concept of continuous passive motion of synovial joints. Clinical Orthop. Rel. Res. 242:12-25; 1989.
86. Salter, R.B.; Field, P. The effects of continuous compression on living articular cartilage. J. Bone Joint Surg. 42A:31-49; 1960.
87. Sasse, J.H.; Vonder Mark, H.; Kuhl, U. Origin of collagen types I, III, and V in cultures of avian skeletal muscle. Dev. Biol. 83:79-89; 1981.
88. Saxane, T.; Heinegard, P.; Wollheim, F.A. Therapeutic effects on cartilage metabolism in arthritis as measured by release of proteoglycan structures into the synovial fluid. Ann. Rheum. Dis. 45:491-497; 1986.
89. Shamos, M.H. Piezoelectric effect in bone. Nature. 197:81-83; 1963.

90. Simkin, P.A. Joints: Structure and function. In: Schumacher, R., ed. Primer on the rheumatic diseases, 9th ed. New York: Raven Press; 1988:27-42.
91. Simkin, P.A.; Huang, A.; Benedict, R.S. Effects of exercise on blood flow to canine articular tissues. J. Orthop. Res. 8:297-303; 1990.
92. Sparrow, M. Regression of skeletal muscle of chicken wing after stretch-induced hypertrophy. Am. J. Physiol. 242:C333-C338; 1982.
93. Stearns, M.L. Studies on the development of connective tissue in transparent chambers in rabbit's ear: II. Am. J. Anat. 67:55-97; 1940.
94. Suominen, H.; Heikkinen, E. Enzyme activities in muscle and connective tissue of M. vastus lateralis in habitually-trained and sedentary 33-to-77-year-old men. Eur. J. Appl. Physiol. 34:249-254;1975.
95. Suominen, H.; Heikkinen, E. Enzyme activities in muscle and connective tissue of M. vastus lateralis in habitually training and sedentary 33 to 70 year old men. Eur. J. Appl. Physiol. 34:249-254; 1975.
96. Suominen, H.; Heikkinen, E.; Parkatti, T. Effects of eight weeks physical training on muscle and connective tissue of the M. vastus lateralis in 69-year old men and women. J. Gerontol. 32:33-37; 1977.
97. Suominen H.; Kiiskinen, A.; Heikkinen, E. Effects of physical training on metabolism of connective tissue on young mice. Acta Physiol. Scand. 108:17-22; 1980.
98. Takala, T.; Vuori, J.; Anttinen, H. Prolonged exercise causes an increase in the activity of galactosylhrdroxylysylglucosyltransferase and in the concentration of type III procollagen aminopropeptide in human serum. Pflugers Arch. 407:500-503; 1986.
99. Thonar, E.J.; Schnitzer, T.J.; Kuettner, K.E. Quantification of keratin sulfate in blood as a marker of cartilage metabolism. J. Rheumatol. 14:23-24; 1987.
100. Tipton, C.M.; James, S.L.; Mergner, W. Influence of exercise on strength of medial collateral knee ligaments of dogs. Am. J. Physiol. 218:894-901; 1970.
101. Tipton, C.M.; Matthes, R.D.; Maynard, J.A. The influence of physical activity on ligaments and tendons. Med. Sci. Sports. 7:165-175; 1975.
102. Tipton, C.M.; Matthes, R.D.; Vailas, A.C. The response of the Galago senegalensis to physical training. Comp. Biochem. Physiol. 63A:29-36; 1979.
103. Tipton, C.M.; Vailas, A.C.; Matthes, R.D. Experimental studies on the influences of physical activity on ligaments, tendons, and joints: A brief review. Acta Med. Scand. [Suppl.]. 711:157-168; 1986.
104. Tozeren, A.; Skalak, R. Interaction of stress and growth in a fibrous tissue. J. Theor. Biol. 130:337-350; 1988.
105. Traub, W.; Piez, K.A. The chemistry and structure of collagen. Adv. Protein Chem. 25:243-248; 1971.
106. Turto, H.; Linday, S.; Halme, J. Protocollagen proline hydroxylase activity in work induced hypertrophy of rat muscle. Am. J. Physiol. 226:63-65; 1974.
107. Vailas, A.C.; Deluna, D.M.; Lewis, L.L. Adaptation of bone and tendon to prolonged hindlimb suspension in rats. J. Appl. Physiol. 65:373-376; 1988.
108. Vailas, A.C.; Pedrini, V.A.; Pedrini-Mille, A. Patellar tendon matrix changes associated with aging and voluntary exercise. J. Appl. Physiol. 58:1572-1576; 1985.
109. Vailas, A.C.; Tipton, C.M.; Laughlin, H.L. The influence of physical activity and hypophysectomy on aerobic capacity of ligaments and tendons. J. Appl. Physiol. 44:542-546; 1978.
110. Vailas, A.C.; Tipton, C.M.; Matthes, R.D. Physical activity and its influence on the repair process of medial collateral ligaments. Connect. Tissue Res. 9:25-31; 1981.
111. Vailas, A.C.; Zernicke, R.F.; Matsuda, S. Adaptation of rat knee meniscus to prolonged exercise. J. Appl. Physiol. 60:1031-1034; 1986.
112. Vasseur, P.B.; Pool, R.R.; Arnoczky, S.P. Correlative biomechanical and histologic study of the cranial cruciate ligament in dogs. Am. J. Vet. Res. 46:1842-1854; 1985.
113. Videman, T.; Eronen, I. Effects of treadmill running on glycosaminoglycans in articular cartilage of rabbits. Int. J. Sports Med. 5:320-324; 1984.
114. Videman, T.; Eronen, I.; Friman, C. Glycosaminoglycan metabolism of the medial meniscus, the medial collateral ligament and the hip joint capsule in experimental osteoarthritis caused by immobilization of the rabbit knee. Acta Orthop. Scand. 50:465-470; 1979.
115. Videman, T.; Nichelsson, J.-E.; Langenskiold, A. The development of radiographic changes in experimental osteoarthritis provoked by immobilization of the knee in rabbits. Int. Res. Comm. Syst. Med. Sci. 5:62-68; 1977.
116. Viidik, A. The effect of training on the tensile strength of isolated rabbit tendons. Scand. J. Plast. Reconstr. Surg. Hand Surg. 1:141-147; 1967.
117. Viidik, A. On the correlation between structure and mechanical function of soft connective tissues. Verh. Anat. Ges. 72:75-89; 1978.

118. Viidik, A. Connective tissues-possible implications of the temporal changes for the aging process. Mech. Ageing Dev. 9:267-285; 1979.
119. Viidik, A. Age-related changes in connective tissue. In: Viidik, A., ed. Lectures on gerontology. Part A. London: Academic Press; 1982:173-207.
120. Viidik, A. Adaptability of connective tissue. In: Saltin, B., ed. Biochemistry of exercise VI. Champaign, IL: Human Kinetics; 16:545-562; 1986.
121. Vogel, H. Correlation between tensile strength and collagen content in rat skin: Effect of age and cortisol treatment. Connect. Tissue Res. 2:177-182; 1974.
122. Williams, P.; Goldspink, G. Connective tissue changes in surgically over loaded muscle. Cell Tissue Res. 221:465-470; 1981.
123. Wolff, J. Das gesetz der transformation der knochen. Berlin: A. Hirschwald; 1892.
124. Wong, M.; Carter, D.R. Theoretical stress analysis of organ culture osteogenesis. Bone. 11:127-131; 1990.
125. Woo, S.L.-Y.; Gomez, M.A.; Amiel, D. The effect of exercise on the biochemical and biomechanical properties of swine digital flexor tendons. J. Biomech. Eng. Trans. ASME. 103:51-56; 1981.
126. Woo, S.L.-Y.; Gomez, T.J.; Sites, P.O. The biomechanical and morphological changes in the medial collateral ligament of the rabbit following immobilization and remobilization. J. Bone Joint Surg. 69A:1200-1211; 1987.
127. Woo, S.L.-Y.; Inone, M.; McGurk-Burleson, E. Treatment of the medial collateral ligament injury: II. Structure and function of canine knees in response to differing treatment regimes. Am. J. Sports Med. 15:22-29; 1987.
128. Woo, S.L.-Y.; Kuei, S.C.; Gomez, M.A. The effect of immobilization and exercise on the strength characteristics of bone-medial collateral ligament-bone complex. Am. Soc. Mech. Eng. Symp. 32:67-70; 1979.
129. Woo, S.L.-Y.; Maynard, J.; Butler, D. Ligament, tendon, and joint capsule: Insertions to bone. In: Woo, S.L.-Y.; Buckwalter, J.A., eds. Injury and repair of the musculoskeletal soft tissues. Park Ridge, IL: American Academy of Orthopaedic Surgeons; 1988:133-166.
130. Woo, S.L.-Y.; Ritter, M.A.; Amiel, D. The biomechanical and biochemical properties of swine tendons: Long-term effects of exercise on the digital extensors. Connect. Tissue Res. 7:177-183; 1980.
131. Wood, T.O.; Cooke, P.H.; Goodship, A.E. The effect of exercise and anabolic steroids on the mechanical properties and crimp morphology of the rat tendon. Am. J. Sports Med. 16:153-158; 1988.
132. Yahia, L.H.; Drouin, G. Microscopic investigation of canine anterior cruciate ligament and patellar tendon: Collagen fascicle morphology and architecture. J. Orthop. Res. 7:243-251; 1989.
133. Young, A.; Stokes, M.; Round, J.; Edwards, R. The effect of light resistance training on the strength and cross sectional area of the human quadriceps. Eur. J. Clin. Invest. 13:411-417; 1983.
134. Zuckerman, J.; Stull, G.A. Effect of exercise on knee ligaments separation force in rats. J. Appl. Physiol. 26:716-720; 1969.

Chapter 24

Physical Activity and Digestive Processes

Frank M. Moses

Gastrointestinal (GI) symptoms are a common source of disability to athletes, particularly those involved in endurance sport. The interaction between physical activity and digestive processes is complex and yet our knowledge is immature. This complexity is due in part to the wide regions encompassed by digestive processes in health and disease: (a) the hollow GI organs from the esophagus to the colon, and (b) the liver, biliary system, and pancreas.

Prior to the last decade scant attention was paid to exercise-associated digestive processes either in health or disease. General statements were expressed that mild exercise improved digestion but that vigorous effort retarded it (1). Literature primarily descriptive in nature has accumulated during the past decade that has paralleled the public's interest in recreational and competitive sports. Much of it suffers from key limitations. Exercise physiologists have previously expressed little interest in GI function and were untrained in appropriate investigative techniques. Similarly, gastrointestinal physiologists were accustomed to evaluating the GI tract at rest, and stressed (if at all) by disease or drugs. The diagnostic instrumentation is designed to function at rest and is not easily converted for use during exercise. The published studies lack standardized or controlled exercise regimens. The use of experimental techniques, although frequently ingenious, are often not validated for the exercising subject.

We lack the fundamental knowledge for much of the basic GI physiology associated with exercise. Individuals fast except for rehydration fluids during most athletic events. However, prolonged events such as the ultramarathon and long-distance triathlons require a functioning GI tract to sustain energy requirements. It has been shown by a variety of methods that blood flow is diverted to exercising muscle groups and away from the visceral system (2,3). GI hormonal changes are known to occur with exercise (4,5,6,7) and could affect motility, absorption, and other functions. Mechanical effects may alter GI function as well.

Reviews of this topic have been published within the past several years (8,9,10,11). This paper will review published literature, concentrating in the past decade, on digestive symptoms associated with exercise, the interaction of digestive organs with exercise, and exercise-associated GI bleeding. Discussion of absorption and metabolism of carbohydrates, proteins, and lipids will be reviewed elsewhere.

Gastrointestinal Symptoms and Physical Activity

Abdominal pain and discomfort, nausea and vomiting, diarrhea, and more severe problems such as gastrointestinal bleeding are commonly seen in athletes. These symptoms infrequently cause severe disability but some are a source of great discomfort and may limit athletic performance. After setting a world record in the marathon, Derek Clayton said, "Two hours later, the elation had worn off. I was urinating quite large clots of blood, and I was vomiting black mucus and had black diarrhea. I don't think too many people can understand what I went through for the next 48 hours" (12). This section will review early reports and surveys of GI symptoms associated with exercise. Publications that deal with more specific symptoms such as diarrhea or GI bleeding will be reviewed in the designated sections.

Reports and Surveys

Publications were uncommon prior to the public's explosive interest and participation in distance running. Beaumont observed the permanent gastric fistula of Alexis St. Martin and noted the differences between moderate and strenuous exercise after meals and seemed aware that fatiguing exercise retarded digestion (13). In the early part of this century the effects of exercise on gastric secretion and digestion were evaluated. It was concluded that exercise that produced no discomfort helped the digestion and that which caused discomfort delayed digestion (1).

The recent literature boom began with *athlete's diarrhea* in two schoolboys during football, a runner with watery diarrhea during long runs, and other members of a runners' club (14). Other reports described a distance runner with abdominal pain and diarrhea; a medical student with bloody diarrhea and pain following hard runs (15); and a runner who suffered abdominal pain and bloody diarrhea who had pale, edematous bowel with small bleeding points on the right colon at laparotomy for suspected appendicitis. A diagnosis of Crohn's disease was made but not confirmed by biopsy. Competitive running was resumed after 3 months without further symptoms (16). Ischemia was the presumed etiology.

The findings of the first survey detailing GI symptoms in a recreational runners' club (17) are summarized in Table 24.1. These studies demonstrate a high prevalence of GI symptoms associated with exercise such as heartburn, abdominal cramps, the urge to have a bowel movement, and a loss of appetite. A larger survey of marathoners found that nearly half occasionally had loose stools and 13% had three or more bowel movements per day (generally considered beyond the clinical norm). The urge to defecate was the most common symptom experienced by runners. Heartburn occurred in up to 9.5% and was prominent during running. Nausea and vomiting were more common with hard runs. Women suffered from GI symptoms more frequently than men. A small percentage reported bloody bowel movements with running (18). Symptoms such as stomachache and intestinal cramps were also substantially greater with the marathon than the shorter race and in those runners who lost greater than 4% body weight or drank the least fluid during the race (19). A similar pattern with predominantly lower GI symptoms, which are more notable in faster runners, has also been reported (20). Multisport competitors experience similar symptoms, though they may suffer more upper abdominal symptoms during competition than runners (21,22,23,24). These surveys were based on large sample populations, which may dilute the inherent reporting bias. Many symptoms are characteristic of the *irritable bowel syndrome* and the surveys were not controlled with a nonrunning group (25). These criticisms are common to all the surveys reviewed.

GI symptoms, particularly those of nausea, vomiting, and abdominal pain, may be manifestations of dehydration, electrolyte disturbances, or hyperthermia and should be treated in an appropriate clinical setting (26,27,28). Some common symptoms such as the *side stitch* are not frequently discussed. Literature on common GI disturbances is summarized in Table 24.1 and is difficult to review and compare. Weaknesses inherent in this type of survey include selection and questionnaire bias and lack of an adequate control group. Several surveys recorded data as *negative* (never/rarely) or *positive* (occasional/frequent). No survey used a linear scale for symptoms.

Some Conclusions Concerning Gastrointestinal Symptoms and Physical Activity

The data summarized in Table 24.1 suggest that GI symptoms are common with exercise. Lower GI symptoms, particularly the urge to defecate, are most common; bowel movements and even diarrhea are frequent and may interrupt runs and affect performance. Bleeding is reported by a small segment of the population. All GI symptoms, particularly lower GI symptoms, are more frequent in women and perhaps younger men and may be proportional to athletic effort. Upper GI symptoms are less prominent but may be more frequent in multisport events such as the triathlon.

The Effects of Physical Activity on the Esophagus

Esophageal disorders manifest as chest pain or heartburn and are pathophysiologically due to gastroesophageal reflux, esophageal dysmotility, or *esophageal angina*. Chest pain, when it occurs in association with exertion, mandates an evaluation for cardiac cause prior to specific investigation of esophageal disease. A review of noncardiac chest pain is too extensive; this section will review specific changes in esophageal function with exercise.

Esophageal Motility

Esophageal motility changes probably occur with exercise. Current diagnostic manometry instrumentation is designed to be used at rest and is unable to filter artifact from movement and increased breathing; however, developing solid-state technology may supersede this difficulty.

Lower esophageal sphincter (LES) pressure increased from 24 to 32 mmHg after a treadmill run and then returned to 27 mmHg at recovery, yet no change was seen in peristaltic amplitude or

Table 24.1 Studies of Gastrointestinal Symptoms Associated With Exercise

Reference	Subjects	Number/total	% Male	Controlled	Method
Sullivan (17)	Running club	57/NS	70	No	Quest
Keeffe et al. (18)	Marathoners	707/1,700	86	No	Quest
Rehrer[e] et al. (19)	25-km racers, marathoners	44/114	73	No	Quest
Halvorsen et al. (20)	Marathoners	279/10%	82	No	Quest
Worobetz[d] and Gerrard (21)	Enduro athletes	70/119	87	No	Quest
Sullivan (22)	Triathletes	110/NS	NS	No	Quest
Worme et al. (23)	Triathletes	64/450	70	No	Quest
Priebe and Priebe (152)	Runners	425/NS	NS	No	Quest
Riddoch and Trinick (153)	Marathoners	471/1,750	92	No	Quest

Reference	Loss of appetite	Heartburn	Chest pain	Belch	Nausea	Vomiting
Sullivan (17)	50[a]	10			6	
Keeffe et al. (18)		9.5[a]			11.6[a]	1.8[a]
Rehrer et al. (26)					11/11[e]	
Halvorsen et al. (20)			16/1[f]		6/5	
Worobetz and Gerrard (21)	11/30[d]	0/11	3/23	7/29	1/20	0/20
Sullivan (22)		24			24	
Worme et al. (23)	12	8	12		6	2
Priebe and Priebe (152)						
Riddoch and Trinick (153)	28[a]				20	4[a]

Reference	Abdominal cramps	Urge to defecate	Defecate with exercise	Diarrhea	Rectal bleeding
Sullivan (17)	25[a]	30			
Keeffe et al. (18)	19.3[a]	36–38	16	10–19	1.2–2.4
Rehrer et al. (26)	0/18[e]	2/25[g]	16/23[h]	0/0	
Halvorsen et al. (20)	19/3			15/6	0/3
Worobetz and Gerrard (21)	3/39	20/34	11/33	6/20	
Sullivan (22)	35		49		
Worme et al. (23)	5	< 5		18	
Priebe and Priebe (152)	67[b]	63[b]	51[b]	30[c]	12
Riddoch and Trinick (153)	31	42		27	

Note. NS = not stated, Quest = questionnaire.

[a]hard run. [b]percentage of 82 subjects with diarrhea. [c]percentage of overall subjects. [d]often/occasionally. [e]with 25 km race/with marathon. [f]abdominal gas. [g]stomachache. [h]sideache.

duration (29). In another study, LES pressure decreased after stationary cycling, abnormal secondary and tertiary contraction appeared, and contraction velocity increased (30). Using solid-state manometry Soffer noted decreases in duration, amplitude, and frequency of esophageal contractions with increasing exercise intensities (31).

Gastroesophageal Reflux

Heartburn is relatively common, and ambulatory esophageal pH monitoring has demonstrated that gastroesophageal reflux (GER) occurs more frequently with exercise, particularly running. GER was more prominent in patients with angina pectoris and low LES pressure while undergoing treadmill testing than in similar patients with normal LES pressures. This suggested that exertional GER accounted for exercise-related chest discomfort in some patients (32). Johnston, O'Connor, Kennon, and Crowe (33) suggested that exercise, by provoking GER in susceptible patients, could be used as an adjunctive test in the diagnosis of GER. However, GER may be provoked in normal subjects who exercise. Furthermore, the nature of the exercise may be important in determining the amount of GER (34). This group then expanded on their observation by performing ambulatory pH monitoring at rest during a 1-hr near-maximal run with and without ranitidine (35). The number of reflux episodes and the acid exposure time increased with running. Most reflux events were associated with belching. Ranitidine decreased the acid exposure time. Antacid and Gaviscon[R] also reduced esophageal acid exposure with running (36). Exercise may also induce GER in children (37). GER is increased with postprandial running (38).

Some Conclusions Concerning Physical Activity and the Esophagus

The clinical relevance of these changes is uncertain and mechanisms are speculative. Hyperventilation and stress can alter esophageal motility. GER may induce reflex changes in pulmonary airway resistance and coronary blood flow (39). While esophageal symptoms are frequent, they are usually not severe. Treatment is usually accomplished with dietary changes, fasting before runs, and occasionally medical therapy with antacids or histamine H-2 antagonists. Kraus, Sinclair, and Castell (35) speculated that chronic exercise-induced GER could lead to esophagitis, but this has not been demonstrated.

The Effects of Physical Activity on the Stomach

Exercise may produce abnormalities of gastric emptying (GE) with nausea, bloating, or vomiting, or changes in acid secretion with mucosal damage and ulceration. Drugs used to alleviate musculoskeletal discomfort may also affect function and mucous damage. Nausea and vomiting occur after racing (40) or during competition (41). GE appears to be a limiting factor in the athlete's ability to hydrate and maintain nutrition requirements during competition, and therefore much work has been undertaken to maximize GE with exercise.

Gastric Emptying

Analysis of GE may be performed by multiple modalities, each with relative strengths and weaknesses that should be recalled during review. Aspiration of gastric residual is minimally invasive and depends upon placement of a tube to remove all fluid. The act of removing the fluid and to some extent the tube itself affect GE. There is a certain variation in results (42), and this method has difficulty accounting for secretion. Dye dilution methods are also tube-dependent but are better able to account for secretion. Radionuclide methods have the advantage of being "tubeless" but are cumbersome unless exercise is stopped while the image is processed. Newer scintigraphy studies demonstrate that cameras are necessary anterior and posterior. This positioning was not done in some older studies. There is a small amount of radiation exposure. Other methods, such as applied potential tomography and ultrasound, have limited availability or reproducibility, may not correlate well with other data, and have been infrequently studied.

The major factors controlling GE are meal characteristics. Liquid emptying differs from solid. Calories and fat progressively delay GE. Temperature, osmolality, and volume also affect emptying (43,44). Comparing different exercise protocols and different meals is difficult. The athlete's hydration and body temperature status may also affect GE (26). Exercising in warm environments has been shown to inhibit GE during exercise (45). Other factors such as sex, menstrual cycle, smoking, and time of day when the study is conducted affect GE (46).

Liquid GE has been investigated more thoroughly (see Table 24.2). Several studies showed little change in water or glucose solutions GE at about 70% of $\dot{V}O_2$max and accelerated GE with light to moderate exercise (47,48,49). It is theorized

Table 24.2 Gastric Emptying (GE) Studies

Reference	Subject	Randomized, blinded	Controlled	GE method
Rehrer et al. (26)	16 male runners	NR	Own vs. rest	Aspiration, 2-sampled
Mitchell and Voss (44)	8 cyclists, competitive	Randomized, not blinded	Own	Aspiration at end
Neufer et al. (48)	10 physically fit males	Randomized, not blinded	Own vs. rest	Aspiration with dye
Marzio et al. (49)	9 male, 8 female nonrunners	Randomized, not blinded	Own vs. rest	Ultrasound and scintigraphy
van den Broek-Evans et al. (50)	8 volunteers	NS	Own vs. rest	Applied potential tomography
Houmard et al. (52)	10 male triathletes	NR	Own vs. rest	Aspiration at end, dye-dilution
Rehrer et al. (154)	9 male triathletes	Randomized and blinded crossover	Own	Aspiration, 2-sampled
Mitchell et al. (157)	10 cyclists, competitive	NR	Own vs. rest	Aspiration at end
Ryan et al. (155)	8 cyclists, trained	Randomized, blinded	Own	Aspiration at end
Soles and Noakes (156)	7 endurance-trained athletes	NR	Own	Aspiration

Reference	Meal	Exercise condition	Result	Conclusion
Neufer et al. (48)	400 ml water	Rest, walk at 28%, 41%, 56%; run at 57%, 65%, 75% $\dot{V}O_2max$	GRV: rest = 181 ml walk = 122 ml/115 ml/ 152 ml run = 99 ml/ 115 ml/160 ml	GE increased with all but run at 75%
Marzio et al. (49)	500 ml mineral water postrun	TM run, 30 min at 50%, 70% MHR	R 50% 70% US 18 9 35′ ST 15 7 30′	GE increases mild and decreases severe exercise
van den Broek-Evans et al. (50)	500 ml, 0.1–0.8 M glucose and 4 sport drink	cycle ergometer at 80% MHR	GE t1/2 exercise > rest	Strenuous exercise delays GE
Houmard et al. (52)	10 ml/kg/hr water, 7% CHO	Rest, run, cycle, 1 hr at 75% $\dot{V}O_2max$	GE rate rest/water > others same	GE run and cycle are equal
Mitchell et al. (157)	150 ml every 15 min, 0%, 6%, 12%, 18% CHO	Rest, 120 min cycle ergometer	GE volume: 1,210 ml/ 1,186 ml/1,049 ml/ 889 ml	Exercise had no effect, only concent
Mitchell and Voss (44)	11, 17, 23 ml/kg/hr, 7.5% CHO	2-hr cycle at 70% $\dot{V}O_2max$	fluid emptied 11 17 23 ml 1.4 1.9 2.3 L	Volume influences GE
Rehrer et al. (26)	8 ml/kg isotonic CHO	Dehydrated and hydrated rest vs. 2-hr, 60% $\dot{V}O_2max^{TM}$ run	GE less when dehydrated and exercise, others NC	Dehydration effects GE and ?sxs

(continued)

Table 24.2 *(continued)*

Reference	Meal	Exercise condition	Result	Conclusion
Rehrer et al. (154)	2 "sport" drinks, isotonic vs. hypertonic	rest vs. 70% $\dot{V}O_2$max run, bike	GE less with hypertonic late in exercise	GE run and cycle are equal
Ryan et al. (155)	350 ml/20 min water, 5% G, 5% GP, 5% GF	3-hr cycle, at 60% $\dot{V}O_2$max in heat	GRV: > 90% empty	Exercise had no effect
Soles and Noakes (156)	7 CHO solution	1.75-hr run at 75% $\dot{V}O_2$max vs. rest	GRV at 30 min: water: exercise < rest 10% GP:NC	Exercise had no effect GE of 10% GP

Note. NS = not stated; NR = not recorded; $\dot{V}O_2$max = maximum oxygen consumption per minute; GRV = gastric residual volume; GE = gastric emptying; TM = treadmill; MHR = maximum heart rate; R = rest; US = ultrasound; ST = scintigraphy; M = molar; GE t1/2 = gastric emptying half-life; CHO = carbohydrate drink; concent = concentration; G = glucose; GP = glucose polymer; GF = glucose plus fructose; NC = no change.

that increased intra-abdominal pressures accelerate emptying. However, others have shown emptying of various glucose solutions and sports drinks is prolonged on a bicycle ergometer (50,51). Most other protocols have found that moderate exercise intensity has little significant effect on GE of water, glucose, or electrolyte solutions (8,10). Surveys have noted that runners are more troubled by gastric symptoms than bicyclists and most other athletes. However, this is not confirmed by all (52).

GE of solids is more complex (53), and exercise might be expected to affect this differently. Accelerated GE of a mixed solid meal with mild exercise on a bicycle ergometer and treadmill walking was noted using scintigraphy (54,55). Another scintigraphy study of a mixed solid meal compared trained distance runners at rest and with a 90-min run with sedentary controls at rest. They found that the runners had significantly accelerated basal GE when compared to controls but that exercise had no effect on their GE (46).

Gastric Secretion

Gastric secretion is probably also affected by exercise. However, the clinical importance is uncertain and it has received relatively little attention. Gastric acid secretion was relatively unchanged in five healthy controls who exercised 45 min on a bicycle at 50% or 70% $\dot{V}O_2$max (56). Others have reported a decrease in basal or meal-stimulated gastric acid secretion with cycling and after exercise (57,58,59). The effect of exercise in duodenal ulcer patients has been contradictory, suggesting increased acid secretion with exercise (60) and improved ulcer healing with exercise (61). The relationship between blood flow and gastric acid secretion is complex and has been reviewed elsewhere (62).

Therapy

Treatment for disorders of GE are primarily preventive. Athletes should avoid fluids and foods in the diet known to adversely effect emptying. The athlete should consume fluid early and often enough to avoid dehydration and hyperthermia. Medications are probably of limited value, although a recent abstract suggested that diocathedral smectite alleviated gastric symptoms in triathletes (63).

Some Conclusions Concerning Physical Activity and the Stomach

Abnormalities of GE and perhaps gastric acid secretion are responsible for at least some of the upper GI (UGI) symptoms that trouble runners and other endurance athletes. GE of liquids is probably unchanged or even accelerated at exercise below 70% $\dot{V}O_2$max. The data for GE of solids is less clear but suggestive of similar changes. GE at levels of exercise above 70% $\dot{V}O_2$max is certainly delayed. Recent reviews have been published (8,10,53,64).

The effects on gastric acid secretion are less clear and the clinical relevance is uncertain. Gastric hypersecretion, if it occurs, is relatively easy to control medically.

The Effects of Physical Activity on the Small Intestine

Exercise-associated small bowel dysfunction may be responsible for *runner's diarrhea,* abdominal bloating, and pain. Physiologic changes could include accelerated or slowed transit time, alterations in permeability, and absorption and secretion of water, electrolytes, and other nutrients. Runners may also be exposed to more calories and fiber, medications, drugs, and infections that could all affect intestinal physiology.

Transit

Small bowel transit may be studied with several different methods. Scintigraphy of nuclear-labeled substances is somewhat cumbersome. Frequent scanning intervals are necessary and can interfere with exercise protocols. A standard, noninvasive and widely used method is the oral–cecal transit time (OCTT) determined by having the subject ingest an incompletely absorbed carbohydrate that is metabolized by cecal bacteria to gaseous hydrogen, absorbed into the blood, exhaled via the lungs, and sampled. However, not all people exhale detectable hydrogen, and methane-producing status is seldom recorded (65). Pulmonary hydrogen excretion is diluted by hyperventilation of exercise, making determination of transit more difficult. While OCTT does correlate with other measures of transit (66,67) reproducibility may be a problem, and there is wide intersubject variability (68).

Ollerenshaw, Norman, Wilson, and Hardy (69) used scintigraphy of labeled resin beads to determine transit with minimal, moderate, and strenuous exercise and concluded that transit was unaffected by daily activity.

Others have used the OCTT to determine transit with exercise and the results have been conflicting (see Table 24.3). OCTT with a solid meal and moderate cycling was nearly 5 hr and unchanged (54). Keeling, Harris, and Martin (70,71) used a novel rebreathing system to surmount the problem of dilution of pulmonary hydrogen excretion with exercise. However, exercise intensity was low and this technique does not allow comparison of the GE component to overall OCTT. This low level of effort has been associated with acceleration of liquid GE. The study by Meshkinpour, Kemp, and Fairshter (72) did not control for menstrual cycle (73) and did not account for hyperventilation-induced breath hydrogen changes. Using more intense 2 hr treadmill running, we found OCTT delayed when compared to standing rest when using a water or glucose polymer meal (74). The mechanism by which change, if any, in small bowel transit occurs is uncertain. GI motility has been felt to influence OCTT results (75). Exercise influences duodenojejunal motor activity and the effect appears to be intensity-dependent (76,77). Hormonal changes occur with exercise but may not correlate with transit (71). Hyperthermia, postulated to influence transit, did not produce an effect when tested (78). As an adaptation to exercise, hyperphagia may alter OCTT (79).

Absorption and Permeability

Small bowel absorption of water, electrolytes, and nutrients may be affected by exercise, mediated perhaps by altered motility, decreased blood flow, or neurohormonal changes. Williams, Mager, and Jacobson (80) found absorption of 3-o-methyl glucose decreased and postulated an abnormality in active but not passive carbohydrate absorption with exercise. Fordtran and Bengt (47), using a triple lumen perfusion technique, found no effect on the absorption rate of water, electrolytes, glucose, xylose, or urea. Another study found no significant change in serum triglyceride concentrations with exercise (56). Isaacs found the small bowel effluent of five marathoning ileostomates compensated supernormally for exercise-induced dehydration and suggested runner's diarrhea was of colonic origin (81). Although it would appear to be an excellent model, no other exercise studies have been done with ileostomates.

The effect of moderate exercise on jejunal absorption was examined in five women and two men using a triple lumen perfusion technique (82). Water and electrolyte absorption was markedly depressed during exercise. Glucose, present in previous test solutions and exercise drinks, was not used in this test solution. In another study the rate of ^{2}H appearance in the plasma was greater at rest than exercise at low, mid, or high intensity (83), and the results were unchanged when corrected for plasma volume. It would appear unlikely that the small change in intestinal transit noted in these studies could exceed the normal absorptive ability (84). A study of carbohydrate absorption with exercise has only been presented in abstract form, and results are inconclusive (85).

Intestinal permeability might be affected by exercise. Urinary PEG-400 excretion increased with exercise in one study indicating a relative increase in permeability with exercise (86). The clinical significance is uncertain but could lead to increased antigen presentation to the gut immune system and contribute to some digestive symptoms and exercise-induced anaphylaxis.

Some Conclusions Concerning Physical Activity and the Small Intestine

Alterations in small intestinal physiology probably occur with exercise, but they are less defined and

Table 24.3 Effects of Exercise on Small Bowel Transit

Reference	Subject	Control	Meal	Exercise
Cammack et al. (54)	1 male, 6 female volunteers	Own R, not B	Solid, 630 kcal, 405 g, no marker	Cycle 60 min at 33 rmp; HR 117
Ollerenshaw et al. (69)	9 male volunteers	Own R, not B	Water, lunch, Nuc-tagged capsules	Varied min-hard up to 5 hr HR to 160
Keeling and Martin (70)	12 male volunteers	Own R, not B	Liquid, 360 kcal, 350 ml lactulose 30 g	TMW 120 min at 5.6 km/hr; HR 109
Meshkinpour et al. (72)	7 male, 14 female volunteers	Own R, not B	Water, 150 ml, lactulose 10 g	TMW 60 min at 4.5 km/hr; HR 106
Moses et al. (74)	10 male volunteers	Own R, not B	1) Water 2) GP polymer lactulose 15 g	TM run 2 hr at 65% $\dot{V}O_2max$
Soffer et al. (77)	8 trained cyclists	Owen R, not B	860-kcal meal, lactulose 10 g	Cycle 20 min at 80% $\dot{V}O_2max$

Reference	Method	Symptoms	Results	Conclude
Cammack et al. (54)	BH_2, each 10 min	NR	~300 min No change	No effect on OCTT
Ollerenshaw et al. (69)	Scint	NR	4.1–5.4 hr No change	No effect on transit
Keeling and Martin (70)	BH_2, each 10 min modified	NR	Rest 66 min Exercise 44 min	Exercise decreases OCTT
Meshkinpour et al. (72)	BH_2, each 10 min	NR	Rest 55 min Exercise 89 min	Exercise increases OCTT
Moses et al. (74)	BH_2, each 10 min	NR	Water GP; Rest 68′ 81; Exercise 102 123	Exercise increases OCTT
Soffer et al. (77)	BH_2, each 10 min	NR	Rest 152 min Exercise 159 min	No effect on transit

R = randomized, B = blinded; kcal = kilocalorie; g = gram; rpm = revolutions per minute; HR = heart rate; ml = milliliter; TMW = treadmill walk; km/hr = kilometer per hour; GP = glucose polymer; $\dot{V}O_2max$ = maximum oxygen consumption per minute; BH_2 = breath hydrogen technique; NR = not recorded; OCTT = oral-cecal transit time; Scint = nuclear scintigraphy.

the clinical significance is uncertain. Low-intensity exercise may modestly accelerate small bowel transit, although the effect may be secondary to GE changes alone and is unlikely to be of clinical significance. Small bowel transit with more intense exercise such as seen in competitive athletics may be delayed but has not been well studied. There may be changes in intestinal absorption as well. However, absorption of electrolytes and water is unchanged when glucose is included. Absorption of more complex materials such as carbohydrates, proteins, and fats with exercise is essentially unknown. Intestinal permeability may increase with exercise.

The Effects of Physical Activity on the Colon

The lower GI symptoms of the urge to defecate, defecation with running, abdominal cramping, and diarrhea are the most frequently noted. A recent survey of a running club disclosed "nervous" diarrhea (43%), defecation with running (62%), diarrhea during racing (often with severe cramps, nausea, and vomiting) (47%), rectal bleeding (16%), and fecal incontinence (12%) (87). These symptoms are probably secondary to exercise effects on the colon; they occur even when fasting and are associated with colonic bleeding.

Method

Colonic physiologic changes with exercise are difficult to evaluate. Transit and motility measurements can require radiation exposure or placement of catheters directly into the colon necessitating cleansing and invasive instrumentation. Furthermore, colonic transit, which encompasses 90% of whole gut transit time, is measured in hours to days and inter- and intrasubject variation is extreme. Multiple environmental stresses can affect colonic symptoms. Endoscopic evaluation of the colon is also more difficult. Evaluation has thus lagged behind that of the esophagus and stomach. Several authors, however, have evaluated the effects of exercise on the colon.

Transit and Motility

Using the *carmine dye estimation*, total GI transit time was measured at the start and again following 6 weeks of training in two groups of volunteers (88). Exercise group transit time decreased from 35 to 24 hr while the control remained at 45 hr. This technique estimates transit but is not adequate for further detail.

In a more controlled setting of a metabolic laboratory during a 9-week training period where diet was rigidly controlled, no change was found in fecal transit time as measured by radioisotope markers, fecal weight, fecal solids or pH, ammonia, or nitrogen (89). However, the training regimen was moderate, the subjects remained asymptomatic and inter- and intrasubject variation was high. Lampe, Slavin, and Apple (90) found no significant change in four groups of women of varying degrees of athletic activity. Marathon racing resulted in a 21% increase in transit time, a 27% decrease in daily stool weight, and a 21% decrease in stool frequency.

In a crossover trial where the subjects either exercised (about 50% of $\dot{V}O_2max$) on a treadmill, on a bicycle ergometer, or rested for 1 hr daily for 1 week, transit (measured by single-dose, radioopaque markers) decreased from 51.2 hr (rest) to 36.6 hr (cycling) and 34 hr (jogging). Stool weight and frequency did not change and no one developed diarrhea with running (91).

In an attempt to determine the mechanism of these changes Dapoigny and Sarna (92) implanted strain gauge transducers in dogs and found that exercise decreased the frequency of migrating motor complexes (MMC) in the fasted state but postprandially disrupted MMCs and increased total duration of contractions. Exercise also induced giant migrating contractions (GMC), defecation, and mass movements. They suggested that the effect of exercise might be to increase fecal mixing and exposure to the colonic mucosa and that runner's diarrhea might be from excessive numbers of GMC in the distal colon.

Therapy

Colonic symptoms may be treated in a variety of ways. "Nervous" prerace diarrhea is generally self-limited and may respond to low-residue diets. Others have used antidiarrheal medications prophylactically. Ultramarathoners report that it is feasible to "train the gut" by reducing exercise duration and intensity to subsymptomatic levels and gradually increase the exercise. Preevent cathartics should be avoided. Severe race-associated diarrhea may respond to reduction in effort.

Some Conclusions Concerning Physical Activity and the Colon

These studies are interesting but do not address the symptoms of severe watery diarrhea runners suffer at extreme exertion, which require intensive investigation of symptomatic runners. Multiple authors have suggested that mild exercise could be beneficial in treating constipated patients but this has yet to be clinically tested. Finally, colonic damage may be produced by medications such as nonsteroidal antiinflammatory drugs (NSAID) occasionally ingested in large quantities to treat musculoskeletal complaints (93). A review of colonic motility has recently been published (94).

The Effects of Physical Activity on the Liver, Biliary System, and Pancreas

The liver, biliary system, and pancreas are rarely a source of clinical problems with exercise. The majority of older literature deals with exercise in the setting of acute hepatitis or other liver diseases. This has been reviewed elsewhere (11). This section will review the usual clinical presentations and interactions of these organ systems with exercise.

Literature Review: Liver

Physically active individuals are most commonly suspected of liver disorders because of incidentally noted abnormal enzymes including bilirubin, aspartate aminotransferase (AST), alanine aminotransferase (ALT), and alkaline phosphatase. They are not uncommon in long-distance runners and may mimic the patterns seen in myocardial infarction or chronic hepatitis (95,96,97,98,99). The abnormalities are usually due to damaged muscle tissue, and liver disease is found coincidentally. Hepatic damage may occur as part of the spectrum of shock, heat, and rhabdomyolysis secondary to prolonged endurance events; however this is rare. Ritland, Foss, and Gjone (100) have suggested that chronic endurance activities are associated with liver hypertrophy, as an adaptation to increased metabolism.

Evaluation of hepatic biosynthetic functions is more difficult and has been performed infrequently in this setting. Galactose elimination capacity, a standard metabolic function, indocyanine green clearance (ICG)—an index of hepatic blood flow, and aminopyrine (AP) metabolism for assessment of hepatic drug metabolism were compared in eight long-distance runners and sedentary medical students (101). No differences were noted between the two groups at rest, and it was concluded that chronic endurance activity had no effect. AP and antipyrine clearance were subsequently evaluated before and after 3 months of aerobic training (102). While $\dot{V}O_2max$ increased 6%, antipyrine and AP clearance increased 12% and 13% respectively, suggesting changes in hepatic drug metabolism with conditioning. Antipyrine clearance was significantly higher in competitive runners than controls, suggesting that alterations in metabolic capability exist with chronic exercise (103).

Hepatic blood flow, as a component of the visceral system, decreases with exercise. Rowell, Blackmon, and Bruce (104) used ICG clearance in 10 men at rest and during severe exertion and found decreases of up to 80% of estimated hepatic blood flow that varied inversely with relative oxygen uptake. Others have used sorbitol clearance and demonstrated decreases with exercise (105). Portal blood flow by Doppler ultrasound is reduced in both normal subjects and patients with cirrhosis, whether they are resting in supine or upright position or are exercising (106).

Caffeine is metabolized by an enzyme system linked to cytochrome P450 in the liver. Exercise increased plasma caffeine concentrations and accelerated the excretion rate of caffeine, and it was postulated that exercise potentiated the cytochrome enzyme system (107). Several animal experiments suggest that exercise may have other effects on hepatic function such as decrease in hepatic glutathione (108), attenuation of alcohol (109), and carbon tetrachloride toxicity (110).

Literature Review: Biliary System and Pancreas

Very little evaluation of changes in the biliary tree or pancreas with exercise has been published. There is some evidence that exercise alters the lithogenicity of bile and reduces the incidence of cholesterol gallstones (111). A letter suggested that *runner's hemolysis* might be associated with pigment gallstones (112). I am unaware of any significant literature of the human exocrine pancreas with exercise.

Some Conclusions Concerning Physical Activity and the Liver

Liver-associated enzyme abnormalities may occur with prolonged strenuous exercise. They do not usually lead to hepatic damage. Exercise does cause a reduction in liver blood flow. Chronic exercise may cause some alterations in hepatic biosynthetic capacity.

Exercise and GI Bleeding

Clinical Manifestations

Gastrointestinal bleeding may be present as: (a) acute upper tract GI bleeding, (b) acute lower tract GI bleeding, or (c) chronic bleeding and incidentally noted stool guaiac tests. Anemia found in runners is frequently multifactorial. *Runner's anemia* may be an artifact caused by plasma volume expansion. It may also be due to blood loss from intravascular hemolysis, hematuria, increased iron loss in the sweat, decreased dietary iron intake or absorption, or GI bleeding. The relative importance of these different factors is difficult to determine. However, GI bleeding has the greatest potential for blood loss.

The incidence of the problem is difficult to ascertain. Examples of acute upper or lower GI bleeding are probably rare and have been published only as isolated case reports or small series. Anemia or iron deficiency is also uncommon but not rare, particularly in women athletes where it may occur in up to one third of the athletes (113,114).

Cases and Surveys

GI bleeding associated with exercise was initially reported in 1980 when a medical student developed recurrent hematochezia after strenuous running (15). The following year two cases of rectal bleeding following running were presented. A presumptive diagnosis of acute appendicitis manifest by abdominal pain in one led to exploratory surgery. The operative findings were consistent with ischemia (16). One presumed cause of death in a survey of joggers was GI hemorrhage (115).

Stimulated by these cases, several groups attempted to determine the incidence of GI bleeding in runners by surveys or prospective evaluations of stool guaiac. The first found 3 of 39 converted to hemoccult (HO) positive following a marathon (116). A survey by Keeffe, Lowe, Goss, and Wayne (18) found a 1.2% to 1.8% incidence of postrace hematochezia (18). Other surveys have shown HO positive rates of 8% to 85% following competitive races (117,118,119,120). Stewart et al. (121) used the Hemoquant[R] assay to demonstrate increases in fecal blood loss in a variety of runners. In addition, they noted a temporal profile of bleeding peaking 24 to 48 hr following the event. This has subsequently been confirmed with ultramarathon racers (122). Bleeding may be proportional to athletic intensity, as was originally suggested by McMahon, Ryan, Larsen, and Fisher (119). Several publications have shown that GI bleeding is more prominent following competition than practice (123,124, 125). The majority of 100-mile ultramarathon runners will become HO positive following races (126). Lampe et al. (90) found increased fecal hemoglobin after a marathon in 5 of 15 women. The effect with running was highly variable and iron status did not correlate with bleeding.

Source of Bleeding

Most cases of GI bleeding associated with running have no locatable source when investigated. Damage to digestive organs from the esophagus to the rectum could be responsible in the individual case. However, several characteristic lesions have been observed.

The stomach has been the most frequently reported location of GI bleeding associated with exercise. The usual lesion is transient hemorrhagic gastritis (HG) spontaneously resolving within 72 hr (127,128,129,130). Cooper, Douglas, Firth, Hannagan, and Chadwick (131) presented a young woman with HG that was endoscopically demonstrated to recur with running and resolved it with either rest or treatment with cimetidine while she continued to run. Gaudin, Zerath, and Guezennec (132) showed histologic changes of submucous hemorrhage and edema in the gastric antrum immediately following running even in the absence of obvious endoscopic damage. A 14-year-old runner with iron deficiency anemia, found to have chronic gastritis when biopsied despite normal endoscopic appearance (133), responded to histamine receptor antagonist therapy and iron supplementation.

Endoscopic surveys of runners have been inadequate to determine the prevalence of gastric mucous lesions associated with exercise. The only published, prospective endoscopic trial to date studied 7 of 9 runners who converted to HO positive following a marathon (134). Unfortunately, only 3 were studied within 48 hr. Two had oozing antral erosions and one had hyperemia and erosion of the splenic flexure. The other examinations 4 to 30 days following the race were unrevealing. The mechanism by which HG develops is also uncertain. Most frequently ischemia has been proposed as the etiology. Experimentally, hemorrhagic shock induces gastric mucosal damage that is mediated, at least in part, by gastric lumenal acid and may be prevented by acid neutralization (135,136).

Prospective trials using cimetidine to prevent GI bleeding in runners have not been conclusive. In an initial trial cimetidine was found to reduce the percentage of HO-positive conversion following an ultramarathon from 85% to 12.5% (126). Subsequent double-blinded trials using similar-dosage cimetidine suggested a reduction in bleeding by either HO or Hemoquant[R] assays following marathon and ultramarathon distance races. However, the trials were not statistically significant (122).

The second most common location of GI bleeding has been the colon. The initial case of exercise-associated GI bleeding was from the colon (15). Several cases were subsequently described of presumed ischemic colitis following strenuous running or other athletic events. A 33-year-old runner developed three episodes of hematochezia following marathon running, and a colonoscopy discovered a small cecal lesion suggesting ischemia (137). Another runner developed hematochezia following a 10-km run at high altitude and was found to have HG, rhabdomyolysis, hematuria, and hemorrhagic colitis (138,139). We described an additional runner who developed bloody diarrhea and abdominal pain following an 8-mile run. Colonoscopy disclosed hemorrhagic colitis of the cecum and ascending colon only (140). Interestingly ischemic colitis may develop after only moderate levels of exertion such as cycling 33 km at a nonstrenuous pace (141). A recent case of ischemic colitis was confirmed operatively (142). A 42-year-old woman developed bloody diarrhea, vomiting, and progressive abdominal pain 3 days after completing a half-marathon in the heat. At laparotomy bloody ascites and an inflamed transverse and right colon were found and a subtotal colectomy performed. Histology demonstrated ischemic colitis.

The etiology of the hemorrhagic colitis is felt by most authors to be ischemia. The proximal colon has been felt to be susceptible to shock-induced ischemia in individuals without underlying vascular lesions (143). Lesions may also develop in the classic "watershed" regions of the splenic flexure and sigmoid colon. NSAIDs, although inconsistently associated with GI blood loss in runners, may contribute to colitis as well. The *cecal slap syndrome* was originally described in a middle-aged runner who developed diarrhea and right lower quadrant pain several days following a marathon, however the syndrome was subsequently ascribed to NSAID use (144,145). Runners may be susceptible to cecal volvulus, which could also cause bleeding and abdominal pain (146).

No instances of esophagitis or esophageal ulcer causing bleeding have been observed to date. Similarly, whereas ischemia has classically been described to affect the small intestine, no cases of hemorrhage or infarction of the small bowel have been reported. Anorectal disorders such as hemorrhoids and fissures are common and may cause bleeding in some runners and bicyclists, although the incidence is unknown. It is probably secondary to local trauma and may be aggravated by sports and altered bowel habits of the athletes.

Etiologies

Exercise induces certain characteristic changes in the GI tract. Prominent among these is the dramatic decrease in blood flow. Investigators using a variety of experimental techniques have demonstrated that visceral blood flow falls to 20% to 50% of baseline values (2,3,147). These values rival those of shock and may last for prolonged periods. Ischemia is felt to be the etiology in the development of exercise-induced hemorrhagic gastritis and colitis. Animal experiments evaluating this mechanism have not been performed.

Digestion of food increases the demand for visceral blood flow. During prolonged endurance events in which the athlete must eat to maintain hydration and energy levels, increased demand may conflict with the decrement in blood flow caused by exercise. This may explain why the majority of ultramarathon runners convert to HO positive (122). Certain individual runners are more susceptible to GI symptoms and bleeding. It has been postulated that these individuals have "design or developmental flaws" in their vascular supply that heighten their response to exercise. This theory, however, has not been investigated. Ultramarathon runners report that eating during training runs is necessary and allows them to compete with fewer symptoms—as if they were training their GI tract.

Trauma may cause bleeding in the GI tract. Running, and to a lesser extent, bicycling and swimming, causes marked pressure changes within the abdomen (148). The diaphragm descends vigorously during high-intensity exercise and could injure the gastric wall. Portions of the colon are free to move within the abdominal cavity and conceivably could cause the cecal slap syndrome or be injured by psoas muscle hypertrophy (149). Trauma could contribute to anal-rectal bleeding lesions.

Medications can cause gastrointestinal mucous lesions. Athletes frequently consume large quantities of NSAID or aspirin that may cause gastric, small intestinal, or colonic inflammation or ulcers (150). The use of NSAIDs or aspirin has not correlated with HO-positive conversion in most series mentioned.

Running and participation in exercise programs is generally considered part of a healthy lifestyle. It does not confer immunity from underlying diseases that may manifest with GI bleeding. This is particularly true if the athlete is older. Standard evaluations such as a search for colon cancer should be performed on individuals at risk for these diseases or any athlete who develops recurrent GI bleeding of an uncertain etiology.

Therapy

The therapy of exercise-associated GI bleeding depends to some degree on the location and severity of the bleed. In an acute condition the athlete is treated as any patient with GI bleeding. Most cases previously cited appear to be self-limited and spontaneously resolve upon cessation of exercise. Some cases of HG may recur repeatedly in individuals. These may be treated by reducing the level of exertion below symptomatic levels and gradually increasing the intensity over time in an attempt to allow the body to make appropriate adjustments. There is now a precedent to treat recurrent HG with an H_2 receptor antagonist or, perhaps, omeprazole. Treatment for hemorrhagic colitis is uncertain. Reduction in the level of exertion and "training through" may be successful in some. This condition appears to recur less often than the gastritis. Bounous and McArdle have recommended an elemental, semihydrolyzed diet, but this has not been tested (151).

Some Conclusions Concerning Exercise and GI Bleeding

GI bleeding is associated with prolonged exercise and is most probably mediated by visceral ischemia. It may produce acute and chronic symptoms, particularly iron deficiency. HG and colitis are the most frequently recognized lesions. HG may be effectively treated with H_2 receptor antagonists but treatment of hemorrhagic colitis is less certain.

References

1. Campbell, J.M.H.; Mitchell, M.D.; Powell, A.T.W. The influence of exercise on digestion. Guy's Hosp. Rep. 78:279-293; 1928.
2. Clausen, J.P. Effective physical training on cardiovascular adjustment to exercise in man. Physiol. Rev. 57:779-815; 1977.
3. Qamar, M.; Reed, A. Effects of exercise on mesenteric blood flow in man. Gut. 28:583-587; 1987.
4. Banks, R.O.; Gallavan, R.H.; Zinner, M.J.; Bulkley, G.D.; Harper, S.L.; Granger, D.N.; Jacobson, E.D. Vasoactive agents in control of mesenteric circulation. Fed. Proc. 44:2743-2749; 1985.
5. Bunt, J.C. Hormonal alterations due to exercise. Sports Med. 3:331-345; 1986.
6. Greenberg, G.R.; Marliss, E.B.; Zinman, B. Effect of exercise on the pancreatic polypeptide response to food in man. Horm. Metab. Res. 18:194-196; 1986.
7. Sullivan, S.N.; Champion, M.C.; Christofides, N.D.; Adrian, T.E.; Bloom, S.R. GI regulatory peptide responses in long-distance runners. Phys. Sportsmed. 12:77-82; 1984.
8. Brouns, F.; Saris, W.H.M.; Rehrer, N.J. Abdominal complaints and gastrointestinal function during long-lasting exercise. Int. J. Sports Med. 8:175-189; 1987.
9. Moses, F.M. The effect of exercise on the gastrointestinal tract. Sports Med. 9:159-172; 1990.
10. Murray, R. The effects of consuming carbohydrate-electrolyte beverages on gastric emptying and fluid absorption during and following exercise. Sports Med. 4:322-351; 1987.
11. Ritland, S. Exercise and liver disease. Sports Med. 6:121-126; 1988.
12. Clayton, D. Runners World. 72; 1979.
13. Beaumont, W. Experiments and observation on the gastric juice and the physiology of digestion. (Reprinted by Andrew Combe, Edinburgh, 1838).
14. Scobie, B.A. Correspondence. N. Z. Fed. Sports Med. 6:31; 1978.
15. Fogoros, R.N. Runners trots: Gastrointestinal disturbances in runners. JAMA. 243:1743-1744; 1980.
16. Cantwell, J.D. Gastrointestinal disorders in runners. JAMA. 246:1494-1495; 1981.
17. Sullivan, S.N. The gastrointestinal symptoms of running. N. Engl. J. Med. 304:915; 1981.
18. Keeffe, E.B.; Lowe, D.K.; Goss, J.R.; Wayne, R. Gastrointestinal symptoms of marathon runners. West J. Med. 141:481-484; 1984.
19. Rehrer, N.J.; Janssen, G.M.E.; Brouns, F.; Saris, W.H.M. Fluid intake and gastrointestinal problems in runners competing in a 25-km race and a marathon. Int. J. Sports Med. 10:S22-S25; 1989.
20. Halvorsen, F.A.; Lyng, J.; Glomsaker, T.; Ritland, S. Gastrointestinal disturbances in marathon runners. Br. J. Sports Med. 24:266-268; 1990.
21. Worobetz, L.J.; Gerrard, D.F. Gastrointestinal symptoms during exercise and enduro athletes: Prevalence and speculations of the etiology. N. Z. Med. J. 98:644-646; 1985.
22. Sullivan, S.N. Exercise-associate symptoms in triathletes. Phys. Sportsmed. 15:105-110; 1987.
23. Worme, J.D.; Doubt, T.J.; Singh, A.; Ryan, C.J.; Moses, F.M.; Deuster, P.A. Dietary patterns, gastrointestinal complaints, and nutritional knowledge of recreational triathletes. Am. J. Clin. Nutr. 51:690-697; 1990.
24. Lopez, A.A.; Preziosi, J.P.; Chateau, P.; Auguste, P.; Plique, O. Digestive disorders in endurance sport competitors: Epidemiological survey covering a triathlon season. Gastroenterology. 100:A11; 1991.
25. Talley, N.J.; Zinsmeister, A.R.; Van Dyke, C.; Melton, J.L. Epidemiology of colonic symptoms and the irritable bowel syndrome. Gastroenterology. 101:927-934; 1991.
26. Rehrer, N.J.; Beckers, E.J.; Brouns, F.; Ten Hoor, F.; Saris, W.H.M. Effects of dehydration on gastric emptying and gastrointestinal distress while running. Med. Sci. Sports Exerc. 22:790-795; 1990.
27. Noakes, T.D.; Norman, R.J.; Back, R.H.; Godlonton, J.; Stenenson, K.; Pittaway, D. The incidence of hyponatremia during prolonged ultraendurance exercise. Med. Sci. Sports Exerc. 22:165-170; 1990.

28. Frizzell, R.T.; Lang, G.H.; Lowane, D.L.; Lathan, S.R. Hyponatremia and ultramarathon running. JAMA. 255:772-774; 1986.
29. Worobetz, L.J.; Gerrard, D.F. Effect of moderate exercise on esophageal function in asymptomatic athletes. Am. J. Gastroenterol. 81:1048-1051; 1986.
30. Peters, O.; Peters, P.; Clarys, J.T.; De Meirleir, K.; Davis, G. Esophageal motility and exercise. Gastroenterology. 94:A351; 1988.
31. Soffer, E.E.; Merchant, R.K.; Deuthman, G.; Launspach, J.; Gisolfi, C. The effect of graded exercise on esophageal motility and gastroesophageal reflux in trained athletes. Gastroenterology. 100:A497; 1991.
32. Schofield, P.M.; Bennett, D.H.; Whorwell, P.J.; Brooks, N.H.; Bray, C.L.; Ward, C.; Jones, P.E. Exertional gastro-oesophageal reflux: A mechanism for symptoms in patients with angina pectoris and normal coronary angiograms. Br. Med. J. 294:1459-1461; 1987.
33. Johnston, P.; O'Connor, B.; Lennon, J.R.; Crowe, J. A comparative evaluation of bicycle exercise testing versus endoscopy plus 24 hour oesophageal pH monitoring in the diagnosis of gastroesophageal reflux. Gastroenterology. 92:A1457; 1987.
34. Clark, C.S.; Kraus, D.; Sinclair, J.; Castell, D. Gastroesophageal reflux induced by exercise in healthy volunteers. JAMA. 261:3599-3601; 1989.
35. Kraus, B.; Sinclair, J.; Castell, D. Gastroesophageal reflux in runners. Characteristics and treatment. Ann. Intern. Med. 112:429-433; 1990.
36. Sears, R.J.; Sears, V.W.; Castell, D.O. Effects of antacids on "runner's reflux." Gastroenterology. 100:A840; 1991.
37. Motil, K.J.; Ostendorf, J.; Bricker, J.T.; Klisch, W.J. Case report: Exercise-induced gastroesophageal reflux in an athletic child. J. Pediatr. Gastroenterol. Nutr. 6:989-991; 1987.
38. Yazaki, E.; Evans, D.F. Long distance running increases post-prandial gastroesophageal reflux. Gastroenterology. 100:A189; 1991.
39. Mellow, M.H.; Simpson, A.G.; Watt, L.; Schoolmeester, L.; Haye, O. Esophageal acid perfusion in coronary artery disease. Gastroenterology. 85:306-312; 1983.
40. Zieve, F.J. Letter. Milit. Med. 151:131-132; 1986.
41. Olivares, C.J. Toughest ironman ever. Triathlete. 52:33-42; 1988.
42. Beckers, E.J.; Rehrer, N.J.; Saris, W.H.M.; Brouns, F.; Ten Hoor, F.; Kester, A.D.M. Daily variation in gastric emptying when using the double sampling technique. Med. Sci. Sports Exerc. 23:1210-1212; 1991.
43. Noakes, T.D.; Rehrer, N.J.; Maughan, R.J. The importance of volume in regulation gastric emptying. Med. Sci. Sports Exerc. 23:307-313; 1991.
44. Mitchell, J.B.; Voss, K.W. The influence of volume on gastric emptying and fluid balance during prolonged exercise. Med. Sci. Sports Med. 23:314-319; 1991.
45. Owen, M.D.; Kregel, K.C.; Wahl, P.T.; Gisolfi, C.V. Effect of ingesting carbohydrate beverages during exercise and heat. Med. Sci. Sports Exerc. 28:568-575; 1986.
46. Carrio, I.; Estorch, M.; Serra-Grima, R.; Ginjaume, M.; Notivol, R.; Calabuig, R.; Vilardell, F. Gastric emptying in marathon runners. Gut. 30:152-155; 1989.
47. Fordtran, J.S.; Bengt, S. Gastric emptying and intestinal absorption during prolonged severe exercise. J. Appl. Physiol. 23:331-335; 1967.
48. Neufer, P.D.; Young, A.J.; Sawka, M.N. Gastric emptying during walking and running: Effects of varied exercise intensity. Eur. J. Appl. Physiol. 58:440-445; 1989.
49. Marzio, L.; Formica, P.; Fabiani, F.; LaPenna, D.; Vecchiett, L.; Cuccurullo, F. Influence of physical activity on gastric emptying of liquids in normal subjects. Am. J. Gastroenterol. 86:1433-1436; 1991.
50. van den Broek-Evans, A.; Lund, J.N.; Lamont, G.L.; Wright, J.W.; Evans, D.F. The effect of exercise on gastric emptying of liquids in man using applied control tomography (APT). Gastroenterology. 94:A476; 1988.
51. Lopes, M.H.; Schwartzman, P.; Estrela, O.; Tondo, C.; Garcia, E.; Ronchetti, F.; Francisconi, C. Delayed gastric emptying of a liquid solution after maximal dynamic exercise. Gastroenterology. 100:A465; 1991.
52. Houmard, J.A.; Egan, P.C.; Johns, R.A.; Neufer, P.D.; Chenier, T.C.; Isreal, R.G. Gastric emptying during 1 h of cycling and running at 75% VO_2max. Med. Sci. Sports Exerc. 23:320-325; 1991.
53. Read, N.W.; Houghton, L.A. Physiology of gastric emptying and pathophysiology of gastroparesis. Gastroenterol. Clin. North Am. 18:359-373; 1989.
54. Cammack, J.; Read, N.W.; Cann, P.A.; Greenwood, D.; Holgate, A.M. Effect of prolonged exercise on the passage of a solid meal through the stomach and small intestine. Gut. 23:957-961; 1982.
55. Moore, J.G.; Datz, F.L.; Christian, P.E. Exercise increases solid meal gastric emptying rates in men. Dig. Dis. Sci. 35:428-432; 1990.

56. Feldman, M.; Nixon, J.V. The effect of exercise on post prandial gastric secretion and emptying in humans. J. Appl. Physiol. Respir. Environ. Exerc. Physiol. 53:851-854; 1982.
57. Markiewicz, K.; Cholewa, M.; Gorski, L.; Chmura, J. Effective physical exercise on gastric basal secretion of healthy men. Acta Hepatogastroenterol. [Stuttg]. 24:377-380; 1977.
58. Markiewicz, K.; Lukin, M.; Jazdzewski, B.; Cholewa, M. Furosemide effect on gastric basal secretion during exercise and post exercise restitution in healthy subjects. Acta Pol. 33:296-304; 1982.
59. Ramsbottom, N.; Hunt, J.N. Effective exercise on gastric emptying and gastric secretion. Digestion. 10:1-8; 1974.
60. Markiewicz, K.; Lukin, M. The effect of physical exercise on gastric secretion and chronic duodenal ulcer patients. Dig. Dis. Sci. 31:344S; 1986.
61. Meeroff, J.C. Aerobic training: An esoteric treatment for ulcer disease? Am. J. Gastroenterol. 80:A843; 1985.
62. Holm, L.; Perry, M.A. Role of blood flow in gastric acid secretion. Am. J. Physiol. 254:G281-G293; 1988.
63. Lopez, A.A.; Preziosi, J.P.; Chateau, P.; Auguste, P. Plique, O. How should gastric disorders in endurance sport competitors be treated? Gastroenterology. 100:A113; 1991.
64. Costill, D.L. Carbohydrates for exercise: Dietary demands for optimal performance. Int. J. Sports Med. 9:1-18; 1988.
65. Cloarec, D.; Bornet, F.; Gouilloud, S.; Barry, J.L.; Saim, B.; Galmiche, J.P. Breath hydrogen response to lactulose in healthy subjects: Relationship to methane producing status. Gut. 31:300-304; 1990.
66. Staniforth, D.H. Comparison of orocaecal transit times assessed by the lactulose/breath hydrogen and the sulfasalazine/sulfapyridine methods. Gut. 30:978-982; 1989.
67. Caride, V.J.; Prokop, E.K.; Troncale, F.J.; Buddoura, W.; Winchenbach, K.; McCallum, R.W. Scintigraphic determination of small intestinal transit time: Comparison with the hydrogen breath technique. Gastroenterology. 86:714-720; 1984.
68. Pressman, J.H.; Hofmann, A.F.; Witztum, K.F.; Gertler, S.L.; Steinbach, J.H.; Stokes, K.; Kelts, D.G.; Stone, D.M.; Jones, B.R.; Dharmsathaphorn, K. Limitations of indirect methods of estimating small bowel transit in man. Dig. Dis. Sci. 32:689-699; 1987.
69. Ollerenshaw, K.J.; Norman, S.; Wilson, C.G.; Hardy, J.G. Exercise and small intestinal transit. Nucl. Med. Commun. 8:105-110; 1987.
70. Keeling, W.F.; Martin, B.J. Gastrointestinal transit during mild exercise. J. Appl. Physiol. 63:978-981; 1987.
71. Keeling, W.F.; Harris, A.; Martin, B.J. Orocecal transit during mild exercise in women. J. Appl. Physiol. 68:1350-1353; 1990.
72. Meshkinpour, H.; Kemp, C.; Fairshter, R. The effect of aerobic exercise on mouth to cecum transit time. Gastroenterology. 96:938-941; 1989.
73. Wald, A.; Van Theil, D.H.; Hoechstetter, L.; Gavaler, J.S.; Egler, K.M.; Verm, R.; Scott, L.; Lester, R. Gastrointestinal transit: The effect of the menstrual cycle. Gastroenterology. 80:1497-1500; 1981.
74. Moses, F.M.; Ryan, C.; DeBolt, J.; Smoak, B.; Hoffman, A.; Villanueva, V.; Deuster, P. Oral cecal transit time during a 2 hr run with ingestion of water or glucose polymer. Am. J. Gastroenterol. 83:1055; 1988.
75. Di Lorenzo, C.; Dooley, C.P.; Valenzuela, J.E. Role of gastrointestinal motility in the variability of gastrointestinal transit time measured by the hydrogen breath test. Gastroenterology. 86:A124; 1987.
76. Evans, D.F.; Foster, G.E.; Hardastle, J.D. Does exercise affect small bowel motility in man. Gut. 24:A1012; 1983.
77. Soffer, E.E.; Summers, R.W.; Gisolfi, C. The effect of exercise on intestinal motility and transit in trained athletes. Am. J. Physiol. 260:G698-G702; 1991.
78. Harris, A.; Keeling, W.F.; Martin, B.J. Identical orocecal transit time and serum motilin in hyperthermia and normothermia. Dig. Dis. Sci. 35:1281-1284; 1990.
79. Harris, A.; Lindeman, A.K.; Martin, B.J. Rapid orocecal transit in chronically active persons with high energy intake. J. Appl. Physiol. 70:1550-1553; 1991.
80. Williams, J.H.; Mager, M.; Jacobson, E.D. Relationship of mesenteric blood flow to intestinal absorption of carbohydrates. J. Lab. Clin. Med. 63:853-862; 1964.
81. Isaacs, P. Marathon without a colon. Salt and water balance in endurance running ileostomates. Br. J. Sports Med. 18:295-300; 1984.
82. Barclay, G.R.; Turnberg, L.A. Effect of moderate exercise on salt and water transport in the human jejunum. Gut. 29:816-820; 1988.
83. Maughan, R.J.; Leiper, J.B.; McGaw, B.A. Effects of exercise intensity on absorption of ingested fluids in man. Exper. Physiol. 75:419-421; 1990.
84. Bo-Linn, G.W.; Santa Ana, C.A.; Morawski, S.G.; Fordtran, J.S. Purging and calorie absorption in bulimic patients and normal women. Ann. Intern. Med. 99:14-17; 1983.

85. Moses, F.M.; Singh, A.; Villanueva, V.; Kelsey, B.; Smoak, B.; Deuster, P. Lactose absorption and transit during prolonged high intensity running. Am. J. Gastroenterol. 84:1192; 1989.
86. Moses, F.M.; Singh, A.; Smoak, B.; Hollander, D.; Deuster, P. Alterations in intestinal permeability during prolonged high intensity running. Gastroenterology. 100:A472; 1991.
87. Sullivan, S.N.; Wong, C. Runners' diarrhea; Different patterns and associated factors. J. Clin. Gastroenterol. 14:101-104; 1992.
88. Cordain, L.; Latin, R.W.; Behnke, J.J. The effects of an aerobic running program on bowel transit time. J. Sports Med. 26:101-104; 1986.
89. Bingham, S.A.; Cummings, J.H. Effect of exercise and physical fitness on large intestinal function. Gastroenterology. 97:1389-1399; 1989.
90. Lampe, J.W.; Slavin, J.L.; Apple, F.S. Iron status of active women and the effect of running a marathon on bowel function and gastrointestinal blood loss. Int. J. Sports Med. 12:173-179; 1991.
91. Oettle, G.J. Effect of moderate exercise on bowel habit. Gut. 32:941-944; 1991.
92. Dapoigny, M.; Sarna, S. Effects of physical exercise on colonic motor activity. Am. J. Physiol. 23:G646-G652; 1991.
93. Stamm, C.P.; Pearce, W.A.; Larsen, B.A.; Willis, S.M.; Kikendall, J.W.; Moses, F.M.; Rosen, H.M.; Wong, R.K.H. Colonic ulcerations associated with non-steroidal anti-inflammatory drug ingestion. Gastrointest. Endosc. 37:260; 1991.
94. Sarna, S.K. Physiology and pathophysiology of colonic motor activity. Dig. Dis. Sci. 36:998-1018; 1991.
95. Apple, F.S.; McGue, M.K. Serum enzyme changes during marathon training. Am. J. Clin. Pathol. 79:716-719; 1983.
96. Bunch, T.W. Blood test abnormalities in runners. Mayo Clin. Proc. 55:113-117; 1980.
97. Holly, R.G.; Bernard, R.J.; Rosenthal, M.; Applegate, E.; Pritikin, N. Triathlete characterization response to prolonged strenuous competition. Med. Sci. Sports Exerc. 18:123-127; 1986.
98. Lignan, P.; Hespel, P.; Vanden Eynde, E.; Amery, A. Biochemical variables in plasma and urine before and after prolonged physical exercise. Enzyme. 33:134-142; 1985.
99. Nagel, D.; Seiler, D.; Franz, H.; Jung, K. Ultra-long-distance running and the liver. Int. J. Sports Med. 11:441-445; 1990.
100. Ritland, S.; Foss, N.E.; Gjone, E. Physical activity and liver disease and liver function in sportsmen. Scand. J. Soc. Med. [Suppl.]. 29:221-226; 1982.
101. Ducry, J.J.; Howald, H.; Zysset, T.; Bircher, J. Liver function in physically trained subjects. Galactose elimination capacity, plasma disappearance of ICG, and aminopyrine metabolism in long distance runners. Dig. Dis. Sci. 24:192-196; 1979.
102. Boel, J.; Anderson, L.B.; Rasmusin, B.; Hanson, S.H.; Dossing, M. Hepatic drug metabolism and physical fitness. Clin. Pharmacol. Ther. 36:121-126; 1984.
103. Orioli, S.; Bandinelli, I.; Birardi, A.; Chieca, R.; Buzzelli, G.; Chiarantini, E. Hepatic antipyrine metabolism in athletes. J. Sports Med. Phys. Fitness. 30:261-263; 1990.
104. Rowell, L.B.; Blackmon, J.R.; Bruce, R.A. Indocyanine green clearance and estimated blood flow during mild to maximal exercise an upright man. J. Clin. Invest. 43:1677-1690; 1964.
105. Zeeh, J.; Lange, H.; Bosch, J.; Pohl, S.; Loesgen, H.; Eggers, R.; Navasa, M.; Chesta, J.; Bircher, J. Steady-state extrarenal sorbitol clearance as a measure of hepatic plasma flow. Gastroenterology. 95:749-759; 1988.
106. Ohnishi, K.; Saito, M.; Nakayama, T.; Iida, S.; Nomura, F.; Koen, H.; Okuda, K. Portal venous hemodynamics in chronic liver disease; Effects of posture change and exercise. Radiology. 155:757-761; 1985.
107. Collomp, K.; Anselme, F.; Audran, M.; Gay, J.P.; Chanal, J.L.; Prefaut, C. Effects of moderate exercise on the pharmacokinetics of caffeine. Eur. J. Clin. Pharmacol. 40:279-282; 1991.
108. Pyke, S.; Lew, H.; Quintanilha, A. Severe depletion and liver glutathione during physical exercise. Biochem. Biophys. Res. Commun. 139:926-931; 1986.
109. Ardies, C.M.; Morris, G.S.; Erickson, C.K.; Farrar, R.P. Effects of exercise and ethanol on liver mitochondrial function. Life Sci. 40:1053-1061; 1987.
110. Day, W.W.; Weiner, M. Inhibition of hepatic drug metabolism and carbon tetrachloride toxicity in Fischer-344 rats by exercise. Biochem. Pharmacol. 42:181-184; 1991.
111. Kato, I.; Nomura, A.; Stemmermann, G.N.; Chyou, P. Prospective study of clinical gallbladder disease and its association with obesity, physical activity, and other factors. Dig. Dis. Sci. 37:784-790; 1992.
112. Leslie, B.R.; Sander, R.N.W.; Gerwin, L.E. Runners' hemolysis and pigment gallstones. N. Engl. J. Med. 313:1230; 1985.
113. Dallongeville, J.; Ledoux, M.; Brisson, G. Iron deficiency among active men. J. Am. Coll. Nutr. 8:195-202; 1989.
114. Nickerson, H.J.; Holubets, M.C.; Weiler, B.R.; Haas, R.G.; Schwartz, S.; Ellefson, M.E.

Causes of iron deficiency in adolescent athletes. J. Pediatr. 114:657-663; 1989.

115. Thompson, P.D.; Funk, E.J.; Carleton, R.A.; Sturner, W.Q. Incidence of death during jogging in Rhode Island from 1975-1980. JAMA. 247:2535-2538; 1982.

116. Porter, A.M.W. Do some marathon runners bleed into the gut? Br. Med. J. 287:1427; 1983.

117. Halvorsen, F.A.; Lyng, J.; Ritland, S. Gastrointestinal bleeding in marathon runners. Scand. J. Gastroenterol. 21:493-497; 1986.

118. McCabe, M.E.; Peura, D.A.; Kadakia, S.C.; Bocek, Z.; Johnson, L.F. Gastrointestinal blood loss associated with running a marathon. Dig. Dis. Sci. 31:1229-1232; 1986.

119. McMahon, L.F.; Ryan, M.J.; Larsen, D.; Fisher, R.L. Occult gastrointestinal blood loss in marathon runner. Ann. Intern. Med. 100:836-837; 1984.

120. Baska, R.S.; Moses, F.M.; Graeber, G.; Kearney, G. Gastrointestinal bleeding during an ultramarathon. Dig. Dis. Sci. 35:276-279; 1990.

121. Stewart, J.F.; Ahlquist, D.A.; McGill, D.B.; Ilstrup, D.M.; Schwartz, S.; Owen, R.A. Gastrointestinal blood loss and anemia in runners. Ann. Intern. Med. 100:843-845; 1984.

122. Moses, F.M.; Baska, R.S.; Peura, D.A.; Deuster, P.A. Effect of cimetidine on marathon-associated gastrointestinal symptoms and bleeding. Dig. Dis. Sci. 36:1390-1394; 1991.

123. Selby, G.; Fram, D.; Eichner, E.R. Effort-related gastrointestinal blood loss in distance runners during a competitive season. Am. Coll. Sports Med. 20:S79; 1988.

124. Dobbs, T.W.; Akins, M.; Ratliff, R.; Eichner, E.R. Gastrointestinal bleeding in competitive cyclists. Am. Coll. Sports Med. 20:S78; 1988.

125. Viala, J.J.; Ville, D. Anemie des coureurs de fond liee a des hemorragies digestives. Presse Med. 20:386; 1991.

126. Baska, R.S.; Moses, F.M.; Deuster, P.A. Cimetidine reduces running-associated gastrointestinal bleeding. A prospective observation. Dig. Dis. Sci. 35:956-960; 1990.

127. Hilpert, G.; Gaudin, B.; Devars Du Mayne, J.F.; Cerf, M. Gastrite ulcereuse chez un coureur de fond. Gastroenterol. Clin. Biol. 8:983; 1984.

128. Papaioannides, D.; Giotis, C.; Karagiannis, N.; Voudouris, C. Acute upper gastrointestinal hemorrhage in long distance runners. Ann. Intern. Med. 101:719; 1984.

129. Scobie, B.A. Recurrent gut bleeding in five long distance runners. N. Z. Med. J. 98:966; 1985.

130. Gaudin, C.; Zerath, E.; Guezennec, C.Y. Gastric lesions secondary to long-distance running. Dig. Dis. Sci. 35:1239-1243; 1990.

131. Cooper, D.T.; Douglas, S.A.; Firth, L.A.; Hannagan, J.A.; Chadwick, V.S. Erosive gastritis and gastrointestinal bleeding in a female runner. Prevention of bleeding and healing of the gastritis with H2-receptor antagonist. Gastroenterology. 92:2019-2023; 1987.

132. Gaudin, C.; Zerath, E.; Guezennec, C.Y. Gastric lesions secondary to long-distance running. Dig. Dis. Sci. 35:1239-1243; 1990.

133. Mack, D.; Sherman, P. Iron deficiency anemia in an athlete associated with campylobacter pylori-negative chronic gastritis. J. Clin. Gastroenterol. 11:445-447; 1989.

134. Schwartz, A.; Vanagunas, A.; Kamel, P. The etiology of gastrointestinal bleeding in runners: A prospective endoscopic appraisal. Ann. Intern. Med. 113:632-633; 1990.

135. Morishita, T.; Guth, P.H. Effect of exogenous acid on the rat gastric mucosal microcirculation in hemorrhagic shock. Gastroenterology. 92:1958-1964; 1987.

136. Yasue, N.; Guth, P.H. Role of exogenous acid and retransfusion in hemorrhagic shock-induced gastric lesions in the rat. Gastroenterology. 94:1135-1143; 1988.

137. Schaub, N.; Spichtin, H.P.; Stalder, G.A. Ischamische kolitis als urs chiner darmblutung bei marathonlauf? Schweiz. Med. Wochenschr. 115:454-457; 1985.

138. Heer, M.; Repond, F.; Hany, A.; Sulser, H. Hemorrhagic colitis, gastritis, hematuria and rhabdomyolysis: Manifestations of multisystemic ischemia? Schweiz. Rundsch. Med. Prax. 75:1538-1540; 1986.

139. Heer, M.; Repond, F.; Hany, A.; Sulser, H.; Kehl, O.; Jager, K. Acute ischemic colitis in a female long distance runner. Gut. 28:896-899; 1987.

140. Moses, F.M.; Brewer, T.G.; Peura, D.A. Running-associated proximal hemorrhagic colitis. Ann. Intern. Med. 108:385-386; 1988.

141. Merlin, P.; Roche, J.F.; Aubert, J.P.; Potet, F.; Gay, G. Ischemic colitis during an unusual effort. Gastroenterol. Clin. Biol. 13:108-109; 1989.

142. Beaumont, A.C.; Teare, J.P. Subtotal colectomy following marathon running in a female patient. J. R. Soc. Med. 84:4339-4340; 1991.

143. Sakai, L.; Keltner, R.; Kaminski, D. Spontaneous and shock associated ischemic colitis. Ann. Surg. 140:755-760; 1980.

144. Porter, A.M.W. Marathon running and the cecal slap syndrome. Br. J. Sports Med. 16:178; 1982.

145. Porter, A.M.W. Non-steroidal anti-inflammatory drugs and ethanol. Br. J. Sports Med. 16:265; 1982.

146. Pruett, T.L.; Wilkins, M.E.; Gamble, W.G. Cecal volvulus: A different twist for the serious runner. N. Engl. J. Med. 312:1262-1263; 1985.
147. Flamm, S.D.; Taki, J.; Moore, R.; Lewis, S.F.; Keech, F.; Maltais, F.; Ahmad, M.; Callahan, R.; Dragotakes, S.; Alpert, N.; Strauss, H.W. Redistribution of regional and organ blood volume and effect on cardiac function in relation to upright exercise intensity in healthy human subjects. Circulation. 81:1550-1559; 1990.
148. Rehrer, N.J.; Meijer, G.A. Biomechanical vibration of the abdominal region during running and bicycling. J. Sports Med. Phys. Fitness. 31:231-234; 1991.
149. Dawson, D.J.; Khan, A.N.; Shreeve, D.R. Psoas muscle hypertrophy: Mechanical cause for "jogger's trots?". Br. J. Med. 291:787-788; 1985.
150. Bjarnason, I.; Zanelli, G.; Smith, T.; Prouse, P.; Williams, P.; Smethurst, P.; Delacey, G.; Gumpel, M.J.; Levi, A.J. Nonsteroidal antiinflammatory drug-induced intestinal inflammation in humans. Gastroenterology. 93:480-489; 1987.
151. Bounous, G.; McArdle, A.H. Marathon runners: The intestinal handicap. Med. Hypotheses. 33:261-264; 1990.
152. Priebe, W.M.; Priebe, J.A. Runners diarrhea—Prevalence and clinical symptomatology. Am. J. Gastroenterol. 79:827-828; 1984.
153. Riddoch, C.; Trinick, T. Gastrointestinal disturbances in marathon runners. Br. J. Sports Med. 22:71-74; 1988.
154. Rehrer, N.J.; Brouns, F.; Beckers, E.J.; Ten Hoor, F.; Saris, W.H.M. Gastric emptying with repeated drinking during running and bicycling. Int. J. Sports Med. 11:238-243; 1990.
155. Ryan, A.J.; Bleiler, T.L.; Carter, J.E.; Gisolfi, C.V. Gastric emptying during prolonged exercise in the heat. Med. Sci. Sports Exerc. 21:51-58; 1989.
156. Sole, C.C.; Noakes, T.D. Faster gastric emptying for glucose-polymer and fructose solutions than for glucose in humans. Eur. J. Appl. Physiol. 58:605-612; 1989.
157. Mitchell, J.B.; Costill, D.L.; Howard; et al. Med. Sci. Sports Exerc. 21:269-274; 1989.

Chapter 25

Physical Activity and Carbohydrate Metabolism

George A. Brooks

It is becoming increasingly evident that carbohydrate-derived fuels provide most of the energy that sustains physical activity, whether the activity lasts a few seconds or a few hours. Maintenance of a blood glucose level within the normal range is one of the principles upon which whole series of physiological responses are coordinated. Because muscle glucose uptake and, therefore, blood glucose utilization increase during exercise, hepatic glucose production and release must increase in coordination with increased blood glucose disappearance. A mismatch between glucose production and utilization during exercise would result in hypoglycemia and central fatigue. During exercise, glycogen in active muscle provides most of the carbohydrate fuel source, but both direct and indirect pathways of glycogen catabolism are utilized. Glycogen in active as well as inactive muscle and possibly other tissues is mobilized to supply substrate for hepatic and renal gluconeogenesis as well as fuel at sites of high cell respiration.

The importance of carbohydrates in sustaining exercise is exemplified by the importance of glucose utilization for good cardiac function during exercise, and the association of skeletal muscle glycogen depletion with fatigue. Phylogenic examination indicates that successful species are often those characterized by sprinting (burst activity) behavior dependent on rapid glycolysis leading to lactic acid formation. Thus, the ability of cells and tissues to store, share, and utilize carbohydrate energy forms is a principal means by which it is possible to sustain physical exercise in daily life and athletic endeavors up to and including the longest of Olympic events, the marathon.

Phylogeny

Dependence on glycolysis is a characteristic that has persisted in evolution from bacteria through invertebrates (5,18,53), cartilaginous and bony fish, amphibians and reptiles, and birds and mammals (7,69). In the case of unicellular organisms capable of existing in the presence or absence of oxygen, lactic acid, the product of glycolysis, can be excreted to the environment. The progression of glycolysis from pyruvate to lactate is necessary to oxidize NADH, thereby providing a reduced cofactor for glyceraldehyde 3 phosphate dehydrogenase. Potential chemical energy is lost from lactate excretion, but rapid glycolytic flux and adenosine triphosphate (ATP) production are possible.

In species not evolved with robust circulatory systems (e.g., some fish, reptiles, and lizards) (28) rapid glycolysis leads to lactate formation and accumulation in skeletal muscle, with in situ reconversion of lactate to glycogen during recovery from burst activity. In humans and other mammals, glycolysis in excess of the pyruvate requirement for oxidative substrate results in cellular lactate efflux and the distribution of carbohydrate in the form of lactate for oxidation and gluconeogenesis at anatomically close or removed sites (8). In this manner, glycogenolysis and glycolysis in one cell can fuel an adjacent cell (8,66-68), one muscle can fuel another, a muscle can fuel the heart (26,27), and a muscle can provide a substrate to gluconeogenic organs. In dogs, glycogenolysis in the liver at exercise onset leads to lactate as well as glucose formation with net release of both carbohydrates for utilization by working muscle (80–82). In all of these cases the shuttling of lactate through the interstitium and vasculature provides a means of distributing carbohydrate potential energy. In mammals, the primary fate of lactate is oxidation during exercise (21,38-40,55,73) as well as recovery (9,14). Although most (70%–80%) lactate is disposed of by direct oxidation during exercise, the remainder, which is disposed of by conversion to glucose, plays an equally important role. Conversion of lactate to glucose during exercise is essential for maintenance of glucose homeostasis (41,77,78).

The phylogeny displayed in Figure 25.1 represents a compilation of results previously published on invertebrates (18) and vertebrates (6,53). As

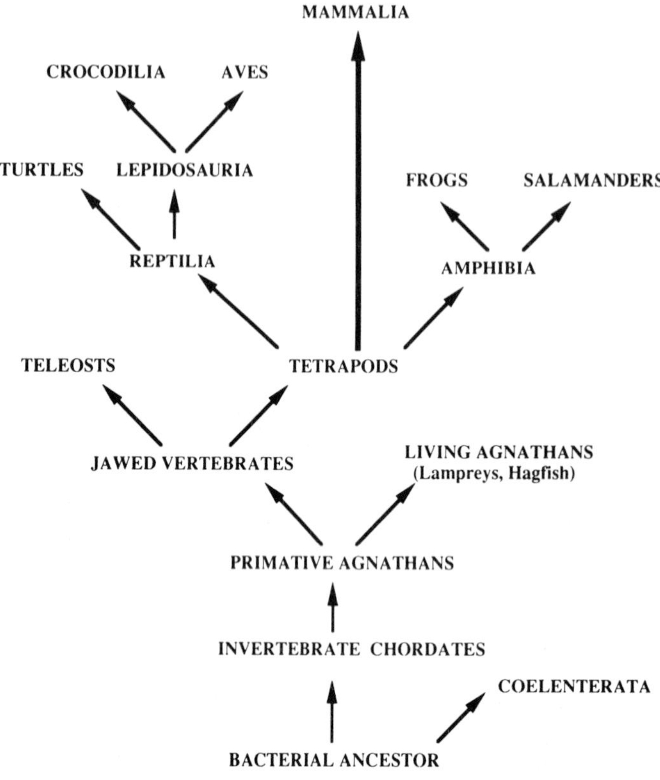

Figure 25.1 Phylogeny tracing the evolution of lactic dehydrogenase (LDH) from unicellular organisms to contemporary mammals including man. As reviewed recently by Bennett (7), high capacity for glycolysis leading to lactic acid formation is a characteristic of species evolved for burst activity (6,7,18,53,69).

discussed previously by Ruben and Bennett (69) and more recently by Bennett (7), vertebrates generally possess a well-developed capacity for lactate formation. This capability has traditionally been interpreted in terms of adaptation to hypoxic environments. However, not all vertebrates evolved to occupy hypoxic environments. Instead, it is more likely that rapid glycolysis leading to lactate formation provides ATP for burst activity. Therefore, the evolution of extensive capacity for glycolytically supported ATP production is closely related to the evolution of vertebrates from chordates, and the biological successes of various vertebrate species.

Cardiac Function, Compartmentation of Function, and Carbohydrate Utilization: The Essential Nature of Glucose Metabolism

Of all forms of mammalian striated muscle, the myocardium is taken as the epitome of an aerobic tissue capable of sustaining high metabolic rates from exogenous substrates. Under resting conditions, the heart operates primarily on circulating free fatty acids (27). In resting individuals, cardiac function as measured by double product is low compared to that during exercise. However, when exercise starts, uptake of glucose and lactate by the myocardium rises, especially when arterial lactate concentration increases and carbohydrate energy sources (i.e., lactate and glucose) become predominant in the heart with lactate supplying most of the oxidizable substrate (26,27). The requirement for increased cardiac function during exercise compared to rest is coincident with increased carbohydrate utilization by the myocardium. In resting individuals lipid supply to the heart is increased by intralipid infusion and cardiac function is depressed. Similarly, in studies on isolated hearts perfused with one of several substrates, cardiac function (dp/dt) is depressed unless exogenous glucose is provided, even if lactate is the predominant fuel (58). In the heart it may be that, as in smooth muscle where enzymes of the glycolytic pathways are contained in the sarcolemma (59), glycolytically produced ATP in the cell membrane is involved in calcium ion flux and the process of excitation-contraction coupling. Whatever the reason, *glucose and glycolytically produced ATP are required for optimal function of the myocardium.* The permissive effect of carbohydrates on lipid metabolism will be discussed later.

Dependence on Glycogen for Burst Activity by Mammalian Muscle

Mammalian muscle clearly depends on glycogen for sprinting and power (burst) activities. In studies on rats run at different intensities (4) as well as in humans engaged in leg cycling of graded power outputs (29,30), the demonstrated pattern of glycogen depletion was predictable based on the size principle (33). This principle states that, as relative exercise intensity increases, the pattern of fiber type recruitment changes to include Type II as well as Type I fibers. Thus, as the muscle force required to perform an activity increases, so does the recruitment of skeletal muscle fibers dependent on glycogen utilization.

The capability for glycogenolysis in muscle is great (72), and the relative efficiency of adenosine diphosphate (ADP) phosphorylation in glycolysis (i.e., about 50%) approximates that of oxidative phosphorylation (16). However, because the free energy change from glycogen to lactate is relatively small, energy capacity of the Embden-Meyerhof Pathway is not great. Rapid glycogenolysis is necessary to support burst activity, but continued exercise is dependent on oxidative catabolism of glycolytic end products, lactate and pyruvate (13).

Maintenance of Euglycemia

Maintenance of blood glucose homeostasis is one of the acknowledged physiological priorities. Precipitous falls in arterial glucose concentration during exercise, or on any other occasion, can lead to severe central nervous system (CNS) dysfunction and cessation of activity. Recently, Galbo and associates (50,71) have contributed greatly to our understanding of the regulation of blood glucose homeostasis during exercise. In contrast to the classic notion of a feedback regulation in which a fall in blood glucose concentration elicits counter-regulatory mechanisms, it is now clear that high- or even moderate-intensity exercises result in elevations in arterial glucose appearance and concentration. Figure 25.2, from Kjaer, Farrell, Chistensen, and Galbo (50), shows the profound rise in arterial glucose that accompanies maximal exercise. In contrast, Figure 25.3 shows a moderate but sustained rise in arterial glucose that results from exercise at 50% $\dot{V}O_2$max (10). Classic feedback mechanisms of glucoregulation, in which a fall in arterial glucose elicits responses of counter-regulatory hormones, do operate during exercise—but mainly when hypoglycemia is imminent (1).

Catecholamines play essential roles in glucoregulation, whether or not the exercise is short-term, high-intensity, or submaximal-intensity for extended periods (10,50,54,61). By means of its β_2 effect on mobilizing peripheral glycogen reserves, epinephrine plays a major role in supplying substrate (lactate) for hepatic gluconeogenesis. In addition, epinephrine promotes hepatic glycogenolysis and gluconeogenesis (50,84). Moreover, epinephrine suppresses pancreatic β-cell function and insulin secretion. In concert, a rise of glucagon and fall of insulin during exercise allows for a fall in the insulin:glucagon ratio. The fall in insulin:glucagon promotes hepatic gluconeogenesis. Norepinephrine, released from hepatic nerves as well as from the systemic circulation, may also stimulate hepatic glucose production during exercise (84). Additionally, norepinephrine may promote muscle glucose uptake (10,11).

Predominance of Muscle Glycogen as a Fuel During Exercise

Net Glycogen Catabolism During Exercise

The classic literature of exercise biochemistry has, in part, origins in biopsy measures of net muscle glycogen change during leg cycle ergometry (36). Subsequently, other forms of leg and arm ergometry (65) and running (17) have been utilized. Today it is widely recognized that muscle glycogen concentration is greatly affected by dietary and exercise history (36). Further, it is becoming recognized that the initial muscle glycogen concentration can affect the rate of muscle net glycogenolysis (61,63), as well as the time subjects can endure at a given submaximal power output (36,86). The onset of muscle fatigue often correlates with muscle glycogen depletion (*vide infra*).

Some of the classic results are necessary inclusions in a review of carbohydrate utilization during exercise. Figure 25.4, modified from Hultman (36), shows that glycogen depletion occurs in active muscle during exercise, and that with rest and adequate nutrition, muscle glycogen repletion can occur usually within 24 hr. Continued rest and

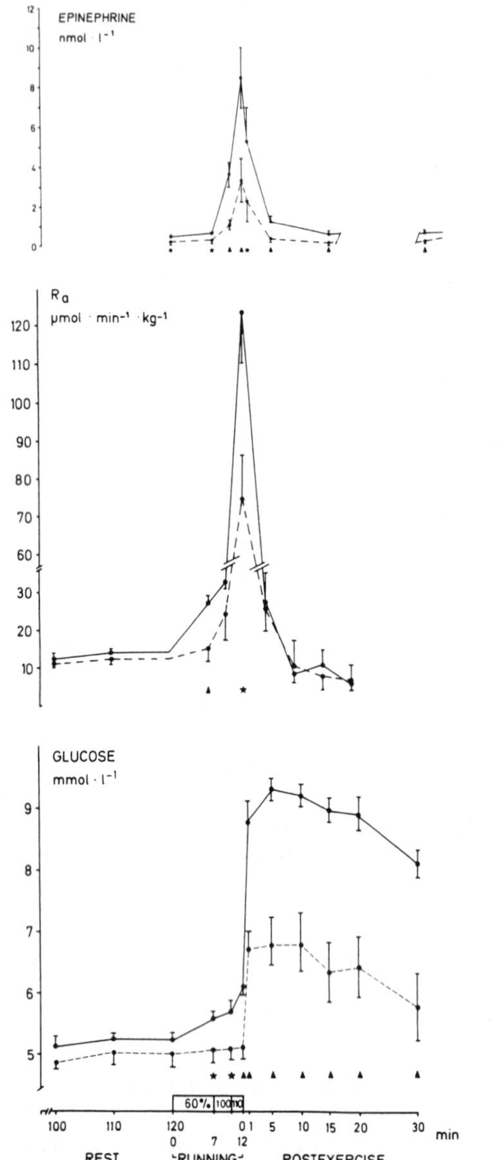

Figure 25.2 Arterial epinephrine (top), glucose appearance rate (middle), and glucose concentration (bottom) in 8 trained and 8 untrained men at rest and during graded exercise (% $\dot{V}O_2$max given at box on the origin). Hepatic glucose production and arterial glucose concentration rise at the start of exercise (reference 50 with permission).

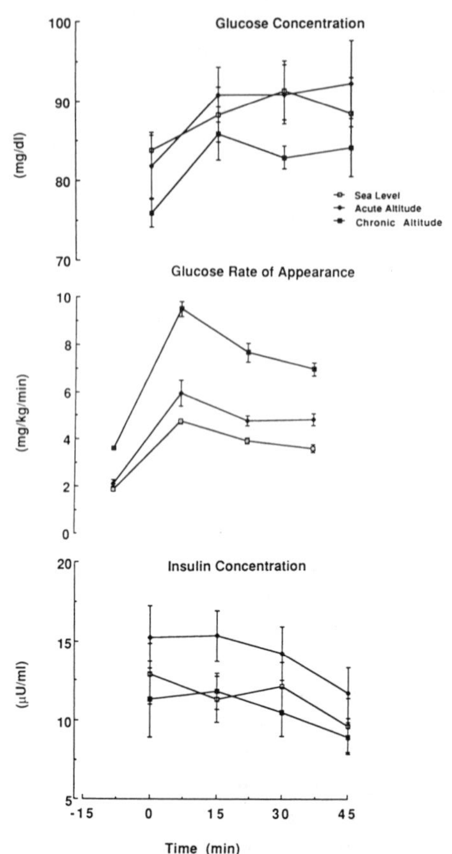

Figure 25.3 Arterial glucose concentration (top), appearance rate (middle), and insulin (bottom) in young exercising at 100 W (50%) of sea level $\dot{V}O_2$max at sea level, upon acute exposure to 4,300 m altitude, and after a 3-week residency at 4,300 m (10).

eating of a "normal" diet rich in complex carbohydrates results in glycogen over ("super") compensation. As a result of these seminal investigations, the nutrition, training, taper, and competition schedules of a generation of athletes have been affected.

Gas Exchange (R) and Relative Effort

The increase in gas exchange (R) ($R = \dot{V}CO_2/\dot{V}O_2$) that accompanies the transition from rest to exercise (Figure 25.5) is a well-known phenomenon that is generally interpreted to mean a shift toward carbohydrate utilization during exercise. Although it has not recently been the custom to correlate and quantitatively compare overall carbohydrate combustion with muscle glycogen catabolism during exercise, the classic efforts of Hultman and associates yielded excellent agreement (36).

When exercise starts, overall carbohydrate combustion, as determined by the rise in $\dot{V}O_2$ and R, increases, although blood insulin falls (10). As already noted, the fall in insulin promotes hepatic glucose production. Additionally, the fall in arterial insulin that accompanies exercise may be a necessary protective mechanism preserving substrate supply for glucose-requiring tissues (e.g., in the CNS where glucose uptake is concentration- and not insulin-dependent). Even though hepatic glucose production rises during exercise (1,10,15), the increase in glucose production is small compared to the overall rise in $\dot{V}O_2$ and CHO combustion as determined from respiratory gas exchange. For instance, during leg cycling exercise at 50% of

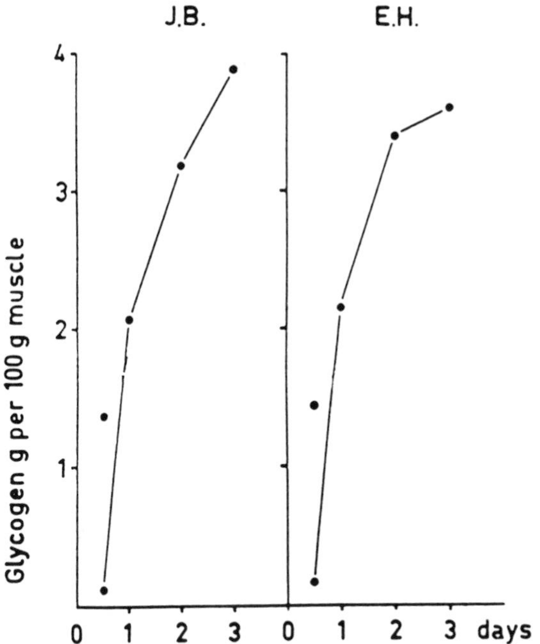

Figure 25.4 Effect of carbohydrate diet on muscle glycogen content after exhaustive, one-leg cycling exercise. Exhaustion coincides with glycogen depletion. Rest and a high carbohydrate diet result in very high human skeletal muscle glycogen levels (reference 36 with permission).

$\dot{V}O_2$max that elicited a tenfold rise in $\dot{V}O_2$, only 50% increments in blood glucose appearance (Ra) and disappearance (Rd) rates have been observed (10,74). It is doubtful that a tenfold rise in hepatic glucose production (Ra) could be achieved or sustained during prolonged exercise, because hypoglycemia would rapidly result if blood glucose disappearance rose tenfold. Therefore, the fall in insulin during exercise spares glucose for the CNS and contracting muscles in which contraction induces insulin-independent glucose uptake.

Although it is generally assumed that contracting skeletal muscle is the site of increased blood glucose disappearance during exercise, surprisingly few attempts have been made to quantitate and compare muscle glucose uptake and hepatic release or blood glucose appearance. What has recently become apparent (15) is that under some circumstances the relative increments in active muscle glucose uptake and whole-body CHO oxidation during exercise can exceed the relative rise in blood glucose Ra and Rd. Therefore, as with the redistribution of cardiac output that occurs during exercise, there is a shunting of blood glucose flux to active muscle during exercise. Implicit in this finding is the realization that nonactive tissues become less glucose-reliant during exercise as compared to rest (15).

Glucose–Lactate Interactions During Exercise

Stanley, Wisneski, Gertz, Neese, and Brooks (74) were the first to study glucose–lactate interactions in exercising humans. Using primed-continuous infusions of radio- and stable carbon isotopes, they showed that during sustained exercise approximately 20% of glucose is converted to lactate prior to disposal. Similarly, they showed that lactate provided a significant fraction: Approximately one fourth of the carbon for glucose production comes from lactate in exercising humans. Moreover, because glucose disposal could only account for a minor fraction (1/5) of lactate production, by inference, muscle glycogen contributed more (4/5) to lactate production than did blood glucose.

Turcotte and colleagues (77,78) infused ^{3}H- and ^{14}C-labeled glucose into running rats and noted marked incorporation of ^{14}C into blood lactate. They estimated that approximately half of blood glucose was disposed of as lactate. These results have been extended by Wasserman, Lacy, Bracy, and Williams (81) who compared lactate and glucose-specific activities in leg venous blood following tracer glucose infusion. They showed that approximately half of the lactate released came from glucose taken by dog leg muscle during rest and treadmill running (Figure 25.6). Because glucose 6 phosphate (G6P) from glycogen is probably metabolized identically as is G6P from glucose, it then follows that glycogen—as well as glucose catabolized in muscle—was converted to lactate prior to disposal.

Using combinations of leg and arm cycle ergometry and arterial–venous (a–v) difference measurements Richter et al. (65) have shown that lactate release from an active (leg) muscle bed can equal glucose uptake (Figure 25.7). Without benefit of a tracer measurement it is difficult to know the proportion of lactate coming from glucose (and that from glycogen). However, data from several laboratories corroborate the finding that during steady-state, submaximal exercise major fractions of glucose and glycogen are converted to lactate prior to metabolism.

Glycogen Turnover During Exercise

In studies on both laboratory rats (56,85) and humans (2) net glycogen catabolism in inactive muscle beds as the result of exercise by other

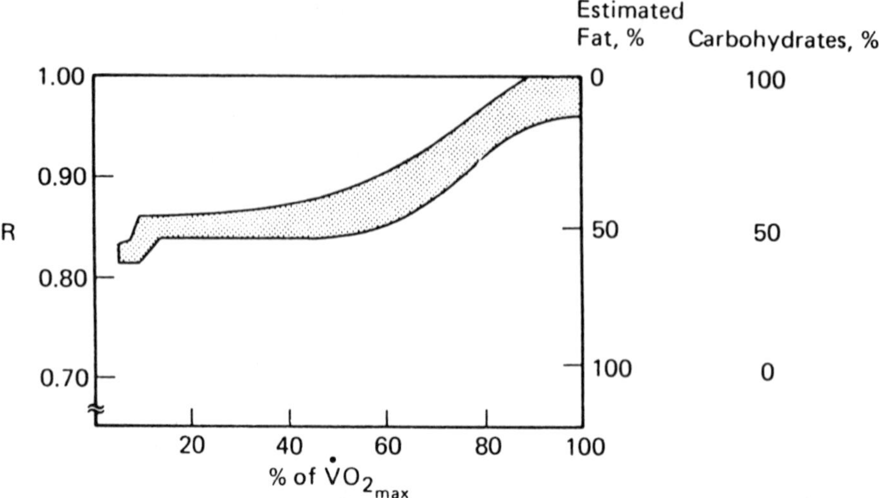

Figure 25.5 Relationships among the ventilatory gas exchange R (= $\dot{V}CO_2/\dot{V}O_2$), relative effort (% $\dot{V}O_2$max), and the balance of carbohydrate and lipid combustion. As the relative effort increases, so does the relative contribution of carbohydrate (13).

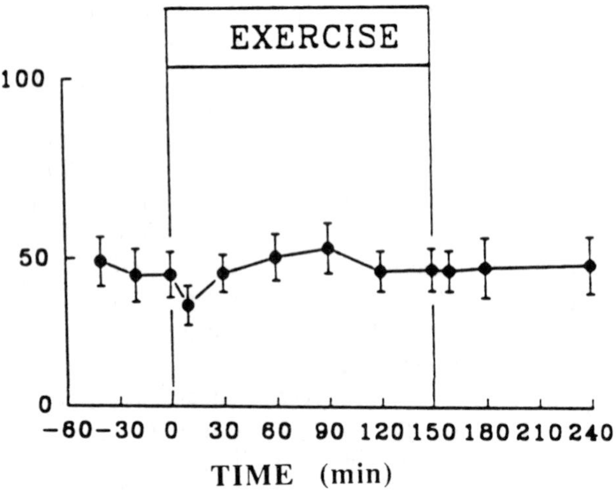

Figure 25.6 Conversion of glucose to lactate as determined by arterial-venous difference across dog limbs during rest and running. Approximately half the glucose taken up by dog muscle is released as lactate during rest and exercise. Because the muscle also takes up lactate on a net muscle basis, most of the glucose taken up by the dog limb is converted to lactate before disposal (reference 82 with permission).

body parts has been demonstrated. Because epinephrine stimulation has a major effect on muscle glycogenolysis, but only a minor, if any, effect on muscle mitochondrial oxygen uptake, it is not surprising that epinephrine stimulation of glycogenolysis leads to lactate release from inactive muscle (11).

Certainly, epinephrine stimulation is only one and not always *the* dominant factor in determining metabolite exchange across a muscle bed. For lactate, and to a more limited extent glucose, arterial concentration is an important determinant of tissue uptake. In results of the 1988 Pikes Peak Study investigators (15) found that on acute exposure to 4,300 m altitude the arms switch from net release to uptake as arterial lactate rises during leg cycling exercise. A similar result was obtained by Richter, Kienes, Saltin, Christensen, and Savard (65), who observed the working leg to switch from net lactate release to uptake as arterial lactate concentration rose in response to the addition of submaximal arm exercise (Figure 25.7).

Until recently, it has not been recognized that skeletal muscle glycogen undergoes turnover (synthesis and degradation) during exercise. However, Hutber and Bonen (37) have shown significant incorporation of label from isotopically infused glucose during exercise. Similarly, Azevedo, Lehman, Linderman, and Brooks (3) infused [6-^{3}H] glucose and [U-^{14}C] lactate into rats at rest and during treadmill running. After exercise or a defined resting control period, blood glucose ^{3}H:^{14}C ratio (precursor) was compared to the muscle glycogen ^{3}H:^{14}C (product) ratio. Large and significant incorporations of tracer into muscle glycogen pools of running rats was observed, which can only mean that muscle glycogen synthesis occurred during exercise. A similar observation has been made on exercising humans infused with tracer glucose (T. Noakes, personal communication). The conclusion to be reached from these reports is that active muscle glycogen turnover (synthesis and degradation) occurs during exercise.

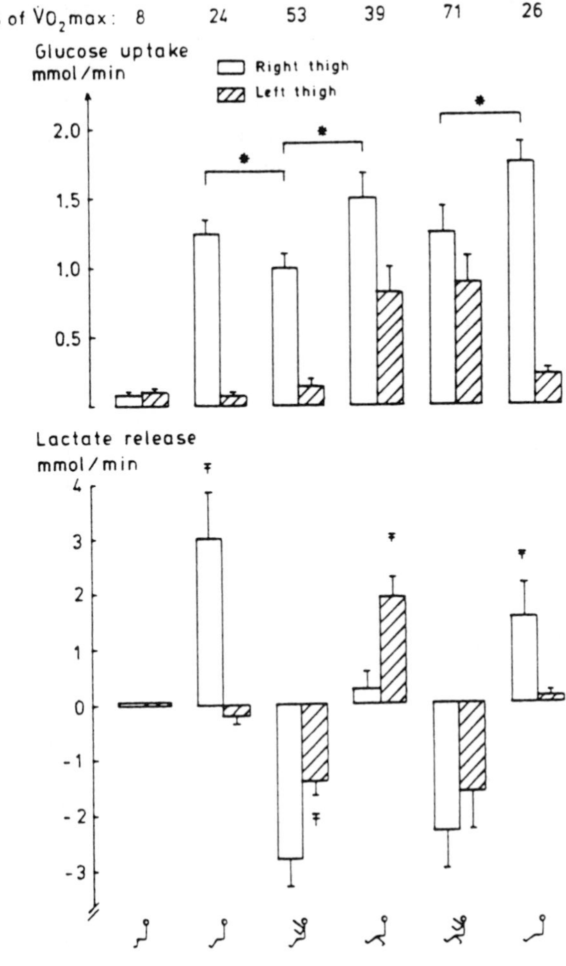

Figure 25.7 Glucose uptake and lactate exchange (net uptake or release) in *left* or *right* thighs at rest and during six different work bouts. The order of work bouts is indicated in the cartoon. At rest (first column), both legs take up glucose and release lactate. During *right* thigh exercise (second column), glucose uptake increases compared to rest and approximates lactate release. The inactive thigh switches from lactate release to uptake. When arm cranking is added to *right* thigh exercise (third column), the arterial lactate concentration rises and both thighs become net lactate consumers. Additionally, glucose uptake by the *right*, exercising thigh is reduced (reference 65 with permission).

The Balance of CHO and Lipid Utilization During Prolonged Exercise

Recent advances have resulted in changes in our understanding of the balance of carbohydrate and fat used during prolonged exercise. Leg muscle glycogen stores have been considered inadequate to allow athletes to complete a marathon, and endurance training results in an expansion of the mitochondrial reticulum (19,34,49). Therefore, previous wisdom has held that endurance training increases the ability to combust fat, and lipid combustion supports endurance activities such as the marathon run. However, this reasoning has assumed that only glycogen in active muscle is available to support exercise, and that training-induced mitochondrial adaptations selectively enhance the ability to combust lipid. However, it is now apparent that glycogen depots within inactive as well as active muscle are available for mobilization to supply fuel for active muscle (*vide supra*). Further, it is realized that training results in proportional increments in the ability of mitochondria to oxidize carbohydrate-derived as well as lipid fuel sources (19,34). Because exhausting exercise leading to glycogen depletion respiratory gas exchange data indicate heavy dependence on lipid oxidation (25), it may be that many of the training-induced adaptations that enhance the ability to utilize fat operate with greatest effect during recovery.

It is unfortunate that few attempts have been made to determine the effects of heavy exercise or exercise training on blood free fatty acid (FFA) or muscle triglyceride (TG) turnover. The single published attempt to measure FFA turnover in heavy (70% $\dot{V}O_2$max) exercise (Figure 25.8) (43) produced results consistent with changes in R; plasma palmitate turnover declined 40% compared to rest in heavy exercise. However, because blood glycerol rose during exercise, the possibility remains that intramuscular TG stores were mobilized and used. It is hoped the future will provide more investigations into the area of lipid utilization during exercise.

In the absence of rigorous attempts to measure lipid utilization in trained versus untrained states (23), investigators have relied on measurements of

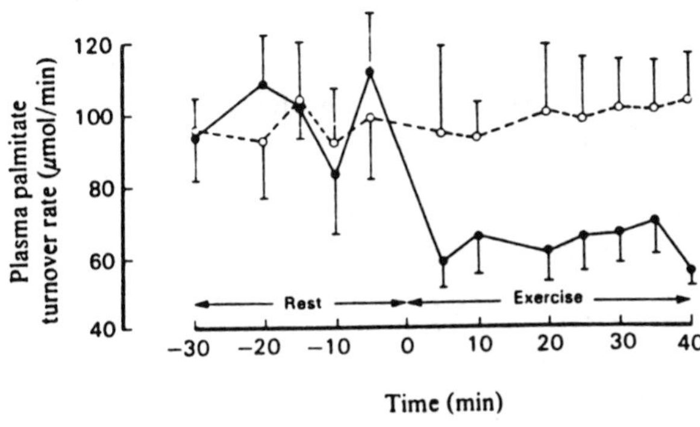

Figure 25.8 Plasma palmitate turnover rates at rest and during light (open circles) and heavy exercise (filled circles); $n = 5$. Heavy exercise was associated with decreased palmitate turnover. These isotope tracer-derived data are consistent with results of indirect calorimetry (Figure 25.6) (reference 43 with permission).

respiratory gas exchange and blood metabolite concentrations before and after training (e.g., 23). Interpretation of such results is compromised by selection of identical power outputs for study before and after training, and by uncertainties about R as a valid measure of the nonprotein RQ during exercise. Because catecholamine, blood glucose, and lactate responses to given power outputs will be dampened after training, the result of a lower gas exchange R from a given absolute exercise power output is to be predicted on the basis of posttraining evaluation at a relatively lower exercise intensity, with lesser perturbation of acid-base balance.

Results of studies on the metabolic response to marathon running provide a good example of the effects of endurance training on the balance of lipid and CHO utilization during prolonged exercise. Table 25.1 summarizes results of completed studies on R during marathon running. With the average reported R of 0.91, predominance of CHO oxidation is indicated. That total-body carbohydrate oxidation during marathon running exceeds the glycogen storage capacity of active muscle requires mobilization of glycogen from diverse pools. For the present, the point suffices that athletes train to compete at both higher absolute and relative power outputs than possible without training. Therefore, demonstration of lower gas exchange Rs for given low- to moderate-intensity exercise power outputs after training possess little practical relevance for application in the real world where athletes strive to perform at high, not low power outputs.

Skeletal Muscle Glycogen and Hepatic Gluconeogenesis: Importance of the Cori Cycle

The role of skeletal muscle glycogen in providing ATP in glycolysis as well as an immediate source of oxidizable substrate for the mitochondrial reticulum in active muscle is widely accepted (*vide supra*). However, until recently the role of muscle glycogen in providing gluconeogenic precursors (lactate mainly, but also pyruvate and alanine) during exercise has not been appreciated. Several technical approaches have allowed assessment of Cori cycle activity during prolonged exercise. As already noted, in laboratory rats studied with dual isotope technique, it has been observed that lactate represents an important source of hepatic glucose production in exercising, postabsorptive rats (9,21,32).

Perhaps the most dramatic demonstration to date of the importance of gluconeogenesis from lactate and other 3-carbon precursors in sustaining blood glucose homeostasis during prolonged exercise comes from experiments on rats with gluconeogenesis blocked by 3-mercaptopicolinic acid (MPA), an inhibitor of the key gluconeogenic enzyme phosphoenolpyruvate-carboxy kinase (PEPCK). John-Alder, McAlister, and Terjung (41) demonstrated that gluconeogenic blockade with MPA results in hyperlactacidemia, hypoglycemia, and increased muscle glycogenolysis in exercising rats. These results were replicated by Turcotte et al. (78) who additionally showed with isotopic tracers that gluconeogenesis-inhibited rats were unable to increase glucose appearance during exercise. In this way the critical importance of gluconeogenesis for hepatic glucose production was illustrated.

In their experiments Turcotte and Brooks (77) demonstrated a profound effect of gluconeogenic blockade with MPA on glucose homeostasis in endurance-trained rats. Untrained adult rats are usually capable of enduring approximately one-half hr running at one mph (26 m/min) on a motorized treadmill. In contrast, endurance-trained rats can

Table 25.1 Summary of Published Studies on Respiratory Gas Exchange During Marathon and Long-Distance Running

Investigation	n	Group	Distance run (miles)	Relative effort (%$\dot{V}O_2$max)	Running time (min)	R
O'Brien et al. (90)	6	Fast	26.2	73	165	0.99
	6	Slow	26.2	65	225	0.90
Bosch et al. (88)	17	Black and white	26.2	78.5	158	0.93
Costill (89)	1	Exhaustion	20.0	69–78	200	0.93
Adams et al. (87)	1	Heat acclimatized	26.2	—	165	0.87
Average						0.91

Note: n = sample size; R = respiratory gas exchange ratio (R = $\dot{V}CO_2/\dot{V}O_2$)

endure for several hours at the same pace. However, when MPA was given to previously endurance-trained rats, they lasted no longer on the treadmill than did untrained animals. Moreover, because arterial lactate concentration was *higher* in exhausted, MPA-blocked, trained than in untrained rats, an effect of training on Cori cycle activity was indicated. As such, the results of Turcotte and Brooks (77) represent probably the first example where endurance-trained mammals demonstrated a greater arterial lactate response to a given submaximal intensity exercise task than did untrained controls.

Perhaps the best data sets available on hepatic metabolite exchange during exercise are those of Wasserman and his colleagues (80,82) on dogs in which portal vein, hepatic vein, and arterial catheters were placed. However, the physiology of carnivorous mammals such as dogs may differ from that of other omnivorous mammals. Wasserman and colleagues observed that when exercise starts, dogs release both glucose and lactate on net bases from the liver, and it is not until considerable time has elapsed that the liver of running dogs switches to net lactate uptake (80). In dogs, alanine is a more significant gluconeogenic precursor than lactate or pyruvate. Therefore, in dogs the Cahill (glucose-alanine) cycle is a more important pathway of gluconeogenesis in submaximal exercise than is the Cori (glucose-lactate + pyruvate) cycle.

Muscle Net Lactate Release and Arterial Lactate Concentration

While it is clear that the site of blood glucose appearance during exercise is the liver, and that both hepatic glycogenolysis and gluconeogenesis are responsible for hepatic glucose production, the tissue sites responsible for blood lactate appearance during exercise are less certain. When exercise starts, arterial lactate concentration rises and stabilizes if the exercise task is constant and submaximal. Figure 25.9 shows mean arterial lactate concentrations (± SEM) of seven men studied at 100 W (50% of SL $\dot{V}O_2$max) at sea level, at the same power output upon acute exposure to 4,300 m and after 3 weeks of acclimatization to altitude (11). Stable lactate levels during exercise are interpreted to represent equivalence between appearance and disappearance (production and removal). In the past it has generally been assumed that increased lactate release from working muscle is responsible for the elevated arterial lactate concentration during exercise. However, attempts to compare arterial lactate concentrations and muscle net release (15) have yielded surprising results. When exercise begins, net lactate release from active muscle beds (net release = blood flow [v–a] lactate) increases (Figure 25.10, top). Furthermore, at 4,300 m altitude initial net lactate release from legs during cycling exercise is greater than at sea level. Increased net lactate release from working muscle beds at exercise onset compared to rest and increased muscle lactate release at altitude compared to sea level is responsible for initial elevations in arterial lactate concentration during exercise (Figure 25.9). However, as exercise continued net lactate release declined over time and varied among subjects (Figure 25.10, top). In some subjects active muscle beds switched from net release to uptake (Figure 25.10, bottom). Additionally, while the initial net lactate release from active muscle for a given exercise intensity at altitude exceeded that at sea level, the response also waned over time while arterial lactate concentration remained constant (11,15,79). Such results indicate that active muscle is not the sole source of lactate during sustained exercise at sea level or high altitude. Skin (42), liver (80), and adipose (57) have been recently identified as sites of net lactate release.

Carbohydrate Depletion and Fatigue

Results of studies on both animals (4,25) and humans (29,30,36) make it clear that muscle glycogen depletion coincides with fatigue during prolonged exercise. The reasons why glycogen depletion results in reduced exercise capacity are not

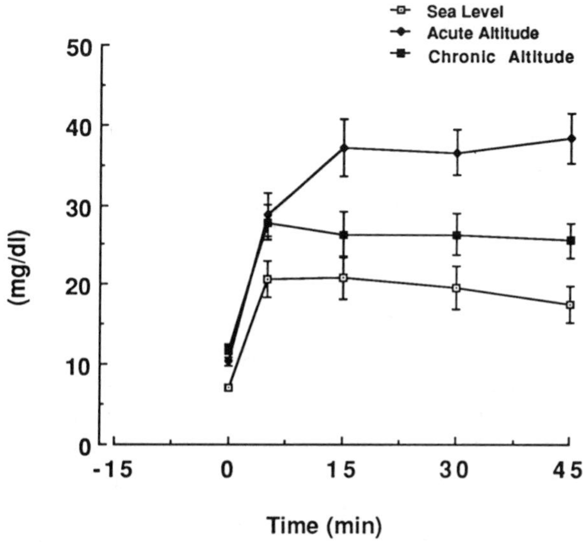

Figure 25.9 Arterial blood lactate concentration as a function of time during exercise at sea level, on acute exposure to 4,300 m altitude, and after a 3-week acclimatization. Values are means ± SEM; $n = 7$. Exercise was at 100 W which elicited 50% of sea level $\dot{V}O_2$max (reference 11).

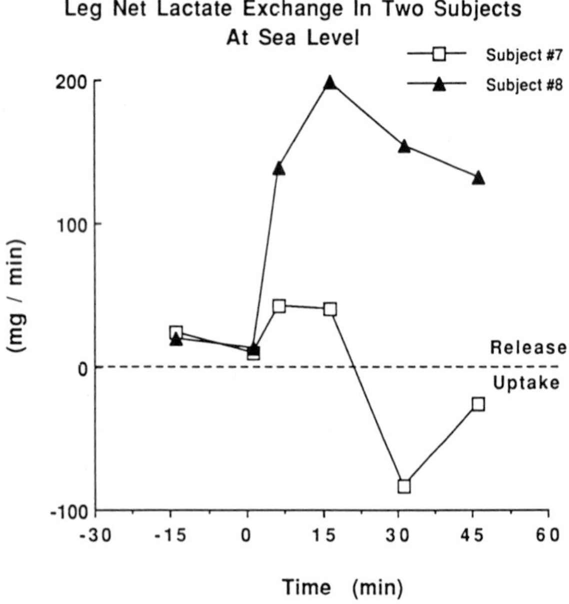

Figure 25.10 Mean (± SEM) net leg lactate release in men during rest and 45 min of exercise at 50% of $\dot{V}O_2$-max at sea level (see Figures 25.3 and 25.9). When exercise started, net lactate release rose initially, but declined over time due to net leg lactate release decline in most subjects, with some switching from release to uptake (bottom) (11,15).

clear. At first brush, the classic results correlating low muscle glycogen and fatigue can be explained as the inability of reducing equivalents from alternative substrates (e.g., blood glucose and FFA, and muscle TG) to sustain mitochondrial ATP production. However, if it is considered that some reasonable exercise capacity is possible after muscle glycogen depletion induced by prior exercise and fasting (86), then the hypothesis of a substrate limitation to explain the low correlation between muscle glycogen and reduced exercise capacity is less tenable.

In addition to supplying the major fuel source for muscle oxidation, glycogen may also provide alternative functions. One mechanism that has been suggested (13) is that rapid tricarboxylic acid cycle (TCA) turnover during exercise results in *cataplerolic* losses (e.g., loss of alphaketoglutarate to form glutamate and glutamine) (14). Though small in quantity, these losses need to be compensated for by addition of *anaplerotic* substrates to the TCA cycle. Malate (via malate dehydrogenase) and oxaloacetate (via pyruvate carboxylase) ultimately derived from carbohydrate sources may be necessary to replenish cataplerotic losses if they occur during exercise. Free fatty acids and triglycerides are not known to possess anaplerotic capabilities and the flux of anaplerotic substrates to the TCA cycle from amino acids in muscle during exercise may be too low to offset cataplerotic losses. For some time, investigators in the nutritional sciences and bioenergetics have believed that "fat burns in a CHO fire" (51). Additionally, as already discussed, glycolytically produced ATP may, for compartmental reasons, provide an essential energy source to sustain muscle contraction.

Regardless of the mechanism, or mechanisms, to explain the link between muscle glycogen depletion and fatigue, the frequency with which the events are correlated under different circumstances in diverse species leads to the conclusion that high rates of carbohydrate utilization are required to sustain prolonged, high-intensity physical exercise. Fatigue by glycogen depletion illustrates the central importance of carbohydrate utilization during exercise.

Cell Membrane Transport Limitations to Carbohydrate Exchange

Traditionally it has been thought that muscle cell glucose metabolism is uptake- (transport-) limited. In the case of untreated Type I diabetes, tissues such as resting skeletal muscle and adipose are largely unable to take up glucose despite greatly elevated levels of circulating glucose. In the case of Type I diabetes, glucose transport (uptake) into insulin-dependent cells limits glycolysis.

In other exercise-related situations the limitations to glucose utilization are less clear. Because glycogen depletion results in fatigue despite the presence of essentially normal levels of arterial glucose (most noticeably in the case of carbohydrate beverage supplementation), and because the increase in blood glucose disposal rate during exercise is far less than the overall increase in CHO oxidation, glycogen is considered to be far more important as a CHO fuel source than blood glucose during exercise. However, although it is apparent that glycogen is a more important precursor for the Embden-Meyerhof pathway (glycolysis) than glucose in muscle, it is less certain what limits glucose utilization; muscle cell uptake and phosphorylation are both considered limiting steps. When contraction starts, intramuscular glucose concentration rises (46). If the level of glucose assayed reflects intracellular, as opposed to interstitial, glucose, then phosphorylation, not transport, may in fact limit glucose entry into the Embden-Meyerhof pathway. Endurance training is known to increase hexokinase activity in skeletal muscle (52). Increased muscle hexokinase activity due to training would facilitate muscle glucose utilization during exercise.

Glucose gains entry into skeletal muscle cells by insulin-dependent as well as independent mechanisms, which may or may not be additive in function (35). In skeletal muscle the major insulin-dependent glucose transport protein is GLUT-4, which is apparently translocated to the sarcolemma from within the cell by the action of insulin. Alternatively, it may be that insulin promotes translocation of GLUT-4 to the T-tubule (24). Nevertheless, it is generally agreed that one of the major effects of insulin is to promote orientation of the transporter protein to a region of the cell surface from which the facilitated transport of glucose can take place. It was initially reported by Kern et al. (47), and subsequently independently confirmed (31), that the greater facility of red skeletal muscle for glucose uptake is associated with higher levels of GLUT-4 transporter protein. Levels and distribution of glucose transporters are probably more affected by exercise and exercise training (60,64) than are insulin receptor number or binding affinity, which are apparently unaffected by exercise or exercise training (76). The effects, if any, of exercise and exercise training on second messengers generated from insulin action need to be determined.

When exercise begins, blood glucose concentration and muscle glucose uptake increase compared to rest (1,15), but arterial insulin falls over time (10). Therefore, muscle contractions increase glucose uptake via insulin-independent mechanisms or greatly enhance the local action of insulin present. Whether or not Ca^{++}, C-AMP, or other second messengers act to facilitate muscle glucose uptake during exercise is an area of active investigation.

Whatever the intracellular factors responsible for the cause or causes of increased insulin action on muscle, exercise is known to result in major effects on glucose tolerance (48). However, the effects of exercise and exercise training on muscle are largely transient. Inactivity for several days results in loss of insulin sensitivity, whereas a single bout of activity largely restores insulin sensitivity (35).

For our present purposes in terms of understanding carbohydrate utilization during exercise, it is possible to reach the following understanding. Muscle cell glucose uptake is, to a limited extent, concentration-dependent. However, insulin and contractions greatly facilitate glucose uptake at any given arterial glucose concentration. As exercise starts, glucose rises transiently in an amount related to exercise intensity and strength of the feed-forward regulatory signals (50,71). In prolonged exercise, arterial glucose may decline over time. Insulin falls over time even if arterial glucose concentration is maintained during sustained exercise. In combination, the fall in circulating insulin and muscle local, active muscle insulin-independent mechanisms operate to shunt the available glucose production to active muscle (15). The rapidity of such effects supports the presence of a translocation or a similar effect that is insulin-independent.

Lactate, like glucose, gains entry into muscle cells by means of a cell membrane transport protein or permease (67,68). Like the family of glucose transporter proteins, there likely exists a family of lactate transporters. Lactate transporters have been shown to exist in mammalian erythrocytes (20,62), cardiocytes (70), kidney brush border cells (5), hepatocytes (22), and intestinal enterocytes (75). Two groups (44,83) have obtained data on isolated muscle tissue that clearly implicates presence of a lactate transporter. Kinetics of lactate transport across human muscle sarcolemmal vesicle preparations indicate presence of a permease (45). The various lactate transporters differ in their kinetics of transport as well as in the cation used to cotransport lactate. For example, in brush border cells, sodium is the favored cation, whereas in erythrocytes and skeletal muscle, hydrogen ion is co-transported with lactate (66–68). The transporters in various tissues differ in other ways, most notably in their sensitivity to inhibitors. The muscle lactate permease activity is apparently unaffected by insulin or any other endocrine factor. Moreover, the sarcolemmal lactate transporter is bidirectional in its action as predicted by its sensitivity to concentration and pH gradients. Therefore, presence of the transporter favors intercellular lactate exchange.

Muscle cell lactate exchange is strongly concentration-dependent. For this reason, lactate efflux from contracting fast glycolytic fibers or other cells to interstitial fluid, venous blood, and adjacent fibers with high respiratory capacity (and low internal lactate and high pH) will be facilitated. As blood courses through active muscle beds, the erythrocyte lactate transporter will facilitate loading of lactic acid into erythrocytes and therefore help to regulate acid-base balance in muscle and blood. At tissue sites of net lactate disposal (i.e., heart and liver), the presence of cell membrane lactate transporters will facilitate efflux of lactate from erythrocytes and plasma to lactate consuming tissues. Thus, the presence of lactate transporters in cell muscle and other cell membranes greatly facilitates the shuttling of lactate from production to utilization sites.

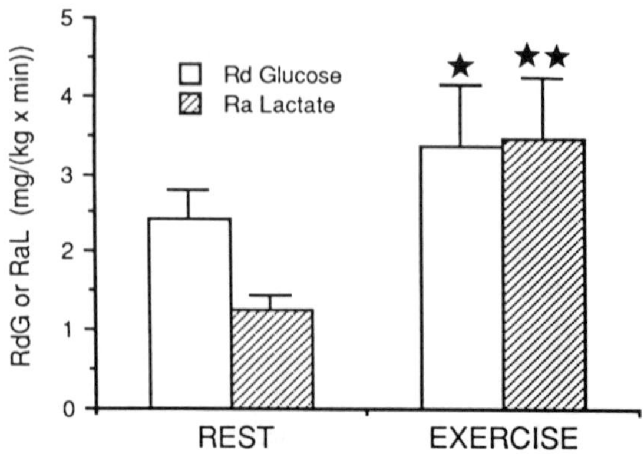

Figure 25.11 Mean values (± SEM) for glucose disappearance (RdG) and lactate appearance (RaL) at rest and after 25-30 min of leg cycling exercise at a power output eliciting 45% $\dot{V}O_2$max. Note that the relative gain in lactate flux exceeds that of glucose even in this mild exercise (74).

Relative and Absolute Magnitudes of Lactate Utilization

Importance of lactate as a fuel and a gluconeogenic precursor that maintains the overall carbohydrate energy flux sustaining exercise is supported by the several lines of evidence already described. Perhaps the most effective means to begin to comprehend the relative importance of lactate as a means of distributing carbohydrate potential energy is to compare blood lactate appearance and disappearance rates with those of glucose determined under similar circumstances, if not simultaneously. Stanley et al. (74) were the first to measure and compare glucose disappearance (Rd) and lactate appearance (Ra) rates in humans during rest and moderate-intensity exercise. These experiments were subsequent to earlier trials on rats (12,21). In resting, fasted young men, glucose Rd per unit body mass was approximately 2 mg/kg/min (74). During sustained (steady-state) exercise at 45% $\dot{V}O_2$max, glucose Rd increased approximately 75%, to about 3.5 mg/kg/min (Figure 25.11). Measured simultaneously, resting lactate Ra was about 1.0 mg/kg/min, but during exercise increased 300% to about 4 mg/kg/min. Thus, during moderate-intensity exercise the relative increase in lactate turnover far exceeded that of glucose, with the absolute rates equal to or exceeding those of glucose (74). Further, as already noted, a significant portion of blood glucose was converted to lactate prior to disposal, and the fraction of lactate disposal directed to gluconeogenesis played a significant role in supporting continued glucose production during exercise.

The initial report of Stanley et al. (74) was subsequently confirmed in the 1988 Pikes Peak experiments (10,11) in which young men were studied at rest and during submaximal exercise, at sea level and upon exposure to 4,300 m altitude. In agreement with Stanley et al., glucose Rd in resting, fasted men studied at sea level exceeded lactate Ra (Figure 25.12, top left). However, upon exposure to 4,300 m altitude, lactate Ra approximated glucose Rd, even though glucose Rd and Ra were increased by altitude exposure (Figure 25.12, top right).

Again, as in the report of Stanley et al. (74), during moderate-intensity (50% $\dot{V}O_2$max) exercise at sea level, lactate Ra approximated glucose Rd (Figure 25.12, bottom left). During exercise at altitude, glucose Rd (and Ra) exceeded that at sea level, indicating an increased dependence in response to hypobaric hypoxia. However, during exercise at 4,300 m altitude, lactate Ra far exceeded glucose Rd (Figure 25.12, bottom right). Because both arterial glucose and lactate levels were constant, it is possible to conclude that while altitude and exercise increased glucose utilization, dependency on lactate as a means of distributing carbohydrate energy was as great as or greater than the dependency on blood glucose.

Summary

In this review two themes have been emphasized. These are the importance of CHO metabolism in facilitating burst as well as prolonged exercise and the integration of CHO metabolism among cells, tissues, and organs during exercise. Cytosolic ATP production from glycolysis supports burst activity. End products of glycolysis provide most of the fuel for mitochondrial respiration. Compartmentation of glycolysis within the cell membranes of smooth and possibly other types of muscle tissues facilitates excitation–contraction coupling. Low blood glucose concentration (hypoglycemia) and

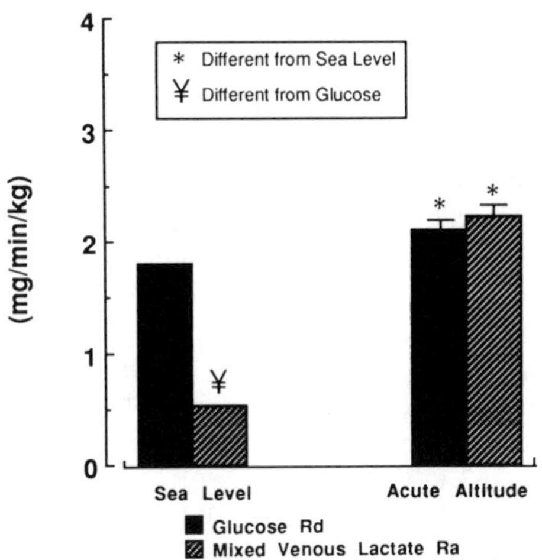

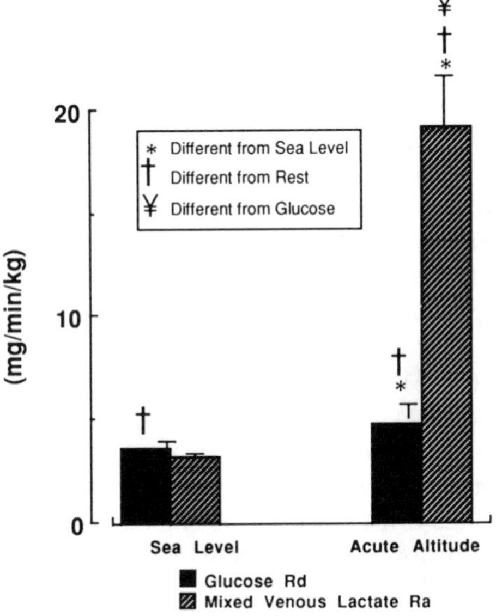

Figure 25.12 Effects of exercise and altitude exposure on blood glucose disappearance (Rd) and lactate appearance (Ra). Resting values (top) are contrasted with those determined during exercise (bottom). Statistical differences as indicated in the figure. Both altitude exposure and exercise cause increased glucose utilization. During rest at sea level, lactate Ra is less than glucose Rd, but at altitude they are not different (top). During exercise at 100 W (50% of $\dot{V}O_2$max) at sea level, glucose Rd and lactate Ra were greater than at rest, and did not differ between each other. During exercise at altitude (bottom), lactate Ra was much greater than glucose Rd, even though glucose Rd increased compared to sea level. Results indicate that during exercise lactate utilization approximates or exceeds glucose utilization (10,11).

skeletal muscle glycogen depletion result in central and skeletal muscle fatigue during exercise.

When exercise starts, hepatic glycogenolysis and gluconeogenesis increase glucose production such that arterial glucose concentration rises. In dogs the liver releases both lactate and glucose for peripheral consumption at exercise onset. Glycogenolysis in muscle and other tissue beds is under both local (contraction-induced) and global (sympathetic) control. Glycogenolysis in excess of that necessary to provide substrate for mitochondrial respiration results in release of lactate from active muscle and other tissue beds. This material then becomes available as a fuel at sites of high respiration as well as a gluconeogenic precursor. Muscle contraction and other local autoregulatory events in diverse tissues, circulating endocrine signals, and the circulation itself all play essential roles in the coordination of carbohydrate metabolism during exercise.

References

1. Ahlborg, G.; Felig, P.; Hagenfeldt, L.; Hendler, R.; Wahren, J. Substrate turnover during prolonged exercise in man. J. Clin. Invest. 53:1080-1090; 1974.
2. Ahlborg, G.; Wahren, J.; Felig, P. Splanchnic and peripheral glucose and lactate metabolism during and after prolonged arm exercise. J. Clin. Invest. 77: 690-699; 1986.
3. Azevedo, J.A.; Lehman, S.L.; Linderman, J.K.; Brooks, G.A. Glycogen turnover during exercise. Med. Sci. Sports Exerc. 24:S93; 1992.
4. Baldwin, K.M.; Campbell, P.J.; Cooke, D.A. Glycogen lactate, and alamine changes in muscle fiber types during graded exercise. J. Appl. Physiol.: Respirat. Environ. Exerc. Physiol. 43:288-291; 1977.
5. Barac-Nieto, M.; Murer, H.; Kinne, R. Lactate-sodium cotransport in rat renal brush border membrane. Am. J. Physiol. 239:F496-F506; 1980.
6. Basaglia, F. Some aspects of isozymes of lactate dehydrogenase malate dehydrogenase and glycosephosphate isomerase in fish. Comp. Biochem. Physiol. 92B:213-226; 1989.
7. Bennett, A.F. The evolution of activity capacity. J. Exp. Biol. 160:1-23; 1991.
8. Brooks, G.A. Lactate: Glycolytic end product and oxidative substrate during sustained exercise in mammals—The "lactate shuttle." In: Gilles, R., ed. Circulation, respiration, and metabolism. Berlin: Springer-Verlag; 1985:208-218.

9. Brooks, G.A.; Brauner, K.E.; Cassens, R.G. Glycogen synthesis and the metabolism of lactic acid after exercise. Am. J. Physiol. 224:1162-1166; 1973.
10. Brooks, G.A.; Butterfield, G.E.; Wolfe, R.R.; Groves, B.M.; Mazzeo, R.S.; Sutton, J.R.; Wolfel, E.E.; Reeves, J.T. Increased dependence on blood glucose after acclimatization to 4,300m. J. Appl. Physiol. 70:919-927; 1991.
11. Brooks, G.A.; Butterfield, G.E.; Wolfe, R.R.; Groves, B.M.; Mazzeo, R.S.; Sutton, J.R.; Wolfel, E.E.; Reeves, J.T. Decreased reliance on lactate during exercise after acclimatization to 4,300m. J. Appl. Physiol. 71:333-341; 1991.
12. Brooks, G.A.; Donovan, C.M. Effect of endurance training on glucose kinetics during exercise. Am. J. Physiol. 244(Endocrinol. Metab. 7):E505-E512; 1983.
13. Brooks, G.A.; Fahey, T.D. Fundamentals of human performance. New York: Macmillan; 1986:76-78.
14. Brooks, G.A.; Gaesser, G.A. End points of lactate and glucose metabolism after exhausting exercise. J. Appl. Physiol.: Respirat. Environ. Exerc. Physiol. 49:1057-1069; 1980.
15. Brooks, G.A.; Wolfel, E.E.; Groves, B.M.; Bender, P.R.; Butterfield, G.E.; Cymerman, A.; Mazzeo, R.S.; Sutton, J.R.; Wolfe, R.R.; Reeves, J.T. Muscle accounts for glucose disposal but not blood lactate appearance during exercise after acclimatization to 4,300m. J. Appl. Physiol.; [In press].
16. Chance, B.; Williams, G.R. The respiratory chain and oxidative phosphorylation. Adv. Enzymol. 17:65-134; 1956.
17. Costill, D.L.; Sparks, K.; Gregor, R.; Turner, C. Muscle glycogen utilization during exhaustive running. J. Appl. Physiol. 31:353-356; 1971.
18. Crawford, D.L.; Constantine, H.R.; Powers, D.A. Lactic dehydrogenase fundulus heteroclitus: Evolutionary implications. Mol. Biol. Evol. 6:369-383; 1989.
19. Davies, K.J.A.; Packer, L.; Brooks, G.A. Biochemical adaptation of mitochondria, muscle and whole-animal respiration to endurance training. Arch. Biochem. Biophys. 209:539-554; 1981.
20. Deuticke, B. Monocarboxylate transport in erythrocytes. J. Membr. Biol. 70:89-103; 1982.
21. Donovan, C.M.; Brooks, G.A. Endurance training affects lactate clearance, not lactate production. Am. J. Physiol. 244:E83-E92; 1983.
22. Fafournoux, P.; Demigne, C.; Remsey, C. Carrier-mediated uptake of lactate in rat hepatocytes. J. Biol. Chem. 260:293-299; 1985.
23. Favier, R.J.; Constable, S.H.; Chen, M.; Holloszy, J.O. Endurance exercise training reduces lactate production. J. Appl. Physiol. 61:885-889; 1986.
24. Friedman, J.E.; Sherman, W.M.; Reed, M.J.; Elton, C.W.; Dohm, G.L. Exercise training increases glucose transporter protein GLUT-4 in skeletal muscle of obese Zucker (fa/fa) rats. FEBS Lett. 268:13-16; 1990.
25. Gaesser, G.A.; Brooks, G.A. Glycogen repletion following continuous and intermittent exercise to exhaustion. J. Appl. Physiol. 49:722-728; 1980.
26. Gertz, E.W.; Wisneski, J.A.; Neese, R.; Bristow, J.A.; Searle, G.L.; Hanlon, J.T. Myocardial lactate metabolism: Evidence of lactate release during net chemical extraction in man. Circulation. 63:1273-1279; 1981.
27. Gertz, E.W.; Wisneski, J.A.; Stanley, W.C.; Neese, R.A. Myocardial substrate utilization during exercise in humans: Dual carbon-labeled carbohydrate isotope experiments. J. Clin. Invest. 82:2017-2025; 1988.
28. Gleeson, T.T. Patterns of metabolic recovery from amphibians and reptiles. J. Exp. Biol. 160:187-207; 1991.
29. Gollnick, P.D.; Armstrong, R.B.; Saubert, C.W.; Sembrowich, W.L.; Shepherd, R.E.; Saltin, B. Glycogen depletion patterns in human skeletal muscle fibers during prolonged work. Pflugers Arch. 33:1-12; 1973.
30. Gollnick, P.D.; Armstrong, R.B.; Sembrowich, W.L.; Shepherd, R.E.; Saltin, B. Glycogen depletion pattern in human skeletal muscle fibers after heavy exercise. J. Appl. Physiol. 34:615-618; 1973.
31. Goodyear, L.J.; Hirshman, M.F.; Smith, R.J.; Horton, E.S. Glucose transporter number, activity, and isoform content in plasma membranes of red and white skeletal muscle. Am. J. Physiol. (Endocrinol. Metab.) 24:E556-E561; 1991.
32. Gregg, S.G.; Mazzeo, R.S.; Budinger, T.F.; Brooks, G.A. Acute anemia increases lactate production and decreases clearance during exercise. J. Appl. Physiol. 67:756-764; 1989.
33. Henneman, E.; Olson, C. Relations between structure and function in the design of skeletal muscles. J. Neurophysiol. 28:581-598; 1965.
34. Holloszy, J.O. Effects of exercise on mitochondrial oxygen uptake, and respiratory enzyme activity in skeletal muscle. J. Biol. Chem. 242:2278-2282; 1967.
35. Horton, E.S. Exercise and physical training effects on insulin sensitivity and glucose metabolism. Diabetes Metab. Rev. 1:1-17; 1986.
36. Hultman, E. Physiological role of muscle glycogen in man, with special reference to exercise. Physiology of muscular exercise. Monograph 15. New York: American Heart

Association; 1967:I99-I112. Circulation. RC 681 A105.

37. Hutber, C.A.; Bonen, A. Glycogenesis in muscle and liver during exercise. J. Appl. Physiol. 66:2811-2817; 1989.
38. Issekutz, B., Jr. Role of β-adrenergic receptors in mobilization of energy sources in exercising dogs. J. Appl. Physiol.: Respirat. Environ. Exerc. Physiol. 44:869-876; 1978.
39. Issekutz, B., Jr. Effect of β-adrenergic blockade on lactate turnover in exercising dogs. J. Appl. Physiol. 57:1754-1759; 1984.
40. Issekutz, B., Jr.; Shaw, W.A.S.; Issekutz, A.C. Lactate metabolism in resting and exercising dogs. J. Appl. Physiol. 40:312-319; 1976.
41. John-Alder, H.B.; McAlister, R.M.; Terjung, R.L. Reduced running endurance in gluconeogenesis-inhibited rats. Am. J. Physiol. 251:R137-R142; 1986.
42. Johnson, J.A.; Fusaro, R.M. The role of skin in carbohydrate metabolism. Adv. Metab. Disord. 6:1-55; 1972.
43. Jones, W.L.; Heigenheuser, G.J.F; Kuksis, A; Matos, C.G.; Sutton, J.R.; Toews, C.J. Fat metabolism in heavy exercise. Clin. Sci. 59:469-478; 1980.
44. Juel, C. Intracellular pH recovery and lactate efflux in mouse soleus muscle stimulated in vitro: The involvement of sodium/protein exchange and a lactate carrier. Acta. Physiol. Scand. 132:363-371; 1988.
45. Juel, C. Human muscle lactate transport can be studied in sarcolemmal giant vesicles mode from needle-biopsies. Acta. Physiol. Scand. 142:133-134; 1991.
46. Katz, A.; Broberg, S.; Sahlin, K.; Wahren, J. Leg glucose uptake during maximal dynamic exercise in humans. Am. J. Physiol. (Endocrinol. Metab.) 14:E65-E70; 1986.
47. Kern, M.; Wells, J.A.; Stephens, J.M.; Elton, C.W.; Friedman, J.E.; Tapscott, E.B.; Pekala, P.H.; Dohm, G.L. Insulin responsiveness in skeletal muscle is determined by glucose transporter (GLUT4) protein level. Biochem. J. 270:397-400; 1990.
48. King, D.S.; Dalsky, G.P.; Staten, M.A.; Clutter, W.E.; Van Houten, D.R.; Holloszy, I.O. Insulin action and secretion in endurance-trained and untrained humans. J. Appl. Physiol. 63:2247-2252; 1987.
49. Kirkwood, S.P.; Packer, L.; Brooks, G.A. Effects of endurance training on a mitochondrial reticulum in limb skeletal muscle. Arch. Biochem. Biophys. 255:80-88; 1987.
50. Kjaer, M.; Farrell, P.A.; Chistensen, N.J.; Galbo, H. Increased epinephrine response and inaccurate glucoregulation in exercising athletes. J. Appl. Physiol. 61:1693-1700; 1986.
51. Kleiber, M. The fire of life: An introduction to animal energetics. New York: Krieger; 1975.
52. Lamb, D.R.; Peter, J.B.; Jeffries, R.N.; Wallace, H.A. Glycogen, hexokinase, and glycogen synthesis adaptation to exercise. Am. J. Physiol. 217:1628-1632; 1969.
53. Long, G.L. The stereospecific distribution and evolutionary significance of invertebrate lactic dehydrogenases. Comp. Biochem. Physiol. 55B:77-83; 1976.
54. Mazzeo, R.S.; Bender, P.R.; Brooks, G.A.; Butterfield, G.E.; Groves, B.M.; Sutton, J.R.; Wolfel, E.E.; Reeves, J.T. Arterial catecholamine responses during exercise with acute and chronic high-altitude exposure. Am. J. Physiol. (Endocrinol. Metab. 24) 261:E419-E424; 1991.
55. Mazzeo, R.S.; Brooks, G.A.; Schoeller, D.A.; Budinger, T.F. Disposal of blood [1-^{13}C] lactate in humans during rest and exercise. J. Appl. Physiol. 60:232-241; 1986.
56. McDermott, J.C.; Elder, G.C.B.; Bonen, A. Nonexercising muscle metabolism during exercise. Pflugers Arch. 418:301-307; 1991.
57. Newby, F.D.; Wilson, L.K.; Thacker, S.V.; DiGorolamo, M. Adipocyte lactate production remains elevated during refeeding after fasting. Am. J. Physiol. (Endocrinol. Metab. 22) 259:E865-E871; 1990.
58. Noakes, T.D.; Opie, L.H. Substrates for maximum mechanical function in isolated perfused working heart. J. Appl. Cardiol. 4:391-405; 1989.
59. Paul, R.J.; Hardin, C.D.; Raeymaekers, L.; Wuytack, G.; Casteels, R. Preferential support of Ca^{++} uptake in smooth muscle plasma membrane vesicles by endogenesis glycolytic cascade. FASEB J. 3:2298-2301; 1989.
60. Plough, T.; Sallkinecht, B.M.; Poders, O.; Kahn, B.B.; Ohkuwa, T.; Vinten, J.; Galbo, H. Effect of endurance training on glucose transport capacity and glucose transporter expression in rat skeletal muscle. Am. J. Physiol. (Endocrinol. Metab. 22) 259:E778-E786; 1990.
61. Podolin, D.A.; Munger, P.A.; Mazzeo, R.S. Plasma catecholamine and lactate response during graded exercise with varied glycogen conditions. J. Appl. Physiol. 71:1407-1433; 1991.
62. Poole, R.C.; Halestrap, A.P. Identification and partial purification of the erythrocyte L-lactate transporter. Biochem. J. 283:855-862; 1992.
63. Richter, E.A.; Galbo, H. High glycogen levels enhance glycogen breakdown in isolated contracting skeletal muscle. J. Appl. Physiol. 61:827-831; 1986.
64. Richter, E.A.; Garetto, L.P.; Goodman, M.N.; Ruderman, N.B. Enhanced muscle glucose metabolism after exercise: Modulation by local

factors. Am. J. Physiol. (Endocrinol. Metab. 9) 246:E476-E482; 1984.
65. Richter, E.A.; Kienes, B.; Saltin, B.; Christensen, N.J.; Savard, G. Skeletal muscle glucose uptake during dynamic exercise in humans: Role of muscle mass. Am. J. Physiol. 254:E555-E561; 1988.
66. Roth, D.A. The sarcolemmal lactate transporter: Transmembrane determinants of lactate flux. Med. Sci. Sports Exerc. 23:925-934; 1991.
67. Roth, D.A.; Brooks, G.A. Lactate transport is mediated by a membrane-borne carrier in rat skeletal muscle sarcolemmal vesicles. Arch. Biochem. Biophys. 279:377-385; 1990.
68. Roth, D.A.; Brooks, G.A. Lactate and pyruvate transport is dominated using a pH gradient-sensitive carrier in rat skeletal muscle sarcolemmal vesicles. Arch. Biochem. Biophys. 279:386-394; 1990.
69. Ruben, J.A.; Bennett, A.F. Antiquity of the vertebrate pattern of activity metabolism and its possible relation to vertebrate origins. Nature. 286:886-888; 1980.
70. Seiler, S.M.; Cragoe, E.J.; Jones, L.R. Demonstration of a Na^+/H^+ exchange activity in purified canine cardiac sarcolemmal vesicles. J. Biol. Chem. 260:4869-4876; 1985.
71. Sonne, B.; Mikines, K.J.; Richter, E.A.; Christensen, N.J.; Galbo, H. Role of liver nerves and adrenal medulla in glucose turnover of running rats. J. Appl. Physiol. 59:1640-1646; 1985.
72. Spriet, L.L.; Soderlund, K.; Bergstron, M.; Hultman, E. Anaerobic energy release in skeletal muscle during electrical stimulation in men. J. Appl. Physiol. 62:611-615; 1987.
73. Stanley, W.C.; Gertz, E.W.; Wisneski, J.A.; Neese, R.A.; Morris, D.L.; Brooks, G.A. Lactate extraction during net lactate release in legs of humans during exercise. J. Appl. Physiol. 60:1116-1120; 1986.
74. Stanley, W.C.; Wisneski, J.A.; Gertz, E.W.; Neese, R.A.; Brooks, G.A. Glucose and lactate interrelations during moderate intensity exercise in man. Metabolism. 37:850-858; 1988.
75. Storelli, C.; Corcelli, A.; Cassano, G.; Hildman, B.; Murer, H.; Lippe, C. Polar distribution of sodium-dependent and sodium-independent transport system for L-lactate in the plasma membrane of enterocytes. Pflugers Arch. 330:11-16; 1980.
76. Treadway, J.L.; James, D.E.; Burcel, E.; Ruderman, N.B. Effect of exercise on insulin receptor binding and kinase activity in skeletal muscle. Am. J. Physiol. (Endocrinol. Metab. 19) 256:E138-E144; 1989.
77. Turcotte, L.P.; Brooks, G.A. Effects of training on glucose metabolism of gluconeogenesis-inhibited, short-term fasted rats. J. Appl. Physiol. 68:944-954; 1990.
78. Turcotte, L.P.; Rovner, A.S.; Roark, R.R.; Brooks, G.A. Glucose kinetics in gluconeogenesis-inhibited rats during rest and exercise. Am. J. Physiol. (Endocrinol. Metab. 21):E203-E211; 1990.
79. Wahren, J.; Felig, P.; Ahlborg, G; Jorfeldt, L. Glucose metabolism during leg exercise in man. J. Clin. Invest. 50:2715-2725; 1971.
80. Wasserman, D.H.; Lacey, D.B.; Green, D.R.; Williams, P.E.; Cherrington, A.D. Dynamics of hepatic lactate and glucose balances during prolonged exercise and recovery in the dog. J. Appl. Physiol. 63:2411-2417; 1987.
81. Wasserman, D.H.; Lacy, D.B.; Bracy, D.; Williams, P.E. Metabolic regulation in peripheral tissues and the transition to an increased gluconeogenic mode during prolonged exercise. Am. J. Physiol. 263 (Endocrinol. Metab. 26):E345-E354; 1992.
82. Wasserman, D.H.; Williams, P.E.; Lacy, D.B.; Goldstein, R.E.; Cherrington, A.D. Exercise-induced fall in insulin and hepatic carbohydrate metabolism during muscular work. Am. J. Physiol. 256:E500-E509; 1989.
83. Watt, P.W.; MacLennan, P.A.; Hundal, H.S.; Kuret, C.M.; Rennie, M.J. L(+)-lactate transport in perfused rat skeletal muscle. Kinetic characteristics and sensitivity to pH and transport inhibitors. Biochim. Biophys. Acta. 944:213-222; 1988.
84. Winder, W.W. Role of cyclic AMP in regulation of hepatic glucose production during exercise. Med. Sci. Sports Exerc. 20:551-560; 1988.
85. Winder, W.W., Fisher, S.R.; Gygi, S.P.; Mitchell, J.A.; Ojuka, E.; Weidman, D.A. Divergence of muscle and liver fructose 2, 6-diphosphate in fasting exercising rats. Am. J. Physiol. (Endocrinol. Metab. 23) 260:E756-E761; 1991.
86. Zinker, B.A.; Britz, K.; Brooks, G.A. Effects of a 36-hour fast on human endurance and substrate utilization. J. Appl. Physiol. 69:1849-1855; 1990.
87. Adams, W.C.; Fox, R.H.; Fry, A.J.; MacDonald, I.C. Thermoregulation during marathon running in cool, moderate, and hot environments. J. Appl. Physiol. 38:1030-1037; 1975.
88. Bosch, A.N.; Goslin, B.R.; Noakes, T.D.; Dennis, S.R. Physiological differences between black and white runners during a treadmill marathon. Evr. J. Appl. Physiol. 61:68-72; 1990.
89. Costill, D.C. Metabolic responses during distance running. J. Appl. Physiol. 28:251-257; 1970.
90. O'Brien, M.J.; Viguie, C.A.; Mazzeo, R.S.; Brooks, G.A. Carbohydrate dependence during marathon running. Med. Sci. Sports Exerc.; (In press).

Chapter 26

Physical Activity, Lipid and Lipoprotein Metabolism, and Lipid Transport

Marcia L. Stefanick
Peter D. Wood

From the moment physical activity is initiated, fuel requirements of working muscle increase significantly from rest. The role and metabolic fate of fat as an energy source for exercise have been described previously in several excellent reviews that serve as references for much of the information presented in this chapter (8,19,22,40,43,60).

Fat, one of the primary energy sources at rest, is oxidized in progressively increasing amounts as total energy expenditure increases with exercise. By this means, lipids (fats) may cover up to 90% of the oxidative metabolism in prolonged exercise of moderate intensity (less than 50% of maximal oxygen intake, $\dot{V}O_2max$). Between 1 and 4 hr of prolonged exercise the uptake of free fatty acids by muscle rises by 70% such that the relative contribution of fatty acids to total oxygen use is twice that of carbohydrates after 4 hours (19). One of the adaptations that characterizes the trained state is an even greater reliance on free fatty acid oxidation during submaximal exercise (27). At high-intensity work (greater than 70% $\dot{V}O_2max$), fat is used in decreasing amounts for energy expenditure and glycogen becomes the predominant energy source. During such efforts, glycogen is quickly depleted and exercise must stop or intensity must be reduced.

Evidence for these changes in fuel sources is found in the respiratory exchange ratio (R-value or the ratio of the rate of carbon dioxide produced metabolically to the rate of oxygen consumed), which is also referred to as the respiratory quotient (RQ). Fat combustion corresponds to an R-value of 0.7, while glucose combustion has an R-value of 1.00. It is worth noting that the R-value of the total body reflects the relative contribution of fat versus carbohydrate as an energy source in all of the body's tissues combined. The RQ of the brain, which generally consumes glucose, is integrated with that of slow-twitch oxidative skeletal muscle and cardiac muscle, for which fatty acids are the preferred energy source, as well as other tissues. A typical R-value of an individual is 0.80 to 0.85 at rest. This decreases with prolonged, mild exercise, as fat is increasingly oxidized in active muscles. The R-value increases as work intensity increases, reflecting greater glucose oxidation.

The class of compounds described as lipids, which are characterized by their general insolubility in water and solubility in organic solvents, is quite diverse; however, the only lipids that serve as important metabolic fuels are free fatty acids (FFA). These are lipids with the basic structure $CH_3(CH_2)_nCOOH$ and their storage form, triacylglycerols, which are generally referred to as triglycerides (TG) and are esters produced by the condensation of three FFA units with glycerol. The concentration of FFA in the blood is quite low at rest and relatively little fat is stored in muscle; therefore, lipids must be mobilized, primarily from adipose tissue, and transported to the working muscle. At least 50% of the fat oxidized during exercise comes from plasma FFA. The remaining fat is thought to be supplied by intramuscular triglyceride stores and circulating plasma triglycerides, the latter being particularly available in the fed state, especially if fat is consumed.

This review of the effects of physical activity on lipid metabolism and transport is organized around the primary tissues involved, focusing first on oxidation of fatty acids in active muscles, utilization of intramuscular and circulating triglycerides, and uptake of circulating FFA, then focusing on the lipolysis, liberation, and transport of FFA from adipose tissue sites, and the balance between muscle utilization and FFA mobilization. Specific roles for given fatty acids (i.e., possible preferential use during exercise) is only briefly mentioned. Dietary factors that influence lipid metabolism during exercise are also only briefly acknowledged;

however, these may be extremely important when interpreting results from cross-sectional studies of active versus sedentary individuals or from longitudinal studies in which diet differs markedly between groups or has not been held constant during the training period. The impact of acute exercise effects or training-induced changes in lipid metabolism on circulating lipoproteins and lipoprotein metabolism is also addressed. This follows a brief discussion of differential effects of sympathetic stimulation and exercise on regional adiposity, which has been repeatedly shown to relate to the lipoprotein profile in sedentary men and women (11,15,61,62,74).

Skeletal and Cardiac Muscle

To utilize lipids as fuel, muscle must take up, activate, and translocate FFA into mitochondria to supply acetyl coenzyme A (CoA) to the citric acid cycle. Sources of FFA for oxidation include intramuscular triglycerides (hydrolyzed within the muscle fiber), circulating triglycerides (hydrolyzed on the surface of the muscle capillary endothelium by lipoprotein lipase [LPL]), and circulating FFA (hydrolyzed by hormone-sensitive lipase within adipose tissue cells, released into the blood, and transported to the active muscle).

Oxidation of Fatty Acids in Muscles

Once located on the inside of the plasma membrane, free fatty acids are converted to fatty acyl-CoA and as such may either be reesterified and stored as triacylglycerol or transported over the mitochondrial membrane into the mitochondrial matrix where they are β-oxidized. For each individual there is a close relationship between arterial FFA concentration and the amount of FFA that is taken up and oxidized in muscles; however, as Hurley et al. (28) pointed out, the rate at which muscles oxidize FFA is determined by the concentration of FFA in the cytoplasm to which the mitochondria are exposed. Therefore increased lipolysis of intramuscular triglycerides or circulating triglycerides could also increase FFA oxidation.

Fat metabolism can only be used under aerobic conditions. The oxidation of FFA is determined by the availability of FFA and the capacity of tissues to oxidize FFA. Both cardiac and skeletal muscle are metabolically oxidative; however, mitochondria are few in number in fast-twitch glycolytic (FG, Type IIb) muscle fiber. It is the slow-twitch oxidative (SO, Type I) muscle fibers that are responsible for most skeletal muscle oxidation of FFA. SO fibers have a large number of mitochondria, are well-vascularized, contain myoglobin, and are primarily activated during exercise of moderate intensity. The relative amount of SO versus FG muscle fiber contributes to an individual's ability to utilize fat metabolism.

It is well known that the primary physiological source of energy for muscle function is adenosine triphosphate (ATP) and that mitochondrial oxidative phosphorylation is quantitatively the most important process supplying ATP to the muscle. The contribution of lipid oxidation to total oxidative metabolism is dependent on the relative work load. If the concentration of ATP in the muscle fiber falls below a certain level, as when muscle contraction commences, a series of events increases the catalytic activity of key enzymes in glycolysis (39). Due to mobilization of lipids from adipose tissue, a rising fatty acid concentration in the blood leads to an increase in fatty acid oxidation in the muscle, which increases the effectiveness of ATP as a feedback inhibitor of glycolysis. Fatty acids inhibit glucose uptake, glycolysis, and glycogenolysis in heart and skeletal muscle. Glucose and glycogen utilization decreases. In the absence of glucose utilization, fat is capable of sustaining only the lowest work intensities. If the demand for energy increases, carbohydrate utilization increases until muscle glycogen stores are depleted, at which point the energy demand must decrease or exercise must stop.

Training Effects

Endurance training enhances the capacity of skeletal muscle to utilize free fatty acids as fuel during heavy exercise. Using the single-leg training method in which the other leg serves as the sedentary control, Henriksson (27) showed that the degree of FFA utilization was higher in the trained leg than in the untrained leg, indicating a difference in preference for substrate. This observation was confirmed by Kiens and Saltin (31), who demonstrated a 40% higher activity of β-OH-acyl CoA-dehydrogenase (HAD), the enzyme needed for β-oxidation of fatty acids. The absolute number and size of mitochondria in skeletal muscle, particularly the slow-twitch red fibers, increases with training, resulting in an increased concentration of enzymes for the citric acid cycle and electron transfer system, as well as for fatty acid oxidation (52). These changes increase the fat oxidation capability and thus the ability to rely on fat as a source of energy during submaximal exercise. Endurance training also results in an increased capillarization of skeletal muscle that (a) increases delivery of oxygen, (b) increases the surface area for transport of FFAs into the muscle, (c) increases exposure of circulating triglycerides to skeletal muscle LPL as well as a number of blood-borne regulatory factors, and (d) facilitates removal of wastes.

Intramuscular Triacylglycerols

A small amount of fat is stored as lipid droplets within the cytosol of muscle cells, ranging from 7 to 25 µmol/g wet muscle. The TG concentration in working muscle decreases during prolonged exercise, particularly in the high-oxidative, red skeletal muscle fibers (60). A 5:1 ratio of TG concentration in SO versus FG muscle fibers was reported in trained subjects before an 85 km skiing race; during the race lipid stores decreased significantly in slow-twitch fibers only (35). Using radiolabeled free fatty acids, Havel, Penrow, and Jones (26) showed that only 50% of the lipid oxidized during exercise is derived from circulating FFA and that only a portion of the FFA taken up by the muscle after exercise was immediately oxidized, suggesting that the rest was used to replenish intramuscular triacylglycerol stores. Inhibition of lipolysis with a nicotinic acid analog, which abolished the rise in plasma FFA during exercise, decreased the rate of lipid oxidation by only 50%, further suggesting that an additional source of lipid such as intramuscular or circulating triglycerides makes a significant contribution to the provision of FFA for exercising muscles (69).

Oscai and Palmer (44) have proposed that an intracellular lipase, generally thought to be the precursor for endothelium-bound lipoprotein lipase (LPL), functions as a mobilizer of free fatty acids from endogenous triglyceride stores. They reported that activity of this lipase increased in the heart after one bout of activity. The increase was related to exercise intensity. Furthermore, free fatty acid levels were elevated in the intracellular fraction of muscle at a time when this intracellular lipoprotein lipase activity was elevated. Adrenaline increased the activity of this enzyme in skeletal and cardiac muscle and glucagon was shown to increase intracellular LPL activity in the heart, with a concomitant reduction in endogenous triglyceride levels (44).

A release of glycerol (reflecting lipolysis) was observed from the quadriceps muscle in men during prolonged exercise, suggesting that TG within muscle was used, but muscle fiber TG was barely changed (31). It was suggested that methodological problems involving contamination from extrafiber TG from fat deposits found within the confines of the muscle, but outside the muscle fiber, may have led to overestimates of intramuscular TG utilization during exercise (22). It may be, however, that intramuscular TG are quickly restored by circulating triglycerides and FFA, including FFA from extrafiber adipocytes, such that the role of intrafiber TG has been underestimated. Methodological issues must be carefully considered in studies that will be designed to resolve this controversy.

Training Effects

Following a strenuous 12-week program of endurance exercise, the decrease in quadriceps muscle triglyceride concentration after prolonged exercise was roughly twice as great relative to the untrained state, and the quantity of fatty acids released by lipolysis of muscle triglycerides could, if completely oxidized, account for the increased proportion (from 35% to 57%) of caloric expenditure derived from fat in the trained state (28). Employing the single-leg training model, Kiens and Saltin (31) reported a greater release of glycerol from the quadriceps muscle in the trained leg than the untrained leg during prolonged exercise, suggesting that TG within muscle was hydrolyzed, which partially accounted for increased lipid utilization observed during exercise in the trained versus untrained muscle.

Circulating Triglycerides and Muscle Lipoprotein Lipase

More than 95% of the triglyceride that circulates through the human bloodstream is carried in chylomicrons, which are produced in the intestine after ingestion of fat, or in very low-density lipoproteins secreted by the liver. Chylomicrons are generally metabolized within hours of ingesting a fat meal and are virtually absent in fasting plasma of normolipemic individuals, as they have a half life of 5 to 15 min in the blood. Plasma triglycerides represent another potential source of fatty acid substrate for moderate exercise. Numerous studies have shown that the circulating TG content can decrease during prolonged exercise (60,64) such as a marathon run (51); however, the time course of the effect of a single exercise bout seems to be critical in demonstrating the role of very low density lipoprotein (VLDL) triglyceride fatty acids as a fuel for exercising muscle. Triglycerides were reduced by 30% immediately following a 70-km cross-country ski race, were still low on the following day, but were restored to normal 2 days after the race (18). An increase in the clearance rate of TG was reduced 1 and 2 days after a 3-hr exercise bout on an ergocycle at 77% $\dot{V}O_2max$, but not within hours of the event (1).

Whereas a 45-min bout of moderate-intensity exercise does not generally bring about decreases in triglyceride concentrations in fasting, normolipemic subjects, such exercise has been shown to temporarily decrease plasma TG concentration in hypertriglyceridemic subjects (45) and to enhance the clearance of triglycerides in people with normal, as well as elevated, fasting triglyceride levels after they have ingested a fat-containing meal (41). Chylomicron fatty acids may be utilized in substantial quantities during the postprandial period (40). A single bout of postprandial exercise at 40% $\dot{V}O_2max$ reduced alimentary lipemia by 34% and was accompanied by higher free-glycerol and FFA concentrations than was found following the meal alone (54).

The clearance rate of exogenous fat increased 76% and fasting triglyceride levels decreased 26% less than 24 hr after a marathon run by elite athletes (relative to levels before the race) (51), and endurance training increased TG disappearance following intravenous administration of fat by 24 ± 24% after 14 weeks and 49 ± 18% after 32 to 48 weeks (65). In studies with elite bicyclists, 70% more fat was oxidized during exercise after consumption of a high-fat diet compared with a low-fat diet (48). High-fat diets increase LPL activity and the TG concentration in quadriceps muscles of trained men (29), suggesting a role for LPL in replenishing intramuscular TG stores. Therefore, in a postprandial state, the circulating TG pool represents a relatively rich source of lipid substrate for oxidation during exercise.

Both myocardium and skeletal muscles, particularly the Type I (SO) fibers, possess a high activity of lipoprotein lipase (LPL), which is synthesized within the muscle fiber, then secreted and localized on the surface of the endothelial cells of capillaries. The degradation of triglyceride-rich particles, largely dependent on the activity of LPL and the uptake of fatty acids from plasma triglycerides, is at rest directly related to the activity of this enzyme. Following cross-sectional observations that endurance-trained men and women had higher skeletal muscle LPL activity than sedentary controls (42), Lithell, Orlander, Schele, Sjodin, and Karlsson reported that a prolonged, exhaustive exercise (an 85-km, 8-hr ski race) was followed by a threefold average increase in muscle LPL activity, in spite of repeated food intake during the exercise (35). The increase in muscle LPL activity was inversely correlated with fitness level ($\dot{V}O_2max$), being as much as sixfold greater in the least fit men.

Similarly, a 20-km run in the fasting state resulted in a twofold increase in skeletal muscle LPL (59). Lithell, Cedermark, Froberg, Tesch, and Karlsson also reported that muscle LPL was increased in men for at least 12 hr after days of heavy work during a 10-day march with heavy packs and decreased after days of rest (34). Adaptation to a high-fat diet increased skeletal muscle LPL activity in the trained leg of a single-leg training program, resulting in a higher capacity for uptake of fatty acids from circulating triglycerides, as well as increased triglyceride content in the trained muscle (29), suggesting that LPL may serve to replete intramuscular TG.

Training Effects

Endurance training increased resting muscle LPL activity in sedentary men of average weight who trained on cycle ergometers for 8 weeks (57). Subjects placed on a metabolic diet during physical exercise conditioning, such that weight loss was prevented, showed a decrease in fasting triglyceride levels and decreased postprandial chylomicron levels by 37% (71). An elegant study by Kiens and Lithell (30) showed significant increases in men in muscle LPL activity of knee extensors of one leg that underwent 8 weeks of dynamic exercise training compared to the other leg that was not exercised. The increase in muscle LPL activity was accompanied by a markedly higher arteriovenous VLDL triglyceride difference in the trained thigh at rest, demonstrating greater VLDL–TG uptake in this leg. Rather than acting as a direct source of fuel during exercise, plasma triglycerides may serve a more important role in restoring intramuscular TG stores after an exercise bout (40). Intramuscular lipid stores are quantitatively larger in physically well-trained than untrained subjects (35).

Uptake of Plasma Free Fatty Acids (FFA)

Uptake of FFA from blood to cells is a simple concentration-dependent process not requiring energy supply. The transfer is rapid. At the very beginning of exercise, the working skeletal muscles preferentially utilize their own glycogen stores (and perhaps endogenous triglycerides) such that the fractional FFA uptake may drop initially; however, the increased blood flow to exercising muscle results in increased FFA uptake by the muscle and an initial decrease in arterial FFA concentration (40). As FFA are mobilized from adipose tissue, arterial FFA concentrations increase such that excessive FFA is offered to the exercising muscle; however, only about 5% of the offered substrate is actually taken up by the muscle (52).

A control system, the glucose-fatty acid cycle, is thought to ensure that when glucose and fatty acids are both available to the muscle, the latter are preferentially used in energy production; any deficit is made up by glucose oxidation (39). The effect of increasing plasma concentration of FFA on substrate utilization in muscle during exercise was recently investigated following infusion of intralipid; the net uptake of FFA and the R-value across the active muscle was unchanged, whereas uptake of ketone bodies was increased (24). The researchers suggested that direct inhibition of glucose transport by increasing lipid and lipid metabolites was responsible for the effects rather than the glucose-fatty acid cycle.

Whether working muscles preferentially take up any specific fatty acids is not clear. When the behavior of plasma free palmitic and oleic acids was studied without use of radioactive tracers in fasting subjects during a vigorous exercise and following rest, the level of total plasma free fatty acids fell during a period of vigorous exercise, and palmitic acid rose and oleic acid fell (76). Further exercise followed by rest led to a considerable increase of total FFA level, and the proportion of oleic acid rose toward that present in the buttock adipose tissue of the particular subject, while the palmitic acid proportion fell. It was proposed that uptake of FFA from plasma during muscular activity proceeded in such a manner that oleic acid had a measurably greater fractional turnover rate than palmitic (76). This may be explained by the greater availability of oleic acid following lipolysis in adipose tissue, which contains twice as much oleic as palmitic acid (37).

Lipid Metabolism in Adipose Tissue

The relationship of physical activity to adipose tissue metabolism is covered in detail in chapter 22; therefore, only a brief overview of major issues will be presented herein as they pertain to mobilization of lipids as an energy source during exercise and to clearance of plasma FFA and circulating TG when exercise ceases.

Adipose tissue represents the largest energy store of the body, containing over 150,000 kcal in nonobese men and women. The two largest fatty regions in humans are the subcutaneous and intra-abdominal (or visceral) fat depots.

Lipolysis and FFA Mobilization

Lipolysis in adipose tissue is a key process in the regulation of the circulating free fatty acid level. In human adipose tissue, norepinephrine and epinephrine are the principal lipolytic hormones. Human adipocytes possess stimulatory β-adrenoceptors and inhibitory alpha-adrenoceptors. The only antilipolytic hormone of physiological importance in human adipocytes is insulin. Increased sympathoadrenal activity and decreased insulin levels with exercise stimulate the activity of a hormone-sensitive lipase (HSL) in adipose tissue, which brings about hydrolysis of stored triglycerides, (i.e., lipolysis). HSL catalyzes the degradation of triacylglycerol to diacylglycerol and monoacylglycerol, while the hydrolysis of the third fatty acid is catalyzed by a specific monoacylglycerol lipase. The rate of lipolysis in adipose tissue can be estimated from plasma glycerol production because glycerol formed by lipolysis cannot be reutilized in adipose tissue due to low concentrations of the enzyme alpha-glycerokinase.

Training Effects

It is well established that the plasma–catecholamine response to moderate exercise is lower after endurance training and that insulin concentrations are reduced. Despres, Bouchard, Tremblay, Savard, and Marcotte (12) demonstrated a significant increase of 66% in men and 46% in women in maximal epinephrine-stimulated lipolysis after a 20-week endurance-training program on an ergocycle. Crampes, Riviere, Beauvill, Marceron, and Garrigues (10), using one tenth the concentration of epinephrine used by Despres, also showed that epinephrine-induced lipolysis was enhanced with training due to an increased efficiency of the β-adrenergic pathway in male and female subjects and a decreased efficiency of the alpha-adrenergic pathway in female subjects. Increased lipolytic sensitivity to β-adrenergic stimulation would increase the lipid mobilizing capacity.

Adipose Tissue Lipoprotein Lipase and Lipid Storage

Adipose tissue lipoprotein lipase, which is synthesized in adipocytes then secreted and localized on the surface of the endothelial cells of capillaries, hydrolyzes circulating triglycerides so that FFA can be taken up and reesterified in adipose tissue for storage. Following cross-sectional observations that endurance-trained men had higher adipose tissue LPL activity than sedentary controls (42), adipose tissue LPL activity was shown to be increased following a 20-km race in the fasting state (59) and to be positively correlated with reported weekly physical activity (38). An intense 90-min bout of exercise on an ergocycle increased suprailiac adipose tissue LPL activity, and this change correlated with work output, but was independent of exercise-induced changes in fat cell lipolysis (53).

Training Effects

A 15-week endurance-training program was shown to increase basal adipose tissue LPL activity significantly (47). The clearance rate of plasma triglycerides following intravenous infusion of a fat emulsion was 92% higher than in sedentary counterparts, and the TG clearance rate was positively correlated with postheparin LPL activity, which includes muscle and adipose tissue LPL from all sites in the body. It was also inversely correlated with fasting TG levels, suggesting that the low TG levels in endurance athletes result at least in part from increased TG removal (50). The ability to replenish TG stores in adipose tissue is improved with training due to changes in insulin sensitivity, adipose tissue LPL activity, and other factors. This is associated with a greater ability to clear diet-derived fats from the circulation.

Lipid Transport

FFA that are released from adipocytes into the blood are bound to the protein albumin and transported to the working muscle. The FFA-carrying capacity is determined by blood albumin concentration, the number of FFA-binding sites on albumin, and blood flow. Each albumin molecule can bind a finite number of fatty acid molecules and does so with decreasing affinity (4); therefore, an increase in the FFA:albumin ratio is accompanied by an increase in the concentration of unassociated or "free" FFA in the blood. At rest, the arterial FFA concentration is about 0.300 mmol/L of plasma. With prolonged light to moderate exercise, FFA concentration reaches 2.0 mmol/L, which is the upper limit of the plasma concentration for albumin-bound FFA. During prolonged exercise, adipose tissue blood flow increases, thus facilitating the removal of fatty acids from the tissue; however, high FFA:albumin ratios in the arterial blood have been shown to increase vascular resistance in adipose tissue (8), which opposes factors acting to increase adipose tissue blood flow.

Re-esterification of Excess FFA

A major fraction of the fatty acids liberated may be reesterified within the adipocyte. Wolfe, Klien, Carraro, and Weber (75) demonstrated the important role of triglyceride–fatty acid (TG–FA) cycling in enabling a rapid response of fatty acid metabolism to major changes in energy requirements caused by starting, maintaining, and stopping exercise in physically active men. At rest, about 70% of all fatty acids released during lipolysis were reesterified; during the first 30 min of exercise (jogging) the value dropped to 25%, whereas total fatty acid release via TG hydrolysis tripled, thereby allowing a sixfold increase in FFA availability for oxidation. Immediately following the cessation of exercise, almost 90% of fatty acids released from lipolysis were reesterified. Thus, a major fraction of the fatty acids liberated may be reesterified within the adipocyte (*intracellular recycling*); the remainder is released into the blood or mobilized either to be taken up by muscle or to be reesterifed elsewhere (e.g., liver) (*extracellular recycling*). It is worth noting that an acylation-stimulating protein (ASP), which promotes FFA uptake and reesterification in various tissues, has been identified (70); however, its role in exercise is unknown.

These biochemical and physiological mechanisms prevent FFA from reaching concentrations that are toxic to cells due to their destabilizing effects on cell membrane structures such as mitochondrial membranes, which can lead to tissue damage. A high concentration of fatty acids could uncouple oxidative phosphorylation, increase platelet aggregation, and lead to fibrillation of the heart. Low concentrations of FFA could lead to increased glucose utilization in muscles and hypoglycemia, resulting in fatigue. Thus hormonal control of lipolysis must be supplemented by a mechanism that provides feedback between rate of energy utilization by muscle and lipolysis.

Balancing Lipid Utilization (Muscle) and Mobilization (Adipose Tissue)

Bulow (8) has proposed that the adjustment of fatty acid mobilization from adipose tissue to fatty acid utilization in working muscle is accomplished by the following sequence of events: lipolysis intensity increases very quickly at the onset of exercise, due to stimulation by sympathoadrenal factors; secondary to this, adipose tissue blood flow increases threefold, promoting the removal of fatty acids from the adipocytes. The rate of lipolysis is stimulated far in excess of the need of the working tissues, and the amount of FFA mobilized from adipose tissue greatly exceeds the simultaneous utilization, as evidenced by an increasing arterial and venous FFA concentration. As the FFA:albumin ratio increases, two feedback mechanisms oppose the excessive mobilization: increased esterification, and rising vascular resistance in adipose tissue. As a result, FFA mobilization is adapted to utilization, but at an increased FFA concentration level, which promotes the FFA uptake in the working muscles. This adjustment is reflected in relatively constant FFA concentrations during the later part of prolonged, constant work. In addition, arterial lactate has been shown to enhance fatty acid reesterification without affecting glycerol release.

Gender and Regional Differences in Lipid Metabolism During Exercise

Gender Differences in Lipid Utilization and Metabolism

Investigations of the effect of gender on exercise substrate have yielded conflicting results, possibly due to differences in maximum oxygen consumption and training status (frequency and duration of training and weekly mileage) of subjects. When men and women were matched for training status (approximately 37 km/wk and 38 min per workout), women had significantly lower R-values throughout a 15.5-km run at 65% $\dot{V}O_2max$ (studied at 30 min intervals), despite the absence of any difference between the sexes in FFA increases or progressive (and significant) glycerol rises during the exercise bout (58). R-value differences appeared to result from less glycogen utilization by the women (58). Similarly, no differences were seen between men and women with the same training status (regularly running 50 km/week in at least four sessions/week) in glycerol or FFA increases in blood samples collected from the earlobe at 4.5 min intervals during incremental graded treadmill tests. Trained individuals, however, had significantly greater glycerol increases and lower FFA:glycerol ratios than men and women who were not endurance-trained (21). Males and females who were equally trained to run 80 to 115 km/week with similar $\dot{V}O_2max$ (60–62 ml/kg/min) and muscle fiber composition, derived similar fractions of their energy from lipids during treadmill running at 70% $\dot{V}O_2max$ (9).

Regional Adiposity

It is well recognized that women generally deposit subcutaneous fat at different sites than do men, such as the upper arms, thighs, buttocks, and breasts, compared to the more common male deposition in the abdominal region. A male-type or *android* (upper body) fat pattern was distinguished from a female-type *gynoid* (lower body) based on skinfold thicknesses (67). Similarly, the subscapular:triceps skinfold ratio (STR) is used to distinguish central or truncal obesity (high STR) from peripheral or extremity adiposity (low STR). Skinfold measurements restrict the discussion of fat depots to subcutaneous fat, which is relatively easy to biopsy. In contrast, the ratio of waist-to-hip circumferences (WHR), which is used to delineate *abdominal* versus *gluteal-femoral* adiposity, includes intra-abdominal adipose tissue, the study of which has generally been associated with surgical procedures for other purposes.

Several noninvasive techniques, in particular, computed axial tomography (CAT) and magnetic resonance imaging (MRI), have been employed recently to study these deep fat stores, as well as subcutaneous depots. These methods have shown that men tend to have a greater ratio of intra-abdominal to subcutaneous abdominal fat than women (5). Although abdominal obesity is not equivalent to the android pattern or central or upper-body obesity, these terms are often used interchangeably because they are all associated with higher WHR and STR values than those in gluteal-femoral obesity, which is commonly interchanged with gynoid pattern, peripheral obesity, or lower-body obesity. The popular press has referred to these as "apple" and "pear" shapes, respectively. The terms are not sex-specific; many women have "male-type" obesity and some men have "female-type" obesity.

Many investigators have demonstrated that abdominal fat deposition is associated with a greater incidence of metabolic abnormalities compared to gluteal-femoral fat in both men and women, particularly with increasing obesity; therefore, one of the most exciting questions to be answered is whether exercise affects lipid metabolism differently in various adipose tissue depots. While this will undoubtedly be addressed in the section on physical activity and adipose tissue metabolism, its potential influence on lipoprotein metabolism warrants consideration here because there is overwhelming evidence that regional adiposity is associated with the lipoprotein profile (11,15,61,62,74), which may partially explain the sex differences commonly found in triglyceride and lipoprotein levels (20).

Regional Differences in Lipid Metabolism

Besides (or perhaps because of) differential effects of sex hormones on adipocytes of different regions, there is mounting evidence that the regulation of subcutaneous fat depots differs from that of intra-abdominal depots and that regulation varies among subcutaneous fat depots. Fatty acid composition differs somewhat between subcutaneous abdominal and buttock fat (particularly with respect to the ratio of saturated versus monounsaturated fatty acids) such that subcutaneous abdominal fat is more semisolid than buttock fat, and the composition of these depots differs from that of deep-seated (perirenal) fat (37). Regional variations in storage and mobilization of fat were found both in the fed and fasted states in obese women: before fasting, lipolytic activity was lower and LPL activity higher in femoral than in abdominal fat; acylglycerol synthesis was similar in the two fat depots before fasting but decreased to a lower level at the abdominal than at femoral site during fasting; and fat cell size decreased in the abdominal but not in the femoral site during fasting (2).

Catecholamines have been shown to be more lipolytic in omental than in subcutaneous fat cells (17,46), and subcutaneous abdominal adipocytes of both sexes have been shown to be four to five times more responsive to norepinephrine than gluteal fat cells (68). Omental fat is also less responsive to the antilipolytic effect of insulin than subcutaneous fat (7). By continuously monitoring glycerol levels (lipolytic index) in the extracellular space of subcutaneous adipose tissue using a microdialysis technique Arner, Kriegholm, Engfeldt, and Bolinder (3) demonstrated that (bicycle) exercise was accompanied by a marked rise in adipose tissue glycerol in the abdominal region and a small increase in the gluteal area, indicating that lipids are mobilized more readily from the former than from the latter region during exercise. These regional differences were more pronounced in women than men; furthermore, women had a higher plasma glycerol level at rest and even higher levels during exercise than men (3).

Aerobic exercise training to bring about weight loss has been shown to result in (a) greater mobilization of trunk fat than extremity fat in men based on skinfolds (13), (b) significant further reduction in waist-to-hip ratio in men and women consuming a low-fat diet (79), and (c) greater loss of deep abdominal fat compared with midthigh adipose tissue in women as determined by computed tomography (CT) (16). A study of trained female runners demonstrated increased sensitivity of the subcutaneous abdominal adipose tissue to the lipolytic action of catecholamines compared to sedentary controls (49), and a 20-week endurance-training program in sedentary women increased suprailiac adipocyte maximal epinephrine-stimulated lipolysis relative to women who remained sedentary throughout this period (12). Women with a male distribution of fat may benefit more from exercise for weight reduction than do women who deposit fat in the more resistant gluteal and thigh areas (33), perhaps because of preferential lipolysis of intra-abdominal fat with stimulation of the sympathetic nervous system during exercise. Abdominal obesity may be associated with fewer SO and more FG muscle fibers, as seen in men and women with a male distribution of excess adipose tissue compared to individuals with gynoid-shaped obesity (33).

It is generally held that omental fat depots release FFA predominantly into the portal circulation, whereas subcutaneous fat depots release their FFA into the systemic circulation; therefore, lipolytic activities in deep abdominal sites should have a greater and more immediate impact on the liver than lipolytic activities in subcutaneous fat including subcutaneous abdominal fat. Although this influx of fatty acids from omental fat stores may play a role in the metabolic complications associated with abdominal obesity—including hypertriglyceridemia and low levels of high-density lipoproteins (see following)—it raises an important question for this discussion. What role do FFA from intra-abdominal fat depots play in exercise if they are released into the portal circulation rather than the systemic circulation? Besides having to pass through the liver, where reesterification is likely, it is well known that splanchnic blood flow decreases during exercise. How readily are omental FFA transported to active muscle?

Details regarding the relative contribution of adipose tissue from various regions of the body as an energy source during exercise are not available at this time. Besides determining the relative mobilization and uptake of FFA from the various subcutaneous versus intra-abdominal adipose tissue sites, it would be interesting to know whether the fat deposited within muscle tissue, yet outside the muscle fibers, plays a special role in providing FFA to the muscle in which it is located. Do local autoregulatory factors favor blood flow or other factors in the active muscle to increase the uptake of FFA from these adipocytes early in the time course of exercise?

Hepatic Lipid Metabolism During Exercise

The liver plays a central role in the regulation of lipid metabolism. Gorski, Oscai, and Palmer (23) have listed three key events that may impact hepatic lipid metabolism during exercise: (a) changed, circulating titers of energy substrates, such as reduced glucose and increased free fatty acids; (b) changed hormonal balance, such that catabolic hormones are increased and insulin secretion is decreased; and (c) reduction of splanchnic blood flow. The liver is virtually the only organ of the body that produces ketone bodies, generally during periods of increased fatty acid oxidation. The concentration of plasma ketone bodies increases during prolonged exercise, presumably due to the abundant delivery of FFA to the liver, and continues to increase for several hours of the postexercise recovery period; this elevation is less pronounced in trained versus untrained individuals both during and after exercise (23). One of the major factors that regulates the rate of fatty acid synthesis in the liver is the insulin:glucagon ratio. When insulin concentrations are high, fatty acid synthesis increases and these acids are largely incorporated into triacylglycerols and secreted as very low density lipoproteins (VLDL). High glucocorticoid concentrations may further facilitate the synthesis of fatty acids and triacylglycerols.

Liver parenchymal cells synthesize a liver triglyceride lipase, hepatic lipase, which has been studied following its release by infusing heparin into subjects. Hepatic lipase activity has been shown to be reduced in trained versus sedentary men (38,73). Furthermore, a 1-year exercise program involving no change in diet significantly reduced postheparin hepatic lipase activity in exercisers versus sedentary controls and was significantly related to weight loss; men undergoing weight loss by caloric restriction with no exercise showed similar significant reductions in hepatic lipase activity versus control during the year (56). Intra-abdominal fat deposition was positively correlated with hepatic lipase activity independent of total adiposity (14).

Effects of Exercise-Induced Lipid Metabolism on Lipoprotein Metabolism

Only a brief overview of the effects of exercise on plasma lipoprotein concentrations will be presented here, as we have reviewed this literature previously (25,77,80). This discussion will emphasize factors relating to lipid metabolism that are likely to have an impact on lipoprotein metabolism.

Plasma Volume

Plasma volume generally decreases during an acute exercise bout because fluid is lost through the breath and sweat. This leads to transient increases in concentrations of all blood constituents unless a concomitant change occurs in their production or removal. Changes in plasma volume differ at various ambient temperatures, being greater at 22 °C than at 0 °C (55). In contrast to acute responses, plasma volume increases with exercise training (65), so that relative concentrations of all blood constituents will appear to decrease unless adjustments occur in production or metabolism. The plasma concentration of many substances is the important physiological variable, yet the absolute amount may also be important for a number of substances. As it is unclear which occurs with respect to plasma lipoproteins, plasma volume changes should be taken into account when interpreting changes in plasma concentrations during acute exercise or in the resting state following training.

Triglycerides, Very Low Density Lipoproteins (VLDL), VLDL Subfractions

Very low density lipoproteins exist as particles covering a wide range of size, density, and flotation rate. The least dense VLDL subfractions are more likely to be converted to high-density lipoprotein through the action of lipoprotein lipase on capillary endothelial surfaces in cardiac, skeletal muscle, and adipose tissue, whereas those carrying less triglyceride are more likely to be converted to intermediate or low-density lipoproteins, which are associated with greater risk for heart disease (6).

As previously discussed, LPL activity is increased in skeletal muscle by acute exercise as well as by exercise training resulting in improved delivery of FFA to the active muscle fibers during exercise as well as possible restoration of intramuscular triacylglycerol stores following exercise cessation. Adipose tissue LPL is also increased by endurance training, which presumably brings about an improved clearance of circulating triglycerides around the clock. Not surprisingly, cross-sectional studies repeatedly show that men and women who report engaging in regular physical activity are much leaner and have lower triglyceride and very low density lipoprotein cholesterol levels than their sedentary counterparts (80) . In addition, they have a distribution of VLDL particles that are associated with a lower risk profile (72,73). In a 1989 meta-analysis of 27 exercise-training studies in women in which serum lipid and lipoprotein concentrations were measured, results showed that exercise reduces triglycerides, and that women most at risk for heart disease (based on elevated preexercise cholesterol concentrations) responded most favorably to exercise training (36).

Although it seems that the exercise-induced increase in skeletal muscle and adipose tissue LPL activity could account for the lower triglyceride levels of trained men and women, it is worth considering the acute impact of exercise with respect to lipid metabolism. Thus, when circulating triglycerides are elevated to a point where they can serve as a major substrate for exercise, it appears that they are utilized. The impact of exercise on postprandial plasma triglyceride clearance may play a more important role in people who regularly exercise within a few hours of a meal as compared to morning runners, for instance, who generally perform their activities in the fasting state.

High Density Lipoproteins (HDL) and HDL Subfractions

Cross-sectional studies repeatedly show that men and women who report engaging in regular physical activity are much leaner and have higher HDL-cholesterol levels than their sedentary counterparts (80). Results from the 1989 meta-analysis of 27 exercise-training studies in women showed that exercise reduces the ratio of total cholesterol to HDL, but did not show significant changes in HDL or LDL levels (36). This is in contrast to data collected in men, where the controversy relates largely to whether exercise-induced weight loss (and metabolic consequences associated with weight loss), rather than a unique feature of exercise physiology, is responsible for HDL-cholesterol increases (63,65,72). Sex differences in fat distribution and lipolytic activities that might minimize weight loss associated with exercise in women, along with the fact that women generally start with higher HDL-cholesterol levels, may explain this difference in the HDL response. It would be particularly interesting to conduct a training study of women who have a male pattern obesity and initial HDL levels within the male range to determine whether the HDL increase is greater than that of women with gynoid obesity and normal female HDL levels.

Generally, most of the studies cited in the section on circulating TG and LPL changes with exercise show inverse effects on HDL such that increased clearance of TG and lower plasma TG levels correspond with higher HDL-cholesterol and mass concentrations. The previously discussed increased clearance rate of exogenous fat following a marathon run, for example, was significantly related to increases in HDL and HDL_2 cholesterol (50), as was the enhanced fat tolerance following endurance training (65). In contrast, strength training was not shown to improve HDL cholesterol or reduce triglyceride levels (32).

Applying the single-leg training method, Kiens and Lithell (30) demonstrated that muscle LPL activity was higher in the trained than the nontrained leg and that HDL- and HDL_2-cholesterol concentrations were increased in venous versus arterial blood in the trained thigh. This suggests that training-induced adaptations in skeletal muscle play a major role in changes in the lipoprotein profile associated with routine exercise. Further evidence of a muscular role in determining the lipoprotein profile was provided by a study showing that the percent of slow-twitch muscle fibers in the quadriceps of 102 men (41 sedentary men, 35 active male joggers, and 26 men with coronary heart disease) correlated positively with HDL cholesterol and negatively with triglycerides; furthermore, the proportion of slow-twitch fibers was higher in joggers than in sedentary controls or coronary heart disease patients (66). Having a high proportion of slow-twitch fibers favors the utilization of fatty acids as fuel and increases the likelihood that LPL activity will be increased with exercise.

We recently studied moderately overweight men and premenopausal women and observed that HDL-cholesterol reductions induced by a hypocaloric National Cholesterol Education Program (NCEP) Step-I diet were offset by addition of aerobic exercise. Results indicated that 39 men and 42 women undergoing weight loss by diet plus exercise showed significant increases in HDL- and HDL_2-cholesterol levels relative to 40 men and 31 women, respectively, undergoing similar weight loss by diet alone (79). In men, the dieting exercisers also increased HDL- and HDL_2-cholesterol levels relative to 40 male controls; whereas, in women, the dieting exercisers did not differ from 39 controls and the significant difference between the diet-only and diet-plus-exercise women resulted from substantial decreases in HDL-cholesterol in the diet-only group (79).

Clearly, significant weight loss (averaging 4.1 kg) achieved by the female dieters was inadequate to maintain HDL-cholesterol levels, whereas the addition of moderate exercise (approximately 10 miles/week of brisk walking and/or jogging), with similar weight loss (averaging 5.1 kg), prevented the diet-induced reduction in HDL cholesterol. Similarly, male dieters failed to increase HDL-cholesterol levels versus control subjects despite significant weight loss equivalent to the amount that resulted in significant HDL-cholesterol elevations versus control subjects in a previous study in which the percentages of calories from fat and carbohydrates were held constant while the total caloric intake was reduced (78). In this earlier study, 47 men who lost weight strictly through exercise with no dietary changes also increased HDL levels relative to the 42 controls, but showed no differences relative to the dieters.

The discrepancy between these two studies is presumably due to the additional effect of the reduced-fat, elevated-carbohydrate diet on lipoprotein metabolism. Therefore, it seems clear that changes in exercise, body fat, and diet composition each influence HDL-cholesterol levels in men and women. From the previous discussion, it might be concluded that the combination of a higher fat diet and greater activity of skeletal muscle and adipose tissue LPL in exercisers will increase hydrolysis of VLDL triglyceride for use as a fuel, thereby promoting the metabolism of very low density lipoproteins to high-density lipoproteins during exercise.

In addition to changes in HDL cholesterol, significant increases in HDL_2 cholesterol (78) and HDL_2 and HDL_3 mass were observed in the men who underwent 1 year of training relative to control, while VLDL mass decreased significantly (72). Because similar changes were seen in men who dieted only, but lost significantly more weight, the discussion focused on whether weight loss was responsible for these changes. An excellent editorial by Thompson (63) convincingly argued for the role of exercise independent of weight loss for the HDL changes generally observed in training studies. That weight loss also contributes to HDL changes seems clear; however, the mechanisms that bring about changes induced by weight loss may be quite different from those underlying exercise-induced changes, particularly when diet composition varies between groups or across the training period.

Hepatic lipase is also involved in the metabolism of high-density lipoprotein, particularly in the conversion of HDL_2 to a denser HDL_3 subfraction of this lipoprotein. Decreases in hepatic lipase activity during a 1-year exercise training program were significantly related to changes in HDL subfractions (56). Although these were equally significant in men undergoing weight loss by diet only, it is worth reemphasizing that exercise was the only intervention in the former group.

Low-Density Lipoproteins (LDL) and LDL Subfractions

Although cross-sectional studies generally show lower LDL-cholesterol levels in trained individuals versus sedentary people, training studies generally are unable to demonstrate a significant reduction in LDL cholesterol. Absence of an effect of exercise on plasma total LDL-cholesterol levels may mask effects on the biologically important LDL subfractions. Runners had significantly lower levels of small, dense LDL particles (73) (the atherogenic component of LDL) (6), than nonrunners, whereas concentrations of larger, more buoyant LDL particles did not differ with training status. This was also seen in our training study of moderately overweight sedentary men who made no changes in diet (72), suggesting that exercise-induced changes in VLDL metabolism can lead to increases in HDL mass and decreases in the more atherogenic LDL fractions. Exercise was the only intervention in these men and weight loss was an exercise-induced effect.

In our recent study of men and women undergoing weight loss with a prudent hypocaloric diet, with versus without exercise, the reduced-fat diet clearly benefited the lipoprotein profile of both diet-only and diet-plus-exercise women, bringing about significantly decreased (by 10%) LDL-cholesterol levels versus control (79). Similar reductions in male diet-only and diet-plus-exercise participants did not reach significance relative to controls who also decreased LDL cholesterol from baseline; however, in both men and women the total cholesterol:HDL-cholesterol ratio was improved when exercise was added to the prudent hypocaloric diet.

Important Research Questions

This discussion has attempted to lay out some of the key features of lipid metabolism during exercise. Many questions have not been answered at this time.

- How is fuel selection regulated during exercise?
- What brings about a transition from predominantly fat to predominantly glycogen utilization as intensity increases, and what underlies the difference in these mechanisms after endurance training?
- What is the stimulus for changes in mitochondria that bring about enhanced oxidation of fatty acids in trained individuals?
- It is clear that endurance athletes are more able to utilize fatty acids during prolonged exercise, but how can they maximize this use to allow intensity to increase for a better performance?
- Is there an optimal work intensity, frequency, or duration of activity that maximizes fat utilization to bring about the greatest benefits for weight regulation and weight-related problems such as lipoprotein disorders, diabetes, etc.?
- What minimum exercise "dose" is necessary to bring about substantial benefits for the masses?
- What is the best nutritional plan to optimize fat utilization during exercise without impairing performance?

- Do individuals with gynoid obesity really differ from individuals with android obesity in their utilization of fuel during exercise, or are there other confounding variables that have influenced these cross-sectional observations?
- Is there a training effect on the preferential use of fat released from one adipose tissue site versus another?
- Which diet and exercise programs maximally increase utilization of centrally deposited fat?
- What happens to FFA release from intra-abdominal fat during moderate-intensity endurance activity?
- Does drainage of omental adipose tissue into the portal circulation influence liver metabolism of lipids differentially from lipolytic events involving release of lipids into the systemic circulation?
- How readily are FFA released from intra-abdominal fat taken up by working muscle?

References

1. Annuzzi, G.; Jansson, E.; Kaijser, L.; Holmquist, L.; Carlson, L.A. Increased removal rate of exogenous triglycerides after prolonged exercise in man: Time course and effect of exercise duration. Metabolism. 36:438-443; 1987.
2. Arner, P.; Engfeldt, P.; Lithell, H. Site differences in the basal metabolism of subcutaneous fat in obese women. J. Clin. Endocrinol. Metab. 53:948-952; 1981.
3. Arner, P.; Kriegholm, E.; Engfeldt, P.; Bolinder, J. Adrenergic regulation of lipolysis in situ at rest and during exercise. J. Clin. Invest. 85:893-898; 1990.
4. Ashbrook, J.D.; Spector, A.A.; Santos, E.C.; Fletcher, J.E. Long chain fatty acid binding to human plasma albumin. J. Biol. Chem. 250:2333-2338; 1975.
5. Ashwell, M.; Dole, T.J.; Dixon, A.K. Obesity: New insight into the anthropometric classification of fat distribution shown by computed tomography. Br. Med. J. 290:1692-1694; 1985.
6. Austin, M.A.; Breslow, J.L.; Hennekens, C.H.; Buring, J.E.; Willett, W.C.; Krauss, R.M. Low density lipoprotein subclass patterns and risk of myocardial infarction. JAMA 260:1917-1921; 1988.
7. Bolinder, J.; Kager, L.; Ostman, J.; Arner, P. Differences at the receptor and post-receptor levels between human omental and subcutaneous adipose tissue in the action of insulin on lipolysis. Diabetes. 32:117-123; 1983.
8. Bulow, J. Lipid mobilization and utilization. In: Poortmans, J.R., ed. Principles of exercise biochemistry. Basel, Karger. Med. Sport Sci. 27:140-163; 1988.
9. Costill, D.L.; Fink, W.J.; Getchell, L.H.; Ivy, L.J.; Witzmann, F.A. Lipid metabolism in skeletal muscle of endurance-trained males and females. J. Appl. Physiol.: Respir. Environ. Exerc. Physiol. 47:787-791; 1979.
10. Crampes, F.; Riviere, D.; Beauvill, M.; Marceron, M.; Garrigues, M. Lipolytic response of adipocytes to epinephrine in sedentary and exercise-trained subjects: Sex-related differences. Eur. J. Appl. Physiol. 59:249-255; 1989.
11. Despres, J.P., Allard, D.; Tremblay, A.; Talbot, J.; Bouchard, C. Evidence for a regional component of body fatness in the association with serum lipids in men and women. Metabolism. 34:967-973; 1985.
12. Despres, J.P., Bouchard, C.; Tremblay, A.; Savard, R.; Marcotte, M. The effect of a 20-week endurance training program on adipose-tissue morphology and lipolysis in men and women. Metabolism. 33:235-239; 1984.
13. Despres, J.P.; Bouchard, C.; Tremblay, A.; Savard, R.; Marcotte, M. Effects of aerobic training on fat distribution in male subjects. Med. Sci. Sports Exerc. 17:113-118; 1985.
14. Despres, J.P.; Ferland, M.; Moorjani, S.; Nadeau, A.; Tremblay, A.; Lupien, P.J.; Theriault, G.; Bouchard, C. Role of hepatic-triglyceride lipase activity in the association between intra-abdominal fat and plasma HDL cholesterol in obese women. Arteriosclerosis. 9:485-492; 1989.
15. Despres, J.P., Moorjani, S.; Ferland, M.; Tremblay, A.; Lupien, P.J.; Nadeau, A.; Pinault, S.; Theriault, G.; Bouchard, C. Adipose tissue distribution and plasma lipoprotein levels in obese women: Importance of intra-abdominal fat. Arteriosclerosis. 9:203-210; 1989.
16. Despres, J.P.; Poulot, M.C.; Moorjani, S.; Nadeau, A.; Tremblay, A.; Lupien, P.J.; Theriault, G.; Bouchard, C. Loss of abdominal fat and metabolic response to exercise training in obese women. Am. J. Physiol. (Endocrinol. Metab. 24) 261:E159-167; 1991.
17. Efendic, S. Catecholamine and metabolism of human adipose tissue. III. Comparison between the regulation of lipolysis in omental and subcutaneous adipose tissue. Acta. Med. Scand. 187:477-483; 1970.
18. Enger, S.C.; Stromme, S.B.; Refsum, H.E. High density lipoprotein cholesterol, total cholesterol and triglycerides in serum after a single exposure to prolonged heavy exercise. Scand. J. Clin. Invest. 40:341-345; 1980.
19. Felig, P.; Wahren, J. Fuel homeostasis in exercise. N. Engl. J. Med. 293:1078-1084; 1975.

20. Freedman, D.S.; Jacobsen, S.J.; Barboriak, J.J.; Sobocinski, K.A.; Anderson, A.J.; Kissebah, A.H.; Sasse, E.A.; Gruchow, H.W. Body fat distribution and male/female differences in lipids and lipoproteins. Circulation. 81:1498-1506, 1990.
21. Friedmann, B.; Kindermann, W.I. Energy metabolism and regulatory hormones in women and men during endurance exercise. Eur. J. Appl. Physiol. 59:1-9; 1989.
22. Gollnick, P.D.; Saltin, B. Fuel for muscular exercise: Role of fat. In: Horton, E.S.; Terjung, R.L., eds. Exercise, nutrition, and energy metabolism. New York: Macmillan; 1988:72-88.
23. Gorski, J.; Oscai, L.B.; Palmer, W.K. Hepatic lipid metabolism in exercise and training. Med. Sci. Sports Exerc. 22:213-221; 1990.
24. Hargreaves, M.; Kiens, B.; Richter, E.A. Effect of increased plasma free fatty acid concentrations on muscle metabolism in exercising men. J. Appl. Physiol. 70:194-201; 1991.
25. Haskell, W.L.; Stefanick, M.L.; Superko, R. Influence of exercise on plasma lipids and lipoproteins. In: Horton, E.S.; Terjung, R.L., eds. Exercise, nutrition, and energy metabolism. New York: Macmillan; 1988:213-227.
26. Havel, R.J.; Penrow, B.; Jones, N.L. Uptake and release of free fatty acids and other metabolites in the legs of exercising men. J. Appl. Physiol. 23:90-99; 1967.
27. Henriksson, J. Training induced adaptation of skeletal muscle and metabolism during submaximal exercise. J. Physiol. 270:661-675; 1977.
28. Hurley, B.F.; Nemeth, P.M.; Martin, W.H.; Hagberg, J.M.; Dalsky, G.P.; Holloszy, J.O. Muscle triglyceride utilization during exercise: Effect of training. J. Appl. Physiol. 60:562-567; 1986.
29. Kiens, B.; Essen-Gastavsson, B.; Lithell, H. Lipoprotein lipase activity and intramuscular triglyceride stores after long-term high-fat and high-carbohydrate diets in physically trained men. Clin. Physiol. 7:1-9; 1987.
30. Kiens, B.; Lithell, H. Lipoprotein metabolism influenced by training-induced changes in human skeletal muscle. J. Clin. Invest. 83:558-564; 1989.
31. Kiens, B.; Saltin, B. Enhanced fat oxidation by exercising skeletal muscle after endurance training. [Suppl. 4]. Clin. Physiol. (Oxf.). 5 86a(Abstr); 1985.
32. Kokkinos, P.F.; Hurley, B.F.; Smutok, M.A.; Farmer, D.; Reece, C.; Shulman, R.; Charabogos, C.; Patterson, J.; Will, S.; Devane-Bell, J.; Goldberg, A.P. Strength training does not improve lipoprotein-lipid profiles in men at risk for CHD. Med. Sci. Sports Exerc. 23:1134-1139; 1991.
33. Krotkiewski, M.; Bjorntorp, P. Muscle tissue in obesity with different distribution of adipose tissue. Effects of physical training. Int. J. Obes. 10:331-341; 1986.
34. Lithell, H.; Cedermark, M.; Froberg, J.; Tesch, P.; Karlsson, J. Increase of lipoprotein lipase activity in skeletal muscle during heavy exercise. Relation to epinephrine excretion. Metabolism. 30:1130-1134; 1981.
35. Lithell, H.; Orlander, J.; Schele, R.; Sjodin, B.; Karlsson, J. Changes of lipoprotein-lipase activity and lipid stores in human skeletal muscle with prolonged heavy exercise. Acta. Physiol. Scand. 107:257-261; 1979.
36. Lokey, E.A.; Tran, Z.V. Effects of exercise training on serum lipid and lipoprotein concentrations in women: A meta-analysis. Int. J. Sports Med. 10:424-429; 1989.
37. Malcom, G.T.; Bhattacharyya, A.K.; Velez-Duran, M.; Guzman, M.A.; Oalmann, M.D.; Strong, J.P. Fatty acid composition of adipose tissue in humans: Differences between subcutaneous sites. Am. J. Clin. Nutr. 50:288-291; 1989.
38. Marniemi, J.; Peltonen, P.; Vuori, I.; Hietanen, E. Lipoprotein lipase of human postheparin plasma and adipose tissue in relation to physical training. Acta. Physiol. Scand. 110:131-135; 1980.
39. Newsholme, E.A. Basic aspects of metabolic regulation and their application to provision of energy in exercise. In: Poortmans, J.R., ed. Principles of exercise biochemistry. Med. Sport Sci. 27:40-77; 1988.
40. Nikkila, E.A. Role of lipoprotein lipase in metabolic adaptation to exercise and training. In: Borensztajn, J., ed. Lipoprotein lipase. Chicago: Evener Publishers, Inc.; 1987:187-199.
41. Nikkila, E.A.; Konttinen, A. Effect of physical activity on postprandial levels of fats in serum. Lancet. 1:1151-1154; 1962.
42. Nikkila, E.A.; Taskinen, M.R.; Rehunen, S.; Harkonen, M. Lipoprotein lipase activity in adipose tissue and skeletal muscle of runners: Relation to serum lipoproteins. Metabolism. 27:1661-1671; 1978.
43. Oscai, L.B.; Palmer, W.K. Cellular control of triacylglycerol metabolism. Exerc. Sport Sci. Rev. 11:1-23; 1983.
44. Oscai, L.B.; Palmer, W.K. Muscle lipolysis during exercise: An update. Sports Med. 6:23-28; 1988.
45. Oscai, L.B., Patterson, J.A., Bogard, D.L.; Beck, R.J.; Rothermel, B.L. Normalization of serum triglycerides and lipoprotein electrophoretic patterns by exercise. Am. J. Cardiol. 30:775-780; 1972.

46. Ostman, J.; Arner, P.; Engfeldt, P.; Kager, L. Regional differences in the control of lipolysis in human adipose tissue. Metabolism. 28:1198-1205; 1979.
47. Peltonen, P.; Marniemi, J.; Hietanen, E.; Vuori, I.; Ehnholm, C. Changes in serum lipids, lipoproteins, and heparin releasable lipolytic enzymes during moderate physical training in man: A longitudinal study. Metabolism. 30: 518-525; 1981.
48. Phinney, S.D.; Bistrian, B.R.; Evans, W.J.; Gervino, E; Blackburn, G.L. The human metabolic response to chronic ketosis without caloric restriction: Preservation of submaximal exercise capacity with reduced carbohydrate oxidation. Metabolism. 32:769-776; 1984.
49. Riviere, D.; Crampes, F.; Beauville, M.; Garrigues, M. Lipolytic response of fat cells to catecholamines in sedentary and exercise-trained women. J. Appl. Physiol. 66:330-335; 1989.
50. Sady, S.P.; Cullinane, E.M.; Saritelli, A.; Bernier, D.; Thompson, P.D. Elevated high-density lipoprotein cholesterol in endurance athletes is related to enhanced plasma triglyceride clearance. Metabolism. 37:568-572; 1988.
51. Sady, S.P.; Thompson, P.D.; Cullinane, E.M.; Kantor, M.A.; Domagala, E.; Herbert, P.N. Prolonged exercise augments plasma triglyceride clearance. JAMA. 256:2552-2555; 1986.
52. Saltin, B.; Gollnick, P.D. Skeletal muscle adaptability: Significance for metabolism and performance. In: Peachy, L.D.; Adrian, R.H.; Geiger, S.R., eds. Handbook of physiology, section 10. Baltimore: Williams & Wilkins; 1983:555-661.
53. Savard, R.; Despres, J.P.; Marcotte, M.; Theriault, G.; Tremblay, A.; Bouchard, C. Acute effects of endurance exercise on human adipose tissue metabolism. Metabolism. 36:480-485; 1987.
54. Schlierf, G.; Dinsenbacher, A.; Kather, H.; Kohlmeier, M.; Haberbosch, W. Mitigation of alimentary lipemia by postprandial exercise—phenomena and mechanisms. Metabolism. 36:726-730; 1987.
55. Sink, K.R.; Thomas, T.R.; Araujo, J.; Hill, S.F. Fat energy use and plasma lipid changes associated with exercise intensity and temperature. Eur. J. Appl. Physiol. 58:508-513; 1989.
56. Stefanick, M.L.; Terry, R.T.; Haskell, W.L.; Wood, P.D. Relationships of changes in postheparin hepatic and lipoprotein lipase activity to HDL-cholesterol changes following weight loss achieved by dieting versus exercise. In: Gallo, L.L., ed. Cardiovascular disease: Molecular and cellular mechanisms, prevention and treatment. New York: Plenum Press; 1987:61-68.
57. Svedenhag, J.; Lithell, H.; Juhlin-Dannfelt, A.; Henriksson, J. Increase in skeletal muscle lipoprotein lipase following endurance training in man. Atherosclerosis. 49:203-207; 1983.
58. Tarnopolsky, L.J.; MacDougall, J.D.; Atkinson, S.A.; Tarnopolsky, M.A.; Sutton, J.R. Gender differences in substrate for endurance exercise. J. Appl. Physiol. 68:302-308; 1990.
59. Taskinen, M.R.; Nikkila, E.A.; Rehunen, S.; Gordin, A. Effect of acute vigorous exercise on lipoprotein lipase activity of adipose tissue and skeletal muscle in physically active men. Artery. 6:471-483; 1980.
60. Terjung, R.L.; Kaciuba-Uscilko, H. Lipid metabolism during exercise: Influence of training. Diabetes Metab. Rev. 2:35-51; 1986.
61. Terry, R.B.; Stefanick, M.L.; Haskell, W.L.; Wood, P.D. Contributions of regional adipose tissue depots to plasma lipoprotein concentrations in overweight men and women: Possible protective effects of thigh fat. Metabolism. 40:733-740; 1991.
62. Terry, R.B.; Wood, P.D.; Haskell, W.L.; Stefanick, M.L.; Krauss, R.M. Regional adiposity patterns in relation to lipids, lipoprotein cholesterol, and lipoprotein subfraction mass in men. J. Clin. Endocrinol. Metab. 68:191-199; 1989.
63. Thompson, P.D. What do muscles have to do with lipoproteins? Circulation. 81:1428-1430; 1990.
64. Thompson, P.D.; Cullinane, E.; Henderson, L.O.; Herbert, P.N. Acute effects of prolonged exercise on serum lipids. Metabolism. 29:662-665; 1980.
65. Thompson, P.D.; Cullinane, E.; Sady, S.P.; Flynn, M.M.; Bernier, D.N.; Kantor, M.A.; Saritelli, A.L.; Herbert, P.N. Modest changes in high density lipoprotein concentration and metabolism with prolonged exercise training. Circulation. 78:25-34; 1988.
66. Tikkanen, H.O.; Harkonen, M.; Naveri, H.; Hamalainen, E.; Elovainio, R.; Sarna, S.; Frick, M.H. Relationship of skeletal muscle fiber type to serum high density lipoprotein cholesterol and apolipoprotein A-I levels. Atherosclerosis. 90:49-57; 1991.
67. Vague, J. The degree of masculine differentiation of obesities: A factor determining predisposition to diabetes, atherosclerosis, gout, and uric calculous diseases. Am. J. Clin. Nutr. 4:20-34; 1956.
68. Wahrenberg, H.; Bolinder, J.; Arner, P. Adrenergic regulation of lipolysis in human fat cells during exercise. Eur. J. Clin. Invest. 21:534-541; 1991.
69. Walker, M.; Cooper, B.G.; Elliott, C.; Reed, J.W.; Orskov, H.; Alberti, K.G.M.M. Role of

plasma non-esterifed fatty acids during and after exercise. Clin. Sci. 81:319-325; 1991.

70. Walsh, M.J.; Sniderman, A.D.; Cianfione, K.I.; Vu, H.; Rodriguez, M.A.; Forse, R.A. The effect of ASP on the adipocyte of the morbidly obese. J. Surg. Res. 46:470-473; 1989.
71. Weintraub, M.S.; Rosen, Y.; Otto, R.; Eisenberg, S.; Breslow, J.L. Physical exercise conditioning in the absence of weight loss reduces fasting and postprandial triglyceride-rich lipoprotein levels. Circulation. 79:1007-1014; 1989.
72. Williams, P.T.; Krauss, R.M.; Vranizan, K.M.; Wood, P.D. Changes in lipoprotein subfractions during diet-induced and exercise-induced weight loss in moderately overweight men. Circulation. 81:1293-1304; 1990.
73. Williams, P.T.; Krauss, R.M.; Wood, P.D.; Lindgren, F.T.; Giotas, C.; Vranizan, K.M. Lipoprotein subfractions of runners and sedentary men. Metabolism. 35:45-52; 1986.
74. Wing, R.R.; Matthews, K.A.; Kuller, L.H.; Meilahn, E.N.; Plantinga, P. Waist to hip ratio in middle-aged women: Associations with behavioral and psychosocial factors and with changes in cardiovascular risk factors. Arterioscl. and Thromb. 11:1250-1257; 1991.
75. Wolfe, R.R.; Klien, S.; Carraro, F.; Weber, J-M. Role of triglyceride-fatty acid cycle in controlling fat metabolism in humans during and after exercise. Am. J. Physiol. (Endocrin. Metab. 21) 258:E382-E389; 1990.
76. Wood, P.D.; Schlierf, G.; Kinsell, L. Plasma free oleic and palmitic acid levels during vigorous exercise. Metabolism. 14:1095-1100; 1965.
77. Wood, P.D.; Stefanick, M.L. Exercise, fitness, and atherosclerosis. In: Bouchard, C.; Shephard, R.J.; Stephens, T.; Sutton, J.R.; McPherson, B.D., eds. Exercise, fitness, and health: A consensus of current knowledge. Human Kinetics; Champaign, IL; 1990:409-423.
78. Wood, P.D.; Stefanick, M.L.; Dreon, D.M.; Frey-Hewitt, B.; Garay, S.C.; Williams, P.T.; Superko, H.R.; Fortmann, S.P.; Albers, J.J.; Vranizan, K.M.; Ellsworth, N.M.; Terry, R.B.; Haskell, W.L. Changes in plasma lipids and lipoproteins in overweight men during weight loss through dieting compared with exercise. N. Engl. J. Med. 319:1173-1179; 1988.
79. Wood, P.D.; Stefanick, M.L.; Williams, P.T.; Haskell, W.L. The effects on plasma lipoproteins of a prudent weight-reducing diet, with or without exercise, in overweight men and women. N. Engl. J. Med. 325:461-466; 1991.
80. Wood, P.D.; Williams, P.T.; Haskell, W.L. Physical activity and high-density lipoproteins. In: Miller, N.E.; Miller, G.J., eds. Clinical and metabolic aspects of high-density lipoproteins. Amsterdam: Elsevier Science; 1984:133-165.

Chapter 27

Physical Activity and Protein Metabolism

Michael J. Rennie
Joanna L. Bowtell
David J. Millward

The effects of physical activity and inactivity on body composition and amino acid and protein metabolism have been subjects of curiosity for many years, but mechanisms to explain the phenomenology have largely been lacking. Despite our development of new concepts (e.g., protein turnover) (80) and a panoply of new techniques (particularly measurement of organ and limb metabolic balance (104) and stable-isotope labeling [5]), we know little about the mechanisms underlying the obvious changes with exercise in nitrogen metabolism.

One aim of this review is to identify those phenomena that we can be reasonably sure exist and for which the accepted mechanisms are reasonable. Wherever possible the examples given will concern people rather than animals, but this implies no judgments about the quality of such work, only its specific relevance.

Intermediary Amino Acid Metabolism in Muscle

Amino acid metabolism in muscle is more limited than in the liver. It includes the transamination of alanine, aspartate, the branched-chain amino acids (BCAA) (70) and glutamate (plus the oxidative deamination of the latter) (35), the oxidation of BCAA via the branched-chain oxo acid dehydrogenase (71), the involvement of aspartate in the purine nucleotide cycle (60), and the synthesis of glutamine (52,79). Glutaminase activity, at least in the rat (45,46,100), is much lower than that of glutamine synthetase. In rat and chicken muscle there are glutamine transminases (100) with activities of the same order as glutamine production; however, their physiological relevance awaits investigation.

Muscle's capacity for amino acid metabolism is demonstrated by the export of glutamine and alanine from human limbs in amounts greater than expected if muscle protein were simply split into its constituent amino acids; they must be synthesized de novo (26,28,79). The BCAA transaminase reaction has a high K_m, that is, transamination is supply-driven (54), and it is likely that all of the nitrogen in alanine and at least half of the α-amino nitrogen in glutamine is transferred simply because of an increase in the availability of the BCAA, which comprises 20% of muscle protein. Supply of BCAA from the blood will complement this.

Human muscle has a high capacity for complete oxidation of the BCAA (22,51) so that only small amounts of oxo acids escape (14,15,23) for oxidation in the liver, which has a much smaller capacity. The source of the NH_3 added as amide into glutamine (i.e., whether from the glutamate dehydrogenase reaction or liberated from the [complete or partial] purine nucleotide cycle) is not yet certain. The provenance of the carbon for alanine and glutamine is not yet completely clear (70).

Blood and Muscle Free Amino Acid Concentrations and Net Uptake or Production by Tissues

The free-amino pool of the body consists of the amino acids in the blood and extracellular space and within the cell water of tissues. The pool size is small compared to amounts in body tissue protein and the quantities involved in protein turnover, dietary intake, and amounts lost in catabolism (94). Thus it is sensitive to changes in the rates of processes adding and withdrawing amino acids from it; for example, it shows acute rises in fasting and falls after insulin treatment (59,69).

In exercise, care should be taken to interpret relatively small changes in whole blood, plasma, and muscle amino acid concentration within the framework of circulatory changes, particularly the shift in blood flow from central to peripheral regions and its large increase, changes in fluid balance between blood and the tissues (e.g., the 10% hemoconcentration that accompanies exercise), and the differences in partition in amino acids between red cells and blood, particularly for glutamate, which is concentrated within the erythrocyte.

Effects of Intense, Short-Duration, Dynamic Exercise and Resistance Exercise

The major metabolic imperative in muscle, which drives most other metabolic changes during short-term exercise, is the homeostatic maintenance of the adenosine triphosphate (ATP):adenosine diphosphate (ADP) ratio after ATP hydrolysis. Any pathways of intermediary amino acid metabolism related to processes involved in the maintenance of myofibrillar ATP availability will inevitably be altered during high-intensity exercise. Thus most prominent should be glycolysis, proton production, and ammonia production (Figure 27.1) which show the biggest relative increase in rate.

Other processes with a smaller metabolic power for resynthesis of ATP (i.e., their power), such as the Krebs cycle, should have little influence. Effects on protein synthesis and breakdown, which are very slow, have little influence on amino acid pool size over the timescale considered here but will be more important in longer term and repeated exercise.

Against this theoretical background, changes observed in the free pools in muscle and plasma (Figure 27.2) and the rates of uptake and production of amino acids fit reasonably well.

Muscle alanine concentrations increase markedly during exercise, presumably due to the increased provision of pyruvate as a substrate for the alanine aminotransferase reaction and the availability of a high concentration of glutamate. Thus 10 to 20 min of exercise at 70% $\dot{V}O_2max$ increases muscle alanine concentration by 60% and decreases muscle glutamate almost stoichiometrically (3,49,50). The transamination of pyruvate to alanine may be advantageous in that (a) it provides a way of exporting a proton in a neutral form, and (b) the other product α-oxoglutarate bypasses the pyruvate dehydrogenase reaction and contributes to the maintenance of the concentration of tricarboxylic acid (TCA) cycle intermediates that help maintain maximal flux through the TCA cycle.

At high intensities of exercise, synthesis of muscle glutamine appears to be minimal over 1 to 4 min, and even over periods of 10 to 20 min its concentration shows only relatively small increases (e.g., compared to alanine). There may also be increases in muscle aspartate concentration in short-term intense exercise (3), arguing against its involvement in the full purine nucleotide cycle, otherwise its concentration ought to fall. There are no other significant changes in concentrations of other muscle amino acids in this type of exercise.

Blood amino acid concentrations appear, to a large extent, to reflect the changes in muscle during short-term intense exercise; two thirds of all

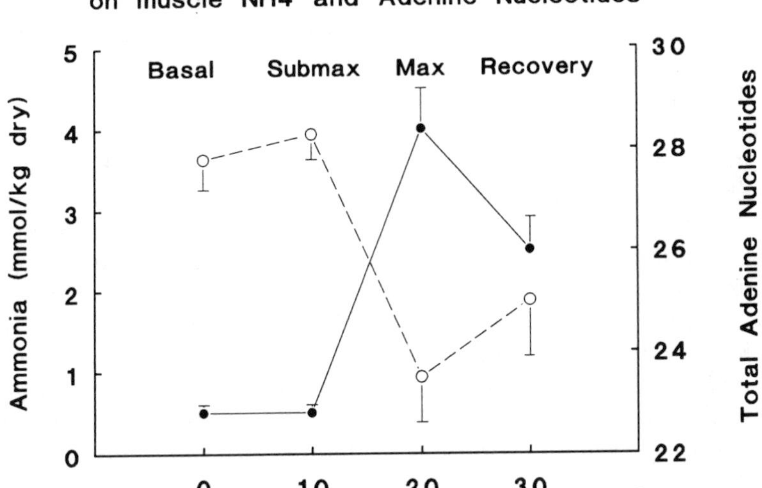

Figure 27.1 Demonstration of stoichiometric relationship between decrease in muscle adenine nucleotides and rise in ammonia production. Data from Katz et al. (49).

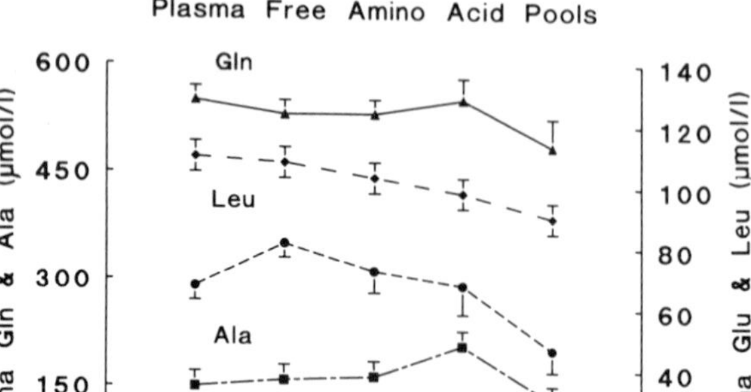

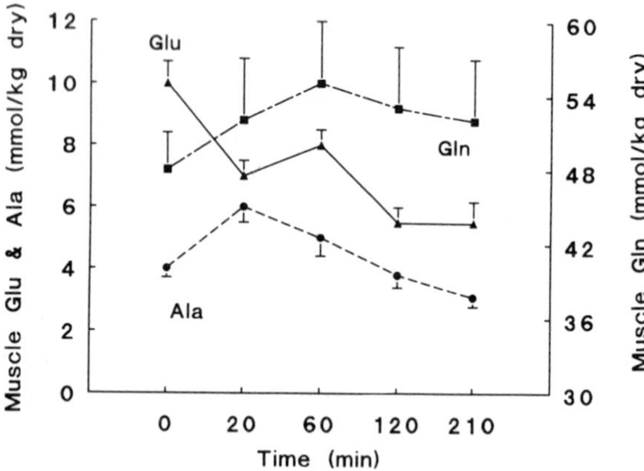

Figure 27.2 Effects of exercise on muscle and plasma free pools of amino acids. Data from Henriksson (43).

α-amino nitrogen released from muscle in the postabsorptive state at rest is in the form of alanine and glutamine, and the most consistent change during short-term, high-intensity exercise is a marked increase in alanine output, which becomes disproportionately greater at higher work loads (e.g., 300% increase at 55% $\dot{V}O_2$max and 900% at 80% $\dot{V}O_2$max) (24).

The increase in the output of glutamine is normally found to be somewhat less than that of alanine, with a variety of responses being reported. Some of the variability may derive from the relative instability of blood glutamine. Nevertheless glutamine released from muscle does appear to increase substantially during exercise of greater than 10 min and this increase must also contribute to the observed fall in intramuscular glutamate from which it is synthesized. The balance of glutamate across muscle is normally marginally positive; this small net uptake has been reported to be either unchanged or markedly elevated in very short-term exercise (24,43,50).

Muscle ammonia production, whether measured as increases in the intramuscular concentration, net efflux from muscle, or in blood concentration is markedly elevated during intense exercise, the increase being exponential in relation to the exercise intensity (24,50). There is still some uncertainty concerning the sources of ammonia during exercise. This could arise simply as a result of adenosine deaminase activity at the expense of adenosine monophosphate (AMP) (44), or the complete operation of the purine nucleotide cycle could result in the oxidative deamination of aspartate to resynthesize AMP with aspartate possibly replenished by the BCAA (91). The extent of the involvement of part or all of the relevant enzymes may depend on the exercise intensity: muscle ammonia production seems to be primarily at the expense of AMP during high-intensity, short-term exercise (37,49,50). However, at lower rates of work, the complete cycle operates in conjunction with BCAA transamination and glutamate dehydrogenase activity (91)—and possibly with glutaminase and glutamine transaminase activity.

During dynamic leg extensor exercise at a rate resulting in exhaustion in 3 min, muscle ammonia concentration increased roughly fourfold, with a near-stoichiometric accumulation of inosine 5′monophosphate (IMP). This strengthens the conclusion that ammonia is derived from AMP deamination (66). In this type of exercise the capacity of the muscle to produce ammonia is greater than the body's capacity to clear it, and the peak blood ammonia concentration only occurs some 2 to 3 min after the cessation of exercise.

Effects of Moderate, Medium-, and Long-Duration Exercise

The most extensive studies in the literature remain those carried out by Felig, Wahren, and their collaborators in the early 1970s (26,28). They first demonstrated the marked preponderance of alanine and glutamine among the amino acids produced by resting muscle in the postabsorptive state; as exercise at 40% $\dot{V}O_2$max progressed, there were sustained, increased muscle uptakes of glutamate and the BCAA and sustained, increased production of alanine and glutamine. Alanine and glutamine concentrations in the arterial blood were elevated early on during exercise (up to 40 min) but returned to near baseline after 4 hr of exercise.

The relatively minor changes in the blood amino acid pattern may result from the facts that only a relatively small muscle mass was involved and the work rate was moderate. Studies of walking or running that involve more muscle, especially at higher work rates, tend to show elevations of blood amino acid concentrations, particularly alanine, glutamine, and the BCAA. These elevations persist for up to about 2 hr, with a progressive fall of the blood amino acid concentration as exercise proceeds beyond this time period (18,73,76,77). The most consistent findings across the various studies are that the longer exercise proceeds, the greater the falls of glutamate and the BCAA, perhaps especially in trained subjects (43).

There is a marked lack of information concerning human muscle amino-acid-concentration changes during long-term exercise. Apart from the expected early increases in alanine and glutamine, decreases in muscle glutamate and increases in muscle tyrosine and phenylalanine are fairly reproducible findings (43,44,77). That muscle tyrosine and phenylalanine concentrations increase during exercise is noteworthy because these amino acids are not extensively metabolized in muscle (although the presence in muscle of the glutamine transaminase L and K types (100) means that there is a possibility of their transamination with branched-chain oxo acids, which should engender caution). Thus, the free-pool size of these amino acids should be inversely proportional to the net balance of protein synthesis and breakdown; a rise should indicate the net release of amino acids from muscle protein or an increase in the import of these amino acids from the blood. Either or both a decrease in protein synthesis or an increase in protein breakdown would have the observed effect (see later).

An amino acid, 3-methylhistidine (3-MeH), is released from myofibrillar protein on its degradation and not reutilized. It therefore provides a possible index of muscle protein degradation rate (21,103). With modern HPLC methods for measurement we ought to be able to discover exactly what happens to 3-MeH in human muscle during exercise, but unfortunately the recent sparse literature is confusing. In a study of walking at 50% of $\dot{V}O_2$max for 3.5 hr we previously found a slight decrease in muscle 3-MeH concentration, although it should be noted that our studies were carried out during the regular hourly ingestion of small amounts of food. We interpreted this as meaning that muscle protein breakdown fell during exercise (77). Henriksson, studying bicycle exercise at a similar rate, found a small increase (25%) in muscle 3-MeH with the opposite conclusion!

Urinary excretion of 3-MeH is not a good measure of the skeletal muscle protein turnover discussed elsewhere (78). The principal objection is the impossibility of distinguishing 3-MeH derived from skeletal and nonskeletal muscle sources such as gut smooth muscle. The recent evidence of increased net protein breakdown in gut during exercise in the dog (93) underlines the difficulty of assigning urinary changes in 3-MeH excretion to changes in skeletal muscle protein turnover.

It is difficult to interpret changes in the muscle branched-chain amino acids during exercise because of the complexity of their metabolism and rate of supply and disposal. That their concentrations are steady or increase less than other nonmetabolized amino acids (such as lysine, tyrosine, threonine, and phenylalanine) (43,61) tends to suggest that although they are being oxidized they are being supplied at an increased rate either by a net increase in the release from protein (by whatever mechanism) or by an increase in delivery from outside muscle.

In long-term aerobic exercise, muscle glycogen makes a major contribution to oxidative fuel metabolism and therefore it ought to be expected that alanine production would, in terms of the direction and approximate size of the changes, more or less match glycogen utilization. This appears to be broadly true and to the extent that trained athletes use more fat and less carbohydrate, alanine production by them is less. Furthermore, in long-term exercise, as glycogen concentrations in muscle progressively fall alanine production rate also falls.

At work rates that can be sustained for substantial periods of time (i.e., up to 2 hr) and that depend on high rates of oxidative metabolism (up to 80% $\dot{V}O_2$max) it appears that the source of muscle ammonia is different from that during intense exercise (Table 27.1).

Wagenmakers, Coakley, and Edwards suggest (91) that degradation of AMP by the purine nucleotide cycle involves the oxidative deamination of BCAA with the transfer of nitrogen successively to α-oxoglutarate to form glutamate and then either to glutamate itself to form glutamine, or to oxalacetate to form aspartate. Lack of α-oxoglutarate (which falls during exercise as Krebs cycle intermediates are lost to other pathways) (39) should lead to the production of increased amounts of free ammonia via the activity of glutamine dehydrogenase. Wagenmakers and co-workers have shown that human muscle branched-chain oxo acid dehydrogenase is progressively activated during exercise and that the extent of the activation is inversely proportional to the muscle glycogen concentration (89,90).

Furthermore the transamination and oxidation of BCAA seem to be accelerated with a greater depletion of glycogen. Wagenmakers has pointed out that the drainage of citric acid cycle intermediates (principally α-oxoglutarate) by branched-chain amino acid transamination, together with

Table 27.1 Effect of Aerobic Exercise (75% $\dot{V}O_2$max) on Human Muscle NH_3, Total Adenine Nucleotides, and Amino Acids

	Rest	Exhaustion (141 min) mmol/kg dry muscle	% change
NH_3	1.21 ± 0.17	2.4 ± 0.37*	+ 1.2
TAN	32.1 ± 1.6	31.7 ± 1.5^{NS}	− 0.4
Asp	1.1 ± 0.09	1.3 ± 0.18^{NS}	+ 0.12
Glu	17.9 ± 2.28	11.1 ± 1.9*	− 6.8
ΣAA	171 ± 27	216 ± 34*	+ 37
ΣBCAA	5.1 ± 1.1	5.8 ± 1.2^{NS}	+ 0.6

Means ± SEM.
*$p < 0.05$ vs. rest

Note. From "Plasma and Muscle Amino Acid and Ammonia Responses During Prolonged Exercise in Humans" by D.A. MacLean, L.L. Spriet, E. Hultman, and T.E. Graham, 1991, *Journal of Applied Physiology*, **70**, pp. 2095-2103. Reprinted by permission.

a reduced inflow from glycolysis as glycogen is depleted, will limit the ability of the Krebs cycle to accept substrate from ω-oxidation of fatty acids. This interpretation is strengthened by the observation by Graham, Kiens, Hargreaves, and Richter (38) that during exercise at 80% of $\dot{V}O_2$max, increasing the availability of free fatty acids inhibits the production of glutamine and alanine as well as that of ammonia. Because it is known that long-chain fatty acids inhibit leucine transamination and oxidation (29) it seems likely that inhibition of branched-chain amino acid oxidation in general would tend to decrease the production of amino acids and ammonia derived from them.

Oxidation of Amino Acids as Metabolic Fuels in Physical Activity

Reviewing the topic in 1925, Cathcart concluded from the substantial amount of evidence available to him even then that there was indeed an increase in urinary nitrogen excretion as the result of exercise (13). He hypothesized that the amino acids are liberated by changes in the balance between protein synthesis and breakdown for which no methods of study were then available.

The work of Ahlborg, Felig, Hagenfeldt, Hendler, and Wahren demonstrated that during long-term exercise muscle increased its production of alanine and glutamine with a substantial contribution of these amino acids to gluconeogenesis (1). As there can be no gluconeogenesis from amino acids without ureagenesis, these results provided indirect evidence for increased complete catabolism of amino acids as a result of exercise. Unfortunately Ahlborg and co-workers did not measure changes in the size of the body urea pool or urinary nitrogen excretion. Nevertheless, other workers were doing just that at roughly the same time (41,74).

However, there are two factors that confounded interpretation of the data: a decrease in renal plasma flow during exercise (12), which caused a decreased urinary nitrogen excretion and resulted in a rebound phenomenon after exercise when urine production is reestablished; and sweating as a route of urea excretion, which if neglected leads to a substantial underestimation of the urea production and of amino acid oxidation (57).

Tracer Studies of Amino Acid Catabolism

The first study using stable isotopes to investigate the effect of exercise on whole-body protein and amino acid metabolism was carried out by our group 10 years ago (76,77). We used ^{15}N glycine as a tracer and carried out our investigations over 2 days, a rest day followed by an exercise day. Because it was a 2-day study we had to feed our subjects (at hourly intervals for 12 hr each day); also, because we were hoping to attain a new steady state during exercise and again afterwards, we used a long period of exercise (3.75 hr at 50% of $\dot{V}O_2$max).

We were able to show that there was substantial exercise-induced increase in amino acid oxidation as judged by increase in blood urea and the urea production, although most of the extra urea nitrogen appeared after exercise because of the diminution of renal filtration during exercise. In one subject we also measured the oxidation of ^{13}C leucine and demonstrated a large increase in the production of $^{13}CO_2$ during exercise, which was confined to the period of exercise alone. We and others have also shown that the extent of whole-body leucine oxidation is proportional to the relative intensity of exercise (58,65), which supports the idea that the site of the increased leucine oxidation is muscle (as expected from its enzymology) (51,90). Studies using the human forearm preparation (Figure 27.3) demonstrate conclusively that there is a substantial rise in $^{13}CO_2$ production from ^{13}C leucine during muscle work (75).

The oxo acid of leucine (α-ketoisocaproate), which muscle produces in small amounts in the resting

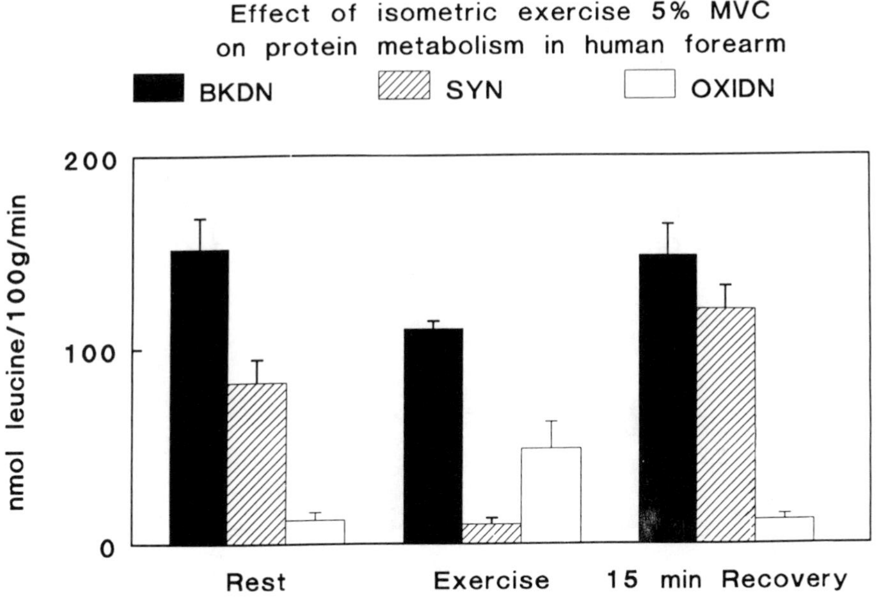

Figure 27.3 Protein turnover in the human forearm before, during, and after aerobic exercise at 5% of maximal voluntary contraction. Notice marked fall in protein synthesis and marked rise in leucine oxidation during exercise with reversal to an anabolic situation in recovery. Data from Rennie (unpublished work).

state, is actually taken up from the circulation during forearm exercise, and this too is oxidized. In human beings, unlike rats, muscle appears to completely oxidize leucine rather than exporting the keto acid to the liver for further oxidation.

One problem in the use of tracer acids using carbon isotopes—whether ^{13}C or ^{14}C—is the extent of carbon dioxide fixation in the body. Many workers use a recovery factor of 0.82 at rest; recent work has suggested that in the postabsorptive state the recovery factor should be about 0.76 and in the fed state about 0.92 (67). During exercise CO_2 turnover increases so that all labeled CO_2 is excreted. No information exists concerning the postexercise period when retention might increase as the result of the fixation of CO_2 via the phosphoenolpyruvate-carboxy kinase (PEPCK) reaction.

Another factor of importance is the small but significant amount of ^{13}C in our diet. This is particularly so for the North American diet, which contains foods (e.g., maize sugars) more highly enriched than the beet sugar eaten by Europeans. Increased carbohydrate oxidation during exercise would lead to an increased production of $^{13}CO_2$ if the glucose or glycogen oxidized contained more ^{13}C than the mix of metabolic fuel oxidized at rest (98). However, in subjects consuming a standard European diet, neither in the whole body nor in the working forearm preparation (Figure 27.4) does exercise cause an increase in $^{13}CO_2$ production in the absence of dietary intake or administration of ^{13}C tracers. It is possible to avoid dietary interference by the use of low (^{13}C) carbohydrates during fed-state experiments.

Wagenmakers and co-workers later showed that 2 hr of exercise at 40% $\dot{V}O_2$max in trained human subjects causes 400% activation of the branched-chain oxo acid dehydrogenase enzyme and that patients with *McArdle's disease* (who lack myophosphorylase and therefore cannot break down muscle glycogen) show a faster enzyme activation on exercise. The link between ammonia production and BCAA oxidation is made strongly by these results: In the McArdle's patients deterioration of exercise performance is associated with increased ammonia production, whereas supplementation with branched-chain oxo acids improved exercise performance and caused a smaller increase in ammonia production. Because BCAA oxidation drains 2-oxo glutarate from the citric acid cycle in the production of glutamate, utilization of BCAA for fuel in patients with McArdle's disease will inevitably increase the production of ammonia. In healthy individuals who exercise sufficiently long to deplete muscle glycogen, metabolism of BCAA would also drain 2-oxo glutarate from the citric acid cycle, thereby impeding the oxidation of glucose and fatty acids and causing reduction in exercise performance.

The evidence that (a) glucose inhibits leucine oxidation (17), (b) urea excretion in urine and sweat is accelerated in glycogen-depleted subjects (56), and (c) the branched-chain oxo acid dehydrogenase is activated to a greater extent in glycogen-depleted rats (48,92) are all consistent with the idea that there

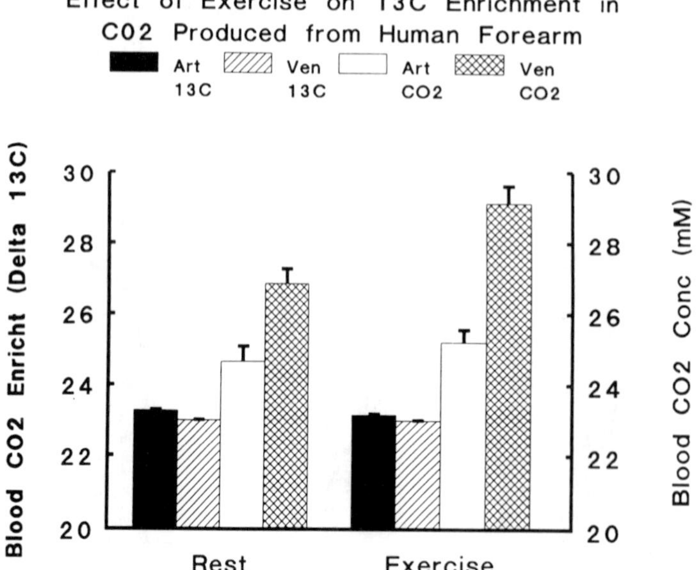

Figure 27.4 Demonstration of lack of perturbation of blood $^{13}CO_2$ enrichment during exercise by the human forearm. Data from Rennie (unpublished work).

is an inverse relationship between the extent of BCAA oxidation and glycogen availability. Direct testing of this hypothesis was made by studying the responses of branched-chain oxo acid dehydrogenase complex and muscle and blood metabolites during exercise in trained subjects after either glycogen depletion or carbohydrate loading. It supports the idea that exercise in the glycogen-depleted condition is associated with more rapid increases of ammonia and lower increases in alanine, glutamate, and glutamine together with a fourfold increase in the activation of the enzyme complex (89). When subjects were carbohydrate-loaded no activation occurred; there was a good correlation between the extent of activation and muscle glycogen concentration (Figure 27.5).

The rise in leucine oxidation observed during exercise is exactly what would be expected from observations of an increased state of activity of the branched-chain oxo acid dehydrogenase in animal and human muscle. Because the K_m for the branched-chain transaminase is high and the K_m for the L-system transporter in muscle is also high (47) leucine oxidation should mainly depend on leucine delivery. Fasting causes increases in plasma leucine concentration (as a result of whole-body protein synthesis falling below the rate of whole-body protein breakdown), and starvation is associated with a fall in insulin and an activation of the branched-chain oxo acid dehydrogenase in muscle. This helps explain why exercise in the fasted state causes a bigger increase in leucine oxidation than in the fed state (53).

The evidence from urinary nitrogen excretion, sweat excretion, and branched-chain amino acid oxidation all tends to bolster the view that exercise is associated with a net increase in amino acid oxidation. Nevertheless there are some difficulties with this interpretation. Wolfe and co-workers claim that exercise is not associated with increases in urea production measured from urine or blood changes, and application of isotopic methods to urea turnover shows no increase in urea production during exercise (97,99). Although artifacts in $^{13}CO_2$ production cannot explain the substantial rise in $^{13}CO_2$ production from ^{13}C leucine (which are matched by similar changes with ^{14}C-labeled leucine) (40), there remains the difficulty of why increased BCAA oxidation does not show up in terms of urea production. Possible difficulties are that the isotopic urea turnover values were methodologically flawed (63), that the work rates examined by Wolfe and colleagues were too low, or that any changes are difficult to see because of the very large urea pool. In chronically catheterized dogs exercise is clearly associated with increased hepatic ureagenesis (i.e., elevated portovenous urea differences) that hardly showed up in the blood urea pool (93).

Selective BCAA oxidation, as an explanation for the mismatch, could only occur if those amino acids liberated from protein during exercise and not oxidized were somehow retained in the body in other forms. One possibility is that synthesis in the liver of acute-phase proteins (which contain less than the bodily average content of the BCAA)

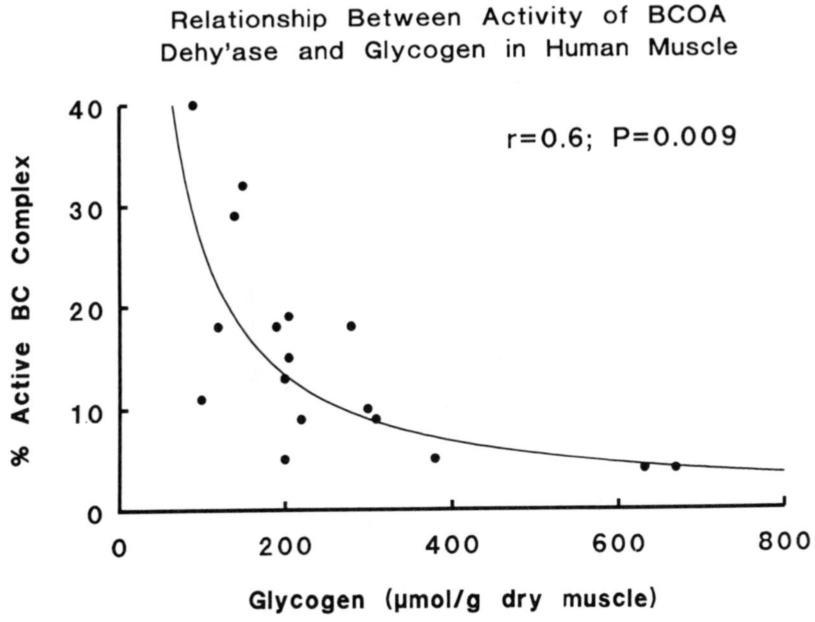

Figure 27.5 Demonstration of the greater extent of activation of branched-chain oxo acid dehydrogenase at low glycogen concentrations in human muscle. Data from Wagenmakers et al. (89).

is stimulated by exercise. Wolfe and colleagues do indeed have evidence that fibronectin and fibrinogen (which are relatively deficient in BCAA) are stimulated as the result of exercise (10) even at low work loads (40% $\dot{V}O_2$max) (Figure 27.6).

Wolfe and colleagues suggest that about one sixth of the amino acids leaving muscle could be taken up by fibrinogen alone. However, this is still a small amount, so other acute phase proteins would have to respond similarly. It is surprising, therefore, that albumin synthesis, which must increase with repeated exercise to accommodate the well-known increase in the vascular pool size, was not stimulated. One would expect the liver itself to be protein-catabolic in exercise, because as glucagon rises, both insulin and arterial blood supply fall—conditions likely to predispose to autophagy (72). Therefore the anabolic effect on acute-phase proteins may be less at higher rates.

Gluconeogenesis From Amino Acids

The work of Ahlborg and collaborators (1) provided strong evidence that at exercise of 40% $\dot{V}O_2$-max there was a net flow of amino acids from muscle to liver associated with increased hepatic glucose production and gluconeogenesis. At the end of 4 hr of exercise amino acids were contributing about 18% of hepatic gluconeogenesis.

In isolated, incubated rat muscle, either pyruvate or glucose is a better source of carbon for alanine synthesis than BCAA (35), suggesting that the supply of glucogenic substrate from muscle proteolysis could be less important than previously hypothesized (27). However the possibility exists that intermediates of BCAA metabolism (3-hydroxyisobutyrate, 2-methylbutyrate and 2-methyl-3-hydroxybutyrate) produced in muscle (83) may be important in interorgan carbon transfer (70). Such intermediates, not being esterified with coenzyme A, could leave mitochondria easily and travel via the plasma to gluconeogenic tissues.

The theory is strengthened by recent findings (7) that of the total flux entering the branched-chain oxo acid pathway in perfused rat heart (measured as the rate of release of labeled carbon dioxide from carboxyl-labeled valine) the rate of complete oxidation of α-ketoisovalerate was only one fifth, four fifths being accounted for by release of hydroxyacids into the medium. Since kidney and liver cells are able to make glucose from such substrates, incomplete valine and possibly isoleucine catabolism in muscle and heart could be important for gluconeogenesis. If so then, as Goldberg and Chang (35) found, pyruvate derived from glycolysis could be a more important immediate source of alanine and glutamine than the carbon chains of the BCAA, however some of the carbon originally could have been part of muscle protein as valine and isoleucine.

The metabolic machinery of the liver is such that increased delivery of amino acids in the portal blood will inevitably result in their uptake by the liver (88). Furthermore, amino acid catabolism in the liver appears to be exacerbated (88) by the

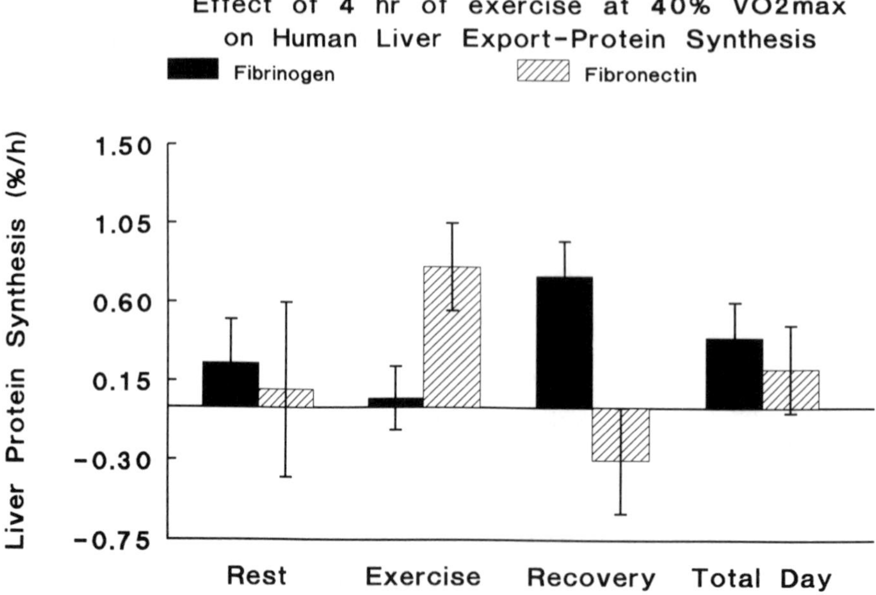

Figure 27.6 Increased acute-phase protein synthesis as a result of exercise may reconcile apparent mismatch between muscle amino acid release and apparent low rate of ureagenesis. Data from Carraro et al. (11).

presence of ammonia in the portal blood, which certainly occurs in exercise. Thus, during exercise hepatic catabolism of amino acids will inevitably be stimulated. The precise extent to which amino acid carbon can be recycled into glucose during exercise and to what extent it is channeled directly to urea is not known.

Careful studies carried out in exercising dogs (93) have increased our knowledge of the role of the viscera during exercise. As well as increasing output of alanine and glutamine by working muscle, exercise causes the gut to become a net exporter of amino acids as a result of increased net protein degradation. Thus a substantial amount of the substrate for gluconeogenesis (e.g., alanine) and oxidation by muscle (e.g., of BCAA) may be derived originally from gut protein. Noting a decrease in visceral protein content in exercising rats and in studies in humans, our group hypothesized that visceral protein breakdown might be accelerated on the basis of the increased 3-MeH excretion associated with exercise.

In exercising dogs hepatic amino acid and ammonia uptake increase with increased delivery to the gut by the hepatic portal vein, although the hepatic urea output oddly did not quantitatively match the uptake of amino acids from the blood. This lends weight to the suggestion that acute-phase protein synthesis may play a part in the disposal of amino acids during exercise.

The glutamine uptake by the gut and liver in exercising dogs was increased more than the delivery of glutamine, that is, the fractional extraction of this amino acid increased. This suggests the involvement of some hormonal effect (possibly glucagon) in stimulating hepatic and gastrointestinal utilization of glutamine.

Protein Turnover

Protein turnover is classically defined as protein synthesis and protein breakdown (95). The concepts are relatively modern and techniques for its measurement are even younger. They are still subject to vigorous debate concerning technical problems related to (a) the choice of precursor pool in which tracer amino acids should be measured, (b) the method of delivery of tracer, and (c) other problems that are particularly important to those using the methods but often confuse those who simply wish to know what happens to the physiology. Readers are referred to work on the subject (4,67,81,82,96).

Effects of Moderate Long-Term Exercise on Whole-Body Protein Turnover

There is now a considerable amount of evidence that supports Cathcart's prediction that there are changes in whole-body protein turnover as the result of exercise. Most of the data suggest that protein synthesis falls during exercise and increases afterwards (6,10,11,20,30,44,65,76,77,84,97).

Some of the conclusions may be suspect to the extent that they are based upon ^{13}C or ^{14}C leucine turnover and leucine oxidation, which may exaggerate both the apparent rise in protein oxidation and the fall in protein synthesis. Nevertheless the work in human subjects does appear to be supported by a substantial array of studies carried out in whole animals and in individual animal tissues (6).

The effects of daily, submaximal exercise have also been examined on whole-body and peripheral tissue amino acid metabolism in healthy subjects who were fed entirely intravenously (2). The results suggested that subjects who exercised for 1 hr/day on a bicycle ergometer had a more positive whole-body balance of protein.

Whether or not whole-body protein breakdown changes during exercise is difficult to discover. In studies with ^{13}C leucine and ^{15}N glycine the results have been contradictory (65,76,77,84). The use of 3-methylhistidine excretion as a measure of myofibrillar protein breakdown has been challenged on the basis that it actually reflects whole-body actin turnover to a greater extent than whole-body myofibrillar protein breakdown. Because actin is in many tissues the results may well be representative only of actin turnover, especially that in smooth muscle (78). Nevertheless whatever the source of the 3-methylhistidine there is good evidence that exercise is associated with an increase in the urinary production of 3-methylhistidine (11,19,20), although whether this occurs as a result of increased breakdown during or after exercise is not easy to discern.

The effects of short-term, intense exercise on whole-body protein turnover in the period after exercise have been studied by Tarnopolsky et al. (86) who were unable to detect any effects on [1-^{13}C] leucine turnover, although the design of their study was not ideal. Accustomed resistance exercise appears to have little effect on whole-body turnover per kilogram of lean body mass (101), although there is a suggestion that it may slightly increase turnover in endurance runners (64) (Table 27.2). Strength training does seem to maintain myofibrillar turnover (and muscle mass) in elderly men compared to their sedentary peers (31).

Little information is currently available concerning the relative size of changes in whole-body protein synthesis in relation to work load, training status, previous nutritional intake, or effects of nutritional supplementation during exercise. The whole area is ripe for research with modern methods.

Changes in Skeletal Muscle and Other Tissues—Effects of Moderate, Medium-, and Long-Term Exercise

It is now common physiological knowledge that the composition of skeletal muscle adapts to repeated aerobic exercise. The principal changes are an increase in mitochondrial volume and increases in the concentration of mitochondrial enzymes and myoglobin in muscle with no increase in muscle mass. Little work has been carried out to investigate the changes in muscle protein turnover during this type of exercise in human muscle. Two possible approaches, the tracer amino acid exchange across a limb and tracer amino acid incorporation into muscle protein (which requires biopsy) both have been applied. The use of the forearm preparation with stable-isotope-labeled leucine (75) suggests that protein synthesis falls during exercise and rises afterwards (Figure 27.4). Certainly a contraction-induced fall in muscle protein synthesis has been seen in perfused rat hind limb muscle (9), the mechanism being ascribed to a fall in muscle ATP:ADP. This is certainly plausible since the protein balance of muscle also falls in hypoxia (75), and in perfused rat muscle hypoxia and ischaemia (which caused a fall in the ratio of creatine phosphate to free creatine) caused a fall in muscle protein synthesis proportionate to that change (62).

Table 27.2 Effect of Endurance Training on Protein Turnover in Young and Middle-Aged Men

	Sedentary	Trained	
	Young	Young	Middle-aged
Turnover (g/kg/day)			
Synthesis	3.1 ± 0.2	3.5 ± 0.2	4.0 ± 0.2
Breakdown	3.0 ± 0.2	3.1 ± 0.2	3.7 ± 0.2

Values are means ± SEM. From (64).

Muscle protein breakdown is insufficiently studied to be sure of what happens, but in forearm muscle it also seems to fall during exercise with a rise afterwards (75). Of course, the fall must be less than with protein synthesis so that a net negative protein balance exists in muscle during exercise with a net positive balance being reinstated afterwards.

In studies carried out in intravenously fed subjects, daily aerobic bicycle exercise was associated with better balance of amino acids across leg tissue, and 3-methylhistidine efflux from the leg was decreased compared to sedentary subjects, suggesting that muscle protein breakdown was diminished (2).

The muscle biopsy-leucine incorporation method for protein synthesis has been applied to the study of muscle protein turnover during and after long-term aerobic exercise by Carrarro, Stuart, Hartl, Rosenblatt, and Wolfe (11) who were able to discern only a slight, insignificant fall in the incorporation of leucine into muscle during 4 hr of exercise at 40% $\dot{V}O_2max$ (Figure 27.6). There was nevertheless a substantial rise in the incorporation of leucine into muscle in the postexercise period.

Effects of Intense, Short-Term Exercise on Muscle Protein Turnover

There is a very large literature concerning changes in muscle protein synthesis in animal muscle (6), and there seems to be little doubt that myofibrillar protein accretion can be induced by increasing contractile activity of muscle in animals. The mechanism of the accretion via substantial increases in muscle protein synthesis is accompanied by smaller increases in muscle protein breakdown that appear to be obligatory for muscle remodeling (55).

Results from work on human subjects are extremely sparse and less common. Some years ago we carried out pilot studies suggesting that exercise increased incorporation of [1-^{13}C] leucine into human quadriceps muscle, but very few subjects were studied and the results were not consistent (76). Recently we were able to detect a marked increase in quadriceps protein synthesis in young men undertaking regular resistance exercise over a period of 12 weeks (101) (Table 27.3). It was noteworthy that treatment with human growth hormone did not increase the accretion of muscle protein or rate of muscle protein synthesis. Also, there are increases of incorporation of [1-^{13}C] leucine into biceps muscle protein of subjects who had previously undertaken high-intensity resistance exercise (16). Two groups of subjects were studied: one group had ^{13}C leucine incorporation measured within 4 hr after exercise; the second group was studied 24 hr afterwards. There was an increase in the rate of muscle protein synthesis of between 10% and 80% within 4 hr that remained elevated for at least 24 hr (Figure 27.7).

That the changes occurred so rapidly after both endurance and resistance exercise suggests they do not necessarily require an increase in transcriptional activity.

We have studied a natural model of chronic resistance exercise by examining protein synthesis in spinal muscle in adolescent children with scoliosis (33). On one side of the spine the muscle is stretched, and the contralateral muscle is flaccid as a result of the spinal curvature. We have shown that in the stretched muscle incorporation of tracer leucine is about twofold higher than in the flaccid muscle.

We have also investigated the effects of limb immobilization by plaster casting on muscle protein synthesis. It is well known that immobilization results in wasting of muscle, and this appears to be associated with a fall in the muscle protein synthetic rate per unit of ribosenucleic acid (RNA), a measure of translational activity (32). The deleterious effects of immobilization on muscle can be prevented or reversed by electrical stimulation of muscle for 1 hr/day (34).

Protein Requirements in Physical Activity—Background and Technical Problems

If protein oxidation increases as the result of exercise either acutely during exercise or immediately afterwards, or if there is muscle damage, then there will be an increased requirement for dietary protein to replace the acute losses. Furthermore, if exercise stimulates muscle growth, then amino acids must either be diverted from other tissues or protein must be ingested. There is remarkably little reliable information in the literature concerning the dietary protein requirements of subjects taking habitual exercise or whose daily work is primarily physical, but nevertheless, physical exercise is usually regarded by expert committees producing recommendations on dietary intake as having little effect on nutritional requirements.

The major difficulty concerns the best method for measurement of protein requirements. The nitrogen-balance method is recognized to have major limitations (42,102), the principal problems being (a) the difficulty of identifying all the routes of nitrogen excretion, (b) the lack of adequate precision, (c) the assumption of linearity between nitrogen retention and protein intake, (d) the problem of how long it takes to adapt at a given experimental intake, and (e) the observed tendency to overestimate positive nitrogen balance.

An alternative approach is to use the extent of amino acid oxidation (indicated with [^{13}C] tracers) to signal saturation of protein accretion, for oxidation of amino acids in excess of requirements should rise linearly with supply (102). This approach leads to the identification of minimum protein requirements for young healthy adults that are much higher than the WHO/FAO/UNN recommended daily amounts (25). Long-term balance studies carried out in Berkeley by Durkin et al. (quoted in [25]) suggest that it is possible for healthy adults to reduce their protein intake to the level of the obligate losses (i.e., about 350 mg protein/kg/day). It is easy to see why there is a

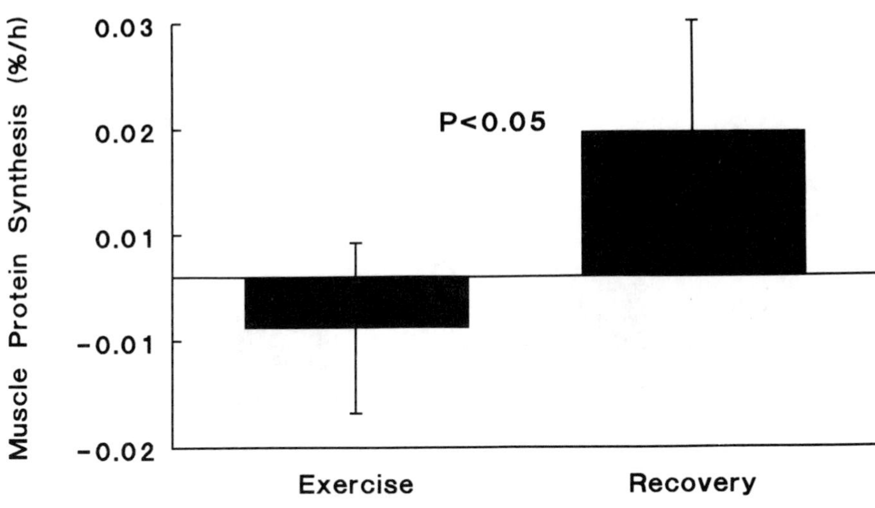

Figure 27.7 Stimulation of human muscle protein synthesis by aerobic exercise. Data from Carraro et al. (10).

Table 27.3 Effect of 12 Weeks Strength Training ± Human Growth Hormone on Muscle Protein Synthesis

	Pre	Post	Δ
	% h'		
Placebo	0.048 ± 0.008	0.066 ± 0.011[a]	+ 38%[a]
HGH	0.048 ± 0.010	0.070 ± 0.004[a,b]	+ 45%[a,b]

[a]Effect of training $p < .01$. [b]Effect of HGH NS.
From (101).

substantial amount of controversy concerning the best methodology to use and the results obtained with it (66).

Until recently there have been no adequate methods to assess the ability to utilize dietary protein for lean tissue gain, a property of obvious interest to athletes and their trainers. A possible solution has been suggested by Millward and coworkers (67,68) who hypothesize that regulation of accretion of body protein occurs to maintain a body-protein full state, which under normal circumstances is never exceeded. They also assume that in response to increasing habitual rates of protein intake, the induction of amino acid catabolic capacity (which is not fixed as in the kinetic approach) (31) leads to increased oxidative losses of amino acids—but at the same body-protein full condition. Over a 24-hr period the nitrogen (N) balance of any subject should oscillate between a period of fasting N loss and feeding N gain, during which protein deposition is accelerated to replace the fasting loss. If the fed-state deposition is measured at different protein intakes, then the slope of the curve of protein gain can be construed as a measure or index of protein deposition efficiency. It might be predicted that any circumstances predisposing to muscle growth will increase this index.

Evidence that the model accurately describes protein metabolism in adults with a range of protein intakes between 0.4 and 1.6 g/kg/day has been obtained using both 12-hr nitrogen balance techniques and leucine turnover techniques (Figure 27.8).

Protein Requirements in Subjects Taking Habitual Exercise

Some years ago it was demonstrated that young healthy men who undertook large amounts of exercise on a fixed protein intake went through a period of negative N balance but then adapted to a near-balance equilibrium (36). Also, the propensity of exercise to increase N accretion on a given protein intake was well demonstrated (8). Nevertheless it has often been pointed out that if repeated exercise is associated with amino acid oxidation then the requirements, particularly for athletes working aerobically, might increase (30,44).

Recently more data has become available on subjects who engage in aerobic exercise and also those who engage in strength training (64,85,87). Meredith, Zackin, Frontera, and Evans (64) used the

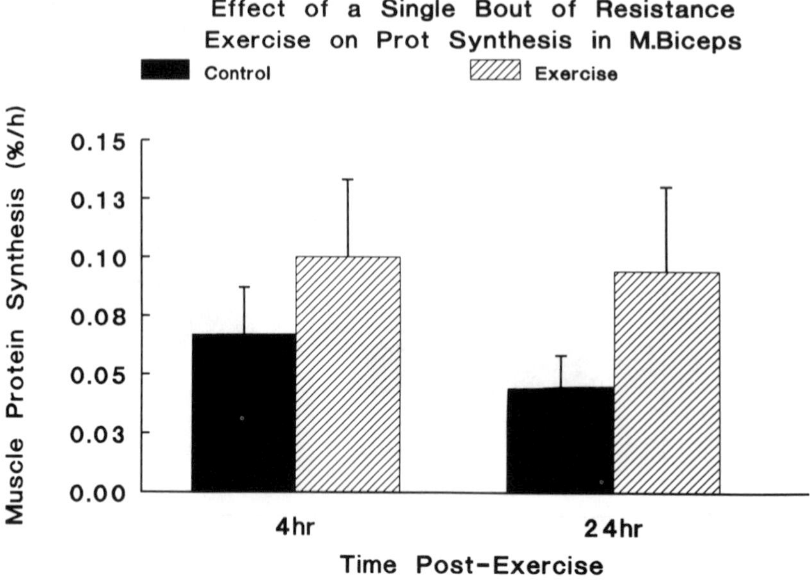

Figure 27.8 Adaptive effect of repeated exercise on N balance at constant nitrogen intake. Data from Gontzea et al. (36).

nitrogen-balance technique and ^{15}N glycine turnover to examine protein requirements in young and middle-aged runners randomly fed three levels of dietary protein. Their results suggested that there were no differences in protein turnover between the two groups (even though the young men exercised substantially more than the middle-aged men and had higher energy expenditures). Both groups had an increased requirement for protein by about 17% above the current U.S. Recommended Dietary Allowance (RDA).

It is difficult to fault the studies in terms of their broad plan of experimental design, except that the adaptation period, even at 10 days, might have been too short for the amino acid catabolizing enzymes to down-regulate. Nevertheless the results seem odd because of the finding of consistent, positive N balance of about 1.4 g per day over the final 5 days of a 10-day period of protein intake of 1.2 g/kg/day. The fact that negative balance was observed at the protein RDA has little meaning unless it can be shown that adaptation was complete, and this may take a substantial time, up to weeks.

Work by Tarnopolsky, MacDougall, and Atkinson (87) using less stringent techniques has come to a similar conclusion concerning endurance runners. They were studied after a period of very high protein intake that followed one already twice the RDA, with no attempt at randomly ordering the treatment. Also, no low-protein diet was examined and no individuals ever experienced negative N balance. The results suggested that endurance athletes required 67% more protein than the RDA to achieve balance, but the impossibly large, sustained, positive balances at high-protein intakes make it hard to accept the conclusions.

Both groups studied subjects who were in a steady state, that is, they had become accustomed to their habitual level of exercise, although protein turnover on a whole-body basis was a little raised over that expected in sedentary subjects. There is no doubt that runners do not show muscle hypertrophy, so their apparently greater protein requirement calculated per kilogram may simply reflect their increased lean body mass per kilogram body weight rather than an increase in protein requirements per se. Because of the imprecision of the methods used it is difficult to be sure that the calculated increase in protein requirements would be real if expressed per kilogram lean body mass (LBM). It seems likely that there is some small extra requirement for protein in those taking habitual aerobic exercise simply because of the imbalance caused by elevated BCAA oxidation. The difficulty is in knowing exactly how much extra is required and if subjects accustomed to low-protein diets (e.g., vegetarians or women on weight-reducing diets) actually suffer in terms of exercise performance or ability to train.

It is also difficult to give a clear answer concerning the protein requirements for weight lifters and bodybuilders. Obviously if muscle growth is occurring then there may be a transitory increase in the requirements for dietary amino acids early on in a period of increased muscular work; for example, as training schedules are intensified and increased efficiency of N accretion occurs. Markedly

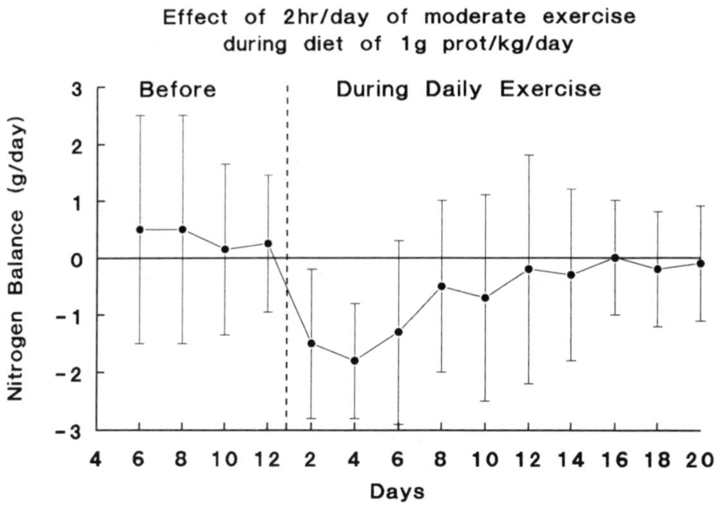

Effect of 2hr/day of moderate exercise during diet of 1g prot/kg/day

Before | During Daily Exercise

Nitrogen Balance (g/day)

Days

Figure 27.9 Stimulation of human muscle protein synthesis by resistance exercise. Data from Chesley et al. (16).

increased muscle protein synthesis has been documented in subjects undergoing increased rates of exercise training (Figure 27.9) (16), but much smaller increases are observed in the fed state after accommodation (Table 27.3) (101). Once steady state has been reached the overall requirements per kilogram of LBM should not be markedly elevated, because whole-body turnover accommodates as demonstrated (101). This is especially so since intense weight-lifting exercise appears to cause little change in whole-body protein turnover in the fasted state (86) and the total amount of exercise may be insufficiently long-lasting to cause much change in the whole-body pool or rates of oxidation of the BCAA.

Nevertheless there are suggestions from two studies by Tarnopolsky and colleagues (85,87) of increases (some very marked) in the protein requirements of strength athletes (Figures 27.10 and 27.11). One study suggested that there were no differences between the requirements of strength athletes and sedentary individuals, whereas in a second study the same authors claimed that zero nitrogen balance can only be achieved at roughly twice the protein intake of a sedentary individual (1.41 g/kg/day vs. 0.69 g/kg/day). These workers recommended an intake of protein of 1.76 g/kg/day as opposed to 0.89 g/kg/day for the sedentary subjects.

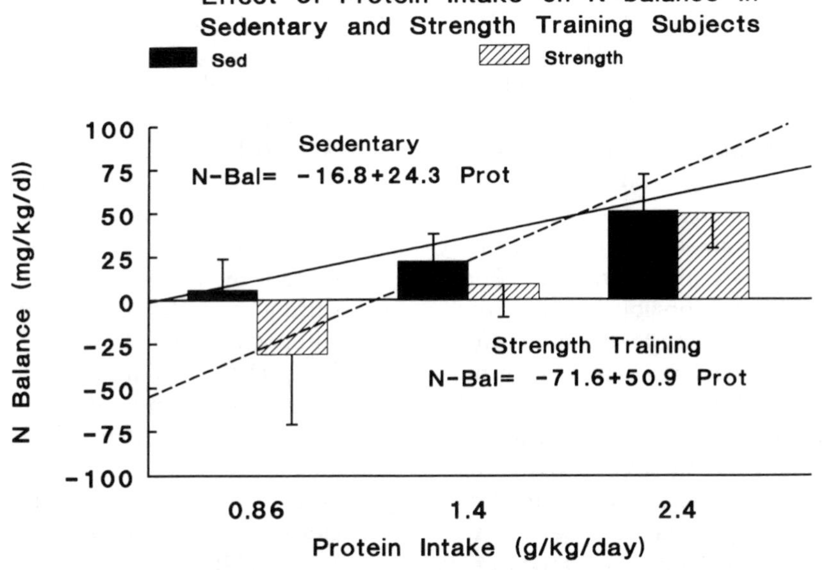

Figure 27.10 Data used to suggest that strength training exercise is associated with a higher requirement than 0.86 g/kg/day of protein intake. Notice very marked apparent positive balance at 1.4 and 2.4 g protein/kg/day and assumption of linearity of relationship between N balance and protein intake.

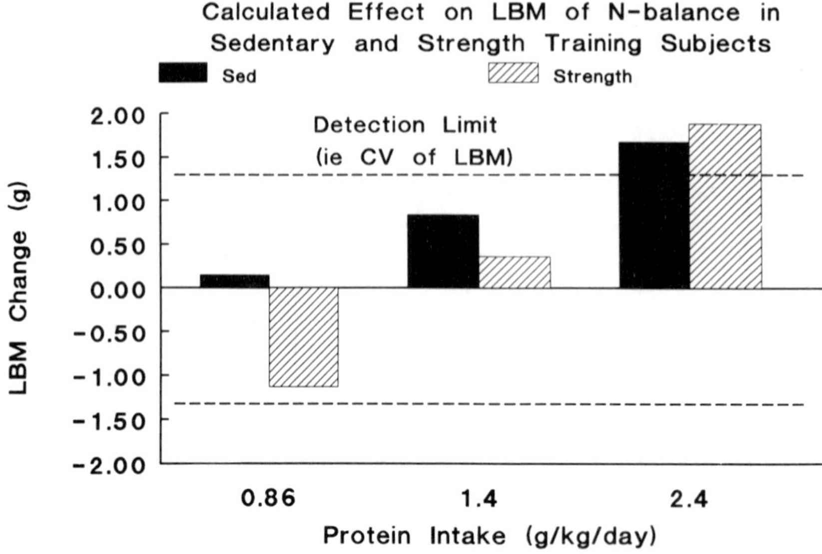

Figure 27.11 Calculated effect on lean body mass of observed N balance at different protein intakes over 13 days of diet. Data calculated from results of Tarnopolsky et al. (87).

Oddly (and perhaps wrongly due to the authors' use of the regression of N balance vs. protein intake to identify N equilibrium) there were no detectable effects of varying protein intake on 24-hr creatinine excretion (i.e., an index of muscle mass) or of lean body mass. These results occurred despite differences in N balance during 13-day periods of low- and high-protein intake of about 6 g N/day equivalent to nearly 2 kg of lean tissue over 13 days. Although the authors suggest that their measures may simply not have been sufficiently sensitive to detect any such changes, this is difficult to accept because the limit of detection was about 1.3 kg LBM in the strength-trained subjects.

Recent work by Butterfield (personal communication) has shown that N balance in weight lifters on increased protein diets was no more positive than usual. It does seem likely that strength training increases muscle and whole-body protein synthesis as lean body mass increases and that oxidation must be elevated to some extent, but the exact requirement cannot be determined from the data presently available. This area obviously needs further work with great care being taken to identify possible sources of error and to counter them by appropriate experimental design.

Because muscular work involves extra energy expenditure and so long as physically active individuals take in sufficient food to achieve neutral energy balance, then because the average protein content of food is about 10%, they will automatically ingest sufficient protein to replenish any losses due to oxidation during exercise. There is certainly no case for protein supplements.

Acknowledgments

We thank SmithKline Beecham plc for funds to support J. Bowtell. Original work by the authors was supported by The Wellcome Trust, MRC, Action Research, The White Top Foundation, Biomedical Research Committee of the SHHD, and University of Dundee.

References

1. Ahlborg, G.; Felig, P.; Hagenfeldt, L.; Hendler, R.; Wahren, J. Substrate turnover during prolonged exercise in man. J. Clin. Invest. 53:1080-1090; 1974.
2. Albert, J.D.; Matthews, D.E.; Legaspi, A.; Tracey, K.J.; Jeevanandam, M.; Brennan, M.F.; Lowry, S.F. Exercise-mediated peripheral tissue and whole-body amino acid metabolism during intravenous feeding in normal man. Clin. Sci. 77:113-120; 1977.
3. Bergström, J.; Fürst, P.; Hultman, E. Free amino acids in muscle tissue and plasma during exercise in man. Clin. Physiol. 5:155-160; 1985.
4. Bier, D.M. Stable isotope methods for nutritional diagnosis and research. Nutr. Rev. 40:129-134; 1982.
5. Bier, D.M. The use of stable isotopes in metabolic investigation. Baillières Clin. Endocrinol. Metab. 1:817-836; 1987.

6. Booth, F.W.; Thomason, D.B. Molecular and cellular adaptation of muscle in response to exercise: Perspectives of various models. Physiol. Rev. 71:541-585; 1991.
7. Brosnan, M.E.; Letto, J. Interorgan metabolism of valine. Amino Acids. 1:29-35; 1991.
8. Butterfield, G.E.; Calloway, D.H. Physical activity improves protein utilization in young men. Br. J. Nutr. 51:171-184; 1984.
9. Bylund-Fellenius, A.-C.; Ojamaa, K.M.; Flaim, K.E.; Li, J.B.; Wassner, S.J.; Jefferson, L.S. Protein synthesis versus energy state in contracting muscle of perfused rat hindlimb. Am. J. Physiol. 246:E297-E305; 1984.
10. Carraro, F.; Hartl, W.H.; Stuart, C.A.; Layman, D.K.; Jahoor, F.; Wolfe, R.R. Whole body and plasma protein synthesis in exercise and recovery in human subjects. Am. J. Physiol. 258:E821-E831; 1990.
11. Carraro, F.; Stuart, C.A.; Hartl, W.H.; Rosenblatt, J.; Wolfe, R.R. Effect of exercise and recovery on muscle protein synthesis in human subjects. Am. J. Physiol. 259:E470-E476; 1990.
12. Castenfors, J. Renal function during exercise. Acta Physiol. Scand. [Suppl. 293]. 70:1-40; 1967.
13. Cathcart, E.P. The influence of muscle work on protein metabolism. Physiol. Rev. 5:225-243; 1925.
14. Cheng, K.N.; Dworzak, F.; Ford, G.C.; Rennie, M.J.; Halliday, D. Direct determination of leucine metabolism and protein breakdown in humans using L–[1–^{13}C,^{15}N]-leucine and the forearm model. Eur. J. Clin. Invest. 15:349-354; 1985.
15. Cheng, K.N.; Pacy, P.J.; Dworzak, F.; Ford, G.C.; Halliday, D. Influence of fasting on leucine and muscle protein metabolism across the human forearm determined using L–[1–^{13}C,^{15}N]leucine as the tracer. Clin. Sci. 73:241-246; 1987.
16. Chesley, A.; MacDougall, J.D.; Tarnopolsky, M.A.; Atkinson, S.A.; Smith, K. Changes in human muscle protein synthesis following resistance exercise. J. Appl. Physiol. 73:1383-1388; 1992.
17. Davies, C.T.M.; Halliday, D.; Millward, D.J.; Rennie, M.J.; Sutton, J.R. Glucose inhibits CO_2 production from leucine during whole-body exercise in man. J. Physiol. 332:41-42P; 1982.
18. Décombaz, J.; Reinhardt, P.; Anantharaman, K.; van Glutz, G.; Poortmans, J.R. Biochemical changes in a 100km run: Free amino acids, urea and creatinine. Eur. J. Appl. Physiol. 41:61-72; 1979.
19. Dohm, G.L.; Israel, R.G.; Breedlove, R.L.; Williams, R.T.; Askew, E.W. Biphasic changes in 3-methylhistidine excretion in humans after exercise. Am. J. Physiol. 248:E588-E592; 1985.
20. Dohm, G.L.; Williams, R.T.; Kasperek, G.J.; van-Rig, A.M. Increased excretion of urea and N_T-methylhistidine by rats and humans after a bout of exercise. J. Appl. Physiol. 52:27-33; 1982.
21. Elia, M.; Carter, A.; Smith, R. The 3-methylhistidine content of human tissues. Br. J. Nutr. 42:567-569; 1979.
22. Elia, M.; Livesey, G. Branched chain amino acid and oxo acid metabolism in human and rat muscle. In: Metabolism and clinical implications of branched chain amino and ketoacids. Walser, M.; Williamson, J.R., eds. New York, Amsterdam, Oxford: Elsevier Science; 1981:257-262.
23. Elia, M.; Livesey, G. Effects of ingested steak and infused leucine on forelimb metabolism in man and the fate of the carbon skeletons and amino groups of branched-chain amino acids. Clin. Sci. 64:517-526; 1983.
24. Eriksson, L.S.; Broberg, S.; Björkman, O.; Wahren, J. Ammonia metabolism during exercise in man. Clin. Physiol. 5:325-336; 1985.
25. FAO, WHO, and UNN. Energy and protein requirements: WHO technical report series no. 74. Geneva: World Health Organization; 1985.
26. Felig, P. Amino acid metabolism in man. Annu. Rev. Biochem. 44:933-955; 1975.
27. Felig, P.; Pozefsky, T.; Marliss, C.; Cahill, G.F. Alanine: Key role in gluconeogenesis. Science. 167:1003-1004; 1970.
28. Felig, P.; Wahren, J. Amino acid metabolism in exercising man. J. Clin. Invest. 50:2703-2709; 1971.
29. Frick, G.P.; Goodman, H.M. Insulin regulation of branched chain α-keto acid dehydrogenase in adipose tissue. J. Biol. Chem. 255:6186-6192; 1980.
30. Friedman, J.E.; Lemon, P.W.R. Effect of chronic endurance exercise on retention of dietary protein. Int. J. Sports Med. 10:118-123; 1989.
31. Frontera, W.R.; Meredith, C.N.; O'Reilly, K.P.; Knuttgen, H.G.; Evans, W.J. Strength conditioning in older men: Skeletal muscle hypertrophy and improved function. J. Appl. Physiol. 64:1038-1044; 1988.
32. Gibson, J.N.A.; Halliday, D.; Morrison, W.L.; Stoward, P.J.; Hornsby, G.A.; Watt, P.W.; Murdoch, G.; Rennie, M.J. Decrease in human quadriceps muscle protein turnover consequent on leg immobilization. Clin. Sci. 72:503-509; 1987.
33. Gibson, J.N.A.; McMaster, M.J.; Scrimgeour, C.M.; Stoward, P.J.; Rennie, M.J. Rates of muscle protein synthesis in para spinal muscles:

Lateral disparity in children with idiopathic scoliosis. Clin. Sci. 75:415-420; 1988.

34. Gibson, J.N.A.; Smith, K.; Rennie, M.J. Prevention of disuse muscular atrophy by means of electrical stimulation: Maintenance of protein synthesis. Lancet. 2:767-770; 1988.
35. Goldberg, A.L.; Chang, T.W. Regulation and significance of amino acid metabolism in skeletal muscle. Federation Proc. 37:2301-2307; 1978.
36. Gontzea, I.; Sutzescu, P.; Dumitrache, S. The influence of adaptation to physical effort on nitrogen balance in man. Nutr. Rep. Int. 22:231-236; 1975.
37. Graham, T.E.; Bangsbo, J.; Gollnick, P.D.; Juel, C.; Saltin, B. Ammonia metabolism during intense dynamic exercise and recovery in humans. Am. J. Physiol. 259:E170-E176; 1990.
38. Graham, T.E.; Kiens, B.; Hargreaves, M.; Richter, E.A. Influence of fatty acids on ammonia and amino acid flux from active human muscle. Am. J. Physiol. 261:E168-E176; 1991.
39. Graham, T.E.; Saltin, B. Estimation of the mitochondrial redox state in human skeletal muscle during exercise. J. Appl. Physiol. 66:561-566; 1989.
40. Hagg, S.A.; Morse, E.L.; Adibi, S.A. Effect of exercise on rates of oxidation, turnover and plasma clearance of leucine in human subjects. Am. J. Physiol. 242:E407-E410; 1985.
41. Haralambie, G.; Berg, A. Serum urea and amino nitrogen changes with exercise duration. Eur. J. Appl. Physiol. 36:39-48; 1976.
42. Hegsted, D.M. Balance studies. J. Nutr. 106:307-311; 1976.
43. Henriksson, J. Effect of exercise on amino acid concentrations in skeletal muscle and plasma. J. Exp. Biol. 160:149-165; 1991.
44. Hood, D.A.; Terjung, R.L. Amino acid metabolism during exercise and following endurance training. Sports Med. 9:23-35; 1990.
45. Hundal, H.S.; Babij, P.; Taylor, P.M.; Watt, P.W.; Rennie, M.J. Effects of corticosteroid on the transport and metabolism of glutamine in rat skeletal muscle. Biochim. Biophys. Acta. 1092:376-383; 1991.
46. Hundal, H.S.; Babij, P.; Watt, P.W.; Ward, M.R.; Rennie, M.J. Glutamine transport and metabolism in denervated rat skeletal muscle. Am. J. Physiol. 259:E148-E154; 1990.
47. Hundal, H.S.; Rennie, M.J.; Watt, P.W. Characteristics of acidic, basic and neutral amino acid transport in perfused rat hindlimb. J. Physiol. 408:93-114; 1989.
48. Kasperek, G.J.; Snider, R.D. Effect of exercise intensity and starvation on activation of branched-chain keto acid dehydrogenase by exercise. Am. J. Physiol. 252:E22-E37; 1987.
49. Katz, A.; Broberg, S.; Sahlin, K.; Wahren, J. Muscle ammonia and amino acid metabolism during dynamic exercise in man. Clin. Physiol. 6:365-379; 1986.
50. Katz, A.; Sahlin, K.; Henriksson, J. Muscle ammonia metabolism during isometric contraction in humans. Am. J. Physiol. 250:C834-C840; 1986.
51. Khatra, B.S.; Chawla, R.K.; Sewell, C.W.; Rudman, D. Distribution of branched-chain α-keto acid dehydrogenases in primate tissues. J. Clin. Invest. 59:558-564; 1977.
52. King, P.A.; Goldstein, L.; Newsholme, E.A. Glutamine synthetase activity of muscle in acidosis. Biochem. J. 216:523-525; 1983.
53. Knapik, J.; Meredith, C.; Jones, B.; Fielding, R.; Young, V.R.; Evans, W. Leucine metabolism during fasting and exercise. J. Appl. Physiol. 70:43-47; 1991.
54. Krebs, H.A. Regulation of fuel supply in animals. Adv. Enzyme Regul. 10:406-413; 1972.
55. Laurent, G.J.; Sparrow, M.P.; Millward, D.J. Turnover of muscle protein in the fowl. Changes in rates of protein synthesis and breakdown during hypertrophy of the anterior and posterior latissimus dorsi muscles. Biochem. J. 176:407-417; 1978.
56. Lemon, P.W.; Mullin, J.P. Effect of initial muscle glycogen levels on protein catabolism during exercise. J. Appl. Physiol. 48:624-629; 1980.
57. Lemon, P.W.R.; Nagle, F.J. Effects of exercise on protein and amino acid metabolism. Med. Sci. Sports Exerc. 13:141-149; 1981.
58. Lemon, P.W.R.; Nagle, F.J.; Mullin, J.P.; Benevenga, N.J. In vivo leucine oxidation at rest and during two intensities of exercise. J. Appl. Physiol. 53:947-954; 1982.
59. Lotspeich, W. The role of insulin in the metabolism of amino acids. J. Biol. Chem. 179:175-180; 1949.
60. Lowenstein, J.M.; Goodman, M.N. The purine nucleotide cycle in skeletal muscle. Federation Proc. 37:2308-2312; 1978.
61. MacLean, D.A.; Spriet, L.L.; Hultman, E.; Graham, T.E. Plasma and muscle amino acid and ammonia responses during prolonged exercise in humans. J. Appl. Physiol. 70:2095-2103; 1991.
62. MacLennan, P.A.; Rennie, M.J. Effects of ischaemia, blood loss and reperfusion on rat skeletal muscle protein synthesis *in vivo*. Biochem. J. 260:195-200; 1989.
63. Matthews, D.E.; Downey, R.S. Measurement of urea kinetics in humans: A validation of stable isotope tracer methods. Am. J. Physiol. 246:E519-E527; 1984.
64. Meredith, C.N.; Zackin, M.J.; Frontera, W.R.; Evans, W.J. Dietary protein requirements and

body protein metabolism in endurance-trained men. J. Appl. Physiol. 66:2850-2856; 1989.

65. Millward, D.J.; Davies, C.T.M.; Halliday, D.; Wolman, S.L.; Matthews, D.E.; Rennie, M.J. Effect of exercise on protein metabolism in humans as explored with stable isotopes. Federation Proc. 41:2686-2691; 1982.
66. Millward, D.J.; Jackson, A.A.; Price, G.; Rivers, J.P.W. Human amino acid and protein requirements: Current dilemmas and uncertainties. Nutr. Res. Rev. 2:109-132; 1989.
67. Millward, D.J.; Price, G.M.; Pacy, P.J.H.; Halliday, D. Whole-body protein and amino acid turnover in man: What can we measure with confidence? Proc. Nutr. Soc. 50:197-216; 1991.
68. Millward, D.J.; Price, G.M.; Pacy, P.J.H.; Quevedo, R.M.; Halliday, D. The nutritional sensitivity of the diurnal cycling of body protein enables protein deposition to be measured in subjects at nitrogen equilibrium. Clin. Nutr. 10:239-244; 1991.
69. Millward, D.J.; Waterlow, J.C. Effect of nutrition on protein turnover in skeletal muscle. Federation Proc. 37:2283-2290; 1978.
70. Palmer, T.N.; Caldecourt, M.A.; Snell, K.; Sugden, M.C. Alanine and inter-organ relationships in branched-chain amino and 2-oxo acid metabolism. Biosci. Rep. 5:1015-1033; 1985.
71. Paxton, R.; Scislowski, P.W.D.; Davis, E.J.; Harris, R.A. Role of branched-chain 2-oxo acid dehydrogenase and pyruvate dehydrogenase in 2-oxo acid metabolism. Biochem. J. 234:295-303; 1986.
72. Poso, A.R.; Wert, J.J., Jr.; Mortimore, G.E. Multifunctional control by amino acids of deprivation-induced proteolysis in liver. J. Biol. Chem. 257:12114-12120; 1982.
73. Refsum, H.E.; Gjessing, R.; Stromme, S.B. Changes in plasma amino acid distribution and urine amino acids excretion during prolonged heavy exercise. Scand. J. Clin. Lab. Invest. 39:407-413; 1979.
74. Refsum, H.W.; Strömme, S.B. Urea and creatinine production and excretion in urine during and after prolonged heavy exercise. J. Clin. Lab. Invest. 33:247-254; 1974.
75. Rennie, M.J.; Babij, P.; Sutton, J.R.; Tonkins, W.W.; Read, W.W.; Ford, C.; Halliday, D. Effects of acute hypoxia on forearm leucine metabolism. Hypoxia, exercise, and altitude: Proc. of 3rd Banff int. hypoxia symp. 1983:317-323.
76. Rennie, M.J.; Edwards, R.H.T.; Davies, C.T.M.; Krywawych, S.; Halliday, D.; Waterlow, J.C.; Millward, D.J. Protein and amino acid turnover during and after exercise. Biochem. Soc. Trans. 8:499-501; 1980.
77. Rennie, M.J.; Edwards, R.H.T.; Krywawych, S.; Davies, C.T.M.; Halliday, D.; Waterlow, J.C.; Millward, D.J. Effect of exercise on protein turnover in man. Clin. Sci. 61:627-639; 1981.
78. Rennie, M.J.; Millward, D.J. 3-Methylhistidine excretion and the urinary 3-methylhistidine/creatinine ratio are poor indicators of skeletal muscle protein breakdown. Clin. Sci. 65:217-225; 1983.
79. Ruderman, N.B.; Lund, P. Amino acid metabolism in skeletal muscle: Regulation of glutamine and alanine release in the perfused rat hindquarter. Isr. J. Med. Sci. 8:295-302; 1972.
80. Schoenheimer, R. The dynamic state of body constituents. Cambridge, MA: Harvard University Press; 1942.
81. Smith, K.; Barua, J.M.; Watt, P.W.; Scrimgeour, C.M.; Rickhuss, P.K.; Rennie, M.J. Preliminary evidence of artefactually high values of muscle protein synthesis obtained by the flooding dose technique compared to the constant infusion method. Clin. Nutr. [Suppl.]. 10, O.21:7; 1991.
82. Smith, K.; Rennie, M.J. Protein turnover and amino acid metabolism in human skeletal muscle. In: Harris, J.B.; Turnbull, D.M., eds. Muscle metabolism, Ballière's Clinical Endocrinology and Metabolism, vol. 4 / number 3. London: Ballière Tindall; 1990:461-499.
83. Spydevold, O.; Hokland, B. Release of leucine and isoleucine metabolites by perfused skeletal muscle and liver of rat. Int. J. Biochem. 15:985-990; 1983.
84. Stein, T.P.; Hoyt, R.W.; Toole, M.O.; Leskiw, M.J.; Schluter, M.D.; Wolfe, R.R.; Hiller, W.D. Protein and energy metabolism during prolonged exercise in trained athletes. Int. J. Sports Med. 10:311-316; 1989.
85. Tarnopolsky, M.A.; Atkinson, S.A.; MacDougall, J.D.; Chesley, A.; Phillips, S.; Schwarcz, H.P. Evaluation of protein requirements for trained strength athletes. J. Appl. Physiol. 73:1986-1995; 1992.
86. Tarnopolsky, M.A.; Atkinson, S.A.; MacDougall, J.D.; Senor, B.B.; Lemon, P.W.R.; Schwarcz, H. Whole body leucine metabolism during and after resistance exercise in fed humans. Med. Sci. Sports Exerc. 23:326-333; 1991.
87. Tarnopolsky, M.A.; MacDougall, J.D.; Atkinson, S.A. Influence of protein intake and training status on nitrogen balance and lean body mass. J. Appl. Physiol. 64:187-193; 1988.
88. Taylor, P.M.; Rennie, M.J. Amino acid fluxes across sinusoidal membranes of perfused rat liver: Relationship with portal ammonia concentrations. In: Soeters, P.B.; Wilson, J.H.P.;

Meijer, A.J.; Holm, E., eds. Advances in ammonia metabolism and hepatic encephalopathy. Amsterdam: Elsevier Science; 1988:45-52.

89. Wagenmakers, A.J.M.; Beckers, E.J.; Brouns, F.; Kuipers, H.; Soeters, P.B.; van der Vusse, G.J.; Saris, W.H.M. Carbohydrate supplementation, glycogen depletion and amino acid metabolism during exercise. Am. J. Physiol. 260:E833-E890; 1991.
90. Wagenmakers, A.J.M.; Brookes, J.H.; Coakley, J.H.; Reilly, T.; Edwards, R.H.T. Exercise-induced activation of the branched-chain 2-oxo acid dehydrogenase in human muscle. Eur. J. Appl. Physiol. 59:159-167; 1989.
91. Wagenmakers, A.J.M.; Coakley, J.H.; Edwards, R.H.T. Metabolism of branched-chain amino acids and ammonia during exercise: Clues from McArdle's disease. Int. J. Sports Med. 11:S101-S113; 1990.
92. Wagenmakers, A.J.M.; Schepens, J.T.G.; Veerkamp, J.H. Effect of starvation and exercise on actual and total activity of the branched chain 2-oxo acid dehydrogenase complex in rat skeletal tissues. Biochem. J. 223:815-821; 1984.
93. Wasserman, D.H.; Geer, R.J.; Williams, P.E.; Becker, T.; Lacy, D.B.; Abumrad, N.N. Interaction of gut and liver in nitrogen metabolism during exercise. Metabolism. 40:307-314; 1991.
94. Waterlow, J.C.; Fern, E.B.; Free amino acid pools and their regulation. In: Nitrogen metabolism in man. England: Applied Science Publishers; 1981:1-16.
95. Waterlow, J.C.; Garlick, P.J.; Millward, D.J. Protein turnover in mammalian tissues and in the whole body. Amsterdam: Elsevier Science; 1978.
96. Watt, P.W.; Lindsay, Y.; Scrimgeour, C.M.; Chien, P.A.F.; Gibson, J.N.A.; Taylor, D.J.; Rennie, M.J. Isolation of aminoacyl tRNA and its labelling with stable isotope tracers: Use in studies of human tissue protein synthesis. Proc. Natl. Acad. Sci. USA. 88:5892-5896; 1991.
97. Wolfe, R.R. Does exercise stimulate protein breakdown in humans? Isotopic approaches to the problem. Med. Sci. Sports Exerc. 19:172-178; 1987.
98. Wolfe, R.R.; Shaw, J.H.F.; Nadel, E.R.; Wolfe, M.H. Effect of substrate intake and physiological state on background $^{13}CO_2$ enrichment. J. Appl. Physiol. 56:230-234; 1984.
99. Wolfe, R.R.; Wolfe, M.H.; Nadel, E.R.; Shaw, J.H.F. Isotopic determination of amino acid-urea interactions in exercise in humans. J. Appl. Physiol. 56:221-229; 1984.
100. Wu, G.; Thompson, J.R.; Baracos, V.E. Glutamine metabolism in skeletal muscles from the broiler chick (Gallus domesticus) and the laboratory rat (Rattus norvegicus). Biochem. J. 274:769-774; 1991.
101. Yarasheski, K.E.; Campbell, J.A.; Smith, K.; Rennie, M.J.; Holloszy, J.O.; Bier, D.M. Effect of growth hormone and reistance exercise on muscle growth in young men. Am. J. Physiol. 262:E261-E267; 1992.
102. Young, V.R.; Bier, D.M. A kinetic approach to the determination of human amino acid requirements. Nutr. Rev. 45:289-298; 1987.
103. Young, V.R.; Munro, H.N. N^t-Methylhistidine (3-methylhistidine) and muscle protein turnover: An overview. Federation Proc. 37:2291-2300; 1978.
104. Zierler, K. Theory of the use of arteriovenous concentration difference for measuring metabolism in steady and non-steady states. J. Clin. Invest. 40:2111-2125; 1961.

Chapter 28

Effects of Exercise on the Immune System

Eric A. Newsholme
M. Parry-Billings

The evidence for an effect of exercise on the immune system is derived from two sources: laboratory-based investigations into specific aspects of immune function and epidemiological studies.

Exercise, particularly low-intensity exercise, appears to be beneficial for the immune system (7,9). Thus, there is evidence that low-intensity exercise enhances the lymphocyte responses to mitogenic stimulation in vitro, and increases the number of natural killer cells and the number of circulating lymphocytes (*leukocytosis*) (9). These effects would be expected to enhance immune function.

In contrast, there is considerable evidence suggesting that exercise of high intensity and long duration is associated with adverse effects on immune function. A period of training may prevent or reduce the magnitude of the postexercise leukocytosis. Although the total number of lymphocytes may increase following exercise, changes in the numbers of lymphocytes in specific subpopulations may not enhance the overall potential immunological activity of the lymphocyte population; thus the ratio of CD4 (T_4) cells (helper): CD8 (T_8) (suppressor) cells is decreased postexercise (9,10). In addition to the effect of exercise on the number of circulating leukocytes, a decrease of immune function by exercise has also been reported. In general, high-intensity exercise and training appear to cause a marked decline in the functioning of cells of the immune system: The response of T-lymphocytes to mitogenic stimulation in vitro may be decreased and antibody synthesis may be impaired (9); immunoglobulin levels in blood and saliva are decreased postexercise in trained subjects (16); training reduces neutrophil and monocyte adherence and monocyte bacteriocidal activity (10); and training is associated with low plasma levels of the complement components C3 and C4 (2).

The exercise-induced decrease in immune function does not appear specific to a particular type of exercise. Indeed, it has been demonstrated in a large number of different types of athletes including runners, swimmers, skiers, and ballet dancers. However, up until now a satisfactory mechanism to explain most if not all aspects of changes in immune function caused by severe exercise or training has not been put forward. We suggest that intense and long-duration exercise, particularly if it is regular, can cause a marked decrease in the plasma glutamine level and this can result in immunosuppression. The importance of glutamine in this mechanism is twofold: It has a specific immunostimulatory role and it is produced for cells of the immune system by muscle (11). In order to understand the evidence in support of this hypothesis it is necessary to consider the nutrition of the immune system.

Nutrition of Cells of the Immune System

Lymphocytes and macrophages play a quantitatively important role in an immune response, during which these cells undergo increased rates of production, recruitment, and activity. It has generally been considered that both lymphocytes and macrophages obtain most of their energy by metabolism of glucose and that lymphocytes, which have not been subjected to an immune response (resting lymphocytes), are metabolically and nutritionally quiescent. This is not so. Recent work has identified glutamine as an extremely important fuel for macrophages and lymphocytes. Thus the rate of glutamine utilization is either similar to or greater than that of glucose. A further important observation is that very little of the glucose and not all of the glutamine is fully oxidized; almost all of the glucose used is converted to lactate and some of the glutamine is converted to lactate, alanine, and aspartate. A high rate of glutamine utilization, but only partial oxidation, is characteristic of other cells (enterocytes, thymocytes, colonocytes, fibroblasts, and possibly endothelial cells) (11), and it has been known for some years that the pathway of glutamine utilization in tumor cells is also only partial.

An interesting point emerges from the quantitative studies into the cellular nutrition of lymphocytes and macrophages. The quantitatively important pathway for glutamine utilization involves only the *left-hand side* of the Krebs cycle, that is, conversion of oxoglutarate to malate or oxaloacetate, despite the fact that the enzymes for the operation of the complete cycle appear to be present in these cells. Why, therefore, is so little of the pyruvate, which is produced from either glutamine or glucose, oxidized via the complete Krebs cycle? At present, basic information is lacking to suggest a testable hypothesis. Nonetheless, a teleological answer can be put forward: Complete oxidation of glutamine or glucose would provide large quantities of adenosine triphosphate (ATP), the concentration would increase, and this, via feedback inhibition, would cause marked decreases in the rates of both glycolysis and glutamine utilization.

Why would this be detrimental to these cells? A theoretically based hypothesis has been put forward that suggests high rates of glycolysis and glutamine utilization provide optimal conditions for the precise regulation of the rate of use of intermediates of these pathways for synthesis of purine and pyrimidine nucleotides during the cell cycle. The high fluxes through these pathways provide a dynamic buffer system to maintain the constant concentration of intermediates despite changes in rates of utilization of the intermediates. This hypothesis predicts that, for example, any significant decrease in the rate of glutamine utilization by lymphocytes should decrease the rate of proliferation in these cells.

Because the K_m for glutamine utilization is higher than the plasma concentration of glutamine, a decrease in the latter would be expected to impair the rate of lymphocyte proliferation. And the problem may be even more severe than this, for the concentration of glutamine in body fluids (e.g., saliva, lymph, alveolar fluid, and peritoneal fluid) may be considerably lower than that in the plasma. And there is now considerable evidence that a decrease in the plasma glutamine level can impair proliferation of lymphocytes and other functions of the immune system (3,4,15,17).

The important point to emerge from this discussion is that glutamine must be used at a high rate by cells of the immune system, even when they are quiescent, in order to be able to function optimally (e.g., in response to an immune challenge). The immune response to invasion by a microorganism, for example, must be rapid. Hence the rate of glutamine utilization must always be high in order to provide optimal conditions for such a rapid response. To delay the response while enzyme concentrations in the cells were increased or contral mechanisms were initiated could be too late for an effective response to the invasion. Consequently, a continuous high rate of glutamine utilization is required. This then raises a further question as to the source of the glutamine considered so essential for the immune system.

Skeletal Muscle and Glutamine Production

Glutamine will be made available in the lumen of the intestine from the digestion of protein. However, little of this glutamine enters the bloodstream; the absorptive cells of the small intestine utilize glutamine at a high rate and probably utilize almost all that is absorbed from the lumen of the gut (14). Hence the body must provide the glutamine to satisfy the high demand by the immune system. There is now considerable evidence that a major tissue involved in glutamine production is skeletal muscle: (a) it contains a high concentration of glutamine (a store of glutamine), (b) it has the enzymic capacity to synthesize glutamine, and (c) it is known to release glutamine at a high rate (11). Thus, glutamine production and release by muscle becomes of considerable physiological and immunological importance.

Furthermore, analysis of the process of glutamine release from muscle and glutamine metabolism from the immune system indicates that glutamine release from muscle is the flux-generating step in the pathway of glutamine utilization by cells of the immune system and other tissues. That is, the rate of release of glutamine by muscle actually regulates the rate of uptake by the cells of the immune system. Thus, the release process is considered to be nonequilibrium and to approach saturation with its subtrate. The pathway of glutamine utilization by cells of the immune system is not saturated with this substrate. Changes in the rate of glutamine release by muscle via changes in the concentration of glutamine in plasma will change the rate of glutamine utilization by immune cells. This emphasizes the important nutritional link between the two tissues.

This information suggests that muscle can now be considered an integral part of the metabolism of the immune system. Consequently, failure of muscle to provide enough glutamine could result in an impairment of the function of the immune system via lack of precision for the regulation of, for example, the rates of purine and pyrimidine nucleotide synthesis for DNA and RNA formation. It would not be surprising, therefore, if muscle contraction and relaxation providing for physical activity might sometimes influence the rate of release of glutamine and hence the plasma level of glutamine, which in turn would influence the function of the immune system. There is considerable evidence in support of the view that prolonged exercise in the rat causes decreased rates of glutamine release from muscle and decreased maximum activity of glutamine synthetase in muscle (6,12,13).

Overtraining and the Immune System

The overtraining syndrome is a complex clinical condition. It may develop in athletes when training periods are too frequent, too intense, or too prolonged, and when training is combined with inadequate nutrition and psychological stress. Such athletes suffer from an increased incidence of viral and bacterial infections and display poor recovery from injury and impaired wound healing. These signs may be caused by a decrease in lymphocyte number and function. However, no large-scale, systematic studies of immune function have been performed on overtrained athletes. It is, however, generally agreed that such athletes experience symptoms indicative of immunosuppression.

In a small study of trained and overtrained athletes, we have shown that the rate of proliferation of peripheral lymphocytes in vitro following mitogenic stimulation and the plasma levels of some cytokines were not affected by overtraining (14). These results suggest that overtraining may not, in fact, affect the function of immune cells under optimal conditions of in vitro culture, but may cause a state of immunosuppresion via change in the plasma level of a fuel or a noncytokine regulator of the immune system in vivo.

What plasma factors could be responsible for this immunosuppression? One possibility is glucocorticoids: The plasma concentration of cortisol is elevated in overtrained athletes, and glucocorticoids are generally considered to be immunosuppressive. However, this adverse effect of glucocorticoids on the immune system may only be evident at supraphysiological concentrations, and a small increase in circulating cortisol levels may in fact stimulate the immune system (8). Another possibility is the amino acid glutamine. We propose that frequent, intense, and long-duration exercise can decrease the plasma glutamine level and this could result in immunosuppression.

Effects of Exercise and Overtraining on the Plasma Concentration of Glutamine

In human subjects the acute response of plasma glutamine to exercise varies according to the duration and intensity. Short-term exercise (sprinting) increases the plasma level of glutamine, whereas endurance exercise (marathon race) decreases the level (Table 28.1).

It is, however, important to distinguish between the acute effect of a single bout of exercise and the chronic effect of a period of training or overtraining on resting plasma amino acid concentrations. Few studies have been performed to examine the chronic effects of training: The plasma glutamine level was decreased following a 6-week training period in rats, but was unchanged in endurance-trained athletes (15). However, use of an automated amino analyzer to measure glutamine concentrations usually involves acidified samples and this leads to degradation of glutamine, which may mask small differences between control and experimental values.

A study that involved a large sample of trained and overtrained athletes was undertaken. The concentrations of glutamine, glutamate, alanine, and the branched-chain amino acids were measured. The concentrations of alanine and branched-chain amino acids were similar in the plasma of trained and overtrained athletes, whereas that of glutamate was increased in overtrained athletes. However, of importance for the present discussion, the plasma concentration of glutamine was lower in overtrained compared to that in trained athletes (14) (Table 28.2). Because samples were taken from resting subjects sometime after performance had been impaired, these results suggest that overtraining has a long-term effect on plasma glutamine and glutamate levels. Although this change in glutamine concentration is small, it is possible that prolonged exercise in overtrained athletes causes a much greater decrease in plasma glutamine level.

It is hypothesized that the decrease in plasma glutamine concentration in overtraining or following prolonged exercise may contribute to the impairment of the immune function observed in these conditions in vivo. This hypothesis is supported

Table 28.1 The Acute Effects of Different Exercise Regimens on Plasma Amino Acid Concentrations

	Plasma amino acid concentration (μM)					
	Glutamine		Alanine		BCAA	
	Pre	Post	Pre	Post	Pre	Post
Marathon race (+placebo)	592 (15) n = 24	495 (18)[c] n = 24	479 (21) n = 15	286 (15)[c] n = 15	489 (22) n = 24	404 (17)[b] n = 24
Marathon race (+BCAA)	581 (17) n = 23	561 (16) n = 23	506 (20) n = 14	410 (20)[b] n = 14	478 (19) n = 23	920 (48)[c] n = 23
30 km Treadmill run	641 (17) n = 12	694 (29) n = 12	328 (14) n = 12	456 (34)[c] n = 12	397 (22) n = 7	378 (21) n = 7
Cycling (73% VO_2max)	567 (16) n = 4	615 (26) n = 4	371 (20) n = 4	539 (35)[b] n = 4	659 (42) n = 4	633 (32) n = 4
Sprints (10 × 6s)	556 (21) n = 10	616 (21)[a] n = 10	319 (38) n = 10	454 (34)[a] n = 10	371 (15) n = 10	374 (13) n = 10

Note. Values are mean (SEM). BCAA = branched-chain amino acids. Pre = preexercise values. Post = postexercise values. (+placebo) = values for subjects receiving placebos. (+BCAA) = values for subjects receiving branched-chain amino acid supplements. The significance of the differences between pre- and postexercise means is indicated by [a]($p < .05$), [b]($p < .01$) and [c]($p < .001$).

Table 28.2 The Effect of Overtraining Syndrome on Plasma Amino Acid Concentrations in Humans

	Plasma amino acid concentration (μM)			
	Glutamine	Glutamate	Alanine	BCAA
Control	550 (14) n = 36	125 (8) n = 35	392 (18) n = 37	398 (16) n = 37
Overtrained	503 (12)[a] n = 40	161 (10)[b] n = 35	379 (14) n = 40	408 (15) n = 40

Values are mean (SEM). BCAA = branched-chain amino acids. The significance of the differences between control and overtrained means is indicated by [a]($p < .02$) and [b]($p < .01$).

by the observation that the overtraining syndrome is rarely seen in sprinters or power athletes, but affects endurance athletes, suggesting that repeated, prolonged exercise is a predisposing factor.

Development of Treatment Strategies

An important extension of this work is the development of treatment strategies to prevent a decline in, or to elevate, the plasma concentration of glutamine. We have shown that supplementation with branched-chain amino acids causes an increase in the plasma concentration of these amino acids and prevents the decrease in plasma glutamine concentration after a marathon race (14). This treatment regimen has been employed by others to maintain plasma and muscle glutamine levels and enhance immune function after injury. In addition, glutamine-containing dipeptides have also been used to maintain muscle and plasma glutamine levels in clinical conditions such as postsurgery. Recently, enteral and parenteral supplements of free glutamine have also been employed to increase plasma glutamine levels and to enhance immune function following injury. These therapeutic interventions have enormous potential in treating patients following surgery, sepsis, trauma, burns, and whole-body irradiation. It is possible that they may also be important in maintaining the functions of the immune system following single bouts of prolonged exercise and during periods of hard training.

Recently, it has been reported that dietary carbohydrate supplementation prevented the decrease in plasma glutamine concentration following prolonged exercise in trained athletes. Similarly, we found that the plasma glutamine concentration was decreased in both humans and rats following exercise that would be expected to deplete glycogen levels in muscle. However, there is no correlation between the concentration of glycogen in skeletal muscle and the rate of glutamine release from this tissue in a range of physiological and pathological conditions. Nevertheless, adequate carbohydrates in the diet may be one factor influencing the rate of glutamine release from muscle and the development of the overtrained state.

References

1. Beecher, G.R.; Puente, F.R.; Dohm, G.L. Amino acid uptake and levels: Influence of endurance training. Biochem. Med. 21:196-201; 1979.
2. Berk, L.S.; Nieman, D.C.; Tan, S.A.; Lee, J.W.; Eby, W.C. Complement and immunoglobulin levels in athletes vs sedentary controls. Proc. int. conf. ex. fitness health; Toronto: 1989.
3. Brambilla, G.; Pardodi, S.; Cavanna, M.; Caraceni, C.E.; Baldini, L. The immunodepressive activity of *E. coli* L-asparaginase in some transplant systems. Cancer Res. 30:2665-2670; 1970.
4. Calder, P.C.; Newsholme, E.A. Glutamine promotes interleukin-2 production by concanavalin-A stimulated lymphocytes. Proc. Nutr. Soc. 51:105A; 1992.
5. Einsphar, K.J.; Tharp, G. Influence of endurance training on plasma amino acid concentrations in humans at rest and after intense exercise. Int. J. Sports Med. 10:233-236; 1989.
6. Falduto, M.T.; Hickson, R.C.; Young, A.P. Antagonism by glucocorticoids and exercise of expression of glutamine synthetase in skeletal muscle. FASEB J. 3:2623-2628; 1989.
7. Fitzgerald, L. Exercise and the immune system. Immunol. Today. 9:337-339; 1988.
8. Jefferies, W.M. Cortisol and immunity. Med. Hypotheses. 34:198-208; 1991.
9. Keast, D.; Cameron, K.; Morton, A.R. Exercise and the immune response. Sports Med. 5:248-267; 1988.
10. Lewicki, R.; Tahorzewski, H.; Majewska, E.; Nowak, Z.; Bag, Z. Effect of maximal physical exercise on T-lymphocyte subpopulations and on interleukin 1 (IL-1) and interleukin 2 (IL-2) production *in vitro*. Int. J. Sports Med. 9:114-117; 1988.
11. Newsholme, E.A. Glutamine metabolism in different tissues: Its physiological and pathological importance. In: Kinney, J.M.; Borum, P.R., eds. Perspectives in clinical nutrition. Baltimore/Munich: Urban & Schwarzenberg; 1989; 71-98.
12. Nie, Z.T.; Lisjo, S.; Karlson, E.; Goertz, G.; Henriksson, J. *In vitro* stimulation of rat epitrochlearis muscle. Contractile activity *per se* affects myofibrillar protein degradation and amino acid metabolism. Acta Physiol. Scand. 135:513-521; 1989.
13. Parry-Billings, M.; Blomstrand, E.; Leighton, B.; Dimitriadis, G.D.; Newsholme, E.A. Does endurance exercise impair glutamine metabolism? Can. J. Sport Sci. 13:27; 1988.
14. Parry-Billings, M.; Budgett, R.; Koutedakis, Y.; Blomstrand, E.; Brooks, S.; Williams, C.; Calder, P.C.; Pilling, S.; Baigrie, R.; Newsholme, E.A. The effect of overtraining on plasma amino acid concentrations and lymphocyte proliferation in man. Med. Sci. Sport. Exerc. 24:1353-1358; 1992.
15. Parry-Billings, M.; Evans, J.; Calder, P.C.; Newsholme, E.A. Does glutamine contribute to immunosuppression after major burns? Lancet. 336:523-525; 1990.
16. Ryan, A.J.; Brown, R.L.; Frederick, E.C.; Falsetti, H.L.; Burke, E.R. Overtraining of athletes. Phys. Sportsmed. 11:1-10; 1983.
17. Schneider, Y.J.; Lavoix, A. Monoclonal antibody production in semi-continuous serum and protein-free culture. J. Immunol. Methods. 129:251-268; 1990.
18. Windmueller, H.C.; Spaeth, A.E. Uptake and metabolism of plasma glutamine by the small intestine. J. Biol. Chem. 249:5070-5079; 1974.

Chapter 29

Physical Activity and Iron Metabolism

Lindsay M. Weight
Timothy D. Noakes

Increased red cell destruction during strenuous physical exercise was first reported in the 19th century (63). Many decades later, the possibility that this accelerated hemolysis could produce a *sports anemia* was suggested (81). The observation that really stimulated the research of the effect of exercise on the hematological status of athletes was the apparently impaired performance of those athletes with low blood-hemoglobin concentrations competing in the 1968 Olympic Games held at high altitude in Mexico City (138). The ensuing plethora of studies has popularized the belief that iron deficiency or sports anemia is a common finding in athletes, both recreational and competitive elite. However, a fundamental issue that has been largely ignored in most of the studies to date is that the diagnostic criteria for sports anemia have not been clearly defined. More particularly, the clinical and physiological significance of changes in the different biochemical indexes of iron status in the athletic population has not been established.

For example, low serum ferritin concentrations have been repeatedly measured in distance runners and other endurance-trained athletes (24,43, 50,53,90,92,94). There are also isolated reports of the absence of bone marrow iron stores in marathon runners (53,91,166,167). In both these conditions, hemoglobin concentrations and other red cell indexes may be entirely normal despite evidence of low iron stores, and could perhaps best be described as a syndrome of apparent iron deficiency without anemia. In contrast, some endurance athletes show a different profile with hemoglobin concentrations and packed cell volumes that are at the lower end of the normal range (3,16,21,50), but with normal values for other indexes of iron status including serum ferritin concentrations and percent transferrin saturation. It is this condition that is usually termed sports anemia (111,170).

The important practical consideration is whether any or all of these conditions are associated with an impaired exercise tolerance. It is clearly established that iron-deficiency anemia lowers the physical work capacity of both rats (14,39,61,115,141) and humans (6,22,66,67,150). However, neither sports anemia nor the syndrome of apparent iron deficiency without anemia has been shown to cause measurable changes in physical work capacity (26,94,121,143,153). It is therefore not surprising that the benefits of oral iron supplementation in athletes with biochemical evidence of iron deficiency but without anemia remains controversial (94,121,127,143,153).

This paper reviews the extensive literature of the hematological status of athletes participating in a wide variety of sports at both the recreational and competitive level. Particular emphasis is placed on stringently defined biochemical and physiological criteria for iron deficiency and anemia; the particular difficulties in characterizing the hematological status of athletes is emphasized (144,152). At least seven different hypotheses have been advanced to explain the apparent hematological aberrations in exercising persons, and these will be discussed. The practical issue of whether athletes should supplement their dietary iron intake with oral iron therapy will also be addressed. To conclude, a critical consideration of the validity of the term *sports anemia* will be presented.

The Hematological Characteristics of Iron Deficiency and Anemia

A state of iron repletion exists when the body iron reserve is in excess of that required for immediate physiological deployment. Iron deficiency develops through several stages, the severity of which determines the degree of functional impairment: (a) Progressive depletion, leads to (b) ultimate exhaustion of available tissue iron stores, causing (c) impairment of erythropoiesis, leading to (d) the development of anemia.

The initial response to a developing iron deficiency is a reduction in body iron stores, reflected by a rise in serum transferrin saturation and a decrease in serum ferritin concentrations (29). As the deficiency progresses, erythropoietic needs cannot be met by the depleted iron reserves. The serum ferritin concentration is characteristically less than 12 µg/L, but transferrin saturation remains normal (± 30%). The serum iron concentrations and percent transferrin saturation fall markedly only when body stores are exhausted. Once the percent transferrin saturation falls below 15%, iron deficiency becomes rate-limiting for erythropoiesis (2) and anemia develops. The diagnosis of anemia is made with reference to age- and gender-appropriate red cell hemoglobin concentrations (169) determined from a representative population (168). The condition is further characterized by microcytosis and hypochromia.

Taken individually, the several biochemical indexes of iron status (namely serum ferritin and red cell protoporphyrin concentrations, the percent transferrin saturation, and blood hemoglobin levels) are of little diagnostic value (29). However, when evaluated in combination they provide a reliable and accurate means of describing the iron status of any individual (12). The essential weakness of the majority of studies on the hematological status of athletes has been the use of too few measures of body iron status. Furthermore, the possibility that the "normal range" for these hematological parameters may in fact be shifted in exercising individuals has often been ignored (143,144).

The Hematological Status of Athletes

Hemoglobin Concentrations

Male Athletes. Hemoglobin concentrations lower than either the population mean or a comparative nonexercising group have been described in male Olympic athletes (26,138), middle-distance runners (3,45), marathon and ultramarathon runners (21,129), competitive cyclists (68), and female Olympic athletes (26,138). However, other workers have found the mean hemoglobin concentrations of distance runners (16,24,27,42,91,93,158,161), swimmers (114,158), and triathletes (158) to be greater than 153 g/L and similar to values in the general population (30,33).

Although the reported mean hemoglobin concentrations of male endurance athletes are for the most part within the normal range (Table 29.1), decreased blood hemoglobin concentrations considered indicative of iron-deficiency anemia have been reported in as many as 59% of the males on the Australian 1968 Olympic team (138), 13% of male recreational runners (82), 11.7% of male distance runners (158), and 9.5% of collegiate swimmers (130). However, in most of these athletes there was no concomitant biochemical evidence of iron deficiency.

Female Athletes. Reported mean hemoglobin concentrations of female distance runners vary from 131 g/L (82) to 139 g/L (94) (Table 29.1). The values are within the normal range for the general population (34). Comparatively higher mean hemoglobin (141 g/L to 155 g/L) concentrations have been measured in female athletes participating in hockey and track-and-field events (42,44,138) (Table 29.1). Subnormal hemoglobin concentrations (less than 120 g/L) have been reported in 64% of female Olympic athletes (138) and 11.7% of female distance and adolescent cross-country runners (99,158). However, in other studies none of the female participants had similarly low blood hemoglobin levels (24,78,124), although a significant proportion had depressed serum ferritin concentrations.

Thus the belief that all persons participating in strenuous sports generally have lower hemoglobin concentrations than their sedentary counterparts reflects a selective interpretation of the literature and is clearly not supported by the bulk of the published data.

Serum Ferritin Concentrations

Male Athletes. The reported mean serum ferritin concentrations in male athletes range widely from 41 µg/L (24) to 256 µg/L (53). In swimmers, mean values of between 97.2 µg/L and 169 µg/L have been reported (43,114). Higher mean values (123.5 µg/L and 422 µg/L, respectively) have been measured in triathletes and professional cyclists (73,158).

Female Athletes. Much lower serum ferritin concentrations, varying between 18 µg/L (27) and 45 µg/L (158) have been reported in female runners, although both Matter et al. (94) and Steenkamp, Fuller, Graves, Noakes, and Jacobs (137) have recorded mean serum ferritin concentrations greater than 120 µg/L in female marathon runners (Table 29.1). The mean serum ferritin concentrations measured in elite swimmers and cross-country skiers were 59 µg/L and 76 µg/L, respectively (109,114). In contrast, the calculated mean value for the general American population, derived from the NHANES II study (33), is 28 µg/L with a normal range of 25 to 32 µg/L (10,29,146).

The Incidence of Low Serum Ferritin Concentrations in Athletes

Male Athletes. Serum ferritin concentrations below 12 µg/L have more recently been documented

Table 29.1 Mean Hematological Values for Athletes Participating in a Variety of Sports

Subjects	Hb g/dl	Hct	MCV fg/L	SF μg/L	% sat	Reference
8 M runners	14.5 ± 1.0	45.0 ± 0.4	93.0 ± 1.0			82
8 M runners	14.9 ± 0.2	42.5 ± 0.8		25.9 ± 5.8		53
11 M distance runners	14.9 ± 1.0	45.1 ± 3.4	90.9 ± 5.8	30.3 ± 6.7		167
15 M ultradistance runners	15.4 ± 1.1	44.9 ± 3.2	90.1 ± 3.5	61.0 ± 29.0	48.0 ± 20.0	48
20 M elite marathoners	15.5 ± 0.9	43.7 ± 2.5	85.9 ± 3.2			93
22 M ultradistance runners	15.3 ± 0.2	43.8 ± 0.5	88.7 ± 0.9	118.6 ± 19.2	25.3 ± 2.9	43
30 M distance runners	15.4 ± 9.0	45.2 ± 2.7		71.3 ± 43.6	28.6 ± 8.1	161
35 M runners	14.8 ± 1.0		91.0 ± 3.0	56.0 ± 35.0	38.0 ± 11.0	3
35 M elite runners	14.8 ± 0.7	41.8 ± 0.2	87.6 ± 3.4	41.1 ± 25.7	24.3 ± 14.1	24
43 M runners	14.6 ± 9.9	41.7 ± 2.5	87.9 ± 7.2	64.3 ± 47.8	31.8 ± 11.6	91,92
60 M distance runners	14.8 ± 1.2	44.0 ± 3.0	92.5 ± 4.7	79.8 ± 55.3	33.2 ± 8.4	158
86 M runners	15.3 ± 0.9			61.4 ± 47.0		27
6 F marathoners	13.7 ± 0.5	39.0 ± 1.0		124.0 ± 41.3	35.8 ± 4.3	137
9 F marathoners				30.0 ± 22.0	22.0 ± 15.0	86
17 F elite runners	13.3 ± 0.9	37.6 ± 3.0	85.2 ± 3.2	27.9 ± 20.0	19.2 ± 10.4	24
32 F runners	13.5 ± 0.9			17.8 ± 8.4		27
37 F runners	13.5 ± 1.3		93.0 ± 4.0	26.0 ± 22.0	24.0 ± 11.0	3
60 F distance runners	13.3 ± 1.2	40.0 ± 4.0	91.9 ± 4.0	45.2 ± 45.1	29.7 ± 13.2	158
11 F distance runners	13.4 ± 0.7	40.1 ± 1.3		15.8 ± 13.6	40.7 ± 15.1	79
11 M swimmers	14.7 ± 0.6	42.8 ± 1.6		20.8 ± 5.8	38.8 ± 9.5	53
12 M swimmers	15.5 ± 0.2	45.3 ± 0.6	90.7 ± 0.6	169.0 ± 13.5	22.8 ± 0.8	43
33 M swimmers	15.4 ± 2.6	49.0 ± 3.5	91.6 ± 2.5	97.2 ± 56.3	32.2 ± 10.3	114
35 F swimmers	14.0 ± 1.8	44.2 ± 2.8	91.2 ± 2.6	58.7 ± 34.1	32.3 ± 11.3	114
60 M triathletes	15.2 ± 0.8	44.0 ± 2.3	90.8 ± 4.2	123.5 ± 105.4	34.0 ± 9.0	158
40 M prof. cyclists	14.2 ± 0.9	40.7 ± 2.7		422 ± 398		73
23 M Olympic athletes	15.8 ± 0.8	44.5 ± 2.0	82.4 ± 5.9			138

(continued)

Subjects	Hb g/dl	Hct	MCV fg/L	SF µg/L	% sat	Reference
136 M Olympic athletes	15.5 ± 1.0	47.5 ± 2.9		32.5 ± 10.0		42
6 F Olympic athletes	15.5 ± 0.3	44.5 ± 1.8	81.4 ± 5.9			138
43 F Olympic athletes	14.4 ± 0.8	43.1 ± 3.1		27.5 ± 11.0		42
29 F athletes (mixed sports)	14.0 ± 1.0	41.1 ± 3.0	89.3 ± 4.3			110
46 F athletes (all sports)	14.6 ± 0.89	40.3 ± 2.5		31.7 ± 15.6		112
13 F hockey players	14.1 ± 0.8	41.2 ± 2.4		23.5 ± 16.0		44
17 M adolescent athletes	14.7 ± 1.0			29.4 ± 17.8		124
9 F adolescent athletes	13.3 ± 0.4			26.6 ± 11.4		124
19 M pro soccer players	14.3 ± 2.0			79.2 ± 42.3	31.7 ± 6.4	120

Note. Data presented = means ± standard deviation. Hb = hemoglobin; Hct = hematocrit; MCV = mean cell volume; SF = serum ferritin; % sat = percent transferrin saturation; M = male; F = female.

in 8% to 9% of male middle- and long-distance runners (3,158). Values below 20 µg/L have been reported in 8% of elite German runners (50), 13% of South African male marathon runners (161), and 29% of Canadian distance runners (24); whereas 22% of competitive cross-country skiers were found to have serum ferritin concentrations below 28 µg/L (78).

Female Athletes. The reported incidence of subnormal serum ferritin (SF) concentrations in female athletes ranges from 9% (SF less than 12 µg/L) to 82% (SF less than 25 µg/L) in American, female distance runners (24,27,79). Lampe, Slavin, and Apple (86) reported that 33% of female marathon runners had serum ferritin concentrations lower than 20 µg/L, with 17% to 25% of female runners having values less than 12 µg/L (3,158). Serum ferritin concentrations less than 20 µg/L have been documented in 40% to 61% of adolescent female athletes (99,124), and 60% of competitive cross-country skiers have had serum ferritin concentrations lower than 28 µg/L (78).

The Incidence of Iron Deficiency

Most of the previous studies have assumed that a reduced serum ferritin concentration or a reduced percent transferrin saturation alone can support a diagnosis of iron deficiency in athletes. Few workers have considered both these parameters in designating an iron deficiency in exercising persons. Magnusson, Hallberg, Rossander, and Swolin (91) were possibly the first to point out that although 18% of the male runners in their study had borderline serum ferritin concentrations (15–25 µg/L), this was not sufficient evidence for an iron deficiency in these athletes. This point has been emphasized by Bothwell (12) and Cook (29,30) and their respective co-workers); the latter showing that a single abnormal hematological value was found in up to 50% of a sample population of American citizens.

Accordingly, when more stringent diagnostic criteria are applied, specifically the requirement that at least two of the designated indexes (eitherserum ferritin and red cell protoporphyrin concentrations or percent transferrin saturation) be abnormal in order to identify an iron deficiency, the true incidence of this condition in the exercising population is considerably lower than that predicted on the basis of single measurements. For example, Weight, Klein, and Jacobs (158) have shown that 3% of male distance runners and none of the triathletes in their study fulfilled these criteria for iron deficiency (SF less than 12 µg/L; percent saturation less than 18%).

The Incidence of Anemia

Male Athletes. The criteria employed in most studies to designate iron-deficiency anemia has been a blood hemoglobin level of less than 140 g/L for males and 120 g/L for females, usually in association with a serum ferritin concentration less than 30 μg/L or a percent transferrin saturation lower than 18%. Accordingly, the reported incidence of iron-deficiency anemia in male runners and elite skiers ranges from 0% to 10% (24,78,91). The research teams of deWijn, de Jongste, Mosterd, and Willebrand (42) and Weight et al. (158) both found that 2.5% of male runners could be classified as anemic, although more rigorous criteria were used in the latter study. In the NHANES II study (34), 0% to 2% of the white American males in a comparable age group had depressed blood hemoglobin (Hb) concentrations (less than 132 g/L) due to iron deficiency or inflammatory disease. Only 0.1% of the total male study population were severely anemic (Hb less than 100 g/L).

Female Athletes. Likewise, iron-deficiency anemia (Hb less than 120 g/L; SF less than 20μg/L) has been recorded in 2% and 4% of Scottish and South African female marathon runners (37,94), in 3% of South African distance runners (158), and in 3% of Scandinavian recreational runners (82). However, other workers have failed to demonstrate this condition in different groups of sportswomen (24,27,44,99,121,124). By comparison, the NHANES II study (34) found 3% to 5% of American women (aged 20–45 years) to have hemoglobin levels less than 117 g/L due to iron deficiency or inflammatory disease, whereas 0.2% of this female population were severely anemic (Hb less than 100 g/L).

These data show that as with iron deficiency, when more stringent criteria for defining iron-deficiency anemia are applied, the condition appears to be much less common among athletes of both sexes than is popularly believed. Indeed, a clinically defined iron-deficiency anemia, occurs no more frequently in female endurance-trained athletes (3,152,158) than it does in the general Western population, most of whose members are not physically active (34). However, the incidence among male athletes may be marginally higher than in the wider population.

Alterations in Iron Metabolism That Could Explain Hematological Aberrations in Athletes

At least seven different hypotheses have been advanced to explain the suboptimal hematological status of some endurance-trained athletes.

Inadequate Dietary Iron Intake

The most common cause of iron deficiency is an inadequate oral intake of iron (12). Considering the correlation between the total energy and iron content of the diet (19), it would seem somewhat paradoxical that trained athletes, who usually consume more kilojoules than sedentary individuals (100), should be at risk of developing iron deficiency (75). The only obvious exceptions would be athletes who do not eat nutritionally adequate diets, either because they are vegetarians or because they choose to maintain low body weights by caloric restriction (134).

The dietary iron intakes of male athletes usually exceed the Recommended Daily Allowance (RDA) for men of 10 mg/day (64), whereas the opposite is true for female athletes, whose daily intake is generally below the RDA of 14 mg/day (64, 100,160). For example, Steel (136) found that the male members of the 1968 Australian Olympic team ingested, on average, twice the the RDA for iron. Similarly, the majority of Canadian Olympic sportsmen (24) and South African marathon runners (160,161) met the RDA (64) for iron, although 29% of the former and 13% of the latter group had low serum ferritin concentrations. Women marathon runners (86,87), cross-country runners (65), and cross-country skiers (57) have all been shown to consume iron-adequate diets.

In contrast, dietary insufficiency was implicated in the iron deficiency experienced by 3% of the male and 7.5% of the female members of the 1968 Dutch Olympic team (42). Likewise, Clement and Asmundsen (24) claim that poor iron intakes accounted for low serum ferritin concentrations in 80% of the Canadian sportswomen they studied, and Deuster et al. (41) have directly related low dietary iron intakes to reduced serum ferritin concentrations in amenorrheic athletes. Risser et al. (121) reported that iron-replete women runners consumed significantly more dietary iron than did their iron-deficient counterparts.

Weight, Noakes, and Jacobs (160) have shown that although the mean iron intake of male marathon runners met the RDA (64), those with apparent iron deficiency (SF less than 20 μg/L; percent transferrin saturation less than 18%) consumed significantly less heme iron than their iron-replete counterparts (0.95 mg/day and 1.96 mg/day, respectively). Female distance runners and nonexercising controls all consumed iron-poor diets (less than 14 mg/day), but there were no differences in the proportion of heme iron in the diets of those females with compromised or normal iron status. In another study (134), women consuming vegetarian-type diets were shown to have significantly lower heme-iron intakes and serum ferritin concentrations than their counterparts who consumed mixed diets containing meat. The total iron content of the vegetarian and mixed diets were not different (134).

Similarly, Haymes and Spillman (79) found that female distance runners consumed less heme iron than female sprinters, although the total iron intake was adequate in both groups. The suggestion that the low iron content of the female athletes' diet could nevertheless be sufficient to maintain body stores derives from the study of Miles, Collins, Holbrook, Patterson, and Bodwell (97) showing that the marginal serum ferritin concentrations of nonexercising women did not decrease over a year despite inadequate iron nutrition.

Thus, although the dietary iron consumption of the majority of athletes of both genders would appear to be entirely adequate (86,100,121), the habitual consumption of vegetarian-type diets with a predominance of proteins not containing heme iron could compromise the nutritional iron status of a small sector of the athletic population, particularly women (79).

Impaired Iron Absorption

The rate of erythropoiesis appears to play a relatively insignificant role in the regulation of iron absorption (12). However, this may not hold true in strenuously exercising persons who experience increased erythroid activity in order to maintain an expanded red cell mass (16,157) in the face of accelerated erythrocyte destruction (35,59,142,156). Possibly, these increased erythropoietic demands are met directly by increased iron absorption—an adaptation that has been described in the rat (89).

Alternatively, it has been suggested that the absorption of dietary iron could be impaired in habitual exercisers (53), although the mechanism is not clear (5). For example, Ehn, Carlmark, and Hoglund (53) found that iron absorption, plasma iron turnover, and red cell incorporation were not accelerated in young male athletes whose bone marrow lacked stainable iron. In contrast, Magnusson et al. (91) found that the absorption of radiolabeled iron was the same in a group of iron-deficient and iron-replete athletes (25.1%). At present, no binding conclusions can be derived from these three studies, which are the only ones so far to employ standardized radiolabeling techniques.

Aberrations in Body Iron Turnover and Storage

Magnusson et al. (91,92) found no evidence of iron-limited erythropoiesis in competitive male distance runners with little or no hemosiderin in their bone marrow. They therefore postulated a shift in senescent red cell catabolism from the reticuloendothelial system to the hepatocytes with increased hepatic iron storage. The serum ferritin concentration, which is regarded as a reliable indicator of bone marrow iron stores (151), would therefore be reduced, and yield incorrect conclusions about the adequacy of body iron stores. This hypothesis is extremely difficult to validate. Although nuclear magnetic resonance imaging techniques are able to provide a semiquantititative assessment of liver iron stores (80), Weight (153) was unable to detect any degree of hepatic iron loading in endurance-trained athletes with this procedure. Possibly because the hepatic iron pool is substantial and turns over rapidly, it would be very difficult to detect any increase in liver iron content, even if a rather substantial fraction of catabolized hemoglobin passed through the hepatocytes (153). Moreover, it may be speculated that there would be little physiological benefit in substantially altering the red cell kinetics of endurance-trained persons.

Increased Iron Losses

Iron excretion in humans is minimal and normally confined to obligatory dermal, gastrointestinal, and menstrual losses (71). Nevertheless, there are some who have argued that physiological iron losses can be substantial in athletes and could contribute to iron deficiency in this population.

Gastrointestinal Losses. Long-distance running, especially competitive racing, may induce gastrointestinal bleeding (31,62,87,95,96,117,139). The extent of the blood loss is apparently related to the intensity of effort (96), therefore this condition is believed to occur only during prolonged strenuous racing—not during training (56). Limited quantitative tests indicate increased fecal blood losses equivalent to 0.4 ml of blood per day (122), or 4 mg of hemoglobin per stool after strenuous racing (139), which is of no clinical consequence (87,122). The iron status of the study groups was also entirely normal. It is therefore debatable as to whether or not the blood loss is a causative mechanism for iron deficiency, although it has been implicated in several case reports of poor iron status in female runners (31,62,128).

Iron Loss in Urine. *Runners hematuria* has been described following physical exertion (9), and is usually attributed to bleeding from the bladder or kidney as a result of either trauma, arteriovenous malformations, or other medical conditions unrelated to exercise (9,11,77). As with occult blood loss, significant hematuria occurs only after prolonged exercise, usually involving repeated footstrikes, and is not likely a feature of daily training. However, it has been suggested that exercise-induced hemolysis may produce large urinary losses in certain predisposed individuals with hereditary spherocytosis (70) or osmotically and mechanically fragile red cells (116,132,170), which could lead to iron deficiency and anemia (4,70).

Iron Loss in Sweat. Iron loss through insensible perspiration and active sweating is generally negligible because the total volume of sweat lost is small (113). However, some have argued that profuse sweating (1 to 3 L/per day) is a likely route for excessive iron loss (0.4 to 1.0 mg/day) in endurance athletes (24,113,149). However, Brune, Magnusson, Persson, and Hallberg (18) have provided contrasting evidence, reporting that 50 L of sweat would need to be lost to account for 1 mg of iron excreted via this route. Earlier, Green et al. (71) and Wheeler, El-Neil, Wilson, and Weiner (163) found that there was no increase in the rate of dermal iron excretion despite considerable sweat losses during physical activity in hot and humid conditions.

Hemolytic Effects of Exercise

Microscopic hematuria and hemoglobinuria after walking and running (*march hemoglobinuria*) was first described over 100 years ago (63) and was ascribed to increased erythrocyte destruction (17) due primarily to mechanical trauma (35,36) compounded by an erythrocyte membrane-protein abnormality (4). Many studies have found depressed levels of various hematologic indexes, including haptoglobin, hemoglobin and hematocrit (47,50,90,133,155,156), and red cell abnormalities (13) following strenuous exercise. This strongly suggests a hemolytic process in distance runners and triathletes after ultradistance events (43,155), in recreational runners (45,82), in competitive middle- and long-distance runners (16,50,54,91–93), in strength-trained males (126), and even in collegiate swimmers (130).

It is debatable whether accelerated erythrocyte breakdown and hemoglobinuria in athletes who train regularly could account for a sufficient degree of hemolysis to cause anemia in the absence of an intrinsic red cell membrane abnormality (35). Godal and Refsum (70) and Banga, Pinder, Gratzer, Linch, and Huehns (4) identified athletes with hereditary spherocytosis who became anemic as a consequence of persistent hemoglobinuria whenever they commenced more intensive training. However, as the iron liberated during accelerated erythrocyte turnover is generally efficiently recycled, it is difficult to understand why a shortened red cell life span should contribute directly to iron deficiency. Nevertheless, there is frequently an increased amount of hemosiderin lost in urine in hemolytic states (12) as the hemoglobin-binding capacity of haptoglobin is exceeded. Thus it is plausible that even a mildly increased rate of erythrocyte catabolism could create and sustain a negative iron balance (55), especially in subjects with an inadequate dietary iron intake and impaired intestinal iron absorption.

Nevertheless, some studies have shown the rate of erythrocyte destruction during exercise is increased only slightly if at all (44,137), particularly in those who wear well-cushioned, shock-absorbing running shoes (55,59). Furthermore, there is also evidence of iron deficiency, anemia, and intravascular hemolysis in athletes participating in nonimpact sports (130), which suggests that mechanisms other than the direct mechanical trauma of footstrike may contribute to this phenomenon, possibly by causing red cells to become osmotically fragile or metabolically vulnerable (13,116,132,135).

A novel observation is that the mean red cell life span of well-trained, male and female marathon runners is on average 42% shorter than that of sedentary persons of similar gender, age, and physique (156). This is comparable to Ashida's finding (1) of a 40% decrease in the erythrocyte life span of exercising rats. It is possible that the increase in erythrocyte turnover could result in excessive amounts of free hemoglobin in the plasma (82,92) that is not effectively reutilized (12) as the catabolized iron is excreted in the urine. This may be sufficient to precipitate an iron deficiency in endurance athletes whose dietary intake or absorption are inadequate to meet the consequently accelerated erythropoietic demand (126,153).

Dilutional Anemia

An overall expansion of blood volume is an early adaptation to aerobic exercise training (125). The rapid increase in plasma and total blood volume occurs independently of changes in hemoglobin concentration or packed cell volume, because the two phenomena are independently controlled (16,28,72,75,123,131). Thus the red cell mass does not expand in parallel with the increase in plasma volume in response to endurance exercise training. Although the former may be normal or even elevated (16,157), the disproportionate changes in plasma volume and red cell mass (16,91,157) could possibly explain the low blood hemoglobin concentrations in athletes (16,21,46,55,91,108,130,157), which therefore would be an essentially functional dilution of a normal or increased red cell mass (46). Magnusson et al. (91,92) have suggested that apparently anemic athletes may simply experience a greater dilutional effect in response to training than that which occurs in those with normal blood hemoglobin levels. However, Weight, Darge, and Jacobs (157) have shown that the plasma volumes of the distance runners who met the standard criteria for iron-deficiency anemia were not different from their iron-replete counterparts.

Eichner (55) notes that the degree of *dilutional anemia* correlates with the amount of exercise performed but does not appear to have any physiological consequence because exercise tolerance was not reduced with increasing hemodilution (46,48, 129,149). Indeed, this hemodilution, together with a right-shift in the oxygen dissociation curve (154), provide important rheological and respiratory advantages due to decreased viscosity (145) and increased hemoglobin desaturation (69,164). Thus a "pseudoanemia" almost certainly accounts for a variable but significant degree of the decreased blood hemoglobin concentrations suggestive of the iron deficiency and anemia observed in endurance-trained subjects.

The Acute Phase Response

Trained athletes exhibit acute changes in plasma protein and trace-metal concentrations, in particular hypoferremia and hypozincemia, after sustained, strenuous exercise (43,49,142,147). This could cause chronic depression of plasma iron (53), ferritin (27,43,53), and zinc (47,76) concentrations. Similarly, the acute biological response to infection and injury involves alterations in plasma protein concentrations and catabolism (85), including acute hypoferremia and hypozincemia (83,84). Moreover, chronic infection, inflammation, and trauma are accompanied by a characteristic disturbance in iron metabolism (88). Sequestration of iron to bone marrow stores results in hypoferremia, hypoferritinemia, and decreased iron binding capacity—the so-called "anemia of chronic disorders" (88).

The similarities between the acute-phase reaction and the physiological responses to exercise suggest that sports anemia and the anemia of chronic disorders might share a common etiology (142). Although formally proposed by Taylor et al. (142), the concept is not new (20,58,74). However, Weight, Alexander, and Jacobs (155) argue that although the metabolic sequelae of strenuous exercise may be similar to those of the inflammatory response in that there are significant increases in C-reactive protein concentrations (51,140,155), creatinine kinase activity (103–106,140,155), plasma fibrinogen, and serum haptoglobin concentrations (155), there are also several inconsistencies, particularly with regard to iron metabolism and plasma protein concentrations. In two recent studies (46,155), serum iron levels, total iron-binding capacity, percent saturation of transferrin, and serum ferritin concentrations of trained athletes did not change after a marathon footrace, nor during any stage of a 20-day road race. Moreover, plasma concentrations of albumin, which is one of the *negative acute-phase reactants* (so named because its production is inhibited in inflammatory states), increase after prolonged exercise (103,104,119,155).

These findings indicate that the acute physiological response to prolonged exercise is not identical to that activated by infection, particularly with respect to changes in hematological indexes. Thus we would suggest that the etiology of sports anemia cannot be directly compared to that of the anemia of chronic disorders.

Effects of Oral Iron Supplementation on Hematological Status and Sports Performance

Iron-deficiency anemia (Hb less than 130 g/L) has been associated with reduced productivity and impaired physical performance in laboratory tests of manual laborers (6,52,66,67,150). Similar limitations to exercise tolerance have been reported for severely iron-deficient and anemic rats (39,59, 60,115,141). Anemia without tissue iron deficiency may limit oxygen transport in maximal exercise (23). Alternatively, tissue iron deficiency affects both maximal and endurance exercise performance of animals even in the absence of anemia (52,60,61). Oral iron therapy has been shown to reverse these symptoms by improving not only the work performance of chronically anemic laborers (6,150), but also the exercise tolerance of untrained men and women (38,107,149), and that of severely iron-deficient rats (39,52,61).

There is no conclusive evidence that the apparent iron deficiency (low serum ferritin concentrations) and anemia (suboptimal blood hemoglobin levels) experienced by athletes is associated with impaired athletic performance (5,25,46,48,65,165), and there is no correlation between hemoglobin concentration and performance in athletes competing in various sports (149). It has been demonstrated that oral iron therapy can enhance the hematological status of athletes with compromised iron stores and reduce peak blood lactate levels after maximal exercise (101,127). However, most workers have been unable to demonstrate measurable changes in physical performance following a period of iron supplementation, even in those athletes whose iron status was improved by the therapy (46,94,118,121,127,143,153,159).

Furthermore, several studies have reported that iron therapy did not cause a significant improvement in iron status or hemoglobin levels among iron-replete athletes in training (32,78,101,112, 143,153,159,162). It is important to note, however, that most studies have used maximal exercise tests to measure performance. Consequently, little is known of the effect of iron supplementation on submaximal exercise tolerance in apparently iron-depleted subjects.

The repeated observation that exercise performance or maximal oxygen uptake was not altered despite correction of the anemia raises the possibility that these athletes are not truly anemic, with a largely dilutional component contributing to the decreased hemoglobin levels (157). Furthermore, there is the possibility that maximum exercise performance may not, as traditionally believed, be limited by a failure of oxygen delivery to the muscle (102). For example, Beard et al. (7) has shown that hemoglobin concentrations lower than the 10th percentile of the population mean did not affect oxygen transport during maximal exercise. Thus an apparent anemia may not cause a decrease in exercise tolerance as predicted by the former hypothesis.

Many exercise physiologists have argued against routine iron supplementation in athletes, unless iron deficiency has been confirmed and the athlete is at risk of developing a clinical anemia (16,46,120,121,143,152,159).

Conclusion

Recent studies (3,158) have shown that iron deficiency with anemia is considerably less prevalent in athletes of both genders than earlier reports would suggest. The most obvious explanation for this discrepancy is that most previous studies considered that reduced serum ferritin concentrations alone indicate iron deficiency. However, clinical criteria for a diagnosis of iron-deficiency anemia require the serum ferritin concentration to be lower than 12 μg/L, the percent transferrin saturation to be less than 18%, and blood hemoglobin levels to be lower than 140 g/L for males and 120 g/L for females (12,30).

Nevertheless, there is good evidence that bone marrow iron stores of endurance-trained athletes may be markedly reduced or entirely lacking (53,91,92,166,167). Although some etiologies proposed that this phenomenon may be discredited, the evidence of an accelerated erythrocyte destruction and turnover due to mechanical trauma (35,59,156), compounded by an adaptational increase in the red cell mass (16,157), is convincing.

An enhanced erythropoietic drive consequent upon these demands is assumed, although not reflected in increased serum erythropoietin levels (8,40,154), plasma iron turnover, or red cell incorporation (53,91). Iron absorption has been shown to be enhanced, at least in male athletes (91,92), in order to meet accelerated erythropoietic requirements. Whereas male athletes are generally able to meet these demands because of their more favorable iron balance (100,160,161), female athletes possibly cannot—given their obligatory iron losses (12) compounded by a greater probability of an inadequate dietary intake (41,44,79,134,160). Moreover, the maintenance of a constantly increased red cell mass, despite an accelerated red cell destruction (36,156), likely places a continual and exaggerated demand on the iron supply. It is therefore improbable that the limited body iron reserve is sequestered in hepatic stores (92) where it is not freely available for erythropoiesis.

Sports anemia, in the sense of its classical definition of a decreased hemoglobin and hematocrit concentration in exercising persons, likely arises from a significantly expanded plasma volume and concomitant but unequal increase in red cell mass, which is reflected peripherally as a pseudoanemia (16,46,126,157). These adjustments, together with a right-shift in the oxygen dissociation curve (15,154), suggest that sports anemia exists only to the degree that it is a favorable physiological adaptation to endurance exercise (75).

Given then the particular hematopoietic demands of exercising persons and the apparent precariousness of their iron balance, it is indeed remarkable that iron deficiency and anemia occur relatively infrequently in athletes (3,158). The further observation that the physical work capacity of athletes is not compromised by an apparent negative iron status (94,153,159) emphasizes the remarkable ability of the human body to meet and adapt to the sometimes excessive physiological demands placed on it.

On the basis of the evidence described herein, it is proposed that sports anemia as a unique entity does not exist and that the suboptimal red cell indexes and negative iron status observed in athletes occur independently of each other (98). Although some athletes experience a frank anemia, it develops for the same reasons as the clinical entity in the nonathletic population and is therefore not related to physical activity per se (3,158). Although oral iron supplementation with ferrous salt is of hematological but not necessarily physiological benefit to these individuals (94,153,159), its indiscriminate use by athletes in positive iron balance is contraindicated (16,46,121,152,159,165). Moreover, in view of the pathological implications of the term "sports anemia" and the contrasting evidence of appropriate hematological and rheological adaptations to endurance exercise, we consider the term to be misleading and would discourage its use.

References

1. Ashida, T. Sports anaemia and protein nutrition. J. Jpn. Soc. Food Nutr. 25:380-384; 1975.
2. Bainton, D.F.; Finch, C.A. The diagnosis of iron deficiency anemia. Am. J. Med. 37:62-70; 1964.
3. Balaban, E.P.; Cox, J.V.; Snell, P.; Vaughan, R.H.; Frenkel, E.P. The frequency of anemia and iron deficiency in the runner. Med. Sci. Sports Exerc. 21:643-648; 1989.
4. Banga, J.P.; Pinder, J.C.; Gratzer, W.B.; Linch, D.C.; Huehns, E.R. An erythrocyte membrane-protein anomaly in march hemoglobinuria. Lancet. 2:1043-1044; 1979.
5. Banister, E.W.; Hamilton, C.W. Variations in iron status with fatigue modelled from training in female distance runners. Eur. J. Appl. Physiol. 54:16-23; 1985.
6. Basta, S.S.; Soerkirman, D.; Kiryadi, D.; Scrimshaw, N.S. Iron deficiency anemia and the productivity of adult males in Indonesia. Am. J. Clin. Nutr. 32:915-925; 1979.
7. Beard, J.L.; Haas, J.D.; Tufts, D.; Spielvogel, H.; Vargas, E.; Rodriguez, C. Iron deficiency anemia and steady-state work performance at high altitude. J. Appl. Physiol. 64:1878-1884; 1988.
8. Berglund, P.; Birgegard, G.; Hemmingson, P. Serum erythropoietin in cross-country skiers. Med. Sci. Sports Exerc. 20:208-209; 1988.
9. Blacklock, N. Bladder trauma in the long-distance runner. '10 000 meters haematuria'. Br. J. Urol. 49:129-132; 1977.
10. Blum, S.M.; Sherman, A.R. The effects of fitness-type exercise on iron status in adult women. Am. J. Clin. Nutr. 43:456-463; 1986.
11. Boileau, M.; Fuchs, E.; Barry, J.; Hodges, C. Stress haematuria: Athletic psuedonephritis in marathoners. Urology. 15:471-474; 1980.
12. Bothwell, T.H.; Charlton, R.W.; Cook, J.D.; Finch, C.A. Iron metabolism in man. Oxford: Blackwell Scientific; 1979.
13. Boucher, J.H.; Ferguson, E.W.; Wilhelmsen, C.L.; Statham, N.; McMeekin, R.R. Erythocyte alterations during endurance exercise in horses. J. Appl. Physiol. 51:131-134; 1981.
14. Bowering, J.; Norton, G.F. Relationships between iron status and exercise in male and female growing rats. J. Nutr. 111:1148-1157; 1981.
15. Braumann, K.M.; Boning, D.; Trost, F. Bohr effect and slope of the oxygen dissociation curve after training. J. Appl. Physiol. 52:1524-1529; 1982.
16. Brotherhood, J.; Brozovic, B.; Pugh, L.G.C. Hematological status of middle and long distance runners. Clin. Sci. Mol. Med. 48:139-145; 1975.
17. Broun, G.O. Blood destruction during exercise. III. Exercise as a bone marrow stimulus. J. Exp. Med. 36:176-188; 1922.
18. Brune, M.; Magnusson, B.; Persson, H.; Hallberg, L. Iron losses in sweat. Am. J. Clin. Nutr. 101:127-128; 1984.
19. Buskirk, E.R. Diet and athletic performance. Postgrad. Med. 61:229-236; 1977.
20. Cannon, J.G.; Kluger, M.J. Endogenous pyrogen activity in human plasma after exercise. Science. 220:617-619; 1983.
21. Casoni, I.; Borsetto, C.; Cavicchi, A.; Martinelli, S.; Conconi, F. Reduced hemoglobin concentration and red cell hemoglobinization in Italian marathon and ultramarathon runners. Int. J. Sports Med. 6:176-179; 1985.
22. Celsing, F.; Ekblom, B. Anemia causes a relative decrease in blood lactate concentration during exercise. Eur. J. Appl. Physiol. 55:74-78; 1986.
23. Celsing, F.; Nystrom, J.; Pihlstedt, P.; Werner, B.; Ekblom, B. Effect of long-term anemia and re-transfusion on central circulation during exercise. J. Appl. Physiol. 61:1358-1362; 1986.
24. Clement, D.B.; Asmundsen, R.C.; Medhurst, C.W. Hemoglobin values: Comparative survey of the 1976 Canadian Olympic team. Can. Med. Assoc. J. 117:614-616; 1977.
25. Clement, D.B.; Asmundson, R.C. Nutritional intake and hematological parameters in endurance runners. Phys. Sportsmed. 10:37-43; 1982.
26. Clement, D.B.; Sawchuk, L.L. Iron status and sports performance. Sports Med. 1:65-74; 1984.
27. Colt, E.; Heyman, B. Low ferritin levels in runners. J. Sports Med. 24:13-17; 1984.
28. Convertino, V.A.; Brock, P.J.; Keil, L.C.; Bernauer, E.M.; Greenleaf, J.E. Exercise training-induced hypervolemia: Role of plasma albumin, renin and vasopressin. J. Appl. Physiol. 48:665-669; 1980.
29. Cook, J.D.; Finch, C.A.; Smith, N. Evaluation of the iron status of a population. Blood. 48:449-455; 1976.
30. Cook, J.D.; Skikne, B.S.; Lynch, S.R.I.; Reusser, M.E. Estimates of iron deficiency in the U.S. population. Blood. 68:726-731; 1986.

31. Cooper, B.T.; Douglas, S.A.; Firth, L.A.; Hannagan, J.A.; Chadwick, V.S. Erosive gastritis and gastrointestinal bleeding in a female runner. Gastroenterology. 92:2019-2023; 1987.
32. Cooter, G.R.; Mowbray, K. Effects of iron supplementation and activity on serum iron depletion and haemoglobin levels in female athletes. Res. Q. 49:114-118; 1978.
33. Dallman, P.R. Biochemical basis for the manifestations of iron deficiency. Annu. Rev. Nutr. 6:13-40; 1986.
34. Dallman, P.R.; Yip, R.; Johnson, C. Prevalence and causes of anemia in the United States 1976-1980. Am. J. Clin. Nutr. 39:437-445; 1984.
35. Davidson, R.J.L. Exertional haemoglobinuria: A case report on three cases with studies on the haemolytic mechanism. J. Clin. Pathol. 17:536-540; 1964.
36. Davidson, R.J.L. March or exertional hemoglobinuria. Semin. Hematol. 6:150-161; 1969.
37. Davidson, R.J.L.; Robertson, J.D.; Galea, G.; Maughan, R.J. Hematological changes associated with marathon running. Int. J. Sports Med. 8:19-25; 1987.
38. Davies, C.T.M.; Van Haaren, J.P.M. Effect of treatment on physiological responses to exercise in East African industrial workers with iron deficiency anemia. Br. J. Ind. Med. 30:335-340; 1973.
39. Davies, K.J.A.; Maguire, J.J.; Brooks, G.A.; Dallman, P.R.; Packer, L. Muscle mitochondrial bionergetics, oxygen supply and work capacity during dietary iron deficiency and repletion. Am. J. Physiol. 242:E418-427; 1982.
40. De Paoli Vitali, E.; Guglielmini, C.; Casoni, I.; Vedovato, M.; Gilli, P.; Farinelli, A.; Salvatorelli, G.; Conconi, F. Serum erythropoietin in cross-country skiers. Int. J. Sports Med. 9:99-101; 1988.
41. Deuster, P.A.; Kyle, S.B.; Moser, P.B.; Vigersky, R.A.; Singh, A.; Schoomaker, E.B. Nutritional intakes and status of highly-trained amenorrheic and eumenorrheic women runners. Fertil. Steril. 46:636-643; 1986.
42. deWijn, J.F.; de Jongste, J.L.; Mosterd, W.; Willebrand, D. Haemoglobin, packed cell volume, serum iron and iron binding capacity of selected athletes during training. J. Sports Med. 11:42-51; 1971.
43. Dickson, D.N.; Wilkinson, R.L.; Noakes, T.D. Effects of ultra-marathon training and racing on hematologic parameters and serum ferritin levels in well-trained athletes. Int. J. Sports Med. 3:111-117; 1982.
44. Diehl, D.M.; Lohman, T.G.; Smith, S.C.; Kertzer, R. Effects of physical training and competition on the iron status of female hockey players. Int. J. Sports Med. 7:264-270; 1986.
45. Dietrick, R.W. Intravascular hemolysis in the recreational runner. Br. J. Sports Med. 25:183-187; 1991.
46. Dressendorfer, R.H.; Keen, C.L.; Wade, C.E.; Claybaugh, J.R.; Timmis, G.C. Development of runners anemia during a 20 day road race: Effect of iron supplements. Int. J. Sports. Med. 12:332-336; 1991.
47. Dressendorfer, R.H.; Sockolov, R. Hypozincemia in runners. Phys. Sportsmed. 8:97-100; 1980.
48. Dressendorfer, R.H.; Wade, C.E.; Amsterdam, E.A. Development of pseudoanemia in marathon runners during a 20-day road race. JAMA. 246:1215-1219; 1981.
49. Dressendorfer, R.H.; Wade, C.E.; Keen, C.L.; Scaff, J.H. Plasma mineral levels in marathon runners during a 20 day race. Phys. Sportsmed. 10:113-118; 1982.
50. Du Faux, B.; Hoederath, A.; Streitberger, I.; Hollman, W.; Assmann, G. Serum ferritin, transferrin, haptoglobin and iron in middle- and long-distance runners, elite rowers and professional racing cyclists. Int. J. Sports Med. 2:43-46; 1981.
51. DuFaux, B.; Hoffken, K.; Hollman, W. Serum C-reactive protein concentrations in well trained athletes. Int. J. Sports Med. 5:102-106; 1984.
52. Edgerton, V.R.; Bryant, S.L.; Gillespie, C.A.; Gardner, G.W. Iron deficiency anemia and physical performance and activity of rats. J. Nutr. 102:381-400; 1972.
53. Ehn, L.; Carlmark, B.; Hoglund, S. Iron status of athletes involved in intense physical activity. Med. Sci. Sports Exerc. 12:61-64; 1980.
54. Eichner, E.R. Runners macrocytosis: A clue to footstrike haemolysis. Runner's anemia as a benefit versus runner's hemolysis as a detriment. Am. J. Med. 78:321-325; 1975.
55. Eichner, E.R. The anemias of athletes. Phys. Sportsmed. 14:122-134; 1986.
56. Eichner, E.R. Gastrointestinal bleeding in athletes. Phys. Sportsmed. 17(5):128-140; 1989.
57. Elsworth, N.M.; Hewwitt, B.G.; Haskell, W.L. Nutrient intake of elite male and female Nordic skiers. Phys. Sportsmed. 13:78-92; 1985.
58. Evans, W.J.; Meredith, C.N.; Cannon, J.G.; Dinarello, C.A.; Frontera, W.R.; Hughes, V.A.; Jones, B.H.; Knuttgen, H.G. Metabolic changes following eccentric exercise in trained and untrained men. J. Appl. Physiol. 61:1864-1968; 1986.
59. Falsetti, H.L.; Burke, E.R.; Feld, R.D.; Frederick, E.D.; Ratering, D. Hematological variations after endurance running with hard- and soft-soled running shoes. Phys. Sportsmed. 11:118-127; 1983.

60. Finch, C.A.; Gollnick, P.D.; Hlastala, M.P.; Miller, L.R.; Dillman, E.; Mackler, B. Lactic acidosis as a result of iron deficiency. J. Clin. Invest. 64:129-137; 1979.
61. Finch, C.A.; Miller, L.R.; Inander, A.R.; Person, R.; Sellar, K.; Mackler, B. Iron deficiency in the rat: Physiological and biochemical studies of muscle dysfunction. J. Clin. Invest. 58:447-453; 1976.
62. Fisher, R.L.; McMahon, L.F.; Ryan, M.J.; Larson, D.; Brand, M. Gastrointestinal bleeding in competitive runners. Dig. Dis. Sci. 31:1226-1228; 1986.
63. Fleisher, R. Uber eine neue form von hamoglobinurie beim menschen. Berl. Klin. Wochenschr. 18:691-695; 1881.
64. Food and Nutrition Board. Recommended dietary allowances, 10th revised ed. Washington, DC: National Academy of Sciences; 1989.
65. Frederickson, L.A.; Puhl, J.L.; Runyan, W.S. Effects of training on indices of iron status in young female cross-country runners. Med. Sci. Sports Exerc. 15(4):271-276; 1983.
66. Gardner, G.W.; Edgerton, V.R.; Barnard, R.J.; Bernauer, E.M. Cardiorespiratory, hematological and physical performance responses of anemic subjects to iron treatment. Am. J. Clin. Nutr. 28:982-988; 1975.
67. Gardner, G.W.; Edgerton, V.R.; Senewiratne, B.; Barnard, R.J.; Ohira, Y. Physical work capacity and metabolic stress in subjects with iron deficiency anemia. Am. J. Clin. Nutr. 30:910-917; 1977.
68. Glass, H.I.; Edwards, R.H.; DeGarreta, A.C.; Clark, J.C. ^{11}CO red cell labelling for blood volume and total hemoglobin in athletes: Effect of training. J. Appl. Physiol. 26:131-134; 1969.
69. Gledhill, N.; Spriet, L.L.; Froese, A.B.; Wilkes, D.L.; Meyers, E.C. Acid base status with induced erythrocythemia and its influence on arterial oxygenation during heavy exercise. Med. Sci. Sports Exerc. [Abstract]. 12:122; 1980.
70. Godal, H.C.; Refsum, H.E. Haemolysis in athletes due to hereditary spherocytosis. Scand. J. Hematol. 22:83-86; 1979.
71. Green, R.; Charlton, R.; Seftel, H.; Bothwell, T.B.; Mayet, F.; Adams, B.; Finch, C.A.; Layrisse, M. Body iron excretion in man. A collaborative study. Am. J. Med. 353-365; 1968.
72. Greenleaf, J.E.; Sciaraffa, D.; Shvartz, E.; Keil, L.C.; Brock, P.J. Exercise-training hypotension: Implications for plasma volume, renin and vasopressin. J. Appl. Physiol. 51:293-305; 1981.
73. Guglielmini, C.; Casoni, I.; Patracchini, M.; Manfredini, F.; Grazzi, G.; Ferrari, M.; Conconi, F. Reduction of Hb levels during the racing season in non-sideropenic professional cyclists. Int. J. Sports Med. 10:352-356; 1989.
74. Haighte, J.S.H.; Keatinge, W.R. Elevation in set point for body temperature regulation after prolonged exercise. J. Physiol. 229:77-85; 1973.
75. Hallberg, L.; Magnusson, B. The etiology of 'sports anaemia': A physiological adaptation of the oxygen-dissociation curve of hemoglobin to an unphysiological exercise load. Acta. Med. Scand. 216:145-148; 1984.
76. Haralambie, G. Electrolytes, trace elements and vitamins in exercise. Medicine sports. Basel, Switzerland: Karger; 1981:134-152.
77. Hayashi, M.; Kume, T.; Nihira, H. Abnormalities of renal venous system and unexplained renal hematuria. J. Urol. 124:12-16; 1980.
78. Haymes, E.M.; Puhl, J.L.; Temples, T.E. Training for cross-country skiing and iron status. Med. Sci. Sports Exerc. 18:162-167; 1986.
79. Haymes, E.M.; Spillman, D.M. Iron status of women distance runners, sprinters and control women. Int. J. Sports Med. 10:430-433; 1989.
80. Hernandez, R.J.; Sarnaik, S.A.; Lande, I.; Aisen, A.M.; Glazer, G.M.; Chenevert, T.; Martel, W. MR evaluation of liver iron overload. J. Comput. Assist. Tomogr. 12:91-94; 1988.
81. Hiramatsu, S. Studies on the cause of erythrocyte destruction in muscular exercise. Acta Haematol. Jpn. 23:843-851; 1960.
82. Hunding, A.; Jordal, R.; Paulev, P.-E. Runners anemia and iron deficiency. Acta Med. Scand. 209:315-318; 1981.
83. Klasing, K. Effect of inflammatory agents and interleukin 1 on iron and zinc metabolism. Am. J. Physiol. 247:R901-R904; 1984.
84. Konijn, A.M.; Hershko, C. Ferritin synthesis in inflammation. Pathogenesis of impaired iron release. Br. J. Haematol. 37:7-16; 1977.
85. Kushner, I. The phenomenon of the acute phase response. Ann. NY. Acad. Sci. 389:39-48; 1982.
86. Lampe, J.W.; Slavin, J.L.; Apple, F.S. Poor iron status of women training for a marathon. Int. J. Sports Med. 7:111-114; 1986.
87. Lampe, J.W.; Slavin, J.L.; Apple, F.S. Iron status of active women and the effect of running a marathon on bowel function and gastrointestinal blood loss. Int. J. Sports Med. 12:173-197; 1991.
88. Lee, G.R. The anaemia of chronic disease. Semin. Hematol. 29:61-80; 1983.
89. Linder, M.C.; Moor, J.R.; Scott, L.E.; Munro, H.N. Mechanism of sex difference in rat tissue iron stores. Biochem. Biophys. Acta. 297:70-80; 1973.

90. Lindermann, R.; Ekanger, R.; Opstad, M.; Nummestad, M.; Ljosland, R. Hematological changes in normal men during prolonged severe exercise. Am. Correct. Ther. J. 32:107-111; 1978.
91. Magnusson, B.; Hallberg, L.; Rossander, L.; Swolin, B. Iron metabolism and 'sports anemia'. I. A study of several iron parameters in elite athletes with differences in iron status. Acta Med. Scand. 216:149-156; 1984.
92. Magnusson, B.; Hallberg, L.; Rossander, L.; Swolin, B. Iron metabolism and 'sports anemia'. II. A hematologic comparison of elite runners and control subjects. Acta Med. Scand. 216:157-164; 1984.
93. Martin, R.O.; Haskell, W.L.; Wood, P.D. Blood chemistry and lipid profiles of elite distance runners. Ann. NY. Acad. Sci. 301:346-360; 1977.
94. Matter, M.; Stitfall, T.; Graves, M.; Myburgh, K.; Adams, B.; Jacobs, P.; Noakes, T.D. The effect of iron and folate therapy on maximal exercise performance in female marathon runners with iron and folate deficiency. Clin. Sci. 72(4):415-422; 1987.
95. McCabe, M.E.; Peura, D.A.; Kadakia, S.C.; Bocek, Z.; Johnson, L.F. Gastrointestinal blood loss associated with running a marathon. Dig. Dis. Sci. 31:1229-1232; 1986.
96. McMahon, L.F.; Ryan, M.J.; Larson, D.; Fisher, R.L. Occult gastro-intestinal blood loss in marathon runners. Ann. Intern. Med. 101:846-847; 1984.
97. Miles, C.W.; Collins, J.S.; Holbrook, J.T.; Patterson, K.Y.; Bodwell, C.E. Iron intake and status of men and women on self-selected diets. Am. J. Clin. Nutr. 40:1393-1396; 1984.
98. Newhouse, I.J.; Clement, D.B. Iron status in athletes: An update. Sports Med. 5:337-352; 1988.
99. Nickerson, H.J.; Tripp, A.D. Iron deficiency in adolescent cross-country runners. Phys. Sportsmed. 11:60-66; 1983.
100. Nieman, D.C.; Butler, J.V.; Pollett, L.M.; Dietrich, S.L.; Lutz, R.D. Nutrient intake of marathon runners. J. Am. Diet. Assoc. 89:1273-1278; 1989.
101. Nilson, K.; Schoene, R.B.; Robertson, H.T.; Escourrou, P.; Smith, N.J. The effect of iron repletion on exercise-induced lactate production in minimally iron-deficient subjects. Med. Sci. Sports Exerc. [Abstract]. 13:92; 1981.
102. Noakes, T.D. Implications of exercise testing for prediction of athletic performance: A contemporary perspective. Med. Sci. Sports Exerc. 20:319-330; 1988.
103. Noakes, T.D.; Carter, J.W. Biochemical parameters in athletes before and after having run 160 kilometers. S. Afr. Med. J. 50:1562-1566; 1976.
104. Noakes, T.D.; Carter, J.W. The responses of plasma biochemical parameters to a 56-km race in novice and experienced ultra-marathon runners. Eur. J. Appl. Physiol. 49:179-186; 1982.
105. Noakes, T.D.; Kotzenberg, G.; McArthur, P.S.; Dykman, J. Elevated serum creatinine kinase MB and creatinine kinase BB-isoenzyme fractions after ultra-marathon running. Eur. J. Appl. Physiol. 52:75-79; 1983.
106. Noakes, T.D.; Nathan, M.; Irving, R.A.; van Zyl Smit, R.; Meissner, P.; Kotzenburg, G.; Victor, T. Physiological and biochemical measurements during a 4-day surf-ski marathon. S. Afr. Med. J. 67:212-216; 1985.
107. Ohira, Y.; Edgerton, V.R.; Gardner, G.W.; Senewirante, B.; Barnard, R.J.; Simpson, D.R. Work capacity, heart rate and blood lactate responses to iron treatment. Br. J. Haematol. 41:365-372; 1979.
108. O'Toole, M.L.; Iwane, H.; Douglas, P.S.; Applegate, E.A.; Hiller, W.D.B. Iron status in ultra-endurance triathletes. Phys. Sportsmed. 16:90-102; 1989.
109. Pakarinen, A. Ferritin in sports medicine. Nordilab Newsl. 4:20-29; 1980.
110. Parr, R.B.; Bachman, L.A.; Moss, R.A. Iron deficiency in female athletes. Phys. Sportsmed. 12:81-86; 1984.
111. Pate, R. Sports anemia: A review of the current research literature. Phys. Sportsmed. 11:115-131; 1983.
112. Pate, R.; Maguire, M.; van Wyk, J. Dietary iron supplementation in women athletes. Phys. Sportsmed. 7:81-86; 1979.
113. Paulev, P.E.; Jordal, R.; Petersen, N.S. Dermal excretion of iron in intensely training athletes. Clin. Chim. Acta. 127:19-27; 1983.
114. Pelliccia, A.; Di Nucci, G.B. Anemia in swimmers: Fact or fiction? Study of hematologic and iron status in male and female top-level swimmers. Int. J. Sports Med. 8:227-230; 1987.
115. Perkkio, M.V.; Jansson, L.T.; Henderson, S.; Refino, C.; Brooks, G.A.; Dallman, P.R. Work performance in the iron deficient rat improved with exercise training. J. Appl. Physiol. 249:E306-311; 1985.
116. Platt, O.S.; Lux, S.E.; Nathan, D.G. Exercise-induced hemolysis in xerocytosis. Erythrocyte dehydration and shear sensitivity. J. Clin. Invest. 68:631-638; 1981.
117. Porter, A.M.W. Do some marathon runners bleed into the gut? Br. Med. J. 287:1427-1429; 1983.
118. Powell, P.D.; Tucker, A. Iron supplementation and running performance in female

cross-country runners. Int. J. Sports Med. 12:462-467; 1991.

119. Reinhart, W.H.; Staubli, M.; Werner Straub, P. Impaired red cell filterability with elimination of old red blood cells during a 100-km race. J. Appl. Physiol. 54:R827-R830; 1983.

120. Resina, A.; Gatteschi, L.; Giamberardino, M.A.; Imreh, F.; Rubenni, M.G.; Vecchiet, L. Hematological comparison of iron status in trained top-level soccer players and control subjects. Int. J. Sports Med. 12:453-456; 1991.

121. Risser, W.L.; Lee, E.J.; Poindexter, H.B.W.; Stewart West, M.; Pivarnik, J.M.; Risser, J.M.H.; Hikson, J.F. Iron deficiency in female athletes: Its prevalence and impact on performance. Med. Sci. Sports Exerc. 20:116-121; 1988.

122. Robertson, J.D.; Maughan, R.J.; Davidson, R.J.L. Faecal blood loss in response to exercise. Br. Med. J. 295:303-305; 1987.

123. Rocker, L.; Kirsch, K.A.; Stoboy, H. Plasma volume, albumin and globulin concentrations and their intravascular protein masses. Eur. J. Appl. Physiol. 36:57-64; 1976.

124. Rowland, T.W.; Black, S.A.; Kelleher, J.F. Iron deficiency in adolescent endurance athletes. J. Adolesc. Health Care. 8:322-326; 1987.

125. Schmidt, W.; Maasen, N.; Trost, T.; Boning, D. Training-induced effects on blood volume, erythrocyte turnover and hemoglobin-oxygen binding properties. Eur. J. Appl. Physiol. 57: 490-498; 1988.

126. Schobersberger, W.; Tschann, M.; Hasibeder, W.; Steidl, M.; Herold, M.; Nachbauer, W.; Koller, A. Consequences of 6 weeks of strength training on red cell O_2 transport and iron status. Eur. J. Appl. Physiol. 60:163-168; 1990.

127. Schoene, R.B.; Escourrou, P.; Robertson, H.T.; Nilson, K.L.; Parson, J.R.; Smith, N.J. Iron repletion decreases maximal exercise lactate concentrations in female athletes with minimal iron-deficiency anaemia. J. Lab. Clin. Med. 102:306-312; 1983.

128. Scobie, B.A. Recurrent gut bleeding in five long-distance runners. N. Z. Med. J. 98:966-969; 1985.

129. Seiler, D.; Nagel, D.; Franz, H.; Hellstern, P.; Leitzmann, C.; Jung, K. Effects of long-distance running on iron metabolism and hematological parameters. Int. J. Sports Med. 10:357-362; 1989.

130. Selby, G.B.; Eichner, E.R. Endurance swimming, intravascular hemolysis, anemia, and iron depletion: New perspectives on athletes anemia. Am. J. Med. 81:791-794; 1986.

131. Sherwood, J.B. The chemistry and physiology of erythropoietin. Vitam. Horm. 41:161-210; 1984.

132. Shiraki, K.; Yamada, T.; Yoshimura, H. Relation of protein nutrition to the reduction of red blood cells induced during physical training. Jpn. J. Physiol. 27:413-421; 1977.

133. Siegal, A.; Hennekens, C.; Solomin, H.; Vanboeck, B. Exercise-related hematuria in a group of marathon runners. JAMA. 241:391-392; 1979.

134. Snyder, A.C.; Dvorak, L.L.; Roepke, J.B. Influence of dietary iron source on measures of iron status among female runners. Med. Sci. Sports Exerc. 21:7-10; 1989.

135. Spodaryk, K.; Berger, L.; Hauke, S. Influences of physical training on the functional changes of young and old red blood cells. Mech. Ageing Dev. 55:199-206; 1990.

136. Steel, J.E. A nutritional study of Australian Olympic athletes. Med. J. Aust. 2:119-123; 1970.

137. Steenkamp, I.; Fuller, C.; Graves, J.; Noakes, T.D.; Jacobs, P. Marathon running fails to influence the red blood cell survival rates in iron-replete women. Phys. Sportsmed. 14:89-95; 1986.

138. Stewart, G.A.; Steel, J.E.; Toyne, A.H.; Stewart, M.J. Observations on the hematology and the iron and protein intake of Australian Olympic athletes. Med. J. Aust. 2:1339-1343; 1972.

139. Stewart, J.G.; Ahlquist, D.; McGill, D.B.; Ilstrup, D.M.; Schwartz, S. Gastrointestinal blood loss and anaemia in runners. Ann. Intern. Med. 101:843-845; 1984.

140. Strachan, A.F.; Noakes, T.D.; Kotzenburg, G.; Nel, A.E.; de Beer, F.C. C-reactive protein concentrations during long distance running. Br. Med. J. 289:1249-1251; 1984.

141. Takamatsu, K. Effects of voluntary running exercise during growing and post-growing periods on iron metabolism and body composition of rats fed on normal and iron deficient diets. Nippn Ika Daigaku Zasshi. 51:441-454; 1984.

142. Taylor, C.; Rogers, G.; Goodman, C.; Baynes, R.D.; Bothwell, T.H.; Bezwoda, W.R.; Kramer, F.; Hattingh, J. Hematological, iron-related and acute phase protein responses to sustained strenuous exercise. J. Appl. Physiol. 62:464-469; 1986.

143. Telford, R.D.; Bunney, C.; Cathpole, E.A.; Deakin, V.; Gray, B.; Hahn, A.G.; Kerr, D. Plasma ferritin concentration and physical work capacity in athletes. Int. J. Sports Nutr. 2:335-342; 1992.

144. Telford, R.D.; Cunningham, R.B. Sex, sport and body-size dependency of hematology in trained athletes. Med. Sci. Sports Exerc. 23:788-794; 1991.

145. Thorling, E.B.; Eslew, A.J. The "tissue" tension of oxygen and its relation to hematocrit and erythropoiesis. Blood. 31:332-343; 1968.
146. Valberg, L.S.; Sorbie, J.; Ludwig, T.; Pellier, D. Serum ferritin and the iron status of Canadians. Can. Med. Assoc. J. 114:417-421; 1976.
147. van Rensburg, J.P.; Kielblock, A.J.; van der Linde, A. Physiological and biochemical changes during a triathlon competition. Int. J. Sports Med. 7:30-35; 1986.
148. Vellar, O.D. Studies on the sweat loss of nutrients. Scand. J. Clin. Invest. 21:157-167; 1968.
149. Vellar, O.D.; Hermansen, L. Physical performance and hematological parameters. Acta Med. Scand. [Suppl. 522]. 1-40; 1971.
150. Viteri, F.E.; Torun, B. Anemia and physical work capacity. Clin. Hematol. 3:609-626; 1974.
151. Walters, G.O.; Miller, F.M.; Worwood, M. Serum ferritin concentrations and iron stores in normal subjects. J. Clin. Pathol. 26:770-772; 1973.
152. Watts, E. Athletes' anemia: A review of possible causes and guidelines in investigation. Br. J. Sports Med. 23:81-83; 1989.
153. Weight, L.M. The hematopoietic response to endurance exercise and the mechanisms of 'sports anemia'. Cape Town, South Africa: University of Cape Town; 1989. Thesis.
154. Weight, L.M.; Alexander, D.; Elliott, T.; Jacobs, P. Erythropoietic adaptations to endurance exercise. Eur. J. Appl. Physiol. [In press, 1992].
155. Weight, L.M.; Alexander, D.; Jacobs, P. Strenuous exercise: Analogous to the acute-phase response? Clin. Sci. 81:677-683; 1991.
156. Weight, L.M.; Byrne, M.J.; Jacobs, P. The hemolytic effects of exercise. Clin. Sci. 81:147-152; 1991.
157. Weight, L.M.; Darge, B.L.; Jacobs, P. Athletes pseudoanemia. Eur. J. Appl. Physiol. 62:358-362; 1991.
158. Weight, L.M.; Klein, M.; Jacobs, P. Sports anemia: A real or apparent phenomenon in endurance-trained athletes? Int. J. Sports Med. 13(4):344-347; 1992.
159. Weight, L.M.; Myburgh, K.H.; Noakes, T.D. Vitamin and mineral supplementation: Effect on running performance of trained athletes. Am. J. Clin. Nutr. 47:192-195; 1988.
160. Weight, L.M.; Noakes, T.D.; Jacobs, P. Dietary iron intake and 'sports anemia.' Br. J. Nutr. 68:253-260; 1992.
161. Weight, L.M.; Noakes, T.D.; Labadarios, D.; Graves, J.; Jacobs, P.; Berman, P. Vitamin and mineral status of trained athletes, including the effects of supplementation. Am. J. Clin. Nutr. 47:186-191; 1988.
162. Weswig, P.H.; Winkler, W. Iron supplementation and hematological data of competitive swimmers. J. Sports Med. 14:112-119; 1974.
163. Wheeler, E.A.; El-Neil, H.; Wilson, J.O.C.; Weiner, J.S. The effect of work level and dietary intake on water balance and the excretion of sodium, potassium and iron in a hot climate. Br. J. Nutr. 30:127-137; 1973.
164. Williams, J.H.; Powers, S.K.; Stuart, M.K. Hemoglobin desaturation in highly trained athletes during heavy exercise. Med. Sci. Sports Exerc. 18:168-173; 1986.
165. Willis, W.T.; Brooks, G.A.; Henderson, S.A.; Dallman, P.R. Effects of iron deficiency and training on mitochondrial enzymes in skeletal muscle. J. Appl. Physiol. 62:2442-2446; 1987.
166. Wishnitzer, R.; Berrebi, A.; Hurwitz, N.; Vorst, E.; Eliraz, A. Decreased cellularity and hemosiderin of the bone marrow in healthy and overtrained competitive distance runners. Phys. Sportsmed. 14:86-98; 1986.
167. Wishnitzer, R.; Vorst, E.; Berrebi, A. Bone marrow iron depression in competitive distance runners. Int. J. Sports Med. 4:27-30; 1983.
168. World Health Organization Technical Report Series No. 503. Nutritional anaemias. Report of the WHO group of experts. Washington, DC: WHO; 1972.
169. Yipp, R.; Johnson, C.; Dallman, P.R. Age-related changes in laboratory variables used in the diagnosis of anemia and iron deficiency. Am. J. Clin. Nutr. 39:427-436; 1984.
170. Yoshimura, H. Anemia during physical training (sports anemia). Nutr. Rev. 28:251-253; 1970.

Chapter 30

Physical Activity, Fibrinolysis, and Platelet Aggregability

Rainer Rauramaa
Jukka T. Salonen

Physical activity has repeatedly been associated with decreased total as well as cardiovascular morbidity and mortality (55). Regular aerobic exercise increases serum high-density lipoprotein (HDL) cholesterol (31), apparently modifies low-density lipoprotein (LDL) particles to less atherogenic forms (77,78), and decreases blood pressure (34,53), thus offering several plausible protective mechanisms. However, because major risk factors explain no more than one third of IHD events (30), and particularly because apparently low-risk populations also experience myocardial infarctions (61), there is an obvious need for uncovering additional mediating mechanisms.

Although knowledge of the key role of platelets in atherosclerosis is by no means new, only since the 1980s has their role been understood more thoroughly. Indeed, along with the plasma lipids, blood platelets are centrally involved in the atherosclerotic process, probably interacting with LDL cholesterol (64). They also play a key role in the acute cardiovascular thrombotic events (11).

According to Morris, Clayton, Everitt, Semmence, and Burgess (48), it is recent physical activity that protects against ischemic heart disease. Thus to reduce risk of IHD one has to exercise on a regular basis. Morris's findings are consistent with the finding that exercise favorably influences platelet function and has antithrombotic effects. Interestingly, the idea that physical exercise may prevent thrombosis was postulated already more than 30 years ago (49). However, as compared to the extensive research carried out regarding the effects of physical activity on plasma lipoproteins, data concerning the effects of regular aerobic exercise on platelet function, blood coagulability, and fibrinolysis are surprisingly sparse.

Physiology of Platelets, Coagulation, and Fibrinolysis

In order to facilitate the understanding of how blood coagulation, fibrinolysis, and platelet function may be interacting with pathological states, particularly atherosclerotic cardiovascular diseases, and how physical activity potentially could play a preventive role, the major reactions in blood coagulation, fibrinolysis, and platelet function are summarized.

Platelets are cytoplasmatic fragments of megacaryocytes, which in normal circumstances circulate as inactive, smooth particles with no tendency to adhere to each other or to endothelial vascular lining. When activated (e.g., in response to hemorrhage), platelets change shape and express two glycoprotein (GP) receptors (GP IIb/IIIa and GP Ia). These changes then allow platelet–platelet and platelet–vessel wall interactions to take place. Platelet activation is accompanied by secretion from alpha granules and from dense bodies of vasoactive substances, particularly thromboxane, adenosine triphosphate (ATP), adenosine diphosphate (ADP), adenosine monophosphate (AMP), cyclic AMP, fibrinogen, and serotonin. Then, more platelets are recruited and adhere to each other. In addition to its powerful proaggregatory function, thromboxane also is a potent vasoconstrictor.

The initial step in the coagulation process is the adhesion of activated platelets to the vascular endothelium at the site of injury. Activated platelets tend to form aggregates of thrombocyte plugs that are stabilized during the active coagulation process by a fibrin net formed from fibrinogen. Due principally to the inadequacy of available methodological tools, the role of initial platelet activation in vascular disease is unclear at the moment. However, future studies on platelet glycoprotein receptors may provide more information in this area. On the other hand, studies on the next step involved in coagulation, platelet aggregation, have provided potentially important information.

Prostacyclin and thromboxane are two prostaglandins intimately involved with platelet function and perhaps the pathophysiology of atherosclerotic vascular diseases. Prostacyclin is a potent antiaggregatory and vasodilating substance released from vascular endothelium, whereas thromboxane is a very potent proaggregator and vasoconstrictor produced by the activated platelets (47). In patients with severe symptomatic peripheral vascular diseases the urinary excretion of prostanoid metabolites is considerably increased, whereas no deviation from normal is found in patients with less severe atherosclerotic cardiovascular disease (18).

Coagulation proteins normally circulate as inert precursors that are transformed into active enzymes and cofactors in a complex, stepwise chain of reactions (intrinsic pathway). For an excellent review on the topic see Furie and Furie (25). Coagulation is initiated by a tissue factor expressed on the cell surface of nonvascular cells that gain access to the blood when tissue is injured (extrinsic pathway). Platelet activation is integral to the hemostatic process. Platelet membrane provides phospholipid surfaces. Platelet factor 3 (PF3) is required for prothrombin and intrinsic factor X activation. Activated factor Xa is the principal component of the prothrombin activator complex, which in turn initiates the conversion of soluble fibrinogen to insoluble fibrin network. Fibrin mesh, which surrounds the platelets, represents the end stage of blood coagulation. Plasma also possesses anticoagulant properties. Antithrombin III and protein C are known for their inhibitory action on most activated coagulation factors, including factors II, VII, IX, XI, and XII.

The fibrinolytic system is comprised of tissue type plasminogen activator (tPA) secreted by the vascular endothelial cells, and its rapid inhibitor, plasminogen activator inhibitor (PAI). These compounds have been shown to demonstrate a circadian fluctuating pattern; tPA activity is lowest in the early morning hours with peak values reached during late afternoon; whereas PAI follows basically an opposite fluctuation pattern in healthy subjects (1).

Hemostatic Function and Cardiovascular Disease

Since platelets are the key elements in thrombogenesis, it is not surprising that their morphological and functional properties have been found to be closely associated with the incidence of cardiovascular disease. Moreover, several large-scale prospective studies also have revealed other coagulation and fibrinolytic factors to be intimately involved in both the chronic forms of atherosclerotic diseases and acute thrombotic sequelae.

Platelet Count and Size

An elevated platelet count in a prospective study in healthy, middle-aged men has been shown to predict the incidence of fatal coronary events independent of age, blood lipid and blood pressure levels, and smoking (69). Platelet size is also claimed to be predictive of future coronary events, with increased platelet volume associated with increased risk of myocardial infarction (8,40,41). Larger circulating platelets originate from larger megacaryocytes, indicating that cardiovascular disease itself may not modify platelets, but instead, hyperactive platelets may contribute to vascular disease.

Platelet Aggregability

Spontaneous platelet aggregation has been postulated as a potential risk marker for thrombosis in otherwise healthy subjects (7). Spontaneous aggregation is also strongly associated with acute cardiac events in patients with previous myocardial infarction who otherwise are at low risk (71). Increased platelet aggregability induced by ADP is also associated prospectively with increased coronary mortality in healthy, middle-aged men independent of their other risk factors (69). Platelet aggregability also is increased in individuals with past myocardial infarction, as well as in those with ischemic electrocardiogram (ECG) changes, but not in patients with stable angina pectoris (20). Such observations indicate the importance of platelet aggregation in acute thrombotic events (i.e., myocardial infarction and sudden cardiac death).

Platelet aggregability displays a diurnal variation, being at its peak during the morning hours (70) following the initial assumption of the upright position (6). This morning increase in platelet aggregability also may be further accelerated when accompanied by increased physical activity such as walking (70). The value of this observation receives more merit when keeping in mind that the incidence of acute myocardial infarction (52) and sudden cardiac death (51) are also highest during the morning hours. However, there is no evidence available of an association of these acute IHD events with everyday physical activities.

Platelet aggregability increases with age and is higher in women than men (44). On the other hand, it is lower in those consuming alcoholic beverages than in those abstaining from them. Smoking, surprisingly, has been reported to be associated with inhibition of platelet aggregation (44); one would expect smoking to increase platelet aggregation because nicotine stimulates catecholamine excretion.

The efficacy of the antiplatelet effects of aspirin has been documented in the large-scale clinical trial involving American physicians (24). Antiatherosclerotic diet also has clearly been shown to exert its beneficial effects on platelet function (17,80). Moreover, serum triglycerides, now often considered to be an independent risk factor for myocardial infarction (3), have been reported to correlate negatively with the plasma level of pros- tacyclin (72), the most potent antiaggregatory substance.

Two separate platelet mechanisms contribute to hemostasis and thrombosis. Proaggregatory compounds such as thrombin activate platelet glycoprotein IIb/IIIa receptors with fibrinogen serving as the ligand. Because the involved cyclooxygenase pathway is aspirin-sensitive, it may help explain the efficacy of aspirin in the primary and secondary prevention of atherosclerotic vascular diseases. The second pathway, shear-induced platelet aggregation, is aspirin-insensitive (54). Shear-induced aggregation is due to changing blood flow patterns (e.g., in bifurcations and bendings of arteries) (27).

In arteries, high shear forces are located adjacent to flow dividers; the blood flow remains laminar, with little tendency fot platelets to adhere to vascular endothelium. Relatively low-shear forces operate at the far wall from the flow divider. At this site the blood flow is no longer laminar, and secondary vortexes are formed. Blood recirculation occurs during systole, hence the particle (platelet) residence time increases, and platelets have more time to be in contact with each other and with vascular endothelium, giving rise to the formation of atherosclerotic plaques.

Blood Coagulation Factors

High levels of factor VII coagulant activity (43) and high plasma levels of fibrinogen (35,43,76) are currently the best documented blood coagulation factors associated with IHD, increased levels appearing to be at least as strong risk factors for IHD as smoking, plasma cholesterol, and hypertension. Cigarette smoking also significantly increases fibrinogen concentration (46,63), whereas physical activity, HDL cholesterol, and social class are inversely associated with fibrinogen levels (46).

Blood levels of the two powerful anticoagulant compounds, antithrombin III and protein C also appear related to IHD. Recently Meade, Cooper, Miller, Howarth, and Stirling (42) observed more deaths from IHD in those with low levels of antithrombin III as well as in those with high levels as compared to those with intermediate concentrations.

Fibrinolysis

Atherosclerotic vessels have decreased fibrinolytic activity, whereas atherosclerosis-free vessels in the same individuals have normal fibrinolytic activity, as evaluated by plasminogen activator activity (38). In atherosclerotic patients prostacyclin has been reported to activate fibrinolysis (13).

Effects of Physical Activity on Platelets

Various aspects of platelet function have been studied during single, acute exercise bouts. Usually the exercise protocols consisted of strenuous, exhaustive, or prolonged dynamic exercise. On the other hand, there have been few studies dealing with the effects of regular, mild to moderate aerobic exercise training on platelet function. For reviews on exercise and various aspects of thrombogenesis see (5,19,33,58,66).

Platelet Size and Count

Physical exercise has been reported in some studies to change the size distribution of circulating platelets. However, divergent results also have been reported. For example, no change in mean platelet volume appeared after prolonged intensive exercise in athletes (37) including long-distance runners (73). On the other hand, moderate (23,26,56) and strenuous (23) exercise in less conditioned nonatheletes (56) and in athletes (26) reportedly induce an increase in mean platelet volume (26,56) and platelet number (23,26). In the latter studies maximal exhaustive exercise caused a further increase in both platelet parameters, whereas increased duration of the test protocol did not elicit such changes. These findings support the theory that exercise intensity is an important determinant of the platelet responses to exercise (26). Platelet number returns to preexercise level soon after cessation of muscular work.

From the preventive point of view it would be important to determine how regular exercise training affects the size distribution and number of circulating platelets. Such data are sparse at the moment. In one of few such studies moderate aerobic exercise three times a week for 1 month diminished the increase in platelet count in response to a strenuous exercise bout compared to the pretraining period (23).

Platelet Activation

Marathon running was reported to cause a significant increase in platelet activation based on measurements of beta-thromboglobulin and platelet factor 4 (62). Further, using platelet shape change as an index of platelet activation, Douste-Blazy et al. (16) observed increased platelet activation during exercise in young men with normal coronary arteries who had suffered a myocardial infarction. However, in these studies platelet activation might not be solely related to exercise or myocardial ischemia. Future studies are needed to determine the effects of different forms and intensities of exercise on platelet activities.

Platelet Adhesiveness

Platelet adhesion to the endothelium is the initial event in platelet activation. Accordingly, any reduction in platelet adhesion in response to vascular injury, whether traumatic or due to rupture of atherosclerotic plaque, would inhibit thrombogenesis. Several studies performed in the 1960s dealt with the effect of exercise on platelet adhesiveness. Prolonged dynamic exercise that does not result in exhaustion seems to reduce in vitro platelet adhesiveness (4,57). Again, no data are available regarding the effect of regular aerobic exercise.

In this regard, of particular interest would be studies on the effects of exercise training on the activities of platelet glycoprotein IIb/IIIa and Ia receptors, which are important in the platelet–platelet and platelet–vessel wall interactions (29). Glycoprotein IIb/IIIa receptor activity also is directly linked to platelet aggregation, the next step in the thrombus formation.

Platelet Aggregation

Strenuous, prolonged physical exercise in trained individuals was found to result in platelet hyperaggregability (14). To our knowledge thus far the only randomized, controlled exercise-training study on platelet aggregation was carried out in our laboratory (60). This study examined the effects of regular dynamic exercise on platelet aggregability. Middle-aged, moderately overweight men with mild hypertension were subjected to a 3-month, low-intensity aerobic exercise program corresponding to about 50% to 60% of their maximal oxygen uptake. To avoid confounding by possible acute effects of exercise on platelet aggregation, blood sampling took place 1 week following determination of maximal oxygen uptake both before and at the end of the intervention period. Significant inhibition of secondary platelet aggregation was observed in the exercise group as compared to the control group, in whom platelet aggregability remained unchanged.

In a cross-sectional study Watts and Weir (74) compared male distance runners with age-matched, less active control subjects. The distance runners were found to have reduced platelet aggregability at rest compared to the control subjects. Long-distance running was associated with a further acute decrease in platelet aggregability; however there were no differences found between running 10 miles and a full marathon. Based on these data the authors concluded that exercise intensity probably is more important than duration.

Prostaglandin Levels

A prolonged, low-intensity, dynamic exercise bout increases prostacyclin levels with no change in thromboxane secretion in healthy subjects (18). On the other hand, in IHD patients short-term walking exercise at maximum tolerable anginal pain caused a less clear increase in prostacyclin, whereas the already increased preexercise level of thromboxane was unaltered.

Following a period of low-intensity aerobic exercise training (walking–jogging), prostacyclin showed a tendency towards increased levels in healthy middle-aged men. The highest increases were observed in those experiencing the greatest increases in serum HDL_2-cholesterol level (59).

Effects of Physical Activity on Blood Coagulation

One of the early reports on the effects of exercise on the blood coagulation system was published by Cohen, Epstein, Cohen, and Dennis (9). In their study involving healthy young men, intense treadmill exercise increased factor VIII activity, apparently due to beta-adrenergic stimulation. Factor VIII levels increase when the subjects are exercising near their maximum levels (12,68), with greatest changes observed immediately postexercise (12). Similar findings have been obtained also immediately after and during recovery from a marathon run (62). The increase in factor VIII complex coagulant activity after maximal dynamic exercise correlates well with the postexercise blood lactate level (75). On the contrary, no association was found in another study between blood coagulation assays and changes in blood lactate or pyruvate following one maximal exercise session (22).

Strenuous physical exercise in healthy untrained (10) or trained subjects (39,62) does not appear to influence plasma fibrinogen concentrations (10,39); it does increase the catabolism of fibrinogen (10) as well as that of fibrin (39). However, exercise does not change the rate of prothrombin consumption (coagulation) in healthy untrained subjects (10,62). In another study involving healthy young men, acute dynamic exercise was found to increase both thrombin and plasmin activities with no effect on fibrinogen or antithrombin III, suggesting that exercise neither leads to the hypercoagulable nor hyperfibrinolytic state (32). Additional studies are needed to confirm these observations.

In contrast to the data on the acute effects of a single exercise bout on blood coagulation, fibrinolysis, and platelet function, the literature is very sparse concerning the effects of aerobic exercise training on these parameters. Moderate aerobic exercise training in a study involving healthy young men diminished the coagulation activity in response to subsequent sessions of strenuous exercise as measured by whole blood clotting time, partial thromboplastin time, and thrombin time; whereas plasma fibrinogen was in fact increased (23).

In another study 6 months of aerobic exercise was found to decrease plasma fibrinogen concentration in older men. No changes were found in young men who had a lower pretrial level of fibrinogen than the older men (67). Exercise training for 6 weeks did not influence plasma fibrinogen levels in either middle-aged, Type II diabetic men or nondiabetic control subjects (65).

Effects of Physical Activity on Fibrinolysis

In spite of the potentially important function of the fibrinolytic system in the prevention of atherothrombotic vascular diseases, there are only limited epidemiological data available on determinants of fibrinolytic activity. White men, low in socioeconomic status but high in occupational physical activity, reportedly have higher resting fibrinolytic activity compared to better educated men in physically less demanding occupations (15).

From the literature it appears that strenuous (as well as moderate-intensity) exercise acutely increases blood fibrinolysis (21,23,45), probably due to increased plasminogen activation. This effect does not appear to be mediated through beta-adrenergic stimulation (9). Postexercise blood lactate levels during maximal treadmill exercise are positively associated with increases in plasma fibrinolytic activity. This relationship is further strengthened by a high preexercise serum HDL-cholesterol level (75). In contrast, submaximal exercise in young, healthy males was found to have only minor changes in fibrinolytic activity, whereas a major increase in fibrinolytic activity again coincided with the maximum exercise level (12). Strenuous exercise in trained subjects also has been associated with increased fibrinolytic activity (39).

Conflicting data exist on the effects of exercise training on fibrinolytic activity. Moderate aerobic exercise training decreased resting fibrinolytic activity (23,79). However, augmentation in fibrinolytic activity during exercise remained unchanged (23) or increased (79). Also, resting antifibrinolysin activity was decreased after conditioning. More recently Ferguson, Bernier, Banta, Yu-Yahiro, and Schoomaker (22) reported that exercise conditioning increases the fibrinolytic response to maximal exercise.

In contrast, another study found that moderate training for 6 months in athletes increased resting fibrinolytic activity and strenuous training for 6 weeks decreased resting activity (36). Middle-aged men exercising up to four times a week had a resting level of fibrinolysis similar to that in sedentary, age-matched men (50). In an uncontrolled study moderate exercise increased the active form of tissue plasminogen activator in older men, but not in young men (67). In diabetic individuals 6 weeks of moderate aerobic exercise improved both resting fibrinolytic activity and the exercise-induced increase (65). Patients with stable angina pectoris generally have reduced fibrinolytic activity at rest, and its improvement during exercise is less than in healthy controls. Furthermore, in patients with stable angina pectoris, it takes longer for the fibrinolytic activity to return to resting level during exercise recovery (28).

Discussion

Early studies dealing with the acute effects of exercise on various aspects of platelet, coagulation, and fibrinolytic activites provide an additional plausible, biological explanation for the apparent preventive potential of a physically active lifestyle against atherosclerotic vascular diseases. However, it also is evident from the preceding literature review that more systematic studies are needed both on the effects of acute and of regular exercise training on platelet function, blood coagulability, and fibrinolytic activity with special emphasis on the basic components of the exercise prescription (i.e., intensity, frequency, duration, and mode of exercise). Furthermore, to avoid conflicting data great attention must be paid to standardize both blood sampling and assay methods.

Prolonged acute exercise as well as regular exercise training appear to increase plasma prostacyclin levels, which could possibly be related to the exercise-induced increase in high density lipoprotein (especially subfraction HDL_2). It has recently been demonstrated that high-density lipoprotein prolongs the half-life of prostacyclin (2). This in turn promotes fibrinolysis, and thus may be the link explaining the acute-exercise-associated increase in fibrinolysis. Evidently, the interactions between platelets, coagulation, fibrinolysis, and lipoprotein lipids are other important areas requiring research in sports and exercise medicine.

Also, the mechanisms for the exercise effects on coagulation and fibrinolysis are important aspects for improving understanding of IHD prevention by regular exercise. This type of information is crucial for an accurate and effective prescription for IHD prevention, a basic requirement for wider acceptance of and more successful compliance with exercise programs.

In conclusion, physical activity is a potential stimulus for proper balance between thrombogenesis and fibrinolysis. However, an accurate prescription of regular exercise for prevention of atherothrombotic states necessitates more systematic studies.

Summary

Research on the relationship between physical activity and platelet function has relatively long traditions. Indeed, early reports on this topic were published in the beginning of this century. However, compared to the extensive research on physical exercise and plasma lipoproteins, for example, there are fewer studies concerning blood coagulation, fibrinolysis, and platelet function. Although dynamic exercise seems to have beneficial effects on blood coagulation and fibrinolysis, there is clearly a need for more extensive research.

There is a close relationship of blood coagulation and fibrinolysis to acute cardiovascular complications. The earliest events initiating the atherosclerotic process are most likely determined by lipid changes such as oxidative modification of low-density lipoproteins rather than by a disturbed balance between blood coagulation and fibrinolysis. However, advanced atherosclerotic lesions may promote thrombus formation, which in a hyperlipidemic environment may not be appropriately counterbalanced by fibrinolytic activity.

Most available data concerning exercise and platelet function is limited to acute responses after a single, dynamic exercise session. Maximal or near-maximal exercise acutely increases the tendency for blood coagulation, whereas more moderate exercise appears to have little effect on thrombogenesis. However, the exercise-induced increase in thrombogenesis is a temporary phenomenon lasting about 1 hr. Such observations are based on studies involving a limited number of healthy subjects that need replication and inclusion of people with various diseases.

In addition, platelet aggregability in a controlled trial has been found to be inhibited following a period of regular, moderate-intensity exercise training in overweight, middle-aged men with elevated blood pressure. However, this potentially significant finding waits to be confirmed in further studies.

Fibrinolysis, the scavenger system for thrombus, is activated even during mild- to moderate-intensity exercise. However, the increase in fibrinolytic activity in response to muscular work disappears within a few minutes postexercise. Thus, one would not expect to see consistently elevated fibrinolytic activity due to exercise training. Instead, frequent, regular bouts of exercise may provide the most efficient prescription for thrombus dissolution. However, no data to support this belief are currently available.

References

1. Andreotti, F.; Davies, G.J.; Hackett, D.R.; Khan, M.I.;, De Bart, A.C.W.; Aber, V.R.; Maseri, A.; Kluft, C. Major circadian fluctuations in fibrinolytic factors and possible relevance to time of onset of myocardial infarction, sudden cardiac death and stroke. Am. J. Cardiol. 62:635-637; 1988.
2. Aoyama, T.; Yui, Y.; Morishita, H.; Kawai, C. Prostaglandin I2 half-life regulated by high density lipoprotein is decreased in acute myocardial infarction and unstable angina pectoris. Circulation. 81:1784-1791; 1990.
3. Austin, M.A. Plasma triglyceride and coronary heart disease. Arterioscl. Thromb. 11:2-14; 1991.
4. Bennett, P.N. Effect of physical exercise on platelet adhesiveness. Scand. J. Haematol. 9:138-141; 1972.
5. Bourey, R.E.; Santoro, S.A. Interactions of exercise, coagulation, platelets, and fibrinolysis—a brief review. Med. Sci. Sports Exerc. 20:439-446; 1988.
6. Brezinski, D.A.; Tofler, G.H.; Muller, J.E.; Pohjola-Sintonen, S.; Willich, S.N.; Schafer, A.I.; Czeisler, C.A.; Williams, G.H. Morning increase in platelet aggregability. Association with assumption of the upright posture. Circulation. 78:35-40; 1988.

7. Burgess-Wilson, E.L.; Green, S.; Heptinstall, S.; Mitchell, J.R.A. Spontaneous platelet aggregation in whole blood: Dependence on age and haematocrit. Lancet. (November 24):1213; 1984.
8. Cameron, H.A.; Phillips, R.; Ibbotson, R.M.; Charson, P.H.M. Platelet size in myocardial infarction. Br. Med. J. 287:449-451; 1983.
9. Cohen, R.J.; Epstein, S.E.; Cohen, L.S.; Dennis, L.H. Alterations of fibrinolysis and blood coagulation induced by exercise, and the role of beta-adrenergic-receptor stimulation. Lancet. (December 14):1264-1266; 1968.
10. Collen, D.; Semeraro, N.; Tricot, J.P.; Vermylen, J. Turnover of fibrinogen, plasminogen, and prothrombin during exercise in man. J. Appl. Physiol. 42:865-873; 1977.
11. Davies, M.J.; Thomas, A. Thrombosis and acute coronary-artery lesions in sudden cardiac ischemic death. N. Engl. J. Med. 310:1137-1140; 1984.
12. Davis, G.L.; Abildgaard, C.F.; Bernauer, E.M.; Britton, M. Fibrinolytic and hemostatic changes during and after maximal exercise in males. J. Appl. Physiol. 40:287-292; 1976.
13. Dembinska-Kiec, A.; Kostka-Trabka, E.; Gryglewski, R.J. Effect of prostacyclin on fibrinolytic activity in patients with arteriosclerosis obliterans. Thromb. Haemost. (Stuttgart). 47:190; 1982.
14. Dimitriadou, C.; Dessypris, A.; Louzou, C.; Mandalaki, T. Marathon run II: Effects on platelet aggregation. Thromb. Haemost. (Stuttgart). 37:451-455; 1977.
15. Dischinger, P.; Tyroler, H.A.; McDonagh, R., Jr.; Hames, C.G. Blood fibrinolytic activity, social class and habitual physical activity—I. A study of black and white men in Evans County, Georgia. J. Chronic. Dis. 33:283-290; 1980.
16. Douste-Blazy, P.; Sie, P.; Boneu, B.; Marco, J.; Eche, N.; Bernadet, P. Exercise-induced platelet activation in myocardial infarction survivors with normal coronary arteriogram. Thromb. Haemost. (Stuttgart). 52:297-300; 1984.
17. Dyerberg, J.; Bang, H.O.; Stofersen, E.; Moncada, S.; Vane, J.R. Eicosapentaenoic acid and prevention of thrombosis and atherosclerosis? Lancet. (July 15):117-119; 1978.
18. Edlund, A.; FitzGerald, G.A.; Sevastik, B.; Wennmalm, Å. Leg exercise increases prostacyclin synthesis without activating platelets in both healthy and atherosclerotic humans. In: Samuelsson, B.; Paoletti, R.; Ramwell, P.W., eds. Advances in prostaglandin, thromboxane, and leukotriene research. New York: Raven Press; 1987:447-449.
19. Eichner, E.R. Antithrombotic effects of exercise. Am. Fam. Physician. 36:207-211; 1987.
20. Elwood, P.C.; Renaud, S.; Sharp, D.S.; Beswick, A.D.; O'Brien, J.R.; Yarnell, J.W.G. Ischemic heart disease and platelet aggregation. The caerphilly collaborative heart disease study. Circulation. 83:38-44; 1991.
21. Ferguson, E.W.; Barr, C.F.; Bernier, L.I. Fibrinogenolysis and fibrinolysis with strenuous exercise. J. Appl. Physiol. 47:1157-1161; 1979.
22. Ferguson, E.W.; Bernier, L.I.; Banta, G.R.; Yu-Yahïro, J.; Schoomaker, E.B. Effects of exercise and conditioning on clotting and fibrinolytic activity in men. J. Appl. Physiol. 62:1416-1421; 1987.
23. Ferguson, E.W.; Guest, M.M. Exercise, physical conditioning, blood coagulation and fibrinolysis. Thrombos. Diathes. Haemorrh. 31:63-71; 1974.
24. Final report on the aspirin component of the ongoing physicians' health study. Steering committee of the physicians' health study research group. N. Engl. J. Med. 321:129-135; 1989.
25. Furie, B.; Furie, B.C. Molecular and cellular biology of blood coagulation. N. Engl. J. Med. 326:800-806; 1992.
26. Gimenez, M.; Mohan-Kumar, T.; Humbert, J.C.; De Talance, N.; Buisine, J. Leukocyte, lymphocyte and platelet response to dynamic exercise. Duration or intensity? Eur. J. Appl. Physiol. 55:465-470; 1986.
27. Glagov, S.; Zarins, C.; Giddens, D.P.; Ku, D.N. Hemodynamics and atherosclerosis. Insights and perspectives gained from studies of human arteries. Arch. Pathol. Lab. Med. 112:1018-1031; 1988.
28. Hamouratidis, N.D.; Pertsinidis, T.E.; Bacharoudis, G.P.; Papazachariou, G.S. Effects of exercise on plasma fibrinolytic activity in patients with ischaemic heart disease. Int. J. Cardiol. 19:39-45; 1988.
29. Hawiger, J. Platelet-vessel wall interactions. Platelet adhesion and aggregation. Atheroscl. Rev. 21:165-186; 1990.
30. Heller, R.F.; Chinn, S.; Tunstall Pedoe, H.D.; Rose, G. How well can we predict coronary heart disease? Findings in the United Kingdom heart disease prevention project. Br. Med. J. 288:1409-1411; 1984.
31. Huttunen, J.K.; Länsimies, E.; Voutilainen, E.; Enholm, C.; Hietanen, E.; Penttilä, I.; Siitonen, O.; Rauramaa, R. Effect of moderate physical exercise on serum lipoproteins. A controlled clinical trial with special reference to serum high-density lipoproteins. Circulation. 60:1220-1229; 1979.

32. Hyers, T.M.; Martin, B.J.; Pratt, D.S.; Dreisin, R.B.; Franks, J.J. Enhanced thrombin and plasmin activity with exercise in man. J. Appl. Physiol. 48:821-825; 1980.
33. Ikkala, E.; Myllylä, G.; Sarajas, H.S.S. Haemostatic changes associated with exercise. Nature. 199:459-461; 1963.
34. Jennings, G.; Nelson, L.; Nestel, P.; Esler, M.; Korner, P.; Burton, D.; Bazelmans, J. The effects of changes in physical activity on major cardiovascular risk factors, hemodynamics, sympathetic function, and glucose utilization in man: A controlled study of four levels of activity. Circulation. 73:30-40; 1986.
35. Kannel, W.B.; Wolf, P.A.; Castelli, W.P.; D'Agostino, R.B. Fibrinogen and risk of cardiovascular disease. The Framingham study. JAMA. 258:1183-1186; 1987.
36. Keber, D.; Stegnar, M.; Keber, I.; Accetto, B. Influence of moderate and strenuous daily physical activity on fibrinolytic activity of blood: Possibility of plasmonigen activator stores depletion. Thromb. Haemost. 41:745-755; 1979.
37. Kishk, Y.T.; Trowbridge, E.A.; Martin, J.F. The effects of exercise on platelet numbers and size. Letters to the editor. Med. Lab. Sci. 42:406-408; 1985.
38. Ljungner, H.; Bergqvist, D. Decreased fibrinolytic activity in human atherosclerotic vessels. Atherosclerosis. 50:113-116; 1984.
39. Mandalaki, T.; Dessypris, A.; Louizou, C.; Bossinakou, I.; Panayotopoulou, C.; Antonopoulou, A. Marathon run I: Effects on blood coagulation and fibrinolysis. Thromb. Haemost. (Stuttgart). 37:444-450; 1977.
40. Martin, J.F.; Bath, P.M.W.; Burr, M.L. Influence of platelet size on outcome after myocardial infarction. Lancet. 338:1409-1411; 1991.
41. Martin, J.F.; Plumb, J.; Kilbey, R.S; Kishk, Y.T. Changes in volume and density of platelets in myocardial infarction. Br. Med. J. 287:456-459; 1983.
42. Meade, T.W.; Cooper, J.; Miller, G.J.; Howarth, D.J.; Stirling, Y. Antithrombin III and arterial disease. Lancet. 338:850-851; 1991.
43. Meade, T.W.; Mellows, S.; Brozovic, M.; Miller, G.J.; Chakrabarti, R.R.; North, W.R.S.; Haines, A.P.; Stirling, Y.; Imeson, J.D.; Thompson, S.G. Haemostatic function and ischaemic heart disease: Principal results of the Nothwick Park heart study. Lancet. (Sept. 6):533-537; 1986.
44. Meade, T.W.; Vickers, M.V.; Thompson, S.G.; Stirling, Y.; Haines, A.P.; Miller, G.J. Epidemiological characteristics of platelet aggregability. Br. Med. J. 290:428-431; 1985.
45. Menon, I.S.; Burke, F.; Dewar, H.A. Effect of strenuous and graded exercise on fibrinolytic activity. Lancet. (April 1):700-703; 1967.
46. Möller, L.; Kristensen, T.S. Plasma fibrinogen and ischemic heart disease risk factors. Arterioscl. Thromb. 11:344-350; 1991.
47. Moncada, S.; Vane, J.R. Arachidonic acid metabolites and the interactions between platelets and blood-vessel walls. N. Engl. J. Med. 300:1142-1147; 1979.
48. Morris, J.N.; Clayton, D.G.; Everitt, M.G.; Semmence, A.M.; Burgess, E.H. Exercise in leisure time: Coronary attack and death rates. Br. Heart J. 63:325-334; 1990.
49. Morris, J.N.; Crawford, M.D. Coronary heart disease and physical activity of work. Br. Med. J. 2:1485-1490; 1958.
50. Moxley, R.T.; Brakman, P.; Astrup, T. Resting levels of fibrinolysis in blood in inactive and exercising men. J. Appl. Physiol. 28:549-552; 1970.
51. Muller, J.E.; Ludmer, P.L.; Willich, S.N.; Tofler, G.H.; Aylmer, G.; Klangos, I.; Stone, P.H. Circadian variation in the frequency of sudden cardiac death. Circulation. 75:131-138; 1987.
52. Muller, J.E.; Stone, P.H.; Turi, Z.G.; Rutherford, J.D.; Czeisler, C.; Parker, C.; Poole, W.K.; Passamani, E.; Roberts, R.; Robertson, T.; Sobel, B.E.; Willerson, J.T.; Braunwald, E.; MILIS Study Group. Circadian variation in the frequency of onset of acute myocardial infarction. N. Engl. J. Med. 313:1315; 1985.
53. Nelson, L.; Esler, M.D.; Jennings, G.L.; Korner, P.I. Effect of changing levels of physical activity on blood pressure and hemodynamics in essential hypertension. Lancet. 2:473-476; 1986.
54. O'Brien, J.R. Shear-induced platelet aggregation. Lancet. 335:711-713; 1990.
55. Paffenbarger, R.S., Jr.; Hyde, R.T.; Wing, A.L. Physical activity and physical fitness as determinants of health and longevity. In: Bouchard, C.; Shephard, R.; Stephens, T.; Sutton, J.; McPherson, B., eds. Exercise, fitness, and health. Champaign, IL: Human Kinetics; 1990:33-48.
56. Peatfield, R.C.; Gawel, M.J.; Clifford-Rose, F.; The effects of exercise on platelet numbers and size. Med. Lab. Sci. 42:40-43; 1985.
57. Pegrum, G.D.; Harrison, K.M.; Shaw, S.; Haselton, A.; Wolff, S. Effect of prolonged exercise on platelet adhesiveness. Nature. 213:301-302; 1967.
58. Rauramaa, R. Physical activity and prostanoids. Acta Med. Scand. [Suppl.]. 711:137-142; 1987.
59. Rauramaa, R.; Salonen, J.T.; Kukkonen-Harjula, K.; Seppänen, K.; Seppälä, E.; Vapaatalo, H.; Huttunen, J.K. Effects of mild physical exercise on

serum lipoproteins and metabolites of arachidonic acid: A controlled randomised trial in middle aged men. Br. Med. J. 288:603-606; 1984.
60. Rauramaa, R.; Salonen, J.T.; Seppänen, K.; Salonen, R.; Venäläinen, J.M.; Ihanainen, M.; Rissanen, V. Inhibition of platelet aggregability by moderate-intensity physical exercise: A randomized clinical trial in overweight men. Circulation. 74:939-944; 1986.
61. Ridker, P.M.; Hennekens, C.H. Hemostatic risk factors for coronary heart disease. Editorial comment. Circulation. 83:1098-1100; 1991.
62. Röcker, L.; Drygas, W.K.; Heyduck, B. Blood platelet activation and increase in thrombin activity following a marathon race. Eur. J. Appl. Physiol. 55:374-380; 1986.
63. Rosengren, A.; Wilhelmsen, L.; Welin, L.; Tsipogianni, A.; Teger-Nilsson, A.-C.; Wedel, H. Social influences and cardiovascular risk factors as determinants of plasma fibrinogen concentration in a general population sample of middle aged men. Br. Med. J. 300:634-638;1990.
64. Ross, R. The pathogenesis of atherosclerosis—an update. N. Engl. J. Med. 314:488-500; 1986.
65. Schneider, S.H.; Kim, H.C.; Khachadurian, A.K.; Ruderman, N.B. Impaired fibrinolytic response to exercise in type II diabetes: Effects of exercise and physical training. Metabolism. 37:924-929; 1988.
66. Sinzinger, H.; Virgolini, I. Effects of exercise on parameters of blood coagulation, platelet function and the prostaglandin system. Sports Med. 6:238-245; 1988.
67. Stratton, J.R.; Chandler, W.L.; Schwartz, R.S.; Cerqueira, M.D.; Levy, W.C.; Kahn, S.E.; Larson, V.G.; Cain, K.C.; Beard, J.C.; Abrass, I.B. Effects of physical conditioning on fibrinolytic variables and fibrinogen in young and old healthy adults. Circulation. 83:1692-1697; 1991.
68. Taniguchi, N.; Furui, H.; Yamauchi, K.; Sotobata, I. Effects of treadmill exercise on platelet functions and blood coagulating activities in healthy men. Jpn. Heart J. 25:167-184; 1984.
69. Thaulow, E.; Erikssen, J.; Sandvik, L.; Stormorken, H.; Cohn, P.F. Blood platelet count and function are related to total and cardiovascular death in apparently healthy men. Circulation. 84:613-617; 1991.
70. Toffler, G.H.; Brezinski, D.; Schafer, A.I.; Czeisler, C.A.; Rutherford, J.D.; Willich, S.N.; Gleason, R.E.; Williams, G.H.; Muller, J.E. Concurrent morning increase in platelet aggregability and the risk of myocardial infarction and sudden cardiac death. N. Engl. J. Med. 316:1514; 1987.
71. Trip, M.D.; Cats, V.M.; van Capelle, F.J.L.; Vreeken, J. Platelet hyperreactivity and prognosis in survivors of myocardial infarction. N. Engl. J. Med. 322:1549-1554; 1990.
72. Viinikka, L.; Ylikorkala, O. An inverse correlation between plasma prostacyclin and serum triglycerides. N. Engl. J. Med. 302:1424-1425; 1980.
73. Watts, E. Platelet size does not change in the thromboscytosis of prolonged exercise. Platelets. 1:89-90; 1990.
74. Watts, E.J.; Weir, P. Reduced platelet aggregation in long-distance runners. Lancet. 1:1013; 1989.
75. Wheeler, M.E.; Davis, G.L.; Gillespie, W.J.; Bern, M.M. Physiological changes in hemostasis associated with acute exercise. J. Appl. Physiol. 60:986-990; 1986.
76. Wilhelmsen, L.; Svardsudd, K.; Korsan-Bengtsen, K.; Larsson, B.; Welin, L.; Tibblin, G. Fibrinogen as a risk factor for stroke and myocardial infarction. N. Engl. J. Med. 311:501-505; 1984.
77. Williams, P.T.; Kraus, R.M.; Vranizan, K.M.; Albers, J.J.; Terry, R.B.; Wood, P.D.S. Effects of exercise-induced weight loss on low density lipoprotein subfractions in healthy men. Arteriosclerosis. 9:623-632; 1989.
78. Williams, P.T.; Kraus, R.M.; Vranizan, K.M.; Wood, P.D.S. Changes in lipoprotein subfractions during diet-induced and exercise-induced weight loss in moderately overweight men. Circulation. 81:1293-1304; 1990.
79. Williams, R.S.; Logue, E.E.; Lewis, J.L.; Barton, T.; Stead, N.W.; Wallace, A.G.; Pizzo, S.V. Physical conditioning augments the fibrinolytic response to venous occlusion in healthy adults. N. Engl. J. Med. 302:987-991; 1981.
80. Willis, A.L. Dihomo-g-linolenic acid as the endogenous protective agent for myocardial infarction. Lancet. (September 22):697; 1984.

Chapter 31

Physical Activity and Free Radicals

E. Randy Eichner

In the past 25 years, oxygen free radicals have come from obscurity to renown in biology and medicine. Free radical research today spawns countless articles every month. Entire scientific journals and periodic international conferences are devoted to free radicals in health and disease. This chapter reviews what we know about physical activity and free radicals.

A *free radical* is generally defined as any molecule, molecular fragment, or other species capable of independent existence and containing one or more unpaired electrons, meaning an electron that is alone in an orbital. As such, free radicals are ubiquitous in biology and, in fact, are normal intermediate products of aerobic metabolism. In short and simple terms, in the normally metabolizing aerobic cell, oxygen undergoes a tetravalent reduction, accepting four electrons to form water. During this process, several free radicals are formed.

The first electron transfer generates the superoxide anion radical. The second transfer generates hydrogen peroxide, not itself a free radical, but capable of spawning free radicals. The third transfer generates the potent hydroxyl radical. Finally, the fourth electron transfer forms a molecule of water.

Free radicals are chemical reactors capable of widespread, unruly oxidation and peroxidation of protein, lipids, and DNA, causing cellular and tissue damage. As such, they may contribute to pathophysiology in a dazzling array of diseases and conditions, including ischemia-reperfusion injury of virtually every organ of the body, as well as heart disease, cancer, stroke, and even aging itself.

In fact, as said in a recent scholarly review, free radicals have been implicated in over 100 conditions, including "excessive exercise." This broad scope, the reviewers note, implies that "free radicals are not esoteric but that their increased formation accompanies tissue injury in most, if not all, human diseases." Sometimes, the reviewers conclude, free radicals contribute to disease pathology; at other times, probably not (20).

It must also be noted that free radicals are not merely detrimental, but are part of normal physiology in, for example: (a) the bacteriocidal action of phagocytes, that is, granulocytes and macrophages; (b) the regulation of smooth muscle tone in blood vessels, in that *endothelium-derived relaxing factor* is the free radical nitric oxide; and (c) the catalytic oxidation of endogenous compounds, drugs, and toxins by way of the heme-protein cytochrome P450 enzyme system (2).

Not all free radicals are equally potent. By far the most potent is the hydroxyl radical, described as "fearsomely reactive . . . can attack all biologic molecules, usually setting off free radical chain reactions" (20). In contrast, the superoxide anion radical is much less reactive. Some of the superoxide anion radical production is a chemical accident due to "leakage" of electrons from mitochondrial electron transport chains onto oxygen (20); this is where aerobic exercise comes in. As mentioned previously, hydrogen peroxide is not a free radical; however, in the presence of traces of transition metals such as iron or copper it can generate the hydroxyl radical (2).

Because free radicals (especially the superoxide anion radical) and other reactive oxygen species (especially hydrogen peroxide) form continuously in vivo, the body has systems both to repair oxidative damage and to prevent it. The latter, known generically as *antioxidant defense systems*, include free radical scavenging enzymes, metal-binding proteins, and antioxidants such as vitamin C, vitamin E, and beta carotene.

A key scavenging enzyme is superoxide dismutase, discovered in 1968; this enzyme converts the superoxide anion radical to oxygen and hydrogen peroxide. The hydrogen peroxide is then removed from the cell by two other scavenging enzymes, catalase and glutathione peroxidase. The study of inborn errors of metabolism suggests that, of the two, glutathione peroxidase is the more important.

Glutathione peroxidase, the only human enzyme that requires the element selenium for its activity, removes hydrogen peroxide by using it to oxidize reduced glutathione (GSH) to oxidized glutathione (GSSG). Catalase, a heme-containing enzyme, transforms hydrogen peroxide into oxygen and water.

As noted, transition metal ions (as in salts of iron or copper) strongly promote free radical reactions.

For example, the ferrous ion transforms hydrogen peroxide into the hydroxyl radical via the Fenton reaction. Hence, metal-binding proteins have antioxidant properties. When it comes to iron, transferrin in the plasma and ferritin and hemosiderin inside the cells ensure that little "free" iron is available to promote free radical reactions. Ceruloplasmin and other proteins do the same for copper.

Other notable antioxidants are vitamin C, vitamin E, and beta carotene. Vitamin C, or ascorbate, seems to be the critical antioxidant in plasma, being the only endogenous antioxidant that completely protects plasma lipids from peroxidative damage induced by aqueous peroxyl radicals (15). Once ascorbate has been consumed in trapping these free radicals, the other water-soluble antioxidants, urate, bilirubin, and the protein thiols, can trap only part of the remaining aqueous peroxyl radicals. Those untrapped diffuse into plasma lipids, where they initiate lipid peroxidation that is inhibited presumably by vitamin E (15).

Lipid-soluble vitamin E thus seems to be a cardinal antioxidant in cell membranes. Vitamin E is a mixture of four tocopherols; alpha tocopherol is the best trapper of peroxyl radicals. Tocopherol transfers a hydrogen atom (with its single electron), thus removing the peroxyl free radical before it can react with adjacent fatty-acid side chains. Hence, tocopherol breaks the "one radical begets another" chain reaction of lipid peroxidation. In the process, tocopherol itself becomes a radical. Because of its molecular structure, however, the tocopherol radical is fairly stable and thus is a good antioxidant. The tocopherol radical may be removed by ascorbate in the plasma or in the aqueous compartment of the cell (2,20). Finally, beta carotene and the carotenoids, although present in lower concentrations than tocopherol, do scavenge free radicals and quench singlet oxygen. Eminently lipid-soluble, the carotenoids seem to be key antioxidants in the most hydrophobic compartments of the cell.

In the human body, then, oxygen free radicals are continuously generated and scavenged during normal aerobic metabolism. Given that physical activity or exercise revs up aerobic metabolism, to what extent does it enhance free radical formation and to what consequence?

Animal Research

Does Physical Activity Increase Free Radical Formation?

Research here is relatively sparse, but in the past 15 years several studies have suggested that certain forms of physical exercise can increase free radical formation, at least in the exercising muscle.

For starters, it is agreed that strenuous exercise can damage skeletal muscle. Along these lines it has been shown in a rat model that exhaustive exercise results in (a) decreased mitochondrial respiratory control, (b) loss of sarcoplasmic reticulum and endoplasmic reticulum integrity, (c) increased levels of lipid peroxidation, and (d) increased free radical concentrations in skeletal muscle. Also, vitamin E deficiency in such rats seems to reduce endurance capacity and accelerate exercise-evoked changes in liver and skeletal muscle (12).

As noted in the introduction, glutathione participates in antioxidant defense in cells. By this framework, when cells are stressed oxidatively, levels of GSH are usually reduced and levels of GSSG are usually increased. Accordingly, in this rat model if the stress to skeletal muscle is oxidative in nature GSH levels should fall during exhaustive exercise; and this has been shown. For example, following exhaustive exercise, the levels of GSH are increased in the plasma, but decreased in the liver and skeletal muscles of rats, whereas levels of GSSG are increased in all three tissues (32).

This result was interpreted as most consistent with the scavenging by glutathione of exercise-induced free radicals in the muscles. It was further proposed that the reduced levels of glutathione in the liver, along with the increased levels in the plasma, might owe to an exercise-induced efflux of GSH from the liver to deliver it to the tissues that need it the most—in this case, skeletal muscle (32).

A confounder in interpreting this research is that the rats were run to exhaustion and so surely incurred muscle damage. Was it the exercise per se that increased free radical formation, or did free radicals stem instead from muscle damage or from neutrophils and monocytes infiltrating the damaged muscle? Another confounder in extrapolating the findings here to humans is that, according to other researchers, human plasma has negligible amounts of GSH and GSSG. In other words, the GSH and GSSG in human blood is thought to come primarily from red cells (17).

Much of the other recent research in animals is perceptively reviewed elsewhere (23). Further support for the hypothesis that exercise generates free radicals comes from a study that used electron paramagnetic resonance, or *electron spin resonance*, to detect free radical signals. The results were interpreted as evidence for the generation of free radicals in rat gastrocnemius muscle that had been stimulated to contract for 30 min (22).

Other researchers have found in animal models that (a) painful stress, (b) a 3-hr swim, (c) injecting adrenaline, or (d) immobilization can notably increase lipid peroxidation (25). Perhaps the general stress of immobilization increases lipid peroxidation, just as that of head-down, hind limb suspension, a rodent model meant to simulate weightlessness, does (16).

In horses, too, acute exercise seems to increase lipid peroxidation. For example, when six horses were run on a sand track for 10 min, blood levels of thiobarbituric acid-reactive substances (TBARS) were increased immediately after exercise but declined to preexercise values within 1 hr. Also, red cell levels of glutathione reductase increased after exercise, as did (24 hr later) red cell levels of GSH, apparently in compensation for changes that occurred during the exercise-induced oxidative stress (49).

In general, then, an acute bout of exercise in untrained animals seems to increase tissue lipid peroxidation. However, the proximate cause may be tissue damage, not the exercise per se. Besides the studies mentioned, two other relevant studies suggest that unaccustomed exercise (swimming to fatigue) in rats increases lipid peroxidation (25), and that, in sedentary rats, acute exercise increases lipid peroxidation in liver and white skeletal muscle (1).

Along these lines exercise has been used as a model to study cellular production of the "heat shock" proteins (45). Cells exposed to various environmental stresses in vitro respond by synthesizing a unique set of polypeptides termed *shock proteins*, or *stress proteins*. The function of such proteins may be to repair incorrectly folded intracellular proteins and to "chaperone" them to their site of membrane insertion. In other words, the naive view that heat denatures proteins and that the role of the heat shock proteins is to renature them may be correct (38).

As a rationale, Salo, Donovan, and Davies (45) argue that exercise per se causes heat shock, that is, muscle temperatures up to 45 °C and core temperatures up to 44 °C. Simultaneously, exercise can cause oxidative stress. Then, too, exercise training promotes mitochondrial biogenesis; that is, it triggers a two- to threefold increase in the content of muscle mitochondria. How might these functions be related?

In a rat model, Salo et al. (45) found that exhaustive exercise (running on a treadmill) spurred the synthesis of heat shock proteins (especially a 70-kDa protein, HSP70) in skeletal and heart muscle. Muscle HSP70 messenger RNA (mRNA) levels peaked 30 to 60 min following exercise and declined slowly toward baseline over 6 hr. This induction of HSP70 is thus "a physiological response to the heat shock and oxidative stress of exercise" (45).

Salo and colleagues argue that the oxidative stress of exercise is largely from its hyperthermia, which uncouples muscle mitochondria, that is, causes them to lose respiratory control and, thereby, to increasingly generate free radicals. Finally, they argue that HSP70, which likely escorts polypeptides from nucleus to mitochondria, may be a link in the molecular mechanism by which exercise spurs the biogenesis of mitochondria (45).

Does Exercise Training Reduce Free Radical Formation?

In general it seems that, in animal models, training may reduce the lipid peroxidation triggered by a given bout of exercise. In a mouse model, for example, 3 weeks of training were shown to reduce the rate of in vitro lipid peroxidation in both white and red muscle (44).

In another study, after a fatiguing swim, rats trained by treadmill running—compared to untrained rats—had less lipid peroxidation in their gastrocnemius muscles (25). A third study showed that exercise increased lipid peroxidation in the liver and white skeletal muscle of untrained rats but not of trained rats (1).

How Might Exercise Training Reduce Free Radical Formation?

If training does reduce lipid peroxidation, it may do so at least in part by increasing the activity of free radical scavenging enzymes. In this light, a study of tissues in rats found a rank order correlation between the oxygen consumption of the tissue (e.g., liver, heart, lung, and muscle) and the tissue enzyme activity of both catalase and superoxide dismutase (24). Alas, as with most other areas reviewed here, the question of an adaptive increase—via exercise training—in muscle content or activity of antioxidant enzymes is fraught with controversy, as reviewed elsewhere (25).

As examples of this controversy, a 3-month training program in rats, sufficient to increase twofold mitochondrial enzymes in leg muscles, did not increase tissue catalase in one study (21). Several other studies found the opposite: Exercise training led to an increase in muscle catalase activity (1,23,27). In one study, however, the training-induced increase in catalase came only after acute exercise, not at rest (1).

The animal research is also mixed on whether training increases muscle content of superoxide dismutase. One group found only a modest increase after exercise training (and only in mitochondrial superoxide dismutase), which they felt was unlikely to be protective (21). Another group found that superoxide dismutase was unaffected by acute or chronic exercise (1). In contrast, two groups found that training increased the activity of superoxide dismutase (23,27). Even so, it has been argued that because the exercise-induced rise in mitochondrial oxidative enzymes may outstrip that in antioxidant enzymes, the rodent may paradoxically be more vulnerable to oxidative stress after training (21).

Conclusions From Animal Research

One may reasonably conclude from the animal research as a whole that a bout of acute, strenuous exercise, especially in untrained animals, tends to increase free radical formation or at least tissue lipid peroxidation. It seems plausible, however, that the proximate cause of the lipid peroxidation is not the exercise per se but the consequences of muscle damage from it. One may also conclude that physical training, in part by inducing scavenging enzymes, offers hope of mitigating the lipid peroxidation from a given bout of exercise.

Interpreting the animal research here is complicated by the (a) expected differences among studies in choice of animals; (b) general experimental design; (c) type, intensity, and duration of the exercise; and (d) state of training or fitness of the animals used. It is further complicated by a vexing lack of a standard assay or even a generally accepted set of assays that seem precise and reliable for measuring the unstable and short-lived free radicals, not to mention their putative tissue effects. All these problems apply also to the human research on physical activity and free radicals.

Human Research

General Trends Parallel Those From Animal Research

Although the results of research with human subjects are relatively sparse and considerably mixed, in general they tend to parallel those with animals: Bouts of exercise tend to increase free radical formation—at least as gauged by indirect assays usually measuring products of lipid peroxidation in blood or breath—and physical training may offer some adaptive protection against free radical formation and its consequences.

A pioneering study examined environmental oxidant effects on man, focusing on ozone toxicity and measuring pentane gas in the expired breath as a gauge of lipid peroxidation. In this study it was unexpectedly found that exercise alone increased production of pentane. The details were these: Six young subjects who exercised for 20 min on a bicycle ergometer at 75% of maximal aerobic capacity averaged a 1.8-fold increase in pentane production during the exercise, as compared with that during rest before and after the exercise (13). The researchers also found that supplementing these well-nourished, healthy subjects with vitamin E, 1,200 IU a day for 2 weeks, reduced expired pentane levels at rest and during exercise (13).

A potential confounder in this study, however, is that with the great increase in ventilation during exercise, the concentration of expired pentane during exercise may well have approached the lower limit of sensitivity of the assay used. Another group, however, recently used similar methods and found similar results. When five healthy men performed graded exercise on a cycle ergometer (10 min at 45%, 5 min at 60%, and 5 min at 75% of maximal oxygen uptake), the mean breath pentane concentration tripled compared to that at rest (40).

Other indirect assays also suggest that physical activity can generate free radicals. One group studied the effect of graded exercise on plasma and blood glutathione status in man. Eight moderately trained men exercised on a cycle ergometer to peak oxygen consumption and for 90 min at 65% of peak consumption. During exercise to peak consumption, blood concentrations of glutathione did not change, but during prolonged submaximal exercise, blood GSH levels decreased 60% from control while GSSG levels increased 100%. These changes were felt to reflect an increased oxygen flux through the blood, giving increased rates of deoxygenation and reoxygenation of red cell hemoglobin, increased formation of methemoglobin, and free radicals generated therefrom. The lack of change in glutathione status during exercise to peak consumption was attributed to a sharp increase in the blood lactate thought to buffer free radical formation; lactic acid in vitro donates hydrogen to reduce methemoglobin in red cells (17).

During recovery from the submaximal exercise, total blood glutathione level and ratio of GSH:GSSG rose from exercise levels and then overshot preexercise levels, peaking in 3 days. It was concluded that prolonged submaximal exercise generates free radicals and that endurance training may enhance the blood's antioxidant potential (17).

The same group studied downhill running with similar results. Ten trained men were exercised to maximal oxygen uptake and for 45 min at 65% of maximum on a treadmill at a –5% grade. Their blood GSH fell 65% from control and GSSG rose 38% in the first 15 min of exercise, suggesting exercise-induced formation of free radicals. It must be noted, however, that with eccentric exercise like downhill running, it is difficult to separate the effects of exercise itself from the muscle damage it causes; serum creatine kinase (CK) levels did increase in this study and, as noted earlier, muscle damage and its consequences can generate free radicals (51).

Most of the other studies in this field tend to agree, at least in part, with the conclusion that exercise—or its attendant muscle damage—seems to generate free radicals in humans. In a cross-sectional study of 12 young men, for example, maximal aerobic capacity correlated with muscle scavenging enzyme activity. Six men with "high aerobic capacity" (i.e., $\dot{V}O_2max$ greater than 60 ml/kg/min), compared to six men with "low aerobic capacity" (i.e., $\dot{V}O_2$ less than 60 ml/kg/min), had greater muscle levels of superoxide dismutase and catalase, as gauged by biopsy of the vastus lateralis. Also, maximal oxygen capacity was linearly related to the muscle activities of superoxide dismutase and catalase (24).

In another study, an 80-km footrace seemed to accelerate free radical formation. When nine middle-aged male runners were tested at rest before the race, serum levels of TBARS correlated with serum levels of creatine kinase (CK) and CK-MB fraction as gauges of muscle damage. After the race all men had higher serum levels of TBARS, which correlated with higher levels of CK and especially CK-MB, suggesting that exercise-induced lipid peroxidation may be related to exertional muscle damage (28).

A similar study yielded similar results. When 16 healthy but untrained young men ran at 75% of age-adjusted maximal heart rate for 45 min down a 12° gradient on a treadmill, muscle enzymes rose in concert with levels of serum TBARS, suggesting a link between free radical generation and the muscle damage induced by eccentric exercise (35).

In another study, when 16 healthy adults ran downhill for 30 min at 65% of maximal heart rate, serum CK peaked 24 hr later when serum levels of vitamins C and E reached their nadirs. These nadirs, however, were not significantly lower than preexercise values (26).

Limited information from muscle biopsies in marathoners also suggests that exercise can generate free radicals. When four runners had biopsies of the vastus lateralis before and after a standard, 42-km marathon, the muscle content of superoxide dismutase did not change, but the muscle level of GSSG tripled. It was concluded that the race may have generated free radicals in the exercising muscles (11).

Bicycle racing also seems to generate free radicals. In a study of 45 bicycle racers and 20 sedentary controls, the effects of training and racing were compared to plasma levels of TBARS and red cell levels of the scavenging enzymes superoxide dismutase, catalase, and glutathione peroxidase. Plasma levels of TBARS were sharply increased by racing 229 km in 5 hr, as well as by the final stage of a 20-day road race. At rest, red cell levels of all three scavenging enzymes in general were higher in cyclists (especially the top cyclists) than in controls. After the 20-day road race, red cell levels of superoxide dismutase rose even further, but levels of catalase fell toward those of control subjects. It was concluded that exercise forms free radicals in top cyclists, and that in compensation such cyclists tend to have elevated red cell activities of scavenging enzymes (36).

What effect has a single bout of exercise on red cell scavenging enzymes among sedentary persons? When 11 sedentary young men rode a cycle ergometer for 30 min at 75% of maximal aerobic capacity, levels of superoxide dismutase and catalase did not change, but levels of glutathione reductase rose—as if to replenish GSH in the face of an oxidant challenge (37).

It might be noted here by way of perspective that red cell glutathione reductase also rose among obese women who underwent a 5-week exercise program of aerobic dance to lose weight. Intriguingly, however, a nearly identical rise in glutathione reductase occurred when such women, instead of exercising, followed for 5 weeks a 1,200-kcal weight-reducing diet. The investigators here attributed the rises in glutathione reductase not so much to exercise or diet, per se, but to riboflavin depletion (4).

Oxidant Stress From Exercise May Be Modest

Recent research suggests that, at least in trained people, the oxidant stress from even strenuous exercise may be modest. When 11 healthy young men (recreational runners or cyclists) were studied during 90 min of submaximal exercise without eccentric muscle contractions (riding a cycle ergometer at 65% of peak oxygen consumption), there was no significant rise in plasma CK levels. However, blood levels of GSH fell and GSSG rose significantly, and plasma ascorbate levels changed in a way interpreted as consistent with release of ascorbate from tissue sites into plasma to help buffer rising levels of free radicals. Despite these suggestions of free radical formation, there was no sign of tissue damage therefrom; that is, no lipid hydroperoxides were found in any plasma sample, and RNA adducts, as measured by urinary 8-hydroxyguanosine content, did not change (52).

When this same submaximal cycling bout was performed 3 days in a row, results suggested that exercise-induced free radical formation is not only modest, but also evanescent and not cumulative. Each day, blood levels of GSH and GSSG tended to return to baseline in 15 min of recovery from the bout of exercise. On the third day, preexercise blood levels of GSH and GSSG were essentially the same as on the first day. In other words, it appears that young, healthy, well-nourished, trained men are well protected against the oxidative stress of exercise (52).

In this study plasma levels of vitamin E did not change during exercise, suggesting that vitamin E was not mobilized from tissues to increase plasma antioxidant capacity during exercise. This contrasts with two studies in which brief, exhaustive ergometric cycling did seem to mobilize tocopherol from tissues. In these two studies, however, the exercise-induced increase in plasma tocopherol level was modest and the values were not corrected for the hemoconcentration of intensive exercise (6,41).

Studies of Antioxidant Vitamin Supplements Are Inconclusive

The few studies here are inconclusive as to whether supplementation with antioxidant vitamins can mitigate exercise-induced muscle damage or free radical formation in man. In one double-blind, placebo-controlled study, 21 sedentary men took either placebo or vitamin E, 800 IU a day for 48 days, and then ran downhill on a treadmill for 45 min at 75% of maximal heart rate. Blood mononuclear cells were assayed for stimulated secretion of three cytokines: interleukin-1, interleukin-6, and tumor necrosis factor. Muscle proteolysis was gauged by urinary excretion of 3-methylhistidine.

Interpretation was difficult because vitamin E supplementation affected each cytokine differently: (a) Secretion of interleukin-6 was decreased overall; (b) exercise-enhanced secretion of interleukin-1 was suppressed, but baseline secretion was not; and (c) secretion of tumor necrosis factor was not affected at all. Urinary 3-methylhistidine excretion correlated roughly with secretion of interleukin-1, suggesting that this cytokine contributes to the regulation of muscle proteolysis.

Because free radicals are said to enhance secretion of interleukin-1, the fact that vitamin E here suppressed exercise-enhanced secretion of interleukin-1 may imply that vitamin E supplementation offers promise in mitigating exertional muscle damage (or delayed-onset muscle soreness). But free radicals are also said to enhance secretion of tumor necrosis factor, yet vitamin E here had no effect on tumor necrosis factor. So this study, although provocative, is inconclusive on vitamin E, physical activity, free radicals, and muscle damage (7).

Other vitamin studies also are mixed and inconclusive. In one well-done study, 20 young men, some trained and some untrained, were randomly assigned to a placebo group or to an antioxidant vitamin group (daily doses of 592 mg alpha tocopherol equivalents, 1,000 mg ascorbic acid, and 30 mg beta carotene). Exercise was 30 min of treadmill running at 60% of maximal oxygen uptake followed by 5 min of running at 90% of maximal uptake. Lipid peroxidation was measured in two ways: (a) by breath pentane and (b) by serum TBARS.

Results were that 6 weeks of vitamin supplementation lowered the baseline but did not reduce exercise-induced lipid peroxidation. In other words, comparing previtamin with postvitamin values showed that vitamin supplementation was associated with lower resting and postexercise values for breath pentane and serum TBARS. This suggests that, when taking antioxidant vitamins, subjects had less ongoing lipid peroxidation. But when the vitamin group was compared to the placebo group, no difference emerged in the rate of increase in levels of breath pentane or serum TBARS during exercise (29).

In another study, 21 healthy male college students performed incremental exercise to exhaustion on a cycle ergometer before and after supplementation with vitamin E, 300 mg/day for 4 weeks. After vitamin supplementation, as compared to before supplementation, the exercise-induced increases in serum TBARS and serum levels of a muscle enzyme, mitochondrial glutamic-oxaloacetic transaminase, were less pronounced. However, the differences were modest, and this study was not counterbalanced, so the results are inconclusive (48).

In another study, eight young men ran for 30 min at 80% of maximal oxygen uptake before and after supplementation with vitamin E, 800 IU a day for 4 weeks. Results were modest and mixed, but they suggested that such running increases levels of certain plasma markers of lipid peroxidation and that vitamin E supplementation can reduce these markers of lipid peroxidation both at rest and after running (18). Whether or not vitamin supplements have a role in the area of physical activity, free radicals, and muscle function remains uncertain and requires more research in humans.

Contradictory Studies Exist

It must also be noted that some studies on physical activity and free radicals in humans contradict, at least in part, the general trends described previously. For instance, when six men cycled at a moderate 40% and then at 100% of maximal aerobic capacity, plasma TBARS increased above the pre-exercise baseline during the maximal exercise but fell slightly below that baseline during the moderate exercise. It was concluded that exhaustive maximal exercise induces free radical formation but that moderate exercise may inhibit it and lipid peroxidation. The differences however, between groups in levels of plasma TBARS, although significant here, were small (33).

Another study compared trained runners to untrained controls. Baseline plasma levels of GSH were higher in the runners. After a bicycle ergometric test, maximal for each subject, plasma levels of GSH, GSSG, and TBARS did not change in the untrained volunteers. Results were different in the runners. Plasma GSH fell, but plasma GSSG did not rise, and plasma TBARS not only failed to rise, but *fell* 40% (31). The authors blamed this fall in TBARS on the oxygen debt that the runners incurred at the end of their all-out exercise; indeed, lactic acid can apparently buffer free radical formation (17). Another confounder here is that measurements were on *plasma*, not red cells, and other researchers find negligible amounts of glutathione in human plasma (17).

Other studies are basically negative. One study of 10 long-distance runners and 10 controls found no difference between groups in mean plasma level of TBARS at rest and no significant increase in the runners during exhaustive exercise on a cycle ergometer. Perhaps the exercise bout was too brief or the lactic acid that resulted from it buffered free radical formation (53).

Another study of 41 healthy men who cycled at 75% of maximal aerobic capacity found that platelet levels of TBARS decreased during the exercise, in contrast to platelet levels of catalase, glutathione peroxidase, and superoxide dismutase, which rose (5).

Assay Methods Questioned

Finally, another recent study questions the common assay for measuring malondialdehyde, long thought to be the principal lipid peroxidation product responsible for the TBARS reaction. When eight men cycled for 6 min at 44% and at 72% of maximal aerobic capacity and to fatigue at 98% of maximal capacity, total glutathione in blood and plasma increased, possibly reflecting free radical formation. But the assay for malondialdehyde was high-performance liquid chromatography (not the older and less specific TBARS assay), and it registered essentially no plasma malondialdehyde during rest or exercise (43).

This study brings us to a statement from a recent national workshop on oxidant stress in humans: "Standardized methods for measuring oxidative stress status are not yet established . . . one of the greatest needs in the field of free radical biology is the development of reliable methods of oxidative stress status" (42).

Indeed, this critique on the state of the art in measuring oxidant stress status in humans lists 43 different assays and decries vagaries in sampling, storing, and interpreting, as well as ignorance of normal ranges and common variables, including, for example, effects of meals and circadian rhythms (42).

Consider the assays most commonly used in the studies reviewed in this chapter. That for plasma, serum TBARS, or malondialdehyde, the method used most is now generally agreed to be nonspecific and capricious. Malondialdehyde is unstable in the presence of hydrogen peroxide (30) and the TBARS reaction varies not only with pH and heating time, but with "standing time," that is, over time a yellow discoloration interferes with reading the pink chromagen (19). The assay for expired pentane gas, sensitive to air pollutants and the products of gut bacteria, appears so variable that some researchers have abandoned it (20). Furthermore, the assay for blood levels of GSH and GSSG surely reflects oxygen flux mainly in red cells, not in muscle or other tissue (17). Elsewhere, experts perceptively review key problems with other assays, including electron spin trapping assays (20).

Conclusions and Implications

It is difficult to compare, one to another, the diverse studies reviewed here. We encounter not only the expected differences in experimental design; selection and fitness of subjects; and type, intensity, and duration of the exercise; but also great uncertainty as to suitability of tissues analyzed and methods of measurement. With these many limitations in mind, it can be concluded fairly that the general trends from human research suggest that physical activity, especially prolonged or intensive exercise, often generates free radicals, or at least lipid peroxidation products, especially in working muscle. It remains unclear whether exercise itself is the culprit, or whether the proximate cause of free radical formation and lipid peroxidation is muscle damage and its consequences. It seems likely that regular, prudent physical activity causes only modest and evanescent oxidant stress, and that healthy, well-nourished people are well suited to counter such stress. It is plausible that aerobic training offers modest, adaptive protection from exercise-induced oxidant stress, and it remains unclear whether antioxidant vitamins, given as supplements to healthy people, can meaningfully reduce exercise-induced muscle damage or soreness.

What are the implications regarding physical activity, fitness, and health? Besides the work of Cannon et al. reviewed herein, other research suggests that muscle damage, reflected by increases in plasma CK levels, may correlate with free radical formation by neutrophils (14). Even if this is true, however, researchers know from recent muscle biopsy studies in young and old men that plasma CK level is a poor predictor of exercise-induced muscle damage (34). And there is no direct proof that free radicals are a key link between exercise stress and consequent muscle damage. Free radicals in damaged muscle may be the cart, not the horse.

Do free radicals play a role in exertional hemolysis? We know that mild intravascular hemolysis can occur in impact sports and nonimpact sports alike (46), and that malondialdehyde in vitro decreases red cell deformability (39). We have, however, no direct evidence that exercise-induced free radicals play any role in hemolysis.

Do exercise-induced free radicals accelerate atherosclerosis? We know that free radicals can oxidize low-density lipoprotein and thus increase its atherogenicity (8,47), but we also know that high-density lipoprotein can scavenge superoxide anion radicals (9). As covered elsewhere in this book, it is found that regular aerobic exercise and its attendant weight loss tends to decrease plasma levels of low-density lipoprotein and increase levels of high-density lipoprotein.

So even if a physically active lifestyle enhances the formation of free radicals, what is the net effect on atherosclerosis? The same can be asked of lifestyle and common drugs, such as, for example, oral contraceptives, which are claimed to increase oxidative stress (10). What about common diseases such as diabetes mellitus, which is modulated not only by lifestyle but also by oxidative stress (3)?

And even if physical activity, by generating free radicals, is somehow detrimental to our health, at what level or frequency of exercise does this become a concern, and can regular, prudent exercise offset this detriment, or by building antioxidant defenses, even make it a benefit? Finally, is there any role for supplements of antioxidant vitamins?

A reasonable consensus summary might be: Because free radicals form during normal aerobic metabolism, they may harm tissues, especially those with high rates of oxygen flux or those subject to ischemia reperfusion during exercise. Clinical research, however, is hampered because assays for free radicals are indirect and unstandardized. The few studies of free radicals in athletes or exercisers show these general trends:

1. Vigorous exercise tends to increase concentrations of breath pentane and serum TBARS and to reduce concentrations of red cell GSH.
2. Increments in serum concentrations of muscle enzymes tend to parallel increments in concentrations of serum TBARS in exercises with an eccentric or tissue-damaging component.
3. Muscle and red cell content of scavenger enzymes may correlate with aerobic fitness.
4. Exercise-induced changes in free radical products tend to be modest and evanescent and tend not to accumulate after repeated days of exercise.

So far, there is no convincing evidence that supplements of antioxidant vitamins can meaningfully mitigate free radical formation.

What we need are reliable and standardized tools to discriminate between oxidative stress and tissue damage from exercise. Such tools are necessary to decide whether physical activity per se increases free radical formation in humans. If physical activity is found to increase free radical formation, we can then examine diverse possible roles for free radicals in the etiology of exercise-induced pathology.

References

1. Alessio, H.M.; Goldfarb, A.H. Lipid peroxidation and scavenger enzymes during exercise: Adaptive response to training. J. Appl. Physiol. 4:1333-1336; 1988.
2. Bast, A.; Haenen, G.R.R.M.; Doelman, C.J.A. Oxidants and antioxidants: State of the art. Am. J. Med. [Suppl. C] 91:2-13; 1991.
3. Baynes, J.W. Role of oxidative stress in development of complications in diabetes. Diabetes. 40:405-412; 1991.
4. Belko, A.Z.; Obarzanek, E.; Roach, R.; et al. Effects of aerobic exercise and weight loss on riboflavin requirements of moderately obese, marginally deficient young women. Am. J. Clin. Nutr. 40:553-561; 1984.
5. Buczynski, A.; Kedziora, J.; Tkaczweski, W.; Wachowicz, B. Effect of submaximal physical exercise on antioxidative protection of human blood platelets. Int. J. Sports Med. 12:52-54; 1991.

6. Camus, G.; Pincemail, J.; Rosegen, A.; et al. Tocopherol mobilization during dynamic exercise after beta-adrenergic blockade. Arch. Int. Physiol. Biochim. 98:121-126; 1990.
7. Cannon, J.G.; Meydani, S.N.; Fielding, R.A.; et al. Acute phase response in exercise. Associations between vitamin E, cytokines, and muscle proteolysis. Am. J. Physiol. 260:R1235-R1240; 1991.
8. Cazzolato, G.; Avogaro, P.; Bittolo-Bon, G. Characterization of a more electronegatively charged LDL subfraction by ion exchange HPLC. Free Radic. Biol. Med. 11:247-253; 1991.
9. Chander, R.; Kapoor, N.K. High density lipoprotein is a scavenger of superoxide anions. Biochem. Pharmacol. 40:1663-1665; 1990.
10. Ciavatti, M.; Renaud, S. Oxidative status and oral contraceptive: Its relevance to platelet abnormalites and cardiovascular risk. Free Rad. Biol. Med. 10:325-338; 1991.
11. Corbucci, G.G.; Montanari, G.; Cooper, M.B.; et al. The effect on mitochondrial oxidative capacity and on some antioxidant mechanisms in muscle from marathon runners. Int. J. Sports Med. 5:135; 1984.
12. Davies, K.J.A.; Quintanilha, A.T.; Brooks, G.A.; Packer, L. Free radicals and tissue damage produced by exercise. Biochem. Biophys. Res. Commun. 107:1198-1205; 1982.
13. Dillard, C.J.; Litov, R.E.; Savin, W.M.; et al. Effects of exercise, vitamin E, and ozone on pulmonary function and lipid peroxidation. J. Appl. Physiol. 45:927-932; 1978.
14. Fielding, R.; Orencole, S.; Fiatarone, M.; et al. Exercise-induced enzyme release and superoxide production: Effects of age and vitamin E. Med. Sci. Sports Exerc. 22:810a; 1990.
15. Frei, B.; England, L.; Ames, B.N. Ascorbate is an outstanding antioxidant in human blood plasma. Proc. Natl. Acad. Sci. USA. 86:6377-6381; 1989.
16. Girter, B.; Oloff, C.; Plato, P.; et al. Skeletal muscle antioxidant enzyme levels in rats after simulated weightlessness, exercise and dobutamine. Physiologist. 32:S-59-S-60; 1989.
17. Gohil, K.; Viguie, C.; Stanley, W.C.; et al. Blood glutathione oxidation during human exercise. J. Appl. Physiol. 64:115-119; 1988.
18. Goldfarb, A.H.; Todd, M.K.; Boyer, B.T.; et al. Effect of vitamin E on lipid peroxidation at 80% VO_2 max. Med. Sci. Sports Exerc. 21:S16; 1989.
19. Hackett, C.; Linley-Adams, M.; Lloyd, B.; Walker, V. Plasma malondialdehyde: A poor measure of in vivo lipid peroxidation. Clin. Chem. 34:208; 1988.
20. Halliwell, B.; Gutteridge, J.M.C.; Cross, C.E. Free radicals, antioxidants, and human disease: Where are we now? J. Lab. Clin. Med. 119:598-620; 1992.
21. Higuchi, M.; Cartier, L.J.; Chen, M.; Holloszy, J.O. Superoxide dismutase and catalase in skeletal muscle: Adaptive response to exercise. J. Gerontol. 40:281-286; 1985.
22. Jackson, M.J.; Edwards, R.H.T.; Symons, M.C.R. Electron spin resonance studies of intact mammalian skeletal muscle. Biochim. Biophys. Acta. 847:185-190; 1985.
23. Jenkins, R.R. Free radical chemistry. Relationship to exercise. Sports Med. 5:156-170; 1988.
24. Jenkins, R.R.; Friedland, R.; Howald, H. The relationship of oxygen uptake to superoxide dismutase and catalase activity in human skeletal muscle. Int. J. Sports Med. 5:11-14; 1984.
25. Jenkins, R.R.; Martin, D.; Goldberg, E. Lipid peroxidation in skeletal muscle during atrophy and acute exercise. Med. Sci. Sports Exerc. 15:93H; 1983.
26. Kanter, M.M.; Eddy, D.E. Effects of eccentric exercise on skeletal muscle damage and serum antioxidant vitamin status. Med. Sci. Sports Exerc. 23:S149; 1991.
27. Kanter, M.M.; Hamlin, R.L.; Unverferth, D.V.; et al. Effect of exercise training on antioxidant enzymes and cardiotoxicity of doxorubicin. J. Appl. Physiol. 59:1298-1303; 1985.
28. Kanter, M.M.; Lesmes, G.R.; Kaminsky, L.A.; et al. Serum creatine kinase and lactate dehydrogenase changes following an eighty kilometer race. Relationship to lipid peroxidation. Eur. J. Appl. Physiol. 57:60-63; 1988.
29. Kanter, M.M.; Nolte, L.A.; Holloszy, J.O. Effects of an antioxidant mixture on lipid peroxidation at rest and post exercise. J. Appl. Physiol.; [In press].
30. Kostka, P.; Kwan, C.Y. Instability of malondialdehyde in the presence of H202: Implications for the thiobarbituric acid test. Lipids. 24:545-549; 1989.
31. Kretzschmar, M.; Muller, D.; Hubscher, J.; et al. Influence of aging, training and acute physical exercise on plasma glutathione and lipid peroxides in man. Int. J. Sports Med. 12:218-222; 1991.
32. Lew, H.; Pyke, S.; Quintanilha, A. Changes in the glutathione status of plasma, liver and muscle following exhaustive exercise in rats. FEBS Lett. 185:262-266; 1985.
33. Lovlin, R.; Cottle, W.; Pyke, I.; et al. Are indices of free radical damage related to exercise intensity? Eur. J. Appl. Physiol. 56:313-316; 1987.
34. Manfredi, T.G.; Fielding, R.A.; O'Reilly, K.P.; et al. Plasma creatine kinase activity and exercise-induced muscle damage in older men. Med. Sci. Sports Exerc. 23:1028-1034; 1991.

35. Maughan, R.J.; Donnelly, A.E.; Gleeson, M.; et al. Delayed-onset muscle damage and lipid peroxidation in man after a downhill run. Muscle Nerve 12:332-336; 1989.
36. Mena, P.; Maynar, M.; Gutierrez, J.M.; et al. Erythrocyte free radical scavenger enzymes in professional bicycle racers: Adaptation to training. Int. J. Sports Med. 12:563-566; 1991.
37. Ohno, H.; Sato, Y.; Yamashita, K.; et al. The effect of brief physical exercise on free radical scavenging enzyme systems in human red blood cells. Can. J. Physiol. Pharmacol. 64:1263-1265; 1986.
38. Pelham, H. Heat-shock proteins: Coming in from the cold. Nature. 332:776-777; 1988.
39. Pfafferott, C.; Meiselman, H.J.; Hochstein, P. The effect of malonyldialdehyde on erythrocyte deformability. Blood. 59:12-15; 1982.
40. Pincemail, J.; Camus, G.; Roesgen, A.; et al. Exercise induces pentane production and neutrophil activation in humans. Effect of propranolol. Eur. J. Appl. Physiol. 61:319-322; 1990.
41. Pincemail, J.; Deby, C.; Camus, G.; et al. Tocopherol mobilization during intensive exercise. Eur. J. Appl. Physiol. 57:189-191; 1988.
42. Pryor, W.A.; Godber, S.S. Noninvasive measures of oxidative stress status in humans. Free Rad. Biol. Med. 10:177-184; 1991.
43. Sahlin, K.; Ekberg, K.; Cizinsky, S. Changes in plasma hypoxanthine and free radical markers during exercise in man. Acta Physiol. Scand. 142:275-281; 1991.
44. Salminen, A.; Vihko, V. Endurance training reduces the susceptibility of mouse skeletal muscle to lipid peroxidation in vitro. Acta Physiol. Scand. 117:109-113; 1983.
45. Salo, D.C.; Donovan, C.M.; Davies, K.J.A. HSP70 and other possible heat shock or oxidative stress proteins are induced in skeletal muscle, heart, and liver during exercise. Free Rad. Biol. Med. 11:239-246, 1991.
46. Selby, G.B.; Eichner, E.R. Endurance swimming, intravascular hemolysis, anemia and iron depletion: A new perspective on athlete's anemia. Am. J. Med. 81: 791-794; 1986.
47. Steinberg, D.; Parthasarathy, S.; Carew, T.E.; et al. Beyond cholesterol: Modifications of low-density lipoprotein that increase its atherogenicity. N. Engl. J. Med. 320:915-924; 1989.
48. Sumida, S.; Tanaka, K.; Kitao, H.; Nakadomo, F. Exercise-induced lipid peroxidation and leakage of enzymes before & after vitamin E supplementation. Int. J. Biochem. 21:835-838; 1989.
49. Ullrey, D.E.; Shelle, J.E.; Brady, P.S. Rapid response of the equine erythrocyte glutathione peroxidase system to exercise. Federation Proc. 36:1095a; 1977.
50. Viguie, C.A.; Frei, B.; Shigenaga, M.K.; et al. Indices of oxidative stress during repeated bouts of submaximal exercise. J. Appl. Physiol.; [In press].
51. Viguie, C.A.; Packer, L.; Brooks, G.A. Muscle trauma does not change blood antioxidant status. Med. Sci. Sports Exerc. 20:S10; 1988.
52. Viguie, C.A.; Packer, L.; Brooks, G.A. Blood glutathione redox status during consecutive days of exercise. J. Appl. Physiol.; [In press].
53. Viinika, L.; Vuori, J.; Ylikorkala, O. Lipid peroxides, prostacyclin, and thromboxane A2 in runners during acute exercise. Med. Sci. Sports Exerc. 16:275-277, 1984.

Chapter 32

The Brain—Regional Cerebral Blood Flow, Metabolism, and Psyche During Ergometer Exercise

Wildor Hollmann
Hans G. Fischer
Kenny De Meirleir
Hans Herzog
Karl Herholz
Ludwig-Emil Feinendegen

The brain is undoubtedly the most mysterious and least explored human organ. It is not only characterized by physicochemical processes similar to all other organs; but it also produces the so-called phenomenon of the "mind being aware of itself." Evolution and selection contain two leaps: the development of life and the formation of consciousness. Homo sapiens sapiens reached the highest stage of consciousness through the mind's feature of self-awareness.

Our knowledge about the physicochemical functions and reactions of the brain during muscular work is very limited. It is not possible to perform needle biopsies as in the muscle before, during, and after a dosed exercise or before and after a training program. On the other hand, modern techniques like positron emission tomography (PET) and the application of radioactive substances enable us to get more information on our brain functions. Supported by electroencephalogram (EEG) investigations and determinations of neurotransmitters and aminoacids, for example, in combination with agonistic or antagonistic functioning of neurotransmitter substances, we can get more information.

In 1985, we began with such combined examinations. The general question was, what are the hemodynamical, metabolic, and psychological reactions of the human brain to a dosed exercise?

Regional Cerebral Blood Flow in Humans During Exercise

Only a few years ago cerebral blood flow (CBF) was said to be constant and independent of rest or muscular work because of the autonomous regulation of the blood support in the brain (26,48, 53,91). In the last years, it has been demonstrated that small limb movements cause an increase of focal blood flow in brain regions that were supposed to be functionally involved in the particular task (46,47,54,62,68).

Therefore, Herholz et al. (37) investigated the effect of ergometer exercise on CBF using intravenous injections of ^{133}Xe.12 on healthy male volunteers aged 22 to 36 years (median age 26.5 years) with a normal maximal oxygen uptake of 3,600 ± 250 ml/min. They performed exercise-load levels of 25 W and 100 W in the supine position. We used the bolus injection method. The activity in the left cerebral hemisphere was measured with a gamma camera in left lateral view, using a specially designed, low-energy, high-efficiency collimator (64, details see 37).

There were significant differences of regional mean CBF between rest and exercise ($p < .001$) and between 25 W and 100 W ($p < .05$). Increase of whole brain mean CBF in the 100 W group was 24.7%, and 13.5% in the 25 W group. Figure 32.1 shows the increase in more detail.

In all probands the gray-matter flow was higher than the white-matter flow; these differences were not statistically significant. In the meantime the results were confirmed by Thomas, Schroeder, Secher, and Mitchell (83). Using the same method of CBF measurement, they reported a constant increase in CBF during increasing intensities of dynamic leg exercises.

Therefore, it is a little surprising that in connection with static exercise no alterations of the re-

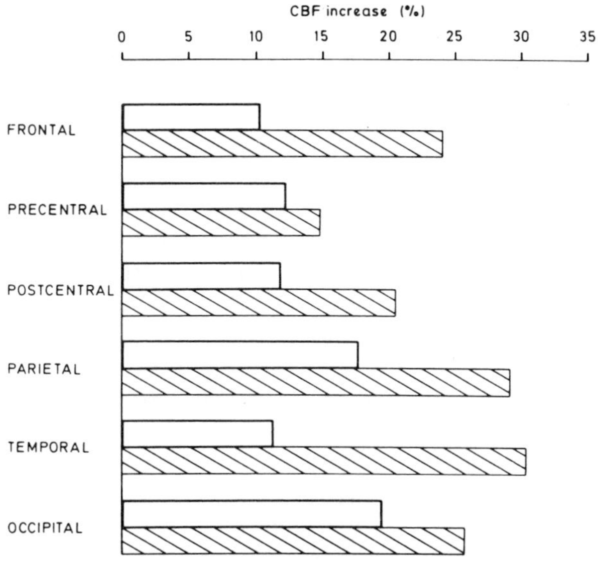

Figure 32.1 Percentage increases of regional mean CBF during 25 (blank bars) and 100 W (hatched bars) exercise intensity (37).

gional cerebral blood flow are to be observed (67). Rogers, Schroeder, Secher, and Mitchell determined CBF in humans at rest and during four consecutive, unilateral, static contractions of the knee extensors. Each contraction was maintained for 3 min, 15 s with the subjects in a semisupine position. The contractions corresponded to 8%, 16%, 24%, and 32% of the individual maximal voluntary contraction and utilized alternate legs. Heart rate and mean arterial pressure increased from resting values of 73 (55–80) and 88 (74–104) mmHg to 106 (86–138) and 124 (102–146) mmHg ($p < .0005$) during the contraction at 32% maximal voluntary contraction. Arterial partial pressure of carbon dioxide (PCO_2) and central venous pressure did not change. The cerebral vascular resistance increased from 1.5 to 2.4 mmHg – 100 $g^{-1}/min^{-1}/ml^{-1}$. There was no difference in CBF between the two hemispheres at rest or during exercise. The conclusion we reach from these studies is that in contrast to dynamic leg exercise, static leg exercise is not associated with an increase in global CBF when measured by the mentioned technique.

A recent review on cerebral circulation (35) concluded that under otherwise constant conditions, a 10 mmHg change in blood pressure causes approximately 6% change in CBF in humans. A more intensive increase of blood pressure is to be observed in connection with the static exercise. Therefore, the behavior of the blood pressure during exercise cannot be the most important factor responsible for the increase of CBF during dynamic work. Some cerebral vasodilation could be expected due to increased brain metabolism. In later described examinations we could not find any augmentation of the brain glucose metabolism; it tended to decrease. The electrical activity is altered in its model but not in the global activity (unpublished results and 78).

Regional CBF increases were frequently observed during specific stimulation tasks involving no or only minor physical work (62,68) and even during pure motor ideation (46). However, measurements during exercise in miniature swine (22) or dogs (29) running on a treadmill using the microsphere method showed constant or slightly decreasing CBF, with an increase only in the cerebellum and sensorimotor cortex, which are functionally activated during exercise. Correspondingly, some studies in humans (26,53,91) showed no increase in CBF during exercise, or even a moderate decrease of –12.5% (48).

In the latest study, however, only a very moderate exercise load increasing the pulse frequency merely from 81 to 87 min^{-1} was applied. In some other studies (34,49,71) CBF increases of 18.5%, 18.4% and 5.4%, respectively, were recorded, but were evaluated as insignificant because of a large variance of data and a small number of observations.

Probably the most important factor is the arterial PCO_2. Depending on the intensity of exercise, PCO_2 decreases in connection with the augmented lactate content in the blood. We measured PCO_2 values of 25 mmHg during exhaustive exercise on the bicycle ergometer. Therefore, constriction of cerebral vessels due to this effect could have counteracted an exercise-induced CBF increase.

The regional distribution of blood flow increase did not show a maximum in the pre- and postcentral region. This lack of evidence for focal neuronal activation is probably due to the arrangement of the detector and regions of interest. The primary motor area for the legs is located close to the interhemispheric fissure and was thus quite distant from the surface of the gamma camera, which was oriented in a lateral view. Furthermore, count rates were not sufficient for usage of smaller regions and, therefore, the central regions represented mainly the sensorimotor areas of the head and the upper limbs, which were not substantially involved in the exercise. Thus, the lack of evidence of focal activation obviously does not indicate its absence.

Also a decrease of the arterial partial pressure of oxygen (PO_2) increases CBF. In our investigations the level of load intensity was too low for a reduction of the arterial PO_2. There was also only a very small increase of epinephrine and norepinephrine as well as lactate. Therefore, these factors cannot play a role in our observation. A comparison of dynamic and static exercise of the leg muscles related to the behavior underlines this statement. It seems that dynamic work could have a vasodilational effect in cerebral regions but the mechanism remains unclear (52). Rogers et al. (67) suggest that the two types of exercise, static and dynamic, are associated with different degrees of cortical activation as indicated by changes in CBF. They did not know our results about the behavior of the glucose metabolism during dynamic exercise, which was constant or even diminished. That means a discoupling between the increased blood flow on the one hand and a constant or decreased glucose metabolism on the other (38).

Despite the performance of unilateral contractions, Rogers et al. (67) did not reveal a difference between hemispheric blood flow to the ipsilateral cortex and the contralateral cortex. Olesen (62), with the use of vigorous hand contractions, showed that despite a 54% focal increase in CBF to the sensorimotor area of the contralateral cortex, the total hemispheric blood flow increased the same amount in both ipsilateral and contralateral hemispheres.

Some authors suggested that the changes occurring in regional CBF are influenced by afferent feedback from the active muscles (23,68). In this case Rogers et al. (67) assume the differences in the response of the CBF to static and dynamic exercise could be the result of stimulation of mechanoreceptors in the exercising muscle or cortical planning of the movement with influences on the effect of central activation.

Beta-Endorphins and Exercise

What should be the objective of an increased cerebral blood flow during dynamic exercise from a teleological point of view? For the following investigations we used the working hypothesis: It might be that muscular work enlarges the production of neuropeptides, and the increased blood flow can support an acceleration and a concentration of the transport of those substances to peripheral aiming points.

At first we investigated the behavior and significance of beta-endorphins. Hughes et al. (44) detected those substances in 1975. The endorphins are neurotransmitters (18,36). So far, 52 different endogenous opioid peptides have been found (6,7,8). The reason for this variety is not known. De Meirleir (8) observed a constancy of beta-endorphins (β-end) during an exercise intensity up to 60% of the individual maximum oxygen uptake. A higher exercise intensity caused an increase of β-end analogous to that of the arterial lactate level (4,8,11). An exercise of longer duration than 50 or 60 min also initiated an increase, if the lactate level did the same. When the maximal O_2-uptake was reached, the β-end level attained threefold of the rest value. De Meirleir et al. described two different reaction types, a rapid and a slow one. Persons of the slow reaction type attained their β-end increase not during exercise but in the recovery time after the exercise (4,8,9).

In order to access the role of endogenous opiates in cardiovascular, respiratory, metabolic, and hormonal response to acute dynamic exercise, De Meirleir used naloxone as a blockade substance for opiates. He described no significant alterations in maximal oxygen uptake, maximal heart rate, maximal minute ventilation and respiratory frequency, lactic acid level, blood pressure, neither in the hormonal reactions of prolactin, gonadotropines, adrenocorticotrophic hormone (ACTH), growth hormone, and thyrotropine hormone (8). This result agrees with that of other authors (30,59,81,82).

Endogenous Opiates, Pain, and Mood

Arentz, De Meirleir, and Hollmann (4) investigated the significance of endogenous opiates on pain and mood. Ten healthy male subjects performed on three different occasions with a 1-week interval using an identical graded bicycle ergometer test until exhaustion. The first test was a control test (C), in the second and third tests either placebo (5 ml saline; P) or 2 mg naloxone (N) was administered 5 min prior to exercise. P and N studies were carried out in a double-blind crossover design. Pain threshold, measured with a technique of dental electrical stimulation, increased after exercise until exhaustion ($p < .01$). N abolished this phenomenon. Psychological questionnaires revealed mood changes to a euphoric state. Pain sensitivity as well as pain tolerance increased significantly ($p < .001$). Results of this study are summarized in Table 32.1 and Figure 32.2.

These results agree with those of Hays, Davies, and Lamb (33) and Shyu, Andersson, and Thoren (74) in examinations of rats. Hair, Quaid, and Mills (31) described a hypoalgesie or a hyperalgesie dependent on the naloxone dosage after an undosed mile run. In our investigations, the application of 2 mg naloxone was sufficient to abolish completely the significant increase of the pain threshold after the end of the ergometer exercise. After naloxone the volunteers felt the slight pressure of the breathing mask was painful. Therefore, it can be concluded that the increased threshold for pain sensitivity and pain tolerance after a normal ergometer exercise was the result of the increased endogenous opiates.

Table 32.1 Pain Sensitivity and Pain Tolerance

	Before		After			
			10 min		60 min	
	x̄	s	x̄	s	x̄	s
Pain tolerance						
No treatment	100		122	18	95	20
Placebo	100		125	16	100	27
Naloxone	100		90	24	95	17
Pain sensitivity						
No treatment	100		126	15	86	22
Placebo	100		131	12	90	18
Naloxone	100		96	16	97	14

Note. Mean values and SD 10 and 60 min after exhaustive physical exercise without drug, with placebo, and with naloxone (4).

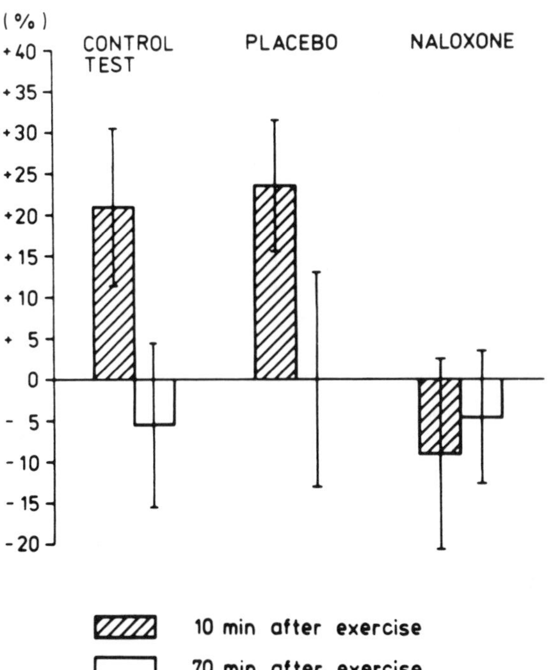

Figure 32.2 Percentage of changes of the pain sensitivity 10 and 70 min after exhaustive physical exercise in the double-blind crossover with placebo and with naloxone (4).

Similar observations were published in connection with births (25), after application of pain (88), and after operations (55). On the other hand no effect was observed after naloxone injections under the conditions of rest (27,28). Therefore, the significance of endogenous opiates seems to be a dynamic function for the regulation of pain threshold related to different environmental conditions. The increasing effect during a submaximal or a maximal exercise load can help to tolerate the task.

In connection with other observations not described here, we suggest that the so-called withdrawal syndrome of top athletes after an acute cessation of any kind of training is caused by the missing production of endogenous opiates.

The higher plasma concentration of opioid peptides in the case of higher exercise levels might contribute to the fact that top-class athletes in certain sports (e.g., rowing, 400-m race, etc.) can tolerate high lactate acidosis relatively well. It may furthermore be assumed that the high lactate concentrations that we could observe during the training of wrestlers and weight lifters can be tolerated better because of the simultaneously high endorphin production. Accidental observations of wrestlers and weight lifters who changed their training led to the conclusion that for these top-class athletes the "stimulus of training" no longer occurred. Consequently, they asked to be permitted to train with higher intensities again.

There is a highly significant positive correlation between the exercise-induced increase in opioid peptides and ACTH (8,9). Both the increase of ACTH and prolactin during exercise seem to be influenced by serotonergic neurotransmission, whereas the increase in growth hormone concentration is controlled by dopaminergic or adrenergic factors (8,9,13). After endurance training there is, at given submaximal load levels, an increase in the exercise-induced rise in ACTH and prolactin and a reduced increase in somatotropin. Thus endurance training seems to change the balance between dopaminergic and adrenergic influences on the one hand and serotonergic influences on the other hand (8,9,10,11,12,13,17,18,45,72). However, a blockade of the peptide effect after naloxone injection does not influence the exercise-induced behavior of the adenohypophyseal hormones.

During exercise, the neurotransmission in the serotonergic, dopaminergic, and opioid areas does not influence the secretion of the luteinizing hormone (LH), follicle-stimulating hormone (FSH), and thyroid-stimulating hormone (TSH) either, nor does the blockade of the opiate effect have an influence on heart rate, systolic blood pressure, oxygen consumption, and respiratory volume. The maximum performance capacity and the rise of the lactate curve also remain unchanged.

There are two other possible mechanisms to increase mood after physical exertion. During exercise the insulin level decreases in order to increase in the recovery phase above the rest value. An increase of insulin in the blood causes an invasion of amino acids into muscle cells, except for the amino acid tryptophan. Therefore, the relative amount of tryptophan in the blood and on the blood-liquor barrier increases. The consequence is a greater chance to find a carrier for the transport into the brain. That also means a greater production of serotonin in the limbic system, as Wurtman et al. (90) showed that an augmented quantity of serotonin in the limbic system improves mood.

Another possibility of enlarging the serotonin amount in the limbic system is an increase of the free tryptophan in the blood during an exercise lasting longer than 30 min, as shown in Figure 32.3. This finding may also be capable of producing more serotonin in the brain in connection with the described mechanism (19,20,21).

Finally, the catecholamines epinephrine, norepinephrine, and dopamine increase during physical exercise. An enlargement of their quantity in the limbic system also causes a positive mood effect (76).

Serotonin, dopamine, and norepinephrine belong to the most important neurotransmitters in the brain. The constellation of these substances in connection with many others like γ-aminobutyric acid (GABA) and with different forms of endogenous opiates in the synapses are responsible for our mood and perhaps for a positive or negative way of thinking (76,90).

Effect of Ketanserin and Pergolide on Biochemical and Biophysical Reactions

Serotonin and dopamine are the decisive neurotransmitters in the so-called rewarding system of the brain. Olds and Milner (61) and De Meirleir et al. (9,11,12,13) investigated the specific role of serotonin and dopamine in connection with ergometer exercise. For the investigation of the serotonin effects, De Meirleir performed a blockade of serotonin with ketanserin. It was demonstrated that oral treatment with ketanserin in normal individuals does not alter heart rate at rest or during exercise, but lowers blood pressure during exercise. The maximal working capacity is not influenced. It elicits a shift to the right of the lactic acid curve during a graded exercise test.

Ketanserin administration did not affect prolactin (PRL) levels before or at 60% of the maximal oxygen uptake. Following placebo, at exhaustion the mean PRL level had increased over baseline. PRL rise continued after stopping exercise and the highest mean value was recorded after ending exercise ($p < .01$). The rise in PRL was significantly impaired by ketanserin. It induced a mean 75% decrease in the serum PRL response ($p < .05$). No statistically significant drug effect could be observed in LH and FSH levels as in growth hormone (GH) level. Ketanserin caused a significant decrease for ACTH and for TSH at exhaustion, the latter also during exercise at 60% of maximal oxygen uptake ($p < .05$) as shown in Figure 32.4.

The alteration of the hemodynamic parameters could be caused by an arteriolar dilation with a lesser systemic vascular resistance (12,16), resulting in reduced lactic acid level by an improved microcirculation in the working muscles as a consequence of the peripheral vasodilative effect of ketanserin (86,87).

The neuroendocrine mechanisms of the exercise-induced increase of PRL concentration in humans remain unclear. Serotonin seems to be involved in

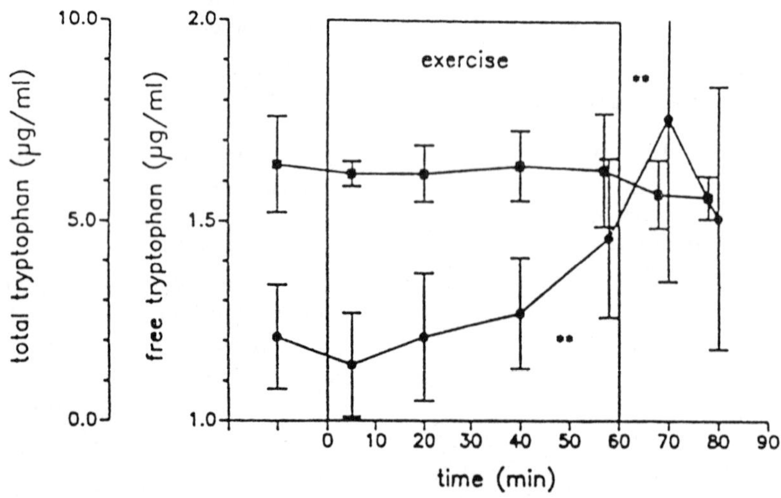

Figure 32.3 Total and free tryptophan in venous blood of healthy male persons before, during, and after a 60 min ergometer exercise performed with 60% of the individual maximal oxygen uptake (n = 10) (20).

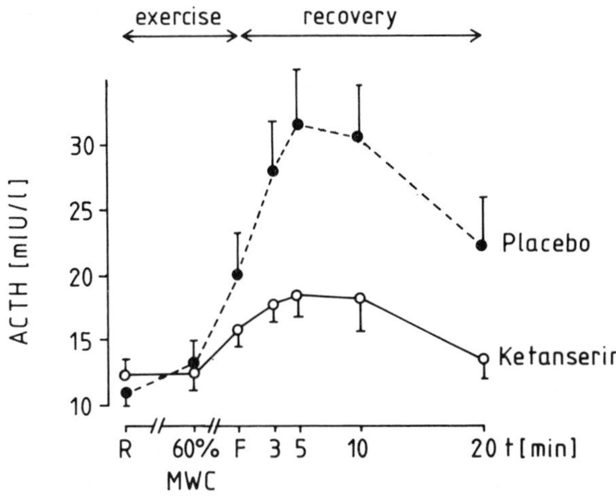

Figure 32.4 Influence of serotonin blockade (ketanserin) on ACTH level in venous blood during 1 hr ergometer exercise with 60% of the individual maximal oxygen uptake followed by increasing exercise intensity until exhaustion and in the recovery phase (n = 10) (12).

human PRL secretion (9,10,12,13), and cyproheptadine blocked this effect in subjects who received 5-hydroxytryptamine (5-HT) orally (8). In the experiments of De Meirleir et al. plasma PRL response to maximal graded exercise was significantly effaced by ketanserin. This suggests that a central serotonergic system, acting through 5-HT receptors, is involved in the stimulation of PRL release during heavy exercise (8), perhaps reacting to the pH alteration. According to unpublished results of our team, serotonin may play a central role in the development of the syndromes of overtraining and sports withdrawal symptoms.

A question of similar interest is the significance of dopamine on the previously described parameters of load intensity and duration during exercise. Because of the different structures of dopamine receptors it is not possible to sufficiently block the dopamine effects. Therefore De Meirleir et al. used a dopamine agonist, the pergylatmesylat pergolide (10). More than half of the content of catecholamines in the brain is dopamine (56). The functional importance in the brain itself and in the periphery remains incompletely understood. Pergolide possesses DA-2 dopamine agonist properties both peripherally and in the brain (43).

Pergolide significantly suppressed ($p < .01$) basal PRL. PRL values also remained unchanged during and after exercise. The gonadotropins were not influenced at rest, but significantly increased LH ($p < .01$) during exercise. The usual observed rise in ACTH during exercise was significantly effaced by pergolide ($p < .01$), as shown in Figure 32.5. The substance also significantly enhanced the increase in GH levels in response to exercise ($p < .01$). It did not alter thyroid-stimulating hormone. Heart rate was significantly lowered at rest and during exercise ($p < .01$), but the maximal heart rate remained unchanged. Also the systolic and diastolic blood pressure decreased at rest and during exercise. The maximal working capacity was significantly enhanced ($p < .05$). At the same time the lactic acid levels were reduced on given submaximal exercise loads ($p < .05$).

The pharmacological properties of the drug as observed in animals (e.g., stimulation of peripheral DA-2 neuronal dopamine receptors, stimulation of central DA-2 receptors, and activation of cardiac prejunctional a2-adrenoceptors) (43) help to explain the observations. De Meirleir emphasizes that the drug's cardiovascular and metabolic effects mimic those induced by endurance training (8).

The mentioned findings indicate an intensive biochemical interlinking of the functions of the brain, the cardiovascular system, and the skeletal muscles. One is reminded of Baron de Coubertin's remark made on the occasion of the revival of the Olympic Games in 1896 that the goal of sport should be "a marriage between mind and muscle."

Brain and Cardiovascular System

This leads to the question of the location and the mechanisms of the possibilities of influencing the cardiovascular system and the skeletal muscles

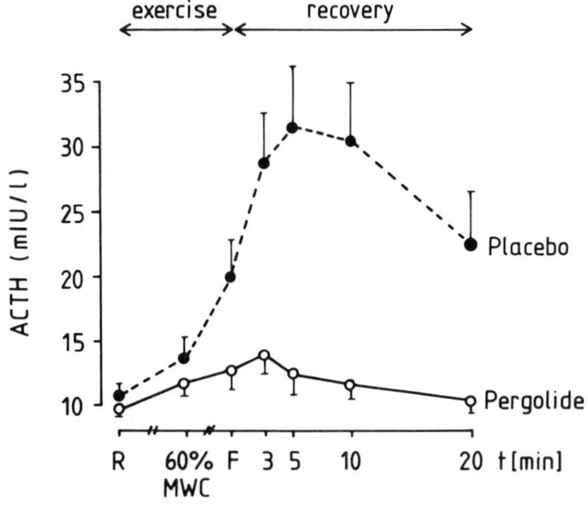

Figure 32.5 Reinforcement of the dopamine influence with pergolide on ACTH during rest, ergometer exercise with 60% of the individual maximal oxygen uptake, and with an increasing exercise intensity until exhaustion (n = 10) (10).

via biochemical aspects of the brain. In past years, the existence of opiate peptides in both the sympathetic and parasympathetic autonomous system have been verified (1,3,6,85,86,87). The connection with the cardiovascular system is particularly close (7,14,24,30,57,63,70,86). Weihe, Nohr, and Hartschuh (87) conclude from their investigations that opioid peptides restrict the release of their cotransmitter noradrenalin by acting on the parasynaptic autoreceptors. This has been demonstrated in connection with the heart in particular. The authors postulate a fundamental significance of the opioid peptides for the regulation of the cardiovascular tonus. The involvement of such peptides might apply both as far as the peripheral and the central primary sensory neurotransmission are concerned.

It might be important to verify opioid peptides in the peripheral cardiovascular regulation of both the endothelium and in the pericytes of capillaries and venules, as well as the arterioles (14,87,88). In contrast to the microvascular segments, macrovascular segments were hardly occupied with peptides if innervated. On the other hand, in individual regions of the heart nerve fibers were found whose neurotransmitters are peptides such as tachykinin, substance E, and neurokinin A, as well as the calcitonin-gene-related peptide and opioid peptides. The release of such substances from peripheral endings of the vagal nerve system also indicates their significance in this branch of the autonomous nerve system. Further influences on primarily sensory functions such as baroreceptors and chemoreceptors are probable (86).

In the brain the opiate receptors are distributed in a typical pattern. An area with a high concentration is the central part of the thalamus. This is the main entrance station to the brain. It filters incoming sensory information and then passes it on to the cortex. A high concentration can also be found in places responsible for the diameter of the pupils of the eye ("pinhead-sized pupils" caused by opiates). An especially high concentration of opiate receptors can be observed in the limbic system. From there nerve pathways travel, for example, to the hypothalamus, which controls hypophysis. So it is understandable that emotional situations are reflected in the hormone concentration behavior in the whole body. This makes "start fright" or "precompetition arousal" explainable.

The connections between thought processes and autonomous reactions such as heart rate are modulated here. The locus ceruleus also sends neuronal projections to the limbic system. The effect of neurotransmitters such as noradrenaline and dopamine can thus be influenced by opiopeptides. An extremely high concentration of opiate receptors can be found in the locus ceruleus itself (76). Thus, a connecting chain can be established from the different structures of the brain via the spinal cord up to the control of the diameter of capillaries and arterioles in the muscles. Hemodynamic and metabolic changes via the peptide system in general, which are expressed especially during muscular exercise, are imaginable. According to this theory, the changes under serotonin blockade or dopamine agonism described herein could be understandable.

It may be assumed that the heart action is also influenced by neuropeptides. Neuropeptide Y (NPY) is the most important peptide in cardiac efferent sympathetic nerves, whereas afferent sympathetic nerves are characterized by the existence of tachykinines, calcitonine-related peptide, and opioide peptide (86). The vagal system of the heart contains mainly tachykinines. The intrinsic peptidergic system in particular consists of vasoactive intestinal polypeptides, whereas the paracrine systems are occupied opioderically to a higher degree. The physiological and pathophysiological significance of these varied peptidergic and nonpeptidergic messenger systems is still largely unknown.

However, recently, a connection between opioide peptides and *silent myocardial ischemia* has been verified. So, today, it is assumed that at least 30% of all cardiac infarctions are silent and that an identical percentage of exercise-induced myocardial ischemias are also silent (14,16). It is not yet well known which stimulus is adequate with regard to coronary pain to trigger the sensation of pain. Chemical substances as well as mechanical stimuli are discussed. The pain information is transmitted to the neocortex via the limbic system. In a patient with coronary insufficiency, both physical and psychological stress can lead to a myocardial ischemia with the possibility of endogenous pain inhibition through an increase in heart work. For individual patients with silent exercise ischemia the administration of naloxone as a morphine antagonist could provoke pain when exercising (14,16). Those patients also showed a higher rest and exercise beta-endorphin value in their blood as compared to patients with the usual symptoms. The possible influence of peptides described earlier explains this behavior.

For centuries clinicians have been familiar with the close connections between psyche and heart. Much has been written about sudden cardiac death or the occurrence of cardiac arrhythmias as a consequence of sudden shock or an extreme or unexpected joy. In these cases there is often a stenosing coronary sclerosis. It is extremely rare that there are no pathological findings. However, fundamentally, the question as to the neurophysiological path arises. In the 1950s and 1960s Raab demonstrated functional and morphological consequences of stress for the heart in experimental animal studies (65,66). It has been known for a long time that concussions of the brain or increases in cerebral pressure can be accompanied by changes in heart function. Using hypothalamic stimulation, Melville (60) caused pathological myocardial alterations including cardiac infarction. Shkhvatsabaya (73) reports similar investigation findings. The enumeration of authors who replicated these results could be continued at great length.

Psychological stress leads to a fluctuation of serum electrolytes (potassium in particular) and can trigger an electrical instability. At the same time, the alpha-adrenergic activity simplifies the excretion of potassium ions leading to hypokalemia. In animal experiments, these adrenalin-controlled changes cause a considerable lowering of the fibrillation threshold. Such mechanisms might also apply to coronary patients. The serotonin concentration in the brain and in the limbic system in particular could be of great significance. An increased amount of serotonin reduces the sympathetic stimulus acting on the heart. In experimental investigations by Lown (57), a highly significant rise of the threshold for triggering cardiac arrhythmias could be observed under these conditions. However, according to earlier presentations, it is exactly this sympathetic activity that is influenced via opioide and other peptides.

It could be observed in animal experiments that the electrical stimulation of the hypothalamus leads to the same change of the terminal electrocardiogram (ECG) segment as in the case in human beings. In dogs with crossed circulation these anomalies could occur in unilateral animals and can be prevented by cross-sectional cutting of the cervical part of the medulla. Therefore a humoral mode of transmission can be ruled out, leaving by deduction a neurogenous mode of transmission. Obviously the mechanism utilizes sympathetic nervous pathways. The connection between psyche and various physical reactions in the form of stress and distress will not be described in detail here (as the related connections between brain, spinal cord, and suprarenal gland with all their consequences for hemodynamics and metabolism have been known in principle for decades) (overview in 65).

High catecholamine concentrations result in an increased myocardial oxygen requirement with its individually different consequences depending on the coronary and myocardial evidence. Further consequences are an aldosterone increase with hypernatremia, hypokalemia and possible effect on the heart, a vasopressin release with a tendency of the coronary arteries to contract, and a thrombocyte aggregation with a tendency to form clots. During physical exercise the atrionatriuretic peptide (ANP) increases in the blood in relation to the exercise intensity (5), and there are influences of the opioid peptides (86).

In migraine headaches there also are often causal relations between psyche, biochemical processes, and vascular system. In the migraine research of today psychological load factors are accepted internationally. Serotonin in particular plays a role in the vascular processes during a migraine attack. However, as far as details are concerned, there are still different views.

For decades, feelings of discomfort have been known that primarily occur if endurance training conducted for years is suddenly stopped. This particularly concerns endurance-trained athletes with an enlarged athlete's heart. The symptoms are unrest, anxiety, sleeplessness, loss of appetite, possible blood pressure instability with a tendency to circulatory collapse, and cardiac arrhythmias. In the past we interpreted these findings as regulation disorders in an organism that has been used to immense stress for years or even decades and that does not succeed in changing to a sudden state of rest as far as morphology and function are concerned (39,40,41,42).

In such cases, all symptoms as well as the anamnestic context suggest that the abrupt abandonment of training has led to hormonal regulation disorders in connection with endogenous opioide peptides. This view is also supported by a depressive attitude. Some symptoms that in the past were explained by the "unharmonious redevelopment of a large athlete's heart" could be explained by regulation disorders on the level of peptides in the central nervous system with consecutive hormonal changes (39).

In experimental investigations on coronary patients and healthy persons causal relations between acute mental stress and myocardial ischemia were described (70). In the case of combined arithmetic and color stress 59% of the patients with secured coronary cardiopathy developed significant reductions of ejection fractions of the left ventricle connected with anomalies of ventricular wall movements. In 83% of all cases the myocardial ischemia took place without symptoms. It occurred at heart rates lower than the heart rates of beginning stress-induced circulatory disturbances. At the same time, there was a significant rise in arterial blood pressure. So it may be correct to call the endogenous peptides "the third messenger system" of our body (39).

Relations Between the Brain, the Nervous System, and the Immune System

In 1964 Solomon and Moos coined the term *psychoimmunology* (overview in 80). Ader extended this term in 1981 to *psychoneuroimmunology* (2). New findings concerned the development of physical diseases and the triggering of immunological disorders in connection with mental stress. Emotional disorders and mental dysfunctions express themselves in quantitative and qualitative changes of immunoglobulins, a reduced immune reaction to antigens, and an increased occurrence of a variety of autoantibodies (84). In cases of schizophrenia, functional anomal lymphocytes are described. Such an enumeration could be continued on the basis of numerous publications (overview in 79).

In animals that were submitted to an immunization through antigens, the impulse rate of neurons, especially in the hypothalamus, increased significantly (50). Neurotransmitters and neuropeptides, whose release is controlled by the central nervous system (CNS), influenced mechanisms of the immune system. Serotonin, for example, delays primary immune reactions and reduces the intensity of primary and secondary antibody reactions (14).

The relations between endogenous peptides and the immune system are extremely complex (84). Beta-endorphin and met-enkephalin increase the natural killer (NK) cell activity (58). Blockade of the endorphin by means of naloxone suppresses NK cell activities. Neuropeptides and neurotransmitters modulate the capacity of macrophages (51). Cells that are competent as far as immunology is concerned possess receptors for neuroendocrines, neurotransmitters, and neuropeptides. Conversely, these regulate areas of the brain and are also given feedback indicated by the following finding: If one infuses radioactive thymosin-alpha, which influences the T-cells, it can later be found in high concentrations in those areas of the brain that participate in the neuroendocrinological regulation (32). The lymphocytes themselves contain gamma-endorphin and ACTH while activated T-helping cells produce met-enkephalin (75,87). Melatonin, which is produced in the pineal gland, plays an essential role in immunoregulation by influencing antigen-activated T-lymphocytes via the endogenous opioid system. The chain of connections between brain, psyche, and immune system could be lengthened by many other details.

Glucose Metabolism in the Human Brain During Exercise

It has been demonstrated that CBF and the cerebral metabolic rate of glucose utilization (CMRglu) are coupled in response to various mental activities (72). The question was whether or not CMRglu is also strictly connected with CBF during physical exercise. Herzog et al. (38) investigated global changes of CMRglu in response to physical exercise using PET and ^{18}F-fluorodeoxyglucose (FDG) in persons prone to migraines.

CMRglu of 10 male patients aged 23 to 61 years with a history of migraine was measured twice at rest and after protocoled bicycle exercise within an interval of 2 days (n = 5), 7 days (n = 4), and 3 weeks (n = 1). The subjects were free of migraine symptoms at each day of the study. Ten minutes after beginning ergometer exercise, FDG was injected and PET scans were started 30 min later. The exercise protocol for each patient assured a level of 1.8 to 2.0 mmol/L of lactate during exercise. Plasma activity of FDG was determined from samples of arterialized earlobe blood.

Images of local CMRglu were calculated using standard rate and lumped constants. Sections were drawn over the cerebellum and several cortical areas in four different slices parallel to the orbitomental line from the cerebellum to the centrum semiovale; because of priority of global changes of CMRglu, the far cranial-located cortical motor region could not be analyzed in this study. The data were statistically tested with matched pair t-tests.

The mean CMRglu of the sum of all sections, weighted according to the size and averaged over all 10 subjects, did not change significantly from 34.1 ± 10.3 mol/min^{-1}/100 g^{-1} during rest to 30.6 ± 4.5 mol/min^{-1}/100 g^{-1} during exercise. The results during and directly after exercise were significantly different from the *rest* values ($p < .05$). Also in single compatible sections averaged over all 10 subjects, there were mean decreases ranging from 4% to 19% in different areas of the cortex and a mean decrease of 6% in the cerebellum during exercise, as shown in Figures 32.6 and 32.7. However, the visual cortex increased by 9%. The interindividual variation in the single sections was reduced by a factor of 1.5 to 3.5 during exercise compared to rest.

In conclusion, in contrast to the reported exercise-induced increase of CBF the present study revealed no related increase of global CMRglu. This indicates uncoupling between CMRglu and CBF under exercise. The reasons could be a reduced neuronal activity during physical exercise (overview in 77) or a metabolic intervention (e.g., by lactate or increased free fatty acids).

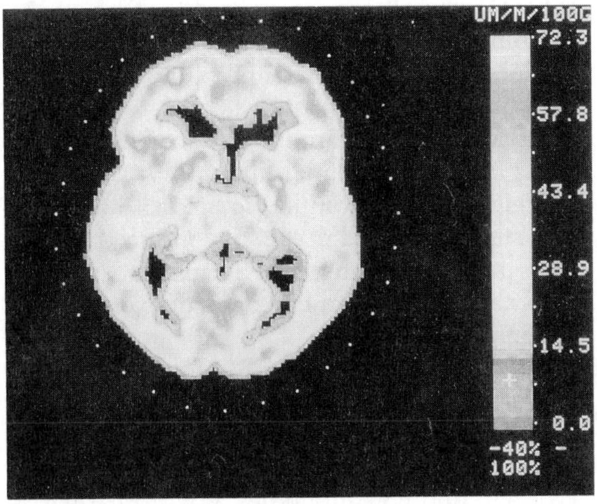

Figure 32.6 Positron emission tomography (PET) at rest. The gray spots are regions with high glucose consumption (38).

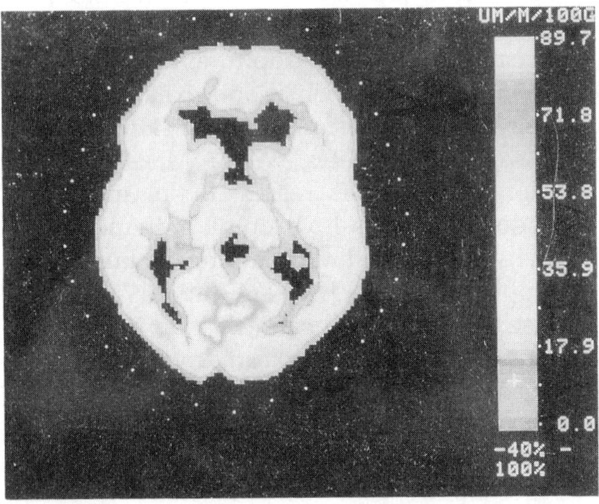

Figure 32.7 The PET of the same person as Figure 32.6 during bicycle ergometer exercise with 80% of the maximal oxygen uptake. Most of the spots disappear (38).

We performed with those migraine patients a 2-month endurance training with jogging. They trained three times weekly with a duration of 60 min for every session. The number and intensity of the migraine attacks were reduced significantly after this period of time ($p < .001$). The mechanisms are unclear.

The connections between brain, mind, and body functions can lead only to the conclusion that for both a preventive and a therapeutic way of thinking in medicine the human being must be considered as a whole concerning his or her sociological, psychological, and physical existence.

Summary and Conclusions

The connected application of (a) positron emission tomography (PET), (b) radioactive isotopes, (c) electroencephalograms (EEG), (d) amino acid and other substrate determinations in the blood, (e) agonistically and antagonistically functioning drugs for neurotransmitter investigations, and (f) psychological tests during and after ergometer exercise give evidence of hemodynamic and metabolic reactions of the human brain, which are combined with psychic alterations. Dynamic, not static, exercise causes an enlargement of cerebral blood flow (CBF). The exercise intensity plays a nonlinear role. Our hypothesis is that the increased blood flow has the task to transport metabolites of the brain as quickly and compactly as possible to peripheral targets.

Endogenous opioid peptides increase in the arterial blood during an incremental ergometer exercise analogous to the lactate curve. A very long-lasting exercise evokes also, for example, a beta-endorphin augmentation. The threshold for pain sensitivity and pain tolerance, measured with a dental stimulation technique, increased significantly after exhaustive exercise ($p < .01$); naloxone abolished this phenomenon. Psychological questionnaires revealed significant mood changes. The endogenous opiate system seems to be directly implicated in provoking a positive mood state.

Ketanserin, an antagonist of serotonin, and pergolide, an agonist of dopamine, cause intense changes in cardiovascular and hormonal reactions during and after ergometer exercise. The most marked alterations are to be seen in anaerobic exercise.

The very close relationships between the brain and the cardiovascular system and their regulation are discussed. Endogenous peptides play an important role. They are called a third messenger system as a connecting link between brain, consciousness, and peripheral body reactions. The withdrawal symptoms experienced after a sudden stop of endurance training that has been conducted for years is explained with hormonal regulation disorders in connection with endogenous peptides. Also, cases of silent myocardial ischemia may belong to this group.

Relations between brain, nervous system, and immune system are sketched. The psychoneuroimmunology has also a significance for sports medicine. There are quantitative and qualitative changes of the immune system in connection with mental or physical stress. PET investigations of the glucose metabolism during ergometer exercise revealed a constancy or even a decrease during ergometer exercise in all regions of the brain except the visual cortex. This indicates uncoupling between local glucose metabolism and cerebral blood flow during exercise. Endurance training with migraine patients invoked a significant reduction in the number and intensity of the migraine attacks.

We conclude that the knowledge of the biochemical and biophysical connections between brain, mind, and body functions during physical exercise can be important for a preventive and a therapeutic way of thinking in medicine.

References

1. Acher, R. Evolution of neuropeptides. Trends Neurosci. 9:225; 1981.
2. Ader, R., editor. Psychoneuroimmunology. New York: Academic Press; 1981.
3. Akil, H.; Watson, S.J.; Young, E.; Lewis, M.E.; Khachaturian, H.; Walker, J.M. Endogenous opioids: Biology function. Annu. Rev. Neurosci. 7:223; 1984.
4. Arentz, T.; De Meirleir, K.; Hollmann, W. Die rolle der endogenen opioiden peptide während fahrradergometerarbeit. Dtsch. Z. Sportmed. 37(7):210; 1986.
5. Bittner, H.; Rippegather, G.; Völker, K.; Hollmann, W.; Forssmann, W.G. Freisetzung kardialer hormone unter ergometrischer Belastung. Dtsch. Z. Sportmed. 11(37):356; 1986.
6. Cavero, I.; Lefevre-Borg, F.; L'Hoste, F.; Sabatier, C.; Richter, C.; Giudicelli, J.F. Pharmacological, hemodynamic and autonomic nervous system mechanisms responsible for the blood pressure and heart rate lowering effects of pergolide in rats. J. Pharmacol. Exp. Ther. 228:779-791; 1984.
7. Chaouloff, F. Physical exercise and brain monoamines: A review. Acta. Physiol. Scand. 137:1; 1989.
8. De Meirleir, K. Studies of cardiovascular drugs and neurohormonal substances in dynamic exercise. Free University of Brussells; 1985. Thesis.
9. De Meirleir, K.; Baeyens, L.; L'Hermite, M.; L'Hermite-Baleriaux, M.; Hollmann, W. Exercise-induced prolactin release is related to anaerobiosis. J. Clin. Endocrinol. Metab. 69:1250; 1985.
10. De Meirleir, K.; Gerlo, F.; Hollmann, W.; Haelst van, L. Cardiovascular effects of pergolide mesylate during dynamic exercise. Br. J. Clin. Pharmacol. 5(23):633; 1987.
11. De Meirleir, K.; L'Hermite-Baleriaux, M.; L'Hermite, M.; Rost, R.; Hollmann, W. Evidence for serotoninergic control of exercise-induced prolactin secretion. Horm. Metab. Res. 7(17):380; 1985.
12. De Meirleir, K.; Smitz, J.; van Steirteghem, A.; Hollmann, W. Serotonine antagonism during exercise in man. Acta Cardiol. (42). 5:360; 1987.
13. De Meirleir, K.; Smitz, J.; van Steirteghem, A.; L'Hermite, M.; Hollmann, W. Dopaminergic and serotoninergic neurotransmitter systems involved in exercise-induced release of adenohypophyseal hormones. 6th internat. symposium biochem. of exercise. Copenhagen: 1985.
14. Devoino, L.V.; Idova, G.V. The influence of some drugs on the immune response IV. Effect of serotonin, 5-hydroxytryptophan, iproniazid, p-chlorophenylalamine on the synthesis of IgM and IgG antibodies. Eur. J. Pharmacol. 22:325; 1973.
15. Diederich, K.W.; Djonlagic, H.; Müller-Eschner, M.; Dageferde, J.; Hoffmann, J. Neurogene endstreckenveränderungen im EKG. Med. Klin. 13(77):411; 1982.
16. Droste, C. Pathophysiologie schmerzhafter und stummer myokardischämie. Herz. 6(12):369; 1987.
17. Farrell, P.A.; Garthwaite, P.L.; Gustafson, A.B. Plasmaadrenacorticotropin and cortisol responses to submaximal and exhaustive exercise. J. Appl. Physiol. 55:1441-1444; 1983.
18. Farrell, P.A.; Gates, W.G.; Maksod, M.G.; Morgan, W.P. Increases in plasma beta-endorphine/beta-lipotrophin in immunoreactivity after treadmill running in humans. J. Appl. Physiol. 52:1245-1249; 1982.
19. Fischer, H.G.; Hollmann, A.; De Meirleir, K. Exercise changes in plasmatryptophan fractions and relationship with prolactin. Int. J. Sports Med. 12(5):487-489; 1991.
20. Fischer, H.G.; Hollmann, W.; De Meirleir, K. Correlation between free plasma tryptophan and prolactine during and after endurance exercise. Int. J. Sports Med. (In press).
21. Fischer, H.G.; Karbach, P.; Lillis, A.; Hollmann, W. Metabolische beziehungen zwischen ammoniak-harnstoff und hypoxanthin-harnsäure bei kraft- und ausdauerbelastungen. Dtsch. Z. Sportmed. (In press).
22. Foreman, D.L.; Sanders, M.; Bloor, C.M. Total and regional cerebral blood flow during moderate and severe exercise in miniature swine. J. Appl. Physiol. 40:191-195; 1976.
23. Friedman, D.B.; Friberg, L.; Mitchell, J.H.; Secher, N.H. Regional cerebral blood flow during isometric handgrip contractions. Clin. Res. 37:260 A; 1989.
24. Ganten, D.; Luft, F.C.; Lang, R.E.; Unger, T. Brain peptides in cardiovascular regulation. In: Kaufmann, W.; ed. Primary hypertension. Berlin-Heidelberg: Springer; 1986.

25. Gintzler, A.R. Endorphine mediated increases in pain threshold during pregnancy. Science. 210:193; 1980.
26. Globus, M.; Melamed, E.; Keren, A.; Tzivoni, D.; Granot, C.; Lavy, S.; Stern, S. Effect of exercise on cerebral circulation. J. Cereb. Blood Flow Metab. 3:287-290; 1983.
27. Grevert, F.; Goldstein, A. Naloxone fails to alter experimental pain or mood in humans. Science. 199:1093-1095; 1978.
28. Grevert, P.; Goldstein, A. Effects of naloxone on experimentally induced ischemic pain and on mood in human subjects. Proc. Natl. Acad. Sci. USA. 74:1291-1294; 1977.
29. Gross, P.M.; Marcus, M.L.; Heistad, D.D. Regional distribution of cerebral blood flow during exercise in dogs. J. Appl. Physiol. 48:213-217; 1980.
30. Grossman, A.P.; Bouloux, P.; Price, P.L.; Drury, K.S.L.; Lam, T.; Turner, J.; Thomas, G.M.; Sutten, J. The role of opioid peptides in the hormonal response to acute exercise in man. Clin. Sci. 67:483-491; 1984.
31. Hair, R.J.; Quaid, A.; Mills, J.S.C. Naloxone alters pain perception after jogging. Psychiatry Res. 5:231-232; 1981.
32. Hall, N.R.; Goldstein, A.L. The thymus-brain connection: Interactions between thymosin and the neuroendocrine system. Lymphokine Res. 211:6; 1983.
33. Hays, G.W.; Davies, J.M.; Lamb, D.R. Increased pain tolerance in rats following strenuous exercise. Med. Sci. Sports Exerc. [Abstract]. 1:56; 1984.
34. Hedlund, S.; Nylin, G.; Regnstroem, O. The behaviour of the cerebral circulation during muscular exercise. Acta Physiol. Scand. 54:316-324; 1962.
35. Heistad, D.D.; Kontos, H.A. Cerebral circulation. In: Handbook of physiology, sec. 2, vol. III. Bethesda, MD: American Physiological Society; 1992:137-182.
36. Henry, J.L. Circulating opioids: Possible physiological roles in central nervous function. Neurosci. Behav. Rev. 6:229-245; 1982.
37. Herholz, K.; Buskies, B.; Rist, M.; Pawlik, G.; Hollmann, W.; Heiss, W.D. Regional cerebral blood flow in man at rest and during exercise. J. Neurol. 234:9; 1987.
38. Herzog, H.; Unger, C.; Kupert, T.; Fischer, H.G.; Scholz, W.; Hollmann, W.; Feinendegen, L.E. Körperliche belastung führt nicht zu erhöhtem zerebralen glukoseverbrauch. Unpublished.
39. Hollmann, W.; De Meirleir, K. Gehirn und sport—hämodynamische und biochemische aspekte. Dtsch. Z. Sportmed. (Special edition). 39:56; 1988.
40. Hollmann, W.; De Meirleir, K.; Herholz, K.; Heiss, W.D.; Bittner, H.; Völker, K.; Forssmann, G. Regional cerebral blood flow, neurohormonal, and cardiac hormonal reactions during exercise. International symposium on exercise physiology (in memoriam Kozlowski, S.; Baranow/Pol); 1987.
41. Hollmann, W.; Rost, R.; De Meirleir, K.; Liesen, H.; Heck, H.; Mader, A. Cardiovascular effects of extreme physical training. Acta Med. Scand. 711:193; 1986.
42. Hollmann, W.; Völker, K.; Heck, H.; Rost, R.; De Meirleir, K. Über das arterielle blutdruckverhalten bei dynamischer und statischer muskelarbeit unter einbeziehung des atrialen natriuretischen peptids (ANP) sowie von neurotransmittern. Z. Kardiol. 7(78):211; 1989.
43. Hornykiewicz, P. Dopamine (3-Hydroythyramine) and brain function. Pharmacol. Rev. 18:925-964; 1966.
44. Hughes, J.; Smith, T.W.; Kosterlitz, H.W.; Fothergill, L.A.; Morgan, M.A.; Morris, H.R. Identification of two related pentapeptides from the brain with potent opiate agonist activity. Nature. 258:577; 1975.
45. Illes, P.; Bettermann, R.; Ramme, D. Brain peptides and catecholamines in cardiovascular regulation. In Buckley, J.P.; Ferrario, G.M., eds. New York: Raven Press; 1987:169-184.
46. Ingvar, D.H.; Philipson, L. Distribution of cerebral blood flow in the dominant hemisphere during motor ideation and motor performance. Ann. Neurol. 2:230; 1977.
47. Ingvar, D.H.; Sjölund, B.; Ardö, A. Correlation between dominant EEG frequency, cerebral oxygen uptake, and blood flow. Electroencephalogr. Clin. Neurophysiol. 41:268; 1976.
48. Kleinerman, J.; Sancetta, S. Effect of mild steady state exercise on cerebral and general hemodynamics of normal untrained subjects. J. Clin. Invest. 34:945-946; 1955.
49. Kleinerman, J.; Sokoloff, I. Effect of exercise on cerebral blood flow and metabolism in man. Fed. Proc. 12:77-81; 1953.
50. Klimenko, V.N. Neural hypothalamic mechanisms in the development of the immune response. In: Korneva, E.A.; Klimenko, V.N.; Shkhinck, E.K., eds. Neurohumoral maintenance of immune homeostasis. Chicago: University Press; 1985:159.
51. Koff, W.C.; Dunegan, M.A. Modulation of macrophagenediated tumoricidal activity by neuropeptides and neurohormones. J. Immunol. 135:350; 1985.
52. Kuschinsky, W.; Wahl, M. Local chemical and neurogenic regulation of cerebral vascular resistance. Physiol. Rev. 58:656; 1985.

53. Lambertsen, C.J.; Owen, S.G.; Wendel, H.; Stroud, M.W.; Lurie, A.A.; Lochner, W.; Clark, G.F. Respiratory and cerebral circulatory control during exercise at .21 and 2.0 atmospheres inspired pO_2. J. Appl. Physiol. 14:966-982; 1959.
54. Lassen, N.A. Control of cerebral circulation in health and disease. Circ. Res. 34:749; 1974.
55. Levine, J.D.; Gordon, N.C.; Jones, R.T.; Fields, H.L. Naloxone enhances clinical pain. Nature. 272:826-827; 1978.
56. Li, C.H. Beta-endorphine: A pituitary peptide with potent morphine-like reactivity. Arch. Biochem. Biophys. 183:595; 1977.
57. Lown, B. Brain, heart, and sudden death. Z. Kardiol. 2(76):1987.
58. Mathews, P.M.; Froelich, C.J.; Sibbit, W.I.; Bankhurst, A.D. Enhancement of natural cytotoxity by beta-endorphin. J. Immunol. 130:1658; 1983.
59. Mayer, G.; Wessel, J.; Knobberling, J. Failure of naloxone to alter exercise induced GH and PRL release in normal men. J. Clin. Endocrinol. 13:413-416; 1980.
60. Melville, K.I. Cardiac ischemic changes induced by central nervous system stimulation. In Raab, W., ed. Prevention of ischemic heart disease. Springfield, IL: Charles C Thomas; 1966.
61. Olds, J.; Milner, P. Positive reinforcement produced by electrical stimulation of septal area and other regions of rat brain. J. Comp. Physiol. Psychol. 47:419; 1954.
62. Olesen, J. Contralateral focal increase of cerebral blood flow in man during arm work. Brain. 93:635-646; 1971.
63. Parati, G.; Pomidossi, G.; Mancia, G. Neural mechanism in human cardiovascular regulation. In: Schmidt, T.H.; Dembroski, T.M.; Blümchen, G., eds. Biological and psychological factors in cardiovascular disease. Berlin-Heidelberg: Springer; 1986.
64. Podreka, I.; Heiss, W.D.; Brücke, T. Atraumatic CBF measurement with the scintillation camera. Comparison with intracarotid rCBF values. Stroke. 12:47-53; 1981.
65. Raab, W. Neurogenic multifocal distraction of myocardial tissue. Ref. Can. Biol. 22:217; 1963.
66. Raab, W., editor. Prevention of ischemic heart disease. Springfield, IL: Charles C Thomas; 1966.
67. Rogers, H.B.; Schroeder, C.; Secher, N.H.; Mitchell, J.H. Cerebral blood flow during static exercise in humans. J. Appl. Physiol. 68(6): 2358-2361; 1990.
68. Roland, P.E.; Lassen, B. Focal increase of cerebral blood flow during stereognostic testing in man. Arch. Neurol. 33:551-558; 1976.
69. Routtenberg, A. Das belohnungssystem des gehirns. In: Spektrum, ed. Gehirn und nervensystem. Heidelberg: Spektrum der Wissenschaft-Verlag; 1985.
70. Rozanski, A.; Bairey, C.N.; Mental stress and the induction of silent myocardial ischemia in patients with coronary artery disease. N. Engl. J. Med. 318(16):1005; 1988.
71. Scheinberg, P.; Blackburn, I.I.; Rich, M.; Saslow, M. Effects of vigorous physical exercise on cerebral circulation and metabolism. Am. J. Med. 16:549-554; 1954.
72. Schwarz, L.; Kindermann, W. Beta-endorphin, cortisol und katecholamine während fahrradergometrischer ausdauerbelastungen und feidtestuntersuchungen. Dtsch. Z. Sportmed. 40(5): 160; 1989.
73. Shkhvatsabaya, I.K. Experimental production of myocardial lesions by disturbing the central nervous system. In: Raab, W., ed. Prevention of ischemic heart disease. Springfield, IL: Charles C Thomas; 1966.
74. Shyu, B.C.; Andersson, S.A.; Thoren, P. Endorphine mediated increase in pain threshold induced by long lasting exercise in rats. Life Sci. 30:833-840; 1982.
75. Smith, E.M.; Blalock, J.E. Human lymphocyte production of corticotrophin and endorphin-like substances: Association with leucocytic interferon. Proc. Natl. Acad. Sci. USA. 78:7530; 1981.
76. Snyder, S.H. Drugs and the brain. New York: Scientific American Books; 1986.
77. Sokoloff, L. Brain imaging and brain function. New York: Raven Press; 1985.
78. Sologub, J.B. Elektroenzephalographie im sport. Leipzig: Barth; 1976.
79. Solomon, G.F. Psychoneuroimmunology: Interactions between central nervous system and immune system. J. Neurosci. Res. 18:1; 1987.
80. Solomon, G.F.; Moos, R.H. Emotions, immunity, and disease. A speculative theoretical integration. Arch. Gen. Psychiatry. 11:657; 1964.
81. Spiler, I.J.; Molitch, M.E. Lack of modulation of pituitary hormone stress response by neural pathways involving opiate receptors. J. Clin. Endocrinol. 50:516-520; 1980.
82. Sutton, J.R.; Brown, G.M.; Kean, P.; Wolker, W.H.C.; Jones, N.L.; Rosenbloom, J.; Besser, G.M. The role of endorphine in the hormonal and psychological responses to exercise. Int. J. Sports Med. 2:19-23; 1982.
83. Thomas, S.N.; Schroeder, T.; Secher, N.H.; Mitchell, J.H. Cerebral blood flow during submaximal and maximal dynamic exercise in man. J. Appl. Physiol. 67:744-748; 1989.

84. Uhlenbruck, G.; Order, U. Perspektiven, probleme und prioritäten: Sportimmunologie—die nächsten 75 Jahre? Dtsch. Z. Sportmed. 28 (Special edition). 4; 1987.
85. Weihe, E. Peripheral innervation of the heart. In: von Arnim, T.; Marx, A., eds. Silent ischemia. Darmstadt: Dr. Steinkopff; 1987.
86. Weihe, E.; Nohr, D.; Gauweiler, B.; Fink, T.; Nowak, E.; Konrad, S. Immunohistochemical evidence for a diversity of opioid coding in peripheral sympathetic, parasympathetic and sensory neurones: A general principle of prejunctional opioid autoinhibition? In: Illes, P.; Farsang, C., eds. Regulatory role of opioid peptides. Weinheim: VCH; 1988.
87. Weihe, E.; Nohr, D.; Hartschuh, W. Immunohistochemical evidence for a co-transmitter role of opioid peptides in primary sensory neurones. Prog. Brain. Res. 74:189; 1988.
88. Willer, J.C.; Dehen, H.; Camwier, J. Stress induced analgesia in humans, endogenous opioids and naloxone-reversible depression of pain reflexes. Science. 212:689-691; 1981.
89. Wise, R. The dopamin synapse and the notion of "pleasure center" in the brain. Trends Neurosci. 4:91; 1980.
90. Wurtman, R.J. Nährstoffe, die gehirnfunktionen fördern. Nervenheilk. 3:33; 1984.
91. Zobl, E.G.; Talmers, F.N.; Christensen, R.C.; Baer, L.J. Effect of exercise on the cerebral circulation and metabolism. J. Appl. Physiol. 20:1289-1293; 1965.
92. Zurabaki, G.; Benedik, M.; Kamb, B.J.; Abrams, J.S.; Zurawski, S.M.; Lee, F.D. Activation of maus T-helper cells induces abundant preproencephalin mRNH synthesis. Science. 232: 772; 1986.

Chapter 33

Physical Activity and Aging: Sensory and Perceptual Processing

George E. Stelmach

For many years there has been speculation as to whether sensorimotor processes are related to physical fitness and well-being. This speculation has led to a great number of research investigations that have sought to establish a relationship between physical activity (PA) and sensory and perceptual processes (34). For this paper the definition of PA provided by Bouchard and Shephard (6) will be used. PA is defined as any body movement produced by the skeletal muscles and resulting in a substantial increase over resting energy expenditure. This broad usage of the term includes active physical leisure, exercise, sport, occupational work, and other physical chores.

This paper is not intended to be a comprehensive review of the benefits of fitness and exercise; rather it is an examination of the available data on the effects of PA on sensory and perceptual processing. No attempt is made to address whether PA is related to good health habits that may produce psychological well-being. In the paper, several important distinctions are made that will hopefully expose researchers in the exercise science area to the importance of isolating specific sensorimotor processing components when making inferences about the effects of PA.

The material covered attempts to find evidence that there is a link between PA and sensation and perception. However, the task of making such an association is not easy. A cursory review of the literature suggests that there are little such data. The most apparent reason for the sparse data is that to perform such research requires precise psychophysical methods that are not so common in exercise science, and because there are few specific hypotheses capable of guiding systematic research. Without specific hypotheses, it would be fatuous for scientists to undertake such a research endeavor on any large scale.

Sensation and perception processes are important to exercise scientists because they are essential for central nervous system integrity that underlies all aspects of perception-action cycle. A primary issue for those interested in physical activity is that skillful human life is dependent on an efficient interaction between the central nervous system and its environment. Such an interaction is accomplished by extracting specific information from the environment and by performing an energy exchange on the information extracted. If PA can be shown to enhance perceptual-motor processing, it provides an additional reason to include regimens of PA as part of daily living.

All sensory receptors share a common function of generating neural activity in response to stimulation; they are involved in transducing or converting the energy of the episodic stimulus from the environment into a neural form. Sensation and perception are areas of inquiry in which cognitive neuroscientists study the link between variation in specified characteristics of environmental stimulation and the attributes and magnitude of subjective experience (29). Thus, the study of sensation and perception is a subset of cognitive-motor processing and requires precise psychophysical methods.

The chapter is divided into several sections. First, I will define the terms *sensation* and *perception*. The point is made that unless investigators in exercise science who study such measures as reaction time (RT), movement time (MT), and response accuracy use component processing research strategies, it is not possible to infer the exact locus of any found relationship between PA and improved sensory and perceptual processing. This section is followed by documenting some of the theoretical postulates that have been suggested as to why PA may lead to improved sensation or perception. As the theoretical rationale is severely limited, I then raise the issue that perhaps a relationship should not be expected. Subsequently, I examine the aging area where there are documented declines in most central and peripheral processing components (26,37). It is an area where the best opportunities lie for attaining a relationship between PA and sensation and perception. Does PA reduce the apparent declines with aging? Can PA reverse the known impairments associated with aging? The final part of the paper raises some methodological issues that should be addressed in future research on PA and perceptual-motor processing.

Sensation and Perception

Many meanings and distinctions have been associated with the terms sensation and perception, but it must be stressed at the beginning of this paper that the taxonomic distinction between the two terms is perhaps of greater relevance for historians than for modern day scientists. As eloquently posited by Schiffman (29), sensation and perception refer to the study of a complex chain of interdependent processes—activated and selectively tuned by sensory receptors.

From a strict psychological view, sensation refers to certain immediate and direct qualitative experiences—such as feedback movement, motion, and pressure, and so on. Typically, these qualitative experiences are formed by the presence of isolated physical stimuli. The study of sensation is thus primarily associated with structure, neural processing, and receptor activity.

In contrast, the study of perception generally refers to psychological processes whereby meaning, past experience, and judgment are involved (29). Perceptions are associated with the organization and integration of sensory attributes. For many, perception means the awareness of things and events rather than simple attributes or qualities. While the study of sensation and perception have a long research history in psychology, they do not have much of an association with exercise science research.

One of the problems of importing psychophysical methods into PA research is that most meaningful sensory interactions between individuals and their environments are not restricted to a single sensory input. Any realistic study of the relationship of PA to sensation and perception must generally take into account the biology and the ongoing activation of more than an isolated sense modality. With current methods and techniques it is not easy to make such explorations.

Mechanistic Postulations of a Relationship Between Physical Activity (PA) and Sensorimotor Processing

Over the years, there have been several hypotheses offered for linking fitness levels with efficient cognitive-motor processing that also apply to the study of sensation and perception. However, none of the hypotheses tendered have received sufficient support for establishing such a relationship. While PA can impact cerebrovascular function, cerebral neurotransmitter ordinance, neuroendocrine and autonomic tone, and brain morphology, there is little evidence that in young or moderately elderly nonpathologic individuals, that changes in any or all of the foregoing really make a difference in cognitive-motor functioning (33). It may be that such a relationship actually exists but that a data base is simply lacking.

It has been accepted for some time that response speed measures and some cognitive functions are impaired by cardiovascular disease (for example, see 40). Similarly, it is known that catecholamine function is influenced by chronic exercise (7). In rats at resting states following exercise training, Spirduso (33) reports that several investigators have observed that brain catecholamine levels and associated neurotransmitter capabilities are enhanced compared to nonexercised animals. Moreover, it has also been demonstrated that vigorous exercise increases the arousal or activation level of the central nervous system (25). As a spinoff the neural activation and stimulation of the reticular activating system may in turn improve attentional focus. Furthermore, there has been some speculation that heightened activation may also extricate some types of information processing (39). A more generalized position has been advocated by Stones and Kozma (38), who propose that exercise creates an enhanced state in the central nervous system by influencing regional blood flow, neuromuscular activity, and biochemical modulations.

As is suggested from the preceding paragraphs, there is some reason to speculate that PA may influence perceptual-motor processes and in turn sensation and perception. The problem with these hypotheses is that they do not predict any localized benefits from PA. For the most part, exercise is thought to have a generalized effect across physiological and psychological domains (22). As a consequence, the offered hypotheses do not suggest that any one function will benefit more from exercise than others.

Physical Activity and Cognitive-Motor Capabilities

In recent years, a great deal of attention has been given to the role of physical fitness and PA in the enhancement of psychological health and well-being. According to Plante and Rodin (22), over 500 articles have been published in scientific journals that attempt to link PA to efficient perceptual-motor processing. In light of the pervasiveness of the fitness phenomenon and the numerous claims made about the benefits of exercise on mental states (22, p. 5), it is surprising that only a small proportion of scientific studies have examined the role of exercise on perceptual, sensory, and motor functions among normal populations.

Tomporowski and Ellis (39) and Spirduso and MacRae (34) have extensively reviewed the evidence on the effects of PA on cognitive functioning. They concluded from the work of Sjoberg (31), Spirduso (32), and others (2,4,5,9,10), that when test performance is compared from individuals who differ in physical fitness levels, or after exercise, there is limited support for the view that cognitive-motor function is enhanced by execution of PA. A similar conclusion was provided by Plante and Rodin (22) due to numerous methodological shortcomings in the research reviewed.

In one of the most extensive experiments in this area, Dustman, Ruhling, and Russell (13) carefully selected young and elderly subjects (exercisers and nonexercisers) and matched them into fitness levels while maintaining equality of intelligence between groups. The authors analyzed the P3 latencies and its amplitude slopes (A/I) from the visual event potentials. They observed that both the young and the older adults that regularly participate in exercise regimens had faster P3s, visual event potentials waves, and more negative A/I slopes than those who did not. While these data may be considered preliminary, they seem to suggest that exercise produces a generalized benefit for brain function (see 33 for more detail).

In a recent study Paas and Adam (21) investigated how physical exercise affects perceptual-motor processing. Subjects performed both a perception and a decision task during two exercise regimens (endurance and interval) as well as during rest conditions. Work load was administered as a fixed percentage of the subject's maximal work load. For the perception task subjects had to identify a briefly presented row of three letters. For the decision task subjects had to localize which of the outer numbers in a row of three digits was larger. The results obtained indicated that increments in physical work load improved performance on the decision task and reduced performance on the perception task. Moreover, decrements in work load reduced performance on the decision task and improved performance on the perception task.

Several important results found in this study are worth noting. Although minimal exercise regimens produced significantly higher heart rates, no differences were found between exercise regimens in perceptual-motor processing. This suggests that substantial changes in PA are required to influence perceptual-motor processing. More importantly, the data demonstrate that it is not possible to make a "pure" link between PA and perceptual-motor processing. As indicated earlier, an increment in exercise improved performance on the decision task but impaired performance on the perception task, whereas decrements in work load reduced performance on the decision task and improved performance on the perception task. Such mixed findings are typical in this research area.

In reviewing the supporting data, a careful analysis will reveal that where such benefits of PA have been obtained, research paradigms and methods are insufficient to localize where the benefit may reside. The exceptions to this statement are several studies that attempted to decompose RT into central and peripheral components (11,17,19). These studies found that when exercisers were compared to nonexercisers, the increased speed of response was localized in the premotor (cognitive) component rather than the motor component. Such data clearly support the view that the benefits of exercise are localized at the higher levels of central nervous system function. Although these paradigmatic efforts are commendable, they do not go far enough.

When a motor output demonstrates improved speed, the benefit of PA may be localized anywhere on a continuum between the onset of sensation and the motor initiation of a response. Heretofore, research methodologies have not employed techniques capable of isolating where such a benefit resides (see 7,10,23,29). As an illustration, it is known that the output of a movement response is the result of a complex set of processes that culminate in a motor action (36). For a dependent measure such as reaction time, any benefit from PA may be associated with changes in one, all, or some combination of the following components (42):

1. Conversion of the stimulus by the sensory receptor into a signal consisting of a series of nerve impulses
2. Transmission of these impulses to the brain
3. Perceptual identification of the episodic sensation
4. Selection of the appropriate motor response
5. Transmission from the brain to the effector muscles making the response
6. Activation of these muscles

Tomporowski and Ellis (39) suggest that methodological problems as well as the fact that most studies were conducted in piecemeal fashion, with little emphasis on theory-based parametric approaches, plague this area of research. For these reasons, the current data fail to provide clear and convincing support for the notion that physical activity improves perceptual-motor functioning.

However, some research suggests that physical activity may improve sensorimotor functioning in elderly subjects.

Aging and Physical Activity: Declines in Perceptual-Motor Processing

An area of study where linkage between PA and sensation and perception might be expected is in the area of advanced aging. Research has made it apparent that age-related impairments are as ubiquitous in the brain as they are in phylogeny: Age-related changes can be detected at practically any level of analysis, from molecular biology to the neuropsychology of perceptual-motor processing (3; also see, 25,26,37). In the elderly there is an abundance of evidence that the perception-action cycle does not operate at optimal levels. These declines in perceptual-motor functioning have been often linked to some types of physical disease, consequently scientists have sought to understand the effects of primary and secondary aging on mental function (33).

Central mechanisms have been implicated in the slowing of performance with age. Welford (46) argues that psychomotor slowing is the result of central or *cognitive* mechanisms rather than peripheral or reflex mechanisms. Thus, RT techniques are used to estimate the time of various cognitive processes. Simple and choice RT tasks have shown that as one ages, central mechanisms are impaired and consequently a slowing of response initiation is seen (8,16). Age deficits are also seen in manipulations of task complexity (18), preparation of movement (15), changes in stimulus-response compatibility (23), speed-accuracy relationships (27), and postural control (20,47). However, it is not clear whether there are generalized deficits in central mechanisms or whether aging has specific effects on one aspect of cognitive-motor processing in particular.

Although a variety of RT techniques have implicated central processing deficits, it is difficult to rule out peripheral problems. Salthouse (28) has proposed several hypotheses that describe and account for the slowness of reaction time. One hypothesis deals with the slowness of transmitting information between the central nervous system and the peripheral output system, which he terms *input or output rate*. The changes in the peripheral system that occur with advanced age are thought to produce the delays in the transmission of information. These peripheral factors may contribute to the slowing, but certainly are not responsible for all slowing observed in older individuals. Weiss (41) and Clarkson (12) fractionated RT into two components to determine whether central or peripheral factors were responsible for the slowing of RT that comes with age. These studies suggest that peripheral processes remain intact with increasing age and the RT deficits in older adults are due to central processing deficits.

A second plausible explanation proposed by Salthouse (28) for aging deficits in speed of processing deals with central mechanism deficits called *hardware differences*, which are internal mechanisms responsible for the operation of the perceptual-motor system. A major theory attributing slowness to hardware differences in older adults is the neural noise hypothesis proposed by Welford (43,44,45). Welford suggests that the signal:noise ratio in older adults is much smaller than the ratio in young people. This could be due to weaker signals, increased noise, or a combination of the two (43), which causes RT to increase because of central transmission deficits.

A final explanation proposed by Salthouse (28) that localizes deficits to one particular aspect of the information processing system is termed *software differences*. These include the sequences of control processes, strategy differences, poor preparation, task complexity, and speed-accuracy trade-offs, which all seem to be affected by age.

Although these hypotheses have helped guide research on the elderly in the cognitive areas, they have not emerged among those studies that have examined the effects of PA in the elderly. However, there are data that have shown that physically fit older adults demonstrate fewer declines in cognitive-motor function compared to sedentary adults (2,10). Spirduso (35) performed the seminal study where reaction times of exercisers and nonexercisers were compared. The findings of the study revealed that the old exercisers were substantially faster at both simple and choice response latency tasks than the old nonexercisers, whose responses also were not significantly slower than subjects 30 years younger. Similar findings have been reported by Hart (17) and Sherwood and Selder (30).

An inspection of these data on older adults reveals that much of the association between fitness and cognition has been obtained from studies that have concentrated on tasks in which response speed was the critical component (e.g., reaction time). The frequency of such studies is in part due to the belief of many scientists that an individuals's reaction time reflects the integrity of the central nervous system (26). For a review of this literature on differences between physically fit and less fit older adults, the reader should inspect Spirduso and MacRae (34) and Chodzko-Zajko (9).

When exercise is used as an intervention strategy in the elderly the results are even less clear (33). A number of studies have found such a relationship, however, they suffer from methodological shortcomings. In reviewing all the work up to 1981, Folkins and Sime (14) concluded that the data from studies that showed a relationship between exercise intervention and cognitive-motor function in the elderly did not employ acceptable research designs.

A more recent study by Dustman et al. (13), which is frequently cited as providing support for the use of PA as an intervention strategy in the elderly, has found that when subjects are matched on socioeconomic and intelligence factors, 4 months of physical training produced improved simple reaction time. Unfortunately, they did not find any evidence that choice reaction latencies were altered. Using correlation methods, Blumenthal and Madden (5) found a relationship between initial levels of fitness and the speed of memory search, however they did not observe a relationship between the improvement in aerobic capacity and changes in postexercise search time. There are few studies that have directly examined the effect of task complexity (intelligence, working memory, and abstract reasoning) on the relationship between physical fitness and cognitive performance (see 9 for review). These studies have produced largely equivocal results.

Methodological Issues and Future Research

There are many methodological issues associated with research on PA that attempt to relate it to perceptual-motor capabilities. Many of these issues have been discussed in other chapters in this volume. For those who may want to inspect other reviews, Chodzko-Zajko (9), Folkins and Sime (14), and Plante and Rodin (22) have detailed the methodological problems that plague research in this area. While these issues have been primarily presented in the context of cognitive performance, they may be appropriately applied to investigations of the sensation and perception area.

As stated by Plante and Rodin (22), methodological flaws strike at both the internal and external validity of the obtained findings. Questions of internal validity include: (a) nonrandom assignment into experimental and control conditions, (b) failure to use any form of control group, (c) examination of a small number of subjects in combination with a large number of dependent variables, and (d) reporting data that do not consider the effect of individuals that dropped from the experimental groups. Questions to external validity include the use of nonstandard measures of exercise, fitness, or psychological constructs as well as the use of atypical exercise regimens (22, p. 18).

However, the current major limitation with respect to this area is that investigators have not utilized the appropriate techniques to isolate component processing. Without using such procedures, research can document at best only the generalized effects of PA on cognitive-motor processing. As a consequence, knowledge will not advance if there are not improvements in research protocols. Another major problem is that it is difficult to produce defensible criteria for assigning subjects to high- and low-fitness groups. This problem makes it difficult to assess the changes, if any, that may occur as the result from any exercise intervention (22, p. 16).

Spirduso (33) describes five factors that make it difficult to know whether PA modulates cognitive-motor function:

(a) Different types of research design, static group comparison (cross-sectional), longitudinal, and quasi-experimental (intervention) designs that have produced divergent results;
(b) Physical fitness that has not been measured adequately, and the questionable criterion used by most investigators;
(c) Stable measures of cognitive or mental function that have not often been obtained;
(d) Cognitive measures used that are substantially correlated with socioeconomic and education factors; and
(e) Selection procedures for age categories that often exaggerate individual differences in older adult groups.

At some point, perhaps this PA area will have to address a more serious methodological challenge. Regardless of whether or not the research uses designs that document the benefits of PA within subjects or between subjects (i.e., exercisers and nonexercisers, or exercise as an intervention strategy), the emerging paradigms will have to address the issue of speed vs. accuracy trade-offs. This term refers to a variety of perception–action situations such as grasping, handwriting, pointing, and typing in which individuals have control of the speed at which they perform, and where it is possible to evaluate the quality or accuracy of the performance (26). For most task situations, there is often a point where the quality or accuracy of the performance begins to suffer if speed is increased. Beyond such a point any increase in speed comes at the cost of reduced accuracy.

This phenomenon is a potential problem for those who are interested in documenting the benefits of exercise by showing improved speed of responding. In such PA experiments, the subjects are often instructed to "respond as rapidly and as accurately as possible." Such ambiguous instructions make it likely that individuals (or groups) will respond differently—some will emphasize speed more than accuracy, while others will emphasize accuracy more than speed. Recognition of this phenomenon suggests that before any comparison between exercise groups, age groups, or pre-versus postcomparisons are made, efforts should be made to assess the speed-accuracy characteristics of the tested individuals or groups.

This can be accomplished by inducing subjects to perform at several different levels of accuracy within a single set of trials (1). The point to be comprehended here is that tests or tasks that assess the speed of responding are uninterpretable unless the performance measures are placed in the context of an individual's or group's speed-accuracy operating characteristics. Some important questions that exercise scientists should keep in mind are:

(a) Do people who exercise perform at different speeds because they have distinct speed-accuracy operating characteristics compared to those who do not, or are they simply operating at noncomparable positions along the same speed-accuracy function?
(b) Do individuals who exercise differ in the slopes of the speed-accuracy functions such that there are differential rates of information processing?

The methodological importance of dealing with the speed-accuracy trade-off phenomenon is derived from the realization that if speed and accuracy are reciprocally related, then it is unlikely that meaningful dependent measures may be derived from comparisons between exercisers and nonexercisers regardless of whether or not within- or between-subject designs are utilized. As posited by Salthouse (1985), those who work with speed-of-responding measures should know that the precision of their time measurement is directly dependent on the associated level of accuracy and the specific parameters of the operating characteristics relating speed to accuracy.

Conclusions

Perhaps this review will expose exercise scientists to the necessity of showing more than a relationship between PA and various sensorimotor processing capabilities. For example, the data on the elderly that suggest the observed decrements may be influenced by PA are particularly interesting. It was shown that changes of movement latency and response speed resemble in many ways those changes associated with brain damage and cardiovascular disease. These data offer stimulating and potentially valuable leads to understanding the causes and processes of change associated with age (42). For these resemblances to become more than superficial antidotes, the mechanisms linking the physiological and psychological findings to behavior and performance need to be systematically documented.

References

1. Bashore, T.R.; Osman, A.; Heffly, E.F. Mental slowing in elderly persons: A cognitive psychophysical analysis. Psychol. Aging. 4:235-244; 1989.
2. Baylor, A.M.; Spirduso, W.W. Systematic aerobic exercise and components of reaction time in older women. J. Gerontol. 43:P121-P126; 1988.
3. Birren, J. Handbook of mental health and aging. Engelwood Cliffs, NJ: Prentice Hall; 1980.
4. Blumenthal, J.A.; Emery, C.F.; Madden, D.J.; Schnieboll, M.; Walsh-Riddle, L.K.; George, C.M.; Dophine, M.B.; Higgenbothan, F.R.; Cobb, Coleman, R.E. Long-term effects of exercise on psychological functioning in older men and women. J. Gerontol: Psychol. Sci. 46:P352-P361; 1991.
5. Blumenthal, J.A.; Madden, D.J. Effects of aerobic exercise training, age and physical fitness on memory search performance. Psychol. Aging. 3:280-285; 1988.
6. Bouchard, C.; Shephard, R. Physical activity and fitness as determinants of health: The general model and basic concepts. In: Bouchard, C.; Shephard, R.; Stephens, T., eds. Physical activity, fitness, and health. Champaign, IL: Human Kinetics: 1992:8-23.
7. Brown, B.; Payne, T.; Kim, C.; Moore, G.; Krebs, P.; Martin, W. Chronic response of rat brain norepinephrine and serotonin levels to endurance training. J. Appl. Physiol. 49:12-23; 1979.
8. Cerella, J. Information processing rates in the elderly. Psychol. Bull. 98:67-83; 1985.
9. Chodzko-Zajko, W. Physical fitness, cognitive performance and aging. Med. Sci. Sport Exerc. 23:868-872; 1991.
10. Chodzko-Zajko, W.J.; Ringel, R.L. Physical fitness measures and sensory and motor performance in aging. Exp. Gerontol. 22:317-328; 1987.
11. Clarkson, P. The effect of age and activity in simple and choice fractionated response time. Eur. J. Appl. Physiol. 40:17-25; 1978.
12. Clarkson, P.M. The effect of age and activity level on simple and choice fractionated response time. Eur. J. Appl. Physiol. 40:17-25; 1978.

13. Dustman, R.; Ruhling, R.; Russell, E. Aerobic exercise training and improved neuropsychological function of older individuals. Neurobiol. Aging. 5:35-42; 1984.
14. Folkins, C.H.; Sime, W.E. Physical fitness and mental health. Am. Psychol. 36:373-389; 1981.
15. Gottsdanker, R. Aging and the maintenance of preparation. Exp. Aging Res. 6:13-27; 1980.
16. Gottsdanker, R. Age and simple reaction time. J. Gerontol. 37:342-348; 1982.
17. Hart, B. The effect of age and habitual activity on the fractionated components of resisted and unresisted response time. Med. Sci. Sports Exerc. 13:78; 1981.
18. Jordan, T.C.; Rabbitt, P.M. Response times to stimuli of increasing complexity as a function of ageing. Br. J. Psychol. 68:189-201; 1977.
19. MacRae, P.; Crum, K.; Giessman, D.; Green, J. The effects of age and fitness level on components of reaction time in women. A presentation at the North American Society for Sport and Physical Activity. Vancouver, BC: 1987.
20. Mankovskii, N.B.; Mints, A.Y.; Lysenyuk, V.P. Regulation of the preparatory period for complex voluntary movement in old and extreme old age. Hum. Physiol. 6:47-50; 1980.
21. Paas, F.G.W.C.; Adam, J.J. Human information processing during physical exercise. Ergonomics. 34:1385-1397; 1991.
22. Plante, T.G.; Rodin, J. Physical fitness and enhanced psychological health. Curr. Psychol. Res. Rev. 9:3-24; 1990.
23. Rabbitt, P.M. How old and young subjects monitor and control responses for accuracy and speed. Br. J. Psychol. 70:305-311; 1979.
24. Randford, C. A role for amines in the antidepressant effect of exercise: A review. Med. Sci. Sports Exerc. 14:1-10; 1982.
25. Rodgers, J. The neurobiology of cerebellar senescence. In: Joseph, J., ed. Central determinants of age-related declines in motor function. New York: Ans. N.Y. Acad. of Sci. 1988:251-267.
26. Salthouse, T. Cognitive aspects of motor functioning. In: Josheph, J., ed. Central determinants of age-related declines in motor function. New York: Ans. N.Y. Acad. of Sci. 1988:33-41.
27. Salthouse, T.A. Adult age and the speed-accuracy trade-off. Ergonomics. 22:811-821; 1979.
28. Salthouse, T.A. Speed of behavior and its implications for cognition. In: Handbook of the psychology of aging. Birren J.E.; Schaie K.W., eds. New York: Van Nostrand Reinhold; 1985:400-426.
29. Schiffman, H. Sensation and perception. New York: Wiley; 1982.
30. Sherwood, D.; Selder, D. Cardiorespiratory health, reaction time, and aging. Med. Sci. Sports Exerc. 11:186-189; 1979.
31. Sjoberg, H. Physical fitness and mental performance during and after work. Ergonomics. 23:977-995; 1980.
32. Spirduso, W. Physical fitness, aging and psychomotor speed: A review. J. Gerontol. 35:850-865; 1980.
33. Spirduso, W. Health, exercise, and mental function. In: Aging and motor performance. Champaign, IL: Human Kinetics; [1993]:254-289.
34. Spirduso, W.; MacRae, P. Motor performance and aging. In: Birren, J.E.; Schaie, K.W., eds. The handbook of the psychology of aging: Third ed. San Diego: Academic Press; 1990: 184-197.
35. Spirduso, W.W. Reaction and movement time as a function of age and physical activity level. J. Gerontol. 30:435-440; 1975.
36. Stelmach, G. Information processing framework for understanding human motor behavior. In: Human motor behavior. New York: Lawrence-Erlbaum; 1982:63-92.
37. Stelmach, G.E.; Worringham, C.G. Sensorimotor deficits related to postural stability. Clin. Geriatr. Med. 1:679-693; 1985.
38. Stones, M.J.; Kozma, A. Age, exercise, and coding performance. Psychol. Aging. 4:190-194; 1989.
39. Tomporowski, P.; Ellis, N. Effects of exercise on cognitive processes: A review. Psychol. Bull. 99:338-346; 1986.
40. Tweit, A.H.; Gollnick, P.D.; Hearn, G.R. Effects of a training program on total body reaction of individuals of low fitness. Res. Q. 34:508-513; 1963.
41. Weiss, A.D. The locus of reaction time change with set, motivation, age. J. Gerontol. 20:60-64; 1965.
42. Welford, A. Reaction time, speed of performance, and age. In: Joseph, J., ed. Central determinants of age-related declines in motor function. New York: Ans. N.Y. Acad. of Sci.; 1988:1-17.
43. Welford, A.T. Signal, noise, performance and age. Hum. Factors. 23:91-109; 1981.
44. Welford, A.T. Motor skills and aging. In: Mortimer, J.; Pirozzolo, F.; Maletta, G. eds. Aging motor system. New York: Praeger; 1982:152-187.
45. Welford, A.T. Between bodily changes and performance: Some possible reasons for slowing with age. Exp. Aging Res. 10:73-88; 1984.
46. Welford, A.T. Psychomotor performance. In: Eisdorfer, C., ed. Annual review of gerontology and geriatrics. New York: Springer; 1984:237-273.
47. Woollacott, M.H.; Shumway-Cook, A.; Nashner, L. Postural reflexes and aging. In: Mortimer, J.; Pirozzolo, F.; Maletta, G., eds. Aging motor system. New York: Praeger; 1982:98-119.

Chapter 34

Nervous System and Sensory Adaptation: Neural Plasticity Associated with Chronic Neuromuscular Activity

V. Reggie Edgerton
Roland R. Roy

Role of Chronic Neuromuscular Activity in Shaping a Learned Motor Task

Although chronic activity-related morphological, electrophysiological, and pharmacologically induced changes in the nervous system have been described in numerous papers, clear evidence of whether or not those changes were obligatory for a known neural function or specific neural pathway is almost always lacking (22). For example, motoneuron soma and axonal size can change in response to chronic exercise (19,20,45), however no one has demonstrated whether these or other similar morphological or physiological changes directly affect any motor task. To demonstrate a cause–effect relationship of cellular changes that are activity-dependent and that underlie the observed changes in motor performance is a formidable problem. Significant progress, however, has been made as a result of the use of more appropriate animal models combined with advances in biological technology that have permitted the execution of more well-defined experiments. Simple as well as complex motor tasks are studied in these animal models.

One of the most productive approaches in defining mechanisms of neuromotor plasticity has been to study a simple motor response in a simple nervous system (e.g., the *Aplysia)* (21). Another strategy has been to simplify the motor and learning tasks by surgically reducing the nervous system (e.g., deafferentation) (49). Another approach has been to study a complex but well-controlled and defined motor task such as the vestibulo-ocular reflex (41,53) or the flexion reflex (14). Functional isolation of the neural pathways involved in a movement, for example, the chronic training of volitional influences on the H-reflex, has been another research strategy (51,52). The present chapter reviews selected studies that represent one or more of the experimental strategies noted herein with the common link being a well-defined motor task that can be closely associated or even directly linked with the observed neural plasticity.

A generally accepted premise is that motor performance can be influenced by the presence or the absence of "practice." This premise, however, does not preclude the possibility that the actual performance of a movement is unnecessary to induce a change in its execution, because there are other neural processes, for example, visualizing and imagining performances, that may also affect a motor task. The present chapter addresses questions related to how motor performance may be influenced by the repetitive use of defined or partially defined neural networks.

Modification of a Well-Defined Neuromotor Pathway in a Normally Behaving Animal

Wolpaw, Lee, and Carp (51,52) have shown that the healthy Rhesus monkey can be trained to modulate a relatively specific neural pathway involved in the output of a specific motor pool. For example, monkeys can increase the amplitude of a Hoffmann reflex (H-reflex, induced by randomly stimulating a peripheral nerve throughout the day by using a food reward) over a period of 70 to 90 days. The average amplitude of the H-reflex is increased when the Rhesus is rewarded for upregulation of the H-reflex in that leg. Similarly, the Rhesus can be trained to down-regulate the H-reflex amplitude to less than half of the pretraining amplitude over a period of 50 days. Further, it was demonstrated that these operant conditioning effects persisted after a complete transection of the spinal cord (T9–T10). Wolpaw and co-workers also found that the amplitude of the H-reflex in the control leg of the down-mode trained animal was larger than the control leg of the up-mode trained animal. This difference was present only after anesthesia and spinal transection. These changes in the contralateral control legs suggest that a functional modification of one neural pathway can induce concomitant and perhaps obligatory changes in the synaptic efficacy associated with the specific motor task.

There are at least two important implications from these studies. First, the results indicate that the monkey provided some chronic bias to neurons that have some link to fast-conducting type Ia fibers that initiate the monosynaptic reflex and that this bias had a net excitatory (up-regulating) or net inhibitory (down-regulating) effect depending on when the food reward was presented by the experimenter. The source of the chronic bias on the synaptic pathways involved seemed to be from supraspinal networks presumably because some interpretation of the occurrence of food reward associated with a correct neural modulation was made. These results show that through some conscious processing the probability of excitation of a specific motor network can be manipulated. Second, the persistence of the conditioned response following spinal cord transection demonstrates that at least some of the manipulated networks are located within the lumbar segments of the spinal cord.

Learning Motor Tasks Without the Cerebellum

Modifications in motor responses following repetitive stimulation have been studied from many different perspectives and may be considered classical conditioning or learned (associative) responses. Whether or not an altered response reflects learning depends on the assumed definition of learning. A modification of a response associated with a time-locked, conditioned stimulus has been considered a learned response. As Patterson (39) has noted, a key question relative to the issue of spinal cord learning is whether the changes in spinal responses are due to associative (hence learned) processes or can it be better classified under nonassociative categories. It seems quite clear that neural networks independent of supraspinal input can be involved in the execution of movements and that the movement can undergo profound changes in response to conditioning training. Although these issues have been reviewed in detail by Patterson (38), a brief examination of some of the studies that bear most directly on the topic of the present chapter will be addressed.

Short-Term Learning

There has been a long controversy over whether the cerebellum is essential for learning a motor task (3,53). It has been shown that learned vestibulo-ocular reflexes can be eliminated by making lesions on or by anesthetizing the cerebellum or selected pathways of the cerebellum (see 53 for a recent review). The extended interpretation of these findings, more than the results of the experiments themselves, seems to have contributed to the controversy related to the essentiality of the cerebellum in motor learning. Although it is apparent that the cerebellum can play a role in the learning of some motor tasks, it seems likely that it does not have a facilitatory or essential role in learning all motor tasks. Bloedel, Bracha, Kelly, and Wu (3) have hypothesized that changes in the cerebellum associated with a learned motor task may be activity-driven, but that these changes may not be substrate-specific for the motor learning. That is, the changes in behavior and the associated neural processing may not be directly involved in the execution of the motor task.

One demonstration that the cerebellum is not essential for the acquisition and extinction of learning all motor tasks was shown by Bloedel et al. (3). In their initial experiments, acutely decerebrated (at the supracollicular level) ferrets or cats were placed over a treadmill belt, supported with a sling, and induced to step by stimulating a locomotor region of the brain stem. Within 5 to 10 steps the forelimb acquired the ability to step over an obstructing object during the swing phase. This adjustment in the motor task consisted of lifting the shoulder and forelimb so that a relatively normal (although exaggerated) swing phase could be executed and thus stepping could continue uninterrupted. After the removal of the obstruction, it took 5 to 15 steps for extinction of the adaptation, that is, for the modified motor task to return to the preobstruction movement pattern. These experiments demonstrated that the learned modification of a motor task could occur without the cerebrum. In additional experiments (3), adaptations to perturbations during stepping were studied in chronic (2–10 months postsurgery) cerebellectomized ferrets and cats. For example, the chronic cerebellectomized animals were acutely decerebrated and the stepping responses with and without an obstacle placed in the path of the foot during the swing phase were studied. The results were essentially identical to that observed with decerebration not preceded by cerebellectomy and are consistent with the interpretation that the cerebellum is not essential for the learning of all motor tasks.

Evidence that the lumbar spinal cord can learn a modified motor task without any supraspinal input has been demonstrated in our laboratory (unpublished observations). An obstacle was placed in the path of the foot during the swing phase of consecutive steps in an adult cat spinalized at vertebral level T12-T13 that had been trained to step on a treadmill belt. The obstacle (a rod) was instrumented with strain gauges so that the impact of the foot on the bar during the swing phase could be estimated. After only a few steps it was apparent that the trajectory of the hind limb was modified during the phase of the swing that preceded contact with the obstacle (Figure 34.1). This observation is important because it has been shown quiteclearly that the chronic spinal cat can modify the swing phase after the dorsum of the foot is stimulated mechanically or electrically (18). Thus, it appears that the response to the presence of and the subsequent withdrawal of the obstacle during the swing phase of stepping is learned in that the experience of the foot contacting the rod in one step modified the neural control of stepping in subsequent steps such that the rod would be less of a disruption. Furthermore, the spinal cord quickly recognized (within a few steps) when the obstacle was no longer present, and the usual trajectories that characterized the swing phase reappeared. Based on these observations we propose that the spinal cord is capable of "short-term learning" and that this neural plasticity in the control of the motor task would appear to be substrate specific. That is, the networks executing the altered motor task were modified.

One of the paradigms for studying conditioned motor responses has been the manipulation of leg position. Horridge (26) reported that an insect with the head removed learned to avoid shock by flexing the legs. Spinal rats (L1–L2) were stimulated (40–60 Hz, 1–4 msec pulse duration and 40–200 V) to flex their legs when a copper wire suspended from their limbs made contact with a electrolytic bath (i.e., the equivalent of an unconditioned stimulus) (5). The period between spinalization and training ranged from 5 days to 6 weeks. After about 16 to 60 min, the frequency of the shock received was reduced substantially during the conditioning period in the leg in which the shock was leg-position-dependent. When the same pattern of stimulus was administered to the leg of another control rat independent of leg position, there was no effect on the leg position and thus the amount of shock received. Further, when the bath was elevated so that the limb was stimulated in a more flexed position, the rat flexed the leg even further.

In a second series of experiments, rats were tested only 2 to 5 hr after spinalization (T12–L1 or T11–T12). This experiment consisted of a similar stimulation paradigm except that one leg served as the experimental (i.e., stimulation dependent on leg position) and the contralateral leg as the control (i.e., stimulation not dependent on leg position). As in the first series of experiments the number of

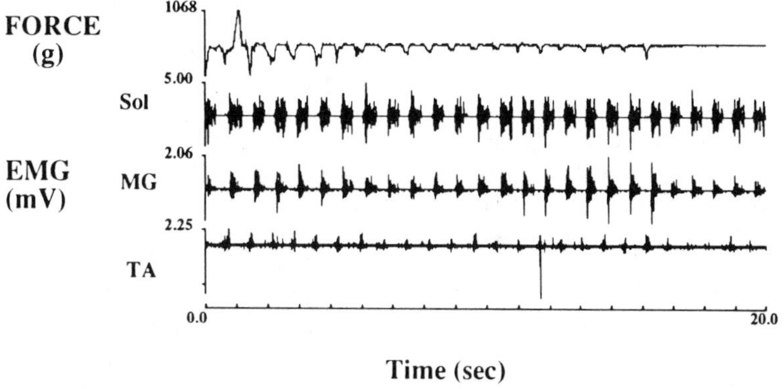

Figure 34.1 Response of a spinalized (T12-T13) cat walking on a treadmill to the imposition of a bar in the path of the foot during swing. The force (top trace) measured by strain gauges on the bar produced by the foot contacting the bar decreases within a few steps after the imposition of the bar. The EMG signals for the medial gastrocnemius (MG) and tibialis anterior (TA) show an increased activation while the bar is present, corresponding to the cat stepping "over" the bar. When the bar is removed (the last four steps), the EMG of the TA and the MG are decreased; soleus (Sol) EMG is unchanged.

leg insertions in the experimental leg was reduced within about 10 min of initiating the experimental paradigm. After a delay of 15 min following the initial training session, a testing session was conducted to compare the responses of the control and experimental legs to position-sensitive stimuli. For the first few minutes of this test the experimental leg had far fewer incidences of shock than the control leg, indicating some retention of the previously acquired learning. After continuing the test session the control leg also became trained. For example, both the experimental and control legs avoided shock by maintaining leg position.

It may be significant that the differences were much more pronounced when separate animals served as control and experimental subjects rather than when ipsilateral and contralateral legs were compared in the same rat. This difference suggests some carryover effect between legs and is consistent with the known interdependence of the neural networks between the two sides of the body (i.e., contralateral, reciprocal inhibition of flexors and extensors during alternating stepping) (34). These results support the view that the spinal cord can learn to execute a modified motor task based on the position of the leg.

As convincing as these data are, there has remained a controversy as to whether these effects are associative or nonassociative. Patterson (39) delivered a conditioned stimulus to the superficial peroneal sensory nerve and an unconditioned stimulus to the skin of the same leg after acute spinal transection (T12-L1) in the cat. The conditioned stimulus intensity produced a small motor response, and the unconditioned stimulus produced a maximal response. The greatest increase in the unconditioned response was found with an interstimulation interval between the conditioned and unconditioned stimuli of 250 ms, a time frame similar to that observed in conditioning experiments in intact animals (cf. 14). Shorter and longer intervals between the two stimuli resulted in a smaller response. These changes in response could not be associated with sensory receptors or changes in the muscle because the animals were curarized. Patterson (39) also reported that motoneuron excitability was not altered in similar preparations and thus concluded that the associative effects of classical conditioning were located in the interneuronal networks of the lumbar spinal cord.

Long-Term Learning

Spinal Cord Fixation

There has been a long history of experiments demonstrating that bilateral asymmetry in posture and locomotion in a range of species (induced by unilaterally lesioning or anesthetizing components of the cerebellum, premotor cortex, motor cortex, sensorimotor cortex, or vestibular nuclei, or by caloric stimulation of the semicircular canals) persists after a complete transection of the spinal cord. Di Giorgio (11–12) and Di Giorgio and Menzio (13) have been some of the primary contributors to the description of these effects and to the efforts to define the mechanisms by which this persistence of asymmetry occurs.

One of the principal objectives of more recent studies has been to define how long the asymmetrical input from supraspinal pathways must last before the spinal cord can be completely transected and the asymmetry persist. A second objective has been to determine how long the asymmetry in the spinal networks can persist in the absence of asymmetric input from supraspinal networks. Although there is some variability in the duration of these periods among species and among the different sites and severities of the spinal cord lesions, the interim between the initial supraspinal lesion that causes the initial asymmetry and the spinal cord transection that eliminates the source of the initial asymmetry seems to be about 30 to 45 min in mammals. Periods as short as 7 min have been reported in pigeons following cerebellectomy, with the asymmetry persisting for days or weeks after spinal transection (35). There is also some evidence that the time course of the asymmetric effects can be modulated pharmacologically. For example, when strychnine was given to dogs that had received a unilateral cerebellar lesion 23 to 24 days earlier, a persistent asymmetry was induced within 30 min after spinalization (12). Following adrenaline administration, the spinal asymmetry occurred within 10 min.

Efforts to identify specific neural pathways that are involved with the behavioral asymmetry have been only partially successful. For example, asymmetry in both monosynaptic and polysynaptic reflex responses have been reported in the postspinal transection stage of asymmetry (50). On the other hand, experiments have also shown that sensory inflow to the spinal cord during the postspinal or prespinal period is not essential for postural asymmetry to occur. Although the severity of the asymmetry was less in bilaterally deafferentated animals, it nevertheless developed following a unilateral supraspinal lesion (7).

These experiments suggest that (a) synaptic efficacy of the networks to motor pools can be modulated by altered activity levels to spinal motor networks that last only minutes or perhaps even seconds, (b) the changes in neural efficacy can persist for days to weeks, (c) some critical interim period must occur between the asymmetry-inducing supraspinal lesion and the elimination of the asymmetric input to the motor pools if the asymmetry is to persist after spinal transection, and (d) there must be sufficient time for RNA and protein modulation to occur if the motor asymmetry is to persist.

Spinal Control of Stepping

It has been known for many years that the hind limbs of mammals can execute organized and effective locomotor movements in the absence of supraspinal input to the spinal networks (see 15,16,24,25,44 for review). The capability of the spinal cord to generate rhythmic locomotor movements was convincingly demonstrated by such pioneers in the field as Brown (4) and Sherrington (46). The dominating concept that evolved from these original studies, however, was that in the absence of supraspinal control the spinal cord only executed stereotypical reflex movements initiated by peripheral excitation. This view, however, has been shown to be very simplistic. First, there have been numerous demonstrations of the ability of central neural networks of the spinal cord to respond differently and purposefully to the same stimulus at different stages of the step cycle (18,43). Secondly, it is clear that in the complete absence of supraspinal control, the spinal cord is capable of generating details of the motor output that are remarkably similar to the output characterizing normal locomotion (2,10,18,32,33). A third factor that provides evidence for spinal cord plasticity is that we (32) and others (2) have demonstrated convincingly that the locomotor capacity of the hind limbs of mammals can be improved with practice. Basically it appears that the spinal cord can "learn" and probably "forget."

The view that daily exercise training was essential to the development and maintenance of the locomotor potential of cats spinalized as neonates was clearly embraced by Forssberg, Grillner, and Halbertsma (18) in the mid-1970s: every spinal cat in their studies was treadmill-trained 10 to 20 min daily. In 1978, we began a series of experiments in cats spinalized at a low thoracic level (T12–T13) to determine if daily treadmill training had an effect on their locomotor potential, and whether or not a cat spinalized at 12 weeks of age (i.e., when the neuromuscular system essentially is completely developed) could step as well as a cat spinalized at 2 weeks of age. In the first series of experiments, spinal cats were treadmill-trained for 3 to 4 months, 5 days per week (16,47,48). Although the overall locomotor performance based on a battery of behavioral and kinetic characteristics was similar in cats spinalized at either 2 weeks or 12 weeks of age, a larger proportion of the cats spinalized at 2 weeks than at 12 weeks of age achieved higher levels of stepping performance.

These results strongly suggested that the treadmill training was more critical for recovery of locomotion in cats spinalized at 12 weeks than those spinalized at 2 weeks of age. Further, these results suggested that stepping could be regained in cats spinalized as adults as well as at a neonatal stage of development. For example, 3 of the 5 cats that were spinalized at 12 weeks of age and trained daily for 3 to 4 months could generate a stepping pattern with occasional to moderate full-weight support of the hind limbs. However, none of the 12-week-old, nontrained, spinalized cats could generate effective treadmill walking 3 to 4 months after spinalization (16).

In a second series of experiments, cats were spinalized at 2 weeks of age and some were trained to walk on a treadmill. Each cat was maintained for about 6 months posttransection. The training regimes were initiated one month postspinalization. During the next 5 months, the spinal cats were assigned either to begin training of the hind limbs on a treadmill for about 30 min per day, 5 days per week or to a nontrained group that only had its hind limbs passively manipulated once a day to maintain adequate range of motion across the joints. Six months postspinalization, all cats were tested for their locomotor potential as defined by the speed at which the hind limbs could step on the treadmill. As observed in the initial experiments, there was a wide range of locomotor capabilities among the cats spinalized at 2 weeks of age 6 months after spinalization although these cats, in general, could walk more effectively than the cats in the initial studies. As in the initial experiments, the results indicated that the probability of achieving higher levels of performance was improved with the treadmill-training program (15,16).

More recently, three groups of adult spinal cats have been studied: nontrained, treadmill-trained (emphasizing full weight-supported stepping), and standing-trained (emphasizing full weight support with no rhythmic movement of the hindlimbs). After 1 month, all spinal cats could fully support the weight of their hind limbs, and thus the training regimes were initiated. Five spinal cats were trained to step on a treadmill for 30 min per day, 5 days per week. The objective during each training session was to accomplish full weight-supported stepping at the maximum speed that each cat could sustain consistently (see 32 for criteria).

Training cats to maintain a standing posture for 30 min per day, 5 days per week was similar in most respects to treadmill training except for a stationary rather than a moving surface. Static standing was initiated and maintained during each 30-min training session by modulating sensory cues from the tail. Efforts to minimize any steplike or alternating weight-support motions and to equalize the weight-support function of each hind leg were made. The untrained spinal cats were treated similarly to the other spinal cats except for the daily training. Observation of cage activity revealed considerable spontaneous oscillatory movements in all spinal cats. Thus, for 23.5 hr each training day and for 24 hr for the 2 nontraining days, the hind limbs of all spinal cats were exposed to similar conditions.

Results from this series of experiments were astounding, particularly for the standing-trained group. The evaluation of individual as well as group mean differences provided considerable insight not only into the potential of the neuronal networks to undergo functional plasticity, but also into the specificity with which this plasticity was manifested. The maximum treadmill speed that could be achieved and maintained while fully supporting the weight of the hind limbs was more than twice as fast for the treadmill-trained than the nontrained cats (i.e., 0.62 and 0.24 m $\cdot$ sec^{-1}, respectively) (32,44,54). In addition, this type of training also seemed to enhance the probability of reaching a higher level of locomotor performance. Even more impressive, however, was the clear difference in the locomotor capability of the standing-trained compared to the treadmill-trained cats. Three of the five cats trained to stand for 5 months could not sustain any stepping pattern, even at the slowest speeds. The other two cats in this group could execute only a few steps at very slow speeds (23,40,44).

The clear differences in the locomotor capacity between the standing-trained and the treadmill-trained adult spinal cats seem to be attributable to some form of neural adaptation. Although there were clear effects of treadmill training on muscle mechanical and metabolic properties (44), it seems unlikely that the inability of three out of five of the standing-trained cats to walk was related to a limited capacity of the musculature. For example, all five standing-trained cats could sustain full weight support for 30 min. Further, there were no differences in the muscle properties between those standing-trained spinal cats that could step very slowly and those that could not walk after 5 months of standing training. In addition, the mean treadmill speed for the nontrained spinal cats was 0.33 m $\cdot$ s^{-1} compared to 0.05 m $\cdot$ s^{-1} for the standing-trained cats, whereas the mechanical and metabolic properties of the muscles were more affected in the nontrained than the standing-trained cats (44). All of these points lead to the conclusion that the differences in the locomotor capability between spinal cats are largely attributable to the neural components of the hind limb neuromuscular apparatus.

To test the ability of the spinal cord to unlearn one motor task and learn a new one, four cats spinalized as adults have been studied in a crossover design in which each cat was trained to walk for 4 or more months following transection and then trained to stand and vice versa. The cats initially trained to walk quickly learned to stand. In contrast, cats initially trained to stand had more difficulty walking at the end of the standing-training period. In addition, the quality of stepping was lower than that observed in cats initially trained to walk (unpublished observations).

In summary, these data on complete spinal-transected cats indicate that the spinal cord has the ability to learn and to forget a motor task. The differential time course in learning and forgetting how to walk or stand suggests that these processes involve complex neural pathways centered in the lumbar spinal cord.

Neuroplasticity in Response to Spaceflight

New neural strategies must be adapted quickly to control mobility and detailed motor tasks when entering the 0G environment. Changes in the vestibular, ocular, and even cognitive functions must be effectively reintegrated in the new gravitational field. Further, the severity and rapidity of the changes that occur in the muscle mass even during short flights (27) represent a further perturbation to which the control of movement must be adjusted. Studying the adaptations of the neural control of movement performed in a weightless environment has a decided advantage over experimental models in which some component of the neuromuscular system is surgically or pharmacologically impaired. For example, neuromuscular adaptations to weightlessness can be studied in a normal, neurally intact animal perturbed only in the kind of motor performance required.

It is now clear that brief (a few days) as well as prolonged space missions (up to a year) result in many adaptations in the neuromotor system and that altered neuromuscular activity may be one of the initiators of many other adaptive motor responses (29–31). For example, marked changes in the functional demands of the lower and upper limbs occur in a 0G compared to a 1G environment. Compared to routine movements at 1G, the upper limbs play a more essential role than the lower limbs in moving from place to place inside the spacecraft as well as during extravehicular activity, whereas the extensor muscles of both the lower and upper limbs are loaded minimally at 0G. In contrast the flexor muscles tend to be more active at 0G compared to 1G. However, there has been little quantification of the muscle activity patterns in a 0G environment.

Postural stability and the control of other movements is moderately to severely impaired in humans after spaceflights, some as short as 2 to 5 days (8). Greater postflight impairment has been evident after flights lasting up to 326 days (9,29,31). The postural instability and decline in movement control is generally characterized and accompanied by

1. slower responses to postural perturbations;
2. less sensitivity to a given postural perturbation;
3. slow, deliberate, wide-based steps during stepping;
4. neuromuscular weakness of the limbs;
5. a feeling of heaviness of the body and head when standing or even rolling around in bed;
6. a reduced amplitude of the monosynaptic tendon reflex;
7. a reduced threshold for initiating a monosynaptic tendon reflex;
8. a reduced H-reflex amplitude;
9. an increased incidence of tremor during upright posture; and
10. an increased sensitivity of the bottom of the feet to vibration.

The perturbations in movement control and related reflexes following spaceflight clearly illustrate that the neural control of movement adapts rapidly to a 0G environment. Presumably, although not necessarily, these changes reflect to some degree the altered functional requirements for movement and the associated changes in neuromuscular activity. It seems evident from the multiple studies of motor control by Kozlovskaya and colleagues (29–31) that a sequence of continuous and extensive compensatory neural adaptations occur throughout flight. One adaptation appears to induce subsequent compensatory adaptations. Serially occurring compensatory processes in the monosynaptic reflex and the H-reflex have been described in cosmonauts who have been in space for a range of periods of time (29). This sequence of continuing adaptations requires careful interpretation of pre- to postflight differences, particularly with respect to flight duration. Few adaptations seem to be related in any linear fashion with respect to time. For example, the absence of a specific adaptation at one point in time may simply mean that other compensatory adaptations had occurred while a de-adaptation of another portion of the neural system was occurring.

Morphological and biochemical changes have been observed in some components of the neuromotor system in response to spaceflight. For example, the soma of selected dorsal root ganglion cells (i.e., the larger cells) appeared to decrease in size in rats exposed to 12 to 14 days of spaceflight (42). McDougal et al. (37) found no effect of 12.5 days of spaceflight (i.e., Cosmos, 1887 flight) on the activity levels of eight different enzymes, including six metabolic enzymes, in hippocampal neurons. Jiang, Roy, Polyakov, Krasnov, and Edgerton (28) reported only a slight decrease in rat soma sizes of the smaller ventral neurons after a 14-day flight. A major limitation in the interpretation of each of these studies, however, is that it is unknown how the activity levels of the neurons were affected during spaceflight.

Mechanisms of Motor Learning

A persistent general question in studying learning of a motor task is, Where does learning occur in the nervous system? Byrne et al. (6, p. 124) state an emerging general principle: "The neural representation of learning and memory is distributed throughout the nervous system." Much of the progress made in understanding the neural components of behavioral plasticity has resulted from studies of simple behavior in invertebrates, for example, nonassociative and associative learning of the gill withdrawal reflex in the mollusk *Aplysia* (6). The gill withdrawal reflex, which serves as one model of long-term plasticity, consists of a tactile or electrical stimulus to the siphon that elicits a withdrawal response. Long-term facilitation of this reflex can be induced by repeated stimuli in an in vitro as well as an in vivo preparation (21). For example, Glanzman , Kandel, and Schacher (21) have shown that long-term facilitation of the synapses involved in the reflex occurs in response to repeated application of serotonin (5-HT or 5-hydroxytryptamine), a neurotransmitter important in behavioral disinhibition and sensitization. When the sensory and motor axons of the *Aplysia* were cocultured, repeated applications of 5-HT induced growth of the sensory neurons that paralleled the long-term enhancement of the synaptic strength observed. No changes in the motoneurons were observed. In subsequent studies using the same model, a down-regulation of cell surface proteins called *neural cell adhesion molecules* occurred when the sensory neurons were exposed repeatedly to 5-HT (36). The down-regulation of surface active proteins seems to have resulted from the endocytosis of these membrane-associated proteins, an internalization process that is dependent on protein synthesis (1). Furthermore, cyclic adenosine monophosphate (AMP) has been implicated in the alteration of synthesis of a number of proteins involved in memory and induction of the long-term effects of repeated stimuli using a classical conditioning paradigm in *Aplysia* (6).

Summary

One of the keys to the rapid progress made over the last decade in the science of motor learning has been the realization that the conceptual framework within which the neural plasticity of a behavior occurs cannot remain confined to a simple Pavlovian paradigm. Secondly, the method of obtaining simplicity has been to study a simple but complete behavior rather than simple, isolated reflexes. Probably the most important strategy, however, has been to match molecular, electrophysiological and morphological plasticity directly with the plasticity of a well-defined behavioral paradigm.

Acknowledgments

This work has been supported by NIH Grant NS16333 and NASA Grant NCC 2-535. The authors thank Dr. Earl Eldred for his contributions to the section on spinal fixation and Dr. John Hodgson, Camille de Guzman, Ray de Leon and Sharlene Lauretz for their contributions in performing the experiments and the data analyses for the chronic spinal cats. We also wish to thank Sharlene Lauretz for the special management of our spinal cats.

References

1. Bailey, C.H.; Chen, M.; Keller, F.; Kandel, E.R. Serotonin-mediated endocytosis of apCAM: An early step of learning-related synaptic growth in *Aplysia*. Science. 256:645-649; 1992.
2. Barbeau, H.; Rossignol, S. Recovery of locomotion after chronic spinalization in the adult cat. Brain Res. 412:84-95; 1987.
3. Bloedel, J.R.; Bracha, V.; Kelly, T.M.; Wu, J. Substrates for motor learning: Does the cerebellum do it all? In: Wolpaw, J.R.; Schmidt, J.T.; Vaughan, T.M., eds. Activity-driven CNS changes in learning and development. New York: New York Academy of Sciences; 1991:305-318.
4. Brown, T.G. On the nature of the fundamental activity of the nervous centres, together with an analysis of the conditioning of rhythmic activity in progression, and a theory of evolution of function in the nervous system. J. Physiol. (Lond.). 48:18-46; 1914.
5. Buerger, A.A.; Fennessy, A. Long-term alteration of leg position due to shock avoidance by spinal rats. Exp. Neurol. 30:195-211; 1971.
6. Byrne, J.H.; Baxter, D.A.; Buonomano, D.V.; Cleary, L.J.; Eskin, A.; Goldsmith, J.R.; McClendon, E.; Nazif, F.A.; Noel, F.; Scholz, K.P. Neural and molecular bases of nonassociative and associative learning in *Aplysia*. In: Wolpaw, J.R.; Schmidt, J.T.; Vaughan, T.M., eds. Activity-driven CNS changes in learning and development. New York: New York Academy of Sciences; 1991:124-149.
7. Cannon, W.B.; Haimovici, H. The sensitization of motoneurons by partial "devervation." Am. J. Physiol. 126:731-740; 1939.
8. Chekirda, I.F.; Bogdashevskiy, R.B.; Yeremin, A.V.; Kolosov, I.A. Coordination structure of walking of Soyuz-9 crew members before and after flight. Kosm. Biol. Med. 5:548-552; 1970.
9. Clement, G.; Lestienne, F. Adaptive modifications of postural attitude in conditions of weightlessness. Exp. Brain Res. 72:381-389; 1988.
10. de Guzman, C.P.; Roy, R.R.; Hodgson, J.A.; Edgerton, V.R. Coordination of motor pools controlling the ankle musculature in adult spinal cats during treadmill walking. Brain Res. 555:202-214; 1991.
11. Di Giorgio, A.M. Persistenza, nell animale spinale, di asimmetrie posturali e motorie di origine cerebellare. Nota II. Richerche intorno al meccanismo funzionale di tali asimmetrie. Arch. Fisiol. 27:543-557; 1929.
12. Di Giorgio, A.M. Persistenza, nell animale spinale, di asimmetrie posturali e motorie di origine cerebellare. Nota III. Sulla possibilita di evocare tali asimmetrie durante lo shock spinale, mediante la stricnina, l'adrenalina e l'iperventilazione. Arch. Fisiol. 27:558-580; 1929.
13. Di Giorgio, A.M.; Menzio, P. Comportamento degli arti posteriori dopo deafferentazione e lesione unilaterale del cervelletto. Boll. Soc. Ital. Biol. Sper. 22:827-828; 1946.
14. Durkovic, R.G.; Damianopolous, E.N. Forward and backward classical conditioning of the flexion reflex in the spinal cat. J. Neurosci. 6:2921-2925; 1986.

15. Edgerton, V.R.; de Guzman, C.P.; Gregor, R.J.; Roy, R.R.; Hodgson, J.A.; Lovely, R.G. Trainability of the spinal cord to generate hindlimb stepping patterns in adult spinalized cats. In: Shimamura, M.; Grillner, S.; Edgerton, V.R., eds. Neurobiological basis of human locomotion. Tokyo: Japan Scientific Societies Press; 1991: 411-423.
16. Edgerton, V.R.; Johnson, D.J.; Smith, L.A.; Murphy, K.; Eldred, E.; Smith, J.L. Effects of treadmill exercises on hindlimb muscles of the spinal cat. In: Kao, C.C.; Bunge, R.P.; Reier, P.J., eds. Spinal cord reconstruction. New York: Raven Press; 1983:435-443.
17. Edgerton, V.R.; Roy, R.R.; Hodgson, J.A.; Gregor, R.J.; de Guzman, C.P. Recovery of full weight-supporting locomotion of the hindlimbs after complete thoracic spinalization of adult and neonatal cats. In: Wernig, A., ed. Restorative neurology, volume 5, chapter 43. Plasticity of motoneuronal connections. New York: Elsevier Science; 1991:405-418.
18. Forssberg, H.; Grillner, S.; Halbertsma, J. The locomotion of the low spinal cat. I. Coordination within a limb. Acta Physiol. Scand. 108:269-282; 1980.
19. Gerchman, L.B.; Edgerton, V.R.; Carrow, R.E. Effects of physical training on the histochemistry and morphology of ventral motor neurons. Exp. Neurol. 49:790-801; 1975.
20. Gilliam, T.B.; Roy, R.R.; Taylor, J.F.; Heusner, W.W.; Van Huss, W.D. Ventral motor neuron alterations in rat spinal cord after chronic exercise. Experientia. 33:665-667; 1977.
21. Glanzman, D.L.; Kandel, E.R.; Schacher, S. Target-dependent structural changes accompanying long-term synaptic facilitation in *Aplysia* neurons. Science. 249:799-802; 1990.
22. Greenough, W.T.; Anderson, B.J. Cerebellar synaptic plasticity: Relation to learning versus neural activity. In: Wolpaw, J.R.; Schmidt, J.T.; Vaughan, T.M., eds. Activity-driven CNS changes in learning and development. New York: New York Academy of Sciences; 1991: 231-247.
23. Gregor, R.J.; Fowler, E.G.; Roy, R.R. Motor output capabilities of adult spinal cats following postural training. Soc. Neurosci. Abstr. 14:64; 1988.
24. Grillner, S. Control of locomotion in bipeds, tetrapods, and fish. In: Brookhart, J.M.; Mountcastle, V.B., eds. Handbook of physiology, the nervous system, motor control, vol. 2, part 1, section 1. Bethesda, MD: American Physiological Society; 1981:1179-1236.
25. Grillner, S.; Buchanan, J.T.; Wallen, P.; Brodin, L. Neural control of locomotion in lower vertebrates: From behavior to ionic mechanisms. In: Cohen, A.H.; Rossignol, S.; Grillner, S., eds. Neural control of rhythmic movements in vertebrates. New York: Wiley; 1988:1-40.
26. Horridge, G.A. Learning of leg position by the ventral nerve cord in headless insects. Proc. R. Soc. Lond. Sec. B. 157:33-52; 1962.
27. Jiang, B.; Roy, R.R.; Navarro, C.; Edgerton, V.R. Absence of a growth hormone effect on rat slows atrophy during a 4-day spaceflight. J. Appl. Physiol. 74:527-531, 1993.
28. Jiang, B.; Roy, R.R.; Polyakov, I.V.; Krasnov, I.B.; Edgerton, V.R. Ventral horn cell responses to spaceflight and hindlimb suspension. J. Appl. Physiol. [Suppl.]. 73:107S-111S; 1992.
29. Kozlovskaya, I.B.; Barmin, V.A.; Stepantsov, V.I.; Kharitonov, N.M. Results of studies of motor functions in long-term space flights. Physiologist. 33:S1-S3; 1990.
30. Kozlovskaya, I.B.; Kirenskaya, A.V.; Dmitrieva, I.F. Gravitational mechanisms in the motor system. Studies in real and simulated weightlessness. In: Gurfinkel, V.S.; Ioffe, M.E.; Massion, J.; Roll, J.P., eds. Stance and motion: Facts and concepts. New York: Plenum Press; 1988: 37-47.
31. Kozlovskaya, I.B.; Kreidich, Y.V.; Oganov, V.S.; Koserenko, O.P. Pathophysiology of motor functions in prolonged manned space flights. Acta Astron. 8:1059-1072; 1981.
32. Lovely, R.G.; Gregor, R.J.; Roy, R.R.; Edgerton, V.R. Effects of training on the recovery of full weight bearing stepping in the adult spinal cat. Exp. Neurol. 92:421-435; 1986.
33. Lovely, R.G.; Gregor, R.J.; Roy, R.R.; Edgerton, V.R. Weight-bearing hindlimb stepping in treadmill-exercised adult spinal cats. Brain Res. 514:206-218; 1990.
34. Lundberg, A. Multisensory control of spinal reflex pathways. In: Granit, R.; Pompeiano, O., eds. Reflex control of posture and movement. (Progress in brain research, vol. 50). Elsevier Science; 1979: 11-28.
35. Manni, E. Fenomeni di eccitamento il stricnico della corteccia cerebellari e loro persistenza dopo taglio del midollo spinale nel piccone. Boll. Soc. Ital. Biol. Sper. 25:440-442; 1949.
36. Mayford, M.; Barzilai, A.; Keller, F.; Schacher, S.; Kandel, E.R. Modulation of an NCAM-related adhesion molecule with long-term synaptic plasticity in *Aplysia*. Science. 256:638-644; 1992.
37. McDougal, D.B., Jr.; Pusateri, M.E.; Carter, J.G.; Krasnov, I.; Ilyina-Kakueva, E.; Manchester, J.; Lowry, O.H. The effect of microgravity and tail suspension on selected enzymes and amino acids of the hippocampus. J. Appl. Physiol. [In press].

38. Patterson, M.M. Mechanisms of classical conditioning and fixation in spinal mammals. In: Riesen, A.; Thompson, R., eds. Advances in psychobiology, vol. 3. New York: Wiley; 1976: 381-426.
39. Patterson, M.M. Mechanisms of classical conditioning of spinal reflexes. In: Thompson, R.F.; Hicks, L.; Shvrykov, V.B., eds. Neural mechanisms of goal-directed behavior and learning. New York: Academic Press; 1980: 263-272.
40. Perell, K.L.; Gregor, R.J.; Fowler, E.G.; Hodgson, J.A.; Roy, R.R. Kinetic and kinematic analysis of locomotor capabilities of posturally trained adult spinal cats. Soc. Neurosci. Abstr. 15:394; 1989.
41. Peterson, B.W.; Baker, J.F.; Houk, J.C. A model of adaptive control of vestibuloocular reflex based on properties of cross-axis adaptation. In: Wolpaw, J.R.; Schmidt, J.T.; Vaughan, T.M., eds. Activity-driven CNS changes in learning and development. New York: New York Academy of Sciences; 1991:319-337.
42. Polyakov, I.V.; Drobyshev, V.I.; Krasnov, I.B. Morphological changes in the spinal cord and intervertebral ganglia of rats exposed to different gravity levels. Physiologist. [Suppl. 1]. 34:S187-S188; 1991.
43. Rossignol, S.; Drew, T. Phasic modulation of reflexes during rhythmic activity. In: Grillner, S.; Forssberg, H.; Stein, P.S.; Stuart, D., eds. Neurobiology of vertebrate locomotion. London: Macmillan; 1986:517-534.
44. Roy, R.R.; Baldwin, K.M.; Edgerton, V.R. The plasticity of skeletal muscle: Effects of neuromuscular activity. In: Holloszy, J., ed. Exercise and sports sciences reviews, vol. 19. Baltimore: Williams & Wilkins; 1991:269-312.
45. Roy, R.R.; Gilliam, T.B.; Taylor, J.F.; Heusner, W.W. Activity-induced morphologic changes in rat soleus nerve. Exp. Neurol. 80:622-632; 1983.
46. Sherrington, C.S. Nervous rhythm arising from rivalry of antagonistic reflexes: Reflex stepping as outcome of double reciprocal innervation. Proc. R. Soc. Lond, Ser. B. 86:233-261; 1913.
47. Smith, J.L.; Edgerton, V.R.; Eldred, E.; Zernicke, R.F. The chronic spinalized cat: A model for neuromuscular plasticity. In: Haber, B.; Perez-Polo, J.R.; Hashim, G.A.; Giuffrida Stella, A.M., eds. Nervous system regeneration. New York: Alan R. Liss; 1983:357-373.
48. Smith, J.L.; Smith, L.A.; Zernicke, R.F.; Hoy, M. Locomotion in exercised and nonexercised cats cordotomized at two or twelve weeks of age. Exp. Neurol. 76:393-413; 1986.
49. Taub, E. Motor behavior following deafferentation in the developing and motorically mature monkey. In: Herman, R.M.; Grillner, S.; Stein, P.S.G.; Stuart, D.G., eds. Neural control of locomotion. New York: Plenum Press; 1976:675-705.
50. Teasdall, R.D.; Villablanca, J.; Magladery, J.W. Reflex responses to muscle stretch in cats with chronic suprasegmental lesions. Bull. Johns Hopkins Hosp. 116:229-242; 1965.
51. Wolpaw, J.R.; Lee, C.L. Memory traces in primate spinal cord produced by operant conditioning of H-reflex. J. Neurophysiol. 61:563-572; 1989.
52. Wolpaw, J.R.; Lee, C.L.; Carp, J.S. Operantly conditioned plasticity in spinal cord. In: Wolpaw, J.R.; Schmidt, J.T.; Vaughan, T.M., eds. Activity-driven CNS changes in learning and development. New York: New York Academy of Sciences; 1991: 338-348.
53. Yeo, C.H. Cerebellum and classical conditioning of motor responses. In: Wolpaw, J.R.; Schmidt, J.T.; Vaughan, T.M., eds. Activity-driven CNS changes in learning and development. New York: New York Academy of Sciences; 1991:292-304.
54. Young, B.C.; Gregor, R.J.; Lovely, R.G.; Roy, R.R. Hindlimb stepping in nonexercised adult spinal cats. Soc. Neurosci. Abstr. 12:685; 1986.

Chapter 35

Exercise and Cognitive Function

Jerry R. Thomas
Daniel M. Landers
Walter Salazar
Jenny Etnier

Exercise has been proposed to produce many psychological benefits including increases in academic performance, assertiveness, confidence, emotional stability, independence, intellectual functioning, internal locus of control, mood, perception, popularity, self-control, sexual satisfaction, well-being, and work efficiency (22). In addition, exercise has been proposed to decrease absenteeism at work, alcohol abuse, anxiety, depression, dysmenorrhea, headaches, hostility, phobias, tension, and work errors (22). Whether exercise directly influences any or all of these characteristics is difficult to determine because so many of the hypothesized benefits simply reflect associations between variables when people who exercise to some extent are compared with people who exercise to a lesser extent.

The purpose of this paper is to focus on whether cognitive function benefits from exercise (defined very broadly to mean physical activity). First, we use a more narrow definition of exercise to evaluate whether moderate to high levels of physical activity (either chronic or acute) improve cognitive function, particularly intelligence. Second, we will take a broader view of exercise that includes engaging in various types of movements (e.g., perceptual-motor training programs) to enhance cognitive function (e.g., academic performance and intelligence). Reviewing this literature is not a novel undertaking as we can identify at least 16 previous reviews that have included the influence of exercise on cognitive function as a section of the overall topic (3,12,13, 18,22,27,30,38,40,41,43,45,47,50,51,52).

Do Moderate to Intense Levels of Exercise Improve Cognitive Function?

Two major (and follow-up) questions are addressed here:

1. Does either (or both) chronic or acute exercise influence cognitive function? If chronic or acute exercise (or both) increases cognitive function, is the effect temporary (only during or just after exercise) or persistent? Given that cognitive function is a multifaceted phenomenon, what aspects of it might exercise improve?
2. Does exercise only affect the processes underlying cognitive function (e.g., allocation of attention)? If so, might effortful rather than automatic processes be influenced? Furthermore, might exercise only have a delaying effect (e.g., prevent the age-related erosion of effortful processing skills) in the elderly?

Before beginning this discussion, we must make clear that nearly all of the data reflect associations from cross-sectional studies between subjects who exercise or those who do not and higher/lower levels of cognitive performance. There are few (if any) good longitudinal studies where experimental groups exercise for reasonable training periods, where controls are used, and where dependent measures reflect the multifaceted aspects of cognitive function.

Does Either (or Both) Chronic or Acute Exercise Influence Cognitive Function?

Findings have been mixed with regard to the influence of exercise (including level of physical fitness) on aspects of cognitive function: Positive benefits have been reported for working memory (e.g., 10,35); mixed findings, both positive and no effects, have occurred for fluid intelligence (e.g., 10,11) and abstract reasoning (e.g., 5,37); and no effects have been reported for crystallized intelligence (e.g., 11). As a result of these mixed findings, Landers and Salazar (31; for a more complete report see 32) have reported an unpublished meta-analysis evaluating the influence of exercise on cognitive function based on over 100 studies yielding just under 700 effect sizes. They divide their overall results by the type of cognitive measure that has been related to exercise. Table 35.1 shows the numbers of cases by the cognitive outcome variables, effect sizes (M) (positive effect size means the physical activity group scores higher than comparison or pretest), standard deviations (SD), and 95% confidence intervals.

Generally the effect sizes are small (0.0 to 0.48) and the standard deviations are large (0.35 to 1.37). In fact the standard deviation for every effect size is larger than the effect size. However, the 95% confidence intervals do not include 0, suggesting reliable effects, for reaction time, math, and acuity. The largest effect size is for math (0.48) but math also has the largest standard deviation (1.37), a value nearly three times as large as the effect size. Landers, Salazar, and Etnier (32) also code a number of study characteristics and relate them to the effect sizes. Table 35.2 includes the coded characteristics and their effect sizes that were significant. Coded characteristics unrelated to effect sizes include (a) whether or not the study was published, (b) number of threats to internal validity, (c) mental level of subjects, (d) length of the acute exercise bout, (e) number of weeks of chronic training, (f) intensity of the exercise, (g) whether or not the supervisor was present during exercise, and (h) whether or not a training effect was found.

When evaluating the combined estimates of cognitive function and comparing them to various coded characteristics, several features emerge:

1. Effects are smaller with male than with female subjects.
2. With acute exercise, one session of exercise produces larger effects than multiple sessions of exercise.
3. Chronic exercise (i.e., a training program) results in larger effects than does acute exercise.

Taken together, these findings suggest that only certain types of cognitive function may be related to exercise—reaction time, math performance, and acuity. If exercise actually influences cognitive function (difficult to determine from mostly cross-sectional designs), the effects are more likely to be observed in female subjects engaging in a chronic exercise program. One session of acute exercise is needed to produce larger effect sizes.

Related but unanswered questions remain. For example, are the effects on cognitive function persistent and related to the level of training? What happens if subjects who show increases in cognitive function associated with physical activity training stop training? Does cognitive function regress, and if so, how far? If we accept that physical activity training does result in a low to moderate increase in cognitive function, is this a threshold or continuous effect? None of these questions have been addressed, probably because the area is somewhat controversial, and the findings have been rather mixed. Even the reliable influences demonstrated by the Landers, Salazar, and Etnier meta-analysis are small and variability is great.

Does Exercise Affect Only the Processes Underlying Intelligence?

Chodzko-Zajko (3) suggested that rather than affecting intellectual functioning directly, chronic

Table 35.1 Effect Sizes for the Relation of Exercise to Various Measures of Cognitive Function

Cognitive measure	Number of cases (*N*)	Effect size (*M*)	Standard deviation (*SD*)	95% confidence interval
Math	28	0.48*	1.37	±0.31
Acuity	59	0.36*	0.47	±0.14
Reaction time	200	0.15*	0.58	±0.04
Short-term/working memory	20	0.36	0.80	±0.47
Fluid intelligence	31	0.27	0.76	±0.27
WAIS digit span	42	0.19	0.36	±0.20
Learning	38	0.00	1.00	±0.06
Crystallized intelligence	6	–0.09	0.36	±3.29

Note. * = reliable effect because 95% confidence interval does not include 0. WAIS = Weehsler Adult Intelligence Scale.

Table 35.2 Coded Variables That Are Significantly Related to Effect Size

Moderator variable	Number of cases (*N*)	Effect size (*M*)	Standard deviation (*SD*)
Subject assignment			
Single group	127	0.16	0.96
Intact groups	221	0.41	0.63
Matching	49	0.47	0.61
Random stratified	14	0.15	0.30
Random	157	0.15	0.49
Equivalent comparison groups			
Not reported	163	0.22	0.59
Yes	438	0.20	0.68
No	98	0.62	0.81
Equivalency determined by			
Not reported	220	0.31	0.72
Pretest	76	0.46	0.67
Random	148	0.11	0.45
Other	255	0.25	0.77
Age groups			
Not reported	54	0.02	0.64
Under 16 years	104	0.45	0.53
17–30 years	336	0.22	0.81
Older than 30 years	205	0.31	0.54
Gender			
Not reported	80	0.35	0.84
Male	407	0.15	0.68
Female	30	0.47	0.59
Mixed	182	0.44	0.62
Measures of physical fitness			
Not reported	347	0.31	0.82
Self-Report	27	0.57	0.39
Submax test	124	0.31	0.62
Max test	201	0.12	0.46
Paradigm used			
Acute	328	0.16	0.74
Training	264	0.32	0.61
Mixed	48	0.07	0.36
Other (athlete vs. nonathlete)	59	0.75	0.76
Type of physical activity			
Not reported	49	0.67	0.93
Cardiovascular (run, bike, etc.)	374	0.21	0.63
Muscular resistance	105	−0.05	0.61
Other	171	0.46	0.70
Type environment for study			
Not reported	30	0.38	0.59
Field	342	0.36	0.63
Laboratory	327	0.16	0.75
Type design			
Between subjects	250	0.32	0.65
Within subjects	409	0.21	0.71
Mixed	40	0.53	0.73
Time cognitive test administered			
Not reported	3	0.25	0.12
Pre- and post	334	0.30	0.56
Pre-during-post	64	−0.01	0.65
Post only	157	0.41	0.87
Other	141	0.15	0.75

exercise might allow the effortful aspect of cognitive processing to occur more efficiently, particularly in elderly subjects. In a review of the literature on cognitive processing, Hasher and Zacks (20) hypothesized that effortful and automatic memory processes should respond differently to stressors or interference. Automatic processes require only that an event be attended to, then processing (a) occurs with little or no additional attention or effort, (b) functions at optimal levels, (c) is not influenced by training and rehearsal, (d) happens without awareness, and (e) does not influence other cognitive processing. Examples of automatic processes include encoding of frequency information and spatial location. Automatic encoding is not influenced by intention, age, arousal, stress, or simultaneous processing (21).

In contrast, effortful processing (a) requires continued attention, (b) responds to training, (c) is influenced by strategy use and imagery, and (d) requires considerable memory capacity (21). If memory capacity is limited (see 24), then effortful processes require some portion of that capacity while automatic processes do not. Because memory performance is typically shown to decrease with aging (see 7,25), Hasher and Zacks (20,21) believe that this decreased performance only reflects effortful, not automatic, processing.

Chodzko-Zajko (3) suggested that if this viewpoint was applied to the influence of exercise on cognitive functioning, data might be better explained. For example, in a conference paper Chodzko-Zajko, Schuler, Solomon, Heinl, and Ellis (4) reported that physical fitness influenced memory performance in older subjects when the memory tasks required effort, but not when the tasks were more automatic. Chodzko-Zajko (3) suggested in a review paper that Spirduso's (43) reaction-time data fit this hypothesis in that more fit elderly subjects, when compared to less fit elderly subjects, have faster choice reaction time (effortful processing). However, he says differences in simple reaction time (closer to automatic processing) were less between fit and unfit older subjects.

A close look at the findings reported by Spirduso (43) do not support Chodzko-Zajko's interpretation. Figure 35.1 is a replot of data from both studies (42,44). As can be observed, none of these interactions are significant. If an interpretation has to be made, the findings from the 1975 paper are exactly opposite of Chodzko-Zajko's interpretation—the difference in the elderly by fitness level is greater in simple reaction time (more automatic task) than in discrimination reaction time (more effortful task). The 1978 paper shows absolutely parallel lines in simple and choice reaction times for the elderly active and inactive subjects. The only reliable effects present in either study are that young subjects have faster reaction times (simple, discrimination, and choice) than old subjects and that active subjects have faster reaction times (simple, discrimination, and choice) than inactive subjects.

The only cross-sectional data remaining to support the application of the Hasher and Zacks model to exercise and cognitive function is a reported but unpublished study by Chodzko-Zajko, Schuler, Solomon, Heinl, and Ellis (4). Chodzko-Zajko (3) says that the "relationship between physical fitness and memory function in old age was found to be task dependent to the extent that the prophylactic effects of fitness on effortfully encoded memory were not found to extend to memory tasks requiring less effortful processing" (p. 870). Given Chodzko-Zajko's previous misinterpretation of Spirduso (43), no presentation of data to support this statement, and the failure to publish the report on which it is based, there seems to be little direct evidence to support the Hasher and Zacks (20) model with regard to exercise preventing the deteriorating effects of aging on effortful, but not automatic, processing.

However, that does not mean that exercise may not deter the negative effects of aging on cognitive function (in fact the Landers, Salazar, and Etnier 1992 meta-analysis suggests that the greatest benefits may be in older and younger subjects). Only the deterring effects may not be differential along the effortful/automatic continuum. In fact, Spirduso's (43) data show that older fit subjects have simple, discrimination, and choice reaction times faster than unfit older subjects and as fast as unfit younger subjects. Stones and Kozma (47) report similar findings. All of these data are from cross-sectional studies contrasting fit and unfit subjects.

Many alternative hypotheses are available to explain these results. For example, fit older subjects may engage (over their lifetime) in more activities requiring quick responses, thus having faster reaction times due to greater numbers of experiences in situations requiring quick responses. Thus, faster reaction times may only reflect more practice, not greater physical fitness. This same explanation is sometimes invoked to explain faster reactions in boys than girls (see 49).

Only a few training studies have been done to evaluate the hypothesis that chronic exercise improves cognitive function in older subjects and the results are mixed. Powell (39) found positive effects of exercise (12 weeks of training) on intellect for one of two measures of memory performance. Dustman et al. (10) also found positive effects of exercise training (4 months) on several psychoneurological tasks. However, Madden, Blumenthal,

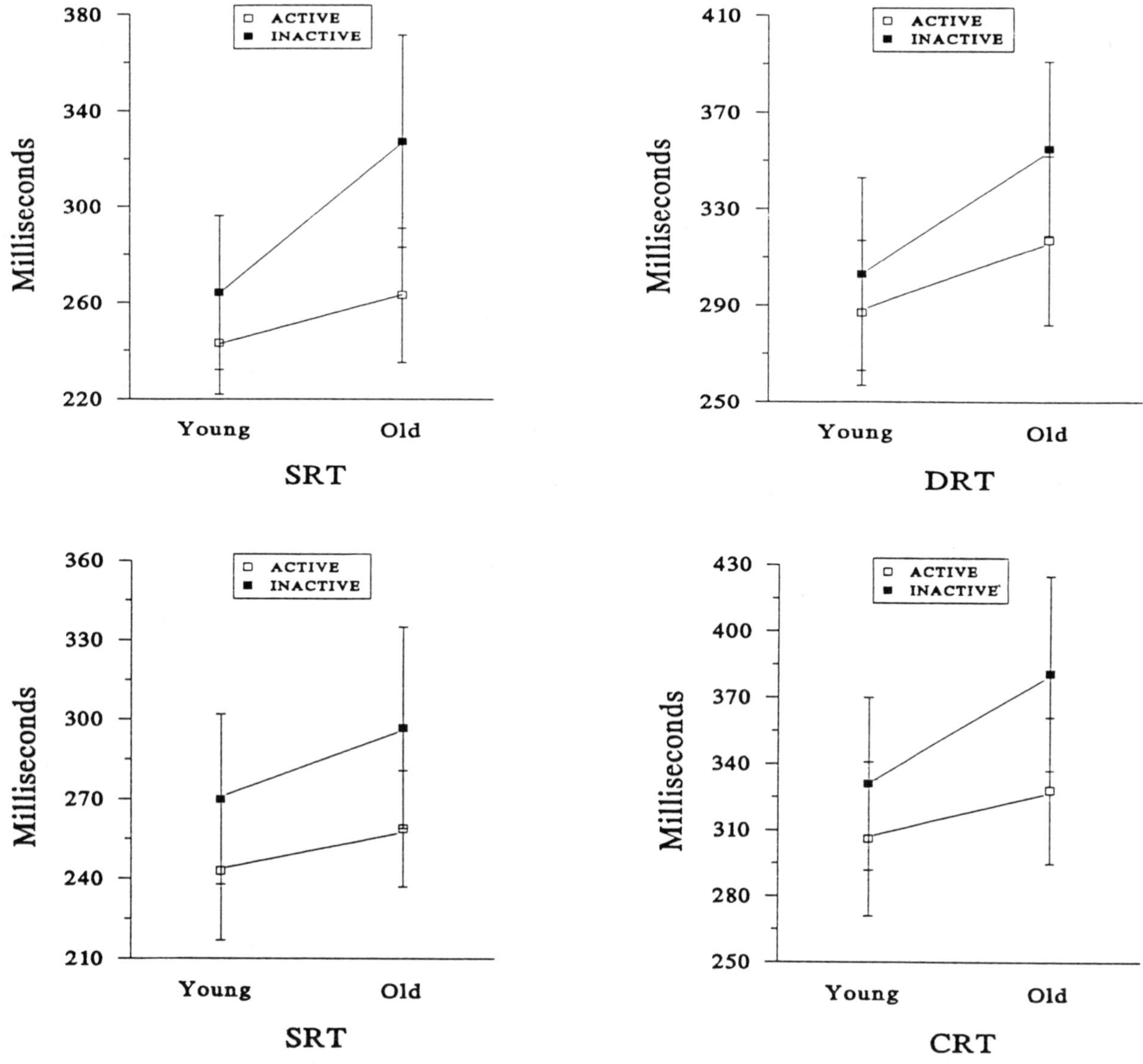

Figure 35.1 Simple and discriminant reaction time by age and activity level (top of figure redrawn from Spirduso [42]); simple and choice reaction time by age and activity level (bottom of Figure redrawn from Spirduso and Clifford [44]).

Allen, and Emery (34) did not find any effects on cognition for 4 months of exercise training, nor did Stamford, Hambacher, and Fallica (46) find exercise effects on memory function (12 weeks of training).

Critical features in exercise studies revolve around issues like, Is it increased physical activity that promotes better cognitive function, or does some threshold of physical fitness have to be reached? The answer to that question is unclear. Dustman et al. (10) reported a 27% change in aerobic capacity and found benefits for cognitive function. Madden et al. (34) reported only an 11% change in aerobic capacity and found no effects. However, the level of exercise intensity was not great in either the Powell (39) (walking) or Stamford et al. (46) (walking) studies, and the outcomes on cognitive function are mixed.

What can be concluded from these data on exercise and cognitive function?

1. The benefits of chronic exercise on cognitive function are small but probably reliable (although variable) for certain tasks—reaction time, math performance, and acuity.
2. Acute exercise bouts have minimal influence on cognitive function.
3. Regular exercise may enhance cognitive function in preadult subjects and may reduce loss of cognitive function in subjects

over 31 years of age, particularly females. This has the potential for the greatest benefit.

4. There is little good longitudinal data (particularly training studies) on any age group, especially children.

Several well-controlled training studies using various age levels (children and adolescents, young and middle-aged adults, and the elderly) need to be conducted to resolve a variety of issues: How large is the effect of exercise on cognitive function? What types of cognitive processing benefit from regular exercise? Are the effects disproportionately greater in the young and elderly? Is the critical issue regular physical activity or specific increases or levels of physical fitness? Do the effects of exercise on cognitive function regress with detraining?

Does Engagement in Movement Performance Enhance Cognitive Function?

Perceptual-motor training has generally focused on children, particularly children with some sort of learning difficulty. Training for these children has generally taken one of three approaches (50, p. 445):

1. Programs that, by training some motor parameter, attempt to improve a specific curriculum area (e.g., by practicing balance the child will read more proficiently)
2. Programs that, by practicing an underlying motor skill(s) related to some specific academic area, attempt to influence the academic area (e.g., practicing fine eye-hand coordination in an attempt to improve handwriting)
3. Programs that use motor tasks to teach academic content (e.g., throwing a ball into a numbered barrel representing the correct answer for an addition problem)

Can Perceptual-Motor Training Improve Cognitive Performance?

Interest in enhancing cognitive function through motor activity is a popular intervention technique, especially for children with learning and intellectual problems (19). Much of the interest in this area has been generated by clinical observations that children with learning problems frequently have motor problems too. Available evidence has shown that associations between varying levels of cognitive or academic performance and motor (often labeled *perceptual-motor*) performance are moderate to high, especially in young children (see 23,48).

However, the relevant question is, Does enhancing motor performance (by training) improve cognitive performance? Many perceptual-motor training programs have been developed (at least 12; e.g., see 1,2,8,9,15,16,29) as well as versions and combinations of these programs. Numerous reviews of these programs have been presented (23 reviews located; e.g., see 6,14,17,28,30,41,50).

Kavale and Mattson (27) have made the most comprehensive and quantitative review yet in which they do a meta-analysis of all the experimental studies where perceptual-motor training has been used to influence intellectual or academic functioning. The only criteria that resulted in a study being automatically excluded was lack of a control group. Kavale and Mattson identified 180 studies meeting their criteria and these studies yielded 637 effect sizes based on a total *N* of 13,000. The average positive effect on all measures of cognitive function for the perceptual-motor training was an effect size of 0.08 (SD = 0.27).

This effect was based on an average of 19 weeks of training for 65 hr of intervention in groups with a 3:1 student to teacher ratio. An effect size this small means very little was gained across periods of training. As a comparison 9 months of reading instruction yields an effect size of about 0.67 (27); decreasing the student teacher ratio from 30:1 to 15:1 results in an effect size gain of 0.15 in achievement, and psycholinguistic training produces a 0.39 effect size change (26). Thus it seems reasonable to conclude that perceptual-motor training has no effect on cognitive function.

Additionally, perceptual-motor training produces no benefits for any of the subcomponents of academic achievement (readiness, reading, arithmetic, language, spelling, or handwriting) or cognitive aptitude (verbal IQ or performance IQ). The lack of effects do not vary by age of the subject (preschool, kindergarten, primary grades, middle grades, junior high school, or high school), subject groupings (normal, educable mentally retarded, trainable mentally retarded, slow learner, culturally disadvantaged, learning disabled, reading disabled, or motor disabled), nor by type of program used in the training (Barsch, Cratty, Delacato, Frostig, Getman, Kephart, combination, or other). The title selected for this paper by Kavale and Mattson (27), "One jumped off the balance beam: . . . " (p. 165, a play on the book and movie, *One Flew Over the Cuckoo's Nest*) indicates the action we should take with regard to these types of programs—we should "jump off" this silly and useless concept.

In fact, Myers and Hammill (36) suggest perceptual-motor programs may be harmful: " . . . they may waste valuable time and money, and they may provide a child with a placebo program when his problems require a real remedial effort" (p. 385). We do not mean to imply that cognition is not important in physical activity—quite the contrary. Clearly, cognitive processing is important in the planning, selection, decisions, knowledge base, and feedback about movement. However, the rule of specificity of training applies: If you want to improve reading or math, practice reading or math, not movement.

Conclusions

Following are conclusions that seem reasonable from the data reported here:

1. The benefits of chronic exercise on cognitive function are small but probably reliable for reaction time, math, and acuity, especially for older (over 30) and younger (under 16) female subjects.
2. Acute exercise bouts have a minimal influence on cognitive function.
3. Regular exercise *may* reduce loss of cognitive function in more elderly subjects.
4. There is little longitudinal data on which to base the cognitive benefits of exercise, especially for children.
5. Perceptual-motor training has no benefit for cognitive function regardless of the subject's age, cognitive ability, or type of perceptual-motor program used as a treatment.

Future Research

The area of greatest interest for future research is whether or not exercise results in benefits for cognitive function. In particular, training studies are needed to identify the following:

1. Is the cognitive benefit of exercise a threshold effect (e.g., some minimal level of physical activity that promotes increased mental functioning) or a continuous effect (more exercise produces greater increases in cognitive function)?
2. Are cognitive benefits of exercise general in nature or specific to certain types of cognitive activity?
3. Is exercise a particularly useful treatment for delaying aging effects on cognitive processing?
4. Do the benefits of exercise on cognitive functioning only continue as long as a program of regular exercise is maintained?
5. Do children show cognitive benefits from regular exercise?
6. Are there really male–female differences in cognitive function as a response to exercise?

We believe there are few good research questions to be asked on the influence of perceptual-motor programs on cognitive function. We would do much better to focus our efforts on topics like the benefits of exercise for physiological and psychological factors and their interaction, and how skilled movements are acquired and controlled.

References

1. Ayres, A.J. Sensory integrative processes and neuropsychological learning disabilities. In: Hellmuth, J., ed. Learning disorders (vol. 3). Seattle: Special Child Publications; 1968.
2. Barsh, R.H. A movigenic curriculum (bulletin no. 25). Madison, WI: Department of Public Instruction, Bureau of the Handicapped; 1965.
3. Chodzko-Zajko, W.J. Physical fitness, cognitive performance, and aging. Med. Sci. Sports Exerc. 23:868-872; 1991.
4. Chodzko-Zajko, W.J.; Schuler, P.B.; Solomon, J.S.; Heinl, B.; Ellis, N. Physical fitness levels and cognitive performance in aging. Paper presented at the 1990 Gatlinburg conference on mental retardation. Brainerd, MN: 1990, April.
5. Clarkson-Smith, L.; Hartley, A.A. Relationship between physical exercise and cognitive performance in aging. Psychol. Aging. 4:183-189; 1989.
6. Cohen, H.J., Birch, H.G.; Taft, L.T. Some considerations for evaluating the Doman-Delacato "patterning method." Pediatrics. 45:302-314; 1970.
7. Craik, F.I.M. Age differences in human memory. In: Birren, J.J., Schaie, K.W., eds. The handbook of the psychology of aging. New York: Van Nostrand Reinhold; 1977:384-420.
8. Cratty, B. Perceptual-motor behavior and educational processes. Englewood Cliffs, NJ: Prentice Hall; 1969.
9. Delacato, C.H. The treatment and prevention of reading problems: The neurological approach. Springfield, IL: Charles C Thomas; 1959.
10. Dustman, R.E.; Ruhling, R.O.; Russel, E.M.; Shearer, D.; Bonekat, H.; Shigeoka, J.; Wood, J.; Bradford, D. Aerobic exercise training and improved neuropsychological function

of older individuals. Neurobiol. Aging. 5:35-42; 1984.

11. Elsayed, M.; Ismail, A.H.; Young, R.J. Intellectual differences in adult men related to age and physical fitness before and after an exercise program. J. Gerontol. 35:383-387; 1980.
12. Falkenberg, L.E. Employee fitness programs: Their impact on the employee and the organization. Acad. Managem. Rev. 12:511-522; 1987.
13. Folkins, C.H.; Sime, W.E. Physical fitness training and mental health. Am. Psychol. 36:373-389; 1981.
14. Footlik, S.W. Perceptual-motor training and cognitive achievement: A survey of the literature. J. Learn. Disabil. 3:40-49; 1971.
15. Frostig, M. A treatment program for children with learning difficulties. In: Bortner, M., ed. Evaluation and education of children with brain damage. Springfield, IL: Charles C Thomas; 1968.
16. Getman, G. How to develop your child's intelligence. Luverne, MN: Getman, G.; 1962.
17. Glass, G.V.; Robbins, M.P. A critique of experiments on the role of neurological organization in reading performance. Read. Res. Q. 3:5-51; 1967.
18. Gutin, B. Exercise-induced activation and human performance: A review. Res. Q. 44:256-268; 1973.
19. Hallahan, D.P.; Cruickshank, W.M. Psycho-educational foundations of learning disabilities. Englewood Cliffs, NJ: Prentice Hall; 1973.
20. Hasher, L.; Zacks, R.T. Automatic and effortful processes in memory. J. Exp. Psychol. [Gen.]. 108:356-388; 1979.
21. Hasher, L.; Zacks, R.T. Automatic processing of fundamental information. Am. Psychol. 39: 1372-1388; 1984.
22. Hughes, J.R. Psychological effects of habitual aerobic exercise: A critical review. Prev. Med. 13:66-78; 1984.
23. Ismail, A.H.; Kane, J.; Kirkendall, D.R. Relationships among intellectual and non-intellectual variables. Res. Q. 40:83-92; 1969.
24. Kahneman, D. Attention and effort. Englewood Cliffs, NJ: Prentice Hall; 1973.
25. Kausler, D.H. Experimental psychology and human aging. New York: Wiley; 1982.
26. Kavale, K. The efficacy of stimulant drug treatment for hyperactivity: A meta-analysis. J. Learn. Disabil. 15:280-289; 1981.
27. Kavale, K.; Mattson, P.D. "One jumped off the balance beam": Meta-analysis of perceptual-motor training. J. Learn. Disabil. 16:165-173; 1983.
28. Keogh, B. Optometric vision training programs for children with learning disabilities: Review of issues and research. J. Learn. Disabil. 7:219-232; 1974.
29. Kephart, N.C. The slow learner in the classroom. Columbus, OH: Charles E. Merrill; 1960.
30. Kirkendall, D.E. Effects of physical activity on intellectual development and academic performance. In: Stull, G.A.; Eckert, H., eds. The academy papers: Effects of physical activity on children. Champaign, IL: Human Kinetics; 1986:49-63.
31. Landers, D.M.; Salazar, W., Effects of exercise on cognitive functioning: A meta-analysis. Paper presented at North American society for psychology of sport and physical activity; 1991; Asilomar, CA; NASPSPA; 1991.
32. Landers, D.M.; Salazar, W.; Etnier, J. Effects of exercise on cognitive function: A meta-analysis. Tempe: Arizona State University; 1993. Unpublished paper.
33. Lehsten, N.G. A study of selected growth and development measures and their relationships to achievement of boys in grades 7-12. Paper presented at AAHPER convention; 1964; Washington, DC; AAHPER; 1964.
34. Madden, D.J.; Blumenthal, J.A.; Allen, P.A.; Emery, C.F. Improving aerobic capacity in healthy older adults does not necessarily lead to improved cognitive performance. Psychol. Aging. 4:307-320; 1989.
35. Milligan, W.L.; Powell, D.A.; Herley, C.; Furchtgott, E. A comparison of physical health and psychosocial variables as predictors of reaction time and serial learning performance in elderly men. J. Gerontol. 39:704-710; 1984.
36. Myers, P.I.; Hammill, D.D. Methods for learning disorders. 2nd ed. New York: Wiley; 1976.
37. Offenbach, S.L.; Chodzko-Zajko, W.J.; Ringel, R.L. The relationship between physiological status, cognition, and age in adult men. Bull. Psychonom. Soc. 28:112-114; 1990.
38. Plante, T.G.; Rodin, J. Physical fitness and enhanced psychological health. Current Psychology: Research & Reviews 9:3-24; 1990.
39. Powell, E. Psychological effects of exercise therapy upon institutionalized geriatric mental patients. J. Gerontol. 29:157-161; 1974.
40. Powell, R.R. Effects of exercise on mental functioning. J. Sports Med. 15:125-131; 1975.
41. Rarick, G.L. Cognitive-motor relationships in the growing years. Res. Q. Exerc. Sport. 51:174-192; 1980.
42. Spirduso, W.W. Reaction and movement time as a function of age and physical activity level. J. Gerontol. 30:435-440; 1975.
43. Spirduso, W.W. Physical fitness, aging, and psychomotor speed: A review. J. Gerontol. 35:850-865; 1980.

44. Spirduso, W.W.; Clifford, P. Neuromuscular speed and consistency of performance as a function of age, physical activity level and type of physical activity. J. Gerontol. 33:26-30; 1978.
45. Spirduso, W.W.; MacRae, P.G. Motor performance and aging. In: Birren, J.E.; Schaie, K.W., eds. The handbook of the psychology of aging: Third edition. San Diego: Academic Press; 1990.
46. Stamford, B.A.; Hambacher, W.; Fallica, A. Effects of daily physical exercise on the psychiatric state of institutionalized geriatric mental patients. Res. Q. 45:35-41; 1974.
47. Stones, M.J.; Kozma, A. Physical activity, age, and cognitive/motor performance. In: Howe, M.L.; Brainerd, C.J., eds. Cognitive development in adulthood: Progress in cognitive development research. New York: Springer-Verlag; 1988:273-321.
48. Thomas, J.R; Chissom, B.S. Relationships as assessed by canonical correlation between perceptual-motor and intellectual abilities for preschool and early elementary age children. J. Mot. Behav. 4:23-29; 1972.
49. Thomas, J.R.; Gallagher, J.D.; Purvis, G.J. Reaction time and anticipation time: Effects of development. Res. Q. Exerc. Sport. 52:359-367; 1981.
50. Thomas, J.R.; Thomas, K.T. The relation of movement and cognitive function. In: Seefeldt, V., ed. Physical activity & well-being. Reston, VA:AAHPERD; 1986:443-452.
51. Tomporowski, P.D.; Ellis, N.R. Effects of exercise on cognitive processes: A review. Psychol. Bull. 99:338-346; 1986.
52. Weingarten, G. Mental performance during physical exertion: The benefit of being physically fit. Int. J. Sport Psychol. 4:16-26; 1973.

Chapter 36

Physical Activity and Other Lifestyle Behaviors

Leonard M. Wankel
Judy M. Sefton

Lifestyle refers to the patterns of behavior that a person adopts from those available in the context of his or her life circumstances. It is a way of living characterized by discernible patterns of behavior that reflect personal attitudes and preferences, an aspect of personal choice. These choices are not boundless, however, but are constrained or influenced by a number of factors. Biological influences (e.g., metabolism, physique), environmental influences (e.g., economic, geographical, climatic conditions), and social influences (e.g., general social norms, influence of significant others, and the level of social support) all help shape lifestyle choices.

Social policies influence the standard of living and basic social conditions (income and educational levels, place of dwelling, and job opportunities) that affect the availability of behavioral options directly, as well as indirectly through effects on other variables (e.g., norms, social support, attitudes). In addition, over time much lifestyle behavior develops a highly learned routine or habitual mode, which is not subject to ongoing conscious decision-making. Hence, lifestyle is a complex concept reflecting a composite of personal and environmental influences. It has meaning in a discernible behavior profile but at the same time it must be recognized that such patterns may be the result of quite different influences.

A "healthy lifestyle" refers to a particular type of lifestyle. It is exemplified when an individual, within the context of his or her individual biological limitations and particular physical and social environment, lives a life that reflects a pattern of ongoing healthy behavior. As with any lifestyle behavior, these health-related behaviors are subject to powerful environmental and social influences. Personal choice and responsibility are important aspects of leading a healthy lifestyle but they occur within a physical and social environment with powerful facilitating and inhibiting influences.

The International Consensus on Physical Activity, Fitness and Health (ICPAFH) basic model includes lifestyle as one of a group of factors that impacts on the interrelationship of physical activity, health-related fitness, and health. The basic model depicts lifestyle as a factor that affects each of the three components directly as well as indirectly through their reciprocal influences. In actuality, with respect to lifestyle the model is more complex than that depicted in Figure 3.1 on page 78 of this book. Each of the directional arrows relating lifestyle to the three basic concepts in the model should be reciprocal. That is, whereas lifestyle behaviors such as diet and smoking may affect physical activity, fitness, and health these three factors in turn may influence lifestyle behaviors.

This chapter focuses on one segment of this proposed reciprocal influence system—the relationship of physical activity involvement to other lifestyle behaviors. This subject differs from many others in this volume in that it addresses the indirect health effects of physical activity. It is proposed that in addition to the direct effects of physical activity on health-related fitness (and in turn health as specified in the direct causal arrows of Figure 3.1) and effects addressed in chapters 17 through 35 of this volume, physical activity involvement may influence other lifestyle behaviors that in turn have been shown to affect fitness and health. As noted by Blair, Jacobs, and Powell (8), "If these indirect effects can be demonstrated, the relationships are of importance not only to epidemiologic research, but also to health education and health promotion programs" (p. 172).

One other aspect of the portrayed ICPAFH model warrants brief mention. Whereas physical activity is included as one of the three central concepts in the model and lifestyle behaviors are depicted as one of a number of distinct influences impacting these variables, in reality level of physical activity involvement is one of the component behaviors of an individual's lifestyle. Thus, in

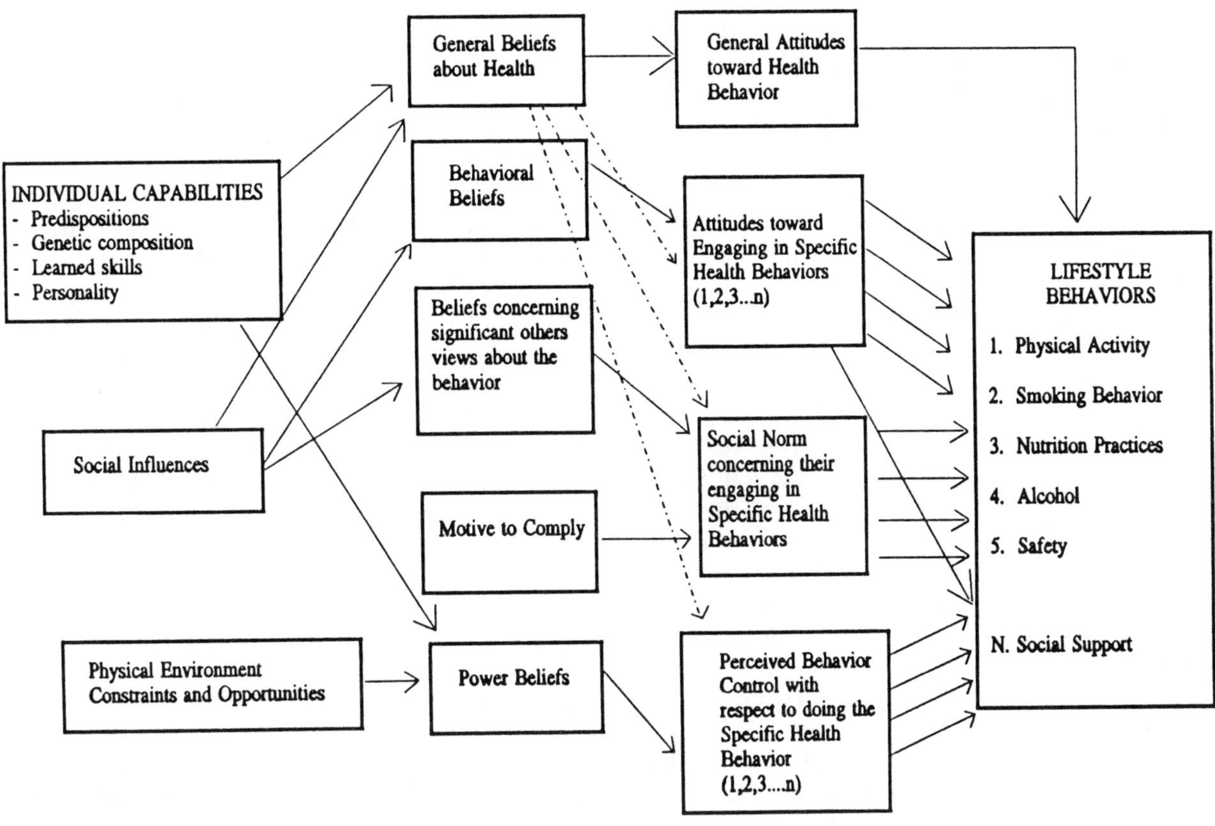

Figure 36.1 An adaptation of the theory of planned behavior to illustrate how an attitude–behavior model might apply to the relationship of physical activity involvement to other lifestyle behaviors.

considering the relationship of regular physical activity to fitness and health, one particular lifestyle behavior is being singled out for attention. The relationship is therefore not of physical activity to lifestyle behaviors but rather physical activity, one lifestyle behavior, to other lifestyle behaviors.

In this chapter, physical activity essentially refers to leisure-time physical activity. Although some lifestyle behavior researchers have utilized physical fitness as an indirect indication of physical activity, that research is given little attention here because performance of physical fitness tests is strongly influenced by factors other than physical activity. Furthermore, because level of occupational physical activity is highly correlated with socioeconomic status, which in turn has a significant influence on health status, little emphasis is placed on this type of physical activity. Although leisure-time physical activity is also influenced by socioeconomic status, this relationship is not uniformly high, and in contrast to occupational physical activity, leisure-time physical activity is largely under volitional control. Hence, leisure-time physical activity is considered the best indicator of physical activity as a health-related lifestyle behavior.

Other health-related lifestyle behaviors included in this chapter are: smoking, diet (in terms of both caloric intake and composition), alcohol intake, and miscellaneous preventive or protective health behaviors. A number of factors included in the Blair, Kohl, and Brill (9) review of physical activity and other health behaviors have not been included in this chapter. Weight control, stress management, sleep patterns, and work output are not included. Consistent with the view of Stephens (60) in the context of the ICPAFH model these additional factors are considered health outcomes rather than health behaviors. Substance abuse and intellectual function have not been included as they are given separate attention in chapters 61 and 35, respectively. Finally, social relationships have not been included due to a lack of research evidence establishing them as an important aspect of health-related behavior.

Methods

The following general procedures were followed in assembling and interpreting the available information. First, searches of the pertinent literature published since 1984 were conducted utilizing the MEDLINE, PSYCH ABSTRACTS, SPORTDISC, Social Science Citation Index, and the Science Citation Index. Both general (e.g., lifestyle behaviors) and specific behaviors (e.g., caloric intake, dietary composition, smoking, alcohol intake) were cross-referenced with physical activity and exercise in the searches. Pertinent articles located by the current searches together with articles referenced in earlier comprehensive reviews using similar methods (8,9,55,60) or in specific articles were reviewed.

After identifying and accessing the pertinent studies the following procedures were used in categorizing and assessing the information. First, the minimal condition for inclusion was that the study had to include a clear definition of how physical activity or exercise and the other relevant lifestyle behavior(s) were operationalized in the study. Beyond this an attempt was made to evaluate the validity, reliability, and generalizability of each study and to use this information in drawing conclusions concerning the research. Although emphasis was placed on the replication of results across studies employing strong research designs, in many cases the quantity and quality of research available dictated that a more flexible and subjective process be employed.

Review of the Evidence for the Relationship of Physical Activity to Other Health-Related Lifestyle Behaviors

Physical Activity Involvement and Smoking

Studies providing evidence pertinent to the relationship of physical activity involvement to cigarette smoking may be grouped into four categories. First, the relationship has been investigated using simple dichotomous smoking status measures (i.e., smokers vs. nonsmokers) related to activity involvement level. Physical activity has been scaled in various ways (e.g., simple dichotomous scale: sedentary vs. active; ordinal category scale: sedentary, mildly active, moderately active, highly active).

Secondly, researchers have examined the relationship of physical activity involvement to cigarette consumption within populations of smokers. Typically smoking consumption is scaled on some index of cigarettes smoked per day. Physical activity may be scaled in various ways, as noted above, or on some type of equal-appearing interval scale (e.g., rated intensity or frequency of activity or energy cost of activity in a certain time). Thirdly, cross-sectional comparisons have been made between selected activity groups. Groups representing different levels of regular activity are compared for smoking status or amount of consumption. Some studies have gathered retrospective self-report data pertaining to changes in smoking and activity behaviors over time, whereas others have monitored activity and smoking levels of comparison groups over time. Finally, a limited number of field studies and experiments have examined physical activity as an intervention for influencing smoking behavior.

Cross-Sectional Studies

Earlier reviews (8,9,55) have noted that, although generally a small negative relation is found between level of involvement in leisure-time physical activity and smoking behavior, there are also a number of studies that report no significant relationship. Those observations are corroborated by the results of more recent research (see Table 36.1).

With respect to large-scale population surveys, although a number of earlier studies reported no difference (17,45,48), this may be due in part to measurement problems. In particular, the manner of assessing physical activity involvement is problematic in a number of studies. The criteria employed to categorize those who are active may markedly influence the results (61). Evidence for this influence is provided in the results of the Folsom et al. (18) study. Smoking behavior was found to be more highly related (negatively) to heavy physical activity involvement than to general physical activity involvement. Similarly, studies of the same population, but with walking (26) and vigorous exercise (52) respectively as the activity variables, resulted in different levels of association with smoking.

The type of activity is also important to the relationship. For example, in the Perrier study (45), it was noted that markedly different motives may underlie participation in different activities and these might be either positively or negatively related to health concerns. Shephard (55) comments that participation in exercise for health-related outcomes would be expected to be more highly related to other health-related behaviors than would participation in activity in general.

Finally, poor measurement characteristics of the research instruments might distort the results. In the majority of cases, instruments without established validity and reliability have been utilized to assess the various lifestyle behaviors. In

Table 36.1 Summary of Evidence for the Relationship of Physical Activity Involvement and Smoking

Study	Sample	Research design/controls	Measurement of physical activity	Measurement of smoking	Results
Kronefeld et al. (29)	N = 663 (220 M, 443 F) insurance company employees; higher education and economic level than general population	Cross-sectional	Index from reported LTPA participation	Cigarettes/day	M: $r = -.16$ F: $r = .04$, N.S.
Marti et al. (35)	N = 8,912 (4,337 M, 4,575 F in initial sample) eastern Finnish adults (aged 30–59 years)	Cross-sectional with replication over 10 years (1972–1982); log linear regression	LTPA: >3 hr/week <3 hr/week OPA: job description Overall activity: low-high	10-level status and amount scale	Smokers less active than nonsmokers at both times Difference increased across years but N.S.
Marti et al. (33) (a) army conscripts	N = 6,592 Swiss M (aged 19 years); random sample of army conscripts	Cross-sectional	6-point activity scale	Cigarettes/day × years of smoking	$r = -.23$
(b) 16-km runners	N = 4,358 of 6,620 participants in Bern, Switzerland 16-km race completed questionnaires	Cross sectional; multiple regression	Weekly kilometers of training	Smoking status and amount smoked	$r = -.10$ for smoking on 16-km running time
Salonen et al. (53)	N = 15,088 eastern Finnish adults (aged 30–59 years)	Cross-sectional; logistic modeling	LTPA: > 5 hr/week < 5 hr/week OPA: four categories	Cigarette consumption	Sedentary Ms and Fs had higher consumption than active Ms and Fs (35% and 36% respectively, $p < .001$)

(continued)

Table 36.1 *(Continued)*

Study	Sample	Research design/controls	Measurement of physical activity	Measurement of smoking	Results
Abel et al. (1)	*N* = 349 M employed by the state of Illinois; stratified sample on "occupational self-direction"	Cross-sectional	LTPA: 4-point scale	4-point status scale	$r = -.06$
Calnan (14)	*N* = 4,224; community survey in southern England	Cross-sectional; representative of adult population	7-point scale (regular daytime activity and sport)	Cigarette consumption	Spearman Rho = –.08 ($p < .001$)
Hovell et al. (26)	*N* = 1,080 (43.4%) response to questionnaire mailed to San Diego residents (Haines Directory)	Relatively inactive group (deleted those who exercise 20 min, 3 ×/week)	Walking	Cigarettes/day	N.S.
Marti et al. (35)	*N* = 636 southwestern Finnish adults (aged 45–64 years)	20-year follow-up	Overall PA based on dichotomous measures of LTPA and OPA at two points to establish four categories: *increasers, maintainers, quitters, sedentary*	Cigarette consumption	*Increasers* smoked less than *sedentary*
Marti & Vartianen (36)	*N* = 1,142 eastern Finnish adolescents (aged 15 years); random sample	Controlled for SES	3-point scale (frequency of exercising for 30 min or more)	Cigarettes/day	M: Spearman Rho = –.16 F: Spearman Rho = –.13
Sallis et al. (52)	*N* = 2,053 (43.4%) random sample of San Diego area; overrepresents affluent, well-educated Caucasians		Number of 20+ min activities/week	Cigarettes/day	$r = -.19$
Blair, Kohl & Brill (9) (a) Cross-sectional	*N* = 10,250 (7,961 M, 2,289 F) self-selected individuals tested at Cooper Clinic; higher education and SES than general population	Cross sectional ANCOVA adjusting for age (all measures transformed to natural log scale to remove skewness)	PA: 5-point scale of activity during past month	Cigarettes/week	Inverse relationship of PA and smoking for both M and F

(b) Longitudinal	*N* = 2,239 M who underwent at least six full medicals at Cooper Clinic	Longitudinal observations study; age × treatment group ANOVA (repeated measures across six time points); data transformation as in (a)	Four exercise exposure groups: *starters, continuers, intermittent, sedentary*	Cigarettes/week	N.S.—no time × treatment effect
Blaxter (10)	*N* = 9,003 (3,905 M, 5,098 F) adult (aged 18+ years) participants in Health and Lifestyle Survey in Great Britain (1984–1985)	Cross-sectional comprehensive study with many control variables (e.g., attitude, geography, SES, education, occupational status, health status); multiple discriminant analysis	Six levels LTPA: energy expenditure for activities in last 2 weeks	Six levels Smoking behavior (none through heavy cigarette use)	N.S. except for young and middle-aged M manual workers
Bofettaet al. (11)	*N* = 5,045 (3,381 M, 1,664 F) hospital-based population (mainly cancer and other chronic illnesses)	Correlation; three age strata	LTPA: dichotomous measure 3 times/week for 1 year	Smoking status	Runners and joggers tended to be nonsmokers
Craig et al. (16)	*N* = 4,000 Canadians (aged 7+ years)	Longitudinal study (initial assessment 1981, retest 1988)	Energy expenditure of 1.5 kcal/kg/day used to classify active vs. inactive in 1981 and 1988 and form four groups: *adherers, starters, lapsers, resisters*	Smoking status	Smoking and adherence inversely related
Reviki et al. (50)	1979 National Survey of Personal Health Practices and Consequences	Correlation	PA: exercise status (exercise, no exercise)	Smoking status (smoker, nonsmoker)	More nonexercisers than exercisers were smokers
Scanlon et al. (53a)	*N* = 36,357 Canadian military personnel	Correlation; stepwise logistic regression	Dichotomous variable: sweats three or more times a week	Dichotomous variable (smoker, nonsmoker)	Odds ratio 1.41 for nonsmokers vs. smokers being active
Summerson et al. (62)	*N* = 270 diabetic adults	ANOVA: activity level × age × sex	Dichotomous activity level (600 kcal/week)	Smoking status	N.S.

(continued)

Table 36.1 *(Continued)*

Study	Sample	Research design/controls	Measurement of physical activity	Measurement of smoking	Results
Intervention studies					
Hill (24)	N = 36 (10 M, 26 F) adults	Experimental study—subjects randomly assigned to control and experimental conditions. Smoking level recorded at initial test, posttest and 1-, 3-, and 6-month follow-up. Control: 2 ×/week smoking cessation counseling program, 5-week duration. Experimental: 2 ×/week combined counseling and aerobic exercise program, 5-week duration. Same instructor for both programs.	PA: recorded on weekly PA form	Cigarettes/day	N.S. treatment effect for both amount of smoking or for number of individuals who quit
Taylor et al. (63)	N = 203 M (mean age 52 ± 9 years) postmyocardial infarction	Pretest–posttest experimental study	Exercise test plus exercise (home or group) (N = 97); exercise test but no training program (N = 26); control (no contact until 26th week) (N = 27)	Cigarettes/day	N.S. treatment effect (although different rates of smoking were evident at pretest. Also may be a social support effect of experimenters [nurses] encouraging smoking cessation as well as activity in exercise program.)
Marcus et al. (32)	N = 20 healthy F (aged 20–50 years); smoked 10 or more cigarettes/day for 3 years	Pretest–posttest experimental study; 8-hour behavior modification smoking cessation program over 4 weeks	Smoking cessation program plus three cycle ergometer training periods/week	Number of individuals who remained abstinent for 24 hours	N.S. but more individuals in exercise condition did remain abstinent over the 12-month period

Note. N = sample size; M = male; F = female; LTPA = leisure-time physical activity; N.S. = not significant; OPA: occupational physical activity; p = probability; min = minutes; PA = physical activity; SES = Socio-economic status; ANCOVA = analysis of covariance; ANOVA = analysis of variance; kcal = kilocalorie; kg = kilogram.

others, the measurement qualities are questionable. The low associations reported between physical activity and other lifestyle behaviors in the Langlie (30) study may be attributable to the unreliable measure of physical activity involvement (Chronbach's $\alpha = .35$) that was utilized.

Recent surveys have been more consistent in reporting negative although modest (e.g., –.10 to –.30) relationships between physical activity and smoking. Some of the most convincing research in this area has been conducted in Finland. A number of studies using carefully constructed measures (although usually single item measures without independent assessments of reliability and validity) across various populations and employing stringent statistical analyses have consistently demonstrated a negative relationship (33–36,53,65). This negative association has been demonstrated in youth populations (33,36) as well as adult populations of varying age levels (33,35,53,65). These Finnish results are paralleled by Norwegian studies indicating similar negative relationships (6,25). Recent results from Canada (61), the United States (50), and Zimbabwe (40) are also generally consistent with these findings.

On the other hand discrepancies are evident. No association of leisure-time physical activity and smoking was evident in a Puerto Rican study (19). In addition, a significant relationship was reported in only 2 of 12 age by sex by occupational type groups in a large study in Great Britain (10). Whether these differences reflect the effects of different measurement instruments or population differences is not clear. It is clear, however, that different factors may influence the interrelation of different lifestyle behaviors. This will be discussed in the closing section of the chapter.

Observational studies of selected comparison groups have indicated that extreme activity groups do differ in smoking behavior. A common observation is that the majority of high-level athletes do not smoke. In a study of participants in the Bern, Switzerland 16-km run, Marti, Abelin, Minder, and Vader (33) report that only 2.0% smoked 20 or more cigarettes per day. Even within this small group of smokers ($N = 65$), a negative relation ($r = -.10$) was observed between weekly training in kilometers and cigarettes consumed per week.

An exploratory, open-ended question to examine the relationship of running behavior and change in smoking status for those who were ex-smokers ($N = 1,041$) revealed that 70% of those who smoked at the time they took up jogging or running subsequently quit smoking as runners. About one half of those ex-smokers stopped smoking within 1 year of taking up running. Further, the proportion of quitters was highly related to the weekly training mileage.

Long-Term Studies to Determine the Effects of Extended Physical Activity Involvement on Smoking Behavior

Marti et al. (34) divided a sample of southwestern Finnish adults into four exercise pattern groups (increasers, maintainers, quitters, and sedentary) on the basis of their reported levels of physical activity involvement at two time points, 20 years apart. They found that increasers smoked less than those who were sedentary.

Follow-up studies on more delimited samples have yielded less positive results. Sedgwick (54), in a 5-year follow-up of participants in an exercise program, found no difference in the smoking behavior of those who remained active and those who were inactive. In a similar study Mackeen, Rosenberger, Slater, Nicholas, and Buskirk (31) in a 13-year follow-up of participants in an 18-month exercise program found no significant effect of activity level on smoking behavior either at baseline or at follow-up. Thus for participants in an exercise program, it would appear that whether or not one maintains activity involvement after the program has little long-term impact on smoking behavior.

Two alternate explanations might be offered for these apparently discrepant results. First, lifestyle behavior changes may have been parallel decisions—when individuals undertook an exercise program they may have already made their decision concerning smoking; that is, they already had stopped smoking prior to joining the exercise program or alternately they were resigned to continue smoking. Second, high-level participants (e.g., serious runners) don't join exercise programs, hence, there are two distinct populations: the highly committed who tend to exercise independently and those who have more difficulty in committing to change on their own and tend to join group programs.

Physical Activity Programs Used as an Intervention as Part of a Smoking Cessation Program

Three intervention studies (24,32,63) were reviewed. None found physical activity to significantly affect smoking behavior. One study (32) reported that more subjects who did participate in an exercise program remained abstinent over 12 months than those who did not. However, these results must be viewed as very tenuous because of the extremely small number of subjects and the potential confounding of social interaction effects. Thus, it must be concluded that at the present time there is no evidence to indicate that physical activity is a useful adjunct to smoking cessation programs.

Physical Activity Involvement and Dietary Practices[1]

Dietary behavior practices that have been studied with respect to physical activity involvement include caloric intake, nutrient composition (essentially percent fat, carbohydrate, protein, etc., of total caloric intake), and various nutritional practice measures such as eating a good breakfast, following food guidelines, or heart-healthy practices. These types of studies parallel those with respect to smoking, and in general the pattern of results are also comparable.

Caloric Intake

With respect to the relation of physical activity to caloric intake the results of population surveys have been mixed. Three studies (2,38,51) reported a positive association; whereas one study (19) reported no relationship.

Observational studies of selected groups provide stronger evidence for the positive association of physical activity and caloric intake. Smith, Mendez, Druckenmiller, and Kris-Etherton (57) compared the caloric intake of two collegiate swimming groups (synchronized and speed) with a sedentary control group of female college students over a 24-week period. The swimmers' energy intake, as recorded by 4-day dietary records, exceeded that of the control group by 21.5%. Blair et al. (7), in a study of long-distance runners versus sedentary controls, found the runners to exceed controls by about one third in total caloric intake. In a study of a less select sample of runners (mean training time = 2.75 hrs/week), Pate, Sargent, Baldwin, and Burgess (44) found the runners' intake marginally greater (1,603.2 kcal vs. 1,538 kcal, $p >$ .05) than that of a control group. Moore, Hartung, Mitchell, Kappus, and Hinderlitter (39), using similar 3-day dietary recall measures, studied the caloric intake of runners (N = 45), joggers (N = 49), and sedentary control (N = 47). Like Pate et al. (44) they reported nonsignificant differences but a trend toward greater intake across the three activity levels.

Two follow-up studies of former exercise class participants (54,31) found no significant differences between continuing exercisers and nonexercisers. This is similar to their results previously reported for smoking behavior.

Nieman, Butler, Pollett, Dietrich, and Lutz (42) conducted a nutritional practices study with 347 volunteers from a random selection of 4,926 runners from the 12,200 applicants for the Los Angeles marathon. Approximately 50% (N = 2,311) of those contacted returned a questionnaire with information on their training habits and demographic characteristics. Eight months later the respondents were asked to participate in a dietary assessment research project. The volunteers were older, more experienced, and better runners than the general population of marathoners, but they were similar on important sociodemographic characteristics. The subjects completed a 3-day food record as well as a questionnaire concerning their training practices. The runners were stratified into three training categories to provide approximately equal groups (less than 32 km/week, N = 102; 32–56 km/week, N = 125; greater than 56 km/week, N = 107). In terms of overall caloric intake, the runners were somewhat higher than the national average (USDA National Food Consumption Survey) for comparable age groups (M = 2,526 vs. 2,428 for males; 1,868 vs. 1,602 for females). Caloric intake for the subjects as a whole did not differ significantly across the three training intensities; however, caloric consumption expressed per kilogram of body weight demonstrated a significant effect across kilometers run per week (M = 32.8, 35.7, 36.7 kcal/kg; F = 3.42, p = .03).

Intervention studies employing self-reports of dietary practices have similarly yielded somewhat conflicting evidence. Wood et al. (67) in a 1-year study of Stanford University employee volunteers, who were assigned to either an exercise program or a sedentary control condition, found no significant difference in caloric intake between the groups. Nieman, Onasch, and Lee (43) used 7-day food records to assess dietary practices of 36 mildly obese women (M = 29.9 years) randomly assigned to an exercise or sedentary control condition. The exercise program involved walking for 45 min, 5 times per week at a prescribed intensity. The exercise group had a significantly higher caloric intake at the 6-week and 15-week (program termination) assessment points. Johnson, Mastropaolo, and Wharton reported opposite findings (28) in a 10-week study of dietary practices of individuals involved in an exercise ergocycle training program (five 30-min sessions/week). The 20 college females reported significantly lower caloric intake after the 10-week program. The absence of a control group raises a question as to whether other factors were involved, given the surprising result in terms of other studies.

The best evidence for the relationship of physical activity and nutrition comes from controlled studies conducted within metabolic wards where energy expenditure and intake can both be carefully

---

[1]A tabular summary of the studies investigating the relationship of physical activity and dietary practices is available from the authors. Space limitations precluded its inclusion in the chapter.

monitored and objectively measured. Pi-Sunyer and Woo (46) have reviewed the research in this area, including a number of their own studies. An interesting result of this research, which was not evident in the field studies using self-report measures, was the importance of subject weight. Whereas, nonobese subjects increase their voluntary food intake levels in proportion to physical-activity-induced energy expenditure, at least in the mild to moderate activity range (i.e., 100% to 125% of baseline energy expenditure); such is not the case with obese subjects. Pi-Sunyer and Woo (46) conclude ". . . studies in overweight volunteers find weight changes associated with exercise that range from loss to gain. Obviously, this lack of consistency strongly suggests that in obese persons, intake is not tightly coupled to expenditure" (p. 85).

The relationships of physical activity and caloric intake reported in carefully controlled studies may not be observed in real life settings. Pi-Sunyer and Woo (46) note that in situations outside the metabolic ward, other factors may override physical activity effects in shaping caloric intake. They report studies in which the palatability of the food was varied as well as energy expenditure. Although voluntary intake in the obese subjects was not affected by energy expenditure, the fixed caloric intake, given the palatable food presented across the energy treatment conditions was at a uniformly high level that exceeded the output demands. According to Pi-Sunyer and Woo (46):

> This observation suggests that the determination of intake in the obese subjects is more related to the sensory characteristics of the diet provided than to any inhibitory or stimulatory signal set up by the exercise programs. Therefore, whatever signals are generated in obese subjects by exercise alone may be attenuated or overwhelmed by other cues which are generated by the foods to be eaten. (p. 89)

Beyond this, when the relation of physical activity and eating practices in everyday life are considered, it is likely that a number of other "inhibitory or stimulatory signals" may be involved. For example, the whole social context is of considerable importance. Leisure-time physical activity is not just moving and eating is not just meeting energy input demands! These are both complex leisure behaviors that satisfy multiple human motives. Once more the importance of motivation to understanding the relationship of different lifestyle behaviors is observed.

Nutritional Practices or Dietary Composition

When dietary composition or the quality of nutritional practices is considered, a number of studies report positive associations with physical activity involvement. Nieman et al. (42) in their study of marathon runners report that the runners exhibited a number of good dietary practices. In comparison to the general population, they consumed a lower percentage of fat (30.9% vs. 37.6% for men; 32.0% vs. 37.2% for women), more carbohydrates (51.8% vs. 44.5% for men; 52.7% vs. 45.4% for women), and more fiber (men +13%, women +49%). Comparisons of marathoners training at different intensity levels indicated no difference in raw intake of different food components. When adjusted for body weight, however, carbohydrate intake increased significantly with level of training. Pate et al. (44), in their study of distance runners compared to a matched sedentary control, report runners to consume less saturated fat, net fat, cholesterol and protein, and more carbohydrates and fiber.

Heinemann and Zerbes (23) in comparing East German national team athletes to a randomly selected control group of the same age noted that the athletes consumed less meat, a higher proportion of polyunsaturated to saturated fat, and more grain and fruit. Female athletes, but not males, had higher carbohydrate and lower overall fat intake. Blair et al. (9) in their cross-sectional study of clients tested at the Cooper Clinic in Dallas, Texas report a positive relationship of level of activity and a number of nutritional practices. Increased activity was associated with lower saturated and net fat intake, lower coffee consumption, and higher polyunsaturated fat intake.

In their longitudinal study of individuals who had undergone a series of six full physical exams over time at the clinic, the authors also found a number of differences between individuals in the four exercise categories established: starters, continuers, intermittent, and sedentary. Continuers, those who were active across their six physical exams, were better than those who were sedentary throughout on saturated, unsaturated, and net fat intake; intermittent, those with a variable activity pattern, were better than the sedentary on unsaturated and net fat; and starters were better than the sedentary on unsaturated fat and coffee consumption.

Other researchers have reported contrary results. Pomrehn, Wallace, and Burmeister (47), in their earlier study of people who had been tested at the Cooper Clinic, found no differences in the nutritional practices of participants classified as improvers and those classified as nonimprovers (considered indirect indicators of activity levels) on their fitness tests. As well, the previously discussed follow-up studies of former participants in exercise programs by Sedgwick (54) and Mackeen et al. (31) found no differences between groups. Smith et al. (57) reported no significant differences in dietary components of their groups of swimmers and college student controls. Similarly, Wood et al. (67) found no difference in the nutritional practices of runners and controls.

In considering these results, two related interpretations are offered. First, nutritional practices and physical activity involvement, as parallel health behaviors, are likely to be more positively related as the level of awareness and knowledge of the population group increases. Thus, as the knowledge of healthy lifestyle behaviors pertaining to these two areas has increased over the years, there is a temporal trend toward higher relationships. This is evident in more positive results in the recent research in contrast to that published 10 years earlier. Secondly, in selected groups (e.g., serious runners) there is likely to be greater attention to all factors that limit health and performance, hence there would be a greater association evident in these groups than in the general population.

A number of studies have reported positive associations of physical activity level with more general indicators of good nutritional practices. National surveys in Canada have found level of activity to be positively associated with eating a nutritious breakfast (15) and with following good nutritional practices (16,61). In the 1988 Campbell Survey on the Well-Being of Canadians, individuals who had been active (greater than 1.5 kcal/kg/day) in both 1981 and 1988 (adherers) were most likely to follow dietary practices consistent with the Canada Food Guide whereas resisters (those not active in either year) were least likely (16). Adherers age 25 years and older were more likely than resisters to restrict their fat consumption. There were no differences between any of the activity pattern groups in their salt and sugar consumption practices.

Earlier studies (e.g., 20,45,66) also report somewhat more healthy dietary practices for active individuals. A U.S. Gallup poll study (cited in Shephard, 55) reported that active individuals ate more fruit and vegetables. A concern with these population surveys is that, unless such factors as education and socioeconomic status are accounted for, the activity-nutrition relationships may simply reflect the common effect of these other variables. Blaxter (10) in her report of the Health and Lifestyle Survey in the United Kingdom controlled for a number of these factors. She found exercise and diet to be positively correlated in women regardless of age and social class. In men, the association was stronger in working-class individuals. The nutrition measure in this study was a composite index based on a number of items combined to reflect good nutrition practices.

Two recent studies based on a random sample of adults in the San Diego district report good nutritional practices to be positively related to walking (r = .20) (26) and running (r = .24) (52).

In conclusion, similar to the relationship of smoking and physical activity, the relationship of physical activity to nutritional practices, both in terms of intake and composition, is somewhat mixed. A number of nonsignificant results are reported but on the whole, the strongest evidence based on more recent research tends to support a positive relationship. Whether these more positive results reflect better measurement approaches or temporal changes is not known.

Alcohol Consumption

Table 36.2 summarizes the research conducted since 1988 to investigate the relationship of physical activity involvement to alcohol consumption. It is evident from this table that most studies have reported a nonsignificant relationship between the two behaviors. The usual measure of drinking behavior employed in these studies is ounces of alcohol or servings of alcohol per week. A question that can be raised in considering these results is whether another measure might yield different results. As the generally recognized negative health effects of alcohol are not linearly related to alcohol consumption but relate to an abuse level, perhaps a measure more sensitive to this might yield different results. One study that employed a criterion of "having four or more drinks at one sitting in previous week" as the alcohol consumption measure (59) did report a small but negative association with activity level.

No recent (i.e., post-1988) studies were located pertaining to the use of physical activity as an adjunct in treatment programs for alcohol abuse. The results of two earlier studies (41,56) are equivocal. Hence, further research is required to determine whether physical activity might serve as a useful intervention modality for reducing alcohol consumption.

Preventive Health Behaviors

Table 36.3 summarizes research examining the relationship of physical activity involvement and such health behaviors as seat belt use, self-examinations, and medical and dental check-ups. This has not been a popular research area as indicated by the fact that only three studies have been published since 1988. In general the results have indicated either small positive associations—or no

Table 36.2 Summary of Evidence for the Relationship of Physical Activity Involvement and Alcohol Consumption

Study	Sample	Research design/controls	Measurement of physical activity	Measurement of alcohol	Results
Kronefeld et al. (29)	N = 663 (220 M, 443 F) insurance company employees; higher education and economic level than general population	Cross-sectional	Index from reported LTPA participation	Drinks in past month	r = .02; N.S.
Marti et al. (33)					
(a) army conscripts	N = 6,592 Swiss M (aged 19 years); random sample of army conscripts	Cross-sectional	Six-point activity scale	Drinks/week	r = −.15
(b) 16-km runners	N = 4,358 of 6,620 participants in Bern, Switzerland 16-km race completed questionnaires	Cross-sectional	Weekly kilometers of training	Consumption/week	N.S.
Abel et al. (1)	N = 349 M employed by the state of Illinois; stratified sample on "occupational self-direction"	Cross-sectional	LTPA: four-point scale	Consumption/week	r = .16
Calnan (14)	N = 4,224; community survey in southern England	Cross-sectional; representative of adult population	Seven-point scale (regular daytime activity and sport)	Frequency and amount	Spearman Rho = .15
Hovell et al. (26)	N = 1,080 (43.4%) response to questionaire mailed to San Diego residents (Haines Directory)	Relatively inactive group (deleted those who exercise 20 min, 3 ×/week)	Minutes of walking for exercise/week	Consumption	N.S.
Sallis et al. (52)	N = 2,053 (43.4%) random sample of San Diego area; overrepresents affluent, well-educated Caucasians	Cross-sectional; regression analysis	PA: frequency of reported activity	Days/week that subjects have a drink	r = −.02

(continued)

Table 36.2 ***(Continued)***

Study	Sample	Research design/controls	Measurement of physical activity	Measurement of alcohol	Results
Blair, Kohl & Brill (9)					
(a) Cross-sectional	N = 10,250 (7,961 M, 2,289 F) self-selected individuals tested at Cooper Clinic; higher education and SES than general population	Cross-sectional ANCOVA adjusting for age (all measures transformed to natural log scale to remove skewness)	PA: five-point scale of activity during past month	Consumption (ounces of alcohol/week)	N.S.
(b) Longitudinal	N = 2,329 M who underwent at least six full medicals at Cooper Clinic	Longitudinal observations study; age × treatment group ANOVA (repeated measures across six time points); data transformation as in (a)	Four exercise exposure groups; *starters, continuers, intermittent, sedentary*	Consumption (ounces of alcohol/week)	N.S.
Blaxter (10)	N = 9,003 (3,905 M, 5,098 F) adult (aged 18+ years) participants in Health and Lifestyle Survey in Great Britain (1984–1985)	Cross-sectional comprehensive study with many control variables (e.g., attitude, geography, SES, education, occupational status, health status); multiple discriminant analysis	Six levels LTPA: energy expenditure for activities in last 2 weeks	Six levels 6-day diary (drinks last week)	Generally N.S. for M; negative for nonmanual but positive for manual workers; consistently negative correlation in F across all ages but only significant for manual workers plus group of nonmanual workers aged 49–59 years
Faulkner & Slattery (17a)	N = 257 (125 M, 132 F) 9th and 10th grade students	Cross-sectional	Three-category scale (hours of various activities/year)	Three-category scale (frequency and amount of drinking/week). Light = <2.5 drinks/month; medium = 2.5–9 drinks/month; heavy = >9 drinks/month	M Tau = .18 F = N.S. 42% of males in most active categories were "heavy drinkers"
Scanlon et al. (53a)	N = 6,537 Canadian military personnel	Cross-sectional; stepwise logistic regression	Vigorous exercise 3+ ×/week	Heavy drinker, not a heavy drinker	N.S.
Summerson et al. (62)	N = 270 diabetic adults	Cross-sectional; ANOVA	PA: > 600 kcal/week < 600 kcal/week no exercise	Ounces/week	N.S.

Note. N = sample size; M = male; F = female; LTPA = leisure-time physical activity; N.S. = not significant, PA = physical activity; SES = socio-economic status; ANCOVA = analysis of covariance; ANOVA = analysis of variance; kcal = kilocalorie.

relationship. Two alternate explanations seem reasonable. One, the small but positive relationships for these behaviors may reflect a broad general value placed on a healthy lifestyle, which has some modest impact on concerns about specific behaviors within such a lifestyle. Different individuals may place different priorities on specific behaviors. Second, the small positive associations may indicate the influence of some other common variable such as socioeconomic status or education level. Given the well-known pervasive influence of such factors, this is a viable explanation in studies where such factors were not controlled (30,37). The fact that comparable results were reported by Stephens (59) and Blair (8) using data sets for which these factors were controlled, however, tends to discount this second interpretation.

The Interrelationship of Multiple Health Behaviors

Limited research has employed multivariate statistical techniques to explore the interrelation of multiple health behavior variables. Reviews of the early research in this area (8,59) revealed little consistency in the results. It was noted that small, nonrepresentative samples and use of different variables in different studies probably contributed to this inconsistency. There has been very little recent research in this area and the results are very tenuous. Lack of consistent results across studies is a common problem in factor analytic studies; so unless stable results are replicated across comparable population groups, the significance of any one reported factor structure must be viewed with some caution.

Recent multivariate research has indicated that the factor structure for the same health behaviors varies markedly across different age levels and even between random samples drawn from the same population group (49,64). Blaxter (10) reported that, in the large Great Britain survey, the relation between different health behaviors including exercise varied considerably between occupational groups, age groups, gender, and within these groupings across geographical areas. On the basis of these results, it must be concluded that although an overall pattern in the relation of different behaviors in the general population may be instructive for comparative purposes, for any practical application it must be recognized that the patterns do vary markedly between different population subgroups.

Conclusions

Consideration of the available evidence leads to the following general conclusions concerning the relationship of physical activity involvement and other lifestyle behaviors:

1. Correlational studies generally indicate that for both smoking status (smoking vs. nonsmoking) and smoking consumption (number of cigarettes/day), there is a negative association with level of leisure-time physical activity involvement.
2. Retrospective and prospective observational studies of selected activity groups indicate that although active groups at baseline generally smoke less than do inactive groups, these differences do not increase appreciably over time.
3. In more highly selected populations (e.g., serious runners, competitive athletes) smoking rates are observed to decline as intensity of training increases. These changes may reflect a desire to remove the performance constraints of smoking.
4. Although the negative relationship of physical activity and smoking has been consistently reported across both male and female populations, the reported relationship is somewhat stronger in males.
5. Controlled, metabolic-ward research indicates that mild and moderate increases in the physical activity levels of nonobese individuals results in corresponding increases in caloric intake. Obese individuals do not appear to make caloric intake adjustments to parallel varying activity levels.
6. There is a trend, especially in the more recent research, for more active individuals to exhibit better nutritional practices (e.g., lower percentage of saturated fat, more balanced diet, eating a good breakfast). The positive association of physical activity involvement and good nutritional practices is most clearly evident in selected groups (e.g., highly active individuals, serious runners).
7. Better nutrition practices are positively related to increased intensity of physical activity training. This is not a linear increase over time with increased training intensity, however, but rather appears as a step-function suggesting a decision-point where better nutrition practices are adopted.
8. No consistent relationship is evident between physical activity involvement and alcohol consumption.
9. The very limited research investigating the association of physical activity involvement with other preventive health behaviors (e.g., wearing a seat belt, regular health checkups) suggests a small positive relationship.

Table 36.3 Summary of Evidence for the Relationship of Physical Activity Involvement and Preventive Health Behavior

Study	Sample	Research design/controls	Measurement of physical activity	Measurement of preventive health behavior	Results
Langlie (30)	*N* = 617; random sample of adults in small New York city (sample somewhat biased toward younger, well-educated F)	Cross-sectional	Four-point scale concerning activity behavior	Four-point scale concerning health actions (e.g., dental check, seat belt use, immunization)	Medical check-up (r = .08); dental check-up (r = .20); miscellaneous health-related examination (r = .14); immunization (r = .13); seat belt use (r = .10)
Mechanic (37)	*N* = 302 adults studied 16 years earlier in Grade 4 in Wisconsin	Cross-sectional	Three-item scale of self-reported exercise in 24 hours	Physical check-up; seat belt use	r = .05; r = .13
Blair, Jacobs, & Powell (8) (a) NSPHPC data	Large representative sample of U.S. population	Cross-sectional; controlled for age, sex, education	Physically active vs. inactive	—	Physical examination (significantly higher); Blood pressure check (significantly higher); breast exam in past 24 months (significantly higher); pap smear (N.S.); seat belt use (significantly higher)
(b) BRFS (1981–1983)	Large representative sample of U.S. population	Cross-sectional	—	Seat belt use	Significantly higher

Stephens (59)	N = 17,726 Canadian adults (aged 20+ years) from Canada Health Survey data (self-completed questionnaire followed by interview)	Cross-sectional; age-adjusted, controlled for gender (income and health status examined, no significant effect)	Dichotomous, measured on various health behavior scales	Dichotomous, measured on various health behavior scales	Recent breast examination (r = –.06); recent pap smear test (r = –.03); breast self-examination (r = –.10); immunization within 5 years (M: r = .06, F: r = .04); regularity of dental visit (M: r = –.02, F: r = –.04; seat belt use (M: r = .10, F: r = .10)
Abel et al. (1)	N = 349 M employed by the state of Illinois stratified sample on "occupational self-direction"	Dichotomous scale	Four-point scale from vigorous participation to no involvement in sport or exercise	Annual physical check-up	r = .11
Summerson et al. (62)	N = 270 diabetic adults	ANOVA: activity level × age × sex	Three groups established based on self-reported weekly calorie energy expenditure	Physical checkup; seat belt use	r = .05; r = .13
Gillis & Perry (21)		Exercise groups vs. wait-list control groups	—	Health responsibility score (subscale of Health Promoting Lifestyle Profile (Walker et al. 66a)	N.S.

Note. N = sample size; F = females; — = not applicable; NSPHPC = National Survey of Personal Health Practices and Consequences; BRFS = Behavioral Risk Factor Survey; N.S. = not significant; M = males; ANOVA = analysis of variance.

Interpretation

The observed relationships of physical activity involvement and other lifestyle behaviors raise questions as to what underlying mechanisms may mediate such relationships. Stephens (60) suggests a number of potential mechanisms. These may be broadly categorized as physiologically based mechanisms (e.g., addiction substitution, sensation habituation, thermodynamic energy expenditure) and psychological mechanisms (e.g., general health belief or health attitude models).

The research indicating that increased physical activity generally results in increased caloric intake, at least for nonobese subjects, is consistent with a thermodynamic energy model. As energy is expended a deficit condition triggers an energy intake-governing mechanism. Why this intake regulatory system works differently in obese than nonobese individuals, however, requires clarification (46). Similarly, such a model cannot account for food composition intake differences between active and inactive individuals. This observed relationship, those for physical activity with smoking, and the weaker association of physical activity with various other preventive health actions are more consistent with a psychological explanation.

We see little justification in the literature for the view that simply initiating an activity program will lead to improvements in other lifestyle behaviors. Although serious runners who wish to maximize their performance may stop smoking because of its counterproductive effect on their goal attainment, this would appear to reflect a conscious decision not an automatic health-gain effect. Further, in broader based populations the positive associations reported would appear to reflect multiple behaviors that show a general increased health consciousness. The temporal patterns suggest that physical activity involvement is generally part of a "positive health behavior package" that is adopted; it is not the cause of other behaviors. In other words, it is our opinion that the most viable explanation for the observed results is an attitude-behavior change model of lifestyle behavior change. Although a number of such models are available (22,58), discussion here will be restricted to the theory of planned behavior.

According to Ajzen (3,4), three principal psychological constructs mediate the effects of all other variables on human behavior. These constructs are: (a) the individual's personal attitudes toward doing the behavior in question, (b) subjective norm (the individual's perception of what other people important to them think about their doing the behavior), and (c) perceived behavioral control (the individual's perception of his or her capability of performing the relevant behavior[2]). These three determinants in turn are the result of the individual's relevant beliefs pertaining to: (a) behavioral beliefs concerning the likelihood of certain outcomes resulting from the behavior weighted by the individual's evaluation of those outcomes, (b) beliefs about significant others' views about the individual engaging in the behavior weighted by the motivation to comply with those views, and (c) power beliefs pertaining to the individual's beliefs about how much power or control he or she has over doing or not doing the behavior. All other variables such as environmental factors, social influences, individual characteristics, and capabilities are posited to influence behavior only through their effect on these more proximal determinants. Figure 36.1 (see page 531) presents a schematic representation of how this model might apply to physical activity involvement and other lifestyle behaviors.

The model suggests that, although each particular lifestyle behavior is subject to its own set of specific attitudes, social norms, and perceived behavioral control determinants, there may be overlap in these determinants. Generalized beliefs about the desirability of leading a healthy lifestyle in general may impact on each specific lifestyle behavior through their relationships to intervening specific determinants. In different populations the degree of relationship is expected to vary. In population groups that are well educated about the benefits of proper nutrition, being active, not smoking, and moderate use of alcohol, the specific predictors of the individual behaviors (and the behaviors themselves) are expected to be positively related. In other populations that have not internalized the holistic, multicomponent, healthy lifestyle message, it would be expected that the specific determinants of the individual behaviors, and in turn, the behaviors themselves, would be less related. We view the observed temporal trends toward greater relationship between the various lifestyle behaviors and the observed higher relationships within more highly committed populations (e.g., serious runners) to be consistent with the model's predictions.

The model can accommodate the noted importance of motivation to the interrelationship of different lifestyle behaviors. To the extent that the underlying beliefs encouraging participation in physical activity and the other lifestyle behaviors

---

[2]Space limitations prevent a complete portrayal of the model. The brief description given is for illustrative purposes to indicate how an attitude–behavior model might be utilized to interpret the observed relationships of physical activity to other lifestyle behaviors.

are similar (e.g., all aimed toward leading a lifestyle compatible with good health outcomes), positive relationships between the various behaviors are expected. On the other hand if the most significant factors underlying physical activity involvement are beliefs concerning other outcomes such as thrill-seeking or escape, then physical activity involvement would not be expected to be related to other lifestyle behaviors.

Future Research

Consistent with the emphasis placed on a cognitive model for interpreting the relationship of different lifestyle behaviors, it is recommended that research be conducted on the personal meanings underlying different behaviors. Why do different individuals engage in the various behaviors? It is clear that there is no simple dichotomy of healthy versus unhealthy lifestyles. Rather, there is a wide variety of specific behavioral patterns for different groups (10). To understand specific subgroups, the meanings underlying these behaviors, and the environmental and social contexts within which they occur must be understood. To obtain such a perspective there is a need for more in-depth, qualitative research (14).

This is not to say that more systematic quantitative research is not also required. We agree with the assessment of Blair et al. (9) that poor measurement techniques have hindered the investigation of the relationship of physical activity involvement to other lifestyle behaviors. Better measurement, however, will not solve all of the problems. The complexity of lifestyles must be acknowledged and greater in-depth attention must be devoted to studying selected population groups. Large, properly controlled surveys will contribute to an overall summary of the interrelationship of lifestyle behaviors within a population. This initial "snapshot," however, should be just a first step to proceeding to a more in-depth examination of the role of physical activity in the lifestyles of specific subgroups.

There is a need for further research into the relationship of physical activity and all of the other lifestyle behaviors reviewed here, although considerably more research has been done on smoking and nutrition than the other behaviors. Other lifestyle behaviors that have not been reviewed here also warrant attention in future research.

The importance of social relationships and social support to health is becoming increasingly well documented (12). In view of the fact that much leisure behavior is of a social nature (27), a question arises as to whether leisure-time physical activity may facilitate health through initiating social relationships. There is a lack of direct evidence on this issue and only limited evidence to suggest that physical activity is an important venue for developing social relationships (5). Recent attention has been drawn to the importance of conducting research into how leisure experiences can be used to facilitate social relationships (13).

The relationship of physical activity behavior to the misuse and abuse of drugs (chapter 61) also warrants additional attention. Another increasingly important health-related lifestyle behavior is that of sexual behavior. What is the relationship of physical activity involvement to sexual behavior?

Finally, from an even broader perspective, as health increasingly becomes an environmental issue, it might be asked whether leisure-time physical activity is systematically related to environmental protection and conservation practices. We would surmise that those who are physically active may tend to rely more on human energy for their transportation than do their inactive counterparts. In addition they may rely less on other energy sources for their leisure entertainment. Do such behavioral relationships in fact occur? Are attitudes about being physically active during leisure linked to broader environmental attitudes?

References

1. Abel, T.; Cockerham, W.C.; Lueschen, G.; Kung, G. Health lifestyles and self-direction in employment among American men: A test of the spillover effect. Soc. Sci. Med. 28:1269-1274; 1989.
2. Aho, K.; Pekkarinen, M. Diet and physical activity of men in east and west Finland in 1969. Annu. Med. 21:241-243; 1969.
3. Ajzen, I. From intentions to actions: A theory of planned behavior. In: Kuhl, J.; Beckman, J., eds. Action-control: From cognition to behavior. Heidelberg: Springer; 1985:11-39.
4. Ajzen, I. The theory of planned behavior. Organizational Beh. Hum. Decision Processes. 50:179-211; 1991.
5. American health: Public attitudes and behavior related to exercise. Princeton, NJ: Gallup Organization; 1985. Cited in: Blair, S.; Kohl, W.; Brill, P. Behavioral adaptation to physical activity. In: Bouchard, C.; Shephard, R.; Stephens, T.; Sutton, J.; McPherson, B., eds. Exercise, fitness, and health: A consensus of current knowledge. Champaign, IL: Human Kinetics; 1990:385-398.

6. Bjartveit, K.; Foss, O.; Gjervig, T. The cardiovascular disease study in Norwegian countries: Results from first screening. Acta Med. Scand. [Suppl.]. 675:95-130; 1983.
7. Blair, S.; Ellsworth, N.; Haskell, W.; Stern, M.; Farquhar, J.; Wood, P. Comparison of nutrient intake in middle-aged men and women runners and controls. Med. Sci. Sports Exerc. 13:310-315; 1981.
8. Blair, S.; Jacobs, D.; Powell, K. Relationships between exercise or physical activity and other health behaviors. Public Health Rep. 100:172-179; 1985.
9. Blair, S.; Kohl, H.; Brill, P. Behavioral adaptation to physical activity. In: Bouchard, C.; Shephard, R.; Stephens, T.; Sutton, J.; McPherson, B., eds. Exercise, fitness, and health: A consensus of current knowledge. Champaign, IL: Human Kinetics; 1990:385-398.
10. Blaxter, E. Health and lifestyles. London: Tavistock/Routledge; 1990.
11. Bofetta, P.; Barone, J.; Wynder, E. Leisure time physical activity in a hospital-based population. J. Clin. Epidemiol. 43:569-577; 1990.
12. Breslow, L. Lifestyle, fitness, and health. In: Bouchard, C.; Shephard, R.; Stephens, T.; Sutton, J.; McPherson, B., eds. Exercise, fitness, and health: A consensus of current knowledge. Champaign, IL: Human Kinetics; 1990:155-163.
13. Burch, W.; Hamilton-Smith, E. Mapping a new frontier: Identifying, measuring, and valuing social cohesion benefits to nonwork opportunities and activities. In: Driver, B.; Brown, P.; Peterson, G., eds. Benefits of leisure. State College, PA: Venture Press; 1991:369-382.
14. Calnan, M. Control over health and patterns of health-related behavior. Soc. Sci. Med. 29:131-136; 1989.
15. Canada Fitness Survey. Fitness and lifestyle in Canada. Ottawa: Fitness Canada; 1983.
16. Craig, C.; Stephens, T.; Landry, F. Fitness, nutrition and health indices: Findings from the 1988 Campbell survey on well-being in Canada. In: Oja, P.; Telema, R., eds. Sport for all. Amsterdam: Elsevier Science; 1991:459-464.
17. Epstein, L.; Miller, G.; Stitt, F.; Morris, J. Vigorous exercise in leisure time, coronary risk factors, and resting electrocardiogram in middle-aged civil servants. Br. Health J. 38:403-409; 1976.
17a. Faulkner, R.; Slattery, C.M. The relationship of physical activity to alcohol consumption in youth, 15-16 years of age. Can. J. Public Health. 81:168-169; 1990.
18. Folsom, A.; Caspersen, C.; Taylor, H.; Jacobs, D.; Luepker, R.; Gomez-Marin, O.; Gillum, R.; Blackburn, H. Leisure time physical activity and its relationship to coronary risk factors in a population-based sample: The Minnesota heart survey. Am. J. Epidemiol. 121:570-579; 1985.
19. Garcia-Palmieri, M.; Costas, R., Jr.; Cruz-Vidal, M.; Sorlie, P.; Havlik, R. Increased physical activity: A protective factor against heart attacks in Puerto Rico. Am. J. Cardiol. 50:749-755; 1982.
20. General Mills. Family health in an era of stress. Minneapolis: General Mills; 1979.
21. Gillis, A.; Perry, A. The relationship between physical activity and health-promoting behaviors in mid-life women. J. Adv. Nurs. 16:299-310; 1991.
22. Godin, G.; Shephard, R. Use of attitude-behavior models in exercise promotion. Sports Med. 10:103-121; 1990.
23. Heinemann, L.; Zerbes, H. Physical activity, fitness, and diet: Behavior in the population compared with elite athletes in the GDR. Am. J. Clin. Nutr. 49:1007-1016; 1989.
24. Hill, J. Effect of a program of aerobic exercise on the smoking behavior of a group of adult volunteers. Can. J. Public Health. 76:183-186; 1985.
25. Holme, I.; Helgeland, A.; Hjermann, I.; Leren, P.; Lund-Larsen, P. Physical activity at work and at leisure in relation to coronary risk factors and social class: A 4-year mortality follow-up. The Oslo study. Acta Med. Scand. 209:277-283; 1981.
26. Hovell, M.; Sallis, J.; Hofstetter, C.; Spry, V.; Faucher, P.; Caspersen, C. Identifying correlates of walking for exercise: An epidemiologic prerequisite for physical activity promotion. Prev. Med. 18:856-866; 1989.
27. Iso-Ahola, S. The social psychology of leisure and recreation. Dubuque, IA: Brown; 1980.
28. Johnson, R.; Mastropaolo, J.; Wharton, M. Exercise, dietary intake, and body composition. J. Am. Diet. Assoc. 61:399-403; 1972.
29. Kronenfeld, J.; Goodyear, N.; Pate, R.; Blair, A.; Howe, H.; Parker, G.; Blair, S. The interrelationship among preventive health habits. Health Educ. Res. 3:317-323; 1988.
30. Langlie, J. Interrelationships among preventive health behaviors: A test of competing hypotheses. Public Health Rep. 94:216-225; 1979.
31. Mackeen, P.; Rosenberger, J.; Slater, J.; Nicholas, W.; Buskirk, E. A 13-year follow-up of a coronary heart disease risk factor screening and exercise program for 40-59 year-old men: Exercise habit maintenance and physiologic status. J. Cardiopul. Rehabil. 5:510-523; 1985.

32. Marcus, B.; Albrecht, A.; Niaura, R.; Abrams, D.; Thompson, P. Usefulness of physical exercise for maintaining smoking cessation in women. Am. J. Cardiol. 68:406-407; 1991.
33. Marti, B.; Abelin, T.; Minder, C.; Vader, J. Smoking, alcohol consumption, and endurance capacity: An anlysis of 6500 19-year-old conscripts and 4100 joggers. Prev. Med. 17:79-92; 1988.
34. Marti, B.; Pekkanen, J.; Nissinen, A.; Ketola, A.; Kivela, S.; Punsar, S.; Karvonen, M. Association of physical activity with coronary risk factors and physical ability: Twenty-year follow-up of a cohort of Finnish men. Age and Aging. 18:103-109; 1989.
35. Marti, B.; Salonen, J.; Tuomilehto, J.; Puska, P. 10-year trends in physical activity in the eastern Finnish adult population: Relationship to socioeconomic and lifestyle characteristics. Acta Med. Scand. 224:195-203; 1988.
36. Marti, B.; Vartiainen, E. Relation between leisure time exercise and cardiovascular risk factors among 15-year-olds in eastern Finland. J. Epidemiol. Community Health. 43:228-233; 1989.
37. Mechanic, D. The stability of health and illness behavior: Results from a 16-year follow-up. Am. J. Public Health. 69:1142-1145; 1979.
38. Montoye, H.; Block, W.; Metzner, H.; Keller, J. Habitual physical activity and serum lipids: Males, age 16-64 in a total community. J. Chronic Dis. 29: 697-709; 1976.
39. Moore, C.; Hartung, G.; Mitchell, R.; Kappus, C.; Hinderlitter, J. The relationship of exercise and diet on high-density lipoprotein cholesterol levels in women. Metabolism. 32:189-196; 1983.
40. Morrison, J.; VanMalsen, S.; Noakes, T. Leisure-time physical activity levels, cardiovascular fitness and coronary risk factors in 1015 white Zimbabweans. S. Afr. Med. J. 65:250-256; 1984.
41. Murphy, T.; Pagano, R.; Marlatt, G. Lifestyle modification with heavy alcohol drinkers: Effects of aerobic exercise and meditation. Addict. Behav. 11:175-186; 1986.
42. Nieman, D.; Butler, J.; Pollett, L.; Dietrich, S.; Lutz, R. Nutrient intake of marathon runners. J. Am. Diet. Assoc. 89:1273-1278; 1989.
43. Nieman, D.; Onasch, L.; Lee, J. The effects of moderate exercise training on nutrient intake in mildly obese women. J. Am. Diet. Assoc. 90:1557-1562; 1990.
44. Pate, R.; Sargent, R.; Baldwin, C.; Burgess, M. Dietary intake of women runners. Int. J. Sports Med. 11:461-466; 1990.
45. The Perrier study: Fitness in America. New York: Perrier; 1979.
46. Pi-Sunyer, F.; Woo, R. Effect of exercise on food intake in human subjects. Am. J. Clin Nutr. 42:983-990; 1985.
47. Pomrehn, P.; Wallace, R.; Burmeister, L. Ischemic heart disease mortality in Iowa farmers: The influence of lifestyle. JAMA. 248: 1073-1076; 1982.
48. President's council on fitness and sports national adult physical fitness survey. Phys. Fitness Res. Digest. 4:1-27; 1974.
49. Rakowski, W.; Lefebvre, R.; Assaf, A.; Lasater, T.; Carleton, R. Health practice correlates in three adult age groups: Results from two community surveys. Public Health Rep. 105:481-491; 1990.
50. Revicki, D.; Sobal, J.; DeForge, B. Smoking status and the practice of other unhealthy behaviors. Fam. Med. 23:361-364; 1991.
51. Rotevatn, S.; Akslen, L.; Bjelke, E. Lifestyle and mortality among Norwegian men. Prev. Med. 18:433-443; 1989.
52. Sallis, J.; Hovell, M.; Hofstetter, C.; Faucher, P.; Elder, J.; Blanchard, J.; Caspersen, C.; Powell, J.; Christenson, G. A multivariate study of determinants of vigorous exercise in a community sample. Prev. Med. 18:20-34; 1989.
53. Salonen, J.; Slater, J.; Tuomilehto, J.; Rauramaa, R. Leisure time and occupational physical activity: Risk of death from ischemic heart disease. Am. J. Epidemiol. 127:87-94; 1988.
53a. Scanlon, L.; Raman, S.; Zitzelsberger, L. Mental health, life-style and physical exercise. In: Oja, P.; Telama, R. eds. Sport for all. Amsterdam: Elsevier, Science; 1991:381-386.
54. Sedgwick, A. Long-term effects of physical training programme on risk factors for coronary heart disease in otherwise sedentary men. Br. Med. J. 232:7-10; 1980.
55. Shephard, R. Exercise and lifestyle change. Br. J. Sports Med. 23:11-22; 1989.
56. Sinyor, D.; Brown, T.; Rostant, L.; Seraganian, P. The role of a physical fitness program in the treatment of alcoholism. J. Stud. Alcohol. 43:380-386; 1982.
57. Smith, M.; Mendez, J.; Druckenmiller, M.; Kris-Etherton, P. Exercise intensity, dietary intake, and high-density lipoprotein cholesterol in young female competitive swimmers. Am. J. Clin. Nutr. 36:251-255; 1982.
58. Sonstroem, R. Psychological models. In: Dishman, R., ed. Exercise adherence: Its impact on public health. Champaign, IL: Human Kinetics; 1988:125-154.
59. Stephens, T. Health practices and health status: Evidence from the Canada health survey. Am. J. Prev. Med. 2:206-215; 1986.

60. Stephens, T. Behavioral adaptation to physical activity. In: Bouchard, C.; Shephard, R.; Stephens, T.; Sutton, J.; McPherson, B., eds. Exercise, fitness, and health: A consensus of current knowledge. Champaign, IL: Human Kinetics; 1990:399-405.
61. Stephens, T.; Craig, C. The well-being of Canadians: Highlights of the 1988 Campbell's survey. Ottawa: Canadian Fitness and Lifestyle Research Institute; 1990.
62. Summerson, J.; Konen, J.; Dignan, M. Association between exercise and other preventive health behaviors among diabetics. Public Health Rep. 106:543-547; 1991.
63. Taylor, C.; Houston-Miller, N.; Haskell, W.; Debusk, R. Smoking cessation after myocardial infarction: The effects of exercise training. Addict. Behav. 13:331-335; 1988.
64. Terre, L.; Drabman, R.; Meydrech, E. Relationships among children's health-related behaviors: A multivariate, developmental perspective. Prev. Med. 19:134-146; 1990.
65. Tuomilehto, J.; Marti, B.; Salonen, J.; Virtala, E.; Lahti, T.; Puska, P. Leisure-time physical activity is inversely related to risk factors for coronary heart disease in middle-aged Finnish men. Eur. Heart J. 8:1047-1055; 1987.
66. U.S. Dept. of Health and Human Services. Highlights from wave I of the national survey of personal health practices and consequences. Vital Health Stat. 15; 1981.
66a. Walker, S.N.; Sechrist, K.R.; Pender, N.J. The health-promoting lifestyle profile: development and psychometric characteristics. Nursing Research. 36:76-81; 1991.
67. Wood, P.; Haskell, S.; Blair, S.; Williams, P.; Krauss, R.; Lindgren, F.; Albers, P.; Ho, P.; Farquhar, J. Increased exercise levels and plasma lipoprotein concentrations: A one-year, randomized, controlled study in sedentary, middle-aged men. Metabolism. 32:31-39; 1983.

Chapter 37

Physical Activity and Psychosocial Outcomes

Edward McAuley

Physical Activity and Psychosocial Outcomes

Whereas exercise and physical activity have been consistently and reliably implicated in the reduction of all-cause mortality (6), cardiovascular disease, and a host of other debilitating conditions (9), their effects on psychological health and well-being are less clear. Although many studies extol the almost intuitive psychological benefits of physical activity, just as many fail to find any association. Apart from a host of methodological and conceptual problems, inherent in this equivocality is the lack of congruence among operational definitions of not only physical activity but also psychosocial outcomes or psychological health. Only one chapter (10) and a commentary (79) from the last consensus proceedings (9) examined the psychological effects of exercise and physical activity. As is relatively typical of the extant literature, these chapters focused primarily on the anxiolytic, stress-dampening, and antidepressant effects of exercise and physical activity. However, the consensus definition of health from the previous symposium specifically identifies the physical, psychological, and social domains of the construct varying along *both* a positive and negative continuum. Therefore, it is encouraging to note that the content of this consensus document reflects a healthy increase in the effects of physical activity on aspects of psychological health and functioning, including anxiety and reduction (42), depression (60), cognitive functioning (85), and psychosocial outcomes.

In Figure 37.1 the psychosocial outcomes associated with exercise and physical activity are organized in terms of the valence of their association. Exercise appears to have a negative relationship with anxiety and depression (i.e., more activity, less stress, depression, anxiety) and positive relationship with self-perceptions (e.g., esteem, mastery, efficacy), mood, and affect. It is the positive psychosocial benefits of physical activity that will be considered in this chapter.

Physical Activity and Self-Perceptions

Psychosocial outcomes as discussed herein are restricted to perceptions of self-esteem, psychological well-being, and self-efficacy. Other than the sheer volume of the literature, the rationale for this decision is based on the following: (a) Self-esteem is commonly acknowledged as the psychological variable having most potential for benefit from physical activity; (b) emotional/psychological well-being, as represented by positive affective responsivity, has received comparatively little attention in the literature; and (c) self-efficacy perceptions are frequently identified as having mediating effects on health behavior but, as it is argued here, are representative of distinct outcomes in and of themselves. Moreover, efficacy cognitions are theorized to be influential in the generation of self-esteem and affective responses.

Exercise, Physical Activity, and Self-Esteem

Although a host of psychological variables have been identified as being influenced by exercise and physical activity, a number of authors and reviewers have suggested that such participation may have the greatest benefit potential for the enhancement of self-esteem (26,37). Self-esteem can broadly be defined as encompassing the favorable views one holds regarding one's self. Although self-esteem is generally considered the evaluative

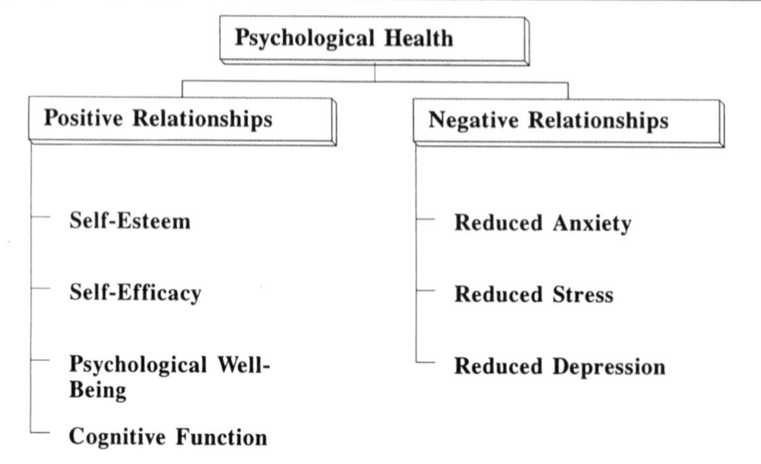

Figure 37.1 Psychosocial outcomes.

component of self-concept (73), the two terms are often used synonymously and will be in this review. As self-esteem is considered a focal aspect of psychological health and well-being (74), it is not surprising that a considerable corpus of literature exists that attempts to establish the link between physical activity participation and self-esteem. However, it should be noted that the majority of this literature has examined *global* self-esteem.

Overview of the Findings From Recent Reviews

Three major reviews published in this area are considered. Sonstroem (80) and Doan and Scherman (19) adopted the traditional approach of the narrative review, whereas Gruber (30) employed meta-analysis to determine the effects of physical activity participation on self-esteem. Each of the reviews employed typical methods for collection of studies (hand and computer searches, personal files, etc.) and the general characteristics of and findings emanating from these reviews are summarized in Table 37.1. It should be noted that these reviews focus primarily (19), if not solely (30, 80), on the physical activity/self-esteem relationship, unlike other reviews that merely include this aspect as one of many psychological effects of physical activity (26, 69).

Study populations across the research reviewed are approximately equally divided between adults (48%) and children (52%), and one review (30) focused entirely on the effect of physical activity on self-esteem development in children. Although all three reviews provide information of varying degrees regarding the nature of the physical activity/exercise intervention, little consistency exists in the presentation of this information. In none of these cases are the results particularly convincing that self-esteem gains are associated with concomitant gains in fitness. In one review (19) only 36% of the studies showed fitness and self-esteem gains. However, the effect size for aerobic activity was twice that for other activities in the case of children's studies (30). Taken together, approximately 60% of the studies reviewed indicate a positive association between physical activity participation and increases in self-esteem.

In Gruber's meta-analysis (30), the positive association between physical activity and self-esteem in children is moderate across studies, appears to be consistent regardless of length of activity program, and is twice as strong in the case of simple controlled studies than in complex, multivariate, multifactorial studies. Sonstroem's review (80), is a very thorough treatment of 16 studies, provides a clear picture of programmatic and subject characteristics, while analyzing findings according to the rigor of methodological design. The Doan and Scherman (19) review is perhaps the weakest for several reasons. First, it reports only one study conducted since 1980. Second, it does not focus entirely on self-esteem but rather on an amalgam of personality/esteem variables, and consequently only self-esteem studies are discussed here. Finally, it is desperately short on details regarding subject and program characteristics, making comparison with other reviews difficult.

Table 37.1 Summary of Characteristics and Conclusions of Previous Reviews of the Effects of Exercise and Physical Activity on Self-Esteem

Authors	*N* of studies and characteristics	Program characteristics	Outcomes
Doan & Scherman (19)	22 studies; 68% with adults, 32% with children	No details were provided of frequency or duration of programs or sample sizes. Fitness gains were demonstrated in 76% of studies reviewed, and 67% of studies had control groups.	Self-esteem increased in 43% of the studies. 36% showed improved self-esteem and fitness, 7% improved self-esteem but not fitness, 41% improved fitness but not self-esteem, and 16% had neither fitness or esteem gains.
Gruber (30)	27 studies; all with children; meta-analysis conducted by multiple categories; *M* of 113 subjects per study	55.6% of programs were gymnastics/motor skill development, 22.2% sports, 22.2% aerobic activity. *M* duration of programs was 15.25 weeks, frequency 2×/week.	Self-esteem was increased in 61% of studies. Overall effect size = .43. Effect sizes similar for short vs. long programs. Larger effect (.89) for physical fitness/aerobic activity than for other activities (.41).
Sonstroem (80)	16 studies; 25% children and 75% adult; 37.5% classified as special populations (e.g., prisoners, rehab, alcoholics, etc.); *M* of 80 subjects per study	44% of programs were aerobic activity only, 37% aerobic plus conditioning/strength training, and 19% classified as other physical activity (for example, military training, strength training). Programs had a duration of 11.75 weeks with a *M* frequency of 3.3×/week.	Self-esteem increased in 75% of the studies. Association was particularly strong in those subjects with initially low self-esteem.

Study Commonalities

Although physical activity is associated with self-esteem in approximately 60% of studies reviewed, the majority of studies have methodological, design, statistical, and conceptual flaws. For example, from a methodological perspective, few studies have employed techniques to control for response distortion or the influence of sociodemographic factors. Statistical treatment of studies ranges from adequate to abysmal. Little effort has been made to statistically control for possible contaminants or external influences (e.g., demographics), to adjust probability levels when multiple analyses are conducted, or to employ multivariate analyses when dependent variables are related (19, 80). Moreover, it would appear that subjects who stand to gain most from physical activity in terms of self-esteem development are those who have poor self-esteem initially. From a conceptual standpoint, the relative stability of global self-esteem is rarely considered, and accordingly the possibility that exercise/activity effects may be better highlighted if measured by domain-specific esteem measures has been ignored.

The conclusions drawn from the reviews reported previously appear to suggest that the robustness of the often-accepted relationship between physical activity and self-esteem is questionable. Methodological and design problems associated with a vast number of studies (19, 80) make conclusive statements difficult. More recent studies demonstrate similar equivocality (e.g., 1,27,49,50). Most research studies reported in the critical reviews, as well as representative recent studies, have at least one singular feature in common: the reliance on global assessment of self-esteem.

Multidimensional Self-Esteem and Physical Activity

Adopting the perspective of Shavelson and his colleagues (78), a number of scholars have called for the adoption of multidimensional assessments of self-esteem (28,51,53,80), in which *physical self-esteem* is one of several first-order dimensions of a higher or second-order factor comprised of global self-esteem. These dimensions are proposed to be influenced by further subareas relevant to the specific dimension.

Marsh and his colleagues (51) have demonstrated that although athletes have a significantly higher self-concept of physical activity than their nonathletic counterparts, they do not significantly differ along other dimensions (e.g., academic, appearance, interpersonal relations) (51). Moreover, Marsh and Peart (53) report physical fitness to be significantly correlated with physical ability self-esteem but not with other dimensions of esteem. In a cross-sectional study comparing athletes and nonathletes (90), physical self-esteem was the only dimension to differentiate between these groups with neither group differing on general self-esteem. Of particular note here was that the authors also assessed the *degree of importance* that subjects placed in the various domains of self-concept and reported athletes to consider physical ability as more important than nonathletes. The role that importance plays in development of self-esteem in the physical domain has largely been ignored.

Fox and Corbin (28) have developed the Physical Self-Perception Profile, which posits that global self-esteem is related to physical self-worth (esteem) at the domain level and that underlying this level are perceptions of physical conditioning, attractive body, physical strength, and sports competence. The measure and the relations theorized among its components have been validated in college-aged samples, and the psychometric properties appear adequate. Finally, Sonstroem and Morgan (81) have recently presented a model of exercise and self-esteem that proposes that physical activity influences perceived physical efficacy, which, in turn, influences perceptions of physical competence. Physical competence is proposed to have a direct effect on global self-worth/esteem and an indirect effect through perceptions of physical acceptance. Like Fox and Corbin (28), Sonstroem and Morgan also underscore the necessity of examining perceived importance of physical activity when testing the proposed relationships.

In conclusion, some evidence suggests that, in spite of a plethora of methodological concerns, a positive association between physical activity and self-esteem exists. It appears that the adoption of multidimensional theoretical frameworks, appropriately robust designs, measures pertinent to domain-specific esteem, and assessment of relative importance of physical activity participation to the individual represent factors likely to enhance our understanding of this relationship.

Exercise and Psychological Well-Being

Psychological well-being (17) is generally acknowledged to comprise both negative and positive emotional or affective states. Traditionally these states are dichotomized in terms of psychological distress (anger, anxiety, depression, negative affect) and psychological well-being (positive affect) (83). However, a review of 81 studies examining the psychological effects of exercise (43) revealed only one study (38) that focused on outcome variables other than anxiety, depression, personality, mood, or self-concept. Similarly, Hughes (37) focused his review on study outcomes of mood, personality, and cognition subsuming under the *mood* category the specific outcomes of depression, anxiety, anger, and irritability; one study (70) assessed morale, an outcome that might liberally be construed as positive. Even the NIMH consensus panel (62) appears to conceive of positive mental health and well-being as largely being the absence or reduction of *negative* symptomology. As noted earlier, the psychological dimension of health has positive, as well as negative, aspects. In keeping with this sentiment, Folkins and Sime (26) have suggested that the extant evidence examining the hypothesis that psychological well-being is associated with exercise and fitness has largely been based on studies examining stress-related emotion, primarily anxiety. To gain an alternative perspective on the physical activity/psychological health relationship, in this chapter studies examining the effects of physical activity on positive affect are reviewed.

Twenty-three published articles are reviewed in this chapter. Two primary criteria for inclusion were employed: (a) Authors clearly identified emotional/psychological well-being as a study outcome, and (b) dependent measures included a measure of affective responsivity other than anxiety, depression, stress reactivity, or a mood-states measure composed primarily of negative scales (e.g., Profile of Mood States [POMS]). The 23 articles are detailed in Table 37.2 and subsequently discussed with respect to subject and program, design, and assessment attributes. It should be noted that the 23 reports actually comprise 27 studies with Stephens (82) detailing findings from 4 population-based studies. In addition, 2 studies (34,75) present very similar findings based on what appear to be the same data in two separate publications. The overall conclusion to be drawn from the collective findings in Table 37.2 is that the majority of the studies (69%) suggest physical activity is positively associated with psychological well-being.

Table 37.2 Effects of Exercise and Physical Activity on Emotional/Psychological Well-Being (PWB)

Authors	*N*	Age	Objective	Program characteristics	Measures of PWB	Outcome
McAuley & Courneya (57)	42 males, 46 females	53.0	Effects of preexisting efficacy on in-task exercise-induced affect	No control group; submaximal bicycle ergometer test	Feeling Scale, self-efficacy	More efficacious individuals reported more positive affect.
McAuley (55)	37 males, 43 females	53.7	Relationship among exercise, efficacy, attributions, and affect	Within subjects design, midpoint of 20-week walking program, 3×/week, 1-hour, 65–75% maximal heart rate	Self-efficacy; positive affect	Exercise participation influenced positive affect through the mediation of self-efficacy and attributions.
Hawkins & Duncan (33)	30 males, 96 females	78.0	Relationship between exercise, sleep, health practices, and quality of life	None; cross-sectional assessment of variables	Quality of life	Quality of life mediated by current and past exercise
Kendzierski & DeCarlo (40)	23 males, 14 females	—	Relationship between choice of physical activity and enjoyment	Jogging on minitrampoline and riding stationary bike for 15 min; 2 sessions	Physical Activity Enjoyment Scale (PACES)	68% of subjects' choices influenced by enjoyment
Blumenthal et al. (7)	50 males, 51 females	67.0	Long-term effects of exercise on psychological function	6-month program of aerobic exercise, 3×/week, 70% MHR	Anxiety; depression; positive affect; negative affect	Significant increase in mood for men and decrease for women
Wiklund et al. (89)	42 males	59.5	Relationship of quality of life and exercise tolerance	Graded exercise test employing Bruce protocol. Patients exercised until they reported chest pain/dyspnea.	General Well-Being Index; quality of life	Treadmill time negatively related to depression; no other relationships
Brown (11)	37 males, 73 females	—	Effects of fitness as a stress buffer	Self-reported physical activity; estimated aerobic capacity	Life stress; negative affect	Less fit and stressed subjects had more visits to health facility than fit and stressed subjects.

(continued)

Table 37.2 *(Continued)*

Authors	*N*	Age	Objective	Program characteristics	Measures of PWB	Outcome
Emergy & Gatz (22)	8 males, 48 females	72.0	Effects of exercise program on psychological function	Random assignment to exercise, social control group, or waitlist control; 12-week conditioning program, 3×/week, 1 hr, 70% MHR	Depression; anxiety; happiness; locus of control	No significant change in any of the variables
Lennox et al. (44)	18 males, 29 females	43.0 47.0	Effects of aerobic activity on nondepressed adults	Random assignment to walk/jog, volleyball/weight-training, or waitlist control group; 13-week program, 50–60 min, 3×/week	Depression; positive affect; negative affect	Fitness gains in the activity groups but no effects on affect or depression
Norris et al. (64)	77 males	20–50	Effects of exercise on life stress and psychological well-being	Nonrandom assignment to aerobic, anaerobic, or control groups; 10 weeks, 3×/week, 30–40 min of activity	Job stress; life quality; general health	Exercise groups had significantly higher life quality and general health than control group. Psychological varibles not related to fitness
Moses et al. (63)	20 males, 55 females	33.8	Effects of exercise training on mental well-being	10-week exercise program randomized to high activity (15–60 min at 60–90% MHR); moderate activity (20 min at 60% MHR); attention group (30 min of flexibility and strength exercise at 50% MHR); or a waitlist control group	Mood (POMS); coping	Enhanced mood and coping responses for moderate- but not high-exercise group. Similar increases in coping at 3-month follow-up
King et al. (41)	60 males, 60 females	48.0	Effects of home-based exercise program on affect and psychological well-being	Random assignment to aerobic exercise or control group; home-based walking program, 5×/week, 65%–77% peak HR, 47-54 min	14-item rating scale of well-being	Exercise reported greater satisfaction with shape, appearance, weight, and perceived fitness

Hardy & Rejeski Study 3 (32)	30 males	19.5	Relationship between affect and perceived exertion during physical work	Acute bout of bicycle ergometry at 30%, 60%, and 90% of maximal aerobic power in three successive 4-min stages	Feeling Scale; RPE; postexercise affect recall	More negative affect as work load increased; no relationship between in-task affect and postaffect recall in 60% work load but related at 30% and 90% work load
Dowall et al. (20)	27 males, 27 females	31.0	Relationship between aerobic fitness, activity level, and psychological well-being	No program; cross-sectional assessment of fitness and affect; assessment of fitness with 12-min walk/run and step test	Positive affect; negative affect	No relationship between well-being and fitness; however fitness and activity were reported as not being important to sample.
Wetzler & Ursano (88)	5,962 males, 356 females	18+	Relationship between health practices and psychological well-being in activity-duty air force personnel	No program; cross-sectional self-report health survey	Positive affect; negative affect	Minor relationships between all health practices and well-being. Active males and less active females had higher well-being.
Seggar et al. (77)	323 females	—	Relationship between physical activity and psychological well-being	No program; cross-sectional known groups survey; all assessments concurrent	Positive affect	Degree of activity participation not related to happiness, contentment, and life satisfaction
Gauvin (29)	54 males, 68 females	32.7	Relationship between activity level and subjective well-being	No program; survey of autonomous exercisers, fitness program members, program dropouts, and nonexercisers	Positive affect; negative affect; life satisfaction	No relationship between activity level and subjective well-being
Stephens (82)	6,913 23,791 3,025 22,250	25-74 15+ 20-64 10+	Validity of the physical activity/mental health relationship in four population studies	No program; secondary data analysis of four large-population surveys	Affect; balance (+/−); depression; general well-being; health opinion; Blue-Cheer Index	Greater levels of physical activity associated with less depression, more positive affect and general well-being, and less negative affect. Relationship stronger for older than younger age groups and females rather than males. Choice of activity or quality of item may influence any psychological benefits of exercise.

(continued)

Table 37.2 *(Continued)*

Authors	*N*	Age	Objective	Program characteristics	Measures of PWB	Outcome
Brown & Siegel (13)	212 females	13.8	Effects of exercise and stress on illness	No program; retrospective recall of activity participation	Stress Illness Rating Scale	Effects of stress on illness moderated by vigorous activity
Ross & Hayes (75)	401	18–83	Relationship between psychological well-being, sociodemographic variables, and exercise	None; telephone survey of an Illinois probability sample	Langner Index of PWB (actually anxiety/ depression items)	Moderate effect of exercise participation patterns on psychological well-being when controlling for sociodemographic influences
Brown & Lawton (12)	220	11–17	Role played by exercise in stress responses of adolescent females	No program; retrospective recall of events and activity participation	Stress; life events; Depression Illness Rating Scale	High stress has negative impact on well-being of low exercisers but no significant effect on high exercisers.
Blumenthal et al. (8)	6 males, 18 females	69.3	Effect of aerobic conditioning on psychological status	No control group; comparison of young-old and old-old; 11-week program, 3×/week, 30 min, 70%–85% MHR	Moods (POMS); temperament; Type A	40% 50% of subjects reported increases in general psychological health.
Carter (14)	216	18+	Relationship between exercise participation and happiness	No program; survey of activity levels	Single-item happiness measure	Level of exercise participation positively correlated with current and global happiness

Subject and Program Characteristics

Approximately 74% of studies include both males and females and sample predominantly adult subjects. In general, few studies clarify whether activity effects on psychological well-being are differentially influenced by sex of subject or age cohort. However, Stephens (82) reports that the exercise/psychological health relationship is stronger for women and older age groups than for men and younger individuals. Whereas a large literature exists examining physical activity effects on self-esteem in children (30), the few studies located (18%) are primarily the work of one author (11,12,13) and concentrate upon the effects of physical fitness as a buffer of stress effects on illness. Of particular note in the studies reviewed here was the obvious attempt to examine the hypothesized relationships in the *normal* population. Much of the extant literature in this area has focused on clinical, and often male, populations (54).

Study Designs

Experimental design varies dramatically across the studies reviewed: 23% comprise large population studies or representative population samples (34,75,82,88), 31% incorporate cross-sectional retrospective survey studies, 31% are intervention studies, and 15% involve acute bouts of activity. Of the eight (31%) studies involving exercise interventions, 62.5% randomly assigned subjects and 75% employed control groups. The majority (69%) of these intervention studies report positive effects of physical activity on psychological well-being; however, it is not clear whether fitness change plays a role in this association or whether vigorous activity is necessary for affective responsivity to take place. Indeed, most of the interventions reporting increases in positive affect do so for moderate-intensity activity programs (41,57,63).

It is tempting to conclude that the diverse methodologies employed in the studies reported here, coupled with relative consistency of findings and support from secondary analysis of large data bases, provide support for the generalizability of the physical activity/psychological well-being relationship. However, even population data, such as those presented by Stephens (82), although appearing impressive, have the typical problems of self-selection and the cross-sectional, correlational data, and such data do not allow for any authoritative statements regarding the temporal nature of causality (79). Only two studies report adequate follow-up data. One (7) reports mixed results, and the other (63) reports continued enhanced function at 3-month follow-up, but only for moderate-intensity activity.

Assessment

In large part there appears to be little conceptual reasoning behind the choice of affective measures, which range from single-item global measures of happiness to multidimensional measures of general psychological health and quality of life. In total, 33 measures are employed to assess aspects of psychological well-being other than depression, anxiety, and mood (POMS). These measures can be categorized as *positive affect* (42.4%), *quality/satisfaction with life* (18.2%), *negative affect* (15.1%), *life stress* (12.1%), *affect balance* (6.1%), *coping* (3%), and *enjoyment* (3%). Of these measures, positive affect does appear to be more consistently linked to physical activity.

Few measures have been developed for, or adequately validated in, the physical activity domain. Measures such as the POMS are too unwieldy and onerous for frequent assessments in normal populations (41), and more importantly they were developed in primarily clinical populations. Moreover, many of the measures employed may simply not be sensitive enough to pick up exercise-induced affective change (21,41). In the present review two measures of exercise-related affect were located, the single-item Feeling Scale (32), which assesses the basic good-bad core of emotion, and the Physical Activity Enjoyment Scale (40).

Affect is comprised of at least two dimensions, positive (PA) and negative (NA) affect, that appear to be both conceptually and empirically orthogonal (87). Watson et al. (87) have developed the Positive and Negative Affect Schedule (PANAS) to assess these constructs; however, this measure awaits application and validation in physical activity settings. Briefer measures of affect, such as the Affect Grid (76), hold promise for multiple assessments of affect, but the nature of the response format does not lend itself particularly well to exercise-testing situations, in which subjects are not free to wield paper and pencil. Finally, McAuley and Courneya (58) have developed a brief three-dimensional Exercise-Induced Affect Scale (EIAS) that assesses NA, PA, and fatigue/energy. Initial psychometric properties are promising, and the fact that the measure is brief and specific to exercise/physical activity may assure sufficient sensitivity to detect meaningful exercise-induced change in psychological well-being in future endeavors.

Exercise, Physical Activity, and Self-Efficacy

Self-efficacy expectations concern the individual's beliefs in his or her capabilities to execute necessary courses of action to satisfy situational demands (4). These judgments of capabilities have been demonstrated to be important determinants of the choice of activities in which people engage, the amount of effort they expend on such activities, and the degree of persistence they demonstrate in the face of failure or aversive stimuli. Efficacy cognitions are also postulated to influence thought processes and affective reactions (4) and have consistently been shown to be important determinants of physical activity and exercise behavior (56), as well as of social, clinical, and health-related behaviors (4,67). Individuals with high self-efficacy expectations tend to approach more challenging tasks, put forth more effort, and persist longer in the face of aversive stimuli. When faced with stressful stimuli, individuals with low self-efficacy tend to give up, attribute failure internally, and experience greater anxiety or depression (3).

As a psychological variable, self-efficacy cognitions, by and large, either have been studied as determinants of exercise behavior or have been identified as potential mediating mechanisms that might explain the effects of exercise on various aspects of psychological functioning (68). Indeed, Rodin (72) has identified a sense of control over the life course as a critical variable influencing physical and psychosocial functioning. Therefore, it is deemed important to determine that exercise and physical activity do indeed enhance perceptions of efficacy as a precursor to suggesting its viability in mediating other physical and psychosocial outcomes.

Several computer and human searches and the personal files of the author resulted in 16 articles being retrieved that met the following conditions: (a) Outcome variable was self-efficacy; (b) study attempted to influence self-efficacy through exercise or physical activity; and (c) mean values were available for efficacy over time (pre- and postintervention).

Table 37.3 details the characteristics of each of these studies in terms of authors, subjects, and exercise stimuli, and Table 37.4 reports study outcomes and provides a brief commentary on each. In general, the effects of information provided by physical activity involvement appear consistent and relatively robust across study designs and populations. That is, exercise participation positively influences perceptions of physical capabilities and both acute bouts of activity and longer term participation appear to have positive effects (24,25,57,59,86).

Study Populations

The majority of the studies (62%) reviewed examined physical activity effects on efficacy perceptions in both males and females primarily of middle age and older. However, only one study (59) reports details regarding difference in responses between males and females; another (57) reports initial differences but statistically controls for them in regression analyses. Forty-four of the studies reviewed focus on clinical populations, two reports (same subjects with long-term follow-up) focus on stressed individuals, and the remainder target apparently healthy, but generally sedentary, adults. Clearly, all of these populations are likely to have reduced percepts of physical/exercise efficacy, and therefore exercise bouts are likely to have strong effects.

Because most adults in North America are either sedentary or intermittently active (18) and the number of impaired and aging individuals is increasing (71), the employment of exercise and physical activity participation to enhance perceptions of personal efficacy appears warranted. Given the consistency with which efficacy is reported as a determinant of *confirmed* exercise and health behavior (57, 67), the reciprocally determining nature of efficacy and behavior appears worthy of future study. Moreover, if exercise is to be championed for its psychological effects, the nature of efficacy as a mechanism influencing psychological health needs to be determined (23,55,68).

Study Designs

Half (50%) of the studies reviewed employed randomized assignment into treatment or control groups and report exercise effects on efficacy that are comparable to the less stringently designed studies. The bulk of the studies without control groups employed within-subjects, pre- and post-exercise stimuli/intervention designs examining exercise effects as a function of relatively short (generally, until the appearance of limiting symptomology) exercise bouts. Given the similarity of results and the diversity of designs, it does appear that information processed as a function of exercise performance has a relatively consistent effect of enhancing one's sense of personal capabilities.

In those studies employing an exercise intervention program (69%), the program length varied from 4 weeks (15) to 20 weeks (59) with a mean

Table 37.3 Exercise and Physical Activity Effects on Perceptions of Self-Efficacy: Subject and Program Characteristics

Authors	Subjects		Objective	Type	Program	
	N	Age			Duration	Control group
McAuley & Courneya (57)	46 males, 42 females	53.4	Effects of acute bout of exercise on efficacy in sedentary middle-aged adults	Bicycle ergometer	Until 70% predicted MHR	None
McAuley et al. (59)	81 males/females	54.0	Efficacy responses as a function of both acute exercise bouts and long-term exercise training	Walking	20 weeks	None
Gulanick (31)	28 males, 12 females	57.7	Comparison of rehab teaching and exercise testing with or without exercise training on the efficacy of post-myocardial infarction or cardiac surgery patients	?	5 weeks	Random assignment to teaching plus exercise testing, teaching plus exercise testing with exercise training, or routine care control group
Oldridge & Rogowski (66)	38 males, 13 females	56.9	Effects of standard education/counseling in combination with exercise rehab on self-efficacy of cardiac patients	Ward walking vs. ergometer/treadmill work	4 weeks	Ward ambulation group or dedicated exercise group; no control
Toshima et al. (86)	87 males, 32 females	62.6	Compared comprehensive rehab program and education control program on exercise endurance, health status, and self-efficacy of COPD patients	Rehab program with exercise component (walking)	8 weeks	Subjects randomized to treatment group or control group
Long & Haney (47)	61 females	40.0	Effects of exercise vs. progressive relaxation on A-trait and self-efficacy	Jogging	8 weeks	Progressive relaxation
Long & Haney (48)	39 females	40.0	Long-term (14-month) follow-up of treatment effects due to exercise and relaxation training	None	None	None
Holloway et al. (36)	27 females	16.0	Effects of strength training on self-efficacy, general confidence, and body attitudes	Strength training	12 weeks	Nonrandom assignment to weight training, mild activity control, or no-activity control groups
Ewart et al. (24)	43 males	55.0	Effects of adding circuit weight training to a jogging program on self-efficacy of subjects with coronary artery disease	Walk/jog plus weight training or volleyball	10 weeks	Subjects randomized to weight-training treatment or volleyball control groups

(continued)

Table 37.3 ***(Continued)***

Authors	Subjects		Objective	Type	Program	
	N	Age			Duration	Control group
Taylor et al. (84)	30 males, 30 females	52.0	To examine effects of treadmill testing on self-efficacy of wives of post-myocardial infarction patients	Graded treadmill testing	Limiting symptomology	Wives randomized to (a) watching husbands engage in exercise test, (b) participating in treadmill walking, or (c) or viewing of husbands treadmill test (control)
Long (46)	10 males, 35 females	—	15-month follow-up of maintenance effects of stress inoculation and aerobic conditioning on stress and efficacy			Random assignment of treatments and waitlist control group
Long (45)	25 males, 48 females	39.9	Compared aerobic conditioning and stress inoculation in the reduction of stress and enhancement of self-efficacy	Walk/jog (90-min sessions)	10 weeks	Random assignment to two treatments or waitlist control group
Hogan & Santomeir (35)	18 males, 20 females	72.3 65.5	Effects of mastering swim skills on older adults' efficacy	Learn-to-swim program	5 weeks	Nonrandomized; no contact
Kaplan et al. (39)	22 males, 38 females	64.8	Effects of specific vs. generalized efficacy on behavior change in COPD patients	Home-based walking program	3 months	Attention control vs. cognitive/behavioral compliance program
Corbin et al. (15)	39 females	29.9	Effects of success-oriented vicarious modeling of exercise	Aerobic dance	4 weeks	Sport slide presentation
Ewart et al. (25)	40 males	52.0	Effects of graded exercise testing on self-efficacy in post-myocardial infarction patients	Treadmill	Limiting symptomology or 10-mm drop in systolic blood pressure	None

Table 37.4 Exercise and Physical Activity Effects on Perceptions of Self-Efficacy: Study Outcomes and Commentaries

Authors	Efficacy outcome	Comment	Follow-up
McAuley & Courneya (57)	Significant increase in efficacy even with relatively short bout of activity	Pretest efficacy predicted in-task affect which, in turn, influenced postexercise efficacy	None
McAuley et al. (55)	Physical efficacy increased as a function of preprogram graded exercise test, long-term exercise program, and postprogram graded exercise test on efficacy	Males initially more efficacious than females; however, postprogram females as efficacious or more so than males	None
Gulanick (31)	All groups improved efficacy from discharge to 4-week recovery and continued to improve over next 5 weeks of intervention. Both treatment groups had significantly higher efficacy than control at 4 weeks and remained higher at 9 weeks	Possible effects of all patient involvement in rehab program, prior to discharge on efficacy; ceiling effects possible on efficacy measures	None
Oldridge & Rogowski (66)	Significant improvement for both groups in efficacy for household and daily activities and returning to work	Not clear whether efficacy effects are due to exercise treatments or simply the resumption of daily activities postdischarge	28-day measurement might be considered as a follow-up
Toshima et al. (86)	Rehabilitation program participants demonstrated significant gains in fitness and efficacy	First randomized experimental trials to show benefits of exercise component in a clinical group beyond 3 months	Efficacy increases for treatment group maintained
Holloway et al. (36)	Greater efficacy in weight-training group than control groups posttest; also increased efficacy with respect to more general capabilities	Small sample size and nonrandomization of subjects weaken results	None
Long & Haney (47)	Both aerobic exercise and relaxation improved efficacy	Assessed general efficacy, therefore would not expect between-group difference	8 weeks, efficacy maintained
Long & Haney (48)	Efficacy increases and anxiety decreases maintained for both groups	Maintenance of treatment effect on general efficacy may have implications for other psychological health outcomes	Results represent 14-month follow-up
Ewart et al. (24)	Initial testing produced significant increases in efficacy specific to the location tested. Weight-training treatment enhanced strength efficacy whereas control group did not. No effects on walk/jog efficacy for either group	Specificity of information effects demonstrated	No follow-up beyond 10-week program
Taylor et al. (84)	Posttreatment wives' efficacy significantly enhanced in treadmill participation group. This, in turn, enhanced the value of cardiac counseling	Exposure to exercise testing may have influence on type and nature of social support being given by spouses of post-MI patients.	Combined efficacy of patients and spouses predictive of exercise performance at 11 and 26 weeks

(continued)

Table 37.4 *(Continued)*

Authors	Efficacy outcome	Comment	Follow-up
Long (45,46)	Efficacy increased in aerobic treatment group and stress-inoculation group but not in control group	Use of an efficacy measure nonspecific to exercise may have masked any unique effects of exercise on efficacy	Efficacy maintained at 3-months and at 15-month follow-up
Hogan & Santomeir (35)	Significant increase in efficacy in treatment group	Difficult to generalize due to design problems	None
Corbin et al. (15)	Treatment increased sport/physical activity confidence	Control lower to begin with	None
Kaplan et al. (39)	Treatment groups (cognitive/behavior modification) made significantly greater gains than control group.	Efficacy gains differential with treatment groups. Behavioral component (goals, behavioral contracts) had greatest efficacy gains.	None
Ewart et al. (25)	Physical efficacy increased post-treadmill performance. Proportionate increase was greater for those tasks similar to exercise. Counseling by a physician and nurse produced a significant additive effect, particularly in dissimilar tasks.	Study findings show support for specific and general effects on efficacy.	Changes in efficacy scores were related to subsequent reports of home-based physical activity.

length of 8.4 weeks. Whereas both acute and long-term effects of exercise on efficacy have been demonstrated, it is unclear how this relationship is affected by changes in physiological function. Only a few of the studies reported here have examined this relationship, and although there appears to be a positive relationship between the two (24,59, 84), such findings need replication and extension in larger, nonclinical, and diverse populations.

Follow-Up

Definitive statements regarding the long-term maintenance of exercise-enhanced efficacy are difficult to make. Three studies report follow-up assessments (46,48,86) and indicate that efficacy was maintained at 4- (86), 15- (46), and 18- (48) month postintervention follow-up. However, no significant increases beyond program termination were reported. At this time the long-term effects of the maintenance of exercise-induced efficacy are not known.

Assessment

Two issues should be briefly addressed with respect to the assessment of self-efficacy and physical fitness. With few exceptions (15, 45, 47), the studies reviewed here have generally measured efficacy cognitions within the basic guidelines proposed by Bandura (3). That is, items that represent generative capabilities with respect to physical tasks (e.g., lifting, walking, jogging) are presented in a hierarchical fashion. The three studies that fail to take this approach measure efficacy as a form of general sport/physical activity confidence (15) or as a form of general confidence across a broad array of domains. Although these latter measures might be criticized from an efficacy perspective, they are still positively influenced by exercise participation. This suggests further testimony to the ability of physical activity to enhance both specific and more generalizable forms of mastery cognitions.

With respect to the measurement of fitness, it is important to examine this aspect in light of whether the study was an exercise intervention, an acute exercise bout, or a follow-up report. Four of eight (50%) interventions report adequate assessment of aerobic capacity, either submaximal or maximal graded exercise testing (24, 39, 59, 86); Toshima et al. (86) also measured endurance at 6-month follow-up. All four studies (24,57,59,84) examining effects of acute bouts of activity used standard graded exercise testing as the exercise stimuli, necessitating only one-time measurement. Moreover, all of these studies report a significant positive relationship between degree of physical capacity and perceived physical capability. Two studies (46,48) were published as long-term follow-up reports, but neither assessed aerobic capacity. This is unfortunate, because any maintenance effects with respect to efficacy could be correlated with maintenance of physiological function.

In conclusion, the evidence suggests that the effects of exercise and physical activity on perceptions of personal efficacy are consistent and robust. Moreover, these effects appear to hold for both acute and long-term activity bouts and across gender and age.

Important Research Questions and Directions

The effects of physical activity participation on self-perceptions of esteem, efficacy, and psychological well-being have been reviewed and documented. Several research questions and directions of importance specific to these relationships need to be addressed over the next decade. First, where it is reliably documented that relationships between physical activity and psychosocial outcomes exist, it will be necessary to determine what factors or processes underlie these relationships. Whereas biological (e.g., changes in body temperature, plasma catecholamine, endorphin, and monoamine levels) explanations have been proposed, limited evidence exists to support such hypotheses. Similarly, psychological variables such as self-efficacy and distraction (2) have been frequently cited as potential mediators, but the empirical confirmation is scant. Although in this review self-efficacy is proposed as a psychosocial outcome of physical activity participation, it has also been demonstrated to be a *determinant* of affective responses to physical activity (55, 57), is proposed to underlie self-esteem development in the physical activity domain (81), and has reliably been shown to mediate levels of depression, stress, and anxiety in other domains of functioning (5). Although self-efficacy expectations are known to be implicated in a broad tapestry of psychobiological function, the challenge for scientists in this area will be to pinpoint the degree of interaction taking place between such cognitive, biological, neurological, and socioenvironmental influences.

Future research efforts must demonstrate consistency in methodology, definitions, and measurement if we are to further understand the physical activity/psychological health relationship. Many of the assumptions and conclusions drawn herein are based on diverse measures and methods, and in spite of recent improvements, we simply are not at the point where we can make conclusive statements about the relationships in question. This dilemma results from too few longitudinal, randomized designs, inadequate follow-up, inconsistent definitions, and conceptually and psychometrically suspect measures. Until such problems are satisfactorily addressed, we will be unable to design appropriate interventions in this area.

The role played by fitness, as opposed to physical activity, in the enhancement of psychosocial functioning is difficult to determine. Whether psychological benefits can result, and what kind of benefits do result, from participation in physical activity that has little or no major effect on physiological condition have yet to be established. If fitness gains are necessary for these benefits, it must be determined whether light to moderate or vigorous physical activity prescriptions are required. Furthermore, the nature and extent to which physical activity influences such outcomes as a function of other external variables (age, sex, ethnicity, etc.) and their interactions with fitness change need to be established. Without the assessment of fitness parameters, we are unable to answer this question. It is wholly conceivable that effects on cardiovascular and psychosocial functioning are orthogonal physical activity outcomes.

Acknowledgments

This chapter was completed while the author was supported by a grant from the National Institute on Aging (#AG07907). Thanks are extended to Kerry Courneya and Steven Petruzzello for their helpful comments on an earlier draft and to Shelly Shaffer for conducting the computer searches.

References

1. Alpert, B.; Field, T.; Goldstein, S.; Perry, S. Aerobics enhances cardiovascular fitness and agility in preschoolers. Health Psychol. 9:48-56; 1990.
2. Bahrke, M.S.; Morgan, W.P. Anxiety reduction following exercise and meditation. Cogn. Ther. Res. 4:323-333; 1978.
3. Bandura, A. Self-efficacy mechanism in human agency. Am. Psychol. 37:122-147; 1982.
4. Bandura, A. Social foundations of thought and action. Englewood Cliffs, NJ:Prentice Hall; 1986.
5. Bandura, A. Self-efficacy mechanism in psychobiological functioning. In: Schwarzer, R.,

ed. Social cognitive mediators of action. [In press.]
6. Blair, S.N. et al. Physical fitness and all-cause mortality: A prospective study of healthy men and women. JAMA. 262:2395-2401; 1989.
7. Blumenthal, J.A.; Emery, C.F.; Madden, D.J.; Schniebolk, S.; Walsh-Riddle, M.; George, L.K.; McKee, D.C.; Higginbotham, M.B.; Cobb, F.R.; Coleman, R.E. Long-term effects of exercise on psychological functioning in older men and women. J. Gerontol. 46:P352-P361; 1991.
8. Blumenthal, J.A.; Schocken, D.D.; Needels, T.L.; Hindle, P. Psychological and physiological effects of physical conditioning on the elderly. J. Psychosom. Res. 26:505-510; 1982.
9. Bouchard, C.; Shephard, R.J.; Stephens, T.; Sutton, J.R.; McPherson, B.D. Exercise, fitness, and health. Champaign, IL: Human Kinetics; 1990.
10. Brown, D. Exercise, fitness, and mental health. In: Bouchard, C.; Shephard, R.J.; Stephens, T.; Sutton, J.R.; McPherson, B.D. eds. Exercise, fitness, and health. Champaign, IL: Human Kinetics; 1990.
11. Brown, J.D. Staying fit and staying well: Physical fitness as a moderator of life stress. J. Pers. Soc. Psychol. 60:555-561; 1991.
12. Brown, J.D.; Lawton, M. Stress and well-being in adolescence: The moderating role of physical exercise. J. Human Stress. 12:125-131; 1986.
13. Brown, J.D.; Siegel, J.M. Exercise as a buffer of life stress: A prospective study of adolescent health. Health Psychol. 7:341-353; 1988.
14. Carter, R. Exercise and happiness. J. Sports Med. 17:307-313; 1977.
15. Corbin, C.B.; Laurie, D.R.; Gruger, C.; Smiley, B. Vicarious success experience as a factor influencing self-confidence, attitudes, and physical activity of adult women. J. Teaching Phys. Educ. 4:17-23; 1984.
16. Crews, D.J.; Landers, D.M. A meta-analytic review of aerobic fitness and reactivity to psychosocial stressors. Med. Sci. Sports Exerc. 19:S114-S120; 1987.
17. Diener, E. Subjective well-being. Psychol. Bull. 95:542-575; 1984.
18. Dishman, R.K. Exercise adherence: Its impact on public health. Champaign, IL: Human Kinetics; 1988.
19. Doan, R.E.; Scherman, A. The therapeutic effect of physical fitness on measures of personality: A literature review. J. Counsel. Dev. 11:28-36; 1987.
20. Dowall, J.R.; Bolter, C.P.; Flett, R.A.; Kammann, R. Psychological well-being and its relationship to fitness and activity levels. J. Hum. Movement Stud. 14:39-45; 1988.
21. Emery, C.F.; Blumenthal, J.A. Effects of physical exercise on psychological and cognitive functioning of older adults. Ann. Behav. Med. 13:99-107; 1989.
22. Emery, C.F.; Gatz, M. Psychological and cognitive effects of an exercise program for community-residing older adults. Gerontologist. 30:184-188; 1990.
23. Ewart, C.K. Psychological effects of resistive weight training: Implications for cardiac patients. Med. Sci. Sports Exerc. 21:683-688; 1989.
24. Ewart, C.K.; Stewart, K.J.; Gillian, R.E.; Kelemen, M.H. Self-efficacy mediates strength gains during circuit weight training in men with coronary artery disease. Med. Sci. Sports Exerc. 18:531-540; 1986.
25. Ewart, C.K.; Taylor, C.B.; Reese, L.B.; DeBusk, R.F. Effects of early post myocardial infarction exercise testing on self-perception and subsequent physical activity. Am. J. Cardiol. 51:1076-1080; 1983.
26. Folkins, C.H.; Sime, W.E. Physical fitness training and mental health. Am. Psychol. 36; 373-389; 1981.
27. Folsom-Meek, S.L. Relationships among attributes, physical fitness, and self-concept development of elementary school children. Perc. Mot. Skills. 73:379-383; 1991.
28. Fox, K.R.; Corbin, C.B. The physical self-perception profile: Development and preliminary validation. J. Sport Exer. Psychol. 11:408-430; 1989.
29. Gauvin, L. The relationship between regular physical activity and subjective well-being. J. Sport Behav. 11:107-114; 1988.
30. Gruber, J.J. Physical activity and self-esteem development in children: A meta-analysis. American academy of physical education papers, 19. Champaign, IL: Human Kinetics; 1986:30-48.
31. Gulanick, M. Is phase 2 cardiac rehabilitation necessary for early recovery of patients with cardiac disease? A randomized, controlled study. Heart Lung. 20:9-15; 1991.
32. Hardy, C.J.; Rejeski, W.J. (1989). Not what, but how one feels: The measurement of affect during exercise. J. Sport Exerc. Psychol. 11:304-317; 1989.
33. Hawkins, W.E.; Duncan, T. Structural equation analysis of an exercise/sleep health practices model on quality of life of elderly persons. Percep. Mot. Skills. 72:831-836; 1991.
34. Hayes, D.; Ross, C.E. Body and mind: The effect of exercise, overweight, and physical health on psychological well-being. J. Health Soc. Behav. 27:387-400; 1986.
35. Hogan, P.I.; Santomier, J.P. Effect of mastering swim skills on older adults' self-efficacy. Res. Q. Exerc. Sport. 55:294-296; 1984.

36. Holloway, J.B.; Beuter, A.; Duda, J.L. Self-efficacy and training for strength in adolescent girls. J. App. Soc. Psychol. 18:699-719; 1988.
37. Hughes. J.R. Psychological effects of habitual aerobic exercise: A critical review. Prev. Med. 13:66-78; 1984.
38. Jasnoski, M.; Holmes, D.S.; Soloman, S.; Aguiar, C. Exercise, changes in aerobic capacity, and changes in self-perceptions: An experimental investigation. J. Res. Pers. 15:460-466; 1981.
39. Kaplan, R.M.; Atkins, C.J.; Reinsch, S. Specific efficacy expectations mediate exercise compliance in patients with COPD. Health Psychol. 3:223-242; 1984.
40. Kendzierski, D.; DeCarlo, K.J. Physical activity enjoyment scale: Two validation studies. J. Sport Exerc. Psychol. 13:50-64; 1991.
41. King, A.C.; Taylor, C.B.; Haskell, W.L.; DeBusk, R.F. Influence of regular aerobic exercise on psychological health: A randomized, controlled trial of healthy middle-aged adults. Health Psychol. 8:305-324; 1989.
42. Landers, D.M.; Petruzzello, S.J. Physical activity, fitness, and anxiety. (Chapter 59 of this volume.)
43. Leith, L.M.; Taylor, A.H. Psychological aspects of exercise: A decade literature review. J. Sport Behav. 13:219-239; 1990.
44. Lennox, S.L.; Bedell, J.R.; Stone, A.A. The effect of exercise on normal mood. J. Psychosom. Res. 34:629-636; 1990.
45. Long, B.C. Aerobic conditioning and stress inoculation: A comparison of stress management interventions. Cogn. Ther. Res. 8:517-541; 1984.
46. Long, B.C. Stress-management interventions: A 15-month follow-up of aerobic conditioning and stress inoculation training. Cog. Ther. Res. 9:471-478; 1985.
47. Long, B.C.; Haney, C.J. Coping strategies for working women: Aerobic exercise and relaxation interventions. Behav. Ther. 19:75-83; 1988.
48. Long, B.C.; Haney, C.J. Long-term follow-up of stressed working women: A comparison of aerobic exercise and progressive relaxation. J. Sport Exerc. Psychol. 10:461-470; 1988.
49. MacMahon, J.R.; Gross, R.T. Physical and psychological effects of aerobic exercise in boys with learning disabilities. Dev. Learn. Pediatr. 8:274-277; 1987.
50. MacMahon, J.R.; Gross, R.T. Physical and psychological effects of aerobic exercise in delinquent adolescent males. Am. J. Delinq. Child. 142:1361-1366; 1988.
51. Marsh, A.W.; Jackson, S.A. Multidimensional self-concepts, masculinity and femininity as a function of women's involvement in athletics. Sex Roles. 15:391-415; 1986.
52. Marsh, A.W.; Parker, J.; Barnes, J. Multidimensional adolescent self-concept: Its relation to age, sex, and academic measures. Am. Educ. Res. J. 22:422-444; 1985.
53. Marsh, H.W.; Peart, M.D. Competitive and cooperative physical fitness training programs for girls: Effects on physical fitness and multidimensional self-concepts. J. Sport Exerc. Psychol. 10:390-407; 1988.
54. Martinsen, E. Benefits of exercise for treatment of depression. Sports Med. 9:380-389; 1990.
55. McAuley, E. Efficacy, attributional, and affective responses to exercise participation. J. Sport Exerc. Psychol. 13:382-393; 1991.
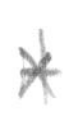
56. McAuley, E. Exercise and motivation: A self-efficacy perspective. In: Roberts, G.C., ed. Motivation in sport and exercise. Champaign, IL: Human Kinetics; 1992.
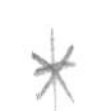
57. McAuley, E.; Courneya, K.S. Self-efficacy relationships with affective and exertion responses to exercise. J. Appl. Soc. Psychol. 22:312-326; 1992.
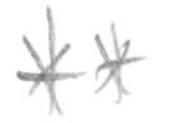
58. McAuley, E.; Courneya, K.S. The exercise-induced affect scale: Preliminary development and validation. Paper presented at the annual meeting of the society of behavioral medicine. New York; Available from the author.
59. McAuley, E.; Courneya, K.S.; Lettunich, J. Effects of acute and long-term exercise on self-efficacy in sedentary middle-aged males and females. Gerontologist. 31:534-542; 1991.
60. Morgan, W.P. Physical activity, fitness, and depression. (Chapter 58 of this volume.)
61. Morgan, W.P. Affective beneficence of vigorous physical activity. Med. Sci. Sports Exerc. 17:94-100; 1985.
62. Morgan, W.P.; Goldstein, S.E. Exercise and mental health. New York: Hemisphere; 1987.
63. Moses, J.; Steptoe, A.; Mathews, A.; Edwards, S. The effects of exercise training on mental well-being in the normal population: A controlled trial. J. Psychosom. Res. 33:47-61; 1989.
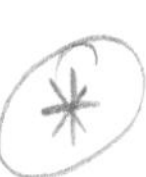
64. Norris, R.; Carroll, D.; Cochrane, R. The effects of aerobic and anaerobic training on fitness, blood pressure and psychological stress and well-being. J. Psychosom. Res. 34:367-375; 1990.
65. North, T.C., McCullagh, P.; Tran, Z.V. Effect of exercise on depression. In: Pandolf, K., ed. Exerc. Sport Sci. Rev. 18:379-415; 1990.
66. Oldridge, N.B.; Rogowski, B.L. Self-efficacy and in-patient cardiac rehabilitation. Amer. J. Cardiol. 66:362-365; 1990.
67. O'Leary, A. Self-efficacy and health. Behav. Res. Ther. 23:437-451; 1985.

68. Petruzzello, S.J.; Landers, D.M.; Hatfield, B.D.; Kubitz, K.A.; Salazar, W. A meta-analysis on the anxiety-reducing effects of acute and chronic exercise. Sports Med. 11:143-182; 1991.
69. Plante, T.G.; Rodin, J. Physical fitness and enhanced psychological health. Cur. Psychol. Res. Rev. 9:3-24; 1990.
70. Prosser, G. et al. Morale in coronary patients following an exercise program. J. Psychosom. Res. 25:587-593; 1981.
71. Ramlow, J.; Kriska, A.; LaPorte, R.A. Physical activity in the population: The epidemiologic spectrum. Res. Q. Exerc. Sport. 58:111-114; 1987.
72. Rodin, J. Aging and health: Effects of the sense of control. Science. 233:1271-1276; 1985.
73. Rosenberg, M. Conceiving the self. New York: Basic Books; 1979.
74. Rosenberg, M. Self-concept and psychological well-being in adolescence. In: Leahy, R.H., ed. The development of the self. Orlando, FL: Academic Press; 1985:205-246.
75. Ross, C.E.; Hayes, D. Exercise and psychological well-being in the community. Am. J. Epidemiol. 127:762-771; 1988.
76. Russell, J.A.; Weiss, A.; Mendelson, G.A. Affect grid: A single-item of scale of pleasure and arousal. J. Pers. Soc. Psychol. 57:493-502; 1989.
77. Seggar, J.F.; McCammon, D.L.; Cannon, L.D. Relations between physical activity, weight discrepancies, body-cathexis, and psychological well-being in college women. Percep. Mot. Skills. 67:659-669; 1988.
78. Shavelson, R.J.; Hubner, J.J.; Stanton, G.C. Self-concept: Validation of construct interpretations. Rev. Educ. Res. 46:407-441; 1976.
79. Sime, W.E. Discussion: Exercise, fitness, and mental health. In Bouchard, C. et al., eds. Exercise, fitness, and health. Champaign, IL: Human Kinetics; 1990:627-633.
80. Sonstroem, R.J. Exercise and self-esteem. In: Terjung, R.L., ed. Exercise and sport sciences reviews (vol.12). Lexington, MA: Collomore Press; 1984:123-155.
81. Sonstroem, R.J.; Morgan, W.P. Exercise and self-esteem: Rationale and model. Med. Sci. Sports Exerc. 21:329-337; 1989.
82. Stephens, T. Physical activity and mental health in the United States and Canada: Evidence from four population surveys. Prev. Med. 17:35-47; 1988.
83. Stewart, A.L.; King, A.C. Evaluating the efficacy of physical activity for influencing quality-of-life outcomes in older adults. Ann. Behav. Med. 13:108-116; 1991.
84. Taylor, C.B.; Bandura, A.; Ewart, C.K.; Miller, N.H.; DeBusk, R.F. Exercise testing to enhance wives' confidence in their husbands' cardiac capability soon after clinically uncomplicated acute myocardial infarction. Am. J. Cardiol. 55:635-638; 1985.
85. Thomas, J.R.; Landers, D.M.; Salazar, W.; Etnier, J. Exercise and cognitive function. (Chapter 35 of this volume.)
86. Toshima, M.T.; Kaplan, R.M.; Ries, A.L. Experimental evaluation of rehabilitation in chronic obstructive pulmonary disease: Short-term effects on exercise endurance and health status. Health Psychol. 9:237-252; 1990.
87. Watson, D.; Clark, L.A.; Tellegen, A. Development and validation of a brief measure of positive and negative affect: The PANAS scales. J. Pers. Soc. Psychol. 54:1063-1070; 1988.
88. Wetzler, H.P.; Ursano, R.J. A positive association between physical health practices and psychological well-being. J. Nerv. Men. Dis. 176: 280-283; 1988.
89. Wiklund, I.; Comerford, M.B.; Dimenas, E. The relationship between exercise tolerance and quality of life in angina pectoris. Clin. Cardiol. 14:204-208; 1991.
90. Zaharopoulus, E.; Hodge, K.P. Self-concept and sport participation. N. Z. J. Psychol. 20:12-16; 1991.

PART V

Physical Activity and Fitness in Disease

Chapter 38

Physical Activity, Fitness, and Atherosclerosis

Sean Moore

When one lists the possible or probable relationships among exercise, fitness, and atherosclerosis, it is appropriate to consider disease initiation, progression, regression, and finally the stenotic and thrombotic or thromboembolic lesions that become manifest as clinical disease. These latter include sudden cardiac death, stable and unstable angina, transient ischemic attacks, lacunar infarcts, stroke, peripheral vascular disease, and renal artery stenosis. Accordingly, it is necessary, in considering these effects of the disease process, to have a theoretical framework of how atherosclerosis begins, progresses, regresses, and leads to significant clinical events.

Current Concepts of Atherosclerosis

Hyperlipidemia

Current thinking on disease initiation is overwhelmingly in favor of hyperlipidemia or dyslipidemia as the most important factor in the initiation of the atherogenic process. In fact, for some, the story is summed up by one word—hypercholesterolemia (84,85).

Although the importance of hyperlipidemia or related disorders of lipoprotein metabolism in the pathogenesis of atherosclerosis seems to be currently widely accepted (55,69), there is continuing debate about whether they are related to initiating events or contribute as secondary or modifying factors, acting upon a lesion initially developed in response to injury (54,55).

However, it is of critical importance to our understanding of atherogenesis to know which of these two factors is of primary importance, in the sense of initiating lesions (57). The current widely accepted concept, that hyperlipidemia or alterations of blood lipids constitute the prime mover in the atherogenic sequence, rests upon experiments in which very high levels of blood lipids are associated with the development of lesions (31). In such lesions, referred to as fatty dots or streaks, lipid-laden macrophages are the main, indeed only, cellular component. However, human fatty streaks, which often constitute the earliest lesions visible to the naked eye, are almost entirely composed of smooth muscle cells (35,39). This has been observed repeatedly (92) and has recently been reemphasized in the PDAY (Pathological Determinants of Atherosclerosis in Youth) study, a large, multicenter study, funded by the U.S. National Institutes of Health) (98,99). Moreover, before any grossly visible lesions occur, human, musculoelastic arteries develop a diffuse, intimal thickening (83,92). On this base eccentric lesions develop at predictable and usual sites (44,83). These lesions are again predominantly composed of smooth muscle cells with a minor contribution of monocyte-macrophage-type cells (82), although the latter are the cellular constituents emphasized as the principal element by those who believe that hyperlipidemia initiates lesions (85). The location of the lesions seems to be related to flow separation and possibly is determined by flow disturbance (44,48,60).

A second problem for proponents of hypercholesterolemia as the initiator of the atherogenic sequence is that macrophages have few or no receptors for low-density lipoprotein (LDL), and these are down-regulated by exposure to LDL (85). This paradox is explained by postulating that LDL is modified in vivo, most likely by oxidation, which makes it acceptable to the scavenger receptor (85). The possibility that LDL may be oxidized after its entry into the intima exists (15,102) but begs the question of why it accumulates in the intima in excess amounts in the first place (57).

In experiments where atherosclerotic lesions are induced by dietary lipid supplement, the blood cholesterol levels are usually very high, in the order of 900 to 1000 mg/dl or more (76). These are the kinds of levels seen in homozygous familial hyperlipidemia, in Watanabe rabbits or the St. Thomas Hospital strain of rabbits (57). The associated lesions are mainly composed of macrophage-type foam cells.

In experiments in swine, monocyte adherence to the endothelium and the accumulation of lipid-laden macrophages in the intima did not occur following feeding of a hyperlipidemic diet for 3 months, even when cholesterol levels in excess of 700 mg/dl were achieved. At 3 months monocyte adherence began first in the coronary arteries (76). Before this, proliferation of smooth muscle cells in the intima was the observed response of the arterial wall (75). These observations further support the view that, at moderate levels of elevation of blood cholesterol, monocyte adherence and migration into the vessel wall are not important aspects of atherogenesis. The corollary is that, in human disease, when cholesterol levels are or are not elevated, and there is a wide overlap in values between those who develop clinical evidence of the disease and those who do not, other mechanisms may not be more significant (36).

Some of the early literature on diet-induced atherosclerosis, especially the articles written by Duff (26,27), indicates that injury to the vessel wall is an important element of diet-induced atherosclerosis and that before lipid accumulation occurs, there is a change in the intimal extracellular matrix. Thus, according to Duff, "Swelling of the subendothelial ground substance appears always to be the forerunner, and it seems entirely probable therefore, that a similar swelling of the intima precedes the earliest deposition of fatty substances" (27). He also observed, "The occurrence of local injury is the primary event, which is followed subsequently by the precipitation of lipoids in the injured area by cellular proliferation in the intima" (26). He linked this pathogenesis to human disease, observing, "There is every reason to believe that local injury to the walls of arteries is an essential factor and the primary event in the development of atherosclerosis in man" (26).

Injury-Induced Lesions

Another way of viewing the initiation of atherosclerotic disease is to consider that the starting point is injury or stimulation of the endothelium, which sets the stage for smooth muscle cell migration from the media and proliferation in the intima. This then serves as the substrate for lipid deposition and accumulation. All the changes that have been considered to be early lesions of atherosclerosis can be induced by injury to the endothelium of arteries in experimental animals, without dietary supplement of lipid (56). These lesions include microthrombi, focal intimal oedema, fatty streaks, and intimal thickenings, composed of smooth muscle cells. The fatty streak lesions appear to be composed of smooth muscle cells.

Recently, as part of the PDAY study of early lesions, platelet microthrombi were identified by scanning electron microscopy on the surface of the aorta and coronary arteries in 4% of specimens and 6% of cases (81). This indicates that focal areas of endothelial damage with platelet adherence may be occurring spontaneously. The sequal to such lesions would presumably be focal, intimal thickening, if the lesion were large enough. Small lesions have been shown to heal by the migration of endothelial cells to cover the denuded area (100). Possibly, repeated injury is needed to induce the development of lesions, and it is possible that the stimulus of repeated injury might modify endothelial function so as to cause the production of endothelial cell-derived growth factor, which then might be the stimulus to smooth muscle cell migration and proliferation in the intima (56).

Experimental Injury-Induced Lesions

It is now clearly established that lipid-containing lesions that resemble morphologically all the known forms of human atherosclerosis can be induced in animals fed a normal diet by either mechanical or immunological damage to the endothelium (54).

The placement of an indwelling polyethylene catheter in the aorta of rabbits is associated with the development of raised lipid-containing lesions in the areas where the catheter repeatedly or continuously comes in contact with the aortic wall and where the thrombus is laid down continuously (53). In some areas fatty streak lesions, which tend to be very transient, develop. In other areas, intimal thickenings composed of smooth muscle cells develop. The raised lesions regress, both in size and lipid content, when the injury stimulus (catheter) is removed (33). Similar lesions are induced by the repeated placement of human serum in a temporarily isolated segment of rabbit carotid artery, and these lesions also regress (32).

A very different type of lesion is induced by removing the endothelium with a Fogarty balloon catheter (59). One removal of the aortic endothelium of rabbits results in an intimal thickening composed of smooth muscle cells that, after periods from several weeks to 3 months, begins to show lipid deposition in both the interstitial tissue and in the smooth muscle cells. These lesions are progressive and continue to grow in thickness, as estimated by the number of layers of smooth muscle cells and the intervening lamellae of elastica above the internal elastic lamina. They also continue to show lipid deposits, which eventually become deeply placed (near the internal elastic lamina) as central lipid pools. These lesions occur in rabbits with normal blood lipid levels, with no dietary lipid supplement.

Mechanism of Lipid Accumulation in Lesions

There is now a fairly extensive literature describing the binding of low-density and very low-density lipoproteins and of apolipoprotein B to proteoglycans, particularly those with chondroitin sulfate side chains (5,8,13,40). Binding of lipoprotein to glycosaminoglycans has long been proposed as a mechanism of lipid accumulation in the vessel wall (40,93).

It has been proposed that an electrostatic binding of positively charged groups on apolipoprotein B to negatively charged groups of the glycosaminoglycans of proteoglycans may facilitate lipid accumulation in the vessel wall (5). The model of endothelial injury, caused by a balloon catheter, has been used to study the content of lipids and proteoglycans in the arterial wall. Chemical analysis of the lipid in lesions shows a very marked increase in cholesteryl ester and a more modest increase in free cholesterol in the lesions (1). Synthesis of glycosaminoglycans was increased in the neointima and was greater in the endothelium-covered areas (white areas) than in the areas remaining uncovered by regenerated endothelium (blue areas, identified by Evans blue dye injected intravenously before killing) (4). When studied in organ culture, synthesized proteoglycan is retained in the white areas but in the blue areas it rapidly equilibrates with the medium. This is paralleled by the kinetics of low-density lipoprotein interaction with the wall in that lipoprotein is retained in the white areas but rapidly equilibrates with that in the bloodstream in the areas uncovered by endothelium (3). Studies using doubly labeled cholesterol in lipoproteins have shown that entry is increased in the white areas compared to the blue areas (22). This is comparable with studies showing greater uptake of LDL by nonconfluent endothelial cells in tissue culture than by confluent cells (94).

In recent years there has been increasing interest in the binding of lipoproteins to proteoglycans in the arterial wall, and it has been demonstrated that there are quantitative and qualitative changes in the proteoglycan molecules, which facilitate this interaction, in the neointima developed in response to injury (4). The binding is particularly avid to chondroitin sulfate glycosaminoglycans, and Camejo has described an extract, rich in these elements, which preferentially binds lipoproteins (14). It has also been shown that dietetically induced elevation of blood lipids results in more avid binding of LDL and very low density lipoprotein (VLDL) to a proteoglycan-enriched fraction than the binding of these elements in normolipemic (on diets not supplemented with lipid) animals (2). The interaction of VLDL seems to be greater than that of LDL. Also the combination of injury-induced changes and hyperlipidemia is synergic (2,3).

Significance of High-Density Lipoprotein Elevation

It is of great interest, especially in considering possible benefits of exercise on the atherogenic process, that there is virtually no binding with high-density lipoprotein (HDL) (2,5). Moreover, in in-vitro studies HDL has been shown to dissociate the complexes of glycosaminoglycans and low-density lipoproteins (9). The reported relative increase in HDL in relation to LDL (17,91,101) in exercise could thus explain some of the favorable effect on atherosclerosis progression and might possibly facilitate regression.

The relatively more avid binding of VLDL, compared to LDL, might be of more importance in diabetes mellitus.

In a recent study (34), immunohistochemistry was used to view the distribution of endogenous apo-B in aortas of normal rabbits and in the aortic wall following the development of a neointima induced by endothelial injury. Protein-A gold labeling showed heavy deposition in the normal endothelium. In areas where endothelium had regenerated, apo-B also accumulated in the endothelium, as well as in the neointimal, interstitial tissue, and was also taken up by smooth muscle cells. Labeling was also seen in deeper, interstitial areas of advanced lesions and was intense in foam cells. These findings are supportive of the concept, derived from previous experiments, of lipid trapping by proteoglycans. These experiments showed lipid accumulation in the neointima developed in response to endothelial injury as shown by increased LDL entry and retention (3), associated with changes in proteoglycan content and composition (4). In the absence of hyperlipidemia or dietary lipid supplement, intimal thickening, occurring in response to injury, can accumulate lipid and progress in the same way as spontaneously occurring human atherosclerosis. The process of lipoprotein binding is, however, greatly facilitated by hyperlipidemia so that both injury and hyperlipidemia combine to cause lesion progression (2).

Whether or not injury and the resulting formation of an intimal smooth muscle cell proliferative lesion is the primary event in atherogenesis, it seems likely that binding of lipoprotein to structural proteins of the arterial intima is an important mechanism of disease progression, if not of initiation. Accordingly, the mechanism is of importance in any event, because it explains more of the relevance of the ratio of the lipoprotein classes to each other as a key factor in disease progression and possibly regression than do other theories.

Complications, Progression, and Regression

It has recently been convincingly shown that when an atherosclerotic plaque ruptures, it does so at the point where there is most stress on the lesion (67); that is, at the point where the fatty central pool or core of the lesion is covered by a relatively thin collagenous cap and where this joins the more solid, compact intima, beside the central lipid pool. Accordingly, regression, induced by drugs (11) or diet, could result in some resorption of the lipid core of lesions, and a rupture might be inhibited or prevented. Some studies appear to have shown decreases in size of plaques in response to lipid-lowering drug therapy (10,11). There are many problems in evaluating the precision of such studies (23). If valid and real reduction in plaque size is, in some instances, achieved, it is still not known which element of the plaque is involved. Possibly nuclear magnetic resonance may give some more precise information concerning this (52). Another consideration may be that decrease in size or some resolution of lesions may relate to decrease in thrombus size. It is well established that lesions grow in size by the incorporation of mural thrombus (57). The influence of various drug regimens on the formation of mural thrombi, developing in response to plaque fissure or rupture, needs to be evaluated (78). The possibility that various lipid-lowering drugs might influence thrombosis seems not to have been much considered.

The relevance of these matters to the relationship of exercise to atherosclerosis initiation and progression is important, but clearly long-term, detailed studies in the clinical trial setting are needed, and determination of some of the end points may be difficult. In effect, studies conducted over long periods of time on many individuals may be needed for conclusive answers.

There are very few animal studies bearing on the influence of exercise on atherosclerosis development. Kramsch showed an effect of exercise on diet-induced atherosclerosis in the coronary arteries of monkeys (43). Moderate conditioning exercise reduced the extent and size of lesions. There have been no experimental studies of the influence of exercise on atherosclerosis induced by endothelial injury. In humans it seems certain that there is an inverse association between physical activity and coronary heart disease (63).

Thrombosis

Modification of the complications of atherosclerosis, especially thrombosis, may be more promising and may be more accessible to meaningful investigation. In assessing the effects of exercise, one needs to determine risks as well as benefits.

Sudden death occurring during or shortly after exercise remains a problem that may not be fully understood (42,79). The mechanism is presumably the same as for sudden death occurring in any individual with coronary heart disease. There is now good evidence that sudden death occurs as a sequel to plaque rupture (16, 20). Mural thrombus forms on the ruptured, plaque material, and fragments of platelet-rich thrombus break off and lodge in the microcirculation of the myocardium (21), setting up foci of arrhythmia. A similar pathogenesis has been demonstrated experimentally and was associated with focal lesions of the myocardium identical to those described in humans dying suddenly of cardiac arrhythmia (58). Any tendency for increased platelet aggregation or coagulation of the blood would theoretically facilitate thrombus formation (29,50,90). In healthy, middle-aged men there are associations between high platelet counts and increased tendency for platelets to aggregate and coronary heart disease mortality to occur (29). Accordingly, changes in these parameters need to be studied to better characterize the risk.

It is known that risk of sudden death during exercise is greater in sedentary subjects who are beginning exercise programs and is greater in the early part of the program (19,79,80). The risk is also higher in the elderly (95) and increases with increasing intensity of exercise (95). Whether these observations relate to an increased tendency to plaque rupture or to changes in coagulation parameters is largely speculative, but there are some observations relating to the latter (28).

Increased blood levels of fibrinogen and factor VII in white men between 40 and 64 years of age, observed for 5 years, were more strongly predictive of ischemic heart disease than were blood cholesterol levels. (50). The risk of high fibrinogen levels was greater in younger men. The association with fibrinogen was strongest. In the follow-up period an increase in one standard deviation for both factor VII and fibrinogen raised the risk of ischemic heart disease (IHD) by about 55% and 67% respectively; neither cholesterol nor systolic blood pressure exerted independent effects. Other studies have confirmed the association of high fibrinogen levels and IHD (86,97). High levels of fibrinogen, apart from favoring the development of a more fibrin-rich thrombus in response to plaque rupture, would facilitate platelet aggregation and increase blood viscosity. Smoking is also relatable to increased fibrinogen levels (50,97) and is therefore of interest in the context of exercise if, for example, participation in an exercise program were also to facilitate withdrawal from smoking.

The effects of exercise on thrombosis are clearly of importance. In general, exercise is viewed by some as antithrombotic; exercise is thought to promote a dilutional pseudoanemia, decrease blood viscosity, decrease platelet aggregability, decrease platelet adhesion to damaged arteries, and activate fibrinolysis (28). Moderate-intensity physical exercise has been shown to inhibit platelet aggregation to adenosine diphosphate in overweight, mildly hypertensive men (64).

Alterations in tissue plasminogen activator (tPA) and tissue plasminogen activator inhibitor (tPA-1) may help explain the reports of increased risk of sudden death (73) early in exercise programs (77) and the benefits of long-term conditioning (30).

In one study, men with symptom-limited exercise were divided into three groups following exercise: normal, those with coronary artery disease (CAD) without exercise-induced ischemia, and those with CAD and transient exercise-induced ischemia. Plasminogen activator inhibitor levels were higher under basal conditions in Group 3 than in Group 1. At peak exercise the first group showed the highest release of tissue plasminogen activator with a related increase in plasminogen activator activity (73). A similar study showed increased plasminogen activator inhibitor in those with exercise-induced ischemia (74) as compared to control subjects.

A study of the effects of 6 months of intensive endurance exercise on tissue-type plasminogen activator activity, plasminogen activator inhibitor type 1 (PAI-1) activity, tPA antigen, and fibrinogen in old men (60 to 82 years) or young men (24 to 30 years) showed a 39% increase in tPA activity, a 141% increase of tPA in the active form, a 58% decrease in PAI-1 activity, and a 13% decrease in fibrinogen in the older subjects (88). The younger men had no significant change in any of the parameters. Although the numbers in the study were small (10 young; 13 old), the results are striking and indicate that sustained physical activity might be beneficial for older men by favorably altering the balance between thrombolysis and thrombosis.

That the effects of exercise on fibrinolysis may be relatively short-lived is indicated by a study of the effects of a marathon race on 16 endurance athletes (68). Tissue plasminogen activator increased 31-fold immediately after the run, but the increased tPA activity and tPA antigen concentration disappeared in the 3 hr following exertion. However, PA1 was not detectable immediately after the race and was significantly reduced 3 hr and 31 hr later.

The long-term effect on tPA in two groups, post-myocardial infarct, showed that it had decreased significantly by 6 months in patients not participating in a rehabilitation program, whereas it had increased slightly in those who did participate (30).

Although plasminogen levels in plasma do not alter with age, fibrinolytic activity becomes lower (89). An association of high levels of tPA inhibitor with hypertriglyceridemia, especially in the elderly, has been noted (51).

No study has yet assessed the role of training on secondary prevention (77), although exercise is part of the regimen of numerous intervention studies (62).

Diabetes and Atherosclerosis

The close association of diabetes mellitus and clinical events that occur as complications of atherosclerosis (41,96) has led to investigation of factors in atherogenesis that might be influenced by the diabetic state. Insulin resistance and hyperinsulinemia, even in the absence of diabetes, are associated with an atherogenic lipid profile, particularly enhanced VLDL synthesis, leading to hypertriglyceridemia (6,65). In studies of the enhanced binding of lipoproteins by the proteoglycans altered in the neointima developed in response to injury, it was observed that the binding of VLDL was more avid than for LDL (3,5). Insulin also enhances the proliferation of smooth muscle cells (87) in culture, as does growth hormone (46), and may augment the synthesis of collagen (24). The accumulation of advanced glycosylation end products on collagen allows covalent binding of LDL (12).

Glycosylated collagen is even more stimulating to platelet aggregation than unmodified collagen (18,47). Platelets from subjects with diabetes are more reactive to agonists and synthesize more thromboxane A_2 (49). Increased production of Von Willebrand factor favors platelet adhesion to damaged vessel walls. Prostacyclin production by the vessel wall is decreased in diabetes (38). In diabetes there is also a change in the proportion of lipoproteins with a decrease in HDL and increase in VLDL (7,45,61).

In Type II diabetes, because many of the changes may relate to insulin resistance (65,66), whether this metabolic feature can be modified by exercise is an important question. There is some evidence that exercise training is associated with improvements in lipid and glucose metabolism that are characterized by enhanced insulin sensitivity, improved glucose tolerance, increased HDL cholesterol levels, and decreased triglyceride levels (37). These aspects are more fully discussed in chapter 45.

An animal model of diabetes, characterized by insulin resistance and hyperlipidemia (25), is associated with the spontaneous development of atherosclerosis and focal myocardial lesions, possibly ischemic in nature (70). The incidence of myocardial lesions is reduced when plasma insulin levels are reduced (70) and are prevented by running (71). The myocardial and vascular lesions are correlated strongly with hyperinsulinemia but not with hyperlipidemia (72). Further study of this model to determine if exercise and other modalities to reduce the hyperinsulinemia also reduce or inhibit atherosclerosis development would clearly be of great interest.

In summary, the development, progression, regression, and complications of atherosclerosis may all be influenced by metabolic changes and by alterations of blood coagulation that accompany exercise.

References

1. Alavi, M.; Dunnett, C.W.; Moore, S. Lipid composition of the rabbit aortic wall following removal of endothelium by balloon catheter. Arteriosclerosis. 3:413-419; 1983.
2. Alavi, M.Z.; Galis, Z.; Li, Z.; Moore, S. Dietary alterations of plasma lipoproteins influence their interactions with proteoglycan enriched extracts from neointima of normal and injured aorta of rabbit. Clin. Invest. Med. 14:419-431; 1991.
3. Alavi, M.; Moore, S. Kinetics of low density lipoprotein interactions with rabbit aorta wall following balloon catheter deendothelialization. Arteriosclerosis. 4:395-402; 1984.
4. Alavi, M.; Moore, S. Glycosaminoglycan biosynthesis in the endothelium covered neointima of de-endothelialized rabbit aorta. J. Exp. Mol. Pathol. 42:389-400; 1985.
5. Alavi, M.Z.; Richardson, M.; Moore, S. The in vitro interactions between serum lipoproteins and proteoglycans of the neointima of the rabbit aorta after a single balloon catheter injury. Am. J. Pathol. 134:287-294; 1989.
6. Barakat, H.A.; Carpenter, J.W.; McLendon, V.D.; Prashaken, K.; Leggett, N.; Heath, J.; Marke, R. Influence of obesity, impaired glucose tolerance and NIDDM on LDL structure and composition. Diabetes. 39:1527-1533; 1990.
7. Barrett-Connor, E.; Grundy, S.M.; Holdbrook, M.J. Plasma lipids and diabetes mellitus in an adult community. Am. J. Epidemiol. 115:657-663; 1982.
8. Berenson, G.S.; Radhakrishnamurthy, B.; Srinivasan, S.R.; Vijayagopal, P.; Dalferes, E.R., Jr. Arterial wall injury and proteoglycan changes in atherosclerosis. Arch. Pathol. Lab. Med. 112:1002-1009; 1989.
9. Bihari-Varga, M. Influence of serum high density lipoproteins on the low density lipoproteins on the low density lipoprotein-aortic glycosaminoglycan interactions. Artery. 4:504-511; 1978.
10. Blankenhorn, D.H.; Nessim, S.A.; Johnson, R.L.; Sanmarlo, M.F.; Azen, S.P.; Casmin-Hemphill, L. Beneficial effects of combined colestipol-niacin therapy on coronary atherosclerosis and coronary venous bypass grafts. JAMA. 257:3233-3240; 1987.
11. Brown, G.; Alberts, J.J.; Fischer, L.D.; Schaefer, B.A.; Lin, J.T.; Kaplan, C.; Zhao, X.-Q.; Bisson, B.D.; Fitzpatrick, V.F.; Dodge, H.T. Regression of coronary artery disease as a result of intensive lipid lowering therapy in men with high levels of apolipoprotein B. N. Engl. J. Med. 323:1289-1298; 1990.
12. Brownlee, M.; Vlassara, H.; Cerami, A. Nonenzymatic glycosylation products on collagen covalently trap low-density lipoprotein. Diabetes. 34:938-941; 1985.
13. Camejo, G. The interaction of lipids and lipoproteins, with intracellular matrix of arterial tissue: Its possible role in atherogenesis. Adv. Lipid Res. 19:1-53; 1982.
14. Camejo, G.; Lalaguna, F.; Lopez, F.; Starosta, R. Characterization of lipoprotein complexing proteoglycan from human aorta. Atherosclerosis. 35:307-320; 1980.
15. Cathcart, M.K.; Morel, D.W.; Chisolm, G.M. Monocytes and neutrophils oxidize low density lipoprotein making it cytotoxic. J. Leukocyte Biol. 38:341-350; 1985.
16. Ciapricotti, R.; Elgamal, M.; Relik, T.; Taverne, R.; Panis, J.; deSwart, J.; van Gelder, B.; Relik-Van Wely, L. Clinical characteristics and coronary angiographic findings of patients with unstable angina, acute myocardial infarction and survivor of sudden ischemic death occurring during and after sport. Am. Heart J. 120:1267-1278; 1990.
17. Chandrashekar, Y.; Anand, L.C. Exercise as a coronary protection factor. Am. Heart J. 122:1723-1739; 1991.
18. Colwell, J.A.; Winocur, P.D.; Lopes-Virella, M.; et al. New concepts about the pathogenesis of atherosclerosis in diabetes mellitus. Am. J. Med. [Suppl. 5]. 75:67-80; 1983.

19. Coplan, N.L.; Gleim, G.W.; Nicholas, J.A. Exercise and sudden cardiac death. Am. Heart J. 115:207-212; 1988.
20. Davies, M.J.; Thomas, A.C. Plaque fissuring: The cause of acute myocardial infarction, sudden ischemic death and crescendo angina. Br. Heart J. 53:363-373; 1985.
21. Davies, M.J.; Thomas, A.C.; Knapman, P.A.; Hangartner, R. Intramyocardial platelet aggregation in unstable angina and sudden ischemic death. Circulation. 73:418-427; 1986.
22. Day, A.J.; Alavi, M.; Moore, S. Influx of $^3H/^{14}C$ cholesterol labelled lipoprotein into re-endothelialized and de-endothelialized areas of ballooned aortas in normal-fed and cholesterol-fed rabbits. Atherosclerosis. 55:339-351, 1985.
23. de Feyter, P.J.; Serruys, P.W.; Davies, M.J.; Richardson, P.; Lubsen, J.; Oliver, M.F. Quantitative coronary angiography to measure progression and regression of coronary atherosclerosis. Value, limitations and implications for clinical trials. Circulation. 84:412-423; 1991.
24. Defronzo, R.A.; Ferrannini, E. Insulin resistance: A multi-facetted syndrome responsible for NIDDM, obesity, hypertension, dyslipidemia and atherosclerotic cardiovascular disease. Diabetes Care. 14:173-194; 1991.
25. Dolphin, P.J.; Stewart, R.; Amy, R.M.; Russell, J.C. Serum lipids and lipoproteins in the atherosclerosis prone LA/N-corpulent rat. Biochim. Biophys. Acta. 919:140-148; 1987.
26. Duff, G.L. Experimental cholesterol atherosclerosis and its relationship to human atherosclerosis. Arch. Pathol. Lab. Med. 20:80-124, 259-304; 1935.
27. Duff, G.L. The nature of experimental atherosclerosis in the rabbit. Arch. Pathol. Lab. Med. 22:161-182; 1936.
28. Eichner, E.R. Antithrombotic effects of exercise. Am. Fam. Physician. 36:207-211; 1987.
29. Elwood, P.C.; Renaud, S.; Sharp, D.S.; Beswich, A.D.; O'Brien, J.R.; Yarnell, J.W.G. Ischemic heart disease and platelet aggregation (the Caerphilly collaborative heart disease study). Circulation. 83:38-44; 1991.
30. Estelles, A.; Aznar, J.; Tormo, G.; Sapena, P.; Tormo, V.; Espana, F. Influence of rehabilitation sports programme on the fibrinolytic activity of patients after myocardial infarction. Thromb. Res. 55:203-212; 1989.
31. Faggiotto, A.; Ross, R.; Harker, L. Studies of hypercholesterolemia in the non-human primate. 1. Changes that lead to fatty streak formation. Arteriosclerosis. 4:323-340; 1984.
32. Friedman, R.J.; Moore, S.; Singal, D.P. Repeated endothelial injury and induction of atherosclerosis in normolipemic rabbits by human serum. Lab. Invest. 30:404-415; 1975.
33. Friedman, R.J.; Moore, S.; Singal, D.P.; Gent, M. Regression of injury-induced atheromatous lesions in rabbits. Arch. Pathol. Lab. Med. 100:189-195; 1976.
34. Galis, Z.S.; Ghitescu, L.D.; Li, Z.; Alavi, M.Z.; Moore, S. Distribution of endogenous apoprotein B-containing lipoproteins in normal and injured aortas of normocholesterolemic rabbits. Lab. Invest. 66:624-638; 1992.
35. Geer, J.C. Fine structure of human aortic intimal thickening and fatty streaks. Lab. Invest. 14:1764-1783; 1965.
36. Ginsburg, G.S.; Safran, C.; Pasternak, R.C. Frequency of low serum high density lipoprotein cholesterol levels in hospitalized patients with "desirable" total cholesterol levels. Am. J. Cardiol. 68:187-192; 1991.
37. Goldberg, A.P. Aerobic and resistive exercise modify risk factors for coronary heart disease. Med. Sci. Sports Exerc. 21:669-674; 1989.
38. Harrison, H.E.; Reece, A.M.; Johnson, M. Decreased vascular prostacyclin in experimental diabetes. Life Sci. 23:351-355; 1978.
39. Haust, M.D. The morphogenesis and fate of potential and early atherosclerotic lesions in man. Hum. Pathol. 2:1-30; 1971.
40. Iverius, P.H. The interaction between human plasma lipoprotein and connective tissue glycosaminoglycans. J. Biol. Chem. 246:2607-2613; 1972.
41. Jarrett, R.J. Diabetes and the heart: Coronary heart disease. Clin. Endocrinol. Metab. 6:389-402; 1977.
42. Koplan, J.P.; Siscovick, D.S.; Goldbaum, G.M. The risks of exercise: A public health view of injuries and hazards. Public Health Rep. 100:189-195; 1985.
43. Kramsch, D.M. Reduction of coronary atherosclerosis by moderate conditioning exercise in monkeys in an atherogenic diet. N. Engl. J. Med. 305:1483-1489; 1981.
44. Ku, D.N.; Gidedems, D.P.; Zarins, C.K.; Glagow, S. Pulsatile flow and atherosclerosis in the human carotid bifurcation position correlation between plaque location and low and oscillating shear stress. Arteriosclerosis. 5:293-302; 1985.
45. Laakso, M.; Barret-Connor, E. Asymptomatic hyperglycemia is associated with lipid and lipoprotein changes favoring atherosclerosis. Arteriosclerosis. 9:665-672; 1989.
46. Ledet, T. Growth hormone stimulating the growth of arterial medial cells in vitro. Absence of effect of insulin. Diabetes. 25:1011-1017; 1976.

47. Le Pape, A.; Gutman, N.; Guitton, J.D.; et al. Non-enzymatic glycosylation increases platelet aggregating potency of collagen from placenta of diabetic human beings. Biochem. Biophys. Res. Commun. 111:602-610; 1983.
48. Liepsch, D.; Moravel, S. Pulsatile flow of a non-Newtonian fluid in distensible models of human arteries. Biorheology. 21:571-586; 1984.
49. McDonald, J.W.D.; Dupre, J.; Rodger, N.W.; et al. Comparison of platelet thromboxane synthesis in diabetic patients on conventional insulin therapy and continuous insulin infusions. Thromb. Res. 28:705-712; 1982.
50. Meade, T.W.; Brozovic, M.; Chakrabarti, R.R.; Haines, A.P.; Imeson, J.D.; Mellows, S.; Miller, G.J.; North, W.R.S.; Stirling, Y.; Thompson, S.G. Haemostatic function and ischemic heart disease: Principal results of the Northwick Park heart study. Lancet. (2)533:537; 1986.
51. Mehta, J.; Mehta, P.; Lawson, D.; Saldeen, T. Plasma tissue plasminogen activator inhibitor levels in coronary artery disease: Correlation with age and serum triglyceride concentrations. J. Am. Coll. Cardiol. 9:263-268; 1987.
52. Mohiaddin, R.H.; Underwood, S.R.; Bogren, H.G.; et al. Regional aortic compliance studied by magnetic resonance imaging: The effects of age, training and coronary artery disease. Br. Heart J. 62:90-96; 1989.
53. Moore, S. Thromboatherosclerosis in normolipemic rabbits. Lab. Invest. 29:478-487; 1973.
54. Moore, S. Injury mechanisms in atherogenesis. In: Moore, S., ed. Vascular injury and atherosclerosis. New York: Marcel Dekker, Inc., 1981:131-148.
55. Moore, S. Pathogenesis of atherosclerosis. Metabolism. 34:13-16; 1985.
56. Moore, S. Thrombosis and atherogenesis—the chicken and the egg. Ann. NY. Acad. Sci. 454:146-153; 1985.
57. Moore, S. Dietary atherosclerosis and arterial wall injury. Lab. Invest. 60:733-736; 1989.
58. Moore, S.; Belbeck, L.W.; Evans, G.; Pineau, S. Effects of complete or partial occlusion of a coronary artery. Lab. Invest. 44:151-157; 1981.
59. Moore, S.; Belbeck, L.W.; Richardson, M.; Taylor, W. Lipid accumulation in the neointima formed in normal-fed rabbits in response to one or six removals of the aortic endothelium. Lab. Invest. 47:32-42; 1982.
60. Nguyen, N.D.; Haque, A.K. Effect of hemodynamic factors on atherosclerosis in the abdominal aorta. Atherosclerosis. 84:33-39; 1990.
61. Nikkilla, E.A. Triglyceride metabolism in diabetes mellitus. Prog. Biochem. Pharmacol. 8:271-299; 1973.
62. Ornish, D.; Brown, S.E.; Scherwitz, L.W.; et al. Can lifestyle changes reverse coronary heart disease? Lancet. 336:129-133; 1991.
63. Powell, K.E.; Thompson, P.D.; Caspersen, C.J.; Kendrick, J.S. Physical activity and the incidence of coronary heart disease. Annu. Rev. Public Health. 8:253-287; 1987.
64. Rauramaa, R.; Salonen, J.T.; Seppanen, K.; Salonen, R.; Venalainen, J.M.; Ihanainen, M.; Rissanen, V. Inhibition of platelet aggregability by moderate-intensity physical exercise: A randomized clinical trial in overweight men. Circulation. 74:939-944; 1986.
65. Reaven, G.M. Role of insulin resistance in human disease. Diabetes. 37:1595-1607; 1988.
66. Reaven, G.M. Resistance to insulin-stimulated glucose uptake and hyperinsulinemia: Role in non-insulin-dependent diabetes, high blood pressure, dyslipidemia and coronary heart disease. Diabete Metab. 17:78-86; 1991.
67. Richardson, P.D.; Davies, M.J.; Born, G.V.R. Influence of plaque configuration and stress distribution on fissuring of coronary atherosclerotic plaques. Lancet. 2:941-944; 1989.
68. Rocker, L.; Thenzer, M.; Drygas, W.K; Lill, H.; Heydvik, B.; Altenkirch, H.V. Effects of prolonged physical exercise on the fibrinolytic system. Eur. J. Appl. Physiol. 60:478-481; 1990.
69. Ross, R. The pathogenesis of atherosclerosis—an update. N. Engl. J. Med. 314:488-500; 1988.
70. Russell, J.C.; Amy, R.M. Myocardial and vascular lesions in the LA/N-corpulent rat. Can. J. Physiol. Pharmacol. 64:1272-1280; 1986.
71. Russell, J.C.; Amy, R.M.; Manickavel, V.; Dolphin, P.J.; Epling, W.F.; Pierce, D.; Boer, D.P. Prevention of myocardial disease in the J.C.R.: LA-corpulent rat by running. J. Appl. Physiol. 66:1649-1655; 1989.
72. Russell, J.C.; Koeslag, D.G.; Amy, R.M.; Dolphin, P.J. Independence of myocardial disease in the J.C.R.: LA-corpulent rat on plasma cholesterol concentration. Clin. Invest. Med. 14:288-295; 1991.
73. Rydzewski, A.; Sakata, K.; Kobayashi, A.; Yamzaaki, N.; Uramo, T.; Takada, Y.; Takada, A. Changes in plasminogen activates inhibitor I and tissue-type plasminogen activator during exercise in patients with coronary heart disease. Haemostasis. 20:305-312; 1990.
74. Sakath, K.; Kurath, C.; Taguchi, T.; Suzuki, S.; Kobayashi, A.; Yamazaki, N.; Rydzewski, A.; Takada, Y.; Takada, A. Clinical significance of plasminogen activator inhibitor activity in patients with exercise-induced ischemia. Am. Heart J. 120:831-838; 1990.
75. Scott, R.F.; Kim, D.N.; Schmee, J.; Thomas, W.A. Atherosclerotic lesions in coronary arteries of

hyperlipidemic swine. Part 2. Endothelial cell kinetics and leukocyte adherence associated with early lesions. Atherosclerosis. 67:1-18; 1986.
76. Scott, R.F.; Reidy, M.A.; Kim, D.N.; Schmee, J.; Thomas, W.H. Intimal cell mass-derived atherosclerotic lesions in the abdominal aorta of hyperlipidemic swine. Part 2. Investigation of endothelial cell changes and leukocyte adherence associated with early lesions. Atherosclerosis. 62:1-18; 1986.
77. Sellier, P.; Corona, P.; Audouin, P.; Payen, B.; Plat, F.; Ourbak, P. Influence of training on blood lipids and coagulation. Eur. Heart J. [Suppl. M]. 49:32-36; 1988.
78. Sherry, S.; Marder, V.J. Thrombosis, fibrinolysis and thrombolytic therapy. Prog. Cardiovasc. Dis. 34:89-100; 1985.
79. Siscovick, D.S.; Laporte, R.E.; Newman, J.M. The disease-specific benefits and risks of physical activity and exercise. Public Health Rep. 100:180-188; 1985.
80. Siscovick, D.S.; Weiss, N.S.; Fletcher, R.H.; Lasky, T. The incidence of primary cardiac arrest during vigorous exercise. N. Engl. J. Med. 311:874-877; 1984.
81. Spurlock, B.O.; Chandler, A.B. Adherent platelets and surface microthrombi of the human aorta and left coronary artery: A scanning electron microscopy study. Scanning Microsc. 1:1359-1365; 1987.
82. Stary, H.C. Evolution and progression of atherosclerosis in the coronary arteries of children and adults. In: Atherosclerosis and aging. New York: Springer-Verlag; 1987.
83. Stary, H.C.; Blankenhorn, D.H.; Chandler, A.B.; Glagov, S.; Insull, W., Jr.; Richardson, M.; Rosenfeld, M.E.; Schaffer, S.A.; Schwartz, C.J.; Wagner, M.D.; Wissler, R.W. A definition of the intima of human arteries and of its atherosclerosis-prone regions. Arteriosclerosis. 12:120-134; 1991.
84. Steinberg, D. Lipoproteins and atherosclerosis: A look back and a look ahead. Arteriosclerosis. 3:283-301; 1983.
85. Steinberg, D. Lipoproteins and the pathogenesis of atherosclerosis. Circulation. 76:508-514; 1987.
86. Stone, M.C.; Thorpe, J.M. Plasma fibrinogen—a major coronary risk factor. J. R. Coll. Gen. Pract. 35:565-569; 1985.
87. Stout, R.W.; Bierman, E.L.; Ross, R. The effect of insulin on the proliferation of cultured primate arterial smooth muscle cells. Circ. Res. 36:319-327; 1975.
88. Stratton, J.R.; Chandler, W.L; Schwartz, R.S.; Cerqveira, M.D.; Levy, W.L; Kahn, S.E.; Larson, V.G.; Cain, K.C.; Beard, J.C.; Abrass, I.B. Effects of physical conditioning on fibrinolytic variables. Circulation. 83:1692-1697; 1991.
89. Takada, A.; Takada, Y. Physiology of plasminogen: With special reference to activation and degradation. Haemostasis. [Suppl. 1]. 18:25-35; 1988.
90. Thaulow, E.; Erikssen, J.; Sandvik, L; Stormorken, H.; Cohn, P.F. Blood platelet count and function are related to total and cardiovascular death in apparently healthy men. Circulation. 84:936-938; 1991.
91. Thompson, P.D.; Cullinane, E.M.; Sady, S.P.; Flynn, M.S.; Chenevert, C.B.; Herbert, P.N. High density lipoprotein metabolism in endurance athletes and sedentary men. Circulation. 84:140-152; 1991.
92. Velican, C.; Velican, D. The precursors of coronary atherosclerotic plaques in subjects up to 40 years old. Atherosclerosis. 37:33-46; 1980.
93. Virchow, R. Hemostatis and thrombosis of the vascular system. In: Collected treatises in medical science. Frankfurt: Medlinger Sohn; 1856:458.
94. Vlodavsky, I.; Fielding, P.E.; Fielding, C.J.; Gospodarowicz, D. Role of contact inhibition in the regulation of receptor mediated uptake of low-density lipoprotein in cultured vascular endothelial cells. Proc. Natl. Acad. Sci. USA. 75:356-360; 1978.
95. Vuori, I. The cardiovascular risks of physical activity. Acta Med. Scand. [Suppl.]. 711:205-214; 1986.
96. West, K.M. Epidemiology of diabetes and its vascular lesions. New York: Elsevier Science; 1963:354-402.
97. Wilhelmsen, L.; Svarsdudd, K.; Korsan-Bengsten, K.; Larsson, B.; Welin, L.; Tibblin, G. Fibrinogen as a risk factor for stroke and myocardial infarction. 311:501-505; 1984.
98. Wissler, R.W.; Vesselinovitch, D.; Komatsu, A. The arterial wall and atherosclerosis in youth from biology of the arterial wall. Satellite meeting, 8th international symposium on atherosclerosis. Siena: 1988, October 7-8.
99. Wissler, R.W.; Vesselinovitch, D.; Komatsu, A. The contribution of studies of atherosclerotic lesions in young people to future research. Ann. NY. Acad. Sci. 598:418-434; 1990.
100. Wong, M.K.; Gotlieb, A.I. In vitro re-endothelialization of a single cell wound. Role of microfilament bundles in rapid filipodia-mediated wound closure. Lab. Invest. 51:75-81; 1984.
101. Wood, P.D.; Stefanick, M.L.; Williams, P.T.; Haskell, W.L. The effects on plasma lipoproteins of a product weight-reducing diet, with or without exercise, in overweight men and women. N. Engl. J. Med. 325:461-466; 1991.
102. Zhang, H.; Basra, H.J.K.; Steinbrecher, V.P. Effects of oxidatively modified LDL on cholesterol esterification in cultured macrophages. Lipid Res. 31:1361-1369; 1990.

Chapter 39

Physical Activity, Fitness, and Coronary Heart Disease

Steven N. Blair

The association between physical activity and coronary heart disease (CHD) has been reviewed by many authors. One of the best of these review papers was published in 1987 by Powell and colleagues (32). They used computerized literature searches, personal files, and a manual review of the tables of contents of the major epidemiological journals to identify an initial list of 121 articles on physical activity and CHD. Each of these articles was reviewed independently and in detail by two of the authors. The application of a list of specific inclusion criteria led to a final list of 43 articles that were selected for the scientific review. These articles were from studies done in several different countries, although a slight majority were from the United States and most of the rest were from Europe, particularly from England and the Nordic countries. The great majority of the studies were limited to men, with only five studies reporting data on women.

A unique feature of the Powell et al. (32) study was the careful evaluation of the quality of each of the studies. They used nine specific criteria to judge the quality of assessment of physical activity, five criteria to evaluate the CHD measure, and six criteria to rate the overall quality of the epidemiological methods used. The application of these criteria led to an evaluation of good, satisfactory, or unsatisfactory for each of the three areas. This evaluation resulted in a ranking of good for 19% of the studies on physical activity assessment, 40% of the studies for CHD measurement, and 35% of the studies for epidemiologic methods. The purpose of rating the quality of study methods was to allow a consideration of study findings stratified by study quality. Overall, 68% of the studies showed an inverse association between physical activity and CHD incidence. However, only 57% of the studies with methods classified as less than good reported a significant inverse association. In contrast, an inverse association between activity and CHD was seen in 73% of the papers that received at least one good evaluation and in 82% of the studies that received two or three good evaluations. These results lead to the conclusion that if physical activity is carefully assessed, CHD is accurately measured, and appropriate epidemiological methods are used, it is virtually certain that a significant inverse association will be found between activity and CHD.

Powell and colleagues conclude that, based on classical criteria established to infer causation from observational studies (15), the relationship between sedentary lifestyle and increased risk of CHD is likely to be causal. Any scientific judgment is subject to change with new data, and most of what we think we know should be tempered with uncertainty and doubt. Scientists always want data from additional studies with improved designs and methods in order to strengthen causal inferences, and the topic considered here is no different. Nonetheless, the review presented here suggests that it is reasonable to conclude that a low level of physical activity is one of the important causes of CHD and that this information should influence public policy and public health initiatives. However, some uncertainty does remain, and there are several important issues for which there are few (or no) data. This chapter provides a review of papers on physical activity or physical fitness and CHD published after the Powell et al. review (32), discusses some additional pertinent issues, and makes recommendations for future research.

Activity, Fitness, and Coronary Heart Disease Studies, 1987-1992

Several population-based studies on the relationship of physical activity or physical fitness to risk of CHD have been published since the Powell et al. review (32). A summary of 14 of these papers is given in Table 39.1. These studies are prospective

Table 39.1 Summary of Studies on Physical Activity or Physical Fitness and Health, 1987-1992

Study group	Design	Physical activity/ fitness measure	End point	Main results
Study group				
1. Representative sample, Alameda County, CA; 4,174 men and women aged 38 years or more at baseline (17)	Prospective, 17-year follow-up	Questionnaire, leisure-time activity	All-cause mortality, 1,219 deaths	RR = 1.38[a] (1.17, 1.62)[b] low/high activity
2. High-risk men in the Multiple Risk Factor Intervention Trial; 12,138 men aged 35–57 years at baseline (20)	Prospective, 7-year follow-up	Questionnaire, leisure-time activity	CHD death, 225 deaths	RR = 0.63[a] (0.43, 0.86) 2nd/1st tertile; RR = 0.64[a] (0.47, 0.88) 3rd/1st tertile
3. Seventh-Day Adventist men; 9,484 men aged 30 years and older at baseline (22)	Prospective, 26-year follow-up	Questionnaire, leisure and work activity	CHD death, 1,351 deaths	Age at crossover (RR = 1.0), 83.9[a] (74.9, 92.8) for moderate/low; 76.5[a] (66.0, 86.9) for high/low
4. British Civil Servants; 9,376 men aged 45–64 years at baseline (23)	Prospective, 9-year follow-up	Questionnaire, leisure-time activity	CHD death, 289 deaths	RR = 0.34[c] (0.18, 0.66) for frequent vigorous aerobic exercise (VE)/no VE
5. Population-based study in southwestern Finland; 636 men aged 40–59 years at baseline (31)	Prospective, 20-year follow-up	Questionnaire, leisure and work activity	CHD death, 106 deaths	RR = 1.3[a], low/high activity
6. Random population samples from eastern Finland; 15,088 men and women aged 30–59 years at baseline (33)	Prospective, 6-year follow-up	Questionnaire, leisure and work activity	CHD death, 102 deaths (90 men, 12 women)	RR = 1.4[a] (1.1, 1.7), low (either leisure or work)/high activity
7. U.S. railroad workers; 2,548 white men (36)	Prospective, 17- to 20-year follow-up	Questionnaire, leisure-time activity	CHD death	RR = 1.28[a] (0.99, 1.63), sedentary/active
8. Japanese-American men in Honolulu; 7,644 men aged 45–69 years at baseline (8)	Prospective, 12-year follow-up	Questionnaire, estimate of total energy expenditure	Fatal and nonfatal CHD, 444 events	RR = 0.69[c] (0.54, 0.88), in active vs. inactive men 45–64 years; RR = 0.42[c] (0.18, 0.96), in active vs. inactive men 65 years and older
9. British Regional Heart Study; 5,714 men aged 40–59 years, free of CHD at baseline (34)	Prospective, 8-year follow-up	Questionnaire, leisure-time activity	Fatal (N = 217) and nonfatal (N = 271) CHD	Men who reported moderate or moderately vigorous activity "experienced less than half the rate seen in inactive men."
Physical fitness				
1. Cooper Clinic patients; 3,120 women, 10,224 men (2)	Prospective, $\bar{x}$ follow-up of slightly more than 8 years	Maximal exercise tolerance, treadmill test	Cardiovascular disease (CVD) death, 73 deaths (7 women, 66 men)	RR = 9.25[c] (–5.1, 0.5)[d] for women; RR = 7.93[c] (–8.8, –3.3)[d] for men, low/high fitness

(continued)

Table 39.1 *(Continued)*

Study group	Design	Physical activity/ fitness measure	End point	Main results
2. Lipid Research Clinics study; 3,106 men, 30–69 years at baseline (10)	Prospective, 8.5-year follow-up	Submaximal exercise test, treadmill	CHD death, CVD death, 45 deaths	RR = 6.5 (1.5, 28.7) for CHD death; RR = 8.5 (2.0, 36.7) for CVD death, least fit quartile/most fit quartile; adjusted RR = 2.8[a] (1.3, 6.1) for CHD; adjusted RR = 3.6[a] (1.6, 5.6) for CVD
3. Cooper Clinic patients; 2,926 men who were hypertensive at baseline (12)	Prospecitve, $\bar{x}$ follow-up of slightly more than 8 years	Maximal exercise tolerance, treadmill test	CVD death, 63 deaths	RR = 2.3[c] (1.3, 3.8) low/high fitness
4. Company or government employees in Oslo; 2,014 men, 40–59 years at baseline (21)	Prospective, 7-year follow-up	Submaximal exercise test, cycle ergometer	CHD death, 58 deaths	RR ≈ 4.8, least fit quartile/most fit quartile
5. U.S. railroad workers; 2,431 white men, 22–79 years at baseline (35)	Prospective, $\bar{x}$ follow-up of approximately 20 years	Submaximal exercise test, treadmill	CHD and CVD death, 258 CHD deaths	RR = 1.45[c] for CHD and 1.51 for CVD; adjusted RR = 1.20[a] (1.10, 1.26) for CHD; low/high fitness

[a]Relative risk (RR) adjusted for age and other major CHD risk factors. [b]Numbers in parentheses are 95% confidence intervals. [c]Relative risk adjusted for age only, although additional adjustments for other factors had a negligible effect. [d]95% confidence interval for linear trend slope.

investigations of the relation of physical activity (nine studies) or physical fitness (five studies) to CHD, cardiovascular disease (CVD), or all-cause mortality. The studies reviewed here probably are methodologically superior as a group compared with the earlier papers reviewed by Powell et al. The evaluation methods used by Powell et al. required subjective judgment and are impossible for me to repeat exactly for the papers listed in Table 39.1. However, I used the same criteria described in their article to evaluate the papers published during 1987 to 1992.

The papers reviewed here used better physical activity assessment methods than the earlier studies. I judge five of the nine (56%) of the prospective physical activity studies to have a good assessment of physical activity and the rest to be satisfactory. The five studies with an objective measurement of physical fitness are all considered to have a good assessment of the exposure variable. Powell et al. assigned a good rating to only 19% of the studies in their review, and 40% were given a satisfactory score (32).

All of the prospective studies described in Table 39.1 used the objective endpoints of CHD, CVD, or all-cause mortality. These outcomes were usually determined from death certificate or central registry analyses or review. The 14 studies reviewed here generally met the criteria for CHD measurement presented by Powell et al. (32). I judge that 11 of the 13 studies (85%) with CHD or CVD end points (1 study only reported all-cause mortality) can be evaluated as having good methods for the measurement of outcomes.

Powell et al. describe five evaluation criteria for epidemiologic methods (32). The random assignment criterion was not met in any of the studies they reviewed, nor in any of the 14 studies in Table 39.1. I believe that the 14 papers reviewed here meet the other evaluative criteria for epidemiologic methods (appropriate time sequence, adjustment for confounders, representativeness, and small loss to follow-up) and are rated good on this dimension.

Physical Activity and Mortality

Nine papers briefly described in Table 39.1 evaluated the relation of physical activity to mortality. All studies had a prospective design, with an assessment of physical activity at baseline and with follow-up intervals ranging from 6 to 26 years. Five of the studies were conducted in the United States (8,17,20,22,36), two in Finland (31,33), and two in Great Britain (23,34). All studies included populations of men; women were represented in two of the studies. Most of the study subjects were probably white, although racial or ethnic identity was not specified in most of the papers. The paper from the Honolulu Heart Program was on a population of Japanese-American men (8). All studies assessed leisure-time physical activity, and the two studies from Finland also measured work-related activity. CHD death was the end point in all the studies except the Alameda County Study (17), where only all-cause mortality was presented. This report was included because it has a representative population sample, and it also reported data on women. CHD is the leading cause of mortality in industrialized populations, and it is reasonable to assume that the all-cause mortality rates in the elderly subjects in the Alameda County Study were heavily influenced by differences in CHD mortality across activity groups.

The reports on physical activity and mortality are consistent with one another and with the conclusion presented by Powell et al. (32). All nine studies demonstrate an inverse gradient for all-cause or CHD mortality across physical activity categories. It is not appropriate to compare directly death rates or relative risks across the studies, due to differences in study methods and different definitions. Nevertheless, the relative magnitude of the effect of sedentary living habits on CHD for the activity papers in Table 39.1 is comparable to the summary statistic (increased relative risk of 1.9 in sedentary compared with active individuals) reported by Powell et al. (32).

The increased mortality in the less active individuals in the studies reviewed here cannot be explained by confounding influences of other established risk factors for CHD. All nine studies took this possibility into account in their designs and analyses. The specific risk factors evaluated varied across studies, due to different data being available, but typically included some combination of age, blood lipids, cigarette-smoking habits, blood pressure, family history of CHD, socioeconomic status, alcohol intake, dietary factors, sleep habits, relative weight, stature, and psychosocial characteristics. Eight of the nine studies excluded from analysis subjects who had cardiovascular disease at baseline, determined by history or clinical examination.

Physical Fitness and Mortality

Table 39.1 presents reviews of five recent investigations on the relationship of physical fitness to mortality. Four of the studies were done in the United States (4,10,12,35), and one was from Norway (21). Only one included women. Physical fitness was assessed in these studies by cycle ergometry or treadmill exercise testing, submaximal tests were used in three of the investigations, and maximal testing was done in two studies. With the exception of the U.S. Railroad Workers Study (35), the fitness studies are from a later generation of studies than the activity studies. The length of follow-up in the fitness studies is 7 or 8 years in four of the reports and is approximately 20 years in the railroad study. Due to generally shorter follow-up intervals, the number of deaths available for analysis tends to be fewer in the fitness studies than in the activity studies.

The fitness studies generally used good epidemiological methods. Potential confounding factors were considered in some detail, and few subjects were lost to follow-up. Subjects with cardiovascular disease were excluded from analyses in four of the investigations. The other study was conducted in hypertensive men to evaluate the relation between fitness and mortality in this special population (12).

All five studies report an inverse gradient for mortality across physical fitness categories. The gradient here is much steeper in healthy men and women (with the exception of the railroad study [35]) than is seen in the investigations on activity and mortality. The latter studies typically have a relative risk of 2.0 or less when the least active are compared with the most active. Age-adjusted relative risks of approximately 5.0 or more are seen when comparing the least fit (defined by quartiles or quintiles) with the most fit in the Oslo (21), Dallas (4,12), and Lipid Research Clinics (10) studies. It is unclear why the relative risk in the railroad study (35) is much lower (less than 2.0) than in the other studies. The follow-up is considerably longer, which might lead to more misclassification on fitness with the passage of time, as workers retire or move to more sedentary jobs.

Summary of Recent Findings on Activity or Fitness and Cardiovascular Disease

Results from three recent studies on physical activity and CHD and from two fitness studies are shown graphically in Figure 39.1. The generally greater reduction in mortality in the fitness studies when compared with activity studies is probably due, at least in part, to the objective measurement of fitness. Our existing methods of physical activity assessment are crude and imprecise and lead to misclassification for many subjects. Physical fitness, as assessed by treadmill or cycle ergometry, is an excellent overall marker of an individual's total physical activity, or the total daily energy expenditure. Thus, physical fitness is a more objective measure of physical activity than are physical activity questionnaires themselves; using physical fitness as a measure leads to less misclassification, (i.e., there is less measurement error). Studies with less measurement error are more likely to detect a relationship, if a true relationship exists, than are studies with higher levels of measurement error. Furthermore, if a high level of random measurement error is present, a study is likely to underestimate the true magnitude of effect. Therefore, the studies on physical activity and mortality are likely to underestimate the true impact of sedentary living habits on CHD; the physical fitness studies provide results that are closer to the true relationships.

A second impression gained by viewing the results in Figure 39.1 is that the mortality reduction curves are generally somewhat steeper on the left side of the figure, although the data from the British Civil Servants are an exception (23). A relatively small change in physical activity or fitness at the lower levels is associated with a relatively greater reduction in mortality than an equivalent change at the higher levels of fitness or activity. Much additional research is needed to more fully characterize the shape of the dose-response relationship between activity or fitness and mortality, but current results suggest that the curve has a curvilinear component. If this observation is correct, it supports an encouraging public health message. Sedentary and high-risk individuals could be told that they do not have to become vigorous exercisers to obtain health benefits and that they can make important gains by simply becoming somewhat more active and fit. The moderate levels of activity and fitness associated with a reduced risk of CHD and CVD mortality as depicted in Figure 39.1 are perhaps best exemplified by a lifestyle that includes 30 to 45 min of brisk walking each day (1,9). Recent research suggests that physical activity (and physical fitness gained) can be accumulated in several bouts spread over the course of the day and does not have to be obtained all in one session (7). Thus, sedentary persons can strive to fit in three or four 10-min walks during the day, which should be an easier exercise plan for many individuals to follow than the traditional prescription and thus may promote better adherence.

Do Sedentary Habits Cause CHD?

Existing evidence supports a causal inference for the inactivity-CHD relationship (32). The studies published during the past 5 years support and reinforce that conclusion. The more recent studies generally used high-quality methods, and the results are consistent in support of the causal hypothesis.

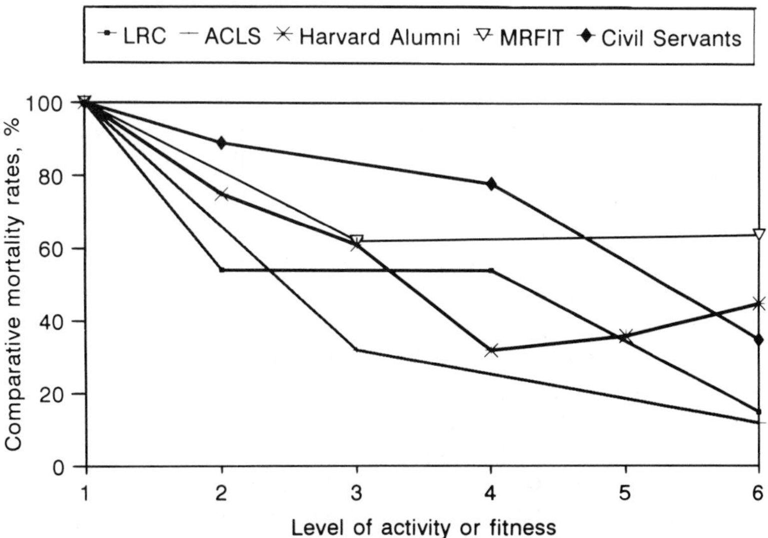

Figure 39.1 Data are presented from five studies on physical activity or physical fitness and CHD or CVD:LRC (10), ACLS (2), Harvard alumni (29), MRFIT (20), civil servants (23). The vertical axis expresses mortality rates in the various activity and fitness categories as percentages of the mortality rates for the least active and fit groups, which are set at 100%. The horizontal axis indicates levels of physical activity or physical fitness. Credit for the concept for Figure 39.1 is given to Dr. William L. Haskell of the Stanford University School of Medicine. The figure is modeled after a slide he presented at the R. Tait McKenzie Lecture at the American Academy of Physical Education.

In addition, large prospective studies on physical fitness and mortality show a strong inverse gradient with cardiovascular disease and add considerable support to the conclusions based on studies of physical activity.

Is the Relationship Causal?

Evidence continues to accumulate that a physically active way of life is associated with improved CHD risk-factor status and may therefore have an indirect pathway of benefit in CHD prevention. Several chapters in this volume present this evidence in detail, and reviews of these studies will not be repeated here. It is sufficient to note that recent studies show that regular physical activity produces a more favorable lipoprotein profile, helps manage body weight, increases insulin sensitivity, increases fibrinolytic activity, decreases blood clotting, lowers blood pressure, is a useful adjunct to smoking-cessation therapy, and may improve the atherogenic body fat pattern. None of the extant population-based studies on activity or fitness and CHD have been able to control for all of these factors in order to isolate the independent impact of activity or fitness on risk of disease. This situation is unlikely to change in the near future, because the ongoing large studies on activity or fitness do not include some of the more recently studied factors such as insulin sensitivity or fibrinolytic capacity. Nonetheless, given the present data it appears that low levels of activity or fitness are independent risk factors for CHD.

However, even if future research shows that they are not related to CHD after additional adjustments are made, sedentary habits are still important in CHD etiology. It is clear from clinical and experimental studies that changing from a sedentary to an active lifestyle produces beneficial changes in several risk factors, and at least part of the mechanism for prevention of CHD by activity must be through change in other risk factors. To cite an analogy, changing to a lower fat diet results in an improved lipoprotein profile. If one were studying the effect of diet on the development of CHD, it would not make sense to adjust for lipid levels in the analysis. The important public health and clinical question is whether or not the disease burden will be decreased if people change from a high-cholesterol, high-fat diet to a prudent diet. Likewise, it is important from a public health and clinical perspective to know if converting from a sedentary to an active way of life reduces risk of CHD, and the answer appears to be in the affirmative. Theoretically, if we completely understood and measured all the mechanisms by which physical activity reduces risk, and if analyses on activity and CHD were adjusted for all these variables, we would find no effect for activity. This conclusion, however, would be incorrect.

Arguments Against a Causal Hypothesis

The arguments against a causal relationship between activity or fitness and CHD frequently focus on the concept of selection bias. Selection bias considers that some other factor (e.g., genetic influences, preexisting disease) causes individuals to be sedentary and also increases risk of CHD. This other characteristic causes persons to be "selected" into sedentary or active categories. For example, undetected subclinical disease might cause a person to feel bad, to not exercise, and thus to self-select into the sedentary group, and these individuals with subclinical disease also would be more likely to have a heart attack or die during a follow-up period. It is impossible to prove a negative hypothesis, and we will never be absolutely certain that selection bias is at least part of the explanation for the reduced death rates in more active individuals. Research does bear on the issue, however, and these studies make the selection bias hypothesis less tenable as an explanation of the main observation.

Preexisting Disease

Most of the studies on activity or fitness and CHD exclude from analysis individuals with cardiovascular disease (and usually other chronic diseases as well) at baseline. The apparently healthy population is then sorted into activity or fitness groups as determined by baseline measurements, and they are followed for disease incidence or mortality. As reviewed earlier, death rates tend to be higher during follow-up in the sedentary and unfit individuals. Skeptics consider that this finding is due to incomplete exclusion of persons with disease at baseline and that these study participants tend to be concentrated in the sedentary category because the disease makes them less active. Investigators have addressed this issue by performing stratified analyses (a) within health status groups and (b) by early and late follow-up.

Results from *early versus late follow-up* analyses are summarized in Table 39.2 for three recent studies on activity or fitness and disease. If undetected chronic diseases at baseline were causing subjects to be more sedentary and also causing increased risk of death, we would expect these individuals to die at a relatively faster rate (earlier in the follow-up period) than the healthy participants. This would increase the difference in death rates between sedentary or unfit participants and the active and fit participants in the early follow-up and

Table 39.2 Morbidity and Mortality by Activity or Fitness Groups by Early Versus Late Follow-Up

Study	Activity or fitness group	Follow-up interval (years) Early	Middle	Late	Results Early	Middle	Late
Aerobics Center Longitudinal Study	Least fit quintile vs. all others	0–3		>3			
10,224 healthy men (2)					1.60[a](1.18, 2.16)		1.45 (1.08, 1.96)
3,120 healthy women (2)					1.47 (0.74, 2.94)		3.0 (1.06, 8.51)
1,832 hypertensive men (4)					2.55[b] (1.48, 4.41)		3.16 (1.93, 5.16)
Harvard Alumni Study (26) 16,936 healthy men	<2,000 kcal/week in physical activity vs. ≥2,000 kcal/week	0–2	3–7	8–12	68%[c]	54%	12%
British Civil Servants Study (23) 9,376 healthy men	Frequent vigorous aerobic exercise vs. no such exercise	0–4		>4	0.41[d](0.22, 0.76)		0.29 (0.13, 0.63)

[a]Age- and risk factor-adjusted increased relative risk in unfit men and women for all-cause mortality (95% confidence interval). [b]Age-adjusted increased relative risk for all-cause mortality in hypertensive men. [c]Percent higher all-cause death rates in sedentary compared with active alumni. [d]Reduced relative risk for CHD attack rates (95% confidence interval) in vigorous aerobic exercisers compared with the rest of the men.

eliminate the difference in later follow-up. Relative risks for all-cause mortality (4,27) or CHD attack rate (23) for early and late follow-up intervals are similar, and in most cases the 95% confidence interval around the relative risks does not include 1.0. The relative risks for all-cause mortality for the healthy men and women in the Aerobics Center Longitudinal Study (4) were adjusted for age and other risk factors (levels of cholesterol and blood pressure, cigarette smoking, body mass index, fasting, blood glucose, and family history of CHD), and the elevated relative risks persisted into the follow-up interval of 3 years and longer. This pattern strengthens the conclusion that the results are not due entirely to confounding by subclinical disease at baseline.

A related issue is the association of activity or fitness to *mortality within various health status strata.* Paffenbarger et al. report similar effects of sedentary habits in hypertensive and normotensive men (27,29,30). Morris and Crawford, in their necropsy study, found an inverse association of CHD across occupational physical activity groups in men who died with hypertension, injuries, infections, cancer, and peptic ulcer (24). Physically fit men and women have lower age-adjusted all-cause death rates across strata of blood pressure (4). We also note lower all-cause (3) and cardiovascular disease (12) death rates in physically fit hypertensive men, so there seems to be a secondary prevention impact. Kohl et al. recently reported an inverse gradient across fitness groups for all-cause and cardiovascular disease mortality by strata of glucose tolerance (19). The results from these papers support the hypothesis that the relationship between activity or fitness and disease is causal and not due to confounding by baseline disease, either detected or undetected.

Another way in which selection bias could affect the activity-disease relationship has been hypothesized for occupational studies. If workers with underlying or overt disease shift to less active jobs, and job-related activity is the measure of exposure, higher death rates seen in workers in sedentary jobs might not be due to their inactivity but to their health status. This issue has been considered in detail by Paffenbarger and his colleagues in their studies of longshoremen (26). Union policy directed that all longshoremen began their employment performing jobs requiring heavy-intensity work. Shifts to less demanding jobs could occur after 5 years of service but did not occur until an average of 13 years. In their analyses, the investigators used the job assignment the man had in the year prior to death (6 months prior to death on the average). Thus, for most of the men, the job assignment used in the analyses was the one over the longer employment period, which would minimize the impact of late job changes due to health problems. The investigators later published an extensive and elegant multifactor logistic analysis on a subset of the longshoremen for whom yearly job assignments were recorded (5). Extensive modeling to account for job changes and various patterns of job changes did not eliminate the inverse association between work-related physical activity and mortality.

Undetected changes in physical activity or physical fitness after the baseline assessment are considered by some to vitiate the findings of these studies. It is true that in our study (4), for example, unfit persons at baseline might follow the intervention advice provided by clinic physicians and begin exercising and thereby improve their physical fitness over the course of follow-up. Such a change would result in a misclassification of that individual throughout much of the follow-up interval. That is, we would consider them unfit because of their baseline treadmill test performance, but they were in fact fit because they changed their exercise habits. Such changes of fitness categories (misclassification) would be likely to reduce the difference in death rates between fit and unfit groups across the follow-up interval.

There are no published reports on the effect of change in physical activity or physical fitness on subsequent mortality rates. Such studies are needed, and a tantalizing early glimpse of work on this topic has been presented in an abstract by Paffenbarger et al. (28). They report on changes in physical activity and other risk factors ascertained during the mid-1960s and mid-1970s, with follow-up for mortality from 1977 to 1985. Initially sedentary college alumni who became physically active had a 28% lower death rate than their peers who did not change. The benefit of starting to exercise in this population of men was comparable to the benefit of stopping smoking. These preliminary findings are of major importance, and we eagerly await the final report.

Genetic Influences

Genetic factors are sometimes mentioned as possible explanations for the inverse gradient of death rates across activity or fitness groups. The rationale is that some individuals are genetically incapable of becoming physically fit or that physical activity is unacceptable to them because of some genetic predisposition. These same individuals, so the argument goes, also have inherited a "weak constitution" and are at a higher risk for morbidity and mortality. Several papers provide data related to this issue. The lower death rates in more active and fit men and women occur in those with a positive family history of early CHD as well as those without such a background (4,23,27). It is clear that CHD has a genetic component, but it is not established that physical activity is determined by inheritance. Other CHD risk factors such as cholesterol level, blood pressure, obesity, and risk for non-insulin-dependent diabetes also have genetic components, but that does not diminish their importance or causal role in the etiology of CHD.

The inheritance factor also can be evaluated via data on participation in competitive sports. It is reasonable to conclude that persons who compete in various sports are endowed with above-average physical prowess and an enhanced ability to perform physical activity. If the inverse relation between physical activity and mortality is due to individuals with inherently superior physical abilities being more likely to exercise and also less likely to develop CHD, one would expect that persons who were athletes in high school or college would have lower CHD rates during follow-up than nonathletes. This is not the case. Paffenbarger et al. report no relation between college sports play and mortality later in life (29); however, both college athletes and nonathletes who were active in middle age had lower death rates than their sedentary peers. Morris et al. also report that previous vigorous exercise is not related to CHD in the British Civil Servants (23); instead it is current activity that is protective. Brill et al. found that former athletes were no more likely to be physically fit or physically active in middle age than men who were not athletic as youth (6). Both groups had similar CHD risk factor profiles as adults. These subjects were given risk factor counseling and advice to start exercising. The rate of adoption of an exercise program was the same in the former athletes and nonathletes, and both groups made comparable improvements in physical fitness and in risk factor profiles. Collectively, these studies suggest that it is unlikely that the lower rates of CHD in active men are due to inherited factors that lead to a more active lifestyle and a simultaneous decrease in disease risk.

Unresolved Issues

Sedentary lifestyle is probably a cause of CHD, but much work remains to be done to more fully describe the relationship and to develop public strategies to promote activity in the population.

Sedentary Habits and CHD in Women

Most of the studies on activity or fitness and CHD have been performed in populations of men. Powell et al. report only five studies with 14 comparisons between sedentary and active women (32). Although a clear majority of studies in men show an inverse gradient for CHD across activity strata, 10 of the 14 comparisons in women show no relationship. In the Framingham study, for example, sedentary men were at increased risk for CHD as determined by a multiple logistic analysis with adjustment for age and other risk factors (16). There was no similar relationship for women, in this same population, with identical methods used in the study.

We find a strong inverse gradient for all-cause and cardiovascular mortality across low, moderate, and high physical fitness groups, and the results are nearly identical in men and women (4). Further analysis in our population shows that when we use self-report of physical activity instead of physical fitness in the analysis, the inverse gradient remains for men and disappears in women (2). These analyses on physical activity were done in exactly the same population of men and women as the fitness analyses, with the same number of deaths and the same analytical methods.

Why are the results congruent between men and women for the fitness analyses but incongruent for activity analyses? The answer is uncertain, but a reasonable hypothesis is that the physical activity questionnaire, which focuses on sports participation and planned fitness activities, is a valid instrument for men and not valid for women. When the objective measure of fitness, determined from a maximal exercise treadmill test, is used as the exposure variable, the same results are obtained for both sexes. One of the primary reasons that many of the published reports on activity and CHD in women find no relationship is perhaps that physical activity was inappropriately and inaccurately measured. Women may expend considerable energy in household and child-care tasks, and these items are typically not covered in current questionnaires. I believe that the relationship between activity or fitness and CHD is comparable in men and women, as applies for other risk factors (11), but additional research is required to confirm or reject this hypothesis.

What Specific Type and Dose of Activity, or of Fitness, Is Required to Protect Against CHD?

We can be confident that sedentary living habits are one of the causes of CHD. Beyond that general conclusion, not enough is known about the specific type, duration, intensity, frequency, pattern, and total dose of physical activity that is required to provide protection against CHD. Some studies, notably those by Morris et al. (23,25), support the conclusion that vigorous exercise (greater than or equal to 7.5 kcal/min) is needed for benefit. In other reports, the role of exercise intensity is unclear, although in some cases this may be because the available data are not sufficient to perform an analysis by intensity strata. Differences in terminology and definitions of activity intensity add confusion to this issue.

I believe that the available evidence suggests that the type of activity is probably not important, although more research on this question is needed. It does not appear to matter whether individuals walk or jog, play sports, or engage in gardening. If the total energy expended is comparable, benefits are likely to be the same.

Low levels of physical fitness are associated with increased risk for mortality (3,4,10,12,19,21,35). Physical fitness in the extant studies has been defined as maximal aerobic power (or some estimate of that variable). Other types of physical fitness also need to be evaluated for their relationship to health. It may be that some type of relative fitness measure—for example, the percentage of maximal aerobic power that can be sustained over long periods without metabolic derangement (lactic acid threshold)—is equally, or perhaps more, important. This endurance capacity is known to be quite responsive to exercise training.

What Is the Optimal Level of Activity or Fitness?

The data illustrate an inverse relationship between physical activity or physical fitness and CHD mortality (see Figure 39.1). The trend is linear for the left side of the distribution and for most studies reaches an asymptote at mid to high levels of activity or fitness. In some studies there is no further benefit beyond the second tertile (the study by Leon et al. (20), for example). Data from the Harvard Alumni Study (26) actually show a slight increase in mortality in the most active men (see Figure 39.1). It is not clear whether or not this elevated risk in the most active is an artifact or if there actually is a point beyond which risk increases. It is theoretically possible that extremely high levels of activity could increase risk for atherosclerosis. Perhaps sustained elevated blood pressure levels during vigorous exercise can have an adverse effect on the arterial wall, risk of sudden death may increase disproportionately at the most vigorous exercise levels, or other mechanisms might be involved. None of the current studies have an adequate amount of follow-up experience in a group of highly active subjects to evaluate properly the hypothesis that it is possible to exercise too much (either too much total energy expenditure or too high an intensity).

It is possible that the optimal amount of physical activity varies with age, gender, ethnic background, presence of other risk factors, family history, genetic factors, presence of other chronic diseases, or environment. Additional studies are needed to investigate these issues.

Recommendations for Research

Much has been learned about the role of sedentary habits in the etiology of CHD, but much remains to be done. The recommendations presented here are broad general topics. Many specific hypotheses can be developed for each recommendation area, and numerous studies can be designed to evaluate these several recommendations.

1. Specify activity dose. Many studies are needed to more fully describe the dose–response relationship between activity or fitness and CHD. There should be efforts to clarify the role of exercise intensity and the optimal dose of exercise within diverse population groups.

2. Studies in women. Most of the extant studies were done with men, and the current studies with women subjects are equivocal. For future studies with women, researchers need to develop new assessment methodologies specifically suited for women. It is important to determine if the dose of exercise required for benefits in women is the same as for men. Different intervention strategies may be required for women.

3. Impact of change in exercise habits. Current observational studies rely on a single assessment of activity or fitness. Mortality follow-up is needed in a group of initially sedentary middle-aged subjects, some of whom remain sedentary and some of whom become active. Because a randomized clinical trial on the effects of activity on CHD mortality is not likely to be mounted due to logistical and cost constraints, observational studies of change in activity or fitness will be the next major test of the causal hypothesis. Researchers also should attempt to characterize the lifetime pattern of physical activity and relate it to disease risk.

4. Physical activity versus physical fitness. Most extant studies have used physical activity as the exposure variable, but a few recent studies have evaluated physical fitness. New studies with assessments of both exposure variables are needed to evaluate the independent and interactive relationships of activity and fitness as they relate to CHD risk.

5. Improved assessment tools. Current studies are hampered by relatively crude and imprecise tools for measuring physical activity. Fitness assessments are more objective than activity measurements, but they are more complicated and expensive. Better field methods for measuring both variables are needed for adoption into large-scale population-based studies.

6. Randomized trial on activity and atherosclerosis. A randomized clinical trial on the primary prevention of clinical manifestations of CHD (heart attack, CHD death, etc.) is not likely to be attempted due to large sample size requirements, complexity, and cost. Development of new methods of quantitative assessment of atherosclerotic disease in humans may allow for a trial of the direct evaluation of physical activity on the atherosclerotic process (37). Ultrasound techniques are being refined and may become sensitive enough for this purpose. Newer imaging techniques including magnetic resonance tomography and scintigraphic approaches may ultimately provide the resolution required for quantitative assessment. A randomized clinical trial of physical activity to evaluate its impact on the atherosclerotic process is urgently needed and may well be feasible in the near future.

7. Development of better intervention strategies. There is enough evidence supporting the health benefits associated with an active way of life that policies and recommendations to promote activity have been developed (14). Traditional methods of promoting physical activity and improving physical fitness involve trained exercise leaders, group classes, and individual exercise prescriptions. These approaches are based on research and will result in improvements in fitness, if the subjects continue the activity. Unfortunately, such programs have high dropout rates. At-home and other lifestyle interventions need to be developed and evaluated (1,18).

Conclusions

This review of the role of sedentary habits in the etiology of CHD confirms and extends previous reviews. Evidence on this issue continues to mount, with accumulation of data from studies with improved designs and methods. The population burden of sedentary living is high: It is estimated that nearly 250,000 deaths per year in the United States are attributed to lack of exercise (13). Additional research is recommended to clarify issues, further refine and define the optimal dose of exercise, and develop better methods for conducting etiological and intervention studies.

Acknowledgments

I thank Laura Becker for manuscript and figure preparation and for proofreading and J.N. Morris, R.S. Paffenbarger, Jr., R.T. Hyde, K.E. Powell, H.W. Kohl, N.F. Gordon, and P. Lloyd for many helpful comments on an early draft of the manuscript.

References

1. Blair, S.N. Living with exercise. Dallas: American Health Publishing Company; 1991.
2. Blair, S.N.; Kohl, H.W.; Barlow, C.E. Physical activity, physical fitness, and mortality in women: Do women need to be active? J. Am. Coll. Nutr. 12:368-371; 1993.
3. Blair, S.N.; Kohl, H.W., III; Barlow, C.E.; Gibbons, L.W. Physical fitness and all-cause mortality in hypertensive men. Ann. Med. 23:307-312; 1991.
4. Blair, S.N.; Kohl, H.W.; III; Paffenbarger, R.S., Jr.; Clark, D.G.; Cooper, K.H.; Gibbons, L.W. Physical fitness and all-cause mortality: A prospective study of healthy men and women. JAMA. 262:2395-2401; 1989.
5. Brand, R.J.; Paffenbarger, R.S., Jr.; Sholtz, R.I.; Kampert, J.B. Work activity and fatal heart attack studied by multiple logistic risk analysis. Am. J. Epidemiol. 110:52-62; 1979.
6. Brill, P.A.; Burkhalter, H.E.; Kohl H.W.; Blair, S.N.; Goodyear, N.N. The impact of previous athleticism on exercise habits, physical fitness, and coronary heart disease risk factors in middle-aged men. Res. Q. Exerc. Sport. 60:209-215; 1989.
7. DeBusk, R.F.; Stenestrand, U.; Sheehan, M.; Haskell, W.L. Training effects of long versus short bouts of exercise in healthy subjects. Am. J. Cardiol. 65:1010-1013; 1990.
8. Donahue, R.P.; Abbott, R.D.; Reed, D.M.; Yano, K. Physical activity and coronary heart disease in middle-aged and elderly men: The Honolulu Heart Program. Am. J. Public Health. 78:683-685; 1988.
9. Duncan, J.J.; Gordon, N.F.; Scott, C.B. Women walking for health and fitness: How much is enough? JAMA. 266:3295-3299; 1991.
10. Ekelund, L-G.; Haskell, W.L.; Johnson, J.L.; Whaley, F.S.; Criqui, M.H.; Sheps, D.S. Physical fitness as a predictor of cardiovascular mortality in asymptomatic North American men: The Lipid Research Clinics Mortality Follow-Up Study. N. Engl. J. Med. 319:1379-1384; 1988.
11. Fair of face and sick at heart. (Editorial). Lancet. 338:1366-1367; 1991.
12. Gibbons, L.W.; Kohl, H.W., III; Cooper, K.H.; Blair, S.N. Physical fitness and lower cardiovascular disease mortality in men with hypertension. [In review].
13. Hahn, R.A.; Teutsch, S.M.; Rothenberg, R.B.; Marks, J.S. Excess deaths from nine chronic diseases in the United States, 1986. JAMA. 264:2654-2659; 1990.
14. Harris, S.S.; Caspersen, C.J.; DeFriese, G.H.; Estes, H., Jr. Physical activity counseling for healthy adults as a primary preventive intervention in the clinical setting: Report for the U.S. Preventive Services Task Force. JAMA. 261:3590-3598; 1989.
15. Hill, A.B. The environment and disease: Association or causation? Proc. R. Soc. Med. 58:295-300; 1965.
16. Kannel, W.B.; Sorlie, P. Some health benefits of physical activity: The Framingham Study. Arch. Intern. Med. 139:857-861; 1979.
17. Kaplan, G.A.; Seeman, T.E.; Cohen, R.D.; Knudsen, L.P.; Guralnik, J. Mortality among the elderly in the Alameda County Study: Behavioral and demographic risk factors. Am. J. Public Health. 77:307-312; 1987.
18. King, A.C.; Haskell, W.L.; Taylor, C.B.; Kraemer, H.C.; DeBusk, R.F. Group- vs home-based exercise training in healthy older men and women: A community-based clinical trial. JAMA. 266:1535-1542; 1991.
19. Kohl, H.W.; Gordon, N.F.; Villegas, J.A.; Blair, S.N. Cardiorespiratory fitness, glycemic status, and mortality risk in men. Diabetes Care. 15:184-192; 1992.
20. Leon, A.S.; Connett, J.; Jacobs, D.R., Jr.; Rauramaa, R. Leisure-time physical activity levels and risk of coronary heart disease and death: The Multiple Risk Factor Intervention Trial. JAMA. 258:2388-2395; 1987.
21. Lie, H.; Mundal, R.; Erikssen, J. Coronary risk factors and incidence of coronary death in relation to physical fitness. Seven-year follow-up study of middle-aged and elderly men. Eur. Heart J. 6:147-157; 1985.
22. Lindsted, K.D.; Tonstad, S.; Kuzma, J. Self-report of physical activity and patterns of mortality in Seventh-day Adventist men. J. Clin. Epidemiol. 44:355-364; 1991.

23. Morris, J.N.; Clayton, D.G.; Everitt, M.G.; Semmence, A.M.; Burgess, E.H. Exercise in leisure time: Coronary attack and death rates. Br. Heart J. 63:325-334; 1990.
24. Morris, J.N.; Crawford, M.D. Coronary heart disease and physical activity of work: Evidence of a National Necropsy Survey. Br. Med. J. 2:1485-1496; 1958.
25. Morris, J.N.; Everitt, M.G.; Pollard, R.; Chave, S.P.W.; Semmence, A.M. Vigorous exercise in leisure-time: Protection against coronary heart disease. Lancet. 2:1207-1210; 1980.
26. Paffenbarger, R.S., Jr.; Hale, W.E. Work activity and coronary heart mortality. N. Engl. J. Med. 292:545-550; 1975.
27. Paffenbarger, R.S., Jr.; Hyde, R.T.; Wing, A.L.; Hsieh, C-C. Physical activity, all-cause mortality, and longevity of college alumni. N. Engl. J. Med. 314:605-613; 1986.
28. Paffenbarger, R.; Hyde, R.; Wing, A.; Jung, D.; Kampert, J. Influences of changes in physical activity and other characteristics on all-cause mortality. Med. Sci. Sports Exerc. [Suppl.]. 23:S82; 1991.
29. Paffenbarger, R.S., Jr.; Hyde, R.T.; Wing, A.L.; Steinmetz, C.H. A natural history of athleticism and cardiovascular health. JAMA. 252:491-495; 1984.
30. Paffenbarger, R.S., Jr.; Wing, A.L.; Hyde, R.T. Physical activity as an index of heart attack risk in college alumni. Am. J. Epidemiol. 108:161-175; 1978.
31. Pekkanen, J.; Marti, B.; Nissinen, A.; Tuomilehto, J.; Punsar, S.; Karvonen, M.J. Reduction of premature mortality by high physical activity: A 20-year follow-up of middle-aged Finnish men. Lancet. 1:1473-1477; 1987.
32. Powell, K.E.; Thompson, P.D.; Caspersen, C.J.; Kendrick, J.S. Physical activity and the incidence of coronary heart disease. Annu. Rev. Public Health. 8:253-287; 1987.
33. Salonen, J.T.; Slater, J.S.; Tuomilehto, J.; Rauramaa, R. Leisure time and occupational physical activity: Risk of death from ischemic heart disease. Am. J. Epidemiol. 127:87-94; 1988.
34. Shaper, A.G.; Wannamethee, G. Physical activity and ischaemic heart disease in middle-aged British men. Br. Med. J. 66:384-394; 1991.
35. Slattery, M.L.; Jacobs, D.R., Jr. Physical fitness and cardiovascular disease mortality: The U.S. Railroad Study. Am. J. Epidemiol. 127:571-580; 1988.
36. Slattery, M.L.; Jacobs, D.R., Jr.; Nichaman, M.Z. Leisure time physical activity and coronary heart disease death: The U.S. Railroad Study. Circulation. 79:304-311; 1989.
37. Wikstrand, J.; Wiklund, O. Frontiers in cardiovascular science: Quantitative measurements of atherosclerotic manifestations in humans. Arteriosclerosis Thrombosis. 12:114-119; 1992.

Chapter 40

Physical Activity and Cardiac Rehabilitation for Patients With Coronary Heart Disease

Susan Quaglietti
V.F. Froelicher

Before the 1970s, the patient who suffered a myocardial infarction (MI) was almost completely immobilized for a minimum of 6 weeks. All activities, including washing, shaving, and feeding, were done for the patient in order to minimize the work load on the heart. It was theorized that this period of immobility would allow the myocardium to form a firm scar. The patient was also told not to expect to return to a normal lifestyle. In contrast, current practice indicates that prolonged immobilization does not speed healing; exposes the patient to the additional risks of venous thrombosis, pulmonary embolism, muscle wasting, lung infections, and deconditioning; and often leads to psychological impairment.

Today, the standard of care for the acute MI patient has completely changed from 20 years ago. A brief stay in the coronary care unit is followed by sitting at the bedside, early mobilization, and carefully graduated exercise. For the patient without complications, discharge from the hospital is usually within 1 week. Randomized trials have demonstrated that early discharge is safe and does not insure cardiac complications.

Though medically safe, the shortened hospital stay dictated by the disease-related groupings (DRG) approach leaves little time for patient education and other rehabilitative services, thus forcing the primary care physician to be responsible for these outpatient services. Certainly, all patients do not need all rehabilitative interventions, but safe exercise programs, educational sessions, group therapy, and psychological and vocational counseling should be available to those who need them.

The Pathophysiology of an Acute Myocardial Infarction

The pathophysiology of acute MI has become better understood. Studies utilizing coronary angiography at the time of infarction have shown that a thrombosis is usually seen acutely, thus disproving that clot formation occurred only in older infarctions. This has led to the current therapeutic approach to lyse clots with streptokinase, urokinase, or thrombolysin plasminogen activator (tPA). Multiple trials have convincingly demonstrated that mortality can be lowered with this approach, particularly when aspirin and heparin are added to stop thrombus from reformation.

Infarct Severity

Myocardial infarctions are generally divided into those that evolve Q-waves and result in transmural myocardial cell death and those that do not evolve Q-waves and only result in subendocardial cell death (64). The electrocardiographic (ECG) pattern can accurately predict the clinical course and outcome of both types of MIs. Subendocardial MI cannot be localized, whereas transmural MI can be roughly localized by the Q-wave pattern. In general, the greater the number of areas with Q-waves and the greater the R-wave loss, the larger the MI. Patients with non-Q-wave MIs who do not have a previous history of MI or a decreased ejection fraction have fewer incidents of congestive heart failure (CHF) or shock and better prognosis. Patients with non-Q-wave MIs are more likely to suffer ischemic events due to available myocardium at risk.

Risk Prediction

It is well known that morbidity and mortality in postinfarction patients who have complicated courses are much higher than in those with uncomplicated MIs. The criteria for a complicated MI are listed in Table 40.1. Patients diagnosed with a complicated MI should not begin progressive ambulation until they reach an uncomplicated status, and further mobilizations should be guided at a slower pace according to clinical signs and symptoms.

Identification of risk for future cardiac events or death and subsequent medical management can be evaluated from clinical features present during the post-myocardial infarction period. Ross and colleagues evaluated a high-risk stratification scheme by studying 1,848 post-myocardial infarction patients and testing 780 patients (86). A patient who manifests spontaneous ischemia during hospitalization has an increased risk of 18% to 20% mortality in the first year post-myocardial infarction and should be referred for diagnostic coronary angiography prior to discharge. Any post-MI patient with evidence of left ventricular failure by clinical or radiographic findings has a projected mortality of 25% in the first year and they should undergo coronary angiography as well. For MI patients who are unable to exercise, a resting radionuclide ventriculogram is necessary to evaluate left ventricular performance. Since ventricular function is the most powerful predictor of prognosis in patients under the age of 70 (2), patients with ejection fractions ranging between 20% to 40% are also classified as high-risk (12% first-year mortality). Evidence of inducible ischemia with ST-segment depression or angina identifies poor left ventricle (LV) perfusion in the predischarge exercise test and is associated with an annual mortality of 11% to 15%. DeBusk reports that for every 100 people who suffer an acute myocardial infarction and survive hospitalization, 50 will be identified as high-risk (10 having spontaneous ischemia/angina, 20 with diminished ventricular function, and 10 with identified ischemia from exercise testing) (21).

Table 40.1 Criteria (One or More) Classifying a Myocardial Infarction as Complicated

- Prior MI
- Continued cardiac ischemic (pain, ST shifts, late enzyme rise)
- Left ventricular failure (congestive heart failure, new murmurs, chest X ray changes)
- Shock (blood pressure drop, pallor, oliguria)
- Important cardiac dysrhythmias (premature ventricular contractions greater than 6/min, atrial fibrillation)
- Conduction disturbances (bundle branch block, atrioventricular block, hemiblock)
- Severe pleurisy or pericarditis
- Complicating illnesses
- Marked creatine kinase rise without a noncardiac explanation
- Age greater than 75
- Stroke

Nicod and associates have recently reconfirmed in a large patient population that the overall 1-year total mortality from admission for patients with a Q-wave myocardial infarction is nearly equal to that of patients who suffer a non-Q-wave infarction (19.5% and 20.4% mortality, respectively) (73). All post-MI patients should therefore undergo similar risk stratification as suggested by Ross and others (86). Klein and colleagues studied 198 patients who survived a myocardial infarction; they performed predischarge submaximal exercise testing and followed the patients for 2 years (58). They found that patients who had exercise-induced ST depression had a risk ratio of two times for suffering reinfarction or death compared to patients without ST depression. However, if the pretest electrocardiogram did not have diagnostic Q-waves, the risk increased to 11 times for an abnormal ST-segment response. This suggests that the predischarge exercise test is an even more powerful predictor of risk in the patient who has suffered an acute non-Q-wave myocardial infarction. This is in agreement with the work done by Krone and co-workers who found that non-Q-wave myocardial infarction patients with exercise-induced ischemia (angina, or ST depression, or both) had a threefold higher incidence of cardiac events in the year following infarction compared to those with a normal predischarge exercise test (60).

Early Mobilization Versus Bed Rest

Prior to 1960, patients with acute MI were thought to require 2 months of prolonged restriction of physical activity, with all activities being performed by nursing personnel. Early ambulation was thought to increase complications such as ventricular aneurysm formation, cardiac rupture, congestive heart failure, dysrhythmias, reinfarction, or sudden death. Animal experiments were designed to challenge portions of this theory and to evaluate the effect of early exercise on late scar formation after MI. The results of scar measurements on rats performing swimming soon after myocardial infarct is equivocal (43,49,59). Despite conflicting animal studies, controlled clinical studies of early mobilization during the early 1980s have not found a greater incidence of death or other complications in patients mobilized early compared to patients who remain at bed rest longer. In contrast, significant deleterious effects have been associated with bed rest. These alterations include 20% to 25% decrease in maximal oxygen consumption, orthostatic hypotension and venous thrombosis resulting from blood volume loss and plasma loss, increased ratio of red blood cells to plasma volume contributing to clot formation, decreased pulmonary function increasing the risk of developing pneumonia, and negative nitrogen and calcium balance. The promising results of these bed rest studies led to recommendations of gradual mobilization during the early post-MI stages. In certain patients, the major cause of decreased exercise capacity is from enforced bed rest. The early exercise prescription for MI patients in the coronary care unit can avoid iatrogenically induced deconditioning.

Researchers have questioned whether the deleterious hemodynamic effects and decreased exercise capacity from bed rest are due to inactivity or to the loss of gravity with the upright exposure. Four primary reasons support the concept that the majority of these alterations are due to loss of upright exposure to gravity: (a) Supine exercise does not prevent the deconditioning effects of being in bed; (b) there is both less and a slower decline in maximal oxygen consumption with chair rest than with bed rest; (c) there is a greater decrease in the maximal oxygen consumption after a period of bed rest when supine exercise is used to prevent deconditioning versus upright exercise; and (d) a lower body positive pressure device used during bed rest decreases the deconditioning effect. Intermittent exposure to gravitational stress such as chair sitting during the bed rest stage of post-MI hospital convalescence appears to obviate much of the iatrogenically induced deterioration in functional capacity (16).

Exercise and Cardiac Changes

Cardiac Changes in Coronary Arteries in Coronary Heart Disease Patients

Many favorable physiological changes have been documented in patients with coronary heart disease who have undertaken an aerobic exercise program. These include lower submaximal and resting heart rate, decreased symptoms, and increased maximal ventilatory oxygen consumption. Peripheral adaptations are at least partially responsible for these changes, and controversy exists concerning the effects of chronic exercise on the heart. In a review of the effects of exercise training on myocardial vascularity and perfusion, Scheuer concluded that strong evidence exists that chronic training promotes myocardial capillary growth and enlargement of extramural vessels in the normal animal heart (87). It is unclear if these changes directly increase perfusion or protect the heart during ischemia. Controversy still remains as to whether or not exercise training can promote coronary collateral circulation in the animal model subjected to chronic ischemia, even though the ischemic pig study of Bloor, White, and Sanders supports this contention (10).

There have been a number of attempts to demonstrate the direct coronary effects of exercise training. Ferguson and colleagues performed coronary angiography on 14 patients (7 patients had documented MI at least 2 years prior to enrollment) before and after 13 months of exercise (29). Despite a 25% increase in maximal oxygen uptake, collateral vessels were observed in only two coronary arteries, and 4 of 14 patients demonstrated progression of disease. Nolewajka and co-workers studied 20 male patients before and after 7 months of exercise training following acute myocardial infarction (74). Neither the 10 exercisers nor the 10 control patients showed any change in collateral circulation or left ventricular function (assessed by coronary angiogram) or improvement in myocardial perfusion (quantified by intracoronary injection of radionuclide). Sim and Neill also failed to demonstrate increased oxygen supply (assessed by myocardial blood flow and myocardial oxygen consumption) in 8 trained angina patients diagnosed with coronary artery disease (92). Whether these negative findings can be explained by limitations in the techniques, patient selection, or inadequate intensity or length of training is uncertain.

Assessment of Cardiac Changes Using Radionuclides

Imaging using radionuclides has been used to evaluate left ventricular performance before and after exercise training in control subjects and cardiac patients. Verani and colleagues used radionuclide ventriculography and thallium scintigraphy to evaluate 16 coronary patients before and after 12 weeks of exercise training (102). Ten patients had a documented MI at least 2 months prior to enrollment, and 15 patients had angiographic documentation of coronary disease. Both posttraining radionuclide exercise studies were performed at the same double product as in the pretraining studies.

For the ventriculography, a multicrystal camera was used, and scintigraphy was accomplished within 10 s of completion of exercise. After the training program, 15 of the 16 patients had improved peak ventilatory oxygen consumption. Resting mean left ventricular ejection fraction increased from 52% to 57%, but no change was noted in exercise ejection fraction or regional wall motion abnormalities. The thallium studies were unchanged, indicating myocardial perfusion was not changed after exercise training.

The Duke group has reported the effects of 6 months of exercise training on treadmill and radionuclide ventriculography performance in 15 patients, all less than 6 months post-MI (14). A training effect was demonstrated by a lower heart rate at a submaximal work load and longer treadmill time in spite of a wide range of resting ventricular function (ejection fractions ranging from 17% to 67%). The mean ejection fraction, end diastolic volume, and wall motion abnormalities during rest and at matched work loads and heart rates were not significantly different after training.

DeBusk and Hung randomized 11 coronary heart disease patients to a home exercise program and 10 to a control group 3 weeks post-myocardial infarction (23). There was no significant difference in resting or exercise ejection fraction or thallium perfusion images between the two groups after 8 weeks.

PERFEXT

PERFEXT (PERFusion, PERFormance, EXercise Trial), a randomized trial of male volunteers with coronary heart disease between the ages of 35 and 65, compared a low-level home walking program to a medically supervised exercise program (33). All patients entered the study 4 months after their cardiac events. The patients were classified by the following criteria: (a) history of myocardial infarction, (b) stable exertional angina pectoris, or (c) coronary artery bypass surgery. Of 146 patients randomized, 72 were in the training group and 74 in the control group.

The patients randomized to the exercise intervention group began training at a minimum of 60% of the estimated maximal oxygen uptake from the initial treadmill test and progressed to 85% of estimated maximal oxygen uptake by Week 8 of training. Patients randomized to the control group were offered a low-intensity walking program. Randomization was successful in equally distributing the clinical, treadmill, radionuclide ventriculography, and thallium imaging parameters between the two groups. No statistically significant differences were found between the groups.

Average intensities for the entire year were as follows: Percent maximal estimated oxygen uptake and percent maximal heart rate by the Karvonen method was approximately 60% ± 10 (ranging from 40% to 100%). Percent of maximal heart rate and measured maximal oxygen uptake was approximately 80%. The mean attendance at exercise sessions was 76% ± 18 (23% to 97%).

A significant training effect (ANOVA statistical testing used) in the intervention group of 59 patients was evident by the decrease in their resting and submaximal heart rates, as well as the significant increase in the measured and estimated maximal oxygen uptake. After 1 year of exercise training, the supervised patient had a significant increase in estimated VO_2 (18%) and measured maximum VO_2 (8.5%). These results are similar to other studies evaluating the influence of exercise training on coronary artery patients after 1 year. The control group showed a significant decrease in exercise capacity, at least partially due to the lower maximal heart rate obtained at 1 year. There was also a small but significant decline in the submaximal heart rate and rate pressure product in the control group, probably due to habituation. No changes were observed in maximal perceived exertion, respiratory quotient, or systolic blood pressure between the two groups initially or at 1 year nor between the initial and 1-year tests.

Analysis of covariance revealed a differential effect of the intervention on stroke volume and cardiac output in patients with and without angina after exercise training. Stage 2 stroke volume was statistically significant where rate pressure product was matched ($p = .02$), at maximal exercise ($p = .03$), and at rest ($p = .06$) for the angina-free group. Exercise tended to increase stroke volume and cardiac output in patients without angina and to decrease them in patients with angina. Similar analysis for heart rate only detected a consistent exercise effect on all but maximal exercise.

There was no significant difference at rest, during the three stages of exercise, or in the percent change from rest to exercise between the control and trained groups at 1 year in ejection fraction, end diastolic volume, stroke volume, or cardiac output. The PERFEXT exercise intervention group experienced a significant improvement in the exercise thallium images following the year using the Atwood scoring system and computer techniques (4). However, comparing thallium scans side by side, which has been done effectively to evaluate surgical intervention, was not successful in the clinical assessment of changes in myocardial perfusion caused by an exercise program. The ST-segment changes did not show an improvement, nor did they agree with the thallium changes.

One criticism might be that our patients did not exercise hard enough and that if they had performed at a higher intensity, definite improvements might have been possible. However, even if we chose those patients who trained the most intensely or had the highest exercise class attendance, we did not find greater changes. There was a surprisingly poor correlation between the intensity or attendance and change in aerobic capacity or the radionuclide changes. In fact, there was a poor correlation between the change in aerobic capacity and changes in the radionuclide tests. A paradox now exists regarding this point concerning maximal exercise in coronary artery disease (CAD) patients. Ehsani and colleagues have reported impressive cardiac changes in a highly selected group of eight cardiac patients with asymptomatic ST-segment depression exercised at very high levels (28). Hossack and Hartwick have reported an increased risk for exercise-induced events in similar CAD patients (52). Two questions still are unanswered: First, can the usual post-MI CAD patient exercise safely at higher levels than in the PERFEXT study (greater than 85% of maximal estimated VO_2 at trained level), and second, can more definite cardiac changes be demonstrated at the higher level?

The Effect of Beta Blockers on Exercise Training

The mechanisms causing hemodynamic changes that occur secondary to regular exercise are poorly understood. High levels of sympathetic stimulation are present during aerobic exercise, and it was concluded from animal studies that catecholamines enhanced myocardial contractility and induced hypertrophy. These observations suggested that repeated, sustained sympathetic stimulation was needed during exercise training to produce a training effect.

If beta-adrenergic stimulation is needed for the effects of exercise training to occur or if beta blockade lessens the ischemia necessary to promote collateralization, then beta blockade might be expected to interfere with the beneficial results of exercise. Beta blockade could also increase perceived exertion and fatigue, thus lessening the tolerance for higher exercise levels and adherence to an exercise program. Therefore, a pharmacologically imposed limitation in heart rate and cardiac output during an exercise program may prohibit obtaining an optimal training effect.

Pratt and colleagues retrospectively studied 35 patients with coronary heart disease who underwent a 3-month walk/jog cycle training program (84). Fourteen patients received no beta blocker, 14 received 30 to 80 mg per day of propranolol, and 7 patients received 120 to 240 mg per day of propranolol at the discretion of their physicians. Each group's estimated oxygen uptake increased after training—by 27% in those not taking beta blockers, by 30% in those on a low dose, and by 46% in those on a high dose.

Vanhees and colleagues compared two groups of post-MI patients without angina pectoris, 15 receiving beta blockers and 14 not receiving beta blocker therapy (101). Exercise training for both groups was at an intensity of between 70% to 90% of maximal capacity for 3 months. Peak measured oxygen uptake increased an average of approximately 35% in both groups, as well as reduced heart rate at rest and at submaximal exercise. Changes in cardiac output, arteriovenous oxygen content difference, stroke volume, and heart rate at peak exercise resulting from the exercise program were not significantly different between the two groups.

We performed an analysis of 59 patients in PERFEXT who exercised for 1 year and control subjects; both groups were placed on beta blockers at the prerogative of their physicians. The exercise records of the patients in the exercise group were reviewed. Average intensities for the year were as follows: Percent maximal estimated oxygen uptake was 60% ± 12 (ranging from 40% to 100%), and percent measured maximal oxygen uptake was 77% ± 14 (ranging from 42% to 100%). There were no significant differences between those who took beta blockers and those who did not. Attendance at exercise sessions was a mean of 76% ± 18 (ranging from 23% to 97%) with no difference between those on beta blockers and those not taking them. The mean attendance was 73% for those taking beta blockers and 78% for those not taking them.

By design, the PERFEXT study demonstrated the effects of exercise training in patients selected by their physicians to be on or off of beta blockers. This clinical question is different than studying the effects of beta blockers on exercise training. However, this latter question has not been resolved, because conflicting results exist as to the effects of being randomized to beta blockade in normal subjects engaged in exercise training. From previous studies it has been demonstrated that the appropriate changes in oxygen uptake, submaximal heart rate, and exercise duration occur in patients on beta blockade who engage in exercise training. Our study supports this but also demonstrates no preferential difference between those patients trained on or off of beta blockers. In addition, this study shows an increase in myocardial perfusion implied by improved thallium scintigrams in angina patients in an exercise program. Our findings and those summarized support the beneficial effects of exercise training in coronary patients taking beta blocker medication.

Patients With Left Ventricular Dysfunction

Squires and colleagues studied 20 patients with left ventricular ejection fractions of less than 25% post-myocardial infarction in a supervised cardiac rehabilitation program (95). There was substantial improvement in exercise capacity in most patients, which was associated with a favorable trend in performing desired activities and returning to work. Conn and associates studied 10 patients with a history of prior myocardial infarction and left ventricular ejection fractions of less than 27% after they enrolled in a supervised cardiac rehabilitation program (15). Exercise capacity increased from a mean of 7.0 METs to 8.5 METs. There was no reported incidence of exercise-related morbidity or mortality. Both of these studies consistently advocate that severely depressed left ventricular function is not an absolute contraindication to cardiac rehabilitation and that these patients can also attain a beneficial cardiovascular training effect safely.

Judgutt and co-workers studied 13 patients with anterior Q-wave myocardial infarctions and 24 matched control patients using echocardiography before and after supervised low-level exercise training versus no intervention (53). Patients were subdivided within each of the treatment groups according to echocardiographic findings. Six patients in the exercise group having ≥ 18% left ventricular asynergy before training had a significant lower global ejection fraction, greater expansion index, lower thinning ratio, larger regional shape distortion indexes, and poor functional class score after exercise training. No change was noted in exercise performance. Left ventricular changes were felt to be secondary to remodeling of an incompletely healed infarct zone. In contrast, the recent preliminary results from the multicenter randomized study, reported by Gianuzzi, evaluating exercise training in anterior myocardial infarction draw contrary conclusions (37). Forty-nine patients with first Q-wave anterior myocardial infarction were randomly assigned to physical training or to a control group for 6 months. The treatment group showed a significant increase in work capacity at 6 months; however, 2D-echo measurements did not change over the 6-month period for either the treatment or control group. When patients were grouped according to ejection fraction (EF) percentage, subjects with less than 40% EF in entry had increased end diastolic volume and greater wall motion abnormalities. Left ventricular function deteriorated after 6 months for both control and treatment patients. These results suggest physical training does not increase spontaneous deterioration for patients with less than 40% EF.

Patients With Right Ventricular Dysfunction

Haines and colleagues studied 61 patients after they had experienced an acute inferior or true posterior myocardial infarction (41). Right ventricular dysfunction was determined to be none, moderate, or severe by blinded, subjective consensus readings of ECG gated equilibrium blood pool imaging at rest. They found no significant difference in exercise tolerance as assessed by treadmill time or METs, at predischarge or 3-month postdischarge testing, between patients with and without right ventricular dysfunction. There also was no difference in exercise-induced ST-segment depression, chest pain, Thallium-201 defects, medically refractory angina, reinfarction rate, or cardiac mortality. No attempt was made to standardize cardiac rehabilitation, other than usual care by the patient's own physicians. Crosby and associates studied 5 patients who had suffered a hemodynamically significant right ventricular infarction and found an improvement in exercise capacity with cardiac rehabilitation was similar for patients with right or left ventricular infarction (18). Patients with right ventricular dysfunction do not appear to be at increased risk for participating in cardiac rehabilitation, and this intervention may be beneficial in improving exercise capacity.

Post-CABS Patients

Coronary artery bypass surgery (CABS) has been shown to prolong life and relieve angina in selected groups of patients with coronary artery disease. Advances in operative techniques, including cardioplegia, the use of the internal mammary artery, and more complete revascularization, have improved operative results. Cardiac rehabilitation can complement surgical advances and improve functional status of both successful and incomplete revascularization patients.

Because of the large number of patients undergoing coronary artery bypass and their potential for rehabilitation, these patients have been included in exercise rehabilitation programs, but the numbers have been small. Less than 200 patients with status post-CABS in postoperative exercise programs in a total of seven studies have been reported. Previous studies have only considered patients with successful surgery that alleviated angina.

Most studies conducted in the 1970s and early 1980s report significant increases in maximum VO_2 levels for post-CABS patients after enrollment in a supervised exercise program (1,27,45,51,79,93). Oldridge found that 90% of the patients' total improvement in functional capacity occurred after 4 months of exercise post-CABS, despite participation over a 32-month period in an exercise program (79).

Fifty-three CABS patients were equally randomized in the PERFEXT study to exercise or routine care, and, in general, exercise training had the greatest effect when implemented soon after surgery. Typical training effects (lower submaximal heart rate [HR], decreased submaximal rate pressure product [RPP], and increased maximal oxygen uptake) were observed, but no significant radionuclide changes accompanied the training effects. A study by Nakai and associates showed that physical exercise improved graft patency rate at 7 weeks post-CABS (98% patency in exercise group vs. 80% patency in control group) documented by coronary angiography (72). Perk et al. demonstrated less medication use and hospitalizations in CABS patients after enrollment into an exercise program (82).

Rehabilitation After PTCA (Percutaneous Transluminal Coronary Angioplasty)

There has been a dramatic exponential growth in PTCA since its first clinical application in 1977 by Andreas Gruentzig; more than 220,000 procedures were performed in 1991 alone. Despite improvements in equipment and technique, late vessel restenosis occurs frequently within 3 to 6 months of the procedure. Depending on the type of patients studied and the definition of restenosis, it occurs in 12% to 48% of patients. Because an average of 30% of patients will have restenosis, a significant number of patients are destined to have recurrence of their ischemia, and cardiac rehabilitation can assist them physically and mentally in coping with their coronary disease.

Ben-Ari and co-workers studied the effects of cardiac rehabilitation in patients post-PTCA and compared them to a group of matched patients who received usual care post-PTCA without rehabilitation (6). They found a higher physical work capacity and ejection fraction in the rehabilitation group compared to control subjects and a lower total cholesterol, lower LDL, and higher HDL as well. There was no difference in the rate of restenosis, though assessed early at 5.5 months of follow-up. Cardiac rehabilitation can also help improve exercise capacity and foster positive coping strategies in patients after PTCA.

Spontaneous Improvement Post-Myocardial Infarction

To document spontaneous improvement in aerobic capacity, the Stanford group has measured VO_2max within the first 3 months after an uncomplicated MI. Forty-six men underwent symptom-limited maximal treadmill tests 3 and 11 weeks after MI. There was a significant increase between the two periods in HR, RPP, and oxygen consumption during submaximal exercise. The mean maximal heart rate increased from 137 to 150, and VO_2max increased from 21 to 27 cc $O_2 \cdot kg^{-1} \cdot min^{-1}$; maximal SBP, double product, and oxygen pulse all increased also.

To evaluate hemodynamic changes after MI, Kelbaek and colleagues measured VO_2max and performed invasive studies at rest and during two submaximal exercise levels (55). Thirty men were studied 2, 5, and 8 months after uncomplicated MI. Fourteen patients participated in an exercise program during the first 3 months of the study, and the other 16 patients attended the training during the second 3-month period. An increase in VO_2max occurred at the 5th month in both groups (16% and 11%, respectively) along with an increase in cardiac index at the same relative submaximal work load. Later in the study, only slight increments in VO_2max and no changes in hemodynamics were recorded within or between the two groups.

In a comprehensive review, Greenland and Chu analyzed eight controlled studies of supervised exercise programs and their effect on physical work capacity (39). In all the studies reviewed, exercise capacity improved in the control or intervention group. The exercise group increased exercise capacity to a higher level, 20% to 25% more than the control group. This suggests that a patient's exercise capacity can be artificially limited by the patient's self-expectations or by the physician's advice based on a low-level predischarge exercise test. It is still unclear how great the spontaneous improvement in exercise capacity post-myocardial infarction can be. Reviewed studies that did not show any benefit may have been limited by exercise programs of inadequate duration (less than 6 months) and by noncompliance with the exercise prescription.

Rehabilitation Models

Types of Programs

Exercise prescription following a myocardial infarction is necessary to ensure safe rehabilitation and prevent deconditioning. Recently, efficacy questions have arisen concerning the type of exercise (circuit weight training vs. aerobic), intensity of exercise (high vs. low) and the format (group supervision vs. home medical supervision).

To evaluate circuit training, Kelemen and colleagues performed a prospective, randomized evaluation of the safety and efficacy of 10 weeks of circuit weight training in coronary disease patients, aged 35 to 70 years (56). Circuit weight training consisted of a series of weight-lifting exercises using a moderate load with frequent repetitions. Patients had participated in a supervised cardiac rehabilitation program for a minimum of 3 months before the study. Control patients (n = 20) continued with their regular exercise consisting of a walk/jog and volleyball program, and the experimental group (n = 20) substituted circuit weight training for volleyball. No sustained arrhythmias or cardiovascular problems occurred in either group. The experimental group significantly increased treadmill time by 12%, whereas there was no change in the control patients. Circuit weight training was safe and resulted in significant increases in aerobic endurance and musculoskeletal strength compared with traditional exercise used in cardiac rehabilitation programs. In a 6-month study of 16 men, Sparling et al. demonstrated that patients achieved a 22% gain in strength without an increase in blood pressure (94). These studies emphasize the safety and efficacy of circuit weight training in cardiac patients.

Goble et al. enrolled 308 men diagnosed with Q-wave myocardial infarction into a randomized study evaluating 8 weeks of group aerobic exercise or group light exercise (38). Patients were then followed for 12 months. There was no significant difference at entry, exit, or 12-month treadmill results for mean resting HR, resting systolic blood pressure, maximal HR, maximal SBP, or RPP. The mean MET was 0.9 MET higher in the high exercise group, but at 12-month review mean MET results were similar (10.8 for high exercise, 10.7 for light exercise). The training effect for transmural MI patients engaging in high or low exercise appears equally beneficial for this patient population.

Because of rising health care costs, varied availability of cardiac rehabilitation programs, and decreased compliance with formal programs, several investigators have proposed home monitoring exercise programs. DeBusk et al. report that patients enrolled in a medically directed home rehabilitation program or in group rehabilitation had similar increases in functional capacity and equal compliance to either program (22). No training complications occurred in either group and low infarction rates were comparable.

It is interesting to note that in the Goble study (38) attendance to either the light or highly supervised exercise program for three quarters of the total classes ranged from 41% to 65%, but more than 90% of all enrolled patients claimed they walked each day for 30 min. Both the DeBusk and Goble studies suggest patients can be made responsible for directing their own exercise program with instruction.

Complications of an Exercise Program

Exercise training after an acute cardiac event can be an important part of cardiac rehabilitation in assisting a patient to return to his or her previous functioning lifestyle. The explicit details of exercise protocols and equipment, absolute and relative contraindications to exercise, warm-up and cool-down periods, and guidelines for terminating exercise are all outlined by the American College of Sports Medicine (3) and should be specifically tailored to each individual patient.

There is a small but definite incidence of cardiac arrest associated with exercise testing of cardiac patients, particularly in the early minutes of recovery. Haskell surveyed 30 cardiac rehabilitation programs in North America using a questionnaire to assess major cardiovascular complications (46). This survey included approximately 14,000 patients for 1.6 million exercise-hours. Eight deaths resulted after a total of 50 cardiopulmonary resuscitations; of 7 MI, 2 resulted in death. Thus, there was 1 nonfatal event per 35,000 patient-hours and 1 fatal event per 160,000 patient-hours. The complication rates were lower in ECG-monitored programs. The current programs reported a 4% annual mortality rate during exercise, a rate not different from that expected for such patients. Other programs have reported rates of cardiopulmonary resuscitations ranging from 1 per 6,000 to 1 per 25,000 man-hours of exercise. Such events are difficult to predict, can occur in patients with only single-vessel disease, can occur at any time after being in a program, and may not be solely related to the exercise prescription. Many of the cardiac events were due to a primary arrhythmic event and not associated with acute MI.

Van Camp and Peterson obtained statistics from 167 randomly selected outpatient cardiac rehabilitation programs and found that the incidence rate for cardiac arrest was 8.9 per million patient-hours (99). Of these cardiac arrests, 86% were successfully resuscitated, giving an incidence rate for death of 1.3 per million patient-hours. This compares favorably with the estimated fatality rate for nonselected joggers at 2.5 per million person-hours of jogging (97). There also was no significant difference in cardiac event rate between rehabilitation programs with or without electrocardiographic monitoring.

The incidence of exertion-related cardiac arrest in cardiac rehabilitation programs is small, and, because of the availability of rapid defibrillation, death rarely occurs. In an earlier review of survival in the CAPRI population, 85% of cardiac arrests took place during exercise classes that the subjects attended for about 3 hours each week. However, the majority of sudden deaths are temporally associated with routine activities of daily life and not with exercise. Therefore, the number of deaths due to strenuous physical exertion is relatively modest. Exertion-related cardiac arrest is usually due to ventricular fibrillation or tachycardia, and exercise may increase its risk of occurrence by 100 times.

Compliance

The success and benefits of any exercise training program are directly related to the patient's compliance with the exercise prescription. Kentala reported that only 13% of his patients carried out the assigned exercise prescription at least 70% of the time (57). Compliance falls as time progresses. At 3 months compliance is 80%, 1 year later compliance is only 45% to 60%, and at 4 years it is only 30% to 55%. Previous health behaviors and current knowledge of illness influence a patient's perception of the importance of exercise rehabilitation and can influence compliance (76). Several options are available to improve compliance behavior—reduce the waiting time, provide expert supervision, tailor the exercise prescription to avoid physical discomfort and frustration, use variable activities including games, incorporate social events, recall absent patients, involve the patient's family or spouse in the program, and involve the patient in monitoring his or her progress.

Risk Factor Modification

Cardiac rehabilitation is defined by the World Health Organization as "the sum of activities required to ensure them the best possible physical, mental, and social conditions so that they may, by their own efforts, resume as normal a place as possible in the life of the community . . . and that . . . rehabilitation cannot be regarded as an isolated form of therapy, but must be integrated into the whole treatment of which it constitutes only one facet" (107). Given the recurrence rate of reinfarction and overall cardiovascular mortality in survivors of myocardial infarction, theoretical benefits of risk-factor modification included in cardiac rehabilitation in this selected high-risk population could be very significant.

Kallio and associates performed a multifactorial intervention combined with cardiac rehabilitation in post-myocardial infarction patients beginning 2 weeks after the event (54). They found in the treated group a decrease in blood pressure, lower body weight, and improved serum cholesterol and triglycerides; smoking decreased by 50% in both the treated and control groups. The National Exercise and Heart Disease Project showed a reduction in low-density lipoprotein (LDL) fractions. The recent analysis of 10-year mortality from cardiovascular disease in relation to cholesterol level by Pekkanen et al. demonstrated the importance of lowering serum cholesterol in men with preexisting cardiovascular disease (81). Previously, it was argued that when atheroma were well established and causing symptoms, alterations in serum cholesterol would have little effect on stenosis size. The findings by Pekkanen are encouraging, because evidence is now beginning to accumulate that the progression of coronary atherosclerosis may be arrested and actually reversed with aggressive dietary and medical therapy. Meta-analysis of the lipid-lowering trials using digital coronary angiography now consistently confirms these findings (88). Recommendations suggest that all patients should have aggressive management to lower LDL cholesterol levels to below 100. The interaction of triglycerides with gene site activity, typing of apo-B, ultracentrifugation of LDL, and other new findings are leading to an exciting new hope that atherosclerosis can be treated more effectively.

Hamalainen and colleagues noted a reduction in sudden deaths by almost 50% in patients enrolled in an aggressive, multifactorial intervention program for 10 years post-myocardial infarction (42). Their interventions included control of smoking, hypertension, and lipids and also the use of antiarrhythmic agents in addition to beta blockers. These studies are promising and emphasize the medical rehabilitation team's responsibility to encourage patients to alter lifestyles that could be deleterious to their health and to institute medical therapy as necessary to control cardiac risk factors.

Prognosis, Efficacy, and Exercise

Meta-Analysis

May and colleagues have presented an excellent review of the long-term trials in secondary prevention after MI (66). Trials reported prior to November 1981 were considered in which both intervention and follow-up were carried out beyond the time of hospital discharge. Random assignment and at least a total sample size of 100 were required. Total mortality was used whenever possible, in order to minimize bias. All patients randomized were included in the mortality estimates to reduce the bias of differential withdrawal. Effectiveness was calculated by considering the percent reduction in deaths that would have occurred if the intervention had been applied to the control group. Though few of the interventions resulted in a significant difference, all of them except for the antidysrhythmics show a trend towards efficacy. This study has been updated by a wave of meta-analyses. Pertinent here are those related to cardiac rehabilitation.

O'Connor and colleagues performed a meta-analysis of 22 randomized trials of cardiac rehabilitation involving 4,554 patients (75). They found a 20% reduction of risk for total mortality, a 22% reduction for cardiovascular mortality, and a 25% reduction in the risk for fatal reinfarction. Criticisms of this analysis are that each evaluated pooled study was not uniform in its treatment of patients and a nonexercise intervention done in the different trials may have biased the results. Oldridge and associates performed a similar meta-analysis with 10 randomized trials including 4,347 patients and found a similar reduction for all-cause death and cardiovascular death in the patients undergoing cardiac rehabilitation (78). Thus, though few trials have demonstrated a significant difference between the groups, the meta-analyses found an average 25% decrease in mortality.

Intervention Studies

Kallio and colleagues were part of a World Health Organization–coordinated project to assess the effects of a comprehensive rehabilitation and secondary prevention program on morbidity, mortality, return to work, and various clinical, medical, and psychosocial factors after MI (54). Kentala studied 298 consecutive males less than 65 years of age admitted to the University of Helsinki Hospital in 1969 with a diagnosis of acute MI (57). Palatsi's study was a nonrandomized trial of 380 patients less than 65 years old recovering from MI (80). The study by Wilhelmson, Sanne, Emfeldt, Grimby, Tibblin, and Wedel included patients born in 1913 or later and hospitalized for MI between 1968 and 1970 in Goteborg, Sweden (105). The Ontario Study included seven Canadian centers that collaborated in this randomized prospective trial. Bengtsson reported 171 MI patients under the age of 65 who were randomized to a control group and an exercise group (7). Carson et al. performed their 3.5-year study in a population of 1,311 male MI patients (12). Vermeulen, Liew, and Durrer described a prospective randomized trial with a 5-year follow-up (103). Mayou and colleagues studied 129 men, 60 years of age or less, admitted with MI (67). The study by Hedback, Perk, and Perski in Sweden was retrospective with a control group of 154 patients and an intervention group of 143 patients; 23 of the control patients and 22 of the exercisers were women (48). These studies are summarized in Table 40.2.

Symptom Control and Quality of Life

In addition to improving oxygen consumption and functional capacity, cardiac rehabilitation may alter quality of life for the coronary artery disease patient. Oldridge and associates investigated the impact of an 8-week cardiac rehabilitation program versus traditional care in 201 post-MI patients (77). A small but statistically significant improvement was seen in exercise tolerance, decreased anxiety state, and improved general emotions after the short intervention in the experimental group. After 12 months, however, similar findings were present in both groups, regardless of intervention. Bethell and Muller randomized 200 post-MI patients to an exercise treatment program supervised by a general practitioner or to an unsupervised exercise program (8). The treatment group (99 patients) reported increased perceived energy (median rise of 41%) associated with a significant rise in predicted maximum oxygen uptake (22 to 27 $ml \cdot min^{-1} \cdot kg^{-1}$) and a significant decrease of the double product at peak exercise. Of the 21 treatment patients who reported angina, 19 patients reported symptoms at the final exercise test. Twenty control patients initially reported angina symptoms, but at the completion of the study, 32 control patients reported angina.

In general, past studies investigating the effect of cardiac rehabilitation on psychosocial variables have been inconsistent. Most patients report improved well-being, but the cause for improvement is difficult to determine. Psychological variables are difficult to quantify, and patients may improve due to close medical contact rather than solely from the cardiac rehabilitation program. Van Dixhoorn et al. have reported that risk of failure in completing an exercise program decreased by half when relaxation therapy was added to the exercise training program (100). For patients with acute high stress levels, intervention used to reduce these levels following MI may reduce the chances of subsequent coronary events occurring, thereby decreasing mortality (31).

Table 40.2 Summary of 13 of the Controlled Intervention Trials of Cardiac Rehabilitation After Myocardial Infarction

		Population randomized					Mean no.			Dropouts (%)		Returned to work (%)		RE-MI (%)		Percent mortality					
																Sudden (%)		Cardiac (%)		Total (%)	
Investigator	Year	Total	Controls	Exercised	Exclusions	% Women	months entry post-MI	Mean age	Years FU	Cntrl.	Exer.	Cntrl.	Exer.	Cntrl.	Exer.	Cntrl.	Exer.	Cntrl.	Exer.	Cntrl.	Exer.
Kentala	72	158	81	77	150		2	53	1			5	8							22	17
Palatsi	76	380	200	180	>65	19.0	2.5	52	2.5		35	33	36	15	12	3	6	14	10	14	10
Wilhelmsen	77	313	157	158	27% > 57	10.0	3	51	4		46					18	16			22	18
Kallio	79	375	187	183	>65	19.0	3	55	3					13	20	14	6	29	19	30	22
NEHDP	81	651	328	323	280	0	14	52	3	31	23			7	5			6	4	7	5
Ontario	82	733	354	379	28. > 54	0	6	48	4	45	46			13	14					7	10
Bengtsson	83	171	90	81	45. > 65	0	1.5	56	1			73	75	4	2					7	10
Carson	83	303	152	151	>70	0	1.5	51	3.5	6	17	81	81	7	7					14	8
Vermeulen	83	98	51	47		0	1.5	49	5					18	9			10	4	10	4
Roman	83	193	100	93		10.0	2	55	9	4	4			5	4	7	4	5	3	6	4
Mayou	83	129	42	44	>60	0	1	51	1.5	25	25	30	57								
Froelicher	84	146	74	76		0	4	53	1	14	17			1	1					0	1
Hedback	85	297	154	143	>65	15.0	1.5	57	1		45	59	66	16.2	5.4			7.8	8.4	7.8	9.1
Averages										21	29	47	54	10	8	11	8	12	8	12	10

Source: Froelicher 1987a; 442.

Note. Cntrl. = controls; Exer. = exercise.

Return to Work

The presumed inability to resume gainful employment can contribute greatly to a patient's loss of self-esteem and perceived economic inadequacy. A concerted effort by the medical/rehabilitation team must be directed to allay these concerns. A normal symptom-limited exercise test can help encourage and reinstill the patient's confidence to resume job-related activities. Fitzgerald and associates have shown that despite the minimal invasiveness of PTCA, many patients have found it difficult to return to work because of low self-confidence despite the lack of any physical contraindications, and only 81% of the PTCA patients actually return to work (30). As previously noted, gradual improvement in exercise capacity can occur even without a formal exercise program. An exercise test showing a lower exercise capacity can also be used to safely gauge a patient's level of activity at work.

Occupational evaluation and counseling were shown to be of benefit by Dennis and co-workers, who decreased the time interval between infarction and return to work by an average of 32% by counseling low-risk, post-MI patients (24). Cost-benefit analysis of these same patients revealed that total medical costs per patient in the 6 months post-myocardial infarction were lower by \$502, and their occupational income was increased during the same time period by \$2,102. The fact that many people are not retiring at age 65 and the fact that 80% of patients under the age of 65 eventually return to work after myocardial infarction underscore that the occupational counseling is beneficial during cardiac rehabilitation.

Predicting Outcome in Cardiac Rehabilitation Patients

It is unclear from the cited literature which variables of a cardiac rehabilitation program will improve mortality, functional capacity, and quality of life. Meta-analysis shows trends toward decreased mortality, but the percentage change is minimal. Individual studies have small sample sizes and different cardiac rehabilitation programs, which make meta-analysis difficult. In addition, other therapies such as revascularization, beta blockers, and anti-coagulation have improved the outcome of the post-myocardial infarction patient without patient enrollment into a cardiac rehabilitation program.

In general, exercise rehabilitation is associated with decreasing submaximal HRs, decreasing resting HR, and increasing maximum VO_2. However, results are equivocal concerning changes in stroke volume, left ventricular function, and ST changes on EKG interpretation. The independent effect of cardiac rehabilitation on cardiac changes has been difficult to prove. Most researchers agree peripheral changes greatly contribute to increasing maximal VO_2.

Most coronary artery patients, including those with left ventricular dysfunction, are able to safely exercise. As noted, previous research suggests that there is a spontaneous improvement in cardiac function without a supervised exercise format. With a supervised approach, patients usually have an additional 15% to 25% increase in functional capacity. The appropriate frequency, duration, and intensity of an exercise program have not been clearly determined. Goble et al. reported similar positive changes in work capacity after high- or low-intensity exercise programs (38). Ehsani's data suggest that cardiac changes can be expected only if patients are exercised beyond 85% of maximum predicted heart rate (28). In general, patients should exercise three times per week to achieve an aerobic effect. Beta blocker therapy does not appear to prevent a training effect.

It has been difficult to assess the independent effect of cardiac rehabilitation. Patients with the lowest baseline functional capacity will obviously show the greatest change in functional capacity from participating in an exercise program. If only low-risk CAD patients are entered 6 months after myocardial infarction, spontaneous improvement will have occurred, and significant changes from program participation are difficult to prove. Subject selection and entrance into a program post-myocardial infarction can bias research results.

Supervised exercise, either in a formal group or monitored by phone, assists the patient's confidence level in his or her exercise capacity level. By 3 to 5 months, most patients have a work capacity of 9 METs, allowing them to return to work. The additional value of counseling helps decrease symptoms, improves the patients' general well-being, and guides risk-factor modification. If light, supervised exercise is beneficial, then medically supervised home monitoring (22) may be a new model for cardiac rehabilitation. Home patient monitoring with counseling can provide close follow-up at probably lower health costs. Compliance with exercise may improve because patients can self-direct their program.

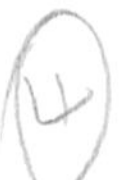

Cardiac rehabilitation programs are expensive and carry a risk. If a patient's success in improving work capacity could be predicted on the basis of initial data, cardiac rehabilitation would be cost-effective as well as efficacious. Considering VO_2max and other indicators of a training effect, we investigated the following questions from the PERFEXT data: (a) Can clinical features prior to training predict whether or not beneficial changes occur with training? (b) Do initial treadmill or radionuclide measurements contribute information to improve this prediction? and (c) Does the intensity of training over the year predict beneficial changes?

Each of the parameters of change with training was regressed against the initial value of those parameters (i.e., resting heart rate, submaximal heart rate, estimated and measured VO_2max, and thallium ischemia) as well as against age, amount of myocardial scar on the thallium scan, and the measures of intensity of training. Our major finding was that a patient's success or failure in improving aerobic capacity following a 1-year aerobic exercise program was poorly predicted on the basis of initial clinical, treadmill, or radionuclide data. Correlations between initial parameters and outcome were poor. Training intensity did not significantly affect outcome. Those with ischemic markers (exercise test–induced angina, ST depression, or decreasing ejection fraction) did not show a different degree of training effect than did patients without ischemia; neither did those with markers of myocardial damage. History of CABS or MI had no influence on whether a patient's work capacity would improve following the training period.

There was a trend for those who initially showed evidence of the poorest state of fitness (high resting or submaximal heart rate, low estimated oxygen consumption) or high thallium ischemia scores to have the most improvement in the same respective parameter. However, initial measured oxygen consumption, the best measure of aerobic capacity on entry, showed no relationship to any measure of training effect at the end of the year of training. Older patients showed only slightly less benefit than younger ones, though Williams and associates (106) report similar improvement in physical capacity despite age group classification. Those with characteristics suggesting larger amounts of scar or ischemia did not have significantly different results from those with less. Multivariate analysis did not greatly improve the ability to predict outcome.

Closing Commentary

There are significant changes evolving in the United States regarding exercise testing and cardiac rehabilitation. Scientific advances are merging with economic and societal forces to alter medical practice dramatically. Some of these advances include the use of meta-analysis to provide accurate study summaries, the demonstration of the regression of coronary artery disease and of cardiac changes due to diet and exercise, the improvement of risk stratification, and the development of the public health recommendation for physical activity rather than physical fitness.

Other global health care changes include care provider assessment by regulatory bodies and reimbursement for efficacy outcome rather than payment for procedures. The Joint Commission on Accreditation of Health Care Organizations (JCAHO) states that hospital accreditation will eventually depend upon the assessment of physician diagnostic and treatment performance. The JCAHO plans to implement quality assessment instead of the current quality assurance (i.e., quality by inspection). The former is aimed at developing a cycle for continuous improvement by establishing acceptable standards, developing a quality-management plan, and measuring patient outcomes. Markers of management performance must be utilized to evaluate quality of care. Examples of this for cardiac rehabilitation have been provided by the American Association of Cardiovascular and Pulmonary Rehabilitation.

In regard to research, molecular biochemistry and genetics are the prime areas for cardiovascular, government-funded research. Clinical areas for research include technological efficacy and outcome assessment. We hope that as data are analyzed, medical practice will reform, quality assessment will improve, and cost containment will occur with less emphasis on procedures.

In an effort to shape these changes, medical associations (such as the American Heart Association, American College of Physicians, American College of Cardiology, American Association of Cardiovascular and Pulmonary Rehabilitation, and the American College of Sports Medicine) are defining and refining guidelines for treatment and the use of technology and are becoming more involved in the accreditation of practitioners. However, these guidelines have not led to adequate changes in practice, and thus governmental actions to effect these needed changes will probably be initiated. With guidelines being developed for the use of procedures and limitations of payments clearly defined, physicians will not have to practice defensive medicine to decrease the fear of litigation.

Health care planners have finally realized that continued increases in health care costs do not improve the general health of our population. DRGs (disease related groupings) and RAM (the VA resource allocation model) have been dismal failures in controlling costs, and in spite of a rising proportion of the U.S. gross national product being allocated for health care, 37 million Americans are denied access to health care for financial reasons. In contrast, the public generally demands access to the most modern technology available, believing that improved technology can prolong life expectancy. A balance between health costs and quality of life must be addressed at a national level.

In order to implement patient outcomes that promote a high quality of life within reasonable health costs, research and clinical practice must combine resources to effectively document the efficacy of new modalities. Much of the medical literature does not have sufficient scientific rigor to recommend findings assimilated into practice. For instance, ECG monitoring for cardiac rehabilitation was recommended unselectively, resulting in unjustifiable costs for exercise training. Electrophysiology studies are now recommended for nearly everyone with syncope, resulting in a threefold increase in billing via Medicare for this diagnosis.

The changes that pertain to exercise testing and cardiac rehabilitation are the following:

1. Exercise testing will be performed more often by family practitioners and internists than by cardiologists. In a recent American College of Physicians survey, 50% of internists were performing exercise tests (104). The test will be used to decide which patients need referral to the cardiologist. Exercise testing will serve as the gatekeeper to more expensive and invasive tests. A key need will be to educate these practitioners to perform and interpret the test properly.
2. Cardiac rehabilitation including risk modification is being accepted as standard practice in the United States. In-hospital programs must be implemented in order for hospitals to be accredited. Physical and occupational therapists are critical in this process. Outpatient programs are being greatly curtailed by declining reimbursement, especially because research findings support rare use of ECG monitoring in Phase II programs. Eventually, centralized cardiac rehabilitation programs responsible for a region will be the best economic approach. Primary care physicians will be more involved with cardiac rehabilitation and risk-factor modification, rather than cardiologists exercising sole management in this area. In addition, research has demonstrated that exercise programs can be safely carried out by selected low-risk patients in the home setting.

The outcome assessment proposed by JCAHO is exciting. Hopefully, this will promote a cycle of continuous improvement. Rather than establishing acceptable thresholds or standards, quality assessment consists of measuring outcomes and utilizing this feedback to improve care. Indicators or markers of performance must be used to evaluate quality of care.

Scientifically, there is a sound basis for these health care delivery changes and support for cardiac rehabilitation. In the United States, we have an opportunity to blend the best parts of current practice with a system that will reach all of our people with an appropriate mix of technology and humanistic concerns.

References

1. Adams, W.C.; McHenry, M.M.; Bernauer, E.M. Long-term physiologic adaptations with special reference to performance and cardiorespiratory function in health and disease. Am. J. Cardiol. 33:765-775; 1974.
2. Ahnve, S.; Gilpin, E.; Ditrich, H.; et al. First myocardial infarction: Age and ejection fraction identify a low-risk group. Am. Heart J. 116:925-932; 1988.
3. American College of Sports Medicine. Guidelines for exercise testing and prescription. 4th ed. Philadelphia: Lea & Febiger; 1991.
4. Atwood, J.E.; Jensen, D.; Froelicher, V.F.; et al. Agreement in human interpretation of analog thallium myocardial perfusion images. Circulation. 64:601-609; 1981.
5. Audet, A.M.; Greenfield, S.; Field, M. Medical practice guidelines: Current activities and future directions. Ann. Intern. Med. 113:709-714; 1990.
6. Ben-Ari, E.; Rothbaum, D.A.; Linnemeir, T.J.; et al. Benefits of a monitored rehabilitation program versus physician care after percutaneous transluminal coronary angioplasty: Follow-up of risk factors and rate of restenosis. J. Cardiopulm. Rehab. 7:281-285; 1989.
7. Bengtsson, K. Rehabilitation after myocardial infarction. Scand. J. Rehabil. Med. 15:1-9; 1983.
8. Bethell, H.; Muller, M. A controlled trial of community-based coronary rehabilitation. B. Heart J. 67:370-375; 1991.
9. Blankenhorn, D.H.; Nessim, S.A.; Johnson, R.L.; Sanmorco, M.E.; Azen, S.P.; Cashin-Hemphill, L. Beneficial effect of combined colestipol-niacin therapy on coronary atherosclerosis and coronary venous bypass grafts. JAMA. 257:3233-3240; 1987.
10. Bloor, C.M.; White, F.C.; Sanders, T.M. Effects of exercise on collateral development in myocardial ischemia in pigs. J. Appl. Physiol. 56:656-665; 1984.

11. Brown, G.; Albers, J.J.; Fisher, L.D.; et al. Regression of coronary artery disease as a result of intensive lipid-lowering therapy in men with high levels of apo-lipoprotein B. N. Engl. J. Med. 323:1289-1298; 1990.
12. Carson, P.; Phillips, R.; Lloyd, M.; et al. Exercise after myocardial infarction: A controlled trial. J. R. Col. Physicians Lond. 16:147-151; 1982.
13. Managing patients and the total cost of health care. Clin. Outcomes. 1:1-8; 1990.
14. Cobb, F.R.; Williams, R.S.; McEwan, P.; Jones, R.H.; Coleman, E.; Wallace, A.G. Effects of exercise training on ventricular function in patients with recent myocardial infarction. Circulation. 66:100-111; 1982.
15. Conn, E.H.; Williams, R.S.; Wallace, R.G. Exercise responses before and after physical conditioning in patients with severely depressed left ventricular function. Am. J. Cardiol. 49:296-300; 1982.
16. Convertino, V.A. Effect of orthostatic stress on exercise performance after bed rest: Relation to in-hospital rehabilitation. J. Card. Rehab. 3:660-663; 1983.
17. Convertino, V.; Hung, J.; Goldwater, D.; DeBusk, R.F. Cardiovascular responses to exercise in middle-aged men after ten days of bed rest. Circulation. 66:134-140; 1982.
18. Crosby, L.; Paternostro-Bayles, M.; Cottington, E.; Pifalo, W.B. Outpatient rehabilitation after right ventricular infarction. J. Cardiopulm. Rehabil. 7:286-291; 1989.
19. DeBusk, R.F. Specialized testing after recent acute myocardial infarction. Ann. Intern. Med. 110:470, 1989.
20. DeBusk, R.F. Why is cardiac rehabilitation not widely used? West. J. Med. 156(2):206-208; 1992.
21. DeBusk, R.F.; Blomquist, C.G.; Kouchos, N.T.; et al. Identification and treatment of low-risk patients after acute myocardial infarction and coronary artery bypass graft surgery. N. Engl. J. Med. 314:161-166; 1986.
22. DeBusk, R.F.; Haskell, W.L.; Miller, N.H.; et al. Medically directed at-home rehabilitation soon after clinically uncomplicated acute myocardial infarction: A new model for patient care. Am. J. Cardiol. 55:251; 1985.
23. DeBusk, R.F.; Hung, J. Exercise conditioning soon after myocardial infarction: Effects on myocardial perfusion and ventricular function. Ann. N.Y. Acad. Sci. 382:343-351; 1982.
24. Dennis, C.; Houston-Miller, N.; Schwartz, R.G.; et al. Early return to work after complicated myocardial infarction: Results of a randomized trial. JAMA. 260:214-220; 1988.
25. Detsky, A.S.; Naglie, I.G. A clinician's guide to cost-effectiveness analysis. Ann. Intern. Med. 113:147-154; 1990.
26. Dodge, H.T. Regression of coronary artery disease as a result of intensive lipid-lowering therapy in men with high levels of apo-lipoprotein B. N. Engl. J. Med. 323:1289-1298; 1990.
27. Dornan, J.; Rolko, A.F.; Greenfield, C. Factors affecting rehabilitation following aortocoronary bypass procedures. Can. J. Surg. 25:677-680; 1982.
28. Ehsani, A.A.; Martin, W.H.; Heath, G.W.; Coyle, E.F. Cardiac effects of prolonged and intense exercise training in patients with coronary artery disease. Am. J. Cardiol. 50:246-254; 1982.
29. Ferguson, R.J.; Petitclerc, R.; Choquette, G.; et al. Effect of physical training on treadmill exercise capacity, collateral circulation and progression of coronary disease. Am. J. Cardiol. 34:764-772; 1974.
30. Fitzgerald, S.T.; Becker, D.M.; Celentano, D.P.; Swank, R.; Brinker, J. Return to work after percutaneous transluminal coronary angioplasty. Am. J. Cardiol. 64:1108-1112; 1989.
31. Frasure-Smith, N. In-hospital symptoms of psychological stress as predictors of long-term outcome after acute myocardial infarction in men. Am. J. Cardiol. 67:121-127; 1991.
32. Froelicher, V.; Jensen, D.; Sullivan, M. A randomized trial of the effects of exercise training after coronary artery bypass graft surgery. Arch. Intern. Med. 145(4):689-692; 1985.
33. Froelicher, V.F.; Jensen, D.; Genter, F.; et al. A randomized trial of exercise training in patients with coronary heart disease. JAMA. 252:1291-1297, 1984.
34. Froelicher, V.F.; Perdue, S.; Pewen, W.; Risch, M. Application of meta-analysis using an electronic spread sheet to exercise testing in patients after myocardial infarction. Am. J. Med. 83:1045-1054; 1987.
35. Froelicher, V.F.; Sullivan, M.; Myers, J.; Jensen, D. Can patients with coronary artery disease receiving beta blockers obtain a training effect? Am. J. Cardiol. 55:155D-161D; 1985.
36. Fuchs, V.F.; Garber, A.M. The new technology assessment. N. Engl. J. Med. 10:673-677; 1990.
37. Gianuzzi, P.; et al. EAMI—exercise training in anterior myocardial infarction: An ongoing multicenter randomized study. Preliminary results on left ventricular function and remodeling. Chest. (May):315S-321S; 1992.
38. Goble, A.; Hare, D.; MacDonald, P.; Oliver, R.; Reid, M.; Worcester, M. Effect of early

programmes of high and low intensity exercise on physical performance after transmural acute myocardial infarction. Br. Heart J. 65:126-131; 1991.

39. Greenland, P.; Chu, J.S. Efficacy of cardiac rehabilitation services. With emphasis on patients after myocardial infarction. Ann. Intern. Med. 109:650-666; 1988.
40. Hadom, D.C. (1990). The future of the American health system. N. Engl. J. Med. 10:752; 1990.
41. Haines, D.E.; Beller, G.A.; Watson, D.D.; Nygaard, T.W.; Craddock, G.B.; Cooper, A.A.; Gibson, R.S. A prospective clinical, scintigraphic, angiographic, and functional evaluation of patients after inferior myocardial infarction with and without right ventricular dysfunction. J. Am. Col. Cardiol. 6:995-1003; 1985.
42. Hamalainen, H.; Luurila, O.J.; Kallio, V.; Knuts, L.R.; Arstila, M.; Hakkila, J.Long-term reduction in sudden deaths after a multifactorial intervention programme in patients with myocardial infarction: Ten-year results of a controlled investigation. Eur. Heart J. 10:55-62; 1989.
43. Hammerman, H.; Schoen, F.J.; Kloner, R.A. Short-term exercise has a profound effect on scar formation after experimental acute myocardial infarction. J. Am. Col. Cardiol. 2:979-982; 1983.
44. Hammond, K.H.; Kelly, T.L.; Froelicher, V.F.; Pewen, W. Use of clinical data in predicting improvement in exercise capacity after cardiac rehabilitation. J. Am. Col. Cardiol. 6:19-26; 1985.
45. Hartung, G.H.; Rangel, R. Exercise training in post-myocardial infarction patients: Comparison of results with high risk coronary and post-bypass patients. Arch. Phys. Med. Rehabil. 62:147-153; 1981.
46. Haskell, W.L. Cardiovascular complications during exercise training of cardiac patients. Circulation. 57(5):920-924; 1978.
47. Haskell, W.L. Restoration and maintenance of physical and psychosocial function in patients with ischemic heart disease. J. Am. Col. Cardiol. 12:1090-1121; 1988.
48. Hedback, B.; Perk, J.; Perski, A. Effect of a post-myocardial infarction rehabilitation program on mortality, morbidity and risk factors. J. Cardiopulm. Rehabil. 5:576-583; 1985.
49. Hochman, J.S.; Healy, B. Effect of exercise on acute myocardial infarction in rats. J. Am. Col. Cardiol. 7:126-132; 1986.
50. Holmes, D.R.; Vliestra, R.E.; Smith, H.C.; et al. Restenosis after percutaneous transluminal coronary angioplasty (PTCA): A report from the PTCA registry of the National Heart, Lung and Blood Institute. Am. J. Cardiol. 53:77C-81A; 1989.
51. Horgan, J.H.; Teo, K.K.; Murren, K.M.; O'Riordan, J.; Gallagher, T. The response to exercise training and vocational counseling in post-myocardial infarction and coronary artery bypass surgery patients. Ir. Med. J. 74:463-469; 1980.
52. Hossack, K.F.; Hartwick, R. Cardiac arrest associated with supervised cardiac rehabilitation. J. Card. Rehabil. 2:402-408; 1982.
53. Judgutt, B.I.; Michorowski, B.L.; Kappagoda, C.T. Exercise training after anterior Q-wave myocardial infarction: Importance of regional left ventricular function and topography. J. Am. Col. Cardiol. 12:363-372; 1988.
54. Kallio, V.; Hamalainen, H.; Hakkila, J.; Luurila, O.J. Reduction in sudden deaths by a multifactorial intervention programme after acute myocardial infarction. Lancet. 2:1091-1094; 1979.
55. Kelbaek, H.; Eskildsen, P.; Hansen, P.F.; Godtfredsen, J. Spontaneous and/or training-induced hemodynamic changes after myocardial infarction. Int. J. Cardiol. 1:205-213; 1981.
56. Kelemen, M.H.; Stewart, K.J.; Gillian, R.E.; et al. Circuit weight training in cardiac patients. J. Am. Col. Cardiol. 7:38-42; 1986.
57. Kentala, E. Physical fitness and feasibility of physical rehabilitation after myocardial infarction in men of working age. Ann. Clin. Res. 4:1-52; 1972.
58. Klein, J.; Froelicher, V.F.; Detrano, R.; Dubach, P.; Yen, R. Does the rest electrocardiogram after myocardial infarction determine the predictive value of exercise-induced ST depression? A 2-year follow-up study in a veteran population. J. Am. Col. Cardiol. 14:305-311; 1989.
59. Kloner, R.A.; Kloner, J.A. The effect of early exercise on myocardial infarct scar formation. Am. Heart J. 106:1009-1014; 1983.
60. Krone, R.J.; Dwyer, E.M.; Greenberg, H.; Miller, J.P.; Gillespie, J.A. The multicenter post-infarction research group. Risk stratification in patients with first non-Q wave infarction: Limited value of the early low level exercise test after uncomplicated infarct. J. Am. Col. Cardiol. 14:31-37; 1989.
61. LaRosa, J.C.; Cleary, P.; Muesing, R.A.; Groman, P.; Hellerstein, H.K.; Naughton, J. Effect of long-term moderate physical exercise on plasma lipoproteins: The national exercise and heart disease project. Arch. Intern. Med. 142:2269-2274; 1982.

62. Levy, R.I.; Breniske, J.F.; Epstein, S.E.; et al. The influence of changes in lipid values induced by cholestyramite and diet on progression of coronary artery disease. Circulation. 69:325-337; 1984.
63. Lipkin, D. Is cardiac rehabilitation necessary? Br. Heart J. 74:34-38; 1991.
64. Maisel, A.S.; Ahnve, S.; Gilpin, E.; et al. Prognosis after extension of myocardial infarction: The role of Q wave or non-Q wave infarction. Circulation. 71:211-217; 1985.
65. Mann, C. Meta-analysis in the breech. Science. 249:476-480; 1990.
66. May, G.S.; Eberlein, K.A.; Furberg, C.D.; Passamani, E.R.; DeMets, D.L. Secondary prevention after myocardial infarction: A review of long-term trials. Prog. Cardiovasc. Dis. 24:331-352; 1982.
67. Mayou, R.A. A controlled trial of early rehabilitation after myocardial infarction. J. Card. Rehabil. 3:397-402; 1983.
68. McGuire, L.B. A long run for a short jump: Understanding clinical guidelines. Ann. Intern. Med. 113:705-708; 1990.
69. McHenry, P.L.; Ellestad, M.H.; Fletcher, G.F.; et al. A position statement for health professionals by the committee on exercise and cardiac rehabilitation of the council on clinical cardiology, American Heart Association. Circulation. 81:396-398; 1990.
70. Meier, B.; Gruentzig, A.R. Return to work after coronary artery bypass surgery in comparison to coronary angioplasty. In Walter, P.J., ed., Return to work after coronary bypass surgery: Psychosocial and economic aspects. New York: Springer-Verlag; 1980:171-176.
71. Miller, N.H.; Haskell, W.L.; Berra, K.; DeBusk, R.F. Home versus group exercise training for increasing functional capacity after myocardial infarction. Circulation. 70:645-649; 1984.
72. Nakai, Y.; Kataoka, Y.; Bando, M.; et al. Effects of physical exercise training on cardiac function and graft patency after coronary artery bypass grafting. J. Thorac. Cardiovasc. Surg. 93:65-72; 1987.
73. Nicod, P.; Gilpin, E.; Dittrich, H.; et al. Short- and long-term clinical outcome after Q wave and non-Q wave myocardial infarction in a large patient population. Circulation. 79:528-536; 1989.
74. Nolewajka, A.J.; Kostuk, W.J.; Rechnitzer, P.A.; et al. Exercise and human collateralization: An angiographic and scintigraphic assessment. Circulation. 60:114-122; 1979.
75. O'Connor, G.T.; Buring, J.E.; Yusuf, S.; et al. (1989). An overview of randomized trials of rehabilitation with exercise after myocardial infarction. Circulation. 80:234-244; 1989.
76. Oldridge, N.; Donner, A.; Buck, C.; et al. Predictors of dropout from cardiac exercise rehabilitation: Ontario exercise heart collaborative study. Am. J. Cardiol. 51:70-74; 1983.
77. Oldridge, N.; Guyatt, G.; Jones, N.; et al. Effects on quality of life with comprehensive rehabilitation after acute myocardial infarction. Am. J. Cardiol. 67:1084-1089; 1991.
78. Oldridge, N.B.; Guyatt, G.H.; Fischer, M.E.; Rimm, A. Cardiac rehabilitation after myocardial infarction. Combined experience of randomized clinical trials. JAMA. 260:945-950; 1988.
79. Oldridge, N.B.; Nagle, F.J.; Balke, B.; et al. Aortocoronary bypass surgery: Effects of surgery and 32 months of physical conditioning on treadmill performance. Arch. Phys. Med. Rehabil. 59(6):268-275; 1978.
80. Palatsi, I. Feasibility of physical training after myocardial infarction and its effect on return to work, morbidity and mortality. Acta. Med. Scand. [Suppl.]. 599; 1976.
81. Pekkanen, J.; Linn, S.; Meiss, G.; et al. Ten-year mortality from cardiovascular disease in relation to cholesterol level among men with and without pre-existing cardiovascular disease. N. Engl. J. Med. 332:1700; 1990.
82. Perk, B.; Hedback, E.; Engvall, G. Effects of cardiac rehabilitation after CABS on readmissions, return to work and physical fitness. Scand. J. Soc. Med. 18:45; 1990.
83. Picard, M.H.; Dennis, C.; Schwartz, R.G.; et al. Cost-benefit analysis of early return to work after uncomplicated acute myocardial infarction. Am. J. Cardiol. 63:1308-1014; 1989.
84. Pratt, C.M.; Welton, D.E.; Squired, W.G, Dirby, T.E.; Hartung, G.H.; Miller, R.R. Demonstration of training effect during chronic beta-adrenergic blockade in patients with coronary artery disease. Circulation. 64:1125-1129; 1981.
85. Rechnitzer, P.A.; Cunningham, D.A.; Andrew, C.M.; et al. Relation of exercise to recurrence rate of myocardial infarction in men. Ontario exercise-heart collaborative study. Am. J. Cardiol. 51:65-69; 1983.
86. Ross, J.; Gilpin, E.A.; Madsen, E.B.; et al. A decision scheme for coronary angiography after acute myocardial infarction. Circulation. 79:292-303; 1989.
87. Scheuer, J. Effects of physical training on myocardial vascularity and perfusion. Circulation. 66:491-495; 1982.
88. Schuler, G.; Rainer, H.; Schlierf, G.; Hoberg, E.; Grunze, M. Progression of coronary stenoses in patients on intensive physical exercise and low fat diet. Circulation. 4:111-238; 1990.

89. Sebrechts, C.P.; Klein, J.L.; Ahnve, S.; Froelicher, V.F.; Ashburn, W.L. Myocardial perfusion changes following one year of exercise training assessed by thallium 201 circumferential count profiles. Am. Heart J. 112:1217-1226; 1986.
90. Shepard, R.J. Exercise regimens after myocardial infarction: Rationale and results. Cardiovasc. Clin. 14:145-157; 1985.
91. Siegel, D.; Grady, P.; Browne, W.S.; Hulley, S.B. Risk modification after myocardial infarction. Ann. Intern. Med. 109:213-218; 1988.
92. Sim, D.N.; Neill, W.A.A. Investigation of the physiological basis for increased exercise threshold for angina pectoris after physical conditioning. J. Clin. Invest. 54:763-770; 1974.
93. Soloff, P.H. Medically and surgically treated coronary patients in cardiovascular rehabilitation: A comparative study. Int. J. Psychiat. Med. 9:93-106; 1980.
94. Sparling, M.; Cantwell, J.; Dolan, R.; Niederman, R. Strength training in a cardiac rehabilitation program: A six-month follow-up. Arch. Phys. Med. Rehabil. 71:148; 1990.
95. Squires, R.W.; Lavie, C.J.; Brandt, T.R.; Gau, G.T.; Bailey, K.R. Cardiac rehabilitation in patients with severe ischemic left ventricular dysfunction. Mayo Clin. Proc. 62:997-1002; 1987.
96. Thompson, P.D. The benefits and risks of exercise training in patients with chronic coronary artery disease. JAMA. 259:1537-1540; 1988.
97. Thompson, P.D.; Funk, E.J.; Carleton, R.A.; Sturner, W.Q. Incidence of death during jogging in Rhode Island from 1975 through 1980. JAMA. 247:2535-2538; 1982.
98. Topol, E.J.; Burek, K.; O'Neill, W.W.; et al. A randomized controlled trial of hospital discharge three days after myocardial infarction in the era of reperfusion. N. Engl. J. Med. 318:1083-1088; 1988.
99. Van Camp, S.P.; Peterson, R.A. Cardiovascular complications of outpatient cardiac rehabilitation programs. JAMA. 256:1160-1163; 1986.
100. Van Dixhoorn, E.; Duivenvoorden, H.; Pool, G. Success and failure of exercise training after myocardial infarction: Is the outcome predictable? J. Am. Col. Cardiol. 15:974-980; 1990.
101. Vanhees, L.; Fagard, R.; Amery, A. Influence of a beta-adrenergic blockade on the hemodynamic effects of physical training in patients with ischemic heart disease. Am. Heart J. 108:270-279; 1982.
102. Verani, M.S.; Hartung, G.H.; Harris-Hoepfel, J.; Welton, D.E.; Pratt, C.M.; Miller, R.R. Effects of exercise training on left ventricular performance and myocardial perfusion in patients with coronary artery disease. Am. J. Cardiol. 47:797-803; 1981.
103. Vermuelen, A.; Liew, K.I.; Durrer, D. Effects of cardiac rehabilitation after myocardial infarction: Changes in coronary risk factors and long-term prognosis. Am. Heart J. 105:798-801; 1983.
104. Wigton, R.S.; et al. Procedural skills of the general internist: A survey of 2500 physicians. Ann. Intern. Med. 111:1023; 1990.
105. Wilhelmsen, L.; Sanne, H.; Emfeldt, D.; Grimby, G.; Tibblin, G.; Wedel, H. A controlled trial of physical training after myocardial infarction. Prev. Med. 4:491-508; 1975.
106. Williams, M.A.; Maresh, C.M.; Esterbrooks, D.J.; Harkbrecht, J.T.; Sketch, M.H. Early exercise training in patients older than age 65 compared with that in younger patients after acute myocardial infarction or coronary artery bypass grafting. Am. J. Cardiol. 55:263-266; 1985.
107. World Health Organization (WHO). Report of expert committee. Rehabilitation of patients with cardiovascular diseases. Technical report no. 270. Geneva; 1964.

Chapter 41

Physical Activity, Fitness, and Stroke

Harold W. Kohl, III
John D. McKenzie

Stroke incidence and mortality is a major public health problem in developed countries. Atherosclerosis of the extra- and intracranial arteries is thought to be the general underlying pathologic basis of both coronary heart disease (CHD) and thromboembolic (ischemic) stroke. Hypertensive disease, although a risk factor for CHD and thromboembolic stroke, is thought to be the major pathologic determinant of hemorrhagic stroke. Although a growing body of literature indicates an inverse causal association between physical activity or physical fitness and CHD, less well studied is the relation between these factors and the risk of ischemic or hemorrhagic stroke. The purpose of this chapter is to review and analyze the evidence that physical activity or physical fitness levels may be a risk factor for the development of stroke. We present data on trends across time, provide a brief discussion of the pathophysiology of stroke, and consider evidence from animal models and human studies on the role that physical activity or fitness may have in the risk of stroke. Finally, we consider difficulties in current data and present suggested directions for future work.

Prevalence, Secular Mortality, and Incidence Trends in Stroke

Stroke is the third leading cause of death in the United States, behind CHD and all cancers (21). It is more commonly disabling than fatal as a neurologic disorder; yet 150,517 deaths due to all strokes were recorded in 1988 in the United States. The overall age-adjusted rate of stroke mortality per 100,000 population in 1988 was 29.7. Ethnic differences exist in stroke mortality in that blacks in 1988 had nearly twice the death rate due to stroke that whites did. Age-adjusted death rates per 100,000 in 1988 due to stroke for black women and men were 46.6 and 57.8 respectively, whereas for white women and men the corresponding figures were 25.5 and 30.0. Rates of stroke death also increase nearly exponentially with age, ranging from 19.2 per 100,000 population aged 45 to 54 years to 1,707.4 per 100,000 population aged 85 years and more in 1988.

Changes in stroke mortality in the United States between 1950 and 1988 for the four race-sex groups are illustrated in Figure 41.1. The downward trend shown in Figure 41.1 has been continuing since the early part of the century and closely mirrors the trends for CHD. Most countries for which adequate data are available also convincingly demonstrate a lowering of the rate of stroke since 1970 (3). Exceptions are most Eastern European countries, where either no change or an increase in stroke mortality has been observed since 1970. The United States and Canada respectively experienced nearly 5.5% and 4.7% per annum decreases in stroke mortality in the 15 years between 1970 and 1985 (3), although the rate of decline, at least in the United States, may be slowing (7). More aggressive and effective detection, treatment, and control of hypertension during this period have been frequently cited as the reason for the decline in stroke incidence and mortality (33), but this hypothesis has recently been called to question (2).

Incidence data for stroke are much more difficult to garner than are mortality statistics because of the worldwide absence of stroke registries. The best available data suggest that the historical decline in stroke mortality has been paralleled by similar declines in incidence, but that incidence may be again increasing in recent years (8). Only one source provides valid stroke incidence data in the United States. Data from the follow-up of residents of Rochester, MN (see Figure 41.2), suggest that between 1945 and 1979, the age-adjusted incidence of stroke in men decreased from 241 strokes per 100,000 population to 141 per 100,000 population (4). The corresponding incidence rate in women fell from 184 per 100,000 population between 1945 and 1949 to a low of 96 per 100,000 between 1975 and 1979. From 1980 to 1984, however, the rates in men and women respectively increased to 168 and 110 per 100,000 population.

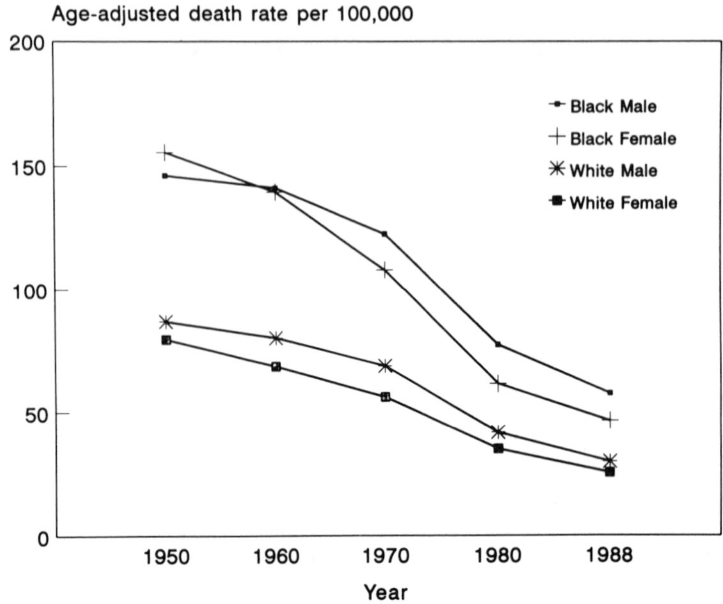

Figure 41.1 Age-adjusted death rates from cerebrovascular diseases by race and sex grouping: United States, 1950-1988. Source: National Center for Health Statistics (21).

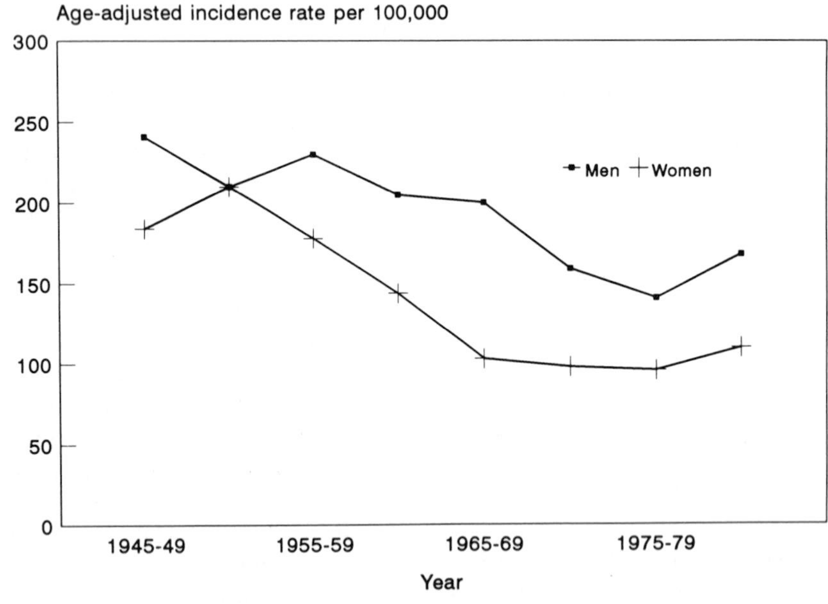

Figure 41.2 Age-adjusted incidence rates of stroke in Rochester, Minnesota by sex, 1950-1988. Adapted from reference 4.

The possible reasons for the recent increase in stroke incidence in Rochester are unclear. Recent improvements in diagnostic capabilities (e.g., computerized tomography) provide for the very real possibility of a temporal shift in stroke diagnosis (e.g., the ability to detect asymptomatic strokes that otherwise would have gone undetected without the technology). In other words, the increased use of computerized tomography may have increased the likelihood of detecting less severe strokes.

It has also been suggested that the increase in stroke incidence could actually be related to the decreasing rates of CHD incidence and mortality. The lower rates of CHD would leave a larger pool of persons at risk for stroke (15). An inverse relation between a high risk of stroke and a low risk of CHD has been observed in the Japanese (26), making this a plausible explanation as well. Extrapolation of findings from the unique population in Rochester requires confirmation and support from nationally representative data, but the rough parallel between historical declines in incidence and mortality, as well as the more recent parallel between the slowdown in stroke mortality and the possibility of a recently increased incidence of stroke, suggests real trends in incidence and mortality due to stroke exist rather than an artifact of increased survival.

Physical Activity Assessment

A major problem in studying the associations of physical activity and fitness with health is the difficulty in the assessment of the exposure (6). This is a pervasive problem in population-based studies where laboratory control and manipulation are not possible. Although the overall objective in the assessment of physical activity is to obtain an accurate estimate of energy expenditure such that it may be related to disease risk, rarely is the problem that straightforward. Several difficulties arise. First, the issue about the type of energy expenditure to assess is important. Changing economic conditions and social environments in the 20th century have allowed industrial societies to develop a preponderance of physically inactive occupations. The 20th century has also been a period in which there was a shift away from occupational demands for energy expenditure so that much of the energy expenditure now results more from leisure pursuits than from job-related tasks for most people in industrialized societies. Thus, estimates of true energy expenditure cannot simply rely on job classifications as they perhaps once could. Accurate estimates of energy expended during leisure time are necessary to avoid misclassification.

Pursuant to estimating the specific type of physical activity is the issue of intraperson variability in energy expenditure. If an accurate profile of energy expenditure is available, how many days or assessments of that profile are necessary to estimate the true habitual level? Issues of intraperson variance and seasonality are important here, and the situation is much the same as in the case of diet assessment (18). Existing studies of physical activity and health, including those to be reviewed in this chapter, have relied on crude, simple-point estimates of physical activity as the exposure. Although the assumption that such crude measures will be correlated with the true level of physical activity and thus grossly classify persons into active or inactive categories, there are few data to support this assumption. Moreover, such crude measures of physical activity increase the risk of misclassification and likely result in an underestimation of the true association between the exposure and the outcome.

A final problem with physical activity assessment, and one that is especially magnified in studies of chronic diseases with long latency periods, is the temporal association of the exposure assessment (physical activity) with occurrence of the outcome (stroke). Prospective population studies typically gather baseline assessments on a variety of clinical features (including physical activity) and then follow the study participants until a predetermined time or the occurrence of an event. In the case of chronic diseases, most prospective studies follow subjects for many years. Rarely, however (and never in the existing studies of physical activity and stroke), are attempts made to reclassify individuals based on changes in physical activity habits during the follow-up period. Available data therefore rely on a single point estimate of physical activity some time distant to the occurrence of the event. Whereas the assumption again is that there is some degree of correlation between physical activity habits across time within individuals, very few data are available to support this contention. This lack of control for changes in exposure during the follow-up is another weakness in the assessment of physical activity that will result in possible misclassification and subsequent underestimation of the association between exposure and disease.

Physical activity assessment is therefore a substantial weakness in studies of physical activity and health. The type of physical activity assessed, the estimate of the true exposure, and issues related to the temporality between exposure and outcome are all factors that can result in misclassification and thus an incorrect estimate of the association being studied. Results of existing studies on physical activity and stroke must be viewed within the constraints of these limitations.

Physical Fitness Assessment

Although no published studies on physical fitness and the risk of stroke are available, several general issues regarding the measurement of fitness as it may be related to health are important to acknowledge. Physical fitness is a physiologic parameter encompassing several constructs (metabolic, cardiorespiratory, musculoskeletal), whereas activity is a behavior, the engagement in which, despite genetic influences, leads to fitness (5). The advantage in using physical fitness (measured by maximal oxygen uptake, physical work capacity, etc.)

as a measure of exposure in studies of health is that it is an objective, tangible measure. The subjective, self-reported format of physical activity assessment in population studies may result in misclassification; the use of an estimate of fitness helps to minimize such errors.

Despite the objectivity of estimates of physical fitness, several disadvantages are evident: the use of submaximal testing (which may not estimate true fitness), a lack of maximal effort in those tests that are designed to be maximal, and the fact that preexisting diseases or conditions may influence fitness levels rather than the fitness levels causally influencing risk of disease.

Pathophysiology of Stroke

Stroke is a general term used by clinicians and others for diseases related to the cerebrovascular system. The World Health Organization defines a stroke as "rapidly developing clinical signs of focal (at times global) disturbance of cerebral function, lasting more than 24 hours or leading to death with no other apparent cause than that of vascular origin" (11). Stroke with a fixed perfusion deficit should be clearly distinguished from other, temporary neurologic deficits related to disturbance of cerebral function. Specifically, a transient ischemic attack (TIA) is characterized by a transient neurologic deficit due to a likewise transient impairment of cerebral perfusion that completely resolves in minutes or hours. Failure of the neurologic deficit to completely resolve within 24 hr is termed a completed stroke.

Subtypes of completed strokes include cerebral infarctions and cerebral hemorrhages (which then further can be classified into subarachnoid or cerebral intraparenchymal hemorrhages). Generally, the several types of stroke can be classified as either hemorrhagic or ischemic. The most common type of stroke in the United States is ischemic and is characterized by a protracted drop in perfusion pressure caused by a thrombus developing in the extracranial carotid system, the large intracranial arterial system, or, most commonly, in the cerebral microcirculation (34). An embolus originating in the extracranial carotid circulatory system or the heart can also lead to ischemic stroke.

Atherosclerosis is the most common underlying cause of ischemic stroke. Despite important and necessary distinctions between the intra- and extracranial arteries and other arterial beds in terms of anatomy and physiology, much of the knowledge about atherosclerosis and the coronary circulation has direct applicability to the cerebral circulation as well. Next we briefly review what is known about the pathogenesis of atherosclerosis and its relation to the occurrence of stroke.

The fibrous plaque precursor for the atherosclerotic lesion is characterized by the proliferation of myointimal cells, increased lipid deposition (primarily cholesterol esters), and increased synthesis of connective tissues (namely, elastin, collagen, and glycosaminoglycans) (27). The process is thought to begin evolution in the first or second decade of life as a fatty streak, a nonraised lesion in the intima, with little or no cell proliferation (33).

There is no generally accepted hypothesis concerning the pathogenesis of atherosclerosis. Two major theories exist to explain this phenomenon (35) and, although different, they share similar features. The lipid infiltration theory relates hypercholesterolemia and cholesterol metabolism to atherosclerosis by suggesting that the higher concentrations of cholesterol-carrying lipoproteins increase the rate at which the lipoproteins are absorbed into the arterial wall (5). It is on this theory that many of the preventive efforts aimed at reducing risk of CHD and atherosclerotic-related stroke have rested—that a reduction in the concentration of circulating lipoproteins will reduce their uptake into the arterial walls and slow the process of atherosclerosis.

The second major theory regarding the pathogenesis of atherosclerosis is based on observations that injury to the endothelial surface, and not just abnormalities in cholesterol concentrations or metabolism, will induce atheromatous lesions (28). Such an injury is thought to increase platelet adherence and aggregation, resulting in a release of platelet-derived growth factor (PDGF). Intimal proliferation follows, resulting in the evolution of an atherosclerotic lesion (33). Although the two hypotheses appear to be uncorrelated, biologic systems rarely act independently, and the actual pathogenesis of atherosclerosis is likely an interaction of the two hypotheses in many people (33).

High blood pressure is a major underlying risk factor in the development of both atherosclerotic-based brain infarctions and hypertensive cerebral hemorrhages. In the case of hypertensive cerebral hemorrhages, the mechanism is thought to be related to elevated arterial or arteriole blood pressure, which results in conditions such as microatheroma, lipohyalinosis, fibrinoid necrosis, and Charcot-Bouchard aneurysms (the pathologic sequelae of uncontrolled systemic blood pressure and rupture of arterial walls with subsequent hemorrhage or in situ thrombosis).

Review of Literature

Animal models. Many animal models of cerebral ischemia exist (13,30), but few studies are available that specifically evaluate the role that physical activity or fitness may play in the occurrence of stroke. Those that do exist rely on the results of studies showing that exercise training decreases resting blood pressure levels in hypertensive animals and humans (9). Thus, the experiments focus on the presence of cerebrovascular lesions and mortality from stroke using exercise to lower blood pressure.

In 1986, Overton et al. reported on the effects of voluntary physical activity on resting pressures, incidence of lesions, and life spans in young, stroke-prone, spontaneously hypertensive rats (22). As part of a larger study, young male (n = 17) and female (n = 15) animals (28 to 35 days old) were assigned either to activity or to sedentary cages, and the animals' frequency, intensity, and duration of running were monitored for 5 weeks. The voluntary exercise performed by the stroke-prone hypertensive rats improved fitness but did not lower resting blood pressure in the rodents. Further, the life span of the exercised animals was no different than that of the nonexercised animals, with or without evidence of cerebrovascular lesions. Thus, voluntary exercise at an intensity high enough to produce a training effect after 5 weeks had no effect on blood pressure or on the occurrence of cerebrovascular lesions in these animals.

As a follow-up to the study by Overton et al., Tipton et al. assessed the effects of moderate exercise training on resting pressures, incidence of cerebral lesions, and life spans in stroke-prone, spontaneously hypertensive rats, with the assumption that the exercise intensity in the previous study was not great enough to produce expected changes (31). Two groups of male and female rats were trained at 40% to 70% of maximal oxygen uptake: One group began training 38 days after birth and the other 134 days after birth.

Results from this study suggest that, regardless of the age at which exercise began, the trained animals were more likely to have cerebrovascular lesions at death than the untrained animals. For both the younger and older groups, the trained animals were 36% and 19% (respectively) more likely to exhibit histological evidence of cerebrovascular lesions (focal hemorrhage or necrosis, or both, or an acute or chronic lesion) during the study than were the comparable untrained animals. No consistent effect of the training on resting blood pressure was noted, and no significant difference between the two groups with respect to life span was noted either. The authors provide several speculations to account for the unexpected findings. The high-sodium diet the animals were on may have inhibited the blood pressure attenuation. Further, the exercise intensity used in this study may actually have been too intense—a liability in this type of experimental animal rather than a benefit.

Human studies. In general, the data relating physical activity or physical fitness to the risk of stroke are equivocal. Existing published studies are listed in Table 41.1. Weaknesses in the design of existing observational studies, including incomplete or nonexistent control for confounding influences, crude and oftentimes temporally incorrect measures of physical activity exposure (as discussed previously), and potentially incomplete case definition and ascertainment are factors that individually and collectively contribute to the equivocal conclusions. No published studies have examined physical fitness as an exposure for the risk of stroke.

The first report providing evidence concerning a possible relation of physical activity to the risk of stroke was contributed by Paffenbarger and Williams in 1967 (25). University of Pennsylvania (n = 15,000 from 1931 to 1940) and Harvard University alumni (n = 35,000 from 1916 to 1950) were followed, and their mortality experience was observed. There were 171 deaths due to stroke in these men, who were then age-matched to four randomly selected surviving classmates who served as a comparison group. Causes of death were abstracted from official death certificates. Physical activity was assessed in 1965 by classifying each man as to whether or not he had participated in varsity athletics during college. For both hemorrhagic (subarachnoid and intracerebral hemorrhages) and ischemic (cerebral thrombi and emboli) strokes, those men who were not varsity athletes as collegians had nearly a twofold increased risk of death due to stroke compared to their more active classmates. The overall rate of varsity athletic participation in the decedents was 7.0 per 100, whereas that in the control group was 15.5 per 100; a similar pattern was seen for both stroke subtypes. No information was available on physical activity exposure after college years in these men, nor were any multivariate analyses to control for possible confounding influences reported.

Paffenbarger also reported on the risk of stroke with lower levels of occupational physical activity in San Francisco longshoremen after an 18.5-year follow-up (23). Men were classified as to whether or not their primary work duties required cargo handling. Cargo handling at the time of the study (1951) was quite strenuous, requiring approximately one-third more energy output than non-cargo-handling (more sedentary) longshoring.

Cargo handlers in this prospective study died at a rate of 23.5 per 10,000 person-years of follow-up, whereas their less active workmates died at

Table 41.1 Summary of Observational Studies Assessing the Relationship Between Physical Activity and Stroke

Study	Population	Definition of exposure	Definition of stroke	Result	Comments
Paffenbarger & Williams (23)	> 50,000 male college alumni survivors aged 30–70 years	Participation in varsity college athletics (yes/no)	Death due to stroke (hemorrhagic and occlusive) (n = 171)	Inverse association	Twofold higher rate of stroke among nonvarsity athletes; no confounding assessment (age only)
Paffenbarger (24)	3,991 longshoremen aged 35 years and over; 18.5-year follow-up from 1951	Occupational activity (cargo handler or not)	Death due to stroke (hemorrhagic and occlusive) (n = 132)	Null association	No difference in risk of death due to stroke in cargo-handling longshoremen compared with more sedentary workmates
Kannel & Sorlie (14)	1,909 men aged 35–64 at fourth biennial examination, Framingham; 14-year follow-up	Physical activity index based on hours/day at specific activity intensity	Cerebrovascular accident (n = 87)	Inverse association	No statistically significant association after controlling for age, systolic blood pressure, serum cholesterol, glucose intolerance, cigarette habit, and left ventricular hypertrophy
Salonen et al. (29)	3,829 women and 4,110 men aged 30–59 years from Eastern Finland; approximately 7-year follow-up	Physical activity at work and during leisure time (low/high)	Cerebral stroke ICD-8 430–437 morbidity and mortality (n = 71 men and 56 women)	Inverse association for women for both leisure time and work; inverse association for men and work; null association for men and leisure time	Statistically signficiant RR (1.6, CI = 1.1–2.5) for men and women (1.7, CI = 1.1–2.7) who were inactive at work; no significant association for leisure-time physical activity; multivariate adjustment for age, serum cholesterol, diastolic blood pressure, body mass index, and tobacco habit
Herman et al. (12)	132 hospital-based stroke cases and 239 age- and sex-matched controls; Dutch men and women aged 40–74 years	Physical activity during leisure time (greatest portion of one's lifetime) ranging from little to regular-heavy	Rapidly developed clinical signs of focal or global disturbance of cerebral function lasting more than 24 hours or leading to death, with no apparent cause other than vascular origin	Inverse association	Statistically significant association (compared to the least active category) with an apparent dose-response across increasing levels of physical activity; adjusted for a variety of possible confounders; relative odds (relative to lowest activity category): light, 0.72 (95% CI = 0.37–1.42); heavy, 0.41 (95% CI = 0.21–0.84)

Paffenbarger et al. (25)	16,936 male college alumni entering college between 1916 and 1950 followed from 1962–1978	Physical activity index (kcal/week) estimated from reports of stairs climbed, city blocks walked, and sports play each week	Death due to stroke (n = 103)	Inverse association	Statistically significant association after adjustment for age, cigarette habit, and physician-diagnosed hypertension; dose-response gradient across physical activity index
Lapidus & Bengtsson (16)	1,462 Swedish women aged 38–60; follow-up between 1968 and 1981	Physical activity at work and during leisure hours, lifetime and during previous years	Fatal and nonfatal stroke (n = 13)	Inverse association	Statistically significant association for work and leisure physical activity in past year; no statistical association for measures of lifetime exposure during work and leisure
Menotti & Seccareccia (20)	99,029 male Italian railroad employees aged 40–59 years; followed for 5 years	Job classification of physical activity at work (heavy, moderate, and sedentary)	Fatal stroke (n = 187)	U-shaped association	Lowest stroke death rate in moderate physical activity category; no control for confounding influences (age only)
Menotti et al. (19)	8,287 men aged 40–59 in six of seven countries from Seven Country Study; 20-year follow-up	Job classification of physical activity at work (heavy, moderate, and sedentary)	Fatal stroke	Null association	No association after statistical adjustment for risk factors

(continued)

Table 41.1 ***(Continued)***

Study	Population	Definition of exposure	Definition of stroke	Result	Comments
Harmsen et al. (10)	7,495 Swedish men aged 47–55 years at baseline and followed an average of 11.8 years	Physical activity at work and leisure hours	Fatal stroke (n = 230)	Null association	No association after adjustment for a variety of risk factors; relative odds = (inactive versus all others) 1.2, 95% CI = 0.8–1.8
Lindsted et al. (17)	9,484 male Seventh-Day Adventists aged 30 years and older; 26 year follow-up	Self-report of level of physical activity in 1960	Fatal stroke (n = 410)	U-shaped association	Risk in moderately active men relative to inactive men = 0.78 (95% CI = 0.61–1.00); risk in highly active men relative to inactive men = 0.94 (95% CI = 0.58–2.01); extensive confounding control
Wannamethee and Shaper (32)	7,735 British men aged 40–59 years; 8.5-year follow-up	Self-report of physical activity at baseline; scale generated based on type and frequency of activity	Fatal and nonfatal stroke (n = 128)	Significant inverse association	Men who were more active had a significantly lower risk of stroke than did their less active counterparts, after researchers controlled for age, social class, smoking, heavy drinking, body mass, and resting systolic blood pressure; risk in vigorously active men compared with inactive men = 0.2 (95% CI = 0.1–0.9)

Note. CI = confidence interval.

From "How Much Physical Activity Is Good for Health?" by S.N. Blair, H.W. Kohl, N.F. Gordon, and R.S. Paffenbarger, Jr., 1992, *Annual Review of Public Health*, **13**, pp. 99-126. Copyright 1992 by Annual Reviews Inc. Adapted by permission.

a rate of 21.2 per 10,000 person-years. Thus, no increased risk of death was associated with occupational physical activity in this group.

As part of the Framingham study, 1,909 men aged 35 to 64 years at their fourth biennial examination were followed for 14 years to determine if physical inactivity predisposed them to a higher risk of stroke (14). A physical activity index was created based on self-reported hours per day that each subject spent at a specific intensity. All cerebrovascular accidents (n = 87) were classified as stroke deaths, and no attempt was made to discern between hemorrhagic and ischemic strokes. Although a univariate inverse association between the physical activity index and risk of stroke was demonstrated among these men, no statistically significant association was observed after multivariate control for age, systolic blood pressure, serum cholesterol, glucose intolerance, cigarette habit, and the presence of left ventricular hypertrophy.

In 1982, Salonen et al. reported on the association of physical activity exposure at work and during leisure time and the subsequent risk of stroke in 3,978 men and 3,688 women as part of the North Karelia study (29). Subjects were 30 to 59 years of age at baseline and were followed approximately 7 years (1972 to 1978) for stroke incidence. There were 71 events in men and 56 in women during the follow-up period. Physical activity, both that acquired during work and that taken during leisure time, was measured as self-reported to a multiple-choice question, and various clinical measures were taken during a field examination. Physical activity at work or leisure was categorized as either low or high based on the responses to the question; 22% of the men and 25% of the women were declared sedentary in their occupations and 33% and 27% of men and women respectively were similarly classified per their leisure-time activities.

After simultaneously controlling for the influences of age, serum cholesterol, diastolic blood pressure, body mass index (weight for height), and tobacco use, researchers found that men and women who were physically inactive at their occupations were respectively at 60% and 70% higher risks of developing a stroke than were their more active counterparts. Men with low physical activity at work had a relative risk (RR) of stroke during the follow-up of 1.6 (90% CI=1.1–2.5), whereas women had a relative risk of 1.7 (90% CI=1.1–2.7). Conversely, relative risks for stroke per low leisure-time physical activity levels did not differ from unity (men: 1.0, 90% CI=0.7–1.5; women: 1.3, 90% CI=0.8–2.0).

A case-comparison design was used to evaluate the possible role that physical activity during leisure time (classified as that taken during the greatest portion of one's lifetime) had in the risk of stroke (12). Dutch stroke patients and hospital-based comparison (nonstroke) subjects were interviewed and examined specifically for the study. There were 49 female and 63 male stroke survivors who developed a stroke during the period October 1978 to July 1981. They were aged 40 to 74 years. Eighty-seven women and 152 men were selected as age- and sex-matched comparison subjects because of hospitalization for nonstroke related conditions. Those with *little* physical activity during leisure time (mainly sitting) were used as the referent category; those men and women who reported regular light activity during leisure time (regularly walking or cycling each week) demonstrated a 51% decreased risk of stroke (RR=0.49, 95% CI=0.31–0.77). Furthermore, those classified as exercising heavily during leisure time were shown to have a further decreased risk of stroke compared with sedentary comparison subjects (RR=0.24, 95% CI=0.10–0.59). The researchers calculated these risk estimates after controlling for effects of sex, age, educational attainment, history of acute myocardial infarction, cardiac arrythmias, hypertension, diabetes mellitus, obesity, history of transient ischemic attacks, and positive Rhesus factor. Not only do these data provide evidence of an inverse association between physical activity and stroke; they also provide evidence of a dose-response gradient across the three physical activity categories.

In an extended follow-up of 16,936 alumni of Harvard University (college age between 1916 and 1950 and recontacted between 1962 and 1978), Paffenbarger et al. reanalyzed the risk of stroke death by level of current physical activity habit, measured by an index encompassing blocks walked, stairs climbed, and time and type of vigorous sports play per week (24). The index was used to express physical activity in kilocalories of energy expended per week in these activities. There were 103 stroke deaths in these men during the time period. When the men were grouped by level of physical activity into those expending less than 500 kcal per week, 500 to 1,999 kcal per week, and 2,000 or more kcal per week, a significant inverse trend in risk of stroke was observed. Men in the lowest category of physical activity died from stroke at a rate of 6.5 per 10,000 man-years, of observation. Men in the middle category died from stroke at a rate of 5.2 per 10,000 man-years, and men who expended 2,000 kcal or more died at a rate of 2.4 per 10,000 man-years. The only confounding controls available in this study were cigarette habit, age, and history of physician-diagnosed hypertension. Much as in the report of Herman et al. (12), a significant inverse dose-response gradient was observed in this study.

In a report from Gothenburg, Lapidus and Bengtsson (16) reported on the fatal and nonfatal stroke risk experience of 1,462 women who were aged 38 to 60 years at baseline and were followed for 14 years. Estimates of physical activity at work, during leisure hours, and during the previous year were used to classify exposure in these women; 13 fatal and nonfatal strokes were observed during the follow-up. There was a statistically significant inverse association of risk of stroke with work and leisure-time physical activity estimates of the past year, but no association for measures of lifetime work and leisure physical activity exposure.

Physical activity exposure at work was used to classify 99,029 male Italian railroad system employees aged 40 to 59 years into three levels of occupational physical activity: heavy work (requiring more than 3,000 kcal per day); moderate work (requiring 2,400 to 3,000 kcal per day), and sedentary (less than 2,400 kcal per day) (20). The men were followed for 5 years, and rates of stroke deaths were tabulated across the three physical activity categories. There were 187 fatal strokes during the follow-up. A U-shaped distribution of the stroke death rates was found after controlling for differences in age. Men in the sedentary category died at a rate of 2.2 per 1,000 in 5 years. Those in the heavy work category died at a rate of 2.21 per 1,000 in 5 years, and those in the moderate work category died at a rate of 1.44 per 1,000 in 5 years. The age-adjusted rate of stroke death in the moderate work category was significantly lower than that in either the sedentary or heavy work category, but no control for other possible confounding influences was carried out in this study.

Menotti et al. reported the 20-year stroke mortality experience in 12 of the 16 cohorts of the Seven Countries Study (19). The 8,247 men in these analyses were aged 40 to 59 years in the late 1950s or early 1960s and represented six of the seven original countries in the study. Self-reported physical activity at work was collected at baseline during the study and formed a three-level exposure variable—sedentary, moderate, and heavy—in much the same manner as was done by Menotti and Seccareccia (20). Neither an ecological analysis using the mean level of physical activity in the individual cohorts and rates of stroke death by country nor an individual-based multivariate model controlling for blood pressure, serum cholesterol, body mass index, cigarette consumption, or age demonstrated a significant association of physical activity at work and the risk of stroke.

Harmsen et al. reported the results of a prospective study of stroke risk factors in 7,495 Swedish men aged 47 to 55 years at baseline who were followed for an average of 11.8 years from 1970 to 1973 (10). In this population-based study, a stroke registry and death certificates were used to identify occurrences of both fatal and nonfatal stroke. Physical activity status, assessed by self-report, was utilized as a four-point scale ranging from sedentary to highly active. One hundred forty-eight first-time strokes were recorded in these men during the follow-up period. No significant association between physical activity and the risk of stroke was evident during follow-up after researchers adjusted for smoking status, known hypertension, diabetes mellitus, family history of stroke, social status, alcohol abuse, marital status, or severe psychological stress. The risk estimates for the lowest category of physical activity relative to the three highest categories for all strokes was 1.2 (95% CI= 0.8–1.8). Furthermore, there was no association seen for any of the four subtypes of stroke (subarachnoid hemorrhage, intracerebral hemorrhage, cerebral infarction, or nonspecified stroke).

Lindsted et al. reported on the association of physical activity habits and patterns of mortality among Seventh-Day Adventist men, a unique study group given the influences of church-based doctrine prohibiting alcohol and tobacco use (17). Based on questionnaire data collected in 1960, 9,484 men aged 30 years and older formed the cohort of Adventists followed for mortality over 26 years. Physical activity exposure was defined by self-report in 1960 to the question "How much exercise do you get (work or play)?" A four-point scale (none, slight, moderate, heavy) was available for responses; for the purposes of the analyses, the two lower categories were combined together to create a three-level physical activity exposure variable (inactive, moderately active, highly active). During the 26-year follow-up there were 3,799 deaths, 410 of which were attributed to cerebrovascular disease. A unique aspect of this study was the ability to evaluate and control (albeit crudely) for potential influences of dietary intake in that a food-frequency section was included on the original questionnaire.

After controlling for any influences associated with ethnicity, smoking habit, educational attainment, personal history of heart disease, hypertension, stroke or cancer, body mass index, marital status, and dietary intake pattern, researchers observed that men who were reportedly moderately active in 1960 had a marginally significant 22% lower risk of death due to stroke, relative to the inactive men (RR=0.78, 95% CI=0.61–1.00). Men in the highly active group had a corresponding risk of stroke death that was 6% lower than that of the sedentary referent group (RR=0.94, 95% CI= 0.58–2.01). As in the report of Italian railroad workers, somewhat of a U-shaped association appears in these data: The moderately active group had a lower estimated risk than either those who were the least or the most active.

Finally, and most recently, Wannamethee and Shaper (32) reported prospective observations of physical activity and the risk of stroke in 7,735 British men who were aged 40 to 59 years at baseline and who were followed for 9.5 years for fatal and nonfatal strokes. Physical activity in these men was evaluated at baseline and was expressed as a summary score of usual activities encompassing regular walking or cycling, recreational activity, and vigorous sporting activities. The score was derived from reported frequency and intensity of each activity. Six categories of activity were created from the score, ranging from inactive to vigorously active. The researchers counted stroke end points using established surveillance procedures, and 128 strokes were recorded in this cohort over the follow-up period.

Men in the most active category (vigorous) at baseline died at a rate that was 84% lower than men in the least active category (inactive rate, 3.1/1,000 per year; vigorous rate, 0.5/1,000 per year). After adjusting for the influences of age, social class, smoking, heavy drinking, body weight, and blood pressure, researchers found that physical activity was inversely associated with the risk of stroke with a significantly protective trend occurring with higher levels of physical activity. This inverse relation was seen both in men with and without previous evidence of ischemic heart disease.

Conclusions and Implications for Future Research

Physical activity and physical fitness are causally related to the risk of death due to CHD. A variety of mechanisms are available to explain this phenomenon, one being that physical activity and fitness either directly or indirectly slow the development of atherosclerotic lesions or contribute to the regression of established lesions, or both. Given the probability of common pathophysiologic mechanisms in CHD and ischemic stroke (namely, atherosclerosis), it follows that physical inactivity and physical unfitness would also adversely affect the risk of stroke. Moreover, physical activity and fitness are known to indirectly and positively influence blood pressure, clotting factors, glucose tolerance, and smoking habits, all factors that have been associated with increased risk of stroke. Although the hypothesis is attractive, the currently available data are equivocal concerning the role that physical activity and physical fitness may play in the risk of stroke. Animal models are scarce and unsupportive, and population studies suffer from design flaws. The U-shaped relation of physical activity and stroke in two studies is intriguing and requires more investigation.

Several directions for future work can be enthusiastically suggested. Perhaps the most urgent need in the study of physical activity, physical fitness, and stroke (indeed for measures of general health as well) is more thorough assessment of physical activity or physical fitness. The existing studies of physical activity and stroke use crude, single-point measures of physical activity, and the potential for misclassification on the exposure, either at the initial assessment or during any follow-up period, is high. Methodological refinements in physical activity assessment, such as the knowledge of the number of days necessary to assess true levels of physical activity and valid ways of assessing historical physical activity levels, are urgently needed. Finally, no published studies on physical fitness and stroke exist. This question must be vigorously pursued.

More studies, with innovative designs, are urgently needed to address the issue of physical activity, physical fitness, and stroke. The ideal would be long-term prospective studies in which persons are enrolled, assessed for risk factors at baseline, periodically and systematically reevaluated, and followed for years for incidence and mortality due to stroke.

In the absence of resources needed to mount such an effort, several alternatives are possible. Particularly well suited to this problem are case-comparison studies in which incident and fatal cases of stroke are identified and matched with an appropriate comparison group and each subject's historical physical activity or fitness exposure is subsequently quantified. Thus, in a uniquely short study period (without having to wait for case accrual), the risk of low activity or fitness in stroke cases and nonstroke cases can be evaluated.

Researchers involved in long-term prospective studies are urged to reanalyze existing data sets to help determine the role that physical activity and fitness may play in the risk of stroke. There are several ongoing studies specifically designed to assess CHD risk factors that could be used to study stroke risk factors (including physical activity habits) relatively quickly. Within the interpretative constraints tied to secondary data analyses, these studies could substantially add to the existing knowledge.

Continued work on, and refinement of, animal models of physical activity, physical fitness, and stroke are needed. Whereas public health experiments (observational studies) can go a long way in helping to determine risk factors and intervention potentials, animal models in many cases are the only way that clues to biologic mechanisms can be uncovered. Experiments are needed not only in the existing rat models, but also in other models that might more closely simulate the human experience.

Acknowledgments

Milton Z. Nichaman and R. Sue McPherson provided constructive criticisms on an early draft of the manuscript. We thank Laura E. Becker for expert secretarial support. This work was supported in part by National Institutes of Health grant AG06945.

References

1. Blair, S.N.; Kohl, H.W.; Gordon, N.F.; Paffenbarger, R.S., Jr. How much physical activity is good for health? Annu. Rev. Public Health. 13:99-126; 1992.
2. Bonita, R.; Beaglehole, R. Increased treatment of hypertension does not explain the decline in stroke mortality in the United States, 1970-1980. Hypertension. [Suppl. I]. 13:I69-I73; 1989.
3. Bonita, R.; Stewart, A.; Beaglehole, R. International trends in stroke mortality: 1970-1985. Stroke. 21:989-992; 1990.
4. Broderick, J.P.; Phillips, S.J.; Whisnant, J.P.; O'Fallon, W.M.; Bergstralh, E.J. Incidence rates of stroke in the eighties: The end of the decline in stroke? Stroke. 20:577-582; 1989.
5. Brown, M.S.; Koranen, P.T.; Goldstein, J.L. Regulation of plasma cholesterol by lipoprotein receptors. Science. 212:628; 1981.
6. LaPorte, R.E.; Montoye, H.J.; Caspersen, C.J. Assessment of physical activity in epidemiologic research: Problems and prospects. Public Health Rep. 100:131-146; 1985.
7. Cooper, R.; Sempos, C.; Hsieh, S-C.; Kovar, M.G. Slowdown in the decline of stroke mortality in the United States, 1978-1986. Stroke. 21:1274-1279; 1990.
8. Frankowski, R.F. Epidemiology of stroke and intracerebral hemorrhage. In: Kaufman, H.H., ed. Intracerebral hematomas. New York: Raven Press; 1992.
9. Hagberg, J.M. Exercise, fitness, and hypertension. In: Bouchard, C.; Shephard, R.J.; Stephens, T.; Sutton, J.R.; McPherson, B.D., eds. Exercise, fitness, and health: A consensus of current knowledge. Champaign IL: Human Kinetics; 1989:455-466.
10. Harmsen, P.; Rosengren, A.; Tsipogianni, A.; Wilhelmsen, L. Risk factors for stroke in middle-aged men in Goteburg, Sweden. Stroke. 21:223-229; 1990.
11. Hatano, S. Experience from a multicenter stroke register: A preliminary report. Bull. WHO. 58:113-130; 1976.
12. Herman, B.; Schmitz, P.I.M.; Leyten, A.C.M.; Van Luijk, J.H.; Frenken, C.W.G.M.; et al. Multivariate logistic analysis of risk factors for stroke in Tilburg, the Netherlands. Am. J. Epidemiol. 118:514-525; 1983.
13. Hossmann, K-A. Animal models of cerebral ischemia. 1. Review of literature. Cerebrovasc. Dis. [Suppl. 1]. 1:2-15; 1991.
14. Kannel, W.B.; Sorlie, P. Some health benefits of physical activity. The Framingham study. Arch. Intern. Med. 139:857-861; 1979.
15. Kuller, L.H. Incidence rates of stroke in the eighties: The end of the decline in stroke? (Editorial). Stroke 20:841-843; 1989.
16. Lapidus, L.; Bengtsson, C. Socioeconomic factors and physical activity in relation to cardiovascular disease and death: A 12 year follow-up of participants in a population study of women in Gothenburg, Sweden. Br. Heart J. 55:295-301; 1986.
17. Lindsted, K.D.; Tonstad, S.; Kuzma, J.W. Self-report of physical activity and patterns of mortality in Seventh-Day Adventist men. J. Clin. Epidemiol. 44:355-364; 1991.
18. Liu, K.; Stamler, J.; Dyer, A.; McKeever, J.; McKeever, P. Statistical methods to assess and minimize the role of intra-individual variability in obscuring the relationship between dietary lipids and serum cholesterol. J. Chronic Dis. 31:399-418; 1978.
19. Menotti, A.; Keys, A.; Blackburn, H.; Aravanis, C.; Dontas, A.; et al. Twenty year stoke mortality and prediction in twelve cohorts of the seven countries study. Int. J. Epidemiol. 19:309-315; 1990.
20. Menotti, A.; Seccareccia, F. Physical activity at work and job responsibility as risk factors for fatal coronary heart disease and other causes of death. J. Epidemiol. Community Health. 39:325-329; 1985.
21. National Center for Health Statistics. Health, United States, 1990. Hyattsville, MD: Public Health Service; 1991.
22. Overton, J.M.; Tipton, C.M.; Matthes, R.D.; Leininger, J.R. Voluntary exercise and its effects on young SHR and stroke-prone hypertensive rats. J. Appl. Physiol. 61:318-324; 1986.

23. Paffenbarger, R.S., Jr. Factors predisposing to fatal stroke in longshoremen. Prev. Med. 1:522-527; 1972.
24. Paffenbarger, R.S., Jr.; Hyde, R.T.; Wing, A.L.; Steinmetz, C.H. A natural history of athleticism and cardiovascular health. JAMA. 252:491-495; 1984.
25. Paffenbarger, R.S., Jr.; Williams, J.L. Chronic disease in former college students XII: Early precursors of fatal stroke. Am. J. Public Health. 57:1290-1299; 1967.
26. Reed, D.M. The paradox of high risk of stroke in populations with low risk of coronary heart disease. Am. J. Epidemiol. 131:579-588; 1990.
27. Ross, R.; Glomset, J. The pathogenesis of atherosclerosis. N. Engl. J. Med. 295:369; 1976.
28. Ross, R.; Glomset, J.; Kariya, B.; Harker, L. A platelet-dependent serum factor that stimulates the proliferation of arterial smooth muscle cells in vitro. Proc. Natl. Acad. Sci. 71:1207; 1974.
29. Salonen, J.T.; Puska, P.; Tuomilehto, J. Physical activity and risk of myocardial infarction, cerebral stroke, and death: A longitudinal study in Eastern Finland. Am. J. Epidemiol. 115:526-537; 1982.
30. Takizawa, S.; Hakim, A.M. Animal models of cerebral ischemia. 2. Rat models. Cerebrovasc. Dis. [Suppl. 1]. 1:16-21; 1991.
31. Tipton, C.M.; McMahon, S.; Leininger, J.R.; Pauli, E.R.; Lauber, C. Exercise training and incidence of cerebrovascular lesions in stroke-prone spontaneously hypertensive rats. J. Appl. Physiol. 68:1080-1085; 1990.
32. Wannamethee, G.; Shaper, A.G. Physical activity and stroke in British middle-aged men. Br. Med. J. 304:597-601; 1992.
33. Wissler, R.W. The evolution of the atherosclerotic plaque and its complications. In: Conner, W.E.; Bristow, J.D., eds. Coronary heart disease: Prevention, complications, and treatment. Philadelphia: Lippincott; 1985: 193-210.
34. Wolf, P.A.; Kannel, W.B. Reduction of stroke through risk factor modification. Semin. Neurol. 6:243-253; 1986.
35. Yatsu, F.M. Atherogenesis and stroke. In: Barnett, H.J.; Stein, B.M.; Mohr, J.P.; Yatsu, F.M., eds. Stroke: Pathophysiology, diagnosis, and management. New York: Churchill Livingstone; 1986:45-56.

Chapter 42

Physical Activity, Fitness, and Claudication

R. James Barnard

Introduction to Peripheral Vascular Disease

Incidence of the Disease

Atherosclerotic peripheral vascular disease (PVD) of the lower extremities is a major clinical problem that results in disability and decreased life expectancy. Boyd (10) reported that the life expectancy of PVD patients was about 10 years less than that of the general population. Patients with PVD also commonly have coronary or carotid atherosclerosis, or both. The incidence of PVD in the Framingham study was reported to be 2.6 per 1,000 for men and 1.1 per 1,000 for women with 25% of patients with coronary disease also possessing symptoms of PVD (47). The true incidence of the disease, however, is not precisely known. Friedman (31) has pointed out that PVD is often overlooked in routine screening of patients and that many patients with PVD are asymptomatic, other than having a reduced exercise tolerance.

Symptoms

Intermittent claudication is the only specific symptom of PVD. Like angina, claudication pain is the result of inadequate delivery of oxygen to muscle cells. The term *claudication* comes from the Latin *claudicare,* which means to limp. This is not an accurate description of the symptoms of PVD because limping is rarely observed. According to Friedman (31), claudication is variable. Some patients feel only a sense of aching or weakness in the legs with walking. In others, a tightening or pressing pain develops in the calves or buttocks, and others experience a sharp, cramping calf pain that may be excruciating.

Risk Factors

Because PVD is a form of atherosclerosis, it is not surprising that risk factors for coronary disease such as hyperlipidemia, smoking, hypertension, and diabetes are also commonly associated with PVD. Diabetes mellitus seems to be the most prominent risk factor. PVD has been reported to be 4 to 11 times more common (and gangrene 40 times more common) in diabetic than in nondiabetic individuals (6,23,47).

Treatment

Medical treatment for PVD ranges from drug therapy to more aggressive procedures, including angioplasty and bypass surgery. In many cases, the medical approach to PVD treatment is short-lived and may be ineffective. In a recent analysis of the medical treatment of PVD in Maryland between 1979 and 1989, it was found that the rate of percutaneous transluminal angioplasty in the lower extremities rose from 1 to 24 per 100,000 population and that the use of bypass surgery rose from 32 to 65 per 100,000. Despite the dramatic increase in these invasive procedures, the rate of lower limb amputation remained stable at about 30 per 100,000 (67). These results might be due to increased diagnosis of PVD or to a lack of success with the invasive procedures. In another study, Veith et al. (68) did report a significant reduction in the number of amputations with increased angioplasty and bypass surgery. Based on a review of the literature, Coffman (18) discouraged the use of invasive treatment for PVD. Coffman stated, "The treatment of patients with intermittent claudication alone should be conservative, because the prognosis for the limb is favorable, because surgical mortality from cardiovascular events is high among such patients, and because the use of interventions has not decreased the rate of amputation in many hospitals" (p. 78). The conservative treatments he suggested included exercise, smoking cessation, and controlling hyperlipidemia, hypertension, and diabetes mellitus.

Exercise Training

Increase in Performance

Numerous studies in patients with PVD have documented that regular exercise can significantly increase performance capacity and reduce or eliminate claudication symptoms (1-4,9,11,13-15,17,19-26,28-30,32,33,37,39,41-46,48-50,52,56,57,61-63,71). Of these 41 studies, only 9 included a control group and only 2 indicated a randomized control group. Most of the studies were of short duration, usually 6 months or less. Although the general conclusion was that training increased performance, not everyone was able to achieve an increase. Some individuals showed no change, and a few got worse and had to drop out of the studies to undergo bypass surgery. Studies with experimental animals (19,27,53,59,66,69,70) have also shown that exercise training can increase performance capacity following acute ligation of iliac or femoral arteries. Table 42.1 lists some of the studies conducted on patients with PVD that document an increase in exercise capacity before the onset of claudication as well as an increase in maximum performance capacity.

A wide variation in the amount of improvement documented is evident from the data in Table 42.1. This variation may be due to differences in tests used to evaluate performance or differences in the exercise training programs. Some programs stressed daily walking, some had subjects exercise only three times per week, some used bicycle ergometry, some employed sports and calisthenics, and others used a combination of activities. The duration of the study was not an important factor. Hall and Barnard (32), using a combination of diet and exercise, reported significant improvements in performance after 3 weeks, whereas Mannarino et al. (52) found no increase in performance until 3 months of training.

Even within studies, significant differences in response to the same training program have been found. For example, Larsen and Lassen (48) studied 7 PVD patients over a 6-month training program consisting of 1 hr of daily walking to the point of severe pain. At the end of 6 months, 2 patients showed no change in performance, and the remaining 5 showed improvements ranging from 50% to 700%. The improvement was unrelated to maximum leg blood flow as assessed by xenon 133 clearance. Carter et al. (14) recently studied 56 PVD patients over a 3- to 6-month training program and found that the walking distance after training was unrelated to the extent of disease as assessed from the ankle/arm pressure index at the start of the study (see Figure 42.1). The mean improvement was 79% to the onset of claudication and 69% for maximum walking. Unfortunately, they did not correlate that amount of improvement with the initial ankle/arm index. The walking distance after training was also unrelated to the location of obstruction (proximal vs. distal or unilateral vs. bilateral). Jonason and Ringqvist (45) also reported no difference in improvement with training between patients with proximal or distal arterial stenosis.

Exercise Prescription

A possible explanation for the variation in improvement may be the actual stress placed on the diseased limb. Walking or jogging is the exercise of choice because it uses the calf muscles and results in the development of lower leg ischemia. According to Scheel (60) ischemia is the stimulus for collateral vessel development and is the reason why Barnard and Hall (3) have emphasized the importance of walking to the point of severe pain. Hall and Barnard (32) reported that emphasizing walking to the point of severe pain on a daily basis resulted in a 61% increase in maximum work capacity after 3 weeks. In a case report, Hall et al. (33) studied a subject with occlusion of both superficial femoral arteries and a walking capacity of less than 100 m with severe pain. With daily walking to the point of severe pain, the subject increased his walking capacity to almost 5 km in 3 weeks. A year later he ran the Chicago Marathon in a little more than 5 hr.

Other investigators have also emphasized the importance of walking to the point of severe pain. Larsen and Lassen (48) told their patients to walk with pain for as long as they could stand it and still found variable results, as discussed earlier. Some individuals may be more willing to endure pain than others and thus create a greater ischemic stimulus. However, Fitzgerald et al. (29) trained 19 patients with daily walking for at least 1 hr per day for 2 years. Despite the fact that it was strongly emphasized that exercise should be stopped as soon as the first symptoms of discomfort were noticed, maximum blood flow and performance were significantly increased, even in patients with severe disease. Whether or not severe ischemia is the stimulus for improvement is still unknown. This point obviously needs to be studied in more detail.

Fitness Level

Most studies have focused on assessing walking or endurance capacity without measuring fitness level or aerobic capacity. Hall and Barnard (32)

Table 42.1 Effect of Training on Exercise Capacity in PVD Patients

Author	No. of subjects	Training duration	% increase in performance: To claudication	Maximum
Larsen & Lassen, 1966 (48)	7	6 months		183
Ericsson et al., 1970 (26)	7	11 months	100	97
Zetterquist, 1970 (71)	9	3–4 months	73	
Sorlie & Myhre, 1978 (63)	10	3–4 months	64	
Ekroth et al., 1978 (25)	148	4–6 months		234
Clifford et al., 1980 (15)	21	6 months		80
Hall & Barnard, 1982 (32)	16	3 weeks		61
Hall et al., 1982 (33)	1	1 year		>1,000
Ernst & Aartrai, 1987 (28)	42	2 months	100	121
Johnson et al., 1989 (43)	10	5 months	86	42
Carter et al., 1989 (14)	56	3–6 months	79	69
Rosfors et al., 1989 (56)	25	6 months	61	143
Mannarino et al., 1989 (52)	8	6 months	87	67
Hiatt et al., 1990 (37)	9	3 months	165	123

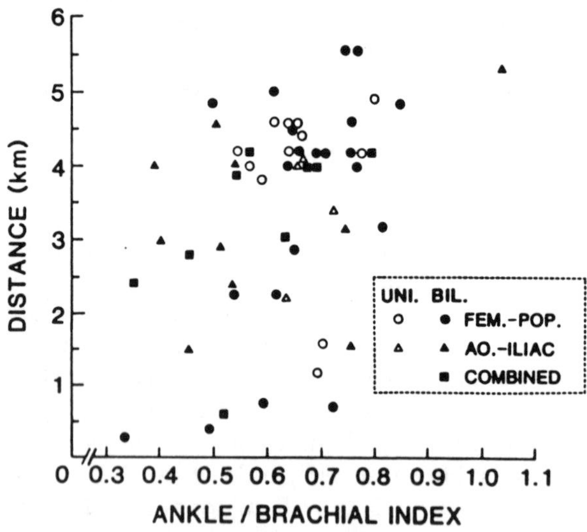

Figure 42.1 Effect of 3-6 months of training on walking distance for patients with various degrees of PVD as assessed from the ankle/arm index obtained before training. From Carter et al. (14), by permission of Mosby-Year Book, Inc.

did report an increase in maximum MET level (4.1 ± 0.4 to 6.6 ± 0.4) in 16 PVD subjects tested using a progressive, multistage treadmill test. More recently Hiatt et al. (37) reported a 30% increase in $\dot{V}O_2$max from 12.8 ± 1.8 to 16.5 ± 1.7 ml · kg^{-1} · min^{-1} after 12 weeks of training.

Comparison of Training With Surgical Procedures

Whereas there has been a tremendous increase in the use of surgical procedures to treat PVD, little documentation has been given for the benefits of surgery as assessed by increases in work capacity. In 1966, Strandness and Bell (64) reported a normalization of ankle pressures in patients following endarterectomy or bypass surgery. Improvement was noted immediately after the surgery and documented for 7 days. Performance capacity, however, was not measured.

More recently, Creasy et al. (20) compared exercise training with percutaneous transluminal angioplasty in a randomized trial. After 3 months the angioplasty group had a better ankle blood pressure index and a greater walking distance to claudication. Maximum walking was higher in the angioplasty group but not statistically significant. After 1 year, the distance to claudication, as well as the maximum walking distance, was significantly greater in the exercise group. These results indicate that regular exercise might be more effective than angioplasty for long-term improvement in functional capacity.

In another randomized trial Lundgren et al. (49) compared training and surgical reconstruction. Three groups were involved in the study: trained (T), bypass surgery (S), and surgery plus training

(S+T). Comparisons were made after 13 months. Symptom-free walking was greatest in the S+T group, and the S group performed better than the T group. Maximum calf blood flow was increased in all three groups, with the changes correlating with the increases in performance. These results indicate that, for at least 13 months, surgery has a greater benefit than exercise, but combining the two gives the best results. This area needs more study.

Whereas invasive procedures may be important for salvaging limbs in cases of severe ischemia, Foley (30) reported on 22 patients with gangrene who were encouraged to stand and walk. In follow-ups ranging from 4 months to 6.5 years, 21 patients healed, and only 1 patient had to have a leg amputation. This patient stopped walking after hospital discharge, whereas the others continued to walk, some up to 4.8 km per day. Jonason and Ringqvist (45) reported that of 8 PVD patients with resting pain, 6 lost their pain after training for 3 months. They also reported that patients without coronary insufficiency were more likely to improve than those with coronary insufficiency.

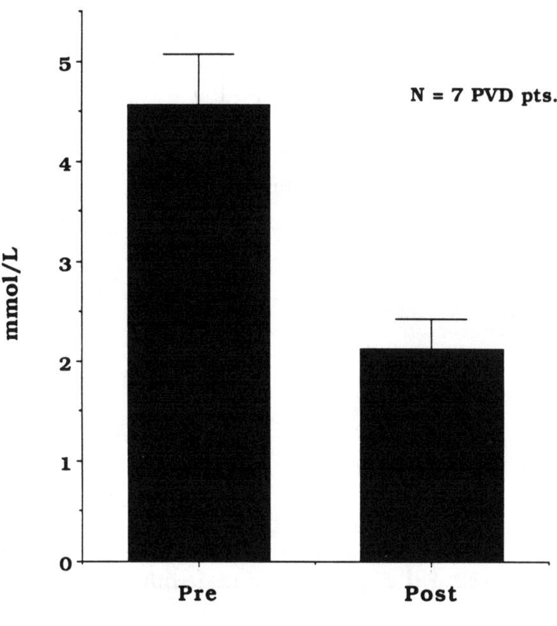

Figure 42.2 Effect of 8 weeks of training on maximum exercise femoral venous lactate concentration. Data taken from Ruell et al. (57).

Mechanisms of Adaptation to Training

Psychological Versus Physiological

Although there is an abundance of evidence showing that regular exercise results in an increase in performance in patients with PVD, the mechanisms involved are far from being completely understood. Part of the improvement might be psychological due to an increased ability to endure pain, but there are well-documented physiological measurements indicating a reduction in the amount of ischemia observed for a given standard work load. A reduction in lactate formation has been reported by Sorlie and Myhre (63) and by Ruell et al. (57) (see Fig. 42.2). In addition, other investigators (32,33) have reported improvements in the ankle/arm pressure index, indicating a reduction in ischemia and the amount of vasodilator metabolites formed during exercise. Figure 42.3 shows the changes reported by Hall and Barnard (32) following 3 weeks of intensive exercise combined with dietary modification. Improvements in the ankle/arm pressure index were observed at rest, immediately after exercise, and during recovery. Similar results were reported by Skinner and Strandness (62) in 1967 using only exercise training. They ascribed the improvements to the development of collateral vessels and an increase in oxygen delivery to the ischemic limbs.

Collateral Vessel Formation

There is little documentation for the formation of collateral vessels in PVD patients following training. One case report by Hall et al. (33) provides angiographic documentation for the formation of collaterals. An initial arteriogram showed occlusion of both superficial femoral arteries distal to the branch of the deep femoral. The subject's walking capacity was limited to less than 100 m, and he experienced severe claudication, as discussed earlier. After 1 year of training, he finished the Chicago Marathon. Before the subject started the exercise program, an initial examination revealed an absence of pulses in both lower legs. An examination conducted after he completed the marathon revealed clear but subnormal pulses in both the posterior tibial and dorsalis pedis arteries in both legs. A second arteriogram still showed occlusion of the superficial femoral arteries in both legs, but large collaterals had developed from small lumbar arteries to perfuse the thigh muscles. Additional collaterals were observed providing flow from the deep femoral to the popliteal artery for lower leg perfusion. Studies with animals have also reported that exercise training enhances collateral development (59).

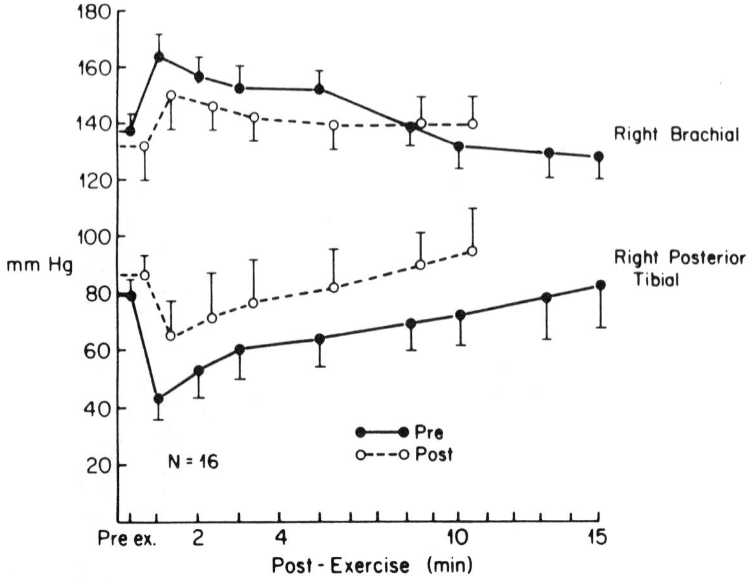

Figure 42.3 Effect of 3 weeks of intensive exercise and diet therapy on blood pressure in PVD patients. From Hall and Barnard (32). Reproduced with permission of the Journal of Cardiopulmonary Rehabilitation.

Maximum Blood Flow

If collateral vessels do develop as a result of exercise training in PVD patients, one would assume there would be an increase in maximum blood flow to the legs. In an initial study, Larsen and Lassen (48) used xenon 131 washout and found maximum blood flow to be increased after 2 months of training but not after 6 months when trained subjects were compared to sedentary control subjects. In a subsequent study (1), they trained 19 PVD patients for 6 months and found an increase in maximum blood flow in 12 of the patients. The increase in maximum blood flow was positively correlated (r = 0.64) with the increase in walking distance. Broomé et al. (11) studied 10 PVD patients who were placed on daily walking but on no organized training program. After 6 months, walking time to the point of claudication increased 140% and maximum blood flow measured by xenon 131 washout increased 113%. In the study by Lundgren et al. (49) where exercise and reconstructive surgery were compared after 13 months, maximal plethysmographic calf blood flow was significantly increased in the trained group (3.0 ± 1.2 ml · 100 ml^{-1} · min^{-1}). A greater increase was observed for the surgery group (7.6 ± 1.5 ml · 100 ml^{-1} · min^{-1}), and the surgery-plus-training group had the greatest increase (9.9 ± 2.4 ml · 100 ml^{-1} · min^{-1}). Hiatt et al. (37) reported a 38% increase in maximum leg flow (plethysmograph) after 12 weeks of training in PVD patients. Peak walking was increased 123%, and pain-free walking was increased 165%.

In total, nine studies (1,2,9,11,26,29,37,48,49) in humans with PVD have reported an increase in maximum blood flow with training; however, eight studies (22,25,39,43,45,52,63,71) reported no change, and one study (17) reported a decrease. In most cases, the reported percent increase in flow was less than the percent increase in performance, which suggests other important adaptations. In the animal studies with arterial insufficiency created by ligation, two studies (59,69) reported an increase in maximum blood flow, and three studies (27,53,70) reported no change with training. Conrad (19) reported that in rats sympathectomy following arterial ligation greatly increased performance and suggested an increase in flow.

Another factor that might be involved in the increased performance and enhanced blood flow observed in PVD patients with training is a decrease in blood viscosity. In an initial study Ernst and Aartrai (28) reported that in a placebo-controlled, double-blind study, hemodilution over 3 weeks lowered hematocrit and blood viscosity while increasing pain-free walking distance. They subsequently exercise-trained PVD patients for 2 months and found a fall in both whole blood and plasma viscosity along with a significant increase in pain-free walking.

Blood Flow Redistribution

In addition to increasing maximum blood flow, exercise training has been shown to result in a redistribution of flow in the involved limb. Sorlie and Myhre (63) and Zetterquist (71) observed no change in maximum blood flow with training in PVD patients, but they did observe an increase in O_2 extraction, which suggests a redistribution of flow within the ischemic limb. Using an animal model, Yang et al. (69) have documented a redistribution of flow from the proximal to the distal segments of the stenosed limb as well as a greater O_2 extraction with training. As can be seen in Figure 42.4, blood flow in control animals, as measured with radioactive microspheres, was almost equally distributed between the upper and lower limb. With acute stenosis, flow to the distal bed was dramatically reduced. With chronic stenosis (approximately 6 weeks), flow to the distal limb had improved without any change in total flow, and with exercise training, it was further improved but not normalized.

In another study, Mathien and Terjung (53) found a redistribution of flow within the distal limb muscle fiber types following training and no increase in maximum flow. Flow from the red portion of the gastrocnemius, mostly fast-twitch oxidative glycolytic fibers, was redistributed to the white portion, mostly fast-twitch glycolytic fibers (see Fig. 42.5). Although the oxidative capacity of the fast-twitch glycolytic fibers is low, increasing blood flow to these fibers, in the face of severely depressed flow, could enhance performance and reduce lactate formation for any standard work load. Thus, a redistribution of flow by mechanisms yet unknown could be, in part, responsible for the improvement in performance seen in patients with PVD.

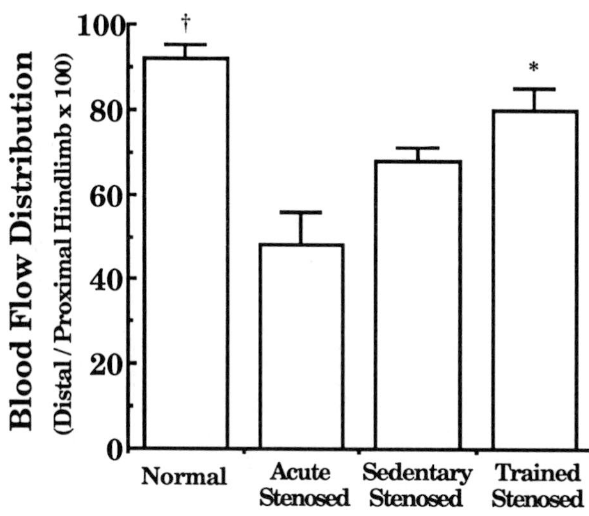

Figure 42.4 Effect of training on blood flow distribution in rats with femoral artery stenosis. Maximum blood flow to the total hindlimb was unchanged with sedentary stenosis but was increased from 78 ± 9 to 94 ± 9 ml · min^{-1} · 100 g^{-1} with training. There also was a significant redistribution of flow from the proximal to the distal limb muscles in both the sedentary stenosis and trained stenosis groups. The control group was significantly different from the three stenosis groups, and the trained stenosis group was significantly different from the sedentary stenosed group. From Yang et al. (70) with permission of the American Physiological Society.

Capillarity

Another adaptation that may increase oxygen utilization is an increase in the number of capillaries. Some studies (16,34,35,51,65) have reported that the capillary-to-fiber ratio is increased in PVD patients. This suggests that local hypoxia may provide the stimulus for vessel formation. Unfortunately, the effect of training on capillarity has not been investigated in humans, but capillaries have been shown to increase following treadmill training in animals with peripheral arterial insufficiency (70).

Metabolic Adaptations

In addition to the reduction in lactate found in PVD patients after training, other metabolic adaptations have been reported. An increase in mitochondrial content and mitochondria marker enzyme activity is commonly found in healthy individuals with intensive training (58). It has been suggested that hypoxia provides the stimulus for enhanced mitochondria production. Kaijser et al. (46) trained healthy volunteers via cycle ergometry. During training, one leg was placed in a pressure chamber to induce ischemia. After 4 weeks, citrate synthase activity was increased to a much greater extent in the ischemic-trained leg. Time to exhaustion was increased in both legs, but the time was significantly greater in the ischemic-trained leg, especially under ischemic conditions. Thus, it is not surprising that an increase in mitochondrial content or marker enzyme activity is found in some PVD patients (12,38,40,49,50). However, PVD patients with severe advanced disease have been found to have a decrease in mitochondria (12, 16,35). With training, an increase in mitochondria has been reported for PVD patients (39,49,50) as well as animals (27,70) with peripheral arterial insufficiency. Lundgren et al. (50) reported that the increase in cytochrome C oxidase after training was correlated with symptom-free walking distance much more than with maximum walking distance. They also found that cytochrome C oxidase decreased following bypass surgery, but the decrease could be prevented with regular training (49).

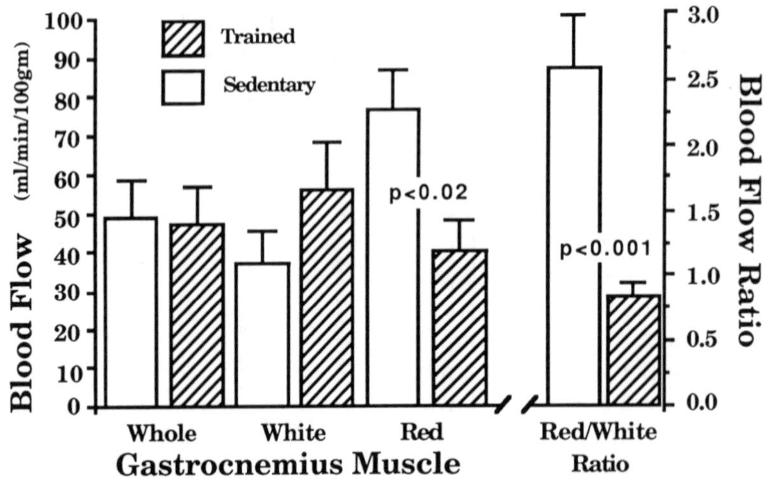

Figure 42.5 Effect of training on blood flow distribution in rats with femoral artery stenosis. Although maximum flow was unchanged, there was a significant redistribution of flow from fast-twitch oxidative glycolytic fibers (red) to the fast-twitch glycolytic fibers (white). From Mathien and Terjung (53), by permission.

One might argue that because oxygen delivery is severely reduced by the disease, an increase in oxidative metabolic capacity should not be important. Terjung et al. (66), however, have offered two possible positive effects resulting from an increase in mitochondria in PVD patients. First, an increase in mitochondrial density could reduce the average path length for oxygen diffusion within the muscle. In addition, more mitochondria could reduce the cytosolic ADP concentration, which would reduce the rate of glycolysis and lactate production (as has been documented). In healthy subjects trained with leg ischemia, Kaijser et al. (46) found that phosphofructokinase activity increased, whereas lactate dehydrogenase activity decreased. Unfortunately, they did not measure glycogen levels.

Whereas Kaijser et al. (46) found that the increase in citrate synthase induced by training correlated with the increase in performance, an increase in glycogen may have been the important factor, especially when performance was measured under ischemic conditions. Holm et al. (39) reported that glucose oxidation, as well as the rate of glycogen formation, was increased in PVD patients. Training further increased the rate of glucose oxidation but had no further effect on the rate of glycogen formation. No human studies could be found in which glycogen levels were measured following training in PVD patients. Clyne et al. (16) found that lactate dehydrogenase and phosphofructokinase activities were increased in patients with mild PVD but decreased in patients with more severe disease. Others (42,50) reported no change in these glycolytic enzymes in PVD patients.

Abnormalities in lipid metabolism have been suggested for PVD patients. Hiatt et al. (36) found an increase in plasma acylcarnitines at rest and after only 10 min of exercise, whereas healthy subjects showed no accumulation at 18 min of exercise. However, at much higher work loads, acylcarnitines increased in healthy subjects. Thus, the observed accumulation of acylcarnitines at lower work loads in PVD patients may not be due to an abnormality in lipid metabolism but merely a response to hypoxia. Based on respiratory quotient measurements, Lundgren et al. (50) concluded that at the point of claudicating pain, the patients were oxidizing mainly fat in spite of a rising lactate output. Lundgren et al. also reported that training resulted in an increase in the activity of hydroxyacyl-CoA dehydrogenase, an enzyme involved in fat metabolism. Hiatt et al. (37) found a decrease in resting plasma acylcarnitines after exercise training. Unfortunately, no measurements were reported immediately after exercise in the trained patients. Thus, whether or not there is any abnormality in lipid metabolism in PVD patients remains to be determined.

Disease Treatment

Risk Factors

Little attention has been focused on treating atherosclerosis by controlling risk factors. Whereas exercise can be effective for controlling many of the risk factors associated with atherosclerosis (as discussed in other chapters), it is not known if the low-level activity done by most patients with PVD has any significant impact on risk factors. Two studies, however, did combine aggressive dietary modification with exercise in an attempt to significantly modify risk factors. Hall and Barnard (32) used a very low-fat (< 10% kcal), high-complex-carbohydrate diet along with daily walking. In just 3 weeks, total serum cholesterol was reduced from 254 ± 18 to 182 ± 12 mg/dl (6.6 ± 0.5 to 4.7 ± 0.3 mmol/L), and triglycerides were reduced from 265 ± 60 to 180 ± 32 mg/dl (3.0 ± 0.7 to 2.1 ± 0.4 mmol/L). Blood pressure dropped from 139 ± 5 to 133 ± 7 mmHg for the systolic and from 81 ± 2 to 76 ± 2 mmHg for the diastolic. Although the decrease in blood pressure was not statistically significant, all 4 patients on antihypertensive drugs were able to discontinue medication. Three cardiac patients were initially taking Inderal: One had the drug discontinued, one had the dosage reduced, and one patient's dosage was unchanged. Similar lipid results were reported by Hutchinson et al. (41) in a 1-year study. Dietary modification combined with exercise can be effective for controlling other risk factors associated with PVD (4).

Atherosclerosis Regression

The fact that more attention has not been focused on treating risk factors is unfortunate. Several studies (5,7,8,26,54,55) have reported regression of lower limb atherosclerosis with treatment of hyperlipidemia by drugs or drugs combined with diet. Although regression was documented with serial angiograms, its affect on performance capacity was not evaluated. Thus, whereas exercise training can have a significant impact on performance in PVD patients, aggressive treatment of risk factors should be combined with exercise because of the well-known progressive nature of atherosclerosis.

Summary

Numerous studies have demonstrated a significant increase in both pain-free and maximum work capacity with exercise training in patients with PVD. Some patients completely lost the symptoms of claudication. The precise mechanisms responsible for the improvements are not clear. A few studies have documented collateral vessel formation. Some studies have reported an increase in maximum blood flow, whereas others found no change in spite of a significant increase in work capacity. Studies with animals have reported a redistribution of flow from the upper leg muscles to the gastrocnemius. Within the gastrocnemius, a redistribution of flow from the red, fast-twitch, oxidative glycolytic fibers to the white, fast-twitch glycolytic fibers was found. A decrease in blood viscosity has also been reported, which could enhance oxygen delivery to the ischemic limb. Capillarity increases in PVD patients and may be further enhanced with training.

A reduction in lactate formation after training and an improvement in the ankle/arm pressure index indicate a reduction in anaerobic metabolism. An increase in O_2 extraction has been reported even without any change in maximum blood flow. Mitochondria and mitochondrial marker enzyme activity increase in PVD patients and may be further increased with training. The activity of hydroxyacyl-CoA dehydrogenase, an enzyme involved in fatty acid metabolism, has been shown to increase with training. The precise significance of the increases in these metabolic factors responsible for aerobic metabolism in the face of a reduction in the oxygen delivery remains to be determined. Whether or not there is any change in glycolytic enzymes or glycogen content with training in PVD patients remains to be determined.

Some patients with severe ischemia are in need of surgical procedures to prevent limb loss, but in less severe cases, exercise may be a better choice. Unfortunately, few studies have focused on the effects of surgery on performance capacity. One study reported that after 1 year of exercise training, exercise tolerance was better in patients given exercise training than in patients undergoing angioplasty. Another study reported that after 1 year bypass surgery was better than exercise alone, but the combination of the two gave the best result. One study reported saving gangrenous feet from amputation by daily exercise. Another study reported major improvement with training in patients with resting pain and severe PVD.

Little attention has been focused on the potential value of exercise in controlling risk factors for the underlying problem of atherosclerosis. Exercise combined with diet has been shown in a few studies to significantly reduce serum cholesterol and triglycerides. Studies with aggressive drug or drug-plus-diet therapy to treat hyperlipidemia have documented regression of atherosclerosis in the lower limb.

The value of treating PVD patients with exercise training has been well established. Early treatment seems to be important for maximum results. Individuals with PVD and coronary disease do show improvement but not as much as do patients with only PVD. Aggressive treatment of atherosclerotic risk factors in addition to regular exercise is especially important for the patient with both PVD and coronary disease.

References

1. Alpert, J.S.; Larsen, O.A.; Lassen, N.A. Exercise and intermittent claudication: Blood flow in the calf muscle during walking studied by the xenon-133 clearance method. Circulation. 39:353-359; 1969.
2. Andriessen, M.P.H.M.; Barendsen, G.J.; Wouda, A.A.; De Pater, L. The effect of six months intensive training on the circulation in the legs of patients with intermittent claudication. Vasa. 18:56-62; 1989.
3. Barnard, R.J.; Hall, J.A. Patients with peripheral vascular disease. In: Franklin, B.A.; Gordon, S.; Timmis, G.C., eds. Exercise in modern medicine. Baltimore: Williams & Wilkins; 1989:107-117.
4. Barnard, R.J.; Pritikin, R.; Rosenthal, M.B.; Inkeles, S. Pritikin approach to cardiac rehabilitation. In: Goodgold, J., ed. Rehabilitation medicine. St. Louis: Mosby; 1988:267-284.
5. Barndt, R.; Blankenhorn, D.H.; Crawford, D.W.; Brooks, S.H. Regression and progression of early femoral atherosclerosis in treated hyperlipoproteinemic patients. Ann. Intern. Med. 86:139-146; 1977.
6. Bell, E.T. Incidence of gangrene of the extremities in nondiabetic and in diabetic persons. Arch. Pathol. 49:469-473; 1950.
7. Blankenhorn, D.H.; Azen, S.P.; Crawford, D.W.; Nessim, S.A.; Sanmarco, M.E.; Selzer, R.H.; Shircore, A.M.; Wickham, E.C. Effects of colestipol-niacin therapy on human femoral atherosclerosis. Circulation. 83:438-446; 1991.
8. Blankenhorn, D.H.; Brooks, S.H.; Selzer, R.H.; Barndt, R. The rate of atherosclerosis change during treatment of hyperlipoproteinemia. Circulation. 57:355-361; 1978.
9. Blümchen, G.; Landry, F.; Kiefer, H.; Schlosser, V. Hemodynamic responses of claudicating extremities. Evaluation of a long range exercise program. Cardiology. 55:114-127; 1970.
10. Boyd, A.M. The natural course of arteriosclerosis of the lower extremities (Section of surgery: Obstruction of the lower limb arteries). Proc. R. Soc. Med. 55:591-593; 1962.
11. Broomé, A.; Cederlund, J.; Eklöf, B. Spontaneous recovery in intermittent claudication. Scand. J. Clin. Lab. Invest. [Suppl.]. 99:157-159; 1967.
12. Bylund, A.C.; Hammarsten, J.; Holm, J.; Schersten, T. Enzyme activities in skeletal muscle from patients with peripheral arterial insufficiency. Eur. J. Clin. Invest. 6:425-429; 1976.
13. Cachovan, M.; de Marees, H.; Kunitsch, G. The effect of oxyfedrine and interval training in intermittent claudication. Z. Kardiol. 67:289-298; 1978.
14. Carter, S.A.; Hamel, E.R.; Paterson, J.M.; Snow, C.R.; Mymin, D. Walking ability and ankle systolic pressure: Observations in patients with intermittent claudication in a short-term walking exercise program. J. Vasc. Surg. 10:642-649; 1989.
15. Clifford, P.C.; Davis, P.W.; Hayne, J.A.; Baird, R.N. Intermittent claudication: Is a supervised exercise class worthwhile? Br. Med. J. 280:1503-1505; 1980.
16. Clyne, C.A.C.; Weller, R.O.; Bradley, W.G.; Silber, D.I.; O'Donnell, T.F.; Callow, A.D. Ultrastructure and capillary adaptation of gastrocnemius muscle to occlusive peripheral vascular disease. Surgery. 92:434-440; 1982.
17. Cochovan, M.; de Marées, H.; Kunitsch, G. Einfluss von intervall training auf die leistungsfähigkeit und periphere duchblutung bie patienten mit claudicatio intermittens. Z. Kardiol. 65:54-67; 1976.
18. Coffman, J.D. Intermittent claudication—be conservative. N. Engl. J. Med. 325:577-578; 1991.
19. Conrad, M.C. Effects of therapy on maximal walking time following femoral ligation in the rat. Circ. Res. 41:775-778; 1977.
20. Creasy, T.S.; McMillan, P.J.; Fletcher, E.W.L.; Collin, J.; Morris, P.J. Is percutaneous transluminal angioplasty better than exercise for claudication?—Preliminary results from a prospective randomized trial. Eur. J. Vasc. Surg. 4:135-140; 1990.
21. Dahllöf, A-G.; Björntorp, P.; Holm, P.; Scherstén, T. Metabolic activity of skeletal muscle in patients with peripheral arterial insufficiency. Eur. J. Clin. Invest. 4:9-15; 1974.
22. Dahllöf, A-G.; Holm, J.; Scherstén, T.; Siverstsson, R. Peripheral arterial insufficiency. Effect of physical training on walking tolerance, calf blood flow and blood flow resistance. Scand. J. Rehabil. Med. 8:19-26; 1976.
23. Dry, T.J.; Hines, E.A., Jr. The role of diabetes in the development of degenerative vascular disease: With special reference to the incidence of retinitis and peripheral neuritis. Ann. Intern. Med. 14:1893-1902; 1941.
24. Duffield, R.G.M.; Lewis, B.; Miller, N.E.; Jamieson, C.W.; Bunt, J.N.H.; Colchester, A.C.F. Treatment of hyperlipidaemia retards progression of symptomatic femoral atherosclerosis. A randomized control trial. Lancet. 2:639-642; 1983.
25. Ekroth, R.; Dahllöf, A-G.; Gunderall, B.; Holm, J.; Scherstén, T. Physical training of patients with intermittent claudication: Indications, methods and results. Surgery. 84:640-643; 1978.

26. Ericcson, B.; Haeger, K.; Lindell, S.E. Effect of physical training on intermittent claudication. Angiology. 21:188-192; 1970.
27. Erney, T.P.; Mathien, G.M.; Terjung, R.L. Muscle adaptations in trained rats with peripheral arterial insufficiency. Am. J. Physiol. (Heart Circ. Physiol. 29). 260:H445-H452; 1991.
28. Ernst, E.E.; Aartrai, A. Intermittent claudication, exercise, and blood rheology. Circulation. 76:1110-1114; 1987.
29. Fitzgerald, D.E.; Keates, J.S.; Macmillan, D. Angiographic and plethysmographic assessment of graduated physical exercise in the treatment of chronic occlusive arterial disease of the leg. Angiology. 22:99-106; 1971.
30. Foley, W. Treatment of gangrene of the feet and legs by walking. Circulation. 15:689-700; 1957.
31. Friedman, S.A. Arteriosclerosis obliterous of the lower extremities. In: Friedman, S.A., ed. Vascular diseases: A concise guide to diagnosis, management, pathogenesis, and prevention. Boston: J. Wright, PSG, Inc.; 1982:1-30.
32. Hall, J.A.; Barnard, R.J. The effects of an intensive 26-day program of diet and exercise on patients with peripheral vascular disease. J. Cardiac Rehabil. 2:569-574; 1982.
33. Hall, J.A.; Dixson, G.H.; Barnard, R.J.; Pritikin, N. Effects of diet and exercise on peripheral vascular disease. Phys. Sportsmed. 10:90-101; 1982.
34. Hammarsten, J.; Bylund-Fellenius, A.C.; Holm, J.; Scherstén, T.; Krotkiewski, M. Capillary supply and muscle fiber types in patients with intermittent claudication: Relationship between morphology and metabolism. Eur. J. Clin. Invest. 10:301-305; 1980.
35. Henriksson, J.; Nygaard, E.; Andersson, J.; Eklöf, B. Enzyme activities, fiber types and capillarization in calf muscles of patients with intermittent claudication. Scand. J. Clin. Lab. Invest. 40:361-369; 1980.
36. Hiatt, W.R.; Nawaz, D.; Brass, E.P. Carnitine metabolism during exercise in patients with peripheral vascular disease. J. Appl. Physiol. 62:2382-2387; 1987.
37. Hiatt, W.R.; Regensteiner, J.G.; Hargarten, M.E.; Wolfel, E.E.; Brass, E.P. Benefit of exercise conditioning for patients with peripheral arterial disease. Circulation 81:602-609, 1990.
38. Holm, J.; Björntorp, P.; Scherstén, T. Metabolic activity in human skeletal muscle. Effect of peripheral arterial insufficiency. Eur. J. Clin. Invest. 2:321-325, 1972.
39. Holm, J.; Dahlöff, A-G.; Björntorp, P.; Scherstén, T. Enzyme studies in patients with intermittent claudication: Effect of training. Scand. J. Clin. Invest. [Suppl.]. 128:201-207; 1973.
40. Holm, J.; Dahlöff, A-G.; Scherstén, T. Metabolic activity of skeletal muscle in patients with peripheral arterial insufficiency. Scand. J. Clin. Invest. 35:81-86; 1975.
41. Hutchinson, K.; O'Berle, K.; Crockford, P.; Grace, M.; Whyte, L.; Gee, M.; Williams, T.; Brown, G. Effects of dietary manipulation on vascular status of patients with peripheral vascular disease. JAMA. 249:3326-3356; 1983.
42. Jansson, E.; Johansson, J.; Sylvën, C.; Kaijser, L. Calf muscle adaptation in intermittent claudication. Side-differences in muscle metabolic characteristics with unilateral disease. Clin. Physiol. Oxf. 8:17-29; 1988.
43. Johnson, E.C.; Voyles, W.F.; Afferbom, H.A.; Pathak, D.; Sutton, M.F.; Greene, E.R. Effects of exercise training on common femoral artery blood flow in patients with intermittent claudication. Circulation. [Suppl. III]. 80:III-59-III-72; 1989.
44. Jonason, T.; Jonzon, B.; Ringqvist, I.; Öman-Rydberg, A. Effect of physical training on different categories of patients with intermittent claudication. Acta. Med. Scand. 206:253-258; 1979.
45. Jonason, T.; Ringqvist, I. Effect of training on the post-exercise ankle blood pressure reaction in patients with intermittent claudication. Clin. Physiol. 7:63-69; 1987.
46. Kaijser, L.; Sundberg, C.J.; Eiken, O.; Nygren, A.; Esbjörnsson, M.; Sylvén, C.; Jansson, E. Muscle oxidative capacity and work performance after training under local leg ischemia. J. Appl. Physiol. 69:785-787; 1990.
47. Kannel, W.B.; Skinner, J.J., Jr.; Schwartz, M.J.; Shurtleff, D. Intermittent claudication incidence in the Framingham study. Circulation. 41:875-883; 1970.
48. Larsen, O.A.; Lassen, N.A. Effect of daily muscular exercise in patients with intermittent claudication. Lancet 2:1093-1095; 1966.
49. Lundgren, F.; Dahllöf, A-G.; Lundholm, K.; Scherstén, T.; Volmann, R. Intermittent claudication—surgical reconstruction or physical training? Ann. Surg. 209:346-355; 1989.
50. Lundgren, F.; Dahllöf, A-G.; Scherstén, T.; Bylund-Fellinius, A.C. Muscle enzyme adaptation in patients with peripheral arterial insufficiency: Spontaneous adaptation, effect of different treatments and consequences on walking performance. Clin. Sci. 77:485-493; 1989.
51. Makitie, J. Skeletal muscle capillaries in intermittent claudication. Arch. Pathol. Lab. Med. 101:500-503; 1977.
52. Mannarino, E.; Pasqualini, L.; Menna, M.; Maragoni, G.; Orlandi, V. Effects of physical training on peripheral vascular disease: A controlled study. Angiology. 40:6-10; 1989.

53. Mathien, G.M.; Terjung, R.L. Influence of training following bilateral stenosis of the femoral artery in rats. Am. J. Physiol. (Heart Circ. Physiol., 19). 250:H1050-H1059; 1985.
54. Olsson, A.G.; Carlson, L.A.; Erikson, U.A.; Helmius, G.; Hemmingsson, A.; Ruhn, G. Regression of computer-estimated femoral atherosclerosis after pronounced serum lipid lowering in patients with asymptomatic hyperlipidaemia. Lancet. 1:1311; 1982.
55. Öst, C.R.; Sténson, T. Regression of peripheral atherosclerosis during therapy with high doses of nicotinic acid. Scand. J. Clin. Lab. Invest. [Suppl.]. 99:241-245; 1967.
56. Rosfors, S.; Bygdeman, S.; Arnetz, B.B.; Lahnborg, G.; Sköldö, L.; Eneroth, P.; Kallner, A. Longterm neuroendocrine and metabolic effects of physical training in intermittent claudication. Scand. J. Rehabil. Med. 21:7-11; 1989.
57. Ruell, P.A.; Imperial, E.S.; Bonar, F.J.; Thursby, P.F. Intermittent claudication: The effect of physical training on walking tolerance and venous lactate concentration. Eur. J. Appl. Physiol. 52:420-425; 1984.
58. Saltin, B.; Gollnick, P.D. Skeletal muscle adaptability: Significance for metabolism and performance. In: Handbook of physiology. Skeletal muscle. Bethesda, MD: Am. Physiol. Soc.; 1983:555-631.
59. Sanne, H.; Sivertsson, R. The effect of exercise on the development of collateral circulation after experimental occlusion of the femoral artery in the cat. Acta Physiol. Scand. 73:257-263; 1968.
60. Scheel, K.W. The stimulus for coronary collateral growth: Ischemia or mechanical factors? J. Cardiac Rehabil. 1:149-153; 1981.
61. Schoop, W. Mechanism of beneficial action of daily walking training of patients with intermittent claudication. Scand. J. Clin. Lab. Invest. [Suppl.] 128:197-199; 1973.
62. Skinner, J.S.; Strandness, D.E., Jr. Exercise and intermittent claudication. II. Effect of physical training. Circulation. 36:23-29; 1967.
63. Sorlie, D.; Myhre, K. Effects of physical training in intermittent claudication. Scand. J. Clin. Lab. Invest. 38:217-222; 1978.
64. Strandness, D.E., Jr.; Bell, J.W. Ankle responses after reconstructive surgery. Surgery. 59:514-516; 1966.
65. Teravainen, H.; Makitie, J. Striated muscle ultrastructure in intermittent claudication. Arch. Pathol. Lab. Med. 101:230-235; 1977.
66. Terjung, R.L.; Mathien, G.M.; Erney, T.P.; Ogilvíe, R.W. Peripheral adaptations to low blood flow in muscle during exercise. Am. J. Cardiol. 62:15E-19E; 1988.
67. Tunis, S.R.; Bass, E.B.; Steinberg, E.P. The use of angioplasty, bypass surgery and amputation in the management of peripheral vascular disease. N. Engl. J. Med. 325:556-562; 1991.
68. Veith, F.J.; Gupta, S.K.; Wengerten, K.R. Changing arteriosclerotic disease patterns and management strategies in lower-limb threatening ischemia. Ann. Surg. 212:402-414; 1990.
69. Yang, H.T.; Dinn, R.F.; Terjung, R.L. Training increases muscle blood flow in rats with peripheral arterial insufficiency. J. Appl. Physiol. 69:1353-1359; 1990.
70. Yang, H.T.; Ogilvie, R.W.; Terjung, R.L. Low-intensity training produces muscle adaptations in rats with femoral artery stenosis. J. Appl. Physiol. 71:1822-1829; 1991.
71. Zetterquist, S. The effect of active training on the nutritive blood flow in exercising ischemic legs. Scand. J. Clin. Invest. 25:101-111; 1970.

Chapter 43

Physical Activity, Fitness, and Hypertension

Robert H. Fagard
Charles M. Tipton

Hypertension is a disease and a risk factor (59,60) that is a serious public health problem in many countries throughout the world. For example, in the United States it is estimated that at least 58 million people have elevated blood pressure (119), whereas in Belgium it is reported that 8% of the men and 12% of the women have resting arterial blood pressures that are greater than or equal to 160 mmHg for systolic and greater than or equal to 90 mmHg for diastolic pressure (110).

Despite the progress made during the last decade, especially in the reduction in number of people who have experienced cerebrovascular lesions (119), the responsible mechanisms for the high morbidity and mortality statistics associated with high blood pressure remain unknown (66,119). Until all the mechanisms are identified, clinicians, researchers, and educators must manage hypertension and reduce its consequences by pharmacological and nonpharmacological means. It is of interest that Horan and Lenfant (59), researchers from the National Institutes of Health concerned with hypertension, have identified the primary risk factors for high blood pressure to be genetic predisposition, age, body mass, excessive sodium intake, increased alcohol consumption, and the lack of exercise. In addition, they have expanded the concept of hypertensive risk factors to incorporate predictors of hypertension (59). This list includes ventricular mass, plasma concentrations of hormones and catecholamines, mental and emotional stressors, and the blood pressure responses to acute exercise. Some of these (and additional) topics are discussed in this chapter.

In this review chapter we discuss the scientific evidence from epidemiological, clinical, and experimental studies from humans and animals on the role and importance of acute and chronic exercise in the regulation of arterial blood pressure and the management of the disease of hypertension. To facilitate these goals, the information pertaining to humans is covered by R.H. Fagard, whereas that pertaining to animals is presented by C.M. Tipton.

The Blood Pressure Response to Acute Exercise

Acute dynamic exercise by healthy humans and animals is associated with sympathoexcitatory events that include elevations in systolic and mean arterial pressures (4). This pressor response involves an interaction between "central command" and an exercise pressor reflex from the skeletal muscles (85). Imaginative studies on acute exercise by investigators (25-27,135) using humans or animals with intact baroreceptors and sinoaortic denervated animals suggest that the operating point of the aortic baroreceptor is reset to higher operating pressures.

Because similar studies have not been conducted in hypertensive animals, we can only speculate that similar processes are active in these animals. Diastolic blood pressure increases slightly during dynamic exercise, whereas the rise in systolic pressure is more pronounced. In general, the changes in pressure are similar in normotensive and hypertensive subjects (32), but they are more variable in the former group. There is some controversy as to whether an exaggerated pressure increase during dynamic exercise will predict the later development of hypertension in normotensive subjects (11,119). In hypertensive patients, blood pressure during exercise does not explain the target organ damage, independent from the pressure at rest (36), nor does it add independent precision to the long-term prognosis (37).

Surprisingly, there are limited data on this subject from animal models (136). When direct measurements were made on spontaneously hypertensive rats (SHR) and normotensive control rats that were performing a $\dot{V}O_2$max test, the SHR group exhibited an exaggerated mean blood pressure response up to 50% $\dot{V}O_2$max that diminished as the intensity of exercise increased (C.M. Tipton, unpublished manuscript). Whether similar responses would occur with stroke-prone hypertensive rats (SHR-SP) is unknown. It is also uncertain whether this pattern is a reflection of the sympathetic nervous system or thermoregulatory adjustments, or both. Static exercise investigations with SHR-SP groups have shown that the pressor response (60 to 100 mmHg in mean arterial pressure) had limited value for inducing strokes or for predicting the magnitude of hypertension that developed with time (127).

Postexercise Blood Pressure

It is well demonstrated in normotensive and hypertensive subjects that the resting pressure after exercise is lower than the preexercise value (69,117,119). This effect can persist for hours and has been implicated as a beneficial mechanism to reduce the rise in pressure that occurs with time. In older subjects, this effect is associated more with a decrease in cardiac output than with a reduction in total peripheral vascular resistance.

Creative animal investigations on this subject by Thoren, Hoffman, and co-workers (56-58) have shown that opioid and serotonin mechanisms are involved. Their studies, as well as those from Arizona (24) (Figure 43.1) demonstrate that the postexercise decrease in blood pressure can be inhibited by naloxone, which has both central and peripheral effects (68). Preliminary results from Arizona suggest that the μ and k-opioid receptors are responding to a central rather than a peripheral effect.

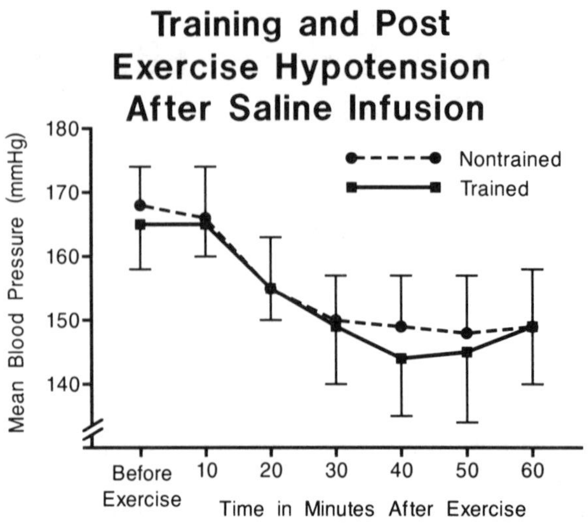

Figure 43.1 The influence of acute exercise (60% to 70% $\dot{V}O_2max$) on mean blood pressure as measured in the carotid artery. Means and standard errors are shown. There were 17 rats in the nontrained group and 18 in the trained group, respectively. These results were obtained from adult males as described in reference 128.

The Influence of Chronic Exercise

Results From Epidemiological Investigations

Some epidemiological studies have analyzed the relationship between blood pressure and physical activity using data from questionnaires and interviews concerning the physical activity of people at work or at leisure, or both. Other studies have used an exercise test to assess physical fitness or performance capacity. Several confounding variables may affect the relationship between physical activity, physical fitness, and blood pressure. Some of these, such as age, weight, and obesity, can be accounted for in analyses; others, such as self-selection and genetic effects, can hardly be controlled.

Several large studies, which allowed for age and anthropometric characteristics, have reported an inverse relationship between blood pressure and either habitual physical activity (21,40,84,87,99,115) or measured physical fitness (19,44,47,52). In addition, exercise (93) and fitness (12) were inversely related to the later development of hypertension. Not all epidemiological studies support this view (35), but the low level of physical activity in Western societies may have hampered the detection of such a relationship. Moreover, in studies that found a significant association, the difference in blood pressure between the most and the least physically active subjects usually amounted to no more than 5 mmHg after adjustment for confounding factors.

It remains difficult, however, to ascribe differences in blood pressure within a population to differences in levels of physical activity or fitness, because of the many possible confounding factors that cannot be accounted for. Therefore, the present review will mainly concern longitudinal intervention studies.

The Use of Animal Models in Hypertension Investigations

To date, the rat has been the most used animal to study the anatomical, biochemical, and physiologic consequences of hypertension; subhuman primates (including baboons), horses, dogs, pigs, rabbits, sheep, calves, and mice have also been employed in various research projects concerned with elevated arterial pressures (45,117,119). Currently, there are genetic and nongenetic rat models available for research purposes (117,119). Perusal of the published literature on genetic models, and especially the genetic model for SHR, suggests that most researchers are using the Japanese strain rather than those from Italy and Australia. During the last decade, a genetic model for borderline hypertension has been used by some for exercise-training purposes (74). This occurs by breeding the SHR and its normotensive control known as the Wistar-Kyoto rat (WKY) (74).

To many (117,119), the swimming of rats is the mode of acute exercise to study the effects of acute and chronic exercise. Even though it is apparent that swimming, cage, and treadmill running will all be associated with exercise adaptations (117,119), we are biased against the swimming of rats as an exercise mode in hypertensive studies because the frequency of bobbing and the duration of submergence create conditions of hypoxia, acidosis, hypercapnia, and diving bradycardia, which are not universal features of treadmill running (111). Rats can be conditioned by avoidance procedures to perform acute bouts of static or isometric exercises (127), although there are not a plethora of studies using this approach with hypertensive animal populations.

To the exercise physiologist, the best single method used to evaluate the acute and chronic effects of exercise is the measurement of maximum oxygen consumption, or $\dot{V}O_2$max (4), an approach which has also been adapted for animals (10,118). The measurement of oxygen consumed during exercise is useful for prescribing acute exercise as well as for evaluating the effects of chronic exercise. Careful animal studies on the prescription of acute exercise for SHR have demonstrated that when the intensity of exercise approaches 90% to 100% of $\dot{V}O_2$max, resting caudal-artery systolic blood pressures become higher, rather than lower, than in the hypertensive control animals (122). In fact, Tipton and associates believe this effect explains the results from other studies using hypertensive rats that show that strenuous exercise causes resting pressures in the trained group to be higher rather than lower than that of the control group (55,113,130). Moreover, Tipton has used these findings, and others from humans, to advocate a chronic exercise prescription for hypertensive subjects that has an intensity between 40% and 70% $\dot{V}O_2$max (119,122). The explanation for this hypertensive effect is obscure, although a central nervous system (CNS) imbalance in the baroreceptive neurons located in the nucleus tractus solitarius (27,100,119) is an attractive hypothesis to test.

The Influence of Endurance Training on Resting Blood Pressure

Data in Humans

Overall results. Many longitudinal studies have assessed the effect of physical training on blood pressure, but essential scientific criteria have not always been observed. Inclusion of a control group or of a control phase is mandatory. To avoid selection bias, allocation to the active or control group or the order of the training and nontraining phases should be determined at random. Ideally the subjects in the control group or in the control phase should be seen regularly, preferably as frequently as those in the training program; some authors included low-level exercise as placebo treatment (46,78).

The present review considers only controlled training studies in normotensive and hypertensive adolescents and adults in whom cardiovascular diseases were reasonably well excluded. Studies are considered only when the actual blood pressures for the training and the control groups or phases, or the pressure changes during the training and control periods, are reported.

We identified 36 papers on the effect of dynamic aerobic, predominantly isotonic, exercise involving large muscle groups (so-called endurance training). Some of these controlled studies involved several groups of subjects or applied different training regimens in the same participants, so that a total of 48 training groups or programs are available for analysis. Table 43.1 summarizes the details of the studies in which allocation to the control group or the order of the phases was determined at random and in which subjects in the control group or phase were followed or contacted regularly. These studies could involve low-level exercise (78), recreational exercise (42), identical visits without exercise (82,83), less frequent visits (23,114,131), or other contacts (13,64,70,89,112,134). In other randomized studies, summarized in Table 43.2, the subjects were only seen at the beginning and at the end of the control period. Table 43.3 lists the controlled studies without randomization procedure.

Most of the participants were men, and the average age of the groups ranged from 16 to 72 years. Duration of training ranged from 4 to 68 weeks (median = 16 weeks), with a frequency of mostly 3 weekly sessions of 15 to 90 min each. The training consisted mainly of walking, jogging, running, or bicycling. Tables 43.1 to 43.3 also give the approximate average training intensity in each group, though this is difficult to compare among studies. From the reported data it can be derived that the average intensity of training varied between 50% and 85% of maximal exercise capacity.

In these 48 groups, the average change of blood pressure in response to training, after adjustment for control observations, ranged from +6 to -20 mmHg for systolic blood pressure and from +5 to -16 mmHg for diastolic pressure. The adjustment

Table 43.1 Effects of Training on Resting Blood Pressure: Data From Randomized Studies With Follow-Up of the Control Group

Authors	Number entered (% analyzed)	Gender	Age of TG	Type of control	Program of training group/phase				
					Dur (we)	Freq (per we)	Time (min)	Intensity	Methods
Gettman et al. (42)	46(67)	m	24	CG[a]	20	3	30	85% (HR_r)	W, J, R
Meredith et al. (83)	10(100)	m + f	21	CG + CP	4	3	40	65% (W_m)	C
Meredith et al. (82)	8(100)	m	36	CG + CP	4	3	40	65% (W_m)	C
Gettman et al. (42)	50(48)	m	25	CG[a]	20	5	30	85% (HR_r)	W, J, R
Gettman et al. (42)	44(50)	m	22	CG[a]	20	1	30	85% (HR_r)	W, J, R
Vroman et al. (134)	11(100)	m	24	CG	12	4	30	80% ($\dot{V}O_{2m}$)	C
Jennings et al. (64)	12(100)	m + f	22	CP	4	3	40	65% (W_m)	C
Jennings et al. (64)	12(100)	m + f	22	CP	4	7	40	65% (W_m)	C
Kukkonen et al. (70)	34(88)	m	39	CG	16	3	50	52% (HR_r)	W, J, R, C, Ski
Suter et al. (112)	61(100)	m	39	CG	16	4	30	80% (HR_m)	W, J, R,
Martin et al. (78)	27(70)	m	44	CG	10	4	30	72% (HR_m)	W, J, R, C
Blumenthal et al. (13)	64(95)	m + f	44	CG	16	3	45	70% ($\dot{V}O_{2m}$)	W, J, R
Nelson et al. (89)	17(76)	m + f	44	CP	4	3	45	65% (W_m)	C
Nelson et al. (89)	17(76)	m + f	44	CP	4	7	45	65% (W_m)	C
Kukkonen et al. (70)	25(96)	m	42	CG	16	3	50	52% (HR_r)	W, J, R, C, Ski
Tanabe et al. (114)	31(100)	m + f	51	CG	10	3	60	LT	C
Urata et al. (131)	20(100)	m + f	51	CG	10	3	70	LT	C
Deplaen & Detry (23)	15(67)	m + f	44	CG	12	3	60	60% ($\dot{V}O_{2m}$)	W, J, R, C, Cal

Authors	n	Results for training group/phase						
		Systolic BP (mmHg)		Diastolic BP (mmHg)		Weight (kg)		PWC
		Control	Active (net Δ)	Control	Active (net Δ)	Control	Active (net Δ)	Δ(%)
Gettman et al. (42)	20	113.7	+5.5	75.6	+0.6	69.6	−1.10	+16% ($\dot{V}O_2$)
Meredith et al. (83)	10	114.0	−8.0	70.0	−5.0	70.2	−0.25	+14% ($\dot{V}O_2$)
Meredith et al. (82)	8	117	−8.0	72.0	−5.0	74.0	+0.4	+15% ($\dot{V}O_2$)
Gettman et al. (42)	13	119.7	+2.6	73.5	−1.8	68.7	−2.00	+21% ($\dot{V}O_2$)
Gettman et al. (42)	11	120.0	−0.8	76.9	−4.8	76.4	−1.20	+12% ($\dot{V}O_2$)
Vroman et al. (134)	6	121.7	−7.2	74.0	+1.9	80.4	−2.70	+20% ($\dot{V}O_2$)
Jennings et al. (64)	12	132.0	−10.0	69.0	−7.0	62.6	+0.10	+11% ($\dot{V}O_2$)
Jennings et al. (64)	12	132.0	−12.0	69.0	−7.0	62.6	+0.20	+24% ($\dot{V}O_2$)
Kukkonen et al. (70)	15	133.0	−1.0	86.0	+5.0	75.2	−0.30	+ 5% ($\dot{V}O_2$)
Suter et al. (112)	39	133.8	+2.5	89.1	−1.7	—	—	—
Martin et al. (78)	10	136.9	−7.6	94.8	−10.3	90.3	−0.80	+4.5% ($\dot{V}O_2$)
Blumenthal et al. (13)	39	141.0	+1.0	95.0	−1.0	82.0	0.00	+15% ($\dot{V}O_2$)
Nelson et al. (89)	13	143.0	−11.0	96.0	−9.0	74.0	+0.10	+17% ($\dot{V}O_2$)
Nelson et al. (89)	13	143.0	−16.0	96.0	−11.0	74.0	−0.10	+19% ($\dot{V}O_2$)
Kukkonen et al. (70)	12	145.0	−9.0	99.0	−4.0	78.2	−1.50	+12% ($\dot{V}O_2$)
Tanabe et al. (114)	21	155.0	−11.6	100.1	−5.4	63.8	−2.60	+22% (LT)
Urata et al. (131)	10	156.3	−14.7	102.8	−4.8	62.4	+0.50	+27% (LT); + 12%
Deplaen & Detry (23)	6	162.0	−2.0	104.0	+3.0	77.0	−4.00	+15% ($\dot{V}O_2$)

Note. Studies are ordered according to the control systolic blood pressure in the trained group/phase. [a]Same control group for each training group. BP: blood pressure; BS: bench stepping; C: cycling; Cal: calisthenics; CG: control group; cont: continuous; CP: control phase; Δ: change; Dur: duration; Ex: aerobic exercises; f: female; Freq: frequency; HR_{ex}: heart rate at submaximal exercise; HR_m: maximal heart rate; HR_r: heart rate reserve; int: interval; J: jogging; Jum: jumping; LT: lactate threshold; m: male; n: number; PWC: physical work capacity; R: running; S: swimming; TG: trained group; $\dot{V}O_{2m}$: maximal oxygen uptake; W: walking; W_m: maximal work load; we: week;—:not reported.

Table 43.2 Effects of Training on Resting Blood Pressure: Data From Randomized Studies Without Follow-Up of the Control Group

Authors	Number entered (% analyzed)	Gender	Age of TG	Type of control	Program of training group/phase: Dur (we)	Freq (per we)	Time (min)	Intensity (%)	Methods
Oluseye (91)	27 (100)	f	35	CG	12	3	50	80 (HR_m)	J, R, Jum, BS (cont)
Oluseye (91)	27 (100)	f	35	CG	12	3	50	80 (HR_m)	J, R, Jum, BS (int)
Van Hoof et al. (132)	30 (87)	m	38	CG + CP	16	3	60	70 (HR_r)	J, R, C, Cal
Mann et al. (76)	133 (62)	m	38	CG	26	3	52	80 (HR_r)	W, J, R, Cal
Myrtek & Villinger (88)	40 (100)	m	23	CG	5	3	15	60 (HR_r)	C
Coconie et al. (18)	—[a] (n = 18)	m + f	72	CG	26	3	31	65 ($\dot{V}O_{2m}$)	W, J, R
Länsimies et al. (73)	100 (90)	m	42	CG	16	3.5	55	53 (HR_e)	W, J, R, C, S, Ski
Duncan et al. (29)	56 (100)	m	30	CG	16	3	60	75 (HR_m)	W, J, R
Coconie et al. (18)	—[a] (n = 11)	m + f	72	CG	26	3	32	65 ($\dot{V}O_{2m}$)	W, J, R
Hagberg et al. (49)	—[b] (—)	m + f	64	CG	37	3	52	77 ($\dot{V}O_{2m}$)	W, J, R, C
Hagberg et al. (49)	—[b] (—)	m + f	64	CG	37	3	60	50 ($\dot{V}O_{2m}$)	W

Authors	n	Results for training group/phase: Systolic BP (mmHg) Control	Systolic BP Active (net Δ)	Diastolic BP (mmHg) Control	Diastolic BP Active (net Δ)	Weight (kg) Control	Weight Active (net Δ)	PWC Δ(%)
Oluseye (91)	15	111.5	–15.1	73.5	–4.1	—	—	—
Oluseye (91)	15	111.9	–16.9	69.9	–4.0	—	—	—
Van Hoof et al. (132)	26	126.0	–4.0	86.0	–5.0	80	–2.0	+17 ($\dot{V}O_2$)
Mann et al. (76)	62	129.0	+2.0	81.0	–2.0	—	—	+16 ($\dot{V}O_2$)
Myrtek & Villinger (88)	20	129.7	–4.5	79.5	+2.5	—	—	+10% (HR_{ex})
Coconie et al. (18)	11	130.0	–4.0	78.0	–5.0	69.6	–0.6	+21 ($\dot{V}O_2$)
Länsimies et al. (73)	44	130.0	–3.0	84.0	–3.0	78.4	–0.2	+15 ($\dot{V}O_2$)
Duncan et al. (29)	44	146.3	–6.2	94.3	–10.0	85.5	–0.7	+13 ($\dot{V}O_2$)
Coconie et al. (18)	6	156.0	–11.0	86.0	–9.0	69.6	–0.6	+21 ($\dot{V}O_2$)
Hagberg et al. (49)	10	157.0	–8.0	99.0	–9.0	79.3	–2.0	+23 ($\dot{V}O_2$)
Hagberg et al. (49)	11	164.0	–20.0	94.0	–10.0	69.2	0.0	+ 5 ($\dot{V}O_2$)

Note. [a]Total number entered = 34; [b]total number entered = 33. See Table 43.1 for abbreviations.

Table 43.3 Effects of Training on Resting Blood Pressure: Data From Nonrandomized Controlled Studies

Authors	Number entered (% analyzed)	Gender	Age of TG	Type of control	Program of training group/phase				
					Dur (we)	Freq (per we)	Time (min)	Intensity (%)	Methods
Gilders et al. (46)	14 (93)	m + f	41	CP	16	3	30	70 ($\dot{V}O_{2m}$)	C
Pollock et al. (96)	24 (96)	m	48.9	CG	20	4	40	70 (HR_m)	W
Seals et al. (105)	24 (83)	m + f	62.0	CG	26	3	37	85 (HR_m)	W, J, R, C
Bonanno & Lies (14)	13 (92)	m	41.3	CG	12	3	47	77 (HR_m)	W, J, R, Cal
Wolfe et al. (137)	33 (67)	m	36.8	CG	26	4	30	80 (HR_m)	J, R
Gilders et al. (46)	15 (53)	m + f	46.0	CP	16	3	30	70 ($\dot{V}O_{2m}$)	C
Pollock et al. (95)	30 (87)	m	55.0	CG	20	3	30	87 (HR_m)	W, J, R
Norris et al. (90)	100 (53)	m	35.0	CG	10	3	35	—	J, R
Cléroux et al. (17)	14 (100)	m + f	37.0	CG	20	3	32	60 ($\dot{V}O_{2m}$)	C
Hagberg et al. (48)	25 (100)	m + f	15.6	CP	26	3	35	62 ($\dot{V}O_{2m}$)	W, J, R, Cal
Cléroux et al. (17)	12 (100)	m + f	32.0	CG	20	3	32	60 ($\dot{V}O_{2m}$)	J, R
Seals & Reiling (106)	34 (76)	m + f	61	CG	26	3.5	41	47 (HR_r)	W
Seals & Reiling (106)	34 (53)	m + f	63	CG	58	3.6	50	57 (HR_r)	W
Somers et al. (109)	20 (80)	m + f	35.0	CP	26	7	30	—	J, R, Ex
Bonanno & Lies (14)	27 (100)	m	41.3	CG	12	3	47	77 (HR_r)	W, J, R, Cal
Schleusing et al. (104)	21 (90)	—	40.0	CG	32	3.5	90	55 (HR_r)	W, J, R, C, S
Baglivo et al. (6)	32 (100)	m + f	50.8	CG	68	3	50	—	C, Ex
Akinpelu (3)	20 (100)	—	55.7	CG	12	3	42	65 (HR_r)	J, R, C
Roman et al. (101)	30 (80)	f	55.0	CP	12	3	30	70 (HR_m)	W, J, R, C, Cal

(continued)

Table 43.3 *(Continued)*

Authors	n	Systolic BP (mmHg) Control	Systolic BP (mmHg) Active (net Δ)	Diastolic BP (mmHg) Control	Diastolic BP (mmHg) Active (net Δ)	Weight (kg) Control	Weight (kg) Active (net Δ)	PWC Δ(%)
Gilders et al. (46)	13	114.5	+1.5	76.5	–0.5	75	—	+11 ($\dot{V}O_2$)
Pollock et al. (96)	15	120.7	–3.6	78.4	–6.4	77.6	–1.3	+28 ($\dot{V}O_2$)
Seals et al. (105)	10	121.0	–13.0	78.0	–13.0	74.0	–2.0	+21 ($\dot{V}O_2$)
Bonanno & Lies (14)	8	123.0	+6.0	84.0	+3.0	86.6	—	+ 5 ($\dot{V}O_2$)
Wolfe et al. (137)	12	126.0	–4.0	—	—	76.1	–0.4	+19 ($\dot{V}O_2$)
Gilders et al. (46)	8	128.0	+2.0	86.0	0	84.0	—	+15 ($\dot{V}O_2$)
Pollock et al. (95)	20	130.3	–2.6	83.9	–2.4	79.1	–1.5	+16 ($\dot{V}O_2$)
Norris et al. (90)	28	131.0	–5.0	79.0	–9.0	—	—	—
Cléroux et al. (17)	7	133.0	–2.0	83.0	–5.0	76.0	0	+13 ($\dot{V}O_2$)
Hagberg et al. (48)	25	138.0	–9.0	79.0	–4.0	74.5	–1.4	+10 ($\dot{V}O_2$)
Cléroux et al. (17)	5	141.0	–9.0	71.0	+2.0	86.0	–2.0	+21 ($\dot{V}O_2$)
Seals & Reiling (106)	14	146.0	–1.0	94	–1.0	76.5	+0.4	+ 6 ($\dot{V}O_2$)
Seals & Reiling (106)	10	146.0	–2.0	93	–2.0	76.4	–1.0	+10 ($\dot{V}O_2$)
Somers et al. (109)	16	148.0	–10.0	82.0	–6.0	—	—	—
Bonanno & Lies (14)	12	148.0	–10.0	97.0	–3.0	86.6	—	+ 5 ($\dot{V}O_2$)
Schleusing et al. (104)	8	153.0	–6.0	106.0	–10.0	—	—	+21 ($\dot{V}O_2$)
Baglivo et al. (6)	17	155.0	–6.0	101.0	–16.0	78.0	–0.6	+24 (W_m)
Akinpelu (3)	10	167.0	–14.0	100.0	–8.0	70.4	–1.5	+16 (HR_{ex})
Roman et al. (101)	27	180.5	–19.5	113.0	–16.0	—	—	+26 ($\dot{V}O_2$)

Note. See Table 43.1 for abbreviations.

took into account the blood pressure changes in the parallel control group or the changes during the nontraining phase in crossover studies. The overall net change of all studies combined averaged -5.3/-4.8 mmHg after adjustment for the control observations and after weighting for the number of trained participants that could be analyzed in each study group. In addition, the training-induced fall in blood pressure became apparent after 2 (83) to 7 (65) weeks of regular exercise; the hypotensive effect did not persist after cessation of training (48,64,82,83,89,101,109,132).

Determinants of the training-induced change of blood pressure.

(1) Level of blood pressure

The 48 study groups were classified into three categories by the average pretraining blood pressure level. According to the 1978 criteria of the World Health Organization (138), 27 groups fell in the normotensive range (systolic blood pressure (SBP) ≤ 140 mmHg and diastolic blood pressure (DBP) ≤ 90 mmHg), 14 had definite hypertension (SBP ≥ 160 mmHg or DBP ≥ 95 mmHg), and 7 could be classified as having borderline hypertension. Table 43.4 summarizes the changes of systolic and diastolic pressure in response to training, after adjustment for control observations and weighting for the number of analyzable trained subjects in each study group. Dynamic aerobic training was associated with a mean net change of systolic/diastolic blood pressure of -3.2/-3.1 mmHg in the groups with a normal average pressure, of -6.2/-6.8 mmHg in borderline hypertensive subjects, and of -9.9/-7.6 mmHg in the hypertensive subjects.

The suggestion that the response of blood pressure is more pronounced in hypertensive persons is corroborated by the results of studies in which normotensive and hypertensive subjects followed the same training program (14-16,18,64,65,70,89). In each of these studies, the blood pressure change was greater in the hypertensive patients than in the normotensive subjects.

(2) Demographic and anthropometric characteristics

Hypertensive patients were on average older than the normotensive subjects, and their training programs were usually less demanding. Therefore the relations between the blood pressure response and various demographic and anthropometric characteristics are looked at in normotensive subjects and hypertensive subjects (including those with borderline hypertension) separately. By use of single regression analysis, weighting for the number of subjects in each trained group, the training-induced changes of systolic and diastolic blood pressure did not seem to depend on age (*P* greater than .25). In addition, Hansen et al. (50) observed in a randomized controlled study that exercise training lowers systolic blood pressure by 4 mmHg in healthy children aged 9 to 11 years. Only two studies (91,101) reported on (hypertensive) women only, and both observed a significant hypotensive effect; analysis of demographic subgroups in the study by Hagberg et al. (48) showed that the blood pressure response was somewhat less in female than in male adolescents. Racial origin did not affect the blood pressure response to training (48); in addition, the blood pressure of African hypertensive subjects responded well to training (3,91).

In several individual studies, the results were not affected by adjustment of the pressure response to the initial weight (13,18,29,90). The net change of body weight during the training period ranged from +0.5 to -4 kg and averaged -0.93 kg. However, the responses of systolic and of diastolic blood pressure were not related to these changes of body weight in either the normotensive or the hypertensive subgroups (*P* greater than .50).

(3) Characteristics of the training program

In weighted, single-regression analysis, the total duration of the program, the weekly frequency, the time per session, and the intensity of exercise did not contribute significantly to explaining the interstudy variance of blood pressure response to training in either the normotensive or the hypertensive subgroups. Gettman et al. (42) compared the effect of one, three, and five weekly training sessions in normotensive subjects, but blood pressure did not change in any subgroup. On the other hand, Jennings et al. (64) (in normotensive subjects) and Nelson et al. (89) (in hypertensive subjects) found that the fall in blood pressure was slightly but significantly greater on a seven-times-per-week schedule than when the participants exercised three times per week; on the three-times-per-week schedule, however, the fall of blood pressure had already reached 70% to 100% of the response achieved with seven-times-per-week exercise. Hagberg et al. (49) claimed that the response of systolic pressure to training was more pronounced when 60- to 69-year-old persons exercised at low intensity (53% of maximal oxygen consumption) than at moderate intensity (73%). However, this difference was not confirmed for the blood pressures measured at the time of the hemodynamic study and during exercise testing; in fact, exercise pressure was only lowered in the moderate-intensity group.

Most studies expressed the effectiveness of the training regimen in terms of increase of maximal oxygen uptake; some employed the change of the maximal work load or of heart rate at submaximal work. The percentage changes of these various expressions of the gain in exercise capacity are more

Table 43.4 The Net Training-Induced Changes of Blood Pressure in Various Groups of Subjects, Classified According to WHO Criteria

WHO classification	Number of trained groups	Net change of blood pressure Systolic	Diastolic
Normotension	27	– 3.2 (+6; -17)	– 3.1 (+5; -13)
Borderline hypertension	7	– 6.2 (-1; -11)	– 6.8 (+2; -10)
Hypertension	14	–9.9 (+1; -20)	– 7.6 (+3; -16)

Note. Values are means, weighted for the number of analyzable trained subjects in each group, and ranges of the average changes in the various groups.

or less similar. In weighted single-regression analysis, the response of diastolic blood pressure was significantly related to the increase of exercise capacity, both in the normotensive (P = .006) and in the hypertensive subgroups (P = .02); more gain in fitness was associated with a larger decrease of diastolic pressure (Figure 43.2). Similar results were obtained in individual studies (13,112).

In weighted multiple-regression analysis, the percent change in exercise capacity and hypertensive status contributed independently ($P \leq .001$) to the variance of the diastolic blood pressure response among studies, and together they explained 46% of the total variance.

(4) The study design

In the randomized studies in which the control subjects were followed in one way or another (Table 43.1), the net weighted training-induced change of blood pressure was -1.6/-2.1 mmHg in the 10 groups of normotensive subjects and -7.2/-4.8 mmHg in the 8 cohorts of hypertensive patients, which included those with borderline hypertension. In the other randomized studies (Table 43.2) blood pressure changes averaged -3.7/-2.7 mmHg in the normotensive subjects (n = 7) and -9.0/-9.8 mmHg in the hypertensive subjects (n = 4). In the controlled studies without randomization (Table 43.3), blood pressure decreased by -4.0/-4.8 mmHg in the 10 normotensive groups and by -9.9/-8.6 mmHg in the 9 groups of hypertensive patients. It appears therefore that the studies that followed the more rigorous scientific criteria showed the smallest decrease of blood pressure.

Data in Animals

In general, the animal training studies support the trends observed in humans. The majority of investigations have been conducted with rats, although it is of interest that when subhuman primates were regularly exercised on a treadmill at a moderate-intensity level, the trained group had significantly lower resting pressures because chronic exercise had delayed the rise in pressure that occurs with aging and inactivity (123).

Treadmill (running) training programs involving adult normotensive rats generally show that the trained rats have resting caudal artery systolic blood pressures that are 5 to 18 mmHg lower than the nontrained control animals (117,119). This difference occurs in weight-matched or non-weight-matched experiments and is due to the fact that the trained rats exhibit very little change in resting pressures during the aging process. This same trend was present in SHR groups. To determine the time course of these observations, Tipton and associates followed the changes in resting pressures of rats between 3 and 16 weeks of age and observed that the trained rats had systolic blood pressures that were lower, with a time-pressure curve that was shifted to the right, after the animals were 8 weeks or older (122).

Using data summarized in previous reviews (117,119) or from other published sources (24,128), we performed an analysis of 16 separate studies lasting 8 weeks or longer. This study involved eight different investigators who had resting data from 219 nontrained and 231 trained hypertensive rats (SHR). We found the nontrained had a mean (201.3 mmHg) that was 10.5 mmHg higher than the trained (190.8 mmHg) animals. Fourteen of these studies, which had both initial and final values, showed that the nontrained rats experienced an increase of 74.3 mmHg during the experimental periods, whereas the trained rats had an increase of 63.6 mmHg. When older SHR groups were inactive for 42 or more weeks and then moderately endurance-trained for 16 weeks, the nontrained rats showed an increase of approximately 14 mmHg,

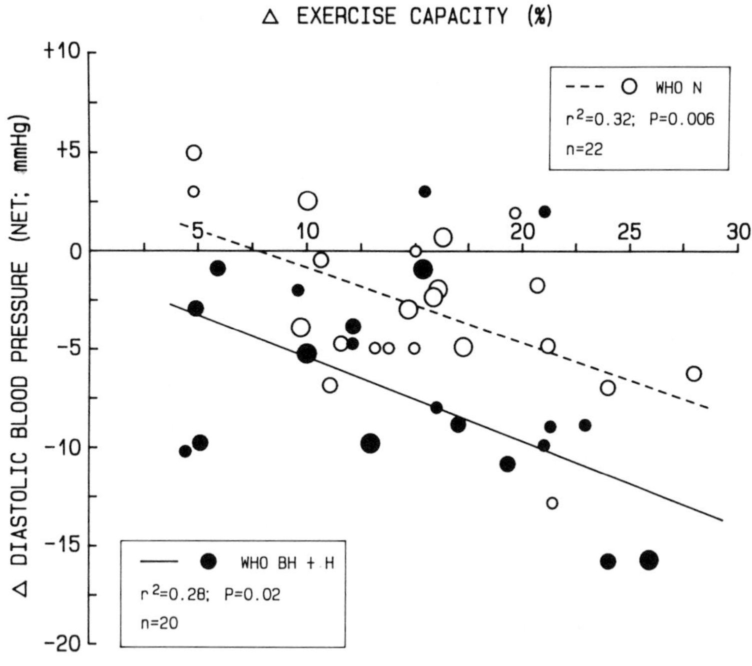

Figure 43.2 Changes of diastolic blood pressure (mmHg) with training, adjusted for control data, versus changes in exercise capacity. An open circle represents the average for a group of normotensive subjects, a closed circle for a group of hypertensives. The 3 sizes of the circles stand for the number of analyzable trained subjects in each group: small for n ≤ 10, medium for n = 11-19 and large for n ≥ 20 subjects. The regression lines are the result of weighted single regression analysis for the normotensive (dotted line) and hypertensive (full line) study groups.

whereas the trained rats had means that were similar to their initial values.

In general, the beneficial effects of endurance training on resting blood pressure are best demonstrated in normotensive and neurogenic hypertensive rats. When other animal models for hypertension have been studied, the results have not been as consistent or impressive.

Several investigators have studied the effect of endurance training on the change in resting blood pressure of Dahl salt-sensitive hypertensive rats, and conflicting results have been reported (102, 107,126). None of the studies used a design that included dose-response components, and the negative results occurred from rats that had a chow containing 8% NaCl and a 1% saline drinking solution that could have masked any beneficial longitudinal effects of training on resting pressure (126). However, there is no controversy concerning the beneficial effects of training on rats that are resistant to salt (107,126).

Salt sensitivity is a key factor in using stroke-prone hypertensive rats (SHR-SP) to study cerebrovascular relationships in any training study because when NaCl is not provided to the animals, the time required to observe mortality and morbidity events is excessive and difficult to quantify. During the initial years when SHR-SP were studied, strokes tended to occur when the resting pressures exceeded 200 mmHg (140). However, this is no longer the situation with the animals currently available for experimental studies, because much higher pressures are recorded with no evidence for changes in morbidity or mortality statistics (119).

Treadmill running studies with adult stroke-prone hypertensive rats have yielded interesting results. In an early study conducted in Japan, the authors observed that the rats running in activity cages appeared to die sooner and to exhibit more extensive histological damage to select regions of the brain than the nontrained control rats (71). Tipton and his students were intrigued by these findings and wondered if the histological results occurred because the strenuousness of the exercise prescribed appeared to be higher than 70% $\dot{V}O_2$max (124). Hence, they initiated a study with male and female SHR-SP groups that exercised between 40% and 70% of $\dot{V}O_2$max until they either exhibited behavioral symptoms of a stroke (140) or died. Using results from only those rats with proven histological evidence for cerebrovascular lesions, they reported that trained rats had strokes earlier and also died sooner than the nontrained control rats (124). The explanation is obscure, but it is possible that the effect was related to a decrease in the influence of the sympathetic nervous system on the tone of the vascular smooth muscles of the cerebral vessels. Research by Heistad and coworkers with SHR-SP populations provides strong support for the concept that the sympathetic nervous system is important for maintaining the integrity of the vascular smooth muscle of cerebral vessels (7,20,38). However, it must be acknowledged that the evidence showing a training effect on the resting sympathetic tone of SHR groups is quite limited.

One frequently used experimental approach with normotensive animals to produce hypertension is constriction of the renal artery with or without removal of the kidney (Goldblatt, two kidney-one clip, one kidney-one clip). This model of renal hypertension is very rapid and effective and has been used extensively by numerous investigators with rats, pigs, and dogs. When this model has been employed in rats (77,103) to determine whether endurance training would significantly alter resting arterial pressures, the results have been negative, thus suggesting that this type of hypertension is not ameliorated by chronic exercise. According to Zambraski, who has been investigating this aspect in pigs (E.J. Zambraski, personal communication), it is possible that the vascular changes are so extensive from the influences of angiotensin that any training benefits are being masked.

Conflicting training results have been reported for rats that have become hypertensive by injections of deoxycorticosterone (DOCA) (22,121). We think the disagreement could be resolved by a careful dose-response study similar to one recommended for the effects of exogenous sodium chloride. When pellets of DOCA, released on a specific time schedule, were placed in pigs who were exercise-trained, negative results were found (E.J. Zambraski, personal communication). Because many of the negative results have occurred in animal models in which the kidney has a major role in the regulation of blood pressure (141), we have speculated that kidney-mediated hypertension is not responsive to the effects of chronic exercise and that its management will require pharmacological approaches.

The Influence of Endurance Training on the Blood Pressure Response During Exercise

The effect of endurance training on blood pressure during exercise can be analyzed, either by considering the data at a fixed work load or by considering the effect at a relative work load—that is, at a certain percentage of the pretraining maximal oxygen uptake and of the usually higher posttraining maximal oxygen uptake. Both approaches have been used.

In normotensive subjects, Martin et al. (79) observed similar blood pressures before and after training, when measured at a work load requiring an oxygen uptake of about 2 L/min. By contrast, Myrtek and Villinger (88) found a significant training-induced net decrease of blood pressure (12/9 mmHg) during cycling at 100 W. Systolic blood pressure decreased by 5 to 7 mmHg at several absolute submaximal work loads in the training study by Van Hoof et al. (132), but the difference in the training and nontraining phases was no longer significant when the work load was expressed in percentage of the prevailing maximal oxygen uptake. Jennings et al. (64) reported a significant training-induced decrease of systolic blood pressure at 25% of maximal work load but not at 50% and 75%; this finding is in agreement with the data from Cléroux et al. (17) that blood pressure was similar before and after training at 60% of predicted maximal oxygen uptake. Training did not affect blood pressure at peak exercise in normotensive subjects (79).

In hypertensive patients, training did not change blood pressure at similar submaximal work loads and at maximal work (13). In other studies, however, the net change of blood pressure at fixed work loads averaged -10 (3,6) and -20 (104) mmHg, respectively, for systolic blood pressure and -5 (3) and -19 (6) mmHg for diastolic pressure. Both systolic and diastolic blood pressures were lower during submaximal exercise at the same absolute work load when older hypertensive subjects trained at moderate intensity, but this was not the case in a low-intensity group (49). The falls of blood pressure were also significant when measured at similar relative work loads (89,101).

In summary, the blood pressure of normotensive subjects remained unchanged or decreased after training when measured at fixed submaximal work, but blood pressure was usually not affected at the same relative work load. In hypertensive patients, most but not all studies found a significant training-induced reduction of blood pressure both at absolute and at relative work loads.

To date, there have been limited studies with animals on this matter, and this area deserves future research.

The Influence of Endurance Training on Ambulatory Blood Pressure

The technique of ambulatory blood pressure measurement has only recently been introduced in training studies. Most of these applied noninvasive automated devices (13,46,63,106,132); only Somers et al. (109) measured ambulatory pressure intra-arterially. Van Hoof et al. (132) trained 26 normal sedentary men for 4 months. Whereas daytime diastolic blood pressure decreased significantly, from 89 to 84 mmHg, the small change in systolic blood pressure, from 131 to 129 mmHg, was not significant. Although the training-induced bradycardia was apparent both during the day and during the night, blood pressure during sleep (control: 105/68 mmHg) remained essentially unchanged after training (107/67 mmHg). Jennings et al. (63) assessed the effect of physical training among expeditioners to Antarctica, who were active in summer and sedentary in winter. The addition of either 3 weeks or 7 weeks of exercise in winter significantly lowered blood pressure. Blood pressure measurements during the working day showed the greatest changes with the exercise training program, which had no effect on blood pressure during sleep. By contrast, Gilders et al. (46) did not observe changes in 24-hour, day- and nighttime blood pressure in 10 trained normotensive subjects; also, in the 7 subjects whose conventional diastolic blood pressure was greater than 85 mmHg, the net change in the 24-hour blood pressure of -5.5/-2 mmHg did not reach statistical significance.

Somers et al. (109) measured intra-arterial (n = 10) or noninvasive (n = 3) ambulatory blood pressure in borderline hypertensive subjects, with an average age of 34 years. Ambulatory pressure averaged 141/89 mmHg in the unfit state and 136/81 mmHg ($P < .01$) in the fit state. However, sleeptime blood pressure, measured in 6 patients, was not significantly different between the unfit state (107/65 mmHg) and the trained state (113/66 mmHg). Seals et al. (106) also observed that the lower systolic blood pressure after 12 months of training was entirely due to a decrease of daytime blood pressure, from 142 to 135 mmHg, whereas nighttime pressure after training (124 mmHg) was not significantly different from the baseline value (128 mmHg); in this study ambulatory pressure was not influenced after the first 6-month period, when the patients had exercised at a lower intensity. Finally, Blumenthal et al. (13) measured ambulatory blood pressure only in the awake period in hypertensive patients and did not find any effect of training on blood pressures overall, during work or at home.

The results of training on blood pressure measured by automated devices, out of the laboratory or clinic environment, agree that nighttime blood pressure is not affected. Some but not all studies observed a significant fall of pressure measured during the day.

The Mechanisms Associated With the Chronic Effects of Endurance Training

Hemodynamic Mechanism

Hypertension is a multifaceted disease that is associated with a variety of physiological and pathological mechanisms. Studies that have examined the hemodynamic relationships in humans are limited and confusing. Until recently, most studies on the hemodynamic effects of endurance training were not controlled, but several controlled studies have now been published. Cardiac output was most often measured by use of the carbon dioxide rebreathing technique (18,48,49,64,82,83,89,106). Others employed dye dilution (67,131), radionuclide techniques (79), imaging (137), or Doppler echocardiography (46).

In normotensive subjects, Jennings et al. (64) and Meredith et al. (82,83) attributed the significant hypotensive effect of physical training to reductions of systemic vascular resistance, ranging from 12% to 22%; cardiac output had consistently increased. Training also resulted in a significant decrease of systemic vascular resistance in the study by Martin et al. (79), although blood pressure had not changed. Blood pressure and the hemodynamic data were not significantly influenced by training in the normotensive subjects studied by Coconie et al. (18), Gilders et al. (46), and Wolfe et al. (137).

Although several controlled studies have now been performed on hypertensive patients, the data remain controversial. Despite a training-induced change of blood pressure, Hagberg et al. (48,49) and Coconie et al. (18) did not observe significant changes of cardiac output and of vascular resistance in adolescent (48) and older hypertensive subjects (18,49). Similarly, Urata et al. (131) could not pinpoint the hemodynamic mechanism of the training-induced reduction of blood pressure, but more recently (67) these authors reported a significant fall of cardiac output, in agreement with the findings by Seals and Reiling (106). In contrast, Nelson et al. (89) ascribed the hypotensive effect of training to a reduction of systemic vascular resistance. Finally, blood pressure and its hemodynamic components remained unchanged in the study by Gilders et al. (46).

In summary, the hemodynamic data in humans are conflicting. This may be due to the different methods that have been used and to the problems inherent to any method for the measurement of cardiac output, particularly when the method is noninvasive.

The number of animal studies that have incorporated hemodynamic measurements are relatively few (119,125), and the results are confusing. When normotensive rats are investigated, resting cardiac output is shown to increase as well as to decrease (128). On the other hand, trained SHR groups have lower resting cardiac output and higher total peripheral resistance means than the nontrained control groups (128) (Table 43.5).

Sympathetic Nervous System

For almost 100 years, the sympathetic nervous system (SNS) has been implicated as an important mechanism for increasing resting blood pressure. Moreover, it is well accepted that the SNS has a central role in essential hypertension (1).

Plasma catecholamines are an expression of the overall activity of the autonomic nervous system. When sedentary normotensive subjects and hypertensive patients were subjected to dynamic training, plasma noradrenalin levels were usually (54,64,82,83,89,114,131) but not consistently (17,18, 29) lowered. Meredith et al. (82) related the decrease of plasma noradrenalin in response to training to a significant reduction in total and renal noradrenalin spillover to plasma, but not in cardiac spillover; noradrenalin clearance was not affected. Plasma adrenalin usually remained unchanged (18,28,64,82,89,131). A decrease in autonomic activity is at least partly responsible for the training-induced reduction in heart rate (31), but we cannot ascertain to what extent it affects blood pressure. Only Urata et al. (131) reported a significant association between the changes in blood pressure and in plasma noradrenalin concentration. In addition, the lack of an effect on blood pressure during sleep (63,106,109,132), when sympathetic activity is low, supports the involvement of the sympathetic nervous system in the hypotensive effect of training.

In the animal model for genetic hypertension, resting sympathetic nerve activity is quite high (129). When experiments were conducted with SHR groups that included chemical sympathectomy, sham injections, adrenal demedullation, and combinations thereof, the trained animals in the sham, chemical-sympathectomized, and demedullated groups had significantly lower resting pressures than the nontrained groups (129). On the other hand, the two subgroups that were chemically sympathectomized and adrenal-demedullated had low, but similar, resting systolic blood pressure means at the end of their experimental periods. These findings indicate that endurance training would be associated with lower resting pressures if either norepinephrine or epinephrine was available. However, if adequate concentrations of either one of these catecholamines were not present, as with conditions of chemical sympathectomy and adrenal demedullation, then a training effect would not occur. Although it is attractive to suggest that a supersensitivity mechanism is involved, there is no plasma or receptor evidence to support this possibility.

Table 43.5 The Influence of Endurance Training on Select Resting Hemodynamic parameters of Unanesthetized Adult Male Hypertensive Rats (SHR)

Parameter	Units	Nontrained	Trained
N		38	38
Caudal artery systolic blood pressure	mmHg	210 ± 3	200 ± 3*
Carotid artery mean blood pressure	mmHg	161 ± 3	151 ± 4*
Cardiac output	ml · min	126 ± 4	112 ± 3*
Cardiac index	$ml \cdot min^{-1} \cdot sq\ cm^{-1}$	0.292 ± 0.011	0.279 ± 0.009
Total peripheral vascular resistance	$mmHg \cdot ml^{-1} \cdot min^{-1}$	1.308 ± 0.040	1.405 ± 0.057
Total peripheral vascular resistance index	$mmHg \cdot ml^{-1} \cdot min^{-1} \cdot kg^{-1}$	3.518 ± 0.146	4.169 ± 0.183*

Note. Mean and standard errors are shown. *Denotes a group difference that was statistically significant at the 0.05 probability level. Data presented have been published in Tipton et al. Reprinted here by permission. See reference 128.

Baroreflexes

There is a vast body of knowledge concerned with the role of the baroreceptors in the regulation of resting blood pressure and in the etiology of hypertension. Moreover, the concept of baroreceptors being reset in hypertensive states is well established (72). On the other hand, the studies on the contributions of chronic exercise on the resting function of baroreceptors in trained hypertensive populations is quite limited.

Somers et al. (109) observed an increased baroreflex sensitivity in the fit state, but this was not related to the training-induced change in blood pressure. In another study baroreflex sensitivity was not different between athletes and control subjects (39).

The limited animal data suggest that changes in baroreceptor functioning do occur. When lower body negative pressure (LBNP) was used to activate the baroreceptors in the cardiopulmonary, carotid sinus, and the aortic sinus of nontrained and trained, sympathectomized, normotensive, and hypertensive rats (94,120), the trained, sympathectomized, and normotensive groups exhibited marked decreases in resting arterial pressures. In contrast to the nontrained control animals, the hypertensive SHR did not. Since the anesthesia (pentobartibal sodium) eliminated the tachycardia associated with the response, minimal credence was given to these results, even though the general trend was similar to that reported for normotensive humans who were trained (98). Bedford and Tipton repeated these types of experiments with tranquilized SHR and observed an elevation in heart rate that is characteristic of the baroreflex response (9). Although they found similar declines in arterial pressures in both groups with LBNP, the trained populations experienced less decline in central venous pressure, suggesting that chronic exercise had altered the interaction between the cardiopulmonary and arterial baroreflexes.

In a related experiment, Bedford and Tipton (8) used an isolated carotid sinus preparation with nontrained and trained normotensive rats and observed that the trained rats exhibited a reduced responsiveness to changes in carotid sinus pressure. DiCarlo and Bishop (25,26) have shown in normotensive rabbits that training will inhibit the afferent contributions to the baroreflex, but these types of baroreceptor experiments have not been performed with select animal models of hypertension. It is known that trained SHR groups have significantly higher resting blood and plasma volumes than the nontrained control groups (120,121), which could be of importance in the resetting process.

The Renin-Angiotensin-Aldosterone System

The renin-angiotensin-aldosterone system is also potentially important through its effects on blood volume and arterial pressure. M'Buyamba-Kabangu et al. (80) found an inverse relationship between plasma renin activity at rest and peak oxygen uptake in 40 young healthy subjects, and Fagard et al. (33) observed a lower plasma renin activity in runners compared to that in sedentary control subjects. Others reported a slightly but not significantly lower resting plasma renin in well-trained subjects compared to nontrained subjects (81,108). Long-term endurance training of normotensive subjects reduced plasma renin activity significantly (43). This was not so in another study (54), but the training-induced change of plasma renin activity was significantly related to the gain in physical working capacity. Jennings et al. (64) observed a fall of plasma renin in the subjects with evidence of decreased sympathetic function after training.

In hypertensive patients, however, plasma renin was not affected by training (49,89,131). Resting plasma angiotensin II also remained unchanged (18,33,54), whereas plasma or urinary aldosterone was lowered (81,108) or unaffected (43,54,131). Hespel et al. (54) observed that plasma aldosterone was reduced in the subjects with the highest gain in exercise capacity. In trained subjects, plasma renin (33,43) and plasma angiotensin II (33) were lower during exercise. However, the lower angiotensin II would not necessarily reduce blood pressure, because the response of blood pressure to exogenous angiotensin II is greatly reduced during acute exercise (34).

As noted earlier, the training of animal models for renal hypertension has reported negative results concerning the effects of endurance training (77,119,141). It is possible that these studies used an inappropriate animal model. On the other hand, it is possible that kidney-mediated forms of hypertension will not be ameliorated by endurance training.

Electrolytes

It is well accepted that an excessive intake of dietary sodium will be associated with an increase in resting pressure. The experimental literature on the influence of endurance training on sodium balance in normotensive and hypertensive subjects is limited.

At the present time, the Dahl salt-sensitive hypertensive rat is the animal model of choice to study this problem. Unfortunately, the training results have been conflicting, and it is difficult to use these studies to gain an insight on the responsible mechanisms.

One dietary practice receiving considerable attention by scientific and commercial groups is the use of supplements to alter the cellular concentration and function of calcium. Although there have been several reports on the benefits of adding calcium to the diet to lower resting blood pressure in SHR groups (119), there have been none concerning its interaction with endurance training.

Preliminary studies conducted by Drummond and co-workers (28) with high- and low-calcium diets that contained sodium concentrations within desirable ranges indicated that training was associated with lower resting pressures in both groups but that high calcium, per se, had no significant effect in reducing the resting pressures in the nontrained animals, regardless of the diet. At the moment, we think the calcium/phosphate ratio of the diet is as important as the concentration of calcium, but additional research is needed to verify this belief.

An interesting recent observation is that intraerythrocyte sodium concentration was reduced when normotensive subjects were trained for 4 months (53). The effect was related to the gain in exercise capacity, but its role in the hypotensive effect could not be clearly established. Adragna et al. (2) had previously observed a small but nonsignificant decrease in intraerythrocyte sodium when a mixed group of hypertensive patients and normotensive volunteers were trained for 12 weeks.

Insulin

Since 1923, changes in body mass have been associated with an increase in resting blood pressure and the development of hypertension (116). In recent years, an insulin theory of hypertension has been proposed to help explain the association between body mass, body fat, and hypertension (75,119). According to this theory, insulin resistance develops in the tissue, causing plasma insulin concentrations to increase, which, in turn, increases sympathetic nervous system activity as well as sodium reabsorption by the kidney tubules (30,119).

Normotensive animals consuming a diet high in fat and sucrose will become hypertensive (125) and will exhibit signs of insulin resistance (92). Interestingly, SHR groups have hyperinsulinemia and evidence for insulin resistance (86). When normotensive rats were fed a high-fat, sucrose diet and exercise-trained, the pressures of the free-eating nontrained animals were higher, and those of the free-eating trained animals were lower. When the trained animals were compared to the food-restricted, weight-matched control animals, the resting pressures were similar. Whether similar results would occur in a genetic model for borderline hypertension is unknown.

Prostaglandins

There is good evidence that the vasodilator prostacyclin, as measured by its metabolite 6-keto-prostaglandin $F_{1\alpha}$, increases with exercise, but the rise is similar in athletes and nonathletic control subjects (33). Also, resting 6-keto-prostaglandin $F_{1\alpha}$ did not differ between runners and appropriate control subjects (133). In a controlled, randomized trial of middle-aged men, regular mild physical exercise tended to increase plasma 6-keto-prostaglandin $F_{1\alpha}$ concentration, but the changes were not different from those in the control group (97).

Structural

One theory of hypertension is that structural changes in the arteries will precede the changes in pressure and that this association can be observed by examining the wall/lumen ratios (119). Detailed studies on the effects of endurance training on wall/lumen ratios of select arteries from nontrained and trained WKY and SHR groups indicate that training had no meaningful effect on the wall thickness; however, it significantly increased the area of the lumen, causing the ratio to decrease (119,129) (Figure 43.3). While this effect of training was new for hypertensive rats, the same effect has been found in dogs (139). One speculation from these changes is that an increase in blood flow would be associated with training and that a rarefaction of vessels could be diminished in hypertensive populations.

With the current interest in the role and function of the endothelium in blood pressure regulation, a training study with hypertensive animals would be interesting to conduct.

The Influence of Weight-Resistive Exercises on Blood Pressure

Eight studies on training that were designed to develop strength, and in which a parallel control group was included, could be identified (5,13,18, 41,51,61,62,90); randomization was applied in three (13,18,51). The training period lasted about 10 (5,41,51,90), 16 (13,61,62), or 26 (18) weeks, training frequency was usually three times per week, and the time of each session ranged from 30 to 60 min. Lower body strength increased by 9% to 33%, and upper body strength by 18% to 50% (18,51,61,62). Maximal oxygen uptake remained unchanged, except for a slight 8% increase in one report (51).

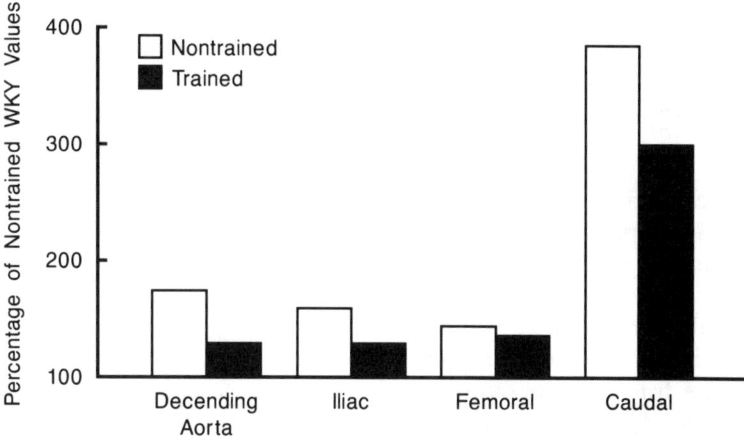

Figure 43.3 The influence of endurance training by male hypertensive rats (SHR) on the wall/lumen ratios of select arteries. Relevant data can be found in references 117 and 129. There were 7-12 animals per group. (© 1991 by Williams and Wilkins, Baltimore. Reprinted by permission. See reference 119.)

In 14- to 17-year-old normotensive male adolescents, a 9-week resistive exercise program did not elicit changes in blood pressure (41). Hurley et al. (61,62) assessed the cardiovascular effects of 16 weeks of high-intensity variable-resistance strength training in healthy 40- to 55-year-old untrained men. Supine diastolic blood pressure decreased significantly, from 84 to 79 mmHg, whereas systolic pressure was not affected. Standing blood pressure as well as pressure measured during treadmill exercise requiring 50% of maximal oxygen uptake were not changed. Coconie et al. (18) randomly assigned 56 healthy men and women (ages 70 to 79 years) to endurance training, strength training, or unchanged activity. Whereas blood pressure decreased from 139/81 mmHg to 135/76 mmHg ($P < .05$ for diastolic blood pressure) with dynamic exercise, pressure did not change significantly in the strength-training group (132/78 mmHg before and after training) and in the control group (137/81 mmHg before and 140/83 mmHg at the end of the control period).

In 28 normotensive men, ages 18 to 26 years, Baechle (5) observed that the blood pressure response to heavy-resistance weight training was not different from the changes in a control group of 14 men, who followed golf classes during the study period; he obtained similar results in young men with borderline hypertension. Harris and Holly (51) studied the effect of circuit weight training, which was defined as the performance of several repetitions using a moderate amount of weight in a continuous fashion. After 9 weeks the training had not changed the systolic blood pressure of 24- to 40-year-old men with moderate hypertension, but the decrease of diastolic blood pressure was significant and was 2.5 mmHg more pronounced than in control subjects. In men and women with moderate hypertension, ages 29 to 59, the blood pressure response to strength training was not significantly different from the observations in the control group (13).

Two studies randomized hypertensive patients to strength training, endurance training, or a control group. Whereas Blumenthal et al. (13) observed that the blood pressure response was similar in the three groups, Coconie et al. (18) found that only endurance training led to a significant decrease of blood pressure. According to Norris et al. (90), however, both endurance and weight training significantly reduce blood pressure; this study can be criticized, however, because of the lack of randomization and the unacceptable 49% dropout rate.

Most studies therefore indicate that strength training does not alter blood pressure, but some have found limited falls of pressure. Any hypotensive effect seems, however, less than what can be achieved with dynamic aerobic training. There is also no evidence from these studies that strength training would increase blood pressure.

The animal studies on this topic have been reviewed elsewhere (119) and provided little insight on training mechanisms. The one study deserving mention is a bar hanging experiment with SHR-SP groups (127). Repeated bouts of static exercise (known to elicit systolic blood pressure increases between 60 to 100 mmHg) were not associated with either higher or lower resting pressures nor with a noticeable incidence of strokes when compared to the nontrained control animals.

Summary

Epidemiological studies suggest an inverse relationship between physical activity or fitness and blood pressure. In a meta-type analysis of controlled longitudinal training studies, the blood pressure response to static training was negligible, whereas the results of dynamic aerobic training seemed to depend on the initial blood pressure status, the efficacy of the training program, and the characteristics of the study. The weighted net change of blood pressure with endurance training averaged -3/-3 mmHg in normotensive subjects, -6/-7 mmHg in borderline hypertensive subjects, and -10/-8 mmHg in hypertensive subjects. In general, the animal training studies support the trends observed in humans. Reductions of blood pressure have also been observed for measurements during exercise and during daytime ambulatory monitoring; sleep blood pressure was, however, not significantly altered. The results on the hemodynamic mechanisms are controversial; it is not clear whether the decrease in blood pressure is related to a lower cardiac output or a lower systemic vascular resistance. Reduced sympathetic activity is most likely involved in the hypotensive response and possibly the renin-aldosterone system, especially in humans.

Acknowledgments

It is a pleasure to acknowledge the secretarial, editing, and proofreading expertise of Ms. Kathleen Wilkin and Ms. Nicole Ausseloos.

References

1. Abboud, F.M. Sympathetic nervous system in hypertension. Hypertension. [Suppl. II]. 4:II-208-II-225; 1982.
2. Adragna, N.C.; Chang, J.L.; Morey, M.C.; Williams, R.S. Effect of exercise on cation transport in human red cells. Hypertens. 7:132-139; 1985.
3. Akinpelu, A.O. Responses of the African hypertensive to exercise training: Preliminary observations. J. Hum. Hypertens. 4:74-76; 1990.
4. Astrand, P.O.; Rodahl, K. Textbook of work physiology. 3rd ed. New York: McGraw-Hill; 1986: 295-340.
5. Baechle, T.R. Effects of heavy resistance weight training on arterial blood pressure and other selected measures in normotensive and borderline hypertensive college men. In: Landry, F.; Orban, W., eds. Sports medicine. Miami: Symposia Specialists; 1978:169-175.
6. Baglivo, H.P.; Fabregues, G.; Burrieza H.; et al. Effect of moderate physical training on left ventricular mass in mild hypertensive persons. Hypertension. [Suppl. I]. 15:I-153-I-156; 1990.
7. Baumbach, G.L.; Dorgin, P.B.; Hart, M.N.; Heistad, D.D. Mechanics of cerebral arterioles in hypertensive rats. Circ. Res. 62:56-64; 1988.
8. Bedford, T.G.; Tipton, C.M. Exercise training and the arterial baroreflex. J. Appl. Physiol. 63:1926-1932; 1987.
9. Bedford, T.G.; Tipton, C.M. Blood pressure responses to LBNP in nontrained and trained hypertensive rats. Med. Sci. Sports Exerc.; [In press].
10. Bedford, T.G.; Tipton, C.M.; Wilson, N.C.; Oppliger, R.A.; Gisolfi, C.V. Maximum oxygen consumption of rats and its changes with various experimental procedures. J. Appl. Physiol. 47:1278-1283; 1979.
11. Benbassat, J.; Froom, P.F. Blood pressure response to exercise as a predictor of hypertension. Arch. Intern. Med. 146:2053-2055; 1986.
12. Blair, S.N.; Goodyear, N.N.; Gibbons, L.W.; Cooper, H. Physical fitness and incidence of hypertension in healthy normotensive men and women. JAMA. 252:487-490; 1984.
13. Blumenthal, J.A.; Siegel, W.C.; Appelbaum, M. Failure of exercise to reduce blood pressure in patients with mild hypertension. JAMA. 266:2098-2104; 1991.
14. Bonanno, J.A.; Lies, J.E. Effects of physical training on coronary risk factors. Am. J. Cardiol. 33:760-764; 1974.
15. Boyer, J.L.; Kasch, F.W. Exercise therapy in hypertensive men. JAMA. 211:1668-1671; 1970.
16. Choquette, G.; Ferguson, R.J. Blood pressure reduction in "borderline" hypertensives following physical training. Can. Med. Assoc. J. 108:699-703; 1973.
17. Cléroux, J.; Péronnet, F.; de Champlain, J. Effects of exercise training on plasma catecholamines and blood pressure in labile hypertensive subjects. Eur. J. Appl. Physiol. 56:550-554; 1987.
18. Coconie, C.C.; Graves, J.E.; Pollock, M.L.; et al. Effect of exercise training on blood pressure in 70- to 79-yr-old men and women. Med. Sci. Sports Exerc. 23:505-511; 1991.

19. Cooper, K.H.; Pollock, M.L.; Martin, R.P.; et al. Physical fitness levels vs selected coronary risk factors: A cross-sectional study. JAMA. 236:166-169; 1976.
20. Coyle, P.; Heisted, D.D. Blood flow through cerebral collateral vessels in hypertensive and normotensive rats. Hypertension. [Suppl.]. 2:II67-II71; 1986.
21. Criqui, M.H.; Mebane, I.; Wallace, R.B.; et al. Multivariate correlates of adult blood pressures in nine North American populations: The lipid research clinics prevalence study. Prev. Med. 11:391-402; 1982.
22. Critz, J.B.; Lipsey, P. Relationships between physical training and DOCA. Proc. Soc. Expl. Bio. Med. 151:552-555; 1976.
23. Deplaen, J.F.; Detry, J.M. Hemodynamic effects of physical training in established arterial hypertension. Acta Cardiol. 35:179-188; 1980.
24. Devine, M.; Sebastian, L.A.; Monnin, K.A.; Tipton, C.M. Training and post-exercise hypotension with hypertensive rats (SHR). Physiologist. [Abstract] 34:267; 1991.
25. DiCarlo, S.E.; Bishop, V.S. Exercise training enhances cardiac afferents inhibition of baroreflex function. Am. J. Physiol. 258:H212-H220; 1990.
26. DiCarlo, S.E., Bishop, V.S. Regional vascular resistance during exercise: Role of cardiac afferents and exercise training. Am. J. Physiol. 258:H842-H847; 1990.
27. DiCarlo, S.E.; Bishop, V.S. Onset of exercise shifts operating point of arterial baroreflex to higher pressures. Am. J. Physiol. 262:H303-H307; 1992.
28. Drummond, H.; Sebastian, L.A.; Edwards, P.K.; Coomes, R.K.; Tipton, C.M. The influence of exercise training and calcium diets on the resting blood pressures of hypertensive rats (SHR). Med. Sci. Sports Exerc. [Abstract] [Suppl. II]. 22:S608; 1990.
29. Duncan, J.J.; Farr, J.E.; Upton, S.J.; et al. The effects of aerobic exercise on plasma catecholamines and blood pressure in patients with mild essential hypertension. JAMA. 254:2609-2613; 1985.
30. Edwards, J.G.; Tipton, C.M. Influences of exogenous insulin on arterial blood pressure measurement of the rat. J. Appl. Physiol. 67:2335-2342; 1989.
31. Ekblom, B.; Kilbom, A.; Soltysiak, J. Physical training, bradycardia and autonomic nervous system. Scand. J. Lab. Invest. 32:251-254; 1973.
32. Fagard, R.; Bielen, E.; Hespel, P.; et al. Physical exercise in hypertension. In: Laragh, J.; Brenner, B., eds. Hypertension: Pathophysiology, diagnosis and management. New York: Raven Press; 1990;1985-1998.
33. Fagard, R.; Grauwels, R.; Groeseneken, D.; et al. Plasma levels of renin, angiotensin II and 6-keto-prostaglandin $F_{1\alpha}$ in endurance athletes. J. Appl. Physiol. 59:947-952; 1985.
34. Fagard, R.; Lijnen, P.; Amery, A. Effects of angiotensin II on arterial pressure, renin and aldosterone during exercise. Eur. J. Appl. Physiol. 54:254-261; 1985.
35. Fagard, R.; M'Buyamba-Kabangu, J.R.; Staessen, J.; et al. Physical activity and blood pressure. In: Bulpitt, C.J., ed. Handbook of hypertension. Vol. 6: Epidemiology of hypertension. Amsterdam: Elsevier Science; 1985:104-130.
36. Fagard, R.; Staessen, J.; Amery, A. Exercise blood pressure and target organ damage in essential hypertension. J. Hum. Hypertens. 5:69-75; 1991.
37. Fagard, R.; Staessen, J.; Thijs, L.; Amery, A. Prognostic significance of exercise versus resting blood pressure in hypertensive men. Hypertension. 17:574-578; 1991.
38. Faraci, F.M.; Mayhan, W.G.; Mayhan, W.H.; Werber, W.H.; Heisted, D.D. Cerebral circulation: Effects of sympathetic nerves and protective mechanisms during hypertension. Circ. Res. [Suppl.] 2:II102-II106; 1987.
39. Fiocchi, R.; Fagard, R.; Vanhees, L.; Bielen, E.; Amery, A. Carotid baroreceptor control of heart rate and physical fitness. In: Fagard, R.H.; Bekaert, I.E., eds. Sport cardiology: Exercise in health and cardiovascular disease. Dordrecht: Martinus Nijhoff Publishers; 1986:129-135.
40. Folsom, A.R.; Caspersen, C.J.; Taylor, H.L.; et al. Leisure time physical activity and its relationship to coronary risk factors in a population-based sample. Am. J. Epidemiol. 121:570-579; 1985.
41. Fripp, R.R.; Hodgson, J.L. Effect of resistive training on plasma lipid and lipoprotein levels in male adolescents. J. Pediatr. 111:926-931; 1987.
42. Gettman, L.R.; Pollock, M.L.; Durstine, J.L.; Physiological responses of men to 1, 3 and 5 day per week training programs. Res. Q. 47:638-646; 1976.
43. Geyssant, A.; Geelen, G.; Denis, C.; et al. Plasma vasopressin, renin activity and aldosterone: Effect of exercise and training. Eur. J. Appl. Physiol. 46:21-30; 1981.
44. Gibbons, L.W.; Blair, S.N.; Cooper, K.H.; Smith, M. Association between coronary heart disease risk factors and physical fitness

in healthy adult women. Circulation. 67:977-983; 1983.

45. Giddens, W.E.; Combos, C.A.; Smith, O.A.; Klein, E.C. Spontaneous hypertension and its equelae in woolly monkeys (lagothrix lagotricha). Lab. Anim. Sci. 7:750-756; 1986.
46. Gilders, R.M.; Voner, C.; Dudley, G.A. Endurance training and blood pressure in normotensive and hypertensive adults. Med. Sci. Sports Exerc. 21:629-636; 1989.
47. Gyntelberg, F.; Meyer, J. Relationship between blood pressure and physical fitness, smoking and alcohol consumption in Copenhagen males aged 40-59. Acta Med. Scand. 195:375-380; 1974.
48. Hagberg, J.M.; Goldring, D., Ehsani, A.A.; et al. Effect of exercise training on the blood pressure and hemodynamic features of hypertensive adolescents. Am. J. Cardiol. 52:763-768; 1983.
49. Hagberg, J.M.; Montain, S.J.; Martin, W.H.; et al. Effect of exercise training in 60- to 69-year-old persons with essential hypertension. Am. J. Cardiol. 64:348-353; 1989.
50. Hansen, H.S.; Froberg, K.; Hyldebrandt, N.; Nielsen, J.R. A controlled study of eight months of physical training and reduction of blood pressure in children: The Odense schoolchild study. Br. Med. J. 303:682-685; 1991.
51. Harris, K.A.; Holly, R.G. Physiological response to circuit weight training in borderline hypertensive subjects. Med. Sci. Sports Exerc.19:246-252; 1987.
52. Hartung, G.H.; Kohl, H.W.; Blair, S.N.; et al. Exercise tolerance and alcohol intake: Blood pressure relation. Hypertension. 16:501-507; 1990.
53. Hespel, P.; Lijnen, P.; Fagard, R.; et al. Changes in erythrocyte sodium and plasma lipids associated with physical training. J. Hypertens. 6:159-166; 1988.
54. Hespel, P.; Lijnen, P.; Van Hoof, R.; et al. Effects of physical endurance training on the plasma renin-angiotensin-aldosterone system in normal man. J. Endocrinol. 116:443-449; 1988.
55. Higuchi, S.; Hashimoto, I.; Yamakawa, K. Effect of exercise training on aortic collagen content of spontaneously hypertensive rats (SHR). Eur. J. Appl. Physiol. 53:330-333; 1985.
56. Hoffmann, P. Endogenous opioid effects elicited by muscle activity: An attempt to explain cardiovascular, analgesic and behavioral mechanisms of exercise. University of Goteborg; 1990. 1-59. Dissertation.
57. Hoffmann, P.; Carlsson, S.; Skarphedinsson, J.O.; Thoren, P. Role of different serotonergic receptors in the long-lasting blood pressure depression following muscle stimulation in the spontaneously hypertensive rat. Acta Physiol. Scand. 129:535-542; 1987.
58. Hoffmann, P.; Friberg, P.; Ely, D.; Thoren, P. Effects of spontaneous running on blood pressure, heart rate and cardiac dimensions in developing and established hypertension in rats. Acta Physiol. Scand. 129:535-542; 1987.
59. Horan, M.J.; Lenfant, C. Epidemiology of blood pressure and predictors of hypertension. Hypertension. [Suppl. I]. 15:I21-I28; 1990.
60. Horan, M.J.; Mockrin, S.C. Hypertension research; The next five years. Hypertension. [Suppl. I]. 15:I25-I28; 1990.
61. Hurley, B.F.; Hagberg, J.M.; Goldberg, A.P.; et al. Resistive training can reduce coronary risk factors without altering $\dot{V}O_2$max or percent body fat. Med. Sci. Sports Exerc. 20:150-154; 1988.
62. Hurley, B.F.; Seals, D.R.; Ehsani, A.A.; et al. Effects of high-intensity strength training on cardiovascular function. Med. Sci. Sports Exerc. 16:483-488; 1984.
63. Jennings, G.L.; Deakin, G.; Korner, P.; et al. What is the dose-response relationship between exercise training and blood pressure? Ann. Med. 23:313-318; 1991.
64. Jennings, G.; Nelson, L.; Nestel, P.; et al. The effects of changes in physical activity on major cardiovascular risk factors, hemodynamics, sympathetic function, and glucose utilization in man: A controlled study of four levels of activity. Circulation. 73:30-40; 1986.
65. Jo, Y.; Arita, M.; Baba, A.; et al. Blood pressure and sympathetic activity following responses to aerobic exercise in patients with essential hypertension. Clin. Exp. Hypertens. [A]. [Suppl. 1]. 11:411-417; 1989.
66. Joint National Committee on Detection, Evaluation, and Treatment of High Blood Pressure. The 1988 report of the joint national committee on detection, evaluation and treatment of high blood pressure. Arch. Intern. Med. 148:1023-1038; 1988.
67. Kinoshita, A.; Urata, H.; Tanabe, Y.; et al. What types of hypertensives respond better to mild exercise therapy? J. Hypertens. [Suppl. 4]. 6:S631-S633; 1988.
68. Kirtisky-Roy, J.A.; Appel, N.M.; Bobbitt, F.G.; Van Loon, G.R. Effects of μ opioid receptor stimulation in the hypothalamic paraventricular nucleus on basal and stress-induced catecholamine secretion and cardiovascular responses. J. Pharmacol. Exp. Ther. 239:814-822; 1986.

69. Kral, J.; Chrąstek, J.; Adamirova, J. The hypotensive effect of physical activity. In: Prevention of ischemic heart disease: Principles and practices. Springfield: Charles C Thomas; 1966:359-371.
70. Kukkonen, K.; Rauramaa, R.; Voutilainen, E.; et al. Physical training of middle-aged men with borderline hypertension. Ann. Clin. Res. 14:139-145; 1982.
71. Kunii, S.; Fukuda, T.; Wakabayashi, K.; Fumino, H.; Hirota, K.; Kita, K. Effect of exercise on blood pressure and attack of cerebrovascular lesions of stroke-prone spontaneously hypertensive rats (SPSHR). Jpn. J. Phys. Educ. 27:35-46; 1982.
72. Kunze, D.L. Rapid resetting of the carotid baroreceptive reflex in the cat. Am. J. Physiol. 241:H802-H806; 1981.
73. Länsimies, E.; Hietanen, E.; Huttunen, J.K.; et al. Metabolic and hemodynamic effects of physical training in middle-aged men. A controlled trial. In: Komi, P.V.; Nelson, R.C.; Morehouse, C.A., eds. Exercise and sport biology. Champaign, IL. Human Kinetics; 1979:199-206.
74. Lawler, J.E.; Barker, G.F.; Hubbard, J.W.; Schaub, R.G. Effects of stress on blood pressure and cardiac hypertrophy in rats with borderline hypertension. Hypertension. 3:496-505; 1981.
75. Lucas, C.P.; Estigarribia, J.A.; Darga, L.I. Insulin and blood pressure in obesity. Hypertension. 7:702-707; 1985.
76. Mann, G.V.; Garrett, H.L.; Farhi, A.; Murray, H.; Billings, F.T. Exercise to prevent coronary heart disease. Am. J. Med. 46:12-27; 1969.
77. Marcus, K.D.; Tipton, C.M. Exercise training and its effects with renal hypertensive rats. J. Appl. Physiol. 59:1410-1415; 1985.
78. Martin, J.E.; Dubbert, P.M.; Cushman, W.C. Controlled trial of aerobic exercise in hypertension. Circulation. 81:1560-1567; 1990.
79. Martin, W.H.; Montgomery, J.; Snell, P.G.; et al. Cardiovascular adaptations to intense swim training in sedentary middle-aged men and women. Circulation. 75:323-330; 1987.
80. M'Buyamba-Kabangu, J.R.; Fagard, R.; Lijnen, P.; Amery, A. Relationship between plasma renin activity and physical fitness in normal subjects. Eur. J. Appl. Physiol. 53:304-307; 1985.
81. Melin, B.; Eclache, J.P.; Geelen, G.; et al. Plasma AVP, neurophysin, renin activity and aldosterone during submaximal exercise performed until exhaustion in trained and untrained men. Eur. J. Appl. Physiol. 44:141-151; 1980.
82. Meredith, I.T.; Friberg, P.; Jennings, G.L.; et al. Exercise training lowers resting renal but not cardiac sympathetic activity in humans. Hypertension. 18:575-582; 1991.
83. Meredith, I.T.; Jennings, G.L.; Esler, M.D.; et al.Time-course of the antihypertensive and autonomic effects of regular endurance exercise in human subjects. J. Hypertens. 8:859-866; 1990.
84. Miall, W.E.; Oldham, P.D. Factors influencing arterial blood pressure in the general population. Clin. Sci. 17:409-444; 1958.
85. Mitchell, J.H. Neural control of the circulation during exercise. Med. Sci. Sports Exerc. 22:141-154; 1990.
86. Mondon, C.E.; Reaven, G.M.; Azhar, S.; Lee, C.M.; Rabkin, R. Abnormal insulin metabolism in rats with spontaneous hypertension. Am. J. Physiol. 257:E491-E498; 1989.
87. Montoye, H.J.; Metzner, H.L.; Keller, J.L.; et al. Habitual physical activity and blood pressure. Med. Sci. Sports Exerc. 4:175-181; 1972.
88. Myrtek, M.; Villinger, U. Psychologische und physiologische wirkungen eines fünfwöchigen ergometertrainings bei gesunden. Med. Klin. 71:1623-1630; 1976.
89. Nelson, L.; Jennings, G.L.; Esler, M.D.; et al. Effect of changing levels of physical activity on blood-pressure and haemodynamics in essential hypertension. Lancet. 2:473-476; 1986.
90. Norris, R.; Carroll, D.; Cochrane, R. The effects of aerobic and anaerobic training on fitness, blood pressure and psychological stress and well-being. J. Psychosom. Res. 34:367-375; 1990.
91. Oluseye, K.A. Cardiovascular responses to exercise in Nigerian women. J. Hum. Hypertens. 4:77-79; 1990.
92. Oscai, L.B. Dietary-induced severe obesity: A rat model. Am. J. Physiol. 242:R212-R215; 1982.
93. Paffenbarger, R.S.; Wing, A.L.; Hyde, R.T.; et al. Physical activity and incidence of hypertension in college alumni. Am. J. Epidemiol. 117:245-257; 1983.
94. Paynter, D.E.; Tipton, C.M.; Tcheng, T.K. Response of immunosympathectomized rats to training. J. Appl. Physiol. 42:935-940; 1977.
95. Pollock, M.L.; Dawson, G.A.; Miller, H.S.; et al. Physiologic responses of men 49 to 65 years of age to endurance training. J. Am. Geriatr. Soc. 24:97-104; 1976.
96. Pollock, M.L.; Miller, H.S.; Janeway, R.; et al. Effects of walking on body composition and cardiovascular function of middle-aged men. J. Appl. Physiol. 30:126-130; 1971.

97. Raumaraa, R.; Salonen, J.T.; Kukkonen-Harjula, K.; et al. Effects of mild physical exercise on serum lipoproteins and metabolites of arachidonic acid: A controlled randomised trial in middle-aged men. Br. Med. J. 288:603-606; 1984.
98. Raven, P.B.; Rohm-Young, D.; Blomqvist, C.G. Physical fitness and cardiovascular response to lower body negative pressure. J. Appl. Physiol. 56:138-144; 1984.
99. Reaven, P.D.; Barrett-Connor, E.; Edelstein, S. Relation between leisure-time physical activity and blood pressure in older women. Circulation. 83:559-565; 1991.
100. Reis, D.J. Experimental evidence in support of a central neural imbalance hypothesis of hypertension. In: Laragh, J.H.; Buhler, F.B.; Sedin, D.W., eds. Frontiers in hypertension research. New York: Springer-Verlag; 1981:341-343.
101. Roman, O.; Camuzzi, A.L.; Villalon, E.; Klenner, C. Physical training program in arterial hypertension. A long-term prospective follow-up. Cardiology. 67:230-243; 1981.
102. Savage, M.V.; Mackie, G.F.; Bolter, C.P. Effect of exercise on the development of salt-induced hypertension in Dahl-S rats. J. Hypertens. 4:289-293; 1986.
103. Scheuer, J.; Malhorata, A.; Hirsch, C.; Capasso, J.; Schaible, T.F. Physiologic cardiac hypertrophy corrects contractile protein abnormalities associated with pathologic hypertrophy in rats. J. Clin. Invest. 70:1300-1305; 1982.
104. Schleusing, G.; Luther, T.; Liebold, F.; Kunadt, F. Der einfluβ des sportlichen trainings auf blutdruckverhalten und leistunsvermögen bei patienten mit hypertonie. Med. Sport. 9:197-201; 1969.
105. Seals, D.R.; Hurley, B.F.; Hagberg, J.M.; et al. Effects of training on systolic time intervals at rest and during isometric exercise in men and women 61 to 64 years old. Am. J. Cardiol. 55:797-800; 1985.
106. Seals, D.R.; Reiling, M.J. Effect of regular exercise on 24-hour arterial pressure in older hypertensive humans. Hypertension. 18:583-592; 1991.
107. Shepherd, R.E.; Kuehne, M.L.; Kenno, K.A.; Durstine, H.L.; Balon, T.W.; Rapp, J.P. Attenuation of blood pressure increases in Dahl salt-sensitive rats by exercise. J. Appl. Physiol. 42:1608-1613; 1982.
108. Skipka, W.; Böning, D.; Deck, K.A.; et al. Reduced aldosterone and sodium excretion in endurance-trained athletes before and during immersion. Eur. J. Appl. Physiol. 42:255-262; 1979.
109. Somers, V.K.; Conway, J.; Johnston, J.; et al. Effects of endurance training on baroreflex sensitivity and blood pressure in borderline hypertension. Lancet. 337:1363-1368; 1991.
110. Staessen, J.; Amery, A.; Fagard, R. Editorial review: Isolated systolic hypertension in the elderly. J. Hypertens. 8:393-405; 1990.
111. Sturek, M.L.; Bedford, T.G.; Tipton, C.M.; Newcomer, L. Acute cardiorespiratory responses of hypertensive rats to swimming and treadmill exercise. J. Appl. Physiol. 57:1328-1332; 1984.
112. Suter, E.; Marti, B.; Tschopp, A.; et al. Effects of self-monitored jogging on physical fitness, blood pressure and serum lipids: A controlled study in sedentary middle-aged men. Int. J. Sports. Med. 11:425-432; 1990.
113. Suzuki, S.; Oshima, S.; Higuchi, M. Influence of physical exercise and nutrition on blood pressure of SHR. Jpn. Heart J. [Suppl. I]. 20:365-370; 1979.
114. Tanabe, Y.; Urata, H.; Kiyonaga, A.; et al. Changes in serum concentrations of taurine and other amino acids in clinical antihypertensive exercise therapy. Clin. Exp. Hypertens. [A]. 11:149-165; 1989.
115. Taylor, H.L. Occupational factors in the study of coronary heart disease and physical activity. Can. Med. Assoc. J. 96:825-831; 1967.
116. Terry, A.H. Obesity and hypertension. JAMA. 31:1283-1284; 1923.
117. Tipton, C.M. Exercise, training and hypertension. In: Terjung, R.L., ed. Exercise and sport sciences. Indianapolis: Benchmark; 1984:245-306.
118. Tipton, C.M. Determinants of $\dot{V}O_2max$: Insights gained from nonhuman species. In: Vollestad, N.K.; Sejersted, O.M., eds. Acta physiol. scand.: Exercise in human physiology. [Suppl. 536]. Blackwell; 1986:128:33-43.
119. Tipton, C.M. Exercise, training and hypertension: An update. In: Holloszy, J.O., ed. Exerc. Sport Sci. Rev. Baltimore: Waverly Press; 1991:19:447-505.
120. Tipton, C.M.; Matthes, R.D.; Bedford, T.G. The influence of training on the blood pressure changes during lower-body negative pressure in rats. Med. Sci. Sports Exerc. 14:81-90; 1982.
121. Tipton, C.M.; Matthes, R.D.; Callahan, A.; Tcheng, T.K.; Lais, T. The role of chronic exercise on resting blood pressure of normotensive and hypertensive rats. Med. Sci. Sports 9:168-177; 1977.
122. Tipton, C.M.; Matthes, R.D.; Marcus, K.D.; Rowlett, K.A.; Leininger, J.R. Influences of exercise, intensity, age and medication on

resting systolic pressure of SHR populations. J. Appl. Physiol. 55:1305-1310; 1983.

123. Tipton, C.M.; Matthes, R.D.; Vailas, A.C.; Schnoebelen, C.L. The response of the Galago senegalensis to physical training. Comp. Biochem. Physiol. [A]. 63:29-36; 1979.

124. Tipton, C.M.; McMahon, S.; Leininger, J.R.; Pauli, E.L.; Lauber, C. Exercise training and incidence of cerebrovascular lesions in stroke-prone spontaneously hypertensive rats. J. Appl. Physiol. 68:1080-1085; 1990.

125. Tipton, C.M.; Monnin, K.; Devine, M.; Drummond, H.; Coomes, R.; Sebastian, L. Endurance training and hemodynamic changes in normotensive rats consuming a diet high in fat and sucrose. Med. Sci. Sports Exerc. 24:S93; 1992.

126. Tipton, C.M.; Overton, J.M.; Pepin, R.B.; Edwards, J.G.; Wegner, J.; Youmans, E.M. Influence of exercise training on resting blood pressures of Dahl rats. J. Appl. Physiol. 63:342-346; 1987.

127. Tipton, C.M.; Overton, J.M.; Pepin, R.B.; Edwards, J.G.; Wegner, J.; Youmans, E.M. Response of hypertensive rats to acute and chronic conditions of static exercise. Am. J. Physiol. 254:H592-H598; 1988.

128. Tipton, C.M.; Sebastian, L.; Overton, J.M.; Woodman, C.R.; Williams, S.B. Chronic exercise and its hemodynamic influences on resting blood pressure of hypertensive rats. J. Appl. Physiol. 71:2206-2210; 1991.

129. Tipton, C.M.; Sturek, M.S.; Oppliger, R.A.; Matthes, R.D.; Overton, J.M.; Edwards, J.G. Responses of SHR to combinations of chemical sympathectomy, adrenal demedullation and training. Am. J. Physiol. 247:H109-H118; 1984.

130. Tomanek, R.J.; Gisolfi, C.V.; Bauer, C.A.; Palmer, P.J. Coronary vasodilator reserve, capillarity and mitochondria in trained hypertensive rats. J. Appl. Physiol. 64:1179-1185; 1988.

131. Urata, H.; Tanabe, Y.; Kiyonaga, A.; et al. Antihypertensive and volume-depleting effects of mild exercise on essential hypertension. Hypertension. 9:245-252; 1987.

132. Van Hoof, R.; Hespel, P.; Fagard, R.; et al. Effect of endurance training on blood pressure at rest, during exercise and during 24 hours in sedentary men. Am. J. Cardiol. 63:945-949; 1989.

133. Viinika, L.; Vuori, J.; Ylikorkala, O. Lipid peroxides, prostacyclins and tromboxane A_2 in runners during acute exercise. Med. Sci. Sports Exerc. 16:275-277; 1984.

134. Vroman, N.B.; Healy, J.A.; Kertzer, R. Cardiovascular response to lower body negative pressure (LBNP) following endurance training. Aviat. Space Environ. Med. 59:330-334; 1988.

135. Walgenbach, S.E.; Donald, D.E. Cardiopulmonary reflexes and arterial pressure during rest and exercise in dogs. Am. J. Physiol. 244:H362-H369; 1983.

136. Weiss, L. Adaptative cardiovascular changes to physical training in spontaneously hypertensive and normotensive rats. Cardiovasc. Res. 12:329-333; 1978.

137. Wolfe, L.A.; Cunningham, D.A.; Rechnitzer, P.A.; Nichol, P.M. Effects of endurance training on left ventricular dimensions in healthy men. J. Appl. Physiol. 47:207-212; 1979.

138. World Health Organization. Report of a WHO expert committee: Arterial hypertension, technical report series 628. Geneva: World Health Organization; 1978.

139. Wyatt, H.L.; Mitchell, J.H. Influences of physical training on the hearts of dogs. Circ. Res. 35:883-889; 1974.

140. Yamori, Y.; Horie, R.; Akguchi, I.; Kihara, M.; Nara, N.; Lovenburg, W. Symptomological classification in the development of stroke in stroke-prone spontaneously hypertensive rats. Jpn. Circ. J. 46:274-283; 1982.

141. Zambraski, E.J. Renal regulation of fluid homeostasis during exercise. In: Gisolfi, C.V.; Lamb, D.R., eds. Perspective in exercise science and sports medicine (vol. 3), fluid homeostasis during exercise. Carmel, IN: Benchmark Press; 1990:247-280.

Chapter 44

Physical Activity, Fitness, and Type I Diabetes

Adria Giacca
Z. Qing Shi
Errol B. Marliss
Bernard Zinman
Mladen Vranic

Type I diabetes affects about 10% of the diabetic population in North America and Europe. It is a disease of the B cells of the pancreatic islets, which are destroyed by an immunologically mediated inflammatory reaction. Although lifestyle factors do not appear to have an obvious role in the etiology and pathogenesis of the disease, physical activity has long been regarded as beneficial to those with Type I diabetes. Joslin considered exercise one of three basic components in the management of Type I diabetes (36). The recommendation of exercise in addition to insulin and diet was based on the observation that it can decrease plasma glucose acutely in people with insulin-treated diabetes (101). Postprandial exercise has also been shown to improve meal-related glucose excursions (62). One would expect these acute responses to have a summation effect on overall glucose control in physically active diabetic patients. However, the American Diabetes Association Position Statement on Diet and Exercise (1990) states, "Exercise programs have not been exclusively shown to improve glycemic control in people with IDDM" (2). It appears from the few studies in the literature that compensatory adjustment in caloric intake or insulin dosage balances the acute hypoglycemic effects of exercise training (see the section "Effect of Training on Glucoregulation and Glycemic Control").

The ADAPSDE encourages people with Type I diabetes to exercise "because of the potential to improve cardiovascular fitness and psychological well-being and for social interaction and recreation" (2), which is essentially why exercise is advised for the general population. Patients with Type I diabetes as members of a younger, more active group than those with Type II, generally choose to exercise. The ADAPSDE recommends that "safe participation in all forms of exercise, consistent with an individual's lifestyle should be a primary goal for people with IDDM." Diet and insulin therapy should be optimized and combined with self-monitoring of blood glucose (SMBG). In the general population, physical activity is increasingly recommended for its potential to provide protection from cardiovascular disease. Although few data are available, current recommendations suggest that exercise training is at least as beneficial for people with Type I diabetes as for the general population (see the section "Effects of Training on the Incidence of Cardiovascular Disease").

Metabolic Response to Exercise

Exercise requires mobilization of metabolic fuels to meet the energy requirements of contracting muscle. In the resting state, skeletal muscle depends almost exclusively on fatty acid oxidation for energy, whereas during exercise carbohydrates are important oxidative fuels. Generation of adenosine triphosphate (ATP) from glycolysis in cytoplasm of the myocyte is more rapid than from fat oxidation in the mitochondria. Under anaerobic conditions, carbohydrates are obligate substrates, and ATP can only be generated from glycolysis. Thus, when rapid regeneration of ATP is required or oxygen is limited, such as at the onset of exercise or during short-term intense exercise, carbohydrate is the prominent fuel. Muscle glycogen is used first, then circulating glucose. With mild to moderate exercise (to 70% $\dot{V}O_2max$), which can be sustained longer, oxidative fuels are used in sequence: Muscle glycogen, then circulating glucose, and finally free fatty acids (FFAs) become the major energy-generating substrate. Twice the energy can be gained from oxidation of triglyceride as from glycogen. Hence, economy of fat storage makes this the most efficient fuel for exercise of long duration (28,86).

Contractile activity may trigger muscle uptake of circulating glucose in the absence of insulin (63). The mechanism has not been clearly elucidated, but there is strong evidence that contraction-related stimulation of myofibrillar ATPase activity represents the principal metabolic event leading to increased muscle glucose uptake (28,86). Contraction per se can also stimulate muscle glycogenolysis in the absence of catecholamines (69). Contractile activity in muscle displaces glucose transporters from an intracellular pool to plasma membrane, as does insulin (24,32). Increased glucose uptake (GU) induced by muscular contraction persists for several hours, both in the presence and in the absence of insulin (27). Postexercise, circulating glucose is utilized to rebuild muscle glycogen stores. Contractile activity and insulin have additive effects on GU during and for 2 hr after muscle contraction in vitro, indicating the two mechanisms are independent (63), although in vivo, the effects are synergistic (22,98). Insulin sensitivity increases 3 hr after in vitro muscle contraction, resulting in a superadditive effect on GU (69), magnified in vivo.

In contrast to carbohydrates, fat stores in muscle are few. Circulating FFAs are thus the main lipid source for contracting muscle. Insulin's antilipolytic effect may regulate muscle GU indirectly during exercise by limiting FFA availability. In dogs, we found a very significant inverse correlation between prevailing FFA levels and metabolic clearance rate (MCR) of glucose during exercise (10). Also, beta-blockade reduced FFA concentrations and normalized glucose MCR in the exercising alloxan-diabetic dog, a model of partial insulin deficiency (95). Beta-blockade did not increase glucose MCR in exercising depancreatized dogs (total insulin deficiency) (10). However, depancreatized dogs had greatly elevated FFA levels, which may have a maximum effect in inhibiting MCR. When available energy from lipids was reduced by combining beta-blockade with an inhibitor of FFA oxidation, GU and MCR markedly increased during exercise despite the total absence of insulin (77,99).

To meet the increased fuel demands of exercise, alterations in the production of energy substrate are essential (28,86). Insulin, glucagon, and catecholamines are primarily responsible for regulating hepatic glucose production (HGP) and FFA mobilization from adipose tissue during exercise. Typically, insulin decreases, and glucagon, catecholamines, growth hormone, and cortisol increase in concentration. Peripheral adrenergic activity (either sympathetic nervous or adrenal medullary) is a regulator of pancreatic hormone secretion. Catecholamines stimulate glucagon secretion in the A cell via α and β-receptors. In contrast, in the pancreatic B cell, α inhibition prevails over β stimulation of insulin release.

During mild to moderate exercise, HGP increases in response to increased glucagon/insulin ratio (93,96,97). In humans, plasma glucagon consistently increases only during hypoglycemic or prolonged exercise, and as a result the glucagon/insulin ratio increases mainly because of suppression of insulin secretion. For the HGP increase, catecholamines are important only during prolonged exercise (59) and perhaps at the onset of exercise (57). Their major role during mild to moderate exercise is as lipid-mobilizing hormones. With this exercise, carbohydrate oxidation increases, but fat remains the predominant substrate utilized. Changes in glucose turnover are moderate (to two-fold). Increased GU is matched by a corresponding increase in HGP primarily from glycogenolysis, whereas gluconeogenesis is more important during prolonged exercise. Thus, plasma glucose concentrations are remarkably stable in nondiabetic individuals (101). Glucose homeostasis is preserved even during exercise after 2 weeks' starvation, since gluconeogenesis seems to respond as rapidly as glycogenolysis to meet the peripheral need for glucose (58). In nondiabetic subjects, hypoglycemia occurs only after prolonged exercise, reflecting greatly diminished carbohydrate stores (8).

During intense exercise, rapid generation of ATP from glycolysis necessitates greater increments in GU, which increases four-fold. Interestingly, the rise in HGP is even greater. Thus, in nondiabetic individuals there is a small hyperglycemic response during exercise, which becomes greater as exhaustion approaches and persists for up to 1 hr. During exercise insulin does not decrease and recovery is associated with hyperinsulinemia. There is a moderate increment in glucagon and an impressive rise in catecholamines (15-fold), which become the principal mediators of the HGP increase (54,55). Exercise in daily life is a combination of periods of different work intensity, often interspersed with periods of rest, and is commonly performed after meal ingestion. In normal subjects, moderate exercise for 30 min after breakfast results in an attenuated rise in both glucose and insulin levels. Meal carbohydrates seem to provide the principal energy source to the contracting muscle, as shown by a respiratory quotient close to unity and an attenuated rise in FFA levels (62).

Metabolic Response to Exercise in Type I Diabetes

In people with Type I diabetes, the body's inability to regulate insulin secretion creates an impediment when it tries to meet the enhanced metabolic requirements of exercise. These needs are met, but often exogenous insulin therapy results in less-than-optimal balance of substrate utilization and consequent large swings in blood glucose during exercise. The metabolic response in the subject with diabetes also varies with exercise intensity.

Mild to Moderate Exercise

During mild to moderate exercise, the main determinant of the metabolic response is the degree of insulinization achieved with therapy (101). The effect of exercise on glucose homeostasis in diabetes has been found to vary under three insulinemic conditions (28,37,86,87): normoinsulinemia, hypoinsulinemia, and hyperinsulinemia.

Normoinsulinemia. When patients with Type I diabetes exercised during a constant insulin infusion that maintained normoglycemia, the HGP response was either insufficient (78) or just adequate (101) to prevent a fall in blood glucose. It is likely that when insulin is infused peripherally, a smaller decrease in insulin delivery is required during exercise than when it is secreted portally, as in nondiabetic subjects. Peripheral insulin infusion generates portal hypoinsulinemia, which may facilitate actions of the counterregulatory hormones to increase HGP during exercise. In practice, normoinsulinization is difficult to achieve with subcutaneous insulin treatment, and therefore patients vary from hypo- to hyperinsulinization.

Hypoinsulinemia. Generally, GU increases similarly in both diabetic and nondiabetic subjects. However, in nondiabetic subjects, this is due to increased MCR, whereas in subjects with inadequately controlled diabetes it is mainly the result of the increased mass action of hyperglycemia, coupled with a smaller increment in MCR (88). In diabetic dogs, we observed a highly significant inverse correlation between prevailing plasma glucose levels and the rise in MCR during exercise (77). Although GU may be normal in hypoinsulinized patients with Type I diabetes, a smaller percentage of glucose utilized is completely oxidized (45,61). Thus, individuals with Type I diabetes in poor control rely to a greater extent on fat metabolism.

Exercise can result in further deterioration of glycemic control in patients with severe insulin deficiency. When subjects with Type I diabetes who were deprived of insulin for a prolonged period (18 to 48 hr) underwent a 3 hr bout of exercise, blood glucose rose further (6). It has been shown that glucose increases during exercise in depancreatized dogs with severe insulin deficiency, because of an attenuated increase in GU and a normal increase in HGP (85,87). It remains unsettled whether the attenuated rise in GU is due to the lack of a direct effect of insulin on glucose transport or of an indirect effect to restrain lipolysis. In severely underinsulinized subjects with Type I diabetes, the exercise-induced increase in FFAs can lead to ketoacidosis (6). The deleterious effects of underinsulinization are not exclusively due to diminished insulin levels; exercise in poorly controlled diabetes (6,81,94,95) is characterized by excessive increases in counterregulatory hormones. The excessive counterregulatory response is normalized by insulin therapy (81).

Hyperinsulinemia. Adequate insulin is important to avoid aggravating the diabetic state during exercise. However, a more common response to exercise in patients with insulin-treated diabetes is a fall in plasma glucose, which in euglycemic patients may proceed to hypoglycemia. Glucose decreases in patients treated with subcutaneous insulin administration because of overinsulinization during exercise. Exercise can accelerate insulin absorption from the subcutaneous tissue, particularly if the injection site is in an exercising part of the body and insulin is injected before or at the onset of exercise (7,37,80,101). A fall in blood glucose, however, may occur during exercise in subjects with Type I diabetes even when insulin mobilization from the injection site is not accelerated (38). The crucial factor seems to be the timing of exercise during the ascending part or peak of the insulin-absorption curve. Sustained insulin levels during exercise may enhance peripheral GU; however, the major effect is attenuation of the rise in HGP. Thus, the release in glucose from the liver cannot match the rate of peripheral GU, and blood glucose concentration falls (37,101).

For people with Type I diabetes, hypoglycemia is a common problem not only during or immediately after exercise but also up to several hours following. This mechanism has not been adequately investigated. It is thought to be mainly a peripheral mechanism, due to increased muscle glucose uptake for glycogen synthesis in the previously exercised muscle groups and to the related increase in insulin sensitivity (28,86). Extent and timing of overinsulinization depend on the modality of insulin treatment (see the subsection "Risks of Exercise and Practical Recommendations").

Intense Exercise

The response of patients with Type I diabetes to intense exercise is an exaggeration of the normal hyperglycemic response (55,56). Only subjects with moderately to well-controlled diabetes have been studied. When patients with Type I diabetes exercised during a constant insulin infusion that maintained normoglycemia, HGP and GU increased during and decreased after exercise similarly to nondiabetic subjects (54,68). Plasma insulin was not different from normal and remained constant during exercise, but it was "clamped" at this level by the constant infusion rate during recovery. The absence of an increase in insulin had marked glucoregulatory implications. Glycemia increased to somewhat higher levels than in nondiabetic subjects and failed to return to preexercise concentrations. This was due to the failure of MCR to remain as elevated as in nondiabetic subjects. In contrast, glucose uptake followed a normal pattern. This was presumably due to a mass effect of hyperglycemia in influencing its own disposal. With continuous subcutaneous insulin infusion kept constant during and after exercise, hyperglycemic responses analogous to those observed with intravenous insulin occur (74). Subcutaneous and intravenous insulin studies suggest that at higher preexercise glucose concentrations, the recovery hyperglycemia is likely to be greater (54). Patients treated with subcutaneous insulin injections have not been studied.

Postprandial Exercise

If patients with Type I diabetes who are treated with a closed-loop artificial pancreas exercise in the postprandial period, the postprandial glycemic excursion is attenuated as in nondiabetic subjects. There is an appropriate 30% decrease in insulin requirements. When the postprandial insulin infusion rate is not decreased, hypoglycemia occurs (62). In patients with Type I diabetes treated with subcutaneous insulin injection, postprandial exercise reduced peak glycemia for breakfast and lunch, when the daily insulin dose was unchanged. However, the effect was variable: Some patients showed improved glucose levels during lunch only, and some showed no improvement at all (16).

Risks of Exercise and Practical Recommendations

Risks of Hypoglycemia and Hyperglycemia

With proper instructions and careful monitoring, most patients with uncomplicated Type I diabetes can exercise safely (2). Specific guidelines vary according to type, intensity, duration of exercise, timing and type of diet and insulin therapy, and glycemic control (28,34). In general, metabolic control is more easily achieved and the risk of hypoglycemia is lessened if exercise can be planned. Patients with diabetes should not exercise when under- or overinsulinized, so SMBG is mandatory before vigorous or unplanned physical activity. If blood glucose is greater than 16.5 mM, or less than 4.0 mM and decreasing, exercise should be postponed and insulin or food should be taken. Exercising people with Type I diabetes should always have glucose-reading strips and a readily absorbable form of carbohydrate available. The exercise-induced increase in catecholamine levels may produce symptoms that could be mistaken for those related to hypoglycemia, and vice versa.

Therefore, SMBG is very important to adjust carbohydrate intake before, during, and after exercise to avoid postexercise hypoglycemia. Although not a safeguard against hypoglycemia, it may be helpful to avoid injecting insulin 60 to 90 min before exercise and to use an injection site (e.g., the abdominal wall) that is not in the area being exercised in order to avoid rapid mobilization of insulin.

Hypoglycemia is more likely to occur when free insulin levels are maximum or rising. Patients with diabetes who are treated with conventional insulin therapy (one or two daily injections of intermediate insulin with or without short-acting insulin) should not exercise at the peak of action of the intermediate insulin, as inferred by the rate of change of blood glucose in the same individual. It has been recommended that exercise should ideally occur 1 to 3 hr after a meal in these patients. If exercise is planned, a reduction of both short- and intermediate-acting insulin may be required according to blood glucose. The disadvantage of a reduction of the insulin dose is underinsulinization if exercise is not carried out.

The overall risk of hypoglycemia is greater with intensive (multiple-injection regimens or continuous subcutaneous insulin infusion [CSII]) than with conventional insulin treatment and is directly proportional to the degree of glycemic normalization (21). However, in the exercise context, these treatment modalities may provide a distinct advantage over standard therapy because they allow for adjustment of the insulin dose before, during, and after exercise. In anticipation of postprandial exercise, depending on timing and duration of exercise and on initial blood glucose concentration, the premeal bolus of insulin may be reduced by one half to two thirds (79). Patients on intensive insulin treatment can safely exercise in postabsorptive and postprandial states, because free insulin levels in these patients are lower postabsorptively than postprandially. With these regimens, the decrease of exogenous insulin concentrations, imitating the exercise-induced decrease of endogenous insulin in nondiabetic subjects, may contribute to the relatively small glycemic decrease induced by exercise in the late postprandial period (about 3 hours after meals) (83,84). For postabsorptive exercise, patients on CSII do not necessarily require adjustment of the basal infusion rate, although for exercise of intermediate to long duration it is prudent to reduce the basal rate by 30% to 50% (29,74). With a multiple-injection regimen featuring insulin boluses at each meal and intermediate insulin at bedtime, and with ultralente-based intensive therapy, free insulin levels between meals are generally less elevated than with CSII. Correspondingly, the risk of hypoglycemia during postabsorptive exercise is even lower (74). With an ultralente-based regimen, the risk of hypoglycemia is less with prebreakfast than with late afternoon exercise (73). Where feasible, exercise earlier in the day is advised for those with Type I diabetes to avoid delayed hypoglycemic events at night.

Exercise with multiple-injection regimens is clearly associated with fewer practical problems than exercise with insulin pumps. Patients on CSII often remove the pumps before exercise, due to vulnerability of the subcutaneous infusion site to trauma. This lessens the risk of hypoglycemia. Administration of a small supplementary dose of insulin before pump removal may or may not be indicated, according to SMBG. With bouts of intense exercise, where the prevalent response in patients with Type I diabetes is an accentuation of the normal hyperglycemic response, consumption of rapidly assimilated carbohydrate may lead to excessive hyperglycemia after exercise. Patients engaged in such activity should probably aim for near normoglycemia before exercise and rigorously self-monitor after each exercise bout to establish patterns. They should also develop flexible strategies to deal with various responses. In these patients, hyperinsulinemia during exercise may not prevent normal glucose mobilization and could indeed be appropriate for the postexercise period. This needs further study before any guidelines can be developed (54).

In summary, many variables affect the metabolic response to exercise in Type I diabetes. Some general guidelines can be suggested, but the ADAP-SDE states: "A uniform recommendation for preventing hypoglycemia and improving metabolic response to exercise cannot be made. Rather, self-monitoring of blood glucose should be incorporated into the exercise program to provide the glycemic information necessary to adjust the patient's diet or insulin dosage" (2).

Exercise in Patients With Complications of Diabetes

The risk of exercise in patients with diabetic complications has not been objectively assessed; however, clinicians generally have been cautious in recommending exercise to patients with more than mild diabetic complications (2,28,34,75). In proliferative retinopathy, high-intensity exercise such as isometric weight lifting, head-down positions, jarring of the head, and all movements that can interfere with venous return from the retina are traditionally contraindicated because of the possibility of developing retinal or vitreous hemorrhages (3) and retinal detachment. For the same reasons, these forms of exercise are contraindicated for a few weeks after laser treatment.

In patients with peripheral neuropathy, pounding movements of the lower extremities such as jogging and running may cause soft-tissue and bone injury of the insensitive foot. Proper footwear should be worn by weight-bearing feet, and non-weight-bearing or arm exercise might be indicated. When neuropathic ulcerations are present, the foot should be kept at rest.

Patients with autonomic neuropathy should maintain proper hydration and electrolyte balance during prolonged exercise in a warm climate, because thermoregulatory responses, including sweating, are often abnormal, and the response to dehydration is reduced. Exercise tolerance is impaired in patients with pronounced autonomic neuropathy; the maximal heart rate is lower, and the resting heart rate is higher. These patients are prone to hypotensive episodes during exercise. However, exercising in water, which facilitates venous return, might still be done. When cardiovascular symptoms are present at rest (i.e., orthostatic hypotension), exercise is traditionally contraindicated because of the risk of syncope and cardiac arrhythmia. Interestingly, in asymptomatic patients with signs of autonomic neuropathy (decreased beat-to-beat variations) and an impaired heart rate response to graded exercise, counterregulatory hormone responses were impaired, but metabolic responses such as the fall in glycemia and increase in lactate levels were similar to those in subjects with Type I diabetes without autonomic neuropathy. The dissociation between hormonal and metabolic responses may be interpreted as either a lack of essential influence of the measured hormones to graded exercise or a change in tissue sensitivity to these hormones (31).

Patients with diabetic nephropathy and heavy proteinuria risk acute renal failure when dehydrated. Besides leading to dehydration, especially when autonomic neuropathy is present, exercise can also increase the protein excretion rate (60). It is unlikely that exercise interferes with the course of diabetic nephropathy, but exercise is poorly tolerated in people with chronic renal failure.

Cardiovascular disease is increased in Type I and Type II diabetes populations and occurs at an earlier age than in nondiabetic people. In patients with coronary heart disease, exercise may precipitate angina pectoris, myocardial infarction, or cardiac arrhythmias. However, in stable coronary heart disease, increased rather than decreased physical activity is recommended for secondary prevention. Supervised exercise training programs are also included in postinfarct rehabilitation. No controlled studies on physical activity in diabetic patients with coronary heart disease have been conducted. Because cardiac damage is generally more extensive, and small vessel disease and cardiomyopathy may be present, more caution is probably advised than in nondiabetic people. Diabetic patients with coronary heart disease are often asymptomatic (64), so screening is essential. An exercise-stress ECG prior to embarking on an exercise program is recommended for all patients older than 35 (75). Exercise is contraindicated in the 6 weeks postinfarct because of the possibility that diabetes-associated increased incidence of arrhythmia after infarct (9) may be further augmented by exercise. It is contraindicated for those with high degrees of heart failure or who have unstable or intractable angina.

Peripheral vessel disease is more extensive, but it is generally asymptomatic in diabetics until ischemic lesions occur. With mild intermittent claudication, increased rather than decreased physical activity is advised. In patients with ulcers, rest of the ischemic foot is one of the mainstays of treatment. In patients with recurrent transient ischemic attacks (TIAs), exercise is traditionally contraindicated because perfusion of the brain may be jeopardized in ischemic areas by exercise-induced lowering of systemic vascular resistance.

Effect of Training on Glucoregulation and Glycemic Control

Several cross-sectional and longitudinal studies have shown that physical training increases insulin sensitivity (42). Insulin action in trained distance runners is enhanced in muscle, liver, and adipose tissue (70). The changes in insulin sensitivity are at least partially independent of changes in body composition. Human studies evaluating the effect of training on insulin binding to blood cells have given mixed results (41), as have the results of animal studies in insulin target tissues (both adipocytes and skeletal muscle) (12,19,92). Postbinding events such as increased glucose transport and changes in intracellular glucose metabolism appear to be the major causes of the increased insulin effect (92). Glycogen synthase activity of skeletal muscle is increased by physical training (82), as are enzymes of oxidative metabolism (33). It has been shown that the increase in insulin sensitivity associated with physical training is in part transient (39). Acute exercise in untrained subjects is also associated with increased insulin sensitivity, which is thought to be related to the depletion of both muscle and liver glycogen stores (11). It was hypothesized that the improvement in insulin action that occurs with training could simply be due to cumulative action of single bouts of exercise (42). However, it is also possible that training may increase the capacity of muscle to utilize glucose by activating slow-onset mechanisms, such as increasing the content of oxidative enzymes. Long-term changes in body composition, such as decreased adiposity and increased muscle mass, could also contribute to improvement in insulin sensitivity (75). The increase in insulin sensitivity that occurs with training may or may not translate into enhanced glucose tolerance in nondiabetic subjects, but it results in decreased insulin levels.

Similarly to nondiabetic subjects, insulin sensitivity, as assessed by the euglycemic clamp technique, is increased following training in patients with Type I diabetes who are on conventional (47,89) or insulin pump (100) treatment. In one study, in which tracer methods were employed in combination with the glucose clamp, hepatic insulin sensitivity, as judged by suppression of HGP at high physiological insulin levels, was not affected by training (100). Insulin binding on circulating erythrocytes was found variably affected (4,100). In skeletal muscle biopsies, binding was not affected, but glycogen synthase activity was increased by training (5). Training also increased the activity of some oxidative enzymes (89).

Also in contrast to what is the case for Type II diabetes, there is no evidence that improvement in insulin sensitivity induced by training results in a beneficial effect on long-term diabetic control. The conclusions of the studies carried out before development of the glycosylated hemoglobin assay, in which control was evaluated by multiple determinations of glycemia or glycosuria, are controversial (1,18,25, 49,51,53). We found 14 studies that evaluated the response of glycosylated hemoglobin (HbA_1 or HbA_{1c}) to training in Type I diabetes. Small sample size and lack of adequate controls characterize most of these studies. Only 4 studies found a significant reduction of glycosylated hemoglobin.

Dahl-Jorgensen et al. (20) first used HbA_1 to assess the metabolic effect of physical training in children with diabetes. They demonstrated a significant fall of 8% in HbA_1 levels following a 5-month exercise program of twice weekly 1-hr sessions in 14 prepubertal children. $\dot{V}0_2$max did not increase, suggesting low-intensity activity. HbA_1 levels were analyzed 5 months after completion of the study and fell in 7 of 8 control subjects. In addition, other indices of metabolic control, such as blood and urinary glucose, did not change. Campaigne et al. (13) carried out a study in 9 children with Type I diabetes subjected to exercise for 25 min three times per week for 12 weeks at about 80% maximum heart rate. $\dot{V}0_2$ max increased 7%, and HbA_1 and fasting blood glucose decreased without changes in insulin dosage. Both studies (13,20), which included sedentary control subjects, were done in subjects who had poorly controlled diabetes with HbA_1 above 13%.

Bak et al. (5) studied 7 adults with Type I diabetes on a 60-min, three-times-per-week exercise program for 6 weeks. $\dot{V}0_2$max increased 7%. They found a 10% reduction in insulin dosage and very minor improvement of HbA_{1c} (7.9% ± 1.4% to 7.7% + 1.5%). In the study of Peterson et al. (66), HbA_1 decreased 40% in adults with Type I diabetes during a 10-month exercise program, but the effects of exercise could not be isolated from those of split-dose insulin treatment and SMBG initiated at the same time. In all other studies no effect was seen with training programs of up to 6 months' duration in either adults or children with Type I diabetes (4,30,35,47, 71,89-91,100,102). In general, body weight was unchanged or increased. Insulin dose was unchanged or decreased. Only three of the studies (35,47,100) included a nontrained control group.

Wallberg-Henriksson et al. (89) studied 9 adult males with Type I diabetes under moderate control (HbA_1 was about 10%) undergoing 60 min of exercise at 150 bpm two to three times per week for 16 weeks. $\dot{V}0_2$max increased 8%. Glycosylated hemoglobin did not change, nor did 24-hr glycosuria despite a 20% increase in insulin sensitivity. Insulin dose did not change significantly, although it was reduced on exercise days in some patients to prevent hypoglycemia. Body weight was unchanged. The same authors (90) studied a group of 10 adult males with Type I diabetes who had similar initial values of HbA_1 and who were submitted to a shorter (8-week) training program (45 min at 150 bpm, three times per week). $\dot{V}0_2$max increased by 13%. HbA_1 and blood glucose were unchanged. Muscle capillary density, which increased with training in control subjects, failed to increase in subjects with diabetes—a probable expression of microangiopathy in this disorder.

Yki-Jarvinen et al. (100) studied 7 adults with Type I diabetes on CSII who underwent training sessions of 60 min at 150 bpm four times per week for 6 weeks. $\dot{V}0_2$max increased 8%. The insulin dose was reduced to prevent hypoglycemia. Body weight was unchanged, but to avoid weight loss during training, exercising patients had an extra snack during each session. HbA_1 was near normal before and did not change, although insulin sensitivity increased. No change occurred in mean daily blood glucose concentrations, *M* values, or glycosuria pre- and posttraining. Zinman et al. showed that the main reason glycosylated hemoglobin is not improved by training in Type I diabetes may be caloric intake readjustment (102). Thirteen adults with Type I diabetes exercised 45 min at 160 bpm three times per week for 12 weeks. $\dot{V}0_2$max increased 28%. The moderately elevated HbA_1 (approximately 10%) and fasting blood glucose were not improved posttraining, despite an acute glucose-lowering effect of exercise throughout the exercise period. Body weight, insulin dose, and frequency of hypoglycemic events were unchanged. Diet histories showed a 280 kcal/day increase in caloric intake. In 9 adolescents with Type I diabetes who were submitted to the same training protocol, which increased their $\dot{V}0_2$max by 9% (Landt et al.) (47), lean body mass increased. Despite increased insulin sensitivity, glycosylated hemoglobin remained at about 12%. The subjects were instructed not to change the insulin dose or caloric intake. There was no apparent increase in caloric intake as judged by dietary records.

To examine the possibility that an exercise program could be effective in glycemic control if carried out for longer periods, 6 adult females with Type I diabetes in a daily training program (20 min cycling at 60% to 90% $\dot{V}0_2$max) for 5 months were studied by Wallberg-Henriksson et al. (91). $\dot{V}0_2$max increased 8%. Daily insulin dose, BMI, and frequency of hypoglycemic events were unchanged. Again, HbA_1 (approximately 10%) and mean blood glucose during training did not change. Rowland et al. (71) studied 13 diabetic children submitted to a 12-week training program three times per week for 1 hr. $\dot{V}0_2$max increased 9%. HbA_1 (approximately 10%), 24-hr glycosuria, and fasting blood glucose were unaffected. Insulin dose and frequency of hypoglycemic events did not change. Body weight increased.

Baevre et al. (4) studied 6 adolescents with Type I diabetes in a 6-month training program of 30 min of exercise, two times per week at 130 bpm. $\dot{V}0_2$max increased 19%. There was no significant change in HbA_1 (approximately 11%) or fasting blood glucose, although a modest decrease was observed. Insulin dose decreased in 2 out of 6 subjects, and body weight increased. A short, intense training period was associated with decreased fasting blood glucose during training (4). However, this decrease did not extend beyond the training period. Glycosylated hemoglobin was unaffected (4,30).

In 16 children and adolescents with Type I diabetes who were submitted to a 3-month exercise program carried out once weekly at 150 bpm for 45 min, $\dot{V}O_2max$ increased 4%. Again, no improvement was seen in HbA_{1C} (approximately 10%), blood glucose, or urinary glucose (35). On the contrary, HbA_{1C} increased in both a sedentary and a trained group, significantly in the latter. When subjects were stratified according to participation in the program, metabolic control was significantly better among subjects with diabetes who participated frequently than among those participating infrequently, regardless of activity. The authors concluded that glycemic control appears to be best among subjects with diabetes who are motivated to participate in any kind of program related to the treatment of the disease.

In summary, most of the studies evaluating the effect of exercise training on glycemic control in Type I diabetes do not meet satisfactory clinical and epidemiologic criteria, mainly because of small sample size and lack of adequate controls. The weight of evidence provided by these studies is negative for a beneficial effect of increased physical activity on glycemic control in Type I diabetes (14). Improvement in glycosylated hemoglobin could be detected in only two studies where starting levels were high in children with badly controlled diabetes. Short duration of diabetes per se was not associated with a positive response to exercise in other studies in children or adolescents. These results appear in contrast to the predominant glucose-lowering effect of acute exercise and to the well-documented increase in insulin sensitivity induced by training in Type I diabetes. Certainly, more extensive, well-controlled studies should be carried out. However, it is not surprising that glycosylated hemoglobin is little affected by increased physical activity, given the importance of diet and insulin therapy as determinants of glycemic control in Type I diabetes. Also, usual levels of physical activity are in general already high in subjects with Type I diabetes. Compensatory adjustments of caloric intake may also occur to obscure the summation effect of the glucose-lowering action of acute exercise and the beneficial effects of increased insulin sensitivity. In Type I diabetes, insulin sensitivity is only secondarily impaired, is normalized by insulin treatment (46), and is only one of the variables affecting long-term glycemic control. In fact, the response to training of subjects with Type I diabetes appears to be similar to that of nondiabetic subjects. That is, whereas insulin sensitivity might be increased following training, control of blood glucose often remains unaltered. The reduction of the insulin dose sometimes observed may be of value from the point of view of diabetic complications.

Effects of Training on the Incidence of Cardiovascular Disease

The incidence of cardiovascular disease, affecting arteries in the heart, brain, and extremities, is two- to threefold greater in the diabetic than the nondiabetic population (52,72). Increased incidence of cardiovascular disease is present not only in Type II but also in Type I diabetes (26).

Almost two thirds of the epidemiological studies have reported a significant association between coronary heart disease and physical inactivity, a graded response, or both (67). The relative risk of coronary heart disease associated with inactivity varies among studies but generally ranges from 1.5 to 2.4. Although higher levels of physical activity seem to confer greater benefit, merely climbing five flights of stairs or walking more than five city blocks daily was associated with reduced incidence of myocardial infarction by 25% in one study (65). There is also indication for an association between physical inactivity and stroke or intermittent claudication, but the studies do not always meet satisfactory epidemiological criteria (76).

Epidemiological data suggest that physical inactivity is probably not as potent an individual risk factor as elevated serum cholesterol, hypertension, or cigarette smoking. Possible direct actions of exercise training on the atherosclerotic process or in tissue response to ischemia have not been investigated. Studies on primates fed an atherogenic diet show that exercise retards development of atherosclerotic lesions (43). Exercise may also lessen known cardiovascular risk factors both directly and through associated weight reduction (23). Physical activity improves the lipid profile and reduces blood pressure. Although the association between total cholesterol and physical inactivity is inconclusive, physically inactive people usually have higher triglyceride and lower HDL cholesterol levels than active people. The atherogenic potential of elevated triglyceride levels, uncertain in the general population, has been established in diabetes. In Type I diabetes, there are a few studies showing an increase in the ratio of HDL-cholesterol to total cholesterol after training (89,100). The effect was insignificant in two other studies (15,91). However, HDL_3 cholesterol was found increased (91), and LDL cholesterol was found decreased

(15). Total cholesterol (4,15,18,50,89,91) decreased significantly in only one study (89). Triglycerides either decreased (18,50) or were not significantly affected (15,91,100). Training programs, although not improving metabolic control as judged by glycosylated hemoglobin, may lead to reduced insulin dosage (see the section "Effect of Training on Glucoregulation and Glycemic Control"). This might reduce hyperinsulinemia, which has been recently associated with atherosclerosis and hypertension. Daily free insulin profiles have not been measured.

Data regarding the relative risk of physical inactivity in the diabetic versus nondiabetic population are few. A recent cohort study examines the relation between glycemic status, physical fitness, and mortality in 8,715 males (40). Blood glucose was stratified into three categories: (a) fasting blood glucose less than 6.4 mM, (b) fasting blood glucose 6.4 to 7.8 mM (n = 509), and (c) fasting blood glucose greater than 7.8 mM or a personal history of Type II diabetes (n = 98). Multivariate estimates of the relative risk of cardiovascular death in the low-fitness group (below 20% of the treadmill time distribution) were 1.62 , 1.43, and 1.80, indicating that the risk associated with low fitness increases with less favorable glycemic status. The level of exercise involved to improve or maintain this level of fitness corresponds to a 30- to 40-min program of moderate-intensity exercise three to five times per week. In another cohort study the incidence of first heart attack was evaluated in male Harvard alumni aged 35 to 74 years (65). The relative risk in people with less than 2,000 kcal/week of physical activity versus people with greater than 2,000 kcal/week was 3.99 in diabetic (2% of the population) and 1.48 in nondiabetic subjects. Subjects were not subdivided into Type I and Type II diabetes.

Although the long-term benefits of increased physical activity in Type I diabetes have not been addressed in well-controlled prospective studies, limited retrospective data are available. An early report from the Joslin Clinic indicates that regular lifetime physical activity was one of the characteristics of a group of 48 diabetic patients with unusually long survival and few diabetic complications (17). In the Pittsburgh Insulin-Dependent Diabetes Mellitus Morbidity and Mortality Study (n = 696), participation in team sports in high school or college was inversely correlated with macrovascular disease (questionnaire-determined) or mortality in males. Such association remained of borderline significance ($p < .1$) on multivariate analysis after adjustment for duration of diabetes and other lifestyle variables (48). A history of higher levels of physical activity was associated with a lower prevalence of diabetic complications (objectively assessed) in males of the same cohort (n = 628) evaluated a few years later. The complications included both microangiopathy and macrovascular disease. Stratification for duration of diabetes did not eliminate the association, except for retinopathy. However, the number of patients with macrovascular disease was small (44). When examined cross-sectionally, low physical activity levels were associated with the presence of all complications, but this might reflect the limitation to physical activity related to the diabetic complications (44,48). In females, physical activity levels were low in most subjects, which might have precluded the detection of any association (44,48). The same authors recently reported an inverse relationship between leisure physical activity and mortality risk 6 years later (44).

In summary, from the limited data available, it appears that increased physical activity is protective against cardiovascular disease in individuals with Type I diabetes. It remains unsettled whether the protective factor is less than, equal to, or more than that of nondiabetic individuals.

Acknowledgments

Adria Giacca has been a fellow of the Istituto Scientifico S. Raffaele Milan, Italy, and she is presently a recipient of a Career Development Award from the Juvenile Diabetes Foundation. Z. Qing Shi is a fellow of the Canadian Diabetes Association. Thanks also to L. Vranic and M. Van Delangeryt for invaluable help in preparing this manuscript.

References

1. Akerblom, H.K.; Koivukangas, T.; Ilkka, J. Experiences from a winter camp for teenage diabetics. Acta Physiol. Scand. 283:50-52; 1980.
2. American Diabetes Association, Diabetes mellitus and exercise: Position statement. Diabetes Care. 13:804-805; 1990.
3. Anderson, B. Activity and diabetic vitreous hemorrhages. Ophthalmology 87:173-175; 1980.
4. Baevre, H.; Sovik, O.; Wisnes, A.; Heiervang, E. Metabolic responses to physical training in young insulin-dependent diabetics. Scand. J. Clin. Lab. Invest. 45:109-114; 1985.
5. Bak, J.F.; Jacobsen, U.K.; Jorgensen, F.S.; Pedersen, O. Insulin receptor function and glycogen synthase activity in skeletal muscle biopsies from patients with insulin-dependent diabetes mellitus: Effects of physical training. J. Clin. Endocrinol. Metab. 69:158-164; 1989.

6. Berger, M.; Berchtold, P.; Cuppers, H.J.; Drost, H.J.; Kley, H.K.; Muller, W.; Wiegelman, W.; Zimmerman-Telschow, H.; Gries, F.A.; Kruskemper, H.L.; Zimmerman, H. Metabolic and hormonal effects of muscular exercise in juvenile type diabetics. Diabetologia. 13:355-365; 1977.
7. Berger, M.; Halban, P.A.; Muller, W.A.; Offord, R.E.; Renold, A.E.; Vranic, M. Mobilization of subcutaneously injected tritiated insulin in rats: Effect of muscular exercise. Diabetologia. 15:113-140; 1978.
8. Bergstrom, J.; Hultman, E.; Saltin, B. Muscle glycogen consumption during cross country skiing (Vasa ski race). Int. Z. Angew. Physiol. 31:71-75; 1973.
9. Bhimji, S.; Godin, D.V.; McNeill, J.H. Coronary artery ligation and reperfusion in alloxan-diabetic rabbits: Ultrastructural and haemodynamic changes. Br. J. Exp. Pathol. 67:851-863; 1986.
10. Bjorkman, O.; Miles, P.; Wasserman, D.; Lickley, L.; Vranic, M. Regulation of glucose turnover in pancreatectomized, totally insulin deficient dogs: Effects of β-adrenergic blockade. J. Clin. Invest. 81:1759-1767; 1988.
11. Bogardus, C.; Thuilliz, P.; Ravussin, E.; Vasquez, B.; Narimiga, M.; Azhar, S. Effect of muscle glycogen depletion on in vivo insulin action in man. J. Clin. Invest. 72:1605-1610; 1983.
12. Bonen, A.; Clune, P.A.; Tan, M.H. Chronic exercise increases insulin binding in muscles but not liver. Am. J. Physiol. 251:E196-E203; 1986.
13. Campaigne, B.; Gillam, T.; Sjenan, M.; Lampman, R.; Schork, M. Effects of a physical activity program on metabolic control and cardiovascular fitness in children with insulin-dependent diabetes mellitus. Diabetes Care. 7:57-62; 1984.
14. Campaigne, B.N.; Gunnarsson, R. The effects of physical training in people with insulin-dependent diabetes. Diabetic Med. 5:429-433; 1988.
15. Campaigne, B.; Landt, K.; Mellies, M.; James, F.; Glueck, C.; Sperling, M. The effects of physical training on blood lipid profiles in adolescents with insulin-dependent diabetes mellitus. Phys. Sports Med. 13:83-89; 1985.
16. Caron, D.; Poussier, P.; Marliss, E.B.; Zinman, B. The effect of postprandial exercise on meal-related glucose intolerance in insulin-dependent diabetic individuals. Diabetes Care. 5:364-369; 1982.
17. Chazan, B.I.; Balodimos, M.C.; Ryan, J.R.; Marble, A. Twenty-five to forty-five years of diabetes with and without vascular complications. Diabetologia. 6:565-569; 1970.
18. Costill, D.L.; Cleary, P.; Fink, W.J.; Foster, C.; Ivy, J.L.; Witzmann, F. Training adaptations in skeletal muscle of juvenile diabetics. Diabetes. 28:818-822; 1979.
19. Crettaz, M.; Horton, E.S.; Wardzala, L.J.; Horton, E.D.; Jeanrenaud, B. Physical training of Zucker rats: Lack of alleviation of muscle insulin resistance. Am. J. Physiol. 244:E414-E420; 1983.
20. Dahl-Jorgensen, K.; Meen, H.D.; Hanssen, F.; Aageneas, O. The effect of exercise on diabetic control and hemoglobin A1(HbA_1) in children. Acta Paediatr. Scand. 283:53-56; 1980.
21. The DCCT Research Group. Diabetes control and complications trial (DCCT): Results of feasibility study. Diabetes Care. 10:1-19; 1987.
22. DeFronzo, R.A.; Ferrannini, E.; Sato, Y.; Felig, P.; Wahren, J. Synergistic interaction between exercise and insulin on peripheral glucose uptake. J. Clin. Invest. 68:1468-1474; 1981
23. Devlin, J. Race for better health: Editorial. Diabetes Care. 13:176-177; 1990.
24. Douen, A.G.; Ramlal, T.; Rastogi, S.; Bilan, P.G.; Cartee, G.D.; Vranic, M.; Holloszy, J.O.; Klip, A. Exercise induces recruitment of the insulin responsive glucose transporter. Evidence for distinct intracellular insulin and exercise-recruitable transporter pools in skeletal muscle. J. Biol. Chem. 265:13427-13430; 1990.
25. Engerbretson, D.L. The effects of exercise upon diabetic control. J. Assoc. Phys. Ment. Rehabil. 19:74-78; 1965.
26. Ganda, O.P. Pathogenesis of macrovascular disease in the human diabetic. Diabetes. 29:931-942; 1980.
27. Garetto, L.P.; Richter, E.A.; Goodman, M.N.; Ruderman, N.B. Enhanced muscle glucose metabolism after exercise in the rat: The two phases. Am. J. Physiol. 246:E471-E475; 1984.
28. Giacca, A.; Vranic, M.; Davidson, J.K.; Lickley, H.L.A. Exercise and stress in diabetes mellitus. In: Davidson, J.K., ed. Clinical diabetes mellitus: A problem oriented approach. New York: Thieme-Stratton, Inc.; 1991:218-265.
29. Gooch, B.R.; Abumrad, N.N.; Robinson, R.P.; Petrik, M.; Campbell, D.; Crofford, O.B. Exercise in insulin-dependent diabetes mellitus: The effect of continuous insulin infusion using the subcutaneous, intravenous and intraperitoneal sites. Diabetes Care. 6:122-128; 1983.
30. Hansen, L.; Jacobsen, B.; Kofoed, P.; Larsen, M.; Tougaard, L.; Johansen, I. Serum fructosamine and HbA_{1c} in diabetic children before and after attending winter camp. Acta Paediatr. Scand. 78:451-452; 1989.

31. Hilsted, J.; Galbo, H.; Christensen, N.J. Impaired responses of catecholamines, growth hormone, and cortisol to graded exercise in diabetic autonomic neuropathy. Diabetes. 29:257-262; 1980.
32. Hirshman, M.; Wallberg-Henriksson, H.; Wardzala, L.; Horton, E.; Horton, E. Acute exercise increases the number of plasma membrane glucose transporters in rat skeletal muscle. FEBS Lett. 238:235-239; 1988.
33. Holloszy, J.O.; Booth, F.W. Biochemical adaptations to endurance exercise in muscle. Annu. Rev. Physiol. 38:273-291; 1976.
34. Horton, E.S. Role and management of exercise in diabetes mellitus. Diabetes Care. 11:201-211; 1988.
35. Huttunen, N.; Lankela, S.; Knip, M.; Lautala, P.; Kaar, M.; Laasonen, K.; Puukka, R. Effect of once-a-week training program on physical fitness and metabolic control in children with IDDM. Diabetes Care. 12:737-740; 1989.
36. Joslin, E.P.; Root, H.F.; White, P., editors. The treatment of diabetes mellitus. Philadelphia: Lea & Febiger; 1959:243-300.
37. Kawamori, R.; Vranic, M. Mechanism of exercise-induced hypoglycemia in depancreatized dogs maintained on long-acting insulin. J. Clin. Invest. 59:331-337; 1977.
38. Kemmer, F.W.; Berchtold, P.; Berger, M.; Starke, A.; Cuppers, H.J.; Gries, F.A.; Zimmermann, H. Exercise-induced fall of blood glucose in insulin treated diabetics unrelated to alteration of insulin mobilization. Diabetes. 28:1131-1137; 1979.
39. King, D.S.; Dalsky, G.P.; Clutter, W.; Young, D.A.; Staten, M.A.; Cryer, P.E.; Holloszy, J.O. Effects of exercise and lack of exercise on insulin sensitivity and responsiveness. J. Appl. Physiol. 64:1942-1946; 1988.
40. Kohl, H.; Gordon, N.F.; Vellegas, J.A.; Blair, S.N. Cardiorespiratory fitness, glycemic status and mortality risk in men. Diabetes Care. 15:184-192; 1992.
41. Koivisto, V.; Soman, V.; Conrad, P.; Hendler, R.; Nadel, E.; Felig, P. Insulin binding to monocytes in trained athletes. J. Clin. Invest. 64:1011-1015; 1979.
42. Koivisto, V.A.; Yki-Jarvinen, H.; DeFronzo, R.A. Physical training and insulin sensitivity. Diab. Metab. Rev. 1:445-481; 1986.
43. Kramsch, B.M.; Aspen, A.J.; Abramowitz, B.M.; Kreimendal, T.; Hood, W. Reduction of coronary atherosclerosis by moderate conditioning exercise in monkeys on an atherogenic diet. N. Engl. J. Med. 305:1483-1489; 1981.
44. Kriska, A.M.; LaPorte, R.E.; Patrick, S.L.; Kuller, L.H.; Orchard, T.J. The association of physical activity and diabetic complications in individuals with insulin-dependent diabetes mellitus: The epidemiology of diabetes complications study - VII. J. Clin. Epidemiol. 44:1207-1214; 1991.
45. Krzentowski, G.; Pirnay, F.; Pallikarakis, N.; Luyckx, A.S.; Lacroix, M.; Mosora, F.; Lefebvre, P. Glucose utilization in normal and diabetic subjects. The role of insulin. Diabetes. 30:983-989; 1981.
46. Lager, I.; Lonnroth, P.; von Schenk, H.; Smith, U. Reversal of insulin resistance in type I diabetes after treatment with continuous subcutaneous insulin infusion. Br. Med. J. 287:1661-1664; 1983.
47. Landt, K.; Campaigne, B.N.; James, F.W.; Sperling, M. Effects of exercise training on insulin sensitivity in adolescents with type I diabetes. Diabetes Care. 8:461-465; 1985.
48. LaPorte, R.E.; Dorman, J.S.; Tajima, N.; Cruickshanks, K.J.; Orchard, T.J.; Cavender, D.E.; Becker, D.J.; Drash, A.L. Pittsburgh insulin dependent diabetes mellitus morbidity and mortality study: Physical activity and diabetic complications. Pediatrics. 78:1027-1033; 1986.
49. Larsson, Y.; Persson, B.; Sterky, G.; Thoren, C. Functional adaptation to rigorous training and exercise in diabetic and non-diabetic adolescents. J. Appl. Physiol. 19:629-635; 1964.
50. Larsson, Y.; Sterky, G.; Persson, B.; Thoren, C. Effect of exercise on blood-lipids in juvenile diabetes. Lancet. 1:350-355; 1964.
51. Larsson, Y.A.A.; Sterky, G.C.G.; Ekengren, K.E.K.; Moller, T.G.H.O. Physical fitness and the influence of training in diabetic adolescent girls. Diabetes. 11:109-117; 1962.
52. Leon, A.S.; Connett, J.; Jacobs, D.R.; Rauramaa, R. Leisure-time physical activity levels and risk of coronary heart disease and death: The multiple risk factor intervention trial. JAMA. 258:2388-2395; 1987.
53. Ludvigsson, J. Physical exercise in relation to degree of metabolic control in juvenile diabetics. Acta Physiol. Scand. 283:45-49; 1980.
54. Marliss, E.B.; Purdon, C.; Miles, P.D.G.; Halter, J.B.; Sigal, R.; Vranic, M. Glucoregulation during and after intense exercise in control and diabetic subjects. In: Devlin, J.; Horton, E.S.; Vranic, M., eds. Diabetes mellitus and exercise symposium. London: Smith-Gordon; 1992: 173-190.
55. Marliss, E.B.; Simantirakis, E.; Miles, P.; Hunt, R.; Gougeon, R.; Purdon, C.; Halter, J.; Vranic, M. Glucose turnover and regulation during intense exercise and recovery in normal male subjects. Clin. Invest. Med. 15:406-419; 1992.
56. Marliss, E.B.; Simantirakis, E.; Miles, P.; Purdon, C.; Gougeon-Reygburn, R.; Field, C.J.;

Halter, J.B.; Vranic, M. Glucoregulatory and hormonal responses to repeated bouts of intense exercise in normal male subjects. J. Appl. Physiol. 71:924-933; 1991.

57. Miles, P.; Finegood, D.; Lickley, L.; Vranic, M. Regulation of glucose turnover at onset of exercise in dogs. J. Appl. Physiol. 72:2487-2494; 1992.
58. Minuk, H.L.; Hanna, A.K.; Marliss, E.B.; Vranic, M.; Zinman, B. Metabolic response to moderate exercise in obese man during prolonged fasting. Am. J. Physiol. 238:E322-E329; 1980.
59. Moates, J.M.; Lacy, D.B.; Goldstein, R.E.; Cherrington, A.D.; Wasserman, D.H. The metabolic role of exercise-induced increment in epinephrine in the dog. Am. J. Physiol. 255:E428-E436; 1988.
60. Mogensen, C.; Vittinghus, E. Urinary albumin excretion during exercise in juvenile diabetes. Scand. J. Clin. Lab. Invest. 35:295-300; 1975.
61. Murray, F.T.; Zinman, B.; McClean, P.A.; Denoga, A.; Albisser, A.M.; Leibel, B.S.; Nakhooda, A.F.; Stokes, E.F.; Marliss, E.B. The metabolic response to moderate exercise in diabetic man receiving intravenous and subcutaneous insulin. J. Clin. Endocrinol. Metab. 44:708-720; 1977.
62. Nelson, J.D.; Poussier, P.; Marliss, E.B.; Albisser, A.M.; Zinman, B. Metabolic response of normal man and insulin-infused diabetics to postprandial exercise. Am. J. Physiol. 242:E309-E316; 1982.
63. Nesher, R.; Karl, I.E.; Kipnis, K.M. Dissociation of the effect(s) of insulin and contraction on glucose transport in rat epitrochlearis muscle. Am. J. Physiol. 249:C226-C232; 1985.
64. Nesto, R.W.; Phillips, R.T.; Kett, K.G.; Hill, T.; Perper, E.; Young, E.; Leland, S. Angina and exertional myocardial ischemia in diabetic and non-diabetic patients: Assessment by exercise thallium scintigraphy. Ann. Intern. Med. 108:170-175; 1988.
65. Paffenbarger, R.S.; Wing, A.; Hyde, R.T. Physical activity as an index of heart attack risk in college alumni. Am. J. Epidemiol. 108:161-175; 1978.
66. Peterson, C.M.; Jones, R.L.; Esterly, J.A.; Wantz, G.E.; Jackson, R.L. Changes in basement membrane thickening and pulse volume concomitant with improved glucose control and exercise in patients with insulin dependent diabetes mellitus. Diabetes Care. 3:586-589; 1980.
67. Powell, K.E.; Thompson, P.D.; Caspersen, C.J.; Kendrick, J.S. Physical activity and the incidence of coronary heart disease. Annu. Rev. Public Health. 8:253-287; 1987.
68. Purdon, C.; Brousson, M.; Nyveen, S.; Miles, P.; Halter, J.; Vranic, M.; Marliss, E. The roles of insulin and catecholamines in the glucoregulatory response during intense exercise and early recovery in insulin-dependent diabetic and control subjects. J. Clin. Endocrin. Metab. 76:566-573; 1993.
69. Richter, E.A.; Garetto, L.P.; Goodman, M.N.; Ruderman, N.B. Muscle glucose metabolism following exercise in the rat. Increased sensitivity to insulin. J. Clin. Invest. 69:785-789; 1982.
70. Rodnick, K.J.; Haskell, W.L.; Swislocki, A.L.M.; Foley, J.E.; Reaven, G.M. Improved insulin action in muscle, liver and adipose tissue in physically trained human subjects. Am. J. Physiol. 253:E489-E495; 1987.
71. Rowland, T.W.; Swadba, L.A.; Biggs, D.E.; Burke, E.J.; Reiter, E.O. Glycemic control with physical training in insulin-dependent diabetes mellitus. Am. J. Dis. Child. 139:307-310; 1985.
72. Ruderman, N.B.; Haudenschild, C. Diabetes as an atherogenic factor. Prog. Cardiovasc. Dis. 26:373-412; 1984.
73. Ruegemer, J.J.; Squires, R.; Marsh, H.; Haymond, M.; Cryer, P.; Rizza, R.; Miles, J.M. Differences between prebreakfast and late afternoon glycemic responses to exercise in IDDM patients. Diabetes Care. 13:104-110; 1990.
74. Schiffrin, A.; Parikh, S.; Marliss, E.B.; Desrosiers, M.M. Metabolic response to fasting exercise in adolescent insulin-dependent diabetic subjects treated with continuous subcutaneous insulin infusion and intensive conventional therapy. Diabetes Care. 7:255-260; 1984.
75. Schneider, S.H.; Ruderman, N.B. Exercise and NIDDM: Technical review. Diabetes Care. 13:785-789; 1990.
76. Schneider, S.H.; Vitug, A.; Ruderman, N.B. Atherosclerosis and physical activity. Diabetes Metab. Rev. 1:513-553; 1986.
77. Shi, Z.; Giacca, A.; Yamatani, K.; Miles, P.; Fisher, S.; Van Delangeryt, M.; Lickely, L.; Vranic, M. Glucose uptake in exercise and stress: The indirect role of insulin. In: Devlin, J.; Horton, E.S., Vranic, M., eds. Diabetes mellitus and exercise symposium. London: Smith-Gordon; 1992:101-112.
78. Simonson, D.C.; Koivisto, V.; Sherwin, R.S.; Ferrannini, E.; Hendler, R.; Juhlin-Dannfeldt, J.; DeFronzo, R. Adrenergic blockade alters glucose kinetics during exercise in insulin-dependent diabetics. J. Clin. Invest. 73:1648-1658; 1984.
79. Sonnenberg, G.E.; Kemmer, F.W.; Berger, M. Exercise in type I (insulin-dependent) diabetic patients treated with continuous subcutaneous insulin infusion. Diabetologia. 33:696-703; 1990.

80. Susstrunk, H.; Morell, B.; Ziegler, W.H.; Froesch, E.R. Insulin absorption from the abdomen and the thigh in healthy subjects during rest and exercise: Blood glucose, plasma insulin, growth hormone, adrenaline, and noradrenaline levels. Diabetologia. 22:171-174; 1982.
81. Tamborlane, W.V.; Sherwin, R.S.; Koivisto, V.; Hendler, R.; Genel, M.; Felig, P. Normalization of the growth hormone and catecholamine response to exercise in juvenile-onset diabetic subjects treated with a portable insulin infusion pump. Diabetes. 28:785-788; 1979.
82. Taylor, A.; Thayer, R.; Rao, S. Human skeletal muscle glycogen synthetase activities with exercise and training. Can. J. Physiol. Pharmacol. 50:411-415; 1971.
83. Trovati, M.; Anfossi, G.; Vitali, S.; Mularoni, E.; Massucco, P.; De Facis, R.; Carta, Q.; Lucchina, P.; Emanuelli, G. Postprandial exercise in type I diabetic patients on multiple daily insulin injection regimen. Diabetes Care. 11:107-110; 1988.
84. Trovati, M.; Carta, Q.; Cavalot, F.; Vitali, S.; Passarino, G.; Rocca, G.; Emanuelli, G.; Lenti, G. Continuous subcutaneous insulin infusion and postprandial exercise in tightly controlled type I (insulin-dependent) diabetic patients. Diabetes Care. 7:327-330; 1984.
85. Vranic, M.; Kawamori, R.; Pek, S.; Kovacevic, N.; Wrenshall, G. The essentiality of insulin and the role of glucagon in regulating glucose turnover during strenuous exercise. J. Clin. Invest. 57:245-255; 1975.
86. Vranic, M.; Wasserman, D.; Bukowiecki, L. Metabolic implications of exercise and physical fitness in physiology and diabetes. In: Rifkin, H.; Porte, D., Jr., eds. Diabetes mellitus: Theory and practice. New York: Elsevier Science; 1990:198-219.
87. Vranic, M.; Wrenshall, G.A. Exercise, insulin and glucose turnover in dogs. Endocrinology. 85:165-171; 1969.
88. Wahren, J.; Hagenfeldt, L.; Felig, P. Splanchic and leg exchange of glucose, amino acids and free fatty acids and ketones in insulin dependent diabetics during exercise. J. Clin. Invest. 55:1303-1314; 1975.
89. Wallberg-Henriksson, H.; Gunnarsson, R.; Henriksson, J.; DeFronzo, R.; Felig, P.; Ostman, J.; Wahren, J. Increased peripheral insulin sensitivity and muscle mitochondrial enzymes but unchanged blood glucose control in type I diabetics after physical training. Diabetes. 31:1044-1050; 1982.
90. Wallberg-Henriksson, H.; Gunnarsson, R.; Henriksson, J.; Ostman, J.; Wahren, J. Influence of physical training on formation of muscle capillaries in type I diabetes. Diabetes. 33:851-857; 1984.
91. Wallberg-Henriksson, H.; Gunnarsson, R.; Rossner, S.; Wahren, J. Long-term physical training in female type I (insulin dependent) diabetic patients: Absence of significant effect on glycemic control and lipoprotein levels. Diabetologia. 29:53-65; 1986.
92. Wardzala, L.J.; Horton, E.S.; Crettaz, M.; Horton, E.D.; Jeanrenaud, B. Physical training of lean and genetically obese Zucker rats: Effect on fat cell metabolism. Am. J. Physiol. 243:E418-E426; 1982.
93. Wasserman, D.H.; Lickley, H.L.A.; Vranic, M. Interactions between glucagon and other counterregulatory hormones during normoglycemic and hypoglycemic exercise. J. Clin. Invest. 74:1404-1413; 1984.
94. Wasserman, D.H.; Lickley, H.L.A.; Vranic, M. Important role of glucagon during exercise and diabetes. J. Appl. Physiol. 59:1272-1281; 1985.
95. Wasserman, D.H.; Lickley, H.L.A.; Vranic, M. Role of β-adrenergic mechanisms during exercise in poorly-controlled insulin deficient diabetes. J. Appl. Physiol. 59:1282-1289; 1985.
96. Wasserman, D.H.; Spalding, J.S.; Bracy, D.; Lacy, D.B.; Cherrington, A.D. Exercise-induced rise in glucagon and ketogenesis during prolonged muscular work. Diabetes. 38:799-807; 1989.
97. Wasserman, D.H.; Williams, P.E.; Lacy, D.B.; Goldstein, R.E.; Cherrington, A.D. Exercise-induced fall in insulin and hepatic carbohydrate metabolism during muscular work. Am. J. Physiol. 256:E500-E509; 1989.
98. Wasserman, D.J.; Geer, R.J.; Rice, D.E.; Bracy, D.; Flakoll, P.J.; Brown, L.L.; Hill, J.O.; Abumrad, N.N. Interaction of exercise and insulin action in humans. Am. J. Physiol. 260:E37-E45; 1991.
99. Yamatani, K.; Shi, Z.; Giacca, A.; Gupta, R.; Fisher, S.; Lickley, L.; Vranic, M. Role of FFA-glucose cycle in glucoregulation during exercise in total absence of insulin. Am. J. Physiol. 263:E646-E653; 1992.
100. Yki-Jarvinen, H.; DeFronzo, R.; Koivisto, V. Normalization of insulin sensitivity in type I diabetic subjects by physical training during insulin pump therapy. Diabetes Care. 7:520-527; 1984.
101. Zinman, B.; Murray, F.T.; Vranic, M.; Albisser, A.M.; Leibel, B.S.; McClean, P.A.; Marliss, E.B. Glucoregulation during moderate exercise in insulin treated diabetics. J. Clin. Endocrinol. Metab. 45:641-652; 1977.
102. Zinman, B.; Zuniga-Guajardo, S.; Kelly, D. Comparison of acute and long-term effects of exercise on glucose control in type I diabetes. Diabetes Care. 7:515-519; 1984.

Chapter 45

Physical Activity, Fitness, and Non-Insulin-Dependent (Type II) Diabetes Mellitus

Uwe Gudat
Michael Berger
Pierre J. Lefèbvre

Medline names 233 articles under the search criteria *non-insulin-dependent diabetes and exercise* between the years 1965 and 1991. Only 27 of these are original articles documenting results of clinical or experimental research directed at ascertaining the metabolic effects of exercise therapy. Even hereunder there is redundancy as several articles are based on one and the same study. Notably, there are 32 reviews and position statements specifically devoted to diabetes and exercise in this period, reflecting either an immense publishing interest or want of information toward this topic. The remaining articles pertain to other topics or general diabetes care.

Non-Insulin-Dependent, or Type II, Diabetes Mellitus

In the United States in 1986, Type II diabetes, or non-insulin-dependent diabetes mellitus (NIDDM), was responsible for $11.6 billion in health care expenditures, including $6.8 billion for diabetic care and $4.8 billion attributable to an excess prevalence of related (principally cardiovascular) conditions. The human toll of non-insulin-dependent diabetes mellitus included 144,000 deaths—about 6.8% of total U.S. mortality—and the disability of 951,000 persons (45). NIDDM is a major health matter, affecting close to 90% of all patients with diabetes. In adult Caucasian populations, reported prevalence rates vary between 3.4% (Australia) and 6.4% (United States) and are 1.4 to 1.8 times higher in women than in men. In non-Caucasian populations, prevalence rates are between 0.0% (Papua New Guinea Highlands) and 24% (Nauru). Incidence rates for NIDDM increase progressively with age. For populations under 30 years of age, the rates are about 5 to 30 per 100,000 individuals, and the rates rise progressively to 572 to 939 per 100,000 for populations between 70 and 79 years of age (60). NIDDM is to a large extent a geriatric condition, an important consideration when one assesses exercise as part of the treatment strategy.

NIDDM is believed to be the result of a genetic-environmental interaction; concordance rates among monozygotic twins are between 55% and 100% (5,77,81). Similar evidence can be derived from prevalence studies on persons of mixed ethnic origin, which show prevalence rates between those expected from the parent populations (56,112). The familial predisposition to NIDDM is possibly inherited by a single major gene in a codominant manner (121). Obesity, particularly if it is associated with a high waist-to-hip ratio, plays a major role in the phenotypic expression of NIDDM (23,52,63,79). However, it must be kept in mind that not all obese people, even the very obese, develop NIDDM. The risk is related to the duration, degree, distribution of obesity (55,73,80, 82,90,103,126,129), and the maximum attained weight at age 25 (73); the intrauterine environment during carriage may be of relevance (91).

Only about 40% of those with impaired glucose tolerance later on manifest NIDDM; at a particularly high risk are subjects who have a first-degree relative with NIDDM and who have high serum insulin levels (103). Furthermore, NIDDM is often an undiagnosed condition. Several epidemiological studies have shown that there is almost one case unknown for every case diagnosed (44).

At present, the pathophysiology of NIDDM remains more or less a mystery. Insulin regulates glucose transport by facilitating translocation of glucose transporters from intracellular microsomal locations to the plasma membrane, prompts glucose metabolism by enzyme activation and protein synthesis, and suppresses lipolysis. NIDDM is a syndrome of impaired insulin sensitivity and relative insulin deficiency. Diagnostic criteria of NIDDM are a fasting hyperglycemia (plasma glucose of at least 140 mg/dl) and a decreased glucose tolerance demonstrated by a plasma glucose level of at least 200 mg/dl within 2 hr of an oral glucose load (76). Fasting hyperglycemia correlates well with the elevated hepatic glucose production found in patients with NIDDM, which is a consequence of an impaired hepatic sensitivity to glucose (69,104), insulin, and glucagon. In addition, islet cell function is impaired. When adjusted for body weight and ambient glycemia, studies show that NIDDM patients have reduced total and blunted first-phase insulin secretion upon an oral glucose challenge (12,15). These observations are paralleled by an impaired acute response of the pancreatic islets to secretagogues such as arginine, secretin, isoproterenol, or sulfonylureas (26,36,85,92,123).

Furthermore, in NIDDM subjects up to 32% of total insulin secretion may be proinsulin compared to 15% in control subjects (125). Basal glucagon levels are elevated with respect to the ambient hyperglycemia, and glucagon release is altered, which suggests a concomitant abnormality in glucose or insulin-mediated regulation of A-cell secretory function (reviews in 65, 66). Histopathologic alterations in islet cell morphology seen in patients with NIDDM include reductions in B-cell mass by 40% to 60% (postmortem examination) compared to nondiabetic subjects' islet cell fibrosis and amyloid deposition (34,127), the latter often being associated with the recently described polypeptide amylin or calcitonin gene-related peptide (CGRP) (17,128). To complicate matters further, increased concentrations of certain peptides such as galanin, pancreastatin, or opiate analogues (1,24,30,35,96), increased diurnal fluctuations of plasma growth hormone concentrations (53), abnormalities of numerous counterregulatory hormones (65,66), and magnesium depletion (88,89) may contribute to the pathophysiology of NIDDM.

Studies utilizing the euglycemic insulin clamp technique have demonstrated that peripheral glucose disposal rates are decreased by up to 55% in NIDDM (58). Critics contend that many of these studies were performed at euglycemia (for an adapted patient with NIDDM an unphysiological condition). Studies on peripheral glucose disposal at levels of hyperglycemia characteristic for NIDDM show peripheral glucose disposal that is close to that of control subjects. This suggests that as insulin sensitivity decreases, this diminution is compensated by the influence of mass action induced by the high blood glucose levels (98). Intracellular glucose utilization of insulin-sensitive tissues (e.g., muscle and fat tissue) is modulated by insulin levels; low levels of insulin predispose to peripheral glucose oxidation, whereas higher levels induce glycogen synthesis. Although both pathways are compromised in NIDDM, peripheral insulin resistance is associated with a more marked reduction of nonoxidative glucose disposal.

Mechanisms suggested to be responsible for an impaired peripheral glucose utilization are a decrease in insulin receptor number, impaired insulin receptor signaling, impaired translocation of glucose transporters from intracellular microsomes to the cell surface, impaired transport capacity of glucose transporters, and impaired activation or modulation of cytoplasmal enzymes. At present there is little evidence for heritable defects in receptor function in NIDDM in which insulin-binding affinity is normal and receptor number is modulated only as a reversible consequence of hyperglycemia (31). Evidence for receptor mutations can be found in only a small subset of the NIDDM population (78). Studies on glucose transporter translocation and synthesis are as yet not conclusive. Recent studies using ^{13}C-NMR spectroscopy in conjunction with [1-^{13}C]-glucose infusion have provided impressive evidence that impaired muscle glycogen deposition is a key feature in the pathophysiology of NIDDM (113).

It thus appears that NIDDM is the result of a variety of phenomena and that considerable heterogeneity is involved in its pathogenesis. Interpretation of any isolated aspect of the glucose homeostatic mechanism cannot be performed without taking into account the interrelationships of islet secretory function, hepatic glucose output, and peripheral glucose uptake at the respective hormone and substrate levels. Glucose is the key regulator of the islet system because it regulates not only insulin and glucagon secretion directly but also modulates responses to other substrates, free fatty acids (FFAs), and amino acids, as well as gut hormones and neural factors. This complicates matters further and makes it difficult to distinguish between primary pathophysiologic phenomena that may cause NIDDM and secondary sequelae.

Substrate Metabolism During Exercise

Specific aspects of substrate metabolism during exercise can be defined in terms of three functional aims: metabolizing the most efficient substrate, preserving glucose homeostasis, and delaying exhaustion. The direct source of energy for muscular contraction (the metabolic currency) is adenosine triphosphate (ATP). Creatine phosphate supplants the immediately accessible intramuscular reserve of high-energy phosphate compounds. Degradation and subsequent oxidation of intramuscular depots of glycogen and triglycerides buffer the rapid depletion of both ATP and creatine phosphate. Thereafter, systemic reserves must be recruited.

During high-intensity work (when ATP hydrolysis is rapid and oxygen availability is limited), carbohydrate oxidation in the cytoplasm can regenerate ATP faster than mitochondrial β-oxidation of fatty acids. In addition, glucose carbon atoms tax less oxygen for complete metabolism because they are already partially oxidized compared with the highly saturated carbon skeleton of fats. In contrast, during sustained periods of medium- to low-intensity exercise and in the postabsorptive resting state, the dynamics of energy supply become secondary to fuel-storage efficiency. Whole-body carbohydrate reserves amount to a caloric equivalent of about 8,000 kJ/1,900 kcal (20 g blood glucose, 80 to 90 g liver glycogen, and 300 to 400 g muscle glycogen); in contrast, adipose tissue offers the equivalent of 600,000 kJ/143,000 kcal (about 15 kg of triglycerides). Differences in the degree of hydration between fatty acids and glucose predict that 2.5 times as many molecules of ATP can be gained from the oxidation of 1 g of triglyceride as from 1 g of glycogen. Thus, with the exception of periods of sudden or strenuous exercise, muscle is a relatively unimportant utilizer of glucose and relies predominantly on FFA oxidation. During exercise at intensities demanding more than 50% to 60% of the maximal oxygen uptake, the sole oxidation of lipids is unable to sustain muscular work, and glycogen once again (this time of mostly hepatic origin) becomes an important fuel source. By releasing gluconeogenic precursors, nonexercising muscle may offer support in substrate recruitment.

Second in importance to the liver with respect to the distribution and maintenance of blood fuel levels is adipose tissue. Hydrolysis of triacylglycerols yields FFA and glycerol. FFA release from adipose tissue is regulated primarily by the actions of insulin, which inhibits, and catecholamines, which stimulate, lipolysis. With a half-life of about 3 min, FFAs constitute a highly dynamic and adaptive system. FFA utilization is regulated by the principle of mass action, the turnover rate being insulin independent and directly proportional to arterial concentrations.

The most significant stimulants for the increased glucose uptake during exercise are muscle contraction and insulin. In vitro studies on isolated rat muscles and hindquarters have demonstrated that in this environment muscle contraction per se may stimulate glucose uptake even independently of the presence of insulin. Despite its potent effects on glucose uptake, contraction alone may be insufficient in vivo, where metabolic events antagonistic to glucose uptake concur (FFA oxidation, catecholamine action), and insulin is thought to be a prerequisite for facilitated muscular glucose uptake during and after exercise.

After an acute bout of exercise, skeletal muscle glucose uptake remains above baseline as glycogen reserves are replenished. Initially, glucose utilization and glycogen synthesis are enhanced, apparently independently of the presence of insulin. Later as the glycogen deficiency becomes progressively less, facilitated glucose uptake requires insulin and is reflected as improved insulin sensitivity. In this process local contraction-induced factors seem to direct glucose uptake predominantly to muscles that have been active. Replacement of muscle and liver glycogen may take up to 48 hr.

In summary, exercise leads to shifts in substrate utilization and cycling. In healthy individuals, muscular work facilitates glucose disposal, systemic insulin levels fall, and peripheral glucose uptake increases. Understandably, improved insulin efficiency is an appealing concept for lowering chronic hyperglycemia in patients with diabetes mellitus. However, as we will note later, work loads that are more or less well tolerated by middle-aged individuals with NIDDM lie at about 50% to 60% $\dot{V}O_2max$, a level at which most energy utilized is derived from FFA and only a smaller part is derived from carbohydrate oxidation.

Physical Exercise and Non-Insulin-Dependent Diabetes

Early evidence in favor of exercise was provided by the study of Björntorp et al. (8) performed on nondiabetic individuals. These authors reexamined 32 of 104 men who participated in an exercise training intervention (1/2 hr per week for 9 months) initiated after a nonfatal myocardial infarction. Only 15 of the 32 men had adhered adequately to the program. Glucose tolerance and insulin levels for adherers, nonadherers, and a control group were compared. In all groups, basal insulin levels fell within the 1-year follow-up. Glucose tolerance was marginally improved only in the adhering exercisers. Devlin, Hirshman, Horton, and Horton (20) assessed the metabolic effects of a single bout of glycogen-depleting exercise (intermittent exercise at 85% $\dot{V}O_2max$ until exhaustion) in 5 patients with NIDDM (age, 37.6 ± 1.8 years; body weight, 106.4 ± 7.7 kg), 6 obese patients, and 6 normal control subject. They found a significantly reduced endogenous glucose production and a fall in fasting plasma glucose 12 hr after exercise in the 5 patients with NIDDM.

Kaplan et al. (47,48) compared the effects of 10 weeks of exercise, exercise and diet, diet only, or standard diabetes teaching only intervention on glucose tolerance in 76 NIDDM patients and lipid metabolism in 65 NIDDM patients. Individualized exercise prescriptions, based on exercise laboratory results, were performed under the supervision of physical education graduate students (1 weekly class—30 min warm-up and stretching followed by 40 to 60 min walking at 60% to 70% $\dot{V}O_2$max). In the exercise-plus-diet intervention, the last half hour of social conversation was replaced by training in dietary behavior modification taught by a graduate student in psychology. The control group was exposed to 10 lectures on diabetes care. All patients were given a 1,200-kcal diet recommendation. In this study, diet alone showed the greatest increase in HDL cholesterol. After promising early results, long-term follow-up 19 months after intervention showed no significant weight loss in any group and only borderline differences in HbA_{1c} in self-selected patients (47).

Barnard, Lattimore, Holly, Cherny, and Pritkin (4) evaluated a combined dietary and exercise intervention of 26 days' duration performed in a health clinic (the Pritkin program) in 60 patients with NIDDM (age, 61.5 ± 12 years; body weight, 83.2 ± 2.5 kg). They reported a significant fall in fasting blood glucose, body weight, and serum lipids and a significant increase in maximum work capacity. Due to the study design, it is impossible to distinguish between exercise effects and those of the dietary measures. Trovati et al. (122) examined the influence of exercise on the bicycle ergometer (1 hr per day, 7 days per week, at 50% to 60% $\dot{V}O_2$max for 6 weeks) on metabolic parameters in 5 NIDDM patients (age, 54.4 ± 4 years; body weight, 115 ± 7% of ideal body weight). To compensate for the additional energy expenditure, patients were told to increase caloric intake by 400 kcal per day. The results showed significant improvement of HbA_1 from 9.6% to 8%, improved intravenous glucose tolerance, and a 28% rise in steady-state infusion rate of glucose under clamp conditions, indicating increased insulin sensitivity.

Rogers et al. (99) assessed the influence of 1 week of exercise (30 min treadmill, 10 min break, then 20 to 30 min bicycle ergometer at approximately 60% to 70% of $\dot{V}O_2$max for 7 days substituted by a 60-min walk on Day 4 [Sunday]) on glucose tolerance in 7 patients with NIDDM and 3 with impaired glucose tolerance (IGT) (age, 53 ± 3 years; body weight, 97.0 ± 3.6 kg). They found a significant decrease in the area under the glucose and insulin curves after an oral glucose tolerance test, and they also found a fall in diastolic blood pressure, serum cholesterol, and serum triglyceride after 7 days of exercise.

Saltin et al. (105) compared the metabolic consequences of exercise (twice weekly, 60 min of light exercise—walking/jogging, football, badminton) and diet, diet only, and exercise only in 48 patients with IGT (age, 47 to 49 years; average body weight, 80.5 kg). They noted a significant weight reduction in patients on diet only and the normalization of oral glucose tolerance in patients on exercise and diet. No significant changes were observed in muscle fiber distribution, muscle capillary density, hexokinase, or succinate dehydrogenase activity.

Ruderman, Ganda, and Johansen (102) investigated the influence of 24 weeks of physical training (bicycle ergometry at home 5 days per week for 20 to 30 min per day with a gradual increase in work load) on glucose tolerance in 6 patients with NIDDM treated by diet only (age, 52 ± 3 years; body weight, 87.3 ± 1.7 kg). They found a significant improvement of intravenous glucose tolerance that was not maintained after 8 days without exercise, a significant fall in serum triglycerides and cholesterol after removing one patient from analysis, no change in fasting blood glucose or insulin, and no improvement in oral glucose tolerance.

Bogardus et al. (10) evaluated the influence of exercise (1 hr per day, 3 days per week under the supervision of a sports physiologist aiming at 75% $\dot{V}O_2$max for at least 20 to 30 min and exercise alone on all other days) or diet on metabolic control over 12 weeks in 18 patients with NIDDM (average age, 45 years; body weight, 96.7 ± 9.8 kg). They could not identify any statistically significant difference between exercise and diet and diet alone on fasting blood glucose, plasma insulin, and C-peptide levels; on intravenous or oral glucose tolerance; or in euglycemic clamp studies.

Schneider et al. (107–109) report on a study on the benefits of exercise in 31 patients with NIDDM (age, 51 ± 2 years; body weight, 78.2 ± 1.5 kg). The exercise prescription encompassed training three times a week under the supervision of a sports physiologist on metered equipment (treadmill, bicycle ergometer, rowing machine) for eight 4-min periods interrupted by 1.5 min of rest. Initial exercise intensity was about 50% $\dot{V}O_2$max and increased after 2 weeks to 70% to 75% $\dot{V}O_2$max. They could achieve a fall in HbA_1 from 12.2% ± 0.5% to 10.7% ± 0.4%, which did not correlate with body weight, age, diabetes duration, initial $\dot{V}O_2$max, or improvement in $\dot{V}O_2$max.

Krotkiewski et al. (62) compared the metabolic effects of 3 weeks of exercise in 24 NIDDM patients (age, 49.8 ± 2.1 years; body weight, 87.5 ± 3.1 kg), 9 IGT patients, and 13 nondiabetic control subjects.

Exercise was composed of warm-ups, walking, jogging, and then alternating strenuous and light-intensity exercise for 50 min. Maximal intensities achieved on the bicycle ergometer were 80% to 90% $\dot{V}O_2$max for approximately 4 min. Subjects who did not show any evidence of physical training as measured by increased $\dot{V}O_2$max or submaximal heart rate were excluded from further evaluation. In the remainder, a significant reduction in the area under the glucose and C-peptide curves was seen in the diabetic patients following an oral glucose load. No change was seen in fasting blood glucose, fasting plasma C-peptide, fasting plasma insulin, and plasma insulin under the curve during the oral glucose load. No change was seen in insulin binding to adipocytes or in antilipolytic response to insulin after physical training. However, insulin-stimulated glucose incorporation into triglycerides after training was increased.

Reitman, Vasquez, Klimes, and Nagulesparan (97) assessed the influence of 6 to 10 weeks of exercise training (five to six times per week, 20 to 40 min of intermittent bicycle ergometer training, 5-min exercise periods interrupted by 2-min rest; intensity, approximately 60% to 90% maximal heart rate) on young American Indians with NIDDM (age, 26.3 years; body weight, 170% of desirable weight). Oral glucose tolerance improved only marginally, but euglycemic clamp studies showed statistically significant positive effects on insulin sensitivity.

Holloszy, Schultz, Kusnierkiewicz, Hagberg, and Ehsani (42) compared the metabolic changes in 21 participants (age, 56 ± 10 years; body weight, 85.4 ± 19 kg) of a coronary care group with NIDDM or IGT after 12 months of endurance exercise. The exercise prescription involved 40 to 45 min at 60% to 70% $\dot{V}O_2$max three times a week for the first 3 months and then a gradual increase to 50 to 60 min at 70% to 90% $\dot{V}O_2$max five times a week. They reported a significant improvement in insulin sensitivity as demonstrated by a decrease in the area under the curve for insulin and glucose during an oral glucose load; they also reported a significant weight loss and improvement in $\dot{V}O_2$max.

Rönemaa, Mattila, Lehtonen, and Kallio (100) compared the influence on glucose metabolism of 4 months of physical training (five to seven times a week of walking, jogging, or skiing for 45 min, equivalent to approximately 70% $\dot{V}O_2$max) in 13 patients with NIDDM to a sedentary control group (25 patients with NIDDM). They reported a significant fall in HbA_{1c} and an improvement in oral glucose tolerance without any changes in fasting plasma glucose or daily urinary glucose. They specifically noted that no metabolic improvement was seen in patients under poor metabolic control.

Jenkins, Furler, Bruce, and Chisholm (46) compared changes in hepatic glucose output (HGO) in healthy control subjects and patients with NIDDM (age, 46 ± 6 years; body weight, 91 ± 10 kg) after 1 hr of exercise at 50% $\dot{V}O_2$max. They observed a significant overall variance in the response of HGO to exercise in the patients with diabetes, summing to a significant decrease compared to healthy control subjects. Overall glucose utilization showed no change after exercise.

The Zuni Diabetes Project (38) documents a significant decrease in fasting blood glucose, a greater weight loss, and a greater decrease in the use of hypoglycemic medications in participants of a community-based exercise intervention compared to nonparticipants at a 2-year follow-up. Interestingly, women were significantly overrepresented among participants. Participant age was 42 ± 10 years, and body weight was 80.0 ± 10 kg. Participants were self-selected, and the study design was retrospective and uncontrolled for dietary measures.

Skarfors, Wegener, Lithell, and Selinus (115) recruited 48 patients with NIDDM out of 2,322 men from a health survey on approximately 60-year-old males. After patients with other major diseases and treatments affecting glucose or lipoprotein metabolism were excluded, 9 patients were eligible for a program involving regular physical exercise, but only 8 consented. Within 2 years, 2 patients had developed coronary heart disease (1 of which had a myocardial infarction), 2 dropped out (1 for personal reasons, 1 due to knee complaints), and 1 patient had a gallbladder operation and thereafter developed Achilles tendinitis. In 2 patients, metabolic control deteriorated even though they were exercising. With the exception of an average improvement in $\dot{V}O_2$max of 15.7% (with a very wide range including one decrease by 6.6%), there were no differences in glycemic control between the control and the exercise groups. Participation rates were low, overall about 53%. The authors conclude contending serious doubts as to the practical feasibility of exercise programs for patients of about 60 years of age with NIDDM (115).

Wing et al. (130), in a study of great practical importance, compared participation in a very low grade intensity exercise group (placebo exercise) over 1 year with participation in a moderate-intensity exercise class. Both interventions seemed to confer much the same effect. It appeared that the placebo exercisers compensated the lower intensity exercise by increasing day-to-day activity. In a follow-up study comparing diet only with strenuous physical activity once again over 1 year, no differences in HbA_{1c} or fasting blood glucose could be found at 0, 10, and 62 weeks, although caloric expenditure by physical activity did differ significantly.

This suggests possibly that the magnitude of the beneficial effect of exercise is but a small one or that emphasis on exercise may distract efforts directed at dietary measures (130).

Erikkson and Lindgärde (27) reported a study performed in 41 subjects with early-stage NIDDM and 181 subjects with impaired glucose tolerance; subjects were recruited from a previously reported screening program of 6,956, 47- to 49-year-old Malmö males. A 5-year protocol, consisting of either dietary treatment or increase in physical activity or training, or both, was completed by 90% of subjects. Data were compared to those of two control groups where nonintervention was made: a group of 79 subjects with IGT and a group of 114 subjects with normal glucose tolerance. Intervention resulted in normalization of glucose tolerance in more than 50% of subjects with IGT. The accumulated incidence of diabetes was 10.6%, and more than 50% of the patients were in remission after a mean follow-up of 6 years. In the nonintervened subjects with IGT, glucose tolerance deteriorated in 67%, and diabetes was found in 28.6%. Improvement in glucose tolerance was correlated to weight reduction (r = .19; p < .02) and increased fitness, as judged by increased $\dot{V}O_2max$ (r = .22; p < .02). It was impossible in this study to separate the effects of diet from those of increased physical activity.

Segal et al. (111) investigated the impact of vigorous training (cycle ergometer, 60-min cycling at 70% $\dot{V}O_2max$, four times a week for 12 weeks) in 10 lean and 10 obese subjects and 6 diet-controlled male NIDDM patients. Body weight and body composition were maintained by refeeding the energy expended in each training session. Cardiorespiratory fitness increased by 27% in all groups. Insulin sensitivity, studied by the euglycemic hyperinsulinemic clamp technique, was not significantly affected by training in any group; however, basal hepatic glucose production was reduced by 22% in the men with diabetes.

Thus, in contrast to promising theoretical considerations, experimental results on the metabolic benefits of exercise in patients with manifest NIDDM have not been unequivocally convincing. Significant improvements in insulin sensitivity and glucose tolerance have been demonstrated 12 hr postexercise (21,100) but were virtually unmeasurable 72 hr after the last bout of exercise (102,107). Carbohydrate feeding may even shorten the period of improved postexercise insulin sensitivity (131). Long-term metabolic improvements have been reliably reported only under training programs that can be assumed to be unacceptable for the majority of patients ($\dot{V}O_2max$ 70% to 90% for 50 to 60 min a day for 5 days a week—equivalent to about 25 to 35 km of running a week) (42). The magnitude of a blood glucose lowering effect of exercise for 30 min at 70% to 75% $\dot{V}O_2max$ was approximately 10% with respect to basal levels (108). On the other hand, in patients with impaired glucose tolerance, experimental results are more promising, suggesting a clinically relevant improvement of glucose tolerance, albeit requiring intensities of approximately 70% $\dot{V}O_2max$ or more.

In summary, caution is warranted against overinterpreting the few (mostly uncontrolled) intervention studies available on physical training and metabolic effects in NIDDM. One often faces difficulties separating dietary influences from exercise effects. Furthermore, recruited patients did not always reflect typical patients with NIDDM but rather selected subgroups (42,97).

Physical Activity and Incidence of Non-Insulin-Dependent Diabetes Mellitus

A few recent studies suggest that regular physical activity has potential in preventing NIDDM. Epidemiological studies based upon the presumption that the major difference between rural and urban populations is the degree of everyday physical activity offer support for this contention (120,132).

Helmrich, Ragland, Leung, and Paffenbarger (39) used questionnaires to examine patterns of physical activity and other personal characteristics in relation to the subsequent development of NIDDM in 5,990 male alumni of the University of Pennsylvania. NIDDM developed in a total of 202 men during 98.524 man-years of follow-up from 1962 to 1976. Leisure-time physical activity, expressed in kilocalories expended per week, was inversely related to the development of NIDDM. The incidence rates declined as energy expenditure increased from less than 500 kcal to 3,500 kcal. For each 500-kcal increment in energy expenditure, the age-adjusted risk of NIDDM was reduced by 6%. The association remained the same when the data were adjusted for obesity, hypertension, and parental history of diabetes. The protective effect of physical activity was strongest in persons at highest risk for NIDDM—defined as those with a high body mass index, a history of hypertension, or a parental history of diabetes. These factors, in addition to weight gain since college, were also independent predictors of the disease. As emphasized by Horton (43), these findings strongly support the position that persons who are at substantial risk for NIDDM should be encouraged to maintain a high level of physical activity in daily life.

In 1991, Manson et al. (71) reported the results of a study in which they examined the association between regular vigorous exercise and the subsequent incidence of NIDDM in a prospective cohort of 87,253 U.S. women (the Nurse's Health Study cohort) aged 34 to 59 years and free of diagnosed diabetes, cardiovascular disease, and cancer in 1980. During 8 years of follow-up, 1,303 cases of NIDDM did occur. Women who had engaged in vigorous exercise at least once per week had an age-adjusted relative risk (RR) of NIDDM of 0.67 ($p < .0001$) compared with women who did not exercise weekly. After adjustment for body mass index, the reduction in risk was attenuated but remained statistically significant (RR = 0.84; $p < .005$). However, among women who exercised at least once per week, there was no clear dose-response gradient according to the frequency of exercise. Multivariate adjustments for age, body mass index, family history of diabetes, and other variables did not alter the reduced risk found with exercise.

Exercise, Non-Insulin-Dependent Diabetes, and Obesity

Over 80% of patients with NIDDM are obese, and their elevated basal insulin levels and diminished insulin sensitivity are at least in part the consequence of their obesity. Obesity is characterized by increased body mass index (greater than 27.2 kg/m^2 in men and greater than 27.8 kg/m^2 in women) and greater accumulation of body fat (greater than 20% of body weight in men and greater than 30% in women). Excess adiposity is secondary to excess caloric intake per se rather than any specific component of the diet, although a diet high in fat content (corresponding to 45% to 50% of total calories) may predispose a person to body fat accumulation. When energy intake exceeds energy use, the excess calories are stored in adipose (fat) tissue as triglycerides. This initially leads to lipid accumulation and cell enlargement and secondarily triggers recruitment of cells from the adipocyte precursor pool (29).

To the dismay of many, weight loss modifies fat cell size but not adipocyte number. Changes in fat cell metabolism associated with obesity include a moderate rise in glucose conversion to glyceride glycerol (enhanced triglyceride reesterification) and an increase in basal lipolysis and lipoprotein lipase activity.

During fasting, 50% to 75% of total glucose metabolized by fat cells is converted to lactate. This lactate represents a significant proportion of precursors for hepatic gluconeogenesis. Increased lactate cycling in the obese may contribute to increased hepatic glucose output in obese diabetic patients (32). FFA elevation from enhanced lipolysis in obesity could contribute to reduced peripheral (mostly muscle) glucose utilization and to hyperinsulinemia by lowering hepatic insulin clearance. In obesity, possibly more so in central obesity (28,124), adipocytes are less sensitive to the insulin's promoting effect on glucose transport, partially due to reduced tissue insulin binding, the latter rapidly compensated by an increase in basal insulin secretion. Furthermore, severe obesity is associated with the development of a postreceptor defect in insulin activity, the magnitude of which correlates with the degree of obesity and plasma insulin levels (49,59,61). Overall basal glucose uptake of adipose tissue seems increased in obesity, from 10% to 20% of circulating glucose in a lean individual up to 30% in the obese (95).

Regular physical activity has been advocated as an adjunct to weight loss, especially in the moderately obese. However, the net caloric expenditure associated with moderate physical activity is often overestimated (walking, 1.15 kcal or 4.7 $kJ^{-1} \cdot kg^{-1} \cdot 1.6\ km^{-1}$; running, 1.71 kcal or 7.16 $kJ^{-1} \cdot kg^{-1} \cdot 1.6\ km^{-1}$; bicycling, 0.6 kcal or 2.5 $kJ \cdot kg^{-1} \cdot 1.6\ km^{-1}$) (33). In addition, in severely obese people, there are definite limitations to the scope of physical exertion possible (64).

Exercise, Non-Insulin-Dependent Diabetes, and Cardiovascular Disease

Diabetes ranks as the seventh leading cause of death in the United States. Ischemic heart disease is 2.8 times more frequent in men with NIDDM and 2.5 times more in women with NIDDM than in the general population and accounts for almost one half of deaths among diabetic men and one third of those among women with diabetes. In Caucasian populations all-cause age-adjusted mortality rates are approximately twice as high in diabetic as in nondiabetic men. Each additional decade of diabetes is associated with a 24% increase in risk for cardiovascular disease death (13,54,86). The most pronounced decrease in life expectancy is found in the young at onset (i.e., 10 to 15 years if NIDDM manifests at an age of 45 to 50 years) (87). In addition, diabetes is associated with a 16-fold higher frequency of extremity amputations; the incidence of cerebrovascular ischemia and the prevalence of arterial hypertension being 2-fold higher than in the general population (40); and the incidence of acquired blindness being 80-fold higher in patients with diabetes than in nondiabetic control subjects (6).

Diabetes care is much more than just blood glucose cosmetics. For most patients with NIDDM, macrovascular disease is responsible for the additional morbidity and mortality associated with the condition. Numerous population studies on physical activity (83,84) and physical fitness (25,116) have documented significantly fewer myocardial infarctions, sudden cardiac deaths, or cases of coronary heart disease in the more fit or more active. In fact, these differences may even be magnified in patients with diabetes (84). Most significant is the fact that a small increment in physical activity in the very sedentary is associated with the most significant change in relative risk of cardiovascular complications (9,68).

Conversely, similar absolute increases in activity in the moderately active may not lead to a measurable decrease in relative risk. Thus one must distinguish between physical fitness (what a person is capable of) and physical activity (what an individual actually does) (93). On a population-based scale, physical activity and fitness are well correlated (25). But this does not necessarily imply that increasing physical activity in the unfit makes them fit or improves disease outcome. For possibly hereditary factors may predispose certain people to be more active and at the same time protect against coronary heart disease (114,117). In general, regular exercise improves physical fitness, typically by about 15% to 20%, in middle-aged men.

There is no controlled intervention study that unequivocally documents the beneficial effect of regular physical activity in curtailing macrovascular disease (110). Circumstantial evidence, however, is highly suggestive. For the individual patient, preventing, delaying, or arresting macrovascular complications is much more meaningful than changes in an abstract concept such as insulin resistance or intermediate substrate cycling. It seems wise to give regular activity the benefit of the doubt. Further positive attributes of regular activity may include improved cardiac dynamics, a reduction of resting blood pressure, and beneficial influences on blood lipid composition or hemorrheological variables. Also, overall psychological well-being has been postulated to be a consequence of an active lifestyle leading to mood benefits and relief of anxiety (93,94). Feeling good about oneself, having an intact sense of coordination, and feeling generally fit are aims many would like to achieve. People with diabetes are unlikely to be an exception. On the contrary, a sense of self-mastery and a more active self-image through regular exercise may be particularly important to an individual confronted with a chronic condition such as non-insulin-dependent diabetes.

Limitations to Exercise and Practical Recommendations in Non-Insulin-Dependent Diabetes

When advocating physical exercise as a therapeutic measure in diabetic patients, one must not overlook the possibility of injury, cardiovascular events, and progression of diabetes-related complications. A recent community-based study in Sweden involving 31,620 individuals found that 17% of all injury-related physician consultations, 3.0% of outpatient and 0.7% of all inpatient care, and 1.2% of all days of compensated sick leave were due to sports and exercise injuries (18,19). Patients with diabetes show a significantly higher prevalence of silent myocardial ischemia, exercise-induced (14) and otherwise (57). Several authors also speculate on an entity distinct from macrovascular, microvascular, and neuropathic disease conferring impaired cardiac response to exercise in patients with NIDDM (11,75,118,119). Furthermore, patients with diabetes may be at a greater risk for cardiac arrhythmias (3), the overall incidence of which increase upon taking up vigorous exercise (114).

In all patients with diabetes, certain precautions are prerequisites to exercise or extended physical exertion. At least moderate metabolic control (blood glucose less than 300 mg/dl and minimal or no ketonuria) must be guaranteed in order to protect against inadvertent ketoacidosis or its progression (7) before the patient begins to exercise. In the case of suspected ketoacidosis, the primary aim is diagnosis. Urine testing is a simple and reliable way to test for ketosis. Symptomatic patients presenting with polyuria, polydipsia, marked weight loss, an acute infection, or muscle weakness would do better to abstain from exercise until metabolic control has stabilized, even if the momentary blood glucose level is acceptable.

Hypoglycemia is the most common specific risk for the physically active patient with diabetes. This is not a complication of the diabetic state but of therapy (oral hypoglycemic agents or insulin). Thus special care should be taken if a person with diabetes is exercising at a time when maximum insulin or oral hypoglycemic drug activity is expected. Warning signs that every person with diabetes, especially the physically active one, should be well aware of are sweating, trembling, unrest, visual disturbances, hunger, feeling weak, difficulty concentrating, dizziness, feeling drunk, and drowsiness (74). If hypoglycemia is suspected, blood glucose self-measurement is a must. The only exception is during a very rapid onset of symptoms, in which case carbohydrate intake may come first. If a patient loses consciousness, elementary steps in first aid involve (a) positioning the patient in such a position that suffocation cannot occur; (b) if available, injecting 1 mg glucagon subcutaneously or intramuscularly. (a possible alternative is placing easily soluble carbohydrate, preferably glucose, in a cheek pocket, ensuring that inadvertent swallowing is impossible), and (c) calling an ambulance or a physician if the condition does not improve rapidly. It is mandatory that those who train with people who have diabetes are aware of appropriate first aid strategies.

Only a few studies have been directed at deriving explicit recommendations toward strategies for consuming additional carbohydrate or adjusting the insulin dose in situations of physical exertion (106). The normoglycemic person whose diabetes is treated with an oral hypoglycemic agent or insulin should take a rapidly assimilated carbohydrate (approximately 0.5 g per minute of moderate exercise or 1 g per minute of vigorous exercise) about 20 to 30 min before exercise. In cases of prolonged exercise, carbohydrate should be taken in 30- to 60-min intervals during exercise and 15 to 30 g should be taken after exercise to prevent hypoglycemia (67). More moderate amounts of additional carbohydrate may be recommended for near-to-normoglycemic patients taking oral hypoglycemic agents (51).

For planned prolonged exercise (hikes, cross-country skiing) in patients on a conventional insulin regimen, reducing the insulin dose by 30% and eating carbohydrates at a rate of approximately 40 g/hr have been recommended (109). Omitting the morning regular insulin dose and reducing the long-acting insulin dose to 20% to 50% of the normal dose are also advised if the patient intends to perform 3 or more hr of moderate exercise after breakfast upon preexisting normoglycemia (50). At blood glucose levels between 200 and 300 mg/dl, a less substantial reduction in insulin dose will be sufficient to prevent hypoglycemia during a 3-hr exercise period. If the patient plans to exercise in the afternoon or evening (and many patients do), he or she should be advised to reduce the evening insulin dose in order to avoid nocturnal hypoglycemic episodes. Postexercise hypoglycemia as a consequence of facilitated peripheral glucose disposal may occur up to 6 to 15 hr after the exercise bout. It appears to be especially common when taking up training after a longer pause (70).

The degree of screening that a patient with diabetes mellitus should be subject to prior to taking up endurance exercise is dependent upon his or her age, duration of diabetes, associated cardiovascular risk factors, and extent of known complications. The patient who reports past symptoms relatable to cardiac disease must be exercise-tested (exercise ECG) irrespective of age. An exercise test is furthermore advisable for patients over 35 years of age with a duration of diabetes of more than 10 years. All patients over the age of 45 should be subject to exercise testing.

When contemplating exercise as part of the therapeutic strategy in the management of patients with NIDDM, one should keep in mind that, in Caucasian populations, the maximal prevalence rates of NIDDM have their peaks at an age of about 60 years for men and 70 years for women. Furthermore, diabetic populations show an impaired cardiovascular reserve and high prevalence of associated illnesses. Thus there are limitations to the degree of physical activity theoretically possible due to the advanced age and the associated prevalence of other diseases and ailments. The European NIDDM Policy Group (2) states : "Objectives and priorities of treatment must be tailored to the individual; particular care must be taken to avoid overtreatment in the elderly."

The following recommendation toward achieving and maintaining cardiovascular fitness applies to healthy populations but may well be extrapolated to the diabetic individual: "exercise which involves large muscle groups in dynamic movement for periods of 20 minutes or longer 3 days or more per week, and which is performed at an intensity of 60% or greater of individual cardiorespiratory capacity" (37). On the other hand, the aforementioned studies on lifetime activity and cardiovascular disease show that a definite lowering of risk is associated with relatively small amounts of additional activity (150 kcal/day). In summary, we can say 20 min at 60% $\dot{V}O_2max$ three times per week would be ideal. If that seems too much, a lower target that the person concerned will actually perform may be much more practical. Lower intensity activities have the added advantage of being more comfortable, more convenient, more affordable, and thus more likely to be done. Light exercise, gardening, cycling, and the like seem to be well tolerated even in elderly patients (72).

Measuring pulse rate before, during, and after maximal exertion is a simple and useful strategy in estimating physical reserve and degree of exertion. However, its use as a measure of exercise intensity may be unreliable in patients with diabetes. A number of studies have reported that during exercise the heart rate of subjects with diabetes was 15 to 30 beats per minute higher at the same percentage of maximal oxygen consumption than that of nondiabetic control subjects. On the other hand, patients with cardiac neuropathy would exhibit a lower heart rate than a healthy control subject at a moderate degree of exertion and also a lower cardiac output and a lower stroke volume (41,101). This should be ruled out prior to regular physical exertion. For those with arterial hypertension, measuring blood pressure before and after (and, if need be, during, especially if symptomatic) an exercise period can be reassuring and protect against unnecessary complications. Contraindications for exercise (and maximal exertion) are systolic blood pressure over 250 mmHg and diastolic over 120 mmHg. In general, it seems wise to recommend abstention from exercise if blood pressure is not near normal.

Although a definite association between sudden increases in abdominal pressure (Valsalva maneuver, push-ups, weight lifting, contact sports, etc.) and retinal hemorrhage or retinal detachment is as yet unproven, it seems prudent to avoid such measures in patients with advanced diabetic retinopathy. Furthermore, exercise should be avoided for about 6 weeks in patients following retinal photocoagulation.

Care also should be taken to ensure proper footwear. Especially in patients with peripheral neuropathy, adequate footwear (soft-cushioned footwear with sufficient support) is mandatory. Trainers, physical education teachers, or physiotherapists should be able to identify pressure marks on a patient's feet and in the shoes. If pressure marks are noted, the patient should be referred to his or her physician. In patients with definite neuropathic ulcerations, immobilization of the involved extremity is the hallmark of treatment. Exercise involving an afflicted foot is contraindicated.

Last, but by far not least, patient compliance is a definite problem. Fitness programs for adults show compliance rates between 40% and 65%. Negative predictors for compliance in one study were a higher percentage of body fat, a higher body weight, and lesser degree of motivation (22). Two out of three of these factors are indeed overrepresented in patients with NIDDM. Similar compliance rates have been reported from cardiac rehabilitation programs and seem typical for counseling programs targeted to other health behaviors such as smoking and dieting (37).

Summary and Conclusions

In patients with established non-insulin-dependent diabetes mellitus (NIDDM), the potential metabolic effects of regular exercise are probably small. If one considers the aforementioned 10% fall in blood glucose levels over baseline after 30 min of moderate exercise (70% to 75% $\dot{V}O_2$) (108) and multiplies this by the expected compliance rate (about 50%), the population-wide benefit of regular physical activity is approximately 5% of basal glucose levels. Such a small decrease will rarely be clinically significant and will hardly influence long-term outcome. With respect to metabolic control and insulin resistance in patients with NIDDM, reducing caloric intake appears to be a more potent tool than regular exercise. With weight loss and an adjusted caloric intake, therapy with oral agents or insulin may be avoided or postponed in many patients with NIDDM. Regular physical activity may be a useful adjunct in maintaining these goals (38). However, exercise seems to have a definite potential in improving glucose tolerance in patients with impaired glucose tolerance (IGT) or very early NIDDM; it is on these subjects that our efforts in advocating exercise therapy should focus. Furthermore, two recent large prospective studies (39,71) indicate that increased physical activity is effective in the primary prevention of NIDDM and that the protective benefit of exercise is especially pronounced in persons with a high body mass index, a history of arterial hypertension, or a parental history of diabetes.

With respect to cardiovascular disease, the relative risk of a sedentary lifestyle for the general population in most studies comes well behind other known risk factors, in particular, cigarette smoking and arterial hypertension (9,83,116). This should be considered when therapeutic priorities are defined. On the other hand, if the majority of the population, patients with diabetes included, had a lifetime physical activity equivalent to a brisk 30-min walk three times per week, we could well see a significant population-wide fall in cardiovascular morbidity and mortality.

Acknowledgment

We acknowledge the expert secretarial help of E. Vaessen-Petit.

References

1. Ahrén, B.; Lindskog, S.; Tatemoto, K.; Efendic, S. Pancreastatin inhibits insulin secretion and stimulates glucagon secretion in mice. Diabetes. 37:281-285; 1988.
2. Alberti, K.G.M.M.; Gries, F.A. Management of non insulin dependent diabetes mellitus in Europe: A consensus view. Diabetic. Med. 5:275-281; 1988.
3. Bakth, S.; Arena, J.; Lee, W.; Torres, R.; Haider, B.; Patel, B.C.; Lyons, M.M.; Regan, T.J. Arrhythmia susceptibility and myocardial composition in diabetes. J. Clin. Invest. 77:382-395; 1986.
4. Barnard, R.J.; Lattimore, L.; Holly, R.G.; Cherny, S.; Pritkin, N. Response of non-insulin-dependent diabetic patients to an intensive program of diet and exercise. Diabetes Care. 5:370-374; 1982.

5. Barnett, A.H.; Eff, C.; Leslie, R.D.G.; Pyke, D.A. Diabetes in identical twins: A study of 200 pairs. Diabetologia. 20:87-93; 1981.
6. Benson, W.E.; Brown, G.C.; Tasman, W. Diabetes and its ocular complications. Philadelphia: Saunders; 1988.
7. Berger, M.; Berchthold, P.; Cüppers, H.J.; Drost, H.; Kley, H.K.; Müller, W.A.; Wiegelmann, W.; Zimmermann-Telschow, H.; Gries, F.A.; Krüskemper, H.L.; Zimmermann, H. Metabolic and hormonal effects of muscular exercise in juvenile type diabetes. Diabetologia. 13:355-365; 1977.
8. Björntorp, P.; Berchtold, P.; Grimby, G.; Lindholm, B.; Sanne, H.; Tibblin, G.; Wilhelmsen, L. Effects of physical training on glucose tolerance, plasma insulin and lipids and on body composition in men after myocardial infarction. Acta. Med. Scand. 192:439-443; 1972.
9. Blair, S.N.; Kohl, H.W., III; Paffenberger, R.S.; Clark, D.G.; Cooper, K.H.; Gibbons, L.W. Physical fitness and all cause mortality. JAMA. 262:2395-2401; 1989.
10. Bogardus, C.; Ravussin, E.; Robbins, D.C.; Wolfe, R.R.; Horton, E.S.; Sims, E.A.H. Effects of physical training and diet therapy on carbohydrate metabolism in patients with glucose intolerance and non-insulin-dependent diabetes mellitus. Diabetes. 33:311-318; 1984.
11. Bouchard, A.; Sanz, N.; Botvinick, E.H.; Phillips, N.; Heilbron, D.; Byrd, B.J.; Karam, B.J.; Karam, J.K.; Schiller, N.B. Noninvasive assessment of cardiomyopathy in normotensive diabetic patients between 20 and 50 years old. Am. J. Med. 87:160-166; 1989.
12. Brunzell, J.D.; Robertson, R.P.; Lerner, R.L.; Hazzard, W.R.; Ensinck, J.W.; Bierman, E.L.; Porte, D. Relationship between fasting plasma glucose levels and insulin secretion during intravenous glucose tolerance tests. J. Clin. Endocrinol. Metab. 42:222-229; 1976.
13. Butler, W.J.; Ostrander, L.D.; Carman, W.J.; Lamphiear, D.E. Mortality from coronary heart disease in the Tecumseh study. Am. J. Epidemiol. 121:541-547; 1985.
14. Callaham, P.R.; Froelicher, V.F.; Klein, J.; Risch, M.; Dubach, P.; Friis, R. Exercise-induced silent ischemia: Age, diabetes mellitus, previous myocardial infarction and prognosis. J. Am. Coll. Cardiol. 14:1175-1180; 1989.
15. Cerasi, E.; Luft, R.; Efendic, S. Decreased sensitivity of the pancreatic beta cells to glucose in prediabetic and diabetic subjects. Diabetes. 21:224-234; 1972.
16. Coon, P.J.; Bleeker, E.R.; Drinkwater, D.T.; Meyers, D.A.; Goldberg, A.P. Effects of body composition and exercise capacity on glucose tolerance, insulin and lipoprotein lipids in healthy older men: A cross sectional and longitudinal intervention study. Metabolism. 38:1201-1209; 1989.
17. Cooper, G.J.S.; Willis, A.C.; Clark, A.; Turner, R.C.; Sim, R.B.; Reid, K.B.M. Purification and characterization of a peptide from amyloid-rich pancreases of type 2 diabetic patients. Proc. Natl. Acad. Sci. 84:8628-8632; 1987.
18. de Loes, M. Medical treatment and costs of sports-related injuries in a total population. Int. J. Sports Med. 11:66-72; 1990.
19. de Loes, M.; Goldie, I. Incidence rate of injuries during sports activity and physical exercise in a rural Swedish municipality: Incidence rates in 17 sports. Int. J. Sports Med. 9:461-467; 1988.
20. Devlin, J.T.; Hirshman, M.; Horton, E.D.; Horton, E.S. Enhanced peripheral and splanchnic insulin sensitivity in NIDDM men after single bout of exercise. Diabetes. 36:434-439; 1987.
21. Devlin, T.; Horton, E.S. Effects of prior high-intensity exercise on glucose metabolism in normal and insulin-resistant men. Diabetes. 34:973-979; 1985.
22. Dishman, R.K.; Ickes, W.; Morgan, W.P. Self-motivation and adherence to habitual physical activity. J. Appl. Soc. Psychol. 10:115-132; 1980.
23. Dowse, G.K.; Zimmet, P.Z.; Gareeboo, H.; Alberti, K.G.M.M.; Tuomilehto, J.; Finch, C.F.; Chitson, P.; Tulsidas, H. Abdominal obesity and physical inactivity as risk factors for NIDDM and impaired glucose tolerance in Indian, Creole, and Chinese Mauritians. Diabetes Care. 14:271-282; 1991.
24. Dunning, B.E.; Ahren, B.; Veith, R.; Böttcher, G.; Sundler, F.; Taborsky, G.J. Galanin: A novel pancreatic neuropeptide. Am. J. Physiol. 251:E127-E133; 1986.
25. Ekelund, L.-G.; Haskell, W.L.; Johnson, J.L.; Whaley, F.S.; Criqui, M.H.; Sheps, D.S. Physical fitness as a predictor of cardiovascular mortality in asymptomatic North American men. N. Engl. J. Med. 319:1379-1384; 1988.
26. Enk, B. Secretin induced insulin response. Acta Endocrinol. 82:312-317; 1976.
27. Eriksson, K.-F.; Lindgärde, F. Prevention of Type 2 (non-insulin-dependent) diabetes mellitus by diet and physical exercise. Diabetologia. 34:891-898; 1991.
28. Evans, D.J.; Hoffmann, R.G.; Kalkhoff, R.K.; Kissebah, A.H. Relationship of body fat topography to insulin sensitivity and metabolic profiles in premenopausal women. Metabolism. 33:68-75; 1984.
29. Faust, I.M.; Johnson, P.R.; Stern, J.S.; Hirsch, J. Diet-induced adipocyte number increase in adult rats: A new model of obesity. Am. J. Physiol. 235:E279-E286; 1978.

30. Feldman, M.; Kiser, R.S.; Unger, R.H.; Li, C.H. Beta-endorphin and the endocrine pancreas. N. Engl. J. Med. 308:349-353; 1983.
31. Flier, J.S. Insulin receptors and insulin resistance. Annu. Rev. Med. 34:145-160; 1983.
32. Foster, D.W. From glycogen to ketones—and back. Diabetes. 33:1188-1199; 1984.
33. Franklin, B.A.; Rubenfire, M. Losing weight through exercise. JAMA. 244:377-379; 1980.
34. Gepts, W.; Lecompte, P.M. The pancreatic islet in diabetes. Am. J. Med. 70:105-115; 1981.
35. Giugliano, D.; Salvatore, T.; Cozzolino, D.; Ceriello, A.; Torella, R.; D'Onofrio, F. Hyperglycemia and obesity as determinants of glucose, insulin, and glucagon responses to β-endorphin in human diabetes mellitus. J. Clin. Endocrinol. Metab. 64:1122-1128; 1987.
36. Halter, J.B.; Porte, D. Mechanisms of impaired acute insulin release in adult onset diabetes: Studies with isoproterenol and secretin. J. Clin. Endocrinol. Metab. 46:952-960; 1978.
37. Harris, S.; Caspersen, C.J.; DeFriese, G.H.; Estes, E.H. Physical activity counseling for healthy adults as a primary prevention intervention in the clinical setting. JAMA. 261:3590-3598; 1989.
38. Heath, G.W.; Leonard, B.E.; Wilson, R.H.; Kendrick, J.S.; Powell, K.E. Community-based exercise intervention: Zuni diabetes project. Diabetes Care. 10:579-583; 1987.
39. Helmrich, S.P.; Ragland, D.R.; Leung, R.W.; Paffenbarger, R.S. Physical activity and reduced occurence of non-insulin dependent diabetes mellitus. N. Engl. J. Med. 325:147-152; 1991.
40. Herman, W.H.; Teutsch, S.M.; Geiss, L.S. Diabetes mellitus. In: Amter, R.W.; Dull, B.H., eds. Closing the gap. Oxford: Oxford University Press; 1984:72-82.
41. Hilsted, J.; Galbo, H.; Christensen, N.J.; Parving, H.-H.; Benn, J. Hemodynamic changes during graded exercise in patients with diabetic autonomic neuropathy. Diabetologia. 22:318-323; 1982.
42. Holloszy, J.O.; Schultz, J.; Kusnierkiewicz, H.; Hagberg, J.M.; Ehsani, A.A. Effects of exercise on glucose tolerance and insulin resistance. Acta Med. Scand. [Suppl.]. 711:55-65; 1985.
43. Horton, E.S. Exercise and decreased risk of NIDDM (Editorial). N. Engl. J. Med. 325:196-197; 1991.
44. Hortulanus-Beck, D.; Lefèbvre, P.J.; Jeanjean, M.F. Diabetes in the Belgian province of Luxembourg: Frequency, importance of the oral glucose tolerance test and of a fasting glycaemia discreetly increased. Diabetes Metab. 16:311-317; 1990.
45. Huse, D.M.; Oster, G.; Killen, A.R.; Lacey, M.; Colditz, G.A. The economic cost of non-insulin dependent diabetes mellitus. JAMA. 262:2708-2713; 1989.
46. Jenkins, A.B.; Furler, S.M.; Bruce, D.G.; Chisholm, D.J. Regulation of hepatic glucose output during moderate exercise in non-insulin-dependent diabetes. Metabolism. 37:966-972; 1988.
47. Kaplan, R.M.; Hartwell, S.L.; Wilson, D.K.; Wallace, J.P. Effects of diet and exercise interventions on control and quality of life in non-insulin-dependent diabetes mellitus. J. Gen. Intern. Med. 2:220-228; 1987.
48. Kaplan, R.M.; Wilson, D.K.; Hartwell, S.L.; Merino, K.L.; Wallace, J.P. Prospective evaluation of HDL cholesterol changes after diet and physical conditioning programs for patients with Type II diabetes mellitus. Diabetes Care. 8:343-348; 1985.
49. Kashiwagi, A.; Bogardus, C.; Lillioja, S.; Hueckstеadt, T.P.; Brady, D.; Verso, M.A.; Foley, J.E. In vitro insensitivity of glucose transport and antilipolysis to insulin due to receptor and postreceptor abnormalities in obese Pima indians with normal glucose tolerance. Metabolism. 33:772-777; 1984.
50. Kemmer, F.W.; Sonnenberg, G.E.; Cüppers, H.J.; Berger, M. Prevention of exercise induced hypoglycemia in diabetes mellitus. In: Serrano-Rios, M.; Lefèbvre, P.J., eds. Diabetes 1985. Amsterdam: Elsevier Science; 1985:963-967.
51. Kemmer, F.W.; Tacken, M.; Berger, M. Mechanisms of exercise-induced hypoglycemia during sulfonylurea treatment. Diabetes. 36:1178-1182; 1987.
52. Kissebah, A.H.; Vydelingum, N.; Murray, R.; Evans, D.J.; Hartz, A.J.; Kalkoff, R.D.; Adams, P.W. Relation of body fat distribution to metabolic complications of obesity. J. Clin. Endocrinol. Metab. 54:254-260; 1982.
53. Kjeldsen, H.; Hansen, A.P.; Lundbaek, K. Twenty four hour serum growth hormone levels in maturity-onset diabetics. Diabetes. 24:977-982; 1975.
54. Kleinman, J.C.; Donahue, R.P.; Harris, M.I.; Finucane, F.F.; Madans, J.H.; Brock, D.B. Mortality among diabetics in a national sample. Am. J. Epidemiol. 128:389-401; 1988.
55. Knowler, W.C.; Pettit, D.J.; Savage, P.J.; Bennett, P.H. Diabetes incidence in Pima indians: Contributions of obesity and parental diabetes. Am. J. Epidemiol. 113:144-156; 1981.
56. Knowler, W.C.; Williams, R.C.; Pettitt, D.J.; Steinberg, A.G. $Gm^{3;5,13,14}$ and type 2 diabetes mellitus: An association in American indians with genetic admixture. Am. J. Hum. Genet. 43:520-526; 1988.
57. Koistinen, M.J. Prevalence of asymptomatic myocardial ischemia in diabetic subjects. Br. Med. J. 301:92-95; 1988.

58. Kolterman, O.G.; Gray, R.S.; Griffin, J.; Burstein, P.; Insel, I. Receptor and postreceptor defects contribute to the insulin resistance in non-insulin-dependent diabetes mellitus. J. Clin. Invest. 68:957-969; 1981.
59. Kolterman, O.G.; Insel, J.; Saekow, M.; Olefsky, J.M. Mechanisms of insulin resistance in human obesity. J. Clin. Invest. 65:1272-1284; 1980.
60. Krolewski, A.S.; Warram, J.H. The epidemiology of diabetes mellitus. In: Joslin, E.P., ed. Joslin's diabetes mellitus. Philadelphia: Lea & Febiger; 1985:12-42.
61. Krotkiewski, M.; Björntorp, P.; Sjöström, L.; Smith, U. Impact of obesity on metabolism in men and women. J. Clin. Invest. 72:1150-1162; 1983.
62. Krotkiewski, M.; Lönnroth, P.; Mandroukas, K.; Wroblewski, Z.; Rebuffé-Scrive, M.; Holm, G.; Smith, U.; Björntorp, P. The effects of physical training on insulin secretion and effectiveness and on glucose metabolism in obesity and type 2 (non-insulin-dependent) diabetes mellitus. Diabetologia. 28:881-890; 1985.
63. Krotkiewski, M.; Sjöström, L.; Björntorp, P.; Smith, U. Regional adipose tissue cellularity in relation to metabolism in young and middle-aged women. Metabolism. 24:703-710; 1975.
64. Lampman, R.M.; Schteingart, D.E.; Foss, M.L. Exercise as a partial therapy for the extremely obese. Med. Sci. Sports Exerc. 18:19-30; 1985.
65. Lefèbvre, P.J. Diabetes: Abnormal secretion of glucagon. In: Samols, E., ed. The endocrine pancreas. New York: Raven Press; 1991:191-205.
66. Lefèbvre, P.J.; Paolisso, G.; Scheen, A. The role of glucagon in non-insulin-dependent (type 2) diabetes mellitus. In: Sakamoto, N.; Angel, A.; Hotta, N., eds. New directions in research and clinical works for obesity and diabetes mellitus. Amsterdam: Elsevier Science; 1991:25-29.
67. Lefèbvre, P.J.; Pirnay, F.; Pallikarakis, N.; Krzentowski, G.; Jandrain, B.; Mosora, F.; Lacroix, M.; Luyckx, A.S. Metabolic availability of carbohydrates ingested during, before, or after muscular exercise. Diabetes Metab. Rev. 1:483-500; 1986.
68. Leon, A.S.; Connet, J.; Jacobs, D.R.; Rauramaa, R. Leisure time physical activity levels and risk of coronary heart disease and death. JAMA. 258:2388-2395; 1987.
69. Liljenquist, J.E.; Mueller, G.L.; Cherrington, A.D.; Perry, J.M.; Rabinowitz, D. Hyperglycemia per se (insulin and glucagon withdrawn) can inhibit hepatic glucose production in man. J. Clin. Endocrinol. Metab. 48:171-175; 1979.
70. MacDonald, M.J. Post exercise late-onset hypoglycemia in insulin-dependent diabetic patients. Diabetes Care. 10:584-588; 1987.
71. Manson, J.E.; Rimm, E.B.; Stampfer, M.J.; Colditz, G.A.; Willett, W.C.; Krolewski, A.S.; Rosner, B.; Hennekens, C.H.; Speizer, F.E. Physical activity and incidence of non-insulin dependent diabetes mellitus in women. Lancet. 338:774-778; 1991.
72. McPhillips, J.B.; Pelletra, K.M.; Barret-Connor, E.; Wingard, D.L.; Criqui, M.H. Exercise patterns in a population of older adults. Am. J. Prev. Med. 5:65-72; 1989.
73. Modan, M.; Karasik, A.; Halkin, H.; Fuchs, Z.; Lusky, A.; Shitrit, A.; Modan, B. Effect of past and concurrent body mass index on prevalence of glucose intolerance and type 2 (non-insulin-dependent) diabetes and on insulin response. Diabetologia. 29:82-89; 1986.
74. Muehlhauser, I.; Heinemann, L.; Fritsche, E.; von Lennep, K.; Berger, M. Hypoglycemia symptoms and frequency of severe hypoglycemia in patients treated with human and animal insulin preparations. Diabetes Care. 14:745-749; 1991.
75. Mustonen, J.N.; Uusituta, M.I.; Tahvanainen, K.; Talwar, S.; Laakso, M.; Länsimies, E.; Kuikka, J.T.; Pyrölää, K. Impaired left ventricular systolic function during exercise in middle aged insulin dependent and non-insulin dependent diabetic subjects without clinically evident cardiovascular disease. Am. J. Cardiol. 62:1273-1279; 1988.
76. National Diabetes Data Group. Classification and diagnosis of diabetes mellitus and other categories of glucose intolerance. Diabetes. 28:1039-1057; 1979.
77. Newman, B.; Selby, J.V.; King, M.-C.; Slemenda, C.; Fabsitz, R.; Friedman, G.D. Concordance for type 2 (non-insulin-dependent) diabetes mellitus in male twins. Diabetologia. 30:763-768; 1987.
78. NIDDM enigma. (Editorial). Lancet. 335:1187-1188; 1990.
79. Ohlson, L.-O.; Larsson, B.; Svärdsudd, K.; Welin, L.; Eriksson, H.; Björntorp, P.; Tibblin, G. The influence of body fat distribution on the incidence of diabetes mellitus. Diabetes. 34:1055-1058; 1985.
80. Ohlson, L.-O.; Larsson, B.; Svärdsudd, K.; Welin, L.; Tibblin, G. Diabetes in Swedish middle-aged men. Diabetologia. 30:386-393; 1987.
81. O'Rahilly, S.; Wainscoat, J.S.; Turner, R.C. Type 2 (non-insulin-dependent) diabetes mellitus. New genetics for old nightmares. Diabetologia. 31:407-414; 1988.
82. O'Sullivan, J.B.; Mahan, C.M. Blood sugar levels, glycosuria, and body weight related

to development of diabetes mellitus. JAMA. 194:117-122; 1965.

83. Paffenbarger, R.S.; Hyde, R.T.; Wing, A.L.; Hsieh, C.-C. Physical activity and all-cause mortality, and longevity of college alumni. N. Engl. J. Med. 314:605-613; 1986.
84. Paffenbarger, R.S.; Wing, A.L.; Hyde, R.T. Physical activity as an index of heart attack risk on college alumni. Am. J. Epidemiol. 108:161-175; 1978.
85. Palmer, J.P.; Benson, J.W.; Walter, R.M.; Ensinck, J.W. Arginine-stimulated acute phase of insulin and glucagon secretion in diabetic subjects. J. Clin. Invest. 58:565-570; 1976.
86. Pan, W-H.; Cedres, L.B.; Liu, K.; Dyer, A.; Schoenberger, J.A.; Shekelle, R.B.; Stamler, R.; Smith, D.; Collette, P.; Stamler, J. Relationship of clinical diabetes and asymptomatic hyperglycemia to risk of coronary heart disease mortality in women. Am. J. Epidemiol. 123:504-517; 1986.
87. Panzram, G. Mortality and survival in type 2 (non-insulin-dependent) diabetes mellitus. Diabetologia. 30:123-131; 1987.
88. Paolisso, G.; Scheen, A.J.; D'Onofrio, F.; Lefèbvre, P. Magnesium and glucose homeostasis. Diabetologia. 33:511-514; 1990.
89. Paolisso, G.; Sgambato, S.; Giugliano, D.; Torella, R.; Varricchio, M.; Scheen, A.J.; D'Onofrio, F.; Lefèbvre, P.J. Impaired insulin-induced erythrocyte magnesium accumulation is correlated to impaired insulin-mediated glucose disposal in type 2 (non-insulin-dependent) diabetic patients. Diabetologia. 31:910-915; 1988.
90. Pell, S.; D'Alonzo, A. Some aspects of hypertension in diabetes mellitus. JAMA. 202:104-110; 1967.
91. Pettit, D.J.; Aleck, K.A.; Baird, R.H.; Carraher, M.J.; Bennett, P.H.; Knowler, W.C. Congenital susceptibility to NIDDM. Diabetes. 37:622-628; 1988.
92. Pfeifer, M.A.; Halter, J.B.; Porte, D. Insulin secretion in diabetes mellitus. Am. J. Med. 70:579-588; 1981.
93. Powell, K.E.; Caspaersen, C.J.; Koplan, J.P.; Ford, E.S. Physical activity and chronic diseases. Am. J. Clin. Nutr. 49:999-1006; 1989.
94. Raglin, J.S. Exercise and mental health. Sports Med. 9:323-329; 1990.
95. Reaven, G.M. Role of insulin resistance in human disease. Diabetes. 37:1595-1607; 1988.
96. Reid, R.L; Yen, S.S.C. Beta-endorphin stimulates the secretion of insulin and glucagon in humans. J. Clin. Endocrinol. Metab. 52:592-594; 1981.
97. Reitman, J.S.; Vasquez, B.; Klimes, I.; Nagulesparan, M. Improvement of glucose homeostasis after exercise training in non-insulin-dependent diabetes. Diabetes Care. 7:434-441; 1984.
98. Revers, R.R.; Fink, R.; Griffin, J.; Olefsky, J.M.; Kolterman, O.G. Influence of hyperglycemia on insulin's in vivo effects in type II diabetes. J. Clin. Invest. 73:664-672; 1984.
99. Rogers, M.A.; Yamamoto, C.; King, D.S.; Hagberg, J.M.; Ehsani, A.A.; Holloszy, J.O. Improvement in glucose tolerance after 1 week of exercise in patients with mild NIDDM. Diabetes Care. 11:613-618; 1988.
100. Rönemaa, T.; Mattila, K.; Lehtonen, A.; Kallio, V. A controlled randomised study on the effect of long term physical exercise on the metabolic control in type 2 diabetic patients. Acta Med. Scand. 220:219-224; 1986.
101. Roy, T.M.; Peterson, H.R.; Snider, H.L.; Cyrus, J.; Broadstone, V.L.; Fell, R.D.; Rothchild, A.H.; Samols, E.; Pfeifer, M.A. Autonomic influence on cardiovascular performance in diabetic subjects. Am. J. Med. 87:382-388; 1989.
102. Ruderman, N.B.; Ganda, O.P.; Johansen, K. The effect of physical training on glucose tolerance and plasma lipids in maturity-onset diabetes. Diabetes. [Suppl. 1]. 28:89-92; 1979.
103. Saad, M.F.; Knowler, W.C.; Pettit, D.J.; Nelson, R.G.; Mott, D.M.; Bennett, P.H. The natural history of impaired glucose tolerance in the Pima indians. N. Engl. J. Med. 319:1500-1506; 1988.
104. Sacca, L.; Hendler, R.; Sherwin, R.S. Hyperglycemia inhibits glucose production in man independent of changes in glucoregulatory hormones. J. Clin. Endocrinol. Metab. 47:1160-1163; 1978.
105. Saltin, B.; Lindgarde, F.; Houston, R.; Hörlin, R.; Nygaard, E.; Gad, P. Physical training and glucose tolerance in middle-aged men with chemical diabetes. Diabetes. [Suppl. 1]. 28:30-32; 1979.
106. Sane, T.A.; Helve, E.; Pelkonen, R.; Koivisto, V.A. The adjustment of diet and insulin dose during long-term endurance exercise in type I (insulin-dependent) diabetic men. Diabetologia. 31:35-40; 1988.
107. Schneider, S.H.; Amorosa, L.F.; Khachadurian, A.K.; Ruderman, N.B. Studies on the mechanism of improved glucose control during regular exercise in type 2 (non-insulin-dependent) diabetes. Diabetologia. 26:355-360; 1984.
108. Schneider, S.H.; Khachadurian, A.K.; Amorosa, L.F.; Gavras, V.; Fineberg, S.E.; Ruderman, N.B. Abnormal glucose tolerance during exercise in type II (non-insulin-dependent) diabetes. Metabolism. 36:1161-1166; 1987.
109. Schneider, S.H.; Kim, H.C.; Khachadurian, A.K.; Ruderman, N.B. Impaired fibrinolytic response to exercise in type II diabetes: Effects of exercise and physical training. Metabolism. 37:924-929; 1988.

110. Sedgwick, A.W.; Brotherhood, J.R.; Harris-Davidson, A.; Tapllin, R.E.; Thomas, D.W. Long-term effects of physical training programme on risk factors for coronary heart disease in otherwise sedentary men. Br. Med. J. 5:7-10; 1980.
111. Segal, K.R.; Edano, A.; Albu, A.; Blando, L.; Tomas, M.B.; Pi-Sunyer, F.X. Effect of exercise training on insulin sensitivity and glucose metabolism in lean, obese, and diabetic men. J. Appl. Physiol. 71:2402-2411; 1991.
112. Serjeantson, S.W.; Owerbach, D.; Zimmet, P.; Nerup, J.; Thoma, K. Genetics of diabetes in Nauru: Effects of foreign admixture, HLA antigens and the insulin-gene-linked polymorphism. Diabetologia. 25:13-17; 1983.
113. Shulman, G.I.; Rothman, D.L.; Jue, T.; Stein, P.; DeFronzo, R.A.; Shulman, R.G. Quantitation of muscle glycogen synthesis in normal subjects and subjects with non-insulin-dependent diabetes by 13C nuclear magnetic resonance spectroscopy. N. Engl. J. Med. 322:223-228; 1990.
114. Siscovick, D.S.; Weiss, N.S.; Fletcher, R.H.; Lasky, T. The incidence of primary cardiac arrest during vigorous exercise. N. Engl. J. Med. 311:874-877; 1984.
115. Skarfors, E.T.; Wegener, T.A.; Lithell, H.; Selinus, I. Physical training as treatment for type 2 (non-insulin-dependent) diabetes in elderly men. A feasibility study over 2 years. Diabetologia. 30:930-933; 1982.
116. Slattery, M.L.; Jacobs, D.R. Physical fitness and cardiovascular disease mortality. Am. J. Epidemiol. 127:571-580; 1988.
117. Sobolski, J.; Kornitzer, M.; De Backer, G.; Dramaix, M.; Abramowicz, M.; Degre, S.; Denolin, H. Protection against ischemic heart disease in the Belgian physical fitness study: Physical fitness rather than physical activity? Am. J. Epidemiol. 125:601-610; 1987.
118. Takahashi, N.; Iwasaka, T.; Sugiura, T.; Hasegawa, T.; Tarumi, N.; Inada, M. Diastolic time in diabetes. Chest. 100:748-753; 1991.
119. Takahashi, N.; Iwasaka, T.; Sugiura, T.; Hasegawa, T.; Tarumi, N.; Matsutani, M.; Onoyama, H.; Inada, M. Left ventricular dysfunction during dynamic exercise in non-insulin dependent diabetic patients with retinopathy. Cardiology. 78:23-30; 1991.
120. Taylor, R.; Ram, P.; Zimmet, P.; Raper, L.R.; Ringrose, H. Physical activity and prevalence of diabetes in Melanesian and Indian men in Fiji. Diabetologia. 27:578-582; 1984.
121. Thomson, G. The genotypic distribution among non-insulin-dependent diabetes mellitus (NIDDM) patients of a restriction fragment length polymorphism. Am. J. Hum. Genet. 36:466-470; 1984.
122. Trovati, M.; Carta, Q.; Cavalot, F.; Vitali, S.; Banaudi, C.; Lucchina, P.G.; Fiocchi, F.; Emanuelli, G.; Lenti, G. Influence of physical training on blood glucose control, glucose tolerance, insulin secretion, and insulin action in non-insulin-dependent diabetic patients. Diabetes Care. 7:416-420; 1984.
123. Varsano-Aharon, N.; Echemendia, E.; Yalow, R.S.; Berson, S.A. Early insulin responses to glucose and to tolbutamide in maturity-onset diabetes. Metabolism. 19:409-417; 1970.
124. Ward, W.K.; Johnston, C.L.W.; Beard, J.C.; Benedetti, T.J.; Porte, D. Abnormalities of islet B-cell function, insulin action, and fat distribution in women with histories of gestational diabetes: Relationship to obesity. J. Clin. Invest. 61:1039-1045; 1985.
125. Ward, W.K.; LaCava, E.C.; Paquette, T.L.; Beard, J.C.; Wallum, B.J.; Porte, D. Disproportionate elevation of immunoreactive proinsulin in type 2 (non-insulin-dependent) diabetes mellitus and in experimental insulin resistance. Diabetologia. 30:698-702; 1987.
126. West, K.M.; Kalbfleisch, J.M. Influence of nutritional factors on prevalence of diabetes. Diabetes. 20:99-108; 1971.
127. Westermark, P.; Wilander, E. The influence of amyloid deposits on the islet volume in maturity onset diabetes mellitus. Diabetologia. 15:417-421; 1978.
128. Westermark, P.; Wilander, E.; Westermark, G.T.; Johnson, K.H. Islet amyloid polypeptide-like immunoreactivity in the islet β cells of type 2 (non-insulin-dependent) diabetic and non-diabetic individuals. Diabetologia. 30:887-892; 1987.
129. Wilson, P.W.; McGee, D.L.; Kannel, W.B. Obesity, very low density lipoproteins, and glucose intolerance over fourteen years. Am. J. Epidemiol. 114:697-704; 1981.
130. Wing, R.R.; Epstein, L.H.; Paternostro-Bayles, M.; Kriska, A.; Nowalk, M.P.; Gooding, W. Exercise in a behavioural weight control programme for obese patients with type 2 (non-insulin-dependent) diabetes. Diabetologia. 31:902-909; 1988.
131. Young, J.C.; Garthwaite, S.M.; Bryan, J.E.; Holloszy, J.O. Carbohydrate feeding speeds reversal of enhanced glucose uptake in muscle after exercise. Am. J. Physiol. 245:R684-R688; 1983.
132. Zimmet, P.; Faaiuso, S.; Ainuu, S.; Whitehouse, S.; Milne, B.; DeBoer, W. The prevalence of diabetes in the rural population of Western Samoa. Diabetes. 30:45-51; 1981.

Chapter 46

Physical Activity, Fitness, and Moderate Obesity

James O. Hill
Holly J. Drougas
John C. Peters

Obesity is a condition of excess body fat that results from energy intake exceeding energy expenditure. Exercise is capable of altering energy intake and energy expenditure, substrate flux, and body composition. Thus, it is an important variable to consider in understanding obesity development and treatment.

In this chapter, we examine the role of physical activity in obesity development, maintenance, and treatment. We focus on moderate obesity, which is distinguished from massive or severe obesity. Moderate obesity is generally associated with a body mass index between 26 and 34, whereas massive obesity is generally associated with a body mass index of 35 or greater. We use the term physical activity to refer to all locomotor activity, planned as well as spontaneous. We distinguish between effects of acute bouts of exercise and effects of exercise training.

The Role of Physical Activity in the Etiology of Obesity

There is little question that physical activity–induced energy expenditure has the potential to play an important role in energy balance. After resting metabolic rate (RMR), physical activity is the largest component of total daily energy expenditure and in most individuals contributes close to half of the daily energy expenditure (16,68). Under extreme conditions of physical labor or athletic training, activity-related energy expenditure may exceed the quantitative contribution of RMR to total daily energy expenditure. Because of the major role played by physical activity in energy expenditure, an attractive hypothesis has been that inactivity is an important contributor to the development of obesity (and, conversely, that vigorous regular physical activity may prevent obesity development).

A relationship between obesity development and reduced physical activity can be hypothesized from epidemiological research. These types of studies include studies of societies undergoing industrial development, studies of aging populations, and comparisons of urban and rural populations. Matsushima, Kriska, Tajima, and LaPorte (48) and Thompson, Jarvie, Lahey, and Cureton (81) have summarized the published literature that provides evidence of an association between reduced physical activity and incidence of obesity.

The relationship between obesity and chronic physical activity can be examined in populations by examining correlations between indices of physical fitness and obesity. A frequently used method of quantifying aerobic physical fitness is the measure of maximum aerobic capacity, or $\dot{V}O_2$max. Although $\dot{V}O_2$max has genetic determinants, it varies directly with aerobic exercise (2,24). $\dot{V}O_2$max shows a strong negative correlation with percentage of body fat and a modest positive correlation with fat-free mass (FFM) (52).

A variety of experimental approaches have been used to quantify potential lean-obese differences in daily physical activity under both natural and controlled settings. Assessment methods using activity diaries, visual observations, and devices such as accelerometers worn on the body have not yielded a consistent picture of whether or not total daily physical activity differs between lean and obese individuals. Some studies support a reduced level of physical activity in the obese, and others do not. Several reviews on this topic are available (48,59,81).

In those studies that have attempted to measure spontaneous activity (separate from exercise, and sometimes referred to as fidgeting) by radar detectors, wide variation has generally been observed between lean and obese individuals (68).

The best evidence for a causal role of physical activity in obesity comes from prospective studies of genetically obese animals or animal strains susceptible to dietary-induced obesity. One of the earliest studies of the potential role of inactivity in obesity was an experiment by Ingle (36) in which rats were given a palatable chow diet and either were allowed to move freely or were placed in cages that restricted activity. The restricted animals gained greater amounts of weight than did their unrestricted counterparts. Although energy intakes were not reported, these data have been taken as evidence that inactivity can cause obesity in rats.

More compelling evidence comes from studies of genetically obese rodents. Both the ob/ob mouse and the obese Zucker (fa/fa) rat are spontaneously less active than their lean littermates (49,78). In the obese Zucker rat, inactivity is evident at weaning and occurs prior to any noticeable obesity. When forced to exercise, both the ob/ob mouse and the fa/fa rat do not become obese as rapidly, although exercise alone does not normalize body weight (50,78,79,89). This latter finding underscores the potential of exercise to prevent or retard the development of obesity, even when food intake is unrestricted.

Additional evidence of the benefit of activity in mitigating against obesity comes from studies of exercise cessation in animals. In both rats (1) and hamsters (85), exercise detraining led to rapid increases in food intake, body weight, and body fat. These responses were accompanied by increased lipogenic enzyme activity and a metabolic pattern that would favor storage of food energy. Thus, although exercise can attenuate the development of obesity, this benefit appears to be rapidly reversed once the stimulus to energy expenditure is removed.

Although there is a relative abundance of prospective data in animals demonstrating the role of inactivity in the development of obesity, relatively few data are available in humans. In a study by Roberts, Savage, Coward, Chew, and Lucas (70) total daily energy expenditure was measured in infants using doubly labeled water. In addition, resting metabolic rate was measured using indirect calorimetry. Infants with the lowest total daily energy expenditure tended to gain the most weight over the subsequent 3 months. However, when RMR was taken into account, it was apparent that much of the weight-gain tendency could be accounted for by differences in spontaneous activity.

In a study of adult Pima Indians, Ravussin et al. (69) measured RMR and total daily energy expenditure. Subjects with the lowest 24-hr total energy expenditure were most likely to gain weight over subsequent months. Although these same individuals also displayed a reduced RMR, the difference between total energy expenditure and RMR was still reduced, suggesting that reduced physical activity was an important factor in obesity development in these individuals.

In summary, although the existing literature provides an indication that some obese humans engage in a reduced amount of physical activity compared to their nonobese counterparts, it is not possible at present to conclude that this low level of physical activity either causes the obesity or contributes to the maintenance of the obese state. Unfortunately, most studies of lean-obese differences in physical activity did not include measures of energy expenditure. Even if some obese individuals engage in less physical activity than their lean counterparts, they may not expend less energy in this activity.

Finally, it may be useful to reconsider the important questions in this area. Much research has focused on the impact on energy expenditure of different levels of physical activity, but energy intake must play an equally important role in determining effects on body weight, because achieving and maintaining overall energy balance depends on matching intake and expenditure. Thus, even if an individual displayed reduced physical activity compared to a matched nonobese control subject, obesity would only develop if energy intake in that same individual were inappropriately high for the actual level of energy expenditure. According to such a model, the defect leading to obesity is not in the activity component, nor is it in the intake component, but rather it is in the mechanism that integrates these components in an attempt to establish a steady state (i.e., balance).

Prospective animal studies provide some support for the hypothesis that inactivity leads to obesity, and there is a great need for more prospective studies in human subjects. A limitation in planning such studies is the unavailability of accurate techniques for quantifying physical activity. A promising technique for quantifying physical activity inside a whole-room calorimeter using a force platform mounted on precision force transducers has recently been described by Sun and Hill (80). The force platform can accurately quantify the work performed by subjects while simultaneous measurements of energy expenditure are made with the calorimeter. An intriguing aspect of this technique is that it allows calculation of work efficiency (the work performed divided by the increase in energy expenditure above RMR due to that work). It is possible that individual differences in work efficiency could be important in obesity development.

Physical Activity in the Treatment of Moderate Obesity

In this section, we examine whether physical activity alone or in combination with food restriction can be an important component of a weight-reduction program for moderately obese humans. In order to do this, it is necessary to consider the effects of physical activity on energy intake, energy expenditure, and body mass.

Exercise Alone as a Treatment for Moderate Obesity

When human subjects increase their level of physical activity, a state of negative energy balance must occur unless there is caloric compensation for the amount and type of energy expended in physical activity. Thus, the first question to consider is whether prescribing exercise in moderately obese humans produces complete caloric compensation. If not, changes in body weight or body composition must occur. The magnitude of these changes will be determined by the degree of negative energy balance. To determine this, the degree of caloric compensation should be subtracted from the effects of exercise on total daily energy expenditure. Clearly, both measures are difficult to quantify accurately, but only on this basis can the true effectiveness of exercise for obesity treatment be evaluated.

Does Exercise Produce Caloric Compensation?

In animal experiments, exercise has been reported to decrease, increase, or have no effect on food intake (57). The specific response seems to depend on the age and sex of the animal, as well as the type, duration, and intensity of the exercise. Generally speaking, in animals, exercise is associated with some food-intake response, and it is rare that intake is increased beyond the level needed to offset the energy expended during exercise. The result is either no change or a reduction in body weight.

In humans, there are relatively few well-controlled studies on this topic. A series of careful studies by Woo, Garrow, and Pi-Sunyer (94,95) have provided evidence that control of energy intake is dissociated from energy expenditure in the obese. They studied the effects of moderate exercise on energy intakes of both nonobese and obese women housed on a metabolic ward and found that whereas nonobese women increased caloric intake when exercise was added to the daily routine, obese women did not. When the palatability of the food offered was enhanced, obese women still did not increase intake in response to exercise. More recent work (37) has confirmed these findings under conditions of moderate- and prolonged-duration exercise in obese women. A similar dissociation of energy intake from energy expenditure was also found in obese men (91). These authors concluded that in obese people, food-related cues more strongly influence control of energy intake than do signals arising from physical activity–induced energy expenditure.

The observation that obese individuals do not increase energy intake when activity is increased suggests that prescribed exercise should be of benefit for either retarding weight gain or causing weight loss. In view of the enhanced responsiveness of some individuals to signals arising from food, the most effective therapeutic measures will likely be combinations of increased physical activity and dietary modification.

Does Exercise Alone Alter Energy Expenditure?

Many investigators have evaluated the effects of exercise on total daily energy expenditure and on various components of energy expenditure. The components are sleeping metabolic rate (SMR), resting metabolic rate (RMR), the thermic effect of food (TEF), and the energy expenditure due to physical activity (EE_{ACT}). The major determinant of RMR is fat-free mass (68). The major quantitative determinants of TEF are not precisely known, but they include the obligatory energy required in processing ingested nutrients. EE_{ACT} consists of the amount of physical activity performed multiplied by the energy cost of each unit of activity. Although the cost of activity is dependent on the amount of body mass being moved (73), this component is highly variable due to individual differences in amount of physical activity performed (16).

It is important to distinguish between the acute effects of a bout of exercise and the effects of chronic exercise on energy expenditure. Three different acute effects of exercise on energy expenditure have been postulated. First, and most obvious, energy expenditure is elevated during a bout of exercise. This will elevate total daily energy expenditure unless the prescribed exercise leads to an equivalent decline in spontaneous physical activity.

Second, it is clear that energy expenditure does not immediately return to preexercise levels following a bout of exercise. However, the period of time during which there is an increase in postexercise energy expenditure may be variable. Some have suggested energy expenditure can be elevated as long as 24 hr after a bout of exercise (6), whereas others have suggested baseline energy expenditure is restored within a few minutes of exercise cessation (25). Furthermore, it appears that the magnitude and duration of the postexercise increase in energy expenditure is related to the intensity and duration of the exercise bout; longer, more intense exercise is likely to produce a more significant postexercise increase in energy expenditure (10). In this regard, it is questionable whether the intensity and duration of exercise usually prescribed for moderately obese humans is sufficient to produce any significant postexercise increase in energy expenditure.

The final mechanism by which exercise could acutely affect energy expenditure is through its interaction with food. Some data suggest a synergistic relationship between the energy expended in physical activity and that due to TEF (53). Segal et al. (74,75) have suggested that obese humans show a smaller increase in energy expenditure in response to the combined effects of a single meal and exercise than do nonobese humans. However, others using a whole-room calorimeter have concluded that, at least with moderate activity, there is little evidence to support a synergistic relationship between energy expenditure due to TEF and that produced by physical activity over a whole day (15,17). Dauncey (16) reviewed this area and concluded that the majority of research suggests the energy cost of human activity is independent of food intake and that there is not a synergistic relationship between the thermic effect of food and that of exercise.

The effects of chronic exercise on energy expenditure are more controversial. Because chronic exercise can alter body composition (41) and because FFM is a major determinant of energy expenditure (68), it is important to assess whether exercise influences energy expenditure directly or via its effects on body composition. Two types of studies exist in the literature: cross-sectional studies examining the relationship between energy expenditure and indices of physical fitness, and longitudinal training studies in which subjects increase physical fitness (usually aerobic fitness).

There are both cross-sectional and longitudinal studies in support of the notion that the effects of chronic exercise are mediated via effects on body composition. The effect of physical fitness on 24-hr sedentary energy expenditure has been assessed in three studies using whole-room indirect calorimetry. Ravussin and Bogardus (67) studied 205 Pima Indians in a whole-room calorimeter and found that $\dot{V}O_2$max did not affect sedentary daily energy expenditure after the known determinants of daily energy expenditure (i.e., FFM, fat mass, age) were accounted for. Sharp, Reed, Abumrad, Sun, and Hill (76) studied 39 men and 39 women for one sedentary day each in a whole-room calorimeter. $\dot{V}O_2$max (measured using a treadmill) and body composition (measured by hydrostatic weighing) were also determined. Although $\dot{V}O_2$max was significantly correlated with total energy expenditure, SMR, RMR, and TEF, when fat-free mass was considered, $\dot{V}O_2$max did not explain a significant amount of the remaining variation in total daily energy expenditure or in any component of energy expenditure. Finally, Schulz, Nyomba, Alger, Anderson, and Ravussin (72) studied sedentary daily energy expenditure in 20 trained and 43 untrained males. They found no difference in daily sedentary energy expenditure between the groups either before or after adjusting for body composition.

Using short-term measures, many investigators (31,43,44,47) have reported that RMR (expressed per unit of FFM or body weight) does not differ in groups of trained versus untrained subjects. Sharp et al. (76) examined the relationships among RMR, $\dot{V}O_2$max, and FFM in a group of 214 weight-stable adult men and women studied over a period of 5 years. All measures were collected in a similar fashion for all subjects. Using a multiple-regression analysis, the researchers found that FFM explained a significant amount of the variation in RMR ($r^2 = .68$), but adding $\dot{V}O_2$max did not significantly increase the amount of the variation in RMR that was explained. This suggests that fitness did not have a direct effect on RMR but rather had an indirect effect via its effect on body composition. Similarly, most investigators have found that exercise training in nonobese subjects has little effect on RMR (7,35,51,66,84). This is not surprising because training in nonobese subjects generally has a very small effect on FFM, the major determinant of RMR.

There are, however, investigators who have reported that exercise can affect RMR independently of effects on body composition. Poehlman and colleagues (63,64) found that RMR is higher in physically fit subjects than in non-physically fit subjects (classified on the basis of $\dot{V}O_2$max) and that the difference is independent of FFM. Similarly, they find a significant positive correlation between $\dot{V}O_2$max and RMR in adults and elderly subjects, even after FFM is taken into account. There are two reports (42,83) in which RMR increased with aerobic exercise training despite no increase in FFM. In one of these (42), 6 nonobese women were subjected to 10 weeks of jogging. RMR was measured every 2 weeks during the study. Although it was reported that exercise training increased RMR, the response was highly variable from measurement to measurement: RMR, as compared to baseline, was increased at Weeks 4 and 10 but not at Weeks 2, 6, and 8.

There are wide discrepancies in the literature regarding whether chronic exercise affects TEF. Some investigators have reported a greater TEF in aerobically fit versus unfit subjects (18,31,47), whereas others have reported no difference in TEF due to aerobic fitness level (58), and still others have reported that TEF is lower in aerobically fit subjects than in unfit subjects (43,44,65,83). The reasons for such discrepant findings are not clear. The effect of chronic exercise on TEF is also unclear; some reports indicate an increase (18), and others show no change (84) in TEF with exercise training.

Very little is known about effects of chronic exercise on EE_{ACT}. It would appear likely that adding exercise to the activities of sedentary subjects increases the total amount of physical activity, but it is possible that the added physical exercise could be offset to some degree by a reduction in other spontaneous activity. It is unclear whether exercise training alters the energy cost of physical activity. It does not appear to do so with non-weight-bearing exercise such as cycling (92), but training may affect the efficiency of weight-bearing exercise such as walking.

Does Exercise Alone Alter Body Weight or Body Composition?

There have been many studies in which the effects of exercise alone on body weight and body composition have been assessed in nonobese as well as in moderately obese humans. These have been comprehensively summarized in review articles by Wilmore (93), Epstein and Wing (23), and Ballor and Keesey (3). In each case, the reviewers concluded that exercise alone can reduce body weight, reduce body fat, and increase fat-free mass. However, it was pointed out that the changes produced by exercise alone are small. Ballor and Keesey (3) identified predictors for changes in body mass and body composition produced by exercise alone. For both men and women, the best predictor for the decrease in body mass was the combination of initial body mass plus the amount of energy expended in exercise. For both men and women, the best predictor for the decrease in fat mass was a combination of initial percentage body fat plus the energy expended in exercise. For both men and women, the best predictor of increase in FFM was the combination of initial percentage body fat and the length of the exercise program. However, this combination accounted for a higher proportion of variance in women than men. Finally, the best predictor of the decline in percentage body fat was the combination of initial percentage body fat plus the amount of energy expended in exercise. Taken together, results of all available studies suggest exercise alone can produce small reductions in body mass, fat mass, and percentage body fat and a modest increase in FFM.

Finally, the data concerning effects of weight training on body mass and body composition are intriguing. Ballor and Keesey (3) also reviewed these studies and found that weight training produced reductions in body fat that were only slightly less than those produced by aerobic exercise and that weight training also produced more substantial increases in FFM. The use of weight training for obesity treatment should be given strong emphasis in the future.

Summary

The majority of research suggests that complete caloric compensation does not occur when moderate exercise is prescribed for obese subjects. Whether or not caloric compensation may be more complete with higher intensity exercise or with long-term exercise training is not clear and needs further attention. It seems likely that obese subjects must experience some degree of negative energy balance when they exercise, and this degree of negative energy balance must produce changes in body weight and body composition. However, with the various types and durations of exercise that have been used previously, the magnitude of both the expected and the observed change was small.

Exercise produces a moderate reduction in body fat and an even smaller increase in FFM. The total reduction in body weight and body fat should be greater in moderately obese than in nonobese subjects and greater in males than females. The type, intensity, and duration of exercise appear to have small effects on these changes, with the total loss of weight and fat varying directly with the total energy expended in exercise.

The strongest data available suggest that the effect of exercise on energy expenditure is small and is mediated by changes in body composition. Finally, when one considers the most common exercise programs used with moderately obese subjects, only small changes in body mass and body composition would be expected. Certainly the expectations of subjects losing weight by exercise alone should be much different than those of subjects losing weight by dieting.

The Combination of Food Restriction and Exercise in Treatment of Moderate Obesity

The literature contains many studies in which the combination of food restriction and exercise for obesity treatment has been compared with food restriction alone. Many reviews have been published on this topic (9,20). The objective here is to briefly review the studies of exercise and food restriction with the intent of identifying particular points of agreement or disagreement among published studies. In Table 46.1 we have summarized the results of 26 studies assessing whether the combined effects of exercise and food restriction differ from effects of food restriction alone on energy expenditure and body mass.

Does Exercise Prevent the Decline in Energy Expenditure That Occurs With Food Restriction?

It is clear that food restriction alone produces a decline in energy expenditure that accompanies the decline in body weight (9). The three major components of energy expenditure—RMR, TEF, and EE_{ACT}—would all be expected to decline as body mass declines. RMR varies directly with FFM and would be expected to decline as FFM declines. TEF varies directly with amount of food eaten so that it would be expected to decline with restricted food intake, and EE_{ACT} is known to vary with total body mass, so it, too, would be expected to decline as body weight is reduced. However, the question remains as to whether the decline in energy expenditure can be totally explained by those three factors or whether an additional adaptive factor plays a role in the decrease in energy expenditure. Additionally, it is necessary to consider the time course of the changes in body mass versus the changes in energy expenditure. For example, Wadden, Foster, Letizia, and Mullen (88) followed subjects for 48 months following weight reduction and found that although RMR declined more rapidly than FFM initially, at 48 months post weight loss RMR was appropriate for FFM.

Seventeen of the studies in Table 46.1 measured the effects of food restriction alone versus exercise and food restriction on RMR. All studies except one (46) found that RMR (expressed in kcal) declined with weight loss. In the vast majority of studies, exercise added to food restriction did not produce a smaller drop in RMR than food restriction alone (5,12,21,29,30,33,34,55,86,90). Additionally, most studies reported that the decline in RMR was explained by the decline in FFM.

In four studies, it was reported that exercise attenuated the decline in RMR seen with food restriction alone (19,46,54,87). In two of these (19,54), all subjects were given exercise early in weight loss, followed by exercise termination. The decline in RMR during the exercise period was compared with the decline in RMR in the no-exercise period. Because weight loss tends to be greater in the early stages of a food-restriction program, this is probably not a valid test of whether exercise affects the decline in RMR. Lennon et al. (46) reported that RMR increased following weight reduction in a group of 65 subjects and that the increase was greater for a group given a prescribed exercise program than for subjects given no exercise. The loss of FFM was minimal in both groups but was slightly greater for exercising subjects than for sedentary subjects. Two studies by Van Dale and colleagues (86,87) provide some support for a beneficial effect of exercise on RMR. In one study (86), although RMR (expressed per kg FFM) was reduced by diet alone and by diet plus exercise, the reduction was less in subjects who exercised during food restriction. In a second study (87), subjects who lost weight by diet alone or by diet plus exercise were studied 42 months after weight loss. RMR (expressed per kg FFM) remained 16% below baseline for subjects dieting alone but was only 4% below baseline values for subjects exercising during food restriction. The latter group also had greater success in sustaining weight reduction.

It has been suggested that the effect of exercise on RMR may depend on the degree of food restriction. Phinney, LaGrange, O'Connell, and Danforth (62) reported that exercise combined with a very low calorie diet (VLCD) led to a greater reduction in RMR than did diet alone. There are, however, reports that exercise plus VLCD increased weight loss without adverse effects on RMR (71) and that resistance exercise plus VLCD may help reduce the drop in RMR (45). With the increased popularity of such diets, it will be important to obtain more information concerning whether exercise provides a benefit to subjects who follow a very low calorie diet.

The question of how TEF is affected by weight loss is unclear, because there is no agreement on whether it is lower in obese subjects before weight loss than in nonobese subjects (14).

It is unclear how EE_{ACT} is altered by weight loss either with or without exercise. Whereas the amount of activity may be relatively independent of body mass and body composition, the energy cost of activity is not (73). Weight reduction is associated with a reduction in the energy cost of physical activity so that even if the amount of activity remains unchanged, EE_{ACT} should decline with weight reduction. Almost no information is available concerning whether the decline in the energy cost of activity with weight reduction is affected by how the weight was lost (i.e., exercise vs. diet).

Does the Addition of Exercise to Food Restriction Affect Body Weight or Body Composition?

Table 46.1 also shows the results of studies examining effects of food restriction alone versus exercise

Table 46.1 Outcomes for Effects of Exercise and Food Restriction on Obesity Treatment

		Does exercise added to food restriction			
Author	Year	Increase weight loss?	Increase body fat loss?	Decrease FFM loss?	Decrease RMR decline?
Buskirk et al. (12)	1963	Trend*	No	No	No
Dudleston & Bennion (22)	1970	Trend			
Kenrick et al. (38)	1972	Trend	Trend		
Zuti & Golding (96)	1976	Trend	Trend	Trend	
Weltman et al. (91)	1980	No	Trend	Trend	
Warwick & Garrow (90)	1981	No	No	No	No
Bogardus et al. (8)	1984	No	No	No	
Donahoe et al. (19)	1984	No			Yes**
Pavlou et al. (61)	1985	No	Yes	Yes	
Lennon et al. (46)	1985	No	Yes (males only)	No	Yes (greater increase)
Sopko et al. (77)	1985	No	Yes		
Hagan et al. (28)	1986	Yes	Yes	No	
Hill et al. (34)	1987	No	Yes	Yes	No
Belko et al. (5)	1987	No	Yes	Yes	No
Van Dale et al. (86)	1987	No	No	No	No
Henson et al. (30)	1987	No			No
Phinney et al. (62)	1988	No	No	No	Greater drop with exercise
Nieman et al. (55)	1988	No	No	No	Trend: RMR/kg of weight increased with weight loss
Hill et al. (33)	1989	Yes	Yes	Yes	No
Mole et al. (54)	1989	No			Yes**
Hammer et al. (29)	1989	Trend	Trend	No	No
Van Dale et al. (87)	1990	Yes	Yes	No	Yes
Wadden et al. (88)	1990	No			No
Ballor et al. (4)	1990	No intensity effect			
Nieman et al. (56)	1990	No	No		
Donnelly et al. (21)	1991	No	No	No	No

*The results of the study were in the expected direction but did not reach statistical significance.

**The study design involved no exercise during early part of weight loss; exercise followed later in study.

plus food restriction on changes in body weight, body fat, and FFM in moderately obese subjects. Few studies have assured that the caloric deficit was similar between conditions, so that adding exercise should produce a greater overall caloric deficit than food restriction alone. The hypotheses to be tested are that exercise added to food restriction produces (a) greater weight loss, (b) greater fat loss, and (c) less FFM loss than food restriction alone. Clearly, the results are mixed. Some studies support some or all of these hypotheses, and some studies do not support them. It is interesting, however, that many of the studies not supporting these hypotheses report effects that are in the expected direction but do not reach statistical significance. This suggests that the results may depend on the total amount of energy expended in the exercise program. Thus, exercise may have produced significant effects on weight loss if the exercise program had been more intense or of longer duration.

In some studies listed in Table 46.1, subjects were studied while living on a metabolic ward, and in some studies subjects were studied as outpatients. The differences in results cannot be explained on this basis; mixed results were obtained in both types of studies. It is also noteworthy that some investigators have reported that exercise can have favorable effects on body composition (i.e., greater loss of body fat and lesser loss of FFM) without having a measurable effect on body weight. Exercise can alter the amounts and proportions of fat and carbohydrate oxidized (i.e., alter respiratory quotient) both during exercise and nonexercise periods (41), and this could be a potential benefit of including exercise with a program of food restriction.

Summary

There is no strong reason from the available data to conclude that the effects of exercise are not additive with the effects of food restriction on energy balance. Thus, the benefit of exercise alone on body weight, body composition, and energy expenditure is preserved when added to a program of food restriction. A major problem with many studies reporting no benefit of exercise has been a failure to evaluate the expected changes (i.e., body weight, body fat, FFM) in relation to the total energy expenditure produced by the exercise.

The Role of Physical Activity in the Maintenance of a Reduced Body Weight

Exercise is one of the few factors that is clearly correlated with success in maintaining a reduced body weight (9,11,40). However, it is unclear from available data whether exercise has distinct value in weight maintenance or whether exercise is simply a marker for identifying subjects who have been compliant with dietary and other lifestyle changes. Many investigators have attempted to identify factors correlated with successful long-term maintenance of a reduced body weight, and exercise is almost always a factor found to correlate with success (13,27,39). Most such studies identified a population of successful subjects (i.e., those who have maintained a reduced body weight for a period of time) and used interviews or questionnaires to assess behavior (13,27). Some studies show that subjects who exercise during weight loss are better at maintaining a weight reduction than subjects who do not exercise during weight reduction (33,60).

A key goal of further research should be to understand why exercise is correlated with successful maintenance of a reduced body weight. In particular, it will be important to determine if there are physiological reasons that explain why exercise helps in weight maintenance. It could be simply that exercise leaves subjects with higher energy requirements than if they were not exercising. This could occur due to the increased energy expended in exercise itself and the effects of exercise on increasing FFM.

Summary

Most available data suggest that many obese humans engage in low levels of physical activity compared to their nonobese counterparts. It is likely that inactivity contributes both to obesity development and maintenance in some individuals. To demonstrate this, prospective research is needed that involves more accurate methods of quantifying physical activity and uses state-of-the-art techniques for measurement of energy expenditure and body composition.

We believe it is erroneous to conclude that exercise itself or in combination with food restriction cannot produce weight loss in the obese. When moderately obese humans increase their physical activity, a state of negative caloric balance is almost certainly produced, at least initially. There is little evidence of complete caloric compensation in moderately obese subjects. This negative energy balance must produce a change in body weight or body composition, or both. Exercise alone appears to lead to reduced body fat and increased FFM. Exercise combined with food restriction appears to enhance fat loss and minimize FFM loss. If exercise continues to create a state of negative energy balance, the loss of body fat will exceed the gain in

FFM, and weight loss will result. Eventually body weight and body composition stabilize at a new level, most likely determined by the beginning body composition of the subject and by the type, intensity, and duration of the exercise. These changes may be rapidly reversed with exercise cessation. Many studies have found benefits of exercise in loss of body weight and body fat, and those that have not may have used insufficient exercise.

Subjects who successfully achieve and maintain a reduction in body weight are highly likely to be exercisers, but it is not clear if exercise provides any advantage beyond the increased energy expenditure produced during exercise itself.

Finally, part of the confusion in assessing the benefits of exercise in obesity treatment may be due to inappropriate comparisons between effects of exercise and food restriction. The degree of negative caloric balance produced by most exercise programs would be small in relation to the degree of negative caloric balance produced by most hypocaloric diets. Thus, it is inappropriate to compare at face value the resulting changes in body weight and body composition produced by exercise with those produced by dieting over the same time period.

References

1. Applegate, E.A.; Stern, J.S. Exercise termination effects on food intake, plasma insulin, and adipose lipoprotein lipase activity in the Osborne-Mendel rat. Metabolism. 36:709-714; 1987.
2. Astrand, P.; Rodahl, K. Textbook of work physiology. New York: McGraw-Hill; 1986.
3. Ballor, D.L.; Keesey, R.E. A meta-analysis of the factors affecting exercise-induced changes in body mass, fat mass and fat-free mass in males and females. Int. J. Obes. 15:717-726; 1991.
4. Ballor, D.L.; McCarthy, J.P.; Wilterding, E.J. Exercise intensity does not affect the composition of diet- and exercise-induced body mass loss. Am. J. Clin. Nutr. 51:142-146; 1990.
5. Belko, A.Z.; Van Loan, M.; Barbieri, T.F.; Mayclin, P. Diet, exercise, weight loss, and energy expenditure in moderately overweight women. Int. J. Obes. 11:93-104; 1987.
6. Bielinski, R.; Schutz, Y.; Jequier, E. Energy metabolism during the postexercise recovery in man. Am. J. Clin. Nutr. 42:69-82; 1985.
7. Bingham, S.A.; Goldberg, G.R.; Coward, W.A.; Prentice, A.M.; Cummings, J.H. The effect of exercise and improved physical fitness on basal metabolic rate. Br. J. Nutr. 61:155-173; 1989.
8. Bogardus, C.; Ravussin, E.; Robbins, D.C.; Wolfe, R.R.; Horton, E.S.; Sims, E.A.H. Effects of physical training and diet therapy on carbohydrate metabolism in patients with glucose intolerance and non-insulin-dependent diabetes mellitus. Diabetes 33:311-318; 1984.
9. Bray, G.A. Exercise and obesity. In: Bouchard, C.; Shephard, R.J.; Stephens, T.; Sutton, J.R.; McPherson, B.D., eds. Exercise, fitness, and health: A consensus of current knowledge. Champaign, IL: Human Kinetics; 1990:497-510.
10. Brehm, B.A.; Gutin, B. Recovery energy expenditure for steady state exercise in runners and nonexercisers. Med. Sci. Sports Exerc. 18:205-210; 1986.
11. Brownell, K.D. Obesity: Understanding and treating a serious, prevalent, and refractory disorder. J. Consult. Clin. Psychol. 50:820-840; 1982.
12. Buskirk, E.R.; Thompson, R.H.; Lutwak, L.; Whedon, G.D. Energy balance of obese patients during weight reduction: Influence of diet restriction and exercise. Ann. NY Acad. Sci. 110:918-940; 1963.
13. Colvin, R.H.; Olson, S.B. A descriptive analysis of men and women who have lost significant weight and are highly successful at maintaining the loss. Addict. Behav. 8:287-295; 1983.
14. D'Alessio, D.A.; Kavle, E.C.; Mozzoli, M.A.; Smalley, K.J.; Polansky, M.; Kendrick, Z.V.; Owen, L.R.; Bushman, M.C.; Boden, G.; Owen, O.E. Thermic effect of food in lean and obese men. J. Clin. Invest. 81:1781-1789; 1988.
15. Dalosso, H.M.; James, W.P.T. Whole-body calorimetry studies in adult men. 2. The interaction of exercise and over-feeding on the thermic effect of a meal. Br. J. Nutr. 52:65-72; 1984.
16. Dauncey, M.J. Activity and energy expenditure. Can. J. Physiol. Pharmacol. 68:17-27; 1990.
17. Dauncey, M.J.; Bingham, S.A. Dependence of 24 h energy expenditure in man on the composition of the nutrient intake. Br. J. Nutr. 50:1-13; 1983.
18. Davis, J.R.; Tagliaferro, A.R.; Kertzer, R.; Gerardo, T.; Nichols, J.; Wheeler, J. Variations in dietary-induced thermogenesis and body fatness with aerobic capacity. Eur. J. Appl. Physiol. 50:319-329; 1983.
19. Donahoe, C.P., Jr.; Lin, D.H.; Kirschenbaum, D.S.; Keesey, R.E. Metabolic consequences of dieting and exercise in the treatment of obesity. J. Consult. Clin. Psychol. 52:827-836; 1984.
20. Donnelly, J.E.; Jakicic, J.; Gunderson, S. Diet and body composition effect of very low calorie diets and exercise. Sports Med. 12:237-249; 1991.

21. Donnelly, J.E.; Pronk, N.P.; Jacobsen, D.J.; Pronk, S.J.; Jakicic, J.M. Effects of a very-low-calorie diet and physical-training regimens on body composition and resting metabolic rate in obese females. Am. J. Clin. Nutr. 54:56-61; 1991.
22. Dudleston, A.K.; Bennion, M. Effect of diet and/or exercise on obese college women. J. Am. Diet. Assoc. 56:126-129; 1970.
23. Epstein, L.H.; Wing, R.R. Aerobic exercise and weight. Addict. Behav. 5:371-388; 1980.
24. Fagard, R.; Bielen, E.; Amery, A. Heritability of aerobic power and anaerobic energy generation during exercise. J. Appl. Physiol. 70:357-362; 1991.
25. Freedman-Akabas, S.; Colt, E.; Kissileff, H.R.; Pi-Sunyer, F.X. Lack of sustained increase in VO_2 following exercise in fit and unfit subjects. Am. J. Clin. Nutr. 41:545-549; 1985.
26. Garrow, J.S. Effect of exercise on obesity. Acta. Med. Scand. 711:67-73; 1986.
27. Gormally, J.; Rardin, D.; Black, S. Correlates of successful response to a behavioral weight control clinic. J. Counsel. Psychol. 27:179-191; 1980.
28. Hagan, R.D.; Upton, S.J.; Wong, L.; Whittam, J. The effects of aerobic conditioning and/or caloric restriction in overweight men and women. Med. Sci. Sports Exerc. 18:87-94; 1986.
29. Hammer, R.L.; Barrier, C.A.; Roundy, E.S.; Bradford, J.M.; Fisher, A.G. Calorie-restricted low-fat diet and exercise in obese women. Am. J. Clin. Nutr. 49:77-85; 1989.
30. Henson, L.C.; Poole, D.C.; Donahoe, C.P.; Heber, D. Effects of exercise training on resting energy expenditure during caloric restriction. Am. J. Clin. Nutr. 46:893-899; 1987.
31. Hill, J.O.; Heymsfield, S.B.; McManus, C.B., III; DiGirolamo, M. Meal size and thermic response to food in male subjects as a function of maximum aerobic capacity. Metabolism. 33:743-749; 1984.
32. Hill, J.O.; Peters, J.C.; Reed, G.W.; Schlundt, D.G.; Sharp, T.; Greene, H.L. Nutrient balance in humans: Effects of diet composition. Am. J. Clin. Nutr. 54:10-17; 1991.
33. Hill, J.O.; Schlundt, D.G.; Sbrocco, T.; Sharp, T.; Pope-Cordle, J.; Stetson, B.; Kaler, M.; Heim, C. Evaluation of an alternating calorie diet with and without exercise in the treatment of obesity. Am. J. Clin. Nutr. 50:248-254; 1989.
34 Hill, J.O.; Sparling, P.B.; Shields, T.W.; Heller, P.A. Exercise and food restriction: Effects on body composition and metabolic rate in obese women. Am. J. Clin. Nutr. 46:622-630; 1987.
35. Hill, J.O.; Thiel, J.E.; Heller, P.A.; Markon, C.; Fletcher, G.; DiGirolamo, M. Effects of exercise training on energy exchange at three levels of caloric intake. Int. J. Obes. 15:169-179; 1991.
36. Ingle, D.J. A simple means of producing obesity in the rat. Proc. Soc. Biol. Med. 72:604-605; 1949.
37. Keim, N.L.; Barbieri, T.F.; Belko, A.Z. The effect of exercise on energy intake and body composition in overweight women. Int. J. Obes. 14:335-346; 1990.
38. Kenrick, M.M.; Ball, M.F.; Canary, J.J. Exercise and weight reduction in obesity. Arch. Phys. Med. Rehabil. 53:323-327; 1972.
39. King, A.C.; Frey-Hewitt, B.; Dreon, D.M.; Wood, P.D. Diet vs exercise in weight maintenance. The effects of minimal intervention strategies on long-term outcomes in men. Arch. Intern. Med. 149:2741-2746; 1989.
40 King, A.C.; Tribble, D.L. The role of exercise in weight regulation in nonathletes. Sports Med. 11:331-349; 1991.
41. Krotkiewski, M.; Mandroukas, K.; Sjostrom, L.; Sullivan, L.; Wetterqvist, H.; Bjorntorp, P. Effects of long-term physical training on body fat, metabolism, and blood pressure in obesity. Metabolism. 28:650-658; 1979.
42. Lawson, S.; Webster, J.D.; Pacy, P.J.; Garrow, J.S. Effect of a 10-week aerobic exercise programme on metabolic rate, body composition and fitness in lean sedentary females. Br. J. Clin. Prac. 41:684-688; 1987.
43. LeBlanc, J.; Diamond, P.; Cote, J.; Labrie, A. Hormonal factors in reduced postprandial heat production of exercise-trained subjects. J. Appl. Physiol. 56:772-776; 1984.
44. LeBlanc, J.; Mercier, P.; Samson, P. Diet-induced thermogenesis with relation to training state in female subjects. Can. J. Physiol. Pharmacol. 62:334-337; 1984.
45. Lemmons, A.D.; Kreitzman, S.N.; Coxon, A.; Howard, A. Selection of appropriate exercise regimes for weight reduction during VLCD and maintenance. Int. J. Obes. [Suppl. 2]. 13:1-200; 1989.
46. Lennon, D.; Nagle, F.; Stratman, F.; Shrago, E.; Dennis, S. Diet and exercise training effects on resting metabolic rate. Int. J. Obes. 9:39-47; 1985.
47. Lundholm, K.; Holm, G.; Lindmark, L.; Larsson, B.; Sjostrom, L.; Bjorntorp, P. Thermogenic effect of food in physically well-trained elderly men. Eur. J. Appl. Physiol. 55:486-492; 1986.
48. Matsushima, M.; Kriska, A.; Tajima, N.; LaPorte, R. The epidemiology of physical activity and childhood obesity. Diabetes Res. Clin. Pract. 10:S95-S102; 1990.
49. Mayer, J. Decreased activity and energy balance in the hereditary obesity-diabetes syndrome of mice. Science. 117:504-505; 1953.

50. Mayer, J.; Marshall, N.D.; Vitale, J.J.; Christensen, J.H.; Mashayekhi, M.B.; Stare, F. Exercise, food intake, and body weight in normal rats and genetically obese mice. Am. J. Physiol. 177:544-548; 1954.
51. Meredith, C.N.; Frontera, W.R.; Fisher, E.C.; Hughes, V.A.; Herland, J.C.; Edwards, J.; Evans, W.J. Peripheral effects of endurance training in young and old subjects. J. Appl. Physiol. 66:2844-2849; 1989.
52. Meredith, C.N.; Zackin, M.J.; Frontera, W.R.; Evans, W.J. Body composition and aerobic capacity in young and middle-aged endurance trained men. Med. Sci. Sports Exerc. 19:557-563; 1987.
53. Miller, D.S.; Mumford, P.; Stock, M. Gluttony. 2. Thermogenesis in overeating man. Am. J. Clin. Nutr. 20:1223-1229; 1967.
54. Mole, P.A.; Stern, J.S.; Schultz, C.L.; Bernauer, E.M.; Holcomb, B.J. Exercise reverses depressed metabolic rate produced by severe caloric restriction. Med. Sci. Sports Exerc. 21:29-33; 1988.
55. Nieman, D.C.; Haig, J.L.; De Guia, E.D.; Dizon, G.P.; Register, U.D. Reducing diet and exercise training effects on resting metabolic rates in mildly obese women. J. Sports Med. 28:79-88; 1989.
56. Nieman, D.C.; Haig, J.L.; Fairchild, K.S.; De Guia, E.D.; Dizon, G.P.; Register, U.D. Reducing-diet and exercise-training effects on serum lipids and lipoproteins in mildly obese women. Am. J. Clin. Nutr. 52:640-645; 1990.
57. Oscai, L.B. The role of exercise in weight control. Exerc. Sports Med. 1:103-123; 1973.
58. Owen, O.E.; Kavle, E.; Owen, R.S.; Polansky, M.; Caprio, S.; Mozzoli, M.A.; Kendrick, Z.V.; Bushman, M.C.; Boden, G. A reappraisal of caloric requirements in healthy women. Am. J. Clin. Nutr. 44:1-19; 1986.
59. Pacy, P.J.; Webster, J.; Garrow, J.S. Exercise and obesity. Sports Med. 3:89-113, 1986.
60. Pavlou, K.N.; Krey, S.; Steffee, W.P. Exercise as an adjunct to weight loss and maintenance in moderately obese subjects. Am. J. Clin. Nutr. 49:1115-1123; 1989.
61. Pavlou, K.N.; Steffee, W.P.; Lerman, R.H.; Burrows, B.A. Effects of dieting and exercise on lean body mass, oxygen uptake, and strength. Med. Sci. Sports Exerc. 17:466-471; 1985.
62. Phinney, S.D.; LaGrange, B.M.; O'Connell, M.; Danforth, E., Jr. Effects of aerobic exercise on energy expenditure and nitrogen balance during very low calorie dieting. Metabolism. 37:758-765; 1988.
63. Poehlman, E.T. A review: Exercise and its influence on resting energy metabolism in man. Med. Sci. Sports Exerc. 21:515-525; 1989.
64. Poehlman, E.T.; McAuliffe, T.L.; Van Houten, D.R.; Danforth, E., Jr. Influence of age and endurance training on metabolic rate and hormones in healthy men. Am. J. Physiol. 259:E66-E72; 1990.
65. Poehlman, E.T.; Melby, C.L.; Badylak, S.F. Resting metabolic rate and postprandial thermogenesis in highly trained and untrained males. Am. J. Clin. Nutr. 47:793-798; 1988.
66. Poehlman, E.T.; Tremblay, A.; Nadeau, A.; Dussault, J.; Theriault, G.; Bouchard, C. Heredity and changes in hormones and metabolic rates with short-term training. Am. J. Physiol. 250:E711-E717; 1986.
67. Ravussin, E.; Bogardus, C. Relationship of genetics, age, and physical fitness to daily energy expenditure and fuel utilization. Am. J. Clin. Nutr. 49:968-975; 1989.
68. Ravussin, E.; Lillioja, S.; Anderson, T.E.; Christin, L.; Bogardus, C. Determinants of 24-hour energy expenditure in man. Methods and results using a respiratory chamber. J. Clin. Invest. 78:1568-1578; 1986.
69. Ravussin, E.; Lillioja, S.; Knowler, W.C.; Christin, L.; Freymond, D.; Abbott, W.G.H.; Boyce, V.; Howard, B.V.; Bogardus, C. Reduced rate of energy expenditure as a risk factor for body-weight gain. N. Engl. J. Med. 318:467-472; 1988.
70. Roberts, S.B.; Savage, J.; Coward, W.A.; Chew, B.; Lucas, A. Energy expenditure and intake in infants born to lean and overweight mothers. N. Engl. J. Med. 318:461-466; 1988.
71. Saris, W.H.M.; van Dale, D. Effects of exercise during VLCD diet on metabolic rate, body composition and aerobic power: Pooled data of four studies. Int. J. Obes. [Suppl. 2]. 13:169-170; 1989.
72. Schulz, L.O.; Nyomba, B.L.; Alger, S.; Anderson, T.E.; Ravussin, E. Effect of endurance training on sedentary energy expenditure measured in a respiratory chamber. Am. J. Physiol. 260:E257-E261; 1991.
73. Schutz, Y.; Ravussin, E.; Diethelm, R.; Jequier, E. Spontaneous physical activity measured by radar in obese and control subjects studied in a respiration chamber. Int. J. Obes. 6:23-28; 1982.
74. Segal, K.R.; Gutin, B.; Albu, J.; Pi-Sunyer, F.X. Thermic effect of food and exercise in lean and obese men of similar lean body mass. Am. J. Physiol. 252:E110-E117; 1987.
75. Segal, K.R.; Pi-Sunyer, F.X. Exercise and obesity. Med. Clin. North Am. 73:217-236; 1989.
76. Sharp, T.; Reed, G.W.; Abumrad, N.N.; Sun, M.; Hill, J.O. Relationship between aerobic fitness level and daily energy expenditure in weight-stable humans. Am. J. Physiol. 263: E121-E128; 1992.

77. Sopko, G.; Leon, A.S.; Jacobs, D.R., Jr.; Foster, N.; Moy, J.; Kuba, K.; Anderson, J.T.; Casal, D.; McNally, C.; Frantz, I. The effects of exercise and weight loss on plasma lipids in young obese men. Metabolism. 34:227-236; 1985.
78. Stern, J.S.; Johnson, P.R. Spontaneous activity and adipose cellularity in the genetically obese Zucker (fa/fa) rat. Metabolism. 26:371-379; 1977.
79. Stern, J.S.; Johnson, P.R. Size and number of adipocytes and their implications. In: Katzen, H.; Mahler, R., eds. Advances in modern nutrition, vol. 2: Diabetes, obesity and vascular disease. New York: Hemisphere; 1978.
80. Sun, M.; Hill, J.O. Measurement of mechanical work and work efficiency in humans. J. Biomech.; [In press].
81. Thompson, J.K.; Jarvie, G.J.; Lahey, B.B.; Cureton, K.J. Exercise and obesity: Etiology, physiology, and intervention. Psychol. Bull. 91:55-79; 1982.
82. Tremblay, A.; Cote, J.; LeBlanc, J. Diminished dietary thermogenesis in exercise-trained human subjects. Eur. J. Appl. Physiol. 52:1-4; 1983.
83. Tremblay, A.; Fontaine, E.; Poehlman, E.T.; Mitchell, D.; Perron, L.; Bouchard, C. The effect of exercise-training on resting metabolic rate in lean and moderately obese individuals. Int. J. Obes. 10:511-517; 1986.
84. Tremblay, A.; Nadeau, A.; Després, J.-P.; St-Jean, L.; Theriault, G.; Bouchard, C. Long-term exercise training with constant energy intake: 2: Effect on glucose metabolism and resting energy expenditure. Int. J. Obes. 14:75-84, 1990.
85. Tsai, A.C.; Rosenberg, R.; Borer, K.T. Metabolic alterations induced by voluntary exercise and discontinuation of exercise in hamsters. Am. J. Clin. Nutr. 35:943-949; 1982.
86. Van Dale, D.; Saris, W.H.M.; Schoffelen, P.F.M.; Ten Hoor, F. Does exercise give an additional effect in weight reduction regimens? Int. J. Obes. 11:367-375; 1987.
87. Van Dale, D.; Saris, W.H.M.; Ten Hoor, F. Weight maintenance and resting metabolic rate 18-40 months after a diet/exercise treatment. Int. J. Obes. 14:347-359; 1990.
88. Wadden, T.A.; Foster, G.D.; Letizia, K.A.; Mullen, J.L. Long-term effects of dieting on resting metabolic rate in obese outpatients. JAMA. 264:707-711; 1990.
89. Walberg, J.L.; Mole, P.A.; Stern, J.S. Effect of swim training on development of obesity in the genetically obese rat. Am. J. Physiol. 242:R204-R211; 1982.
90. Warwick, P.M.; Garrow, J.S. The effect of addition of exercise to a regime of dietary restriction on weight loss, nitrogen balance, resting metabolic rate and spontaneous physical activity in three obese women in a metabolic ward. Int. J. Obes. 5:25-32; 1981.
91. Weltman, A.; Matter, S.; Stamford, B.A. Caloric restriction and/or mild exercise: Effects on serum lipids and body composition. Am. J. Clin. Nutr. 33:1002-1009; 1980.
92. Whipp, B.J.; Bray, G.A.; Koyal, S.N. Exercise energetics in normal man following acute weight gain. Am. J. Clin. Nutr. 26:1284-1286; 1973.
93. Wilmore, J.H. Body composition in sport and exercise: Directions for future research. Med. Sci. Sports Exerc. 15:21-31; 1983.
94. Woo, R.; Garrow, J.S.; Pi-Sunyer, F.X. Voluntary food intake during prolonged exercise in obese women. Am. J. Clin. Nutr. 36:478-484; 1982.
95. Woo, R.; Garrow, J.S.; Pi-Sunyer, F.X. Effect of exercise on spontaneous calorie intake in obesity. Am. J. Clin. Nutr. 36:470-477; 1982.
96. Zuti, W.B.; Golding, L.A. Comparing diet and exercise as weight reduction tools. Phys. Sports Med. 4:49-53; 1976.

Chapter 47

Physical Activity, Fitness, and Severe Obesity

Richard L. Atkinson
Janet Walberg-Rankin

The quantity of literature available on exercise in severe obesity depends on the definition of the term *severe obesity*. The 1991 NIH Consensus Development Conference on Surgical Treatment of Obesity defined severe obesity as a body mass index (BMI) of 40 or above, or if significant medical complications of obesity are present, a BMI of 35 or above is considered severely obese (33). However, the number of papers involving exercise in individuals with a BMI of 35 or above is extremely limited. A Medline literature search using the terms *morbid obesity* and *exercise or physical fitness* produced only four references since 1966, although some appropriate references were not captured from the data base, as noted later in this chapter.

The National Health and Nutrition Evaluation Survey (NHANES) defined *overweight* and *severely overweight* as a BMI above 27.8 and 31.1, respectively, for men, and above 27.3 and 32.3, respectively, for women (33). Because the available literature is so limited for individuals fitting the NIH definition of severe obesity, for the purposes of this review, a BMI of 31 or greater will be considered severe obesity.

The rationale for separating severe obesity from lesser degrees of obesity is that there is evidence that there may be physiological differences. At a BMI of 35, which corresponds to a body weight about 70% over ideal (37), adipocyte size reaches a maximum, and further increases in adipose tissue mass are due to adipocyte hyperplasia (4). There is some evidence that severely obese individuals at this level are different from lean and moderately obese individuals in anatomy, adipocyte metabolism, hormone and substrate physiology and biochemistry, and response to treatment. Severe obesity is associated with a higher incidence of the major complications of obesity. These complications include diabetes mellitus and insulin resistance, hypertension, hyperlipoproteinemia, atherosclerotic disease (including myocardial infarction and cerebrovascular accidents), gallbladder disease, and sleep apnea (50,53). Although there is an increased incidence of several types of cancer with obesity—including breast, uterine, prostate, and colon cancer (50,53)—it is not clear that their incidence is enhanced in severely obese individuals.

There is good evidence that reduction of body weight in obese individuals results in reduction or elimination of the complications of obesity listed above. However, there also is evidence that severely obese individuals are remarkably resistant to treatment. Drenick, Bale, Seltzer, and Johnson (17) found that virtually 100% of severely obese patients who had lost large amounts of weight during an inpatient starvation program returned to their initial weight during long-term follow-up. However, the success of treatment of lesser degrees of obesity also is very poor. Wadden, Sternberg, Letizia, Stunkard, and Foster (54) found a success rate of only 5% after 5 years of follow-up in obese patients treated with a comprehensive program of diet, exercise, and behavior modification. Clearly, more effective methods of obesity treatment must be found.

This review will focus on the changes with exercise in the following variables in severely obese individuals: (a) body weight; (b) body composition; (c) exercise performance, including changes in $\dot{V}O_2$max; exercise heart rate, or endurance; (d) metabolic rate; (e) glucose and insulin metabolism; and (f) other hormone and substrate dynamics and metabolism. Most of the discussion will be concerned with the changes in these variables with obesity treatment over differing periods of time, but the effects of acute bouts of exercise on some of these and other variables will also be covered.

Body Weight

Obesity is an excess of adipose tissue. Body weight is not the most reliable indicator of the obese state, because body composition, including fat and lean body mass, may vary in individuals of the same weight. However, body weight and changes in weight are the variables most easily measured in a clinical setting and in many studies are the only assessments of obesity that are given. Exercise increases energy expenditure, which theoretically should enhance weight loss. Twenty-two of the studies in this review evaluated weight loss with exercise in the treatment of severely obese individuals. Eight studies used exercise alone, nine studies were controlled trials comparing diet alone with diet and exercise, and the remainder of the studies used both diet and exercise with no controls, lean subjects as controls, or baseline weight as a control. In contrast to expectations, many of these studies did not find an enhancement of weight loss by exercise in the severely obese population. This review will focus on the controlled studies of exercise alone and diet with or without exercise for the treatment of severe obesity. Other references will be briefly discussed.

Exercise Treatment Alone

It is clear that exercise alone, without reduction in calories, is not effective as a method of losing significant amounts of weight. Several investigators have prescribed exercise alone in severely obese patients and found only a very modest weight loss or none at all (8,9,10,15,29,31,49,51).

Bjorntorp and co-workers (7,8,9,10,31) and Sullivan (51) reported a series of four studies of exercise alone in severely obese individuals and found no significant effect of exercise on weight loss. Exercise included calisthenics, walking/jogging, and bicycle ergometry for 1 hr three times weekly for up to 6 months. In three of the studies, body weight increased over the 6 months of training, and there was no change in weight in the fourth.

Depres et al. (15) studied the response of 13 obese women (BMI, 34.5; body fat, 47%) to exercise treatment without dietary intervention over 14 months. The subjects participated in a variety of aerobic activities (walking, cycling, swimming, aerobic dance), 4 to 5 days per week, at 55% $\dot{V}O_2max$, up to 90 min per session. Weight loss occurred but was very slow—3.7 kg by the 14th month.

Krotkiewski et al. (29) studied 20 women whose mean BMI was 31, slightly below the level defined as severe obesity for the purposes of this review. Subjects trained in a gymnasium for 55 min three times weekly. The first 15 min were at 60% of maximum work capacity, a period of intense exercise at a level 10 to 15 bpm below measured maximum heart rate followed, and the session ended with 15 min of light exercise. Body weight increased by almost 2 kg (p = NS) over the 3 weeks of the study. A similar study with 38 women produced comparable results (31).

Schwartz, Jaeger, Veith, and Lakshminarayan (49) exercised 18 subjects for 3 months with an endurance program of walking/jogging for about 40 min five times weekly at 70% to 85% of maximum heart rate. They found a difference in body weight of 2.3 kg from baseline ($p < .01$ by paired t test). In comparison, diet alone resulted in a loss of 13.2 kg in this study.

These studies suggest that if the only intervention is an increase in energy expenditure via activity, weight loss will occur, but it will be modest. However, as will be discussed later, other metabolic and physiological abnormalities of these patients may be improved through this regular exercise training in spite of only modest weight loss.

Uncontrolled Studies of Exercise With or Without Diet

The studies in this section either compared obese subjects with lean control subjects or had all subjects on both diet and exercise. Foss et al. (18-20) and Lampman, Schteingart, and Foss (34) evaluated massively obese individuals participating in the residential weight-reduction program at the University of Michigan, which consists of an extensive regimen of diet, exercise, and behavior modification. Weight losses of 27 kg to as high as 127 kg are reported from this program, but it is not possible to determine the importance of exercise in these losses. Moore, Oddou, and Leklem (38) compared adult-onset versus childhood-onset obesity in individuals matched for age and weight in a diet-and-exercise program. There were no significant differences in weight loss between the two groups (3.3 kg vs. 5.7 kg). Again, the role of exercise in this weight loss cannot be distinguished.

Controlled Studies of Diet With or Without Exercise

There were nine references from eight controlled studies that contrasted dietary treatment alone to the combination of diet and exercise in severely obese subjects (16,22,23,26,32,41,42,47,57) (Tables 47.1 and 47.2). There were wide differences among studies in subjects (initial body weight, sex, age), diet intervention (degree of caloric restriction, degree of control, macronutrient content), exercise intervention (type, frequency, intensity, duration), and overall length of the treatment.

Table 47.1 Characteristics of Exercise for the Treatment of Severe Obesity

Ref. No.	Author	No. of subjects	Length of study	Daily diet	Exercise type	Exercise frequency (days per week)	Exercise duration	Exercise intensity
Exercise only								
7	Bjorntorp et al. (1973a)	3M 5F	6 month	None	C, J, Ca	3	35 min	5 min submax × 3
8	Bjorntorp et al. (1970)	2M 8F	8 week	None	C, ST, R, Ca	3–5	3–4 hr	4 min max × 4
9	Bjorntorp et al. (1973)	2M 3F	8 week	None	C, ST, R, Ca	3	45 min	5–10 min submax × 2
10	Bjorntorp et al. (1977)	4M 4F	6 week	None	C, J, Ca	3	50 min	5 min max × 3
15	Depres et al. (1991)	0M 13F	14 month	None	W, C, A, S	4–5	90 min	55% VO_2max
29	Krotkiewski et al. (1983)	0M 30F	3 month	None	C, J, Ca	3	55 min	hi submax
31	Krotkiewski et al. (1979)	0M 38F	6 month	None	J, Ca	3	55 min	hi submax
49	Schwartz et al. (1990)	18M 0F	3 month	None	W, J	3–5	40 min	70%–80% HRmax
Diet with or without exercise								
16	Donnelly et al. (1990)	0M 69F	90 days	2,184 kJ	Diet only	None	—	—
					End, W, C, R	4	20–60 min	70% HRmax
					ST	4	20–60 min	70%–80% IRM
					End, ST	4	>20–60 min	As above
22	Hammer et al. (1989)	0M 26F	16 week	800 kcal	W, J	5	1.6 km up to 4.8 km	60%–85% HRmax
23	Hill et al. (1987)	0M 3F (NoEx) 5F (Ex)	5 week	800 kcal	W	Daily	1.6 km to 5.6 km	Variable
26	Kenrick et al. (1972)	12 (sex NA)	26 week	1,000–1,500 kcal	W, Ca	Daily	30 min	HR:120–140
32	Krotkiewski et al. (1981)	0M 18F	3 week	1,650 kcal	C, J, Ca	3	55 min	Variable
41	Pavlou et al. (1989)	72M 0F	8 week	420–1,000 kcal	End, W, Ru, Ca	3	60 min	69.15 HRmax
41	Pavlou et al. (1989)							
	Pilot study	21M 0F	12 week	1,000 kcal (balanced, PSMF)	W, J, Ru, Ca	3	35–60 min	70%–85% HRmax
	Main study	110M 0F	12 week	1,000 kcal for balanced and PSMF diets; 420 kcal for DPC-70; 800 kcal for DPC-800	W, J, Ru, Ca	3	35–60 min	70%–85% HRmax
47	Saris & Van Dale (1989)	9M (NoEx) 8M (Ex) 25F (NoEx) 20F (Ex)	5 week	3.0 MJ	A, Ca, J, S	5	1 hr	No data

(continued)

Ref. No.	Author	No. of subjects	Length of study	Daily diet	Exercise type	Exercise frequency (days per week)	Exercise duration	Exercise intensity
57	Wirth et al. (1987)							
	Experiment 1	10M 10F	4 week	300 kcal	C	6	10–20 min	50% HRmax
	Experiment 2	10M 10F	4 week	300 kcal	C	6	10–20 min	50% HRmax

Note. M = male; F = female; C = cycling; J = jogging; Ca = calesthenics; min = minute; submax = submaximal exercise; ST = strength training; R = rowing; hr = hour; max = maximal exercise; W = walking; A = aerobics; S = swimming; VO_2max = maximal oxygen consumption; HRmax = heart rate maximum; kJ = kilojoule; End = endurance exercise; kcal = kilocalorie; NoEx = no exercise group; Ex = exercise group; NA = not available; HR = heart rate; Ru = running; PSMF = protein sparing modified fast; DPC-70 = commercial formula diet with 420 kcal/day and 70 g/day protein; DPC-800 = commercial formula diet with 800 kcal/day; O = other.

Donnelly, Pronk, Jacobsen, Pronk, and Jakicic (16) gave 69 obese females a very low calorie liquid formula diet (VLCD). Subjects did either no exercise, endurance exercise only, weight training only, or both endurance exercise and weight training. There were no differences in weight loss or body composition among groups.

In a 2 × 2 factorial design study, Hammer, Barrier, Roundy, Bradford, and Fisher (22) had 26 women follow an 800-kcal diet or a low-fat, ad libitum carbohydrate diet, with or without exercise (walking or jogging 5 days/week). Exercise produced an additional 1-kg weight loss and fat mass loss, but these were not statistically significantly different ($p < .10$).

Hill, Sparling, Shields, and Heller (23) studied 8 female inpatients for 5 weeks on an 800-kcal diet with or without a progressive, supervised daily walking program (up to 5.6 km/day). Exercising subjects lost only an additional 0.2 kg ($p <$ NS).

Kenrick, Ball, and Canary (26) matched 12 super-obese inpatient subjects into two groups and used a 1,000- to 1,500-kcal/day diet with or without treadmill walking and mat exercises. The goal was to maintain the subjects' pulse rates at 120 to 140 bpm. Weight loss did not differ among the two groups, although exercise enhanced body fat loss.

Krotkiewski, Toss, Bjorntorp, and Holm (32) found no significant differences in weight loss, fat loss, or lean body mass loss in 18 obese women on a 500-kcal/day VLCD with or without 55-min exercise sessions three times per week. This study must be interpreted with caution because the subjects were not randomized to exercise but were allowed to choose, and the program lasted only 3 weeks.

Pavlou et al. (41,42) published two studies from the same population of Boston police officers. The subjects were randomized into eight groups and followed a balanced, low-calorie diet (1,000 kcal/day), a high-protein, low-carbohydrate, protein-sparing modified fast (1,000 kcal/day), or one of two very low calorie liquid formula diets (420 and 800 kcal/day). Some subjects following each diet exercised, and some did not. The exercise program was 8 weeks long and consisted of walking/jogging at 70% of maximum heart rate (MHR) for 2 weeks and then exercising at 85% of MHR for 6 weeks, for a total distance increasing to 5 miles. The walking/jogging was followed by a series of calisthenics. The nonexercising subjects on the balanced, low-calorie diet lost significantly less weight than the other groups, but there was no difference in weight loss among the groups following the other three diets. There were differences in body composition due to exercise.

Saris and Van Dale (47) combined four similar studies with a total of 62 subjects (45 females, 17 males) and compared VLCD alone with a 5-week exercise program of 5 hours per week of aerobics, fitness, jogging, and swimming. The authors reported a significant difference ($p < .05$) in weight loss (9.6 kg, -10.5% vs. 11 kg, -11.6%), but the standard deviations and methods of statistical analysis were not given.

Wirth, Vogel, Schomig, and Schlierf (57) hospitalized 40 subjects (20 males, 20 females) for 4 weeks and placed them on a diet of 300 kcal/day. Some subjects did not exercise, and others followed an exercise program of 10 to 20 min of cycling on a bicycle ergometer 6 times daily, 6 days per week, at 50% of maximum capacity. The subjects were divided into two experiments of 20 subjects each. Weight loss was reported as 8.8 kg and 9 kg in the diet-alone groups and 11.1 kg and 11 kg in the diet-plus-exercise groups, respectively, for the two studies. No error measurements or statistical analyses were given for the first experiment, and weight loss in the second experiment

Table 47.2 Effects of Exercise for the Treatment of Severe Obesity

Ref. No.	Author	Body mass index Wt/(Ht)^2	Body weight (kg)	Body fat (kg)	Fat-free mass (kg)	$\dot{V}O_2max$ (L/min)
Exercise only						
7	Bjorntorp et al. (1973a)	NA	B—111.6 A—112.6	B—42.0 A—39.0	NA	B—2.52 A—NA
8	Bjorntorp et al. (1970)	NA	B—106.2 A—109.2	B—39.5 A—42.8*	NA	B-2.48 A—NA
9	Bjorntorp et al. (1973)	NA	B—127.5 A—129.3	B—54.0 A—52.8	NA	B—2.63 A—NA
10	Bjorntorp et al. (1977)	NA	B—113.8 A—115.0	B—49.5 A—50.4	NA	B—2.68 A—NA
15	Depres et al. (1991)	B—34.5 A—33.1*	B—90 A—86.3*	B—42.6 A—38.9	B—47.4 A—48.3	B—2.19 A—2.52*
29	Krotkiewski et al. (1983)	B—30.8 A—31.4	B—84.4 A—86.2	B—36.8 A—37.1	B—29.6 A—27.9	
31	Krotkiewski et al. (1979)	NA	B—78.8 A—80.0	B—34.1 A—34.1	B—44.7 A—45.9	NA
49	Schwartz et al. (1990)	NA	B—98.7 A—96.5**	B—30.4 A—27.5	B—68.3 A—68.9	NA
Diet with or without exercise						
16	Donnelly et al. (1990)	B—38.2 A—NA	B—105.3 A—84.9*	B—47.9 A—33.8*	B—55.3 A—50.6*	B—2.10 A—2.00
		B—37.5 A—NA	B—99.9 A—78.5*	B—46.6 A—30.0*	B—53.3 A—48.5*	B—2.36 A—2.33
		B—38.2 A—NA	B—101.7 A—80.8*	B—46.9 A—30.8*	B—54.7 A—50.0*	B—2.25 A—2.13
		B—38.3 A—NA	B—100.3 A—77.4*	B—46.9 A—28.9*	B—53.3 A—49.2*	B—2.18 A—2.38
22	Hammer et al. (1989)	NoEx—33.8	B—92.3 A—85.2*	B—38.9% A—34.5%*	B—55.6 A—55.1	B—2.17 A—2.03
		Ex—31.3	B—85.6 A—77.6*	B—37.5% A—31.6%*	B—52.8 A—52.3	B—2.22 A—2.39
23	Hill et al. (1987)	NoEx: B—34.8 A—32.0	B—96.6 A—88.7	B—44.3% A—43.2%	B—53.8 A—50.4	NA NA
		Ex: B—36.0 A—32.9	B—98.6 A—90.3	B—44.5% A—41.8%	B—54.7 A—52.6†	NA NA
26	Kenrick et al. (1972)	NA	Weight—NA Wt loss: NoEx: 33.9 kg Ex: 40.3 kg	Fat loss: NoEx—25 Ex—31.4†	FFM loss: NoEx: 0.9 Ex: 1.3	NA
32	Krotkiewski et al. (1981)	NA	NoEx: B—101 A—95	NoEx: B—46.6 A—44.0	NoEx: B—30.9 A—28.9	NA
			Ex: B—103 A—96.1	Ex: B—49.2 A—47.3	Ex: B—30.5 A—27.7	NA
41	Pavlou et al. (1989) Pilot study					
	Balanced	NoEx: B—31.9 A—29.1	NoEx: B—99.2 A—90.5*†	NA NA	NA NA	NoEx: B—2.9 A—3.0
		Ex: B—31.7 A—27.2	Ex: B—102.3 A—87.6*	NA NA	NA NA	Ex: B—3.0 A—3.8*

(continued)

Ref. No.	Author	Body mass index Wt/(Ht)^2	Body weight (kg)	Body fat (kg)	Fat-free mass (kg)	$\dot{V}O_2$max (L/min)
41 (p)	PSMF	NoEx: B—30.4	NoEx: B—97.3	NA	NA	NoEx: B—3.1
		A—25.6	A—81.6*	NA	NA	A—2.9
		Ex: B—31.1	Ex: B—101.7	NA	NA	Ex: B—2.9
		A—26.6	A—86.8*	NA	NA	A—3.7*
41	Pavlou et al. (1989) Main study					
	Balanced	NoEx: B—32.4	NoEx: B—105.0	NA	NA	NoEx: B—3.1
		A—30.2	A—97.9*†	NA	NA	A—3.2
		Ex: B—32.5	Ex: B—103.1	NA	NA	Ex: B—3.1
		A—28.7	A—91.0*	NA	NA	A—3.5*
	PSMF	NoEx: B—31.5	NoEx: B—98.8	NA	NA	NoEx: B—2.8
		A—28.1	A—88.2*	NA	NA	A—2.8
		Ex: B—32.1	Ex: B—100.8	NA	NA	Ex: B—2.8
		A—28.1	A—88.3*	NA	NA	A—3.4*
	DPC-70	NoEx: B—34.8	NoEx: B—103.0	NA	NA	NoEx: B—3.1
		A—30.3	A—89.8*	NA	NA	A—2.7
		Ex: B—30.1	Ex: B—96.1	NA	NA	Ex: B—3.1
		A—25.6	A—81.8*	NA	NA	A—3.2
	DPC-800	NoEx: B—33.8	NoEx: B—105.7	NA	NA	NoEx: B—2.8
		A—30.7	A—96.1*	NA	NA	A—2.8
		Ex: B—31.9	Ex: B—100.8	NA	NA	Ex: B—2.9
		A—28.1	A—88.7*	NA	NA	A—3.4*
41	Pavlou et al. (1989)	NoEx: B—31.7	NoEx: B—100.8	NoEx: B—37.5	NoEx: B—62.7	NoEx: B—3.0
		A—28.8	A—91.6*	A—32.5*	A—59.4*	A—2.9
		Ex: B—31.5	Ex: B—99.3	Ex: B—36.5	Ex: B—63.2	Ex: B—2.9
		A—27.5	A—87.5*†	A—25.0*†	A—62.6	A—3.5*
						ml·min^{-1}·kg^{-1} LBM
						NoEx: B—48.1
						A—49.4
						Ex: B—45.7
						A—55.2*†
47	Saris & Van Dale (1989)	NoEx: 32.6	NoEx: B—90.4	NoEx: B—34.5	NoEx: B—55.9	NoEx: B—26.9
		Ex: 33.1	A—80.8*	A—27.2*	A—53.6	A—28.3
			Ex: B—93.9	Ex: B—36.4	Ex: B—57.5	Ex: B—27.6
			A—82.9*†	A—27.4*†	A—55.5	A—31.8*
57	Wirth et al. (1987)					
	Experiment 1	NoEx: B—36	NoEx: B—102.5	NoEx: B—29.9	NoEx: B—72.6	NA
		A—32	A—93.7	A—24.3	A—69.4	NA
		Ex: B—34	Ex: B—95.7	Ex: B—25.6	Ex: B—70.1	NA
		A—30	A—84.6	A—18.3	A—66.3	NA
	Experiment 2	NoEx: B—39	NoEx: B—113.0	NA	NA	NA
		A—35	A—103.6			
		Ex: B—38	Ex: B—107.2	NA	NA	NA
		A—34	A—96.5			

Note. Wt = weight; Ht = height; kg = kilogram; $\dot{V}O_2$max = maximal oxygen consumption; L/min = liters/minute; NA = not available; B = before treatment; A = after treatment; NoEx = no exercise group; Ex = exercise group; FFM = fat-free mass; Balanced = balanced diet; PSMF = protein sparing modified fast; DPC-70 = commercial formula diet with 420 kcal/day and 70 g/day protein; DPC-800 = commercial formula diet with 800 kcal/day.

*$p < .05$ versus baseline. **$p < .01$ versus baseline. †$p < .05$ versus no exercise group or other groups.

was compared only with initial weight, not between groups. It is not clear that these differences are statistically significant.

Only two of these eight controlled studies found a statistically significant benefit of exercise for increasing total body weight loss during obesity treatment, and in these, the differences were small (41,42,47). Because exercise increases energy expenditure acutely, an enhancement of weight loss with exercise during a weight-reduction regimen might have been expected. Possible explanations for why significant weight loss was not found include the following: (a) Exercise intensity and duration in these severely obese subjects may not cause a large enough increase in energy expenditure to perturb body weight control, (b) variability between individuals, coupled with low subject numbers, may obscure the results, and (c) there may be compensation for the energy expenditure of exercise with a lower energy expenditure at other times.

With severe caloric restriction, the rate of weight loss may approach a maximum, and the effect of additional energy expenditure is lost. Garrow (21) reviewed the evidence that exercise enhances metabolic rate and concluded that there was little or no additional energy expenditure on exercise days, suggesting that metabolic rate may fall below the level that is maintained on nonexercise days, thus canceling the increased energy expenditure due to the exercise. In support of this hypothesis, Phinney, LaGrange, O'Connell, and Danforth (43) reported that in moderately obese subjects the addition of exercise to a restricted diet caused a drop of resting metabolic rate of a greater magnitude than diet alone. This compensation may only occur during severe energy restriction and could limit additional weight loss with exercise.

There is a suggestion of a sex difference in weight loss in response to exercise. Studies that compared men and women observed a more positive effect of exercise in men, although the data are very skimpy. This possible interaction of sex with weight-loss treatment has been suggested by other researchers (5,52).

Finally, the wide variation in body weight loss, even when treatment was tightly controlled, is striking (11). This variation emphasizes the need for high numbers of subjects to produce the statistical power to adequately test the hypothesis that exercise is a beneficial component in weight-reduction treatment programs. In the controlled studies, all but one of the diet-plus-exercise groups had a higher average weight loss than those groups on diet alone. It is possible that studies with small numbers of subjects are committing Type II errors due to the variability and subject number. However, the very small additional weight losses with exercise and the necessity for such large numbers of subjects to achieve statistical differences points out the limited clinical utility for exercise to enhance weight loss. There may be additional benefits of exercise in severely obese people, but the cost-benefit ratio for weight loss is not favorable.

An important point concerning body weight loss and exercise is that the most benefit may only be obvious over a period longer than that followed by most studies. The value of exercise may be most important in helping patients maintain weight lost by dietary restriction. For example, Pavlou, Steffee, Lerman, and Burrows (42) followed subjects for up to 18 months after their 8-week formal diet, exercise, or diet-and-exercise treatment. Only those individuals who exercised during the follow-up period were successful in maintaining weight lost during treatment.

In summary, there is insufficient data to generalize from the limited number of studies available, and it is clear that additional research in large numbers of subjects will be necessary to address the role, if any, of exercise in the initial treatment of severe obesity.

Body Composition

Change in weight is not a good indicator of successful treatment of obesity. Because excess adipose tissue is associated with complications of obesity such as glucose intolerance, hypertension, and cardiovascular disease, the object of treatment is to reduce adipose tissue mass while preserving lean body mass as much as possible. Nineteen of the references reviewed measured changes in body composition. As noted above, eight of these studies were controlled trials of diet with or without exercise (16,22,23,26,32,41,42,47,57), and eight studies evaluated exercise alone for obesity (7,8,9,10,15, 29,31,49). A summary of these controlled trials is presented in Tables 47.1 and 47.2, and in the following discussion.

Body Fat

The results of studies that evaluated the effects of exercise on body fat were similar to those on body weight. Six of the 8 studies of exercise alone (7,8,9,10,29,31) and 4 of the 8 controlled studies of diet with and without exercise (16,22,32,57) found no statistically significant effect or an increase of body fat with exercise in severely obese subjects. However, of the 10 negative studies, 4 observed a nonsignificant decrease in body fat (7,9,16,22). If these are added to the 6 trials that did show a significant decrease in body fat (15,23,27,41,47,49), the majority of studies suggest that exercise may have a beneficial effect in reducing body fat. As with changes in body weight, the reductions are small and may not be clinically significant, and the small numbers of subjects in most of the trials may obscure the true effect of exercise.

Bjorntorp et al. (7) reported a loss of 3 kg (p = NS) of body fat over a 6-month treatment period of exercise alone, but in three other studies of 6 to 8 weeks (8,9,10), two showed a gain in fat and the other showed a loss of 1.2 kg (p = NS). Depres et al. (15) reported a 4.6-kg average reduction in body fat of obese women (BMI = 34.5) who were not given dietary intervention but who regularly participated in aerobic exercise 4 to 5 days/week over 14 months. Schwartz et al. (49) found a loss of 2.9 kg (2.3%) of body fat during 3 months of exercise alone ($p < .001$) and a loss of 8.9 kg of fat ($p < .001$) from diet alone. Krotkiewski et al. (31) found no change in body fat in a 6-month study of exercise alone. However, taken together, these findings suggest that longer term studies may show an effect of exercise on body fat, reinforcing the idea that for exercise to be effective, it must represent a long-term change in lifestyle.

Aerobic exercise typically increases the reliance on fat for ATP resynthesis. Thus, if food consumption remains constant, regular exercise would be expected to diminish fat stores. This is typically, although not always (10), observed when very obese individuals add aerobic activity to their routines (55). Because the actual fat utilization during a typical exercise bout may be small if the exercise is brief, a clinically significant drop in body fat will require long-term exercise participation.

Respiratory quotient (R ratio) gives an indication as to the fuels being utilized by the body to produce ATP. R ratio tends to decrease over time with prolonged aerobic exercise, reflecting increased fat utilization. Thus, the shift toward fat utilization during aerobic exercise will tend to decrease body fat stores with long-term exercise training. The importance of this shift in fuel use was discussed by Keim, Barbieri, and Van Loan (25). They found that the blood's free fatty acid and glycerol concentrations immediately following an exercise bout predicted total fat loss in obese women undergoing dietary treatment for obesity. This suggests that individuals who can more easily switch to fat utilization from carbohydrate during exercise will be more successful at body weight and fat loss. One way to accelerate the shift to fat utilization during exercise is through regular aerobic exercise training. Chronic exercise enhances the use of fat at any aerobic exercise intensity compared to before training.

Reduction of body fat during exercise treatment has been shown by Depres et al. (15) to occur more rapidly in some fat depots than others. For example, during 14 months of aerobic exercise treatment, there was more depletion of fat from abdominal adipocytes than from gluteal fat cells. This could result in an alteration in overall body fat distribution. Because a high waist-to-hip ratio is considered a risk for health problems such as hypertension, diabetes, and heart disease, this change would tend to reduce the risk or severity of these diseases. As discussed below, some studies have shown that exercise, even without weight or fat loss, results in lower insulin levels and improved glucose tolerance.

Some investigators have suggested that childhood-onset obesity is more resistant to treatment than adult-onset obesity. Moore et al. (38) tested this hypothesis in two groups of extremely obese individuals. Seven subjects were categorized as having childhood-onset obesity (BMI = 36.6, body fat = 45%), and 8 had a similar degree of obesity (BMI = 34.2, body fat = 46%) but had developed obesity during adulthood. A combined treatment of modest dietary restriction (500 kcal less than maintenance) plus walking 3 days/week for 40 min caused significant weight and fat loss in both groups over 9 months but did not indicate a difference between the groups. Thus, they suggest that age of obesity did not affect the effectiveness of the treatment.

As mentioned previously, gender may be a possible factor in influencing magnitude of body fat loss during treatment. The studies summarized in Tables 47.1 and 47.2 that included men in the population tended to show an enhancement of fat loss with exercise treatment. Tremblay, Despres, Leblanc, and Bouchard (52) has previously shown that 20 weeks of regular aerobic exercise reduced body weight, body fat, and fat cell size in men buthad no similar effect in women. Bjorntorp (5) has reviewed this topic and points out that women not only have more relative fat but they have approximately 50% more fat cells than men do. In addition, women store more body fat in the gluteal-femoral region, which is resistant to fat emptying. Thus, adipose cells of men may be more responsive to lipolytic activation with exercise. Elucidating the mechanisms of the differences between the sexes in response of adipose tissue to exercise may be a fruitful area for future research.

Fat-Free Mass

A commonly held belief is that it is desirable to prevent any loss of fat-free mass with weight loss.

It is very unlikely that there will be no loss of lean body mass with the amount of weight that must be lost in severely obese individuals (27). Some studies have found no change in lean body mass (LBM) with exercise during weight loss, but the reduction in body weight was modest (15,22,38). Most studies report some reduction of LBM if weight loss is substantial. The composition of the lost LBM is unknown but may consist of body water, skeletal muscle, and protein pools in the liver and gut with a rapid turnover (27).

The issue of whether the addition of exercise during dieting can preserve LBM better than dieting alone in severely obese patients is unsettled. Krotkiewski et al. (32) and Donnelly et al. (16) did not find any sparing of lean mass in severely obese patients when exercise was added to a VLCD. Several other investigators observed a lower LBM loss in the exercise-plus-diet groups compared to those in the diet-alone treatments (23,42,47).

If exercise does preserve LBM during a weight-loss regimen, the mechanisms might be a relatively higher body water due to increased glycogen storage, increased protein synthesis, or decreased protein degradation. Muscle growth secondary to exercise is possible even during energy restriction and weight loss (3). Also, studies measuring the excretion of 3-methyl histidine, an index of muscle contractile protein breakdown, suggest that muscle protein degradation is reduced during negative energy balance. For example, Hoffer and Forse (24) reported a 25% to 30% decrease in 3-methyl histidine excretion of obese women when they consumed a 360 kcal/day diet. This suggests a tendency to protect muscle tissue during energy restriction. Collection of nitrogen balance data in the very obese population during a variety of treatments would help to differentiate sources of the change in LBM.

Exercise Capacity ($\dot{V}O_2max$)

$\dot{V}O_2max$ reflects the aerobic fitness of the cardiovascular system (central) as well as that of the muscles (peripheral) that extract oxygen from the blood. Severely obese individuals typically have a low $\dot{V}O_2max$ due to low central and peripheral aerobic fitness and the burden of carrying excess body fat. This very low level of fitness may severely limit the ability to exercise. For example, Foss, Lampman, Watt, and Schteingart (20) studied the aerobic fitness of 16 extremely obese patients (BMI = 61.2 for women and 63.4 for men) who were entering a weight-reduction program. They asked all patients to walk 1 mile on a treadmill, setting it to their fastest pace. Although this test was completed by 3 of the 16 individuals, others were able to complete as little as 0.1 mile before fatigue, dyspnea, or other symptoms forced them to stop. The average distances covered for women and men were 0.2 and 0.6 miles, respectively. This report emphasizes the potential for a very low initial exercise capacity in extremely obese individuals as well as the wide variation among individuals. Thus, exercise prescriptions may have to begin very modestly and must be tailored to each individual's fitness.

Weight loss alone, regardless of how it is accomplished, will usually increase the ability of the obese individual to perform aerobic exercise. Foss, Lampman, and Schteingart (19) documented the changes in aerobic exercise tolerance in a group of 11 extremely obese men and women (body weight = 189 kg) during a residential weight-reduction program that included a 600-kcal/daily diet and aerobic exercise 3 days per week. The average time required prior to treatment to cover 1 mile on a treadmill was 20.6 min. This fell to 15.8 min after weight loss of approximately 30 kg. Exercise tolerance clearly improved in these patients. However, because all individuals received the same combination of exercise and dietary treatment, it is unclear how much of the improvement is due to weight loss per se as opposed to regular exercise training.

Exercise tolerance may improve after weight loss due to the smaller amount of work necessary to move the lower body mass. Improvement in cardiovascular function also may contribute to an improved exercise capacity. There may be other metabolic changes with weight reduction that contribute to an improved exercise endurance. Scheen, Pirnay, Luyckx, Lefebvre (48) observed impaired fatty acid mobilization into the bloodstream in obese individuals during a 3-hr exercise bout and suggested that the elevated blood insulin concentration that often accompanies obesity may be responsible. Since both weight loss and exercise tend to reduce hyperinsulinemia, the lower insulin levels after obesity treatment may enhance fatty acid mobilization and thus increase aerobic exercise tolerance.

Changes in exercise tolerance are expressed as changes in $\dot{V}O_2max$. However, $\dot{V}O_2max$ may be expressed either on an absolute basis (L/min) or on a relative basis ($ml \cdot kg^{-1} \cdot min^{-1}$). The method of expressing the data is a critical factor when one compares studies. Reduction of body weight alone, without any exercise training, will mathematically increase relative $\dot{V}O_2max$, implying that exercise tolerance has improved. Examination of absolute $\dot{V}O_2max$ changes may be more instructive. Weight loss through dieting alone has been reported by most researchers to have no effect on absolute $\dot{V}O_2$max (22,32,42), although the studies of Davis and Phinney (14) and Pavlou, Krey, and Steffee (41) suggest that treatment with some diets, especially those with very low energy and protein levels, may result in a reduction in this measurement. Both research groups found that a diet containing 420 kcal and 70 g protein per day caused a significant deterioration of $\dot{V}O_2$max when diet was the only treatment (14,41).

The addition of aerobic exercise to dietary treatment of severely obese individuals consistently improves absolute $\dot{V}O_2$max in almost all cases (7,8,10, 18-20,22,23,26,30,34,41,42,47,49,57), although rare studies do not find an effect (9,16). Depres et al. (15) reported a 15% increase in $\dot{V}O_2$max after a 14-month exercise-only study, and Pavlou et al. (42) reported a 17% increase in absolute aerobic capacity in men after an 8-week diet-plus-exercise program. A later study by Pavlou et al. (41), using the same exercise program in men, found gains between 12% and 21%, depending on the diet utilized. Hammer et al. (22) reported gains in absolute $\dot{V}O_2$max of smaller magnitude, approximately 9%, for women consuming either an 800-kcal or 1,450-kcal daily diet while doing aerobic exercise 5 days per week for 16 weeks. Saris and Van Dale (47) found a 15% increase over only 5 weeks of exercise versus a 5% increase in the diet-only group ($p < .01$).

Thus, it appears clear that even severely obese individuals can show improvement in $\dot{V}O_2$max and aerobic exercise tolerance if a regular exercise program is included in treatment. The type of exercise does not appear to be critical, perhaps due to their very low initial levels of fitness.

Muscle Function

The quality of muscle tissue from obese individuals has been reported to be different from that of lean individuals. Landin, Lindgards, Saltin, and Wilhelmsen (35) reported that skeletal muscle from obese men had more fat and less potassium than did samples from control subjects. This finding suggests a possible disturbance in the sodium potassium pump activity across the muscle cell membrane. Lennmarken, Sandstedt, Von Schenk, and Larsson (36) found reduced concentrations of the fuels ATP, CP, and glycogen in muscle in obese subjects. These differences could be associated with a reduced ability to do power-type contractions that rely on these fuels. Histological analysis of a muscle biopsy taken from each of 11 men by Wade, Marbut, and Round (55) revealed a significant negative correlation between percent body fat and proportion of slow-twitch (ST) fibers in the muscle sample. They suggested that the low proportion of ST fibers, which are well adapted for fat utilization, could contribute to the storage of excess body fat. Their follow-up study on 50 men supported this hypothesis, showing that the lower the percentage of ST fibers in a muscle biopsy, the lower the utilization of total fat during a standard exercise bout (55). It should be noted that although there was a range of percent body fat among subjects, only 1 subject had above 25% body fat. However, Krotkiewski, Aniansson, Grimby, Bjorntorp, and Sjostrom (28) added evidence in support of this hypothesis. They observed a relatively higher percentage of Type IIB (fast-twitch) fibers and a lower proportion of Type I (ST) fibers in obese versus lean individuals.

A difference in muscle fiber type distribution and concentration of substrates and electrolytes could influence various aspects of muscle function. Lennmarken et al. (36) confirmed a reduction in muscle strength in very obese (body weight = 123 kg) versus normal-weight women by testing the electrically stimulated force of contraction of the adductor pollicis muscle. They did not find a difference in muscle endurance between groups.

Several research groups have followed the changes in muscle function during weight-reduction treatment. Although Pavlou et al. (41,42) found no reduction in muscle strength as measured by peak torque at 30 degrees/second on a Cybex apparatus, Krotkiewski, Grimby, Holm, and Szczepanik (30) and Russell, Leiter, Whitwell, Marliss, and Jeejeebhoy (44) reported that weight loss via dietary restriction reduced maximum strength. Krotkiewski et al. (30) assessed strength in very obese women (BMI = 36.9) before, after 2 weeks, and after 4 weeks of a 544-kcal/day diet. Peak torque from maximal effort contractions at 30, 60, and 180 deg/s on a Cybex apparatus was reduced within 2 weeks of energy restriction. This reduction in strength was positively correlated to an observed reduction in area of Type II (FT) fibers and to the reduction in muscle glycogen. Russell et al. (44) tested strength using electrical stimulation of the adductor pollicis in women consuming 400 kcal/day for 2 weeks followed by 2 weeks of fasting. Davis and Phinney (14) reported that peak quadriceps torque varied with the diet fed to produce weight loss. A significant decrease in muscle strength occurred following a 17-kg weight loss in women consuming a 420-kcal, 70-g protein formula VLCD (initial BMI = 31.9) but was unchanged if the diet was of a similar energy value but consisted of meat, fish, and poultry (initial BMI = 33.5).

No consensus exists concerning the effect of weight reduction on muscle endurance. Krotkiewski et al. (28) observed an increase in muscle endurance as measured by percent change in torque from the initial repetition to the final of 50 repetitions on a Cybex apparatus at 180 deg/s. Davis and Phinney (14) reported no change in muscle endurance in the obese subjects they studied. Russell et al. (44) found that the adductor pollicis was quicker to fatigue after the dietary treatment.

Few studies have been performed using resistance weight training in treatment of the very obese. Krotkiewski et al. (28,29) were interested in characterizing the changes in muscle and adipose morphology following 5 weeks of strength training in obese women (mean body fat = 31%). Strength training caused changes in muscle and adipose quality and quantity similar to those that have been observed in nonobese people. For example, muscle hypertrophy, an increase in area of Type II (FT) fibers, and an increase in anaerobic enzymes were noted in the muscles of the obese women after regular weight training. This was reflected by a 14% to 26% increase in strength of the quadriceps. No change in body fat or fat cell size occurred. This is not surprising because weight training is an anaerobic activity that does not depend on fat as fuel.

Pavlou et al. (41,42) did not have resistance weight training as part of their treatment program, but they did include calisthenics designed to stress various skeletal muscles. Both studies reported that the combination of diet with aerobic exercise and calisthenics increased muscle strength 22% to 25% as assessed by peak torque at 30 deg/s on a Cybex apparatus. The later study also assessed muscle endurance and reported a 50% increase in the exercise-and-diet combination group.

Although the evidence is limited, it appears that obese people are likely to have no change or an impairment of muscle function during weight loss by dieting unless muscle-stressing exercise is incorporated into the treatment regimen. The evidence thus far suggests that in obese patients, exercise that specifically overloads the muscles will improve function and muscle size in a manner similar to that seen in lean individuals.

Resting Metabolic Rate

A limited number of studies have evaluated the effects of exercise on resting metabolic rate (RMR) in severely obese patients (16,22,23,47,49). Donnelly et al. (16) fed subjects a diet of 2,184 kJ per day for 90 days, with or without exercise, and noted a decrease in RMR with weight loss ranging from 7% to 12% of baseline. Hammer et al. (22) also found no effects of 16 weeks of exercise on RMR as compared to diet only. Hill et al. (23) kept the diet constant at 800 kcal/day during a 5-week study of diet with or without exercise. The finding that there was no difference in RMR between the groups despite a higher daily energy expenditure suggested that exercise kept the RMR higher than it otherwise might have been. Saris and Van Dale (47) fed 3.0 MJ per day to 62 subjects and found decreases in sleeping metabolic rate of 17.3% in the diet-only group and 16.6% in the diet-and-exercise group (p = NS). Schwartz et al. (49) prescribed either diet (1,200 kcal/day) or an endurance exercise program for 3 months and measured the number of kilocalories necessary to maintain weight stability. They found that the diet group needed 247 fewer kcal per day to maintain a weight loss of 13.2 kg. The exercise group lost only 2.3 kg but required an increase of 202 kcal/day to maintain body weight stability at the lower level.

All of these studies suggest that weight loss decreases energy requirements and may decrease resting metabolic rate and that exercise does not prevent this decline. However, as Hill et al. (23) point out, if diet is kept constant, a further decrease in RMR would be expected because the diet-plus-exercise regimen requires a greater daily energy expenditure than diet alone. Thus it seems likely that exercise may help decrease or prevent the drop in metabolic rate associated with an energy deficit.

Glucose and Insulin Metabolism

Obesity has profound effects on glucose and insulin metabolism. Insulin resistance has been implicated in producing some of the complications of obesity and may play a role in the etiology of obesity. Numerous studies have shown that glucose tolerance is decreased in obesity and that there is resistance to the action of insulin (39,40,50,53). With increasing obesity and fat cell size, there is in vivo and in vitro resistance to the action of insulin (39,40,45). Conversely, weight loss reduces plasma glucose and insulin levels (2,39,40,46). Bjorntorp et al. (7,8,9,10) and Sullivan (51) performed a series of studies in severely obese individuals in which they measured glucose and insulin before and after an exercise program during which diet was held constant. As described previously, there was no significant weight loss, but glucose and insulin levels, and the associated insulin resistance, decreased significantly. This occurred without changes in body composition, or even with increases in fat mass. However, others have not confirmed these studies. Depres et al. (15) treated 13 obese women with exercise alone for 14 months and did not see a reduction in glucose or insulin levels, although C-peptide and glucose/insulin ratio during a glucose tolerance test were reduced. Weight loss in this study was 3.7 kg, and body fat loss was 4.6 kg. The researchers noted that the women with the greatest reduction in deep abdominal fat had the greatest improvements in glucose tolerance with training.

After 3 months of physical training in obese subjects, Krotkiewski et al. (29) found no changes in fasting glucose, but a significant ($p < .01$) decrease in fasting insulin, and decreases in both glucose and insulin levels stimulated by an oral glucose load. In a second study comparing VLCD with or without exercise, Krotkiewski et al. found a deterioration of plasma glucose with diet alone and no change with diet and exercise combined (32). In a third study with 38 women treated with exercise alone for 6 months, Krotkiewski et al. (31) found no change in glucose and insulin levels.

Wirth et al. (57) studied 40 obese subjects on diet-alone or diet-and-exercise programs for 4 weeks. They found a reduction in insulin and in C-peptide levels with diet and exercise but no change in glucose levels.

These studies present a mixed picture and suggest that the severely obese individual often does not have an improvement in insulin and glucose tolerance with exercise, especially in the absence of weight loss.

Other Hormone and Substrate Metabolism

Exercise in the severely obese alters a variety of other hormones and substrates (10,15,23,32,41,49, 51,57). Bjorntorp, Sullivan, and colleagues (10,51) found that, at baseline, urinary cortisol was higher in 8 severely obese subjects (4 men, 4 women) versus matched lean controls and that urinary cortisol fell significantly ($p < .05$) into the normal range after six weeks of treatment with exercise alone (diet held constant). Growth hormone was low in the obese subjects and did not change with exercise. Urinary norepinephrine (NE) excretion was higher in the obese subjects than in lean control subjects at baseline, but it did not decrease with exercise. Plasma NE did not differ between the groups at any time period. Free fatty acids (FFA) and glycerol also were elevated in the obese subjects but did not change with exercise. Serum triglycerides fell in both lean and obese subjects with exercise.

Depres et al. (15) noted significant reductions in total cholesterol, LDL cholesterol, and apoprotein B with a 14-month exercise-only program (diet held constant). HDL-apoprotein A-1 rose with exercise, as did the ratios of HDL_2-cholesterol/HDL_3-cholesterol and HDL-apoprotein A-1/LDL-apoprotein B. Post heparin hepatic triglyceride lipase fell significantly over the 14-month period of exercise.

Hill et al. (23) compared diet to diet and exercise and found a decrease in T3 in both groups but no change in T4, free T4, or TSH in either group after 5 weeks. Total cholesterol declined significantly in both groups, but there was no difference between groups. There were no significant changes in HDL, triglycerides, or total cholesterol/HDL ratio.

Krotkiewski et al. (32) measured a variety of hormones in a 3-week, nonrandomized study of diet versus diet and exercise. In both groups T3 fell and reverse T3 increased, but there were no differences between groups. Testosterone rose in both groups, although not significantly. Sex hormone binding globulin had highly significant increases in both groups, and the final values were identical. In another study of exercise alone for 6 months, Krotkiewski et al. (31) noted a significant fall in triglycerides and a fall in resting blood pressure that correlated with changes in insulin levels.

Despite significant increases in $\dot{V}O_2max$, Pavlou et al. (41) did not see improvements in triglycerides, cholesterol, or HDL levels with a 12-week course of diet and exercise.

Schwartz et al. (49) compared obese subjects on a 1,200-kcal/day diet versus an extensive exercise program without dietary restriction over 3 months and found that diet alone reduced arterial norepinephrine (NE) appearance rate. There were no differences in plasma NE and epinephrine levels or in NE clearance rate, and there were no significant differences between the groups.

Wirth et al. (57) compared diet versus diet and exercise and noted that levels of free fatty acids (FFA) at rest and after exercise increased with both groups over time but were greater in the diet-plus-exercise group. A similar pattern was seen with serum glycerol levels. At baseline, plasma epinephrine levels were increased, and they fell over time (diet, -45%; diet plus exercise, -74%). With maximal work on an exercise test at the end of the treatment period, the changes in the two groups were opposite: Plasma concentrations decreased in the diet-only group and increased in the diet-plus-exercise group. The pattern of NE levels was similar: Resting levels of NE fell 48% in the diet-plus-exercise group and only 9% in the diet-only group. The rise in NE at maximal exercise occurred only in the diet-plus-exercise group.

Exercise and Other Variables in Severely Obese People

Depres et al. (15) evaluated the regional distribution of fat in severely obese women who exercised over 14 months. They found that exercise selectively reduced abdominal fat more than femoral fat. Furthermore, the selective decrease in abdominal fat came predominantly from the subcutaneous depot. The deep abdominal depot decreased in proportion with fat losses in the rest of the body. Bjorntorp (5) has reviewed the differences between men and women in the regulation of energy balance with exercise. Differences in levels of adipose tissue lipoprotein lipase in femoral versus abdominal fat depots may contribute to these sex differences. Further studies are indicated to determine if this selective loss of fat from the abdominal depot is associated with severe obesity in both sexes or with the female sex alone.

The preceding portion of this review has concentrated on references that used exercise in the treatment of severe obesity. A number of nontreatment studies have dealt with biochemical, physiological, anatomical, and pathological aspects of exercise in severely obese people.

Alpert et al. (1) performed exercise tests in morbidly obese subjects (twice ideal body weight) and evaluated left and right ventricular function. They concluded that right ventricular dysfunction occurred in 23% of subjects at rest, but with exercise, the incidence of RV dysfunction rose to 50%. A similar pattern was seen when LV function was tested with exercise. This suggests that exercise testing in severely obese individuals would be useful to uncover ventricular dysfunction that is not apparent at rest. They also noted, "There is an accumulating body of evidence that obesity may produce left ventricular dysfunction in the absence of systemic hypertension or underlying organic heart disease." Severely obese people are likely to be at greater risk for this type of heart disease.

Bray, Whipp, Koyal, and Wasserman (12) compared the effects of exercise in lean versus obese (BMI = 33.7) men and noted a number of differences. At comparable external work, obese men required more oxygen. When O_2 intakes were matched, obese men were doing less work than lean men. Blood pressure rose more in the obese men than in the lean men with exercise. There were no differences between groups in efficiency of work, changes in lactate and bicarbonate levels, and growth hormone response to exercise.

Burstein, Epstein, Shapiro, Charuzi, and Karnieli (13) compared response to a euglycemic clamp with and without an acute bout of exercise among obese diabetic subjects, nondiabetic subjects, and lean control subjects. They found that exercise increased the metabolic clearance rate (MCR) of glucose at higher insulin levels in the two obese groups but did not affect the MCR in lean subjects. They concluded that an acute bout of exercise markedly reduces, but does not reverse, the insulin resistance of severe obesity.

A number of papers raised the possibility that exercise is more difficult for severely obese people, and that such individuals are more difficult when asked to exercise. Foss, Lampman, and colleagues (18-20,34) reported that severely obese individuals have a marked variation in exercise ability and respond to exercise very differently. Severely obese individuals perceive increases in exercise work load to be more severe than they are, especially later in the course of a maximal exercise test (19). These subjects were described as being more immature, requiring more time, complaining more, and being more resistant to a new experience (18). Kenrick et al. (26) echoed these comments and noted that their severely obese patients became apathetic, bored, and hostile during the course of their exercise program. With increasing weight loss and over time, it became difficult to keep the patients in the program, and a great deal of time was required to convince them to exercise. At times the patients would refuse to exercise.

The reasons for this behavior are probably multifactorial, but there is some evidence that severely obese people may be different from lean individuals and potentially may suffer more discomfort with exercise than lean people do. Krotkiewski et al. (29,30) and Wade et al. (55) performed muscle biopsies in obese individuals and noted differences in the distribution of fiber types. Obese people have fewer slow-twitch (Type I) fibers, and the proportion of Type I fibers is inversely related to the percentage of body fat (55). Krotkiewski et al. (29) noted a decrease in fast-twitch Type B fibers and an increase in fast-twitch Type A fibers in obese individuals during an exercise program. Type B fast-twitch fibers have a higher glycolytic capacity, and Type A fibers have a higher oxidative capacity. Thus the change with exercise favors the utilization of fatty acids. These authors also showed that there was increased capillary density around the Type A fast-twitch fibers with exercise, which might allow greater oxidation of fatty acids with training.

Scheen et al. (48) compared severely obese subjects with lean control subjects during a 3-hour bout of treadmill exercise. They found that at a similar heart rate and level of oxygen consumption, ventilation was significantly lower in the obese subjects. Plasma FFA levels were higher initially in the obese subjects, but did not rise as much with exercise. Plasma lactate levels were higher in the obese subjects, and blood glucose levels were significantly decreased. Glucagon levels did not rise as much in the obese subjects, which could reduce lipolysis. All these findings suggest that obese people may use more carbohydrate and build up more lactate during exercise, which potentially may cause more discomfort than in lean people. Scheen et al. (48) postulate that this may represent a metabolic limitation for performing prolonged exercise in severely obese patients.

Discussion

The studies evaluating effects of exercise in severely obese subjects on body weight, body composition, and metabolic rate are conflicting. The degree of obesity, length of study, and the type, intensity, and duration of exercise were not standardized across the published studies, making interpretation difficult. The limitation of the ability of severely obese individuals to exercise at a sufficient intensity or duration of exercise may have limited the effects on body weight, composition, or metabolic variables. Other accompanying treatments and diets may have affected the results.

Many severely obese people have remarkably poor levels of physical fitness. Habitual lack of exercise is the most likely explanation for the poor exercise tolerance of severely obese people. However, anecdotal data in humans regarding the physical discomfort of exercise, coupled with data on pain sensitivity in obese animals and the alterations in lactate metabolism with exercise in obese humans, suggest that strenuous exercise may be more uncomfortable for the very obese. This could affect adherence to an exercise regimen. The occurrence of arthritis, venous stasis lesions, thermal stress, skin rashes, and so forth in severely obese people also may limit exercise tolerance. Some data suggest differences in muscle fiber types in severely obese versus lean individuals. This could influence substrate utilization and ability to perform prolonged exercise.

All of these data suggest that there may be differences between severely obese and moderately obese individuals. There has been insufficient data collected to be able to draw any conclusions as to differences in severely obese people and whether exercise plays the same role in these individuals as it does in moderately obese people. Therefore, we suggest the following potential areas for further research involving exercise with severe obesity:

1. Additional studies comparing changes in severely obese versus lean or moderately obese subjects. Are severely obese people a separate subgroup?
2. Evaluation of special barriers to exercise in severe obesity. Can compliance to an exercise regimen be improved?
3. Are there differences in muscle types or amounts in severely obese versus lean or moderately obese individuals, and does this affect substrate utilization and exercise tolerance?
4. What is the relative importance of the various components of the exercise prescription for severely obese people, including mode, intensity, duration, and frequency?
5. Can exercise be used for long-term maintenance of weight loss in severely obese people? Is there a role for a combination of exercise and drugs in weight loss or maintenance?
6. How do dietary energy and macronutrient content affect ability to exercise, outcome of weight-loss programs, and complications of obesity?
7. Determination of body composition is difficult in severely obese people, and this compromises the ability to assess alterations due to exercise. Better methods are needed.
8. There are no studies on exercise and obesity surgery. Does pre- or post-surgery exercise alter outcome in any way?

References

1. Alpert, M.A.; Singh, A.; Terry, B.E.; Kelly, D.L.; Sharaf El-Deane, M.S.; Mukerji, V.; Villarreal, D.; Artis, A.K. Effect of exercise and cavity size on right ventricular function in morbid obesity. Am. J. Cardiol. 64:1361-1365; 1989.
2. Atkinson, R.L.; Kaiser, D.L. Effects of calorie restriction and weight loss on glucose and insulin levels in obese humans. J. Am. Coll. Nutr. 4:411-419; 1985.
3. Ballor, D.L.; Katch, V.L.; Beque, M.D.; Marks, C.R. Resistance weight training during caloric restriction enhances lean body weight maintenance. Am. J. Clin. Nutr. 47:19-25; 1988.
4. Bjorntorp, P. Adipocyte precursor cells. In: Bjorntorp, P.; Cairella, M.; Howard, A., eds.

Recent advances in obesity research: III. London: John Libbey Publishers; 1981:58-69.

5. Bjorntorp, P. Sex differences in the regulation of energy balance with exercise. Am. J. Clin. Nutr. 49:958-961; 1989.
6. Bjorntorp, P.; Berchtold, P.; Grimby, G.; Lindholm, B.; Sanne, H.; Tibblin, G.; Wilhelmsen, L. Effects of physical training on glucose tolerance, plasma insulin and lipids on body composition in men after myocardial infarction. Acta Med. Scand. 192(5):439-443; 1972.
7. Bjorntorp, P.; De Jounge, K.; Krotkiewski, M.; Sullivan, L.; Sjostrom L.; Stenberg, J. Physical training in human obesity. III. Effects of long-term physical training on body composition. Metabolism. 22:1467-1475; 1973.
8. Bjorntorp, P.; De Jounge, K.; Sjostrom, L.; Sullivan, L. The effect of physical training on insulin production in obesity. Metabolism. 19(8): 631-638; 1970.
9. Bjorntorp, P.; De Jounge, K.; Sjostrom, L.; Sullivan, L. Physical training in human obesity. II. Effects on plasma insulin in glucose-intolerant subjects without marked hyperinsulinemia. Scand. J. Clin. Lab. Invest. 32:41-45; 1973.
10. Bjorntorp, P.; Holm, G.; Jacobsson, B.; Schiller-de Jounge, K.; Lundberg, P-A.; Sjostrom, L.; Smith, U.; Sullivan, L. Physical training in human hyperplastic obesity. IV. Effects on the hormonal status. Metabolism. 26(3):319-328; 1977.
11. Bouchard, C.; Tremblay, A.; Nadeau, A.; Dussault, J.; Depres, J-P.; Theriault, G.; Lupien, P.J.; Serresse, O.; Boulay, M.R.; Fournier, G. Long-term exercise training with constant energy intake. 1: Effect on body composition and selected metabolic variables. Int. J. Obes. 14:57-73; 1990.
12. Bray, G.A.; Whipp, B.J.; Koyal, S.N.; Wasserman, K. Some respiratory and metabolic effects of exercise in moderately obese men. Metabolism. 26:403-412; 1977.
13. Burstein, R.; Epstein, Y.; Shapiro, Y.; Charuzi, I.; Karnieli, E. Effect of an acute bout of exercise on glucose disposal in human obesity. J. Appl. Physiol. 69:299-304; 1990.
14. Davis, P.G.; Phinney, S.D. Differential effects of two very low calorie diets on aerobic and anaerobic performance. Int. J. Obes. 14:779-787; 1990.
15. Depres, J.; Pouliot, M-C.; Moorjani, S.; Nadeau, A.; Tremblay, A.; Lupien, P.J.; Theriault, G.; Bouchard, C. Loss of abdominal fat and metabolic response to exercise training in obese women. Am. J. Physiol. 261:E159-E167; 1991.
16. Donnelly, J.E.; Pronk, N.P.; Jacobsen, D.J.; Pronk, S.J.; Jakicic, J. Effects of a very-low calorie diet and physical-training regimens on body composition and resting metabolic rate in obese females. Am. J. Clin. Nutr. 54:56-61; 1991.
17. Drenick, E.J.; Bale, G.S.; Seltzer, F.; Johnson, D.G. Excessive mortality and causes of death in morbidly obese men. JAMA. 243:443-445; 1980.
18. Foss, M.L.; Lampman, R.M.; Schteingart, D. Physical training program for rehabilitating extremely obese patients. Arch. Phys. Med. Rehabil. 57:425-429; 1976.
19. Foss, M.L.; Lampman, R.M.; Schteingart, D.E. Extremely obese patients: Improvements in exercise tolerance with physical training and weight loss. Arch. Phys. Med. Rehabil. 61:119-123; 1980.
20. Foss, M.L.; Lampman, R.M.; Watt, E.; Schteingart, D.E. Initial work tolerance of extremely obese patients. Arch. Phys. Med. Rehabil. 56:63-67; 1975.
21. Garrow, J.S. Effects of exercise on obesity. Acta. Med. Scand. [Suppl.]. 711:67-73.
22. Hammer, R.L.; Barrier, C.A.; Roundy, E.S.; Bradford, J.M.; Fisher, A.G. Calorie-restricted low-fat diet and exercise in obese women. Am. J. Clin. Nutr. 49:77-85; 1989.
23. Hill, J.O.; Sparling, P.B.; Shields, T.W.; Heller, P.A. Effects of exercise and food restriction on body composition and metabolic rate in obese women. Am. J. Clin. Nutr. 46:622-630, 1987.
24. Hoffer, L.J.; Forse, R.A. Protein metabolic effects of a prolonged fast and hypocaloric refeeding. Am. J. Physiol. 258:E832-E840; 1990.
25. Keim, N.L.; Barbieri, T.F.; Van Loan, M. Physiological and biochemical variables associated with body weight loss in overweight women. Int. J. Obes. 15:283-293; 1991.
26. Kenrick, M.M.; Ball, M.F.; Canary, J.J. Exercise and weight reduction in obesity. Arch. Phys. Med. Rehabil. 53:323-340; 1972.
27. Kreitzman, S.N. Lean body mass, exercise and VLCD. Int. J. Obes. [Suppl. 2]. 13:17-25; 1989.
28. Krotkiewski, M.; Aniansson, A.; Grimby, G.; Bjorntorp, P.; Sjostrom, L. The effect of unilateral isokinetic strength training on local adipose and muscle tissue morphology, thickness, and enzymes. Eur. J. Appl. Physiol. 42:271-281; 1979.
29. Krotkiewski, M.; Bylund-Fallenius, A-C.; Holm, J.; Bjorntorp, P.; Grimby, G.; Mandroukas, K. Relationship between muscle morphology and metabolism in obese women: The effects of long-term physical training. Eur. J. Clin. Invest. 13:5-12; 1983.
30. Krotkiewski, M.; Grimby, G.; Holm, G.; Szczepanik, J. Increased muscle dynamic endurance associated with weight reduction on a very-low-calorie diet. Am. J. Clin. Nutr. 51:321-330; 1990.

31. Krotkiewski, M.; Mandroukas, K.; Sjostrom, L.; Sullivan, L.; Wetterqvist, H.; Bjorntorp, P. Effects of long-term physical training on body fat, metabolism, and blood pressure in obesity. Metabolism. 28:650-658; 1979.
32. Krotkiewski, M.; Toss, L.; Bjorntorp, P.; Holm, G. The effect of very-low-calorie diet with and without chronic exercise on thyroid and sex hormones, plasma proteins, oxygen uptake, insulin and c peptide concentrations in obese women. Int. J. Obes. 5:287-293; 1981.
33. Kuczmarski, R.J. Prevalence of overweight and weight gain in the United States. Am. J. Clin. Nutr. 55:495S-502S; 1992.
34. Lampman, R.M.; Schteingart, D.E.; Foss, M.L. Exercise as a partial therapy for the extremely obese. Med. Sci. Sports Exerc. 18(1):19-24; 1986.
35. Landin, K.; Lindgards, F.; Saltin, B.; Winhelmsen, L. Decreased skeletal muscle potassium in obesity. Acta Med. Scand. 223:507-513; 1988.
36. Lennmarken, C.; Sandstedt, S.; Von Schenck, H.; Larsson, J. Skeletal muscle function and metabolism in obese women. J. Parent. Ent. Nutr. 10:583-587; 1986.
37. Metropolitan Life Insurance Co. Statistical bulletin. 40:1-4; 1959.
38. Moore, J.M.; Oddou, W.E.; Leklem, J.E. Energy need in childhood and adult-onset obese women before and after a nine-month nutrition education and walking program. Int. J. Obes. 15:337-344; 1991.
39. Olefsky, J.; Reaven, G.M.; Farquhar, J.W. Effects of weight reduction on obesity. J. Clin. Invest. 53:64-76; 1974.
40. Olefsky, J.M.; Kolterman, O.G. In-vivo studies of insulin resistance in human obesity. In: Bjorntorp, P.; Cairella, M.; Howard, A.N., eds. Recent advances in obesity research:III. London: John Libbey; 1981:254-267.
41. Pavlou, K.N.; Krey, S.; Steffee, W.P. Exercise as an adjunct to weight loss and maintenance in moderately obese subjects. Am. J. Clin. Nutr. 49:1115-1123; 1989.
42. Pavlou, K.N.; Steffee, W.P.; Lerman, R.H.; Burrows, B.A. Effects of dieting and exercise on lean body mass, oxygen uptake, and strength. Med. Sci. Sports Exerc. 17:466-471; 1985.
43. Phinney, S.D.; LaGrange, B.M.; O'Connell, M.; Danforth, E. Effects of aerobic exercise on energy expenditure and nitrogen balance during very low calorie dieting. Metabolism. 37:758-765; 1988.
44. Russell, D.McR.; Leiter, L.A.; Whitwell, J.; Marliss, E.B.; Jeejeebhoy, K.N. Skeletal muscle function during hypocaloric diets and fasting: A comparison with standard nutritional assessment parameters. Am. J. Clin. Nutr. 37:133-138; 1983.
45. Salans, L.B.; Knittle, J.L.; Hirsch, J. The role of adipose cell size and adipose tissue insulin sensitivity in the carbohydrate intolerance of human obesity. J. Clin. Invest. 47:153-165; 1968.
46. Samaan, N.; Brown, J.; Fraser, R.; Trayner, I. Effect of obesity and of starvation on insulin activity. Med. J. 1:1153-1156; 1965.
47. Saris, W.H.M.; Van Dale, D. Effects of exercise during VLCD diet on metabolic rate, body composition and aerobic power: Pooled data of four studies. Int. J. Obes. [Suppl. 2]. 13:169-170; 1989.
48. Scheen, A.J.; Pirnay, F.; Luyckx, A.S.; Lefebvre, P.J. Metabolic adaptation to prolonged exercise in severely obese subjects. Int. J. Obes. 7:221-229; 1983.
49. Schwartz, R.S.; Jaeger, L.F.; Veith, R.C.; Lakshminarayan, S. The effect of diet or exercise on plasma norepinephrine kinetics in moderately obese young men. Int. J. Obes. 14:1-11; 1990.
50. Simopoulos, A.P.; Van Itallie, T.B. Body weight, health and longevity. Ann. Intern. Med. 100:285-295; 1984.
51. Sullivan, L. Metabolic and physiologic effects of physical training in hyperplastic obesity. Scand. J. Rehabil. Med. [Suppl.]. 5:1-38; 1976.
52. Tremblay, A.; Despres, J.P.; Leblanc, C.; Bouchard, C. Sex dimorphism in fat loss in response to exercise-training. J. Obes. Weight Regul. 3:193-203; 1984.
53. Van Itallie, T.B. Obesity: Adverse effects on health and longevity. Am. J. Clin. Nutr. 32: 2723-2733; 1979.
54. Wadden, T.A.; Sternberg, J.A.; Letizia, K.A.; Stunkard, A.J.; Foster, G.D. Treatment of obesity by very low calorie diet, behavior therapy, and their combination: A five year perspective. Int. J. Obes. [Suppl. 2]. 13:39-46; 1989.
55. Wade, A.J.; Marbut, M.M.; Round, J.M. Muscle fibre type and aetiology of obesity. Lancet. 335:805-808; 1990.
56. Walberg, J. Aerobic exercise and resistance weight-training during weight reduction: Implications for obese persons and athletes. Sports Med. 47:343-356; 1989.
57. Wirth, A.; Vogel, I.; Schomig, A.; Schlierf, G. Metabolic effects and body fat mass changes in obese subjects on a very-low-calorie diet with and without intensive physical training. Ann. Nutr. Metab. 31:378-386; 1987.

Chapter 48

Physical Activity, Fitness, and Osteoarthritis*

Richard S. Panush

Former President Carter attracted national attention when he collapsed while competing in a 10K footrace during September 1979. Former President Bush, too, recently required medical attention when he was unable to complete a jog. Three patients serve further to introduce and focus this presentation. One was a gentleman aged 71 years when evaluated, a former Boston Marathon champion, Olympian, and world-record holder at several distances, who developed angina pectoris in his eighth decade. Another was a former all-pro (American football) linebacker who suffered knee injuries during his career and consulted colleagues at our institution for recurrent effusions, crepitation, and degenerative changes. The third was a general surgeon, a former Kansas state high school quarter-mile-run champion, who was seen at age 44 in consultation for several years of inflammatory polyarthritis; resumption of running, including competitive marathons, was associated with complete remission of arthritis. Was physical exercise beneficial or detrimental to the health of these individuals (121,123–139)?

These incidents illustrate the current wave of popularity of recreational activities in the United States and also raise the question as to their value. Millions of persons have taken up running for its potential benefits to health. Many more regularly participate in tennis, skiing, cycling, dancing, soccer, football, basketball, baseball, and other activities (79,80). The possible benefits attributed to regular recreational activity include retardation or prevention of coronary atherosclerosis, improved cardiovascular fitness, psychological well-being, and weight control (79). It is well documented that regular physical activity may cause a variety of short-term, acute injuries. These are generally related to the degree of fitness and intensity and the quantity of exercise (117,143). There is a large body of literature describing these injuries for many activities and recommending means of preventing and managing them; they will not be discussed here (143). This review will focus on information relevant to determining long-term effects of exercise on the musculoskeletal system. Is exercise a risk for the development of osteoarthritis? Can the circumstances of the previously described patients be explained?

Osteoarthritis

Osteoarthritis (OA) is the most common type of arthritis. This syndrome also has been termed degenerative joint disease or osteoarthrosis. OA refers to a process of multifactorial etiology, not yet well understood, that leads to cartilaginous degeneration and that is associated with clinical symptoms. A variety of factors are important in its pathogenesis, including genetic predisposition, trauma, inflammation, biochemical and metabolic pathways, possible immunologic events, occupational and environmental influences, and—the subject of this discussion—certain recreational factors. A uniform view of the clinical, radiologic, and pathologic criteria that can be used to define OA has not yet been reached (7-10,59,60). This has limited understanding of OA and has created difficulties in analyzing the effects of sport-related activities on the development of OA. Radiologic criteria for diagnosis of OA were used for a number of years. More recently the American College of Rheumatology has supported development of preliminary criteria for clinical, laboratory, and radiographic classification of OA. Important clinical features are painful range of motion, morning stiffness not exceeding 30 min in duration, crepitance, and bony enlargement. Radiographic findings include osteophytes, subchondral cysts or sclerosis, joint-space narrowing, malalignment, or attrition of normal bone mineralization (7-10, 60,72).

*Portions of this chapter excerpted from *Topics in Geriatric Rehabilitation*, 4(3):23-31, with permission of Aspen Publishers, Inc., © 1989.

OA is considered to be quite common, particularly among an aging population (50). One survey estimated radiographic evidence of OA to exist in as many as 40 million Americans, not all of whom were symptomatic. Of a population between ages 70 and 79, as many as 85% had OA (46). This disease can affect virtually any joint but has a particular predilection to the knees, hips, spine, distal interphalangeal joints, and first carpometacarpal joints. Symptoms are usually pain and stiffness without associated inflammatory or systemic complaints. The disease is not inexorably progressive, disabling, or crippling and generally can be managed satisfactorily with supportive analgesia (105,127,128).

Relationship of Physical Activity to OA

Factors Important in the Pathogenesis of OA

Ligamentous instability, abnormal joint motion, and prior injury may be important in the premature development of OA and of OA associated with regular exercise. Studies of individuals with cruciate, collateral ligament, and meniscal injuries have supported the concept that unstable or damaged knees were associated with development of premature OA (5,13,22,24,27,32,39,40,47,48,69,70, 74,96,101,114,116,151,156).

An interesting long-term follow-up study reviewed 86 patients at an average of 4.5 years after surgery (161). Most of the patients (81%) had sustained sports injuries to the anterior cruciate and medial collateral ligaments (28 from downhill skiing and 20 from football). It was found that 42% of the subjects had chondromalacia patellae, and 20% to 52% had radiologic abnormalities. A retrospective study (100) made at 10-year and 14-year follow-up periods of patients with untreated anterior cruciate ruptures found that almost all of these injuries had occurred during sports participation, and 86% of the patients had undergone removal of one or both menisci. Seventy-five percent of these patients had continued at the same level of sports participation without a change in their symptoms. Through radiographs, one third of the knees demonstrated cartilage loss or evidence of arthritic changes. It was concluded that development of arthritis may be associated with varus deformity, previous meniscectomy, and relative body weight.

Correlation of simultaneous meniscal injury and anterior collateral ligamentous reconstructive surgery by the iliotibial band procedure was studied (96). A 42% incidence of meniscal tears was detected at initial evaluation. If the patient deferred reconstructive surgery during the first year and continued to participate in sports, the incidence of meniscal tears doubled. Both partial and total meniscectomies were associated with degenerative changes. It was concluded that early joint stabilization and direct meniscus repair surgery may decrease the incidence of premature OA. Menisci are important for weight bearing, stabilization, and protection against premature OA of the knee (28, 40,48,69,70,151). A 10% incidence of OA of the knee was noted during long-term follow up of 440 patients who underwent meniscectomies (13). These observations all support biomechanical abnormality as an important—perhaps necessary—factor predisposing to development of sports-related OA.

Immobilization may hasten articular degeneration. The biochemical factors important in osteoarthritis are under investigation (38,119,120,161). The effects of chronic exercise on joint lubrication, local inflammation, microfractures, and aging of cartilage are unknown.

Other factors considered important in the development of sports-related OA include certain physical characteristics of the participant, biômechanical and biochemical factors, age, gender, hormonal influences, nutrition, characteristics of the playing surface, unique features of particular sports, and duration and intensity of exercise participation. These factors have been reviewed extensively elsewhere (121,123–128). Increasingly, it is recognized that biomechanical factors have an important role in the pathogenesis of OA.

Occupational Observations

Is osteoarthritis caused in part by mechanical stress? One analytical approach to determining a possible relationship between exercise and joint disease is to consider the epidemiological evidence that degenerative arthritis may follow repetitive trauma, such as might occur with certain occupations. Most discussions of the pathogenesis of osteoarthritis include a role for stress (29,62-64,71,93,119,134,138). Stamm wrote that "osteoarthritic changes in a joint are always and only of mechanical origin" (149). Several studies have suggested an increased prevalence of osteoarthritis of elbows and knees in miners (73,90); of shoulders and elbows in pneumatic drill operators (25,71); of intervertebral disks in dock workers (90); of hands in cotton workers (91), diamond cutters (91), and garment makers (152); and of hand joints in textile workers (53,54). Studies of skeletons of several populations have suggested that "age of onset, frequency, and location of degenerative changes are directly related to the nature and degree of environmentally associated stress" (71), which is consistent with previous observations associating hand osteoarthritis and usage patterns (1). However, not all of these studies were carried out to contemporary standards, nor have they been confirmed. A more recent report, for example, failed to find an increased incidence of osteoarthritis in pneumatic drillers (25). These authors criticized inadequate sample sizes, lack of statistical analyses, and omission of appropriate control populations in previous reports. They further commented that earlier work was "frequently misinterpreted" and that studies from their groups suggested that "impact, without injury or preceding abnormality of either joint contour or ligaments, is unlikely to produce osteoarthritis." Wear and tear may indeed predispose a joint to osteoarthritis, but this notion should be considered tentative and not accepted uncritically (53,54).

Epidemiologic Observations

Do epidemiologic studies of OA implicate physical or mechanical factors pertaining to predisposition or development of disease? The first national Health and Nutrition Examination Survey of 1971 to 1975 (HANES 1) and the Framingham study explored cross-sectional associations between radiologic OA of the knee with possible risk factors (12,41). These and other recent studies noted strong associations between knee OA and obesity and those occupations involving stress of knee bending (42,43,55), but not all habitual physical activities and leisure-time physical activities (running, walking, team sports, racket sports, and others) were linked with knee OA (31,60,77,94,136,142) (Table 48.1).

Table 48.1 Occupational Physical Activity and Possible Associations With Osteoarthritis

Occupation	Involved joints	Risk of OA	References
Miners	Elbow, knee	Increased	73,90
Pneumatic drillers	Shoulder, elbow	Increased None	71 25
Dock workers	Intervertebral discs	Increased	90
Cotton workers	Hand	Increased	91
Diamond workers	Hand	Increased	91
Garment makers	Hand	Increased	152
Textile workers	Hand	Increased	54
Occupations requiring knee bending	Knee	Increased	41,43

Note. From Panush & Brown (125). Reprinted with permission.

Clinical Observations

Is regular participation in physical activity associated with degenerative arthritis? Several animal studies suggested, but did not prove, a possible relationship between exercise and OA (20,62,137, 146,158,160,163). There are some, but not many, pertinent observations in human studies (Table 48.2) (19,66,67,115,121-129,140,150). Wrestlers were reported to have an increased incidence of osteoarticular lesions of the spine (141), cervical spine, knees, and elbows (92); boxers of the carpometacarpal joints (68); baseball pitchers of shoulders and elbows (18,34); parachutists of knees, ankles, and spine (108,109); cyclists of the patella (16); cricketers of fingers (2); and gymnasts of shoulders, elbows, and wrists (2). Some of these reports are largely anecdotal (2), and not all reflect confirmed, valid associations. Studies of ballet dancers (23,30) noted OA of talar joints as well as other chronic lower extremity problems; criteria for osteoarthritis were not specified (23).

Talar joint osteoarthritis was also reported in 33 of 34 football players (23). Klunder, Rud, Hansen, and Sondegaard compared the clinical and radiological findings in knees and hips of 57 retired football (soccer) players with those in control subjects and found a significant increase of OA of the hip (49% compared to 25% in the control subjects) (76). These conclusions contrasted with others that found frequent OA of knees (28%) and ankles (92%), but not of hips (0%), in amateur soccer players. Frequent ankle (astragalotibia) abnormalities were suggested among association football players (21). A careful examination of knees of 51 association football players found osteoarthrosis in only 7 individuals (2). Degenerative changes of the cervical spine were noted in former national team association football players in Norway; onset of changes preceded those of a control population by 10 to 20 years (148).

Few studies of American football players have been reported. Three hundred fifty former University of Missouri players were questioned 10 to 30 years after participation, and radiographs of their knees were reviewed. Among the 44 respondents, 83% had radiological evidence of OA (139). A study comparing 23 American high school football

Table 48.2 Sports Participation and Alleged Associations With Osteoarthritis

Sport	Site (joint)	References
Ballet	Talus	23,30,102,118
	Ankle	37,162
	Cervical spine	37,162
	Hip	37,162
	Knee	162
	Metatarsophalangeal	11
Baseball	Elbow	3,56
	Shoulder	18
Boxing	Hand (carpometacarpal)	68
Cricket	Finger	157
Cycling	Knee	16
Football (American style)	Ankle	159
	Feet	159
	Knee	139
	Spine	6,44,104
Gymnastics	Elbow	22
	Shoulder	22
	Wrist	15,22
	Hip	107
Lacrosse	Ankle	153
	Knee	153
Martial arts	Spine	141
Parachuting	Ankle	108
	Knee	108
	Spine	109
Rugby	Knee	144
Running	Knee	100
	Hip	33,78,84–89,100, 121–129,135
	Ankle	78,98
Skiing (downhill)	Thumb	49
Soccer	Ankle-foot	130,131
	Cervical spine	148
	Hip	76
	Knee	76,131,147
	Talus	23,147
	Talofibular	21
Weight lifting	Spine	4,45,81,106
Wrestling	Cervical spine	92
	Elbow	92
	Knee	92

Note. From Panush & Brown (125). Reprinted with permission.

players 20 years after high school graduation with 11 age-matched control subjects found no significant increase in OA—radiographically, subjectively, or objectively. However, a significant increase in knee joint OA was found in the subgroup of football players who had sustained a knee injury while playing football (104). Ninety percent of football players (average age, 23 years) competing for a place on a professional team had radiological abnormalities of the foot or ankle, compared with 4% of an age-matched control population; linemen had more changes than ball carriers or linebackers, who, in turn, had more changes than flankers or defensive backs. All those who had played football for 9 years or longer had abnormal findings on radiography (159). Eighty-six patients were reviewed, most of whom (81%) had sports injuries (skiing, 28; football, 20) to the anterior cruciate and medial collateral ligaments. At an average of 4-1/2 years after operation, 42% had chondromalacia patellae, and 20% to 52% had radiological abnormalities (161).

Most of these studies, which are few in number, suffer in several respects. It was not always possible to determine the sport studied; criteria for OA (osteoarthrosis, degenerative joint disease, or abnormality) were not always clear, specified, or consistent; duration of follow-up was often not indicated or was inadequate to determine the risk of musculoskeletal problems at a later age; intensity and duration of physical activity were variable and difficult to quantify; selection bias toward individuals exercising or not exercising was not weighted; other possible risk factors and predisposition to musculoskeletal disorders were rarely considered; studies were not always properly controlled and examinations not always blind; little information regarding the nonprofessional, recreational athlete was available; and little clinical information about functional status was provided.

Medical problems of performing artists and dancers have recently been recognized. As for athletes, these are frequent and may have long-term consequences to joints, such as development of OA (23,30,37,52,61,95,102,111,118,162).

Clinical Studies of Runners

Several studies have now examined a possible relationship between running and OA. Uncontrolled observations generally suggest that runners without underlying biomechanical problems of the lower extremity joints do not appear to develop arthritis at a rate different from nonrunner, normal populations (145). Those individuals who had underlying articular biomechanical abnormalities do appear to be at greater risk of subsequent development of OA (100), and these observations seem to be valid for other sports activities as well. We examined groups of long-duration, high-mileage runners and nonrunning control subjects. We found a comparable (and low) prevalence of OA in both runners and nonrunners and concluded that running need not lead inevitably to OA (129). These observations generally have now been confirmed by others (see Table 48.3).

Our study compared 17 male runners (average age, 56 years) with age-matched and weight-matched sedentary controls. Running subjects (53% marathoners) ran a mean of 28 miles per week for 12 years. We did not find an increased prevalence of OA among runners. Our observations suggested, within the limits of the study, that long-duration, high-mileage running need not be associated with premature degenerative joint disease in the lower extremities (129).

Similar observations were reported by others. Lane and colleagues studied 41 distance runners and matched control subjects (50 to 72 years old). The runners were noted to have 40% more bone mineral, whereas female runners had more sclerosis and spurs; no differences were noted between groups in loss of cartilage, crepitation, joint stability, or OA (87). These authors have now provided additional pertinent information (84,86,88,89). A comparison of 498 distance runners with 365 con-

Table 48.3 Studies of Running and Risk of Developing Osteoarthritis

Reference	No. runners	Age (years, mean)	Years run (mean)	Miles per week (mean)	Comments
Murray & Duncan (107)	319	NA	NA	NA	OA was noted more frequently in former runners (with underlying anatomic tilt abnormality [epiphysiolysis]) than in nonathletes.
Puranen et al. (135)	74	56	21	NA	Champion distance runners had no more hip OA than nonrunners in their sixth decades.
de Carvalho & Long Feldt (33)	32	NA	NA	NA	X rays of runners' hips and knees were similar to those of control subjects.
McDermott & Freyne (100)	20	35	13	48	OA occurred in those runners with underlying anatomic (biomechanical) abnormalities.
Sohn & Micheli (145)	504	57	9–15	18–29	"No association [was found] between moderate long-distance running and the future development of OA" (of hips and knees).
Panush et al. (129)	17	53	12	28	Comparable low prevalence of OA of lower extremities was found in runners and nonrunners.
Lane et al. (87)	41	58	9	5 hr/week	No differences were found between runners and control subjects in cartilage loss, crepitation, joint stability, or symptomatic OA.
Lane et al. (88)	498	59	12	27	"No differences were found between groups in conditions thought to predispose to OA and musculo-skeletal disability."
Marti et al. (98,99)	27	42	NA	61 (reference year)	More radiologic changes of hip OA were found in former Swiss national team long-distance runners than in bobsledders and control subjects; few runners had clinical symptoms of OA. No differences were noted in ankle joints.
Konradsen et al. (78)	30	58	40	12–24	No clinical or radiographic differences of hips, knees, and ankles were found between runners and nonrunners.
Lane et al. (89)	35	60	10–13	23–28 (3–4 hr/week)	"Running did not appear to influence the development of radiologic OA (with the possible exception of spur formation in women)."

Note. NA = not available.

trol subjects indicated that runners had less physical disability, greater functional capacity, and better cardiovascular fitness; runners also weighed less, sought medical services less often, and developed musculoskeletal disability at a lower rate than nonrunners (88). More recent information from these investigators corroborated the original observations—runners maintained greater bone density and, with the possible exception of spur formation in women, running did not appear to influence development of OA (86,89).

Former college varsity long-distance runners were compared with former college swimmers (145). Questionnaires were sent to 1,153 former athletes. Respondents included 504 runners and 287 swimmers; average age was 57 years. Swimmers had a 2.4% incidence of severe pain of the hips or knees and a 19.5% incidence of moderate pain, compared with a 2% incidence of severe pain in the hips and knees and 15.5% incidence of moderate pain for runners. Eventually 2.1% of the swimmers and 1% of the runners underwent surgery (the difference was not statistically significant). Runners averaged 25 miles per week for 12 years. There was no correlation between the onset of pain and the number of miles run per week or the number of years of running. The authors concluded that there was no association between moderate levels of running or number of years running and the development of symptomatic OA. Twenty middle-aged long-distance runners complained of knee pain. Six of the 20 had clinical and radiographic evidence of osteoarthritis, 4 had a history of knee trauma, and all 6 had anatomical variances. This group ran an average of 62 miles per week for 20 years, whereas unaffected runners averaged 41 miles per week for 12 years. The authors concluded that running alone did not cause OA, but rather prior injuries and anatomical variances were directly responsible for some of the changes (100). Several additional reports have found that runners are not at risk of developing premature OA of knees or ankles (33,78,98,145).

We are aware of two studies that examined degenerative hip disease in former athletes. One found that former champion distance runners had no more clinical or radiologic evidence of OA than did nonrunners (135); a second study reported more radiologic changes of degenerative hip disease in former Swiss national team long-distance runners than in bobsled competitors and control subjects, although few of the former runners had clinical symptoms of OA (99). These observations were interpreted as suggesting that long-term, high-intensity, high-mileage running should not be dismissed as a potential risk factor for premature hip OA.

These studies generally suggest that runners without underlying biomechanical problems of the lower extremity joints do not appear to develop arthritis at a rate different from nonrunner, normal populations. Those individuals who had underlying articular biomechanical abnormalities did appear to be at greater risk for subsequent development of OA, and these observations seemed to be valid for other sports activities as well. Conflicting studies regarding the development of radiologic degenerative hip changes in former athletes suggest that long-term, high-intensity, high-mileage running perhaps should not be entirely dismissed as a potential risk factor for premature hip OA.

Benefits

Are there any potential long-term benefits of physical activity to the musculoskeletal system? Prolonged exercise has been found to increase bone density (65,81,112). Increased bone density was found not only in athletes of highest international class, but also in ordinary athletes and exercising control subjects; in all of these groups bone density exceeded that of sedentary individuals. Among athletes, average bone density was highest in weight lifters and was progressively lower in throwers, runners, soccer players, and swimmers (112).

Are there other factors that might pertain to the musculoskeletal consequences of regular exercise? It is now appreciated that physical conditioning induces secretion of endorphins—endogenous opioid peptides with diverse functions, including effects on energy balance, appetite, lipolysis, reproduction, thermoregulation, and psychological well-being (14,26). It is also known that psychological or environmental stress can influence immunological responsiveness (82) as well as manifestations of musculoskeletal disease (155). Furthermore, several studies have shown alterations in immunological homeostasis in conditioned athletes or following stress (51,57). It is therefore possible, but still highly speculative, that physical conditioning, endorphin elaboration, and immune responsiveness—and perhaps other pathways—may interrelate to affect the development of musculoskeletal disease, either adversely or favorably, through yet uncertain mechanisms.

There is little documentation of clinical benefit for patients with arthritis from traditional exercise and physical therapy programs (17). Indeed some long-held concepts relating to exercise and arthritis are now being challenged (127). Several investigative groups have begun to study the therapeutic effects of aerobic exercise programs for patients with arthritis. Most of these observations remain preliminary; however, there are reports that the condition of patients with inflammatory (rheumatoid) arthritis has improved (by subjective and objective criteria) with participation in aerobic dance, aquatic, cycling, t'ai chi, treadmill exercise programs, Nautilus, and other exercise programs (35,36,54,58,75,83,97,103,110,113, 132,133,156,159). Although these observations are of considerable interest, they are limited and experimental; it would be premature to attempt to generalize therapeutic exercise recommendations for arthritis patients.

Summary

Clearly, recreational physical exercise is popular. The possible short-term and long-term psychological and cardiovascular benefits of regular exercise have been well publicized, although not necessarily well documented. Millions of adults now exercise, as do large numbers of school-age children. The injury rate among participants is high, ranging from 20% to 66% in football players to 90% in runners. Fortunately, most injuries appear to be limited, although some may lead to chronic disability, especially if they result in joint or ligamentous instability. The sports medicine community is focusing considerable attention on the management of these training and overuse injuries and to the identification of factors predisposing to them. However, there has been surprisingly little information on the possible long-term consequences of regular exercise on the musculoskeletal system.

Some studies suggest, but do not prove, that vigorous and prolonged participation in certain activities (such as ballet, soccer, football, boxing, parachuting, and possibly others) may predispose individuals to degenerative joint disease; however, other studies have found little risk of degenerative arthritis from soccer, long-distance running, or certain occupations and have pointed out serious flaws and misinterpretations in prior reports. The difficulties in interpreting the available information have been emphasized.

Further studies are needed, ideally including contributions from orthopedics, rheumatology, biomechanical engineering, biochemistry, radiology, and possibly other disciplines. The studies would need to carefully define and quantify physical stress, include appropriate study and control populations, and be of sufficient duration and sample size to provide definitive information. They also should use standardized clinical and radiologic assessments of joint degeneration, quantify the patient's functional status, and assess the contributions of other risk factors. These would be difficult studies to conduct, and they may never be done. We need more information about the consequences of exercise on the musculoskeletal system, however, so that physicians can confidently advise the millions of participants about the beneficial and deleterious effects of regular exercise.

And what of the patients presented in the introductory paragraph? Former President Carter had heat exhaustion, President Bush had arrhythmia, the marathon champion had well-preserved joints and was long-lived, the linebacker developed sports-related knee OA, and the surgeon's inflammatory arthritis may have benefited from aerobic exercise; all of these outcomes are consistent with themes developed in this presentation.

Conclusions

Recreational exercise has achieved great popularity. Possible benefits to participants include increased longevity, decreased risk of cardiovascular disease, improved psychological well-being, and greater fitness. An important but yet unanswered concern is whether exercise or physical overuse conditions play a role in the pathogenesis of OA.

In humans, anecdotal observations have suggested relationships between certain recreational activities and degenerative joint disease. The few controlled studies that exist, however, have indicated that exercise need not be deleterious to joints. Available data may be interpreted to suggest that reasonable recreational exercise—carried out within limits of comfort, putting joints through normal motions, and without underlying joint abnormality—need not inevitably lead to joint injury, even over many years.

Also we are witnessing thoughtful reevaluation of physical exercise as a therapeutic modality for arthritis patients. It is possible that certain patients may achieve psychological and clinical benefit from selected exercise programs.

Acknowledgments

The author gratefully acknowledges the superb assistance of Pat Palma in the preparation of the manuscript. This work was supported in part by the Saint Barnabas Research Foundation. Portions of this manuscript were reproduced from Panush, R.S., Recreational activities and the risk of musculoskeletal disease. Arthritis in Society, The Impact of Musculoskeletal Disease edited by N.M. Hadler and D.B. Gillings, eds., Butterworth, 1985, pp 65-71 (121); Panush, R.S.; Brown, D.G.: Exercise and arthritis, Sports Medicine 4:54-64, 1987 (125);

Panush, R.S.: Exercise and arthritis, Topics in Geriatric Rehabilitation 4:23-31, 1989 (122); and Panush, R.S.: Does exercise cause arthritis? Long-term consequences of exercise in the musculoskeletal system, Rheumatic Disease Clinics of North America 16:827-836, 1990 (123). All reprinted by permission.

References

1. Acheson, R.M.; Chan, Y.K.; Clemett, A.R. New Haven survey of joint diseases. XII. Distribution and symptoms of osteoarthrosis in the hands with reference to handedness. Ann. Rheum. Dis. 29:275-286; 1970.
2. Adams, I.D. Osteoarthritis and sport. Clin. Rheum. Dis. 2:523-541; 1976.
3. Adams, J.E. Injury to the throwing arm; a study of traumatic changes in the elbow joints of boy baseball players. Cal. Med. 102:127-129; 1965.
4. Aggrawal, N.D.; Kaur, R.; Kumar, S.; Mathur, D.N. A study of changes in the spine in weight lifters and other athletes. Br. J. Sports Med. 13:58-61; 1965.
5. Aichroth, P. Osteochronditis dessicans of the knee; a clinical survey. J. Bone Joint Surg. 53B:440-447; 1971.
6. Albright, J.P.; Moses, J.M.; Feldick, H.G.; Dolan, K.D.; Burmeister, L.F. Non-fatal cervical spine injuries in interscholastic football. JAMA. 13:1243-1245; 1976.
7. Altman, R.; Alarcon, A.; Appelrough, D.; et al. The American College of Rheumatology criteria for the classification and reporting of osteoarthritis of the hand. Arthritis Rheum. 30:1601-1610; 1990.
8. Altman, R.; Alarcon, G.; Appelrough, D.; et al. The American College of Rheumatology criteria for the classification and reporting of osteoarthritis of the hip. Arthritis Rheum. 34:505-514; 1991.
9. Altman, R.; Asch, E.; Bloch, D.; Bole, G.; Borenstein, D.; et al. Development of criteria for the classification and reporting of osteoarthritis. Arthritis Rheum. 29:1039-1049; 1986.
10. Altman, R.D.; Bloch, D.A.; Bole, G.G., Jr.; et al. Development of clinical criteria for osteoarthritis. J. Rheumatol. [Suppl. 14]. 14:3; 1987.
11. Ambre, T.; Nilson, B.E. Degenerative changes in the first metatarsophalangeal joint of ballet dancers. Acta Orthop. Scand. 49:317-431; 1978.
12. Anderson, J.J.; Felson, O.T. Factors associated with osteoarthritis of the knee in the first national health and nutrition examination survey (HANES I). Evidence for an association with overweight, race, and physical demands of work. Am. J. Epidemiol. 128:179-189; 1988.
13. Appel, H. Late results after meniscetomy in the knee joint. Acta Orthop. Scand. [Suppl.] 133:1; 1970.
14. Appenzeller, O. What makes us run? N. Engl. J. Med. 305:578-579; 1981.
15. Auberge, T.; Zenny, J.C.; Duvallet, A.; Godefroy, D.; Horreard, P.; et al. Bone maturation and osteoarticular lesions in top level sportsmen. J. Radiol. 65:555-561; 1984.
16. Bagneres, H. Lesions osteo-articulaires chroniques des sportifs. Rheum. Halneol. Allergiol. 19:41-50; 1967.
17. Basmrajian, J.V. Therapeutic exercise in the management of rheumatic diseases. J. Rheumatol. [Suppl. 15]. 14:22; 1987.
18. Bennett, G.E. Shoulder and elbow lesions of the professional baseball pitcher. JAMA. 117:510-514; 1941.
19. Blazek, O.; Streda, A.; Cermak, V.; Skallova, O. Degenerative changes in the spine of top sportsmen. Cesk. Radiol. 37:383-388; 1983.
20. Bollet, A.J. An essay of the biology of osteoarthritis. Arthritis Rheum. 12:152-163; 1969.
21. Bourel, M.; Cormier, M.; Lenoir, P.; Dagorne, J.N.; Delahaye, D. Les complications locomotrices due footbal et des maladies osteoarticulaires. Rev. Rheum. 7/8:297-303; 1960.
22. Bozdech, Z. Chronic injury-gymnastics. In: Larson, L.A., Encyclopedia of sports sciences and medicine. New York: Macmillan; 1971:616.
23. Brodelius, A. Osteoarthrosis of the talar joints in footballers and ballet dancers. Acta Orthop. Scand. 30:309-314; 1961.
24. Brown, A.R.; Rose, B.S. Familiar precocious polyarticular osteoarthrosis of chrondroplastic type. N. Z. Med. J. 65:449-461; 1966.
25. Burke, M.J.; Fear, E.C.; Wright, V. Bone and joint changes in pneumatic drillers. Ann. Rheum. Dis. 36:276-279; 1977.
26. Carr, D.B.; Bullen, B.A.; Skinar, G.C.; Arnold, M.A.; Rosenblatt, M.; Bettins, I.Z.; Martin, J.B.; McArthur, J.W. Physical conditioning facilitates the exercise-induced secretion of beta-endorphin and beta-lipotropin in women. N. Engl. J. Med. 305:560-563; 1981.
27. Carter, C.; Wilkinson, J. Persistent joint laxity and congenital dislocation of the hip. J. Bone Joint Surg. 46B:40-45; 1964.
28. Charnely, R.K. Late joint changes as a result of internal derangement of the knee. Am. J. Surg. 76:496; 1948.
29. Cooke, T.D.V.; Dwosh, I.; Cossairt, J. Clinical pathologic osteoarthritis workshop. J. Rheumatol. [Suppl.]. 9:1-118; 1983.
30. Coste, F.; Desoille, H.; Illouz, G.; Chavy, A.L. Apareil locomoteur et danse classique. Rev. Rhum. 28: 259-267; 1960.

31. Croft, P.; Cooper, C.; Wilkham, C.; Loggon, D. Physical activity and osteoarthritis of the hip in men. Arthritis Rheum. 34:S87; 1991.
32. Dandy, D.J.; Jackson, R.W. The diagnosis of problems after meniscectomy. J. Bone Joint Surg. 57B:349-352; 1975.
33. de Carvalho, A.; Long Feldt, B. Lobetraening og arthrosis de formans. En radiologisk vurdering (Running practice and arthrosis deformans. A radiological assessment). Ugeskr. Laeger. 139:2421-2422; 1977.
34. Dively, R.L.; Meyer, P.W. Baseball shoulder. JAMA. 171:1659-1661; 1969.
35. Ekbloom, B.; Lovgren, O.; Alderin, M.; Frodstrom, M.; Satterstrom, G. Effect of short-term physical training on patients with rheumatoid arthritis. A six-month follow-up study. Scand. J. Rheumatol. 4:87-91; 1975.
36. Ekdahl, C.; Andersoon, S.I.; Moritz, U.; Svensson, B. Dynamic versus static training in patients with rheumatoid arthritis. Scand. J. Rheumatol. 19:17-26; 1990.
37. Ende, L.S.; Wickstrom, J. Ballet injuries. Phys. Sportsmed. 10:101-118; 1982.
38. Enneking, W.F.; Horowitz, M. The intra-articular effects of immobilization on the human knee. J. Bone Joint Surg. 54A:973-985; 1972.
39. Fahmy, N.R.M.; Williams, E.A.; Noble, J. Meniscal pathology and osteoarthritis of the knee. J. Bone Joint Surg. 65B:24-28; 1983.
40. Fairbank, T.J. Knee joint change after meniscetomy. J. Bone Joint Surg. 30B:664; 1948.
41. Felson, D.J.; Anderson, J.J.; Naimark, A.; Walker, A.M.; Meenan, R. Obesity and knee osteoarthritis. The Framingham study. Ann. Intern. Med. 109:18-24; 1988.
42. Felson, D.T.; Hannan, M.T.; Anderson J.J.; Naimark, A. Occupational physical demands (phys), knee bending (bend) and x-ray knee osteoarthritis (OA): The Framingham study. Arthritis Rheum. 33:S10; 1990.
43. Felson, D.T.; Hannan, M.J.; Naimark, A.; Berkeley, J.; Gordon, G.; Wilson, P.W.F.; Anderson, J. Occupational physical demands, knee bending, and knee osteoarthritis: Results from the Framingham study. J. Rheumatol. 18:1587-1592; 1991.
44. Ferguson, R.J.; McMaster, J.H.; Stanitski, C.L. Low back pain in college football lineman. J. Sports Med. 2:63-69; 1975.
45. Fitzgerald, B.; McLatchie, G.R. Degenerative joint disease in weight lifters, fact or fiction? Br. J. Sports Med. 13:97-101; 1980.
46. Forman, M.D.; Malamet, R.; Kaplan, D. A survey of osteoarthritis of the knee in the elderly. J. Rheumatol. 10:282-287; 1983.
47. Funk, J.F. Osteoarthritis of the knee following ligamentous injury. Clin. Orthop. 172:154-157; 1983.
48. Gear, M.W.L. Thelate results of meniscectomy. Br. J. Surg. 54:270; 1967.
49. Gerber, C.; Senn, E.; Matter, P. Skier's thumb; surgical treatment of recent injuries to the ulnar collateral ligament of the thumb's metacarpophalangeal joint. Am. J. Sports Med. 9:171-177; 1981.
50. Gordon, T. Osteoarthrosis in U.S. adults. In: Bennett, P.H.; Wood, P.H.N., eds. Population studies of the rheumatic diseases, 19. Amsterdam: Excerpta Medica Foundation; 1968:391.
51. Green, R.L.; Kaplan, S.S.; Rabin, B.S.; Stanitski, C.L.; Zdziarski, V. Immune function in marathon runners. Ann. Allergy. 47:73-75; 1981.
52. Greer, J.M.; Panush, R.S. Rheumatic problems in performing artists. Postgrad. Adv. Rheum. 3(2):1; 1988.
53. Hadler, N.M. Industrial rheumatology. Clinical investigations into the influence of the pattern of usage on the pattern of regional musculoskeletal disease. Arthritis Rheum. 20:1019-1025; 1977.
54. Hadler, N.M.; Gillings, D.B.; Imbus, H.R.; Levittin, P.M.; Makuc, D.; Utsinger, P.D.; et al. Hand structure and function in an industrial setting. The influence of the three patterns of stero-typed, repetitive usage. Arthritis Rheum. 21:210-220; 1978.
55. Hannan, M.J.; Felson, D.J.; Anderson, J.J.; Naimark, A. Habitual physical activity and knee osteoarthritis (OA) in the Framingham study. Arthritis Rheum. 34:S171; 1991.
56. Hansen, N.M. Epiphyseal changes in the proximal humerus of an adolescent baseball pitcher. Am. J. Sports Med. 10:380-384; 1982.
57. Hanson, P.G.; Flaherty, D.K. Immunologic responses to training in conditioned runners. Clin. Sci. 60:225-228; 1981.
58. Harkcom, T.M.; Lampman, R.M.; Blanwell, B.F.; Caston, C.W. Therapeutic value of graded aerobic exercise training in rheumatoid arthritis. Arthritis Rheum. 28:32-39; 1985.
59. Hochberg, M.C. Osteoarthritis. Postgrad. Adv. Rheum. 3(3):1; 1988.
60. Hochberg, M.C. Epidemiologic considerations in the primary prevention of osteoarthritis. J. Rheumatol. 18:1438-1439; 1991.
61. Hoppmann, R.A.; Patrone, N.A. A review of musculoskeletal problems in instrumental musicians. Semin. Arthritis Rheum. 19:117-124; 1989.
62. Howell, D.S.; Altman, R.D.; Pita, J.C.; Woessner, J.F., editors. The pathogenesis of osteoarthritis. Kalamazoo, MI: Upjohn; 1983:5-53.
63. Howell, D.S.; Sarolsky, A.I.; Pita, J.C.; Woessner, F. The pathogenesis of osteoarthritis. Semin. Arthritis Rheum. 5:365-383; 1976.
64. Howell, D.S.; Woessner, J.F.; Jimenez, S.; Seda, H.; Schumacher, H.R. A view on the

pathogenesis of osteoarthritis. Bull. Rheum. Dis. 29:996-1001; 1979.

65. Huddleston, A.L.; Rockwell, D.; Kulund, D.N.; Harrison, R.B. Bone mass in lifetime tennis athletes. JAMA. 244:1107-1109; 1980.
66. Hughston, J.C. Acute knee injuries in athletes. Clin. Orthop. 3:31-35; 1962.
67. Hussey, H.H. Cervical spine injuries in football. JAMA. 11:1274; 1976.
68. Iselin, M. Importance de l'arthrose dans le syndrome 'main fragile' des boxeurs. Rev. Rhum. Mal. Osteoartic. 7-8:242-243; 1960.
69. Jackson, J.P. Degenerative changes in the knee after meniscectomy. Br. Med. J. 2:525; 1968.
70. Jones, R.E.; Smith, E.C.; Reisch, J.S. Effects of medical meniscectomy in patients older than forty years. J. Bone Joint Surg. 60A:73; 1978.
71. Jurmain, R.D. Stress and the etiology of osteoarthritis. Am. J. Phys. Anthropol. 46:353-365; 1977.
72. Kellgren, J.H.; Lawrence, J.S. Radiological assessment of osteoarthrosis. Ann. Rheum. Dis. 16:494-501; 1957.
73. Kellgren, J.H.; Lawrence, J.S. Osteoarthritis and disk degeneration in an urban population. Ann. Rheum. Dis. 12:5-15; 1958.
74. Kirk, J.A.; Anse, B.M.; Bywater, E.G.L. The hypermobility syndrome. Ann. Rheum. Dis. 26:419-425; 1967.
75. Kirsteins, A.E.; Dietz, F.; Hwang, S-M. Evaluating the safety and potential use of a weight-bearing exercise, tai-chi chuan, for rheumatoid arthritis patient. Am. J. Phys. Med. Rehabil. 70:136-141; 1991.
76. Klunder, K.B.; Rud, B.; Hansen, J. Osteoarthritis of the hip and knee joints in retired football players. Acta. Orthop. Scand. 51:925-927; 1980.
77. Kohutson, N.D.; Schurman, D.J. Risk factors for the development of osteoarthrosis of the knee. Clin. Orthop. 261:242-246; 1990.
78. Konradsen, L.; Hansen, E.M.; Sondegaard, L. Long distance running and osteoarthritis. Am. J. Sports Med. 18:379-381; 1990.
79. Koplan, J.P.; Powell, K.E.; Sikes, R.K.; Shirley, R.W.; Campbell, C.C. An epidemiologic study of the benefits and risks of running. JAMA. 248:3118-3121; 1982.
80. Koplan, J.P.; Siscovick, D.S.; Goldbaum, G.M. The risks of exercise: A public health view of injuries and hazards. Public Health Rep. 100:188-195; 1985.
81. Kotani, P.T.; Ichikawa, N.; Wakabayashi, W.; Yoshii, T.; Koshimune, M. Studies of spondylosis found among weight-lifters. Br. J. Sports Med. 6:4-8; 1970.
82. Kusnecov, A.W.; Sivyer, M.; Kiny, M.G.; Hushand, A.J.; Cripps, A.W.; Clancy, R.L. Behaviorally conditioned suppression of the immune response by antilymphocytic serum. J. Immunol. 130:2117-2120; 1983.
83. Labowitz, R.J.; Challman, J.; Palmeri, S. Aerobic exercise in the management of rheumatic diseases. Del. Med. J. 60:659-662; 1988.
84. Lane, N.E. Does running cause degenerative joint disease? J. Musculoskel. Med. 4:17; 1987.
85. Lane, N.E. Exercise and osteoarthritis. Bull. Rheum. Dis. 41:5-7; 1992.
86. Lane, N.E.; Bloch, D.A.; Hubert, H.B.; Jones, H.; Simpson, U.; Fries, J.J. Running, osteoarthritis, and bone density: Initial 2-year longitudinal study. Am. J. Med. 88:452-459; 1990.
87. Lane, N.E.; Bloch, D.A.; Jone, H.H.; Marshall, W.H., Jr.; Wood, P.D.; Fries, J.J. Long-distance running, bone density and osteoarthritis. JAMA. 255:1147-1151; 1986.
88. Lane, N.E.; Bloch, D.A.; Wood, P.D.; Fries, J.J. Aging, long distance running, and the development of musculoskeletal disability. Am. J. Med. 82:772; 1987.
89. Lane, N.; Micheli, B.; Bjorkengren, A.; Oehlert, J.; Bloch, D.; Shi, H.; Fries, J. The risk of osteoarthritis with running and aging: A 5 year longitudinal study. Rheum. 20:461-468; 1993.
90. Lawrence, J.S. Rheumatism in coal mines. III. Occupational factors. Br. J. Ind. Med. 12:249-261; 1955.
91. Lawrence, J.S. Rheumatism in cotton operatives. Br. J. Ind. Med. 18:270-276; 1961.
92. Layani, F.; Roeser, J.; Nadaud, M. Les lesion osteoarticulaires des catcherus. Rev. Rhum. Mal. Osteoartic. 7-8:244-248; 1960.
93. Lee, P.; Rooney, P.J.; Sturrock, R.D.; Kennedy, A.C.; Dick, W.C. The etiology and pathogenesis of osteoarthrosis; a review. Semin. Arthritis Rheum. 3:189-218; 1974.
94. Lindberg, H.; Montgomery, F. Heavy labor and the occurrence of osteoarthrosis. Clin. Orthop. 214:235-236; 1987.
95. Lockwood, A.H. Medical problems of musicians. N. Engl. J. Med. 320:221-227; 1989.
96. Lynch, M.A.; Henning, C.E.; Glick, K.R., Jr. Knee joint surface changes. Clin. Orthop. 172:148-153; 1983.
97. Lyngberg, K.; Danneskiod-Samsoe, B.; Halskov, O. The effect of physical training on patients with rheumatoid arthritis: Changes in disease activity, muscle strength and aerobic capacity. A clinically controlled minimized cross-over study. Clin. Exp. Rheumatol. 6:253-260; 1988.
98. Marti, B.; Biedert, R.; Howald, H. Risk of arthrosis of the upper ankle joint in long distance runners: Controlled follow-up of former elite athletes. Sportverletzung Sportschaden. 4(4):175-179; 1990.

99. Marti, B.; Knobloch, M.; Tschopp, A.; et al. Is excessive running predictive of degenerative hip disease? Controlled study of former elite athletes. Br. Med. J. 229:91; 1989.
100. McDermott, M.; Freyne, P. Osteoarthrosis in runners with knee pain. Br. J. Sports Med. 17:84-87; 1983.
101. McDonald, W.J., Jr.; Dameron, T.B., Jr. The untreated anterior cruciate ligament rupture. Clin. Orthop. 172:158-163; 1983.
102. Miller, E.H.; Schneider, H.J.; Bronson, J.L.; McLain, D. A new consideration in athletic injuries; the classical ballet dancer. Clin. Orthop. 3:181-191; 1975.
103. Minor, M.A.; Hewett, J.E.; Webel, R.R.; Anderson, S.K.; Kay, D.R. Efficacy of physical conditioning exercise in patients with rheumatoid arthritis and osteoarthritis. Arthritis Rheum. 32:1396-1405; 1989.
104. Moretz, J.A.; Harlan, S.D.; Goodrich, J.; Walters, R. Long-term follow-up of knee injuries in high school football players. Am. J. Sports Med. 12:298-300; 1984.
105. Moskowitz, R. Management of osteoarthritis. Bull. Rheum. Dis. 31:31; 1981.
106. Muenchow, H.; Albert, H., editors. The spine in weight-lifters. Medizine and Sport No. 1, Berlin, 1969.
107. Murray, R.O.; Duncan, C. Athletic activity in adolescence as an etiological factor in degenerative hip disease. J. Bone Joint Surg. 53B:406-419; 1971.
108. Murray-Leslie, C.F.; Lintott, D.J.; Wright, V. The knees and ankles in sport and veteran military parachutists. Ann. Rheum. Dis. 36:327-331; 1977.
109. Murray-Leslie, C.F.; Lintott, D.J.; Wright, V. The spine in sport and veteran military parachutists. Ann. Rheum. Dis. 36:332-342; 1977.
110. Nath, A.; Webel, R.R.; Kay, D.; Minor, M. Training effect of aerobic exercise in arthritis patients. Clin. Res. [Abstract]. 35:566A; 1987.
111. Nikolaev, I.A.; Najdenov, S. Osteo-arthropathies professionelles et danse classique. Arch. Mal. Prof. Med. Trav. Secur. Soc. [Paris]. 31:39-42; 1980.
112. Nilsson, B.E.; Westlin, N.E. Bone density in athletes. Clin. Orthop. 77:179-182; 1971.
113. Nordemar, R.; Ekblom, B.; Zuchrisson, L.; Lundqrist, K. Physical training in rheumatoid arthritis: A controlled long-term study. I. Scand. J. Rheumatol. 10:17-23; 1981.
114. Noyes, F.R.; Matthews, D.S.; Mooar, P.A.; Grood, E.S. The symptomatic anterior cruciate-deficient knee. J. Bone Joint Surg. 65A:163-173; 1983.
115. O'Carroll, P.F.; Sheehan, J.M.; Gregg, T.M. Cervical spine injuries in rugby football. Ir. Med. J. 12:377-379; 1981.
116. O'Donoghue, D.H.; Frank, G.H.; Jeter, G.L.; Johnson, W.; Zeiders, J.W.; Kenyon, R. Repair and reconstruction of the anterior cruciate ligament in dogs; factors influencing long-term results. J. Bone Joint Surg. 53A:710-718; 1971.
117. Orava, S.; Saarela, J. Exertion injuries to young athletes. Am. J. Sports Med. 6:68-74; 1978.
118. Ottani, G.; Betti, R. Studio radiologico deue alterazioni osteoarticolari nei giocatori di calico. Stud. Med. Chir. Sport. 4:3-14; 1953.
119. Palmoski, M.J.; Brandt, K.D. Running inhibits the reversal of atrophic changes in canine knee cartilage after removal of a leg cast. Arthritis Rheum. 24:1329-1337; 1981.
120. Palmoski, M.J.; Perricone, E.; Brandt, K.D. Development and reversal of a proteoglycan aggregation defect in normal canine knee cartilage after immobilization. Arthritis Rheum. 22:508-517; 1979.
121. Panush, R.S. Recreational activities and the risk of musculoskeletal disease. In: Hadler, N.M.; Gillings, D.B., eds. Arthritis and society. The impact of musculoskeletal diseases. London: Butterworth Co.; 1985:65-71.
122. Panush, R.S. Exercise and arthritis. Top. Geriatr. Rehabil. 4:23-31; 1989.
123. Panush, R.S. Does exercise cause arthritis? Long-term consequences of exercise on the musculoskeletal system. Rheum. Dis. Clin. 16:827-836; 1990.
124. Panush, R.S.; Brown, D. Exercise, the musculoskeletal system and arthritis. Postgrad. Adv. Rheum. 2(6):3-20; 1987.
125. Panush, R.S.; Brown, D.G. Exercise and arthritis. Sports Med. 4:54-64; 1987.
126. Panush, R.S.; Brown, D.G. Exercise and osteoarthritis. Patient Man. 11:199-213; 1987.
127. Panush, R.S.; Lane, N., editors. Exercise and arthritis. Bailliere's clinical rheumatology. [In press].
128. Panush, R.S.; Panush, D.M. Short consensus proposal for 1992 international consensus symposium on physical activity, fitness and health. [In press].
129. Panush, R.S.; Schmidt, C.; Caldwell, J.; Edwards, N.L.; Longley, S.; et al. Is running associated with degenerative joint disease? JAMA. 255:1150-1154; 1986.
130. Pellegrini, P.; Nibbio, N.; Piffaneli, A. Atropatie croniche da attivita sportiva: Il piede e il ginocchio del calciatore professionista. Arch. S. Anna. Ferr. Ist. Radiol. 17:879-910; 1964.
131. Pellissier, M.; Bruschet, J.; Levere, F.; Leenhardt, P. Le pied des footballeurs. Fil. lit. Mediterr. (23 Novembre):403-404; 1952.
132. Perlman, S.G.; Connell, K.; Alberti, J.; et al. Synergistic effects of exercise and problem-

solving education for rheumatoid arthritis. Arthritis Rheum. [Abstract]. 30:S13; 1987.

133. Perlman, S.B.; Connell, K.J.; Clark, A.; Robinson, M.S.; Conlon, P.; Gecht, M.; Caldron, P.; Singcore, J.M. Dance-based aerobic exercise for rheumatoid arthritis. Arthritis Care Res. 3:29-35; 1990.

134. Peyron, J.G. Epidemiologic and etiologic approach of osteoarthritis. Semin. Arthritis Rheum. 8:288-306; 1979.

135. Puranen, J.; Ala-Ketola, L.; Peltokalleo, P.; Saarela, J. Running and primary osteoarthritis of the hip. Br. Med. J. 1:424-425; 1975.

136. Radin, E.L.; Burr, D.B.; Caterson, B.; Fyhrie, D.; Brown, T.D.; Boyd, R.D. Mechanical determinants of osteoarthritis. Semin. Arthritis Rheum. [Suppl. 2]. 21:12-21; 1991.

137. Radin, E.L.; Eyre, D.; Schiller, A.L. Effect of prolonged walking on concrete on the joints of sheep. Arthritis Rheum. [Abstract]. 22:649; 1979.

138. Radin, E.L.; Paul, I.L.; Rose, R.M. Role of mechanical factors in pathogenesis of osteoarthritis. Lancet. 5:519-522; 1972.

139. Rall, K.L.; McElroy, G.L.; Keats, T.E. A study of the long term effects of football injury to the knee. Mo. Med. 61:435-538; 1964.

140. Robey, J.M.; Blyth, C.S.; Mueller, F.O. Athletic injuries; application of epidemiologic methods. JAMA. 217:184-189; 1977.

141. Rubens-Duval, A.; Bellin, A.; Ficheuz, M.; Villiaumey, J.; Souchet, B. Le rachis des ceinturs noives. Rev. Rhum. Mal. Osteoartic. 7-8:233-241; 1960.

142. Salaff, F.; Cavaliere, F.; Nolli, M.; Ferraccioli, G. Analysis of disability in knee osteoarthritis. Relationship with age and psychological variables but not with radiographic score. J. Rheumatol. 18:1581-1586; 1991.

143. Sheehan, G.A. An overview of overuse syndromes in distance runners. Ann. NY Acad. Sci. 301:877-880; 1977.

144. Slocum, D.B. Overuse syndrome of the lower leg and foot in athletes. Instructor's lecture at American Academy of Orthopedic Surgery. 17:359; 1960.

145. Sohn, R.S.; Micheli, L.J. The effect of running on the pathogenesis of osteoarthritis of the hips and knees. Clin. Orthop. 198:106-109; 1985.

146. Sokoloff, L. Natural history of degenerative joint disease in small laboratory animals. Arch. Pathol. 62:118-128; 1956.

147. Solonen, K.A. The joints of the lower extremities of football players. Ann. Chir. et Gynaecol. Fenn. 55:176-180; 1966.

148. Sortland, D.; Tysvaer, A.T.; Storli, O.V. Changes in cervical spine association of football players. Br. J. Sports Med. 16:80-84; 1982.

149. Stamm, T.T. Aetiology and treatment of osteo-arthritis. Lancet. 2:754-756; 1939.

150. Stenstrom, C.H.; Lindell, B.; Swanberg, E.; Harms-Rindahl, K.; Nordemar, R. Functional and psychosocial consequences of disease and experience of pain and exertion in a group of rheumatic disease patients considered for active training. Results of a survey in Bollnas medical district. I. Scand. J. Rheumatol. 19:374-382; 1990.

151. Tapper, E.M.; Hooever, N.W. Late results after meniscectomy. J. Bone Joint Surg. 51:517-526; 1969.

152. Tempelaar, H.H.G.; Van Breeman, J. Rheumatism and occupation. Acta Rheum. 4:36-38; 1932.

153. Thomas, R.B. Chronic injury; lacrosse. In: Larson, L.A., ed. Encyclopedia of sports sciences and medicine. New York: Macmillan; 1971:621.

154. Tork, S.C.; Douglas, V. Arthritis water exercise program evaluation. A self-assessment survey. Arthritis Health Care Res. 2:28-31; 1989.

155. Trentham, D.E. Collagen arthritis as a relevant model for rheumatoid arthritis. Arthritis Rheum. 25:911-916; 1982.

156. Troyer, H. The effect of short-term immobilization in the rabbit knee joint cartilage. Clin. Orthop. 107:249-257; 1975.

157. Vere Hodge, N. Chronic injury; cricket. In: Larson, L.A., ed. Encyclopedia of sports sciences and medicine. New York: Macmillan; 1971:606.

158. Videman, T. The effect of running on the osteoarthritic joint; an experimental matched-pair study with rabbits. Rheum. Rehabil. 21:1-8; 1982.

159. Vincelette, P.; Laurin, C.A.; Levesque, H.P. The footballer's ankle and foot. Can. Med. Assoc. J. 107:873-877; 1972.

160. Walton, M. Naturally occurring osteoarthrosis in the mouse and other animals. In: Ali, S.Y.; Elves, M.W.; Leaback, D.H., eds. Normal and osteoarthrotic articular cartilage. London: Institute of Orthopedics; 1974:285.

161. Warren, R.F.; Marshall, J.L. Injuries of the anterior and medial collateral ligaments of the knee; a long-term follow-up of 86 cases. II. Clin. Orthop. 136:198-211; 1978.

162. Washington, E.L. Musculoskeletal injuries in theatrical dancers; site, frequency and severity. Am. J. Sports. Med. 2:75-98; 1978.

163. Williams, J.M.; Brandt, K.D. Exercise increases osteophyte formation but protects against fibrillation following iodoacetate-induced cartilage damage. J. Anat. 139:599-611; 1984.

Chapter 49

Physical Activity, Fitness, and Osteoporosis

Barbara L. Drinkwater

Weight-bearing physical activity is an essential requirement for bone health. Without the beneficial effect of gravitational or mechanical loading on the axial and appendicular skeleton, there is a rapid and marked loss of bone. Whether the generalized decrease in physical activity as one ages has a cumulative negative impact on bone mass is unknown. However, there is ample evidence that active individuals have a greater skeletal mass than those who are inactive. There are also data to support the concept that those who are sedentary can increase bone mass by becoming more active. However, the role habitual physical activity may play in the prevention of *osteoporosis* (defined as a disease characterized by low bone mass and microarchitectural deterioration of bone tissue leading to enhanced bone fragility and a consequent increase in fracture risk) is still uncertain.

Although several recent studies (12,21,49) have reported that a low bone mineral density (BMD) is associated with an increase in fracture risk, there are no prospective studies to document the effect of increased physical activity with a resultant increase in bone mass on the incidence of osteoporotic fractures. Without those studies, designed and conducted with the same scientific rigor that is demanded of other intervention studies, no firm conclusions can be drawn regarding the role of physical activity in the prevention of osteoporosis.

Exercise as an Intervening Variable

For the purposes of this review, *physical activity* will include both exercise and sport. In prospective studies, *exercise* will be defined as structured physical activity for the specific purpose of increasing bone mass. In cross-sectional studies the term *exercise* encompasses a broad range of activities that vary from one study to another but have in common a history of sustained participation over a period of months or years. Sport is included as a specific category of exercise and includes both competitive and noncompetitive activities pursued voluntarily toward the achievement of a specific goal.

Exercise is broadly categorized by type (aerobic, anaerobic, strength, etc.) and as acute or chronic. Within each category, it is further defined by duration, frequency, and intensity. Most in vivo studies of exercise and bone examine the chronic category (the cumulative effect of a series of exercise sessions over a period of time). Investigators interested in the immediate effect of exercise on bone metabolism may use a single (or acute) bout of exercise.

Experimental Design and Protocol in Exercise Studies

The method of choice in determining the effect of exercise on bone in an unselected population is the randomized prospective cohort study. Since true random selection of subjects is seldom feasible, the nonrandomized prospective cohort design is more common with random assignment of subjects to either the control or experimental group. A control group is considered essential. Cross-sectional studies may provide some interesting information about differences in BMD between two or more groups that differ in activity patterns or about an association between some measure of activity and bone mass, but such studies are notoriously weak in establishing causation.

To overcome the bias introduced by nonrandom selection of subjects, confounding variables must be identified and measured. Among potential confounding factors in osteoporosis studies are age, weight, medications, menstrual cycle irregularities, use of oral contraceptives, diet, and prior medical problems. Not only must sources of bias be identified, but consideration must be given to how they are to be controlled.

Tables 49.1 and 49.2 evaluate the design and protocol of a number of exercise and bone mass studies using criteria suggested by Loucks (29) plus additional factors relevant to the present topic. For example, the technique for measuring bone density should be described clearly along with an anatomical identification of the sites measured. Both short-term and long-term precision of the technique in the laboratory where the measurements were done should be included in the methods. In addition, the exercise protocol should be quantified in terms of frequency, duration, and intensity of exercise. Failing to quantify the protocol makes it impossible to verify the results in a subsequent study or to effectively use the protocol in a clinical setting. The statistical treatment of the data should be described in sufficient detail for the reader to evaluate the meaning of the results. This should include an indication of the power of the statistical tests.

Application of Training Principles

General principles of physical training that affect the training responses of other physiological systems may also apply to the skeletal system. Very few studies have considered the application of these principles to bone in spite of their potential importance to understanding the role of exercise in maintaining skeletal health.

Principle of Specificity

Exercises should stress the specific physiological system being trained. Many studies investigating the effect of exercise on bone have used aerobic activities designed to stress the cardiovascular system, not the skeletal system. Because the effect of exercise on bone appears to be a localized effect, the specificity principle would suggest that the exercise program involve activities that add mechanical stress to those areas where osteoporotic fractures occur most frequently—the spine, the femoral neck, the distal radius, and the humerus. Unless the purpose of the study is to test the systemic effect of exercise on bone, BMD should be measured at the skeletal site subjected to increased mechanical loading or gravitational force.

Principle of Overload

To effect change, the training stimulus must slowly but consistently increase. If the demand on the system does not increase, no further training effect will occur. With the exception of strength-training protocols, few studies have made an attempt to apply this principle to bone. Whether progressive overload is best achieved by increasing the intensity, frequency, or duration of activities designed to increase bone mass is not known at this time.

Principle of Reversibility

The positive effect of exercise on bone will be lost if the exercise program is discontinued. Bone mass gained through physical activity will revert to pretraining levels if the activity ceases (13). Consideration of this principle raises other important questions: How much exercise is required to maintain the BMD gained through activity? Is maintenance dependent upon the duration, frequency, or intensity of the exercise? Can drug or hormone therapy maintain the higher BMD gained through exercise?

Principle of Initial Values

Those at the lowest levels of fitness have the greatest percent improvement in training studies; those with average or above-average fitness have the least. If this principle also applies to bone, studies that enroll only sedentary women may be optimizing results and overestimating the potential benefit for the population as a whole. Subject selection can thus affect the magnitude of the outcome independently of the exercise protocol.

Principle of Diminishing Returns

There is a biological ceiling to exercise-induced improvements in the functioning of any physiological system. As this ceiling is approached, more and more effort is required to obtain smaller gains. The question is, How much increase in bone mass can be expected in young women whose BMD is in the lowest quartile of the normal range? Is the potential benefit enough to decrease the risk of osteoporosis later in life?

Physical Activity and Bone Mass in the Young Adult

It has been suggested that habitual physical activity during adolescence and the young adult years is important in ensuring that each individual will attain her or his biological potential for peak bone mass. This section examines the evidence that exercise can increase bone mass during this period and examines how calcium and estrogen interact with the osteogenic effect of exercise. This review is limited to studies of women's skeletal response to physical activity because women have a greater

Table 49.1 Characteristics of the Design and Protocol of Longitudinal Studies of Exercise and Bone Mass

	Reference numbers											
	1	9	13	19	25	31	33	34	38	41	43	50
Design												
Random	0	+	0	0	0	0	0	+	0	+	0	−
No. of subjects	9	33	17	34	16	300	18	9	40	120	10	52
No. of control subjects	9	15	18	38	15	0	18	11	19	42	7	21
Confounding factors												
Age	+	+	+	+	+	+	−	+	+	+	+	+
Weight	0	+	+	0	+	+	−	+	+	0	+	+
Height	0	+	+	0	+	+	−	+	+	0	+	+
Calcium intake	−	−	+	−	0	+	+	+	0	+	0	0
Hormonal status	+	+	<	<	<	<	+	+	<	+	+	<
Medications	0	+	+	+	−	+	+	0	+	−	+	0
Medical history	+	+	−	0	−	+	−	0	−	−	−	0
Activity history	−	0	−	−	0	0	−	0	−	0	+	0
Sex steroid use	0	+	<	<	<	+	+	+	−	+	+	<
Race	+	+	+	+	0	+	+	0	0	+	+	+
Exercise program												
Frequency	+	+	+	+	+	0	+	+	+	+	+	+
Duration (min, hr)	+	+	+	+	+	0	+	+	+	+	+	0
Intensity	−	+	+	+	0	−	+	−	+	0	+	0
Length (months, years)	+	+	+	+	+	+	+	+	+	+	+	+
Activity	−	−	+	+	−	+	+	+	+	−	+	−
Progressive	+	+	+	+	0	0	+	+	+	0	+	+
Compliance	0	+	+	+	+	0	+	+	+	+	+	+
Outcome variable												
Bone mass/density												
Method	+	+	+	+	+	+	+	+	+	+	+	+
Site	+	+	+	+	+	+	+	+	+	+	+	+
Precision	+	+	+	+	0	+	+	+	+	+	+	+
Statistics												
Type I error	0	+	+	+	+	+	+	+	0	+	0	0
Power	0	+	0	0	0	0	0	0	0	0	0	0
Analysis	0	+	+	+	+	+	+	+	+	+	+	0

Note. + = adequate control, description, or measurement; − = imprecise control, measurement, or description; 0 = not measured or not described for all groups; < = potential bias.

Table 49.2 Characteristics of the Design and Protocol of Cross-Sectional Studies of Exercise and Bone Mass

	Reference numbers										
	6	10	14	20	22	24	35	36	42	48	54
Design											
No. of subjects	42	17	18	40	120	19	41	40	29	83	123
No. of control subjects	38	14	9	18	46	19	41	—	13	—	—
Confounding factors											
Age	+	+	+	+	−	+	+	+	+	+	+
Weight	< +	< +	+	+	0	+	+	+	+	+	+
Height	+	0	+	+	0	+	+	+	+	+	+
Calcium intake	0	−	+	+	0	+	+	−	+	0	0
Hormonal status	−	−	+	+	0	+	−	+	< +	0	0
Medications	0	−	+	0	0	0	−	0	+	−	0
Medical history	+	+	+	0	−	−	−	0	+	−	−
Activity history	+	+	+	+	−	−	−	+	+	+	−
Sex steroid use	0	+	−	+	< −	−	−	−	< +	0	−
Race	+	+	0	0	0	+	0	0	+	+	0
Exercise program											
Frequency	0	+	0	+	−	0	+	+	−	0	0
Duration (min, hr)	0	0	0	+	−	0	0	+	0	0	+
Intensity	−	0	0	0	0	0	0	−	−	0	0
Length (months, years)	+	0	−	+	−	+	+	0	0	0	0
Activity	+	0	+	+	+	+	+	+	+	−	+
Outcome variable											
Bone mass/density											
Method	+	+	+	+	+	+	+	+	+	+	+
Site	+	+	+	+	+	+	+	+	+	+	+
Precision	+	0	+	0	0	0	0	+	+	+	0
Statistics											
Type I error	0	0	+	+	0	0	0	0	+	+	0
Power	0	0	0	0	0	0	0	0	0	+	0
Analysis	+	+	+	+	0	+	+	+	+	+	−

Note. + = adequate control, description, or measurement; − = imprecise control, measurement, or description; < = potential bias; 0 = not measured or not described for all groups.

incidence of osteoporosis and the majority of studies on this topic include only females.

Cross-Sectional Studies

The majority of studies in the young adult population compare the BMD of athletes or active women with that of sedentary control subjects. Although measurements have been made at the humerus, radius, and calcaneus, the most common sites are the lumbar vertebrae and the femoral neck. Overall, active women and athletes have a higher BMD than their sedentary peers (20,22,42,52). Swimmers are the exception; two studies have reported lower vertebral BMD for collegiate swimmers than for other athletes and control subjects (22,42).

The apparent benefit of weight-bearing activities to the spine of young women ranges from 1.6% to 14.8% (*Mn* = 7.8%). When one considers the strenuous training program of these competitive athletes (an average of 2.5 hr per day at least 5 days per week), a difference of 7.8% between the athletes' vertebral BMD and that of sedentary women seems relatively small. The average lumbar BMD for this age group is 1.20 g/cm^2 (Lunar Corporation). For a young woman whose BMD is 2 standard deviations below the mean (0.96 g/cm^2), an increase of 10% would still leave her spinal density well below average.

Longitudinal Studies

There are relatively few prospective studies in this age group, so the question of whether exercise can aid in maximizing peak bone mass is still unanswered. In the largest study to date (n = 292), Mazess and Barden (31) found no relationship between moderate activity levels and the percent change in BMD at the spine, proximal femur, or radius over a 2-year period. Nor were there any differences in vertebral, femoral neck, or radial BMD between women stratified into quartiles of activity (km/day) based on pedometer and accelerometer data for two 48-hr periods. However, these 4 days may not have reflected the overall activity pattern of the women nor have included activities other than locomotion that might have exerted a mechanical stress on the skeleton.

The most surprising report (19) was the lack of a significant effect on spinal and os calcis BMD following a 12-month Nautilus weight-lifting program. Strength training is, after all, one activity where there can be a gradual but continuous increase in training stimulus. Yet whereas the weight-lifting group had an overall increase in strength of 83%, they had only a 0.8% increase in vertebral BMD and a 0.3% decrease in os calcis BMD. Additional studies are needed to determine whether free weights might be more effective in transmitting the increase in loading to the axial skeleton.

Hormonal Status

Bone hypertrophy resulting from exercise is blunted in the absence of normal levels of endogenous estrogen in young women. A number of studies (7, 17,27,30) have found that amenorrheic female athletes have lower vertebral BMD than do their eumenorrheic peers with similar training regimens. Although women who resume normal menses do regain some bone (18,28), women with a history of menstrual irregularities have a lower vertebral density than women who have always had regular periods (16). Apparently, the osteogenic stimulus of physical activity is most effective in a normal hormonal milieu.

Physical Activity and Bone Mass in the Mature Adult

Perhaps the most important factor in determining a woman's risk of an osteoporotic fracture in her later years is her bone mass at the time she reaches menopause. Therefore, the emphasis during this period of a woman's life (35 to 50 years) in regard to skeletal health should be on maintaining or increasing BMD at those sites where osteoporotic fractures are most likely to occur—the spine, femoral neck, and distal radius. The few studies that have examined the effect of physical activity in this age group report that active women have a higher BMD than do sedentary women and that an exercise training program does increase bone mass. How effective the exercise is in achieving this goal depends on the activity selected and the design of the study.

Cross-Sectional Studies

Although active women in this age group also have a higher BMD than do sedentary women, other factors can affect that relationship. Brewer, Meyer, Keele, Upton, and Hagan (6) found that runners had higher values for the midshaft of the radius (+4.7%) and the middle phalanx of the fifth finger (+12.3%) compared to sedentary women, but the runners had a lower os calcis density (–6.8%) than did inactive women who weighed 7.5 kg more. The significance of these observations is a bit uncertain because the sites where BMD was higher in runners do not receive the benefit of mechanical loading during running, whereas the site where runners' BMD was lower would be the area expected to benefit from the impact as the foot strikes the ground. Apparently, weight was more effective than running in determining the BMD of this weight-bearing bone.

Aloia, Vaswani, Yeh, and Cohn (2) correlated total body calcium (TBCa) and vertebral density with activity measured by a motion sensor in a small group of women (n = 24). Although they reported a significant relationship between TBCa (r = .51) and lumbar BMD (r = .41) with estimates of physical activity, the correlations accounted for only 16% to 25% of the variablity in BMD among the women. The mean activity level of these women (28.2 counts/h) was low, which may explain the relatively low association with bone density.

Longitudinal Studies

The only study (43) to examine the skeletal response of premenopausal women in this age group to a structured training program reported that there was a decrease in lumbar (–4.0%) and femoral neck (–1.0%) BMD following 9 months of weight training, even as strength increased by 57%. Notelovitz, Martin, Tesar, McKenzie, and Fields (34) also used women in this age group for a weight-training study, but their subjects were surgically menopausal women with or without hormone replacement therapy and therefore more comparable to postmenopausal women.

The similarity of the results of Rockwell et al. (43) to those of Gleeson, Protas, LeBlanc, Schneider, and Evans (19) for younger women raises questions about the role of weight training in increasing bone mass. In cross-sectional studies, both male and female weight lifters have significantly greater BMD than do other athletes or sedentary control subjects (14,20). It may be that a longer training period is required to effect change or that one must reach a point where the training intensity is higher in order to achieve bone hypertrophy. Because both the Rockwell et al. and the Gleeson et al. studies (19,43) enrolled naive subjects, one might assume that the initial weights or resistance was relatively low. It is also possible that the positive effects of weight training are first apparent at sites other than the spine and femoral neck, the humerus or radius perhaps.

When one considers the importance of preserving bone mass during these premenopausal adult years, it is surprising that there is only one prospective study examining the effectiveness of physical activity in maintaining BMD. Nevertheless, until definitive results are available from well-designed prospective studies that clearly define the role of exercise in maintaining or increasing bone mass in the mature adult female, all women should be encouraged to incorporate some form of moderate activity into their lives. Any increase in physical activity may have a positive effect on bone mass for those women who have been sedentary.

Physical Activity and Bone Mass in the Postmenopausal Woman

It is tempting to prescribe exercise to postmenopausal women as a means of preventing osteoporosis on the basis of the many studies that have shown that active older women have better bones and that sedentary women can increase bone density by becoming more active. However, it is important to differentiate between women who are most at risk for osteoporotic fractures and those who enter menopause with a vertebral and proximal femur BMD in the low-risk area. There are two questions to be answered: (a) How effective is physical activity in increasing bone mass? and (b) How effective must it be to protect women from an osteoporotic fracture? The answer to the first question depends on whether the data comes from a cross-sectional or longitudinal study and on the type of activity (Figures 49.1 and 49.2). The answer to the second question depends upon the BMD a woman has when she enters menopause *and* whether she has elected hormone replacement therapy (HRT). Women who are 2 standard deviations (SD) below the mean of the young adult female are entering an at-risk area. They are twice as likely to have a fracture as women only 1 SD below the mean for young women. The risk doubles for each SD below the mean, and each SD represents about a 10% change in BMD. Therefore, the woman 2 SD below the young adult mean, who has a fourfold increase in risk, must increase her BMD 20% to get above the at-risk area. The results from the longitudinal training studies of postmenopausal women who are not on HRT suggest that this amount of improvement will be difficult to attain (Figure 49.1).

At present there is no evidence that exercise can offset the detrimental effect that the decrease in endogenous estrogen production has on bone mass. On the contrary, studies of Masters athletes and the experience of the young amenorrheic athlete indicate that prolonged, intensive training programs do not protect the skeleton from the effect of decreased levels of endogenous estrogen.

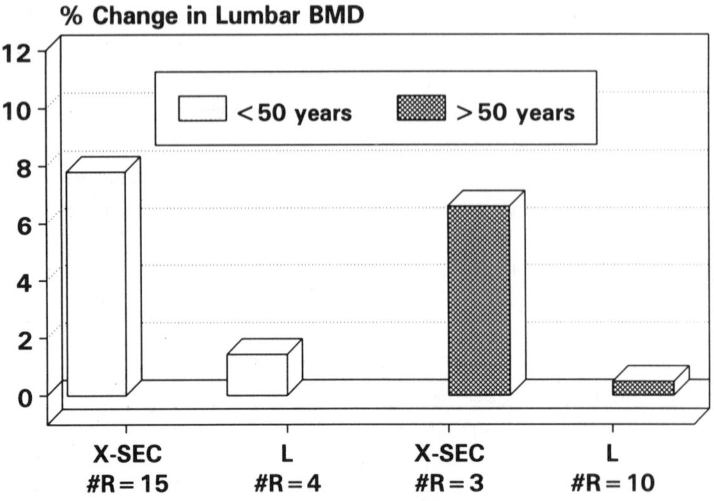

Figure 49.1 The effect of physical activity on lumbar BMD of women by age and design of study. X-Sec = cross-sectional; L = longitudinal; #R = reference cited.

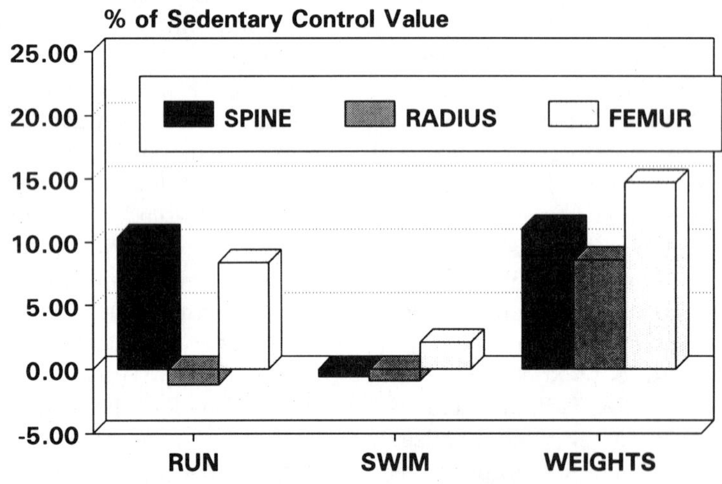

Figure 49.2 BMD as a percentage of sedentary control values at three skeletal sites for runners, swimmers, and weight-lifters.

Cross-Sectional Studies

The emergence of the Masters Sports Program in recent years has made it possible to identify serious athletes in the postmenopausal age group. The results from studies of Masters runners are mixed. Using computed tomography (CT), Lane et al. (26) reported a lumbar vertebral density of 139 mg/cm^3 for 6 runners and 103.2 mg/cm^3 for matched control subjects, a 35% advantage for the active women. However, Michel, Bloch, and Fries (32) found an average lumbar density of 112.5 mg/cm^3 for 28 female runners from the same association, which represented only a 9.2% difference between runners and control subjects. In each study the vertebral BMD values are well below those of young women measured by the same CT technique (165.8 mg/cm^3) (7), suggesting that running had not completely prevented bone loss even though both studies included some women who were using HRT. Five of the women in the Michel et al. (32) study who exercised at least 5 hr per week had very low vertebral BMD (94 mg/cm^3). This finding led the authors to suggest that "extremely vigorous exercise . . . may be detrimental to bone density in individuals after age 50." Actually there was no measure of intensity; the term *vigorous* referred to hours per week spent in weight-bearing exercise.

A comparison of postmenopausal runners with young runners and a sedentary age-matched group provided further evidence that running does not protect women from either vertebral or radial bone loss following menopause (24). There was no difference in BMD at either site between the older runners and control subjects. There were, however, large differences between the older and younger runners, 39% and 16% lower BMD at the spinal and radial sites respectively for the Masters runners (Figure 49.3).

The vertebral bones of female Masters swimmers did not appear to benefit from activity unless the swimmers were on HRT (35). Non-HRT swimmers had a 0.9% greater BMD than nonexercisers, whereas swimmers on HRT had a 4% advantage over nonswimmers using HRT. The spinal BMD of the estrogen-replete swimmers was 11% higher than the estrogen-deficient swimmers. Vertebral BMD dropped from 155 mg/cm^3 for premenopausal swimmers (age = 46) to 121 mg/cm^3 for postmenopausal swimmers on HRT to 109 mg/cm^3 for postmenopausal swimmers not using HRT.

Chow, Harrison, Brown, and Hajek (10) recruited women ages 50 to 59 years from the general population and divided them into an average fitness group and an above-average fitness group on the basis of estimated aerobic power ($\dot{V}O_2max$). The more fit women had an 18% higher calcium bone index (CaBI) measured at the trunk and proximal femur by neutron activation. In a similar study, Oyster, Morton, and Linnell (36) divided women ages 60 to 69 years into two groups based on a physical activity profile. The cortical width of the second metacarpal was 18% greater in the more active group. The differences between groups in these two studies are much larger than those reported between Masters athletes and their sedentary control subjects. This may be due to differences in the skeletal site measured, the measurement techniques, selection bias, type of activity, or some other as yet unidentified factor.

Strength training satisfies many of the training principles discussed earlier. Mechanical loading can be directed to specific skeletal sites, and the work load (intensity) can be slowly but consistently increased. Training can be individualized so that each woman can progress at her own pace. Theoretically, this type of activity has the potential to have a positive effect on bone mass. As noted in earlier sections, changes in BMD with weight training in younger women have been disappointing. When the strength of various muscle groups are correlated with BMD in the postmenopausal age group, the results are mixed. Some studies report a significant association (39,46), others (8) have failed to find that weight training increases BMD, and still others (5) have reported mixed results. In one study, an association that was significant for premenopausal women was not significant for postmenopausal women (39). A fact often overlooked in evaluating the interaction of strength

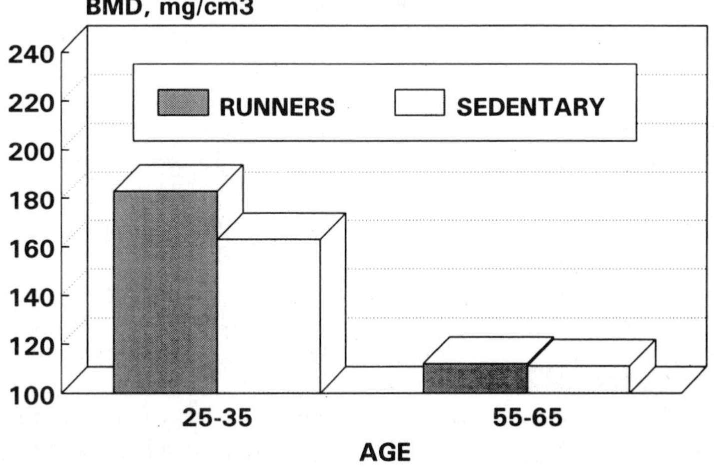

Figure 49.3 The lumbar BMD of young (ages 25 to 35) and Masters (ages 55 to 65) runners compared to sedentary control subjects of the same age. Adapted from Kirk et al. (24).

with bone mass is that strength is directly related to muscle mass, which in turn is related positively to two other factors that are significantly associated with BMD, body weight and age. Caution is warranted in considering the results of any study that does not take these factors into consideration in the experimental design or statistical analysis.

Longitudinal Studies

The results of prospective studies in this age group clearly illustrate the need for an effective exercise prescription for enhancing bone health of postmenopausal women (Figure 49.1). The changes in vertebral BMD across time range from −12% to +8%, vary from one activity to another, and usually apply only to women not on HRT. The results from four studies (8,33,44,50) suggest that walking, the most commonly prescribed activity for older women, does not prevent bone loss in women with an average age in the mid to late 50s. In two studies (44,50) that measured changes in BMD at the radius, the negative result may represent an application of the specificity principle. One would expect walking to be more effective in increasing BMD in the spine and legs. However, Cavanaugh and Cann (8) reported a loss of even greater magnitude (−5.6%) in the trabecular area of the lumbar vertebrae. Changes at the proximal femur were no more encouraging (33). Only when Nelson, Fisher, Dilmanian, Dallal, and Evans (33) combined walking with a daily calcium intake of 1,462 mg/day was there an increase in both vertebral and femoral BMD. Prince et al. (41) also examined the interaction of exercise and calcium supplementation and reported a slower rate of radial bone loss in the group receiving a 1,000 mg/day calcium supplement than in the exercise-only group. It should be noted, however, that the exercise consisted of one supervised session of low-impact aerobics per week plus two 30-min walks and that compliance was very poor.

Walking is a popular choice of exercise for many older women and a relatively safe exercise prescription because the risk for musculoskeletal injuries is low. The value of this weight-bearing activity for preserving bone mass needs to be investigated in more detail. Would walking hills be more effective in protecting hip BMD? What might be the effect on vertebral BMD of wearing a weighted backpack during the walk?

Other studies have used a more varied exercise program that included aerobics (9), calisthenics (1,25), stair climbing (13), weight lifting (4,9,34), or dancing (38). The results of these studies are more positive. The mean increase in lumbar BMD from all studies has been 5.8%. The largest increase (+8.4%) was reported by Notelevitz et al. (34), who were the only group to look at the additive effect of exercise plus estrogen and the effect of a resistance circuit weight-training program. Both of these variables—the effect of estrogen plus exercise and the value of resistance training—need to be examined further.

Fracture Incidence, Bone Mass, and Physical Activity

An osteoporotic fracture is an extremely serious event in a woman's life. Vertebral fractures can result in disability, pain, deformity, and a marked decrease in the quality of life. Among women who have a hip fracture, about 15% to 20% may die as a result of complications within 6 months, and about 50% of those surviving cannot return to independent living. The disease is a serious public health problem as well as a personal tragedy for the woman and her family. Current estimates place the cost at close to $10 billion per year in the United States. As our populations age, this problem can only worsen, unless a way can be found to prevent this disease.

Physical activity is an attractive candidate as a prophylaxis. It is inexpensive and available to all, and the side effects of a well-planned exercise program can be improved cardiovascular health; improved flexibility, coordination, and balance; and increased muscular strength and endurance. The question is, Is exercise effective in preventing fractures?

Several epidemiological studies (3,11,37,51) are unanimous in reporting that the physical activity levels of women with fractures are lower than those of women without fractures. Astrom, Ahnqvist, Beertema, and Jonsson (3) examined the level of physical activity in groups of older women with and without a femoral neck fracture and found that nonfracture women had been significantly more active between ages 15 and 45 than had the fracture group. A similar result was reported by Wickham et al. (51), who found that women who scored highest on an index of outdoor activity had the lowest odds ratio (1.0) for a hip fracture whereas those who scored lowest had the highest risk (3.9). Another study from the same group (11) reported that the risk of a hip fracture was greatest in women who reported less frequent muscle loading, less productive activity, slower walking speeds, and shorter periods on their feet. Outdoor activity was also a significant discriminator in a study of a retirement community in southern California (37). Women who spent more than 1 hr per day in active outdoor activities had a relative risk of 0.68 for hip fracture compared to those who spent less than 30 min in outdoor exercise.

A negative finding from a study of former college athletes (53) found no difference in fracture rate between the athletes (29%) and nonathletes (32%) in the postmenopausal age groups. This held true even when other risk factors were accounted for and in spite of the fact that 73.5% of the former athletes were currently exercising regularly compared to 57% of the nonathletes. One might question the definition of *athlete* in this study, but there is no doubt that these former athletes were more active than the comparison group.

Physical Activity and Bone Mass Across Age Categories

A number of investigators have examined the relationship between BMD and physical activity across a wide age range. Some have used an activity profile questionnaire to divide subjects into active and sedentary groups; others have related BMD to some measure of physical fitness such as aerobic power ($\dot{V}O_2$max), activity profiles, or activity monitors. There are problems with all these techniques. $\dot{V}O_2$max, a measure of cardiorespiratory fitness, may not represent participation in activities that load the skeleton. When expressed as liters per minute, its relationship to bone mass is confounded by its association with body size, which is also related to bone mass. The problem is exacerbated when submaximal tests are used to predict $\dot{V}O_2$max; prediction error can be unacceptably high.

Activity habits, determined by questionnaire or motion sensors, are generally used to categorize women into high- and low-activity groups but are seldom validated. Activity has been quantified as hours per day or energy expenditure per hour with no attempt to discriminate between activities that do or do not place mechanical stress on the specific skeletal sites being measured.

The results of studies in this category are inconclusive. Pocock, Eisman, Yeates, Sambrook, and Eberl (40) found a significant association between predicted $\dot{V}O_2$max in liters per minute and both femoral neck (r = .60) and lumbar spine (r = .54) BMD in women ages 20 to 75 years. A later report from this group (39) did not find an association between $\dot{V}O_2$max and lumbar BMD when aerobic power was expressed relative to body weight. They did, however, find a significant association between $\dot{V}O_2$max and BMD at the femoral neck (r = .49), trochanter (r = .40), and Ward's triangle (r = .56). One other study (5) also failed to find a significant association between spinal density and $\dot{V}O_2$max—measured directly and expressed relative to body weight (ml · kg^{-1} · min^{-1})—in postmenopausal women.

Two other studies (47,48) also suggest that the beneficial effect of exercise on bone may be somewhat attenuated in older women. Stillman, Lohman, Slaughter, and Massey (48) reported that the BMD of the radius and ulna, adjusted for age and menstrual status, were higher for premenopausal women in the high-activity group (0.68) than in the low- (0.62) or moderate- (0.65) activity groups. When the women, ages 30 to 85, were divided into pre- and postmenopausal groups, the association of BMD to activity habits was not significant in the postmenopausal group. In the only longitudinal study involving a wide range of ages (35 to 65 years) (47), women who exercised 45 min, 3 days a week, for 4 years continued to lose bone at the radius, ulna, and humerus, although the rate of loss was significantly less than in the sedentary group. The rate of loss per year was less for premenopausal women (–0.32%) than for postmenopausal women not on hormone replacement therapy (–1.24%); this suggests that the exercise routines were unable to prevent an increased rate of bone loss following menopause.

Even when the association between BMD and fitness or activity profiles is significant, the results may be physiologically meaningless. For example, a correlation of .23 between lumbar BMD and hours spent walking each day was significant in a large group of women 24 to 79 years of age (54). However, r^2, the amount of variation in BMD that could be predicted from walk time, was only 5%. In other words, 95% of the variability in lumbar density in this group of 123 women could not be explained by the number of hours they spent walking. As noted earlier, other investigators (8,33, 44,50) have been unable to document a positive effect on bone from walking programs in early postmenopausal women.

Related Benefits of Physical Activity

Whereas a sedentary lifestyle is considered one of the risk factors for osteoporosis, it also results in a downward spiral in other physiologic functions. The loss of strength and aerobic capacity in many older adults leads to a further decrease in activity and an inability to continue the types of activities that provide an adequate load-bearing stimulus to maintain bone mass. Studies indicate, for example, that 40% of women in the United States between the ages of 55 and 64 cannot lift 4.5 kg. As strength continues to decline, this number increases to 65% by age 75 (23). Many of these same women cannot sustain even light aerobic activities for more than a few minutes at a time.

It has been estimated that the minimum fitness level required for an older individual to live independently is a $\dot{V}O_2max$ of 1 L/min, a figure equal to an energy expenditure of 5 kcal/min (45). Simply walking at a normal pace on a hard surface would require a maximal effort for a 62-kg woman at this minimal level of fitness. Unfortunately, the average fitness level of women in their early 70s (a $\dot{V}O_2max$ of 1.3 L/min) is already close to this threshold, and it is probable that many women over the age of 75 could not even follow the usual prescription for bone health—brisk walking (16). Fortunately, much of this loss in strength and overall fitness can be reversed through a carefully planned and progessive exercise program. Until the ability of the underlying physiologic systems essential for load-bearing activity are restored, it will be impossible for many older individuals to maintain a level of activity essential for protecting the skeleton from further bone loss.

Summary

Physical activity is essential for the maintenance of bone health. However, further research is necessary to understand the role exercise can play in preventing osteoporosis. There is no evidence at present that exercise is an alternative to hormone replacement therapy for the postmenopausal woman. However, any increase in bone mass during the postmenopausal years has to be considered a benefit. Even though the relative increase is modest, the gain must be weighed against the continued loss of bone mass in the respective control groups. The effect of this attenuation in bone loss on the probability of an osteoporotic fracture in this age group is not known. However, if an osteoporotic fracture can be delayed by even a few years, the result may be fewer years of dependency. Perhaps the most important contribution of an active lifestyle in preventing osteoporotic fractures will be to enable women to remain active as they age and to decrease the incidence of falls by increasing muscular strength and improving balance and coordination.

References

1. Aloia, J.F.; Cohn, S.H.; Ostuni, J.A.; Cane, R.; Ellis, K. Prevention of involutional bone loss by exercise. Ann. Intern. Med. 89:356-358; 1978.
2. Aloia, J.F.; Vaswani, A.N.; Yeh, J.; Cohn, S.H. Premenopausal bone mass is related to physical activity. Arch. Intern. Med. 148:121-123; 1988.
3. Astrom, J.; Ahnqvist, S.; Beertema, J.; Jonsson, B. Physical activity in women sustaining fracture of the neck of the femur. J. Bone Joint Surg. 69-B:381-383; 1987.
4. Ayalon, J.; Simkin, A.; Leichter, I.; Raifmann, S. Dynamic bone loading exercises for postmenopausal women: Effect on the density of the distal radius. Arch. Phys. Med. Rehabil. 68:280-283; 1987.
5. Bevier, W.C.; Wiswell, R.A.; Pyka, G.; Kozak, K. C.; Newhall, K.M.; Marcus, R. Relationship of body composition, muscle strength, and aerobic capacity to bone mineral density in older men and women. J. Bone Miner. Res. 4:421-432; 1989.
6. Brewer, V.; Meyer, B.M.; Keele, M.S.; Upton, S.J.; Hagan, R.D. Role of exercise in prevention of involutional bone loss. Med. Sci. Sports Exerc. 15:445-449; 1983.
7. Cann, C.E.; Martin, M.C.; Genant, H.K.; Jaffe, R.B. Decreased spinal mineral content in amenorrheic women. JAMA. 251:626-629; 1984.
8. Cavanaugh, D.J.; Cann, C.E. Brisk walking does not stop bone loss in postmenopausal women. Bone. 9:201-204; 1988.
9. Chow, R.; Harrison, J.E.; Notarius, C. Effect of two randomised exercise programmes on bone mass of healthy postmenopausal women. Br. Med. J. 295:1441-1444; 1987.
10. Chow, R.K.; Harrison, J.E.; Brown, C.F.; Hajek, V. Physical fitness effect on bone mass in postmenopausal women. Arch. Phys. Med. Rehabil. 67:231-234; 1986.
11. Cooper, C.; Barker, D.J.P.; Wickham, C. Physical activity muscle strength, and calcium intake in fracture of the proximal femur in Britain. Br. Med. J. 297:1443-1446; 1988.
12. Cummings, S.R.; Black, D.; Arnaud, C.; Browner, W.S.; Cauley, J.A.; Genant, H.K.; Mascioli, S.; Nevitt, M.C.; Scott, J.; Seeley, D.; Sherwin, P.; Steiger, P.; Vogt, T. Appendicular densiometry predicts hip fractures. J. Bone Miner. Res. [Suppl 1]. 4:S327; 1989.
13. Dalsky, G.; Stocke, K.S.; Eshani, A.A.; Slatopolsky, E.; Lee, W.C.; Birge, S.J. Weight-bearing exercise training and lumbar bone mineral content in postmenopausal women. Ann. Intern. Med. 108:824-828; 1988.
14. Davee, A.M.; Rosen, C.J.; Adler, R.A. Exercise patterns and trabecular bone density in college women. J. Bone Miner. Res. 5:245-250; 1990.
15. Drinkwater, B.L. Assessing fitness and activity patterns of women in general population studies. In: Drury, T., ed. Assessing physical fitness

and physical activity in population-based surveys. DHHS pub. no. (PHS) 89-1253. Washington, DC: U.S. Government Printing Office; 1989:261-271.

16. Drinkwater, B.L.; Bruemmer, B.; Chesnut, C.H., III. Menstrual history as a determinant of current bone density in young athletes. JAMA. 263:545-548; 1990.
17. Drinkwater, B.L.; Nilson, K.; Chesnut, C.H., III; Bremner, J.; Shainholtz, S.; Southworth, M.B. Bone mineral content of amenorrheic and eumenorrheic athletes. N. Engl. J. Med. 311:277-281, 1984.
18. Drinkwater, B.L.; Nilson, K.; Ott, S.; Chesnut, C.H., III. Bone mineral density after resumption of menses in amenorrheic women. JAMA. 256:380-382; 1986.
19. Gleeson, P.B.; Protas, E.J.; LeBlanc, A.; Schneider, V.S.; Evans, H.J. Effects of weight lifting on bone mineral density in premenopausal women. J. Bone Miner. Res. 5:153-158; 1990.
20. Heinrich, C.H.; Going, S.B.; Parmenter, R.W.; Perry, C.D.; Boyden, T.W.; Lohman, T.G. Bone mineral content of cyclically menstruating female resistant and endurance trained athletes. Med. Sci. Sports Exerc. 22:558-563; 1990.
21. Hui, S.L.; Slemenda, C.W.; Johnston, C.C. Baseline measurement of bone mass predicts fracture in white women. Ann. Intern. Med. 111:355-361; 1989.
22. Jacobsen, P.C.; Beaver, W.; Grubb, S.A.; Taft, T.N.; Talmage, R.V. Bone density in women: College athletes and older athletic women. J. Orthop. Res. 2:328-332; 1984.
23. Jette, A.M.; Branch, L.G. The Framingham disability study: II. Physical disability among the aging. Am. J. Public Health. 71:1211-1216; 1981.
24. Kirk, S.; Sharp, C.F.; Elbaum, N.; Endres, D.B.; Simons, S.M.; Mohler, J.G.; Rude, R.K. Effect of long-distance running on bone mass in women. J. Bone Miner. Res. 4:515-522; 1989.
25. Krolner, B.; Toft, B.; Nielsen, S.P.; Tondevold, E. Physical exercise as prophylaxis against involutional vertebral bone loss: A controlled trial. Clin. Sci. 64:541-546; 1983.
26. Lane, N.E.; Bloch, D.A.; Jones, H.H.; Marshall, W.H.; Wood, P.D.; Fries, J.F. Long-distance running, bone density, and osteoarthritis. JAMA. 255:1147-1151; 1986.
27. Lindberg, J.S.; Fears, W.B.; Hunt, M.M.; Powell, M.R.; Boll, D.; Wade, C. Exercise-induced amenorrhea and bone density. Ann. Intern. Med. 101:647-648; 1984.
28. Lindberg, J.S.; Powell, M.R.; Hunt, M.M.; Ducey, D.E.; Wade, C.E. Increased vertebral bone mineral in response to reduced exercise in amenorrheic runners. West. J. Med. 146:39-42; 1986.
29. Loucks, A.B. Does exercise training affect reproductive hormones in women? Clin. Sports Med. 5:535-557; 1986.
30. Marcus, R.; Cann, C.; Madvig, P.; Minkoff, J.; Goddard, M.; Bayer, M.; Martin, M.; Gaudiani, L.; Haskell, W.; Genant, H. Menstrual function and bone mass in elite women distance runners. Ann. Intern. Med. 102:158-163; 1985.
31. Mazess, R.B.; Barden, H.S. Bone density in premenopausal women: Effect of age, dietary intake, physical activity, smoking, and birth-control pills. Am. J. Clin. Nutr. 53:132-142; 1991.
32. Michel, B.A.; Bloch, D.A.; Fries, J.F. Weight-bearing exercise, overexercise, and lumbar bone density over age 50 years. Arch. Intern. Med. 149:2325-2329; 1989.
33. Nelson, M.E.; Fisher, E.C.; Dilmanian, F.A.; Dallal, G.E.; Evans, W.J. A 1-y walking program and increased calcium in postmenopausal women: Effects on bone. Am. J. Clin. Nutr. 53:1304-1311; 1991.
34. Notelovitz, M.; Martin, D.; Tesar, R.; McKenzie, L.; Fields, C. Estrogen therapy and variable resistance weight training increases bone mineral in surgically menopausal women. J. Bone Miner. Res. 6:583-590; 1991.
35. Orwell, E.S.; Ferar, J.; Oviatt, S.K.; McClung, M.R.; Huntington, K. The relationship of swimming exercise to bone mass in men and women. Arch. Intern. Med. 149:2197-2200; 1989.
36. Oyster, N.; Morton, M.; Linnell, S. Physical activity and osteoporosis in post-menopausal women. Med. Sci. Sports Exerc. 16:44-50; 1984.
37. Paganini-Hill, A.; Chao, A.; Ross, R.K.; Henderson, B. Exercise and other factors in the prevention of hip fracture: The leisure world study. Epidemiology. 2:16-25; 1991.
38. Peterson, S.E.; Peterson, M.D.; Raymond, G.; Gilligan, C.; Checovich, M.M.; Smith, E.L. Muscular strength and bone density with weight training in middle-aged women. Med. Sci. Sports Exerc. 23:499-504; 1991.
39. Pocock, N.; Eisman, J.; Gwinn, T.; Sambrook, P.; Kelly, P.; Freund, J.; Yeates, M. Muscle strength, physical fitness, and weight but not age predict femoral neck bone mass. J. Bone Miner. Res. 4:441-448; 1989.
40. Pocock, N.A.; Eisman, J.A.; Yeates, M.G.; Sambrook, P.N.; Eberl, S. Physical fitness is a major determinant of femoral neck and lumbar spine bone mineral density. J. Clin. Invest. 78:618-621; 1986.
41. Prince, R.; Smith, M.; Dick, I.M.; Price, R.I.; Webb, P.G.; Henderson, K.; Harris, M. Prevention of osteoporosis: A comparative study of exercise, calcium supplementation, and hormone-replacement therapy. N. Engl. J. Med. 325:1189-1195; 1991.

42. Risser, W.L.; Lee, E.J.; LeBlanc, A.; Poindexter, H.B.; Risser, J.M.H.; Schneider, V. Bone density in eumenorrheic female college athletes. Med. Sci. Sports Exerc. 22:570-574; 1990.
43. Rockwell, J.C.; Sorensen, A.M.; Baker, S.; Leahey, D.; Stock, J.L.; Michaels, J.; Baran, D.T. Weight training decreases vertebral bone density in premenopausal women: A prospective study. J. Clin. Endocrinol. Metab. 71:988-993; 1990.
44. Sandler, R.B.; Cauley, J.A.; Hom, D.L.; Sashin, D.; Kriska, A.M. The effects of walking on the cross-sectional dimensions of the radius in postmenopausal women. Calcif. Tissue Int. 41:65-69; 1987.
45. Shephard, R.J. Physical activity and aging. London: Croom Helm Ltd.; 1978.
46. Sinaki, M.; Offord, K.P. Physical activity in postmenopausal women: Effect on back muscle strength and bone mineral density of the spine. Arch. Phys. Med. Rehabil. 69:277-280; 1988.
47. Smith, E.L.; Gilligan, C.; McAdam, M.; Ensign, C.P.; Smith, P.E. Deterring bone loss by exercise intervention in premenopausal and postmenopausal women. Calcif. Tissue Int. 44:312-321; 1989.
48. Stillman, R.J.; Lohman, T.G.; Slaughter, M.H.; Massey, B.H. Physical activity and bone mineral content in women aged 30 to 85 years. Med. Sci. Sports Exerc. 18:576-580; 1986.
49. Wasnich, R.D.; Ross, P.D.; Heilbrun, L.K.; Vogel, J.M. Prediction of postmenopausal fracture risk with use of bone mineral measurements. Am. J. Obstet. Gynecol. 153:645-751; 1985.
50. White, M.K.; Martin, R.B.; Yeater, R.A.; Butcher, R.L.; Radin, E.L. The effects of exercise on the bones of postmenopausal women. Int. Orthop. 7:209-214; 1984.
51. Wickham, C.A.C.; Walsh, K.; Cooper, C.; Parker, D.J.P.; Margetts, B.M.; Morris, J.; Bruce, S.A. Dietary calcium, physical activity, and risk of hip fracture: A prospective study. Br. Med. J. 299:889-892; 1989.
52. Wolman, R.L.; Faulmann, L.; Clark, P.; Hesp, R.; Harries, M.G. Different training patterns and bone mineral density of the femoral shaft in elite, female athletes. Ann. Rheum. Dis. 50:487-489; 1991.
53. Wyshak, G.; Frisch, R.E.; Albright, T.E.; Albright, N.L.; Schiff, I. Bone fractures among former college athletes compared with nonathletes in the menopausal and postmenopausal years. Obstet. Gynecol. 69:121-126; 1987.
54. Zylstra, S.; Hopkins, A.; Erk, M.; Hreshchyshyn, M.M.; Anbar, M. Effect of physical activity on lumbar spine and femoral neck densities. Int. J. Sports Med. 10:181-186; 1989.

Chapter 50

Physical Activity, Fitness, and Back Pain

Fin Biering-Sørensen
Tom Bendix
Kurt Jørgensen
Claus Manniche
Henrik Nielsen

The relationship between physical activity and back pain (BP) should be considered in a wide perspective, but in this chapter the focus is on pathophysiological factors because the major impact of literature is related to this field.

In our delimitation of BP we exclude neck pain and primarily consider low-back trouble or pain (LBP) including radiating pain.

This presentation concentrates on studies published since the last consensus symposium was held in 1988, where Nachemson (103) and Mayer (92) reviewed the field of BP (although for obvious reasons in various contexts it will be necessary to use older publications as references as well).

Pathoanatomical Considerations

Physical activity strengthens the vertebrae and the disks, as has been shown in cadaveric studies (117). The increase in the motion segment's compressive strength with physical activity is in agreement with the observed increase of bone mineral content in vertebral bodies of Swedish power lifters (47).

In a study of 86 male cadavers, Videman, Nurminen, and Troup (140) found that symmetrical disk degeneration was associated with sedentary work, whereas vertebral osteophytosis was related to heavy work. The onset of degeneration in a sedentary lifestyle can be seen in the light that disk nutrition depends on movement (58,139). However, other factors like smoking also influence disk degeneration, as was demonstrated in an MRI study with identical twins (8).

Kalimo, Rantanen, Viljanen, and Einola (67) reviewed studies on lumbar muscles and found that selective atrophy of the fast-twitch fibers seems to ensue from inactivity, not only in patients with BP but also in sedentary control subjects. Both the fiber-type composition and degree of atrophy may well influence a person's susceptibility to LBP.

Gordon (46) hypothesized that for LBP the sedentary lifestyles of modern industrialized countries "create disuse changes beginning with muscle, which ultimately causes interference with the adaptive and structural dynamics of specialized connective tissue," i.e. bone, cartilage, ligaments, and tendons.

Occupational Exposure

In recent years, several reports have reviewed the available literature regarding the relationship between work load and LBP (2,21,24,25,56,85,104, 116,118,136,148). The risk factors for LBP that are especially emphasized are hard physical work and heavy lifting, forward-bent working positions and other static work, torsions or other awkward movements, and whole-body vibrations.

The more frequently heavy lifts are performed, the more often problems will arise in the musculoskeletal system (104). This corresponds with the findings of Kelsey, Githens, and White (70), who demonstrated that there is an increased risk of acute lumbar slipped disk with lifts performed at increased frequencies during a working day. Kumar (77) demonstrated that cumulative compression and shear were significantly associated with pain. In a study on nearly 13,000 twin pairs (10), the occurrence of BP was strongly associated with workload, especially among male twins. Twin concordance regarding BP was considerably higher in monozygotic (MZ) than in dizygotic (DZ) twins, supporting the possibility that a relationship exists between genetic factors and the occurrence of BP.

Thus heavy physical load clearly appears to be correlated to LBP. The role of sedentary occupations, however, is more unclear and often not properly analyzed in epidemiological studies.

In the classical study of Magora (84), a U-shape was observed approximately as illustrated in Figure 50.1a. However, the left rise associated with a sedentary lifestyle was not observed by either Riihimäki, Sakari, Videman, and Hänninen (119) or Svensson, Vedin, Wilhelmsson, and Andersson (130). The reviews discussed earlier could not address the U-shape controversy, because most epidemiological studies categorize people as either *hard* or *light* physical workers (Figure 50.1b), or they use linear regression (Figure 50.1c); in either case a possible U-shape response may be overlooked.

A slight U-shape would be expected from a healthy-worker effect: Those having LBP early in life may tend to choose sedentary occupations.

Leisure-Time and Sports Activities

The relationship between exercise and health has been of growing interest. Strong data link high-level physical activity to decreased risk of cardiovascular disease, normalization of blood pressure, body weight reduction, improvement of mood, and so forth. In part because of these findings, running and other fitness activities in general have become important. There is a lack of epidemiological data regarding the correlation of physical activity to BP. Gyntelberg (51) observed a moderate difference in favor of those practicing sport; Mälkiä (85) also observed a small inverse correlation. The possibility of selection bias has to be considered; among 1,715 schoolchildren the prevalence of BP was significantly higher in the group participating in competition sports than in those doing less intense physical activities (4). Likewise, other studies have primarily concentrated on the negative effect of sports activities on the back.

In a review over a 10-year period of 4,790 college athletes, the back injury rate was 7% (68), with significant highest rates in football players and gymnasts. Eighty percent of the back injuries occurred during practice, 6% during competition, and 14% during preseason conditioning. The nature of the injury was acute in 59%, overuse in 12%, and an aggravation of a preexisting condition in 29%. Among 739 apparently healthy and physically fit orienteers (average age, 32.7 years) the lifetime prevalence for LBP was 47.1% and for thoracic back problems, 14.6% (82). The lifetime prevalence of LBP was 59% among retired wrestlers, compared to 23% among retired heavy-weight lifters and 31% in a slightly younger, control group (48).

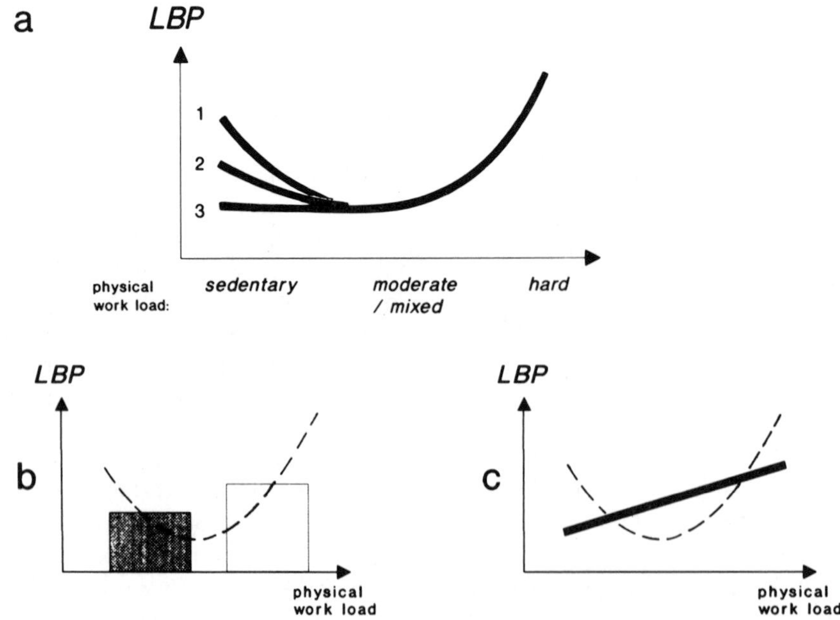

Figure 50.1 a. The relation between physically hard work and LBP (low back pain) seems evident, whereas the significance of sedentary occupations is unclear. In part a, '1' reflects the observation of Magora (84) from a population of 3,316, '2' that of Videman et al. (140) (n = 88), and '3' those of Svensson et al. (130) (n = 940), and Riihimäki et al. (119) (n = 1,911). Parts b and c show two ways of possibly overlooking a U-shape—if present (dotted line).

In triathletes the most frequently injured area of the body was the back; 72% of the athletes reported either LBP or sciatica during the previous year of training (112). LBP is also frequent among rowers (13) and has been reported to affect as many as 82.2% of them (60). In a prospective study of 82 high-performance, young fast bowlers in cricket, 11% sustained a stress fracture to one or more vertebrae, and 27% sustained a soft-tissue injury to the back during the season (38). Professional golfers over a 1-year period had an incidence of back injury of 34% (20). Correspondingly, 82% of professional tennis players have missed tournaments because of BP (23); 43 of 143 players reported chronic LBP (52). Other sports of risk are reviewed by Watkins and Dillin (146). Unfortunately, these studies are primarily anecdotal and lack proper control groups.

According to Stanish (128), ideopathic scoliosis, particularly involving the thoracolumbar region, increases the risk for LBP in athletes.

Spondylolysis, present in about 3% to 5% of the Caucasian population, is normally asymptomatic, but it can become painful during athletic activities, particularly in hyperextension but also in forced flexion or rotation (61,65,95). Spondylolysis may lead to instability of the lumbar segment that may be exacerbated by sporting activities (128). Female gymnasts appear to be at specific risk. After X-ray analysis of the lumbar spine of 100 females, aged 6 to 24 years, Jackson, Wiltse, and Cirincione (65) reported a fourfold higher risk among gymnasts. All of these stress-related defects were found in the lower lumbar region. Similar defects have been reported in football players (95), butterfly swimmers (101), divers, wrestlers, and weight lifters (120).

Intervertebral disks as well as bony structures may be vulnerable to the excessive range of motion associated with certain sports activities. In a study by Tertti et al. (132) of 35 competitive young gymnasts (mean age, 12), 11 had suffered from episodes of LBP during exercise, and 8 were found to have evidence of back trauma. Three of the 35 gymnasts had MRI evidence of degenerated disks, and in all 3 it was associated with Scheuermann's manifestation or spondylolysis. The authors concluded that the intervertebral disk itself seems to adapt to physical stress, but the presence of osseous abnormalities needs attention, because it may lead to disk degeneration later on. Pure mechanical derangement of a lumbar disk seems to be an unusual problem in the skeletally immature athlete (65). Until athletes reach early adulthood, isolated disk herniation does not become a factor of significance (132). Various reports indicate that immature athletes with LBP have structural problems (e.g., spondylolysis) or postural abnormality directly or indirectly related to intervertebral disk dysfunction (76,90,128,131).

Treatment

Physiotherapy, in terms of exercise alone or in combination with other treatment modalities, is probably the most widely prescribed treatment for LBP. During the last few years, information on back exercises has increased as a result of several controlled clinical trials that demonstrated the efficacy.

Indication for Exercises

Acute Back Pain

In simple acute LBP, back exercises have been shown to be an effective treatment (100), whereas bed rest for more than 2 days increased the risk for chronicity (29).

Patients with acute herniated disks may also improve from an exercise program. Follow-up reports seem to indicate that exercises can be as effective as disk surgery (75,121). At least, a physical exercise program performed with a preset number of repetitions and without regard to pain severity succeeded in preventing chronicity and work absenteeism (37,89).

Chronic Back Pain

It has been shown in several randomized studies that chronic LBP can be treated succesfully with back exercises (30,74,87,88). Some patients with chronic LBP have a mixture of symptoms and signs often attributable to psychological and behavioral issues (144). As a consequence, some back centers offer a multidisciplinary treatment including behavioral support, back exercises, general fitness training, and ergonomic education (35,55,83, 93,94,98,111,115,122) to chronic BP patients if BP has hampered working capability. No randomized studies have demonstrated the superiority of the multidisciplinary treatment in comparison with exercise alone. This implies that, unfortunately, we don't know which patients will benefit from which of these treatments.

Design of Exercise Programs

Selection of exercise programs has often been based on tradition (63,64,108,135). Many studies with insignificant results have been published

(36,73,74,91). The review by Koes, Bouter, Beckerman, van der Heijden, and Knipschild (74) indicates the methodological difficulties that clinical studies of back training encounter.

Dose

Manniche, Hesselsøe, Bentzen, Christensen, and Lundberg (87) showed in a randomized study that it seems to be the high-dose exercise programs over longer periods of time that provide positive treatment results in chronic LBP patients.

With exercise twice weekly the program has to be extended for 1 to 3 months before improvement can be expected (86). Many trials with insignificant results (74) have used neither high-dose exercises nor an intervention period of more than a few weeks, thus not providing the opportunity to improve a chronic BP condition (30,88). On the other hand, remarkable improvements were shown using daily high-dose exercise programs in a 3-week period (55,93,122). Data from Hansen, Bendix, and Skov (54) indicate that intensive back exercises seem most effective for those with sedentary job functions.

It has been indicated that use of electromyographic biofeedback during the exercise program improves the training result (3).

Isometric and Dynamic Exercises

It has been recommended for many years to use isometric back exercises and to avoid dynamic forceful exercises (102). However, recently controlled trials showed significant benefit due to dynamic exercises (34,87,88,109), at least for women (54).

Flexion and Extension Exercises

Flexion exercises can be effective in chronic LBP (71,80), but extension exercises have proved effective as well (87,88,109). Elnaggar, Nordin, Sheikhzadeh, Parnianpour, and Kahanovitz (34) demonstrated no difference between a flexion program and an extension program. Donelson, Grant, Kamps, and Medcalf (33) showed that 40% of individuals with nonspecific LBP had a preference for extension and 7% for flexion exercises.

Flexibility Exercises

In chronic LBP patients, hip flexion/extension ranges were found to have an inverse correlation with pain (97), but spinal hypo- as well as hyperflexibility may be risk indicators for LBP (11,17), although this was not observed by Battié, Bigos, Sheehy, and Wortley (5). Several back exercise programs have been shown to improve the flexibility of the spine (34,74,109,129), but this may partly reflect the simultaneous decrease in pain. However, in a randomized trial full-range exercises resulted in better flexibility than exercises not using the full range (86).

Side Effects of Exercise Programs

The potential risk of eliciting spinal bone fractures or aggravating spondylolisthesis (15,61) indicates that patients with radiological findings of spondylolysis or halisteresis should be excluded from intensive training programs. Few patients have claimed aggravation of back or leg pain during clinical trials using intensive exercises (74,88), but many studies don't give information about reasons for dropout (74).

Prevention in Relation to Physical Activity and Fitness

Because of the multifactorial etiology to BP and the poorly understood mechanisms for its occurrence, prevention can be very difficult. Generally, specific prevention is feasible only if the risk factors are known; this is applicable in the present relationship as well. Although prevention of BP directed toward physical activity and fitness will not be sufficient (39), this chapter concentrates on the available information regarding this relationship.

Primary Prevention in Occupational Settings

Lifting

Hard physical work (in particular, heavy lifting) is the single factor that most epidemiological studies have demonstrated to represent a risk factor for BP. Therefore, adaptation of lifting jobs to the person performing the lift seems to be relevant. A major problem in this kind of prevention program is the lack of detailed scientific evidence about which factors in the lifting procedure are the most important in terms of prevention.

The present knowledge of the strains exposing the spinal column during lifting has been used to define limits and guidelines for maximum acceptable weights to be lifted in different circumstances in order to limit job-related LBP (1,26,104). It has been concluded that even under the most optimal conditions, a single bimanual lift of a compact load close to the body and from midthigh to shoulder height should not exceed approximately 50 kg. Snook and Ciriello's (127) tables based on the psychophysical methodology also support that the maximum acceptable weights be of this magnitude. Genaidy, Asfour, Mital, and Waly (42) have developed a model for manual lifting tasks based on a combination of the latest research and additional task parameters. This may be a useful tool for practitioners of safety and health prevention. Our current problem related to the statement regarding maximum acceptable load is that the underlying evidence is indirect in nature, making it very difficult to prove the statement even in prospective studies. This ought to be solved by randomized intervention studies, in which one or more factors are investigated at a time. In addition, Nicholson (105) has pointed out that the different methods for establishing load-handling capabilities do provide several inconsistent results.

Prevention of back injuries may be possible by using the National Institute for Occupational Safety and Health lifting guide (104). This is indicated in the study of Liles and Mahajan (81) utilizing extensive job, injury, and industrial data collected over a period of several years. In addition, an intervention study by Videman et al. (141) demonstrated that specific ergonomic training regarding patient-handling skills in a population of nurses was able to prevent some back injuries.

Muscle Function

Some studies indicate that back and abdominal muscle strength is reduced in persons with LBP (11,78,79). However, this finding may primarily indicate that BP is responsible for reduced muscle strength. Isometric endurance of the back extensors may be reduced in persons with LBP (59,106). Two prospective studies (11,12,138) have shown that reduced isometric and dynamic trunk flexion strength is a possible indicator of recurrent or continous BP. In addition, men with relatively reduced muscle endurance of the back extensors had a greater risk of experiencing first-time LBP during a 1-year follow-up period (11,12). Paradoxically, for women the trend was the opposite.

A physical training program directed toward specific manual lifting tasks may be a tool to control overexertion injuries of the back (41,43). In addition, Graves et al. (50) found that a training frequency as low as one time per week increased lumbar extensor strength. Furthermore, a worker's likelihood of sustaining a back injury or musculoskeletal illness increased when job lifting requirements approached or exceeded the strength capability demonstrated by that individual on an isometric simulation of the job (22).

The prospective studies of Cady et al. (18,19) and Keyserling, Herrin, and Chaffin (72) show that isometric trunk muscle tests may be valuable for the selection of workers, in order to reduce the number of back injuries resulting from hard physical work.

On the other hand, in a 10-year follow-up study no association was found between muscle function at baseline and the development of LBP (79). Likewise, in a 4-year follow-up study, Battié et al. (7) did not observe any predictive value for future back problems of isometric lifting strength in industrial workers when they controlled for the effects of age.

Other Factors

Along the line of preventing back injury and reducing time loss from work, Walsh and Schwartz (145) have shown that education (back school) plus wearing a custom-molded lumbosacral orthosis decreased lost time due to injuries among male warehouse workers. It did not cause adverse effects on abdominal muscle strength.

The studies of Cady et al. (18,19) support the hypothesis that greater cardiovascular fitness is associated with fewer back problems in the physically demanding job of fire fighting. On the other hand, Lehto, Helenius, and Alaranta (78) found no association between ergometer test performance and the 1-year prevalence of LBP and disability among dentists. Likewise, Battié et al. (6) found no evidence of cardiovascular fitness being predictive of future back injury reports for blue-collar workers. For comparison, those who reported smoking at the time of the premorbid examination were significantly more likely to report a subsequent back problem than were nonsmokers. Furthermore, Kellett, Kellett, and Nordholm (69) did not find any change in cardiovascular fitness during their LBP-reducing intervention.

The significance of individual behavioral factors to the prevalence of LBP has been stressed (137, 143). In their national survey, Deyo and Bass (28) found that smoking and obesity contributed independent risks for LBP, even after age, education, exercise level, and employment status were controlled for. In addition, they found a dose-response relationship for both of these factors. The authors state, "Our data suggest that programmes for improving these unhealthy lifestyles may have financial impact far beyond that related to heart disease alone." In another study on risk indicators, persons with either recurring or first-time LBP had more health problems and probably lived under a higher psychosocial pressure than those without LBP in the follow-up year (12).

Primary Prevention in Leisure-Time and Sports Activities

The previous remarks regarding occupational prevention to a large extent apply to leisure-time activities as well, but regarding to BP among athletes, certain specific considerations have to be taken into account as well. The considerations were reviewed by Deusinger (27). It is usually easier to avoid the damaging activities during leisure time than during working hours, where a specific task is demanded. It is important to recognize structural causes early, especially in skeletally immature athletes (53). In the older generation it is important to be aware of the normal aging process and the resultant structural changes that occur in the spine. Moreover, the sports medicine clinician should have an overall appreciation of the patient and realize that pain may frequently be neglected, due to enthusiasm during the competition, particularly by professional athletes.

Secondary Prevention

Frymoyer (39) states: "Once a patient has LBP, the most important prevention measures should be directed to the restoration of function and returning the person to work."

Linton, Bradley, Jensen, Spangfort, and Sundell (83) present a controlled study of nurses and nursing aides, who had been sick-listed for BP during the previous 2-year period but who were currently working. The intervention group underwent a 5-week program with physical and behavioral intervention involving activities at least 8 hr/day on weekdays, including various exercise activities (walking, swimming, jogging, cycling, etc.) at least 4 hr/day. There were significantly greater improvements in the treatment group than the control group for pain intensity, anxiety, sleep quality and fatigue ratings, observed pain behavior, activities, mood, and helplessness. The differences were generally maintained at a 6-month follow-up. For the treatment group, a trend toward increasing amounts of pain-related absenteeism because of musculoskeletal problems was reversed. However, the effect on BP separately cannot be evaluated from this study. Likewise, the study cannot elucidate the specific effect of the exercise activities itself, but the authors concluded that the results suggest that a secondary prevention program aimed at altering lifestyle factors may represent an effective method for dealing with musculoskeletal pain problems.

Donchin, Woolf, Kaplan, and Floman (32) demonstrated that trunk flexion and pelvic tilt exercises for 45 min biweekly for 3 months could reduce the number of recurrent LBP episodes significantly in hospital employees, when compared to a back school and a control group, respectively. It was found that the improvement in forward flexion, as well as in abdominal muscle strength, was inversely correlated with the number of episodes.

Following an exercise program 1 hour a week for 1-1/2 years during paid working hours, combined with exercise at least once a week during leisure, reduced the number of episodes of BP and the number of sick-leave days attributable to BP more than 50% during the intervention period (69). Absenteeism attributable to BP increased in the control group. Cardiovascular fitness, as estimated from a submaximal exercise test, showed no significant change from pre- to postintervention. McQuade, Turner, and Buchner (96) found that the higher the aerobic work capacity, the more generally active were the individuals with chronic LBP. Reports of pain intensity, however, were not affected by fitness (aerobic capacity, strength, and flexibility).

Thus, the multifactorial nature of LBP makes multivariable models necessary for the prediction of outcome (16).

Physiological and Biomechanical Methods for Evaluation of Back Function

The previous sections of this chapter discussed studies in which various physiological and biomechanical methods were performed and used in occupational, treatment, and prevention perspectives, as well as in the possible prediction of future BP. In this section we evaluate the reproducibility of these methods.

Muscle Performance

Strength

Muscle strength has been classified with respect to the parameter that is controlled. In *isometric* contractions the length of muscle is kept constant. In *isokinetic* and *isotonic* contractions the velocity of the movement or the tension in the muscle, respectively, is kept constant. The contractions are performed either during shortening (*concentric*) or lengthening (*eccentric*) of the muscle. Finally, in *isoinertial* contractions the inertia of the load is kept constant throughout the range of motion.

When one evaluates the capacity of the trunk muscles, it is important that capacity be measured in an easy, applicable, and reproducible way. This can be accomplished by optimizing the trunk muscle performance measurements by (a) standardization of testing position, including stabilization of the pelvis, minimization of the contribution from hip and leg muscles, and control of the influence of gravitational forces during testing; and (b) measuring either dynamically through the full range of motion or isometrically at defined trunk angles (49).

Beimborn and Morrissey (9) reviewed the literature concerning the testing of trunk muscle strength in more than one muscle synergy. Fifty papers were included, and 56% of the studies were based on isometric measurements, 36% on isokinetic measurements, and 8% on isotonic measurements. The majority of studies included only trunk extensor-flexor measurements. Recently, isoinertial trunk muscle studies have appeared (113). Relatively few reports of trunk muscle testing include sufficient information concerning evaluation of the methods. The reproducibility of trunk muscle strength seems to be less in patients than in control subjects and more so in flexors than extensors (57). In isometric contractions it is generally agreed that the test-retest reliability is excellent; that is, the coefficient of reliability (r) varies from .89 to .99 when the test is performed in a neutral position (45,49,59,133) and the coefficient of variation (CV) is normally less than 10% (11,45,57).

A trunk performance device (Kin-Com) was systematically studied by Smidt et al. (124,125) in isometric as well as concentric and eccentric contractions at relatively slow velocities (20° per second) from -15° extension to 30° flexion. They found that kinetic variables (e.g., peak torque, torque rise rate, torque time integral) were highly reliable ($r > .90$). The angle where peak torque occurred, however, showed quite low r values (50% with $r < .60$). At higher velocities (30°, 60°, 90°, 120° per second), the kinetic parameters showed lower r values between .76 and .90 in test-retest trials (126). To our knowledge, no reproducibility studies of the isoinertial methods have been published yet. It seems that the reproducibility of trunk muscle strength corresponds to that from other skeletal muscle synergies, if the standardization is properly controlled (134,142,147). It is worthwhile to stress that moderate to fast contraction velocities of the trunk muscles still remain to be investigated. The clinical tests for trunk muscle performance (e.g., leg lowering and sit-ups) in general were poor discriminators of trunk flexor strength (123). These clinical tests are not able to discriminate within the normal human strength capability (123).

Endurance

The endurance tests show less reliability than trunk muscle strength tests, probably due to motivational factors. Two different tests for isometric trunk extensor endurance have been evaluated (11,66). They corresponded to a trunk extensor load of 35% and 60% of the maximal voluntary contraction (MVC); the r values were .89 and .82, respectively, and CV was 19% (62,66). Nordin et al. (107) found a CV of less than 10%. Similarly, Holmström, Moritz, and Andersson (59) found $r = .91$ and CV for three consecutive contractions of 4% to 7%.

Flexibility

The methods measuring movements of the spine may be categorized according to their sophistication (114) as (a) one-dimensional measures, giving a linear measure of some aspects of body movement; (b) two-dimensional measurements, most often providing a rotation within one plane with inclinometers, spondylometer, flexicurves, or photographic technique; or (c) three-dimensional techniques including radiological, vector-stereographical, and optical methods.

The three-dimensional methods are expensive, technically difficult, and some of them even ethically questionable (X rays) and are therefore not easily applicable in large-scale clinical investigations.

Gill, Krag, Johnson, Haugh, and Pope (44) studied the reproducibility of five methods for determining the lumbar spinal sagittal motion: a photometric technique, two inclinometer methods, fingertip-to-floor distance, and the modified Schober methods. They found that the Schober method was superior to the others. The use of the inclinometer or Schober test has also proved most reliable according to Frymoyer, Nelson, Spangfort, and Waddell (40). Reproducible measurements of flexion and extension (CV < 10%) (11,31,57), (r = .67) (31) and lateral bend ($r = .78$) (31) are available, but axial rotation measurements other than with sophisticated three-dimensional tracking devices are unreliable (14) ($r < .5$) (31,40). Hyytiäinen, Salminen, Suvitie, Wickström, and Pentti (62) found the modified Schober test to have intra- and interobserver test-retest reliability coefficients of .88 and .87 respectively, but the interobserver difference was significant. Similar r-values were reported by Öhlén, Spangfort, and Tingvall (110) with Debrunners kyphometer, and the CV was 4.4%. Surprisingly, flexibility measured by sophisticated equipment has a poorer reliability and utility (more time-consuming) (31). Therefore, the modified Schober test is recommended if spinal flexibility measurements are performed in large-scale clinical settings, although this method has been questioned in a recent study (99).

References

1. Andersson, G.; Bjurvall, M.; Bolinder, E.; et al. Modell för bedömning av ryggskada i enlighet med arbetsskadeförsikringen. Lakartidningen. 78:2765-2767; 1981.
2. Andersson, G.B.J. Epidemiologic aspects on low-back pain in industry. Spine. 6:53-60; 1981.
3. Asfour, S.S.; Khalil, T.M.; Waly, S.M.; Goldberg, M.L.; Rosomoff, R.S.; Rosomoff, H.L. Biofeedback in back muscle strengthening. Spine. 15:510-513; 1990.
4. Balgué, F.; Dutoit, G.; Waldburger, M. Low back pain in schoolchildren. Scand. J. Rehabil. Med. 20:175-179; 1988.
5. Battié, M.C.; Bigos, S.J.; Sheehy, A.; Wortley, M.D. Spinal flexibility and individual factors that influence it. J. Am. Phys. Ther. Assoc. 67:48-53; 1987.
6. Battié, M.C.; Bigos, S.J.; Fisher, L.D.; et al. A prospective study of the role of cardiovascular risk factors and fitness in industrial back pain complaints. Spine. 14:141-147; 1989.
7. Battié, M.C.; Bigos, S.J.; Fisher, L.D.; Hansson, T.H.; Jones, M.E.; Wortley, M.D. Isometric lifting strength as a predictor of industrial back pain reports. Spine. 14:851-856; 1989.
8. Battié, M.C.; Videman, T.; Gill, K.; et al. Smoking and lumbar intervertebral disc degeneration: An MRI study of identical twins. Spine. 16:1015-1021; 1991.
9. Beimborn, D.S.; Morrissey, M.C. A review of the literature related to trunk muscle performance. Spine. 13:655-660; 1988.
10. Bengtsson, B.; Thorson, J. Back pain: A study of twins. Acta Genet. Med. Gemellol. 40:83-90; 1991.
11. Biering-Sørensen, F. Physical measurements as risk indicators for low-back trouble over a one-year period. Spine. 9:106-119; 1984.
12. Biering-Sørensen, F.; Thomsen, C.E.; Hilden, J. Risk indicators for low back trouble. Scand. J. Rehabil. Med. 21:151-157; 1989.
13. Boland, A.L.; Hosea, T.M. Rowing and sculling and the older athlete. Clin. Sports Med. 10:245-256; 1991.
14. Boline, P.D.; Keating, J.C.; Haas, M.; Anderson, A.V. Interexaminer reliability and discriminant validity of inclinometric measurement of lumbar rotation in chronic low-back pain patients and subjects without low-back pain. Spine. 17:335-338; 1992.
15. Brinckmann, P.; Biggemann, M.; Hilweg, D. Fatigue fracture of human lumbar vertebrae. Clin. Biomech. [Suppl. 1]. 3:S1-S23; 1988.
16. Burton, A.K.; Tillotson, K.M. Prediction of the clinical course of low-back trouble using multivariable models. Spine. 16:7-14; 1991.
17. Burton, A.K.; Tillotson, K.M.; Troup, J.D.G. Variation in lumbar sagittal mobility with low-back trouble. Spine. 14:584-590; 1989.
18. Cady, L.D.; Bischoff, D.P.; O'Connell, E.R.; Thomas, P.C.; Allan, J.H. Strength and fitness and subsequent back injuries in firefighters. J. Occup. Med. 21:269-272; 1979.
19. Cady, L.D.; Thomas, P.C.; Karwasky, R.J. Program for increasing health and physcial fitness of fire fighters. J. Occup. Med. 27:110-114; 1985.
20. Callaway; Jobe. Injuries on the Professional Golfers Association tour of 1985 to 1986. (Cited in Watkins, R.G.; Dillin, W.H. Lumbar spine injury in the athlete. Clin. Sports Med. 9:419-448; 1990.)
21. Chaffin, D.B. Manual materials handling and the biomechanical basis for prevention of low-back pain in industry—An overview. Am. Ind. Hyg. Assoc. J. 48:989-996; 1987.
22. Chaffin, D.B.; Herrin, G.D.; Keyserling, W.M. Preemployment strength testing. An update position. J. Occup. Med. 20:403-408; 1978.
23. Chard, M.D.; Lachmann, S.M. Racquet sports—patterns of injury presenting to a sports injury clinic. Br. J. Sports Med. 21:150-153; 1987.
24. Clemmer, D.I.; Mohr, D.L. Low-back injuries in a heavy industry II. Labor market forces. Spine. 16:831-834; 1991.
25. Clemmer, D.I.; Mohr, D.L.; Mercer, D.J. Low-back injuries in a heavy industry I. Worker and workplace factors. Spine. 16:824-830; 1991.
26. Community Ergonomics Action. Guidelines for manual handling in the coal industry. European coal and steel community. Report No. 14 - series 3. Luxembourg: Bureau of Information and Coordination of Community Ergonomics Action; 1990.
27. Deusinger, R.H. Biomechanical considerations for clinical application in athletes with low back pain. Clin. Sports Med. 8:703-715; 1989.
28. Deyo, R.A.; Bass, J.E. Lifestyle and low-back pain. The influence of smoking and obesity. Spine. 14:501-506; 1989.
29. Deyo, R.A.; Diehl, A.K.; Rosenthal, M. How many days of bed rest for acute low back pain? A randomized clinical trial. N. Engl. J. Med. 315:1064-1070; 1986.
30. Deyo, R.A.; Walsh, N.E.; Martin, D.C.; Schoenfeld, L.S.; Ramamurthy, S. A controlled trial of transcutaneous electrical nerve

stimulation (TENS) and exercise for chronic low back pain. N. Engl. J. Med. 322:1627-1634; 1990.

31. Dillard, J.; Trafimow, J.; Andersson, G.B.J.; Cronin, K. Motion of the lumbar spine. Reliability of two measurement techniques. Spine. 16:321-324; 1991.
32. Donchin, M.; Woolf, O.; Kaplan, L.; Floman, Y. Secondary prevention of low back-back pain. A clinical trial. Spine. 15:1317-1320; 1990.
33. Donelson, R.; Grant, W.; Kamps, C.; Medcalf, R. Pain response to sagittal end-range spinal motion. A prospective, randomized, multicentered trial. Spine. 16:S206-S212; 1991.
34. Elnaggar, I.M.; Nordin, M.; Sheikhzadeh, A.; Parnianpour, M.; Kahanovitz, N. Effects of spinal flexion and extension exercises on low-back pain and spinal mobility in chronic mechanical low-back pain patients. Spine. 16:967-972; 1991.
35. Estlander, A.-M.; Mellin, G.; Vanharanta, H.; Hupli, M. Effects and follow-up of a multimodal treatment program including intensive physical training for low back pain patients. Scand. J. Rehabil. Med. 23:97-102; 1991.
36. Evans, C.; Gilbert, J.R.; Taylor, W.; Hildebrand, A. A randomized controlled trial of flexion exercises, education, and bed rest for patients with acute low back pain. Physiother. Can. 39:96-101; 1987.
37. Fordyce, W.E.; Brockway, J.A.; Bergman, J.A.; Spengler, D. Acute back pain: A control-group comparison of behavioral vs traditional management methods. J. Behav. Med. 9:127-140; 1986.
38. Foster, D.; John, D.; Elliott, B.; Ackland, T.; Fitch, K. Back injuries to fast bowlers in cricket: A prospective study. Br. J. Sports Med. 23:150-154; 1989.
39. Frymoyer, J.W. Back pain and sciatica. N. Engl. J. Med. 318:291-300; 1988.
40. Frymoyer, J.W.; Nelson, R.M.; Spangfort, E.; Waddell, G. Clinical tests applicable to the study of chronic low-back disability. Spine. 16:681-682; 1991.
41. Genaidy, A.M. A training programme to improve human physical capability for manual handling jobs. Ergonomics. 34:1-11; 1991.
42. Genaidy, A.M.; Asfour, S.S.; Mital, A.; Waly, S.M. Psychophysical models for manual lifting tasks. Appl. Ergonomics. 21:295-303; 1990.
43. Genaidy, A.M.; Bafna, K.M.; Sarmidy, R.; Sana, P. A muscular endurance training program for symmetrical and asymmetrical manual lifting tasks. J. Occup. Med. 32:226-233; 1990.
44. Gill, K.; Krag, M.H.; Johnson, G.B.; Haugh, L.D.; Pope, M.H. Repeatability of four clinical methods for assessment of lumbar spinal motion. Spine. 13:50-53; 1988.
45. Gomez, T.; Beach, G.; Cooke, C.; Hrudey, W.; Goyert, P. Normative database for trunk range of motion, strength, velocity and endurance with isostation B-200 lumbar dynamometer. Spine. 16:15-21; 1991.
46. Gordon, G.A. A molecular basis for low back pain in Western industrialized cultures. Med. Hypotheses. 33:251-256; 1990.
47. Granhed, H.; Jonson, R.; Hansson, T. The loads on the lumbar spine during extreme weight lifting. Spine. 12:146-149; 1987.
48. Granhed, H.; Morelli, B. Low back pain among retired wrestlers and heavyweight lifters. Am. J. Sports Med. 16:530-533; 1988.
49. Graves, J.E.; Pollock, M.L.; Carpenter, D.M.; et al. Quantitative assessment of full range-of-motion isometric lumbar extension strength. Spine. 15:289-294; 1990.
50. Graves, J.E.; Pollock, M.L.; Foster, D.; et al. Effect of training frequency and specificity on isometric lumbar extension strength. Spine. 15:504-509; 1990.
51. Gyntelberg, F. One year incidence of low back pain among male residents of Copenhagen aged 40-59. Dan. Med. Bull. 21:30-36; 1974.
52. Haas, S.S.; MacCartee, C.C.; Wells, J.R. Medical aspects of the men's professional tennis tour. (Cited in Marks, M.R.; Haas, S.S.; Wiesel, S.W. Low back pain in the competitive tennis player. Clin. Sports Med. 7:277- 287; 1988.)
53. Halpern, B.C.; Smith, A.D. Catching the cause of low-back pain. Phys. and Sportsmed. 19:71-79; 1991.
54. Hansen, F.R.; Bendix, T.; Skov, P.; et al. Intensive dynamic back-muscle exercises, conventional physiotherapy, or placebo-control treatment in chronic low-back pain—a randomized, observer-blinded trial. Spine. 18:98-107; 1993.
55. Hazard, R.G.; Fenwick, J.W.; Kalisch, S.M.; et al. Functional restoration with behavioral support. A one-year prospective study of patients with chronic low-back pain. Spine. 14:157-161; 1989.
56. Heliövaara, M. Risk factors for low back pain and sciatica. Ann. Med. 21:257-264; 1989.
57. Hirsch, G.; Beach, G.; Cooke, C.; Menard, M.; Locke, S. Relationship between performance on lumbar dynamometry and Waddell score in a population with low-back pain. Spine. 16:1039-1043; 1991.
58. Holm, S.; Nachemson, A. Variations in the nutrition of the canine intervertebral disc induced by motion. Spine. 8:866-874; 1983.

59. Holmström, E.; Moritz, U.; Andersson, M. Trunk muscle strength and back muscle endurance in construction workers with and without low back disorders. Scand. J. Rehabil. Med. 24:3-10; 1992.
60. Howell, D.W. Musculoskeletal profile and incidence of musculoskeletal injuries in lightweight women rowers. Am. J. Sports Med. 12:278-281; 1984.
61. Hutton, W.C.; Stott, J.R.R.; Cyron, B.M. Is spondylolysis a fatigue fracture? Spine. 2:202-209; 1977.
62. Hyytiäinen, K.; Salminen, J.J.; Suvitie, T.; Wickström, G.; Pentti, J. Reproducibility of nine tests to measure spinal mobility and trunk muscle strength. Scand. J. Rehabil. Med. 23:3-10; 1991.
63. Jackson, C.P.; Brown, M.D. Is there a role for exercise in the treatment of patients with low back pain? Clin. Orthop. 179:39-45; 1983.
64. Jackson, C.P.; Brown, M.D. Analysis of current approaches and a practical guide to prescription of exercise. Clin. Orthop. 179:46-54; 1983.
65. Jackson, D.W.; Wiltse, L.L.; Cirincione, R.J. Spondylolysis in the female gymnast. Clin. Orthop. 117:68-73; 1976.
66. Jørgensen, K.; Nicolaisen, T. Two methods for determining trunk extensor endurance. Eur. J. Appl. Physiol. 55:639-644; 1986.
67. Kalimo, H.; Rantanen, J.; Viljanen, T.; Einola, S. Lumbar muscles: Structure and function. Ann. Med. 21:353-359; 1989.
68. Keene, J.S.; Albert, M.J.; Springer, S.L.; Drummond, D.S.; Clancy, W.G. Back injuries in college athletes. J. Spinal Dis. 2:190-195; 1989.
69. Kellett, K.M.; Kellett, D.A.; Nordholm, L.A. Effects of an exercise program on sick leave due to back pain. Phys. Ther. 71:283-293; 1991.
70. Kelsey, J.L.; Githens, P.B.; White, A.A., III; et al. An epidemiological study of lifting and twisting on the job and risk for acute prolapsed lumbar intervertebral disc. J. Orthop. Res. 2:61-66; 1984.
71. Kendall, P.H.; Jenkins, J.M. Exercises for backache: A double-blind controlled trial. Physiotherapy. 54:154-157; 1968.
72. Keyserling, W.M.; Herrin, G.D.; Chaffin, D.B. Isometric strength testing as a means of controlling medical incidents on strenous jobs. J. Occu. Med. 22:332-336; 1980.
73. Klein, R.G.; Eek, B.C. Low-energy laser treatment and exercise for chronic low back pain: Double-blind controlled trial. Arch. Phys. Med. Rehabil. 71:34-37; 1990.
74. Koes, B.W.; Bouter, L.M.; Beckerman, H.; van der Heijden, G.J.M.G.; Knipschild, P.G. Physiotherapy exercises and back pain: A blinded review. Br. Med. J. 302:1572-1576; 1991.
75. Kopp, J.R.; Alexander, A.H.; Turocy, R.H.; Levrini, M.G.; Lichtman, D.M. The use of lumbar extension in the evaluation and treatment of patients with acute herniated nucleus pulposus. Clin. Orthop. 202:211-218; 1986.
76. Kraus, D.R.; Shapiro, D. The symptomatic lumbar spine in the athlete. Clin. Sports Med. 8:59-69; 1989.
77. Kumar, S. Cumulative load as a risk factor for back pain. Spine. 15:1311-1316; 1990.
78. Lehto, T.U.; Helenius, H.Y.M.; Alaranta, H.T. Musculoskeletal symptoms of dentists assessed by a multidisciplinary approach. Community Dent. Oral Epidemiol. 19:38-44; 1991.
79. Leino, P.; Aro, S.; Hasan, J. Trunk muscle function and low back disorders: A ten-year follow-up study. J. Chronic. Dis. 40:289-296; 1987.
80. Lidström, A.; Zachrisson, M. Physical therapy on low back pain and sciatica. Scand. J. Rehabil. Med. 2:37-42; 1970.
81. Liles, D.H.; Mahajan, P. Using NIOSH lifting guide decreases risks of back injuries. Occup. Health Saf. 54:57-60; 1985.
82. Linden, S.M.v.d.; Fahrer, H. Occurrence of spinal pain syndromes in a group of apparently healthy and physically fit sportsmen (orienteers). Scand. J. Rheumatol. 17:475-481; 1988.
83. Linton, S.J.; Bradley, L.A.; Jensen, I.; Spangfort, E.; Sundell, L. The secondary prevention of low back pain: A controlled study with follow-up. Pain. 36:197-207; 1989.
84. Magora, A. Investigation of the relation between low back pain and occupation. 3. Physical requirements: Sitting, standing and weight lifting. Indus. Med. 41:5-9; 1972.
85. Mälkiä, E. The physical activity of Finnish adults suffering from low back disorders and symptomes. Finland: Institute of Occupational Health, SF-00250; 1991.
86. Manniche, C.; Asmussen, K.; Lauritsen, B.; et al. Intensive dynamic back exercises for chronic low back pain after first time discectomy with or without use of hyperextension: A clinical trial. Spine. 18:560-567; 1993..
87. Manniche, C.; Hesselsøe, G.; Bentzen, L.; Christensen, I.; Lundberg, E. Clinical trial of intensive muscle training for chronic low back pain. Lancet. 2:1473-1476; 1988.
88. Manniche, C.; Lundberg, E.; Christensen, I.; Bentzen, L.; Hesselsøe, G. Intensive dynamic back exercises for chronic low back pain: A clinical trial. Pain. 47:53-63; 1991.

89. Manniche, C.; Skall, H.F.; Braendholt, L.; et al. Clinical trial of postoperative dynamic back exercises after first lumbar diskectomy. Spine. 18:92-97; 1993.
90. Marks, M.R.; Haas, S.S.; Wiesel, S.W. Low back pain in the competitive tennis player. Clin. Sports Med. 7:277-287; 1988.
91. Martin, P.R.; Rose, M.J.; Nichols, P.J.R.; Russell, P.L.; Hughes, I.G. Physiotherapy exercises for low back pain: Process and clinical outcome. Int. Rehabil. Med. 8:34-38; 1986.
92. Mayer, T.G. Discussion: Exercise, fitness, and back pain. In: Bouchard, C.; Shephard, R.J.; Stephens, T.; Sutton, J.R.; McPherson, B.C., eds. Exercise, fitness, and health. Champaign, IL: Human Kinetics; 1990:541-546.
93. Mayer, T.G.; Gatchel, R.J.; Kishino, N.; et al. Objective assessment of spine function following industrial injury. A prospective study with comparison group and one-year follow-up. Spine. 10:482-493; 1985.
94. Mayer, T.G.; Gatchel, R.J.; Mayer, H.; Kishino, N.D.; Keeley, J.; Mooney, V. A prospective two-year study of functional restoration in industrial low back injury. JAMA. 258:1763-1767; 1987.
95. McCaroll, J.R.; Miller, J.M.; Ritter, M.A. Lumbar spondylolysis and spondylolisthesis in college football players. Am. J. Sports Med. 14:404-406; 1986.
96. McQuade, K.J.; Turner, J.A.; Buchner, D.M. Physical fitness and chronic low back pain. Clin. Orthop. 233:198-204; 1988.
97. Mellin, G. Correlations of hip mobility with degree of back pain and lumbar spinal mobility in chronic low-back pain patients. Spine. 13:668-670; 1988.
98. Mellin, G.; Hurri, H.; Härkäpää, K.; Järvikoski, A. A controlled study on the outcome of inpatient and outpatient treatment of low back pain. Scand. J. Rehabil. Med. 21:91-95; 1989.
99. Miller, S.A.; Mayer, T.; Cox, R.; Gatchel, R.J. Reliability problems associated with the modified Schöber technique for true lumbar flexion measurement. Spine. 17:345-348; 1992.
100. Mitchell, R.I.; Carmen, G.M. Results of a multicenter trial using an intensive active exercise program for the treatment of acute soft tissue and back injuries. Spine. 15:514-521; 1990.
101. Mutoh, Y. Low back pain in butterfliers. In: Eriksson, B.; Furber, B., eds. Swimming medicine IV. Baltimore: University Park Press; 1977:115-123.
102. Nachemson, A. Work for all. For those with low back pain as well. Clin. Orthop. 179:77-85; 1983.
103. Nachemson, A. Exercise, fitness, and back pain. In: Bouchard, C.; Shephard, R.J.; Stephens, T.; Sutton, J.R.; McPherson, B.C., eds. Exercise, fitness, and health. Champaign, IL: Human Kinetics; 1990:533-540.
104. National Institute for Occupational Safety and Health (NIOSH), Department of Biomedical and Behavioral Science. Work practices guide for manual lifting. Cincinnati: U.S. Department of Health and Human Services; 1981.
105. Nicholson, A.S. A comparative study of methods for establishing load handling capabilities. Ergonomics. 32:1125-1144; 1989.
106. Nicolaisen, T.; Jørgensen, K. Trunk strength, back muscle endurance and low-back trouble. Scand. J. Rehabil. Med. 17:121-127; 1985.
107. Nordin, M.; Kahanovitz, N.; Verderame, R.; et al. Normal trunk muscle strength and endurance in women and the effect of exercises and electrical stimulation. Part 1: Normal endurance and trunk muscle strength in 101 women. Spine. 12:105-111; 1987.
108. Nutter, P. Aerobic exercise in the treatment and prevention of low back pain. Occup. Med. 3:137-145; 1988.
109. Nwuga, V.C.B. Relative therapeutic efficacy of vertebral manipulation and conventional treatment in back pain management. Am. J. Phys. Med. 61:273-278; 1982.
110. Öhlén, G.; Spangfort, E.; Tingvall, C. Measurement of spinal sagittal configuration and mobility with Debrunners's kyphometer. Spine. 14:580-583; 1989.
111. Oland, G.; Tveiten, G. A trial of modern rehabilitation for chronic low-back pain and disability. Spine. 16:457-459; 1991.
112. O'Toole, M.L.; Hiller, W.D.B.; Smith, R.A.; Sisk, T.D. Overuse injuries in ultraendurance triathletes. Am. J. Sports Med. 17:514-518; 1989.
113. Parnianpour, M.; Li, F.; Nordin, M.; Kahanovitz, N. A database of isoinertial trunk strength tests against three resistance levels in sagittal, frontal, and transverse planes in normal male subjects. Spine. 14:409-411; 1989.
114. Pearcy, M. Measurement of back and spinal mobility. Clin. Biomech. 1:44-51; 1986.
115. Peters, J.L.; Large, R.G. A randomised control trial evaluating in- and outpatient pain management programmes. Pain. 41:283-293; 1990.
116. Pope, M.H. Risk indicators in low back pain. Ann. Med. 21:387-392; 1989.
117. Porter, R.W.; Adams, M.A.; Hutton, W.C. Physical activity and the strength of the lumbar spine. Spine. 14:201-203; 1989.
118. Riihimäki, H. Low-back pain, its origin and risk indicators. Scand. J. Work Environ. Health. 17:81-90; 1991.

119. Riihimäki, H.; Sakari, T.; Videman, T.; Hänninen, K. Low-back pain and occupation. Spine. 14:204-209; 1989.
120. Rossi, F. Spondylosis, spondylolisthesis and sports. Ital. J. Sports Med. Phys. Fitness. 18:317-340; 1978.
121. Saal, J.A.; Saal, J.S. Nonoperative treatment of herniated lumbar intervertebral disc with radiculopathy. An outcome study. Spine. 14:431-437; 1989.
122. Sachs, B.L.; David, J.-A.F.; Olimpio, D.; Scala, A.D.; Lacroix, M. Spinal rehabilitation by work tolerance based on objective physical capacity assessment of dysfunction. Spine. 15:1325-1332; 1990.
123. Smidt, G.L.; Blanpied, P.R.; Anderson, M.R.; White, R.W. Comparison of clinical and objective methods of assessing trunk muscle strength—An experimental approach. Spine. 12:1020-1024; 1987.
124. Smidt, G.L.; Blanpied, P.R.; White, R.W. Exploration of mechanical and electromyographic responses of trunk muscles to high-intensity resistive exercise. Spine. 14:815-830; 1989.
125. Smidt, G.; Herring, T.; Amundsen, L.; Rogers, M.; Russell, A.; Lehmann, T. Assessment of abdominal and back extensor function. Spine. 8:211-219; 1983.
126. Smith, S.S.; Mayer, T.G.; Gatchel, R.J.; Becker, T.J. Quantification of lumbar function. Part 1. Isometric and multispeed isokinetic trunk strength measures in sagittal and axial planes in normal subjects. Spine. 10:757-764; 1985.
127. Snook, S.H.; Ciriello, V.M. The design of manual handling tasks: Revised tables of maximum acceptable weights and forces. Ergonomics. 34:1197-1213; 1991.
128. Stanish, W. Low back pain in athletes: An overuse syndrome. Clin. Sports Med. 6:321-344; 1987.
129. Stankovic, R.; Johnell, O. Conservative treatment of acute low-back pain. A prospective randomized trial: McKenzie method of treatment versus patient education in "mini back school." Spine. 15:120-123; 1990.
130. Svensson, H.-O.; Vedin, A.; Wilhelmsson, C.; Andersson, G.B.J. Low-back pain in relation to other diseases and cardiovascular risk factors. Spine. 8:277-285; 1983.
131. Swärd, L.; Hellstrom, M.; Jacobsson, B.; Nyman, R.; Peterson, L. Acute injury of the vertebral ring apophysis and intervertebral disc in adolescent gymnasts. Spine. 15:144-148; 1990.
132. Tertti, M.; Paajanen, H.; Kujala, U.M.; Alanen, A.; Salmi, T.T.; Kormano, M. Disc degeneration in gymnasts. Am. J. Sports Med. 18:206-208; 1990.
133. Thorstensson, A.; Arvidson, Å. Trunk muscle strength and low back pain. Scand. J. Rehabil. Med. 14:69-75; 1982.
134. Thorstensson, A.; Nilsson, J. Trunk muscle strength during constant velocity movements. Scand. J. Rehabil. Med. 14:61-68; 1982.
135. Tollison, C.D.; Kriegel, M.L. Physical exercise in the treatment of low back pain. Part I: A review. Orthop. Rev. 17:724-729; 1988.
136. Troup, J.D.G. Causes, prediction and prevention of back pain at work. Scand. J. Work Environ. Health. 10:419-428; 1984.
137. Troup, J.D.G.; Foreman, T.K.; Baxter, C.E.; Brown, D. The perception of back pain and the role of psychophysical tests of lifting capacity. Spine. 12:645-657; 1987.
138. Troup, J.D.G.; Martin, J.W.; Lloyd, D.C.E.F. Back pain in industry. A prospective survey. Spine. 6:61-69; 1981.
139. Urban, J.P.G.; Holm, S.; Maroudas, A.; Nachemson, A. Nutrition of the intervertebral disc. Effect of fluid flow on solute transport. Clin. Orthop. 170:296-302; 1982.
140. Videman, T.; Nurminen, M.; Troup, J.D.G. Lumbar spinal pathology in cadaveric material in relation to history of back pain, occupation, and physical loading. Spine. 15:728-740; 1990.
141. Videman, T.; Rauhala, H.; Asp, S.; et al. Patient-handling skill, back injuries, and back pain. An intervention study in nursing. Spine. 14:148-156; 1989.
142. Viitasalo, J.T.; Era, P.; Leskinen, A.-L.; Heikkinen, E. Muscular strength profiles and athropometry in random samples of men aged 31-35, 51-55 and 71-75 years. Ergonomics. 28: 1563-1574; 1985.
143. Waddell, G. A new clinical model for the treatment of low-back pain. Spine. 12:632-644; 1987.
144. Waddell, G.; Pilowsky, I.; Bond, M.R. Clinical assessment and interpretation of abnormal illness behaviour in low back pain. Pain. 39:41-53; 1989.
145. Walsh, N.E.; Schwartz, R.K. The influence of prophylactic orthosis on abdominal strength and low back injury in the workplace. Am. J. Phys. Med. Rehabil. 69:245-250; 1990.
146. Watkins, R.G.; Dillin, W.H. Lumbar spine injury in the athlete. Clin. Sports Med. 9:419-448; 1990.
147. Westing, S.H. Skeletal muscle strength in man. Stockholm, Sweden: Department of Physiology III, Karolinska Institutet; 1990. Thesis.
148. Yu, T.; Roht, L.H.; Wise, R.A.; Kilian, D.J.; Weir, F.W. Low-back pain in industry. An old problem revisited. J. Occup. Med. 26:517-524; 1984.

Chapter 51

Physical Activity, Fitness, and Chronic Lung Disease

Brian J. Whipp
Richard Casaburi

In order to meet the increased demands for pulmonary gas exchange during muscular exercise, the lungs must replenish the O_2 extracted from the alveoli by the increased flow of more desaturated mixed venous blood. This preserves alveolar and hence arterial O_2 partial pressure (PaO_2). The lungs must also provide the alveoli with diluting quantities of CO_2-free (atmospheric) air at rates commensurate with the increased delivery rate of CO_2 in the mixed venous blood. This maintains alveolar and hence arterial CO_2 partial pressure ($PaCO_2$). However, the metabolic (chiefly lactic) acidosis of high-intensity exercise requires that alveolar CO_2 concentration be diluted more in order to reduce alveolar and arterial PCO_2 in order to provide a component of respiratory compensation that constrains the fall of arterial pH.

The pulmonary system is therefore confronted by different demands for blood-gas and acid-base regulation during exercise. There are competing ventilatory demands for alveolar $PO_2(P_AO_2)$ and $PCO_2(P_ACO_2)$ regulation when the respiratory exchange ratio (R) differs from unity and also for arterial PCO_2 and pH regulation when the exercise results in a metabolic acidosis.

In patients with lung disease this process is further complicated by pulmonary gas exchange inefficiencies that result in often-marked differences between alveolar (either *ideal* or *real*) and arterial gas partial pressures. Consequently, the impaired pulmonary gas exchange in patients with chronic lung disease further increases the ventilatory demand during exercise; the impaired pulmonary mechanics, however, constrain or even limit the ability to meet the demands.

The demands for increased respiratory flow of inspiratory O_2 and diluting flow of CO_2-free gas to the alveoli during exercise require increased inspiratory-muscle work and power in order to generate the pressure necessary (Pmusc) to overcome the elastic, resistive, and inertial components of the total pulmonary impedance; that is,

$$\text{Pmusc} = E \cdot V + R \cdot \dot{V} + I \cdot \ddot{V} \qquad [51.1]$$

where E, R, and I are the pulmonary system elastance, resistance, and inertia, respectively, and V, $\dot{V}$, and $\ddot{V}$ are the volume, air (and pulmonary tissue) flow, and acceleration, respectively. The inertial component, however, is normally only a small fraction of the total pulmonary impedance. This is because, although the acceleration of the air can be large, its mass is so small, and although the mass of the thorax is relatively large, its acceleration is small.

In patients with obstructive pulmonary disease, the impairment is predominantly in the resistive component, whereas in patients with restrictive lung disease the impairment is predominantly of the elastic component. We shall therefore consider these categories separately, with the fundamental requirements for blood-gas and acid-base regulation as the frame of reference.

Ventilatory Determinants During Exercise

The alveolar PO_2 is determined by the inspired $PO_2(P_IO_2)$ and the proportionality between the pulmonary O_2 uptake ($\dot{V}O_2$) and the effective alveolar ventilation ($\dot{V}_A$). That is,

$$PaO_2 = P_IO_2 \cdot N - 863 \cdot \dot{V}O_2/\dot{V}A \qquad [51.2]$$

where N is the small and variable correction factor needed to account for the inequality of inspired and expired N_2 partial pressure that results when inspired and expired gas volumes are not the same; 863 is the constant that allows the relationship to be described in partial pressures rather than fractional concentrations, with $\dot{V}O_2$ and $\dot{V}_A$ expressed in terms of standard temperature and pressure, dry (STPD) and body temperature and pressure, saturated (BTPS), respectively. However, as the body is required also to ventilate the physiological dead space (V_D) to effect alveolar ventilation

$$P_AO_2 = P_IO_2 \cdot N - 863\ \dot{V}O_2/[\dot{V}_E \cdot (1 - V_D/V_T)] \quad [51.3]$$

where $\dot{V}_E$ is the total pulmonary ventilation, and V_D/V_T is the physiologic dead space fraction of the breath. As $\dot{V}CO_2/\dot{V}O_2 = R$, then

$$P_AO_2 = (P_IO_2 \cdot N) - (P_ACO_2/R). \quad [51.4]$$

Similarly, alveolar PCO_2 is given by

$$P_ACO_2 = 863 \cdot (\dot{V}CO_2/\dot{V}_A) \quad [51.5]$$

or

$$P_ACO_2 = 863 \cdot \dot{V}CO_2/[\dot{V}_E \cdot (1 - V_D/V_T)]. \quad [51.6]$$

Notice that in these relationships it is necessary to be able to determine accurately either P_ACO_2, $\dot{V}_A$, or V_D/V_T to allow rigorous evaluation of these mass balance equations. This proves to be extremely difficult in reality. For example, alveolar PCO_2 varies continuously during inspiration and expiration by amounts that differ in different parts of the lung (being most marked in patients with lung disease) and that are represented at the mouth only during expiration after regional delays that also vary in an unknown manner. It is important to recognize that the expedient used to make these relationships tractable has significant implications for understanding both ventilation and gas exchange in patients with lung disease (35).

The expedient is the seemingly simple replacement of arterial PCO_2 for P_ACO_2 in Equation 51.6. This procedure results in a series of necessary consequences. If P_ACO_2 is substituted for $PaCO_2$, then

- the P_AO_2 that is calculated from Equation 51.4 is an ideal alveolar PO_2; that is, one with no gas exchange abnormalities—which in reality would make P_ACO_2 and $PaCO_2$ differ;
- $\dot{V}_A$ is not the real ventilation of the alveolar spaces, but that which would provide an alveolar PCO_2 equal to $PaCO_2$; this of course can be appreciably less than the real ventilation of the alveoli in patients with lung disease; and
- it will appear that there is alveolar dead space (i.e., a ventilated space that is not perfused) even when there may not be (e.g., in patients with an increased dispersion of regional $\dot{V}_A/\dot{Q}$ or right-to-left shunt).

If these limitations are acknowledged, Equation 51.6 may be modified to

$$\dot{V}_E(\text{BTPS}) = 863 \cdot \dot{V}CO_2(\text{STPD})/[PaCO_2 \cdot (1 - V_D/V_T)]. \quad [51.7]$$

This demonstrates that, if we wish to understand the ventilatory demands of patients with lung disease, then it is necessary to establish the factors influencing the three determining variables (i.e., $\dot{V}CO_2$, $PaCO_2$, and V_D/V_T) such as the work of breathing or blood lactate elevation, hypoxic ventilatory drive, and increased $\dot{V}_A/\dot{Q}$ dispersion, respectively.

The collective influence of all three variables can be illustrated, as shown in Figure 51.1. Note that although it may be possible to predict the $\dot{V}O_2$ cost of a particular activity such as walking or cycling, it is not possible to predict the $\dot{V}_E$ cost (43). As shown in Figure 51.1, the $\dot{V}_E$ cost of the same task can easily vary by three- to fourfold depending on the current loads of $\dot{V}CO_2$, $PaCO_2$, and V_D/V_T.

It is important to point out that, in the final quadrant of Figure 51.1, $\dot{V}_E$ has been established with no consideration of the pulmonary mechanical costs of achieving that level of $\dot{V}_E$. Killian and Jones (23) have presented a graphical scheme, also a four-quadrant diagram, that extends the $\dot{V}_E$ response as shown in Figure 51.2 and proceeds via the fraction of the maximum inspiratory pressure that is utilized (by the measured or estimated pressure developed by the inspiratory muscles) and on to the perceptual consequence of shortness of breath or dyspnea. This is useful also because it clearly depicts the notion of the ratio of the ventilatory demand to the subject's ventilatory capacity as a determinant of exercise limitation in patients with lung disease (42).

We shall therefore consider the extent to which the ventilatory demands of muscular exercise encroach on the limit of pulmonary function in patients with chronic obstructive and also restrictive lung disease.

Chronic Obstructive Pulmonary Disease (COPD)

The "obstructive" of COPD by definition refers to a condition of impaired airflow ($\dot{V}$) generation. Although, conceptually, physiologists can separate COPD into categories of predominantly reduced lung recoil (emphysematous or Type-A COPD) and predominantly increased airways resistance (bronchitic or Type-B COPD), in practice there is often considerable overlap. Bronchial asthma will be considered separately below.

As shown in Equation 51.8, impaired expiratory airflow can be a result of increased airways resistance (Raw) or reduced recoil pressure (Prec) of the lung or thorax. Reduced expiratory effort (pleural pressure, Ppl) can also contribute to reduced airflow; that is,

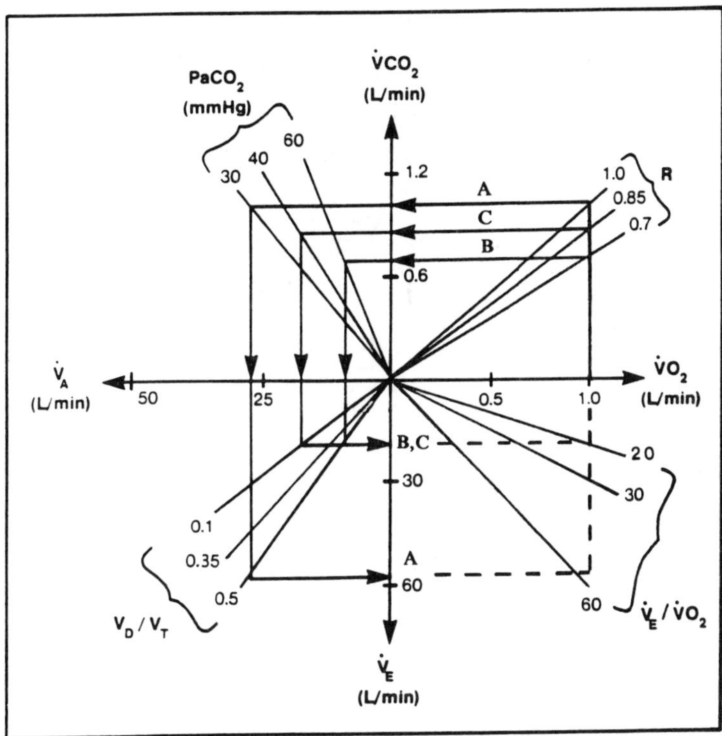

Figure 51.1 Schematic representation of the influence of CO_2 output ($\dot{V}CO_2$), arterial PCO_2 ($PaCO_2$) and the dead space fraction of the breath (V_D/V_T) on the ventilatory ($\dot{V}_E$) requirement for exercise. The particular combination of these determining variables can substantially alter the $\dot{V}_E$ requirement at a given O_2 uptake ($\dot{V}O_2$), relative to normal (**C**). For example, the typically low $PaCO_2$ setpoint (*hyperventilation*) and elevated V_D/V_T of the Type A COPD patient (**A**) serve to increase the $\dot{V}_E$ requirement, and this can be exacerbated if carbohydrate is the predominant metabolic substrate (R = 1.0). In contrast, the Type B patient (**B**) evidences a $\dot{V}_E$ requirement that may be normal or even low; that is, the influence of an elevated V_D/V_T is offset by an increased $PaCO_2$ setpoint (*CO_2 retention*) and also by a reduction in metabolic R.Q. See text for further details.

$$\dot{V} = Palv/Raw = (Prec + Ppl)/Raw. \qquad [51.8]$$

Each of these factors plays a role in establishing the ventilatory and breathing pattern response to exercise as shown in Figure 51.3.

As a result of the increased Raw or reduced Prec, maximum expiratory airflow and maximum voluntary ventilation (MVV) are reduced in patients with COPD (20,42). Consequently, the effective operating range of the subject's $\dot{V}_E$ during exercise is reduced. The ventilatory demands, however, are most commonly greater than normal (see Equation 51.7 and Figures 51.1-3). This is a result of a dispersion of ventilation:perfusion ($\dot{V}_A/\dot{Q}$) ratios in the lung causing V_D/V_T to be high (20,41); often the ventilatory equivalent for CO_2 ($\dot{V}_E/\dot{V}CO_2$) is further increased as a result of the consequent arterial hypoxemia (20, 41,42). However, some patients with COPD, predominantly of the bronchitic type, can have higher-than-normal $PaCO_2$.

The combination of increased ventilatory demands during exercise and decreased maximum attainable $\dot{V}_E$ leads to the *breathing reserve* (BR)—defined as the difference between the resting MVV and the maximum $\dot{V}_E$ attained during exercise—being close to or even less than zero (Figure 51.4) in patients with COPD (42). This results in the predominant symptom limiting exercise tolerance in COPD: dyspnea (3,20,23,42). Healthy, moderately fit subjects, even at maximum exercise

- do not achieve spontaneously generated airflows that reach the levels attained during a forced expiratory maneuver (Figure 51.5),
- attain $\dot{V}_E$ greater than 80% of MVV only rarely and almost never attain values of 90% of MVV (Figure 51.4),
- do not increase end-expiratory lung volume (EELV)—it is comonly reduced below resting levels (Figure 51.5), and
- only rarely report dyspnea as the cause of the exercise limitation (Figure 51.2).

Subjects with COPD on the other hand commonly

- achieve spontaneous expiratory airflows that equal or even exceed (2,43) that achieved at a

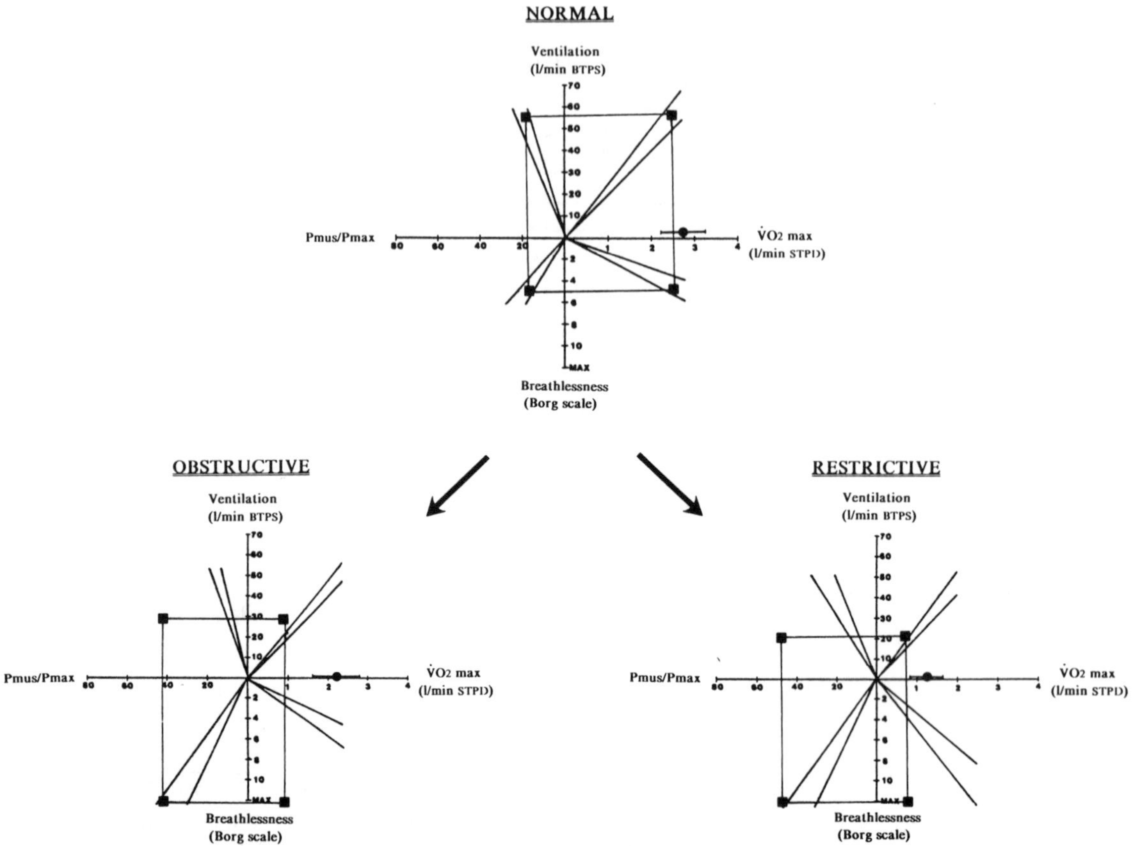

Figure 51.2 Schematic representation of the influence of ventilation ($\dot{V}_E$) and inspiratory muscle force (expressed as a percentage of the maximal inspiratory muscle force that can be generated volitionally) (Pmus/Pmax) on breathlessness (Borg scale) for maximal exercise (• represents predicted maximal $\dot{V}O_2 \pm 1$ SD). **Upper panel**: healthy subject; **lower left panel**: patient with obstructive pulmonary disease; **lower right panel**: patient with restrictive pulmonary disease. Note that, for the healthy subject, all responses lie within the normal prediction bands. However, the impaired pulmonary-mechanical function of both the obstructive and restrictive patients exacerbates the inspiratory muscle force requirement and, in turn, the intensity of breathlessness. See text for further details. Modified with permission from Killian and Jones. Clin. Chest Med. **5**: 99-108; 1984.

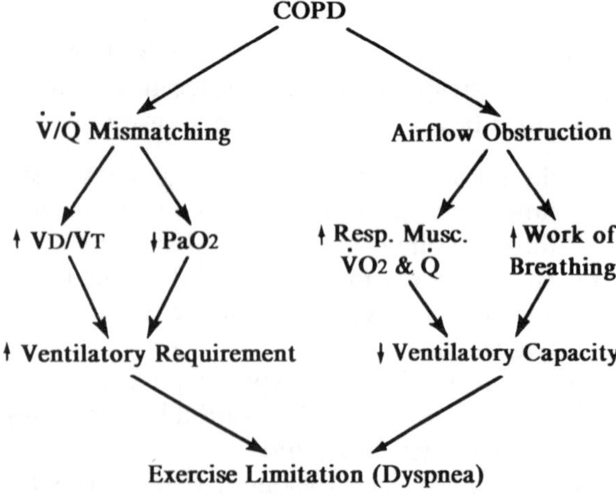

Figure 51.3 Factors leading to exercise limitation in the COPD patient. See text for further details. Modified with permission from Wasserman et al. Principles of exercise testing and interpretation. Philadelphia: Lea & Febiger; 1987.

given lung volume during a maximal flow-volume maneuver (Figure 51.5);

- approach closely or even exceed (2,43) the MVV during exercise (Figure 51.4);
- increase EELV (25,43) (Figure 51.5), although this may not be apparent when there is also significant impairment in inspiratory airflow; and
- cite dyspnea as the cause of exercise termination (20,42), but not invariably (20) (Figure 51.2).

There are three reasons, which potentially interplay, that explain the seeming paradox of expiratory airflow during exercise exceeding that generated during a maximal expiratory effort at rest (2,43):

1. some bronchodilatation can occur during the exercise as a result of increased concentrations of circulating catecholamines;
2. during the forced maneuver from total lung capacity (TLC), the fast time-constant units

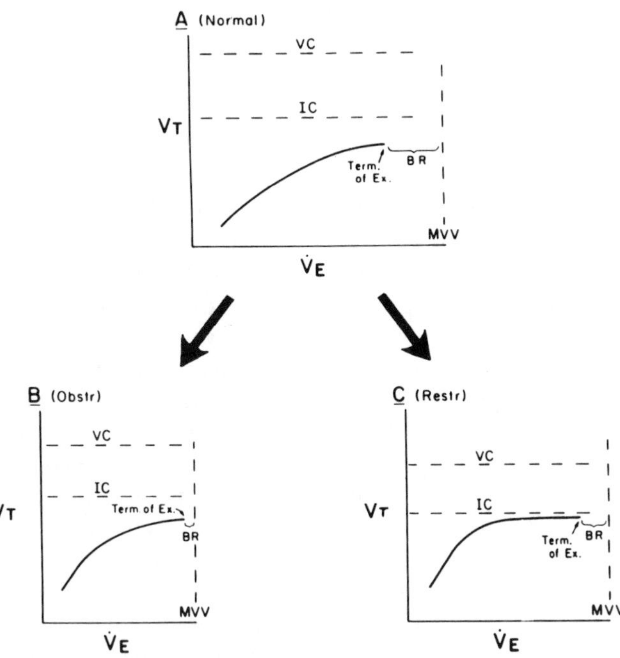

Figure 51.4 Tidal volume (V_T) as a function of ventilation ($\dot{V}_E$) during maximal incremental exercise for a normal subject (**A**), a patient with obstructive pulmonary disease (**B**), and a patient with restrictive pulmonary disease (**C**). Note that V_T at the termination of exercise is less than the inspiratory capacity (IC) for the normal subject and the obstructive patient, but approaches IC in the restrictive patient. In contrast, while both the normal subject and the restrictive patient attain a maximum exercise $\dot{V}_E$ that is well below the corresponding maximum voluntary ventilation (MVV), the maximum exercise $\dot{V}_E$ approaches MVV in the obstructive patient (i.e., the breathing reserve approaches zero). Modified with permission from Wasserman et al. Principles of exercise testing and interpretation. Philadelphia: Lea & Febiger; 1987.

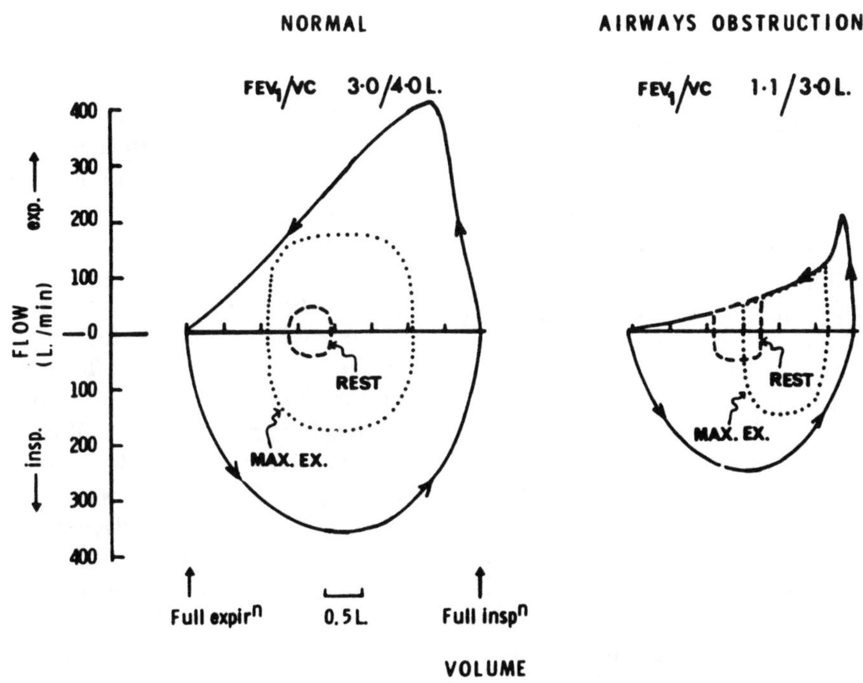

Figure 51.5 Spontaneous flow-volume curves from a normal subject (**left**) and a COPD patient (**right**) at rest (dashed lines) and at maximal exercise (dotted lines). Note that for the COPD patient the maximal exercise curve impacts on the volitionally generated maximal flow-volume curve; this is not the case for the normal subject. See text for further details. From Leaver and Pride. Scand. J. Respir. Dis. [Suppl.]. 77:23-27; 1971. Used by permission.

of the lung empty at high lung volumes, leaving the longer time-constant units to empty at lower lung volumes. When these less-than-maximum lung volumes are attained during spontaneous breathing during exercise, the fast time-constant units can now begin to empty at the lower lung volumes, resulting in greater airflow—at *that* lung volume. This is likely significant because similarly greater airflows are generated in such patients when the forced exhalation is begun at less than TLC (i.e., when a "partial flow-volume curve" is generated); and

3. in patients with COPD, the maximum expiratory airflow is not achieved with a maximum expiratory effort—this is especially the case at low lung volumes. This is a consequence of dynamic airway compression and even closure, in some cases, during the forced maneuver.

The following question and its answer may prove illustrative in this regard: What is the maximum frequency of breathing that would allow a subject to exhale passively to the normal end-expiratory lung volume, without having to accelerate expiratory airflow by contraction of expiratory muscles? To answer the question, the notion of the time constant for the passive thoracic recoil (τrec) and its determinants is crucial. First the thorax, having been distended to a higher volume by inspiratory muscle contraction, will passively recoil (i.e., neither accelerated by expiratory muscle action nor braked by inspiratory muscle action) to its equilibrium position at functional residual capacity (FRC) (assumed here to equal EELV) in approximately four time constants. That is, in one time constant it will recoil 63% of the way back to FRC, in two it will recoil 86.5%, in three 95%, and in four 98.2%. The value for the thoracic mechanical time constant, however, is determined by the thoracic compliance (C) and resistance (R) of the airways and a small component of tissue flow resistance. That is,

$$\tau(s) = R(\text{cm } H_2O \cdot L^{-1} \cdot s) \cdot C(L \cdot \text{cm } H_2O^{-1}) = s \qquad [51.9]$$

Normal values for R and C are about 2 cm $H_2O \cdot L^{-1} \cdot s$ and about 0.2 L · cm H_2O^{-1}, respectively, giving τrec about or equal to 0.4 s. To empty the lung passively back to FRC therefore takes (4 × 0.4) s or 1.6 s. Assuming inspiratory and expiratory durations (T_I and T_E, respectively) to be approximately equal, then the required total breath duration (Ttot) is about or equal to 3 s or the breath frequency about or equal to 20 min^{-1}.

Imagine that τrec in the patient with COPD is doubled. This of course will represent only the average of values for τrec from different lung regions, but for illustrative purposes we choose the average as being doubled—either because of an increase in R, C, or both. Thus, clearly if τrec = 0.8 s, then (4 × 0.8) or 3.2 s is needed for T_E, requiring Ttot to be about or equal to 6 s or f about or equal to 10 min^{-1} (i.e., close to resting levels).

At even modest levels of exercise, therefore, either the expiratory muscles must accelerate airflow or EELV must increase. The latter begins at relatively low work rates, and the former can be sufficiently marked so that expiratory airflow limitation can occur (2,44). It appears, however, that such patients do not develop pleural pressures in excess of those needed to attain this limiting flow (13,25,34), which would increase respiratory muscle work without further increasing expiratory flow. Another strategy to reduce the need for the problematic, positive pleural pressures in such patients is to conserve a large portion of the breath for exhalation by shortening inspiratory duration, that is, reducing the inspiratory duty cycle, T_I/Ttot. This is indeed a strategy adopted during exercise by subjects with COPD, although surprisingly it is only invoked in relatively severe cases (44), T_I/Ttot falling to 0.3–0.4 and in some extreme cases as low as 0.2. T_I/Ttot in patients with mild to moderate COPD has repeatedly been demonstrated to be within the normal range of 0.4 to 0.5 (6,39,43).

The reduction in T_I in these conditions results in an increase in mean inspiratory flow (V_T/T_I) and hence increased inspiratory work and power. Consequently, the increased V_T/T_I associated with an increased EELV (which tends to reduce the mechanical advantage of the inspiratory muscles) imposes greater energy demands on the inspiratory muscles during exercise thereby increasing their propensity to fatigue. This is the basis for the apparently anomolous strategy of attempts to improve *inspiratory* muscle function to benefit patients with impairment of *expiratory* flow generation. However, in addition to the increased energy demands on the inspiratory muscles during exercise, patients with COPD have inspiratory muscle weakness (16,38). In fact, unloading the inspiratory muscles during exercise by means of continuous airway positive pressure (CPAP) in COPD patients was found to improve the tolerable duration of submaximal exercise (29) (for discussion see 16). Petrof, Calderini, and Gottfried (33) have demonstrated that CPAP actually does unload the inspiratory muscles in such patients.

Other factors can also contribute to reduced exercise tolerance in patients with COPD, including coexistent heart disease, impaired venous return, pulmonary hypertension, nutritional deficiencies, and detraining as a result of low-activity patterns of daily living.

As the attainment of limiting expiratory airflow and maximal ventilation and associated dyspnea sets the upper limit for exercise tolerance, other of the body's energy supply systems may not be stressed to their limits (20,42). Consequently, maximum heart rate and O_2-pulse are often markedly less than predicted in such patients despite the tendency for arterial hypoxemia to increase these functions. That is, the *heart rate reserve* (HRR), defined as the difference between the predicted maximum HR and that actually measured at the limit of exercise tolerance (42), is greater than normal. The resting hypoxemia is predominantly a consequence of mismatching of $\dot{V}_A$ and $\dot{Q}$ in patients with COPD (20,41), with an additional hypoventilatory component in those who also retain CO_2. Although the pattern of blood-gas response to muscular exercise is highly variable in these subjects (41), in many cases the resting levels of PaO_2 can even be maintained with no further hypoxemia (42). There is no clear evidence that the degree or pattern of the $\dot{V}_A/\dot{Q}$ inequality becomes worse during the low levels of exercise attainable in these patients (11,37,41). What does appear clear in this patient group is that O_2 diffusion limitation across the alveolar-capillary bed is not a significant contributing factor to the hypoxemia either at rest or during exercise (41) even in those patients whose carbon monoxide diffusing capacity (D_LCO) is reduced. Furthermore, in those patients who are capable of generating a metabolic acidosis by increasing blood lactate during high-intensity exercise, there is little or no respiratory compensation owing to the obstructive constraint on ventilation (10,42).

It is, of course, only part of the challenge to determine—through appropriate strategies of exercise testing—the cause of the exercise intolerance in patients with COPD. It is also important to improve where possible both physiological function and the range of tolerable physical activities.

If a subject performs a range of particular high-intensity work rates (W) to the limit of tolerance (t) on a cycle ergometer, then a power-duration curve may be constructed. This relationship has been shown to be hyperbolic, of the form

$$(W - \Theta F) \cdot t = W' \qquad [51.10]$$

where ΘF is the asymptote on the power axis and W' is a constant with the units of work. ΘF, or the fatigue threshold, therefore represents the demarcation between the range of power outputs for which there is no fatigue (i.e., less than ΘF) of the kind that limits the tolerable duration in the fatiguing range (i.e., greater than ΘF). Consequently, ΘF, which may be considered to represent the upper limit of sustainable power generation for this kind of exercise, has been shown to represent the highest work rate at which $\dot{V}O_2$ and the increased blood lactate can be stabilized. All higher work rates are associated with inexorable increases in these variables toward their maximal values.

A similar series of tests can be imposed on the respiratory muscles. This is typically achieved by having the subject match a target ventilation by volitional hyperpnea for as long as possible, with precautions taken to prevent hypocapnia by adding appropriate amounts of CO_2 to the inspirate. This results in a basically similar pattern of response.

And so, despite the recognition (24,43) that

- the level of ventilation may not be a good index of respiratory muscle work rate being performed,
- there is a complex pattern of recruitment and efficiency of contraction of the respiratory muscles during this test, and
- this pattern may not cohere with that spontaneously adopted to produce that level of $\dot{V}_E$ during exercise,

the assumption that the respiratory system compliance and airways resistance are reasonably similar under the two conditions allows the upper limit for sustainable exercise ventilation to be defined by this resting ventilation-duration curve (see Figure 51.6b).

The horizontal asymptote of this ventilation-duration curve (Figure 51.6b) therefore represents the greatest ventilation that is sustainable for prolonged periods by volitional effort; by inference it is also considered the upper limit of $\dot{V}_E$ sustainable for prolonged exercise. This asymptote has been termed the *maximum sustainable ventilatory capacity* or MSVC (5,7). In normal subjects of moderate fitness the MSVC is approximately 55% to 80% of the MVV (15,22,32). This fraction can be higher than normal in patients with COPD (32); furthermore, it represents a very small absolute range of $\dot{V}_E$ owing to the markedly reduced MVV.

When exercise requires ventilations in the range between MSVC and MVV, it is likely to involve a component of respiratory muscle fatigue (3,8, 26,27). Spectral analysis of the diaphragmatic electromyogram during high-intensity exercise has demonstrated patterns consistent with fatigue in patients with COPD (18,30). It is important to recognize that respiratory muscles begin to fatigue above MSVC. However, it is only when they have operated in this zone long enough for the *total* respiratory work above MSVC to reach the value of the curvature constant of the relationship between maximal $\dot{V}_E$ and tolerable time (i.e., the limiting amount of inspiratory work) that respiratory muscle fatigue actually limits the exercise.

This concept is schematized in Figure 51.6. As shown in Figure 51.6c, time zero for the putative onset of respiratory muscle fatigue is when the $\dot{V}_E$ attained during the incremental exercise test starts to exceed MSVC. When $\dot{V}_E$ actually reaches the fatigue curve (i.e., point [i]), the fatigue is not limiting. This is because the limit of fatigue would only occur at this $\dot{V}_E$ had it been sustained at this level for this time; that is, $\dot{V}_E$ = (area Y + area X). But the actual $\dot{V}_E$ above MSVC during the exercise is only area X. $\dot{V}_E$ can continue until area Z = area Y. At this point, the $\dot{V}_E$ attained is greater than that on the MSVC curve, but the total $\dot{V}_E$ in this fatiguing region would end at a time equivalent to point (ii) on the resting MSVC curve.

Attempts to train the respiratory muscles using isocapnic, target hyperpnea techniques and increased resistive loads have proved successful at improving both respiratory muscle strength and endurance (manifest as an increased MSVC) in subjects with COPD. However, the benefits in terms of improved exercise tolerance are not as clear, where some investigators find improvements and others do not (see 3,44 for discussion). The differences may reflect differences in the training protocols and also the use of appropriate control groups.

The use of more traditional forms of physical training to improve skeletal muscle (i.e., nonrespiratory, at least by design) and cardiovascular function in patients with COPD is traditionally considered of limited benefit because

- the training does not significantly alter lung mechanics (i.e., the limits are unchanged);
- there is only a small component, if any, of metabolic trainability as evidenced by the low blood lactate and heart rate at maximum exercise; and
- there is a lack of improvement in aerobic enzyme profiles as a result of endurance training (4) (i.e., such patients are unable to train at an intensity sufficient to elicit a training response).

Recently, however, Casaburi et al. (10) have provided evidence that challenges this conventional wisdom. They demonstrated (confirming a previous report by Sue, Wasserman, Moricca, and

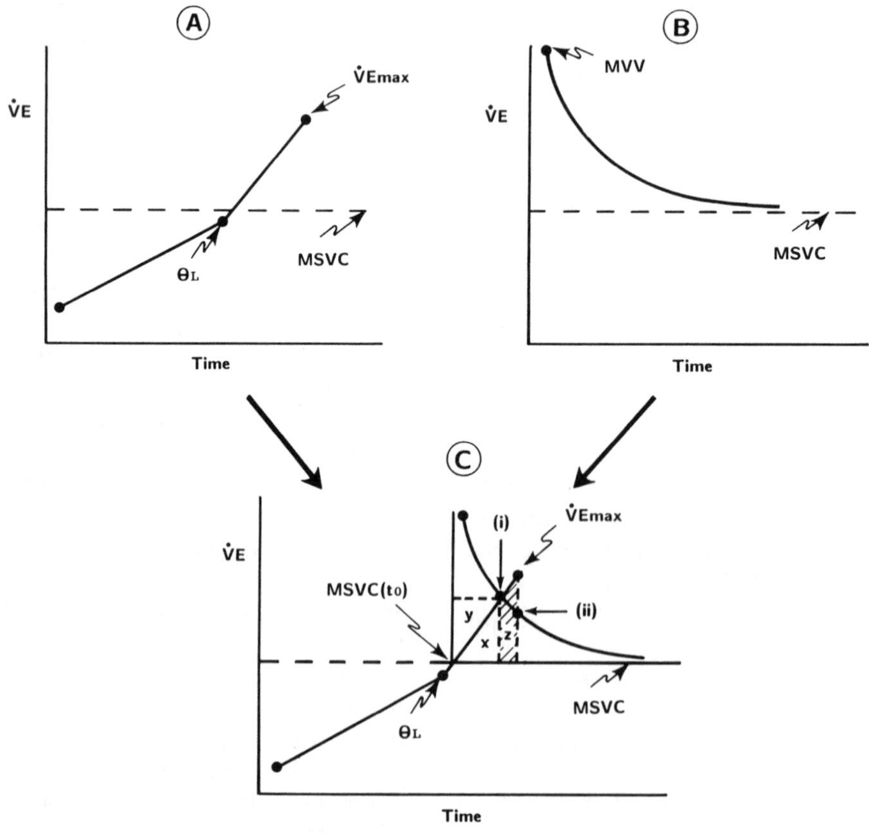

Figure 51.6 Influence of the temporal profile of the ventilatory ($\dot{V}_E$) response to incremental exhausting exercise (**panel A**) and the relationship between maximal $\dot{V}_E$ and tolerable time (**panel B**) in determining the relationship between the onset of respiratory muscle fatigue and the maximal sustainable ventilatory capacity (MSVC). θ_L represents the lactate threshold. See text for further details.

Casaburi [40]) that many of their patients with COPD did increase blood lactate appreciably, beginning at "surprisingly low levels of exercise," and achieving values up to 10 mEq $\cdot$ L^{-1} in some cases at the highest tolerated work rates, often resulting in arterial pH below 7.30. (Gallagher [16] presents evidence of several other studies that support this notion.) The magnitude of this lactate increase, however, was not well related to the subjects' forced expiratory flow in 1 s (FEV_1). This is presumably one important factor in explaining why the FEV_1 is a relatively good predictor of both MVV and of maximal $\dot{V}_E$ during exercise in such patients, yet so poor an index of actual exercise tolerance. Some subjects with a particular FEV_1 might generate high blood lactate and require additional ventilation; this brings them to their $\dot{V}_E$ limit sooner. Others do not, and therefore can tolerate a higher work rate before their limiting ventilation is attained.

When the subjects in this study underwent a physical-training program, which required participation for 5 days per week for 8 weeks, ventilation for a standardized exercise task was decreased by an amount that correlated significantly ($r = .73, p < .005$) with the training-induced reduction in blood lactate. Exercise tolerance was consequently increased both for maximal-incremental and high constant-load exercise (Figure 51.7). This study further showed that high-intensity training produced strikingly greater training effects than low-intensity training, even though the total work performed during the training period was the same.

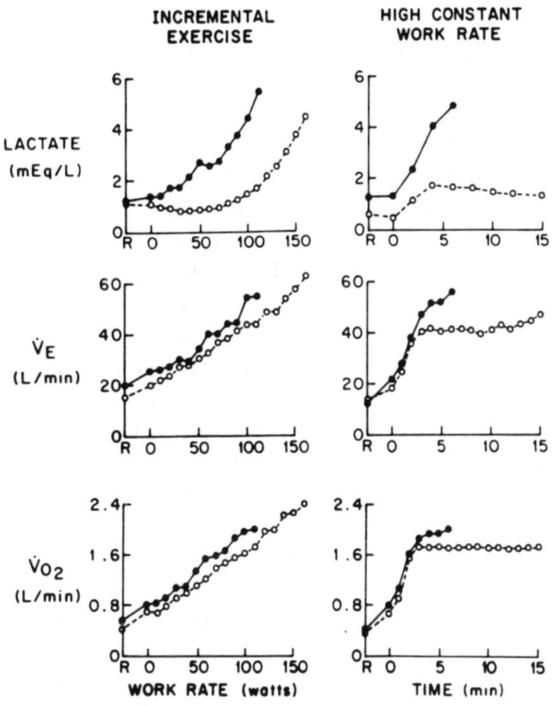

Figure 51.7 Temporal response profiles of arterial [lactate], ventilation ($\dot{V}_E$), and O_2 uptake ($\dot{V}O_2$) of a COPD patient to incremental exhausting exercise (10 Watts $\cdot$ min^{-1}) (**left panel**) and high-intensity constant-load exercise (**right panel**) before (•) and after (o) participation in an exercise training program. See text for further details. Modified with permission from Casaburi et al. Am. Rev. Respir. Dis. **143**:9-18; 1991.

One inference of this study is that such training would be of most benefit in the subgroup of COPD patients who can exercise to levels that engender a significant metabolic acidosis. It may also help explain differences between previous training studies, very few of which demonstrated physiologic benefits of training in COPD patients (9).

Jones and Killian (20) have stressed that an increase in exercise tolerance is a primary objective in the management of such patients, and suggest the following options for a particular patient:

- Reduced respiratory impedance (e.g., use of bronchodilators)
- Reduction in ventilation (endurance training, O_2 therapy)
- Increased respiratory muscle strength and endurance (ventilatory muscle training, use of xanthines) and
- Changes in the pattern of force deployment (education)

The options listed by Belman (3) are virtually identical: intensity of exercise, type of exercise, oxygen administration, energy-saving techniques, and breathing retraining.

The goal, therefore, is to try to achieve the possible functional improvements that will allow patients with chronic lung disease to enjoy the lifestyle benefits of a wide range of physical activities. For further discussion of appropriate physical-training strategies in patients with COPD the reader is referred to Farinearz and Mahler (14) and Patessio, Ioli, and Donner (31).

Restrictive Lung Disease

Pulmonary diseases such as diffuse interstitial fibrosis result in increased pulmonary and hence thoracic elastance (Equation 51.1); that is, reduced compliance. This requires greater inspiratory muscle force development, more negative pleural pressures, and greater respiratory work to effect the same inspiratory volume. The increased elastance leads to total lung capacity (TLC), vital capacity (VC), FRC, and residual volume (RV) all being low. This both predisposes to and, in fact, effects a typical pattern of low tidal volume response to exercise. Jones and Rebuck (21) have reported that the maximum V_T attained during exercise in patients with diffuse fibrosing alveolitis is reduced in proportion to the reduced vital capacity. In six patients who increased their vital capacity as the alveolitis improved, so did the maximum exercise V_T. These authors (21) and others (17) therefore suggest that the lung appears to behave more as if it is small rather than intrinsically "stiff." This in turn results in high breathing frequencies and consequently more-rapid, shallow breathing, which compounds the $\dot{V}_A/\dot{Q}$ effects on V_D/V_T (41), leading to overall ventilation being high at a given metabolic rate in restrictive lung disease (23,42,44).

Although V_T is relatively low during exercise in patients with restrictive lung disease, the tidal volume-to-inspiratory capacity ratio, V_T/IC (where IC is measured at rest), is markedly high; at maximum exercise, it approaches 1.0 (see Figure 48.4) with respiratory frequencies of greater than 50 min^{-1} being common (42). This can be achieved because respiratory muscle strength is not reduced in this disease state (12,44). Maximum exercise $\dot{V}_E$ often approximates MVV (42) and, in addition to the effects of the hypoxemia, results in dyspnea, which is the dominant symptom in such patients (23,42). The breathing reserve is therefore low and the heart rate reserve high in such patients at maximum exercise. We stress that IC is that measured at rest, as the effects of exercise on EELV in restrictive lung disease have not been well characterized.

As the disease is nonuniform, there can be significant pulmonary gas exchange abnormalities during exercise. Arterial hypoxemia typically worsens as the work rate increases—not, it appears, because the $\dot{V}_A/\dot{Q}$ maldistribution (which is the predominant cause of the hypoxemia in this condition) worsens further (41), but because of the diffusional component of the alveolar-to-arterial PO_2 difference, (A-a)PO_2. This results in the typical progressive hypoxemia as work rate increases in patients with restrictive lung disease (41,42). resulting in (A-a)PO_2 rising to 60 mmHg or more at maximum exercise. This can also be exacerbated as Wagner and Gale (41) point out by abnormally large decreases in mixed venous PO_2 consequent to an inadequate cardiovascular response to exercise. CO_2 retention, however, is not a common consequence, although it can be seen in advanced cases.

Abnormalities of airflow generation are not an inherent feature of restrictive lung diseases, but they can occur in patients with coexistent COPD. The net effect is that exercise tolerance can be markedly affected in this condition, with severe dyspnea at relatively low work rates (see Figure 51.2).

Asthma

Bronchial asthma is also a chronic obstructive lung disease, but unlike the categories discussed above it is not in most cases chronic and persistent; rather, it is most often chronic and spasmodic. That is, the acute exacerbation of the disease is triggered by a wide range of intrinsic and extrinsic factors, with exercise falling into the latter category. During the asthmatic "attack," the consequent airways obstruction—the result of inflammation, bronchoconstriction, and the secretion of copious, sticky mucus that plugs or narrows the bronchioles—limits both inspiratory and expiratory airflow, reducing the maximum achievable ventilation and predisposing to dyspnea. In extreme cases, it is life-threatening.

However, unlike the pulmonary emphysematous and chronic bronchitic forms of COPD for which the condition itself is not made worse by exercise, significant exacerbation of the asthma can be triggered by the exercise itself (1,19,28). Importantly, the exercise-induced bronchoconstriction can occur in subjects who do not have a history or even a recognition of airway hyperreactivity (19). Exercise-induced asthma (EIA) is considered to be present when there is a reduction of 10% to 20% or more in forced expiratory flow indexes, such as FEV_1 or peak expiratory flow rate (PEFR) as a result of muscular exercise.

The bronchoconstriction triggered by high-intensity exercise is typically a postexercise phenomenon reaching a peak of intensity at some 5 to 15 min of recovery and not resolving for as much as 1 hr. During this period the reduction in forced expiratory airflow is associated with arterial hypoxemia (41), which is a consequence of increased dispersion of $\dot{V}_A/\dot{Q}$. It is not unusual for actual improved airflow in the early recovery period thought to be mediated by the increased concentration of circulating catecholamines. Interestingly, following the resolution of the bronchospastic episode, many patients actually become relatively refractory to the effects of subsequent exercise for a short period (19). It has also been demonstrated that a prior exercise warm-up at moderate levels is useful in ameliorating the intensity of EIA provoked by subsequent high levels of exercise (36).

The most widely held theory for the mechanism of the exercise-induced component of the bronchospasm is the loss of bronchiolar heat and water as a result of a failure of the upper airways to humidify and heat the inspired air to body temperature at high levels of airflow. The precise mechanism whereby increased bronchiolar heat and water loss triggers the EIA remains a topic of debate. The interested reader is referred to the work of McFadden (28) and Anderson, Daviskas, and Smith (1) for insightful analyses of the issue. There is little disagreement, however, that the important predisposing conditions involve high levels of ventilation (with the consequent hypocapnia also a possible contributing factor) and breathing of cold, dry air.

Exercise itself is, of course, the most appropriate challenge to determine the presence and severity of EIA; however, other techniques of bronchoprovocation are standardly used to assess the bronchial hyperreactivity thought to predispose to the EIA. The most common challenge is to inhale histamine or methacholine. Using the methacholine bronchoprovocation test Huftel, Gaddy, and Busse (19) found an appreciably higher incidence of bronchial hyperresponsiveness in college athletes than could be predicted on the basis of a history of asthma. The importance of these findings is that more athletes might benefit from appropriate preexercise medication than are actually aware of it.

Although postexercise bronchospasm naturally reduces the functional capacity to perform a subsequent bout of high-intensity exercise, any bronchospasm prior to or during exercise similarly leads to reduced exercise tolerance. Medications are therefore commonly used prior to exercise. However, considerable care should be exercised in the choice of this ameliorating medication prior to athletic competition; some asthma drugs are approved for this use—at least at the international level—whereas others are prohibited (19). For example, inhaled beta$_2$-adrenergic agonists are permitted, whereas in ingested form they are not. Inhaled corticosteroids are permitted, but in oral, intramuscular, or intravenous forms they are not. Nonnarcotic analygesics and antitussives are approved, but narcotic analgesics (including codeine) and antitussives are banned.

Many asthmatic subjects have controlled their condition and attained great success in international athletic competition and serve as stimulating role models for others with this condition.

Conclusion

Subjects manifest work (or, more properly, power) intolerance when they are unable to sustain a given work rate sufficiently long for the successful completion of the task. The physiological systems, whose interactions sustain the energy transfer processes, need to function appropriately in order to allow a sufficiently wide range of physical activities to be undertaken to provide a satisfying lifestyle.

The tolerable range of work rates in patients with lung disease is constrained by a combination of factors, chief of which are

1. impaired pulmonary-mechanical and gas exchange function that increases the demand for airflow and ventilation;
2. limitations in response capabilities, either of airflow generation or of lung distention;
3. increased physiological costs of meeting the ventilatory responses, in terms of respiratory muscle work, blood flow, and O_2 consumption;
4. predisposition to shortness of breath or dyspnea as a consequence of the high fraction of the achievable ventilation demanded by the work rate, and commonly exacerbated by arterial hypoxemia; and
5. the often-marked reduction in the range of spontaneously selected daily activities that results from the dyspnea and further reduces the state of physical training.

Strategies designed to increase exercise tolerance in such patients should therefore attempt to increase (where possible) the ventilatory limits, reduce the demand for ventilation, and reduce the intensity of, or attempt to desensitize the subject to, the consequent dyspnea.

References

1. Anderson, S.D.; Daviskas, E.; Smith, C.M. Exercise-induced asthma: A difference in opinion regarding the stimulus. Allerg. Proc. 10:215-226; 1989.
2. Beck, K.C.; Staats, B.A.; Hyatt, R.E. Dynamics of breathing during exercise. In: Whipp, B.J.; Wasserman, K., eds. Pulmonary physiology and pathophysiology of exercise. New York: Dekker; 1991:67-97.
3. Belman, M.J. Exercise in chronic obstructive pulmonary disease. In: Ryan, A.J.; Allman, F.L., Jr., eds. Sports medicine. New York: Academic Press; 1989:647-669.
4. Belman, M.J.; Kendregan, B.A. Exercise training fails to increase skeletal muscle enzymes in patients with chronic obstructive pulmonary disease. Am. Rev. Respir. Dis. 123:256-261; 1981.
5. Belman, M.J.; Mittman, C. Ventilatory muscle training improves exercise capacity in chronic obstructive pulmonary disease patients. Am. Rev. Respir. Dis. 121:273-280; 1980.
6. Bradley, G.W.; Crawford, R. Regulation of breathing during exercise in normal subjects

and in chronic lung disease. Clin. Sci. Mol. Med. 51:575-582; 1976.

7. Bradley, M.E.; Leith, D.E. Ventilatory muscle training and the oxygen cost of sustained hyperpnea. J. Appl. Physiol. 45:885-892; 1978.
8. Bye, P.T.P.; Farkas, G.A.; Roussos, C. Respiratory factors limiting exercise. Ann. Rev. Physiol. 45:439-451; 1983.
9. Casaburi, R. Exercise training in chronic obstructive lung disease. In: Casaburi, R.; Petty, T.L., eds. Principles and practice of pulmonary rehabilitation. Philadelphia: Saunders; [1992].
10. Casaburi, R.; Patessio, A.; Ioli, F.; Zanaboni, S.; Donner, C.F.; Wasserman, K. Reductions in exercise lactic acidosis and ventilation as a result of exercise training in patients with obstructive lung disease. Am. Rev. Respir. Dis. 143:9-18; 1991.
11. Dantzker, D.R.; D'Alonzo, G.E. The effect of exercise on pulmonary gas exchange in patients with severe chronic obstructive pulmonary disease. Am. Rev. Respir. Dis. 134:1135-1139; 1986.
12. DeTroyer, A.; Yernault, J.-C. Inspiratory muscle force in normal subjects and patients with interstitial lung disease. Thorax. 35:92-100; 1980.
13. Dodd, D.S.; Brancatisano, T.; Engel, L.A. Chest wall mechanics during exercise in patients with severe chronic airflow obstruction. Am. Rev. Respir. Dis. 129:33-38; 1984.
14. Farinearz, K.; Mahler, D.A. Writing an exercise prescription for COPD patients. J. Respir. Dis. 11:638-644; 1990.
15. Freedman, S. Sustained maximum voluntary ventilation. Respir. Physiol. 8:230-244; 1970.
16. Gallagher, C. Exercise and chronic obstructive pulmonary disease. Med. Clin. North Am. 74:619-641; 1990.
17. Gibson, G.J.; Pride, N.B. Pulmonary mechanics in fibrosing alveolitis. The effects of lung shrinkage. Am. Rev. Respir. Dis. 116:637-647; 1977.
18. Grassino, A.; Gross, D.; Macklem, P.T.; Roussos, C.; Zagelbaum, G. Inspiratory muscle fatigue as a factor limiting exercise. Bull. Eur. Physiopathol. Respir. 15:105-111; 1979.
19. Huftel, M.A.; Gaddy, J.N.; Busse, W.W. Finding and managing asthma in competitive athletes. J. Respir. Dis. 12:1110-1112; 1991.
20. Jones, N.L.; Killian, K.J. Exercise in chronic airway obstruction. In: Bouchard, C.; Shephard, R.J.; Stephens, T.; Sutton, J.R.; McPherson, B.D., eds. Exercise, fitness, and health. Champaign, IL: Human Kinetics, 1990:547-559.
21. Jones, N.L.; Rebuck, A.S. Tidal volume during exercise in patients with diffuse fibrosing alveolitis. Bull. Eur. Physiopathol. Respir. 15:321-327; 1979.
22. Keens, T.G.; Krastins, I.R.B.; Wannamaker, E.M.; Levison, H.; Crozier, D.N.; Bryan, A.C. Ventilatory muscle endurance training in normal subjects and patients with cystic fibrosis. Am. Rev. Respir. Dis. 116:853-860; 1977.
23. Killian, K.J.; Jones, N.L. The use of exercise testing and other methods in the investigation of dyspnea. Clin. Chest Med. 5:99-108; 1984.
24. Klas, J.V.; Dempsey, J.A. Voluntary versus reflex regulation of maximal exercise flow: Volume loops. Am. Rev. Respir. Dis. 139:150-156; 1989.
25. Leaver, D.J.; Pride, N.B. Flow-volume curves and expiratory pressures during exercise in patients with chronic airway obstruction. Scand. J. Respir. Dis. [Suppl.]. 77: 23-27; 1971.
26. Leith, D.E.; Bradley, M. Ventilatory muscle strength and endurance training. J. Appl. Physiol. 41:508-516; 1976.
27. McFadden, E.R., Jr. Hypothesis: Exercise-induced asthma as a vascular phenomenon. Lancet. 335:880-883; 1990.
28. Macklem, P.T.; Roussos, C. Respiratory muscle fatigue: A cause of respiratory failure. Clin. Sci. Mol. Med. 53:419-422; 1977.
29. O'Donnell, D.E.; Sanii, R.; Younes, M. Improvement in exercise endurance in patients with chronic airflow limitation using continuous positive airway pressure. Am. Rev. Respir. Dis. 138:1510-1514; 1988.
30. Pardy, R.L.; Rivington, R.N.; Despas, P.J.; Macklem, P.T. The effects of inspiratory muscle training on exercise performance in chronic airflow limitation. Am. Rev. Respir. Dis. 123:426-433; 1981.
31. Patessio, A.; Ioli, F.; Donner, C.F. Exercise prescriptions. In: Casaburi, R.; Petty, T.L., eds. Principles and practice of pulmonary rehabilitation. Philadelphia: Saunders; [1992].
32. Peress, L.; McLean, P.; Woolf, C.R.; Zamel, N. Ventilatory muscle training in obstructive lung disease. Bull. Eur. Physiopathol. Respir. 15:91-92; 1979.
33. Petrof, B.; Calderini, E.; Gottfried, S.B. Continuous positive airway pressure (CPAP) improves respiratory muscle performance and dyspnoea during exercise in severe chronic obstructive pulmonary disease (COPD). Am. Rev. Respir. Dis. 139:A343; 1989.
34. Potter, W.A.; Olafsson, S.; Hyatt, R.E. Ventilatory mechanics and expiratory flow limitation during exercise in patients with obstructive lung disease. J. Clin. Invest. 50:910-919; 1971.
35. Rahn, H.; Fenn, W.O. A graphical analysis of the respiratory gas exchange. The O_2-CO_2 diagram. Washington, DC: American Physiological Society; 1955.

36. Reiff, D.B.; Choudry, N.B.; Pride, N.B.; Ind, P.W. The effect of prolonged submaximal warm-up exercise on exercise-induced asthma. Am. Rev. Respir. Dis. 139:479-484; 1989.
37. Roca, J.; Montserrat, J.M.; Rodriguez-Roisin, R.; Guitart, R.; Torres, A.; Agusti, A.G.N.; Wagner, P.D. Gas exchange response to naloxone in chronic obstructive pulmonary disease with hypercapnic respiratory failure. Bull. Eur. Physiopathol. Respir. 23:249-254; 1987.
38. Rochester, D.F.; Braun, N.M.T. Determinants of maximal inspiratory pressure in chronic obstructive pulmonary disease. Am. Rev. Respir. Dis. 132:42-47; 1985.
39. Schanning, J. Respiratory cycle time during exercise in patients with chronic obstructive lung disease. Scand. J. Respir. Dis. 59:313-318; 1978.
40. Sue, D.Y.; Wasserman, K.; Moricca, R.B.; Casaburi, R. Metabolic acidosis during exercise in patients with chronic obstructive pulmonary disease. Chest. 94:931-938; 1988.
41. Wagner, P.D.; Gale, G.E. Ventilation-perfusion relationships. In: Whipp, B.J.; Wasserman, K., eds. Pulmonary physiology and pathophysiology of exercise. New York: Dekker, 1991:121-142.
42. Wasserman, K.; Hansen, J.E.; Sue, D.Y.; Whipp, B.J. Principles of exercise testing and interpretation. Philadelphia: Lea & Febiger; 1987.
43. Whipp, B.J.; Pardy, R. Breathing during exercise. In: Macklem, P.; Mead, J., eds. Handbook of physiology, respiration (pulmonary mechanics). Washington, DC: American Physiological Society; 1986:605-629.
44. Younes, M. Determinants of thoracic excursions during exercise. In: Whipp, B.J.; Wasserman, K., eds. Pulmonary physiology and pathophysiology of exercise. New York: Dekker, 1991:1-65.

Chapter 52

Physical Activity, Fitness, and Kidney Disease

Andrew P. Goldberg
Herschel R. Harter

The quality of life and survival of patients with end-stage renal disease (ESRD) is limited by inadequate rehabilitation and the accelerated development of atherosclerosis and its cardiovascular complications (11,20,31). A survey of 2,481 patients on maintenance dialysis indicated that only 60% of nondiabetic and 23% of diabetic patients were capable of participation in physical activity beyond that requiring self-care (20). In another survey, fewer than 50% of dialysis patients worked, more than 80% could not participate in vigorous activities, and most had a poor quality of life, with one third living below the poverty level (11).

The reduced functional capacity of patients with chronic renal failure is caused by the accumulation of uremic toxins in the blood and the development of abnormalities in cardiovascular, endocrine-metabolic, musculoskeletal, neurological, and hematological function. These patients frequently have hypertension, left ventricular hypertrophy, hyperlipidemia, glucose intolerance, and hyperinsulinemia, all risk factors for the development of atherosclerotic cardiovascular disease (CVD) (14). The longer patients with chronic renal failure require maintenance dialysis, the more limited their functional capacity and quality of life become. After 10 years of hemodialysis the rate of CVD complications in dialysis patients approaches that of nonuremic subjects with multiple risk factors for atherosclerosis (14,31).

Exercise training reduces risk factors for CVD in nonuremic individuals by (a) lowering blood pressure; (b) improving lipoprotein lipid profiles, glucose tolerance, and insulin sensitivity; and (c) enhancing cardiovascular function indexed by a rise in maximal aerobic capacity ($\dot{V}O_2$max) (30). The prevalence of these conditions and the exceedingly sedentary lifestyle of patients with ESRD led to measurement of their $\dot{V}O_2$max and evaluation of the physiological effects of exercise training (21,23,33).

Although most studies were of short duration in small numbers of patients, the improvement in $\dot{V}O_2$max and psychosocial functioning and the reduction in risk factors for CVD suggested that exercise training has the potential to reduce morbidity and mortality and improve the quality of life in patients with chronic renal failure. The purpose of this chapter is to examine the relationship of physical activity and physical fitness to physiological and psychological function in patients with chronic renal failure and to determine the health-related benefits of exercise training in this chronically ill, debilitated population.

Physiology of Exercise in Patients With Chronic Renal Failure

Chronic renal failure (CRF) results from damage to the kidney as a result of a number of diseases including hypertension, chronic infections, diabetes mellitus, autoimmune processes, interstitial disease, and the attendant syndromes of glomerular hyperfiltration. The rate of decline in the glomerular filtration rate can be modified by (a) adequate treatment of hypertension; (b) reducing protein intake; (c) normalizing calcium, phosphate, parathyroid hormone, and vitamin D metabolism; (d) correcting hyperlipidemia; and (e) treating comorbid diseases such as diabetes mellitus and vasculitis. Nevertheless, despite these interventional maneuvers, CRF often progresses to ESRD and necessitates dialysis, transplantation, or intensive medical treatment for long-term survival. Unfortunately, many of these treatments actually may enhance the risk for comorbid events in these patients. The multisystemic effects of CRF cause organ function to decline leading to comorbidity that modifies the rehabilitative potential and exercise capacity of dialysis patients (Table 52.1).

The quantity of aerobic muscular work that can be achieved during maximum physical exertion is measured as the $\dot{V}O_2$max, an index of the ability

Table 52.1 Multisystem Dysfunction in End-Stage Renal Disease

Cardiovascular
- Atherosclerotic heart disease
- Hypertension, left-ventricular hypertrophy
- Cardiomyopathy
- Conduction abnormalities, arrhythmias
- Pericarditis with or without effusion
- Congestive heart failure (volume overload)

Endocrine-metabolic
- Insulin resistance (glucose intolerance, hyperinsulinemia)
- Dyslipoproteinemias
- Abnormal bone, mineral, and vitamin D metabolism
- Hyperparathyroidism
- Sexual dysfunction

Electrolyte and acid-base imbalance
- Abnormal volume (hyper- and hypovolemia)
- Abnormal acid-base metabolism (acidosis)
- Abnormal cation metabolism (calcium, magnesium)
- Hyperkalemia
- Hyperphosphatemia

Neurological
- Neuropathy
- Myopathy
- Uremic encephalopathy
- Autonomic dysfunction
- Cerebrovascular disease
- Progressive dementia

Hematological
- Anemia
- Coagulopathy with bleeding diathesis
- Neutrophil dysfunction (infections)
- Impaired, delayed hypersensitivity

Psychological
- Cognitive-motor dysfunction
- Depression, hostility, anger
- Anxiety, hopelessness

of the cardiovascular system to deliver oxygen and blood to working muscles and for these muscles to use oxygen and energy to perform work. The $\dot{V}O_2max$ is determined by the product of cardiac output and the extraction of oxygen per unit of blood by muscle and other tissues during exercise, the arteriovenous oxygen, $(a\text{-}v)O_2$, difference. In patients with ESRD the pathologic and metabolic consequences of uremia impair cardiovascular and muscular responses to exercise, reducing $\dot{V}O_2max$ (Figure 52.1). In these patients volume overload reduces cardiac output and the delivery of oxygen and nutrients to peripheral tissues; furthermore, a high-output cardiac state caused by anemia, hypoxemia, and the arteriovenous fistula itself impairs cardiac function by increasing intravascular pressure and volume overload to cause hypertension. Hypertension and increased vascular resistance raise intravascular pressure and along with volume overload cause left ventricular hypertrophy and abnormal systolic and diastolic ventricular function. Insulin resistance, hyperlipidemia, abnormalities of carbohydrate metabolism, and dyslipoproteinemia coupled with hypertension accelerate the development of atherosclerosis promoting coronary insufficiency and leading to development of a cardiomyopathy in these patients.

A reduction in cardiac output caused by the metabolic acidosis, hyperkalemia, hypercalcemia, hypermagnesemia, and autonomic dysfunction in patients with ESRD worsens left ventricular function by decreasing left ventricular contractility and increasing the risk of lethal arrhythmias. Volume overload and increased left atrial pressure cause pulmonary vascular pressure to rise, which further reduces cardiac output. All of these factors aggravate the already existent cardiac disease seen in these patients, increasing susceptibility to pulmonary congestion and congestive heart failure.

The abnormalities in cardiac function in patients with ESRD are further aggravated during acute exercise because of a blunted heart rate and myocardial contractile response to catecholamines released during acute exercise. This reduces stroke volume and maximal cardiac output, leading to early muscular fatigue because of reduced blood flow and substrate and oxygen delivery to peripheral tissues. Reduced levels of oxyhemoglobin and substrate transport across the cytosol—due to decreased tissue levels of carnitine acyl transferase—further impair oxygen and substrate delivery to muscle during exercise. Thus, the physical work capacity of patients with ESRD also is impaired by abnormalities in muscle metabolism, which lead to weakness and decreased exercise tolerance.

The in vivo evaluation of muscle metabolism in man is difficult, therefore several in vitro muscle preparations have been used to elucidate the abnormalities in muscle metabolism in uremia. These studies used either isolated muscle preparations or isolated, perfused hindquarters from uremic rats to show that uremia is associated with an increased release of the noncatabolic amino acids, phenylalanine, and tyrosine indicative of an increase in muscle protein catabolism (24). In contrast, protein synthesis is not affected by uremia (13). Uremic toxins were proposed as the primary mechanisms responsible for the increased catabolism of muscle protein in uremia, but recent data show that decreased protein intake, metabolic acidosis, altered vitamin D and parathyroid hormone metabolism, and insulin resistance all contribute to the markedly increased protein catabolism and muscle wasting in uremia. This increase in muscle protein catabolism

Factors Affecting Maximal Aerobic Capacity ($\dot{V}O_2max$) in Chronic Renal Disease

$\dot{V}O_2max$ = Cardiac Output$_{max}$ x Tissue O_2 Extraction [(A-V)O2 Difference$_{max}$]

Cardiovascular

1. Pathology
   - Atherosclerosis
   - Hypertension
   - Cardiomyopathy
   - Pericardial Disease
2. Hemodynamic Abnormalities
   - LV Systolic/Diastolic function
   - High Output State
   - Arrhythmias
   - ↓Perfusion/O_2 transport
3. Hormone/Metabolic Dysfunction
   - Uremic Toxins
   - Autonomic Dysfunction
   - Acidosis
   - Electrolyte Imbalance

Musculoskeletal

1. Pathology
   - Myopathy
   - Neuropathy
   - Degenerative Changes
2. Fuel/Substrate Abnormalities
   - ↓Perfusion
   - ↓Oxidative Enzymes
   - Acidosis
   - ↓Oxyhemoglobin
   - ↑Protein Catabolism
   - Insulin Resistance
   - ↓Substrate/Fuel Homeostasis
3. Malnutrition
   - Vitamin Deficiency
   - Amino Acid Deficiency
   - Cachexia

Figure 52.1 Cardiovascular (central) and muscle (peripheral) factors affect maximal aerobic exercise capacity in patients with chronic renal failure.

causes degeneration of muscle fibers and alterations in oxidative enzyme capacity and leads to myopathy, neuropathy, muscle wasting, and weakness (12), further reducing the exercise capacity and $\dot{V}O_2max$ of patients with ESRD.

In addition to the central (cardiac) and peripheral (muscular) abnormalities limiting the exercise capacity of patients with ESRD, their psychological state affects compliance to exercise and influences motivation for rehabilitation. In the only study that examined behavioral habits in dialysis patients who were offered participation in an exercise program, only 14 of 50 eligible hemodialysis patients volunteered for the exercise program and only 7 attended more than half of the classes (40).

Although self-perceived health status, cardiovascular function, medications, anemia, and duration on dialysis were comparable in the patients at the onset of exercise training, only the more compliant patients increased their treadmill duration and $\dot{V}O_2$max with training. The best predictors of compliance were lower levels of anxiety, hostility, and depression. More compliant patients were better adjusted psychologically and had a higher intellectual capacity than those with poor adherence to the program. However, none of the measures of psychological function improved after training. In contrast, in a longer 24-week exercise-training program the increase in $\dot{V}O_2max$ in dialysis patients was associated with an improvement in Beck Depression Scores and psychosocial function (3).

Exercise in Patients With End-stage Renal Disease

Evaluation Prior to Exercise

Many factors related to CRF and its treatment affect exercise testing and training the dialysis population. Prior to consideration for entry into an exercise program, the patient's dialysis regimen should be optimized. Interdialytic weights and chemistries, especially potassium and creatinine, and medications should be adjusted to ensure that the patient is medically stable. Attention should be paid to the timing of dialysis to exercise, interdialytic weight gains, medication changes, dietary compliance, and drugs that affect cardiovascular performance to limit possible complications.

The high prevalence of CVD and comorbidity in patients with ESRD makes it important to perform a careful medical evaluation prior to exercise testing and training (Table 52.2). It is important to screen for symptoms of ischemic heart disease, congestive heart failure, cardiomyopathy, and retinopathy, as well as to evaluate hypertension, dialysis control, and electrolyte and fluid balance. The presence of uremic complications, such as pericardial and pleural friction rubs, hyperkalemia or hypocalcemia, and cardiovascular complications, including recent myocardial infarction, severe hypertension, pulmonary congestion, or peripheral edema are contraindications to exercise. Individuals with severe diabetes, with or without retinopathy, or those with a recent cerebrovascular accident or residual weakness and balance disturbance after a stroke should be excluded from participation in a vigorous exercise program.

The low functional capacity and reduced maximal heart rate during exercise can obscure whether a treadmill test provides a sufficient evaluation of cardiovascular function in a patient with ESRD. Patients with equivocal hemodynamic and electrocardiographic (ECG) responses during exercise should be referred to a cardiologist for evaluation. Left ventricular hypertrophy is present in many dialysis patients and is not an absolute contraindication to exercise; however, left ventricular strain in the hypertensive patient may cause ECG changes consistent with ischemia and result in a false-positive exercise test. The thallium scan increases the sensitivity of treadmill exercise tests to diagnose coronary artery disease in this patient population. The presence of diastolic and systolic dysfunction, valvular abnormalities, and pericardial disease can be diagnosed by doppler echocardiography and radionuclide ventriculography.

Hyperkalemia is a major risk factor for cardiac arrhythmias in patients with ESRD and may be exaggerated by exercise. Exercise causes a similar efflux of potassium from muscle both in healthy individuals and in patients with ESRD. Because serum potassium levels may be elevated in patients with ESRD, persistent acidosis and exercise will augment potassium shifts from cells. This increases the risk of these patients for hyperkalemia-related arrhythmias and myocardial conduction abnormalities. Therefore, careful attention must be made to evaluate plasma potassium levels and the fluid-electrolyte status of the ESRD patient prior to exercise testing and training. We avoid exercise in patients with predialysis potassium levels consistently greater than 5.5 meq/L, metabolic acidosis typified by bicarbonate levels less than 18 meq/L, or excessive fluid weight gains of more than 2.5 kg between dialysis.

When there is concern about the cardiovascular, electrolyte, or health status of the ESRD patient despite a thorough medical evaluation, one can perform a submaximal exercise test to 75% of maximal heart rate. If the hemodynamic and electrocardiogram (ECG) responses and the patient's perceived exertion and symptoms during the test are normal, the investigator can then measure $\dot{V}O_2max$ and maximal heart rate during a maximal treadmill exercise test. This comprehensive evaluation may prevent medical complications during exercise testing and training of patients with ESRD, identify patients at high risk for cardiovascular decompensation, and alert personnel to precautions required in the dialysis population during exercise.

Table 52.2 Evaluation of Patients With CRF Prior to Exercise

1. Medical and dietary history
2. Review of medications, especially antihypertensive drugs
3. Medical and cardiovascular examination
4. Review dialysis schedule and adequacy
5. Blood chemistries (potassium, bicarbonate, urea)
6. Resting pre- and postdialysis blood pressures
7. Exercise electrocardiogram with blood pressure
8. If medical or cardiovascular concerns, submaximal exercise test by cardiologist

Exercise Testing of Patients with ESRD

The Balke or a modified Bruce protocol are appropriate for exercise testing of patients with ESRD because they require a $\dot{V}O_2$ in the range of 3 to 4 metabolic equivalents (METs) in the third minute of exercise. If the Bruce test is modified to start at 1.7 miles per hour on a level grade, it elicits a $\dot{V}O_2$ of approximately 2 to 3 METs during the first stage. The treadmill speed is increased gradually over the next 3 to 5 min to raise $\dot{V}O_2$ 1 MET every 2 min before increasing the incline until the patient is exhausted. Another effective testing protocol begins with a constant, comfortable walking speed on the treadmill and increasing the grade every 2 min to raise $\dot{V}O_2$ by 1 MET until the patient is exhausted.

The treadmill is the most reproducible and effective manner for exercise testing. However, some investigators feel tests are safer on bicycle ergometers where postural hypotension and fluid volume changes during exercise will have a smaller effect on hemodynamic responses. During cycle tests the initial work rate should be in the range of 20 W and increased by 10 to 20 W or 1 MET every 2 min to a maximum of 75 to 100 W. The increments during exercise should be sufficient to ensure adequate time to assess heart rate, blood pressure, and heart rate responses, yet progressively intensive enough to increase cardiac work in a gradual fashion so that patients reach $\dot{V}O_2max$ after 7 to 9 min of exercise.

Using these protocols most investigators report an impaired exercise capacity in patients with

ESRD (Table 52.3). On the average, the physical work capacity of carefully screened and perhaps somewhat "healthier" selected patients with ESRD was 15 to 28 ml·kg^{-1}·min^{-1} or 30% to 65% of normal; yet some patients had a $\dot{V}O_2$max as low as 7 ml·kg^{-1}·min^{-1}. The $\dot{V}O_2$max of patients treated with peritoneal dialysis does not seem to differ from hemodialysis patients, and the $\dot{V}O_2$max of renal transplant recipients with normal renal function and hematocrit averages 25% below normal (34).

Patients with ESRD have lower chronotropic responses to exercise, presumably due to reduced beta-agonist stimulation of the heart; however, glucose, lactate, and hemodynamic responses are similar to healthy controls during 1 hr of treadmill exercise at the same relative percentage of $\dot{V}O_2$max (26). This suggests that substrate metabolism may not be the limiting factor in the responses of patients with ESRD during acute exercise. However, when cardiovascular and metabolic responses to exercise in hemodialysis patients are compared to healthy control subjects at the same absolute work rate, lactic acid levels rise quickly and tachycardia and hypertension occur (1). Thus, when the exercise is adjusted appropriately for the low $\dot{V}O_2$max of patients with ESRD, their physiological responses are comparable to healthy control subjects exercising at the same relative work load.

Exercise Training of Patients With ESRD

The goal of endurance exercise training is to stimulate the cardiovascular system and major muscle groups by repetitive exercise at an ample stress to produce sufficient energy over a prolonged period of time. This will usually elicit a sufficient increase in heart rate (HR) to stimulate the hemodynamic responses necessary to achieve the desired intensity required for aerobic conditioning. Exercise at an intensity greater than 60% to 75% of $\dot{V}O_2$max that involves repetitive movement of the largest muscle groups is appropriate for training because it elicits significant increases in $\dot{V}O_2$max when performed for 30 to 45 min at least three times a week for 3 to 6 months.

The most convenient way to determine the training prescription is based on the linear relationship between heart rate and relative exercise intensity. The target heart rate (THR) is maintained at the prescribed percentage of heart rate reserve (HRR) as described by the Karvonen equation: THR = (percent HRR desired)(HRmax – HRrest) + HRrest. Because dialysis patients have lower maximal heart rates, exercise intensity should be based on a percentage of the measured HRmax or $\dot{V}O_2$max, not on estimates of the maximal heart rate from age and gender using available equations.

Table 52.3 Exercise Capacity ($\dot{V}O_2$max) in Patients With Chronic Renal Failure

Study	Number of patients	Age (years)	Treatment/duration (years)	$\dot{V}O_2$max ml·kg^{-1}min^{-1}
Beasley et al. (2)	18	52	PD/1.6	14.6 ± 5.5
Diesel et al. (10)	10	38	HD/4.4	17.7 ± 3.6
Goldberg et al. (18)	6	37	HD/3.0	18.1 ± 3.7
Goldberg et al. (16)	25	38	HD/2.5	20.0 ± 7.0
Kettner et al. (27)	18	31	HD/10.0	14.7 ± 2.2
Kettner et al. (26)	9	37	CRF/8.3	19.0 ± 5.0
Latos et al. (28)	9	40	HD/1.5	20.0 ± 3.1
Lennon et al. (29)	10	48	HD,PD/3.6	18.5 ± 5.9
Lundin et al. (32)	10	33	HD/8.4	28.6 ± 5.6
Painter et al. (34)	18	45	HD/4.6	19.1 ± 5.8
Painter et al. (34)	12	36	PD/1.0	21.1 ± 5.4
Painter et al. (35)	14	42	HD/3.8	19.6 ± 4.1
Robertson et al. (36)	19	47	HD/6.7	15.3 ± 5.4
Ross et al. (38)	12	62	HD/3.5	17.7 ± 4.0
Sagiv et al. (39)	10	30	CRF/15.0	22.6 ± 3.5
Shalom et al. (40)	14	46	HD,PD/5.0	15.4 ± 5.8
Zabetakis et al. (42)	10	45	HD/6.0	18.9 ± 3.6
	224	43 years	4.9 years	19.9 ± 5.3

Note. ml·kg^{-1}min^{-1} = milliliters per kilogram per minute; HD = Hemodialysis; PD = Peritoneal Dialysis; CRF = Chronic Renal Failure. Data are mean ± SD.

Cycle ergometry is the most efficacious initial mode of exercise for patients with ESRD. It permits accurate measurement of heart rate and blood pressure responses to known work rates to determine the relative intensity of exercise necessary to achieve the requisite increase in $\dot{V}O_2$. Cycle ergometry also is non-weight-bearing, and in patients with musculoskeletal problems due to myopathy, neuropathy, and osteomalacia there is an increased risk of muscle and bone pain, as well as fractures and other skeletal injuries. Once patients become familiar with heart rate palpation and the rationale underlying the exercise prescription and demonstrate that they are capable of self-monitoring heart rates and subjective responses to exercise, it is safe to proceed to walking and then gradually increase the exercise intensity by incorporating jogging into the program (Figure 52.2).

Effects of Exercise Training in End-Stage Renal Disease

Initial interest in the study of the effects of exercise in patients with ESRD was stimulated during the evaluation of a 44-year-old dialysis patient who worked part-time, jogged, played racquetball, swam, and scuba dived. This patient had a normal hematocrit, blood pressure, and lipid profile including high-density lipoprotein cholesterol of 48 mg/dl with no evidence of glucose intolerance or hyperinsulinemia. Early studies by Jette, Posen, and Cardarelli (25) also suggested that exercise might have salutary effects on the functional capacity, metabolism, and cardiovascular function of hemodialysis patients. This led to preliminary studies that examined the physiological effects of exercise training in seven hemodialysis patients (17,18,23).

There are now approximately 10 studies that report improvements in the exercise capacity, measured as $\dot{V}O_2$max, or exercise intensity of approximately 100 patients with ESRD after as few as 10 weeks of aerobic training (Table 52.4). Only one study was of sufficient duration (more than 6 months) to show improvements in blood pressure, glucose, and lipid metabolism as well as in anemia and the psychological profiles of hemodialysis patients (3,15-18,22).

The improvements in functional status, subjective sense of well-being, and enthusiasm in dialysis patients who participated in exercise programs (3) and the potential for reduction in risk factors for CVD (14) supports the need for further research in this area. A multicenter longitudinal study will be needed to determine the mechanisms by which exercise training improves physiological function and to assess the long-term effects of exercise on morbidity, mortality, and quality of life in these patients.

Exercise, Cardiovascular, and Muscular Function in ESRD

Endurance exercise training induces adaptations in the cardiovascular and musculoskeletal systems to raise $\dot{V}O_2$max and increase the ability of trained individuals to exercise more efficiently and for a

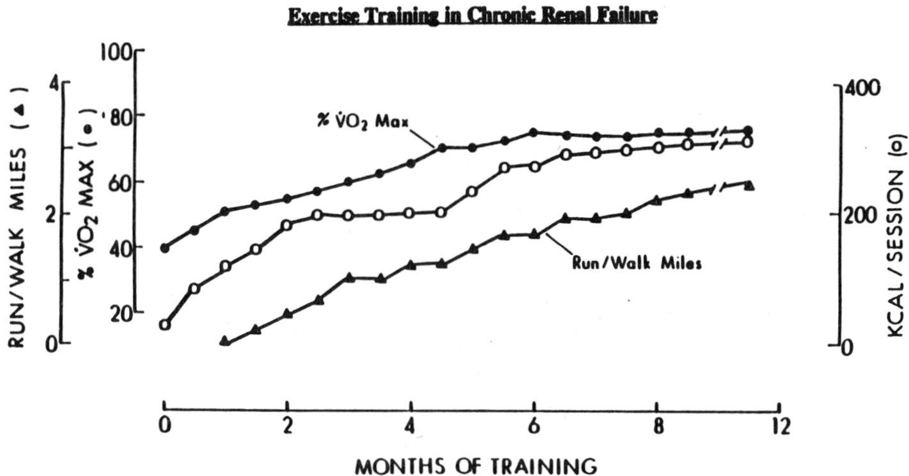

Figure 52.2 Exercise training progression in chronic renal failure is at an exercise intensity of energy expended (o, kilocalories/session) based on a relative percentage of maximal aerobic capacity ($\dot{V}O_2$max, •). Patients initially cycle at low work rates until they are capable of walking and then jogging (▲) at a gradually increasing intensity based on objective (target heart rate) and subjective (fatigue, musculoskeletal symptoms) criteria.

Table 52.4 Effects of Exercise Training in Patients With Chronic Renal Failure

Reference	Clyne et al. (5)	Goldberg et al. (16,18)	Lennon et al. (29)	Painter et al. (35)	Roseler et al. (37)	Ross et al. (38)	Shalom et al. (40)	Stephens et al. (41)	Zabetakis et al. (42)
Patients									
•Exercisers	10	20	10	12	13	9	14	10	5
•Controls	9	11	0	6	0	0	0	0	4
•Age (years)	47	37	48	42	47	62	45	52	45
•Duration HD (years)	CRF	2.5	3.6	3.8	CRF	3.5	5	2.8	6
•Health	Good	Good	Good	Good	Good	Good	Good	Good	Good
Exercise									
•Type	W,J strength	C,W,J	Cycle	Cycle	Cycle	C,W	Cycle	W,J	Treadmill
•Intensity	Moderate	Moderate	Low	Low	Low	Low	Low	Low	Low
•Duration (months)	3	9–12	2	6	3	3	3	8	2.5
•Compliance	80%	>65%	NR	>75%	Good	>80% <50%	>63%(7) <23% (7)	NR	Good
•$\Delta\dot{V}O_2max$	↑10%	↑22%	↑24%	↑40%	NR	↑17%	↑42% (7) NC (7)	NR	↑21%
•ΔPWC	↑46%	↑30%	NR	↑26%	↑34%	↑18%	NR	NR	↑21%

Note. HD = Hemodialysis; CRF = Chronic renal failure; W = walk; J = jog; C = cycle; NR = Not Reported; NC = No Change; PWC = Physical work capacity (intensity of exercise).

longer duration of time. In the ESRD patients enrolled in exercise-training programs, their baseline $\dot{V}O_2max$ was approximately 50% below that of healthy individuals (absolute value), but increased by 20% within only 3 months of regular exercise training. In a subset of eight patients who exercised for more than 12 months, there was a 40% increase in $\dot{V}O_2max$ (15). Such a dramatic change would be highly unlikely in otherwise healthy individuals, but in dialysis patients the relative change was magnified because the initial $\dot{V}O_2max$ was so much lower than baseline values in healthier individuals. In absolute terms, however, the increase in $\dot{V}O_2$max averaged only 6 $ml \cdot kg^{-1} \cdot min^{-1}$.

Exercise training alters the balance between sympathetic and parasympathetic activity, and at the same work rate vagal tone is usually greater and plasma catecholamines lower in trained individuals. In one study, after only 3 months of exercise training there was a decrease in heart rate, blood pressure, stroke volume, lactate levels, and cardiac output in hemodialysis patients during exercise at the same submaximal work rate (37). These results suggest there was an increase in cardiovascular reserve, whereas the decline in blood lactate levels implied increased oxygen extraction and substrate utilization by muscle. This indicated that peripheral adaptations such as increased skeletal muscle capillary density, oxidative enzyme capacity, and myoglobin content—as well as reduced peripheral vascular resistance—may have improved blood flow and oxygen extraction by exercising muscle. Thus, an increase in both maximal cardiac output and arteriovenous oxygen difference contributed to raise the $\dot{V}O_2max$ of these dialysis patients.

The most mechanistic data examining the effects of exercise on muscle metabolism have been obtained from in vitro experimental models. Utilizing an isolated muscle preparation from uremic, sedentary, and exercise-trained animals, these studies showed that exercise-training a uremic animal decreases muscle protein catabolic rates as reflected by the decreased release of the nonmetabolizable amino acids phenylalanine and tyrosine from muscle in vitro (6). This decrease in amino acid release (catabolism) was presumably due to increased insulin sensitivity induced by the exercise-training program; and recent studies have confirmed an increase in insulin sensitivity by a shift to the left in the insulin dose–response curve (7). The same group also demonstrated that exercise training enhanced glucose uptake and glycogen production in muscle preparations from both healthy and uremic animals (8). Exercise training decreases protein catabolism and increases glucose uptake by muscle from uremic animals due to enhanced insulin sensitivity. Consequently, endurance exercise should increase aerobic capacity, reduce glucose intolerance, insulin resistance, and dyslipoproteinemia in dialysis patients, thereby reducing their risk for CVD.

Hypertension is another medical condition seen frequently in patients with ESRD and is a major risk factor for CVD in these patients. Three studies reported a decrease in resting blood pressure and the reduction in the dosages of antihypertensive medications in hypertensive dialysis patients after exercise training (18,22,35). Blood pressure and catecholamine levels also were lower at submaximal work rates, even after a reduction in the dose of antihypertensive medications (15). Although plasma volume and body weight did not change in the patients, total blood volume rose due to an increase in red blood cell mass (16). To elucidate the mechanisms by which exercise lowers blood pressure in patients with ESRD will involve studies determining cardiac volumes, peripheral vascular resistance, and the response of hormones regulating blood pressure to acute and chronic exercise.

Exercise and Lipoprotein Metabolism in ESRD

The high prevalence of lipid abnormalities in patients with ESRD is important in the pathogenesis of accelerated atherosclerosis. Hemodialysis patients with CVD tend to have higher triglyceride (TG) and reduced high-density lipoprotein cholesterol (HDL-C) levels; and in one study heightened cardiovascular mortality in white males on hemodialysis was attributed to low HDL_2 and high plasma TG levels (19). The mechanisms responsible for dyslipoproteinemia in patients with ESRD are related to impaired clearance of TG-rich lipoproteins and reduced formation of HDL_2 due to reduced activity of lipoprotein lipase and impaired reverse cholesterol ester transfer (9).

Exercise training lowers plasma TG, raises HDL-C, and increases lipoprotein lipase activity in healthy individuals (30). However, significant improvements in the lipoprotein metabolism of hemodialysis patients were observed only in the patients who completed exercise training for greater than 9 months' duration (16,18,23). In these patients plasma TG levels decreased by 35% and HDL-C levels increased by 25%, but neither total nor low-density lipoprotein (LDL) cholesterol levels changed. The increase in lipoprotein lipase activity and the decrease in TG production rates and hepatic lipase activity occurred without change in the body weights or diets of the exercising hemodialysis patients. A deterioration in the lipid profiles of the sedentary controls suggested that the improvements in the lipoprotein metabolism with exercise training were mediated by an increase in TG clearance and HDL_2 formation. These were due to an increase in the enzyme lipoprotein lipase and a decrease in HDL catabolism caused by a reduction in the activity of the enzyme hepatic lipase.

Exercise and Glucose Metabolism in ESRD

Abnormalities in glucose metabolism characterized by insulin resistance and hyperinsulinemia, impaired glucose tolerance, delayed glucose clearance after insulin administration, and reduced insulin-stimulated glucose transport occur in patients with CRF. The relationship of insulin resistance to a sedentary lifestyle, hyperlipidemia, hypertension, and atherosclerosis in nonuremic individuals suggests that treatment of abnormal glucose metabolism in patients with ESRD should also reduce their risk for CVD.

Exercise training improves glucose metabolism and insulin sensitivity in healthy subjects by reducing fasting and postprandial hyperinsulinemia and increasing insulin-mediated glucose disposal, with no change or a slight improvement in glucose tolerance. The same exercise-training studies that demonstrated improved lipoprotein metabolism in hemodialysis patients after 9 months of aerobic training also showed improved glucose tolerance and insulin sensitivity (16,18,23). In those studies an increase in relative insulin receptor binding affinity was associated with a 25% increase in total specific insulin receptor binding, with no change in insulin receptor number. There was a decrease in plasma insulin levels and an increase in the glucose disappearance rate (16), consistent with an increase in insulin sensitivity. These in vivo data were confirmed by the finding of an increase in glucose transport in response to insulin stimulation in isolated muscle preparations from exercise-trained, uremic rats (8). Furthermore, glycogen levels rose significantly in muscles from exercising uremic rats and documented the increase in insulin sensitivity.

These improvements in glucose metabolism and insulin sensitivity in uremia would suggest that exercise training could (a) reduce hepatic TG synthesis, (b) raise HDL-C by increasing lipoprotein lipase activity and thus HDL synthesis, and (c) improve glucose metabolism, leading to a reduced risk for atherosclerosis in dialysis patients. Additional studies will be necessary to determine the site in the glucose transport process where exercise enhances insulin sensitivity and the mechanisms by which the improvements in glucose metabolism and insulin sensitivity affect lipoprotein metabolism.

Exercise and Hematologic Function in ESRD

Anemia almost always accompanies CRF and contributes to the morbidity associated with the disease. Inadequate erythropoiesis and blood loss as well as decreased utilization of iron and red blood cell fragility are major reasons for anemia in ESRD. Administration of human recombinant erythropoietin to hemodialysis patients has alleviated these problems. This increased hematocrit and red cell mass leads to an increase in energy, activity levels, and strength as well as a rise in the $\dot{V}O_2$max of dialysis patients (36). Exercise training usually is associated with a rise in both red cell mass and plasma volume in healthy individuals. Thus, hematocrit and hemoglobin values may not change in these individuals.

Chronic exercise training was associated with a twofold rise in the reticulocyte count and a 46% increase in red blood cell survival, but no change in plasma volume of dialysis patients (23). This raised hematocrit, hemoglobin concentration, and red cell mass by more than 20% in these patients. The changes in hematocrit and reticulocyte count were related to $\dot{V}O_2$max, suggesting that exercise training either increased red blood cell synthesis, reduced red cell destruction, or both simultaneously. This may be due to an exercise-induced increase in erythropoietin, because the rise in hematocrit after erythropoietin administration also raised $\dot{V}O_2$max and muscle strength in hemodialysis patients (36). Whether or not there would be a complementary or synergistic effect of exercise and erythropoietin in hemodialysis patients is not known.

Exercise and Psychological Function in ESRD

Renal failure and the need for chronic dialysis have profound psychosocial effects on patients with ESRD. The stresses are often severe and overwhelming, with patients demonstrating significant elevations on the depression, hypochondriasis, anxiety, and hysteria scales of the Minnesota Multiphasic Personality Inventory. The relationship between depression scores and $\dot{V}O_2$max suggests that the low physical conditioning status of hemodialysis patients reflects the severity of illness, hopelessness, and limited functional capacity beyond that of self-care in these patients (4,11,20).

Favorable preliminary findings of reduced depression, anxiety, and hostility and increased participation and enjoyment in social activities in four hemodialysis patients after exercise training (17) led to a controlled study of the effects of exercise training on psychological and social functioning in a larger study group (3). Although the exercise group was sufficiently motivated and psychologically stable enough to exercise regularly, their psychological profile at baseline did not differ from that of the control subjects. After 6 months of exercise training there was a subjective and objective improvement in measures of depression in the exercisers, but a deterioration or no change was observed in the control subjects receiving regular psychotherapy. Six months after the formal exercise and psychotherapy groups had ceased, the exercise group still reported greater participation and enjoyment in social and leisure-time activities and an improved quality of life; furthermore, several exercisers had secured part-time employment. There was either no change or a slight deterioration in the psychological profiles of the control subjects. Thus, exercise training seemed to have improved the psychosocial functioning and helped rehabilitate some hemodialysis patients.

The internal sense of reward from accomplishment during exercise was probably sufficient to improve the psychological status and social functioning of hemodialysis patients. However, this intensive exercise program also improved their metabolic, hematologic, and cardiovascular function, making them feel physically and mentally stronger. Antihypertensive medications were reduced, fewer transfusions were necessary, and fluid balance was stabilized in many of the dialysis patients who exercised regularly. Other patients reported increased appetite and were allowed to liberalize their fluid and salt intake to prevent hypotension during exercise, as sweating was induced by the exercise. This may have increased their feelings of self-efficacy and independence, encouraging them to continue regular exercise. These results suggest there is potential for regular exercise to improve the metabolic and psychological status and successfully rehabilitate some patients with ESRD to a more functional lifestyle.

Conclusions and Future Considerations

Exercise has significant physiological and psychosocial benefits in healthy populations and in patients with atherosclerotic cardiovascular disease, hypertension, diabetes mellitus, obesity, and lung disease. The studies in patients with ESRD on hemodialysis illustrate the potential benefit of exercise in a much more chronically ill population. There are only 10 prospective studies examining the effects of exercise training on the functional capacity of patients with ESRD (Table 52.4).

These studies involved 103 patients, and most of the studies lasted for a relatively short duration. Despite these limitations, exercise programs of mild to moderate intensity were associated with a 20% increase in $\dot{V}O_2max$. This can be attributed to the low level of exercise capacity of the patients at entry into the program, yet nearly all investigators reported dramatic improvements in the functional capacity and attitude of dialysis patients participating in the exercise programs.

The benefits of exercise for patients with ESRD are very encouraging; however, there is need for further study. The multisystemic nature of chronic renal disease and the complexity of treatment to sustain life make it necessary to develop new technology to improve the quality of life of this depressed, poorly rehabilitated, functionally limited patient population. The documented improvements in cardiovascular function, lipid and glucose metabolism, hematological, and psychological status of dialysis patients with exercise training could have far-reaching implications. It would be of major socioeconomic benefit if dialysis patients could maintain employment, reduce their medications, and have lower medical costs due to fewer disease-related complications.

Despite the dramatic responses described here in selected patients, it is not known how many patients with ESRD would benefit from exercise training and what the long-term socioeconomic and health-related implications of such programs would be for this patient population. The potential for exercise to delay disability, improve psychosocial function, enhance attitude and participation in pleasant events—as well as to reduce medications and medical complications—may be sufficient incentive for patients with chronic renal disease to become involved in exercise training.

Once the basic physiology of exercise and its metabolic, cardiovascular, and psychological effects are understood in patients with chronic renal disease, then programs can be designed to optimize adherence and determine the long-term effects of exercise in preventing disability and reducing risk factors for comorbid diseases in this population. Further studies are needed to determine the mechanisms by which exercise (a) improves cardiovascular, metabolic, and musculoskeletal function; (b) reduces risk factors for CVD; and (c) enhances psychological status to improve the quality of life in patients with chronic renal disease.

These studies will need the cooperation of the patients, their families, their physicians, exercise physiologists, and other allied health professionals to provide the optimal environment to ensure compliance so that the maximal benefits of exercise training can be realized for patients with ESRD. Only with more knowledge of the physiological and psychological effects of exercise in patients with ESRD can we gain insight into its potential to enhance the quality of life and reduce the medical complications and socioeconomic and psychological consequences of renal disease.

References

1. Barnea, N.; Drory, Y.; Iania, A.; Lapidot, C.; Reisin, E.; Eliahou, H.; Kellermann, J.J. Exercise tolerance in patients on chronic hemodialysis. Isr. J. Med. Sci. 16:17-21; 1980.
2. Beasley, C.R.; Smith, D.A.; Neale, T.J. Exercise capacity in chronic renal failure patients managed by continuous ambulatory peritoneal dialysis. Aust. N. Z. J. Med. 16:5-10; 1986.
3. Carney, R.M.; Templeton, B.; Hong, B.A.; Harter, H.R.; Hagberg, J.M.; Schechtman, K.G.; Goldberg, A.P. Exercise training reduces depression and increases the performance of pleasant activities in hemodialysis patients. Nephron. 47:194-198; 1987.
4. Carney, R.M.; Wetzel, R.D.; Hagberg, J.M.; Goldberg, A.P. The relationship between depression and aerobic capacity in hemodialysis patients. Psych. Med. 48:143-147; 1986.
5. Clyne, N.; Ekholm, J.; Jogestrand, T.; Lins, L.E.; Pehrsson, S.K. Effects of exercise training in predialytic uremic patients. Nephron. 59:84-89; 1991.
6. Davis, T.A.; Karl, I.E.; Tegtmeyer, E.D.; Osborne, D.F.; Klahr, S.; Harter, H.R. Muscle protein turnover: Effects of exercise training and renal insufficiency. Am. J. Physiol. 248:E337-E345; 1985.
7. Davis, T.A.; Klahr, S.; Karl, I.E. Insulin-stimulated protein metabolism in chronic azotemia and exercise. Am. J. Physiol. 253:E337-E345; 1985.
8. Davis, T.A.; Klahr, S.; Karl, I.E. Glucose metabolism in muscle of sedentary and exercised rats with uremia. Am. J. Physiol. 252:F138-F145; 1987.
9. Dieplinger, H.; Schoefeld, P.Y.; Fielding, C.J. Difference between treatment by hemodialysis or peritoneal dialysis. J. Clin. Invest. 007:1071-1083; 1986.
10. Diesel, W.; Noakes, T.; Swanepoel, C.; Lambert, M. Isokinetic muscle strength predicts maximum exercise tolerance in renal patients on chronic hemodialysis. Am. J. Kidney Dis. 16:109-114; 1990.
11. Evans, R.W.; Manninen, D.L.; Garrison, L.P.; Hart, L.G.; Blagg, C.R.; Gutman, R.A.; Hull, A.R.; Lowrie, E.G. The quality of life of patients with end-stage renal disease. N. Engl. J. Med. 312:553-559; 1985.
12. Floyd, M.; Ayyar, D.R.; Barwick, D.D.; Hudgson, P.; Weightman, D. Myopathy in chronic renal failure. Q. J. Med. 43:509-524; 1974.
13. Garber, A.J. Skeletal muscle protein and amino acid metabolism in experimental chronic uremia in the rat: Accelerated alanine and glutamine formation and release. J. Clin. Invest. 62:623-632; 1978.
14. Goldberg, A.P. A potential role for exercise training in modulating coronary risk factors in uremia. Am. J. Nephrol. 4:132-133; 1984.
15. Goldberg, A.P. Effects of exercise training on lipid and carbohydrate metabolism in hemodialysis patients. Final report, N01-AK-3-9-2221F. U.S.P.H.S.: Chronic Renal Disease Program. National Institutes of Health; 1984.
16. Goldberg, A.P.; Geltman, E.M.; Hagberg, J.M.; Gavin, J.R.; Delmez, J.A.; Carney, R.M.; Naumowicz, A.; Oldfield, M.H.; Harter, H.R. Therapeutic benefits of exercise training for hemodialysis patients. Kidney Int. 24:S303-S309; 1983.
17. Goldberg, A.P.; Hagberg, J.M.; Delmez, J.; Carney, R.M.; McKevitt, P.M.; Ehsani, A.A.; Harter, H.R. The metabolic and psychological effects of exercise training in hemodialysis patients. Am. J. Clin. Nutr. 33:1620-1628; 1980.
18. Goldberg, A.P.; Hagberg, J.M.; Delmez, J.A.; Haynes, M.E.; Harter, H.R. Metabolic effects of exercise training in hemodialysis patients. Kidney Int. 18:754-761; 1980.
19. Goldberg, A.P.; Harter, H.R.; Patsch, W.; Schechtman, K.B.; Province, M.; Weerts, C.; Kuisk, I.; McCrate, M.M.; Schonfeld, G. Racial differences in plasma high-density lipoproteins in patients receiving hemodialysis. N. Engl. J. Med. 308:1245-1252; 1983.
20. Gutman, R.A.; Stead, W.W.; Robinson, R.R. Physical activity and employment status of patients on maintenance dialysis. N. Engl. J. Med. 304:309-313; 1981.
21. Hagberg, J.M. Patients with end-stage renal disease. In: Franklin, B.A.; Gordon, S.; Timmis, G.C., eds. Exercise in modern medicine. Baltimore: Williams & Wilkins; 1989:146-155.
22. Hagberg, J.M.; Goldberg, A.P.; Eshani, A.A.; Heath, G.W.; Delmez, J.A.; Harter, H.R. Exercise training improves hypertension in hemodialysis patients. Am. J. Nephrol. 3:209-212; 1983.

23. Harter, H.R.; Goldberg, A.P. Endurance exercise training: Effective therapeutic modality for hemodialysis patients. Med. Clin. North Am. 69:159-175; 1985.
24. Harter, H.R.; Karl, I.E.; Klahr, S.; Kipnis, D.M. Effects of reduced mass and dietary protein intake on amino acid release and glucose uptake by rat muscle in vitro. J. Clin. Invest. 64:513-523; 1979.
25. Jette, M.; Posen, G.; Cardarelli, C. Effects of an exercise program in a patient undergoing hemodialysis treatment. J. Sports Med. Phys. Fitness. 17:181-186; 1977.
26. Kettner, A.; Goldberg, A.P.; Hagberg, J.M.; Delmez, J.; Harter, H.R. Cardiovascular and metabolic responses to submaximal exercise in hemodialysis patients. Kidney Int. 26:66-71; 1984.
27. Kettner-Melsheimer, A.; Weib, M.; Huber, W. Physical work capacity in chronic renal disease. Int. J. Artif. Organs. 10:23-30; 1987.
28. Latos, D.L.; Strimel, D.; Drews, M.; Allison, T.G. Acid-base and electrolyte changes following maximal and submaximal exercise in hemodialysis patients. Am. J. Kidney Dis. 10:439-445; 1987.
29. Lennon, D.; Shrago, E.; Madden, M.; Nagle, F.; Hanson, P.; Zimmerman, S. Carnitine status, plasma lipid profiles, and exercise capacity of dialysis patients: Effects of submaximal exercise program. Metabolism. 25:728-735; 1986.
30. Leon, A. Physical activity levels and coronary heart disease: Analysis of epidemiologic and supporting studies. Med. Clin. North Am. 69:3-20; 1985.
31. Lindner, A.; Charra, B.; Sherrard, D.J.; Scribner, B.H. Accelerated atherosclerosis in prolonged maintenance hemodialysis. N. Engl. J. Med. 290:697-701; 1974.
32. Lundin, A.P.; Stein, R.A.; Frank, F.; LaBelle, P.; Berlyne, G.M.; Krasnow, N.; Friedman, E.A. Cardiovascular status in long-term hemodialysis patients: An exercise and echocardiographic study. Nephron. 28:234-238, 1981.
33. Painter, P.L. Exercise in end-stage renal disease. Exerc. Sport Sci. Rev. 16:305-339; 1988.
34. Painter, P.L.; Messer-Rehak, D.; Hanson, P.; Zimmerman, S.W.; Glass, N.R. Exercise capacity in hemodialysis, CAPD, and renal transplant patients. Nephron. 42:47-51; 1986.
35. Painter, P.L.; Nelson-Worel, J.N.; Hill, M.M.; Harrington, A.R.; Weinstein, A.B. Effects of exercise training during hemodialysis. Nephron. 43:87-92; 1986.
36. Robertson, H.T.; Haley, N.R.; Guthrie, M.; Cardenas D.; Eschbach, J.W.; Adamson, J.W. Recombinant erythropoietin improves exercise capacity in anemic hemodialysis patients. Am. J. Kidney Dis. 15:325-332; 1990.
37. Roseler, E.; Aurisch, R.; Precht, D.; Strangfeld, D.; Priem, F.; Siewert, H.; Lindenam, K. Haemodynamic and metabolic responses to physical training in chronic renal failure. Proc. EDTA. 17:702-706; 1980.
38. Ross, D.L.; Grabeau, G.M.; Smith, S.; Seymour, M.; Knierim, N.; Pitetti, K.H. Efficacy of exercise for end-stage renal disease patients immediately following high-efficiency hemodialysis: A pilot study. Am. J. Nephrol. 9:376-383; 1989.
39. Sagiv, M.; Rudoy, J.; Rotstein, A.; Fisher, N.; Ben-Ari, J. Exercise tolerance end-stage renal disease patients. Nephron. 57:424-427; 1991.
40. Shalom, R.; Blumenthal, J.A.; Williams, R.S.; McMurray, R.G.; Dennis, V.W. Feasibility and benefits of exercise training in patients on maintenance dialysis. Kidney Int. 25:958-963; 1984.
41. Stephens, R.; Williams, A.; McKnight, T.; Dodd, S. Effects of self-monitored exercise on selected blood chemistry parameters of end-stage renal disease patients. Am. J. Phys. Med. Rehabil. 70(3):149-153; 1991.
42. Zabetakis, P.M.; Gleim, G.W.; Pasternack, F.L.; Saranti, A.; Nicholas, J.A.; Michelis, M.F. Long-duration submaximal exercise conditioning in hemodialysis patients. Clin. Nephrol. 18:17-22; 1982.

Chapter 53

Physical Activity, Fitness, and Bladder Control

Kari Bø

Lack of bladder control or urinary incontinence is defined as "a condition in which involuntary loss of urine is a social or hygienic problem and is objectively demonstrable" (1). The condition is a major clinical problem and a significant cause of disability and dependency. Lack of bladder control is common in the elderly but may affect all age groups. It is estimated that at least 10 million adult Americans suffer from urinary incontinence, including 15% to 30% of community-dwelling older people and one half of all nursing home residents. The monetary costs of managing urinary incontinence are estimated at $10.3 billion annually (58).

Although lack of bladder control also seems to be prevalent in many women performing sport and fitness activities (13,19,62), there is little information available on this topic.

The reason for the paucity of research in this field may be that lack of bladder control is a problem most people do not want to talk about (33,62). Only 25% of those reporting the problem in surveys are seeking help for the problem (33,76). Many women believe that urinary leakage is a normal and inevitable consequence of childbirth and aging (47,67), and they do not know that they can be cured or greatly improved by simple means (47,79). That research into lack of bladder control has been conducted by health personnel outside the exercise sciences may in part also explain why the studies have focused so little on the problem during physical activity.

This chapter is divided into two parts. Part I focuses on the mechanisms behind bladder control during physical activity and stress urinary incontinence in particular. In Part II pelvic floor muscle exercises to treat female stress urinary incontinuence (SUI) are discussed.

This chapter is based on papers written in the English language compiled from a computerized search, original papers found in review articles (11,80,82), and a manual review of the proceedings from International Continence Society (ICS) annual meetings from 1984 to 1991.

I. Bladder Control

Bladder control implies the ability to store urine until the appropriate place and time for voluntary micturition occurs. Continence requires adequate urethral closure, and this is achieved by an integrated spinal and cerebral nervous control. A higher urethral than bladder pressure is termed *positive closure pressure*, and a lower urethral than bladder pressure is termed *negative closure pressure*.

Urethral factors affecting the closure mechanism are the condition of the mucosa, the submucosa, the collagen and elastic fibers, as well as striated and smooth muscle activity within the urethral wall. In addition, voluntary and reflex *pelvic floor muscle* (PFM) contractions contribute to closure during sudden rise in intraabdominal pressure (52).

Incontinence

Incontinence may be caused by any pathologic, anatomic, or physiologic factor that make the intravesical pressure higher than the maximum urethral pressure. The most common types of urinary incontinence that may occur during physical activity are *urge incontinence*, *stress urinary incontinence* (SUI), and a combination of the two (*mixed incontinence*).

Urge incontinence is defined as the involuntary loss of urine associated with a strong desire to void (urgency) (1). Implicit in this definition is the assumption that the strong desire to void is caused by a detrusor contraction that the patient is unable to inhibit. Causes of urge incontinence are central nervous system lesions (stroke, demyelinating disease) and urinary infections or bladder tumors. However, in many cases no specific etiology can be identified (58).

SUI is involuntary urinary leakage during physical exertion (e.g., coughing, sneezing, laughing, running, jumping, and lifting). When the intravesical pressure exceeds the urethral pressure in absence of a simultaneous detrusor contraction the condition is termed *genuine stress incontinence* (GSI) (1). This diagnosis implies urodynamic assessment.

Enhørning (32) explained the mechanism behind SUI as hypermobility of the bladder and the urethra during a rise in intraabdominal pressure. Normally the ligaments and the PFM keep the bladder and the urethra within the intraabdominal cavity. If these supporting tissues are too elastic, descent of the urethra may occur. Such movements have been visualized by ultrasonography (7,53). For a short period of time the bladder pressure is higher than the urethral pressure and leakage may occur.

A quick and strong reflex contraction of the PFM may prevent descent of the bladder base and the urethra (22,23) and constrict the urethra, pressing it against the pubic symphysis and thereby raising the urethral pressure (24,25). Any disturbance in the function of the PFM and the smooth and striated muscles of the urethra may cause SUI.

Prevalence of Stress Urinary Incontinence

The prevalence of incontinence is higher in females than in males (58). Most males have such problems after cerebrovascular and neurological diseases or after prostatectomy—problems out of the scope of this article. There are no studies in the literature dealing with incontinence in men during physical activity. SUI is the type of incontinence most frequently affecting women (33,39) and will be the focus of this analysis.

Prevalence studies of female SUI show a variation from 8% (43) to 52% (59) (Table 53.1). The huge variation in prevalence may be explained by different populations investigated, low response rate (62), and the use of different definitions of incontinence used in the questionnaires and interviews. According to ICS criteria of incontinence, the condition should be experienced as a hygienic or social problem. When this aspect is included in the questions, the prevalence tends to decrease (31,70).

Etiology

Age, Menopause

The National Institutes of Health (NIH) Consensus Statement on Urinary Incontinence in Adults states that there is a persistent myth that urinary incontinence is a normal consequence of aging (58). Thomas, Plymat, Blannin, and Meade (76) showed that there was an increasing prevalence of incontinence with age. However, in three studies (20,41,78) (see Table 53.1) a lower prevalence was found in persons older than age 60 years than in younger age groups seen in other studies. Fall, Frankenberg, Frisen, Larson, and Petren (33) observed that the highest prevalence of SUI was in the group between 40 to 49 years of age. This may reflect a higher activity level at this age, a factor supported by the results found in other studies (47).

There are controversies about the influence of estrogen depletion on SUI. Iosif and Becassy (41) found a prevalence of 29% in 1,200 women age 61 years. This prevalence is not higher than what is found in other age groups (see Table 53.1). Thomas et al. (76) and Hørding, Pederssen, Sidenius, and Hedegaard (39) found that the frequency of urinary incontinence was not higher in postmenopausal women. Bennes, Abbott, Cardozo, Saavas, and Studd (8) asked 248 women about urinary problems. One hundred women had been on continuous estrogen therapy for 10 years and 148 had never been on such therapy. The results demonstrated that SUI was significantly more common in the estrogen-therapy group. However, the two groups were not similar concerning important background variables, which may confound the results.

Conclusion. Normal aging may not be a cause of urinary incontinence. However, age-related changes in lower urinary tract dysfunction in addition to common diseases in the elderly may predispose for the condition (58). Based on the present knowledge, age and age-related diseases seem to be more important factors than menopause in development of SUI.

Pregnancy and Childbirth

SUI is often considered a problem primarily occurring after childbirth. A higher prevalence has been demonstrated in parous than in nulliparous women (62,70,76). SUI after parturition has been explained as being the result of peripheral nerve damage (4,68).

Allen and Warrell (4) demonstrated a significant fall in vaginal squeeze pressure from mean 15 cm H_2O antenatally to 4.6 cm H_2O postpartum. Two months postnatally the mean value was 9.8 cm H_2O. However, many of the women were still breastfeeding, which may have influenced the results. In addition no check of the women's ability to perform a correct PFM contraction was performed. The results should therefore be interpreted with

Table 53.1 Prevalence Studies of Female Stress Urinary Incontinence (SUI)

Study	Methods/ response rate	*N*	Population	Operational definition	Prevalence	Questions on physical activity
Nehmir & Middleton (59)	Questionnaire, 100%	1,327	Nulliparous college students aged 17 to 21 years	Coughing, laughing, sneezing, excitement	52% SUI	No
Beck & Hsu (6)	Interview (?), 100% (?)	1,000	Outpatient gynecology clinic patients, age unknown	No information given	31% SUI	Unknown
Wolin (85)	Questionnaire, interview, 100% (?)	4,211	Nulliparous nursing students aged 17 to 25 years	Coughing, laughing, sneezing, excitement	51% SUI, 16% every-day leakage	No
Yarnell & Leger (78)	Interview, 98%	388	Samples from medical practice over 65 years of age	No information given	17% incontinence	Unknown
Thomas et al. (76)	Postal survey, 89%	20,398	General practitioner's patients over 5 years of age	2 or more episodes per month	< 65 years: 8% > 65 years: 11.6% incontinence	No
Stanton et al. (72)	Postal survey, 100% (?)	181	Healthy pregnant women aged 25.8 and 27.7 years (nulli/multipara)	Loss of urine on physical effort	Postnatally: 6%, 11% nulli/multipara	Unknown
Iosif et al. (43)	Questionnaire (physicians office) (?)	512	Municipality service gynecology program participants aged 20 to 70 years	Coughing, physical activity, heavy lifting, walking stairways, rapid movements	8.2% SUI	Yes

Iosif (42)	Postal survey, 94.1%	1,500	Newly delivered women, age unknown	Coughing, physical activity, heavy lifting, walking stairways, rapid movements	22% SUI	Yes
Yarnell et al. (78)	Interview, 95%	1,060	Geographical area residents over 18 years of age	At any time (e.g., coughing, laughing, sneezing)	22% SUI	No
Iosif & Ingemarsson (44)	Postal survey, 77.3%	204	Women delivering by elective cesarean section, age unknown	No information given	9% SUI	Unknown
Iosif & Bekassy (41)	Postal survey, 75%	1,200	Geographical area residents aged 61 years	Coughing, laughing, lifting, climbing and descending stairs, rapid movements	29% incontinence, 11% SUI	Yes
Fall et al. (33)	Postal survey, 74%	10,000	Swedish population aged 20 to 74 years	Laughing, sneezing, physical exercise	8% incontinence (male and female)	Yes
Campbell et al. (20)	Interview, 94.9%	559	Community members over 65 years of age	Do you ever wet yourself/always get to toilet in time?	11% incontinence, > 80 years: 22%	Unknown
Hørding et al. (39)	Interview, 85%	515	Health survey respondents aged 45 years	Laughing, sneezing, running, jumping	22% incontinence (75% of which was SUI)	Yes
Jolleys (47)	Postal survey, 89%	973	Rural practice patients over 25 years of age	Coughing with full bladder, laughing, on exercise, lifting, climbing stairs	41% incontinence	Yes
Elving et al. (31)	Postal survey, 85%	3,114	Town inhabitants aged 30 to 79 years	Have you ever in adult life experienced one or more episodes of incontinence on physical stress?	26% incontinence (SUI predominated)	No

(continued)

Table 53.1 *(Continued)*

Study	Methods/ response rate	N	Population	Operational definition	Prevalence	Questions on physical activity
Bø et al. (13)	Postal survey, 84%	116	Physical education students aged 19 to 37 years	Do you ever experience urinary leakage on coughing, laughing, sneezing, running, jumping (feet together), jumping (feet apart), lifting, throwing, ab-off, landing?	26% SUI	Yes
Sommer et al. (70)	Postal survey, 72%	432	National register aged 20 to 79 years	Unknown	40% incontinence, 15% SUI	No
Simeonova et al. (67)	Questionnaire (physicians office), 82%	451	Health center patients over 18 years of age	Incontinence on effort	44% incontinence (33% of which was SUI)	No
Nygaard et al. (62)	Postal survey, 51.7%	326	Private gynecologic practice patients aged 17 to 68 years	Have you ever leaked urine? (Operational definition on several forms of exercise)	47% incontinence	Yes

Note. N = number; M = male; F = female.

some caution. Those mothers with a long second stage (more than 1 hr) and those who delivered larger babies (over 3.5 kg) had significantly longer motor unit potential duration.

Snooks, Swash, Mathers, and Henry (69) followed their patients for 5 years, and persistent and worsening pudendal neuropathy was found.

Both Stanton, Kerr-Wilson, and Harris (72) and Allen and Warrell (4) found that the prevalence of SUI rose during pregnancy and then declined after childbirth, indicating that the increased pressure from the fetus on the bladder may cause leakage temporarily during pregnancy. When the increased weight of the fetus is removed at delivery, incontinence may disappear in some women. However, Allen and Warrell (4) demonstrated a higher prevalence of SUI after delivery than before gestation.

Nygaard, DeLancey, Arnsdorf, and Murphy (62) and Jolleys (47) found a higher prevalence with higher parity, and Beck and Hsu (6) reported that the incontinence was progressively worse with successive pregnancies. On the other hand, Thomas et al. (76) could not demonstrate any differences within parity ranges of 1 to 3. However, the prevalence was increased in women having four or more children.

Iosif (42) concluded that incontinence more often begins during the first pregnancy than during subsequent pregnancies. Demonstrating a prevalence of 9% in women delivered with cesarean section, Iosif and Ingemarsson (44) concluded that the pregnancy itself and hereditary factors may predispose more than parturition trauma in some women.

In correspondence with the above-mentioned hereditary factor, Nehmir and Middleton (59) and Wolin (85) found a prevalence of more than 50% in nulliparous college women. Wolin reported that 16% of nursing students experienced daily leakage (85). Both Bø, Maehlum, Oseid, and Larsen (19) and Jolleys (47) have found a prevalence of 31% in young nulliparous women.

Conclusion. Apparently SUI is often caused by pregnancy and childbirth. However, there is a high prevalence of SUI also in young nulliparous women. Pregnancy and childbirth may worsen the condition considerably for women already having the problem.

Obesity and SUI

Many authors consider obesity a risk factor for developing SUI (2,63,71). However, very few studies have actually looked into this. In three studies an association between obesity and incontinence has been found (30,54,67). Conversely, Wilkie (81) could not demonstrate any difference in urethral function in overweight women with and without SUI. However, in each of these studies obesity was defined differently, and the results cannot be directly compared.

Conclusion. The question of whether or not there is an association between obesity and SUI is not answered. More studies comparing matched groups of continent and incontinent women are needed to resolve this.

Exercise and SUI

There has been a general belief that physically fit women also have strong PFM, thus preventing SUI. However, Nichols and Milley (60) suggested that the cardinal and uterosacral ligaments, PFM, and the connective tissue of the perineum may be damaged chronically because of repeatedly increased intraabdominal pressure due, for example, to such phenomena as hard manual work and chronic cough. According to this theory, strenuous exercise raising the intraabdominal pressure may also be a contributing factor in development of SUI in some women.

The most frequently applied operational definition of physical exertion used in surveys is coughing, laughing, and sneezing (see Table 53.1). In eight studies questions about leakage during different forms of physical activity have been incorporated. However, only Bø et al. (19) and Nygaard et al. (62) have investigated the activity level of the subjects studied. This may be a crucial point in estimating true prevalence of SUI. Women who exercise raise the intraabdominal pressure more frequently than sedentary women. They are therefore more likely to experience leakage than physically inactive women.

On the other hand, both Nygaard et al. (62) and Jolleys (47) found that leakage was less common during exercise than during daily activities. This implies that if SUI is present, it should be detected during daily activities. However, it may be more frequent and experienced more often as a problem in women exercising regularly.

Bø et al. (19) studied female physical education students and found a prevalence of SUI of 26%. The question was "Do you ever experience urinary leakage in one or more of these activities: coughing and sneezing, laughing, take off, landing, throwing, situps, running, jumping up and down with feet together, jumping with feet apart, and lifting?" Comparing students exercising more than three times a week to sedentary students, there was a significantly higher prevalence (p = .02) in physically active students.

Nygaard et al. (62) studied the relationship between exercise and incontinence in 326 women attending a gynecological practice. Eighty-nine percent of the women were exercising at least once a week, and 33% of the exercisers experienced some degree of incontinence during at least one type of exercise.

Conclusion. There is a high prevalence of SUI in women exercising regularly. Thus, general exercise does not seem to prevent or treat female SUI. Whether some movements or exercises strengthen the PFM and thereby prevent SUI is not yet known. The question of whether or not strenuous physical exercise (e.g., long-distance running and weight lifting) may cause SUI in some women cannot be answered with the data available today.

Social Impact of SUI During Exercise

Urinary incontinence may lead to withdrawal from social activities and to reduction of well-being (40). Norton, MacDonald, and Stanton (61) reported that urinary leakage frequently interfered with daily lives in more than 50% of their study group. Fall et al. (33) reported that 42% of the women with incontinence had problems in connection with sport and physical activities. Bø, Hagen, Kvarstein, and Larsen (13) demonstrated that two thirds of sedentary SUI women reported urinary leakage to be the cause of inactivity. Twenty-seven out of 52 women had tried to participate in specific sport and fitness activities, but had withdrawn from one or more activities because of leakage.

Most women (19 out of 27) had withdrawn from aerobic and dance activities. They all reported that the major urinary leakage occurred during high-impact activites in the aerobic session, and especially when jumping with legs in subsequent ab- and adduction (jumping jacks). After specific strength training of the PFM, 17 out of 22 women had improved during jumping and running and 15 during lifting.

Nygaard et al. (62) found that 20% of those women who were incontinent during a particular activity stopped doing it solely because of incontinence. Eighteen percent changed the way they performed an exercise because of incontinence. Frequency, time spent per session, and duration of the exercise had no significant impact on the prevalence.

Conclusion. High-impact activities, especially jumping with legs apart, is problematic for women with SUI. Many women change the way they exercise or withdraw from regular physical activity because of SUI. Low-impact activities (always one foot on the floor) enable many women with SUI to continue exercising. Bicycling, fast walking, swimming, and low-impact aerobics can therefore be recommended.

Assessment of Bladder Control During Exercise

Usually the diagnosis of SUI is settled by urodynamic assessment during coughing in a half-sitting, lithotomy position. The validity of this evaluation, however, can be questioned, as most women do not leak in a sitting or lying position (45).

The criterion of GSI is that the bladder and urethral pressure should be measured simultaneously demonstrating a negative closure pressure. Very few such studies have been performed during exercise. The most commonly used pad test, a 1 hr test, did not originally involve physical activity (5). It was later developed to also involve activities such as stair climbing and jumping (1). Another criticism of this commonly used test has been that it does not include the use of a standardized bladder volume, and it has been shown to have low reproducibility (55,57).

Henalla, Kirwan, Castleden, Hutchins, and Breeson (37) designed a test with some degree of physical exercise such as jumping and lifting during the test. Hagen, Kvarstein, Bø, and Larsen (35) designed an exercise test involving running, jumping jacks, standing up and laying down, and abdominal curls. This latter test was found to be nine times as provocative as the ICS 1-hr test involving daily activities. The authors concluded that assessment of the degree of SUI has to be physically provocative to detect SUI.

Few studies have been conducted to describe the bladder and the urethral function during physical activity. James (45) claimed that many women experienced SUI only during exercise, arguing that assessment of SUI should be performed in standing and working positions. Applying ambulatory bladder pressure measurements, he demonstrated that the peaks of bladder pressure rise during running and jumping occurred when the feet touched the floor. Although pressure rise was higher during coughing, some women were only leaking during exercise.

These early studies of James (45) did not involve urethral pressure. In addition, the standing measurement during exercise without proper fixation of the catheter can be questioned, as the force of gravity and the exercises tend to move the catheters. Kulseng-Hanssen and Klevmark (56) improved the methodology by placing the bladder and urethral transducer catheters in a silicon cuff that was sutured to the external urethral opening. The patients were doing vigorous coughing and 20 jumping jacks in standing position, after which they were encouraged to perform daily activities for 45 min.

Tracings from a stress incontinent patient during jumping and coughing is seen in Figure 53.1. In 16 of the patients, 115 leakage episodes were seen in 45 min. In 92 of these episodes the maximum urethral pressure decrease was larger than the detrusor pressure increase. However, some patients complained of urinary leakage during strenuous exercise (running and jumping for longer periods of time), although leakage was undetected even in this test. As SUI may be due to fatique of the pelvic floor and the urethral wall muscles, some women may need even more vigorous and continuous activities to provoke leakage.

Conclusion. Due to methodological problems, very few studies have been conducted to describe the function of urethral closure during exercise. There is a need for development of a better methodology and comparison between nulliparous stress-incontinent and continent women during exercise.

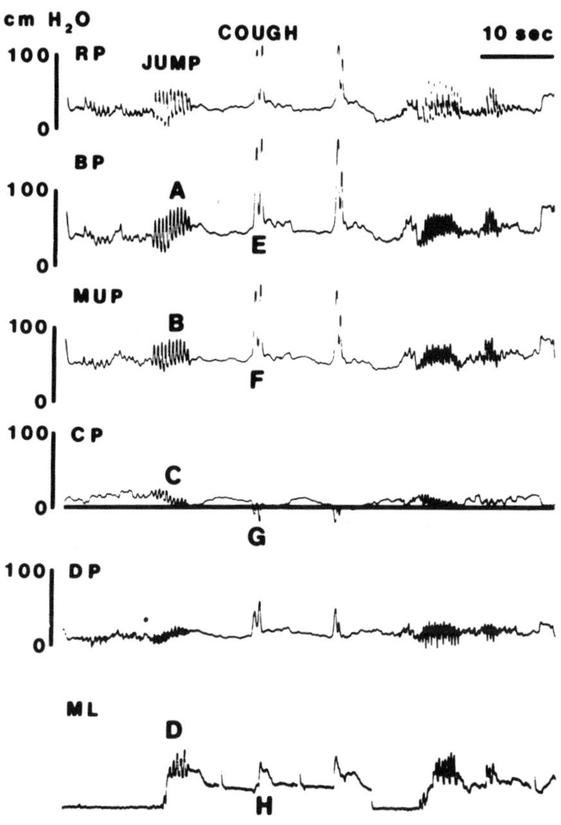

Figure 53.1 Tracings from a stress-incontinent patient during jumping and coughing. The intraabdominal pressure increase is more effectively transmitted to the bladder (A,E) than to the urethra (B,F), and the closure pressure (C,G) becomes negative, whereupon the patient leaks urine (D,H). Shortly after the incontinence is indicated by the leak indicator, the patient signals leakage by means of the push button. RP = rectal pressure; BP = bladder pressure; MUP = maximum urethral pressure; DP = detrusor pressure; ML = leakage.
From Kulseng-Hanssen and Klevmark: Ambulatory Urethro-Cysto-Rectometry: A New Technique. Neurourol. Urodyn.7:119-130, p. 127: 1988. Reprinted by permission.

II. Pelvic Floor Muscle (PFM) Exercise to Treat Female SUI

Kegel (49) was the first to introduce PFM exercise to treat female SUI. He reported an 84% cure rate after a course of PFM strength training. However, in spite of the good results observed, surgery soon took over as the first choice of treatment, and not until the last decade was there a renewed interest in PFM exercise (see Table 53.2).

The overall trend of the results indicate that strength training of the PFM is effective to treat female SUI. However, there is a general lack of reliable and valid methods to measure both PFM strength and degree of SUI, and the outcome variables vary between studies. In addition there is a huge variability in research designs, diagnostic criteria, duration of the exercise period, and frequency and intensity of the training. These are all factors known to influence the effect of an intervention. The results are therefore both difficult to compare and to interpret. This paper will discuss the exercise regimens designed to develop PFM strength and the clinical results obtained after strength training.

Exercise Regimens

The two main factors that contribute to development of muscle strength—specificity and overload (26)—must be given special attention when it

Table 53.2 Pelvic Floor Muscle Exercise Regimens

Study	Technique	Evaluation of correct PFM contraction	Measurement of PFM strength	Exercise period	Exercise design
Kegel (49)	20 min., 3 times a day or 300 contractions	Vaginal palpation	Perineometer, PFM strength results not reported	Unknown	Home exercise, single group
Hendrickson et al. (36)	20 min., 3 times a day, hold each contraction for 2 s	Vaginal palpation	No	3 weeks	Hospitalized, single group
Shepherd et al. (66)	Technique not described	No	Pelvic exerciser, PFM strength 1. 6.4 → 19.3 cm H_2O 2. 7.1 → 11.2 cm H_2O	3 months	Home exercise, randomized: 1. with pelvic exerciser 2. without pelvic exerciser Weekly assessment
Castleden et al. (21)	4 to 5 contractions a day, interruption of micturition	No	Perineometer, PFM strength increase = 2 (cm H_2O or mmHg not reported)	4 weeks	Home exercise, single group
Sandri et al. (65)	2 weeks with instructor, regimen not described	No	Perineometer 8.3 → 15.1 cm H_2O	4 months	Home exercise, single group
Klarskov et al. (51)	5 times with instructor, regimen not described	No	No	4 months	Randomized: 1. surgery 2. PFM home exercise

Burgio et al. (10)	1 hr with instructor every 2 weeks: 24 contractions, hold for 10 s; home exercise: 17 contractions, 3 times a day	Vaginal palpation	External anal sphincter squeeze results not reported	2 months	1 month pretreatment bladder training, randomized: 1. with bladder-sphincter biofeedback 2. with verbal feedback
Benvenuti et al. (9)	30 min with instructor 5 days a week for 2 weeks, then once a week: hold for 30 s; home exercise: 10 times every hour, stop urine stream	Vaginal palpation	Urethral squeeze pressure, anal EMG, PFM strength 56 → 74 cm H_2O	3 months	Mixed bladder and PFM exercise, hospital and home exercise, single group
Wilson et al. (84)	1. Progression to 10 times every 30 min, stop urine stream; 2. 2 times a week with instructor and perineometer, 6 contractions, 3 times, hold contraction for 15s	No	Perineometer 1. 5.8 → 6.9 cm H_2O 2. 7.1 → 15.7 cm H_2O	6 weeks	Randomized: 1. home PFM 2. hospital PFM 3. PFM plus fardism 4. PFM plus interferential therapy
Henalla et al. (37)	Home exercise: 10 min every hour, hold for 5 s (fast contractions were also performed)	Vaginal palpation	No	3 months	Home exercise, single group, weekly assessment
Tshou et al. (77)	30 min with instructor twice a week, home exercise, overflow exercise of other muscles	No	No	4 weeks	Instructor-conducted exercise, single group
Tapp et al. (75)	Technique not described	Vaginal palpation	Perineometer results not reported	3 months	Home exercise (?), single group

(continued)

Table 53.2 *(Continued)*

Study	Technique	Evaluation of correct PFM contraction	Measurement of PFM strength	Exercise period	Exercise design
Ferguson et al. (34)	Technique not described	Not stated	Vaginal squeeze pressure, custom-fitted vaginal balloon 1. 23.2 → 33.4 cm H_2O 2. 38.3 → 46.5 cm H_2O	6 weeks	Randomized: 1. with intravaginal balloon 2. without intravaginal balloon
Bø et al. (14)	HE: 8 to 12 contractions 3 times a day, as hard as possible; IE: HE regimen plus instruction in maximum contraction during group exercise 45 min, once a week (use of 6- to 8-s contractions with 3–4 fast contractions on top, positions with legs abducted, strong verbal encouragement)	Vaginal palpation plus inward movement of balloon catheter	Vaginal squeeze pressure (balloon, microtip transducer) HE: 7.2 → 15.2 cm H_2O IE: 7.0→ 22.5 cm H_2O	6 months	Randomized: 1. home exercise 2. intensive exercise with weekly instructor-conducted exercise
Ramsey and Thou (64)	PFM: 4 maximum isometric contractions, held for 4 s every hour, 10-s rest between contractions; Placebo: 4 maximum isometric contractions in abduction with crossing feet	No	Perineometer results not reported	3 months	Randomized: 1. PFM at home 2. abduction of legs with crossing feet

Note. PFM = pelvic floor muscle; EMG = electromyogram; HE = home exercise; IE = instructor exercise.

comes to PFM exercise. Because the muscles and the muscle contractions are invisible from the outside, PFM strength training is difficult to instruct. The instructor is unable to control and assess the force of the contraction by observation.

Specificity

Benvenuti et al. (9), Bø et al. (18), and Hesse, Schussler, Frimberger, Obernitz, and Senn (38) have demonstrated that about 30% of SUI women, although thoroughly taught in PFM anatomy and function of the muscles, are unable to perform a correct voluntary PFM contraction at their first attempt.

A correct PFM contraction has been described as an inward lift and squeeze of the muscles, and is not externally visible. Ability to correctly contract the PFM can be evaluated by vaginal palpation (16,49) and observation of movement of the perineum or a vaginal catheter (16,24,46,50).

According to Bø et al. (18) the most common errors are to contract abdominal, gluteal, and hip adductor muscles instead of the PFM. In addition 9 out of 60 women in their study were performing a Valsalva maneuver, stretching the muscles instead of strengthening them. After 6 months of exercise 4 out of 52 women still were not able to contract the PFM correctly (14). This corresponds with Hesse et al. (38) who reported that 3 women needed up to 16 weeks to become aware of a correct contraction. In the latter study electrical stimulation was combined with exercise to enhance muscle awareness.

In eight of the quoted studies in Table 53.2, control of correct PFM contraction has not been performed, and the contractions may have been ineffective. Thus the results of these studies must be regarded with caution.

Overload, Intensity

Even if women are able to contract the PFM correctly, studies have shown that most women with SUI perform very weak contractions (14). Because close to a maximum contraction is required to create a high tension, the best way to achieve this is to stimulate women to contract as hard as possible and try to sustain the contraction for several seconds. Many authors do not describe the holding periods of the PFM contraction. The ones described vary between 2 s (36) and 30 s (9). As these authors have not visualized the contraction by recordings, it is impossible to know whether such long holding periods are possible.

Bø, Hagen, Kvarstein, Jørgensen, and Larsen (14) combined the three following principles in order to stimulate high-intensity contractions:

1. Six to 8 s sustained high-intensity contractions with 3 to 4 fast contractions at the top.
2. Use of initial positions with legs in abduction (see Figure 53.2).
3. Strong verbal encouragement by the instructor to motivate for high-intensity contractions.

By allowing contraction of outer pelvic muscles such as abdominal, hip adductor, and gluteal muscles, the PFM contraction is masked, and the women perceive a strong contraction although they are actually only performing a weak PFM contraction. Bø, Kvarstein, Hagen, and Larsen (16) and Dougherty, Abrams, and McKey (27) have demonstrated that synergistic contraction of other muscles does not add significant vaginal pressure above that registered from attempts of PFM contraction alone. The way women perceive their contraction and the awareness of the pelvic floor must be considered a crucial factor in achieving maximum tension. Positions with legs in abduction make contraction of other muscles difficult. In this way the women have to work hard to create and perceive the PFM contraction.

Duration of the Exercise Period

The length of the PFM exercise periods varies between 3 weeks (77) and 6 months (14). During the first weeks of strength training there may be a 20% to 40% increase in strength without a noticeable increase of cross-sectional area of the muscle involved (26). The explanation for this strength improvement is a more effective recruitment of motor units and increased frequency of excitation. However, the increase in cross-sectional area is a much slower process. In order to reveal the real potential for PFM exercise to treat SUI, the duration of the treatment periods should be at least 5 months.

Frequency

Kegel (49) recommended performing many contractions with no or low load. In fact he applied as many as 3 to 400 repetitions per day, most likely an amount impossible to perform for most of today's active, working women. The recommendation for strength training of other skeletal muscles are 3 to 4 sets of 8 to 12 high-resistance, slow-velocity contractions 3 times a week (26).

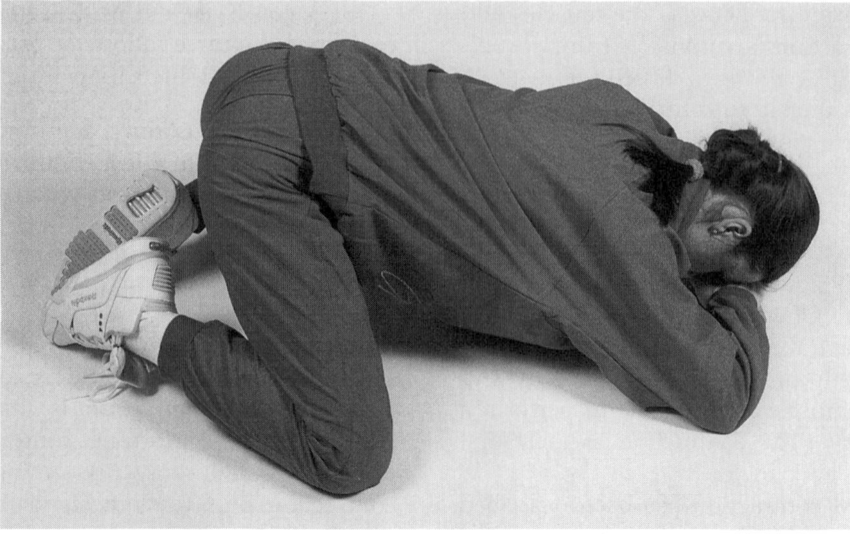

Figure 53.2 Example of a position to exercise the pelvic floor muscles effectively.

Most researchers apply the Kegel concept, but some have applied fewer repetitions (10,14). Performing close to maximum contractions, it may be possible to achieve the same effect with even fewer repetitions, for example, performed only every second day. In addition this may be more motivating for the patients.

PFM Training and the Effect on Increased Muscle Strength

The use of different methodology to measure PFM strength makes it impossible to draw any conclusions on what exercise program is the most effective in increasing PFM strength. The most common method applied is the perineometer. This method developed by Kegel (29,48) measures vaginal squeeze pressure during PFM contraction. Today more sensitive pressure transducers and more accurate printers have been developed (3,15,27,74). These devices have been found to be reproducible (15,27,83).

However, vaginal squeeze pressure has met a lot of criticism because rise in intraabdominal pressure also can be measured at the same time. Hence, a Valsalva maneuver can incorrectly be registered as a PFM contraction. However, as a correct contraction involves inward movement of the perineum, Bø et al. (16) combined clinical observation of inward movement of the perineum or the catheter with pressure registration to secure valid measurement. Only contractions involving an inward movement are registered as correct contractions.

In many studies (21,34,51,64,66,77,84) control of correct contractions has not been performed. In four studies (36,37,51,77) PFM strength has not been measured. In addition there is no report of strength development in four studies (36,49,64,75). Burgio, Robinson, and Engel (10) measured anal sphincter strength instead of isolated PFM strength. Hence, many researchers have not measured or reported the actual PFM strength before and after treatment (Table 53.2). However, without strength measurement it is impossible to conclude whether the intervention has been effective or not. Failure to monitor the treatment directly is therefore a serious flaw in many studies.

Bø et al. (16) have concluded that pressure measurement of PFM strength is not valid without simultaneous use of other methods (observation of inward muscle action) to ensure correct contraction. Very few studies satisfy these requirements.

Benvenuti et al. (9) demonstrated a significant improvement in urethral squeeze pressure during PFM contraction after 3 months of PFM exercise in combination with bladder training. This must be considered a very valid method to measure PFM strength, as it measures the pressure rise exactly where it is essential for prevention of urinary leakage.

Bø et al. (14) is the only group who has applied other methods simultaneously with measurement of vaginal squeeze pressure to secure valid measurements. They described development of muscle strength following two different exercise regimens throughout a 6-month exercise period (Figure 53.3).

The intensive exercise group (IE) was followed closely. They performed weekly group training of PFM exercises in addition to home exercises involving 8 to 12 contractions 3 times a day. Close

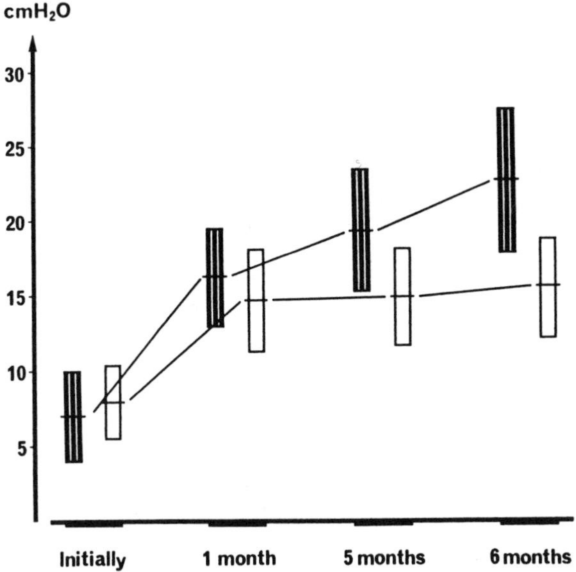

Figure 53.3 Maximum pelvic floor muscle strength before, after 1, 5 and 6 months of exercise. Columns illustrate 95% confidence intervals of the means. Means are given as horizontal lines. Dark bars = intensive exercise group; light bars = home exercise group. Both groups had increased the muscle strength significantly at 1 month ($p < 0.01$). At 5 months there was a significant difference in muscle strength between the two groups ($p < 0.03$).
From Bø et al: Pelvic floor muscle exercise for the treatment of female stress urinary incontinence: III. Effects of two different degrees of pelvic floor muscle exercises. Neurourol. Urodyn. 9:489-502, p. 496: 1990. Reprinted by permission.

to maximum contractions were emphasized using positions with legs apart to prevent simultaneous contraction of other muscles than the PFM. The home exercise group (HE) learned how to perform a correct contraction and were asked to perform 8 to 12 contractions 3 times a day. They had no further instruction of how to achieve a maximum contraction. However, they met once a month for strength measurement and motivation.

Both groups started at the same level of muscle strength and both increased their strength by 100% during the first month (Figure 53.3). This is a considerable strength gain, which may be explained because the PFM, in contrast to other skeletal muscles, most likely are totally untrained. After the first month of exercise, although exercise compliance was at the same level, the HE group did not gain further strength. The IE group, however, exercising according to the principles described previously, continued to increase their strength. After 5 months there was a significant difference between the two groups.

Instructor-Conducted Exercise

Wilson, Sammarai, Deakin, Kolbe, and Brown (84) and Bø et al. (14) have both demonstrated that PFM exercise has to be instructor-conducted to be effective. Bø et al. (14) led the exercises in groups throughout the 6-month exercise period. Group exercise may be more motivating for both participants and the instructor, and it reduces both time and cost of the treatment. In addition it may change the view of SUI as a disease that needs treatment in hospitals to one that is addressed in a preventive health approach. However, group exercise can never substitute the first important individual training with vaginal palpation.

Conclusion

More research is required to decide the optimal intensity, frequency, and duration of PFM exercise to develop PFM strength. However, certain principles are effective in increasing PFM strength:

1. The need of thorough individual instruction of PFM function
2. Palpation or observation with feedback of the correctness of the contraction
3. Performance of close to maximum high-intensity contractions
4. Isolation of PFM contractions by use of positions with legs apart
5. Instructor-conducted exercises and close follow-up with motivation during the exercise period
6. Long exercise periods (at least 5 months)

Clinical Results

The results of PFM exercise to treat female SUI will be discussed according to diagnostic criteria of SUI, research design, sample size, dropout and compliance rates, and the methods applied to measure treatment outcome.

Diagnostic Criteria of SUI

According to ICS, SUI should be demonstrated objectively. In all but four of the published studies (21,36,51,64), the diagnosis of SUI has been made by urodynamic measurements such as stress tests, urethral pressure profilometry, or pad tests (Table 53.3).

Table 53.3 Clinical Outcome of Pelvic Floor Muscle Strength Training

	Material and methods				Results					
Study	*N*	Age (years)	Design	Urodynamic assessments	Women's own assessment	MUCP (rest)	MUCP (stress)	Pad test	Micturition chart	Stress test
Hendrickson (36)	13	40–60	Pre-posttest	—	Score on questionnaire 11.9 → 1.6	—	—	—	—	—
Shepherd et al. (66)	22	23–67	Randomization: 1. $N = 11$ with pelvic exerciser 2. $N = 11$ without pelvic exerciser; pre-posttest; follow-up after 3 months	Cystometry, urethral pressure profile	1. 8 cured 2 improved 1 unchanged 2. 3 cured 2 improved 5 unchanged	Only measured before treatment	Only measured before treatment	—	Only measured before treatment	—
Castleden et al. (21)	19	23–85	Randomization: 1. PFM alone 2. with perineometer; Pre-posttest crossover	Cystometry (only 8 patients)	14 continent/improved (77%) VAS score: 1. +6.7 2. +23.9	—	—	—	—	—
Klarskov et al. (51)	50	31–66	Randomization: 1. $N = 26$, surgery 2. $N = 24$, PFM exercise; pre-posttest crossover; follow-up after 8 months	Cystometry	1. 16 cured 7 improved 2 unchanged 1 worse 2. 3 cured 14 improved 7 unchanged 42% satisfied after PFM exercise	—	—	Only measured after treatment, and only in some patients	Number of incontinence episodes per 3 days: 6 → 0, $p < .01$ 6 → 2, $p < .05$	—

Sandri et al. (65)	24	Mean age 50	Pre-posttest	Colpocys-tourethrography	12% unchanged 12% slightly improved 35% markedly improved 41% cured	—	—	65% "essen-tially dry"	—	—
Burgio et al. (10)	24	29–64	Randomization: 1. PFM, verbal feedback 2. PFM, anal pressure measure-ments; pre-posttest	Stress test with 350 ml saline in the bladder	—	—	—	—	Frequency of in-continence epi-sodes per week: 5.8 → 2.5, $p < .01$ 6.9 → 1.8, $p < .01$	Number with positive test 1. 4 2. 6
Benvenuti et al. (9)	22	36–65	Pre-posttest; follow-up by questionnaire	Micturition cys-tourethrography (15 patients), cys-tometry, urethral closure pressure profilometry	32% cured all improved	39–56 cm H_2O $p < .01$	(FUPL mm 27 → 31 $p < .01$)	—	Weekly reduction of incontinence episodes: 10.2 → 0.3 $p < .01$	—
Wilson et al. (84)	60	19–79	Randomization: 1. PFM in hospital 2. PFM plus faradism 3. PFM plus in-terferential therapy 4. PFM at home Pre-posttest; follow-up after 4 1/2 months	Synchroneous video pressure-flow cystour-ethrography	In all groups: 33% unchanged 33% improved 33% much improved (66% improved)	49.6 → 51.5 cm H_2O (NS), 56.1 → 58.0 (NS), 50.7 → 56.0 ($p < .05$); 49.8–5.3 (NS); OBS! only 45 patients	Only mea-sured in 45 pa-tients, and only after treatment	—	Yes, but no mea-surements of incontinence episodes	—
Henalla et al. (37)	58	27–77, 26–74	Same study in two different hospitals; pre-posttest	Cystometry, ure-thral pressure "studies"	—	—	—	22 cured/im-proved 17 cured/im-proved (bladder vol-ume not stan-dardized)	—	—
Tschou et al. (77)	14	33–67	Pre-posttest	Static urethral pressure profile, stress test, cys-tometry	—	51.6 → 48.9 mmHg (NS)	FUPL 2.5 → 2.6 mm (NS)	—	—	9 negative after treat-ment

(continued)

Table 53.3 ***(Continued)***

	Material and methods				Results					
Study	*N*	Age (years)	Design	Urodynamic assessments	Women's own assessment	MUCP (rest)	MUCP (stress)	Pad test	Micturition chart	Stress test
Tapp et al. (75)	45	—	Pre-posttest	Video-cystourethrography, urethral pressure profilometry	VAS: 12 cured	Values not reported	Values not reported	Values not reported	—	—
Ferguson et al. (34)	20	Mean age 36	Randomization 1. with vaginal balloon 2. without vaginal balloon	Cystometry, rest and stress pressure profile	—	—	NS increase in MUCP, significant increase in FUPL by 0.1 in group without balloon	1. –3.4g 2. –6.9g	—	—
Bø et al. (14)	52	24–64, mean age 45.9	Randomization 1. home exercise 2. intensive exercise, instructor-conducted	Cystometry, flowmetry, rest and stress pressure profile	1. 17% cured/almost cured, leakage index: from 3.1 to 2.6 ($p < .01$), social activity index: NS 2. 60% cured/almost cured, leakage index: from 3.0 to 1.9 ($p < .01$), social activity index: from 7.7 to 9.3 ($p < .01$)	4.6 cm H_2O increase ($p < .01$)	—	From 27 g to 7 g ($p < .01$)	—	60% cure
Ramsey & Thou (64)	44	—	Randomization: 1. PFM 2. isometric abduction of legs	—	1. 14 improved 2 unchanged 6 worse 2. 14 improved 6 no change 2 worse	—	—	1. Significantly worse by 1.5 g 2. Significantly improved by 2.1 g	—	—

Note. N = number; MUCP = maximum urethral closure pressure; — = unknown; PFM = pelvic floor muscle; *p* = probability; FUPL = functional urethral profile length; NS = not significant.

Research Design

With the exception of some cases developed during pregnancy and after childbirth, SUI is not a self-improving condition. Therefore, the patients may act as their own control subjects. However, randomized studies comparing different methods will to a certain degree eliminate the Hawthorne effect (i.e., no matter what is done, the patients will improve), and they are therefore stronger designs. The research designs vary between single group studies and randomized, controlled studies comparing the efficacy of two or more treatment methods.

In five studies (10,21,28,34,66) the effect of adding biofeedback (vaginal or anal feedback systems) to PFM exercise has been compared to regular PFM exercises. The results differ, hence today, no conclusion can be drawn as to whether or not the addition of biofeedback provides better results. Susset and Galea (73) applied biofeedback therapy combining audio and visual signals in 15 women with mixed stress and urge incontinence and reported complete cure in 12 women after 6 weeks of treatment. Thirteen demonstrated dryness as evaluated with a pad test with standardized bladder volume. Although promising, the results of adding biofeedback are controversial and need further research.

Klarskov et al. (51) and Wilson et al. (84) randomly assigned patients to PFM exercise or to other treatments. Klarskov et al. found that surgery was superior to PFM exercise measured by the number of self-reported incontinence episodes per day and subjective statement of being cured, improved, unchanged, or worse. However, 42% of the patients treated with PFM exercise were satisfied with the treatment outcome. Wilson et al. (84) found no significant differences between PFM alone, PFM plus faradism or PFM plus interferential therapy measured as self-reported micturitions, pad changes per 24 hr, perineometry, and maximal urethral closure pressure (MUCP) plus PFM contraction. In-hospital treatment was superior to home exercises.

Bø et al. (14) demonstrated that a specially designed PFM exercise program aimed to produce maximum contractions and conducted partly as group exercise for 6 months was significantly more effective than exercises conducted at home with no instruction of how to produce maximum contractions.

Ramsey and Thou (64) performed a double-blind, randomized, placebo study in which PFM exercises were compared to exercises of hip abduction with crossed legs. The placebo group improved more than the PFM-exercise group measured by pad test. This may seem convincing. However, there was no assessment of ability to perform correct contractions. Therefore, the group performing abduction of the gluteal muscles may have obtained a better training stimulus to the PFM than the actual exercise group. In addition compliance to the exercise program was very low.

To evaluate the effect of the instructor, Henalla et al. compared the effect of the same PFM exercise regimen conducted by two physiotherapists at two different hospitals. They found no significant difference in treatment outcome (pad test) when the exercises were taught by two different instructors.

Sample Size

The sample size is crucial when testing statistical significance and may be one of the reasons for not finding such differences (66,84). The sample size varies between 13 (36) and 60 (84). However, Wilson et al. divided his sample into 4 groups leaving only 15 women in each group. Only Klarskov et al. (51), Henalla et al. (37), and Bø et al. (14) have conducted randomized studies comparing two groups with a sample size of more than 50.

Dropout and Compliance Rates

Dropout rates as reported in these studies vary between 13% (36) and 29% at a 4-month follow-up (65). In 10 out of 14 studies there were no dropouts from pre- to posttest. Compliance to the exercise program is a key factor when evaluating the effect of PFM exercise. A thorough registration of compliance therefore has to be obtained, reported, and analyzed.

The compliance rates are reported in very few studies. Bø et al. (14) had close to 100% compliance as reported in a training diary both for the home-exercise and the intensive-exercise group. The high compliance rate of the home-exercise group in this study may be explained by the monthly follow-up with personal motivation and measurement of PFM strength. However, Ramsey and Thou (64) reported that their exercise groups had performed only 15% of the requested level of exercise. The patients had no follow-up during the 3-month exercise period.

Subjective Cure and Patient's Effect Evaluation

The methods applied to evaluate the patient's opinion of the treatment effect are simple scales (cured, improved, unchanged, worse). However, such scales do not relate to the daily activities and concrete situations where leakage occurs. Thus the answers give only limited information about individual cure or improvement.

The success rate as evaluated by the women varies between 32% (9) and 84% (49). Bø et al. (14) have operationalized "subjective cure," and have constructed two instruments to assess the women's evaluation of how they perceive the condition of SUI before and after tretment (12). The results after PFM exercise assessed by these two methods are given in Table 53.3 again demonstrating that intensive exercise was more effective than home exercise.

Objective Cure

The term *objective measurements* is too often used to describe evaluation tools that simply involve figures and numbers instead of methods tested for reproducibility (inter- and intravariability), validity, and sensitivity. Interpreted in this context, some pad tests and urethral pressure measurements do not fulfill the criteria of being objective measures of SUI. Reliable, valid, and sensitive measurements of SUI are difficult to obtain, and there is no agreement of which parameters to use.

Only Benvenuti et al. (9), Wilson et al. (84), and Bø et al. (14) have demonstrated significant improvement in resting urethral pressure. Benvenuti et al. (9) demonstrated improvement after a combination of bladder training and PFM exercise and Wilson et al. (84) after a combination of PFM exercise and interferential therapy. However, the clinical significance of such an increased resting urethral pressure in SUI is not clear.

Benvenuti et al. (9) and Ferguson et al. (34) demonstrated significant increase in functional urethral profile length (FUPL). In the study of Tshou, Adams, Varner, and Denton (77) 9 out of 14 women demonstrated a negative stress test after treatment. Bø et al. (14) demonstrated a 60% cure rate after intensive PFM exercise (cure defined as positive closure pressure during cough).

Sandri, Magnaghi, Fanciullacci, and Zanollo (65), Henalla et al. (37), Tapp, Cardozo, Hills, and Barnic (75), Ferguson et al. (34), and Bø et al. (14) have applied pad tests to assess improvement after PFM exercise. Tapp et al. (75) did not report the results, and Sandri et al. (65) and Henalla et al. (37) did not apply a standardized bladder volume. Bladder volume will affect the reproducibility of the test (55,57). Ferguson et al. (34) and Bø et al. (14) both demonstrated significant reduction of urine loss measured by pad tests with standardized bladder volume.

Limitations of PFM Exercise in Treatment of SUI

Wilson et al. (84), Henalla et al. (37), Tapp et al. (75) and Bø, Larsen, Kvarstein, and Hagen (17) have all analyzed their data in order to predict which patients will benefit from PFM exercises. Wilson et al. (84) found that treatment success was more likely in younger women, in those with lesser degree of urethral sphincter incompetence, and in those who had no history of pelvic floor surgery. Similar results were found by Tapp et al. (75). Those who benefited most from PFM exercises were premenopausal women with a shorter duration of symptoms and better urethral function during stress.

In contrast, Henalla et al. (37) and Bø et al. (17) found that neither the severity of symptoms, nor the age, nor previous surgery influenced treatment outcome. Age may be a limiting factor for strength development and may be confounded with more severe SUI. In the study of Bø et al. (17) the responders to intensive PFM exercise were significantly older (mean age 48.4 years vs. 38.3 years), had a longer history of SUI, a higher body mass index score, lower resting urethral pressure, stronger PFM, and more severe SUI. A discriminant function classified the responders according to a combination of the following pretreatment parameters: low flow rate, moderate PFM strength, long incontinence history, and severe SUI measured by a leakage index.

The controversy in results may be due to the small sample sizes, and further studies based on high-compliance, long-lasting, and intensive PFM exercises should be conducted to settle the question about limitations in treatment outcomes for special groups.

There are no reports of complications or side effects after PFM exercise.

Conclusions

1. PFM exercise has no known side effects and should be considered the first choice of treatment for SUI.
2. Assessed by patient opinion and reliable, sensitive, and valid measurements, cure and satisfying improvement rate after isolated PFM exercise may reach 60%.
3. High cure rate is dependent on 5 to 6 months of intensive exercise conducted partly under supervision and with a close follow-up. The patients should not be left alone with a written explanation on how to perform PFM exercises.
4. More research is required to further assess the efficacy of different exercise regimens.

5. Motivation is a key factor in all methods involving patient participation.
6. Group exercise may be more motivating for both instructor and participants.

References

1. Abrams, P.; Blaivas, J.G.; Stanton, S.L.; Andersen, J.T. The standarisation of terminology of lower urinary tract function. Scand. J. Urol. Nephrol. [Suppl.]. 114:5-19; 1988.
2. Abrams, P.; Fenely, R.; Torrens, M. Urodynamics. Berlin, Heidelberg, New York: Springer-Verlag; 1983.
3. Abrams, R.M.; Batich, C.; Dougherty, M.C.; McKey, P.L.; Chang Lin, Y.; Parker, J. Custom-made vaginal balloons for strengthening circumvaginal musculature. Biomat. Med. 14(3,4): 239-248; 1986.
4. Allen, R.E.; Warrell, D. The role of pregnancy and childbirth in partiel denervation of the pelvic floor. Neurourol. Urodyn. 6:183-184; 1987.
5. Bates, P.; Bradley, W.; Glen, E. Quantification of urine loss. Fifth report on the standardization of terminology of lower urinary tract function. International Continence Society Committee for Standardization of Terminology; 1983.
6. Beck, K.P.; Hsu, N. Pregnancy, childbirth, and the menopause related to the development of stress incontinence. Am. J. Obstet. Gynecol. 91:820-823; 1965.
7. Beco, J.; Sulu, M.; Schaaps, J.P.; Lambotte, R. A new approach to the troubles of urinary incontinence in women: Urodynamic ultrasound examination by the vaginal route. J. Gynecol. Obstet. Biol. Reprod. 16:987-998; 1987.
8. Bennes, C.; Abbott, D.; Cardozo, L.; Savvas, M.; Studd, J. Lower urinary tract dysfunction in postmenopausal women—the role of estrogen deficiency. Neurourol. Urodyn. 10(4):315-316; 1991.
9. Benvenuti, F.; Caputo, G.M.; Bandinelli, S.; Mayer, F.; Biagini, C.; Somavilla, A. Reeducative treatment of female genuine stress incontinence. Am. J. Phys. Med. 66(4):155-168; 1987.
10. Burgio, K.L.; Robinson, J.C.; Engel, B.T. The role of biofeedback in Kegel exercise training for stress urinary incontinence. Am. J. Obstet. Gynecol. 154:58-64; 1986.
11. Bø, K. Pelvic floor muscle exercise for the treatment of female stress urinary incontinence. Methodological studies and clinical results. Oslo, Norway: The Norwegian University of Sport and Physical Education; 1990.
12. Bø, K. Reproducibility of instruments designed to measure women's subjective assessment of stress urinary incontinence. Neurourol. Urodyn. 10(4):424-426; 1991.
13. Bø, K.; Hagen, R.; Kvarstein, B.; Larsen, S. Female stress urinary incontinence and participation in different sport and social activities. Scand. J. Sports Sci. 11(3):117-121; 1989.
14. Bø, K.; Hagen, R.H.; Kvarstein, B.; Jørgensen, J.; Larsen, S. Pelvic floor muscle exercise for the treatment of female stress urinary incontinence: III. Effects of two different degrees of pelvic floor muscle exercises. Neurourol. Urodyn. 9:489-502; 1990.
15. Bø, K.; Kvarstein, B.; Hagen, R.; Larsen, S. Pelvic floor muscle exercise for the treatment of female stress urinary incontinence: I. Reliability of vaginal pressure measurements of pelvic floor muscle strength. Neurourol. Urodyn. 9:471-477; 1990.
16. Bø, K.; Kvarstein, B.; Hagen, R.; Larsen, S. Pelvic floor muscle exercise for the treatment of female stress urinary incontinence: II. Validity of vaginal pressure measurements of pelvic floor muscle strength and the necessity of supplementary methods for control of correct contraction. Neurourol. Urodyn. 9:479-487; 1990.
17. Bø, K.; Larsen, S.; Kvarstein, B.; Hagen, R.H. Classification and characterization of responders to pelvic floor muscle exercise for female stress urinary incontinence. Neurourol. Urodyn. 9(4):395-397; 1990.
18. Bø, K.; Larsen, S.; Oseid, S.; Kvarstein, B.; Hagen, R.; Jørgensen, J. Knowledge about and ability to correct pelvic floor muscle exercises in women with urinary stress incontinence. Neurourol. Urodyn. 7(3):261-262; 1988.
19. Bø, K.; Maehlum, S.; Oseid, S.; Larsen, S. Prevalence of stress urinary incontinence among physically active and sedentary female students. Scand. J. Sports Sci. 11(3):113-116; 1989.
20. Campbell, A.J.; Reinken, J.; McCosh, L. Incontinence in the elderly: Prevalence and prognosis. Age Ageing. 14:65-70; 1985.
21. Castleden, C.M.; Duffin, H.M.; Mitchell, E.P. The effect of physiotherapy on stress incontinence. Age Ageing. 13:235-237; 1984.
22. Constantinou, C.E.; Faysal, M.H.; Rother, L.; Govan, D.E. The impact of bladder neck suspension on the mode of distribution of abdominal pressure along the female urethra. In Female incontinence. New York: Alan R. Liss; 1981:121-132.
23. Constantinou, C.E.; Govan, D.E. Contribution and timing of transmitted and generated pressure components in the female urethra. In Female incontinence. New York: Alan R. Liss; 1981:113-120.

24. DeLancey, J.O.L. Anatomy and mechanics of structures around the vesical neck: How vesical neck position might affect its closure. Neurourol. Urodyn. 7(3):161-162; 1988.
25. DeLancey, J.O.L. Videoproduction on pelvic floor muscle contraction. 1990. Available from: University of Michigan Medical Center. 1500 E. Medical Center Drive. Dept. of Ob/Gyn—D2230 MPB. Ann Arbor, MI 48109-0718.
26. DiNubile, N.A. Strength training. Clin. Sports Med. 10(1):33-62; 1991.
27. Dougherty, M.C.; Abrams, R.; McKey, P.L. An instrument to assess the dynamic characteristics of the circumvaginal musculature. Nurs. Res. 35(4):202-206; 1986.
28. Dougherty, M.C.; Abrams, R.M.; Battich, C.D.; Bishop, K.R.; Gimptty, P. Effect of exercise on the circumvaginal muscles (CVM). Neurourol. Urodyn. 6(3):189-190; 1987.
29. Dubin, L.; Morales, P. Perineometer testing of the bulbocavernous reflex. J. Urol. 93(1):57-59; 1965.
30. Dwyer, P.L.; Lee, E.T.C.; Hay, D.M. Obesity and urinary incontinence in women. Br. J. Obstet. Gynaecol. 95:91-96; 1988.
31. Elving, L.B.; Foldspang, A.; Lam, G.W.; Mommsen, S. Descriptive epidemiology of urinary incontinence in 3100 women age 30-59. Scand. J. Urol. Nephrol. [Suppl.]. 125:37-43; 1989.
32. Enhørning, G. Simultaneous recording of intravesical and intra-urethral pressure. Acta Chir. Scand. Suppl:276; 1961.
33. Fall, M.; Frankenberg, S.; Frisen, M.; Larson, B.; Petren, M. 456000 svenskar kan ha urininkontinens. Endast var fjarde søker hjalp før besvaren. [456000 Swedes may have incontinence. Only one out of four seeks help for the problem.] Läkartidningen. 82:2054-2056; 1985.
34. Ferguson, K.L.; McKey, P.L.; Bishop, K.R.; Kloen, P.; Verheul, J.B.; Dougherty, M.C. Stress urinary incontinence: Effect of pelvic muscle exercise. Obstet. Gynecol. 75:671-675; 1990.
35. Hagen, R.H.; Kvarstein, B.; Bø, K.; Larsen, S. A simple pad test with fixed bladder volume to measure urine loss during physical activity. Papers to be read by title: International continence society 18th annual meeting; Oslo; 1988:88-89.
36. Hendrickson, L.S. The frequency of stress incontinence in women before and after the implementation of an exercise program. Issues Health Care Women. 3:81-92; 1981.
37. Hennalla, S.M.; Kirwan, P.; Castleden, D.M.; Hutchins, C.J.; Breeson, A.J. The effect of pelvic floor muscle exercises in the treatment of genuine stress incontinence in women at two hospitals. Br. J. Obstet. Gynaecol. 95:81-92; 1988.
38. Hesse, U.; Schussler, B.; Frimberger, J.; Obernitz, N.V.; Senn, E. Effectiveness of a three step pelvic floor reeducation in the treatment of stress urinary incontinence: A clinical assessment. Neurourol. Urodyn. 9(4):397-398; 1990.
39. Hørding, U.; Pederssen, K.H.; Sidenius, K.; Hedegaard, L. Urinary incontinence in 45-year-old women. Scand. J. Urol. Nephrol. 20:183-186; 1986.
40. Hunskaar, S.; Vinsnes, A. The quality of life in women with urinary incontinence as measured by the sickness impact profile. JAGS. 39:378-382; 1991.
41. Iosif, C.S.; Becassy, Z. Prevalence of genito-urinary symptoms in the late menopause. Acta Obstet. Gynecol. Scand. 63:257-260; 1984.
42. Iosif, S. Stress incontinence during pregnancy and puerperium. Int. J. Gynaecol. Obstet. 19:13-20; 1981.
43. Iosif, S.; Henriksson, L.; Ulmsten, U. The frequency of disorders of the lower urinary tract, urinary incontinence in particular, as evaluated by a questionnaire survey in a gynecological health control population. Acta Obstet. Gynecol. 60:71-76; 1981.
44. Iosif, C.S.; Ingemarsson, I. Prevalence of stress incontinence among women delivered by elective cesarian section. Int. J. Gynecol. Obstet. 20:87-89; 1982.
45. James, E.D. The behaviour of the bladder during physical activity. Br. J. Urol. 50:387-394; 1978.
46. James, E.D.; Shaldon, C.S.; Niblett, P.G. Vaginal pressure: Its role in urodynamic studies and in re-educating pelvic floor muscles. Proc. int. cont. sos.; Innsbruck; 1984:150-151.
47. Jolleys, J.V. Reported prevalence of urinary incontinence in women in a general practice. Br. Med. J. 296:1300-1302; 1988.
48. Kegel, A.H. Progressive resistance exercise in the functional restoration of the perineal muscles. Am. J. Obstet. Gynecol. 56:238-249; 1948.
49. Kegel, A.H. Physiologic therapy for urinary incontinence. JAMA. 146:915-917; 1951.
50. Kegel, A.H. Stress incontinence and genital relaxation. Ciba Found. Symp. 2:35-51; 1952.
51. Klarskov, P.; Belving, D.; Bischoff, N.; Dorph, S.; Gerstenberg, T.; Okholm, B.; Pedersen, P.H.; Tikjøb, G.; Wormslev, M.; Hald, T. Pelvic floor exercise versus surgery for female urinary stress incontinence. Urol. Int. 41:129-132; 1986.
52. Klevmark, B.; Kulseng-Hanssen, S. Continence mechanism in the female. Scand. J. Urol. Nephrol. [Suppl.]. 138:35-40; 1991.
53. Koelbl, H.; Bernascheck, G.; Wolf, G. A comparative study of perineal ultrasound scanning and urethro cystography in patients with genuine stress incontinence. Arch. Gynecol. Obstet. 244:39-45; 1988.

54. Koelbl, H.; Riss, P. The significance of the body mass index for genuine stress incontinence. Neurourol. Urodyn. 6:186-187; 1987.
55. Kralj, B. Comparative study of pad tests-reliability and repetiveness. Neurourol. Urodyn. 8(4):305-306; 1989.
56. Kulseng-Hanssen, S.; Klevmark, B. Ambulatory urethro-cysto-rectometry: A new technique. Neurourol. Urodyn. 7:119-130; 1988.
57. Lose, G.; Rosenkilde, P.; Gammelgaard, J.; Schroeder, T. Pad weighing test performed with standardized bladder volume. Urology. 32(1):78-80; 1988.
58. National Institutes of Health. Urinary incontinence in adults. Medical applications of research, National Institutes of Health. Medical Applications of Research. 7:1-11; 1988.
59. Nemir, A.; Middleton, R.P. Stress incontinence in young nulliparous women. Am. J. Obstet. Gynecol. 68:1166-1168; 1954.
60. Nichols, D.H.; Milley, P.S. Functional pelvic anatomy: The soft tissue supports and spaces of the female pelvic organs. In: The human vagina. Reprod. Med. 2:21-37; 1978.
61. Norton, P.; MacDonald, L.; Stanton, S.L. Distress associated with female urinary complaints and delay in seeking treatment. Neurourol. Urodyn. 6(3):170-171; 1987.
62. Nygaard, I.; DeLancey, J.O.L.; Arnsdorf, L.; Murphy, E. Exercise and incontinence. Obstet. Gynecol. 75:848-851; 1990.
63. Ostergaard, D.R. Gynecologic urology and urodynamics. Theory and practice. Baltimore/London: Williams & Wilkins; 1980.
64. Ramsey, I.N.; Thou, M. A randomized, double blind, placebo controlled trial of pelvic floor exercises in the treatment of genuine stress incontinence. Neurourol. Urodyn. 9(4):398-399; 1990.
65. Sandri, S.D.; Magnaghi, C.; Fanciullacci, F.; Zanollo, A. Pad controlled results of pelvic floor physiotherapy in female stress incontinence. Proceedings of third joint meeting: Boston; 1986:233-235.
66. Shepherd, A.; Montgomery, E.; Anderson, R.S. A pilot study of a pelvic exerciser in women with stress urinary incontinence. J. Obstet. Gynecol. 3:201-202; 1983.
67. Simeonova, Z.; Bengtsson, C. Prevalence of urinary incontinence among women at a Swedish primary health care centre. Scand. J. Prim. Health Care. 8:303-306; 1990.
68. Snooks, S.J.; Setchell, M.; Swash, M.; Henry, M.M. Injury to innervation of pelvic floor sphincter musculature in childbirth. Lancet. (Sept.):546-550; 1984.
69. Snooks, S.J.; Swash, M.; Mathers, S.E.; Henry, M. M. Effect of vaginal delivery on the pelvic floor: A 5 year follow up. Br. J. Surg. 77:1358-1360; 1990.
70. Sommer, P.; Bauer, T.; Nielsen, K.K.; Kristensen, E.S.; Hermann, G.G.; Steven, K.; Nordling, I. Voiding patterns and prevalence in women. Br. J. Urol. 66:12-15; 1990.
71. Stanton, S.L. Clinical gynecologic urology. St. Louis: Mosby; 1984.
72. Stanton, S.L.; Kerr-Wilson, R.; Harris, V.G. The incidence of urological symptoms in normal pregnancy. Br. J. Obstet. Gynaecol. 87:897-900; 1980.
73. Susset, J.G.; Galea, G.; Read, L. Biofeedback therapy for female incontinence due to low urethral resistance. Neurourol. Urodyn. 143(6):1205-1208; 1990.
74. Taher, A.L.-H.I.; Sudherst, J.R.; Richmond, D.N.; Brown, M.C. Vaginal pressure as an index of intra-abdominal pressure during urodynamic evaluation. Br. J. Urol. 59:529-531; 1987.
75. Tapp, A.J.S.; Cardozo, L.; Hills, B.; Barnic, C. Who benefits from physiotherapy? Neurourol. Urodyn. 7(3):260-261; 1988.
76. Thomas, T.M.; Plymat, K.T.; Blannin, J.; Meade, T.W. Prevalence of urinary incontinence. Br. Med. J. 281:1243-1245; 1980.
77. Tschou, D.C.H.; Adams, C.; Varner, R.E.; Denton, B. Pelvic-floor musculature exercises in treatment of anatomical urinary stress incontinence. Phys. Ther. 68:652-655; 1988.
78. Yarnell, J.G.; St. Leger, A.S. The prevalence, severity and factors associated with urinary incontinence in a random sample of the elderly. Age Ageing. 8:81-85; 1979.
79. Yarnell, J.G.; Voyle, G.J. The prevalence and severity of urinary incontinence in women. J. Epidemiol. Community Health. 35:71-74; 1981.
80. Wells, T.J. Pelvic (floor) muscle exercise. JAGS. 38:333-337; 1990.
81. Wilkie, D.H.L. Stress incontinence and obesity: A study of the effect of obesity on urethral function. Neurourol. Urodyn. 6:184-185; 1987.
82. Wilson, P.D. Conservative management of urethral sphincter incompetence. Clin. Obstet. Gynecol. 33(2):330-345; 1990.
83. Wilson, P.D.; Herbison, G.P.; Heer, K. Reproducibility of perineometry measurements. Neurourol. Urodyn. 10(4):389-394; 1991.
84. Wilson, P.D.; Sammarai, T.A.L.; Deakin, M.; Kolbe, E.; Brown, A.D.G. An objective assessment of physiotherapy for female genuine stress incontinence. Br. J. Obstet. Gynaecol. 94:575-582; 1987.
85. Wolin, J.H. Stress incontinence in young healthy nulliparous female subjects. J. Urol. 101:545-549; 1969.

Chapter 54

Physical Activity, Fitness, and Infection

David C. Nieman

Infection in Athletes

Several types of infectious diseases affect athletes, often because they perform in an environment in which certain pathogenic microorganisms are particularly widespread or, due to the type of sport, abrasions or other tissue injury are more likely (15). Athletes may be at increased risk for various infections because of cross-infection from others with whom they are in close contact. In addition, exposure to alien environmental pathogens during foreign travel may result in infection due to lack of specific immunity (34). There is also the potential for immunosuppression from both psychosocial and physiological stress that can arise during periods of heavy training and competition (66–68).

Skin Infections

Athletic clothing and footwear provide a warm, moist environment for several types of bacteria and viruses. During athletic participation, frictional trauma can damage the skin, increasing adherence and penetration of these microorganisms (15). Skin infections that can be acquired by person-to-person contact in such sports as wrestling and rugby (especially in the scrum) include streptococcal impetigo, folliculitis, erysipelas, herpes simplex, and tinea barbae. These infections have been appropriately termed "scrumpox." Abrasions and the wearing of facial stubble facilitate the inoculation of the infecting agent during grinding physical contact. Prevention of the spread of such infections is best achieved by the combined efforts of the athletes and medical personnel. Newly acquired cuts and abrasions should be treated with soap, water, and topical antiseptics. Oral and topical antibiotics are effective against mild infections. Open wounds should be covered, and athlete-to-athlete skin contact should be discontinued until healing has occurred.

Herpes simplex is a viral infection characterized by a localized, primary lesion, latency, and a tendency to localized recurrence (5). Cutaneous and ocular infection with herpes simplex virus Type I (HSV-1) was initially recognized as a health risk for wrestlers and rugby players in the 1960s and labeled *herpes gladiatorum* (4). Herpes is highly infectious, spreading rapidly from person to person by droplets, where skin surfaces are directly opposed, as in contact sports, or indirectly by the sharing of eating utensils, infected towels, clothing, and equipment (92). In 1989, researchers from the Centers for Disease Control and the Minnesota Department of Health investigated a large outbreak of herpes gladiatorum among high school wrestlers attending a 4-week intensive-training camp (4). HSV-1 infection was diagnosed in 34% of the wrestlers, with lesions found on all parts of the body where skin-to-skin contact was effected. Constitutional symptoms were common, including fever, chills, sore throat, and headache. The researchers concluded that control efforts should emphasize the early identification of skin lesions and the prompt exclusion of potentially infected wrestlers. Routine skin examinations by coaches or trainers may be helpful because some athletes are reluctant to report skin lesions that would bar them from competition.

Infections can also be acquired from the environment of changing facilities; the most frequently occurring are the superficial dermatophyte skin infections *tinea pedis* ("athlete's foot"), and *tinea cruris* ("jock rot") (34). Several species of fungi survive well in the moist environment present in dressing and shower rooms, and fungal infections are more prevalent in hot, humid climates and during warm seasons (84). Definitive diagnosis can be made with a potassium hydroxide preparation, a test quickly and easily performed in most physicians' offices. Treatment is usually simple and consists of antifungal medication and alteration of the warm, moist environment of the affected area. For prevention, athletes are encouraged to keep the skin area as cool and dry as possible, wear loose, absorbent clothing rather than tight garments or those made of synthetic fabrics, and not share towels, soaps, or sports equipment with other athletes.

Viral Hepatitis B

Viral hepatitis B occurs worldwide, with particularly high rates of infection occurring in Africa and Asia (5). Approximately 5% of the adult population of the United States has serologic evidence of previous infection, with 0.2% to 0.9% being chronic carriers of the hepatitis B virus (HBV). Severity ranges from inapparent cases detectable only by liver function tests to fulminating, fatal cases of acute hepatic necrosis. HBV may be the cause of up to 80% of all cases of hepatocellular carcinoma worldwide. HBV has been found in virtually all body secretions and excretions; however, only blood, saliva, semen, and vaginal fluids have been shown to be infectious (107). Transmission occurs by percutaneous and permucosal exposure to infective body fluids, as may occur in sexual and perinatal exposure, contamination of skin lesions, or by exposure of mucous membranes to infective blood. The incubation period of hepatitis B is long, averaging 6 weeks to 6 months. Effective vaccines are available that afford immunity to infection, and regimens of immune globulin and vaccination can prevent infection in an exposed individual if begun soon after exposure.

Detecting the asymptomatic carrier has proven to be virtually impossible; thus, one should be aware of the need for overall good hygiene. For example, communally used razors and toothbrushes have been implicated as occasional transmitters of HBV. Protection of open wounds and avoidance of unsafe sexual contact are essential. HBV vaccination is recommended for various high-risk groups such as people living or working with HBV patients or carriers or travelers staying more than 6 months in high-level HBV areas (5).

The United States Olympic Committee has emphasized that because the HBV is more easily transmitted than the human immunodeficiency virus (HIV), overall risk of HBV infection in athletic settings is substantially higher (105). The USOC recommends that prophylactic hepatitis B vaccine be considered for athletes in high-risk sports such as boxing, tae kwon do, and wrestling and in moderate-risk sports such as basketball, field hockey, ice hockey, judo, soccer, and team handball. The USOC also recommends that

1. voluntary testing for HBV and educational information be made available to all athletes in high- and moderate-risk sports,
2. gloves be worn when contact with blood or other body fluids is anticipated and skin surfaces washed and cleaned with soap and a diluted solution of household bleach (1:100 bleach:water dilution) immediately if contaminated,
3. all athletes in the high-risk sports be required to wear mouthpieces,
4. matches be interrupted when an athlete has a wound where a large amount of exposed blood is present to allow the blood flow to be stopped and the area and athletes cleaned,
5. open wounds be covered with dressings to prevent contamination, and
6. athletes and officials in the high-risk sports wear protective eyewear to reduce the possibility of bloody body fluids entering the eyes.

HIV Infection

Acquired immune deficiency syndrome (AIDS) is a major public health problem of this generation, first recognized as a distinct syndrome in 1981 (5). Within several weeks to several months after infection with the *human immunodeficiency virus* (HIV), many individuals develop an acute, self-limited mononucleosis-like illness lasting for a week or two. Most persons infected with HIV develop detectable antibodies within 1 to 3 months, although occasionally there may be a more prolonged interval. HIV-infected persons may be free of clinical signs or symptoms for many months to years before onset of clinical illness, which starts with a constellation of nonspecific symptoms (*AIDS-related complex* or ARC) and proceeds to AIDS. Fully developed AIDS infection also includes more than a dozen additional opportunistic infections and several cancers. The proportion of HIV-infected persons who will ultimately develop AIDS is not precisely known. Although the vast majority of HIV-infected persons is projected to develop AIDS within 15 to 20 years, with modern therapy the incubation period is expected to be considerably longer. Without specific therapy, the case fatality rate of AIDS has been very high, with 80% to 90% of patients dying within 3 to 5 years after diagnosis.

The primary target of this virus is the T-helper/inducer cell because it binds directly to the CD4 surface membrane receptor and kills the cell as replication proceeds. As a result, AIDS patients have a marked reduction in the number of CD4 cells, the most evident hallmark of disease progression, with symptoms usually rare until the count falls below 400 to 500 cells/mm^3 (normal counts range from 600 to 1200 cells/mm^3). When CD4-cell counts fall below 50 cells/mm^3, most patients develop the most serious of the opportunistic infections associated with AIDS. The Centers for Disease Control has proposed that HIV-infected patients with CD4-cell counts below 200 cells/mm^3 be diagnosed with AIDS. Other immunologic abnormalities that develop in AIDS patients include (a) a deficiency in ability to mount an appropriate antibody response, (b) defects in monocyte function, (c) a reduction in natural killer (NK)-cell activity, and (d) a marked decrease in T-cell proliferative response to mitogens (2).

Pertinent questions have been raised regarding HIV transmission during sports that require close physical contact. Most patients diagnosed with active AIDS are acutely and chronically ill and are not likely to participate in athletic endeavors. For each patient with clinically apparent AIDS, however, there are many more who are HIV-infected but are free of clinical manifestations or present with nonspecific symptoms (ARC) and who may be capable of normal participation in sports (10).

Routine social or community contact with an HIV-infected person carries no risk of transmission; only sexual exposure and exposure to blood or tissues carries a risk. Although the HIV has been found in saliva, tears, urine, and bronchial secretions, there is no evidence that the virus can be transmitted after contact with these secretions. HIV has not been found in eccrine sweat (111).

There are several situations, however, in which the transmission of HIV is of concern in athletic settings. In sports in which athletes can be cut such as boxing or wrestling or other contact sports such as football, basketball, and baseball, risk of HIV transmission exists when the mucous membranes of a healthy athlete are exposed to the blood of an infected athlete. At present, the feeling is that testing all athletes prior to sport participation is impractical, unethical, and unrealistic. Therefore, the team physician and athletic trainer are urged to provide information about the transmission of HIV, recommended behavior to reduce risks, and referral for care or diagnosis (107).

These concerns and concepts have been summarized by several consensus reports from the World Health Organization and International Federation of Sports Medicine (110), the USOC (105), and the American Academy of Pediatrics (1). These three organizations have made recommendations concerning HIV infection in the athletic setting, and these are summarized in the next several paragraphs.

- No evidence exists for a risk of transmission of HIV when infected persons, without bleeding wounds or skin lesions, engage in sports. Thus, athletes infected with HIV should be allowed to participate in all competitive sports unless future research documents that transmission of HIV is found to occur in the sport setting. Additionally, there is no medical or public health justification for testing or screening for HIV infection prior to participation in sport activities.

- There is a very low risk of HIV transmission during combative sports when an infected athlete with a bleeding wound or a skin lesion with exudate comes in contact with another athlete who has a skin lesion or an exposed mucous membrane. Olympic sports with the greatest risk include boxing, tae kwon do, and wrestling. Basketball, field and ice hockey, judo, soccer, and team handball, however, pose only moderate risk. There is one report of a possible transmission of HIV involving a collision between soccer players (103). However, this report from Italy remains undocumented. It should be the responsibility of any athlete participating in a combative sport who has a wound or other skin lesion to report it immediately to a responsible official and seek medical attention. Athletes who know they are HIV-infected should seek medical counseling about further participation in sports, especially in sports such as wrestling or boxing that involve a high theoretical risk of contagion to other athletes.

- Sport organizations, sport clubs, and sport groups have special opportunities to educate athletes and ancillary personnel about AIDS and should ensure that each are aware of the major issues involved.

- Each coach and athletic trainer should receive training in how to clean skin and athletic equipment surfaces exposed to blood or other body fluids. These procedures are the same as outlined previously in this chapter for HBV.

Can exercise training be used as a method to delay the progression from HIV infection to AIDS? Few investigators have published results in this area (51,86,100). One descriptive study of long-surviving persons with AIDS found that nearly all engaged in physical fitness or exercise programs (99). However, many other factors may explain this association.

Rigsby, Dishman, Jackson, Maclean, and Raven (86) studied the effects of an exercise program (three 1-hr sessions per week of strength training and aerobic exercise) on 37 HIV-infected subjects who spanned the range of HIV disease progression from asymptomatic to a diagnosis of AIDS (CD4 counts ranged from 9 to 804 cells/mm^3). Subjects were randomly assigned to either a 12-week exercise-training group or to a counseling control group. Although exercise training had the expected effect in improving both strength and cardiorespiratory fitness in exercise subjects, no significant change in CD4-cell counts or the CD4:CD8 ratio was found for either condition. The exercise group experienced an average increase of 58 CD4 cells/mm^3 during the study compared to no change in the counseling group, but the heterogeneous nature of the relatively small study group weakened the likelihood of the change being statistically significant (Figure 54.1). The increase in strength with weight training, which has also been reported by Spence, Galantino, and Mossberg (100) in AIDS subjects, is noteworthy in that muscle atrophy and nervous system disorders are common among ARC and AIDS patients. Weight training may provide one means of retarding the wasting syndrome that accompanies AIDS and improving the quality of life for these individuals.

LaPerriere et al. (49–51) randomly assigned asymptomatic, healthy homosexual males to 10 weeks of either an aerobic exercise-training or a measurement-only control group. The subjects included 12 seronegative exercisers, 10 seropositive exercisers, 11 seronegative controls, and 6 seropositive controls. The aerobic exercise training involved 45 min of stationary bicycle ergometry exercise three times per week, at an intensity of 70% to 80% of age-predicted maximum heart rate and resulted in significant improvement of cardiorespiratory endurance. Both HIV-seronegative and -seropositive subjects in the exercise group showed an increase in CD4 cells, with the magnitude greater in the seronegative group (220 vs. 115 cells/mm^3, respectively). Seropositive exercisers experienced a smaller decrease in NK cells than seropositive control subjects (38 vs. 170 cells/mm^3, respectively). Results of this study suggest that exercise training in asymptomatic HIV-positive subjects (with CD4 counts in the healthy range) may attenuate the usual decrements seen in immune status and function. However, longer term studies with greater numbers of subjects are needed before any definitive conclusions can be drawn.

One tentative conclusion that can be made from these studies is that appropriately supervised exercise training does not appear to adversely affect HIV-infected individuals. Several potential benefits of both aerobic and strength training by HIV-infected individuals, especially when initiated early in the disease state, include improvement in psychological coping, maintenance of health and physical function for a longer period, and attenuation of negative immune system changes. LaPerriere, Antoni, Fletcher, and Schneiderman (49) have recommended that exercise prescriptions for all HIV-infected individuals should be made on an individual basis with appropriate initial screening. The exercise prescription should emphasize both cardiorespiratory and musculoskeletal training components.

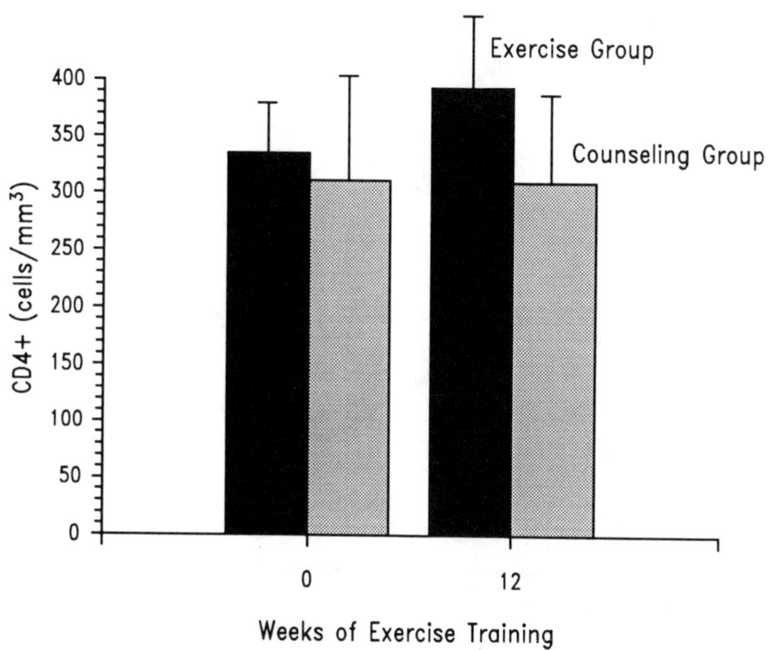

Figure 54.1 CD4 response to 12 weeks of exercise training or counseling (control) among men seropositive for the HIV-1 virus. Data from Rigsby et al. (85).

Physical Activity and Upper Respiratory Tract Infection

The Centers for Disease Control has estimated that the 429 million colds and flus occurring annually in the United States result in $2.5 billion in lost school and work days and medical costs (73). The National Center for Health Statistics has reported that acute respiratory conditions have an annual incidence rate of 90 per 100 persons (73). In response, much attention has recently been focused on various measures (including physical activity) to reduce the public health burden of upper respiratory tract infection (URTI) (48,68). There is a common belief among the general and athletic populations alike that regular exercise training decreases the risk of acquiring a cold or flu, whereas severe exertion may increase risk. For example, in a 1989 *Runner's World* survey, 60.7% of 700 subscribers reported that they had caught fewer colds since beginning to run, but only 4.9% claimed they had caught more. Understanding the relationship between physical activity and URTI has potential public health implications and for the athlete may mean the difference between being able to compete or missing the event due to illness.

The relationship between physical activity and URTI may be modeled in the form of a *J* curve (Figure 54.2). This model suggests that although the risk of URTI may decrease below that of a sedentary individual when one engages in moderate exercise training, risk may rise above average during periods of excessive amounts of exercise. The evidence for and against this model is summarized in Table 54.1 and will be reviewed in the next section. There are relatively few studies that have explored the relationship between physical activity and URTI. Of the 10 studies outlined in Table 54.1, 8 are epidemiologic in design (evenly divided between prospective and retrospective), and only 2 employed a randomized, controlled experimental design.

Heavy Exertion and Infection

Many athletes feel that although their regular training programs promote resistance to URTI, the actual competitive event itself increases their risk (62). There is considerable anecdotal information from coaches and physicians of athletic teams in support of the belief that severe exertion, especially when coupled with mental stress, places athletes at increased risk for URTI (28,43). It has been reported that at the 1988 Olympic Games, some of the world's best athletes were unable to compete due to infectious illness (28). The URTI that afflicted British Olympic gold medalist Sebastian Coe, for example, during the British Olympic trials in August so affected his running that he failed to qualify for the Olympic team. At the 1992 Winter Olympic Games, a sizable number of athletes reported that they were unable to compete or had subpar performances because of URTI.

Epidemiological Evidence

Several epidemiological reports suggest that athletes engaging in marathon-type events or very heavy training are at increased risk of URTI. Nieman, Johanssen, Lee, and Arabatzis (65) researched the incidence of URTI in a group of 2,311 marathon

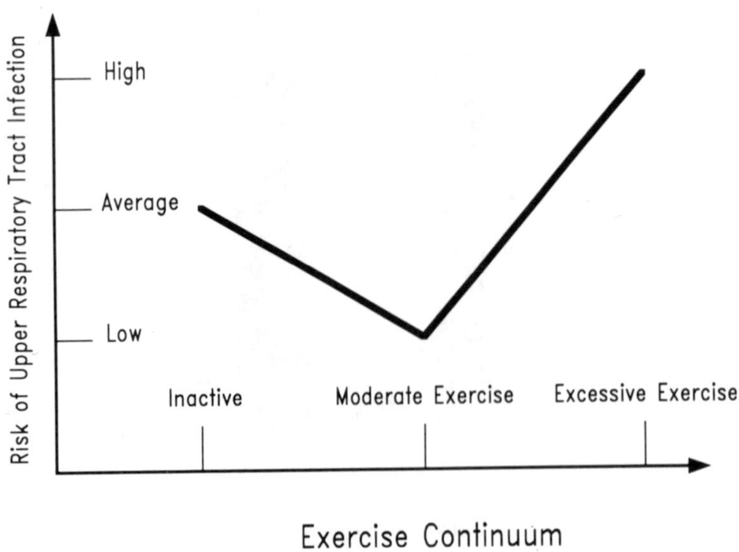

Figure 54.2 *J*-shaped model of relationship between varying amounts of exercise and risk of URTI. This model suggests that moderate exercise may lower risk of URTI whereas excessive amounts may increase the risk.

Table 54.1 Epidemiological and Experimental Research on the Relationship Between Physical Activity and Upper Respiratory Tract Infection (URTI)

Study	Subjects	Research design; statistical method	Method of determining URTI	Major finding
Peters & Bateman (80)	141 South African marathon runners vs. 124 live-in controls	2-week recall of URTI after race, retrospective; chi-square analysis	2-week recall of URTI incidence and duration using self-reported questionnaire	URTI incidence twice as high in runners after race vs. controls (33.3% vs. 15.3%)
Linde (54)	44 Danish elite orienteers vs. 44 matched nonathletes	12-month prospective; Mann Whitney statistical test	URTI symptoms self-recorded in daily log	Orienteers vs. controls had 2.5 vs. 1.7 URTIs during year
Osterback & Qvarnberg (74)	137 Finnish children (62 in and 75 not in athletics)	12-month prospective; descriptive statistics and univariate t-test	Nurse contacted parents every 2 months to recall all URTI	No differences between two groups of children
Schouten et al. (90)	199 Dutch nonathletic young adults (92 M and 107 F)	6- and 3-month retrospective for URTI and physical activity, respectively, aerobic power; correlation statistics	6-month recall of URTI incidence and duration of symptoms by self-report questionnaire	No significant correlation between physical activity or fitness with URTI
Strauss et al. (101)	84 Ohio State University athletes (34 wrestlers, 25 swimmers, 25 gymnasts)	8-week prospective during winter; chi-square statistical analysis	Team physician interviewed each team member weekly	URTI incidence: 92% wrestlers, 84% swimmers, 80% gymnasts; no group differences
Nieman et al. (64)	294 Californian runners	2 months before and 1 week after March 5K, 10K, half-marathon race, retrospective; chi-square analysis	2-month recall of URTI incidence during training for race, 1-week recall after race, self-report	Training 42 vs. 12 km per week associated with lower URTI, no effect of race on URTI
Nieman et al. (65)	2,311 Los Angeles Marathon runners	2 months before and 1 week after March marathon race, retrospective; multiple logistic regression model	2-month recall of URTI incidence during training for race, 1-week recall after race, self-report	Runners training ≥ 97 vs. < 32 km per week at higher URTI risk, odds ratio 5.9 for participants vs. nonparticipants
Nieman et al. (70)	36 mildly obese, inactive women, Loma Linda University	Subjects randomized to walking and sedentary control groups, five 45-min walking sessions per week for 15 weeks, late January to May; t-test statistic	Daily log using self-reported, precoded, URTI symptoms	Walking group reported fewer days with URTI symptoms than controls (5.1 vs. 10.8)
Heath et al. (37)	530 runners, South Carolina	12-month prospective; multiple logistic regression model	Daily log using self-reported, precoded, URTI symptoms	Increase in running distance positively related to increased URTI risk
Nieman et al. (67)	44 elderly women (32 inactive, 12 highly conditioned), Appalachian State University	Subjects randomized to walking and sedentary control groups, five 37-min walking sessions per week for 12 weeks, September to November; chi-square analysis	Daily log using self-reported, precoded, URTI symptoms	Incidence of URTI 8% in highly conditioned, 21% in walkers, 50% in controls

Note. M = male; F = female.

runners who varied widely in running ability and training habits. Using a pilot-tested questionnaire, runners self-reported demographic, training, and URTI episode and symptom data for the 2-month period (January, February) prior to and the 1-week period immediately following the race.

An important finding was that 12.9% of Los Angeles Marathon (LAM) participants reported an infectious episode during the week following the race in comparison to only 2.2% of similarly experienced runners who had applied but did not participate (for reasons other than sickness). Controlling for important demographic and training data by using logistic regression, it was determined that the odds were 6 to 1 in favor of sickness for the LAM participants versus the nonparticipating runners (Figure 54.3).

Forty percent of the runners reported at least one URTI during the 2-month winter period prior to the LAM. Controlling for important confounders, it was determined that runners training more than 60 miles per week (over 96 km per week) doubled their odds for sickness compared to those training less than 20 miles per week (under 32 km per week). Although the lowest odds of sickness were in the group running less than 20 miles per week, the odds ratio did not increase significantly until 60 miles per week were exceeded (Figure 54.4). The researchers concluded that runners may

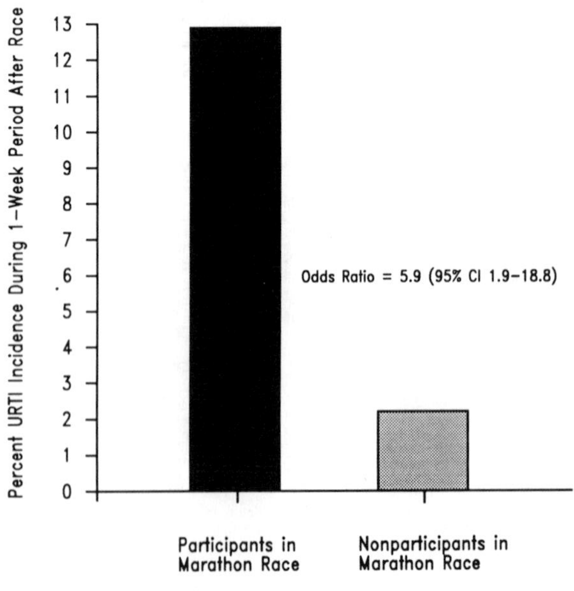

Figure 54.3 Self-reported URTI in 2,300 Los Angeles Marathon runners during the week following the 1987 Los Angeles Marathon. CI = confidence interval. Data from Nieman et al. (65).

experience increased risk for URTI during heavy training or following a marathon race event.

Other epidemiological data support these findings. Peters and Bateman (80) studied the incidence of URTI in 150 randomly selected runners who took part in a 56-km race in comparison to matched controls who did not run. Symptoms of URTI occurred in 33.3% of runners compared with 15.3% of controls during the 2-week period following the race and were most common in those who achieved the faster race times (Figure 54.5). The most prevalent symptoms after the race were sore throats and nasal symptoms. Of the total number of symptoms reported by the runners, 80% lasted for longer than 3 days, suggesting an infective origin.

Linde (54) studied URTI in a group of 44 elite orienteers and 44 nonathletes of the same age, sex, and occupational distribution during a 1-year period. The orienteers experienced significantly more infectious episodes during the year in comparison to the control group (2.5 vs. 1.7 episodes, respectively). Whereas one third of the controls reported no URTI during the yearlong study period, this applied to only 10% of the orienteers. The average duration of symptoms in the group of orienteers was 7.9 days compared to 6.4 days in the control group. The control group had the expected seasonal variation with the peak incidence in winter and relatively few cases in summer; the orienteers tended to show a more even distribution.

Heath et al. (37) followed a cohort of 530 runners who self-reported URTI symptoms daily for 1 year. The average runner in the study was about 40 years of age, ran 32 km per week, and experienced a rate of 1.2 URTI per year. Controlling for various confounding variables using logistic regression, the lowest odds ratio for URTI was found in those running less than 16 km per week. The odds ratio more than doubled for those running more than 27 km per week. This study is somewhat difficult to interpret for several reasons. In contrast to other studies (65), living alone and a low body mass index (kg/m^2) were found to be risk factors for developing a URTI within this group of runners. When included within the logistic regression model, these two factors may have altered the running distance threshold at which the odds ratio for URTI became significant. Nonetheless, this study demonstrated that total running distance for a year is a significant risk factor for URTI, with risk increasing as the running distance rises. The threshold at which running distance becomes a risk factor awaits further investigation.

In a 1-year prospective study of URTI in 137 children (average age 12.7 years), participation in sports (gymnastics, swimming, or ice hockey) did

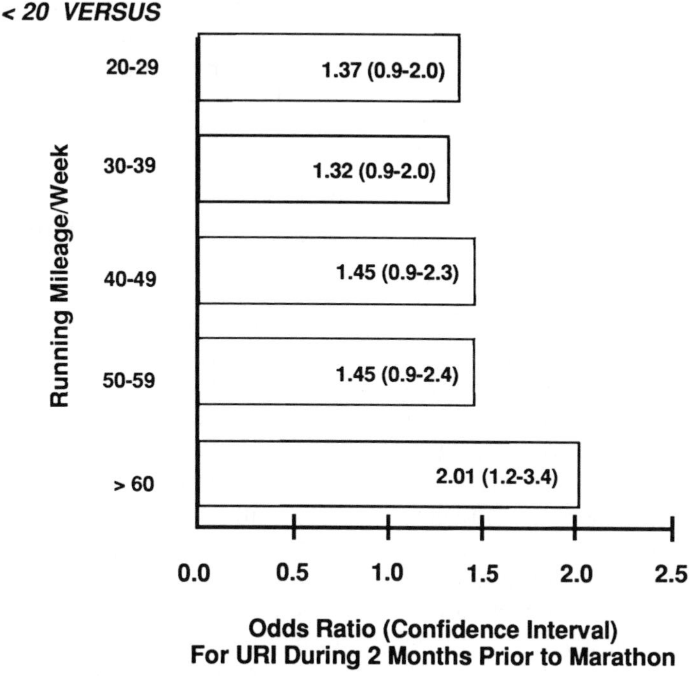

Figure 54.4 Self-reported URTI in 2,300 Los Angeles Marathon runners during the 2-month period (January, February) prior to the 1987 Los Angeles Marathon. Runners self-reported training distances in miles per week. Data from Nieman et al. (65).

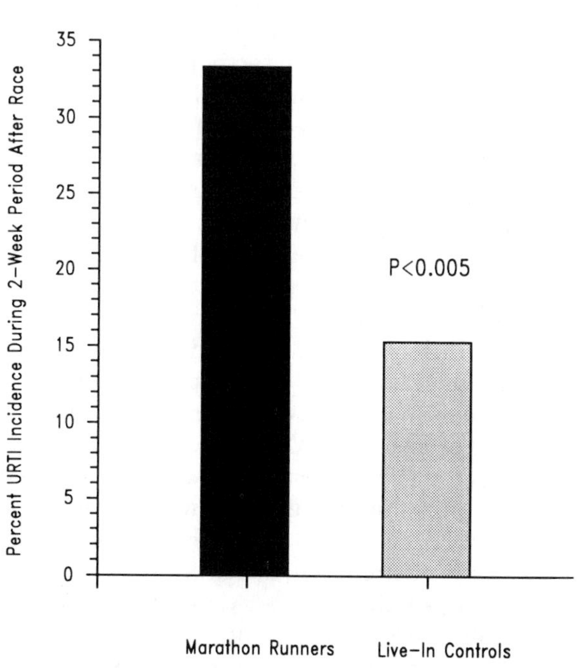

Figure 54.5 URTI in runners versus controls during a 2-week period following a 56-km race in South Africa. Data from Peters and Bateman (79).

not have an effect on the occurrence of illness (74). This study is difficult to interpret, however, in that duration and intensity of exercise were not quantified. The control students (those not engaging in supervised sport training) were enrolled in physical education classes and were allowed to take part in extracurricular physical activities. Thus although sports participation by children appeared to have no effect on occurrence of URTI, data from this study cannot be used to answer the question as to whether or not varying levels of physical activity have an effect.

Although there have been other published reports on the relationship between exercise or sport participation and URTI, the methods used in these investigations make it difficult to draw conclusions or make comparisons with other studies (8,90, 91,101). For example, Schouten, Verschuur, and Kemper (90) conducted a 6-month retrospective study of 199 young adults and concluded that the incidence and duration of URTI was not significantly related to physical activity and fitness levels. However, in this study no attempt was made to control for potential confounding factors, and the accuracy with which young adults are able to recall the incidence and duration of URTI from the previous 6 months is questionable. Strauss, Lanese, and Leizman (101) compared incidence of URTI in three different athletic teams during an 8-week period, but no sedentary control groups were followed for comparison or minutes of physical activity calculated.

Clinical Evidence and Possible Mechanisms

The epidemiological studies reviewed thus far suggest that heavy acute or chronic exercise is associated with increased risk of URTI. This interpretation is consistent with both human and animal experimental evidence (66–68).

Changes in Immunity From Physiological Stress. Several researchers have reported that various aspects of immune function are depressed following intense, prolonged endurance exercise (6,62,67). Heavy exertion is a form of physiological stress that causes large increases in epinephrine and cortisol levels—hormones that have been consistently associated with a suppression of immune function—and rapid perturbations in circulating levels of leukocyte and lymphocyte subsets.

Nieman et al. (62) and Berk et al. (6) ran 10 seasoned marathoners at their fastest marathon pace on treadmills for 3 hr. Cortisol rose 59% above baseline levels after the 3-hr run, remaining elevated for 1.5 hr of recovery before falling to normal daytime levels. This increase in cortisol correlated inversely with a 25% to 46% decrease in NK-cell activity at 1.5 hr of recovery, which persisted for nearly 6 hr (Figure 54.6). Pedersen et al. (75,77,78) and Kappel et al. (45) have carefully demonstrated that the postexercise suppression of NK-cell activity is also related to increased levels of prostaglandins released from monocytes.

Eskola et al. (23) and Gmünder et al. (35) have reported a significant decrease in T-cell proliferative response for several hours after a marathon (42.2 km). MacNeil et al. (56) have demonstrated that the T-cell proliferative response is decreased for at least 2 hr following cycle ergometer exercise, especially after high-intensity exercise by athletes. Following 1 hr of cycling at 80% $\dot{V}O_2max$ by untrained individuals, Tvede, Heilmann, Halkjaer-Kristersen, and Pedersen (104) found suppression of B-lymphocyte function for at least 2 hr because of an inhibitory effect of activated monocytes. Smith, Telford, Mason, and Weidemann (96) have determined that neutrophil killing capacity is decreased in elite athletes engaging in prolonged periods of intensive training in comparison to untrained controls.

Nieman, Tan, Lee, and Berk (71) and Smith, Chi, Krish, Reynolds, and Cambron (97) have reported significantly lower serum complement in long-distance runners relative to sedentary controls. A significant decrease in salivary immunoglobulin concentrations following 2 hr of intense cycling or 50 km of cross-country ski racing has been described by two groups of investigators (55,102). Israel, Buhl, Krause, and Neumann (41) have reported that serum immunoglobulins fall 10% to 28% for at least 1 day after athletes run 45 or 75 km at high intensity. Russian investigators have related that exhaustion of immune reserves can be observed during periods of important competitions manifested by lowered immunoglobulin levels and suppression of phagocytic activity of neutrophils (79,81,82).

Results from animal studies have rather consistently supported the viewpoint that heavy acute and chronic exertion are related to negative changes in immune function. Several researchers have reported that exhaustive single bouts of exercise by both trained and untrained animals or 6 days to 4.5 months of heavy exercise training are linked to increased splenic epinephrine and cortisol levels and decreased splenic NK- and T-cell lymphocyte function (26,38,57,94). Thus both circulating immune cells and those found in secondary lymphoid tissues may have their function suppressed because of the increase in cortisol and catecholamine levels that occur following heavy exertion.

These data, however, must be balanced against the findings of other researchers who have come to alternate conclusions. Pedersen et al. (76) have reported significantly higher basal NK-cell activity in 27 elite Danish cyclists relative to untrained subjects, suggesting that as a result their resistance to infection was improved. Nieman et al. (63) have also reported higher NK-cell activity in highly conditioned versus sedentary elderly women. The highly conditioned subjects (mean age 73 years) exercised an average of 1.6 hr a day and regularly competed in state and national senior games and road race endurance competitions. Fehr, Lötzerich, and Michna (25) have related that the enzyme content and phagocytic activity of connective tissue macrophages increase when competitive sportsmen run 15 km at high intensity. Macrophages from the lung, however, may respond differently than those from connective tissue areas following exercise. For example, Wong, Thompson, Thong, and Thornton (109) have established that the antimicrobial function of alveolar macrophages is strongly suppressed for 3 days in horses following single bouts of strenuous exercise.

Further research is warranted to better elucidate the clinical significance of exercise-induced changes in immune status and function (many of which are transient in nature) and which variables best predict potential changes in host protection. The data at present are not consistent enough between studies to even suggest thresholds for various immune system markers that may indicate increased risk of URTI.

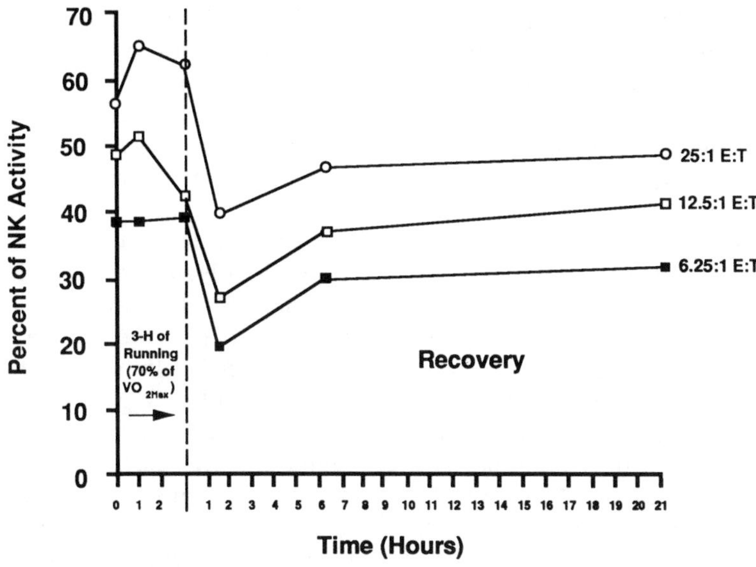

Figure 54.6 Changes in percent NK-cell activity in 10 male marathon runners at three E:T ratios in response to a 3-hr run at 70% $\dot{V}O_2$max. E:T = effector:target ratios (effector cells = peripheral blood mononuclear cells; target cells = K562 cells derived from patient with myelogenous leukemia). * = $p < .05$, contrast with baseline. Data from Berk et al. (6).

Interaction Effect of Psychological Stress. Psychological factors may also play an important role in the relationship between exercise and URTI. Exercise is a form of physiological and psychological stress varying according to the intensity and duration of the training program. Interestingly, the acute response of the immune system to psychological stressors alone is in many ways similar to those that occur in response to acute exercise (59).

If the exercise-training program is deemed stressful by the athlete, the combined psychological and physiological impact may overwhelm the ability of the immune system to protect the host (68). Mental stress alone has been related to a wide variety of negative changes in immunity (44). Bereavement, major depression, loneliness, schizophrenia, marital discord, and other forms of mental stress have all been associated with suppression of immune function (42,46).

A biochemical basis for bidirectional communication between the immune system and neuroendocrine system has been established (7). These systems produce and use many of the same signal molecules in the form of hormones, lymphokines, and monokines for inter- and intrasystem communication and regulation. Lymphoid organs are innervated by the autonomic nervous system, and lymphocytes have receptors for the various stress hormones. In the other direction, for example, products of leukocytes have been shown to alter neuronal activity in certain areas of the brain.

Thus stress of any form may decrease host protection from infection through both autonomic nervous system and hormonal mechanisms. Research by Graham, Douglas, and Ryan (36), for example, has demonstrated that during a given 6-month period of time, highly stressed individuals have twice as many days with URTI symptoms as compared with low-stressed people. Cohen, Tyrrell, and Smith (14) gave nasal drops containing respiratory viruses to 394 subjects and reported that psychological stress was associated in a dose–response manner with an increased risk of URTI. Although specific research in this area has not yet been conducted, it would seem logical to assume that athletes around the time of competition, when both physiological and psychological stress are high, would be most vulnerable to respiratory infections.

The Acute Phase Response. Another factor that may prove to be important with respect to risk of URTI in athletes is the involvement of the immune system in the tissue repair process that occurs following strenuous exercise. It has been well established that both heavy acute and chronic exertion are associated with muscle cell damage, local inflammation, and the stereotyped sequence of host defense reactions known as the acute-phase response (24).

The acute-phase response following long endurance exercise involves the complement system, neutrophils, macrophages, various cytokines, and acute-phase proteins and can last for several days, promoting clearance of damaged tissue and setting the stage for repair and growth. Lymphocytes, neutrophils, and macrophages are attracted to the injured muscle cells and invade the area to aid in the process. Neutrophils phagocytize tissue debris and release a wide variety of factors that aid in the digestion of adjacent dead tissue cells (98). Macrophages have surface receptors that allow them to react nonspecifically to a variety of substances, a process enhanced by the presence of opsonins (primarily complement and antibody). Macrophages also are a prime source of cytokines that mediate most of the physiological and inflammatory reactions accompanying muscle cell injury. Dufaux and Order (22) have shown that plasma elastase-alpha 1-antitrypsin, neopterin, tumor necrosis factor, and soluble interleukin-2 receptor increase during recovery from a 2.5-hr running test, supporting the concept of a functional involvement of polymorphonuclear neutrophils and an activation of macrophages and T-lymphocytes. Dufaux and Order (21) have also provided evidence for complement activation after 2.5 hr of running.

Could the active enmeshment of the immune system in the muscle tissue repair and inflammation process mean that protection from URTI is compromised? Research to answer this question is certainly warranted and may greatly increase our understanding as to how and why athletes appear to be more susceptible to URTI during periods of heavy training.

Management of the Athlete During Infection

If an athlete experiences sudden and unexplained deterioration in performance during training or competition, viral infection should be suspected (87,88). It is well established that various measures of physical performance capability are reduced during an infectious episode (19,29–33,40). Several case histories have been published demonstrating that sudden and unexplained deterioration in athletic performance can in some individuals be traced to either recent URTI or subclinical viral infections that run a protracted course (87,88). Daniels et al. (19), for example, concluded that during a mild fever state there is a marked effect on the ability or willingness of some individuals to perform both cardiorespiratory and musculoskeletal exercise. Other researchers have reported decrements in measurements of muscle strength, including Friman et al. (30,33) who have shown that isometric muscle strength in both the upper and lower extremities is reduced to 85% to 95% of late convalescent values in patients who were hospitalized with various acute infectious diseases. Although studies consistently show decrements in measurements of exercise performance, the mechanism for these decreases is not completely known. Friman, Ilbäck, Crawford, and Neufeld (32) have suggested that infection-induced degradation of various performance-related muscle enzymes may be one important factor.

Should athletes exercise when they have a viral infection? Most clinical authorities in this area recommend that if the athlete has symptoms of a common cold with no constitutional involvement, then regular training may be safely resumed a few days after the resolution of symptoms (88,93). Mild exercise during sickness with the common cold does not appear to be contraindicated but there is insufficient evidence at present to say one way or the other. However, if there are symptoms or signs of systemic involvement (fever, extreme tiredness, muscle aches, swollen lymph glands, etc.), then 2 to 4 weeks should probably be allowed before resumption of intensive training. These precautions are advised because of the well-documented relationship between intensive exercise and risk of developing viral cardiomyopathy and other severe forms of viral infection (92).

Clinicians since the 1940s have observed that certain patients with paralytic poliomyelitis give a history of severe exertion immediately preceding or during the onset of paralysis (39). Levinson, Milzer, and Lewin (52) found that the incidence and severity of paralysis was greater in monkeys subjected to exhausting exercise than in control animals. Weinstein (108) concluded that participation in strenuous sport late in the incubation period increased the risk of extensive and severe paralysis in schoolboys during an epidemic of poliomyelitis in Greenwich, Connecticut.

Several studies have demonstrated that exhaustive exercise after contracting an infection may be detrimental. In particular, the virulence of the Coxsackie virus, which has a predilection for the heart muscle, has been shown to be increased by intense exercise. Reyes and Lerner (85), for example, showed that when weanling Swiss albino mice are inoculated with the Coxsackie virus and subsequently forced to swim vigorously daily, a dramatic increase in virus multiplication occurred in the hearts as compared to that observed in the inactive control mice.

It has been known for several decades that many types of viral infections can produce myocarditis or pericarditis (9). Respiratory infections, including the common cold and flu syndromes are all potentially serious; the patient may be prone to develop cardiac damage and sudden death through acute arrhythmias. Patients who develop viral cardiomyopathy are usually previously healthy young people who have stressed themselves with vigorous, prolonged physical exercise during the height of a viral infection or soon thereafter. Furthermore, these subjects usually have continued with stressful exercise, while ignoring the early onset of dyspnea, palpitation, weakness, fatigability, and general ill feeling—all symptoms and signs also observed in persons suffering cardiac damage. It is recommended that strenuous physical stress be avoided for at least 2 weeks postinfection.

There are numerous case reports of death in young healthy people who engaged in vigorous exercise during an acute viral illness (3,47, 87,88,92). Phillips et al. (83) reviewed the clinical and autopsy records of the 19 sudden cardiac deaths that occurred among 1.6 million Air Force recruits during basic training. Strenuous physical exertion was associated with sudden death in 17 of 19 cases, and the most frequent underlying etiology was myocarditis. Because viral illness is endemic in barrack-residing recruits, the authors conjectured that exertion may have exacerbated subclinical cases of myocarditis leading to sudden death in 7 of 8 recruits that had myocarditis. Drory, Kramer, and Lev (20) in their study of 20 male soldiers in the Israel Defense Forces (1974–1986) who had died suddenly and unexpectedly within 24 hr of strenuous exertion also concluded that febrile disease may have been a cause of death in some of the subjects.

Moderate Exercise Training and Infection

What about the common belief that moderate physical activity is beneficial in decreasing risk of URTI and improving immune function? Very few studies have been carried out in this area and more research is certainly warranted to investigate this interesting question (Table 54.1).

Epidemiological Evidence

The Run Through Redlands race in Redlands, California is conducted in March of each year drawing nearly 1,200 runners to its 5K, 10K, and half-marathon courses. Nieman, Johanssen, and Lee (64) studied the incidence of URTI in these runners during the 2-winter-month period prior to the race evaluating the impact of varying levels of training. In addition, the effect of the race experience on URTI was studied. In this group of recreational runners, 25% of those running 25 km or more per week (average of 42 km per week) reported at least one URTI episode during January and February as opposed to 34.3% training less than 25 km per week (average of 12 km per week) (chi-square 2.83, $p = .092$). During the week following the road race, runners did not report an increase in URTI episodes as compared to the week prior to the race. These findings suggest that running an average of 42 km versus 12 km per week is associated with a slight reduction in URTI incidence, and racing 5 to 21.1 km is not related to an increased risk of URTI during the ensuing week.

Clinical Evidence and Possible Mechanisms

The influence of exercise training on resistance to infection has been investigated using animal models since the turn of the century. Cannon and Kluger (11,12) have reviewed the animal literature and concluded that moderate exercise prior to infection may increase resistance to infection, but that exhaustive exercise after contracting an infection may be detrimental. In accordance with this viewpoint, Slubik, Levin, Mashneva, and Pulkov (95) have reported that moderate physical exercise preceding irradiation diminishes radiation injury in animals, whereas intensive exercise and stress may aggravate the damage.

Smith, Telford, Mason, and Weidemann (96) have shown that 1 hr of cycling at 60% $\dot{V}O_2max$ may increase resistance to infection by improving the "killing capacity" of neutrophils, an effect that persists for at least 6 hr of recovery. Because neutrophils are the body's best phagocyte, these findings suggest that regular episodes of moderate exercise may increase resistance to infection.

In a randomized, controlled study by Nieman et al. (70) and Nehlsen-Cannarella et al. (60), the effects of walking on immune response and URTI were measured on a group of sedentary, mildly obese women (Table 54.1). The exercise subjects walked 45 min per session, 5 times per week, for 15 continuous weeks on a measured course under supervision. Subjects recorded health problems and symptoms in a daily log book.

Exercise subjects experienced half of the days with URTI symptoms during the 15-week period compared to that of the sedentary control group (5.1 ± 1.2 vs. 10.8 ± 2.3 days, $p = .039$). The number of separate URTI episodes did not vary between groups (1.0 ± 0.2 vs. 1.1 ± 0.2 for exercise and sedentary groups, respectively, $p = .693$) but the number of symptom days per URTI episode was significantly lower in the exercise group ($p = .049$) (Figure 54.7). Moderate exercise training led to a 20% net increase in each of the three serum immunoglobulins and was significantly correlated with fewer URTI symptoms days (66). Moderate exercise training also led to a significant increase in NK-cell activity, which was correlated with a decrease in the duration of URTI symptoms per episode. These results are similar to those of Crist,

Mackinnon, Thompson, Atterbom, and Egan (17) who moderately exercised elderly women for 16 weeks and measured a 33% higher NK-cell activity at rest and a heightened increase following maximal testing.

The relationship between cardiorespiratory exercise, immune function, and URTI in 32 sedentary elderly women was recently explored using a 12-week randomized, controlled clinical design with cross-sectional comparisons at baseline with a group of 12 highly conditioned elderly women who were active in state and national senior game and road race endurance events (63). The highly conditioned elderly women (average VO_2max of 31 ml · kg^{-1} · min^{-1}) had been physically active for an average of 11 years and had trained moderately an average of 1.6 hr daily during the past year. The intervention group walked 30 to 40 min 5 days per week for 12 weeks at 60% heart rate reserve.

At baseline, the highly conditioned subjects exhibited superior NK- (119 ± 13 vs. 77 ± 8 lytic units, $p < .01$) and T- (33.3 ± 4.9 vs. 21.4 ± 2.1 cpm × 10^{-3} using phytohemagglutinin, $p < .05$) cell function compared to the 32 sedentary elderly women. Twelve weeks of moderate cardiorespiratory exercise improved the VO_2max of the sedentary subjects 12.6%, but did not result in any improvement in immune function relative to the control group. Figure 54.8 compares the incidence of URTI in the highly conditioned, walking, and calisthenic control groups during the 12-week study (September through November). Half of the elderly women in the calisthenic group obtained an URTI during the study as compared with 3 of 14 in the walking group and 1 of 12 in the highly conditioned group (chi-square = 6.36, $p = .042$). The percentages shown in Figure 54.8 suggest that elderly women not engaging in cardiorespiratory exercise are more likely than those who do exercise regularly to experience an URTI during the fall season.

Taken together the studies reviewed in this chapter suggest that the response of the immune system to exercise and the degree of protection from URTI may have much to do with the level of intensity and total exertion load and corresponding changes in concentrations of cortisol and epinephrine. Both of these hormones have been associated with many negative effects on immune function (13,16,18). Lymphocytes have ß-adrenergic receptors, and the presence of epinephrine during exercise increases receptor number on T-suppressor/cytotoxic and NK cells, which are the major lymphocyte subsets that increase in response to an exercise challenge (27,58,106). The degree to which these lymphocyte subsets increase in the peripheral blood as they are

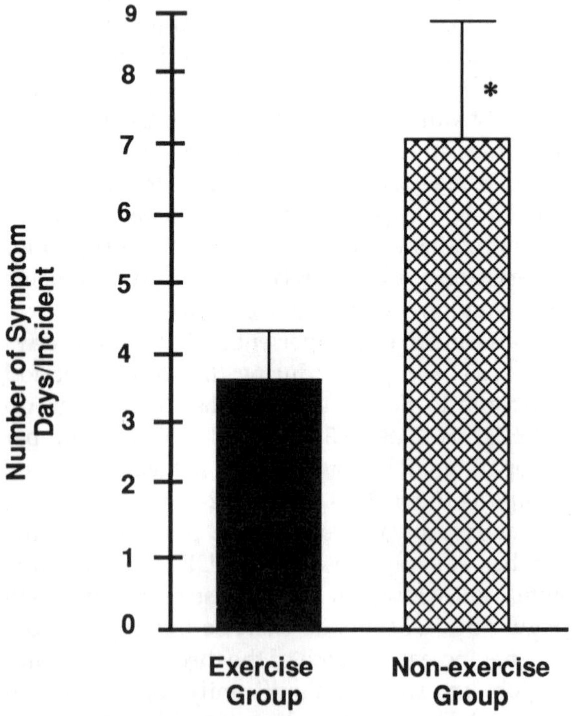

Number of Symptom Days/Incident
0 1 2 3 4 5 6 7 8 9
*
Exercise Group
Non-exercise Group

Figure 54.7 Moderate exercise training effects on the duration of symptoms from URTI during a 15-week period in 18 walkers versus 18 sedentary controls. * = $p < .05$. Data from Nieman et al. (70).

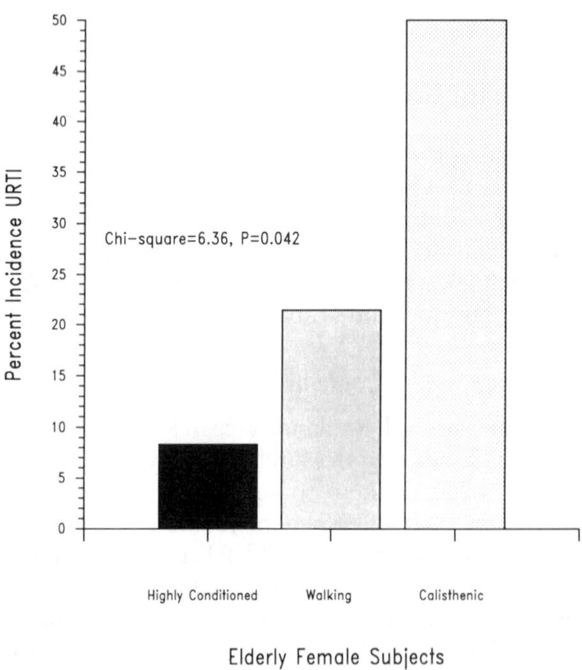

Figure 54.8 Incidence of URTI during a 12-week study period (September through November) in highly conditioned, walking, and calisthenic groups of elderly women (chi-square = 6.36, $p = .042$). Data from Nieman et al. (66).

recruited from lymphoid tissue pools is highly dependent on the magnitude of change in epinephrine. Additionally, the effect on lymphocyte function is also dependent on the change in both epinephrine and cortisol.

Moderate exercise such as walking does not increase the concentration of these two hormones in the blood, but results in a small lymphocytosis in contrast to intense exercise where levels of both hormones increase and a much larger perturbation in circulating levels of lymphocyte subsets occurs (61,69). Thus it may be argued that moderate exercise induces a small increase in NK and T-cytotoxic/suppressor cells without the potential suppressive effect of epinephrine or cortisol and creates a milieu that may be favorable for host protection. There are only a finite number of lymphocytes that are specific to any particular antigen. Theoretically, by recruiting lymphocytes from the periphery, moderate exercise may increase the rate of lymphocyte circulation through the body, improving the potential for interaction of lymphocyte and antigen without the attending negative effects of stress hormones (68,69). Pedersen (75), for example, has reported that moderate physical activity increases circulating NK-cell number and activity, but does not cause the usual postexercise suppression of NK-cell activity by monocytes that has been measured after heavy exertion.

Summary

In general, the data reviewed in this chapter suggest that unusually heavy training or intense exercise bouts lead to several negative changes in immunosurveillance, many of which are probably related to the effects of cortisol and epinephrine. These changes may lead to an infectious illness, especially when psychological stress is a contributing factor. Regular, moderate exercise training, on the other hand, may decrease the individual's risk of acquiring an infection. There are several immune system changes that occur during moderate exercise that may improve host protection.

There is an interesting similarity in the metabolic and immunologic responses to intense endurance exercise and an infectious challenge (53,72,89). In both conditions (a) the number of circulating leukocytes increases, (b) lymphopenia occurs (especially T cells that shift to peripheral tissues), (c) the lymphocyte responses to in vitro mitogens decrease, (d) body core temperature rises, (e) plasma levels of acute-phase proteins increase, and (f) degranulation of neutrophils develops. Because endurance exercise is associated with muscle cell damage and an increased intake of potential pathogens through heightened ventilation, it is logical that in preparation for such a challenge, the immune system receives a signal from the neuroendocrine network that activates the immune system.

Why then do epidemiological data and clinical experience point toward an increased risk of URTI in some athletes? The mass of evidence favors the view that psychosocial variables play an important role in affecting immunologic competence. The net effect of combined psychological and physiological stress from unusually heavy endurance exercise, especially during times of competition, may lead to suppression of the immune system.

For those athletes who must exercise intensely for competitive reasons, several precautions can help decrease the risk of sickness. These include spacing vigorous workouts and race events as far apart as possible, eating a well-balanced diet, keeping other life stresses to a minimum, avoiding overtraining and chronic fatigue, and obtaining adequate sleep. Before and following intense race events, the athlete should try to avoid contact with sick people if at all possible. If the athlete is competing during the winter months, a flu shot is highly recommended. Because of the proposed connection between muscle soreness and immune system involvement (which may reduce the ability of the immune system to successfully ward off viruses) the athlete should avoid unusual amounts of muscle soreness from heavy training.

For the fitness enthusiast the area of concern is not so much the harm that may come from overexertion, but the benefits that may derive from engaging in regular, moderate forms of exercise. At this time, even though investigative evidence suggests improved host protection and immunosurveillance from moderate physical activity, more research is needed to improve our understanding of the work load threshold below or above which exercise becomes protective versus detrimental.

References

1. American Academy of Pediatrics, Committee on Sports Medicine and Fitness. Human immunodeficiency virus (acquired immunodeficiency syndrome [AIDS] virus) in the athletic setting. Pediatrics. 88:640-641; 1991.
2. Antoni, M.H.; Schneiderman, N.; Fletcher, M.A.; et al. Psychoneuroimmunology and HIV-1. J. Consult. Clin. Psychol. 58:38-49; 1990.
3. Baron, R.C.; Hatch, M.H.; Kleeman, K.; MacCormack, J.N. Aseptic meningitis among

members of a high school football team. JAMA. 248:1724-1727; 1982.
4. Belongia, E.A.; Goodman, J.L.; Holland, E.J.; et al. An outbreak of herpes gladiatorum at a high-school wrestling camp. N. Engl. J. Med. 325:906-910; 1991.
5. Benenson, A.S. Control of communicable diseases in man. Washington, DC: American Public Health Association; 1990.
6. Berk, L.S.; Nieman, D.C.; Youngberg, W.S.; et al. The effect of long endurance running on natural killer cells in marathoners. Med. Sci. Sports Exerc. 22:207-212; 1990.
7. Blalock, J.E. A molecular basis for bidirectional communication between the immune and neuroendocrine systems. Physiol. Rev. 69:1-32; 1989.
8. Budgett, R.G.M.; Fuller, G.N. Illness and injury in international oarsmen. Clin. Sports Med. 1:57-61; 1989.
9. Burch, G.E. Viral diseases of the heart. Acta Cardiol. 34(1):5-9; 1979.
10. Calabrese, L.H.; Kelley, D. AIDS and athletes. Phys. Sportsmed. 17(1):127-132; 1989.
11. Cannon, J.G.; Kluger, J.J. Endogenous pyrogen activity in human plasma after exercise. Science. 220:617-619; 1983.
12. Cannon, J.G.; Kluger, J.J. Exercise enhances survival rate in mice infected with salmonella typhimurium. Proc. Soc. Exp. Biol. Med. 175: 518-521; 1984.
13. Cavallo, R.; Dartori, M.L.; Gatti, G.; Angeli, A. Cortisol and immune interferon can interact in the modulation of human natural killer cell activity. Experientia. 42:177-179; 1986.
14. Cohen, S.; Tyrrell, D.A.; Smith, A.P. Psychological stress and susceptibility to the common cold. N. Engl. J. Med. 325:606-612; 1991.
15. Conklin, R.J. Common cutaneous disorders in athletes. Sports Med. 9:100-119; 1990.
16. Crary, B.; Hauser, S.L.; Borysenko, M.; et al. Epinephrine-induced changes in the distribution of lymphocyte subsets in peripheral blood of humans. J. Immunol. 131:1178-1181; 1983.
17. Crist, D.M.; Mackinnon, L.T.; Thompson, R.F.; Atterbom, H.A.; Egan, P.A. Physical exercise increases natural cellular-mediated tumor cytotoxicity in elderly women. Gerontology. 35:66-71; 1989.
18. Cupps, T.R.; Fauci, A.S. Corticosteroid-mediated immunoregulation in man. Immunol. Rev. 65:133-155; 1982.
19. Daniels, W.L.; Sharp, D.S.; Wright, J.E.; et al. Effects of virus infection on physical performance in man. Milit. Med. 150:8-14; 1985.
20. Drory, Y.; Kramer, M.R.; Lev, B. Exertional sudden death in soldiers. Med. Sci. Sports Exerc. 23:147-151; 1991.
21. Dufaux, B.; Order, U. Complement activation after prolonged exercise. Clin. Chim. Acta. 179:45-49; 1989.
22. Dufaux, B.; Order, U. Plasma elastase-alpha 1-antitrypsin, neopterin, tumor necrosis factor, and soluble interleukin-2 receptor after prolonged exercise. Int. J. Sports Med. 10:434-438; 1989.
23. Eskola, J.; Ruuskanen, O.; Soppi, E.; et al. Effect of sport stress on lymphocyte transformation and antibody formation. Clin. Exp. Immunol. 32:339-345; 1978.
24. Evans W.J.; Cannon J.G. The metabolic effects of exercise-induced muscle damage. Exerc. Sport Sci. Rev. 19:99-125; 1991.
25. Fehr, H.G.; Lötzerich, H.; Michna, H. Human macrophage function and physical exercise: Phagocytic and histochemical studies. Eur. J. Appl. Physiol. 58:613-617; 1989.
26. Ferry, A.; Weill, B.L.; Rieu, M. Immunomodulations induced in rats by exercise on a treadmill. J. Appl. Physiol. 69:1912-1915; 1990.
27. Field, C.J.; Gougeon, R.; Marliss, E.B. Circulating mononuclear cell numbers and function during intense exercise and recovery. J. Appl. Physiol. 71:1089-1097; 1991.
28. Fitzgerald, L. Overtraining increases the susceptibility to infection. Int. J. Sports Med. [Suppl. 1]. 12:S5-S8; 1991.
29. Friman, G. Effects of acute infectious disease on circulatory function. Acta Med. Scand. [Suppl.]. 592:5-62; 1976.
30. Friman, G. Effect of acute infectious disease on isometric muscle strength. Scand. J. Clin. Lab. Invest. 37:303-308; 1977.
31. Friman, G.; Ilbäck, N.G.; Beisel, W.R. Effects of streptococcus pneumoniae, salmonella typhimurium and francisella tularensis infections on oxidative, glycolytic and lysosomal enzyme activity in red and white skeletal muscle in the rat. Scand. J. Infect. Dis. 16:111-119; 1984.
32. Friman, G.; Ilbäck, N.G.; Crawford, D.J.; Neufeld, H.A. Metabolic responses to swimming exercise in streptococcus pneumoniae infected rats. Med. Sci. Sports Exerc. 23:415-421; 1991.
33. Friman, G.; Wright, J.E.; Ilbäck, N.G.; et al. Does fever or myalgia indicate reduced physical performance capacity in viral infections? Acta Med. Scand. 217:353-361; 1985.
34. Girdwood, R.W.A. Infections associated with sport. Br. J. Sports Med. 22:117; 1988.
35. Gmünder, F.K.; Lorenzi, G.; Bechler, B.; et al. Effect of long-term physical exercise on

lymphocyte reactivity: Similarity to spaceflight reactions. Aviat. Space Environ. Med. 59:146-151; 1988.

36. Graham, N.M.H.; Douglas, R.M.; Ryan, P. Stress and acute respiratory infection. Am. J. Epidemiol. 124:389-401; 1986.
37. Heath, G.W.; Ford, E.S.; Craven, T.E.; et al. Exercise and the incidence of upper respiratory tract infections. Med. Sci. Sports Exerc. 23:152-157; 1991.
38. Hoffman-Goetz, L.; Keir, R.; Thorne, R.; Houston, M.E.; Young, C. Chronic exercise stress in mice depresses splenic T lymphocyte mitogenesis *in vitro*. Clin. Exp. Immunol. 66:551-557; 1986.
39. Horstmann, D.M. Acute poliomyelitis: Relation of physical activity at the time of onset to the course of the disease. JAMA. 142:236-241; 1950.
40. Ilbäck, N.G.; Friman, G.; Crawford, D.J.; Neufeld, H.A. Effects of training on metabolic responses and performance capacity in streptococcus pneumoniae infected rats. Med. Sci. Sports Exerc. 23:422-427; 1991.
41. Israel, S.; Buhl, B.; Krause, M.; Neumann, G. Die konzentration der immunglobuline A, G und M im serum bei trainierten und untrainierten sowie nach verschiedenen sportlicken ausdauerleistungen. Med. Sport. 22:225-231; 1982.
42. Jemmott, J.B.; Locke, S.E. Psychosocial factors, immunologic mediation, and human susceptibility to infectious diseases: How much do we know? Psychol. Bull. 95:78-108; 1984.
43. Jokl, E. The immunological status of athletes. J. Sports Med. 14:165-192; 1974.
44. Kaplan, H.B. Social psychology of the immune system: A conceptual framework and review of the literature. Soc. Sci. Med. 33:909-923; 1991.
45. Kappel, M.; Tvede, N.; Galbo, H.; et al. Evidence that the effect of physical exercise on NK cell activity is mediated by epinephrine. J. Appl. Physiol. 70:2530-2534; 1991.
46. Khansari, D.N.; Murgo, A.J.; Faith, R.E. Effects of stress on the immune system. Immunol. Today. 11(5):170-175; 1990.
47. Krikler, D.N.; Zilberg, B. Activity and hepatitis. Lancet. 2:1046-1047; 1966.
48. Landmann, R.M.A.; Müller, F.B.; Perini, Ch.; et al. Changes in immunoregulatory cells induced by psychological and physical stress: Relationship to plasma catecholamines. Clin. Exp. Immunol. 58:127-135; 1984.
49. LaPerriere, A.; Antoni, M.; Fletcher, M.A.; Schneiderman, N. Exercise and health maintenance in AIDS. In: Galantino, M.L., ed. Clinical assessment and treatment in HIV: Rehabilitation of a chronic illness. Thorofare, NJ: Slack; [1992].
50. LaPerriere, A.R.; Antoni, M.H.; Schneiderman, N.; et al. Exercise intervention attenuates emotional distress and natural killer cell decrements following notification of positive serologic status for HIV-1. Biofeedback Self Regul. 15:229-241; 1990.
51. LaPerriere, A.R.; Fletcher, M.A.; Antoni, M.H.; et al. Aerobic exercise training in an AIDS risk group. Int. J. Sports Med. [Suppl. 1]. 12:S53-S57; 1991.
52. Levinson, S.O.; Milzer, A.; Lewin, P. Effect of fatigue, chilling and mechanical trauma on resistance to experimental poliomyelitis. Am. J. Hyg. 42:204-213; 1945.
53. Lewis, D.E.; Gilbert, B.E.; Knight, V. Influenza virus infection induces functional alterations in peripheral blood lymphocytes. J. Immunol. 137: 3777-3781; 1986.
54. Linde, F. Running and upper respiratory tract infections. Scand. J. Sport Sci. 9:21-23; 1987.
55. Mackinnon, L.T.; Chick, T.W.; van As, A.; Tomasi, T.B. The effect of exercise on secretory and natural immunity. Adv. Exp. Med. Biol. 216A:869-876; 1987.
56. MacNeil, B.; Hoffman-Goetz, L.; Kendall, A.; et al. Lymphocyte proliferation response after exercise in men: Fitness, intensity, and duration effects. J. Appl. Physiol. 70:179-185; 1991.
57. Mahan, M.P.; Young, M.R. Immune parameters of untrained or exercise-trained rats after exhaustive exercise. J. Appl. Physiol. 66:282-287; 1989.
58. Maisel, A.S.; Harris, T.; Rearden, C.A.; Michel, M.C. ß-adrenergic receptors in lymphocyte subsets after exercise: Alterations in normal individuals and patients with congestive heart failure. Circulation. 82:2003-2010; 1990.
59. Naliboff, B.D.; Benton, D.; Solomon, G.F.; et al. Immunological changes in young and old adults during brief laboratory stress. Psychosom. Med. 53:121-132; 1991.
60. Nehlsen-Cannarella, S.L.; Nieman, D.C.; Balk-Lamberton, A.J.; et al. The effects of moderate exercise training on immune response. Med. Sci. Sports Exerc. 23:64-70; 1991.
61. Nehlsen-Cannarella, S.L.; Nieman, D.C.; Jessen, J.; et al. The effects of acute moderate exercise on lymphocyte function and serum immunoglobulins. Int. J. Sports Med. 12:391-398; 1991.
62. Nieman, D.C.; Berk, L.S.; Simpson-Westerberg, M.; et al. Effects of long endurance running on immune system parameters and lymphocyte function in experienced marathoners. Int. J. Sports Med. 10:317-323; 1989.

63. Nieman, D.C.; Henson, D.A.; Gusewitch, G.; et al. Superior immune function in highly conditioned versus unconditioned elderly women. Med. Sci. Sports Exerc. 25:823-831; 1993.
64. Nieman, D.C.; Johanssen, L.M.; Lee, J.W. Infectious episodes in runners before and after a roadrace. J. Sports Med. Phys. Fitness. 29:289-296; 1989.
65. Nieman, D.C.; Johanssen, L.M.; Lee, J.W.; Arabatzis, K. Infectious episodes in runners before and after the Los Angeles Marathon. J. Sports Med. Phys. Fitness. 30:316-328; 1990.
66. Nieman, D.C.; Nehlsen-Cannarella, S.L. The effects of acute and chronic exercise on immunoglobulins. Sports Med. 11:183-201; 1991.
67. Nieman, D.C.; Nehlsen-Cannarella, S.L. Effects of endurance exercise on immune response. In: Shephard, R.J.; Astrand, P.O., eds. Endurance in sport. Oxford, England: Blackwell Scientific; 1992.
68. Nieman, D.C.; Nehlsen-Cannarella, S.L. Exercise and infection. In: Eisinger, M.; Watson, R.W., eds. Exercise and disease. Boca Raton, FL: CRC Press; 1992.
69. Nieman, D.C.; Nehlsen-Cannarella, S.L.; Donohue, K.M.; et al. The effects of acute moderate exercise on leukocyte and lymphocyte subpopulations. Med. Sci. Sports Exerc. 23:578-585; 1991.
70. Nieman, D.C.; Nehlsen-Cannarella, S.L.; Markoff, P.A.; et al. The effects of moderate exercise training on natural killer cells and acute upper respiratory tract infections. Int. J. Sports Med. 11:467-473; 1990.
71. Nieman, D.C.; Tan, S.A.; Lee, J.W.; Berk, L.S. Complement and immunoglobulin levels in athletes and sedentary controls. Int. J. Sports Med. 10:124-128; 1989.
72. Northoff, H., Berg, A. Immunologic mediators as parameters of the reaction to strenuous exercise. Int. J. Sports Med. [Suppl. 1]. 12:S9-S15; 1991.
73. Office of Disease Prevention and Health Promotion, The. U.S. Public Health Service. U.S. Department of Health and Human Services. Disease prevention/health promotion: The facts. Palo Alto, CA: Bull; 1988.
74. Osterback, L.; Qvarnberg, Y. A prospective study of respiratory infections in 12-year old children actively engaged in sport. Acta Paediatr. Scand. 76:944-949; 1987.
75. Pedersen, B.K. Influence of physical activity on the cellular immune system: Mechanisms of action. Int. J. Sports Med. [Suppl. 1]. 12:S23-S29; 1991.
76. Pedersen, B.K.; Tvede, N.; Christensen, L.D.; et al. Natural killer cell activity in peripheral blood of highly trained and untrained persons. Int. J. Sports Med. 10:129-131; 1989.
77. Pedersen, B.K.; Tvede, N.; Hansen, F.R.; et al. Modulation of natural killer cell activity in peripheral blood by physical exercise. Scand. J. Immunol. 27:673-678; 1988.
78. Pedersen, B.K.; Tvede, N.; Klarlund, K.; et al. Indomethacin in vitro and in vivo abolishes post-exercise suppression of natural killer cell activity in peripheral blood. Int. J. Sports Med. 11:127-131; 1990.
79. Pershin, B.B.; Kuz'min, S.N.; Suzdal'nitskii, R.S.; Levando, V.A. Reserve potentials of immunity. Zh. Mikrobiol. Epidemiol. Immunobiol. 6:59-64; 1985.
80. Peters, E.M.; Bateman, E.D. Respiratory tract infections: An epidemiological survey. S. Afr. Med. J. 64:582-584; 1983.
81. Petrova, I.V.; Kuz'min, S.N.; Kurshakova, T.S.; et al. The phenomenon of the formation of universal rosette-forming cells under superextreme loads. Zh. Mikrobiol. Epidemiol. Immunobiol. 2:72-76; 1985.
82. Petrova, I.V.; Kuz'min, S.N.; Kurshakova, T.S.; et al. Neutrophil phagocytic activity and the humoral factors of general and local immunity under intensive physical loading. Zh. Mikrobiol. Epidemiol. Immunobiol. 12:53-57; 1983.
83. Phillips, M.; Robinowitz, M.; Higgins, J.R.; et al. Sudden cardiac death in air force recruits: A 20-year review. JAMA. 256:2696-2699; 1986.
84. Ramsey, M.L. How I manage jock itch. Phys. Sportsmed. 18(8):63-72; 1990.
85. Reyes, M.P.; Lerner, A.M. Interferon and neutralizing antibody in sera of exercised mice with coxsackievirus B-3 myocarditis. Proc. Soc. Exp. Biol. Med. 151:333-338; 1976.
86. Rigsby, L.W.; Dishman, R.K.; Jackson, A.W.; Maclean, G.S.; Raven, P.B. Effects of exercise training on men seropositive for the human immunodeficiency virus-1. Med. Sci. Sports Exerc. 24:6-12; 1992.
87. Roberts, J.A. Loss of form in young athletes due to viral infection. Br. J. Med. 290:357-358; 1985.
88. Roberts, J.A. Viral illnesses and sports performance. Sports Med. 3:296-303; 1986.
89. Schaefer, R.M.; Kokot, K.; Heidland, A.; Plass, R. Jogger's leukocytes. N. Engl. J. Med. 316:223-224; 1987.
90. Schouten, W.J.; Verschuur, R.; Kemper, H.C.G. Physical activity and upper respiratory tract infections in a normal population of young men and women: The Amsterdam

growth and health study. Int. J. Sports Med. 9:451-455; 1988.

91. Seyfried, P.L.; Tobin, R.S.; Brown, N.E.; Ness, P.F. A prospective study of swimming-related illness I. Swimming-associated health risk. Am. J. Public Health. 75:1068-1070; 1985.
92. Sharp, J.C.M. Viruses and the athlete. Br. J. Sports Med. 23:47-48; 1989.
93. Simon, H.B. Exercise and infection. Phys. Sportsmed. 15(10):135-141; 1987.
94. Simpson, J.R.; Hoffman-Goetz, L. Exercise stress and murine natural killer cell function. Proc. Soc. Exp. Biol. Med. 195:129-135; 1990.
95. Slubik, V.M.; Levin, M.I.; Mashneva, N.I.; Pulkov, V.M. The combined effect of ionizing radiation and physical exercises on some indices of nonspecific protection and immunity. Radiobiologiia. 27:548-550; 1987.
96. Smith, J.A.; Telford, R.D.; Mason, I.B.; Weidemann, M.J. Exercise, training and neutrophil microbicidal activity. Int. J. Sports Med. 11:179-187; 1990.
97. Smith, J.K.; Chi, D.S.; Krish, G.; Reynolds, S.; Cambron, G. Effect of exercise on complement activity. Ann. Allergy. 65:304-310; 1990.
98. Smith, L.L. Acute inflammation: The underlying mechanism in delayed onset muscle soreness? Med. Sci. Sports Exerc. 23:542-551; 1991.
99. Solomon, G.F. Psychosocial factors, exercise, and immunity: Athletes, elderly persons, and AIDS patients. Int. J. Sports Med. [Suppl. 1]. 12:S50-S52; 1991.
100. Spence, D.W.; Galantino, M.L.A.; Mossberg, K.A. Progressive resistance exercise: Effect on muscle function and anthropometry of a select AIDS population. Arch. Phys. Med. Rehabil. 71:644-648; 1990.
101. Strauss, R.H.; Lanese, R.R.; Leizman, D.J. Illness and absence among wrestlers, swimmers, and gymnasts at a large university. Am. J. Sports Med. 16:653-655; 1988.
102. Tomasi, T.B.; Trudeau, F.B.; Czerwinski, D.; Erredge, S. Immune parameters in athletes before and after strenuous exercise. J. Clin. Immunol. 2:173-178; 1982.
103. Torre, D.; Sampietro, C.; Ferraro, G.; Zeroli, C.; Speranza, F. Transmission of HIV-1 infection via sports injury. Lancet. 335:1105; 1990.
104. Tvede, N.; Heilmann, C.; Halkjaer-Kristensen, J.; Pedersen, B.K. Mechanisms of B-lymphocyte suppression induced by acute physical exercise. J. Clin. Lab. Immunol. 30:169-173; 1989.
105. United States Olympic Committee, Sports Medicine and Science Committee. Transmission of potentially lethal infectious agents during athletic competition. [Unpublished internal memorandum]. 1991.
106. Van Tits, L.J.; Michel, M.C.; Grosse-Wilde, H.; Happel, M. Catecholamines increase lymphocytebeta 2-adrenergic receptors via a veta 2-adrenergic, spleen-dependent process. Am. J. Physiol. 258:E191-E202; 1990.
107. Walker, E. Herpes simplex, hepatitis B and the acquired immune deficiency syndrome. Br. J. Sports Med. 22:118; 1988.
108. Weinstein, L. Poliomyelitis: A persistent problem. N. Engl. J. Med. 288:370-371; 1973.
109. Wong, C.W.; Thompson, H.L.; Thong, Y.H.; Thornton, J.R. Effect of strenuous exercise stress on chemiluminescence response of equine alveolar macrophages. Equine Vet. J. 22:33-35; 1990.
110. World Health Organization and International Federation of Sports Medicine. AIDS and sports. [Unpublished statement]. 1990.
111. Wormser, G.P.; Bittker, S.; Forseter, G.; et al. Absence of infectious human immunodeficiency virus type 1 in "natural" eccrine sweat. J. Infect. Dis. 165:155-158; 1992.

Chapter 55

Physical Activity, Fitness, and Cancer

I-Min Lee

The hypothesis that increased physical activity may prevent cancer development is not a new idea. In 1922 Cherry (21) noticed lower cancer rates in primitive societies, that toiled continuously for food, than in more civilized cultures. He then examined cancer rates for pairs of towns located within 50 miles of each other in Europe and the United States that housed similarly sized populations. Within each pair, the more industrialized town had the higher rate. Finally, he noted that the amount of physical activity required on the job was inversely correlated with cancer mortality in men, as did Sivertsen and Dahlstrom (101) in the same year. Findings from subsequent investigations appear to support these initial observations, with the refinement that perhaps only certain site-specific cancers are affected. The aim of this chapter is to summarize what is currently known about the relation between physical activity, fitness, and cancer and to highlight unknown aspects of the relation where further research needs to be conducted.

Current Status of Knowledge

Physical Activity and Cancer

Cancer of All Sites

Initially, investigators tended to regard cancer as a single disease entity rather than a series of diseases of different sites. Findings from these studies have been equivocal. Taylor et al. (104) followed a cohort of white men working in the United States railroad industry (85,112 person-years of clerks—deemed least active, 61,630 of switchmen, and 44,867 of section men—deemed most active) for 2 years. Section men had a lower cancer mortality rate (1.47 per 1,000) than either clerks or switchmen (2.23 and 2.19 per 1,000, respectively), but the statistical significance of the differences was not determined. An opposite finding was published by Rook (95) when comparing the mortality experience of 710 nonsportsmen and 772 sportsmen attending an English university. Death certificates, from which the cause of mortality was determined, were obtainable for only half the men. Somewhat lower proportions of deceased nonsportsmen had died from cancer (12.3% to 12.8%) than sportsmen (10.1% to 18.4%). Again, the significance of these differences was not determined.

Subsequently, some investigators who studied site-specific cancers also examined all cancers (Table 55.1; 3,35,82,87,115). Paffenbarger, Hyde, and Wing (82) observed a gradient of decreasing cancer mortality with increased activity level among college alumni (cancer mortality rates for three categories of alumni of increasing activity level: 28.9, 20.0, and 19.6 per 10,000 person-years, respectively), but no association between energy expended by longshoremen on the job and cancer mortality. Garfinkel and Stellman (35) also reported that cancer mortality was inversely related to amount of exercise. However, among men who smoked and among women, those exercising heavily had higher cancer mortality rates than those exercising moderately. Albanes, Blair, and Taylor (3) noted that low levels of nonrecreational activity increased cancer risk in men (relative risk = 1.8, 95% confidence interval, 1.4–2.4, comparing most sedentary with most active men), but not in women. In addition, the adverse effect of little recreational activity in men was of borderline significance.

Waterbor, Cole, Delzell, and Andjelkovich (115), who followed 958 white, professional baseball players in the United States from 1925 to 1984, observed that among those playing appreciably more games (men whose death certificates listed "baseball player" as their occupation) there was a substantially lower cancer mortality rate than players whose death certificate listed other occupations (no figures given). On the other hand, Polednak (87) noted that major athletes had a significantly higher cancer mortality rate (14.8 per 100) than nonathletes (11.8 per 100). These men were followed until more than 86% had died, thus the high cancer mortality rates, as these figures almost reflect the proportion of deceased who had died from cancer.

Although methodological problems (see page 824) may in part have led to these discrepant findings, inconsistencies would also be expected if physical activity influences the risk of only certain site-specific cancers and their distribution had differed in the various studies.

Still, it remains plausible for physical activity to influence risk of all cancers. Immediately following submaximal or maximal graded exercise protocols, investigators consistently have shown significant, transitory increases in the percentage of circulating natural killer cells—cells that exhibit spontaneous cytotoxicity against a variety of tumor cells (48,49)—and in their activity (28,70,76,84). However, the effect of long-term physical training on natural killer cells has been less clear (24,75,77,83,116), and exhaustive endurance exercise such as marathon running may even be associated with transient decreases in the number and activity of such cells (11).

Colon Cancer

Much of the research to date on physical activity and site-specific cancers has focused on colon cancer. These studies are summarized in Table 55.1. Only statistically significant findings are reported. Investigators generally have used an alpha level of .05 for statistical significance, except for three studies where .10 was used instead (37,62,102).

The consistency of observations, despite different methodologies employed and different populations studied, makes it unlikely for chance to explain the findings. Of the 25 publications listed in Table 55.1 (describing 27 studies), the authors of all except 6 (3,35,61,82,87,113) noted a significant, inverse association between physical activity level and colon cancer risk. Studies documenting an inverse relation have been of different designs: Cohort, case-control, and proportional mortality study designs have been employed. Physical activity in these studies has been assessed using occupational activity alone (17,18,29,34,37,58,68,72,86, 110,111), leisure-time activity alone (121), or both (5,36,38,62,100,102,119). Where investigators assessed only occupational activity, activity level has been inferred from occupation recorded either at a single time (17,18,29,34,37,58,68,72,86) or over a lifetime (110,111). In studies that reported a beneficial effect of occupational and leisure-time activity, investigators have used a variety of assessment techniques. These techniques have ranged from the simple, such as use of a single, multiple-choice question (36,38,100), to more detailed, such as estimation of energy expenditure from self-reported activities (5,62,100,102).

Investigators have assessed physical activity at only one time in all but two studies, where activity assessment over decades was attempted (38,62). Where individuals have been classified into more than two levels of physical activity, a significant trend of increasing risk with decreasing activity level sometimes has been observed (17,18,34,121). In one other study, this trend was of borderline significance (5). Although not formally evaluated, a trend seemed apparent in several other studies (29,38,58,72,102,110,111). Lack of trend was reported in three studies (62,86,100). Because of the myriad techniques used to assess physical activity, it is difficult to compare results across studies. With this caveat, available data suggest that those most sedentary have 1.2 to 3.6 times the colon cancer risk of those most active.

The majority of the studies described have been conducted in the United States. An inverse association also has been observed for populations from Denmark (68), Japan (58), Sweden (29, 36–38), and Switzerland (72). For the most part, investigations have been of white subjects. An inverse relation also has been documented in the few studies of blacks (34), Chinese (119), Hispanics (34), and Japanese (58,100). The data appear to be more consistent for men than women. Six of the 25 publications in Table 55.1 that investigated men reported no significant association (3,35,61,82,87,113), compared with 5 of the 14 studying women (3,5,35, 82,113). Two studies of women described inverse trends that were not significant (121) or not tested for significance (61).

Although the inverse relation between physical activity and colon cancer risk is likely to be real, we should explore alternative explanations. Case-control studies are more susceptible to bias than cohort studies, because in the former, activity is assessed after colon cancer already has been diagnosed. Cases may report a lower level of activity prior to the onset of illness than in truth. Case-control studies utilizing hospital controls may be subject to an opposite bias: Cases are compared with a control group that may be unusually inactive. Nevertheless, inverse associations have been documented with both study designs.

Not allowing for a lag period between activity assessment and ascertainment of colon cancer raises further concern. A spurious inverse relation may arise if individuals with as yet undiagnosed disease had decreased their activity levels. One might also transfer to a physically less demanding job with the onset of illness; thus relating occupational activity at the time of diagnosis to colon cancer risk may reflect illness instead. Most investigators did not allow for a lag period. Of those who did (37,38,62,102,119), all documented an inverse relation between physical activity and colon cancer risk. It is unclear how much lag time is required.

Table 55.1 Summary of Published Epidemiological Studies on Physical Activity and Colon Cancer

Reference	Study design	Study subjects	Outcome studied	Assessment of physical activity	Potential confounders accounted for	Main results
Polednak (87)	Cohort study	8,393 men born 1860 to 1889 who attended a U.S. college, followed from college to 1967	Fatal colon cancer (n = 131)	Based on college athleticism: Men were classified as nonathletes, minor (non-"lettered") athletes, or major ("lettered") athletes.	Age	No significant differences in colon cancer mortality between the three groups
Garabrant et al. (34)	Population-based case-control study	2,950 male residents of Los Angeles County, California, aged 20 to 64 years, diagnosed with colon cancer from 1972 to 1981. Controls were 31,724 male residents, same age range, with nonbowel cancer during the same period.	Incident colon cancer, subsites within colon also studied	Based on occupation: Men were classified as having sedentary, moderate-, or high-activity level jobs.	Age, race	Men in sedentary jobs had 1.6 times the risk of those in jobs requiring high activity; dose–response relation present; findings consistent across socioeconomic and racial groups; strongest effect for descending colon
Vena et al. (111)	Hospital-based case-control study	210 white men aged 30 to 79 years, admitted with colon cancer to a U.S. hospital from 1957 to 1965. Controls were 1,431 white men, same age range, admitted with nonneoplastic, nondigestive diseases during the same period.	Incident colon cancer; subsites within colon also studied	Based on lifetime occupation: Men were classified into three or four categories according to time spent in sedentary/light activity jobs.	Age, socioeconomic status	Gradient of increasing risk with increasing time spent in sedentary/light-activity jobs; the most sedentary category had about twice the risk of the most active; strongest effect for multiple and unspecified sites within the colon
Gerhardsson et al. (37)	Cohort study	1.1 million Swedish men aged 20 to 64 years in 1960, followed from 1961 to 1979	Incident colon cancer (n = 5,100); subsites within colon also studied	Based on occupation: Men were classified as having sedentary or physically active jobs.	Age, marital status, population density, social class, region	Sedentary men had 1.3 times the risk of men in physically active jobs; strongest effect for transverse colon and flexures
Paffenbarger et al. (82)	Three cohort studies	6,351 U.S. longshoremen aged 35 to 74 years, followed for 12 or 22 years until 1972	Fatal colorectal cancer (n = 21)	Based on energy expended on the job: Men were classified as having light, moderate, or high work-activity levels.	Age	No significant differences in colorectal cancer mortality between the three groups
		51,977 men and 4,706 women entering two U.S. colleges from 1916 to 1950, followed from college to 1978	Incident colon cancer (n = 201)	Based on sports played in college: Subjects were classified as playing sports < 5 hr/week or ≥ 5 hr/week.	Age, gender	No significant difference in colon cancer incidence between the two groups
		16,936 men aged 35 to 74 years who had attended one of the above U.S. colleges, followed for 12 or 16 years, until 1978	Fatal colon cancer (n = 44)	Based on climbing stairs, walking, and playing sports in contemporary time: Men were classified as expending < 500, 500 to 1,999, or ≥ 2,000 kcal/week.	Age, cigarette smoking, body mass index	No significant differences in colon cancer mortality between the three groups

Vena et al. (110)	Proportional mortality study	430,000 white men who died between 1950 and 1979 in Washington state, USA, and 25,000 white women who died between 1974 and 1979 in the same state	Fatal colon cancer (n = 6,459 for men, 604 for women)	Based on usual occupation for most of working life: Subjects were classified into one of five activity levels by gender.	Age, year of death	For men and women, a gradient of decreasing risk with increasing activity level
Wu et al. (121)	Cohort study	11,644 men and women from a U.S. retirement community, followed from 1981 or 1982 until 1985	Incident colorectal cancer (n = 58 for men, 68 for women); subsites within colon also studied	Based on time per day engaged in physical activity: Subjects were classified as spending < 1, 1 to 2, > 2 hr/day in physical activity.	Age, alcohol intake, cigarette smoking, body mass index	For men, but not women, a gradient of decreasing risk with increasing time spent in physical activity; seen for both right- (cecum to splenic flexure) and left-sided (descending colon to rectum) cancer
Vlajinac et al. (113)	Hospital-based case-control study	88 men and women diagnosed with colon cancer from 1984 to 1986 at five hospitals in Yugoslavia. Two sets of controls were 88 patients from the same hospital with unknown malignancies and 88 men and women from the same neighborhood.	Incident colon cancer	Based on subject's own assessment of occupational activity: Subjects were classified as having sedentary or active jobs.	Age, gender, residence	No significant difference in colon cancer incidence between the two groups
Slattery et al. (102)	Population-based case-control study	110 male and 119 female residents of Utah, USA, diagnosed with colon cancer from 1978 to 1981. Controls were 180 male and 204 female residents identified by random-digit telephone dialing.	Incident colon cancer	Based on occupational and leisure-time activity: Subjects were classified into quartiles of total energy expenditure by gender. Intense and nonintense activities were examined separately.	Age, body mass index, diet	Women in the most active quartile had 0.48 times the risk of those in the least active; findings in men were nonsignificant for total energy expenditure, but intense activity was significantly and inversely related to risk
Garfinkel et al. (35)	Cohort study	372,336 men and 496,284 women from the United States, aged ≥ 30 years, followed from 1982 to 1984	Fatal colorectal cancer (n = 150 for men, 133 for women)	Based on subject's own assessment of activity level at work or during leisure time: Subjects were classified as having no, slight, moderate, or heavy amount of exercise.	Age, cigarette smoking	For men and for women, no significant difference in colorectal cancer mortality between those with moderate or heavy amount of exercise; findings for the other groups not reported
Lynge et al. (68)	Cohort study	2 million Danish men and women aged 20 to 64 years who were economically active in 1970, followed from 1970 to 1980	Incident colon cancer	Based on occupation: Subjects were classified as having sedentary or nonsedentary occupations.	Age	Sedentary men had 1.38 times the risk of all men in the cohort; sedentary women had 1.73 times the risk of all women in the cohort

(continued)

Table 55.1 *(Continued)*

Reference	Study design	Study subjects	Outcome studied	Assessment of physical activity	Potential confounders accounted for	Main results
Gerhardsson et al. (36)	Cohort study	16,477 twin individuals (men and women) born 1886 to 1925 who were identified from the Swedish twin registry, followed from 1969 to 1982	Incident colon cancer (n = 121)	Based on subject's own assessment of activity level at work and during leisure time: Subjects were classified into three and two activity levels, respectively.	Age, gender, geographic region, degree of urbanization, diet	No significant differences between work activity categories; those inactive during leisure time had 1.6 times the risk of those active; those most sedentary both at work and during leisure time had 3.6 times the risk of those most active
Severson et al. (100)	Cohort study	7,925 Japanese men born 1900 to 1919 living in Hawaii, USA, followed from between 1965 and 1968 to 1986	Incident colon cancer (n = 192); subsites within colon also studied	Three assessments used: (1) Based on time per 24 hr spent in activities of different intensity, men were classified into tertiles of a summary physical activity index; (2) based on the men's own assessment, they were classified into two activity levels at work, and during leisure time; (3) based on resting heart rate.	Age, body mass index	Men in the middle and most active tertiles had 0.56 and 0.71 times the risk, respectively, of those in the least active; strongest effect for ascending colon; active men at work and during leisure time had 0.66 and 0.72 times the risk, respectively, of inactive men; gradient of increasing risk with increasing heart rate
Brownson et al. (18)	Population-based case-control study	1,993 white men diagnosed with colon cancer from 1984 to 1987 in Missouri, USA. Controls were 9,965 white men with other cancers during the same period in the same state.	Incident colon cancer; subsites within colon also studied	Based on occupation: Men were classified as having sedentary, moderate-, or high-activity level jobs.	Age	Sedentary men had 1.4 times the risk of men in high-activity jobs; gradient of increasing risk with decreasing activity level; effect limited to men aged ≥ 75 years; strongest effect for cecum
Albanes et al. (3)	Cohort study	5,141 men and 7,413 women aged 25 to 74 years from the United States, followed from between 1971 and 1975 to between 1982 and 1984	Incident colorectal cancer (n = 62 for men, 67 for women)	Based on subject's own assessment of activity level at work and during leisure time: Subjects were classified into three activity levels for work and for leisure time.	Age, race, economic status, cigarette smoking, body mass index, dietary fat	No significant differences in colorectal cancer incidence between the three levels of work activity or the three levels of leisure-time activity
Fredriksson et al. (29)	Population-based case-control study	156 male and 156 female residents of three counties in Sweden, aged 30 to 75 years, diagnosed with colon cancer from 1980 to 1983, who were alive at the time of data collection in 1984 to 1986. Controls were 306 men and 317 women from the same counties.	Nonfatal colon cancer; subsites within colon also studied	Based on occupation: Subjects were classified as having sedentary, intermediate activity, or physically active jobs. Three categories of an index, reflecting both duration and intensity of physical activity on the job, also were created.	Age, county	Men and women in physically active jobs had 0.82 and 0.68 times the risk, respectively, of those in sedentary jobs; using the index, strongest effect observed for the descending and sigmoid colon

Peters et al. (86)	Population-based case-control study	147 white male residents of Los Angeles County, California, USA, aged 25 to 44 years, diagnosed with colon cancer from 1974 to 1982. Controls were 147 white men from the same neighborhood.	Incident colon cancer; subsites within colon also studied	Based on occupation: Using the longest held job, men were classified as sedentary, moderately active, or very active. Tertiles of a score reflecting both duration and intensity of physical activity on the job between age 18 to 28 years also were created.	Age, race, residence, body mass index, diet, occupational exposures	Men in sedentary jobs had a threefold increased risk for transverse and descending colon cancer compared with those in moderately active jobs; no significant differences between tertiles of job activity score
Marti et al. (72)	Population-based case-control study	1,995 Swiss men aged 15 to 79 years, dying of colon cancer, 1979 to 1982. Controls were 1.9 million Swiss men of the same age identified from the 1980 census.	Incident colon cancer	Based on occupation: Men were classified as having low-, moderate-, or high-activity level jobs.	Age	Men with low-activity jobs had 1.3 times the risk of those with high-activity jobs, gradient of increasing risk with decreasing job activity
Ballard-Barbash et al. (5)	Cohort study	1,906 men and 2,308 women from Framingham, Massachusetts, USA, aged 30 to 62 years in 1954, followed for up to 28 years	Incident colorectal cancer (n = 73 for men, 79 for women)	Based on time spent per 24 hr in activities of different intensity: Subjects were classified into tertiles of a summary physical activity index.	Age, education, alcohol intake, cigarette smoking, body mass index, height, serum cholesterol, (for women) parity, menopausal status	Men in the least active tertile had 1.8 times the risk of those in the most active; no significant differences between tertiles for women
Gerhardsson de Verdier et al. (38)	Population-based case-control study	163 men and 189 women born 1907 to 1946 residing in part of Stockholm County, Sweden, who were diagnosed with colon cancer from 1986 to 1988. Controls were 512 men and women residing in the same part of the county.	Incident colon cancer; subsites within colon also studied	Based on subject's own assessment of activity level at work and during leisure time every 5 years from 1950 to 1985: Subjects were classified as being sedentary, fairly active, or very active. Combining assessments from 1950 to 1985, subjects were further categorized into three levels.	Age, gender, body mass index, diet	Using 1980 assessment, inverse relation with physical activity limited to left (descending and sigmoid) colon, sedentary subjects had 3.2 times the risk of very active subjects; gradient of increasing risk with decreasing physical activity; using combined assessment, middle and least active categories had 1.9 and 2.7 times, respectively, the risk of most active category
Kato et al. (58)	Population-based case-control study	1,716 men aged ≥ 20 years from Aichi Prefecture, Japan, who were diagnosed with colon cancer from 1979 to 1987. Controls were 16,000 men aged ≥ 20 years from the same prefecture with other cancers during the same period.	Incident colon cancer; subsites within colon also studied	Based on occupation: Men were classified as having low-, moderate-, or high-activity level jobs.	Age, residence, marital status, beer intake, cigarette smoking, family history of colorectal cancer	Men in low- and moderate-activity level jobs had 1.87 and 1.79 times the risk, respectively, of those in high-activity level jobs; similar results for proximal (cecum to transverse colon) and distal (descending colon to rectosigmoid junction) colon cancer

(continued)

Table 55.1 ***(Continued)***

Reference	Study design	Study subjects	Outcome studied	Assessment of physical activity	Potential confounders accounted for	Main results
Whittemore et al. (119)	Population-based case-control study	179 male and 114 female Chinese residents of Los Angeles and San Francisco, California, USA, and Vancouver, British Columbia, Canada, aged ≥ 20 years, 95 male and 78 female Chinese residents of Hangzhou and Ningbo, China, aged 20 to 79 years diagnosed with colon cancer 1981 to 1986. Controls were 698 male and 494 female Chinese-Americans, 678 male and 618 female Chinese residing in China from the same neighborhood.	Incident colon cancer; subsites within colon also studied	Three assessments used: (1) Based on time per day spent in activities of different intensity, subjects were classified as having a sedentary or active lifestyle; (2) based on occupation, subjects were classified as sedentary or active; (3) based on daily distance walked and flights of stairs climbed (North America) or distance cycled (China).	Age, gender, residence, body mass index, diet, (for Chinese-Americans) time in North America	Chinese-Americans with sedentary lifestyle had 1.6 times the risk of those with active lifestyle; no significant differences for Chinese in China; Chinese-American men in sedentary jobs had 2.5 times the risk of those in active jobs but no significant differences for Chinese-American women or Chinese in China; similar findings for right- (cecum to splenic flexure) and left-sided (descending and sigmoid) colon; risk not related to distance walked, flights climbed, or distance cycled
Kune et al. (61)	Population-based case-control study	202 men and 190 women from Melbourne, Australia, diagnosed with colon cancer from 1980 to 1981. Controls were 398 men and 329 women from the same community.	Incident colon cancer	Based on activities carried out in an average day: Interviewers subjectively classified subjects into one of five activity levels.	Age, body mass index, diet	No significant differences in colon cancer incidence between the activity groups for men or women
Brownson et al. (17)	Population-based case-control study	1,838 white men aged ≥ 20 years, diagnosed with colon cancer from 1984 to 1989 in Missouri, USA. Controls were 15,309 white men aged ≥ 20 years with other cancers during the same period in the same state.	Incident colon cancer; subsites within colon also studied	Based on occupation: Men were classified as having low-, moderate-, or high-activity level jobs.	Age, cigarette smoking	Men holding moderate- and low-activity level jobs had 1.1 and 1.2 times, respectively, the risk of those in high-activity level jobs; gradient of increasing risk with decreasing activity level; strongest effect for cecum
Lee et al. (62)	Cohort study	17,148 men aged 30 to 79 years who were alumni of a U.S. college, followed for up to 24 years	Incident colon cancer (n = 225)	Based on climbing stairs, walking, and participating in sports or recreational activities: Men were classified as inactive, moderately active, or highly active. Activity level was assessed at two points in time separated by 11 or 15 years.	Age, body mass index	Activity level assessed at one point in time did not predict risk; men moderately active or highly active at both points in time had about half the risk of those inactive at both periods

Investigators have used a lag period ranging from 1 (37,38) to 3 years (62). The importance of a lag period diminishes with longer follow-up, because any bias will be diluted by the increasing weight of unbiased data.

Few investigators have simultaneously evaluated potential confounding by body mass index (2,65) and diet (120,123). Physically active individuals tend to be thinner and may be more healthy in their diet habits, two traits associated with lower colon cancer incidence (65,120,123). Of those who did consider both factors, five reported an inverse relation between activity level and colon cancer risk (36,38,86,102,119), one noted a similar trend in men only that did not achieve statistical significance (3), and investigators of the remaining study did not formally test the apparent inverse trend that was observed in women but not men (61).

Six of the publications in Table 55.1 reported findings at variance with the majority (3,35, 61,82,87,113), and Whittemore et al. (119) noted an inverse association for Chinese living in America, but not China. Albanes et al. (3) observed a nonsignificant inverse trend with nonrecreational activity, but no effect of recreational activity on colorectal cancer risk in men. Both types of activity were unrelated to risk in women. Besides the small number of cases studied, use of colorectal rather than colon cancer as the outcome of interest may have contributed to the lack of statistical power. Rectal cancer (*see below*) appears to be unaffected by physical activity; thus combining the two outcomes may dilute the effect of activity. Paffenbarger et al. (82, longshoremen) and Garfinkel and Stellman (35), who also did not distinguish between colon and rectal cancer, observed no relation between activity level and colorectal cancer mortality. In another study (61) there appeared to be a trend of decreasing colon cancer incidence with increasing activity level in women, but an opposite trend in men. Neither trend was formally tested. Paffenbarger et al. also noted an opposite, nonsignificant trend of increasing colon cancer mortality with increasing activity level in college alumni (82). In the remaining studies, physical activity was unrelated to colon cancer risk (82 [college students], 87,113).

Is it plausible for physical activity to reduce colon cancer risk? Some have postulated that decreased intestinal transit time may reduce large bowel cancer incidence (4,19,20) by decreasing contact between colonic mucosa and potential carcinogens in the fecal stream (93). However, no consensus exists (41,71). Exercise has been shown to decrease oral-anal transit time in some (23,50,81), but not all (13) studies. It is possible that increased activity may shorten transit time within certain gut segments without affecting total transit time. Indeed, total transit time is not a good indicator of transit rate through particular gut segments of the rat (67).

A second mechanism may operate via prostaglandins. Prostaglandin $F2_{\alpha}$ inhibited colon cancer growth when injected into rats (107). Strenuous exercise may increase plasma prostaglandin $F2_{\alpha}$ (25). In addition, human colon cancer cells in tissue culture release more prostaglandin E than surrounding normal tissue (9,10), and inhibitors of prostaglandin synthesis appear to suppress colon cancer development (74,78,88–90,92,106). Exercise may reduce prostaglandin-E levels: Physical training somewhat decreased prostaglandin-E levels among men in one study (91), but not in another (25). Prostaglandins may also affect intestinal transit—prostaglandin $F2_{\alpha}$ strongly increased and prostaglandin E decreased intestinal motility in fasted dogs (105).

Finally, exercised mice have been reported to have significantly higher levels of antioxidant enzymes in the blood (57), and antioxidants may protect against large bowel cancer (123).

Rectal Cancer

Many who investigated the relation between physical activity and all cancers (115) or colon cancer (Table 55.1;3,5,17,34-36,38,58,61,62,68,72,82,100,110,111,119, 121) also studied rectal cancer. For the most part, no significant association was observed (17,34-36,38,61, 62,68,72,82 [longshoremen], 100,111,115). Jarebinski, Adanja, and Vlajinac (56), utilizing the study base described by Vlajinac, Jarebinski, and Adanja (113; Table 55.1), also reported no association with occupational activity.

Some investigators who did not distinguish between colon and rectal cancer described a significant, inverse relation between physical activity and colorectal cancer risk (5,121), or a nonsignificant, inverse trend with nonrecreational activity (3) in men but not in women. In two other studies of rectal cancer alone, investigators also noted increased activity to significantly decrease risk (relative risk = 0.46, no confidence interval given, comparing active with sedentary college students) (82), or conversely, decreased activity to significantly increase risk (relative risk = 1.38, 95% confidence interval of 1.17–1.62, comparing most sedentary with most active subjects) (58). Vena et al. (110) reported an overall inverse trend in men, but not in women, that was not consistently observed for each decade under study. Whittemore et al. (119) observed an adverse effect of inactivity among Chinese living in America (relative risk = 1.6, 95% confidence interval of 1.1–2.4, comparing sedentary with active subjects), but not in China. In addition, Huseman, Neubauer, Duhme (53), who conducted a hospital-based case-control study of 59 men and 46 women with rectosigmoid cancer in Germany, noted that the proportion holding sedentary occupations was significantly higher in cases than in either control group. The two control groups were comprised of 55 patients with stomach cancer and 99 patients with cholelithiasis. Finally, a single study (82) noted a direct relation between activity level and rectal cancer mortality based on 14 deaths (rectal cancer mortality rates for three categories of college alumni of increasing activity level: 1.8, 2.0, and 2.5 per 10,000 person-years, respectively).

The weight of evidence suggests no relation between physical activity and rectal cancer risk, although the number of rectal cancers studied has sometimes been small (e.g., fewer than 100; see 56,62,82,100) or unreported (36,68,115). A lack of association has been observed for studies conducted in Australia (61), China (119), Denmark (68), Sweden (36,38), Switzerland (72), the United States (17,34,35,62,82 [longshoremen], 100,110,111, 115), and Yugoslavia (56). Studies generally have been conducted in white populations. A nonrelation also has been documented in two studies of Chinese (119) and Japanese (100). The lack of association holds for both men (17,34-36,38,56, 61,62,68,72,82,100,111,115,119) and women (3,5,35, 36,38,56,61,68,110,119,121). Why does physical activity influence colon but not rectal cancer risk? Although increased peristalsis may decrease contact between fecal matter and colonic mucosa, it may not greatly affect contact between fecal material and rectal mucosa, as the rectum is only intermittently filled with feces.

Prostatic Cancer

Epidemiologic data on physical activity and risk of prostatic cancer have been confusing, with various studies showing an inverse, a direct, or no effect with increased activity. A significant inverse relation was reported by Vena et al. (110) in their study of 8,116 fatal cases (proportional mortality ratios for four categories of men of increasing activity level: 109, 103, 103, and 93, respectively). Brownson, Chang, Davis, and Smith (17) who studied 2,878 fatal prostatic cancers also described a similar relation (relative risk = 1.5, 95% confidence interval of 1.2–1.8, comparing most sedentary with most active men) as did Albanes et al. (3) in a study of 95 incident occurrences of prostatic cancer (relative risk = 1.8, 95% confidence interval of 1.0–3.3, comparing recreationally most sedentary with most active men; no effect of nonrecreational activity). Lee, Paffenbarger, and Hsieh (63) found increased activity to decrease risk in men aged 70 years and older (relative risk = 0.53, 95% confidence interval of 0.29–0.95, comparing most active with most sedentary men). The authors followed a cohort of 17,719 college alumni aged 30 to 79 years for up to 27 years, during which 419 prostatic cancers developed.

On the other hand, Polednak (87) found physical activity to significantly increase prostatic cancer risk in a study of 198 fatal prostatic cancers (prostatic cancer mortality rates for three categories of men of increasing activity level: 2.2, 2.3, and 3.6 per 100, respectively) as did Paffenbarger et al. (82), who studied 154 fatal occurrences (relative risk = 1.66, no confidence interval given, for active compared with sedentary college students). Le Marchand, Kolonel, and Yoshizawa (64) conducted a population-based, case-control study between 1977 and 1983 of 452 incident cases of prostatic cancer and 899 control subjects in the United States. A direct association also was reported, especially among those aged 70 years and older (relative risk = 0.5, 95% confidence interval of 0.3–0.9 for men spending more than 54% of their life in sedentary or light jobs compared with those never holding such jobs).

Severson, Nomura, Grove, and Stemmermann (100) in their study of 206 incident occurrences of prostatic cancer found no effect of occupational activity or resting heart rate, but an almost significantly reduced risk with increased recreational activity. Garfinkel and Stellman (35) noted no relation, based on a small (unspecified) number of fatal prostatic cancers (Table 55.1). In a case-control study of 1,162 prostatic cancer patients diagnosed between 1969 and 1984 in several hospitals in the United States and 3,124 control subjects, a lack of association also was observed (122).

The biological basis for a protective effect of increased activity on prostatic cancer development seems plausible. Most (44,45,73,103,117,118) though not all (69) studies show basal testosterone levels to be depressed in trained athletes. In animals, testosterone appears to play a role in prostatic cancer development (16,51,79). In humans, withdrawal of androgens was first reported to be effective in treating advanced disease in 1941 (52). Today, antitestosterone therapy still remains the mainstay of treatment for advanced prostatic cancer (40). Prostatic levels of testosterone may be higher in carcinomatous tissues than healthy tissues or tissues undergoing benign hyperplasia (43,46,60). Investigators of some (1,39,54) but not all (1,7,8,47,54,55,94,99) studies have observed higher levels of circulating testosterone in men with prostatic cancer than in healthy men. Still others have attributed the twofold difference in prostatic cancer rates between black and white men in the United States to be almost entirely due to a 15% higher testosterone level in the former (96). However, investigators examining prediagnostic plasma or serum testosterone did not find higher hormone levels to be associated with increased risk of subsequent prostatic cancer (6,80). We can further argue that testosterone is unlikely to play an important role because prostatic cancer rates increase sharply at older ages (124) when testosterone levels are declining (42). This apparent contradiction nonetheless would be compatible with a long induction period for the effect of testosterone or a long latent period of the cancer.

Breast Cancer in Women

Frisch et al. (31, 32) reported a significantly higher risk of subsequent breast cancer in college nonathletes than athletes after taking into account age, leanness, smoking status, age at menarche, number of pregnancies, use of oral contraceptives and postmenopausal hormones, and family history of cancer (relative risk = 1.86, 95% confidence interval of 1.00–3.47). Their study investigated a random sample of 2,776 nonathletes, and 2,622 athletes from 10 colleges or universities in the United States. Living alumnae aged 21 to 80 years responded to a questionnaire inquiring about sociodemographic characteristics, athletic training in college, and medical and reproductive history, and reported 69 prevalent breast cancers. Vena et al. (110) in their study of 791 fatal breast cancers also documented an inverse relation with occupational activity (proportional mortality ratios for three categories of women of increasing activity level: 115, 83, and 85, respectively). However, Paffenbarger et al. (82) found no effect of increased activity when investigating 46 incident occurrences of breast cancer among college alumnae. A lack of association was further noted by Garfinkel et al. (35) studying few (unspecified) fatal breast cancers, and by Albanes et al. (3) who investigated 122 incident occurrences.

Although epidemiologic data have been inconclusive, it is biologically plausible for increased activity levels to decrease breast cancer risk. Strenuous physical training can delay menarche (30,33,114), and late menarche appears to decrease breast cancer risk (59). The substantial weight loss experienced by some women athletes may lead to hypothalamic dysfunction (109,112), which could potentially alter hormonal milieu and affect risk. Interestingly, the study by Frisch et al. (31,32) noted an independent effect of college athleticism after statistical adjustment for age at menarche and leanness.

Cancers of Other Sites

Studies examining cancers of other sites all have been described previously (3,17,31,32,35,82,87, 100,115). With these limited data it seems unlikely that physical activity is strongly associated with other cancers.

Lung cancer was investigated in five studies. Severson et al. (100) found a significant trend of decreasing risk with increasing activity level. In addition, men in the middle and upper tertiles of resting heart rate (presumably those less active) had increased risk compared with those in the lower tertile (relative risks = 1.50, 95% confidence interval of 1.02–2.19 and 1.42, 95% confidence interval of 0.98–2.06, respectively). Albanes et al. (3) documented an inverse association with nonrecreational activity (relative risk = 2.0, 95% confidence interval of 1.2–3.5, comparing most sedentary with most active men), but no effect of recreational activity. Paffenbarger et al. (82) noted a similar relation of borderline significance among college alumni. No significant association was observed for the other two cohorts studied, although the relative risks associated with inactivity were greater than one (82). On the other hand, Brownson et al. (17) noted decreased occupational activity to significantly decrease lung cancer incidence (relative risk = 0.8, 95% confidence interval of 0.6–0.9, comparing most sedentary with most active men), whereas Garfinkel and Stellman (35) observed activity to be unrelated to lung cancer risk in men and women.

Investigators of all four studies on pancreatic cancer (17,35,82,115) observed no relation with physical activity. Of three groups examining stomach cancer, one (100) described significant, direct associations with nonrecreational (relative risk = 1.45, 95% confidence interval of 1.07–1.97, comparing active with sedentary men) and recreational (relative risk = 1.74, 95% confidence interval of 1.08–2.81, comparing active with sedentary men) activity, but no association with resting heart rate. The remaining two studies (17,82 [college students]) reported no influence of physical activity.

Frisch et al. (31,32) noted that women nonathletes in college later faced a significantly higher risk of reproductive cancers than athletes (relative risk = 2.53, 95% confidence interval of 1.17–5.47). Albanes et al. (3) documented a significant, adverse effect of decreased nonrecreational activity on cervical cancer (relative risk = 5.2, 95% confidence interval of 1.4–14.5, comparing most sedentary with most active women). Meanwhile, Garfinkel and Stellman (35) reported no association with uterine cancer risk. All three studies were based on small numbers.

Scant data exist for remaining site-specific cancers. Polednak (87) observed no relation between college athleticism and mortality from the following cancers: buccal cavity or pharynx, digestive, respiratory, genitourinary, and lymphatic or hemopoietic. Paffenbarger et al. (82) found nonfatal and fatal cancers of the kidney, bladder, testis, brain, malignant melanoma, Hodgkin's disease, non-Hodgkin's lymphoma, and leukemia in college students to be unaffected by activity level. Among college alumni, risks of fatal bladder cancer, Hodgkin's disease, non-Hodgkin's lymphoma, and leukemia were similarly unrelated to physical activity. Risk of incident bladder cancer was described by Severson et al. (100) to be uninfluenced by occupational or leisure-time activity, or resting heart rate. Brownson et al. (17) noted an adverse effect of inactivity on incident testicular cancer (relative risk = 2.2, 95% confidence interval of 1.3–3.7, comparing most sedentary with most active men), but not other cancers (buccal cavity, esophagus, larynx, kidney or other urinary organs, bladder, brain or other nervous system components, malignant melanoma, non-Hodgkin's lymphoma, and leukemia).

Methodological Problems

Inconsistent findings from studies presented may partly stem from methodological issues, some of which have been discussed in the section on colon cancer.

Physical activity assessment at times has been imprecise: Instead of measuring activity in each individual, some investigators inferred amount of activity based on membership in a particular group. In two studies (87,95), college men who had distinguished themselves in sports were classified as *active*, and their less remarkable colleagues were considered *inactive*. Such a classification scheme would erroneously categorize individuals who, although not excelling in sports, still might have been physically active. Frisch et al. (31,32) also categorized women according to athletic status in college, but tried to minimize misclassification by including in the athlete group women nonathletes who had trained regularly during college. Physical activity was inferred using occupation alone in several studies (17,18,29,34,37,58,68,72,82 [longshoremen], 86,104,110,111,113). Because avocational activity was not assessed, misclassification again may have occurred. Garfinkel and Stellman (35) assessed physical activity using a single multiple-choice question with several graded responses. Others (3,36,38,100) adopted a similar format, using one question each for nonrecreational and recreational activity. Such an assessment technique requires subjective interpretation. All these errors in classification tend to bias toward a null result; that is, an observation of no association between activity and cancer risk. This would be of special concern with rectal cancer, as the majority of investigators reported no relation with physical activity. In a case-control study (61), interviewers listened to subjects describe their typical daily activities, then they categorized subjects into an activity level the interviewers deemed appropriate. If these interviewers were unblinded to the case or control status of subjects, they could have made biased assessments.

Use of a single assessment of physical activity, rather than several assessments, may not validly reflect an individual's true activity level, especially over the long term. An attempt was made to combine activity assessments from different measurements over time in only three studies (38,62,63). The specific time frame during which physical activity might influence cancer risk is unknown. In studies with discrepant findings, perhaps physical activity was assessed at an inappropriate time. The importance of a lag period between activity assessment and ascertainment of cancer has been discussed previously. Few studies have taken into account a lag period (37,38,62,63,102,119). The maximum period considered was 3 years (62,63), which may or may not have been sufficient to overcome bias. A lag period is less relevant for studies where activity was assessed early in life, such as during college (31,32,82 [college students], 87,95), because most cancers tend to occur late in life.

On several occasions fatal rather than incident cancer was the outcome of interest (35,82 [longshoremen, college alumni], 87,95,104,110,115). Findings from these studies, instead of predicting cancer, may reflect survival patterns. Frisch et al. (31,32) on the other hand examined only nonfatal female cancers. The authors state that their findings are unlikely to be due to greater cancer mortality among athletes, because the differential in nonfatal cancer rates between nonathletes and athletes was consistently observed for every age group. Comparing the proportions of deceased men who died from cancer (95,110) rather than actual cancer mortality rates may potentially bias results. If the overall mortality of physically active men were lower than that of inactive men because of decreased mortality from coronary heart disease (12), the proportion of deceased men who died from cancer may be inflated in the active group (95). The number of cancers studied was occasionally small; for example, fewer than 100 in some studies of colon cancer (82 [longshoremen, college alumni], 113), rectal cancer (56,62,82,100), and breast cancer (31,32,35,82 [college alumnae]), thus yielding low statistical power. On the other hand, investigators who examined multiple outcomes (3,17,35,82,87,100) might have detected by chance alone a significant association between activity and one or more outcomes.

Cigarette smoking, alcohol consumption, and dietary habits may confound the relation between physical activity and cancer risk (27). Few studies of all cancers evaluated the role of smoking (3,35,82) or diet (3), and none took alcohol into account. A high body mass index (65) and a diet high in animal fat (120,123) have been implicated to increase colon cancer risk. Neither factor was controlled for in many of the colon cancer studies (17,18,29,34,35,37,58,68,72, 82,87,110,111,113). Dietary factors may also play a role in the development of rectal cancer (123) and prostatic cancer (124), although its role in breast cancer development has been controversial (66). Again, few studies examining rectal cancer (3,36,38,61,119), prostatic cancer (3,64), or breast cancer (3) evaluated potential confounding by diet.

Physical Fitness and Cancer

There is a paucity of data on physical fitness as it relates to cancer risk. In the one study of this topic (14), investigators found physical fitness to be inversely related to mortality from all cancers. Physical fitness, assessed by a maximal treadmill test, was determined for 10,224 men and 3,120 women. Subjects were followed on average for 8 years during which 64 cancer deaths occurred in men, 18 in women. Age-adjusted cancer mortality rates for three categories of subjects of increasing fitness levels were 20.3, 7.3, and 4.7 per 10,000, respectively for men; 16.3, 9.7, and 1.0 per 10,000, respectively for women. After adjustment for potential confounders, including smoking habit, the trend was still apparent.

To the extent that heart rate is an adequate surrogate for physical fitness, two other studies also examined the relation between physical fitness and cancer risk. Persky et al. (85) followed three cohorts of 1,233, 1,899, and 5,784 white, male employees for 18, 17, and 5 years, respectively. During follow-up, 99, 78, and 95 cancer deaths, respectively, occurred. After taking into account differences in age, relative weight, cigarette smoking, and systolic blood pressure, men in the first cohort who died from any cancer and from colon cancer were observed to have had a significantly higher mean heart rate than those alive. Heart rate was not associated with lung or upper gastrointestinal cancer deaths. Investigators observed no significant association between pulse rate and cancer mortality in the second cohort. In the third cohort, those who died from any cancer had a significantly higher mean heart rate than those alive; but heart rate was not related to lung cancer, upper gastrointestinal cancer, colon cancer, or sarcoma deaths. When investigators allowed for a 2-year lag period, only results for the first cohort remained significant. Severson et al. (100) also investigated resting heart rate and risks of colon, rectal, prostatic, lung, stomach, and bladder cancers. Their results have been discussed previously.

These findings should be considered preliminary. Generally, small numbers—especially of site-specific cancers—were investigated. Another concern is whether heart rate serves as an adequate proxy for physical fitness. In addition, none of these studies took into account potential confounding by dietary factors or alcohol consumption (27).

Further Research Questions

Because humans can modify their physical activity behavior, it is important to clarify the nature of the relation between physical activity and cancer. Available data suggest that increased activity confers protection against colon cancer but does not influence rectal cancer. Data regarding other site-specific cancers have been inconclusive, and clarification is needed. Special attention should be given to cancers of the prostate in men and of the breast and reproductive system in women, as the biological basis for a protective relation is plausible. Moreover, these cancers represent some of the most commonly occurring cancers (15). Since physical activity influences physical fitness, it would also be relevant to pursue the relation between physical fitness and cancer. Future studies should attempt to avoid methodological problems discussed previously.

Although data for an inverse relation between physical activity and colon cancer risk have been rather convincing, there are other aspects of the relation requiring elucidation. These issues also should be addressed for other site-specific cancers. We need more data on minority populations. Much of the research to date has focused on white subjects and on men. Investigators need to develop and validate instruments specifically designed to measure physical activity in women. The energy cost of carrying out household tasks seems especially difficult to assess. In previous studies that included women, homemakers were (a) asked to subjectively assess their own activity level (3,35,36,38), (b) assumed to be moderately active (29), or (c) excluded altogether (68,110). We should measure total physical activity in each individual rather than inferring activity from athletic status or occupation.

We need to determine the appropriate induction period for the effect of physical activity. That is, when should an individual be physically active in order to accrue benefit? Inconsistent findings from previous studies may have resulted partly from activity assessment at different times in life. In order to determine the induction period, several assessments over time are needed. Assuming an inverse relation between physical activity and the cancer of interest, the activity assessments associated with the largest reduction in cancer risk would reflect the appropriate window of time during which increased activity is beneficial (97). Having several assessments of activity may also enable investigators to assess an individual's true activity level more accurately. Multiple assessments over time could perhaps clarify whether one needs to be active over the long term in order to accrue any benefit, as suggested by Lee et al. (62). In a related vein, it is important to ascertain whether a sedentary individual can gain any benefit when taking on a more active lifestyle. Conversely, will an individual who changes from an active to a sedentary lifestyle lose some or all of the protection conferred by previous activity? Only one group of investigators has examined changes in physical activity over time with inconclusive results (62,63).

The kinds of activity that may be of benefit in preventing cancer are unknown. Slattery, Schumacher, Smith, West, and Abd-Elghany (102) have suggested that in men, intense activity might confer greater protection against colon cancer risk than nonintense activity. More data are required. In addition, we need to assess how much activity is needed and whether the frequency, duration, and constancy of physical activity have any relevance.

For colon cancer specifically, some have suggested that physical activity may affect various subsites of the colon differently. The proximal colon was sometimes found to be most influenced by increased activity (18,37,100), at other times, the distal colon (17,29,34,38,86). Yet others have noted both proximal and distal colon to be equally affected (58,119,121). Again for colon cancer specifically, preliminary data exist that suggest body mass index (3,5), dietary fat (38,102,119), fiber (38), and protein (38,102) may modify the physical activity-cancer relation. Clarification of these issues could help us gain further insight into the biological mechanisms underlying this relation.

Finally, there has been virtually no research on the role of exercise in the treatment of human patients with cancer. Data from as far back as 1944 suggest that exercise may retard growth of tumors in animals (22,98), although heavy-intensity exercise (108) or exercise in later stages of tumor development (26) may be detrimental. We need to determine whether we can extrapolate these findings to humans.

In conclusion, although knowledge regarding the relation between physical activity, fitness, and cancer has advanced much since Cherry published his treatise in 1922, much still remains unknown.

Acknowledgments

This work was supported by Public Health Service grants CA-44854 and CA-09001 from the National Cancer Institute, National Institutes of Health, Department of Health and Human Services.

References

1. Ahluwalia, B.; Jackson, M.A.; Jones, G.W.; Williams, A.O.; Rao, M.S.; Rajguru, S. Blood hormone profiles in prostate cancer patients in high-risk and low-risk populations. Cancer. 48:2267-2273; 1981.
2. Albanes, D. Potential confounding of physical activity risk assessment by body weight and fatness. Am. J. Epidemiol. 125:745-746; 1987.
3. Albanes, D.; Blair, A.; Taylor, P.R. Physical activity and risk of cancer in the NHANES I population. Am. J. Public Health. 79:744-750; 1989.
4. Baker, A.R.; Ward, J.M.; Simon, R.M.; Stinson, S.F.; Devereux, D.F. Intestinal transit time as an important factor in the pathogenesis of dimethyl-hydrazine-induced rat colon cancer. Surg. Forum. 29:491-492; 1978.
5. Ballard-Barbash, R.; Schatzkin, A.; Albanes, D.; Schiffman, M.H.; Kreger, B.E.; Kannel, W.B.; Anderson, K.M.; Helsel, W.E. Physical activity and risk of large bowel cancer in the Framingham study. Cancer Res. 50:3610-3613; 1990.
6. Barrett-Connor, E.; Garland, C.; McPhillips, J.B.; Khaw, K.-T.; Wingard, D.L. A prospective, population-based study of androstenedione, estrogens and prostatic cancer. Cancer Res. 50:169-173; 1990.
7. Bartsch, W.; Horst, H.-J.; Becker, H.; Nehse, G. Sex hormone binding globulin binding capacity, testosterone, 5α-dihydrotestosterone, oestradiol, and prolactin in plasma of patients with prostatic carcinoma under various types of hormonal treatment. Acta Endocrinol. 85:650-664; 1977.
8. Bartsch, W.; Steins, P.; Becker, H. Hormone blood levels in patients with prostatic carcinoma and their relation to the type of carcinoma growth differentiation. Eur. Urol. 3:47-52; 1977.

9. Bennett, A.; Del Tacca, M. Prostaglandins in human colonic carcinoma. Gut. 16:409; 1975.
10. Bennett, A.; Del Tacca, M.; Stamford, I.F.; Zebro, T. Prostaglandins from tumours of human large bowel. Br. J. Cancer. 35:881-884; 1977.
11. Berk, L.S.; Nieman, D.C.; Youngberg, W.S.; Arabatzis, K.; Simpson-Westerberg, M. The effect of long endurance running on natural killer cells in marathoners. Med. Sci. Sports Exerc. 22:207-212; 1990.
12. Berlin, J.A.; Colditz, G.A. A meta-analysis of physical activity in the prevention of coronary heart disease. Am. J. Epidemiol. 132:612-628; 1990.
13. Bingham, S.A.; Cummings, J.H. Effect of exercise and physical fitness on large intestinal function. Gastroenterology. 97:1389-1399; 1989.
14. Blair, S.N.; Kohl, H.W., III; Paffenbarger, R.S., Jr.; Clark, D.G.; Cooper, K.H.; Gibbons, L.W. Physical fitness and all-cause mortality. A prospective study of healthy men and women. JAMA. 262:2395-2401; 1989.
15. Boring, C.C.; Squires, T.S.; Tong, T. Cancer statistics, 1991. CA. 41:19-36; 1991.
16. Brown, C.E.; Warren, S.; Chute, R.N.; Ryan, K.J.; Todd, R.B. Hormonally induced tumors of the reproductive system of parabiosed male rats. Cancer Res. 39:3971-3975; 1979.
17. Brownson, R.C.; Chang, J.C.; Davis, J.R.; Smith, C.A. Physical activity on the job and cancer in Missouri. Am. J. Public Health. 81:639-642; 1991.
18. Brownson, R.C.; Zahm, S.H.; Chang, J.C.; Blair, A. Occupational risk of colon cancer. An analysis by anatomic subsite. Am. J. Epidemiol. 130:675-687; 1989.
19. Burkitt, D.P. Epidemiology of cancer of the colon and rectum. Cancer. 28:3-13; 1971.
20. Burkitt, D.P.; Walker, A.R.P.; Painter, N.S. Effect of dietary fibre on stools and transit-times, and its role in the causation of disease. Lancet. 2:1408-1411; 1972.
21. Cherry, T. A theory of cancer. Med. J. Aust. 1:425-438; 1922.
22. Cohen, L.A.; Choi, K.; Wang, C.-X. Influence of dietary fat, caloric restriction, and voluntary exercise on N-nitrosomethylurea-induced mammary tumorigenesis in rats. Cancer Res. 48:4276-4283; 1988.
23. Cordain, L.; Latin, R.W.; Behnke, J.J. The effects of an aerobic running program on bowel transit time. J. Sports Med. 26:101-104; 1986.
24. Crist, D.M.; Mackinnon, L.T.; Thompson, R.F.; Atterbom, H.A.; Egan, P.A. Physical exercise increases natural cellular-mediated tumor cytotoxicity in elderly women. Gerontology. 35:66-71; 1989.
25. Demers, L.M.; Harrison, T.S.; Halbert, D.R.; Santen, R.J. Effect of prolonged exercise on plasma prostaglandin levels. Prostaglandins Med. 6:413-418; 1981.
26. Deuster, P.A.; Morrison, S.D.; Ahrens, R.A. Endurance exercise modifies cachexia of tumor growth in rats. Med. Sci. Sports Exerc. 17:385-392; 1985.
27. Doll, R.; Peto, R. The causes of cancer. New York: Oxford University Press; 1981.
28. Fiatorone, M.A.; Morley, J.E.; Bloom, E.T.; Benton, D.; Solomon, G.F.; Makinodan, T. The effect of exercise on natural killer cell activity in young and old subjects. J. Gerontol. 44:M37-M45; 1989.
29. Fredriksson, M.; Bengtsson, N.O.; Hardell, L.; Axelson, O. Colon cancer, physical activity, and occupational exposures. A case-control study. Cancer. 63:1838-1842; 1989.
30. Frisch, R.E.; Gotz-Welbergen, A.V.; McArthur, J.W.; Albright, T.; Witschi, J.; Bullen, B.; Birnholz, J.; Reed, R.B.; Hermann, H. Delayed menarche and amenorrhea of college athletes in relation to age of onset of training. JAMA. 246:1559-1563; 1981.
31. Frisch, R.E.; Wyshak, G.; Albright, N.L.; Albright, T.E.; Schiff, I.; Jones, K.P.; Witschi, J.; Shiang, E.; Koff, E.; Marguglio, M. Lower prevalence of breast cancer and cancers of the reproductive system among former college athletes compared to non-athletes. Br. J. Cancer. 52:885-891; 1985.
32. Frisch, R.E.; Wyshak, G.; Albright, N.L.; Albright, T.E.; Schiff, I.; Witschi, J.; Marguglio, M. Lower lifetime occurrence of breast cancer and cancers of the reproductive system among former college athletes. Am. J. Clin. Nutr. 45:328-335; 1987.
33. Frisch, R.E.; Wyshak, G.; Vincent, L. Delayed menarche and amenorrhea in ballet dancers. N. Engl. J. Med. 303:17-19; 1980.
34. Garabrant, D.H.; Peter, J.M.; Mack, T.M.; Bernstein, L. Job activity and colon cancer risk. Am. J. Epidemiol. 119:1005-1014; 1984.
35. Garfinkel, L.; Stellman, S.D. Mortality by relative weight and exercise. Cancer. 62:1844-1850; 1988.
36. Gerhardsson, M.; Floderus, B.; Norell, S.E. Physical activity and colon cancer risk. Int. J. Epidemiol. 17:743-746; 1988.
37. Gerhardsson, M.; Norell, S.E.; Kiviranta, H.; Pedersen, N.L.; Ahlbom, A. Sedentary jobs and colon cancer. Am. J. Epidemiol. 123:775-780; 1986.
38. Gerhardsson de Verdier, M.G.; Steineck, G.; Hagman, U.; Rieger, Å.; Norell, S.E. Physical activity and colon cancer: A case-referent

study in Stockholm. Int. J. Cancer. 46:985-989; 1990.

39. Ghanadian, R.; Puah, C.M.; O'Donoghue, E.P.N. Serum testosterone and dihydrotestosterone in carcinoma of the prostate. Br. J. Cancer. 39:696-699; 1979.
40. Gittes, R.F. Carcinoma of the prostate. N. Engl. J. Med. 324:236-245; 1991.
41. Glober, G.A.; Klein, K.L.; Moore, J.O.; Abba, B.C. Bowel transit-times in two populations experiencing similar colon cancer risks. Lancet. 2:80-81; 1974.
42. Gray, A.; Berlin, J.A.; McKinlay, J.B.; Longcope, C. An examination of research design effects on the association of testosterone and male aging: Results of a meta-analysis. J. Clin. Epidemiol. 44:671-684; 1991.
43. Habib, F.K.; Lee, I.R.; Stitch, S.R.; Smith, P.H. Androgen levels in the plasma and prostatic tissue of patients with benign hypertrophy and carcinoma of the prostate. J. Endocrinol. 71:99-107; 1976.
44. Hackney, A.C.; Sinning, W.E.; Bruot, B.C. Reproductive hormonal profiles of endurance-trained and untrained males. Med. Sci. Sports Exerc. 20:60-65; 1988.
45. Hackney, A.C.; Sinning, W.E.; Bruot, B.C. Hypothalamic-pituitary-testicular axis function in endurance-trained males. Int. J. Sports Med. 11:298-303; 1990.
46. Hammond, G.L. Endogenous steroid levels in the human prostate from birth to old age: A comparison of normal and diseased tissues. J. Endocrinol. 78:7-19; 1978.
47. Harper, M.E.; Peeling, W.B.; Cowley, T.; Brownsey, B.G.; Phillips, M.E.A.; Groom, G.; Fahmy, D.R.; Griffiths, K. Plasma steroid and protein hormone concentrations in patients with prostatic carcinoma, before and during oestrogen therapy. Acta Endocrinol. 81:409-426; 1976.
48. Herberman, R.B. Natural killer cells. Annu. Rev. Med. 37:347-352; 1986.
49. Herberman, R.B.; Ortaldo, J.R. Natural killer cells: Their role in defenses against disease. Science. 214:24-30; 1981.
50. Holdstock, D.J.; Misiewicz, J.J.; Smith, T.; Rowlands, E.N. Propulsion (mass movements) in the human colon and its relationship to meals and somatic activity. Gut. 11:91-99; 1970.
51. Hovenanian, M.S.; Deming, C.L. The heterologous growth of cancer of the human prostate. Surg. Gynecol. Obstet. 86:29-35; 1948.
52. Huggins, C.; Hodges, C.V. Studies on prostatic cancer. I. The effect of castration, of estrogen and of androgen injection on serum phosphatases in metastatic carcinoma of the prostate. Cancer Res. 1:293-297; 1941.
53. Husemann, B.; Neubauer, M.G.; Duhme, C. Sitzende tätigkeit und rektum-sigmakarzinom. Onkologie. 4:168-171; 1980.
54. Jackson, M.A.; Kovi, J.; Heshmat, M.Y.; Ogunmuyiwa, T.A.; Jones, G.W.; Williams, A.O.; Christian, E.C.; Nkposong, E.O.; Rao, M.S.; Jackson, A.G.; Ahluwalia, B.S. Characterization of prostatic carcinoma among blacks: A comparison between a low-incidence area, Ibadan, Nigeria, and a high-incidence area, Washington, DC. Prostate. 1:185-205; 1980.
55. Jacobi, G.H.; Rathgen, G.H.; Altwein, J.E. Serum prolactin and tumors of the prostate: Unchanged basal levels and lack of correlation to serum testosterone. J. Endocrinol. Invest. 3:15-18; 1980.
56. Jarebinski, M.; Adanja, B.; Vlajinac, H. Case-control study of relationship of some biosocial correlates to rectal cancer patients in Belgrade, Yugoslavia. Neoplasma. 36:369-374; 1988.
57. Kanter, M.M.; Hamlin, R.L.; Unverferth, D.V.; Davis, H.W.; Merola, A.J. Effect of exercise training on antioxidant enzymes and cardiotoxicity of doxorubicin. J. Appl. Physiol. 59:1298-1303; 1985.
58. Kato, I.; Tominaga, S.; Ikari, A. A case-control study of male colorectal cancer in Aichi Prefecture, Japan: With special reference to occupational activity level, drinking habits and family history. Jpn. J. Cancer Res. 81:115-121; 1990.
59. Kelsey, J.L.; Gammon, M.D. The epidemiology of breast cancer. CA. 41:146-165; 1991.
60. Krieg, M.; Bartsch, W.; Voight, K.D. Binding, metabolism and tissue level of androgens in human prostatic carcinoma, benign prostatic hyperplasia and normal prostate. Excerpta Med. ICS. 494:102-104; 1979.
61. Kune, G.A.; Kune, S.; Watson, L.F. Body weight and physical activity as predictors of colorectal cancer risk. Nutr. Cancer. 13:9-17; 1990.
62. Lee, I-M.; Paffenbarger, R.S., Jr.; Hsieh, C-C. Physical activity and risk of developing colorectal cancer among college alumni. JNCI. 83:1324-1329; 1991.
63. Lee, I-M.; Paffenbarger, R.S., Jr.; Hsieh, C-C. Physical activity and risk of prostatic cancer among college alumni. Am. J. Epidemiol. 135:169-179; 1992.
64. Le Marchand, L.; Kolonel, L.N.; Yoshizawa, C.N. Lifetime occupational physical activity and prostate cancer risk. Am. J. Epidemiol. 133:103-111; 1991.

65. Lew, E.A.; Garfinkel, L. Variations in mortality by weight among 750,000 men and women. J. Chronic Dis. 32:563-576; 1979.
66. London, S.; Willett, W. Diet and the risk of breast cancer. Hematol. Oncol. Clin. North Am. 3:559-576; 1989.
67. Lupton, J.R.; Meacher, M.M. Radiographic analysis of the effect of dietary fibers on rat colonic transit time. Am. J. Physiol. 255:G633-G639; 1988.
68. Lynge, E.; Thygesen, L. Use of surveillance systems for occupational cancer: Data from the Danish national system. Int. J. Epidemiol. 17:493-500; 1988.
69. MacConnie, S.E.; Barkan, A.; Lampman, R.M.; Schork, M.A.; Beitins, I.Z. Decreased hypothalamic gonadotrophin-releasing hormone secretion in male marathon runners. N. Engl. J. Med. 315:411-417; 1986.
70. Mackinnon, L.T. Exercise and natural killer cells. What is the relationship? Sports Med. 7:141-149; 1989.
71. MacLennan, R.; Jensen, O.M. Dietary fibre, transit-time, faecal bacteria, steroids, and colon cancer in two Scandinavian populations. Report from the international agency for research on cancer intestinal microecology group. Lancet. 2:207-211; 1977.
72. Marti, B.; Minder, C.E. Physische berufsaktivität und kolonkarzinommortalität bei Schweizer männern 1979-1982. Soz. Praventivmed. 34:30-37; 1989.
73. Morville, R.; Pesquies, P.C.; Guezennec, C.Y.; Serrurier, B.D.; Guignard, M. Plasma variations in testicular and adrenal androgens during prolonged physical exercise in man. Ann. Endocrinol. 40:501-510; 1979.
74. Narisawa, T.; Sato, M.; Tani, M.; Kudo, T.; Takahashi, T.; Goto, A. Inhibition of development of methylnitrosourea- induced rat colon tumors by indomethacin treatment. Cancer Res. 41:1954-1957; 1981.
75. Nehlsen-Cannarella, S.L.; Nieman, D.C.; Balk-Lamberton, A.J.; Markoff, P.A.; Arabatzis, K.; Chritton, D.B.W.; Gusewitch, G.; Lee, J.W. The effects of moderate exercise training on immune response. Med Sci. Sports Exerc. 23:64-70; 1991.
76. Nieman, D.C.; Nehlsen-Cannarella, S.L.; Donohue, K.M.; Chritton, D.B.W.; Haddock, B.L.; Stout, R.W.; Lee, J.W. The effects of acute moderate exercise on leukocyte and lymphocyte subpopulations. Med. Sci. Sports Exerc. 23:578-585; 1991.
77. Nieman, D.C.; Nehlsen-Cannarella, S.L.; Markoff, P.A.; Balk-Lamberton, A.J.; Yang, H.; Chritton, D.B.W.; Lee, J.W.; Arabatzis, K. The effects of moderate exercise training on natural killer cells and acute upper respiratory tract infections. Int. J. Sports Med. 11:467-473; 1990.
78. Nigro, N.D.; Bull, A.W.; Boyd, M.E. Inhibition of intestinal carcinogenesis in rats: Effect of difluoromethylornithine with piroxicam or fish oil. JNCI. 77:1309-1313; 1986.
79. Noble, R.L. The development of prostatic adenocarcinoma in Nb rats following prolonged sex hormone administration. Cancer Res. 37:1929-1933; 1977.
80. Nomura, A.; Heilbrun, L.K.; Stemmermann, G.N.; Judd, H.L. Prediagnostic serum hormones and the risk of prostate cancer. Cancer Res. 48:3515-3517; 1988.
81. Oettlé, G.J. Effect of moderate exercise on bowel habit. Gut. 32:941-944; 1991.
82. Paffenbarger, R.S., Jr.; Hyde, R.T.; Wing, A.L. Physical activity and incidence of cancer in diverse populations: A preliminary report. Am. J. Clin. Nutr. 45:312-317; 1987.
83. Pedersen, B.K.; Tvede, N.; Christensen, L.D.; Klarlund, K.; Kragbak, S.; Halkjær-Kristensen, J. Natural killer cell activity in peripheral blood of highly trained and untrained persons. Int. J. Sports Med. 10:129-131; 1989.
84. Pedersen, B.K.; Tvede, N.; Hansen, F.R.; Andersen, V.; Bendix, T.; Bendixen, G.; Bendtzen, K.; Galbo, H.; Haahr, P.M.; Halkjær-Kristensen, J. Modulation of natural killer cell activity in peripheral blood by physical exercise. Scand. J. Immunol. 27:673-678; 1988.
85. Persky, V.; Dyer, A.R.; Leonas, J.; Stamler, J.; Berkson, D.M.; Lindberg, H.A.; Paul, O.; Shekelle, R.B.; Lepper, M.H.; Schoenberger, J.A. Heart rate: A risk factor for cancer? Am. J. Epidemiol. 114:477-487; 1981.
86. Peters, R.K.; Garabrant, D.H.; Yu, M.C.; Mack, T.M. A case-control study of occupational and dietary factors in colorectal cancer in young men by subsite. Cancer Res. 49:5459-5468; 1989.
87. Polednak, A.P. College athletics, body size, and cancer mortality. Cancer. 38:382-387; 1976.
88. Pollard, M.; Luckert, P.H. Prolonged antitumor effect of indomethacin on autochthonous intestinal tumors in rats. JNCI. 70:1103-1105; 1983.
89. Pollard, M.; Luckert, P.H. Effect of piroxicam on primary intestinal tumors induced in rats by N-methylnitrosourea. Cancer Lett. 25:117-121; 1984.
90. Pollard, M.; Luckert, P.H.; Schmidt, M.A. The suppressive effect of piroxicam on autochtho-

nous intestinal tumors in the rat. Cancer Lett. 21:57-61; 1983.

91. Rauramaa, R.; Salonen, J.K.; Kukkonen-Harjula, K.; Seppänen, K.; Seppälä, E.; Vapaatalo, H.; Huttunen, J.K. Effects of mild physical exercise on serum lipoproteins and metabolites of arachidonic acid: A controlled randomized trial in middle-aged men. Br. Med. J. 288:603-606; 1984.
92. Reddy, B.S.; Maruyama, H.; Kelloff, G. Dose-related inhibition of colon carcinogenesis by dietary piroxicam, a nonsteroidal anti-inflammatory drug, during stages of rat colon tumor development. Cancer Res. 47:5340-5346; 1987.
93. Reddy, B.S.; Wynder, E.L. Metabolic epidemiology of colon cancer. Fecal bile acids and neutral sterols in colon cancer patients and patients with adenomatous polyps. Cancer. 39:2533-2539; 1977.
94. Robinson, M.R.G.; Thomas, B.S. Effect of hormonal therapy on plasma testosterone levels in prostatic carcinoma. Br. Med. J. 4:391-394; 1971.
95. Rook, A. An investigation into the longevity of Cambridge sportsmen. Br. Med. J. 1:773-777; 1954.
96. Ross, R.; Bernstein, L.; Judd, H.; Hanisch, R.; Pike, M.; Henderson, B. Serum testosterone levels in healthy young black and white men. JNCI. 76:45-48; 1986.
97. Rothman, K.J. Modern epidemiology. Boston: Little, Brown; 1986.
98. Rusch, H.P.; Kline, B.E. The effect of exercise on the growth of a mouse tumor. Cancer Res. 4:116-118; 1944.
99. Saroff, J.; Kirdani, R.Y.; Chu, T.M.; Wajsman, Z.; Murphy, G.P. Measurements of prolactin and androgens in patients with prostatic disease. Oncology. 37:46-52; 1980.
100. Severson, R.K.; Nomura, A.M.Y.; Grove. J.S.; Stemmermann, G.N. A prospective analysis of physical activity and cancer. Am. J. Epidemiol. 130:522-529; 1989.
101. Sivertsen, I.; Dahlstrom, A.W. The relation of muscular activity to carcinoma. A preliminary report. J. Cancer Res. 6:365-378; 1922.
102. Slattery, M.L.; Schumacher, M.C.; Smith, K.R.; West, D.W.; Abd-Elghany, N. Physical activity, diet and risk of colon cancer in Utah. Am. J. Epidemiol. 128:989-999; 1988.
103. Strauss, R.H.; Lanese, R.R.; Malarkey, W.B. Weight loss in amateur wrestlers and its effect on serum testosterone levels. JAMA. 254: 3337-3338; 1985.
104. Taylor, H.L.; Klepetar, E.; Keys, A.; Parlin, W.; Blackburn, H.; Puchner, T. Death rates among physically active and sedentary employees of the railroad industry. AJPH. 52:1697-1707; 1962.
105. Thor, P.; Konturek, J.W.; Konturek, S.J.; Anderson, J.H. Role of prostaglandins in control of intestinal motility. Am. J. Physiol. 248:G353-G359; 1985.
106. Thun, M.J.; Namboodiri, M.M.; Heath, C.W., Jr. Aspirin use and reduced risk of fatal colon cancer. N. Engl. J. Med. 325:1593-1596; 1991.
107. Tutton, P.J.M.; Barkla, D.H. Influence of prostaglandin analogues on epithelial cell proliferation and xenograft growth. Br. J. Cancer. 41:47-51; 1980.
108. Uhlenbruck, G.; Order, U. Can endurance sports stimulate immune mechanisms against cancer and metastasis? Int. J. Sports Med. 12:S63-S68; 1991.
109. Veldhuis, J.D.; Evans, W.S.; Demers, L.M.; Thorner, M.O.; Wakat, D.; Rogol, A.D. Altered neuroendocrine regulation of gonadotropin secretion in women distance runners. J. Clin. Endocrinol. Metab. 61:557-563; 1985.
110. Vena, J.E.; Graham, S.; Zielezny, M.; Brasure, J.; Swanson, M.K. Occupational exercise and risk of cancer. Am. J. Clin. Nutr. 45:318-327; 1987.
111. Vena, J.E.; Graham, S.; Zielezny, M.; Swanson, M.K.; Barnes, R.E.; Nolan, J. Lifetime occupational exercise and colon cancer. Am. J. Epidemiol. 122:357-365; 1985.
112. Vigersky, R.A.; Andersen, A.E.; Thompson, R.H.; Loriaux, D.L. Hypothalamic dysfunction in secondary amenorrhea associated with simple weight loss. N. Engl. J. Med. 297:1141-1145; 1977.
113. Vlajinac, H.; Jarebinski, M.; Adanja, B. Relationship of some biosocial factors to colon cancer in Belgrade (Yugoslavia). Neoplasma. 34:503-507; 1987.
114. Warren, M.P. The effects of exercise on pubertal progression and reproductive function in girls. J. Clin. Endocrinol. Metab. 51:1150-1157; 1980.
115. Waterbor, J.; Cole, P.; Delzell, E.; Andjelkovich, D. The mortality experience of major-league baseball players. N. Engl. J. Med. 318:1278-1280; 1988.
116. Watson, R.R.; Moriguchi, S.; Jackson, J.C.; Werner, L.; Wilmore, J.H. Modification of cellular immune functions in humans by endurance exercise training during β-adrenergic blockade with atenolol or propranolol. Med. Sci. Sports Exerc. 18:95-100; 1986.
117. Wheeler, G.D.; Wall, S.R.; Belcastro, A.N.; Cumming, D.C. Reduced serum testosterone and prolactin levels in male distance runners. JAMA. 252:514-516; 1984.

118. Wheeler, G.D.; Wall, S.R.; Conger, P.; Belcastro, A.N.; Cumming, D.C. Reduced testosterone levels in high mileage and competitive distance runners. [Abstract]. Can. J. Appl. Sports Sci. 8:225-226; 1983.
119. Whittemore, A.S.; Wu-Williams, A.H.; Lee, M.; Shu, Z.; Gallagher, R.P.; Deng-ao, J.; Lun, Z.; Xianghui, W.; Kun, C.; Jung, D.; Teh, C-Z.; Chengde, L.; Yao, X.J.; Paffenbarger, R.S., Jr.; Henderson, B.E. Diet, physical activity, and colorectal cancer among Chinese in North America and China. JNCI. 82:915-926; 1990.
120. Willett, W.C.; Stampfer, M.J.; Colditz, G.A.; Rosner, B.A.; Speizer, F.E. Relation of meat, fat, and fiber intake to the risk of colon cancer in a prospective study among women. N. Engl. J. Med. 323:1664-1672; 1990.
121. Wu, A.H.; Paganini-Hill, A.; Ross, R.K.; Henderson, B.E. Alcohol, physical activity and other risk factors for colorectal cancer: A prospective study. Br. J. Cancer. 55:687-694; 1987.
122. Yu, H.; Harris, R.E.; Wynder, E.L. Case-control study of prostate cancer and socioeconomic factors. Prostate. 13:317-325; 1988.
123. Zaridze, D.G. Environmental etiology of large-bowel cancer. JNCI. 70:389-400; 1983.
124. Zaridze, D.G.; Boyle, P. Cancer of the prostate: Epidemiology and aetiology. Br. J. Urol. 59:493-502; 1987.

Chapter 56

Physical Activity, Fitness, and Recovery from Surgical Trauma

Tom Christensen

The review of this topic in 1988 in Toronto underlined the need for studies of people undergoing elective surgical procedures with measurements of muscle strength and endurance and for the description and evaluation of the syndrome of postoperative fatigue. In addition studies of postoperative exercise testing and training both before and after surgery especially in old age were called for.

What Do We Know About Activity, Muscle Performance, and Fitness After Surgical Trauma?

Normal Activity After Surgery

Surgery and trauma are followed by decreased physical activity, although only a few studies are available (43,52). Activity (lying, sitting, standing, and walking) was measured in 97 patients employing a lightweight recorder and sensors to monitor posture and movement over 24 hr-periods before, 2, 4, 6, and 12 weeks after surgery (52). Seventy-nine patients had major surgery and 18 patients minor surgery. Even 1 month after the operation, at the time when many patients are expected to return to work and daily activities, there was a decrease in physical activity in both groups. The patients walked less and spent more time lying down. The patients who had major surgery, and therefore a greater surgical stress, had the most pronounced decrease in activity, although both groups returned to preoperative levels 6 weeks after surgery. Sakamoto, Nakano, Hashimoto, and Nagamachi (42) assessed a physical index from a 24-hr heart rate ratio in 15 patients before and 1, 3, 6, and 12 months after gastrectomy. The index remained significantly lower even 3 months after surgery compared to before. Between 6 and 12 months the index was restored to preoperative level (42).

Fitness

Fitness related to health refers to those components of fitness that are favorably influenced by habitual physical activity and characterized by an ability to perform daily activities with vigor. After surgery and trauma patients do not complain about lack of fitness but rather about increased feelings of fatigue (8).

Postoperatively, patients still in the hospital complain of fatigue from walking in the ward and climbing stairs (8). After coming home many patients realize how tired they really are after doing minor tasks such as cooking and shopping (8) and they often feel the need to lie down, which agrees with the important study of Stock, Clague, and Johnston (52).

By the use of a fatigue scale constructed in the descriptive studies of Christensen et al. (8,10-17) it has been found that uncomplicated major surgery is followed by increased feelings of fatigue after 1 month in about one third of patients (11) and that feelings of fatigue return to preoperative levels 2 months postoperatively (23). Postoperative fatigue was found to be related to postoperative deterioration in nutritional parameters (12) and impaired adaptability of heart rate during exercise (15,16), but not to any preoperative factors (11)

Strength

Decreases in hand grip force from 5% or 6% (30) to 12% (47) have been measured during the first 8 days after major abdominal surgery. On the other hand, no decrease in hand grip force was found in 10 patients 3, 10, 20, and 30 days (37) and 1, 2, 4, and 8 days (49) after elective cholecystectomy compared to preoperative hand grip force.

Muscle force of elbow flexors was assessed before, 10, and 20 days after uncomplicated, elective abdominal surgery in 20 patients (17). The maximum force was 21 to 24 kg preoperatively and had decreased by approximately 10% by day 10 and

7% by day 20 after surgery. To distinguish between the central and peripheral components in the postoperative decline in muscle function, objective measurements of the contractile force can be made after nerve stimulation; the effects of motivation and central drive are eliminated and only the peripheral component is measured by this technique.

The force of maximal voluntary isometric contractions of the *adductor pollicis* (a small muscle with an unusual distribution of fiber types) and this force, when stimulated through the ulnar nerve at the wrist, was measured before and after major abdominal surgery (31,34,47,58). There was a decrease in voluntary muscle force, but no difference in skeletal muscle function after nerve stimulation on day 3 (58), day 4, 7, and 10 (31,34,47) or day 14, 30, and 90 (47) after surgery.

Endurance

In 20 patients (17) endurance at a force adjusted to 30% of maximum force of elbow flexors had decreased about 30% both on day 10 and 20 after major abdominal surgery compared to the endurance at the same force preoperatively. Edwards, Rose, and King (18) also found a 30% deterioration of endurance of hip muscles after surgery including both minor and major operations.

The muscles lose force after the surgical trauma when used voluntarily, but not when stimulated through the ulnar nerve. But maybe the adductor pollicis muscle (40) is not the perfect muscle to render signals of physical deterioration and fatigue from the body. On the other hand, there was no change of clinical importance in the function of *musculus quadriceps femoris* when stimulated through large, damp electrodes before and after surgery (34).

Thus it appears that the subjective feeling of weakness in postoperative patients cannot be related to any objective measure of neuromuscular dysfunction, although electromyographic findings 10 days after surgery suggested activation of fewer motor units compared to preoperative findings during a force of 2 kg and a force of 30% of maximum elbow flexion (17).

Oxygen Consumption

Surgical trauma has little influence on respiratory gas exchange during exercise (8,56,58). Twelve patients performed an exercise test on a treadmill at a work rate of 20 and 56 kpm/min before and 3 days after elective abdominal surgery (58). Oxygen consumption increased significantly from rest during exercise, but there was no difference between the pre- and postoperative values (0.61 L/min versus 0.66 L/min) when steady-state conditions were reached 3 min after the commencement of exercise.

Ten, 20, and 30 days after major abdominal surgery six patients had oxygen consumption during a comparable exercise load on a bicycle ergometer 2% lower on all postoperative days than preoperatively (8). This is consistent with the unchanged values found by others following abdominal surgery (56) or meniscectomy (3). Thus oxygen uptake at each given level of work performance does not change after surgery.

Pulse Rate

Pulse rates were increased in 16 patients 10, 20, and 30 days after elective, uncomplicated, abdominal surgery compared to preoperative rates during an orthostatic stress test (8). Pulse rate differences between pre- and postoperative tests were only significant on day 10, maybe because ortostatic work represents only a minor operation. Three days after abdominal surgery the heart rate was significantly higher compared to before surgery, both at rest and after exercise on a treadmill at a work rate of 20 and 56 kpm/min (58). In bicycle ergometer tests performed at 65% of preoperative work capacity, the heart rate was significantly higher day 20 postoperatively (15,16) compared to that preoperatively.

Energy Expenditure and Muscular Effiency

In the treadmill exercise test mentioned previously (58), energy expenditure and muscular efficiency were measured. Energy expenditure was calculated from oxygen consumption and carbon dioxide production and muscular efficiency as the ratio of the net change in work rate divided by the net change in energy expenditure. During the same work on the treadmill 3 days after surgery the muscular efficiency was 12% lower postoperatively and accompanied by a 19% rise in net energy expenditure. Thus, after surgical trauma there is a deterioration in cardiovascular function during exercise along with lower muscular efficiency and a rise in net energy expenditure.

Factors That May Influence Physical Activity and Fitness in Recovery After Surgery

Preoperative Factors

Daily Activity of the Patient

From the study of Stock et al. (52) patients who were determined most active preoperatively by walking a number of steps equal to or greater than the median preoperative value for all patients were also most active after surgery (5,050 vs. 935 steps walked 2 weeks after surgery and 8,020 vs. 4,500 steps walked at 4 weeks after surgery, $p < .01$).

Muscle-Force

On the other hand there is no evidence that stronger patients have any advantage preoperatively, because there was no relation between preoperative muscle force in 20 patients and postoperative fatigue 10 and 20 days after major abdominal surgery (17).

Anxiety and Fatigue

Neither anxiety, measured by the State-Trait Anxiety Inventory (51), nor preoperative feelings of fatigue (8) related to degree of fatigue postoperatively (10,11). However, patients who complained most of symptoms from their disease preoperatively also were most inactive 2 and 12 weeks after surgery ($p < .05$) (52).

Therapeutic Measures: Preoperative Training. In Adolfsson's study (1) 6 week's worth of preoperative running and gymnastics to music (two, 30-min sessions a week) in 58 female gallstone patients resulted in a preoperative improvement in their general condition and physical working capacity. Nevertheless, the effect of the training disappeared in the course of the first postoperative week, and the working capacity 4 weeks after surgery was no different than that of 30 untrained patients in the control group.

Thus, preoperative training alone at a low intensity has no influence on postoperative physical working capacity, and the effect of a more intense training or a combination with behavioral preparation for surgery is unknown. Elective surgery patients who prepared for surgery with training in muscle relaxation and information about the sensations they would experience had a reduced hospital stay and feelings of increased strength and energy postoperatively (55).

Perioperative Factors

Surgical Trauma and Anesthesia

Surgery and trauma initiate well-known changes in endocrine and metabolic function such as loss of body protein and negative nitrogen balance (26). Feelings of fatigue increase after major but not minor surgery, although mean duration of surgery and anesthesia is similar in the two groups (11). The length of surgery was related to reduction in postoperative activity (reduction in time spent standing), but peroperative blood loss was not (52). Thus, the magnitude of the trauma and not the duration of anesthesia may be important for postoperative fitness and degree of physical activity.

Therapeutic Measures: Modify Stress Response. The stress response has been considered a defense mechanism by which the body protects itself against injury; however other effects of surgery such as pulmonary complications, myocardial infarction, pain, inability to work, and increased fatigue in convalescence are undesirable. Therefore, a "stress-free anaesthesia and surgery" seems reasonable (27).

An afferent neurogenic blockade by analgesia is known to reduce the catabolic response to hip and pelvic surgery (7,35,54) and causes partial reduction in patients undergoing upper abdominal surgery (47). Administered into the epidural space, it may therefore have a positive influence on fitness and activity after surgery. In the meantime, no studies have been performed on physical activity and fitness in patients undergoing lower body procedures where epidural analgesia very effectively inhibits the surgical stress response.

Schultze, Roikjaer, Hasselstrøm, Jensen, and Kehler (49) could not modify the postoperative increase in fatigue from 1 to 8 days after upper abdominal surgery with epidural analgesia. On the other hand a single preoperative high-dose glucocorticoid in combination with epidural analgesia and indomethacin reduced fatigue and complications postoperatively (48,50). Further controlled trials are needed in which the effect of preoperative, high-dose glucocorticoid, epidural analgesia, and indomethacin on physical activity and fitness in patients undergoing surgical procedures is investigated.

Postoperative Factors

Pain

The most effective regimen to provide pain relief postoperatively combines epidural bupivacaine with morphine plus systemic indomethacin (49). Yet no significant effect was seen on postoperative fatigue, and the influence on physical activity was not measured. In the study of Schroeder and Daker (45) continuous interpleural infusion of bupivacaine for analgesia after cholecystectomy resulted in a significantly lower pain score and better ventilatory capacity compared to the control group. No evidence of shortened postoperative hospitalization and postoperative fatigue was found in the two groups.

Nutrition

The postoperative period is characterized by an insufficient nutritional intake (20,22). In a Danish nutritional study of 21 abdominal patients admitted for a colonic resection (22) 75% of the patients consumed less energy per day than the basal metabolism + 30% during the entire postoperative stay in the hospital. The same pattern was found in English patients (20).

Therapeutic Measures: Improve Postoperative Nutrition. Impairment in nutritional status with loss in body weight after major abdominal surgery is significantly correlated to development of postoperative fatigue during the first month after the operation (12,13,16). Likewise, different peri- and postoperative nutritional support systems may be valuable in preventing decreased postoperative exercise capacity and fitness.

Fifty-five patients were assigned to four different nutrition groups (57): (a) 90 g amino acids plus 3,000 calories of glucose per day, (b) 100 g glucose per day, (c) 90 g amino acids per day, and (d) 90 g amino acids and 60 g glucose plus 1,600 calories of fat per day in 8 days after major surgery. Group (a) also received parenteral nutrition 2 weeks prior to surgery. All groups lost weight postoperatively, but the net nitrogen retention was significantly better in groups receiving a caloric supplement (groups [a] and [d]), and body cell mass determined from total exchangable potassium improved at the expense of extracellular mass in the same two groups.

Thus the postoperative weight loss in Groups (a) and (d) was an overall decrease in total body water, which reflected loss of extracellular fluid. The patients performed an exercise test before and 10 days after surgery on a bicycle ergometer with loads varying from 25 to 175 W depending on their work capacity. Postoperative exercise capacity was only 4% lower in Groups (a) and (d) in contrast to a 13% decrease in Groups (b) and (c). Thus by receiving a caloric supplement postoperatively, and thereby preserving body cell mass, postoperative exercise capacity can be maintained (57).

A clinical value of early postoperative feeding with elemental diet was found in 15 patients (41) who had less weight loss and a shorter stay in the hospital than 15 patients allocated to conventional postoperative feeding. Bastow, Rawlings, and Allison (5) also found a considerable shortening in rehabilitation time by nutritional regimen in patients being undernourished at admission to the hospital. However, enteral nutrition during 4 days (1,200 kcal/day) had no influence on postoperative fatigue and decrease in body weight (46).

Immobilization

Postoperative patients experience an impaired cardiovascular adaptability to exercise (15,16) similar to the increased heart rate during submaximal exercise shown in patients after bed rest (43) and detraining (19). Although most patients are encouraged to mobilize soon after surgery, patients are not mobilized 1 month after surgery (52).

Therapeutic Measures: Exercise and Training.
Abdominal Surgery

Studies with exercise during general surgery are very scanty. In the old study of Adolfsson (1), five training evenings of 30 minutes each after cholecystectomy had no effect on exercise capacity in 20 patients on a bicycle ergometer compared to 30 patients without any training at all. In patients receiving both pre- and postoperative training, however, recovery of working capacity during convalescence was more rapid, and 4 weeks after the operation the physical capacity was 20% to 25% above the initial value.

Cardiac Surgery: Coronary Bypass Surgery.

For most cardiac patients, exercise training has become an integral part of the rehabilitation process. Two groups of nine male patients after coronary bypass surgery started training 24 and 26 days after surgery for 3-1/2 weeks (32). One group was trained by the interval method (work and interval each 1:1 min) and the other trained continuously by increasing physical performance on a bicycle ergometer. Training was 20 min and 25 min per day the first 5 days in the week and 25 min per day during the weekend. The exercise training intensity was set at 86% of individual maximum heart rate. The results after training suggest that interval training was superior to continuous training: Physical performance was higher, heart rate was lower at rest and at 75 W, and lactate rate was lower at 75 W after interval training compared to continuous training (32).

Hydraulic circuit training utilizes cylinders to provide concentric exercise for both agonist and antagonist muscle groups. Eight weeks of hydraulic training in eight patients (21) resulted in an increase in both muscular strength and endurance during knee and shoulder exercise compared to cycle training in eight other patients after coronary bypass surgery. Following training there was a significant reduction in the heart rate responses to submaximal exercise in both groups in contrast to the results in eight patients who served as a nonexercising control group (21).

Training on a bicycle ergometer for 12 weeks after coronary artery bypass surgery also had a positive effect 1 and 5 years after the operation on increased working capacity in the training group compared to the nontraining group (2). Concomitantly there was a fast, significant decrease in plasma triglycerides during the first postoperative year in the training group (2). These results show the effect of exercise during the first months after surgery.

Cardiac Surgery: Transplantation.

It is known that physical work performance is impaired after cardiac transplantation (44). In human cardiac transplants nerve regeneration does not occur (5), but despite this persistent total denervation, the donor heart has a response to exercise. After surgery the resting heart rate is elevated (90–110 beats/min) (25) in part due to loss of vagal tone. The resting cardiac output is normal and systolic and diastolic pressures higher, maybe as a result of elevated norepinephrine levels (6).

During submaximal exercise, cardiac output is increased by an initial elevation of stroke volume and gradual rise in heart rate (44). The *Starling mechanism* may be responsible for the increased stroke volume, and increased secretion of catecholamines, or increased myocardial sensitivity to catecholamines may be due to the increased heart rate. The effectiveness of a 2-year (16 + 7 months) walk/jog exercise program was studied on 36 male orthotopic cardiac transplant patients 2 to 23 months after surgery (25).

The effect of training resulted in increased power output during submaximal exercise with a significantly reduced rate of perceived exertion, but unchanged mechanical efficiency and submaximal cardiac output. In eight highly compliant patients with a weekly training distance of 32 km, the effect of training on heart rate at rest and during exercise was a greater decrease and peak power output, a greater increase than in the other 28 patients with a training distance of 24 km.

Before training the patients had a lesser lean body mass than age-matched healthy men (56 + 7 kg vs. 63 + 8 kg) ($p < .001$), but after training body mass had incresed by 4 kg without any increase in body fat. Thus it seems as though the training effect in the transplant patients comes from the strengthening of the peripheral muscles and not from a central improvement, because the cardiac outputs over the period of training were unchanged.

This finding that cardiac transplant patients are able to attain jogging distances between 24 and 32 km per week implies that exercise training has considerable potential for improving the quality of life of such patients (25), especially when no similar changes are observed spontaneously in cardiac function after cardiac transplantation (39).

Renal Transplantation.

In 13 renal transplant patients aerobic capacity increased 42% from a preoperative exercise test and was shown to increase 4 months after surgery without any exercise training in the postoperative period (36). Supervised exercise sessions in 10 patients began about 2 weeks after renal transplantation and continued for a mean of 5-1/2 weeks (33). The exercise capacity was improved about 90% after the 5-week exercise sessions on the treadmill and cycle ergometer, which corresponds to 100% of predicted mean exercise capacity of healthy persons of similar age.

An additional 12% improvement was found 2 years after surgery among 7 of the 10 patients who had continued regular exercise training. In 16 renal transplant recipients (28), ventilation, oxygen consumption, and respiratory exchange ratios were unchanged, whereas the blood lactate concentrations decreased at submaximal work loads after 24-weeks of exercise training. After training, the muscle power and endurance of *musculus quadriceps* was increased between 12% and 26%.

Thus in renal transplant patients as well as in cardiac patients (25) skeletal muscle contractile function increases with training and is concomitant with a metabolic adaptation in muscles, which is explained by the reduced blood lactate concentrations during submaximal exercise after training.

Lower Limb Amputation.

Fifteen weeks of aerobic training exercise in 10 subjects who had an amputation of the lower limb or limbs resulted in an increase of 25% in the maximum capacity for exercise and lower values for heart rate and consumption of oxygen. The duration of training was about 20 to 25 min every second day (38). Isokinetic strength increased significantly in the amputated leg after training of knee extensor muscles in eight patients after knee amputation, and the cross-sectional area of the muscle fibers increased in the amputated leg in all patients except one. The patients estimated their ability to walk after training to be more than double the distance compared to before training (29).

Breast Cancer Surgery.

The effect of active shoulder exercises from the first postoperative day was evaluated against exercises started on the eighth postoperative day in 144 patients with breast cancer after auxiliary lymph node dissection. No difference between groups was found in shoulder function 6 months after surgery (24).

Thus after cardiac surgery renal transplantation, and lower limb amputation the same positive effect of exercise training is found as in other sedentary individuals who start training.

Blood Loss

The big increase in exercise capacity in renal patients may be related partly to a 45% increase in oxygen-carrying capacity (33). In 7 male subjects loss of 1 L of blood resulted in a decrease in maximal oxygen uptake from 4.00 L/min to 3.54 L/min and an increase in submaximal heart rate from 125 beats/min to about 135 beats per minute. Values returned to preoperative levels after 3 weeks. In 16 abdominal patients (14) hematocrit values 20 days after surgery were significantly lower both at rest and during submaximal exercise. This agrees with the results of the Adolfsson study (1).

Unanswered Questions and Future Directions for Studies of Physical Activity and Fitness After Surgery

Studies evaluating effective epidural analgesia on physical activity and fitness after surgery are needed.

Preoperative training prevented postoperative functional capacity from dropping below the initial pretraining level (1), but the effect of more intensive pre- and postoperative training on recovery are needed. No studies are available on the effect of postoperative exercise on the fatigue syndrome.

Complete postoperative pain relief after cholecystectomy using epidural analgesia in combination with systemic morphine and indomethacin did not influence postoperative fatigue (48). However, the effect of complete postoperative pain relief on physical activity and fitness has not been measured. The difference between voluntary and nerve-stimulated force postoperatively may indicate that muscle fatigue is of central origin. The endocrine metabolic response to exercise after abdominal surgery (16) was unchanged compared to preoperative response apart from serum lactate with significantly higher values after surgery both at rest and during work. An insignificant positive correlation was found between fatigue and noradrenaline after surgery (15), but not between fatigue and increased lactate. Further studies are needed.

The negative nitrogen balance characteristic after the surgical trauma can be altered by administration of human growth hormone. In seven patients growth hormone improved protein economy and increased fat oxidation after major gastrointestinal surgery (53). Further studies to evaluate the effect of growth hormone on the clinical outcome and physical activity and fitness after surgery should be interesting.

Conclusions

Surgical trauma is followed by a convalescence period with decreased physical activity and increased feeling of fatigue extending at least through the first postoperative month. There is a loss in voluntary muscle force, whereas nerve-stimulated involuntary muscle function is unchanged. During postoperative convalescence a decline in physical condition with impaired adaptability of heart rate to submaximal work loads has been demonstrated, whereas oxygen uptake at a given level of work performance is unchanged. During indentical work before and 20 days after surgery s-lactate concentration is significantly higher postoperatively.

Decrease in physical activity and exercise capacity after surgery correlates to loss in body weight postoperatively. Increased fatigue after surgery correlates to the magnitude of the trauma, the decrease in voluntary force, increased pulse rate during bicycle exercise postoperatively, and loss in body weight postoperatively. Postoperative fatigue is independent of age, sex, general anesthesia, duration of surgery, postoperative pain relief, and increased s-lactate concentration during postoperative exercise tests.

Important mechanisms to these postoperative changes may be the endocrine-metabolic response to the surgical trauma, immobilization, and decreased nutritional intake. Important research problems on the physical activity and fitness after surgery may therefore be the effect of effective epidural analgesia, the effect of intensive pre- and postoperative training, the influence of enteral nutrition, and the effect of complete pain relief after surgery. It seems likely that the problem of recovery is multifactorial and therefore studies combining the different therapeutic possibilities may be most important.

References

1. Adolfsson, G. Circulatory and respiratory function in relation to physical activity in female patients before and after cholecystectomy. Acta Chir. Scand. [Suppl.]. 401:8-106; 1969.
2. Ågren, B.; Olin, C.; Castenfros, J.; Nilsson-Ehle, P. Improvements of the lipoprotein profile after coronary bypass surgery: Additional effect of an exercise training program. Eur. Heart J. 10:451-458; 1989.
3. Bassey, E.J.; Benett, T.; Birmingham, A.T.; Fantem, P.H.; Fitton, D.; Goldsmith, R. Effects of surgical operation and bedrest on cardiovascular responses to exercise in hospital patients. Cardiovasc. Res. 7:588-592, 1973.
4. Bassey, E.J.; Fentem, P.H. Extent of deterioration in physical condition during postoperative bed rest and its reversal by rehabilitation. Br. Med. J. 4:194-196; 1974.

5. Bastow, M.D.; Rawlings, J.; Allison, S.P. Benefits of supplementary tube feeding after fractured neck of femur: A randomised controlled trial. Br. Med. J. 287:1589-1592, 1983.
6. Borow, K.M.; Neumann, A.; Arensman, F.W.; Yacoub, M.H. Left ventricular contractility and contractile reserve in humans after cardiac transplantation. Circulation. 71:866-872; 1985.
7. Brandt, M.B.; Fernandes, A.; Mordhorst, R.; Kehlet, H. Epidural analgesia improves postoperative nitrogen balance, Br. Med. J. 1:1106-1108; 1978.
8. Christensen, T.; Bendix, T.; Kehlet, H. Fatigue and cardiorespiratory function following abdominal surgery. Br. J. Surg. 69:417-419; 1982.
9. Christensen, T.; Christensen, G. The effects of blood loss on the performance of physical exercise. Eur. J. Appl. Physiol. 39:17-25; 1978.
10. Christensen, T.; Hjortsø, N.C.; Mortensen, E.; Riis-Hansen M.; Kehlet, H. Fatigue and anxiety in surgical patients. Acta Psychiatr. Scand. 73:76-79; 1986.
11. Christensen, T.; Hougård, F.; Kehlet, H. Influence of pre- and intraoperative factors on the occurrence of postoperative fatigue. Br. J. Surg. 72:63-65, 1985.
12. Christensen, T.; Kehlet, H. Postoperative fatigue and changes in nutritional status. Br. J. Surg. 71:473-476; 1884.
13. Christensen, T.; Kehlet, H.; Vesterberg, K.; Vinnars, E. Fatigue and muscle amino acids during surgical convalescence. Acta Chir. Scand. 153:567-570; 1987.
14. Christensen, T.; Nygaard, E.; Kehlet, H. Skeletal muscle fiber composition, nutritional status and subjective feeling of fatigue during surgical convalescence. Acta Chir. Scand. 154:335-338; 1988.
15. Christensen, T.; Nygaard, E.; Stage, J.G.; Kehlet, H. Skeletal muscle enzyme activities and metabolic substrates during exercise in patients with postoperative fatigue. Br. J. Surg. 77:312-315; 1990.
16. Christensen, T.; Stage, J.G.; Galbo, H.; Christensen, N.J.; Kehlet, H. Fatigue and cardiac and endocrine metabolic response to exercise after abdominal surgery. Surgery. 105:46-50; 1989.
17. Christensen, T.; Wulff, C.H.; Fuglsang-Frederiksen, A.; Kehlet, H. Electrical activity and arm muscle force in postoperative fatigue. Acta Chir. Scand. 151:1-5; 1985.
18. Edwards, H.; Rose, E.A.; King, T.C. Postoperative deterioration in muscular function. Arch. Surg. 117:899-901; 1982.
19. Galbo, H. Hormonal and metabolic adaptation to exercise. Stuttgart: Georg Thieme Verlag; 1983. Thesis.
20. Hacket, A.F.; Yeung, C.K.; Hill, G.L. Eating patterns in patients recovering from major surgery—a study of voluntary food intake and nergy balance. Br. J. Surg. 66:415-418; 1979.
21. Haennel, R.G.; Quinney, H.A.; Kappagoda, C.T. Effects of hydraulic circuit training following coronary artery bypass surgery. Med. Sci. Sports Exerc. 23:158-165; 1991.
22. Hessov, I.; Wara, P. Energy and protein intake in bowel resected patients during hospitalization. Ugeskr. Laeger. 140:1469-1473; 1978.
23. Hjortsø, N.-C.; Andersen, T.; Frøsig, F.; Kehlet, H. A controlled study of the effect of epidural analgesia with local anaesthetics and morphine on morbidity after abdominal surgery. Acta Anaesthesiol. Scand. 29:790-796; 1985.
24. Jansen, F.M.; van Geel, A.N.; de Groot, H.G.W.; Rottier, A.B.; Olthuis, G.A.A.; van Putten, W.L.J. Immediate versus delayed shoulder exercises after axillary lymph node dissection. Am. J. Surg. 160:481-484; 1990.
25. Kavanagh, T.; Yacoub, M.H.; Mertens, D.J.; Dennedy, J.; Campbell, R.B.; Sawyer, P. Cardiorespiratory responses to exercise training after orthotopic cardiac transplantation. Circulation. 77:162-171; 1988.
26. Kehlet, H. The stress response to anaesthesia and surgery: Release mechanisms and modifying factors. Clin. Anaesthesiol. 2:315-339; 1984.
27. Kehlet, H. Modifications of responses to surgery by neural blockade: Clinical implications. In: Cousins, M.J.; Bridenbaugh, P.O., eds. Neural blockade in clinical anesthesia and management of pain. Philadelphia: Lippincott; 1987: 145-188.
28. Kempeneers, G.; Noakes, T.D.; van Zyl-Smit, R.; Myburgh, K.H.; Lambert, M.; Adams, B.; Wiggins, T. Skeletal muscle limits the exercise tolerance of renal transplant recipients: Effects of a graded exercise training program. Am. J. Kidney Dis. 1:57-65; 1990.
29. Klingenstierna, U.; Renström, P.; Grimby, G.; Morelli, B. Isokinetic strength training in below-knee amputees. Scand. J. Rehabil. Med. 22:39-43; 1990.
30. Maxwell, A. Muscle power after surgery. Lancet. 1:420-421; 1980.
31. McCue, J.; Newham, D. Postoperative muscle strength. Ann. R. Coll. Surg. Engl. 72:291-295; 1990.
32. Meyer, K.; Lehmann, M.; S nder, G.; Keul, J.; Weidemann, H. Effects of interval vs continuous exercise training on physical performance, cardiac function, metabolism, and catecholamines in selected patients after coronary bypass ssurgery. Z. Kardiol. 79:697-705; 1990.

33. Miller, T.D.; Squires, R.W.; Cau, G.T.; Ilstrup, D.M.; Frohnert, P.P.; Sterioff, S. Graded exercise testing and training after renal transplantation: A preliminary study. Mayo Clin. Proc. 62:773-777; 1987.
34. Newham, D.J.; Harrison, R.A.; Clark, C.G. Skeletal muscle function after major abdominal surgery. Clin. Nutr. 41C:363-371; 1987.
35. Nistrup Madsen, S.; Brandt, M.R.; Engquist, A.; Badawi, I.; Kehlet, H. Inhibition of plasma cyclic AMP, glucose and cortisol response to surgery by epidural analgesia. Br. J. Surg. 64:669-671; 1977.
36. Painter, P.; Zimmerman, S.W. Exercise in end-stage renal disease. Am. J. Kidney Dis. 7:386-394; 1986.
37. Petersson, B.; Wernerman, J.; Waller, S.-O.; von der Decken, A.; Vinnars, E. Elective abdominal surgery depresses muscle protein synthesis and increases subjective fatigue: Effects lasting more than 30 days. Br. J. Surg. 77:796-800; 1990.
38. Pitetti, K.H.; Snell, P.G.; Stray-Gundersen, J.; Gottschalk, F.A. Aerobic training exercises for individuals who had amputation of the lower limb. J. Bone Joint Surg. 69A:914-921; 1987.
39. Pope, S.E.; Stinson, E.B.; Daughters, G.T.; Schroeder, J.S.; Ingels, N.B.; Alderman, E.L. Exercise response of the deervated heart in longterm cardiac transplant recipients. Am. J. Cardiol. 46:213-218; 1980.
40. Round, J.M.; Jones, D.A.; Chapman, S.J.; Edwards, R.H.T.; Ward, P.S.; Fodden, D.L. The anatomy and fibre type composition of the human adductor pollicis in relation to its contractile properties. J. Neurol. Sci. 66:263-292; 1984.
41. Sagar, S.; Harland, P.; Shields, R. Early post-operative feeding with elemental diet. Br. Med. J. 1:293-295; 1979.
42. Sakamoto, K.; Nakano, G.; Hashimoto, I.; Nagamachi, Y. Potential usefulness of a physical activity index in the assessment of quality of life of patients after gastrointestinal surgery. Acta Chir. Scand. 155:305-312; 1989.
43. Saltin, B.; Blommquist, B.; Mitchell, J.H.; Johnson, R.L.; Wildenthal, K., Jr.; Chapman, C.B. Response to submaximal and maximal exercise after bedrest and training. Circulation. 38:1-78; 1968.
44. Savin, W.M.; Haskell, W.L.; Schroeder, J.S.; Stinson, E.B. Cardiorespiratory responses of cardiac transplant patients to graded, symptomlimited exercise. Circulation. 62:55-60; 1980.
45. Schroeder, D.; Daker, P. Interpleural catheter for analgesia after cholecystectomy: The surgical perspective. Aust. N.Z.J. Surg. 60:689-694; 1990.
46. Schroeder, D.; Gillanders, L.; Mahr, K.; Hill, G.L. Effect of immediate postoperative enteral nutriton on body composition, muscle function, and wound healing. JPEN. 15:376-383; 1991.
47. Schroeder, D.; Hill, G.L. Postoperative fatigue: A prospective physiological study of patients undergoing major abdominal surgery. Aust. N.Z.J. Surg. 61:774-779; 1991.
48. Schultze, S.; Møller, I.W.; Bang, U.; Rye, B.; Kehlet, H. Effect of combined prednisolone, epidural analgesia and indometahcin on pain, systemic response and convalescence after cholecystectomy. Acta Chir. Scand. 156:203-209; 1990.
49. Schultze, S.; Roikjaer, O.; Hasselstr–m, L.; Jensen, N.H.; Kehlet, H. Epidural bupivacaine and morphine plus systemic indomethacin eliminates pain but not systemic response and convalescence after cholecystectomy. Surgery. 103:321-327; 1988.
50. Schultze, S.; Sommer, P.; Bigler, D.; Honnens, M.; Shenkin, A.; Bukhave, K.; Kehlet, H. Effect of epidural analgesia, indomethacin and methylprednisolone on pain, cytokines, acute phase and pulmonary response to colonic surgery. Arch. Surg. [In press, 1992].
51. Spielberger, C.D.; Gorsuch, R.L.; Lushene, R.E. Manual for the state-trait anxiety inventory. Palo Alto, CA: Consulting Psychologists Press; 1970.
52. Stock, S.E.; Clague, M.B.; Johnston, D.A. Postoperative fatigue—a real phenomenon attributable to the metabolic effects of surgery on body nutritional stores. Clin. Nutr. 10:251-257; 1991.
53. Ward, H.C.; Falliday, D.; Sim, A.J.W. Protein and energy metabolism with biosynthetic human growth hormone after gastrointestinal surgery. Ann. Surg. 206:56-61; 1987.
54. Wilmore, D.W.; Long, J.M.; Mason, A.D.; Pruitt, B.A. Stress in surgical patients as a neurophysiological reflex response. Surg. Gynecol. Obstet. 142:257-269; 1976.
55. Wilson, J.F. Behavioral preparation for surgery: Benefit or harm? J. Behav. Med. 4:79-102; 1981.
56. Wood, C.D. Postoperative exercise capacity following nutritional support with hypotonic glucose. Surg. Gynecol. Obstet. 152:39-42; 1981.
57. Wood, C.D.; Glover, J.; McCune, M.; Hendricks, J.; Johns, M.; Pollard, M. The effect of intravenous nutrition on muscle mass and exercise capacity in perioperative patients. Am. J. Surg. 158:63-67; 1989.
58. Zeiderman, M.R.; Welchew, E.A.; Clark, R.G. Changes in cardiorespiratory and muscle function associated with the development of postoperative fatigue. Br. J. Surg. 77:576-580; 1990.

Chapter 57

Physical Activity, Fitness, and the Physically Disabled (Neuromuscular Disorders)

Neil McCartney

There are many anatomical, physiological, and psychological causes of physical disability, which may be viewed as a reduced exercise capacity when compared with others of similar age, gender, and stature (47). In the past two decades there has been greater recognition of the importance of regular exercise and sports participation for many of those with disabilities, but despite this growing awareness there is limited research data on the activity patterns and exercise capacities of many of those with physical impairments. The effects of exercise training have not been examined systematically in many groups with disabilities, despite the attractive possibility of improved function in daily activities that may accompany gains in strength and cardiorespiratory endurance. Perhaps the best studied are those cases involving spinal cord injuries. Notable reviews on this population already exist (36) and will not be duplicated here.

The present review will critically examine the research on exercise capacity and strength and the effects of training in patients with selected neuromuscular disorders (NMD). This will include disorders that are classed as myopathies (e.g., the muscular dystrophies) and others that originate in the nervous system (e.g., motor neurone disease).

Evaluation of Functional Capacity in Neuromuscular Disorders

Laboratory exercise tests for the assessment of functional capacity have been used extensively in healthy subjects, in patients with cardiorespiratory diseases (47), and in those with effort syndromes and muscle pain (65,67). This approach has been adopted sparingly in the evaluation of NMD, however, despite evidence that it is useful in distinguishing different categories of patients (15). Assessment has focused more on manual muscle testing, gait analysis, and the timing of simple tasks (26). Many patients are too weak and uncoordinated to take part in exercise testing, and there has been a traditional concern that strenuous exertion may cause overwork weakness and possible muscle damage. Nevertheless, the data that do exist suggest that exercise testing may be of significant value in our understanding of limiting factors in NMD and as a means of monitoring the effectiveness of therapeutic interventions (56).

Exercise Capacity in NMD

The Muscular Dystrophies

Muscular dystrophy is an umbrella term for a group of so-far incurable, inherited disorders characterized by the progressive degeneration of the voluntary muscles (35). The age at the onset of symptoms and the rate of decline in muscle strength varies markedly among the different entities. Undoubtedly the most severe is the *Duchenne* type, which affects 1 in every 3,000 to 3,500 males at birth and has a population prevalence of approximately 3/100,000 (35). The disease is rapidly progressive throughout childhood, and death usually occurs from respiratory complications before the age of 25 years. Other forms such as *facioscapulohumeral dystrophy* (FSH) have a reduced incidence and prevalence. The symptoms usually appear in the second or third decade and progress to severe disability in 20 years. Comprehensive reviews of the distinguishing features of the muscular dystrophies can be found elsewhere (27,35,64).

With the inherent variability in the severity of symptoms and the rate of disease progression one would expect diverse exercise responses in patients with dystrophic disorders, and this appears to be the case. As may be anticipated, the lowest dynamic exercise performance among the dystrophies has been reported in children with the Duchenne form. The only systematic investigation of maximum oxygen uptake ($\dot{V}O_2max$) in 13 boys with this condition aged 6 to 11 years (86) reported values of 14.4 ± 5.4 ml · min^{-1} · kg^{-1} (4.1 METs), corresponding to 36% of the level achieved by age- and weight-matched controls. The maximal heart rate of 136 ± 13 beats per minute (bpm) (67% predicted) was 72% of control values, and the $(a-\bar{v})O_2$ difference of 7.7 ± 5.0 vol% was also lower than in controls (11.8 ± 3.1 vol%). Maximum cardiac output was only 53% of controls, due mainly to the reduced heart rate. Although the maximum values were uniformly low, the relation between increases in cardiac output and increases in oxygen uptake was appropriate and consistent with reports of healthy muscle blood flow (14,75) and oxidative metabolism (73).

In a study of patients with assorted NMD, Carroll, Hagberg, Brooke, and Schumate (17) reported a similar value for $\dot{V}O_2max$ of 13 ml · min^{-1} · kg^{-1} in an 11-year-old boy with Duchenne dystrophy. Their data indicated that his performance was lower than subjects with more benign forms of dystrophy and was most likely the result of reduced muscle mass and greater muscle weakness. Although there has been no systematic study, it is diminished muscle mass and strength that probably restricts aerobic exercise capacity in this population, rather than any inherent deficits in oxygen transport or utilization. The markedly low power outputs of boys with Duchenne dystrophy in the 1930s Wingate cycling test (4,5) may also be attributed to reduced muscle mass and strength in addition to deficits in glycogenolytic and glycolytic enzymes among all fiber types (18).

There is also scarce information on the exercise capacities of patients with less severe forms of muscular dystrophy. Data on 6 males with FSH have been reported (17,32,39). Combining the results revealed a $\dot{V}O_2max$ in cycle ergometry of 23.4 ± 6.4 ml · min^{-1} · kg^{-1}, or approximately 70% of control values. As with patients with Duchenne dystrophy, the circulatory adjustments to increasing exercise were within healthy limits.

Information on 5 patients with limb-girdle dystrophy was also contained in the previous three studies. The $\dot{V}O_2max$ ranged from 5.5 (17) to 21.6 ml · min^{-1} · kg^{-1} (32), or from 15% to 66% of the respective control values. Isolated descriptions of maximum exercise capacity in Becker's (17,39), myotonic (17), and congenital dystrophy (32) have reported variations in $\dot{V}O_2max$ ranging from 21 to 36 ml · min^{-1} · kg^{-1}.

Effects of Endurance Training in the Muscular Dystrophies

One male patient with limb-girdle dystrophy, and 1 with the congenital form, were included in a study investigating the effects of 12 weeks of cycle ergometry training in assorted NMD (32). Although the individual responses were not identified, the 6 myopathy patients improved their $\dot{V}O_2max$ (range) from approximately 13% to 47%, and reductions in heart rates at two levels of submaximal exercise ranged from 9 bpm to 31 bpm. These changes were comparable to those in matched control subjects. Despite these encouraging findings, 1 patient with limb-girdle and 1 with congenital dystrophy demonstrated 30% increases in resting plasma concentrations of creatine kinase and myoglobin, so the possibility of training-induced muscle damage could not be discounted in these individuals.

Summary

There is a paucity of information on the dynamic exercise performance of patients with muscular dystrophy. Research in this population is extremely difficult due to the low prevalence of the disease, and there is a long-standing concern that exercise may exacerbate muscle damage and weakness. The majority of studies in the literature have been hampered by (a) small sample sizes, (b) heterogeneity of disease entities, (c) wide variations in subjects' ages and physical dimensions, (d) marked differences in the time of disease onset and duration, and (e) difficulty in matching control subjects. Despite these problems, the evidence suggests a reduced maximum exercise capacity in the dystrophies with a positive relation between residual muscle mass and function. A report of a healthy training response in 2 patients with slowly progressive disease is encouraging and worthy of follow-up. Evidence suggestive of muscle damage does not appear to be a generalized finding, but further investigations are needed.

Exercise Capacity in Other Myopathies

Congenital Myopathies

There are other congenital myopathies such as nemaline myopathy and central core disease that result in abnormal muscle fiber structure (27), but the exercise responses of individuals with such disorders have been rarely documented. In 2 patients with nemaline myopathy the peak values for $\dot{V}O_2$ ranged from 22.4 (32) to 27.6 ml · min^{-1} · kg^{-1} (17), or approximately 76% of control subjects. The $\dot{V}O_2$max of 3 patients with central core disease was lower, averaging 17.8 ml · min^{-1} · kg^{-1} (54% of control) (17,32,38).

Effects of Endurance Training in Congenital Myopathies

Central core disease is nonprogressive, and the rate of decline in muscle strength associated with nemaline myopathy is extremely slow, so exercise training could theoretically be of some value in these patients. There have been two reports of exercise training in central core disease and one in nemaline myopathy. Hagberg, Carroll, and Brooke (38) demonstrated that 9 months of cycle ergometry training in a 36-year-old male with central core disease produced significant improvement in functional capacity. Resting heart rate decreased by 26 bpm, whereas $\dot{V}O_2$max and maximum power output increased by 44% and 53%, respectively. In another study from the same laboratory (32) which did not identify individual patients, 12 weeks of cycle ergometry training improved the peak $\dot{V}O_2$ of a subject with central core disease by anywhere from 13% to 47%. This was also the case for a patient with nemaline myopathy.

Metabolic Myopathies

A common finding in patients with metabolic myopathies is relatively well preserved muscle strength but variably diminished dynamic exercise capacity. Genetic defects in the glycolytic pathway, in mitochondrial enzymes, and in the electron transport chain all result in impairment of muscle energy metabolism. The nature of these disorders has been reported in detail elsewhere (see 27 for references), and the current emphasis will be on the interactions with exercise performance.

Disorders of mitochondrial oxidative metabolism include deficiencies in specific cytochromes of the electron transport chain (72,92), deficiencies in pyruvate oxidation (53,57), and uncoupling disorders such as Luft's syndrome (59). Electron transport defects result in severe effort intolerance associated with lactacidosis, excessive exercise tachycardia and cardiac output during submaximal exercise (28), dyspnea, and palpitations (55). There does not appear to be a primary cardiac limitation to exercise, but impaired tissue oxygen extraction may restrict peak $\dot{V}O_2$ to less than 50% of that predicted (10,40), and at any level of submaximal $\dot{V}O_2$ the cardiac output may be threefold greater than expected (40).

Disorders of pyruvate oxidation result in similar findings of lactacidemia and a hyperkinetic circulation during exercise (53,57), with some amelioration of the condition following the administration of a high-fat diet (27). The $\dot{V}O_2$max in these patients is often restricted to less than 1 L · min^{-1} (27).

Luft's syndrome was first described in 1962 (59) and is a condition of partially uncoupled mitochondrial metabolism; only one other case has been reported (25). This disorder is characterized by hypermetabolism at rest, a very low dynamic exercise performance, together with a disproportionately high cardiac output response (59).

Disorders of fat metabolism were first reported only 2 decades ago (13,30). It is now recognized that a deficiency in carnitine, or *carnitine parmityltransferase* (CPT), interferes with the β-oxidation of fatty acids by reducing their translocation into the mitochondria (27). Carnitine deficiency is often associated with muscle weakness and a reduced exercise capacity that may be improved with oral carnitine (3); reliance on glycogen as a fuel source promotes lactacidosis. CPT deficiency causes muscle pain during exercise, and elevated levels of plasma creatine kinase and myoglobinuria are indicative of muscle damage (27).

Haller, Lewis, Estabrook, Nunally, and Foster (39) studied two young men with CPT deficiency and reported that the cardiorespiratory responses during maximum cycle ergometry were the same as in matched controls. Subjects may exhibit a high respiratory quotient and elevated plasma lactate concentrations during moderate exercise consistent with a dependence on carbohydrate fuel sources (54). It appears that the extent of muscle glycogen stores is the primary determinant of exercise capacity in these individuals.

There are at least seven enzyme defects of carbohydrate metabolism that affect muscle (27). The best studied in relation to exercise performance are *myophosphorylase deficiency* (McArdle's disease) and *phosphofructokinase* (PFK) *deficiency* (Type-7 glycogenosis). Patients with either syndrome have adequate muscle strength at rest and they can perform light exercise, but heavy exertion causes pain, muscle contractures, and evidence of muscle damage. The $\dot{V}O_2$max in 17 patients with McArdle's disease, and 5 patients with PFK deficiency ranged from 13 to 30 ml · min^{-1} · kg^{-1} (29% to 66% of that predicted) in the review by Lewis and Haller (56). Circulatory values were within the expected range, but the $(a-\bar{v})O_2$ difference increased only slightly. The lack of intramuscular glycogen as a substrate for oxidative metabolism appears to be the reason for the reduced oxygen extraction and low $\dot{V}O_2max$ in both conditions. This is consistent with the observation that increasing the levels of blood-borne substrates by intravenous infusion (76), fasting (16), or previous light exertion (76) may increase exercise endurance and $\dot{V}O_2max$ quite significantly. As expected in conditions where the intramuscular glycogen stores are unavailable, anaerobic exercise capacity is severely restricted and may result in electrically silent contractures. Despite the presence of contractures, however, there is relatively little depletion of muscle adenosine triphosphate (ATP) content (79).

Effects of Endurance Training in Metabolic Myopathies

Lewis and Haller (56) have speculated that training-induced increases in cardiac output could be of value in McArdle's disease and PFK deficiency by increasing substrate delivery to muscle, but as yet there are no training data available. The training responses of individuals with other metabolic myopathies are also unknown at this time.

Summary

Isolated reports of patients with nemaline myopathy and central core disease have documented reduced maximum exercise capacities and significant potential for improvements after training. Patients with metabolic myopathies tend to have relatively well-preserved muscle strength, but a variably diminished dynamic exercise capacity depending on the nature of the defect. Information on the potential benefits or hazards of endurance training is lacking.

Neurogenic Atrophies and Neuromuscular Junction Disease

There is little known about the dynamic exercise capabilities of individuals with these disorders. Among the neurogenic atrophies there have been isolated reports of exercise capacity in *juvenile spinal muscular atrophy* (32,39), in *Kugelberg-Welander disease* (60), in *amyotrophic lateral sclerosis* (ALS) (81), and in *Charcot-Marie-Tooth disease* (32); values for maximum oxygen uptake have ranged from approximately 11 to 41 ml · min^{-1} · kg^{-1}.

The only systematic evaluation was in 35 middle-aged patients (32 males, 3 females) with ALS by Sanjak et al. (81). They demonstrated reductions in maximum work capacity and $\dot{V}O_2max$ (range approximately 12 to 37 ml · min^{-1} · kg^{-1}), with a quadratic relationship to the decrease in functional ALS score. The heart rates, ventilation, and oxygen consumption during submaximal exercise were significantly elevated above control values, a finding that was attributed to an inefficient additional recruitment of accessory muscles. Previous work in ALS and Charcot-Marie-Tooth disease (49) also demonstrated increased resting oxygen consumption and lactate production in forearm muscles associated with augmented utilization of blood-borne glucose and free fatty acids. Regional muscle ischemia secondary to impaired autoregulation of blood flow was proposed as the mechanism for the increased metabolism.

As with the majority of NMD, the stage and rate of disease progression appear to be the primary determinants of dynamic exercise capacity in neurogenic disorders.

In recent years there has been a growing awareness of symptomatic complications in late survivors of acute poliomyelitis (44). It is estimated (41) that from 75,000 to 120,000 survivors of polio in the United States will develop *postpolio syndrome* (PPS), which is associated with muscular atrophy and symptoms of weakness, fatigue, and effort intolerance (2). Several etiologies have been proposed to account for the apparent deterioration in neuromuscular function (for review see 48), and reports of exercise capacity and especially muscular strength are becoming more frequent.

Maximum dynamic exercise capacity in PPS has been documented in two studies and was at a level one might expect in healthy, deconditioned subjects. In the report by Owen and Jones (74) the maximum functional capacity ranged from 3.6 to 8.7 METs. A later study (46) in 37 patients with PPS reported a mean maximum power output and $\dot{V}O_2max$ in cycle ergometry of 123.7 W, and 1.53 L · min^{-1}, respectively. Subjects' ages ranged from 30 to 60 years, and, as results for each were not listed, the data cannot be compared directly to standards of healthy individuals.

Included among disorders of the neuromuscular junction are *myasthenia gravis* and *myotonias* (27). Very mild aerobic exercise has been used in myasthenia to investigate serum enzyme changes (51), but there have been no studies that systematically attempted to quantify maximum functional capacity. The emphasis in this group of patients has been on electrophysiological measurement and assessment of muscle strength and fatigue. This has also been the case in myotonic syndromes (31,37,77,87) except for two isolated reports on individual male subjects with myotonia congenita.

In one 24-year-old patient (17) the $\dot{V}O_2max$ during progressive incremental cycle ergometry was 36.4 ml · min^{-1} · kg^{-1}, or 78% of that predicted (47). The patient studied by Brooke, Carroll, Davis, and Hagberg (15) was 34 years old, and achieved a $\dot{V}O_2max$ of 2 L · min^{-1}; the subject's weight was not reported.

Effects of Endurance Training in Neurogenic Atrophies and Neuromuscular Junction Disease

As with most NMD there are few reports of exercise training in neurogenic syndromes. One 32-year-old female, and one 19-year-old male with Charcot-Marie-Tooth disease were included in the study by Florence and Hagberg (32). After 12 weeks of cycle ergometer training, the increases in $\dot{V}O_2max$ in the 2 subjects were approximately 3% and 17%. These improvements were less than in 5 patients with assorted myopathies, and their heart rates at two specified, submaximal exercise intensities actually increased by approximately 9 to 20 bpm rather than showing the usual post-training reduction.

Jones, Speier, Canine, Owen, and Stull (46) trained 16 patients with PPS for 16 weeks; training was done 3 times per week on a cycle ergometer at approximately 70% of maximum heart rate. The exercise group displayed classic training adaptations: reductions in resting heart rate, systolic and diastolic pressures of up to 7%, and increases in $\dot{V}O_2max$ and peak power output of 15% and 17.8%, respectively. None of the patients exhibited signs or symptoms of overwork muscle damage, and, in fact, the 4 subjects with preexisting atrophy demonstrated relative increases in $\dot{V}O_2max$ that were almost twice the group average.

Summary

There has been little systematic research on the dynamic exercise capabilities of patients with neurogenic atrophies and even less in patients with neuromuscular junction disease. The majority of available data were collected in individual subjects who were studied as part of a larger cohort with assorted NMD. One investigation in 35 patients with ALS confirmed that the primary determinant of exercise capacity was the stage and rate of disease progression, and this is likely the case in other NMD. Training data from 2 individuals with Charcot-Marie-Tooth disease suggested that some patients with neurogenic syndromes may respond differently than those with myopathies; increases in $\dot{V}O_2max$ were accompanied by substantial elevations in heart rate during submaximal exercise, the opposite of what would be expected. Limited observations suggest that PPS patients have markedly reduced functional capacities but a relatively good potential to improve with training.

Future Directions in the Study of NMD

There is a considerable need for well-controlled, systematic studies of dynamic exercise capacity in NMD. With the lack of effective pharmacologic management in most NMD, endurance training as a potential therapeutic modality is particularly deserving of investigation. Future studies must include adequate sample sizes and well-matched control subjects; case studies are interesting, but will not effect changes in the management of NMD. For this to happen, any benefits of exercise training must also be shown to translate into improved function in activities of daily living and enhanced quality of life. It seems likely that in order to generate large enough sample sizes, future studies will need to be organized as multicenter trials.

Muscular Strength in Neuromuscular Disorders

The most common complaint in patients with NMD is skeletal muscle weakness and fatigue (64). Whereas there are standardized, objective techniques of exercise testing that allow comparison of NMD patients' performance to healthy standards and comparison among trials, there is no universally accepted method of quantifying muscle strength. The most widely used approach in clinical practice has been some adaptation of the Kendall system (6) of manual muscle testing, which is subject to considerable intra- and intertester variability (19). It is only in recent years that objective methods of measuring isometric and dynamic strength have been applied to patients with NMD, but reports are few in number and the majority feature individuals with muscular dystrophy in trials of therapeutic strength training (see the following section).

Edwards (26) reported that the maximum isometric contraction force of the hip flexors and ankle dorsiflexors in 30 boys with Duchenne dystrophy rarely exceeded the fifth percentile of values for healthy children. The utility of serial measurements to follow the progressive deterioration in strength that occurs in the natural history of progressive NMD has also been demonstrated (26).

Edwards (26) further highlighted the need to consider the interactions among quadriceps strength, body weight, and functional capacity. Over a 3-1/2-year period, a female patient with the Kugelberg-Welander form of spinal muscular atrophy suffered a loss in quadriceps strength of 6.5% per year, but because she also reduced her body weight by 24 kg, her quadriceps strength:body weight ratio actually increased. This resulted in restoration of the ability to raise her heels from the floor and improved ambulation.

Fowler and Gardner (33) gave perhaps the best example of quantitative strength measurement in NMD. They recorded the isometric strength of 13 muscle groups in 43 boys with Duchenne dystrophy and in 32 patients with myotonic, limb-girdle, and facioscapulohumeral dystrophy; results were compared to those of age-matched control subjects. In addition to the cross-sectional data, serial measurements were made over a 2-year period in 11 of the Duchenne patients and over 3 years in 20 of the remainder.

Differences in strength between the boys with Duchenne dystrophy and control subjects increased with age. At age 5 to 6 years the average upper and lower limb strength in the boys with Duchenne dystrophy was 39.6% and 30%, respectively, of that in the healthy control subjects; by age 15 to 16 years these values had decreased to 8.6% and 5.6%. Serial measurements in 11 subjects with Duchenne dystrophy demonstrated rapid, progressive reductions in strength from the time of initial evaluation, thus yielding a bleaker picture than that suggested from the mean cross-sectional data. In patients with one of the more slowly progressive dystrophies, the average upper and lower limb strength was approximately 78% of control values from age 5 to 14 years, but had deteriorated to only 29% by age 25 to 34 years. However, serial determinations over 3 years demonstrated minimal changes in strength.

Other work in 25 patients with myotonic dystrophy (8) and 20 patients with the limb-girdle form (65) demonstrated reductions in maximum plantarflexor and dorsiflexor torques to about 55% of control levels. It was also reported that some patients were unable to achieve complete motor unit activation initially, but this could be improved with practice during the same testing session. Such an observation is of practical significance as it suggests that voluntary strength may be underestimated in patients with dystrophies unless several repetitions are made.

Additional observations from studies of muscle strength in NMD (33,65) show that marked variations in strength occur among patients with the same clinical diagnosis and that retention of strength among different muscle groups may vary considerably within the same subject. McComas, Belanger, Garner, and McCartney (65) cited 1 patient with limb-girdle dystrophy in whom voluntary dorsiflexion and plantarflexion torques were 5% and 90% of the respective control mean values. Despite possibly severe reductions in strength, many patients with NMD have normal fatigue properties.

Effects of Strength Training in NMD

It is well documented in healthy individuals that physical inactivity associated with bed rest (52), trauma (82), and limb immobilization (61) results in muscle fiber atrophy and losses in strength; adverse effects of enforced inactivity have also been reported in patients with Duchenne dystrophy (24). In contrast, whereas muscle strength and size are known to improve in healthy subjects with overload training (21,66), the efficacy of this approach in NMD is a matter of debate (22,34,89,90). There are many anecdotal reports of apparent overwork weakness in NMD (9,42,45,50,58), and these have probably served to deter others from undertaking rigorous, controlled trials of strength training. The majority of studies have been in patients with muscular dystrophy, especially the Duchenne form, and there is hardly any information on strength training in the neurogenic atrophies. As a consequence the following discussion of the effects of strength training will not be separated into individual sections for myopathic and neurogenic disorders.

Early studies of resistive exercise, mostly in patients with Duchenne dystrophy (1,43,93), produced equivocal results. One study (1) claimed a modest improvement in 50% of patients, and no change in the remainder after 7 months of moderate resistance exercise. In two other investigations (43,93), the authors reported no actual gains in strength except an attenuated rate of decrease compared to the period before the program began. The problems inherent in the early studies are common to many subsequent investigations of strength training in NMD: There was no systematic application of the principle of progressive overload in the training regimen; manual muscle testing was used to evaluate strength; there were no control subjects; subjects' ages ranged from 2 to 20 years; some patients were ambulatory whereas others were confined to wheelchairs and had probably lost more than 50% of their muscle mass (90); and contractures were present in the majority of patients.

Recognizing many of the limitations of earlier trials, Vignos and Watkins (91) conducted a 12-

month study of weight training in 14 children with Duchenne dystrophy, 6 subjects with limb-girdle dystrophy, and 4 with the facioscapulohumeral form. Subjects exercised five muscle groups for a total of 30 min daily, performing 10 repetitions of each exercise. Gains in strength occurred during the first 4 months of training in each class of dystrophy, and thereafter strength remained stable. Improvements in strength and in speed during functional activities were greatest in patients with the slowly progressive forms of disease. Within individual subjects the improvements in maximum weight lifted by the trained muscles were positively correlated to their initial capacity; those muscles that started out stronger improved the most, on average by 50%. The increased dynamic strength in the patients with Duchenne dystrophy was in contrast to matched control subjects in whom strength had declined progressively throughout the 12 months.

De Lateur and Giaconi (20) made perhaps the best controlled study of resistive exercise in Duchenne dystrophy. They used a Cybex isokinetic dynamometer to train the knee extensors of a single limb in 4 boys; the contralateral limb served as a within-subject control. Training comprised 30 submaximal contractions repeated 4 or 5 days per week for 6 months. Measurements of maximum torque were made monthly during the training period and up to 12 months, and then at 18 and 24 months. Between months 1 and 6 the maximum torques in the control limb were, on average, 18.9% lower than in the exercising leg, but the differences were only significant at month 5. After the intervention period, and up to 24 months, the control leg remained 14.3% weaker than the trained leg, but the only significant difference was in month 9. This study confirmed that formal resistance training was feasible in patients with Duchenne dystrophy and resulted in some improvements in strength until the progression of the disease reduced muscle contractile force to zero.

Other approaches to improving muscle strength in these patients have included direct electrical stimulation and inspiratory maneuvers to stress the respiratory muscles. The effects of respiratory muscle training are equivocal. There is one report of exceptional improvements in ventilatory endurance in a group of patients with assorted NMD after only 6 weeks of training (23), and other studies in patients with Duchenne dystrophy either showed small increases (62) or no change (78,85). Chronic low-frequency stimulation of the ankle dorsiflexors (84) and knee extensors (83) 3 hr per day for up to 11 weeks has been effective in increasing the maximum voluntary contraction force of boys with Duchenne muscular dystrophy. As in the majority of studies, intervention in the early stages of the disease was most beneficial.

It seems obvious that patients with slowly progressive NMD, who retain a larger proportion of their muscle mass, would benefit the most from strength training, and the limited research data support this contention. Milner-Brown and Miller (70) studied the effects of high-intensity, progressive resistance weight-lifting training in 16 adult patients (aged 20 to 53 years) with gradually deteriorating disorders. Among the muscular dystrophy patients were 6 with facioscapulohumeral, 1 with limb-girdle, 4 with myotonic, and 1 with Becker; neurogenic disorders were represented by 3 individuals with spinal muscular atrophy and 1 with polyneuropathy. Training of the elbow flexors and knee extensors was done up to 4 days per week for a mean time of 13 months. In some subjects the contralateral limb was not exercised and served as a within-subject control.

The training resulted in ($\bar{x} \pm$ SD) increases in isometric strength of the knee extensors and elbow flexors of 77 ± 40% and 83 ± 60%, respectively. In 4 subjects, the nonexercised elbow flexors demonstrated improvements in strength of 19 ± 3%. The data confirmed previous findings (91) as the absolute gains in strength were positively correlated to the initial muscle strength. Even weak muscles with an initial capacity ranging from 15% to 25% of healthy values (68) were able to improve their maximum values by more than 100%; individuals with baseline strength of less than 10% of healthy values showed no change with training.

This study highlighted that patients with assorted NMD can increase strength with resistance training, but it did not identify the underlying mechanisms. The observation of significant strength gains in a contralateral control limb suggests that a neural adaptation may have been a contributing factor (80). The results of two other investigations also suggest that a neural mechanism may be responsible for much of the training-induced gains in strength in NMD. After 8 months of combined electrical stimulation and weight training in 10 patients with slowly progressive NMD, isometric strength of the knee extensors increased by more than 100% in the exercised limb and also by 25% in the contralateral control limb (69).

Similar findings were reported in a 9-week trial of weight-lifting training in 5 patients with spinal muscular atrophy, limb-girdle, and facioscapulohumeral muscular dystrophy (63). The maximum load that could be lifted once only increased by up to 34% in the trained arm and up to 25% in the control arm. Also in this study, the interpolated twitch technique (7) applied to the elbow flexors of both arms confirmed that motor unit activation was submaximal prior to training but increased to full activation after the training period. This was interpreted to mean that training had resulted in the descending motor pathways becoming more efficient in exciting lumbosacral motoneurones.

There are only isolated reports of resistance training in other NMD. One study of 12 patients with PPS (29) who engaged in 6 weeks of combined isometric and isokinetic training demonstrated a mean increase in knee extensor strength of 27%. Case studies of single patients with PPS (88) and ALS (11) also support the use of carefully monitored strength training.

Summary

Patients with NMD have variably reduced muscle strength in accordance with disease severity. The worst afflicted are those with Duchenne dystrophy, and the rapidly progressive nature of this disease offers little hope for long-term improvements in strength with resistance training. Studies of strength training in this population have suffered from many methodological and design flaws, but have generally documented limited increases in strength with no attendant evidence of overwork weakness. Patients with more slowly progressive NMD are better candidates for resistance training programs, and their capacity for improvement appears to be dependent on the initial strength of individual muscles. Part of the increases in muscle strength with resistance exercise appear to be due to neural adaptations. This being the case, it offers the possibility that resistance training can effect rapid, meaningful increases in strength in patients with NMD in the absence of muscle hypertrophy. The relation of gains in muscle strength to performance in daily activities has not been established but is an important question for future research efforts.

Conclusions and Further Questions

Research to date on exercise capacity and muscle strength in NMD has been nonsystematic with (a) a preponderance of case-control studies; (b) small sample sizes; (c) patients who were different in the stage and rate of progress of their disease process; (d) wide variations in ages, strength, and muscle mass; (e) poorly matched control subjects, or none at all; and (f) nonstandardized testing procedures with questionable validity and reliability. Future research in this area must be more rigorously standardized, with larger sample sizes most likely in multicenter trials. Important questions include:

1. Which NMD patients can benefit from endurance and resistance training in terms of activities of daily living and quality of life?
2. Are conventional methods of exercise prescription appropriate for NMD patients?
3. What are the appropriate physiological and psychological tests to assess changes in performance in daily activities and quality of life?
4. What is the relation of endurance exercise and strength training to overwork weakness in the various NMD?
5. Can either endurance or resistance training counter the deleterious effects associated with various progressive NMD?
6. What are the relationships between medications, exercise, and NMD?

Until such time as the answers to these questions are known, the balance of available evidence suggests that health care practitioners would be prudent to prescribe carefully monitored exercise regimens for their NMD patients, especially those with slowly progressive disorders.

References

1. Abramson, A.S.; Rogoff, J. An approach to rehabilitation of children with muscular dystrophy. Proceedings of the first and second medical conferences of the MDAA, Inc. New York: Muscular Dystrophy Association of America, Inc.; 1953:123-124.
2. Agre, J.C.; Rodriquez, A.A.; Tafel, J.A. Late effects of polio: Critical review of the literature on neuromuscular function. Arch. Phys. Med. Rehabil. 72:923-931; 1991.
3. Angelini, C.; Lucke, S.; Cantarutti, F. Carnitine deficiency of skeletal muscle: Report of a treated case. Neurology. 26:633-637; 1976.
4. Bar-Or, O. Pediatric sports medicine for the practitioner. New York: Springer-Verlag; 1983.
5. Bar-Or, O. Pathophysiological factors which limit the exercise capacity of the sick child. Med. Sci. Sports Exerc. 18:276-282; 1986.
6. Beasley, W.C. Quantitative muscle testing: Principles and applications to research and clinical service. Arch. Phys. Med. Rehabil. 42:398-425; 1961.
7. Belanger, A.Y.; McComas, A.J. Extent of motor unit activation during effort. J. Appl. Physiol. 51:160-167; 1981.

8. Belanger, A.Y.; McComas, A.J. Contractile properties of muscles in myotonic dystrophy. J. Neurol. Neurosurg. Psychiatry. 46:625-631; 1983.
9. Bennett, R.L.; Knowlton, G.C. Overwork weakness in partially denervated skeletal muscle. Clin. Orthop. 12:22-29; 1958.
10. Bogaard, J.M.; Busch, H.F.M.; Arts, W.F.M.; Heijsteeg, M.; Stam, H.; Versprille, A. Metabolic and ventilatory responses to exercise in patients with a deficient O_2 utilization by a mitochondrial myopathy. Adv. Exp. Med. Biol. 191:409-417; 1984.
11. Bohannon, R.W. Results of resistance training on a patient with amyotrophic lateral sclerosis: A case report. Phys. Ther. 6:965-968; 1983.
12. Bonsett, C.A. Pseudohypertrophic muscular dystrophy: Distribution of degenerative features as revealed by anatomical study. Neurology. 13:728-738; 1963.
13. Bradley, W.G.; Hudgson, P.; Gardner-Medwin, D.; Walton, J.N. Myopathy associated with abnormal lipid metabolism in skeletal muscle. Lancet. 1:495-498; 1969.
14. Bradley, W.G.; O'Brien, M.D.; Walder, D.N.; Murchison, D.; Johnson, M.; Newell, D.J. Failure to confirm a vascular cause of muscular dystrophy. Arch. Neurol. 32:466-473; 1975.
15. Brooke, M.H.; Carroll, J.E.; Davis, J.E.; Hagberg, J.M. The prolonged exercise test. Neurology. 29:636-643; 1979.
16. Carroll, J.E.; DeVivo, D.C.; Brooke, M.H.; Planer, G.J.; Hagberg, J.H. Fasting as a provocative test in neuromuscular diseases. Metabolism. 28:683-687; 1979.
17. Carroll, J.E.; Hagberg, J.M.; Brooke, M.H.; Shumate, J.B. Bicycle ergometry and gas exchange measurements in neuromuscular disease. Arch. Neurol. 36:457-461; 1979.
18. Chi, M.M.Y.; Hintz, C.S.; McKee, D.; Felder, S.; Grant, N.; Kaiser, K.K.; Lowry, O.H. Effect of Duchenne muscular dystrophy on enzymes of energy metabolism in individual muscle fibers. Metabolism. 36:761-767; 1987.
19. Cook, J.D.; Glass, D.S. Strength evaluation in neuromuscular disease. Neurol. Clin. 5:101-123; 1987.
20. De Lateur, B.J.; Giaconi, R.M. Effect on maximal strength of submaximal exercise in Duchenne muscular dystrophy. Am. J. Phys. Med. 58:26-36; 1979.
21. DeLorme, T.L. Restoration of muscle power by heavy resistance exercises. J. Bone Joint Surg. 27:645-667; 1945.
22. Demos, J. Early diagnosis and treatment of rapidly developing Duchenne de Boulogne type myopathy. Am. J. Phys. Med. 50:271-284; 1971.
23. DiMarco, A.F.; DiMarco, M.S.; Jacobs, I.; Shields, R.; Altose, M.D. The effects of respiratory resistive training on respiratory muscle function in patients with muscular dystrophy. Muscle Nerve. 8:284-290; 1985.
24. Dubowitz, V.; Heckmatt, J. Management of muscular dystrophy: Pharmacologic and physical aspects. Br. Med. Bull. 36:139-144; 1980.
25. Edelman, N.H.; Santiago, T.V.; Conn, H.L. Luft's syndrome: O_2 cost of exercise and chemical control of breathing. J. Appl. Physiol. 39:857-859; 1975.
26. Edwards, R.H.T. Studies of muscular performance in normal and dystrophic subjects. Br. Med. Bull. 36:159-164; 1980.
27. Edwards, R.H.T.; Jones, D.A. Diseases of skeletal muscle. In: Peachy, L.D.; Adrian, R.H.; Geiger, S.R., eds. Handbook of physiology: Skeletal muscle. Bethesda, MD: American Physiological Society; 1983:633-672.
28. Edwards, R.H.T.; Wiles, C.M.; Gohil, K.; Krywawych, S.; Jones, D.A. Energy metabolism in human myopathy. In Schotland, D.L., ed. Disorders of the motor unit. New York: Wiley; 1982:715-735.
29. Einarsson, G. Muscle conditioning in late poliomyelitis. Arch. Phys. Med. Rehabil. 72:11-14; 1991.
30. Engel, W.K.; Vick, N.A.; Glueck, C.J.; Levy, R.I. A skeletal muscle disorder associated with intermittent symptoms and a possible defect of lipid metabolism. N. Engl. J. Med. 282:697-704; 1970.
31. Estenne, M.; Borenstein, S.; De Troyer, A. Respiratory muscle function in myotonia congenita. Am. Rev. Respir. Dis. 130:681-684; 1984.
32. Florence, J.M.; Hagberg, J.M. Effect of training on the exercise responses of neuromuscular disease patients. Med. Sci. Sports Exerc. 16:460-465; 1984.
33. Fowler, W.M.; Gardner, G.W. Quantitative strength measurements in muscular dystrophy. Arch. Phys. Med. Rehabil. 48:629-636; 1967.
34. Fowler, W.M., Jr.; Taylor, M. Rehabilitation management of muscular dystrophy and related disorders: 1 role of exercise. Arch. Phys. Med. Rehabil. 63:319-321; 1982.
35. Gardner-Medwin, D. Clinical features and classification of the muscular dystrophies. Br. Med. Bull. 36:109-115; 1980.
36. Glaser, R. Exercise and locomotion for the spinal cord injured. Exerc. Sport Sci. Rev. 13:263-303; 1985.
37. Gutman, L.; Riggs, J.E.; Brick, J.F. Exercise-induced membrane failure in paramyotonia congenita. Neurology. 36:130-132; 1986.

38. Hagberg, J.M.; Carroll, J.E.; Brooke, M.H. Endurance exercise training in a patient with central core disease. Neurology. 30:1242-1244; 1980.
39. Haller, R.G.; Lewis, S.F.; Cook, J.D.; Blomqvist, C.G. Hyperkinetic circulation during exercise in neuromuscular disease. Neurology. 33:1283-1287; 1983.
40. Haller, R.G.; Lewis, S.F.; Estabrook, R.W.; Nunally, R.; Foster, D.W. A skeletal muscle disorder of electron transport associated with deficiency of cytochromes aa3 and b and abnormal cardiovascular regulation in exercise. Clin. Physiol. [Suppl. 7]. 5:34; 1985.
41. Halstead, L.S.; Wiechers, D.O.; Rossi, C.D. Late effects of poliomyelitis: A national survey. In Halstead, L.S.; Wiechers, C.O. eds. Late effects of poliomyelitis. Miami, FL: Symposia Foundation; 1985:11-31.
42. Herbison, G.J.; Jaweed, M.M.; Ditunno, J.F., Jr. Exercise therapies in peripheral neuropathies. Arch. Phys. Med. Rehabil. 64:201-205; 1983.
43. Hoberman, M. Physical medicine and rehabilitation: Its value and limitations in progressive muscular dystrophy. Am. J. Phys. Med. 34:109-115; 1955.
44. Holman, K.G. Post-polio syndrome: The battle with an old foe resumes. Postgrad. Med. 79:44-53; 1986.
45. Johnson, E.W.; Braddom, R. Overwork weakness in facioscapulohumeral muscular dystrophy. Arch. Phys. Med. Rehabil. 52:333-336; 1971.
46. Jones, D.R.; Speier, J.; Canine, K.; Owen, R.; Stull, A. Cardiorespiratory responses to aerobic training by patients with postpoliomyelitis sequelae. JAMA. 261:3255-3258; 1989.
47. Jones, N.L. Clinical exercise testing. 3rd ed. Philadelphia: Saunders; 1988.
48. Jubelt, B.; Cashman, N.R. Neurological manifestations of the post-polio syndrome. Rev. Neurobiol. 3:199-220; 1987.
49. Karpati, G.; Klassen, G.; Tanser, P. The effects of partial chronic denervation on forearm metabolism. Can. J. Neurol. Sci. 6:105-112; 1979.
50. Knowlton, G.C.; Bennett, R.L. Overwork. Arch. Phys. Med. Rehabil. 38:18-20; 1957.
51. Kolins, J.; Gilroy, J. Serum enzyme levels in patients with myasthenia gravis after aerobic and ischemic exercise. J. Neurol. Neurosurg. Psychiatry. 35:34-40; 1972.
52. Kottke, F.J. The effects of limitation of activity upon the human body. JAMA. 196:117-122; 1966.
53. Larsson, L.E.; Linderholm, H.; Muller, R.; Ringqvist, T.; Sornas, R. Hereditary metabolic myopathy with paroxysmal myoglobinuria due to abnormal glycolysis. J. Neurol. Neurosurg. Psychiatry. 27:361-380; 1964.
54. Layzer, R.B.; Havel, R.J.; McIlroy, M.B. Partial deficiency of carnitine palmityltransferase: Physiologic and biochemical consequences. Neurology. 30:627-633; 1980.
55. Layzer, R.B.; Lewis, S.F. Clinical disorders of muscle energy metabolism. Med. Sci. Sports Exerc. 16:451-455; 1984.
56. Lewis, S.F.; Haller, R.G. Skeletal muscle disorders and associated factors that limit exercise performance. Exerc. Sport Sci. Rev. 17:67-113; 1989.
57. Linderholm, H.; Muller, R.; Ringqvist, T.; Sornas, R. Hereditary abnormal muscle metabolism with hyperkinetic circulation during exercise. Acta Med. Scand. 185:153-166; 1969.
58. Lovett, R.W. The treatment of infantile paralysis. JAMA. 64:2118; 1915.
59. Luft, R.; Ikkos, D.; Palmieri, G.; Ernster, L.; Afzelius, B. A case of severe hypermetabolism of nonthyroid origin with a defect in the maintenance of mitochondrial respiratory control: A correlated clinical, biochemical, and morphological study. J. Clin. Invest. 41:1776-1801; 1962.
60. Lyager, S.; Noerra, N.; Pedersen, O.F. Cardiopulmonary response to exercise in patients with neuromuscular diseases. Respiration. 45:89-99; 1984.
61. MacDougall, J.D.; Elder, G.C.B.; Sale, D.G.; Moroz, J.R.; Sutton, J.R. Effects of strength of training and immobilization of human muscle fibres. Eur. J. Appl. Physiol. 43:25-34; 1980.
62. Martin, A.G. Respiratory muscle training in Duchenne muscular dystrophy. Dev. Med. Child Neurol. 28:314-318; 1986.
63. McCartney, N.; Moroz, D.; Garner, S.H.; McComas, A.J. The effects of strength training in selected neuromuscular disorders. Med. Sci. Sports Exerc. 20:362-368; 1988.
64. McComas, A.J. Neuromuscular function and disorders. London: Butterworths; 1977:3-364.
65. McComas, A.J.; Belanger, A.Y.; Garner, S.A.; McCartney, N. Muscle performance in neuromuscular disorders. In Jones, N.L.; McCartney, N.; McComas, A.J., eds. Human muscle power. Champaign, IL: Human Kinetics; 1986:309-324.
66. McDonagh, M.J.N.; Davies, C.T.M. Adaptive response of mammalian skeletal muscle to exercise with high loads. Eur. J. Appl. Physiol. 52:139-155; 1984.
67. Mills, K.R.; Edwards, R.H.T. Investigative strategies for muscle pain. J. Neurol. Sci. 58:73-88; 1983.
68. Milner-Brown, H.S.; Mellenthin, M.; Miller, R.G. Quantifying human muscle strength, endurance and fatigue. Arch. Phys. Med. Rehabil. 67:530-535; 1986.

69. Milner-Brown, H.S.; Miller, R.G. Muscle strengthening through electric stimulation combined with low-resistance weights in patients with neuromuscular disorders. Arch. Phys. Med. Rehabil. 69:20-24; 1988.
70. Milner-Brown, H.S.; Miller, R.G. Muscle strengthening through high-resistance weight training in patients with neuromuscular disorders. Arch. Phys. Med. Rehabil. 69:14-19; 1988.
71. Milner-Brown, H.S.; Miller, R.G. Increased muscular fatigue in patients with neurogenic muscle weakness: Quantification and pathophysiology. Arch. Phys. Med. Rehabil. 70:361-366; 1989.
72. Morgan-Hughes, J.A.; Darveniza, P.; Kahn, S.N.; Landon, D.N.; Sheratt, R.M.; Land, J.M.; Clark, J.B. A mitochondrial myopathy characterized by a deficiency in reducible cytochrome b. Brain. 100:617-640; 1977.
73. Olson, E.; Vignos, P.J.; Woodlock, J.; Perry, T. Oxidative phosphorylation of skeletal muscle in human muscular dystrophy. J. Lab. Clin. Med. 71:220-231; 1968.
74. Owen, R.R.; Jones, D. Polio rediduals clinic: Conditioning exercise program. Orthopedics. 8:882-883; 1985.
75. Paulson, O.B.; Engel, A.G.; Gomez, M.R. Muscle blood flow in Duchenne type muscular dystrophy, limb-girdle dystrophy, polymyositis, and in normal controls. J. Neurol. Neurosurg. Psychiatry. 37:685-690; 1974.
76. Porte, D., Jr.; Crawford, W.D.; Jennings, D.B.; Aber, C.; McIlroy, M.B. Cardiovascular and metabolic responses to exercise in a patient with McArdle's syndrome. N. Engl. J. Med. 275:406-412; 1966.
77. Riggs, J.E.; Gutmann, L.; McComas, C.F.; Morehead, M.A.; Louden, M.B.; Martin, J.D. Exercise-induced weakness in paramyotonia congenita: Exacerbation with thyrotoxicosis. Neurology. 34:233-235; 1984.
78. Rodillo, E.; Noble-Jamieson, C.M.; Aber, V.; Heckmatt, J.Z.; Muntoni, F.; Dubowitz, V. Respiratory muscle training in Duchenne muscular dystrophy. Arch. Dis. Child. 64:736-738; 1989.
79. Rowland, L.P.; Araki, S.; Carmel, P. Contracture in McArdle's disease. Stability of adenosine triphosphate during contracture in phosphorylase-deficient human muscle. Arch. Neurol. 13:541-544; 1965.
80. Sale, D.G. Neural adaptation to resistance training. Med. Sci. Sports Exerc. [Suppl.] 20:S135-S145; 1988.
81. Sanjak, M.; Paulson, D.; Sufit, R.; Reddan, W.; Beaulieu, D.; Erickson, L.; Shug, A.; Brooks, B.R. Physiologic and metabolic response to progressive and prolonged exercise in amyotrophic lateral sclerosis. Neurology. 37:1217-1220; 1987.
82. Sargeant, A.J.; Davies, C.T.M. The effect of disuse muscular atrophy on the forces generated in dynamic exercise. Clin. Sci. Mol. Med. 53:183-188; 1977.
83. Scott, O.M.; Hyde, S.A.; Vrbova, G.; Dubowitz, V. Therapeutic possibilities of chronic low frequency stimulation in children with Duchenne muscular dystrophy. J. Neurol. Sci. 95:171-182; 1990.
84. Scott, O.M.; Vrbova, G.; Hyde, S.A.; Dubowitz, V. Responses of muscles of patients with Duchenne muscular dystrophy to chronic electrical stimulation. J. Neurol. Neurosurg. Psychiatry. 49:1427-1434; 1986.
85. Smith, P.E.M.; Coakley, J.H.; Edwards, R.H.T. Respiratory muscle training in Duchenne muscular dystrophy. Muscle Nerve. 11:784-785; 1988.
86. Sockolov, R.B.; Irwin, B.; Dressendorfer, R.H.; Bernauer, E.M. Exercise performance in 6-to-11-year old boys with Duchenne muscular dystrophy. Arch. Phys. Med. Rehabil. 58:195-201; 1977.
87. Subramony, S.H.; Wee, A.S. Exercise and rest in hyperkalemic periodic paralysis. Neurology. 36:173-177; 1986.
88. Twist, D.J.; Ma, D.M. Physical therapy management of the patient with post-polio syndrome: A case report. Phys. Ther. 9:1403-1406; 1986.
89. Vignos, P.J., Jr. Physical models of rehabilitation in neuromuscular disease. Muscle Nerve. 6:323-338; 1983.
90. Vignos, P.J., Jr. Exercise in neuromuscular disease: Statement of the problem. In Serratrice, G., ed. Neuromuscular diseases. New York: Raven Press; 1984:565-569.
91. Vignos, P.J.; Watkins, M.P. The effect of exercise in muscular dystrophy. JAMA. 197:843-848; 1966.
92. Willems, J.C.; Manneis, L.A.H.; Trijbels, J.M.F.; Verrkaps, J.H.; Meyer, A.E.R.H.; Van Dam, D.; Van Haeslit, V. Leigh's encephalomyopathy in a patient with cytochrome c oxidase deficiency in muscle tissue. Pediatrics. 60:850-857; 1977.
93. Wratney, M.J. Physical therapy for muscular dystrophy children. Phys. Ther. Rev. 38:26-32; 1958.

Chapter 58

Physical Activity, Fitness, and Depression

William P. Morgan

The efficacy of psychotherapy and pharmacological therapy in the treatment of depression is well documented. However, it has been estimated that 21% of individuals who experience major depressive disorders are not seen in any service settings, and as many as 56% are seen by their physicians without receiving mental health services. There is also evidence that those individuals who receive treatment may not be well served. In one large, multisite study, over 50% of individuals with depressive disorders had previously been treated with anxiety-reducing drugs rather than antidepressants, and only 1 in 10 depressives who received antidepressants were given adequate doses. Antidepressant agents are also known to have side effects, and it is important that patients be monitored carefully. When one considers the cost and potential side effects of antidepressant drugs, a search for nonpharmacological interventions is understandable. Psychotherapy can be particularly effective in the treatment of "nonbiological" depression and an effective adjunct when used in concert with biological interventions, but it requires time and money. Finally, because of the pandemic nature of depression, neither drug therapy nor psychotherapy offers an acceptable solution. The best solution is prevention, not treatment, and one potential coping strategy is exercise.

Early Research

Much of the research literature dealing with the relationship between physical fitness and emotional health prior to 1970 was restricted to psychiatric samples or comparisons of psychiatric patients with nonhospitalized controls. Furthermore, in most of this research the psychiatric samples were comprised of schizophrenic patients. Samples consisting of patients diagnosed as psychoneurotics were studied in a few investigations. Furthermore, the published research in this area was principally of a cross-sectional nature, and most of the reports were restricted to selected components of physical fitness; that is, fitness was not conceptualized as a multidimensional construct in this early work (21).

Despite the fact that much of this research was characterized by numerous methodological problems, consistent patterns of findings emerged over a period of some four decades (1930–1970). This research was summarized by Morgan (21) in a 1969 paper, and the general finding was that psychopathology and physical fitness were inversely correlated. In other words, schizophrenic patients scored lower on measures of physical fitness than patients diagnosed as psychoneurotics or personality disorders, and these groups in turn were less fit than nonhospitalized controls (21). However, there are at least two problems associated with this cross-sectional research. First, it is possible that performance of physical fitness tests was impaired or dampened in the psychiatric patients studied because of psychological problems involving motivation or cognition. In other words, it is likely that psychiatric patients may not understand test instructions because of cognitive impairments and it is equally possible that many patients may simply lack the desire or drive necessary to perform well on fitness tasks. Unless alternative hypotheses of this nature can be refuted, it would be questionable to conclude that psychiatric patients, in fact, have lower levels of physical fitness. Furthermore, it is not appropriate to generalize about the relationship between physical fitness and affective states in nonhospitalized controls from research carried out on psychiatric samples. Although this principle of external validity may seem rather obvious, reviewers often overlook this important methodological issue.

This initial review by Morgan (21) involving physical fitness and mental health has been expanded and updated in a series of articles and chapters by the author and his associates over the past 2 decades (25,26,28,29,30,31,35,36,38). These reviews have each demonstrated that physically active individuals are characterized by lower levels of depression in comparison with sedentary individuals. Furthermore, the limited experimental and quasi-experimental research in this area has been interpreted in these reviews as demonstrating that adoption of aerobic exercise is associated with decreased depression in individuals judged as moderately depressed at the outset of these exercise programs.

The conclusions reached in these reviews are in agreement with anecdotal reports that exercise is effective in reducing depression in hospitalized, manic-depressed patients (7), as well as nonhospitalized college students (6,12). It also agrees with epidemiological research showing that exercise is associated with decreased symptoms of depression (55,57). Furthermore, the previously cited reviews are also in general agreement with subsequent narrative reviews by Martinsen (17), Raglin (51), and Taylor, Sallis, and Needle (61), as well as quantitative reviews (meta-analysis) by McDonald and Hodgdon (19) and North, McCullagh, and Tran (45).

There have been at least three authors who have not reached the same conclusions advanced in the aforementioned reviews. In the first of these three papers, Weinstein and Meyers (65) concluded that ". . . definitive conclusions regarding the antidepressant properties of running are currently unwarranted" (p. 288). These authors arrived at this conclusion on the basis of conceptual and methodological shortcomings of published research on this topic. The statement by Weinstein and Meyers (65) that "... there is little clear evidence to support running as a strategy for modifying depression" (p. 296) is not in agreement with most of the published reviews prior to or following the appearance of their paper in 1983. Nevertheless, the recommendation by Weinstein and Meyers (65) that improved methodology was needed in this area of inquiry persists to the present time.

In a subsequent review, Hughes (14) concluded that little evidence exists for the claim that exercise improves depression. This conclusion is not surprising since only twelve of the 1,100 published articles met the inclusion criteria deemed necessary by Hughes (14). In other words, 99% of the studies dealing with the psychological effects of habitual aerobic exercise failed to satisfy the inclusion criteria adopted for this review. Hughes (14) dismissed 99% of the published literature as being unacceptable for one or more methodological reasons (e.g., absence of randomization, small sample size, inadequate psychological measures, experimenter/subject biases). While it is clear that improved experimental design and methodology is needed in this area of inquiry, it is remarkable that investigators have tended to observe antidepressant responses following exercise interventions that have varied in (a) duration (i.e., several weeks to several months), (b) method of assessing depression, (c) type of exercise program, (d) experimental design, and (e) small sample sizes. In other words, it could be argued that the observed antidepressant effect of exercise must be reasonably powerful since the effect has occurred despite elevated variance due to experimental error in concert with inadequate statistical power.

The position expressed by Hughes (14) represents a minority point of view, but it received limited support in a review paper published in the following year by Simons, McGowan, Epstein, Kupfer, and Robertson (56). These authors argued that early research dealing with the effects of exercise on depression was characterized by ". . . conceptual confusion and methodological problems" (p. 553). Simons et al. (56) went on to conclude, however, that more recent research ". . . provides grounds for cautious optimism regarding the potential therapeutic effects of exercise" (p. 553). The cautious optimism called for by Simons et al. (56) in 1985 has been supported by experimental research and subsequent reviews during more recent years.

In an effort to overcome some of the problems associated with the earlier research in this area, Morgan (20) conducted a study of the physiological and psychomotor correlates of depression in a group of 69 male psychiatric patients within 48 hr of admission to a psychiatric facility. All testing was carried out prior to the administration of medication in order to minimize performance suppression or facilitation due to drug effects. Furthermore, in order to overcome problems associated with reliability and validity inherent in psychiatric diagnoses, objective measures of depression were employed for quantitative purposes. Depression was measured by the MMPI Depression scale (MMPI) and the Self-Rating Depression scale (SDS). Twenty-five of these patients scored in the depressed range, and they were compared with a subgroup of 22 nondepressed patients, as well as a second group of 22 patients who scored between the two extremes. Assessments of body fat, small muscle reaction time, large muscle reaction time, strength of grip, and muscular endurance were obtained following the psychological assessments. The only dependent variable on which the three groups differed was finger ergometer endurance as measured by a modified Mosso ergograph, and these results are illustrated in Figure 58.1. The depressed group was found to score significantly lower ($p < .05$) than the nondepressed group on performance (39 J vs. 68 J), but neither sample differed from the intermediate group. In some respects these observations support the earlier research summarized by Morgan (21); that is, the lowest level of muscular endurance was associated with the greatest psychopathology. However, the finger ergometer endurance task may represent more of a psychological construct because it seems to involve a motivational component. At any rate, the absence of differences in body fat, reaction time, and muscular strength implies that psychomotor retardation in depressed patients may mirror affective states to a greater degree than actual physical competence.

In order to overcome the problem associated with volitional efforts of the type described in the previous study, two additional pilot studies involving male and female psychiatric patients were performed by Morgan (22,23). In the first investigation 17 male psychiatric patients ranging in age from 20 to 50 years (M = 36, SD = 11.4) completed the SDS (66) during the first week of admission to a regional mental health center. Physical working capacity (PWC) was assessed during this same period, and PWC was defined as the length of time the patient could exercise before reaching a heart rate of 150 beats per min (bpm) on a standardized bicycle ergometer test (PWC-150). A Quinton bicycle ergometer was pedaled at a rate of 50 revolutions per minute (rpm) for 5 min at a work load of 300 kpm, and this work load was increased by 300 kpm every 5 min until the patient's heart rate reached 150 bpm. Ten of the patients scored 53 or higher on the SDS, the cutoff for depression of clinical significance, and they were compared with the remaining seven patients who scored in the nondepressed range.

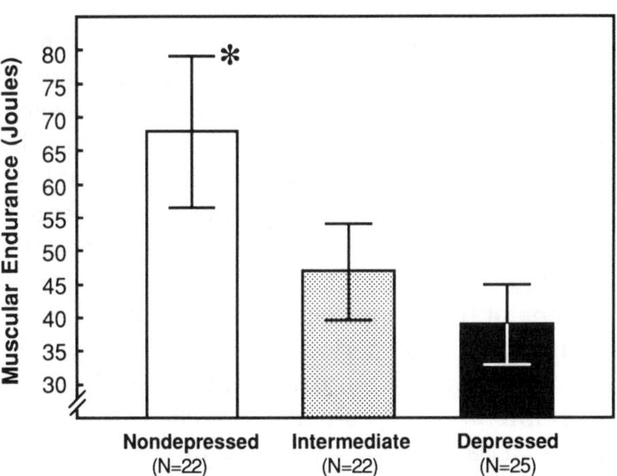

Figure 58.1 Muscular endurance of psychiatric patients differing in depression as measured by the Self-Rating Depression scale (66). This figure has been adapted from an article by Morgan (20).

This design affords a stronger test of the fitness–psychopathology hypothesis because an autonomic response (exercise heart rate) presumably would not be subject to differences in motivation or cognitive function. The depressed patients scored significantly lower than the nondepressed patients on the PWC-150, and a significant negative correlation (r = –.50) was observed between depression on the one hand and PWC on the other. This finding served to confirm results of earlier research suggesting that an inverse relationship exists between physical fitness and psychopathology. However, since it is known that physical fitness and psychopathology are both influenced by heritability, these results should be viewed as simply demonstrating an association.

A similar protocol was employed in a study of 15 female psychiatric patients with an age range of 16 to 46 years (M = 31, SD = 9.7). Pilot work revealed that many of the female patients on this psychiatric service were unable to cycle the ergometer at a work load above 300 kpm. Therefore, this study (23) differed from the previous one (22) in that patients pedaled the ergometer at a work load of 300 kpm for 5 min. Otherwise, there were no differences in the test protocol. Nine patients scored above 53 on the SDS, and the mean exercise heart rate of this group at the end of 5 min was 143 bpm, which did not differ from the value of 144 bpm observed for the nondepressed group. Although these findings are not in agreement with those of the previous study involving male patients (22), the results do confirm the general report of lowered physical fitness in psychiatric patients as compared with nonhospitalized controls. Indeed, the predicted $\dot{V}O_2max$ (1) for these patients was 1.6 L/min, which falls substantially (i.e., 24%) below the expected value of 2.1 L/min for females of this age group (10). These findings serve to confirm the view that physical fitness of psychiatric patients falls below that of the normal population, and this study extends the principle to include females.

The findings of this exploratory work have been replicated and extended by Martinsen, Strand, Paulson, and Kaggestad (18) who administered a bicycle ergometer test to 90 patients meeting the DSM-III criteria for anxiety or unipolar depressive disorders shortly after admission to a psychiatric facility. These investigators employed submaximal as well as maximal tests of physical working capacity (PWC). It was found that PWC values were dramatically reduced in these patients compared with nonhospitalized controls—for both direct and indirect measurements of maximum. Martinsen et al. (18) point out that these findings should not be interpreted within a causal context. These investigators point out that sedentary and less fit individuals may become depressed, but it is also possible that depression leads to sedentary lifestyles and lowered fitness.

Irrespective of the relationship between physical fitness and depression at a given point in time, it is possible that fitness at the time of a psychiatric episode might influence recovery. This hypothesis was tested by Morgan (24), who compared the muscular strength and endurance at the time of admission in 20 male patients who experienced short ($N = 10$) or long ($N = 10$) hospital stays. All patients completed the MMPI depression scale and the SDS within 48 hr of admission, as well as tests of muscular strength and endurance (24). The short-term group consisted of 10 patients who were hospitalized for an average period of 61 days, and this group was compared with 10 additional patients who were still hospitalized a year later. The two groups did not differ at the outset on the standardized measures of depression, and therefore, degree of depression at the time of admission was not of prognostic value.

Note in Figure 58.2 that the total work output was significantly greater (79 J vs. 33 J) at the outset in those patients who subsequently experienced short-term hospitalizations, and these patients also scored significantly higher on strength of grip (51 kg vs. 45 kg) at the outset as well. Furthermore, significant negative correlations were observed between hospitalization (days) and muscular strength (–.44) and endurance (–.53). Conversely, a zero-order correlation was observed between depression at the time of admission and length of hospitalization. These results suggest that recovery, once hospitalization occurs in connection with a psychiatric episode, is influenced in part by the patient's physical fitness at the time of admission. Again, however, one should keep in mind that expression of physical performance is influenced in part by motivation, not merely capacity.

The research appearing between 1940 and 1970 was almost entirely of a cross-sectional nature and was restricted to individuals who were hospitalized for various psychiatric disturbances. Beginning in the early 1970s investigators began to study the psychological effects of exercise interventions on nonhospitalized controls as well as cardiac and psychiatric patients. One of the first investigations designed to quantify the psychological and physiological effects of involvement in a regular program of physical activity has been summarized in companion papers by Morgan, Roberts, Brand, and Feinerman (42) and Roberts and Morgan (54). A quasi-experimental design was employed in this study, and participants consisted of 140 male faculty members at the University of Missouri, Columbia. The test subjects ranged in age from 22 to 62 years ($M = 39.1$, $SD = 9.3$). Physical working capacity was assessed by means of standardized treadmill and bicycle ergometer tests at the beginning and close of a 6-week exercise program.

The subjects volunteered to participate in one of eight exercise programs, and a group of 16 individuals who were unable to exercise at any of the scheduled times served as controls. There were three running groups, two cycling groups, two swimming groups, and one circuit-training group. Exercise intensity was maintained at approximately 85% of predicted maximal heart rate, but frequency ranged from 2 to 3 days per week in selected groups. It was found that improvement in physical working capacity was dependent on mode and frequency of exercise, with running being the most effective form of exercise (54). Furthermore, all of the exercise groups had greater gains than the control group, and four of these differences were statistically significant.

The psychological effects of this intervention were reported by Morgan et al. (42), and depression served as the dependent variable. Depression was measured by the SDS (66) in this study. All of the groups fell within the normal range on the SDS at the outset, and none of the groups experienced a change in depression following 6 weeks of exercise. Designs of this nature are admittedly open to criticism for a number of reasons. First, it would be preferable to randomly select individuals from a target population, and once this selection was completed, it would then be desirable to randomly assign the subjects to various groups. It is always possible that problems associated with volunteerism might occur otherwise. However, the use of volunteers is not only more realistic in a democratic society, but a study based on volunteerism possesses greater external validity. That is, individuals are not normally forced to exercise, nor are they customarily forced to perform a specific form of exercise. At any rate, it is important to recognize that the exercise groups and the control group, although formed on the basis of self-selection, were remarkably similar at the outset of the study. Indeed, it would not have been possible to generate more comparable groups on the depression variable had these volunteers been randomly assigned to the various groups.

None of the groups changed on depression following the 6-week period, and none of the exercise groups improved more than the control group. Therefore, it is unlikely that expectancies and demand characteristics influenced the results. More to the point is the fact that subsequent research over the next two decades, some of which relied on more rigorous experimental designs, has failed to refute these results. A number of investigators have since reported that gains in aerobic power

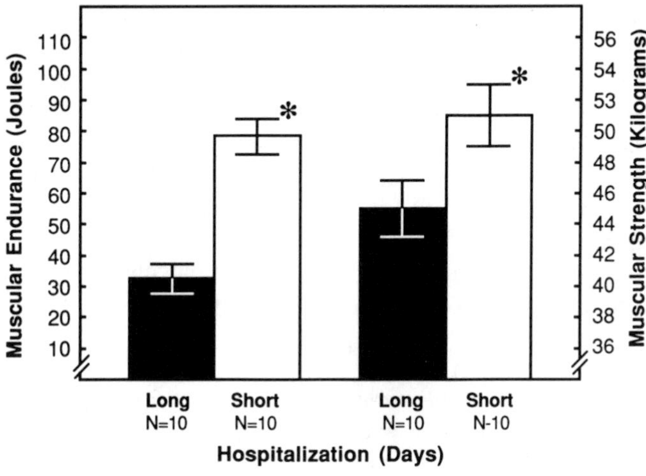

Figure 58.2 Muscular strength and muscular endurance at the time of admission in psychiatric patients who subsequently experienced short or long hospitalizations. This figure was adapted from an article by Morgan (24).

are not associated with reduced depression in exercisers who are nondepressed at the outset of a training program (17,41,44,59). This is not a very profound observation, and although it reflects what one would intuitively expect, some authors have persisted in asserting that programs of aerobic exercise will lead to reduced depression in nonhospitalized controls (45).

There is one additional point that should be made regarding this exploratory study. Zung (66) has reported that individuals scoring above 53 on the SDS possess depression of clinical significance. It was found that 11 of the exercisers scored above 53 on the SDS at the outset of this study (42). Inspection of the change scores for this subgroup revealed that a significant decrease in depression occurred, and furthermore, each of the subjects experienced a decrease in depression. This improved affect was independent of the mode or frequency of exercise because the 11 exercisers represented each of the exercise groups. This finding suggests that improvement in depression is most likely to occur in those individuals who are mildly depressed at the outset. It should also be noted that none of the nondepressed exercisers became depressed following the intervention. Despite the observation that significant decreases in depression were not observed for any of the exercise groups, many of the test subjects reported that they felt better as a consequence of participating in the exercise study. Indeed, 85% of the subjects volunteered to take part in future exercise studies.

The findings reported by Morgan et al. (42) have been replicated by Morgan and Pollock (41) and Morgan and Vogel (44). While these subsequent investigations (41,44) differed from each other, as well as differed from the initial study (42) in terms of overall design, the general findings provided convergent evidence for the view that exercise interventions do not lead to reduced depression in nonhospitalized controls. Morgan and Pollock (41) randomly assigned a group of healthy adult males (N = 54) to a control group or aerobic exercise performed at an intensity of 85% to 90% of maximum heart rate 3 days per week for 15, 30, or 45 min per day for 20 weeks. All subjects completed a $\dot{V}O_2$max test before and after the 20 weeks of training. The control group did not improve, whereas the cardiorespiratory fitness of the exercise groups improved in direct proportion to the exercise duration (50). The greatest increase occurred in the group that trained 5 days per week followed by the 3-day group, and the smallest increase was observed for the 1-day group. Depression was measured before and following training with the Profile of Mood States (POMS). A repeated measures analysis of variance (ANOVA) revealed that none of the groups differed at any point on this measure of depression, nor was depression found to decrease following 20 weeks of training.

In a related investigation Morgan and Pollock (41) randomly assigned healthy adult males to a minimal treatment (placebo) group or to a group performing aerobic exercise at 85% to 90% of maximum heart rate, 30 min per day, for 1, 3, or 5 days per week. Otherwise, the procedures were identical with those described for the first experiment. The placebo group did not experience a change in aerobic power, whereas aerobic power increased in direct proportion to the frequency of exercise. None of the groups differed on depression at any point, nor was there a decrease in depression for any group following the 20-week period.

The third study involved a quasi-experimental design in which healthy adult males ($N = 100$) were administered a $\dot{V}O_2max$ test before and following a 5-month jogging program in which subjects ran 2 to 4 miles per day, 5 days per week, at a pace of approximately 6 to 8 mph (44). These subjects experienced a significant improvement in $\dot{V}O_2max$ (49), and the posttraining value exceeded that of controls who were assessed prior to embarking on the same training program. These subjects also completed the POMS before and following the 5-month training program (44). The mean depression score on the POMS did not change (44) even though a significant gain in aerobic power was noted (49). Approximately 20% of the subjects in this study were characterized by response distortion as measured by the Eysenck Personality Inventory (EPI) Lie scale, and these individuals were deleted from the study a priori.

It is possible that investigators who have reported that nondepressed, nonhospitalized controls who experience reductions in depression with exercise training have failed to consider response distortion. It is obvious, however, that most subjects who participate in such experiments may be influenced by demand characteristics. At any rate, the four studies reviewed here indicated that nondepressed individuals do not experience decreases in depression following programs of aerobic training (41,42,44), even though significant gains in aerobic power have been noted (49,50,54). Such a finding is not very profound, and although it makes sense from a theoretical and logical standpoint, some researchers have reported that exercise reduces depression in nonhospitalized controls as well as depressed individuals.

It is possible that exercise is associated with transient shifts in depression that return to baseline levels within hours or perhaps a day or so. This sort of transitory change has been consistently found in studies involving state anxiety (31,36,43,52). One study involving the effect of acute physical activity on depression was carried out by Morgan, Roberts, and Feinerman (43). Adult males were randomly assigned to bicycle ergometer ($N = 60$) or treadmill ($N = 60$) exercise, and fifteen subjects in each category were randomly assigned to exercise bouts that would result in heart rates of 150, 160, 170, or 180 beats per minute (bpm). A posttest-only design (8) was employed in order to avoid behavioral artifacts due to expectancy effects and pretest sensitization. Form A of the Depression Adjective Check List (DACL) (16) was administered to the test subjects 5 min following exercise. It can be assumed that a posttest-only, randomized-groups design (8) of the type employed in this study generated groups that did not differ on depression prior to exercise. The depression scores were contrasted with those of a control group ($N = 214$), and the results are summarized in Figures 58.3 and 58.4.

It will be noted in Figure 58.3 that depression scores for each of the treadmill exercise groups fell below the control or norm value, and the greatest antidepressant effect occurred for the group that exercised to a heart rate of 160 bpm. The results for the bicycle ergometer group are summarized in Figure 58.4. It will be noted that depression

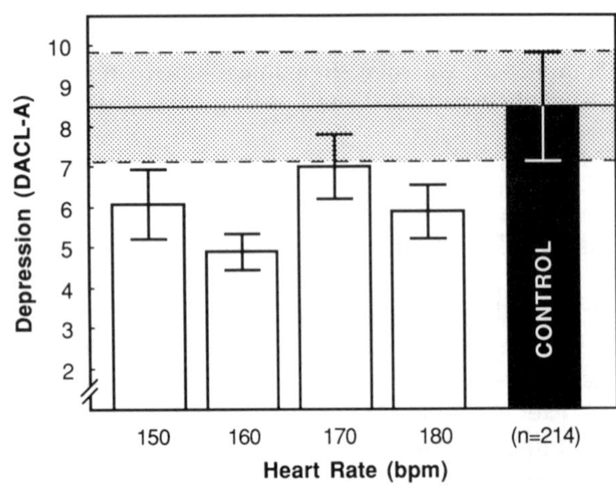

Figure 58.3 Depression scores of normal adult males following exercise of varying intensities on a treadmill protocol. This figure was adapted from an article by Morgan et al. (43).

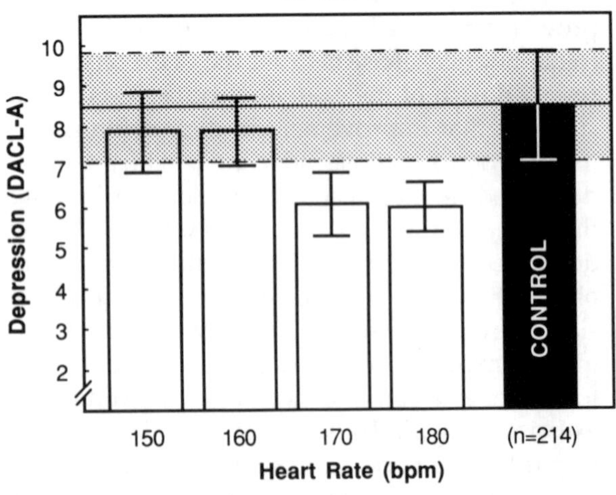

Figure 58.4 Depression scores of normal adult males following exercise of varying intensities on a bicycle ergometer protocol. This figure was adapted from an article by Morgan et al. (43).

scores fell below the norm value for each group, and the lowest scores were noted for the groups that exercised to heart rates of 170 and 180 bpm. The findings of these experiments suggest that depression falls below population norm values following acute physical activity in nondepressed individuals. These effects are probably transient since reduced depression is not observed in nonhospitalized controls following chronic physical activity (43).

The aforementioned study by Morgan and Pollock (41) was conducted over 20 years ago, and there is a need to replicate these findings as well as elucidate the mechanisms responsible for this apparent antidepressant effect.

Due to restrictions on the scope of this paper it is simply not possible to cite each investigation that has been conducted on the topic of exercise and depression. However, the work of Greist et al. (12), Martinsen (17), and Martinsen et al. (18) warrants attention.

It is fair to say that the work by Greist et al. (12) served as the stimulus for much of the research on exercise and depression during the past decade. In this seminal work psychiatric outpatients were assigned to time-limited psychotherapy, time-unlimited psychotherapy, or running therapy. It was found that exercise was associated with a significant reduction in depression, and the antidepressant effect was equal to that observed for time-unlimited psychotherapy and superior to that observed for time-limited psychotherapy. This study was unique in the sense that exercise was contrasted with traditional forms of therapy rather than being compared with nothing (i.e., a control group). It is also noteworthy that patients in the exercise group were found to be nondepressed at 12 months of follow-up whereas half of the patients in the psychotherapy groups were depressed at the time of follow-up. In other words, exercise was associated with a longer lasting antidepressant effect than was psychotherapy.

The work by Greist et al. (12) is significant for one additional reason. It has been estimated that approximately 22% of the 1.7 million persons receiving psychiatric treatment during a given year have a principal diagnosis of affective disorder. Most of these individuals (84%) receive outpatient care, as did the patients who participated in the study by Greist et al. (12). Furthermore, during 1988 there were 8.3 million patient care episodes generated by 4,930 mental health organizations in the United States. There has also been a major shift in patient care episodes since 1955 when 77% were provided by inpatient care compared to 28% in 1988. The increase in ambulatory care has implications for health psychologists and behavioral medicinists concerned with selected wellness and prevention strategies such as exercise.

The subsequent work by Martinsen (17) has served to confirm the earlier work by Greist et al. (12), but it has differed systematically in one important way. Martinsen (17) has relied primarily on the testing of inpatients and important findings have emerged. First, exercise can be safely performed by patients with mild depression who are also receiving antidepressant medications. That is, exercise is not contraindicated for patients with unipolar depression who are receiving antidepressant medications, providing the exercise and medication are titrated under the supervision of a physician. Second, exercise has consistently been observed to be associated with reduced depression in patients suffering from unipolar depression of a modest nature. However, the mechanisms underlying this antidepressant effect remain to be elucidated.

The research by Greist et al. (12) and Martinsen (17) has shown that depressed inpatients suffering from unipolar depression of a moderate nature experience a consistent and significant decrease in depression following chronic aerobic exercise performed for periods ranging from 2 to 6 months. There is no evidence, however, that exercise is effective in the treatment of patients with major depression or patients with bipolar depression.

Earlier Reviews

In some respects it can be argued that we do not need additional reviews dealing with the influence of physical activity and fitness on psychological states and traits in general and depression in particular. That is, a case can be made for rigorous, well-designed experimental research. Unfortunately, while there is a plethora of reviews available, both the qualitative and quantitative reviews tend to be of a noncritical nature. Reviewers have usually examined published literature in a matter-of-fact manner with little if any attention paid to important issues such as validity (internal or external) and behavioral artifacts. Two examples will be presented in order to illustrate the point.

In a widely cited paper by Jankowski et al. (15) reviewers have reported that exercise was found to be superior or equivalent to psychotherapy and drug therapy. Although this paper is often regarded as providing compelling support for the exercise–mental health hypothesis, inspection of the methodology reveals a number of problems. First of all, the study involved a comparison of drug therapy with fitness activities and psychotherapy in adolescent males engaged in outpatient or inpatient therapy. Hence, the proposal that findings of the study (15) can be generalized to adult males and females, healthy or depressed, is simply preposterous. There are many additional problems with this particular study, and some of the more significant shortcomings are listed:

- Patients were not randomly assigned to treatments.
- Raters were not blinded to the patients' treatments.
- There were no statistical analyses.
- Some of the rating scales were not validated.
- Measures of physical fitness were not defined.
- Kinetic therapy (i.e., exercise) did not improve the fitness of inpatients.
- Fitness improved in the outpatients receiving kinetic therapy and psychotherapy.
- Psychotherapy was more effective than kinetic therapy in reducing depression in the outpatients.
- The kinetic therapy and waiting-list controls became more neurotic during the intervention period.

The paper by Jankowski et al. (15) has been cited in a number of review articles as demonstrating that fitness or sport activity (kinetic therapy) is equivalent to psychotherapy or drug therapy. However, kinetic therapy was actually inferior to psychotherapy in the outpatient cohort. Also, the apparent positive effect of kinetic therapy with the inpatients may have reflected the influence of "any treatment" versus "no treatment" (i.e., *placebo effect*). At any rate, generalizability of these results to healthy individuals or psychiatric outpatients is not warranted. It is probable that authors who have cited the paper by Jankowski et al. (15) in a noncritical manner have simply accepted the English translations provided by other authors.

The second example to be cited actually consists of three papers by Stern and associates (58,59,60). These papers are not only cited uncritically in the published literature, but members of the 1992 Consensus Panel actually felt that it would be an oversight not to include these investigations in a review of exercise and depression. However, this work is characterized by a number of fatal flaws, and it will be considered here primarily for the purpose of illustrating one of the reasons why there is controversy in this area.

In the first investigation in the series, Stern and Cleary (58) studied 784 males with documented myocardial infarction (MI) during the past 3 years. There were a number of methodological problems with this study, but even if the design had been sound any findings or conclusions would not be generalizable to healthy or depressed individuals; that is, generalizability would be restricted to post-MI males. The subjects were randomly assigned to an exercise group or a control group, and all subjects were first required to participate in a 6-week exercise program. The authors reported that this preinvestigation exercise program was performed in order to have the subjects become familiar with the exercise and equipment in the study. This paper focused on the psychosocial effects of the exercise familiarization in all of the subjects, as well as characterization of those subjects who dropped out before randomization to the control and exercise conditions.

It was reported that 19% of the subjects were depressed at the outset as measured by the MMPI compared with 13% following the 6 weeks of low-level exercise. Stern and Cleary (58) noted that the reduction of the mean depression score from 22.1 to 21.3 was statistically significant ($p < .05$). Although the reduction of 0.8 raw score units on the MMPI may have been statistically significant, a difference of this magnitude is not of clinical or practical significance. The reason for the significance of this trivial reduction stems from the size of the sample ($N = 651$). This study is often cited as evidence for the view that exercise can reduce depression in nonhospitalized controls as well as depressed patients, however this position is inappropriate for the following reasons:

1. The study dealt with post-MI patients, and generalizability to other groups is not justifiable.
2. There is no reason to think that the modest reduction in depression was not due to one or more of the many behavioral artifacts known to plague research of this nature such as demand characteristics, pretest sensitization, placebo effect, and so on (38).
3. It is probable that a combination of statistical regression and large sample size was responsible for the reduced depression rather than exercise per se.

The 651 post-MI subjects who participated in the second part of the study (59) were randomly assigned to a control or exercise group and followed for 2 years. Assessments of depression at baseline, 6 months, and 24 months with the MMPI revealed that the control and exercise groups did not differ at any point on depression. This study is often cited as one of the few randomized trials using large samples of exercise and control subjects that failed to support the view that exercise can function as an antidepressant intervention. There are, however, at least two additional explanations for the failure of Stern and Cleary (59) to observe an antidepressant effect for exercise in this study. First, the subjects were not depressed to begin with, and hence, one would not expect them to experience a reduction in depression. Second, it is possible that the modest improvement in depression observed in the earlier prerandomization trial (58) eliminated the likelihood of further reductions in depression during the 2-year study. At any rate, it is quite inappropriate to cite this study (59) as evidence that exercise will not reduce depression in depressed individuals, because the participants were post-MI subjects, not depressives.

In a somewhat related study Stern, Gorman, and Kaslow (60) compared the relative effectiveness of exercise therapy and group counseling in 106 post-MI patients. This study differed from the earlier reports by Stern and Cleary (58,59) in that Zung's SDS was used in place of the MMPI. This is a significant difference, for it has been shown that the two scales only share about 50% of the common variance (19). In this study (60) exercise was associated with a significant reduction in depression. However, the mean reduction in depression for the exercise group was merely 1.4 raw score units, and the baseline mean was slightly lower than the population average. It is certainly possible that the observed reduction in depression for this nondepressed group may have reflected demand characteristics or the *Hawthorne effect* (37). Furthermore, the statistical analyses were inappropriate for the most part. Rather than using a repeated measures ANOVA for multifactor experiments in order to test for group, time, and group-by-time interaction, a simple one-way ANOVA was carried out at each point to test for group differences. The group therapy and exercise groups did not differ at 3, 6, and 12 months of treatment, but both groups were found to differ from the controls. While baseline differences were not analyzed, inspection of Figure 2 in this paper (60) suggests that the controls scored higher than the group therapy and exercise groups at the outset. Indeed, the baseline differences between the control and exercise group are just as great as the decreases reported for the exercise group following the training intervention.

The research by Stern and Cleary (58,59) and Stern et al. (60) has been selectively cited to both support and refute the view that exercise possesses antidepressant qualities. In point of fact, however, the methodological deficiencies in this research are so extensive that the results simply are not interpretable. This would be the case for both narrative and quantitative reviews in the sense that meta-analysis cannot eliminate the many design problems in this work. Nevertheless, this research (58,59,60) is of interest from a historical perspective, and it continues to be instructive from a design standpoint. However, this research is of little value in attempting to understand the influence of exercise on depression.

One of the most recent reviews dealing with the influence of exercise and depression is based on a meta-analysis by North, McCullagh, and Tran (45). Although the conclusions presented in this chapter are in general agreement with those previously reached by the NIMH Consensus Panel on Exercise and Mental Health (33), the chapter by North et al. (45) is characterized by numerous methodological and interpretive problems. Some of these problems are merely symptomatic of the inherent shortcomings associated with meta-analysis, whereas others stem from an apparent rejection of fundamental canons of science. At any rate, the conclusions and recommendations presented by North et al. (45) should be viewed with caution.

There are many potential pitfalls associated with both qualitative (i.e., narrative) and quantitative (i.e., meta-analysis) review methods. Authors who rely extensively on meta-analysis either imply or state explicitly that meta-analysis is a superior methodology because of its objectivity. However, there have been a number of concerns raised regarding the efficacy of this procedure. Shortcomings involving the use of meta-analysis in attempting to understand the effect of exercise on anxiety and depression have been presented by Blumenthal (4) and Dunn and Dishman (11). It appears that a principal problem associated with the use of meta-analysis in efforts to understand the link between physical activity and depression has involved the disregard for issues of a methodological nature. However, as Dunn and Dishman (11) correctly point out: "Contrary to the assumptions of meta-analysis, the methodological problems of past research cannot be resolved by any type of review of the existing human literature on exercise and depression" (p. 48).

The initial review by Morgan (21) in 1969 dealing with the relationship between physical fitness and emotional health has been updated by Morgan and his colleagues a number of times over the succeeding two decades (25,26,28,29,30,31,35,36,38). Also, the summary of conclusions reached by the NIMH Consensus Panel on Exercise and Mental Health have been published in an edited volume titled *Exercise and Mental Health* (34). Several of the panel's conclusions are relevant to the present review, and these consensus statements follow:

1. Physical fitness is positively associated with mental health and well-being.
2. Exercise is associated with the reduction of stress emotions.

3. Anxiety and depression are common symptoms of failure to cope with mental stress, and exercise has been associated with a decreased level of mild to moderate depression and anxiety.
4. Severe depression usually requires professional treatment, which may include medication, electroconvulsive therapy, or psychotherapy, with exercise as an adjunct.
5. Physically healthy people who require psychotropic medication may safely exercise when exercise and medications are titrated under close medical supervision.

It is important to recognize that the NIMH Consensus Panel agreed that exercise was associated with reduced depression, but this group of experts did not feel there was sufficient evidence to conclude that exercise was actually an antidepressant. This represents an important reservation because it is known that personality structure (13) as well as physical capacity and adaptability (5) are influenced to a substantial degree by genetic factors. There are additional reasons for advancing associational versus causal views at this point in time. The statistical, design, and methodological inelegancies characteristic of inquiry in this area have been so numerous that causal explanations are simply not possible. A summary of some of the more significant problems will be presented next in the hope that such shortcomings can be eliminated or minimized in future research.

Methodological Issues

It has been noted in earlier reviews that most investigations dealing with the efficacy of exercise as an antidepressant have relied on preexperimental or quasi-experimental designs (8). While this criticism is an accurate one, there have been far more fundamental and significant problems associated with research studies in this area (38). Furthermore, it is unlikely that true experimental designs (8) are possible in this area with the exception of those investigations where animal models are employed. Unless one were to experimentally produce depression in a subset of randomly selected individuals, an ethically indefensible intervention, it would be necessary to adopt less powerful designs (i.e., volunteers who already differ on levels of depression). Hence, our concern should not be with the recognized weaknesses associated with quasi-experimental designs, but rather our concern should be with maximizing internal and external validity. A discussion of several principles that can and should be adopted follows.

In a number of investigations the influence of regular exercise on depression has been compared with depression levels in nonexercise controls. Investigators have often reported that the exercise group experienced a greater decrease in depression than did the nonexercise controls. It matters little that participants in the studies were not randomly selected from the target population, nor does it matter that they were not randomly assigned to exercise and control conditions. Indeed, even if both randomization principles were employed, the finding that the exercise group experienced a greater decrease in depression would not be persuasive for many reasons. First, a number of investigators have reported that affective improvement occurs even though the exercise did not produce an improvement in fitness. Second, even where a fitness gain has accompanied the exercise intervention, it is not very profound to report that "exercise is better than nothing" (i.e., control). In other words, rather than comparing exercise treatments with nonexercise controls, there is a need to draw contrasts with (a) traditional therapy, (b) minimal treatment, or (c) placebo groups (2).

The need for alternative paradigms has been recognized by some investigators (12,13,28,57,58) in this field, but the use of contrasts that exceed mere control groups has been the exception rather than the rule. This is an important consideration because most of the published literature does not permit the conclusion that reduced depression following an exercise program exceeds or is equivalent to antidepressant effects one might see with other treatments such as psychotherapy or drug therapy. Also, such findings do not permit one to conclude that exercise is superior to a placebo. It has been recognized for many years that the "special attention" or Hawthorne effect can play an important role in most behavioral studies, and this is particularly true where the dependent variables are subjective as opposed to objective. It is not always possible to eliminate the Hawthorne effect, but it is possible to quantify the magnitude of this influence by employing a placebo plot.

It is recognized that double-blind paradigms should be employed, if possible, and where this is not possible, a single-blind design should be employed. It is common in this area of inquiry for the investigators, who evaluate the level of depression in patients participating in these studies, to be aware of the patients' group affiliation. This can result in another behavioral artifact known as the *Halo effect*, and it is simply imperative that evaluators not be aware of the individual's treatment status (e.g., exercise, drug, placebo, or psychotherapy) at the time of performing assessments on the dependent measure(s). This applies to both the administration of self-report depression questionnaires as well as clinical assessments. It is not only possible for investigators to be intentionally or unintentionally influenced when performing the assessments of depression, but it is also possible for the test administrator to communicate expectancies to the person being tested. This can result in *demand characteristics* that can be quite problematic given the transparent nature of most self-report measures of depression. Furthermore, efforts to detect response distortion (i.e., faking) is essentially nonexistent in this area of research.

It is also known that pretest sensitization effects can influence the outcome of many studies. The administration of a pretest can often serve to alert a test subject to the hypothesis under study, and it is relatively easy for such a person to respond on the posttest in the manner he or she feels is desired. One solution to this problem is to employ what is known as a posttest-only, control group design (8). The ideal approach is use of the Solomon Four-Group Design (8). However, the author is unaware of any study involving exercise and psychological effects in which the Solomon Four-Group Design has been employed.

There has also been an absence of psychometric rigor in some investigations dealing with the influence of exercise on depression, and therefore, internal validity has been absent in some studies. It is imperative that individuals with appropriate training be involved in the diagnosis and assessment of depression. In this context it should also be noted that the appropriate measure of depression in a given study will be governed by the question being asked. In addition to problems with internal validity, there have also been shortcomings associated with external validity. The use of inferential statistics implies that an investigator intends to infer from the sample he or she has studied to the population from which the sample has been drawn. This principle is widely accepted in psychology, yet investigators and reviewers often generalize far beyond the appropriate population where the influence of exercise on depression is concerned. In other words, research carried out with psychiatric inpatients cannot be generalized to nonhospitalized controls, and conversely, studies involving nonhospitalized controls should not be generalized to psychiatric patients.

A welcome exception to the generalization that reviewers have often neglected important methodological issues in discussing earlier work is the recent monograph by McDonald and Hodgdon (19) titled *Psychological Effects of Aerobic Fitness Training: Research and Theory*. The authors devote an entire chapter to experimental design and methodological issues, and attention is paid to the important consideration of how depression is assessed. The interpretation of research evidence relies on meta-analysis in this review, but unlike most investigators who employ this method, McDonald and Hodgdon (19) address both the strengths and weaknesses of this approach. The final chapter in this monograph deals with theory and conclusions, and this also represents a valuable addition to this literature because many of the earlier reviews have been atheoretical in nature. This comprehensive review led to the conclusion that "The combined effect of all studies in this group indicated that there was a statistically significant decrease in depression scores, independent of instrument used to measure depression" (p. 119).

These investigators also reported that reduced depression following aerobic exercise was observed in (a) female and male groups, (b) all adult age groups, and (c) survey and experimental reports, and that the antidepressant effect was approximately 40% greater in depressed versus healthy groups. It is reassuring to note that these conclusions are in complete agreement with those of the NIMH Consensus Panel (34) published in 1987. It is also noteworthy that similar conclusions were reached with a meta-analysis (45) and a narrative review (17). One would not expect otherwise, of course, where competent scientists perform the respective reviews.

Assume for a moment that a given set of studies dealing with the influence of exercise on depression are influenced in one way or another by problems involving (a) the Hawthorne Effect, (b) the Halo Effect, (c) pretest sensitization, (d) lack of appropriate comparison groups, (e) inadequate sample size, (f) demand characteristics, (g) response distortion, (h) volunteerism, (i) absence of randomization (selection and group assignment), (j) improper statistical models, (k) lack of replication, (l) internal validity, and (m) external validity. Furthermore, assume that a reviewer ignores these methodological shortcomings and proceeds to perform a meta-analysis. The result would be what computer aficionados call GIGO or "garbage-in, garbage-out." Design issues must be taken into account by reviewers, and this applies to both narrative reviews as well as those based on meta-analysis. There is no substitute for critical analysis of the experimental literature, and in any case, meta-analysis cannot make behavioral artifacts disappear.

Negative Effects of Exercise

Despite the observation that habitual physical activity is associated with reduced depression in moderately depressed individuals, there are two additional findings that warrant attention. First, a number of investigators have reported that individuals engaged in aerobic training programs experience reduced depression in the absence of an increase in aerobic power. This has led some authors to maintain that the reduction in depression is not dependent on the physical activity per se because the antidepressant response was not associated with a gain in physical fitness. While this proposal is plausible, it is also possible that various cardiovascular, histochemical, and enzymatic changes can occur in the absence of improvements in aerobic power. Similarly, increased muscular strength and endurance, muscle tone, and flexibility along with reduced sense of effort and improved self-esteem can also occur in regular exercisers even though aerobic power may not increase. Therefore, the failure to find changes in $\dot{V}O_2max$ does not mean that regular exercise does not have other physiological and psychological concomitants that may underlie the reduced depression.

A second finding in this research area that has been largely ignored by all but a few reviewers (32,35,36,52), is the paradoxical observation that healthy, nondepressed individuals often become depressed as a result of high training loads. In other words, while habitual physical activity is associated with reduced depression in depressed individuals, it also results in the elevation of depression in nondepressed individuals when the volume of training exceeds a given level (i.e., overtraining). A brief summary of this research literature follows. It is remarkable that meta-analysts, who argue that narrative reviews suffer from subjective decisions about inclusion and exclusion of selected studies, have uniformly failed to incorporate any of the overtraining studies in their reviews. This would be analogous to a drug researcher not incorporating any study involving the effect of a given antidepressant drug in a review if a given dose led to undesired effects. There is also limited evidence that some individuals become exercise-addicted or exercise-dependent (27,63). At any rate, any review dealing with the influence of exercise on fitness and depression must certainly consider negative as well as positive findings.

The effect of overtraining on selected mood states has been described by a number of investigators in recent years. In the first report involving this issue, Morgan, Brown, Raglin, O'Connor, and Ellickson (32) summarized the effect of overtraining on 200 female and 200 male swimmers studied over a 10-year period. It was found that mood disturbance occurred in a dose–response manner, and mood states were predictably worsened or improved by increasing or decreasing training volumes.This dose–response observed by Morgan et al. (32) with swimmers has also been reported for speedskaters, wrestlers, and rowers (52). Furthermore, it was found that 80% of the swimmers who were judged to experience staleness exhibited depression of clinical significance (32). It should be noted that staleness is a syndrome characterized by various signs and symptoms such as decreased performance, inability to train at customary levels, chronic fatigue, muscle soreness, hypertension, increased perception of effort for standard work loads, hormonal dysregulation, hypothalamic dysfunction, insomnia, loss of appetite, and disturbed mood. However, athletes who experience staleness do not have all of these symptoms, and although most stale athletes do experience mood disturbance, depression is not present in every case. In other words, it is a mistake to conclude that staleness and depression are synonymous. Staleness should be conceptualized as a complex psychobiologic response to overtraining, and this independent construct warrants syndromic status.

It is widely agreed that the best treatment for staleness is rest, and athletes may need to cease training for several weeks once this syndrome is diagnosed (51). It is also necessary to supplement rest with medical and psychological treatment in some cases, and Barron, Noakes, and Levy (3) have reported that the effects of staleness sometimes persist for up to 6 months following the initial episode. While the incidence of staleness in athletes exposed to overtraining has not been established, there is indirect evidence involving the occurrence of this problem in elite distance runners. It has been reported by Morgan et al. (37,39) that 64% of elite female and male distance runners have experienced staleness at some point in their careers.

The initial report by Morgan et al. (32) demonstrating mood disturbance with increased training has since been replicated by Morgan et al. (33), O'Connor et al. (46,47), and Raglin et al. (51). Also, in the paper by O'Connor, Morgan, Raglin, Barksdale, and Kalin (47) it was reported that those athletes who experienced staleness were characterized by significant elevations in resting levels of salivary cortisol in comparison with other athletes who were exposed to overtraining but did not develop staleness. Since hypercortisolism has been associated with some forms of depression, cortisol measures may prove of use as a marker in the study of staleness. At any rate, it is important to recognize that habitual physical activity is associated with mood disturbance as well as mood enhancement. The extent to which physical activity has euphoric as opposed to dysphoric effects seems to be dependent in part on exercise volume.

Although exercise has been recognized as possessing mood-enhancing qualities for centuries (11), it is remarkable that contemporary authors have generally made no reference to the "dark side" of exercise. This has been true for summaries based on meta-analysis (45) as well as more traditional narrative reviews (17). An exception to this generalization are the reviews by Morgan and O'Connor (35,36) and Raglin (51) who have summarized research indicating that exercise can lead to mood disturbance in healthy young men and women. It has been demonstrated in a systematic manner that mood disturbance can be provoked in a predictable, dose–response manner. Increases in the training volume of swimmers, for example, results in mood disturbance, and reductions in training volume (i.e., tapering) results in improved mood (32,46,52). Furthermore, it has been shown that samples of college students who are not engaged in rigorous training do not experience altered mood states during the same period when significant fluctuations in mood take place in athletes exposed to increased and decreased training (32). These findings suggest that titration of exercise volume is linked to mood state in a causal manner.

The most common approach to the study of threshold effects is to randomly assign individuals to selected doses of a drug, for example, and then attempt to quantify the optimal dose in mg/kg for the desired effect. There are potential problems associated with the use of such an approach in the study of exercise volume because it would be ethically indefensible to experimentally produce depression, for example, in healthy individuals. One alternative to the production of depression in healthy individuals would be to adopt an animal model, and this possibility will be reviewed in the next section.

Animal Models

The efficacy of using animal models in the study of psychopathology has been addressed at some length by Dunn and Dishman (11). Also, Morgan, Olson, and Pedersen (40) have presented an animal model of psychopathology for use in the exercise and sport sciences. The rationale for the use of comparative models is based on ethical and experimental considerations, and there are several excellent examples of animal models of human psychopathology in the literature. Furthermore, the use of animal models enables one to address selected mechanisms that cannot be directly tested with human models (e.g., brain monoamine hypothesis) (53).

One of the first demonstrations of how animal models can be used in exercise psychology was presented by Weber and Lee (64). These investigators randomly assigned 48 prepubertal Sprague-Dawley rats to a sedentary control, voluntary exercise, or forced exercise condition. These animals were exposed to a novel stress, the open-field test, postpuberty following 35 days of the intervention. Emotionality levels of the three groups, as measured by the open-field test, were found to be superior for the forced exercise group followed by the voluntary exercise group, and the sedentary controls were found to be the most emotional. The research by Weber and Lee (64) was replicated and extended by Tharp and Carson (62) who randomly assigned rats to one of the following exercise groups: (a) wading, (b) swimming, (c) walking, or (d) running. It was found that the lowest levels of emotionality existed in the running and swimming groups, and while these groups did not differ, both were significantly less emotional than the walking or wading groups.

The work by Weber and Lee (64) and Tharp and Carson (62) is exemplary in many ways, but neither report attempts to elucidate the mechanisms responsible for the exercise-emotionality link. In a related paper by Olson and Morgan (48), Sprague-Dawley rats were classified as emotional or stable using the same open-field test employed in the earlier papers (62,64). The animals were then sacrificed, and whole-brain concentrations of dopamine, norepinephrine, and serotonin were determined. All assays were performed by personnel who were blinded to the animal's group affiliation. The results are presented in Figure 58.5, and it will be noted that whole-brain norepinephrine levels were significantly ($p < .01$) lower in the stable animals, but the two groups did not differ on whole-brain levels of dopamine or serotonin.

If one were to hypothesize that depressed animals would traverse fewer squares in the open-field test than nondepressed animals, the above results can be interpreted to mean that depressed animals have higher whole-brain levels of norepinephrine. Although this study has not been replicated, it does suggest that rats differing in exploratory behavior also differ in whole-brain levels of norepinephrine. This study sets the stage for an experiment in which exercise is employed as an intervention. It would be hypothesized on the basis of earlier research that depressed animals would become less depressed with training (i.e., enhanced open-field score). The monoamine hypothesis could also be tested in such a study in an effort to elucidate the mechanisms

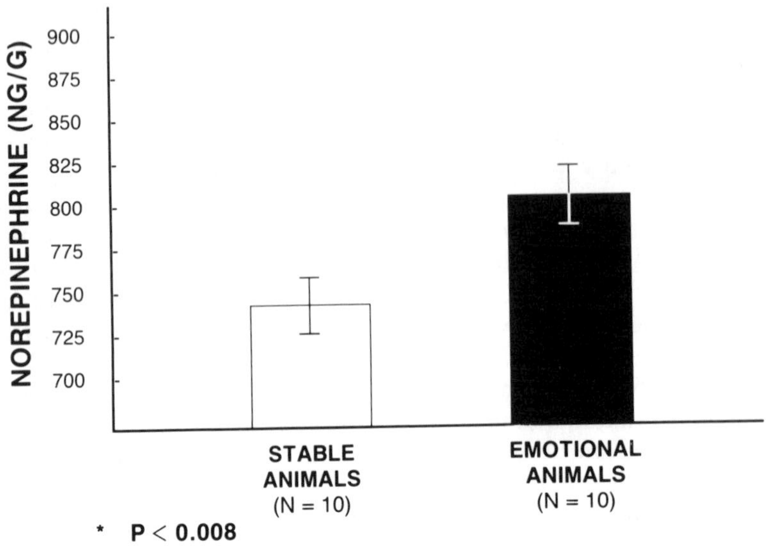

Figure 58.5 Brain norepinephrine in stable and emotional rats. This figure was adapted from an article by Olson and Morgan (48).

underlying the antidepressant effect. It would be appropriate to also examine regional levels of brain monoamines in future research, and Dishman et al. (9) have recently taken such an approach in a study dealing with exercise and brain chemistry using a rat model.

Conclusions

Physical fitness is positively associated with mental health and well-being. Depression is a common symptom of failure to cope with mental stress, and exercise has been associated with a decreased level of mild to moderate depression. Severe depression usually requires professional treatment, which may include medication, electroconvulsive therapy, or psychotherapy, with exercise as an adjunct. Current clinical opinion holds that exercise has beneficial emotional effects across all ages and in both sexes. Physically healthy people who require psychotropic medication may safely exercise when exercise and medications are titrated under close medical supervision.

There is compelling evidence in support of the *association* noted in the preceding statements, but there is an absence of *causal evidence*. There is a need for rigorous research designed to elucidate the mechanisms underlying the hypothesized antidepressant effect of exercise, for much of the research in this area has been characterized by serious design problems and behavioral artifacts.

Important Research Questions

1. Is the reduction in depression observed in depressed individuals following programs of chronic physical activity caused by the physical activity?
2. If so, what is/are the mechanism(s) responsible for the antidepressant effect?
3. If vigorous physical activity reduces depression, are there conditions that maximize this effect (e.g., mode, intensity, duration, frequency)?
4. If excessive exercise (i.e., overtraining) causes mood disturbance, what is/are the mechanism(s) responsible for these affective changes?
5. How can exercise models be employed to understand the prevention, onset, and treatment of depression within an overall therapeutic milieu?
6. How would the efficacy of an exercise intervention compare with traditional drug therapy or psychotherapy in the treatment of depressed patients suffering from various depressive disorders?

References

1. Åstrand, I. Aerobic work capacity in men and women with specific reference to age. Acta Physiol. Scand. [Suppl.]. 49:169; 1960.

2. Bahrke, M.S.; Morgan, W.P. Anxiety reduction following exercise and meditation. Cogn. Ther. Res. 2:323-334; 1978.
3. Barron, J.L.; Noakes, T.D.; Levy, W. Hypothalamus dysfunction in overtrained athletes. J. Clin. Endocrinol. 60:803-806; 1985.
4. Blumenthal, J.A. Response to Abbot and Peters. Psychosom. Med. 51:219-221; 1989.
5. Bouchard, C. Gene-environment interactions in human adaptability. In: Malina, R.M.; Eckert, H.M., eds. Physical activity in early and modern populations. Champaign, IL: Human Kinetics; 1988:56-66.
6. Brown, R.S.; Ramirez, D.E.; Taub, J.M. The prescription of exercise for depression. Phys. Sportsmed. 6:35-45; 1978.
7. Campbell, D.D.; Davis, J.E. Report of research and experimentation in exercise and recreational therapy. Am. J. Psychiatry. 96:915-933; 1940.
8. Campbell, D.T.; Stanley, J.C. Experimental and quasi-experimental designs for research. Chicago: Rand McNally; 1966.
9. Dishman, R.K.; Renner, K.J.; White, J.E.; Bunnell, B.N.; Youngstedt, S.D.; Armstrong, R.B. Effects of treadmill training on locus coeruleus monoamines following running and immobilization. Med. Sci. Sports Exerc. 24:S25; 1992.
10. Drinkwater, B.; Horvath, S.; Wells, C. Aerobic power of females, ages 10 to 68. J. Gerontol. 30:385-394; 1975.
11. Dunn, A.D.; Dishman, R.K. Exercise and the neurobiology of depression. In: Holloszy, J.O., ed., Exercise and sport sciences reviews. Baltimore: Williams & Wilkins; 1991:41-98.
12. Greist, J.H.; Klein, M.H.; Eischens, R.R.; Faris, J.; Gurman, A.S.; Morgan, W.P. Running as treatment for depression. Compr. Psychiatry. 20:41-54; 1979.
13. Holden, C. The genetics of personality. Sci. 237:598-601; 1987.
14. Hughes, J.R. Psychological effects of habitual aerobic exercise: A critical review. Prev. Med. 13:66-78; 1984.
15. Jankowski, K.; Andrejewska, E.; Endicott, J.; Fraczek, A.; Jankowska, K.; Kozlowski, S.; Markiewicz, L.; Reykowski, J. Effect of psychotherapy, pharmacotherapy and sporttherapy on emotionally disturbed adolescents. Z. Klin. Psychother. 24:251-255; 1976.
16. Lubin, B. Manual for the depression adjective check list. San Diego: Educational and Industrial Testing Service; 1967.
17. Martinsen, E.W. Benefits of exercise for the treatment of depression. Sports Med. 9:380-389; 1990.
18. Martinsen, E.W.; Strand, J.; Paulson, G.; Kaggestad, J. Physical fitness level in patients with anxiety and depressive disorders. Int. J. Sports Med. 10:58-61; 1989.
19. McDonald, D.G.; Hodgdon, J.A. The psychological effects of aerobic fitness training: Research and theory. New York: Springer-Verlag; 1991.
20. Morgan, W.P. Selected physiological and psychomotor correlates of depression in psychiatric patients. Res. Q. 39:4, 1037-1043; 1968.
21. Morgan, W.P. Physical fitness and emotional health: A review. Am. Corr. Ther. J. 23:124-127; 1969.
22. Morgan, W.P. A pilot investigation of physical working capacity in depressed and non-depressed psychiatric males. Res. Q. 40:859-861; 1969.
23. Morgan, W.P. Physical working capacity in depressed and non-depressed psychiatric females: A preliminary study. Am. Corr. Ther. J. 24:14-16; 1970.
24. Morgan, W.P. Physical fitness correlates of psychiatric hospitalization. In: Kenyon, G.S., ed. Contemporary psychology of sport. Chicago: Athletic Institute; 1970:297-300.
25. Morgan, W.P. Exercise and mental disorders. In: Ryan, A.J.; Allman, F.L., Jr., eds. Sports medicine. New York: Academic Press; 1974.
26. Morgan, W.P. Psychological consequences of vigorous physical activity and sport. In: Scott, M.G., ed. Academy papers. Iowa City, IA: American Academy of Physical Education; 1977.
27. Morgan, W.P. Negative addiction in runners. Phys. Sportsmed. 7:57-70; 1979.
28. Morgan, W.P. Psychological benefits of physical activity. In: Nagle, F.J.; Montoye, H.J., eds. Exercise, health, and disease. Springfield, IL: Charles C Thomas; 1981:299-314.
29. Morgan, W.P. Psychological effects of exercise. Behav. Med. Update. 4:25-30; 1982.
30. Morgan, W.P. Physical activity and mental health. In: Eckert, H.; Montoye, H.J., eds. The academy papers. Champaign, IL: Human Kinetics; 1984:132-145.
31. Morgan, W.P. Affective beneficence of vigorous physical activity. Med. Sci. Sports Exerc. 17:94-100; 1985.
32. Morgan, W.P.; Brown, D.R.; Raglin, J.S.; O'Connor, P.J.; Ellickson, K.A. Psychological monitoring of overtraining and staleness. Br. J. Sports Med. 21:107-114; 1987.
33. Morgan, W.P.; Costill, D.L.; Flynn, M.G.; Raglin, J.S.; O'Connor, P.J. Mood disturbance following increased training in swimmers. Med. Sci. Sports Exerc. 20:408-414; 1988.
34. Morgan, W.P.; Goldston, S.E., editors Exercise and mental health. Washington, DC: Hemisphere Publishing; 1987.

35. Morgan, W.P.; O'Connor, P.J. Exercise and mental health. In: Dishman, R.K., ed. Exercise adherence and public health. Champaign, IL: Human Kinetics; 1987:91-121.
36. Morgan, W.P.; O'Connor, P.J. Psychological effects of exercise and sports. In: Ryan, A.J.; Allman, F., eds. Sports medicine. 2nd ed. New York: Academic Press; 1989.
37. Morgan, W.P.; O'Connor, P.J.; Ellickson, K.A.; Bradley, P.W. Personality structure, mood states, and performance in elite male distance runners. Int. J. Sport Psychol. 19:247-263; 1988.
38. Morgan, W.P.; O'Connor, P.J.; Koltyn, K.F. Psychological benefits of physical activity through the lifespan: Methodological issues. In: Telama, R., ed. Movement and sport: A challenge for lifelong learning. Jyväskylä, Finland: Proceedings of the Jyväskylä Sport Congress; 1990:65-72.
39. Morgan, W.P.; O'Connor, P.J.; Sparling, B.P.; Pate, R.R. Psychological characterization of the elite female distance runner. Int. J. Sports Med. [Suppl.]. 8:124-131; 1987.
40. Morgan, W.P.; Olson, E.G., Jr.; Pedersen, N.P. A rat model of psychopathology for use in exercise science. Med. Sci. Sports Exerc. 14:91-100; 1982.
41. Morgan, W.P.; Pollock, M.L. Physical activity and cardiovascular health: Psychological aspects. In: Landry, F.; Orban, W., eds. Physical activity and human well-being. Miami, FL: Symposia Specialists; 1978:163-181.
42. Morgan, W.P.; Roberts, J.A.; Brand, F.R.; Feinerman, A.D. Psychological effect of chronic physical activity. Med. Sci. Sports. 2:213-217; 1970.
43. Morgan, W.P.; Roberts, J.A.; Feinerman, A.D. Psychologic effect of acute physical activity. Arch. Phys. Med. Rehabil. 52:422-425; 1971.
44. Morgan, W.P.; Vogel, J.A. Psychological states and traits before and following a military training program. Unpublished report. Natick, MA: U.S. Army Research Institute of Environmental Medicine; 1975.
45. North, T.C.; McCullagh, P.; Tran, Z.V. Effects of exercise on depression. In: Pandolf, K.B., ed. Exercise and sport sciences reviews. Baltimore: Williams & Wilkins; 1990:379-415.
46. O'Connor, P.J.; Morgan, W.P.; Raglin, J.S. Psychobiologic effects of three days of increased training in female and male swimmers. Med. Sci. Sports Exerc. 23:1055-1061; 1991.
47. O'Connor, P.J.; Morgan, W.P.; Raglin, J.S.; Barksdale, C.M.; Kalin, N.H. Mood state and salivary cortisol level following overtraining in female swimmers. Psychoneuroendocrinology. 4:303-310; 1989.
48. Olson, E.B., Jr.; Morgan, W.P. Rat brain monoamine levels related to behavioral assessment. Life Sci. 30:2095-2100; 1982.
49. Patton, J.F.; Morgan, W.P.; Vogel, J.A. Perceived exertion of absolute work during a military training program. Eur. J. Appl. Physiol. 36:107-114; 1977.
50. Pollock, M.L.; Gettman, L.R.; Milesis, C.A.; Bah, M.D.; Durstine, L.; Johnson, R.B. Effects of frequency and duration of training on attrition and incidence of injury. Med. Sci. Sports. 9:31-36; 1977.
51. Raglin, J.S. Exercise and mental health: Beneficial and detrimental effects. Sports Med. 6:323-329; 1990.
52. Raglin, J.S.; Morgan, W.P.; O'Connor, P.J. Changes in mood states during training in female and male college swimmers. Int. J. Sports Med. 12:585-589; 1991.
53. Ransford, C.P. A role for amines in the antidepressant effect of exercise: A review. Med. Sci. Sports Exerc. 14:1-10; 1982.
54. Roberts, J.A.; Morgan, W.P. Effect of type and frequency of participation in physical activity upon physical working capacity. Am. Corr. Ther. J. 25:99-104; 1971.
55. Ross, C.E.; Hayes, D. Exercise and psychologic well-being in the community. Am. J. Epidemiol. 127:762-771; 1988.
56. Simons, A.D.; McGowan, C.R.; Epstein, L.H.; Kupfer, D.J.; Robertson, R.J. Exercise as a treatment for depression: An update. Clin. Psychol. Rev. 5:553-568; 1985.
57. Stephens, T. Physical activity and mental health in the United States and Canada: Evidence from four population surveys. Prev. Med. 17:35-47; 1988.
58. Stern, M.J.; Cleary, P. Psychosocial changes observed during a low-level exercise program. Arch. Intern. Med. 141:1463-1467; 1981.
59. Stern, M.J.; Cleary, P. The national exercise and heart disease project: Long-term psychosocial outcome. Arch. Intern. Med. 142:1093-1097; 1982.
60. Stern, M.J.; Gorman, P.A.; Kaslow, L. The group counseling v exercise therapy study: A controlled intervention with subjects following myocardial infarction. Arch. Intern. Med. 143: 1719-1725; 1983.
61. Taylor, C.B.; Sallis, J.F.; Needle, R. The relation of physical activity and exercise to mental health. Public Health Rep. 100:195-202; 1985.
62. Tharp, G.D.; Carson, W.H. Emotionality changes in rats following chronic exercise. Med. Sci. Sports Exerc. 7:123-126; 1975.
63. Veale, D.M.W. Psychological aspects of staleness and dependence on exercise. Int. J. Sports Med. [Suppl. 1]. 12:19-22; 1991.

64. Weber, J.C.; Lee, R.A. Effects of differing prepuberty exercise programs on the emotionality of male albino rats. Res. Q. 39:748-751; 1968.
65. Weinstein, W.S.; Meyers, A.W. Running as treatment for depression: Is it worth it? J. Sport Psychol. 5:288-301; 1983.
66. Zung, W.W.K. Self-rating depression scale. Arch. Gen. Psychiatry. 12:63-70; 1965.

Acknowledgments

The preparation of this paper was supported in part by a generous gift from Donald and Diane Masterson of Boise, Idaho. Appreciation is expressed to Gernot Presting and Patrick J. O'Connor for translating the paper by Jankowski et al. (15) from German to English.

Chapter 59

Physical Activity, Fitness, and Anxiety

Daniel M. Landers
Steven J. Petruzzello

In the United States, anxiety has become a pervasive social problem. According to very recent statistics, *panic attack* is now the most frequent type of psychopathology. Because of the fast-paced lifestyles that people live, this has been referred to by some as the Age of Anxiety. Estimates from earlier reports (16,56) suggest that 30 million U.S. citizens have their "normal" lifestyles disrupted by anxiety or anxiety-related problems, and from 30% to 70% of the patients seen by general practitioners and internists have problems managing stress.

Health care providers continue to use psychotropic drugs or psychotherapeutic interventions (e.g., meditation, biofeedback, relaxation, group therapy) to treat anxiety disorders. However, there is growing interest among many health care professionals in the role that physical activity plays in preventing the onset of emotional problems and in serving as a treatment modality once such problems have developed (60,105). For example, among 1,756 primary care physicians, 60% of those surveyed indicated that they routinely prescribed exercise for patients with anxiety disorders (82). Of course, psychotropic drugs are also prescribed, but their administration can produce adverse effects (e.g., withdrawal following termination of treatment, potential negative side effects or interaction with other drugs, or financial expense associated with prolonged use).

Considering that many health care providers believe that exercise can have benefits similar to those of prescribed drugs, scientific evidence for the anxiolytic (i.e., anxiety-reducing) effect of exercise would further promote the use of exercise in preventing the onset of anxiety-related problems. The heightened clinical awareness of the anxiolytic role of exercise has prompted the National Institutes of Mental Health to identify this topic of immediate concern (60).

Since the 1950s, data-based research on the topic of physical activity/fitness and anxiety reduction has been conducted. Currently, some 29 reviews of this literature have been located. The purposes of the present review are to (a) discuss the general conclusions derived from these narrative and meta-analytic reviews, (b) examine the research evidence for some of the variables that reviewers have suggested as moderating the relationship between physical activity/fitness and anxiety reduction (i.e., duration and intensity of exercise needed to produce the effect), and (c) review literature on physical fitness and anxiety and the recent research literature since January 1989 on the effects of training on anxiety. Before discussing the main conclusions of these reviews, it is first necessary to define *anxiety* and *physical activity/fitness*, which in turn will determine the scope of the present review.

Definition of Terms and Scope of the Present Review

Anxiety and Its Measurement

The time-honored, inverted-U relation between arousal level and performance indicates that an intermediate level of arousal is necessary for optimal behavioral functioning. The degree of arousal is dependent on task characteristics and individual differences. Arousal, considered an energizing function responsible for harnessing the body's resources for intense and vigorous activity (83), can range from a comatose state at one extreme to a panic attack at the other. Arousal and stress are to some degree related notions (20) and are typically measured with physiological (i.e., autonomic or central nervous system) or biochemical (e.g., cortisol, catecholamines) measures. In many of the studies examining the anxiolytic effect of exercise, anxiety reduction has been inferred from physiological or biochemical measures of arousal (69).

In this review anxiety is associated with arousal but is also differentiated from it. Anxiety is associated with the downturn on the right side of the inverted-U. Coincident with moderate to high arousal levels where the individual's behavior begins to become disrupted (i.e., performance drops, perception, retention, and decision making are degraded) is the emergence of a negative form of cognitive appraisal typified by worry, self-doubt, and apprehension. This negative cognitive appraisal is termed *anxiety*. It arises because the individual perceives a high degree of uncertainty or lack of control over task demands, available resources, behavioral consequences and their meaning, and bodily reactions (20). With more understanding and certainty about a situation or about life in general, individuals perceive having a greater degree of control and are thus less anxious about a specific situation or about life in general.

Because anxiety is fundamentally a cognitive phenomenon, it is measured by a number of questionnaire instruments (69). A common distinction in this literature is between trait and state measures of anxiety. *Trait* anxiety is the general predisposition to respond across many situations with high levels of anxiety. *State* anxiety, on the other hand, is much more specific and refers to the subject's anxiety at a particular moment. The instructions for the questionnaire convey the set in which subjects should respond to the question; for example, "how I feel in general" (trait) versus "how I feel at this moment" (state). Although trait and state aspects of anxiety are conceptually distinct, the available operational measures for these (37) and other partitions of anxiety (i.e., *cognitive-somatic* anxiety) are not statistically independent (92).

Physical Activity/Fitness

The emphasis here will be on cardiovascular efficiency because this is generally agreed to be the best indicator of fitness and health. In this sense, this review will include studies that examine prolonged engagement in physical activities at an intensity and duration that have the potential for improving aerobic or anaerobic capacity. Studies of overtraining were not included. Therefore, data-based studies that examine physical activity and fitness in relation to an anxiety-reduction effect following acute exercise or following an exercise-training program will be examined. This includes studies of (a) trait anxiety of fit and unfit individuals, (b) state anxiety response before and after an acute bout of exercise, and (c) state and trait anxiety before and after a longitudinal exercise-training program.

Excluded from this review are studies of skill development to overcome anxiety regarding a particular physical skill (e.g., swimming instruction to reduce fear of the water). Also excluded were studies on trait anxiety of athletes and nonathletes, because these studies typically have no objective description of fitness levels or of the amounts of physical activity. Finally, studies were also excluded if they were not data-based, if they combined another treatment modality along with exercise, if they exposed subjects to a situational stressor during the postexercise recovery period, or if they used exercise for experimental purposes other than to create anxiety reduction following exercise. A listing of the excluded references are available upon request from the primary author.

Methods

Procedures for Literature Search

The 104 published and unpublished studies reported between 1960 and January 1989 on acute and chronic exercise (69) formed the primary empirical basis for this review. These studies were identified through a computerized search of ERIC and PsychINFO, using *anxiety, exercise, physical activity, physical fitness, mood,* and *tension* as key terms. References were also cross-checked in the relevant studies, literature reviews, and relevant journals (*Medicine and Science in Sports and Exercise, Journal of Sports Medicine and Physical Fitness, Health Psychology, Psychosomatic Medicine, Research Quarterly for Exercise and Sport, Journal of Sport and Exercise Psychology,* etc.) and unpublished sources (e.g., *Dissertation Abstracts, Completed Research in Health, Physical Education, Recreation and Dance,* etc.).

In addition, the search was broadened to include: (a) some of the studies that were excluded from the Petruzzello, Landers, Hatfield, Kubitz, and Salazar review (69) because of insufficient information (e.g., standard deviations) for calculation of effect sizes (ES), (b) additional references reported from January 1989 to June 1992 that employed trait or state measures of anxiety, and (c) studies comparing trait anxiety in physically fit and unfit individuals. This search procedure resulted in 55 additional studies beyond the 104 studies in the meta-analytic review (69). Tables containing effect sizes and study characteristics for physical fitness and anxiety studies (1,5,37,44,64,75,79,87,100,110,111) and studies examining the effects of training on anxiety (2,4,6,7,8,14,21,22,27,30,31,40,41,42,45,47,48,49,51,54,61,63,65,66,67,68,71,77,78,80,81,84,86,91,93,94,95,96,97,98,104,106,109,111) are available from the primary author.

Methods Employed in Previous Reviews

The reviews dealing with this topic included 27 narrative reviews and two meta-analytic reviews

(52,69) (see Table 59.1). Only five of these reviews described procedures for conducting a systematic review of literature. In many cases, the reviews simply described the author's own research program (12,13,15). Only five reviews had identifiable criteria for inclusion of studies. Therefore, it was very common to find studies included in these reviews that did not meet the typical definitions for physical activity/fitness effects on anxiety reduction (e.g., stress reactivity, moods other than anxiety, other variables combined with exercise) mixed in with the studies meeting the definition. Studies with the strictest inclusion criteria (39) reviewed very few of the available studies (i.e., four), whereas the meta-analytic reviews (52,69) did not on a priori grounds exclude any of the studies reviewed. This means that studies deemed to have weak methodologies (e.g., intact group, no control group, etc.) were included in the meta-analytic reviews.

These meta-analytic investigators adopted the rationale (32) that (a) whether or not study quality makes a difference in the findings is a question that should be examined statistically by blocking studies into categories on the basis of relevant moderating variables (e.g., subjects assigned to conditions randomly vs. intact groups), and that (b) parsimony demands acceptance of the idea that flawed research can converge on a true conclusion. Only by including all studies, flawed or not, can it be ascertained whether or not study quality affected the outcome. However, if it is determined that study quality does not affect the findings, it does not logically follow that it is acceptable to conduct poorly designed studies. This simply permits an empirical test to determine if study quality has influenced the results of research done to date.

The practice of excluding studies also leaves open the possibility of the author's personal bias coloring the findings. This could result in an inaccurate reflection of the entire area under review. The potential for bias in the narrative review is heightened since it is difficult to quantify the magnitude of the effect in question. Reviewers often conclude that the results are contradictory, needing better quality research to clarify the findings. If there is an effect, it is impossible for the narrative reviewer to determine the magnitude of the effect unless the effect is very large.

For behavioral science variables, which yield small to moderate effects, narrative reviewers will invariably find contradictory results. Some study findings are statistically significant and others are not. Although most investigators use the conventional .05 alpha level to determine statistical significance, the studies on this topic typically have very low statistical power. For example, summed across 207 comparisons (69), the average ES for studies using self-reported state anxiety was 0.24. For this small ES 105 subjects would be needed in each group (or for each comparison) to achieve statistical power of .80 at an alpha level of .05 (46). Only 5 of the 64 studies using measures of state anxiety (69) had sample sizes that provided adequate statistical power.

Similarly, only 19% of 41 studies using measures of trait anxiety (69) had suitable statistical power (for ES = 0.34 at least 51 subjects per cell or comparison are needed for alpha = .05, beta = .80). The number of subjects could be reduced by designing studies with moderating variables that have larger ES. Despite the fact that the group means may indicate that physically fit individuals have lower anxiety than unfit individuals, the lack of statistical power will often result in nonsignificant alpha levels. This lack of power presents a problem for narrative reviewers who rely totally on whether the study findings were significant at the .05 level.

The present review relied on the Petruzzello et al. (69) meta-analytic review because it used similar criteria for study inclusion, had far more moderator variables, and had more ES for each level of the moderator variables. As in other reviews (69), ES was calculated by subtracting the mean for the treatment group from the mean of the comparison group (or posttest mean from the pretest mean) and dividing this difference by the pooled standard deviation (69). When means and standard deviations were unavailable, F, t, r, z, or p values were used to estimate ES (38,76). The resultant ES was then corrected for sample size.

For interpretive purposes, ES are categorized as small (low meaningfulness, < 0.41), moderate (0.41–0.70), and large (high meaningfulness, > 0.70). To provide greater consistency among the correlations and ES, the sign (+ or –) of the ES in the Petruzzello et al. (69) review was reversed. Thus, all correlations, ES, and mean differences reported in this review indicate that higher levels of physical activity/fitness are related to lower levels of anxiety.

Considering these issues, the methods in the present review will include (a) initial inclusion of all relevant studies regardless of study quality, (b) comparison of the overall findings with studies considered to have more methodological sophistication (adequate sample size, design, subject assignment, etc.), and (c) reliance on statistics unaffected by sample size (e.g., either ES corrected for sample size or the direction of mean differences in the absence of reported standard deviations).

To better judge the general conclusions of previous reviewers, an "index of surety" was used (70). This index provides a way of rating how sure or

Table 59.1 Reviews Dealing with Physical Activity/Fitness and Anxiety

Author	Systematic literature search procedures identified	Identifiable criteria for study inclusion	Number of other areas reviewed	Number of anxiety studies reviewed	Anxiety measured	General correlational support for: Acute effects	General correlational support for: Chronic effects	Estimated duration of acute anxiolytic effect	Estimated intensity necessary to produce effect	Effect present for state or trait anxiety	Results stronger for low-fit subjects	Results stronger for clinically anxious subjects	Exercise as good as or better than other interventions
Cattell (9)	No	No	0	2	Self-report physiological	—	2+	—	—	Both	—	—	—
Cureton (12)	No	No	2	3	Self-report physiological	—	2+	—	—	—	—	—	—
Cureton (13)	No	No	2	4	Self-report physiological	—	2+	—	—	—	—	—	—
Hammett (34)													
Franks & Jette (28)	No	No	0	11	Self-report physiological	—	1+	—	Moderate	Trait	Yes	Yes	—
Layman (50)	No	No	14	11	Self-report	—	1+	—	Moderate-vigorous	Trait	—	Yes	—
Folkins & Amsterdam (23)	No	No	2	11	Self-report	—	2+	—	—	—	—	—	—
Morgan (56)	No	No	0	15	Self-report physiological	2+	—	—	Vigorous	Both	—	No	As good as
deVries (15)	No	No	0	9	Self-report physiological	2+	2+	—	Low-moderate[j]	—	—	No	Better than
Folkins & Sime (25)	No	Yes[a-d]	5	9	Self-report physiological	—	2+	—	—	—	Yes	Yes	—
Morgan (57)	No	Yes[b]	3	13	Self-report physiological	2+	2+	4–6 hr	Vigorous[k]	State	—	—	As good as
Dishman (16)	No	No	20	1[f]	Self-report physiological	2+	—	4–6 hr	Vigorous	State	—	—	As good as
Mihevic (55)	No	No	1	19[g]	Self-report physiological	2+	1+	—	Vigorous	—	—	—	As good as

(continued)

Morgan (58)	No	No	2	8	Self-report physiological	2+	—	4–6 hr	Vigorous	—	—	—	As good as
Hughes (39)	Yes	Yes[a-e]	3	4	Self-report	—	1+	—	—	—	—	No	—
Sime (89)	No	No	2	9	Self-report	—	2+	—	—	—	—	—	—
Van Andel & Austin (103)	No	Yes[c]	5	12	Self-report physiological	—	2+	—	—	—	Yes	—	As good as
Dishman (17)	No	No	7	42	Self-report physiological behavior	2+	2+	4–6 hr	Moderate-vigorous	State	Yes	Probably	As good as
Goff & Dimsdale (33)	No	No	4	12	Self-report physiological	2+	2+	—	Vigorous	—	Yes	Yes	—
Morgan (59)	No	No	2	6	Self-report physiological	2+	2+	2–5 hr	—	Both	—	No	—
Raglin & Morgan (73)	No	No	0	17[h]	Self-report physiological	2+	2+	2–5 hr	Moderate-vigorous	—	—	No	As good as
Dishman (18)	No	No	8	32	Self-report	2+	2+	1–6 hr	Moderate	State	Yes	No	As good as
Doan & Scherman (19)	Yes	No	5	14	Self-report	—	1+	—	—	Both	—	—	—
					Behavioral physiological				Vigorous				
Hatfield & Landers (36)	No	No	6	24	Physiological	1+	2+	—	Moderate	—	—	—	—
Phelps (70)	No	No	16	3[i]	Self-report	—	1+	—	—	—	—	—	—
McDonald & Hodgdon (52)	Yes	Yes	4	22	Self-report	—	2+	—	—	Yes	—	—	—
Petruzzello et al. (69)	Yes	Yes	0	104	Self-report physiological	2+	2+	2–5 hr	Low-vigorous	Both	—	Yes	As good as
Simono (90)	No	No	2	21	Self-report	2+	2+	—	Vigorous	—	Yes	Yes	As good as
Tuson & Sinyor (102)	Yes	Yes	5	50	Self-report physiological	2+	—	—	—	—	No	No	As good as

[a]Excluded comparisons of fit/unfit people. [b]Excluded comparisons of athletes/nonathletes. [c]Excluded studies that assessed anxiety for an exercise group once (case study) or twice (pre-post design for single group). [d]Excluded studies not showing a training effect. [e]Excluded studies not published in scientific journals. [f]Most citations were from a previous review by Morgan (57). [g]Some of the studies were not independently published, but were cited in review articles. [h]Studies cited as "in preparation" were not included in this total. [i]Only cited previous review. [j] = 33% of max. [k] = 70%–80% of max. [l] = lower intensity for psychophysiological measures and higher intensity for state/trait anxiety. [m]"0 = data are mixed, no point of view is favored; 1+ = most data are supportive but a significant fraction of reports (significant either in number or quality of results) does not support the claim; 2+ = established, little or no conflicting data" Phelps (70).

certain each reviewer was in regard to physical activity/fitness affecting anxiety reduction. If the reviewer concluded that the results of the studies were mixed and no point of view was favored, this would constitute a surety index rating of 0. If most of the findings were supportive of the hypothesized relationship, but there were some significant (in number or quality) divergent results, the review would receive a surety index of 1+. Finally, if the reviewer concluded that physical activity/fitness was related to anxiety reduction following exercise and there was little or no conflicting data presented in the review, a surety index rating of 2+ was given.

Results

Trait Anxiety in Physically Fit/Unfit Individuals

Information on this topic was derived from six reviews (9,12,13,28,34,50). The doctoral (43,107) and master's theses (2,5,42) contained in these reviews were part of Cureton's research program at the University of Illinois. Trait anxiety in these studies was typically measured with Cattell's tense/composed (Q_4) factor from the Sixteen Personality Factor Questionnaire (16 PF) and the Taylor Manifest Anxiety Scale. In previous reviews (28,50), this literature has been summarized as showing:

> . . . an inverse relationship between manifest anxiety and physical fitness measures. The correlations have been low to moderate, seldom higher than 0.35 (thus accounting for no more than 10-15% common variance). . . . In addition, the correlations between physiological measures that have been used to measure anxiety such as heart rate and blood pressure range from 0.15 to 0.45. (p. 49)

Although this summary of results may be correct, it is difficult to verify. The primary problem is the lack of an acceptable measure of fitness. For example, manifest anxiety scores are correlated with 30 to 50 fitness measures ranging from blood pressure to trunk extension to dip-ups. With so many correlations, in which the direction of the relationship is not always consistent with expectations, it is nearly impossible to determine if higher levels of fitness are related to lower levels of anxiety.

When cardiovascular measures of fitness are emphasized, the studies are supportive of the low correlations just noted. For example, Wells (107) compared 80 subjects' all-out treadmill run times with the 16 PF (Q_4) and found a significant ($p < .05$) negative correlation of –.224. In addition, Jette (43) found that subjects who had lower heart rate response to a 5-min bicycle ergometer ride had less manifest anxiety ($p < .10$). This is consistent with other studies (1,44) that, for both cardiovascular and questionnaire measures of physical activity/fitness, found that better fitness was significantly correlated with lower levels of trait anxiety (*r*s ranging from –.24 to –.63).

These results are supported by 11 other studies (summary information available upon request from the primary author). Of the 30 ES that could be derived from these studies, all but 4 of them showed lower anxiety being associated with higher levels of physical fitness. The average ES for this set of studies was –0.38, which is a small to moderate effect. The 15 mean differences also show lower anxiety in the physically fit subjects. The only mean differences having the reverse direction were those showing a slight tendency for active people engaged in aerobic activity other than running to have less anxiety than committed runners (37). In this study people who knew the subjects well also rated their anxiety lower. The close correspondence between subject and informant ratings for both the exercise and sedentary groups give additional credence to these findings.

In a large-scale, multivariate study of 4,351 patients from a preventive medicine clinic (10), 23 clinical risk factors of coronary heart disease (CHD) were examined along with 29 psychological characteristics. In their study, cardiorespiratory fitness was measured from a maximal treadmill test and anxiety was measured by the Clinical Anxiety Questionnaire. The canonical correlations having the highest loadings revealed that people who were fit and who exercised were less likely to have somatic complaints or nervous tension.

Although these studies are cross-sectional and correlational in nature, they are strikingly consistent in showing that physically fit people have less anxiety than unfit people. Although the small to moderate ES indicates that this effect is meaningful, it does not suggest that exercise or fitness per se is the cause of these anxiety differences. It may be that fit people live more healthy lifestyles (better nutrition, education, occupation, etc.) and thus tend to be less anxious. In order to better determine if exercise is responsible for changes in anxiety, it is necessary to examine studies comparing changes in anxiety either before and after an acute bout of exercise or before and after a longitudinal exercise-training program.

Trait Anxiety and Chronic Exercise

Comparing the anxiety scores before and after subjects participate in an exercise program, it is evident that on average subjects report lower anxiety scores following an aerobic exercise program (69). The magnitude of this difference was about one third of a standard deviation for the 62 ES (69). The 51 ES in the current review that relate to trait anxiety represent an average of –0.40. (Summary information for these studies is available upon request from the primary author.) In addition, 63% of the 46 trait anxiety comparisons in studies where ES could not be computed showed mean differences consistent with the ES findings. Although some reviewers (16,17,18,57) have suggested that trait anxiety would not be expected to change much from pretest to posttest, these findings show that trait anxiety scores are influenced by exercise.

State Anxiety and Chronic Exercise

Several studies have employed state anxiety measures before and after an exercise-training program. Similar to the results found for trait anxiety, the state anxiety measures have shown that subjects report less anxiety after participating in an exercise program. This is supported by the 88 ES with an average of –0.25 (69). In the current review, the 30 ES derived from the exercising subjects show a small to moderate ES of –0.38 (available upon request). All 11 of the mean differences for which ES could not be computed were negative. It is evident that both state and trait anxiety measures, which are typically correlated with one another to a moderate degree, show similar anxiety reductions following an exercise program.

State Anxiety and Acute Exercise

Investigators have also examined whether or not anxiety is reduced following a single bout of exercise. Most of these studies have measured aerobic exercise requiring that subjects cycle or run continuously for 20 to 30 min at greater than 50% of maximal aerobic capacity. Petruzzello et al. (69) report that with 119 ES from studies of this type, the pre-post reduction in anxiety is small (ES = –0.23). The 25 ES derived from studies where subjects performed acute exercise show an ES of –0.53 and negative mean differences for a study (21) in which ES could not be computed. For a wrestling match (61), which is neither clearly aerobic or anaerobic, the ES ranged from –0.38 to –0.53 when the early season anxiety scores are compared to the postmatch scores. Effect sizes are even larger when more aerobic activities are employed (22,47,68,71,77,78,81,109).

This acute effect is perhaps best illustrated in the Roth (77) study. He randomly assigned 40 subjects to an exercise group (20 min cycling at a heart rate of 120–160 beats per minute) and 40 subjects to a nonexercising control group. Although the control subjects did not appreciably change their state anxiety scores (ES = 0.04), the aerobic exercise group showed much less anxiety postexercise than they did prior to the exercise (ES = –0.58).

Regardless of the kind of anxiety measure employed (state or trait) and the exercise paradigm employed (acute vs. chronic), the results are remarkably consistent in showing that exercise is associated with a reduction in anxiety. These results are not surprising, for this is a typical conclusion in the 29 reviews on this topic. These results do not support hypotheses (72) that would predict the opposite result. Although these results are clear, the moderating variables relating to the physical activity–anxiety-reduction relationship are not as readily recognized. In other words, which variables make this relationship stronger and which make it weaker? Answering this question may help to further clarify the finding and may be a first step in the eventual explanation of its occurrence.

Suggested Variables Moderating the Relationship

Are the Findings Highly Influenced by Study Quality?

In spite of Glass's caveat concerning parsimony, it would seem that studies having better designs might be more apt to show stronger or at least more consistent effects. Although this has been examined to some extent (69), not all methodological considerations were undertaken. Of course, study quality is relative as none of the 159 studies identified for this review are without problems. For example, none of the studies have selected subjects randomly from the population at large, most have low statistical power, and training studies usually have dropouts.

In order to determine if study quality is an important consideration, methodological variables in which there was considerable variability among the various studies have been coded (69). The results were very similar for state and trait anxiety measures when comparing exercise to either a motivational control group or to a no-treatment control group. There was a tendency for larger ES in studies employing within-subjects designs, which are known to provide more statistical power.

Although the way in which subjects were assigned to groups did not matter for state anxiety measures, it did influence ES for trait anxiety studies (69). Effect sizes were larger when subjects were randomly assigned to treatment conditions than when they were part of an intact group. This may account for the larger ES among the 55 studies in this review where the use of random assignment has increasingly been employed in the more recent studies. In general, the results appear to be quite robust as evidenced by the fact that 84% of the findings in this review show the predicted relationship. For example, comparable ES can be found in studies of higher methodological quality (77,96) as well as in studies with relatively few subjects and no control groups (8,26). These results suggest that methodological considerations may be more important for understanding the relationship between exercise and anxiety reduction than they are for producing the effect.

Are the Findings Different for Anaerobic and Aerobic Forms of Exercise?

Very few studies have examined activities that are clearly more anaerobic. Petruzzello et al. (69) only located 15 ES where exercise was not of an aerobic nature (e.g., strength training). These ES were very small and in the opposite direction from the predicted anxiolytic effect. There is some evidence for this among the five nonaerobic studies in the present review. Whereas a wrestling match produced results similar to those found in aerobic studies (61), activities like handball (31) and strength/flexibility training (51,63,67,93) are associated with slight increases in anxiety (ES = 0.019). There may be something associated with the nature of aerobic activities that is conducive to producing anxiolytic effects. Future research systematically investigating the key elements that make aerobic and nonaerobic activities different is needed to determine why anxiolytic effects are primarily linked to aerobic activities.

What Is the Time Course of the Anxiolytic Effect?

The main consideration here is the time course of the anxiety reduction following an acute bout of exercise. Several reviewers (see Table 59.1) have indicated that anxiety is reduced for up to 4 to 6 hr following exercise. Unfortunately, these estimates are based on only one unpublished study (85). This study only measured anxiety at a few time points following exercise. Thus, the only conclusion may be that somewhere between 4 to 6 hr after exercise anxiety returned to preexercise levels.

Few other studies have measured state anxiety beyond 20 min following exercise. The nine ES derived from these studies confirm Seemann's (85) finding by showing a small ES of –0.27 (69). Effect sizes of similar magnitude are also found between 0 to 5 min following acute exercise. Subsequent time periods of 5, 10, and 20 min also show ES ranging from –0.27 to –0.49 (69). These results show that the anxiolytic effects of exercise begin almost immediately after exercise and continue for at least 2 hr.

In some studies (73), anxiety is reduced following conditions of either quiet rest or exercise, but relative to the quiet rest group, the exercise group has lower blood pressure and state anxiety up to 3 hr after exercise. Future research is needed to determine the point in time when anxiety levels begin to return to preexercise (baseline) levels. That anxiety is reduced for a time after a bout of exercise has led to the suggestion that "the benefits of regular exercise may reside in its ability to reduce anxiety on a daily basis and, hence, *prevent* the development of chronic anxiety" (57, p. 306).

Is the Length of the Training Program a Factor in Producing This Effect?

In examining the results of several studies, training programs have ranged from 4 weeks to more than 15 weeks (69), most programs being between 7 and 12 weeks. Although only four ES were derived from studies with training programs lasting more than 15 weeks (69), the postprogram anxiety reduction in these studies was much greater (ES = –0.90) than for exercise training of less than 9 weeks (ES < –0.18). Similar results are observed from the aerobic-training studies contained in the present review. With nonclinical subjects, the average ES for training programs less than 9 weeks was –0.183 (n = 10). Likewise, training programs greater than 15 weeks yielded an ES of –0.51 (n = 6). Therefore, based on these results, it appears that anxiety is reduced much more if the length of the training program is at least 10 weeks and preferably greater than 15 weeks.

There is also some evidence that trait anxiety is still reduced from 6 weeks to 52 weeks following the training program (4,49,80,86,91). However, very little can be concluded from this finding because most of these studies fail to report whether subjects were still exercising at the time of follow-up assessment.

Are the Findings Influenced by Exercise Intensity or Duration?

This is perhaps the most controversial question among the previous reviews of this area. With older subjects (15), low to moderate exercise was sufficient to reduce tension levels, as measured by electromyography and Hoffman reflex. With trait anxiety measures (28), moderate exercise reduced trait anxiety better than vigorous exercise. However, the majority of the reviewers adopted the position of Morgan (56,57) that exercise needed to be at 70% to 80% of $\dot{V}O_2max$ to elicit anxiolytic effects.

This conclusion was based on walking exercise at 55% to 72% maximal heart rate (HRmax) (62) and treadmill exercise (HR = 100–110 bpm) (88). Although exercise intensity was attributed to the failure to find anxiety reductions in these acute exercise studies, there were confounding factors that could explain these findings. For example, both studies had very low statistical power and one study (88) involved subjects anticipating an acute mild stressor.

Examination of the intensity of the exercise stimulus (% HRmax or % $\dot{V}O_2$) across several studies (69) showed no significant differences in state anxiety for exercise intensities ranging from 40% to greater than 80%. There were also no differences in trait anxiety for intensities ranging from 70% to greater than 80%. Inspection of 55 studies contained in this review also reveals several instances of low-intensity exercises like walking and jogging being related to meaningful reductions in posttest anxiety (30,49,71,86,91). Within studies where exercise intensity has been varied, moderate exercise (50%–60% HRmax) is sometimes better (63) and sometimes worse (67) than higher intensity exercise (70%–75% HRmax).

Similar results were reported by Franks and Jette (28), which led them to conclude that training should be at an intensity at which subjects can adjust. From an examination of these 159 studies in their entirety, it does not appear that there is a clearly established exercise intensity that is necessary to lower anxiety. Dose–response studies, where exercise intensity is systematically varied, are needed to clarify if there are exercise intensity effects on postexercise anxiety reduction.

For both state and trait anxiety, inspection of the ES would at first glance suggest that exercise durations less than 20 min do not yield anxiolytic effects (69). Upon closer inspection of these studies with exercise durations of less than 20 min, Petruzzello et al. (69) found that most of these ES were confounded with other design or methodological characteristics that were associated with negligible ES (e.g., comparing exercise with known anxiety-reducing treatments like relaxation or meditation). When the ES from these confounded comparisons were eliminated, the ES for exercise durations between 5 and 20 min were increased from −0.12 to −0.22. Thus, it may not be necessary to insist that people exercise longer than 20 min to achieve anxiety-reducing effects (18). To specify more precisely the minimum duration needed to reduce anxiety, experimental studies are needed so that exercise duration can be manipulated within the 0- to 20-min time frame (e.g., 5, 10, 15, or 20 min).

Are the Results Influenced by Initial Levels of Fitness and Anxiety?

Although the meta-analytic review (69) does not address this issue, some of the narrative reviewers have suggested that less fit individuals, who are prone to be more anxious, should benefit the most from a physical-training program (33,90). The law of initial values would suggest that this is true. If physical activity/fitness and anxiety are related as the evidence suggests, then subjects initially scoring low on fitness should with proper training be able to make rapid improvements in fitness and thus lower their anxiety levels. Likewise, highly anxious subjects, who are typically less fit, can conceivably make more rapid fitness gains than highly fit subjects and this change should produce greater reductions in anxiety.

In examining the narrative reviews for initial levels of fitness, there is very meager evidence that less fit people experience greater anxiety reductions. Folkins, Lynch, and Gardner (24) found that although male and female college students improved in fitness, only the women showed significant anxiety reductions after a 12-week jogging program. The authors subsequently discovered that prior to the beginning of the exercise program the women were less fit and more anxious than the men. Similar results were found by Wilfley and Kunce (108). When they subdivided their sample into those above or below the mean, they found that improvements in anxiety occurred only for those below the sample mean on fitness and anxiety before the start of the exercise program.

There is much more evidence regarding initial levels of anxiety than initial levels of fitness. Comparisons within and across trait anxiety studies reveal that compared to nonclinical subjects there is a tendency for higher ES for cardiac rehabilitation patients, psychiatric patients, and highly anxious subjects (69). The same trends are not seen however with state anxiety measures. There are very few ES for clinical subjects, so caution needs to be exercised in interpreting these results. However, additional evidence is contained in the studies in the present review. For instance, Jette (42) found larger mean differences for highly anxious subjects than subjects with low anxiety levels. Likewise, other investigators (86,93) showed very meaningful differences for walking/jogging (ES > −1.48) in pre-post anxiety scores of symptomatic neurotics and previously inactive, anxious adults. Mean pre-post anxiety differences of −4.50 have been found for myocardial infarct patients undergoing treadmill running for 23 weeks. These results are consistent with the earlier reported low to moderate correlations between physical fitness and trait anxiety. Although more studies are needed comparing subjects on initial levels of fitness or anxiety, the results to date suggest that initially low-fit and highly anxious individuals have the most to gain psychologically from an exercise-training program.

Are the Results for Exercise Better Than Other Anxiety-Reducing Treatments?

With one exception (15), most of the reviewers of this literature have concluded that exercise is no better than traditional interventions used to alleviate stress and anxiety (e.g., meditation, relaxation, quiet rest, or reading). deVries (15) was not referring to psychological interventions, but instead compared exercise to a tranquilizer drug (meprobamate). He concluded that "exercise of an appropriate type and intensity had significantly greater effect on resting musculature than did meprobamate" (p. 49). There is some support for deVries's conclusion in the trait anxiety literature (69). Here there is a meaningful difference among 15 comparisons between exercise and some other anxiety-reducing treatment (ES = −0.32).

Although exercise may differ from tranquilizer drugs, in most of the state anxiety studies, exercise has not been shown to be any different from other known anxiety-reducing interventions. This is evident in the meta-analysis (69). When exercise is compared to other anxiety-reducing treatments, the ES is nearly zero (ES = −0.04). One of the first studies (3) to demonstrate this found that whether subjects exercised, meditated, or rested quietly while reading an article, anxiety was significantly reduced. The results from the present review were mixed. Compared to exercise, group counseling (96) reduced anxiety more, eating a lunch (109) reduced it to the same extent, and relaxation by yoga training (6,21,80) reduced anxiety less than exercise. Considering these studies together with other studies (69), it is not clear at this time that exercise consistently produces larger anxiety reductions following exercise than other anxiety-reducing interventions.

Morgan (57) has suggested that these results can best be explained by a "time-out" hypothesis. This explanation is similar to other explanations (29) that activities (e.g., exercise, meditation, and quiet reading) unrelated to the cause of the stress divert or distract the person's attention away from the stress cues. This explanation is consistent with the failure to find reduced anxiety following acute exercise when subjects are exposed to high-distraction conditions (21). This may be correct for state anxiety, but other explanations like subject's expectancy regarding the benefits of exercise and the other anxiety-reducing interventions may affect their anxiety reports during the posttest. Unfortunately, none of the more elegant experimental designs (e.g., pretest-posttest randomized groups) can totally control for expectancy effects (99).

Are Similar Results Found When Behavioral and Physiological Measures Are Used to Infer Anxiety/Tension Levels?

Although this review has focused on self-report measures, anxiety can also be inferred from physiological measures of arousal or behavioral measures of emotionality. Consistent with the early observations (12,28), physiological measures generally show larger ES than self-report measures. Petruzzello et al. (69) have shown that the average for 138 ES is −0.56, with the largest ES for skin resistance, electromyogram (EMG), and central nervous system measures. Blood pressure results are somewhat smaller (ES = −0.33 to −0.38), however the postexercise hypotension is consistent across the human and animal literature in showing a similar time course to the postexercise anxiety reductions (11,101). It is difficult to conceive of a strictly psychological explanation (e.g., "time-out" hypothesis) for improvements in anxiety following exercise when these more unobtrusive, physiological measures are showing the same effects.

Behavioral studies have been done with albino rats. The idea is that exercise training would make rats less emotional when confronted with the stress of a novel environment. More emotional rats would be likely to freeze and exhibit less exploratory behavior than less emotional rats. Weber and Lee (106) found that rats who were forced to exercise for 35 days traversed more squares on a marked open field than sedentary rats. Similar results were found (98) for rats forced to run or swim for 8 weeks. Moderate ES were found between the forced exercise groups and the control (no exercise) rats. Interestingly, comparisons between attentional control groups for the runners (i.e., walkers) and the swimmers (i.e., waders) still showed improved emotionality in the exercising groups (ES ranging from −0.16 to −0.47). It is hard to imagine that rats would consider the exercise a "diversion" as they were in their more natural state of actively exploring their environment. If time-out were an all-encompassing explanation for the anxiety-reducing effects of exercise, there should not be meaningful differences between exercisers and walkers or waders. In this case it appears that exercise per se may have more to do with these findings. Considering the unobtrusiveness of the physiological and behavioral measures and their consistency with the findings derived from self-report measures, parsimony would suggest that exercise may be responsible for the reductions in anxiety.

Is Exercise the Cause of These Findings?

Many of the more contemporary studies have reported measured fitness gains and at the same time have demonstrated improvement in anxiety following a training program. However, few investigators have correlated the fitness gains with pre-post changes in anxiety. Those that have have found mixed results. Most studies did not find that fitness gains were correlated with anxiety levels (48,51,86,91,93,104). Other studies (1,45,81) found significant correlations between anxiety reduction and perceived ratings of fitness, but did not find similar relationships with objective measures of fitness (e.g., $\dot{V}O_2$). These results would seem to suggest that aerobic fitness is independent of emotional state. It may be that factors associated with exercise (e.g., decreased body weight and satisfaction with body shape and appearance) are more important for anxiety reduction (45).

However, before concluding that exercise is not directly related to anxiolytic effects, it should be pointed out that even though the fitness gains in these studies were statistically significant, they were relatively small gains (i.e., 5% to 17%). Thus, with this greatly restricted range of fitness and anxiety-change scores, the variability necessary to find significant correlations between fitness gains and changes in anxiety may be insufficient. There is some support for this interpretation (97). With 23 weeks of training given to 52 unfit myocardial infarct patients, fitness gains of 35% functional capacity (i.e., peak work load in METs) were demonstrated. These investigators found that changes in anxiety between 3 and 26 weeks were significantly correlated with change in peak treadmill heart rate for the same period of time ($r = -.25$, $p < .0001$). These results suggest that perhaps more prolonged training that is strenuous enough to produce fitness gains of greater than 20% is needed to provide a reasonable test of exercise causing an anxiety reduction.

The question of causation in the exercise–anxiety-reduction relationship is of primary importance since it may shed light on the plausible explanations for this relationship. Determining if $\dot{V}O_2max$ is related to pre-post exercise changes in anxiety will go a long way in eliminating several of the rival psychological and physiological explanations (35,36,53,90,102).

Conclusions

Based upon the 159 studies meeting the criteria for inclusion in this review, the following conclusions seem warranted.

1. There is a small to moderate relationship showing physically fit people to have less trait anxiety than unfit people.
2. Compared to no-treatment control groups, state anxiety is reduced following an aerobic exercise-training program or following an acute bout of aerobic exercise.
3. Research designs that maximize statistical power (i.e., within-subject designs or optimal sample size) and equality among groups (i.e., randomized) are associated with larger anxiety differences between exercise and a no-treatment control group.
4. For state anxiety, anxiolytic effects of exercise begin almost immediately after acute exercise and continue for at least 2 hr.
5. Trait anxiety is reduced more if the length of the training program is beyond 10 weeks.
6. Reductions in state and trait anxiety are associated with activities involving continuous, rhythmical exercise (i.e., more aerobic) rather than resistive, intermittent exercise (i.e., less aerobic).
7. Regardless of exercise intensity or duration, anxiety reduction occurs following acute or chronic exercise.
8. Individuals who are initially low-fit or high-anxious achieve the greatest reductions in anxiety from an exercise-training program.
9. In most of the state anxiety studies, exercise has not been shown to reduce anxiety any more or less than other known anxiety-reducing treatments (e.g., relaxation, meditation, and quiet rest).
10. The relationship between anxiety change and physical fitness change is equivocal.
11. Reductions in anxiety following exercise are observed irrespective of whether self-report, behavioral, or physiological measures are employed.

Suggested Questions

1. What are the key task elements (e.g., continuous vs. resistive activities, social context) that make various exercise modes different in their anxiolytic effects?
2. What is the time course (i.e., beyond 2 hr) of anxiety reduction following acute exercise, and how long is anxiety reduced following an exercise program?
3. Will prolonged aerobic training that is strenuous enough to produce a wide range of fitness gains result in a significant correlation between fitness gains and changes in anxiety?
4. What are the explanations underlying the anxiety reduction following exercise that best account for these effects?

References

1. Abadie, B.R. Relating trait anxiety to perceived fitness. Percept. Mot. Skills. 67:539-543; 1988.
2. Babka, J. Effects of swimming and basic movement on selected measures of fitness in college women. Champaign-Urbana, IL: University of Illinois; 1969. Thesis.
3. Bahrke, M.; Morgan, W.P. Anxiety reduction following exercise and meditation. Cogn. Ther. Res. 4:323-333; 1978.
4. Bargman, E.P.; Stucky-Ropp, R.C.; Vieth, A.; LaFontaine, T.; Frensch, P.; Sellers, D.M.; DiLorenzo, T.M. Long-term effects of exercise-induced fitness change on mood. Paper presented at the annual convention of the American Psychological Association. San Francisco; 1991 August.
5. Betz, R.L. A comparison between personality traits and physical fitness tests in males. Urbana, IL: University of Illinois; 1953. Thesis.
6. Blumenthal, J.A.; Emery, C.F.; Madden, D.J.; George, L.K.; Coleman, R.E.; Riddle, M.W.; McKee, D.C.; Reasoner, J.; Williams, R.S. Cardiovascular and behavioral effects of aerobic exercise training in healthy older men and women. J. Gerontol. 44:M147-M157; 1989.
7. Blumenthal, J.A.; Emery, C.F.; Madden, D.J.; Schiebolk, S.; Walsh-Riddle, M.; George, L.K.; McKee, D.C.; Higginbotham, M.B.; Cobb, F.R.; Coleman, R.E. Long-term effects of exercise on psychological functioning in older men and women. J. Gerontol.: Psychol. Sci. 46:352-361; 1991.
8. Buccola, V.A.; Stone, W.J. Effects of jogging and cycling programs on physiological and personality variables in aged men. Res. Q. 46:134-139; 1975.
9. Cattell, R.B. Some psychological correlates of physical fitness and physique. In: Staley, S.C.; Cureton, T.K.; Huelster, L.J.; Barry, A.J., eds. Exercise and fitness. Chicago: Athletic Institute; 1960.
10. Collingwood, T.R.; Bernstein, I.H.; Hubbard, D.; Blair, S.N. Canonical correlation analysis of clinical and psychologic data in 4,351 men and women. J. Card. Rehabil. 3:706-711; 1983.
11. Cononie, C.C.; Graves, J.E.; Pollock, M.L.; Phillips, M.I.; Sumners, C.; Hagberg, J.M. Effect of exercise training on blood pressure in 70- to 79-yr-old men and women. Med. Sci. Sports Exerc. 23:505-511; 1991.
12. Cureton, T.K. Anatomical, physiological and psychological changes induced by exercise programs (exercises, sports, games) in adults. In: Staley, S.C.; Cureton, T.K.; Huelster, L.J.; Barry, A.J., eds. Exercise and fitness. Chicago: Athletic Institute; 1960.
13. Cureton, T.K. Improvement of psychological states by means of exercise-fitness programs. J. Assoc. Phys. Ment. Rehabil. 17:14-17; 1963.
14. de Geus, E.J.C.; van Doornen, L.J.P.; de Visser, D.C.; Orlebeke, J.F. Existing and training induced differences in aerobic fitness: Their relationship to physiological response patterns during different types of stress. Psychophysiology. 27:457-478; 1990.
15. de Vries, H.A. Tranquilizer effect of exercise: A critical review. Phys. Sportsmed. 9(11):47-55; 1981.
16. Dishman, R.K. Contemporary sport psychology. Exerc. Sport Sci. Rev. 10:120-159; 1982.
17. Dishman, R.K. Medical psychology in exercise and sport. Med. Clin. North Am. 69(1): 123-143; 1985.
18. Dishman, R.K. Mental health. In: Seefeldt, V., ed. Physical activity and well-being. Reston, VA: AAHPERD; 1986:303-341.
19. Doan, R.E.; Scherman, A. The therapeutic effect of physical fitness on measures of personality: A literature review. J. Counsel. Dev. 66:28-36; 1987.
20. Druckman, D.; Swets, J.A. Enhancing human performance: Issues, theories, and techniques. Washington, DC: National Academy Press; 1988.
21. Felts, W.M.; Vaccaro, P. The effect of aerobic exercise on post-exercise state anxiety and psychophysiological arousal as a function of fitness level. Clin. Kinesiol. (Nov.-Dec.):89-96; 1988.

22. Fillingim, R.B.; Roth, D.L.; Haley, W.E. The effects of distraction on the perception of exercise-induced symptoms. J. Psychosom. Res. 33:241-248; 1989.
23. Folkins, C.H.; Amsterdam, E.A. Control and modification of stress emotions through chronic exercise. In: Amsterdam, E.A.; Wilmore, J.H.; DeMaria, A.N., eds. Exercise and cardiovascular health and disease. New York: Yorke; 1977.
24. Folkins, C.H.; Lynch, S.; Gardner, M.M. Psychological fitness as a function of physical fitness. Arch. Phys. Med. Rehabil. 53:503-508; 1972.
25. Folkins, C.H.; Sime, W.F. Physical fitness training and mental health. Am. Psychol. 36:373-389; 1981.
26. Franks, B.D. Effects of different amounts and kinds of training on selected fitness measures. In: Cureton, T.K., ed. Exercise and fitness. Chicago: Athletic Institute; 1969.
27. Franks, B.D.; Cureton, T.K. Effects of training on time components of the left ventricle. J. Sports Med. Phys. Fitness. 9:80-88; 1969.
28. Franks, B.D.; Jette, M. Manifest anxiety and physical fitness. National College Physical Education Association Men annual proceedings 1970 December; Chicago.
29. Gal, R.; Lazarus, R.S. The role of activity in anticipating and confronting stressful situations. J. Human Stress. (December):4-20; 1975.
30. Gayle, R.C.; Spitler, D.L.; Karper, W.B.; Jaeger, R.M.; Rice, S.N. Psychological changes in exercising COPD patients. Int. J. Rehabil. Res. 11:335-342; 1988.
31. Gettman, L. Effects of different amounts of training on cardiovascular and motor fitness of men. Champaign-Urbana, IL: University of Illinois; 1967. Thesis.
32. Glass, G.V. Integrating findings: The meta-analysis of research. Rev. Res. Educ. 5:351-379; 1978.
33. Goff, G.; Dimsdale, J.E. The psychologic effects of exercise. J. Cardiopulm. Rehabil. 5:234-240; 1985.
34. Hammett, V.B.O. Psychological changes with physical fitness training. Can. Med. Assoc. J. 96:764-769; 1967.
35. Hatfield, B.D. Exercise and mental health: The mechanisms of exercise-induced psychological states. In: Diamant, L., ed. Psychology of sports, exercise, and fitness: Social and personal issues. New York: Hemisphere; 1991:17-49.
36. Hatfield, B.D.; Landers, D.M. Psychophysiology within exercise and sport research: An overview. Exerc. Sport Sci. Rev. 15:351-387; 1987.
37. Hayden, R.M.; Allen, G.L. Relationship between aerobic exercise, anxiety, and depression: Convergent validation by knowledgeable informants. J. Sports Med. 24:69-74; 1984.
38. Hedges, L.V.; Olkin, I. Statistical methods for meta-analysis. New York: Academic Press; 1985.
39. Hughes, J.R. Psychological effects of habitual aerobic exercise: A critical review. Prev. Med. 13:66-78; 1984.
40. Ismail, A.H.; Young, J. The effect of chronic exercise on the personality of middle-age men by univariate and multivariate approaches. J. Hum. Ergol. 2:47-57; 1973.
41. Jasnoski, M.L.; Holmes, D.S. Influence of initial aerobic fitness, aerobic training and changes in aerobic fitness on personality functioning. J. Psychosom. Res. 25:553-556; 1981.
42. Jette, M. Progressive physical training on anxiety in middle-age men. Urbana, IL: University of Illinois; 1967. Thesis.
43. Jette, M. The long-term effects of an exercise program on selected physiological and psychological measures in middle-aged men. Champaign-Urbana, IL: University of Illinois; 1969. Dissertation.
44. Jette, M. Habitual exercisers: A blood serum and personality profile. J. Sports Med. 3:12-17; 1975.
45. King, A.C.; Taylor, C.B.; Haskell, W.L.; DeBusk, R.F. Influence of regular aerobic exercise on psychological health: A randomized, controlled trial of healthy middle-age men. Health Psychol. 8:305-324; 1989.
46. Kraemer, H.C.; Thiemann, S. How many subjects: Statistical power analysis in research. Beverly Hills, CA: Sage; 1987.
47. Kraemer, R.R.; Dzewaltowski, D.A.; Blair, M.S.; Rinehardt, K.F.; Castracane, V.D. Mood alteration from treadmill running and its relationship to beta-endorphin, corticotropin, and growth hormone. J. Sports Med. Phys. Fitness. 30:241-246; 1990.
48. Kugler, J.; Dimsdale, J.E.; Hartley, H.; Sherwood, J. Hospital supervised vs home exercise in cardiac rehabilitation: Effects on aerobic fitness, anxiety, and depression. Arch. Phys. Med. Rehabil. 71:322-325; 1990.
49. Labbe, E.E.; Welsh, M.C.; Delaney, D. Effects of consistent aerobic exercise on the psychological functioning of women. Percept. Mot. Skills. 67:919-925; 1988.
50. Layman, E.M. Psychological effects of physical activity. Exerc. Sport Sci. Rev. 2:33-70; 1974.
51. Martinsen, E.W.; Hoffart, A.; Solberg, O.Y. Aerobic and non-aerobic forms of exercise in

the treatment of anxiety disorders. Stress Med. 5:115-120; 1989.

52. McDonald, D.G.; Hodgdon, J.A. The psychological effects of aerobic training. New York: Springer-Verlag; 1991.
53. McMurray, R.G. Exercise, mood states, and neuroendocrinology. In: Diamant, L., ed. Mind-body maturity: Psychological approaches to sports, exercise and fitness. New York: Hemisphere; 1991:237-253.
54. McPherson, B.D.; Paivio, A.; Yuhasz, M.S.; Rechnitzer, P.A.; Pickard, H.A.; Lefcoe, N.M. Psychological effects of an exercise program for post-infarct and normal adult men. J. Sports Med. Phys. Fitness. 7:95-102; 1967.
55. Mihevic, P.M. Anxiety, depression, and exercise. Quest. 33(2):140-153; 1982.
56. Morgan, W.P. Anxiety reduction following acute physical activity. Psychiatr. Ann. 9(3):141-147; 1979.
57. Morgan, W.P. Psychological benefits of physical activity. In: Nagel, F.J.; Montoye, H.J., eds. Exercise in health and disease. Springfield, IL: Charles C Thomas; 1981.
58. Morgan, W.P. Physical activity and mental health. Am. Acad. Phys. Educ. Papers. 17:132-145; 1983.
59. Morgan, W.P. Affective beneficence of vigorous physical activity. Med. Sci. Sports Exerc. 17:94-100; 1985.
60. Morgan, W.P.; Goldston, S.N., editors. Exercise and mental health. Washington, DC: Hemisphere; 1987.
61. Morgan, W.P.; Hammer, W.M. Influence of competitive wrestling upon state anxiety. Med. Sci. Sports. 6:58-61; 1974.
62. Morgan, W.P.; Roberts, J.A.; Feinerman, A.D. Psychological effect of acute physical activity. Phys. Med. Rehabil. 52:422-425; 1971.
63. Moses, J.; Steptoe, A.; Mathews, A.; Edwards, S. The effects of exercise training on mental well-being in the normal population: A controlled trial. J. Psychosom. Res. 33:47-61; 1989.
64. Naughton, J.; Bruhn, J.G.; Lategola, M.T. Effects of physical training on physiologic and behavioral characteristics of cardiac patients. Arch. Phys. Med. Rehabil. 49:131-137; 1968.
65. Negy, S.; Frazier, S. The impact of exercise on locus of control, self-esteem and mood scales. J. Soc. Behav. Pers. 3:263-268; 1988.
66. Netz, Y.; Tennenbaum, G.; Sagiv, M. Pattern of psychological fitness as related to pattern of physical fitness among older adults. Percept. Mot. Skills. 67:647-655; 1988.
67. Norris, R.; Carroll, D.; Cochrane, R. The effect of physical activity and exercise training on psychological stress and well-being in an adolescent population. J. Psychosom. Res. 36:55-65; 1992.
68. Petruzzello, S.J. An examination of proposed physiological and psychological mechanisms for exercise-related reductions in anxiety. Tempe, AZ: Arizona State University; 1991. Dissertation.
69. Petruzzello, S.J.; Landers, D.M.; Hatfield, B.D.; Kubitz, K.A.; Salazar, W. A meta-analysis on the anxiety-reducing effects of acute and chronic exercise. Sports Med. 11:143-182; 1991.
70. Phelps, J.R. Physical activity and health maintenance—Exactly what is known? West. J. Med. 146:200-206; 1987.
71. Pistacchio, T.; Weinberg, R.; Jackson, A. The development of a psychobiologic profile of individuals who experience and those who do not experience exercise related mood enhancement. J. Sport Behav. 12:151-165; 1989.
72. Pitts, F.N.; McClure, J.N., Jr. Lactate metabolism in anxiety neurosis. N. Engl. J. Med. 277:1329-1336; 1967.
73. Raglin, J.S.; Morgan, W.P. Influence of vigorous exercise on mood states. Behav. Ther. 8:179-183; 1985.
74. Raglin, J.S.; Morgan, W.P. Influence of exercise and quiet rest on state anxiety and blood pressure. Med. Sci. Sports Exerc. 19:456-463; 1987.
75. Renfrow, N.E.; Bolton, B. Personality characteristics associated with aerobic exercise in adult males. J. Pers. Assess. 43:261-266; 1979.
76. Rosenthal, R. Meta-analytic procedures for social research. London: Sage; 1991.
77. Roth, D.L. Acute emotional and psychological effects of aerobic exercise. Psychophysiology. 26:593-602; 1989.
78. Roth, D.L.; Bachtler, S.D.; Fillingim, R.B. Acute emotional and cardiovascular effects of stressful mental work during aerobic exercise. Psychophysiology. 27:694-701; 1990.
79. Roth, D.L.; Holmes, D.S. Influence of physical fitness in determining the impact of stressful life events on physical and psychological health. Psychosom. Med. 47:164-173; 1985.
80. Roth, D.L.; Holmes, D.S. Influence of aerobic exercise training and relaxation training on physical and psychologic health following stressful life events. Psychosom. Med. 49:355-365; 1987.
81. Rubenstein, L.K.; May, T.M.; Bonn, M.B.; Batts, V.A. Physical health and stress in entering dental students. J. Dent. Educ. 53:545-547; 1989.
82. Ryan, A.J. Exercise is medicine. Phys. Sportsmed. 11:10; 1983.

83. Sage, G. Motor learning and control. Dubuque, IA: Brown; 1984.
84. Scharr, P. Effects of training on the physique and cholesterol of women. Urbana, IL: University of Illinois; 1969. Thesis.
85. Seemann, J.C. Changes in state anxiety following vigorous exercise. Tucson, AZ: University of Arizona; 1978. Thesis.
86. Sexton, H.; Maere, A.; Dahl, N.H. Exercise intensity and reduction in neurotic symptoms. Acta Psychiatr. Scand. 80:231-235; 1989.
87. Sharp, M.W.; Reilley, R.R. The relationship of aerobic physical fitness to selected personality traits. J. Clin. Psychol. 31:428-430; 1975.
88. Sime, W.E. A comparison of exercise and meditation in reducing physiological response to stress. Med. Sci. Sports. 9:55; 1977.
89. Sime, W.E. Psychological benefits of exercise training in the healthy individual. In: Herd, J.A.; Miller, N.E.; Weiss, S.M., eds. Behavioral health: A handbook of health enhancement and disease prevention. New York: Wiley; 1984:488-508.
90. Simono, R.B. Exercise and mental health: The mechanisms of exercise-induced psychological states. In: Diamant, L., ed. Psychology of sports, exercise, and fitness: Social and personal issues. New York: Hemisphere; 1991:51-66.
91. Simons, C.W.; Birkimer, J.C. An exploration of factors predicting the effects of aerobic conditioning on mood state. J. Psychosom. Res. 32:63-75; 1988.
92. Smith, R.E. Conceptual and statistical issues in research involving multidimensional anxiety scales. J. Sport Exerc. Psychol. 11:452-457; 1989.
93. Steptoe, A.; Edwards, S.; Moses, J.; Mathews, A. The effects of exercise training on mood and perceived coping ability in anxious adults from the general population. J. Psychosom. Res. 33:537-547; 1989.
94. Stern, M.J.; Cleary, P. National exercise and heart disease project: Psychosocial changes observed during a low-level exercise program. Arch. Intern. Med. 141:1463-1467; 1981.
95. Stern, M.J.; Cleary, P. The national exercise and heart disease project: Long-term psychosocial outcomes. Arch. Intern. Med. 142:1093-1097; 1982.
96. Stern, M.J.; Gorman, P.A.; Kaslow, L. The group counseling v exercise therapy study: A controlled intervention with subjects following myocardial infarction. Arch. Intern. Med. 143:1719-1725; 1983.
97. Taylor, C.B.; Houston-Miller, N.; Ahn, D.K.; Haskell, W.; DeBusk, D.K. The effects of exercise training programs on psychosocial improvement in uncomplicated postmyocardial infarction patients. J. Psychosom. Res. 30:581-587; 1986.
98. Tharp, G.D.; Carson, W.H. Emotional changes in rats following chronic exercise. Med. Sci. Sports. 7:123-126; 1975.
99. Thomas, J.R.; Nelson, J.K. Research methods in physical education. 2nd ed. Champaign, IL: Human Kinetics; 1990.
100. Tillman, K. Relationship between physical fitness and selected personality traits. Res. Q. 36:483-489; 1965.
101. Tipton, C.M. Exercise, training and hypertension: An update. Exerc. Sport Sci. Rev. 19:447-505; 1991.
102. Tuson, K.M.; Sinyor, D. On the affective benefits of acute aerobic exercise: Taking stock after twenty years of research. In: Seraganian, P., ed. Exercise psychology: The influence of physical exercise in psychological processes. New York: Wiley; 1992:80-121.
103. Van Andel, G.E.; Austin, D.R. Physical fitness and mental health: A review of the literature. Adapt. Phys. Educ. Q. 1:207-220; 1984.
104. van Dixhoorn, J.; Duivenvoorden, H.J.; Pool, J.; Verhage, F. Psychic effects of physical training and relaxation therapy after myocardial infarction. J. Psychosom. Res. 34:327-337; 1990.
105. Walsh, R.; Davidson, G.P. Desensitization to lactic acid as a possible mechanism mediating the therapeutic effect of physical exercise on anxiety neurosis. J. Sports Med. 20:158-160; 1980.
106. Weber, J.C.; Lee, R.A. Effects of differing prepuberty exercise programs on the emotionality of male albino rats. Res. Q. 39:748-751; 1968.
107. Wells, H.P. Relationship between physical fitness and psychological variables. Urbana, IL: University of Illinois; 1958. Dissertation.
108. Wilfley, D.; Kunce, J. Differential physical and psychological effects of exercise. J. Counsel. Psychol. 33:337-342; 1986.
109. Wilson, V.E.; Berger, B.G.; Bird, E.I. Effects of running and of an exercise class on anxiety. Percept. Mot. Skills. 53:472-474; 1981.
110. Wilson, V.E.; Morley, N.C.; Bird, E.I. Mood profiles of marathon runners, joggers and non-exercisers. Percept. Mot. Skills. 50:117-118; 1980.
111. Young, R.J.; Ismail, A.H. Personality differences of adult men before and after a physical fitness program. Res. Q. 47:513-519; 1976.

Chapter 60

Physical Activity, Fitness, and Compulsive Behaviors

Janet Polivy

Most of the chapters in this volume document the physical and psychological benefits of exercise. However, there are a number of reports that correlate embarking on a fitness program with a compulsive or driven quality to the activity and the possible harmful effects of excessive exercising. Compulsive behavior usually refers clinically to behavior that is done to relieve intense anxiety and that the individual feels unable to control. That definition is appropriate for what has been termed a *negative addiction* to exercising, in which the person continues to exercise at what many consider an excessive level, often despite injury, inconvenience, or interference with other aspects of one's life.

Morgan (39) was one of the first to point out that sports medicine specialists have been seeing an increasing number of overuse injuries, and that for some the benefits of running or other exercise may be somewhat offset by what appears to be a negative addiction. De Coverley Veale (14) proposed that exercise dependence be included as a dependence syndrome in DSM-IV because it meets the usual criteria for dependence or addiction. This negative addiction syndrome has been contrasted with a more popular view of compulsive exercising as a positive addiction because of its salutary effects on self-esteem and mood. Many case studies and several experiments have documented the appearance of withdrawal symptoms, self-destructive exercising because the individual cannot go without an exercise "fix," and other evidence of an addiction or compulsion to exercise.

These studies will be reviewed and evaluated to facilitate conclusions about the threat posed by such a negative addiction to physical activity. It should be noted that short-term experimental studies wherein exercise is introduced in one group of subjects but not in a control group frequently find improvements in general well-being and other measures in the exercise group. Such studies will not be reviewed here, however, because their short duration is insufficient to detect an addictive or compulsive process. Addiction to activity presumably takes some time to build and become problematic.

Another focus of research on compulsive fitness training has been the hyperactive behavior of many eating disorder patients, particularly those with *anorexia nervosa*. These patients are frequently observed to drive themselves to exercise in a compulsive manner, presumably in order to burn calories and lose weight. The question of causality (Does exercise cause anorexia nervosa, or does anorexia nervosa induce hyperactivity?) has been discussed and investigated and will be reviewed here as well.

It should be remembered that the question being addressed here is whether or not physical activity contributes to the development of dysfunctional compulsive behavior in *some* of those who pursue fitness. This is not to say that fitness should be discouraged or is dangerous for the majority of people. Both anorexia nervosa patients and compulsive exercisers or "negative addicts" represent a pathological extreme. In all studies of these populations it is clear that there are individuals who exercise to lose weight or to achieve elevated mood and self-esteem, but who do not become compulsive about their activity. There is thus a range of compulsiveness connected to physical activity, with some individuals crossing a hypothetical line between what is normal and acceptable and what is destructive or pathological. This review will attempt to evaluate the extent of this pathology.

The studies to be reviewed here were collected through computer searches and scanning of recent Current Contents. They can be divided into three types: (a) true experiments, (b) questionnaire studies, and (c) case studies. In addition, there are a number of conceptual and empirically based review papers.

Studies of Addiction to Exercising

Experimental Studies

The initial experiment on addiction to exercising began as an attempt to study the effects of exercise deprivation in regular exercisers (1). Baekeland (1) was struck by the difficulty he encountered in trying to find regular exercisers willing to deprive themselves of exercise for 1 month. He finally convinced 14 college students who exercised 3 to 4 days per week to participate for money. (Those who exercised 5 to 6 days a week refused to be in the study because they were unwilling to stop exercising for the month of study.) Sleep was studied during an exercise period and during restriction from activity. Subjective reports and sleep recordings both indicated that exercise abstinence was stressful for subjects; there was evidence of increased anxiety and arousal. This was the first time anyone had noted what seemed to be a compulsive need to exercise and the presence of physical and psychological symptoms when exercise was prevented.

The next experimental study of the effects of running and abstinence from regular (5 days a week) exercise was reported more than a decade later in habitual runners (61). One day (24 hr) of deprivation was compared with no deprivation on anxiety, depression, fatigue, and vigor. Unfortunately, the pretesting of half of the 33 faculty, staff, and student volunteers on the galvanic skin response (GSR) test appeared to have influenced the results not only on GSR, but mood as well. The nonpretested group, however, showed the expected deleterious effects of 24 hr of deprivation of running on mood (and elevated GSR). Interestingly, the author interpreted this to indicate that running should be used to treat obsessive-compulsives, to reduce their anxiety and provide "a productive outlet for compulsiveness." Some might argue, however, that running is contraindicated for such subjects as it might encourage their compulsiveness.

The unpleasant withdrawal symptoms associated with exercise deprivation were manipulated by prohibiting and then allowing exercise (to produce and then alleviate withdrawal) (42). Expectations of how easy it would be to stop running for 2 weeks, how much this would affect subjects' lives, how addicted they thought they were, and other cognitions were assessed for each subject along with questionnaires and an exercise diary. Scores on the General Health Questionnaire (GHQ), somatic symptoms, anxiety and insomnia, and social dysfunction scales were all elevated in the deprived group during deprivation weeks. The deprived group also reported feeling more depressed and anxious after their second week of not running. Thus, stress and physical symptoms appeared right away but emotional disturbance appeared only after a longer period of deprivation.

This suggests that the results are not just a demand effect and supports the notion that withdrawal of exercise leads to both immediate and more delayed withdrawal symptoms. It is possible that this represents merely a return to the "prerunning" state, insofar as deprivation removes the benefits of running. Running may have been used as an antidepressant or anxiolytic, which gradually wears off when the activity ceases; the observed effects on depression and anxiety support this interpretation. It took a little time for the depression and anxiety to subside when running was resumed, though there was no longer a significant elevation after one week. Avoidance of withdrawal symptoms may thus motivate continued running.

Controlled experiments have been performed to assess the effects of fitness and exercise on psychological state, but evidence for addiction and compulsive behavior was neither sought nor apparently found (e.g., 43,44).

Questionnaire and Interview Studies of Addiction to Exercising

Investigators have conducted many questionnaire studies comparing exercisers with nonexercisers on personality and demographic variables. Such studies generally find little difference between athletes and nonathletes at worst, and healthier personalities in the athletes (usually runners) at best (e.g., 17,33,40,41,49; see 16 or 22 for reviews), although one study on young long-distance runners found some causes for concern (45). The subjects chosen for study were usually small convenience samples that were not truly representative of the full population of athletes and nonathletes of various ages and sexes, the studies were mostly cross-sectional rather than longitudinal, and the selection of personality measures was fairly arbitrary. As a result, these studies are not especially informative. Furthermore, these studies did not address compulsive or addictive aspects of exercising.

An interesting series of clinical studies predated and anticipated the current interest in addiction to physical activity. Little (36,37) noted that male neurotic psychiatric patients seemed to fall into two categories, overvaluers of athletics (*athletic neurotics*) and nonathletes. He compared these patients with matched nonneurotic males. The neurotic athletic personality was found in 39% of the neurotic patients but only 9% of controls. The athletic neurotics differed from the nonathletic neurotics in the precipitant of their neurosis—athletic neurotics had usually succumbed to some sort of threat to physical well-being (illness or injury), whereas this was rarely a precursor in nonathletes. Although the two neurotic groups had similar depressive and anxiety syndromes, the athletes were more likely to have panic attacks and hypochondriacal symptoms. Little notes that the premorbid personalities of the neurotic athletes were significantly more healthy than those of the nonathletic neurotics, and not different from the normal controls. It seems as if the exaggerated athleticism was masking or replacing neurotic characteristics until around midlife when an injury or illness interfered with this coping mechanism.

Little also notes that the prevalence of this athletic neurosis in his general psychiatric practice was 9% of all male patients, a figure comparable to that for schizophrenia or depression. The prognosis for these patients was also poorer than that for nonathletic neurotics. Little concluded that this syndrome is neither rare nor trivial and represents a deprivation or bereavement reaction to the loss of a significant aspect of one's identity. He suggests that athleticism in and of itself is not problematic, but overvaluation of physical prowess may make individuals vulnerable to this neurotic syndrome in the course of natural aging as approaching mortality is faced.

As early as 1970 it was recognized that exercise could have addictive qualities for some (1). Whereas such addiction was initially seen as positive because exercise had beneficial effects on the individual (25), it was soon noted that being addicted to physical activity could also have negative consequences (38). Aspects of addiction to exercising were assessed in a large sample of runners (9) with a commitment to running scale. Both euphoria or "spinning free" and withdrawal or discomfort when a run was missed correlated with commitment to running.

An epidemiologic study of the benefits and risks of running identified quitting smoking and weight loss as benefits, and injuries, dog bites, collisions with vehicles, and being hit by thrown objects as risks encountered by their sample (30). People continued to run despite these risks.

A recent study (27) compared people with temporary and chronic injuries to healthy people on determinants of walking and exercise. A random sample of residences in San Diego, California, surveyed by mail, produced 2,053 usable questionnaires. A reasonable number (39%) reported vigorous exercise at least 3 times per week. The amount and nature of activity performed by the ill or injured was compared to that of healthy subjects. As expected, healthy people reported doing the most aerobic exercise, followed by those with a temporary injury. But subjects who must constrain their activity because of illness or injury still reported a considerable amount of physical activity and walking. This supports De Coverley Veale's (14) observation that exercise-addicted individuals remain active even when they are injured or ill and are most likely to be identified through a persistent sport injury.

In the last decade, investigations into the psychological and addictive effects of running and other physical activity have become more common. For example, the experience of euphoria or *runner's high* and the less pleasant *hitting the wall* phenomenon have been taken beyond anecdotal reports through questionnaire assessments of large samples of marathon runners (e.g., 59,60). These studies also indicated that more than 35% of such high-activity subjects report negative effects of their exercise, but persisted nonetheless. Marital strain, injuries, psychological problems such as irritability and obsession with running, interference with work, and lack of time for other activities were reported by significant numbers (36%) of marathon runners (59), and 82% acknowledged at least some level of addiction to running. Females were even more likely to report being addicted than were male runners. These authors speculated that the pain of running long distances may be utilized as some sort of narcissistic, masochistic way to improve self-esteem and gain social approval.

Others have tried to identify personality characteristics that would predict who would become addicted to physical activity (53,54), but level of addiction did not seem to be strongly correlated with any of the investigated personality variables. Frequency of jogging was actually found to be associated with a less addictive personality profile on an addictiveness questionnaire (joggers were comparable to controls and scored lower than alcoholics or gamblers), but joggers did score higher on a compulsiveness scale, particularly the subscales measuring order and regularity, and detail and perfectionism (28). Frequent joggers thus appeared to be compulsive rather than addictive persons.

An attempt to quantify specifically the negative addiction to exercise was made (26). Scores on a negative addiction scale increased with length of running history, indicating a possible progression through stages of addiction. It should be noted however that even among the runners who had run the longest, some scored low on the negative addiction scale. It is thus important to identify what produces negative addiction and who is most likely to develop the problem.

A more recent attempt at a negative addiction scale (52) developed and tested two forms, leading to a final form with 17 3-choice Likert items. A sample of 244 male and 244 female marathon runners were sent questionnaires, and 202 (98 men, 104 women) completed all items. About half had been running 5 years or longer. Addiction level correlated negatively with self-esteem and positively with anxiety. The authors divided addiction scores into tertiles and looked at injury rates and found them also to be significantly related to addiction.

Thompson and Blanton's (62) review of the literature demonstrated that energy balance mechanisms are affected by food restriction and exercise, leading them to propose a model of exercise dependence based on sympathetic arousal. Reductions in sympathetic output to exercise might mediate dependence, requiring heightened levels of training to produce the same arousal or output as at pretraining. This theory still needs to be tested and confirmed empirically, as the current evidence is somewhat contradictory. (Table 60.1 summarizes these studies.)

Case Studies of Addiction to Exercise

Case reports provide some illustrative data on both the compulsive nature of addicted exercisers and potential causal factors. Morgan used eight case studies to illustrate the negative aspects of exercise addiction (39). He defined addiction as present if the person feels compelled to exercise daily and feels unable to live without it and when deprived of exercise, experiences withdrawal symptoms including anxiety, irritability, and depression. Negative addiction also leads to deterioration of interpersonal relations at home, work, and social settings. Other symptoms often present include restlessness, insomnia, fatigue, tics, muscle tension and soreness, decreased appetite, and irregularity; in other words, a reversal of the usual benefits of exercise. The true addict continues to exercise despite medical, social, and vocational contraindications. As with drug addiction, the exercise addict also must increase the "dosage" or amount of activity to get the same high. Morgan concludes that it is excessive activity that promotes addiction and cautions moderation in exercising.

Sacks (55) provides a case that suggests that periods of emotional stress may provoke addiction to exercise. Physical activity is described as a coping response to losses to self-esteem or emotional distress that may become obsessive when stress increases (e.g., Little's athletic neurotics). In a similar vein two cases were reported of obsessive exercising becoming full-blown psychotic episodes (15). In these two women, running had been used to shore up shaky self-concepts and to defend against serious depression. When these attempts at pseudoidentity failed or the stress of particularly strenuous running was unendurable, these women lost control of themselves and became psychotic. Overexercising thus may not be an ideal long-term solution to life stress.

Yates (68,69) presents cases of exercise addiction based on a large number of in-depth interviews. She encountered a number of runners who seemed obliged or compelled to run. They were attempting to control their bodies through exercise, but became obsessed with physical activity. Their lives revolved around doing the activity, thinking about it, reevaluating past performances of it, and planning future occasions. These athletes continued exercising despite discomfort from bad weather or physical pain, injuries from car accidents or thrown objects, job and interpersonal losses because of time spent exercising, or activity-induced injury. When prevented from exercising by serious illness or injury, these athletes described serious depressive reactions, anxiety, and sensations that their bodies were deteriorating or fragmenting. Yates did note, though, that these pathological, obligatory runners are a minority of the committed runners she interviewed over a period of about 7 years. The obligatory runners also seem to perceive benefits from their activity that compensate for the costs and keep them involved in exercising.

Finally, Waldstreicher (64) told of a patient who was seen in the hospital for a suspicious hip fracture for which the doctor wanted to do a bone biopsy. The real cause of the patient's injury and pain was 2 to 3 hr per day of exercise, which she did not stop even when she (a nurse!) knew she was injured. Her fear of gaining weight motivated this excessive exercising, although the patient was normal weight. The author concluded that the patient's excessive exercising and fear of fatness actually reflected anorexia nervosa.

Negative Addiction to Exercise: Conclusion

Some athletes apparently feel compelled to exercise, even when they acknowledge that the activity is harmful to them. Case reports, surveys, and studies of committed athletes all concur that significant numbers of exercisers report continuing with their exercise despite pain, interference with significant relationships or work, lack of time for other leisure pursuits, recognized obsession with the activity, and other psychological problems. In addition, those who seem addicted to activity also show compulsive behaviors around this activity, maintaining rigid schedules of training, ritualized

Table 60.1 Studies of Negative Addiction to Exercise

Study	Sample	Type	Measures	Findings
Baekeland (1)	14 college-age male runners	Experimental: 30-day exercise deprivation	Anxiety, arousal, REM, sexual tension, sleep, appetite	All worsened when exercise withdrawn
Thaxton (61)	33 faculty, staff, and students	Experimental: 24-hr exercise deprivation	GSR, anxiety, depression, fatigue, vigor	All worsened when exercise withdrawn
Morris et al. (42)	Marathon runners	Experimental: 2-week exercise deprivation	Anxiety, depression, GHQ, exercise diary	GHQ scores worse during deprivation; anxiety, depression worse after second week of deprivation
Little (36,37)	Male neurotic psychiatric patients	Correlational	Interviews	Athletic neurotics = 9% of patients; poorer prognosis
Carmack & Martens (9)	Runners	Correlational	Commitment to running scale	Euphoria and withdrawal related to commitment
Sachs (53)	Regular exercisers	Correlational	Personality scales, level of addiction scale	No relation found between personality and level of addiction
Hailey & Bailey (26)	Male runners in 5-mile race	Correlational	Length of running, negative addiction scale	History of running related to negative addiction symptoms
Summers et al. (59,60)	Male and female marathon runners	Correlational	Questionnaires	36% report negative effects of exercise (marital strain, injury, psychological problems, no time for others) and addiction
Kagan (28)	Joggers	Correlational	Addictive personality scale, compulsiveness scale	Frequency of jogging related to less addictive personality, jogging related to compulsiveness
Rudy & Estok (52)	98 male, 104 female marathon runners	Correlational	17-item, 3-choice Likert negative addiction scale, self-esteem scale, anxiety, injury	Addiction level correlated negatively with self-esteem, positively with anxiety; positively related to injury rates
Hofstetter et al. (27)	2,053 respondents to random survey	Correlational	Questionnaire on injury, illness, amount and nature of activity	Healthy subjects exercised most, followed by temporarily injured. Even those with illness or injury did physical activities

Note. REM = rapid eye movement; GSR = galvanic skin response; GHQ = general health questionnaire.

warm-up routines, obsessive record keeping about activity levels, and guilt about missing a scheduled activity session. This obviously represents compulsive behavior, but little information is available about it. More investigations into this sort of compulsivity around exercise are needed.

There is a greater tendency for exercise abuse in some who are probably predisposed to psychological disturbance, especially those without a strong self-identity (16). Cross-sectional studies do not show an increase in psychopathology though, so the incidence of this may be low, or it may be specific to a small number of individuals. Exercise can, despite its generally salutary effects, become a compulsive activity for some individuals.

Studies Relating Exercise and Symptomatology of Eating Disorders

Some have argued that addiction to exercise is merely a variant of anorexia nervosa (e.g., 69) whereas others (e.g., 14) distinguish between primary exercise dependence and that which is secondary to a preexisting eating disorder. Excessive exercise may be the presenting feature of an eating disorder, but this seems to represent secondary dependence, with the eating disorder the primary diagnosis. Self-induced weight or fat loss is also present in many dependent exercisers as a means of improving performance, but no morbid preoccupation with weight is present in these individuals, distinguishing them from those with an eating disorder. Social pressure to reduce fat in young athletes may, however, contribute to the development of anorexia nervosa (14). Questionnaire and case studies have been used to explore these issues.

Questionnaire Studies of Obligatory Exercise and Eating Disorder Symptomatology

Increased physical activity has for some time been recognized as a feature of anorexia nervosa during the dieting and weight loss stage of the disorder (32) and is usually explained as part of the patient's conscious effort to lose weight. One early study (32) tried to assess the prevalence and nature of hyperactivity in anorexics before, during, and after hospitalization for the disorder using patients' hospital charts; they then followed up all anorexics discharged more than 1 year previously. The charts probably underreported hyperactivity insofar as an intake physician would not have been looking for this at intake. The lack of opportunity for sports or formal activity in the hospital may also make the chart notes an inadequate reflection of true activity level—pacing may be seen as aimless rather than exercise, and actual exercising in the patient's room may not be seen. The authors assumed if no mention of hyperactivity appeared in the chart, no abnormality was present. There was no control group of normal women to which to compare patients' activity, and nothing but subjective reporting was used.

Despite these potential underreporting biases, 25 out of 33 patients were described as hyperactive before or during hospitalization, whereas only 1 was noted to have an unremarkable activity level. No correlation was found between reported activity level and weight or amount of weight lost. Of the 25 hyperactive patients, 21 were described as extremely active before they had ever even dieted or lost weight. In all 15 of the patients followed after discharge, hyperactivity during hospitalization had been marked; 11 were still hyperactive at follow-up (1 who died had had an unknown activity level). Three had recently subsided to normal activity levels but described this as exhaustion, not real normalization. Only 1 felt her currently normal activity level was due to total improvement in her eating disorder.

The patients described their activity both before and after their weight loss as usually goal-directed, organized, and planned (tightly scheduled and rigidly carried out). Activity during active weight loss, though, was described as intense and driven, but more disorganized, less goal-directed, and done alone. At that time they reported feeling unable to sit still or to sleep. The authors concluded that starvation produces abnormal increased motor behavior that is poorly organized on top of a prior hyperactivity in anorexic patients. Hyperactivity may thus be one of the earliest signs of anorexia nervosa and one of the last to remit. It seemed to be independent of denial, starvation, or a conscious attempt to work off calories. Beumont, Booth, Abraham, Griffiths, and Turner (2) supported this to some extent in their examination of the symptoms of their anorexic patients. They looked at the temporal sequence of symptoms and found that dieting came first and increased activity was usually next, very early in the development of the disorder.

A team of researchers interested in anorexia nervosa discovered an elevated incidence of it in ballet dancers (23,24). They looked in particular at dancers who are required to exercise a great deal and pay attention to their body size and shape. It was predicted that more anorexia nervosa would be found in these dancers. Higher mean scores were indeed found on an eating disorder pathology questionnaire, and almost 30% of the dancers scored in the anorexic range. Competition was also a factor, with more pathology found in the more competitive dance schools. These were the first studies to find a connection between anorexia nervosa and exercise by looking at the exercisers; however, not all women exposed to these pressures to be thin, to exercise, and to compete develop anorexia nervosa. The connection is more complex than a simple, causal one.

Athletes in sports that do or do not emphasize leanness were compared to nonathletes to investigate the degree of preoccupation with weight and other tendencies toward eating disorders (5). There were no differences between athletes and nonathletes on either measure when athletes were combined into one group, but when those in sports emphasizing thinness were separated from those whose sports did not focus on body size, the "lean" athletes were significantly more likely to show weight preoccupation or potential eating disorder pathology.

Looking only at the presence of the specific eating disorder symptom of *amenorrhea* in female athletes (which is reviewed more completely as a separate topic in this symposium) (see 8 for a review), many studies have documented that female athletes heavily involved in any type of athletic activity are at significant risk of developing menstrual irregularities.

Female ballet dancers were assessed on menstrual cycles, weight, height, on measures of eating pathology, and self-image (7). Thirty-three percent reported having had an eating problem (17% had had anorexia nervosa, 21% had had bulimia nervosa). Dancers with oligomenorrhea, amenorrhea, or normal cycles were compared to each other. The amenorrheic dancers weighed less and were leaner than the oligomenorrheic or normal-cycle dancers, had higher eating pathology scores, were more likely to have had anorexia nervosa, and had a more labile emotional tone and greater psychopathology than the other two groups. The authors concluded that these correlations support the idea that amenorrhea in athletes also seems to be associated with eating problems and dieting behavior, especially for athletes in events where low body weight is desirable.

Similarly, a comparison of adolescents who engaged in three sports differing in the body size and shape preferred in each and in the amount of energy expended in training examined the effect of exercise on dieting, weight concerns, menarcheal age, and self-image (6). Figure skating and ballet have weight requirements (extreme thinness) but swimming does not. Female athletes aged 14 to 18 years (elite competitive figure skaters, ballet dancers, and swimmers) were compared to female nonathletes from private schools. Eating pathology, perfectionism, and age of menarche were assessed. Dancers and skaters were lighter than the others, as well as shorter and leaner. Dancers and skaters had higher scores for dieting, bulimia, perfectionism, menarcheal age, and oral control, and dancers had higher dieting and lower oral-control scores than did skaters. Swimmers did not differ from nonathletic control subjects on these variables. Sports emphasizing thin body shape thus seem more likely to engender compulsive dieting behaviors.

The weight-control techniques used by competitive female intercollegiate athletes from two midwestern universities in the United States were investigated (50). The authors assessed vomiting, use of laxatives, diuretics, and diet pills for weight loss, binges, weight loss below goal, injuries, and perceived performance compared to teammates. Vomiting and laxative abuse were reported by 14% and 16% of the women; diet pills were used by 25%. Use of at least one of these pathogenic weight-control techniques was acknowledged by 32% of the subjects. Continued weight loss was mostly a result of a fear of losing control of one's eating.

Most of the 30 athletes who completed a follow-up survey said that their concern about weight was related to athletic performance rather than toward enhancing appearance. The athletes did not realize that these pathogenic weight-control techniques could lead to adverse physical consequences for them. Older athletes and coaches were frequently role models who encouraged these techniques and reassured the athletes that no harm would result from their use. It should be noted that it was not only gymnasts and distance runners who showed these behaviors—one golfer, a swimmer, tennis players, field hockey players (1/2 the team), and softball players all acknowledged using one or more of these pathogenic weight-control techniques. The authors conclude that any feedback to an athlete that she is too fat may trigger these sorts of pathological dietary practices.

Similar results were found with competitive swimmers aged 9 to 18 years (19), who revealed themselves as likely to misperceive themselves as overweight (especially the girls) and who based their decisions to change their weights on these misperceptions and on others' opinions of their weights. A number (15.4%) of the girls and even some of the boys (3.6%) used pathogenic weight-loss techniques. Weight concerns were prevalent among the female swimmers, even among those who were normal or underweight and were more tied to appearance than to performance. Compulsive dieting is thus prevalent among athletes even when thin body shape is not a focus of the sport.

A recent study examined both amenorrhea and disturbed eating practices in female bodybuilders (presumably motivated to manipulate their diet and exercise to minimize fat and maximize muscle mass) (63) to see if there is a tendency for higher menstrual irregularity in this group. Weight lifters were more likely to have menstrual disorders than were college student controls, particularly competitive lifters, although this was not related to percent body fat. Eating Disorder Inventory scores were all normal, but weight lifters scored significantly higher on drive for thinness than did controls. Eating behavior also did not differ between the three groups, although there were significantly more former anorexics among the weight lifters than among controls. Overall, there was little report of drastic weight control behavior in these subjects despite the fact that 67% of the competitors acknowledged being terrified of fat and 58% reported that they were obsessed with food. (These percentages were also higher in noncompetitive weight lifters than controls.) Laxative use was also higher in weight lifters than in controls, but no diagnosable eating disorders were found in any of the subjects. This finding accords with other reports of drastic dieting measures in athletes.

Eating disorder patients have disturbed body images as well as eating disturbances, so these characteristics were investigated in male and female obligatory runners, weight lifters, and sedentary controls (47). Runners and controls overestimated their body size more than did weight lifters. Runners and weight lifters had more drive for thinness (on the Eating Disorder Inventory) than did controls, and females scored higher than males. Females also had higher body dissatisfaction scores, and female runners and controls were higher than the males in those groups. Female runners were more dissatisfied with their general appearance than were male runners. Weight lifters were more accurate at size estimation (but saw themselves more often in mirrors in lifting rooms than did the other subjects). Females were not significantly worse than males at size estimation.

There has also been an upsurge of interest in (and studies on) a direct comparison of the personality characteristics of athletes and eating disorder patients. This was sparked by an article (69) that combined a questionnaire survey with case history reports to study the thesis presented earlier (57) that male obligatory runners resemble anorexia nervosa patients in many respects. This article was heavily criticized as having no pertinent data, poor methodology, no relevance to the majority of runners, an overreliance on extreme individuals, and overstating the similarities between the groups (31,34,58,66). Yates replied (67) that this article was meant to be only a preliminary study suggesting the need for further research. Many more case studies were presented in response (see section later in this chapter), and many questionnaire studies were conducted comparing athletes, particularly runners, to eating disorder patients.

One of the first responses to Yates and colleagues' proposal tested their notion that obligatory runners and anorexics share personality traits (3,4) by comparing anorexia nervosa patients and obligatory runners. The patients were examined in their first 2 weeks of hospitalization, and the runners were recruited from campus newspapers and local races and assessed on the Obligatory Running Scale. Patients differed from runners on 8 of 10 clinical Minnesota Multiphasic Inventory subscales (scoring higher) and were lower than runners on an ego-strength scale. More patients also had at least one score in the abnormal range than did runners; the runners generally had normal profiles, but among the patients only 5 of 24 did so.

So no support was found here for the contention that runners resemble anorexia nervosa patients psychologically. Patients had almost four times the level of psychopathology that runners evidenced. In fact, the data from the runners supported the contention that those who exercise regularly are essentially well-adjusted and cope with stress well. Even when the data were reanalyzed to examine only the most dedicated group of runners, no evidence of psychopathology or abnormal personality was discovered (4). The authors acknowledge (3) that there may have been a somewhat biased sample of runners in this study since there were several world class runners in the sample. Also, none had ever been referred for treatment of any kind. Finally, the authors point out that for anorexic patients, exercise most likely is a means to an end (weight control), but for obligatory runners it is an end in itself.

This study was criticized (18) on the grounds that the original paper (69) proposed four areas of similarity between anorexia nervosa and obligatory running, but Blumenthal, O'Toole, and Chang (3) examined only one of these, which is not sufficient to allow for rejecting the analogy. Moreover, the selection bias in the Blumenthal et al. (3) study may be more serious than the authors acknowledge. Not only were these world class runners, but they were healthy, well-functioning individuals being compared to hospitalized psychiatric patients. Also the long-distance runners selected were not necessarily pathological or obligatory runners. Just as not all dieters become anorexic, not all runners become addicted to running; so the patients should be compared to addicted runners.

Female runners were compared with college student controls on measures of eating disorder pathology to find the incidence of anorexia nervosa (65). There were no group differences overall. High eating pathology scores were most prevalent in an elite marathon subgroup and lowest in general marathoners; however these differences were not reliable. Among the high scorers 89% had moderate to high mass:height ratios, so it was concluded that running may be a substitute for anorexia nervosa and may help some individuals to avoid the full clinical syndrome. It must be remembered, however, that the incidence of anorexia nervosa was no higher among these competitive runners than in the general population.

A set of studies by Davis (12,13) examined the relation of exercise to body image and weight- and diet-preoccupation in college women. One study looked at avid female exercisers to see if they are more narcissistic about their bodies and if they emphasize their appearance more than do comparable nonexercisers (12). Few differences were found, although exercisers reported that the way they feel about their body is important to the way they feel about themselves, and their emotional well-being was correlated with body dissatisfaction and weight and diet concerns. The pattern of relations among the variables differed for nonexercisers and exercisers. Weight and diet concerns were related to emotional reactivity in both groups, but actual weight was more important for nonexercisers and perceived body size was more so for exercisers. Greater weight and diet concerns and body dissatisfaction were related to poorer emotional well-being only in exercisers. Regular exercise thus seems related to body narcissism, although the direction of causality has yet to be established.

The second study by Davis (13) focused more directly on the role of the addictive nature of exercise in the development of eating disorders. She found addictiveness to be correlated with all weight and diet variables as well as perfectionism among exercising women only. It is not entirely clear what these data mean, however, because there were no differences in absolute level of addictiveness or any other critical variable between the two groups. These two studies are thus similar but inconclusive.

Mallick, Whipple, and Huerta (38) tested whether athletes have psychological traits similar to those of eating disorder patients. They studied females with eating-disorders, athletes, and teenage students. They found that menstrual and diet patterns fell along a continuum, with eating disorder patients having the worst patterns and students having the best. The patients had the poorest self-image, especially with respect to emotional tone and social relationships, and the athletes had the highest. Grades and health were also best for athletes and worst for patients. Overall, the athletes looked best psychologically and did not resemble eating disorder patients.

Another recent study (46) compared female bulimic patients with male runners (volunteers recruited in a park) and normal-weight male controls who had never had an eating disorder. The runners scored as compulsive exercisers and as fitness-preoccupied on an Obligatory Running Questionnaire. The bulimics scored significantly higher on the eating symptom scales than either group of males, who were not different from each other and were within the nonclinical range on all subscales. On size estimation, the male runners did not differ from either bulimics or controls. Thus male runners did not resemble these eating disorder patients but scored as significantly better adjusted. The authors do acknowledge, however, that comparing randomly selected, (presumably) normally functioning male runners with patients seeking therapy may not be fair. They point out that there are likely to be different motivations behind male running than females with eating disorders—the males looking for physical effectiveness or competition and achievement, and the female patients looking to raise lowered self-esteem or improve physical appearance.

This study (46) also attempted to compare *continued running* and *stop running* groups, but none of the runners would agree to random assignment into the stop running group; running was too important to them. If running is being used as a coping mechanism, then comparing those for whom this mechanism is temporarily unavailable with eating disorder patients might provide a more balanced comparison. There was no control for gender effects, either. It is thus still possible that female runners or runners prevented from masking their distress with running would resemble bulimic patients.

Case Studies Relating Exercise and Eating Disorder Symptoms

Case descriptions have been presented to make three main arguments concerning physical activity and eating disorders:

1. Anorexia nervosa and bulimia nervosa may be precipitated by exercising, just as they are thought to be triggered by restrictive dieting (as, for example, Rowley [51] speculated).
2. Eating disorders and compulsive exercising are related variants of a similar pathological

process and may even be mistaken for each other (as in the Waldstreicher case [64]).
3. Hyperactivity in eating disorder patients is merely a technique for losing weight by burning off calories (although some [32] disagree).

Support for the first thesis is provided by Katz (29) who described two case studies of patients where long-distance running clearly preceded the development of anorexia nervosa and seemed to play a role in its onset. Forced reduction of running in these patients was associated with depression and bulimia. It seems then that exercise and weight loss can trigger anorexia nervosa just as extreme dieting and weight loss can. Exercise might lead to anorexia by causing weight loss, which in turn causes increased investment in the body (*narcissism*), truly diminished appetite, and elevated production of endorphins. The depression that appeared in these two men when their running had to be decreased might have resulted from reduced endorphins or from running having been used to mask depression (for which both had positive family histories).

Support for the second argument is provided by Smith (56), who presents a case study of a rower to illustrate his thesis that high school and college athletics promote an emphasis on thinness or loss of fat that can result in excessive activity and weight loss resembling anorexia nervosa. Both sexes are at equal risk, given the demand for extreme reductions in body fat in many varsity sports. Fatness can be a handicap by reducing speed, quickness, and endurance, and by increasing fatigue. Fatness is thus used as a means to evaluate the fitness of an athlete for competition. Compulsive training schedules, conditioning routines, and obsessive care of equipment are admired and reinforced by both parents and coaches. Aversion to food and subsequent weight loss are frequent results despite hunger from the excessive activity. The author points out that athletes further resemble eating disorder patients in that they often have eating binges at the end of a tournament or season. The high-performing athlete is also likely to be a competitive student and to set unrealistic goals, again, like anorexics. Finally, he notes that amenorrhea is common among competing female athletes as well as anorexics.

Both of the latter two arguments about exercise and eating disorders are supported by Chalmers, Catalan, Day, and Fairburn (10) in a report of a woman who exercised compulsively despite serious leg injuries and amenorrhea (she wanted children). The exercising took all her spare time, she felt fat (at 81% of normal weight), she even took a day off work after Christmas to exercise off the calories she consumed on the holiday. She was diagnosed as having anorexia nervosa, although exercise was the dominant symptom, rather than eating or dangerously low weight. The authors note that increasing societal attention to exercise may lead to greater use of this approach instead of dieting to regulate body shape, mood, and self-esteem. When exercising gets out of control as it did for this patient, it is a sign of pathology.

Yates' interviews (69) of obligatory runners generated three case histories that illustrated the similarities between anorexia nervosa in adolescent females and obligatory running or exercising in 30- to 40-year-old males. Runners obsess about running the way anorexics obsess about eating and both negate or neglect their physical needs (ignore pain or hunger) in a quest for a physical ideal. Both are grim ascetics and share backgrounds, values, and personal characteristics (anorexics even tend to be athletic). A tentative explanation offered for the sex difference and that in age of onset of these two disorders is that both are responses to life or identity challenges, but that these challenges occur at different times for males and females. Gender difference may also reflect cultural values—looks are emphasized for women, athleticism for men. This emphasis would become especially important where the sense of self is weak, as it seems to be both for anorexics and these obligatory runners. The timing of the emphasis or focus on these different characteristics differs, too—for girls, adolescence is when appearance counts most (for dating), but for men, athleticism becomes more important when their bodies pass their physical peaks and start to decline. Unfortunately, no evidence beyond the case histories is offered for these speculations.

Patel, Andrews, and Bowman (48) responded to Yates' description (69) of male obligatory runners with a similar case history of an obligatory runner whose blood profile was like that of an anorexic and who was also impotent and very thin. Yates (67) replied that this case may reflect how running, as a response to impotence and divorce, may be used as a coping mechanism. She goes on to speculate that the increase in Iron Man events is the male analogue of the rise in anorexia nervosa in females.

Liberman and Palek (35) looked at the hematology of an obligatory male athlete and found identical abnormalities to those seen in anorexic patients. The patient also had other physiological features of anorexia nervosa. The patient's self-confidence depended on his exercising. He became anxious when he didn't exercise, was diet-conscious, counted calories, and weighed himself every morning. He denied any fear of being obese, but wanted to be perfectly fit. His weight was less than 10% below the minimal normal weight for his height. It is difficult to distinguish a diagnosis of anorexia nervosa from obligatory exercising for this patient.

Review Papers and Conclusions About Exercise Addiction and Eating Disorders

Several review articles have proposed explanations for this disparate literature on exercise addiction and eating disorders. Eisler and LeGrange (20) proposed four models to link excessive exercise and eating disorders.

1. Exercise addiction and anorexia nervosa (AN) form distinct groups. Exercise in anorexics, due to their preoccupation with weight and shape, is solely a means to reach the goal of thinness. These patients are seen as very different from excessive exercisers (EXE), and the similarities noted are only superficial.
2. AN and EXE overlap and EXE can lead to AN: EXE develops from normal healthy exercising, but high levels of exercise lead to AN through addiction to starvation or food-reduction brought on by heavy exercise.
3. AN and EXE are both related to another underlying disorder: Both disorders are manifestations of an obsessive-compulsive or affective disorder or some other disorder. The similarities between these two are just artifacts of the real underlying disorder. A weaker version of this model is that another illness is a predisposing factor for both AN and EXE. The data support this thesis better; however, this tells us little about links between AN and EXE and explains even less.
4. EXE is a variant of an eating disorder: The etiological process leading to AN sometimes produces EXE instead (the same disorder with different manifestations). This is said to explain the female:male ratio in eating disorders. It is, however, the least clear and most controversial of the four models. Is a further explanation for the female:male ratio needed beyond cultural and developmental pressures? Because men get EXE at a later age than women get AN, researchers must also posit that the debilitating pressures hit each sex at different times. This is not parsimonious and makes the argument somewhat circular.

The first three models seem to explain most of the data reasonably well. The authors make some interesting points in critiquing the literature. They note that studies looking for a high prevalence of eating disorder symptoms in avid exercisers are not really relevant, because one wouldn't expect to find much pathology in a random group of non-dysfunctional exercisers. A more appropriate comparison group for exercisers is committed dieters, not eating disorder patients. Looking at different levels of performance also misses that dysfunction is the issue. Furthermore, studies comparing athletes with and without variables related to eating disorders is circular, as this may predate exercise and not be related at all to activity. Finally, they point out that methodological problems abound in this literature, including an overreliance on self-report questionnaire data and small sample sizes for the problem under investigation. They suggest several alternative research strategies for distinguishing among their proposed models.

1. Study EXE in a broad range of subjects with follow-up to see the course of the disorder where it has been identified.
2. If EXE subjects are identified, compare them with AN and exercising anorexics, and control for age, sex, and duration of disorder. They object to comparing adolescent female anorexics with older male EXEs.
3. Investigate attitudes about eating and exercise in nonclinical populations at risk for both AN and EXE (e.g., models, dancers, gymnasts, swimmers, and runners) and see if all get both disorders (supporting model 4), or if some get only one disorder (supporting model 1). These individuals could be followed up over time to see if one disorder leads to the other as well.

Crisp (11) hypothesized that the hyperactivity of anorexia nervosa is merely a side effect of the arousal produced by weight loss. A more specific and detailed biobehavioral perspective was taken by Epling and Pierce (21). They reviewed evidence from animals and humans indicating that strenuous exercise such as running suppresses appetite and decreases the reinforcing value of food, resulting in decreased eating and weight reduction. As weight goes down, an increased motivation for activity leads to a further escalation in exercise, additionally reducing the value of food in a self-perpetuating loop. In this way, excessive exercising could cause anorexia nervosa. Unfortunately, no explanation is offered here for why, in identical environments, some individuals develop anorexia nervosa and others do not. Exercise and desire for thinness alone do not seem to be enough to produce the disorder.

Conclusions

The models and theories proposed to account for the presence of symptoms of eating disorder pathology in excessive exercisers or similarities between eating disorder patients and obligatory or excessive exercisers have yet to be tested. Although the literature needs to be directed and unified with an explanatory theory and tends to be spread around a variety of questions, some points do emerge.

Questionnaire studies of individuals who exercise a great deal do not find many similarities in personality or pathology with eating disorder patients. This is not surprising, because the subjects in the former group tend to be well-functioning individuals, whereas the latter group consists of identified psychiatric patients. When only the most extreme exercisers are examined, certain symptoms are commonly found in both eating disorder patients and excessive exercisers. These include a desire to be thinner than is normal, either for the sake of appearance or performance, but in both cases in the service of an unrealistic ideal. Both groups use drastic measures to lose weight. Females who engage in either activity tend to develop menstrual irregularities and amenorrhea. Case studies indicate that both eating disorders and excessive exercising tend to be found in individuals who are under stress, who often have low self-esteem, who use these means to cope with distress, and who attempt to bring a measure of personal control into their lives. If prevented from exercising, both groups become dysphoric and distressed. The literature thus does not provide answers for questions such as whether excessive exercising is a variant or a cause of eating disorders, or even if it is related at all. It simply indicates that similarities do exist on some dimensions and that both forms of excess are harmful to the individual.

As Nudelman stated, "Like weight control, exercise could be viewed as falling along a continuum from reasonable efforts to maintain fitness to a lifestyle of exercise and preoccupation with fitness that is out of proportion to the expected benefits of exercise" (46, p. 626). The current review supports Dishman's conclusion (16) that there does seem to be a syndrome of unhealthy exercise addiction where one will exercise despite medical, social, work, or other reasons not to do so.

What is not known at this time is the etiological mechanism that converts some people from normal exercisers into addicted, compulsive ones, or individuals with eating disorders. Some have argued that this is to some degree inherent in the activity, and, with time and degree of exertion, most will fall prey to the pathology. The causal mechanism is far from clear; however, those studies that have attempted to blame the activity have been correlational, not experimental or even quasi-experimental. At this time, we do not have accurate figures on the prevalence of pathological compulsive exercising. We have thus identified the existence of problematic excessive exercising or exercise addiction that affects some physically active individuals. Now we must discover who these susceptible people are, how they develop the problem, and how to prevent it.

Research Questions

This review suggests some much needed research:

1. More correlational and experimental investigations are needed to identify the factors responsible for compulsive exercising to the point of injury, social disruption, or vocational interference. We need to understand the etiology and to be able to determine which individuals will develop this disorder.
2. Personality factors associated with development of an exercise compulsion need to be identified so that those most at risk can be monitored.
3. More needs to be understood about why some individuals appear to be able to exercise vigorously over a period of years *without* becoming addicted or negatively affected.
4. The similarities and differences between compulsive exercising manifesting as anorexia nervosa and that manifesting as chronic sports injuries should be delineated.
5. Experimental studies wherein individuals are randomly assigned to undergo fitness training or not are needed to strengthen causal modeling. In particular, once risk factors are identified, it would be useful to randomly assign those with and without the risk factor and assess the degree to which each manifests symptoms of impending addiction (assuming, of course, that this can be reversed).
6. Identified exercise addicts should be studied to determine what factors contributed to their developing the addiction.
7. Treatment programs need to be developed to help those who are addicted to exercising return to a comfortable level of activity.

References

1. Baekeland, F. Exercise deprivation—Sleep and psychological reactions. Arch. Gen. Psychiatry. 22:365-369; 1970.
2. Beumont, P.J.V.; Booth, A.L.; Abraham, S.F.; Griffiths, D.A.; Turner, T.R. A temporal sequence of symptoms in patients with anorexia nervosa: A preliminary report. In: Darby, P.L.; Garfinkel, P.E.; Garner, D.M.; Coscina, D.V., eds. Anorexia nervosa: Recent developments in research. New York: Alan R. Liss; 1983: 129-136.
3. Blumenthal, J.A.; O'Toole, L.C.; Chang, J.L. Is running an analogue of anorexia nervosa? An empirical study of obligatory running and anorexia nervosa. JAMA. 252:520-523; 1984.
4. Blumenthal, J.A.; Rose, S.; Chang, J.L. Anorexia nervosa and exercise: Implications from recent findings. Sports Med. 2:37-247; 1985.
5. Borgen, J.S.; Corbin, C.B. Eating disorders among female athletes. Phys. Sportsmed. 15: 89-95; 1987.
6. Brooks-Gunn, J.; Burrow, C.; Warren, M.P. Attitudes toward eating and body weight in different groups of female adolescent athletes. Int. J. Eat. Disord. 7:749-757; 1988.
7. Brooks-Gunn, J.; Warren, M.P.; Hamilton, L. The relation of eating problems and amenorrhea in ballet dancers. Med. Sci. Sports Exerc. 19:41-44; 1987.
8. Brownell, K.D.; Steen, S.N.; Wilmore, J.H. Weight regulation practices in athletes: Analysis of metabolic and health effects. Med. Sci. Sports Exerc. 19:546-556;1987.
9. Carmack, M.A.; Martens, R. Measuring commitment to running: A survey of runner's attitudes and mental states. J. Sport Psychol. 1:25-42; 1979.
10. Chalmers, J.; Catalan, J.; Day, A.; Fairburn, C. Anorexia nervosa presenting as morbid exercising. Lancet. 1:286-287; 1985.
11. Crisp, A. Arousal, physical activity and energy balance in eating and body weight and shape disorders. Int. J. Eat. Disord. 4:627-649; 1985.
12. Davis, C. Weight and diet preoccupation and addictiveness: The role of exercise. Pers. Indiv. Diff. 11:823-827; 1990.
13. Davis, C. Body image and weight preoccupation: A comparison between exercising and non-exercising women. Appetite. 15:3-21; 1990.
14. De Coverley Veale, D.M.W. Exercise dependence. Br. J. Addict. 82:735-740; 1987.
15. DeFries, Z. "Running madness": A prelude to real madness. In: Sacks, M.H.; Sachs, M.L., eds. Psychology of running. Champaign, IL: Human Kinetics; 1981:261-266.
16. Dishman, R.K. Medical psychology in exercise and sport. Med. Clin. North Am. 69:123-143; 1985.
17. Dowd, R.; Innes, J.M. Sport and personality: Effects of type of sport and level of competition. Percept. Mot. Skills. 53:79-89; 1981.
18. Dresser, R. Obligatory running and anorexia nervosa. JAMA. 253:979-980; 1985.
19. Dummer, G.M.; Rosen, L.W.; Heusner, W.W.; Roberts, P.J.; Counsilman, J.E. Pathogenic weight-control behaviors of young competitive swimmers. Phys. Sportsmed. 15:75-84; 1987.
20. Eisler, I.; le Grange, D. Excessive exercise and anorexia nervosa. Int. J. Eat. Disord. 9:377-386; 1990.
21. Epling, W.F.; Pierce, W.D. Activity-based anorexia: A biobehavioral perspective. Int. J. Eat. Disord. 7:475-485; 1988.
22. Folkins, C.H.; Sime, W.E. Physical fitness training and mental health. Am. Psychol. 36:373-389; 1981.
23. Garfinkel, P.E. Some recent observations on the pathogenesis of anorexia nervosa. Can. J. Psychiatry. 26:218-223; 1981.
24. Garner, D.M.; Garfinkel, P.E. Socio-cultural factors in the development of anorexia nervosa. Psychol. Med. 9:605-609; 1980.
25. Glasser, W. Positive addiction. New York: Harper & Row; 1976.
26. Hailey, B.J.; Bailey, L.A. Negative addiction in runners: A quantitative approach. J. Sport Behav. 5:150-154; 1982.
27. Hofstetter, C.R.; Hovell, M.F.; Macera, C.; Sallis, J.; Spry, V.; Barrington, E.; Callender, L.; Hackley, M.; Rauh, M. Illness, injury, and correlates of aerobic exercise and walking: A community study. Res. Q. Exerc. Sport. 62:1-9; 1991.
28. Kagan, D.M. Addictive personality factors. J. Psychol.121:533-538; 1987.
29. Katz, J.L. Long-distance running, anorexia nervosa, and bulimia: A report of two cases. Compr. Psychiatry. 27:74-78; 1986.
30. Koplan, J.P.; Powell, K.E.; Sikes, R.K.; Shirley, R.W.;Campbell, G.C. An epidemiologic study of the benefits and risks of running. JAMA. 248:3118-3121; 1982.
31. Krelstein, M. Is running an analogue of anorexia nervosa? N. Engl. J. Med. 309:48; 1983.
32. Kron, L.; Katz, J.; Gorzynski, G.; Weiner, H. Hyperactivity in anorexia nervosa: A fundamental clinical feature. Compr. Psychiatry. 19:433-440; 1978.
33. Kukla, K.J.; Pargman, D. Comparative perceptions of psychological well-being as influenced

by sport experience in female athletes. Res. Q. 47:75-380; 1976.
34. Larsen, K.D. Is running an analogue of anorexia nervosa? N. Engl. J. Med. 309:47; 1983.
35. Liberman, R.B.; Palek, J. Hematologic abnormalities simulating anorexia nervosa in an obligatory athlete. Am. J. Med. 76:950-952; 1984.
36. Little, J.C. The athlete's neurosis—A deprivation crisis. Acta Psychiatr. Scand. 45:187-197; 1969.
37. Little, J.C. Neurotic illness in fitness fanatics. Psychiatr. Ann. 9:49-56; 1979.
38. Mallick, M.J.; Whipple, T.W.; Huerta, E. Behavioral and psychological traits of weight-conscious teenagers: A comparison of eating disordered patients and high- and low-risk groups. Adolescence. 22:157-168; 1987.
39. Morgan, W.P. Negative addiction in runners. Phys. Sportsmed. 7:57-70; 1979.
40. Morgan, W. P. Affective beneficence of vigorous physical activity. Med. Sci. Sports Exerc. 17:94-100; 1985.
41. Morgan, W.P.; Costill, D.L. Psychological characteristics of the marathon runner. J. Sports Med.12:42-46; 1972.
42. Morris, M.; Steinberg, H.; Sykes, E.; Salmon, P. Effects of temporary withdrawal from regular running. J. Psychosom. Res. 34:493-500; 1990.
43. Moses, J.; Steptoe, A.; Mathews, A.; Edwards, S. The effects of exercise training on mental well-being in the normal population: A controlled trial. J. Psychosom. Res. 33:47-61; 1989.
44. Norris, T.; Carroll, D.; Cochrane, R. The effects of aerobic and anaerobic training on fitness, blood pressure, and psychological stress and well-being. J. Psychosom. Res. 34:367-375; 1990.
45. Nudel, D.B.; Hassett, I.; Gurian, A.; Diamant, S.; Weinhouse, E.; Gootman, N. Young long distance runners. Clin. Pediatr. 28:500-505; 1989.
46. Nudelman, S. Dissimilarities in eating attitudes, body image distortion, depression, and self-esteem between high-intensity male runners and women with bulimia nervosa. Int. J. Eat. Disord. 7:625-634; 1988.
47. Pasman, L.; Thompson, J.K. Body image and eating disturbance in obligatory runners, obligatory weightlifters, and sedentary individuals. Int. J. Eat. Disord. 7:759-769; 1988.
48. Patel, S.B.; Andrews, A.T.; Bowman, H.S. Is running an analogue of anorexia nervosa? N. Engl. J. Med. 309:47-48; 1983.
49. Renfrow, N.E.; Bolton, B. Physiological and psychological characteristics associated with women's participation in intercollegiate athletics. Percept. Mot. Skills. 53:90; 1981.
50. Rosen, L.W.; McKeag, D.B.; Hough, D.O.; Curley, V. Pathogenic weight-control behavior in female athletes. Phys. Sportsmed. 14:79-86; 1986.
51. Rowley, S. Psychological effects of intensive training in young athletes. J. Child Psychol. Psychiatry. 28:371-377; 1987.
52. Rudy, E.B.; Estok, P.J. Measurement and significance of negative addiction in runners. West. J. Nurs. Res. 11:548-558; 1989.
53. Sachs, M.L. Running addiction. In: Sacks, M.H.; Sachs, M.L., eds. Psychology of running. Champaign, IL: Human Kinetics; 1981:116-126.
54. Sachs, M.L.; Pargman, D. Running addiction: A depth interview examination. J. Sport Behav. 2:143-155; 1979.
55. Sacks, M.H. Running addiction: A clinical report. In: Sacks, M.H.; Sachs, M.L., eds. Psychology of running. Champaign, IL: Human Kinetics; 1981:127-130.
56. Smith, N.J. Excessive weight loss and food aversion in athletes simulating anorexia nervosa. Pediatrics. 66:139-142; 1980.
57. Sours, J.A. Running, anorexia nervosa, and perfection. In: Sacks, M.H.; Sachs, M.L., eds. Psychology of running. Champaign, IL: Human Kinetics; 1981:80-91.
58. Stewart, J.D. Is running an analogue of anorexia nervosa? N. Engl. J. Med. 309:47; 1983.
59. Summers, J.J.; Machin, V.J.; Sargent, G.I. Psychosocial factors related to marathon running. J. Sport Psychol. 5:314-331; 1983.
60. Summers, J.J.; Sargent, G.I.; Levey, A.J.; Murray, K.D. Middle-aged, non-elite marathon runners: A profile. Percept. Mot. Skills. 54:963-969; 1982.
61. Thaxton, L. Physiological and psychological effects of short-term exercise addiction on habitual runners. J. Sport Psychol. 4:73-80; 1982.
62. Thompson, J.K.; Blanton, P. Energy conservation and exercise dependence: A sympathetic arousal hypothesis. Med. Sci. Sports Exerc. 19:91-99; 1987.
63. Walberg, J.L.; Johnston, C.S. Menstrual function and eating behavior in female recreational weight lifters and competitive body builders. Med. Sci. Sports Exerc. 23:30-36; 1991.
64. Waldstreicher, J. Anorexia nervosa presenting as morbid exercising. Lancet. 1:987; 1985.
65. Weight, L.M.; Noakes, T.D. Is running an analog of anorexia?: A survey of the incidence of eating disorders in female distance runners. Med. Sci. Sports Exerc. 19:213-217; 1987.
66. Wells, R.J. Is running an analogue of anorexia nervosa? N. Engl. J. Med. 309:47; 1983.

67. Yates, A. Is running an analogue of anorexia nervosa? N. Engl. J. Med. 309:48; 1983.
68. Yates, A. Compulsive exercise and the eating disorders. New York: Brunner/Mazel; 1991.
69. Yates, A.; Leehey, K.; Shisslak, C.M. Running—An analogue of anorexia nervosa? N. Engl. J. Med. 308:251-255; 1983.

Chapter 61

Physical Activity, Fitness, and Substance Misuse and Abuse

Melvin H. Williams

A healthy lifestyle involves a number of personal behaviors that may enhance the quality and possibly the quantity of life. The major focus of this conference is the effect of exercise and fitness on health, but other personal behaviors such as proper nutrition are also important considerations. A major area of increasing concern is the misuse or abuse of both licit and illicit substances that may adversely influence health status. Senay (175) reviewed the evidence of substance abuse from a global perspective and indicated that the use of agents with liability for abuse is widespread and associated with public health and social problems of great magnitude.

In general, health professionals use the collective terms *substance misuse* or *substance abuse* when referring to the use of certain substances in ways that may negatively affect health. Although myriad substances may be misused or abused, these terms are most commonly associated with chemicals, particularly drugs. Since the primary focus of this paper is on drugs, the terms *drug misuse* and *drug abuse* will be used interchangeably.

Individuals who are physically active may use drugs for a variety of reasons, and in each case may misuse or abuse these drugs as well. First, physically active individuals may use drugs for legitimate medical purposes, such as nonsteroidal antiinflammatory drugs (NSAIDS) to relieve the pain of inflamed tissues aggravated by exercise; however, an improper drug protocol may predispose the individual to gastrointestinal bleeding (46). Second, physically active individuals may use so-called recreational drugs, such as alcohol, for social purposes; however, excessive alcohol intake may predispose an individual to an array of health problems (204). Third, physically active individuals may use drugs for ergogenic purposes in attempts to enhance athletic performance; however, although a variety of drugs may be effective ergogenics, they may also cause serious health sequelae (104).

Unfortunately, space does not permit a discussion of all substances or drugs that may negatively impact health. Thus, the major focus of this chapter will be those drugs whose negative potential for health is of such magnitude that their reduction in use has been targeted by the United States Public Health Service in *Healthy People 2000: National Health Promotion and Disease Prevention Objectives* (193), including alcohol, nicotine (cigarette smoking, smokeless tobacco), marijuana, cocaine, and anabolic steroids. Although the health implications of each drug will be discussed individually, it is important to note, with the exception of anabolic steroids, that a substantial amount of covariance exists in the use of these drugs (71,175,200), and thus users of multiple drugs may be exposed to multifarious risks. The final section of this chapter will focus on the potential for exercise or fitness to serve a preventive role in substance misuse and abuse.

Alcohol (Ethanol)

Alcohol misuse is a major drug problem throughout the world (1,59,130,143,193). Associated health problems are numerous and varied (134,192), contributing substantially to health care costs. For example, in the United States, Burke (23) indicated that 1 in every 10 deaths is alcohol-related, and the economic cost would approximate $150 billion in 1995. Concerted efforts to reduce alcohol consumption and related health risks have been implemented worldwide.

Extensive experimental research with animal models has been used to determine mechanisms underlying the adverse health effects of alcohol, and some experimental studies with humans have also examined the effects of alcohol on various health risk factors. However, most of the available evidence is epidemiological in nature. Camargo (24) identified some of the possible methodologic issues underlying inconsistent results relative to the association between alcohol consumption and health status, including the validity of self-reported drinking, failure to differentiate non-drinking status as abstainers versus ex-drinkers, the drinking pattern (e.g., binges), lack of uniformity in expressing usual alcohol intake, and failure to control for possible confounders.

Addiction and Psychological Disorders

Alcohol is one of nine psychoactive drugs listed by the American Psychiatric Association (9) that is associated with a high potential for abuse and dependence. Data from western countries suggest approximately 10% of the adult population are at risk for alcoholism (1,9); it is interesting to note that these 10% account for about 50% of the alcohol consumed.

Epidemiologic data have indicated increased levels of psychiatric distress and psychotic experiences with alcohol abuse (45,189). Some of the psychological effects accompanying intoxication, such as increased aggressiveness and irritability (9), may be associated with the increased homicides observed in both victims and suspects (111,140), while other effects such as depression and impaired judgment may be associated with suicidal tendencies, particularly in those aged 15 to 24 years (117,180).

Psychomotor Abilities and Health

Alcohol depresses brain function, and the effects are dose-dependent, ranging from reduced tension to death. Although there is considerable interindividual variation, blood alcohol concentrations (BAC) ranging from 0.05 to 0.10 will impair judgment and fine motor coordination. Gross motor coordination, visual functioning, and consciousness are also affected with increasing BAC.

These perturbations to normal brain function are associated with increased risks for injury and trauma (132), including occupational injury (5), recreational injuries (149), and motor vehicle injuries (194). Accidental death is coincident with alcohol misuse.

Alcoholic Liver Disease

Alcoholic liver disease covers a spectrum from mild asymptomatic fatty liver to life-threatening cirrhosis (66). Smart and Mann (182) note cirrhosis is one of the most significant consequences of alcohol abuse, indicating that an extensive body of literature documents the strong relationship between population levels of alcohol consumption and cirrhosis rates. Alcohol also appears to potentiate the effect of viral hepatitis implicated in the etiology of primary liver cancer (191).

Cancer

Tuyns (191) noted that although alcohol has never been shown to cause cancer in animals, it is nevertheless clearly implicated in the etiology of some human cancers. In vitro research has shown that alcohol and acetaldehyde could cause changes in DNA comparable to changes elicited by carcinogens (56), and alcohol may suppress natural killer cell activity in mice (17), two factors that may predispose to cancer. Additional factors may be operating such as (a) the nitrosamine content in beer (162), (b) the nonalcoholic contents of dark distilled liquor (166), (c) confounding by diets with a high fat content (72), or (d) displacement of possible dietary cancer inhibitors when alcohol displaces other food sources of energy (185).

Oral, Pharyngeal, and Esophageal Cancer

One of the most common sites associated with alcohol-induced cancer is the aerodigestive tract. In a review of earlier epidemiologic studies, Tuyns (191) noted that both cohort and case-control studies have supported a relationship between alcohol intake and cancer of the mouth, hypopharynx, larynx, and esophagus. These earlier findings have been supported by recent epidemiologic data from around the world (121,136,208,212). Although alcohol has been cited as a causal factor independent of tobacco smoking (21), the effect is multiplicative when combined with smoking (191,212). Adjusted for smoking, Maier, Dietz, Gewelke, Seitz, and Heller (121) reported a relative risk (RR) of 21.4 in heavy drinkers (greater than 100 g ethanol/day) for developing oropharyngeal cancer; the synergistic effect of heavy smoking and drinking increased the RR to 146.2.

Gastric Cancer

Boeing (18) reviewed 4 cohort and 16 case-control studies conducted between 1980 and 1990 relative to the etiology of stomach cancer. Prospective studies did not support a relationship between alcohol consumption and gastric cancer, whereas the case-control studies showed divergent results.

Colorectal Cancer

Longnecker, Orza, Adams, Vioque, and Chalmers (115) recently conducted a meta-analysis of 27 studies relative to the association of alcoholic beverage consumption to risk of colorectal cancer. Their overall analysis revealed a weak association; on the average, the RR for consumption of two drinks daily was 1.10. They also noted some slight differences supporting beverage specificity, as the

RR for beer was 1.26 compared to wine and liquor, 1.11 and 1.13, respectively. They concluded that because of the small degree of association there are inconclusive data to support a causal role of alcohol consumption on colorectal cancer. Additional research by Longnecker (113) revealed that a prolonged history (20 years) of heavy drinking (five or more drinks/day) was associated with a RR of 1.8 for cancer of the rectum. Two other studies reported a significant relationship between beer consumption and rectal cancer (164,185), the RR of rectal cancer in male beer drinkers being 1.73 (164); the nitrosamine content of beer might be involved.

Pancreatic Cancer

In 1986, Velema, Walker, and Gold (198) reviewed the epidemiologic studies from the preceding 15 years to evaluate the association between alcohol consumption and pancreatic cancer and concluded the available evidence was insufficient to support a causal relationship. Contrarily, Olsen, Mandel, Gibson, Wattenberg, and Schuman (150) reported that heavy alcohol consumption (four or more drinks/day), even when adjusted for confounding variables, was positively associated with pancreatic cancer, the reported odds ratio (OR) being 2.69. They suggested alcohol may contribute to the development of pancreatic cancer, possibly by causing calcifying pancreatitis, which may interact with other risk factors.

Breast Cancer

The association between alcohol consumption and breast cancer has received considerable research attention, and a variety of reviews have attempted to analyze the epidemiological data collected over the past 25 years. Longnecker, Berlin, Orza, and Chalmers (114), using a meta-analysis technique—with rigid criteria for selection of studies reported from 1967 to 1988 to study a dose–response relationship—reported that the risk of breast cancer at a daily alcohol intake of 1 oz (two drinks) relative to nondrinkers was 1.4 for the case-control studies reviewed and 1.7 for the follow-up data. They indicated the findings provided strong support for an association between alcohol consumption and cancer risk, but were not proof of causality. However, in a recent review of six case-control studies that adjusted for possible diet-related confounders such as fat and fiber, Howe et al. (84) reported an absence of an association between consumption of up to 40 g of alcohol per day and risk of breast cancer, but a highly statistically significant and consistent elevated risk for drinkers of 40 g or more daily. Compared to nondrinkers, the RR was 1.69.

Osteoporosis

Because chronic alcoholics experience disturbances in bone metabolism and histology (110) and a higher prevalence of bone fractures (30), excessive alcohol intake is postulated as one of the many factors that may contribute to osteoporosis. This impaired bone metabolism may be reversible; chronic alcoholics who abstained from alcohol consumption for at least 2 years had bone formation and turnover rates similar to social drinkers (110).

Cardiovascular Disease and Related Risk Factors

The effect of alcohol on cardiovascular disease and related risk factors has received considerable research attention not only because alcohol may exert direct toxic effects on the heart, but also because of a reported *J* or *U* effect, suggesting that small or moderate amounts of alcohol may decrease mortality due to cardiovascular disease.

Body Composition

A review of 31 carefully selected epidemiological studies revealed many studies actually found alcohol consumers weighed less than nondrinkers; but, the data were inconsistent between sexes, diverse populations, and other factors suggesting that patterns of intake may be influential. This led the reviewers to conclude that the role of alcohol in determining adiposity in the general population remains inconclusive (74).

Diabetes

Epidemiologic studies have suggested alcohol may be a risk factor for diabetes. Holbrook, Barrett-Connor, and Wingard (80) followed 524 individuals for 12 years, and found that males, but not females, who developed diabetes reported greater alcohol intake; the highest rate of diabetes was in those classified as heavy drinkers. They suggested alcohol appears to be associated with risk of non-insulin-dependent diabetes mellitus (NIDDM); chronic alcoholism is often associated with insulin resistance (153). Compared to a normoglycemic group, Balkau, Eschwege, Ducimetiere, Richard, and Warnet (14) found that although the RR of both overall death and coronary heart disease (CHD) death increased to about 1.6 and 2.3 for glucose intolerant and diabetic groups respectively, the RR for alcohol and cirrhosis deaths increased to 7.0 in the glucose intolerant and 13.3 in the diabetic. Several mechanisms might be operative, including increased waist:hip ratio (WHR)

(155) or obesity and serum triglycerides, which impair glucose utilization and elicit hyperinsulinemia (98). Animal models have provided evidence of decreased insulin binding sites and subsequent postreceptor events such as decreased glucokinase activity (153).

Blood Pressure

Reviews emanating from the Canadian Consensus Conference on Nonpharmacological Approaches to the Management of High Blood Pressure (53) and the National Institutes of Health (82) have identified excessive alcohol intake as a risk factor for hypertension. Possible mechanisms involve the interactions among alcohol, sodium, and calcium intake (67) and metabolism, for alcohol has been shown to decrease urinary excretion of sodium (100) or lead to an increased concentration of calcium in vascular smooth muscle, leading to vasoconstriction and increased peripheral vascular resistance (34).

Several investigators have reported a J-shaped dose–response association between alcohol intake and blood pressure, indicating that the blood pressure of moderate drinkers appears to be slightly lower than nondrinkers and heavy alcohol consumers (70,138). Both studies indicated heavy alcohol consumption was a risk factor for hypertension.

Serum Lipids

Both low (30 g) and high (70 g) dosages of alcohol may acutely increase triglyceride-rich lipoproteins (38,197), whereas chronic alcoholism is associated with hypertriglyceridemia and, in liver damage, is associated with subnormal levels of high-density lipoproteins (HDL), both risk factors for cardiovascular disease (184).

Contrarily, a large number of both epidemiologic and experimental studies have supported a positive association between alcohol intake and serum HDL levels. Recent epidemiologic studies have shown that moderate alcohol intake was positively associated with total HDL cholesterol (20) and its subfractions (11,20,29,44). The effect of short-term abstinence from alcohol in habitual users revealed significant decreases in HDL, HDL-2, and HDL-3 after 3 weeks abstinence and significant increases after subjects resumed drinking for 3 weeks (69).

The increase in HDL cholesterol appears to be related to the effect of alcohol on liver metabolism, possibly by increasing plasma lecithin:cholesterol acyltransferase (79) or the cholesteryl ester transfer protein (170).

Cerebrovascular Disease

The association between alcohol intake and stroke has been the subject of considerable epidemiologic research, and the major reviews available (24,78, 126) have concluded that alcohol abuse increases the risk for both ischemic and hemorrhagic stroke. Research subsequent to these reviews has been supportive of these conclusions, indicating heavy alcohol intake was associated with a RR of stroke of 3.8 in men without previously diagnosed cardiovascular disease (177). The effects of moderate alcohol intake are less consistent. In one of the most extensive reviews, Camargo (24) concludes that moderate drinking (less than 60 g/day) increases the risk of intracerebral and subarachnoid hemorrhage in diverse populations; whereas moderate drinking and ischemic stroke have a complex association that might be explained by race. Predominantly white populations have a J-shaped association, whereas little association has been found among Japanese.

Gorelick (64) suggested alcohol could increase the risk for ischemic stroke by several mechanisms including activation of the clotting cascade, and for hemorrhagic stroke by prolongation of the bleeding time. Gorelick (64) also suggested that moderate doses of alcohol could exert a protective effect against ischemic stroke via increased prostacyclin levels, which may induce vasodilation and inhibition of platelet aggregation.

Coronary Heart Disease (CHD)

Several major reviews (37,139,161) have indicated that alcohol may exert a direct toxic effect on the heart. Acute doses may induce idiopathic atrial arrhythmias in some individuals (99,103), and chronic intake can lead to cardiomyopathy and heart failure (37,139,161).

Moderate drinking, however, has been associated with reduced mortality from CHD. Several reviews of clinical, cohort, case-control epidemiologic research have indicated that moderate alcohol consumption is associated with lower risk of CHD (88,156,171). Compared to nondrinkers, examples of some of the RR reported in epidemiologic studies include 0.5 for men consuming 5 to 14 drinks per week (133), 0.6 and 0.4 for women who consume 5 to 24 g per day and more than 25 g per day, respectively (183), and even 0.6 for individuals who consumed five or more drinks daily (86).

The U-shaped association between alcohol consumption and CHD has been challenged because many of the nondrinkers who serve as the baseline may actually be ex-drinkers who abstain because of accumulating ill health (176). However, three studies subsequent to this report did control for the nature of the nondrinker and supported the inverse relationship between alcohol intake and CHD or CHD mortality (19,85,165).

Summary

Although some of these findings suggest the moderate use of alcohol may confer some health benefits in relation to cardiovascular disease, the potential for abuse and the possible adverse effects on other aspects of health preclude a recommendation for individuals to increase their alcohol intake or to initiate drinking if they currently abstain (144).

Cigarette Smoking

The inhalation of smoke from cigarette tobacco introduces a number of compounds into the body, most notably nicotine, tar, and carbon monoxide, that may substantially increase health risks. Cigarette smoking is a major risk factor for all-cause mortality (54,195). The Surgeon General of the United States Public Health Service has identified smoking as the single most important preventable source of morbidity and mortality and has enumerated the health benefits of smoking cessation (147). The number of health risks associated with cigarette smoking is extensive. Space does not permit coverage of all these conditions, so only several will be discussed.

Addiction

Nicotine elicits a psychological state of alertness and excitation or, paradoxically, a sense of relaxation. These psychological effects of nicotine are the basic reasons individuals continue to smoke even when they are aware of potential health risks (204).

Nicotine is an addictive drug, the American Psychiatric Association (9) notes that the most common form of nicotine dependence is associated with inhalation of cigarette smoke. Although its liability for addiction is not equal to that of other agents such as cocaine (36,75), nicotine's health effects are significant because of the large number of individuals who smoke.

Cancer

Cigarette smoke may contain a number of carcinogens. The causal effect of cigarette smoking on cancer has been reported worldwide. Findings from the new American Cancer Society prospective study indicate that mortality risks among smokers have increased substantially for most of the eight major cancer sites causally associated with cigarette smoking (178). Similar findings have been reported in Europe (107), Japan (3), and China (58).

Oropharyngeal and Laryngeal Cancer

In a review Boyle et al. (21) noted that oropharyngeal cancer was the sixth most common site of cancer and a causal role has been established for tobacco use. Smoking appears to be the primary cause of laryngeal cancer, chronic smoking of more than 30 cigarettes per day increasing the relative risk to 59.7 (212).

Gastric Cancer

In a major review, Forman (55) indicated that gastric cancer is associated with tobacco use, but even in heavy smokers the risk does not exceed twofold, although a study subsequent to this review revealed an RR of 2.6 (96).

Lung Cancer

Recent reviews of worldwide epidemiologic data have noted that the appearance of lung cancer, with an appropriate time lag, parallels changes in cigarette consumption (58,97,107,116,209), and reviewers note that the epidemiologic evidence linking cigarette smoking to lung cancer is unequivocal (102,159).

Pancreatic Cancer

Cigarette smoking has previously been identified as one of the major risk factors involved in the etiology of pancreatic cancer (120), and three recent case-control studies have reported RR ranging from 1.76 to 6.52 (61,83,150).

Breast Cancer

Research in general shows little or no association between breast cancer and cigarette smoking (50,131,196) or a slightly elevated risk, a RR of 1.2 (33,151), although the RR increased to 1.7 to 1.8 or higher for women who were heavy smokers and started smoking before 16 years of age (151).

Osteoporosis

Not all investigators have shown an association between cigarette smoking and osteoporosis (31,158), but several studies have reported significantly lower bone mineral content (BMC) in spinal bone and a tendency toward decreased BMC at other sites in women smokers (101,127,181). Possible mechanisms underlying this association are smoking-induced changes in hepatic metabolism of estrogen (27) or decreases in calcium absorption (101).

Chronic Obstructive Lung Disease (COLD)

In a recent review Higgins (77) noted that death rates from COLD are about 10 times greater in smokers compared to nonsmokers, and cigarette use accounts for approximately 80% of all COLD deaths in the United States.

Cardiovascular Disease and Related Risk Factors

In a recent review, McGill (129) noted the well-established relationship between cigarette smoking and atherosclerosis. He noted that there are many physiologic responses to cigarette smoking that can mediate its effects on atherosclerosis; although there is little evidence of the importance of these effects, two possibilities are regional fat distribution and serum cholesterol.

Body Composition

Although some research has shown that smokers may have lower estimated body fat than former smokers or those who never smoked (95,163), other studies have reported a significant association between cigarette smoking and the waist:hip ratio (WHR) (92,160,173), even when other potential confounders such as physical activity were controlled (172,190).

Serum Cholesterol

Epidemiologic research has indicated that chronic cigarette smoking is related in a dose–response manner to depressed HDL cholesterol levels (68,135). The smoking-induced reduction of the serum ratio of high- to low-density lipoproteins (HDL:LDL ratio) was also one of the major conclusions in the extensive review by Anthony (12).

Coronary Heart Disease (CHD)

Cigarette smoking is generally recognized worldwide as a major risk factor for CHD. In the United States, cigarette smoking accounts for 21% of all CHD deaths and 40% for individuals under age 65 years (193). A review of 10 epidemiologic studies has indicated that passive smoking also increases the risk of CHD (62).

Summary

The research literature supporting a causal association between cigarette smoking and lung cancer and CHD is voluminous, yet some contend that genetic factors may predispose certain individuals to smoking and disease. However, recent data from the Finnish Twin Cohort study with monozygotic (MZ) twins revealed a RR for first death of 13.0 in MZ twins who smoked compared to the nonsmoking twin (89), supportive of causal effects.

Smokeless Tobacco (ST)

Smokeless tobacco (ST) is commonly used as either chewing tobacco, a packed form of tobacco leaves, or snuff, a preparation of fine-cut, powdered tobacco. Its use is predominantly a behavior characteristic of young, white males (122), particularly baseball players (49).

ST contains nicotine in quantities somewhat similar to cigarettes, and the total amount of nicotine consumed daily is comparable between ST users and cigarette smokers (32). The overall health risks appear to be less because ST use is confined to the mouth and other toxic substances found in cigarette smoke are not inhaled into the body (15).

Oral Disease

The most documented health threat of ST use is oral disease. Chewing tobacco and snuff are normally held in one place in the mouth, and the most serious damage occurs at that spot. The most common observation is leukoplakia, white spots or patches in the mucous membrane of the tongue or cheek (32,40,91). In the study with baseball players, the RR for leukoplakia in users was 60 (49).

Leukoplakia caused by ST may become malignant. Several consensus conferences, including the National Institutes of Health Consensus Conference on the Health Implications of Smokeless Tobacco, have agreed that the available data support a causal relationship between ST and oral cancer (206).

Summary

Given these potential health risks, one of the major objectives listed by the United States Public Health Service in *Healthy People 2000* is the reduction of the proportion of males in the 12 to 24 years age group who use ST on a regular basis (193).

Marijuana (Marihuana)

Marijuana contains the shredded, dried leaves, flowers, and stems from the plant *cannabis sativa*. *Cannabis sativa* contains over 400 different chemical entities, 60 of these being cannabinoids (43), but only delta-9-tetrahydrocannabinol (THC) has psychoactive properties in significant amounts (2). Martin (125) and Dewey (43) note that THC exerts a relatively nonselective, complex mixture of excitatory and depressant effects on the central nervous system, indicating that the effects may be dose-dependent with excitatory, euphoric effects associated with lower doses and depressive effects with higher ones. The behavioral responses to marijuana are influenced by a variety of factors such as personality, expected outcomes, and preexisting mood. Marijuana is the most widely used illicit psychoactive substance in the United States (9), particularly among those aged 12 to 35 years. Its effect on health has been studied extensively, but Hollister (81) noted several methodological difficulties in such research, such as the confounding effect of multiple drug use, particularly alcohol and cigarette smoking.

Psychological Disorders

The American Psychiatric Association (9) characterizes *cannabis dependence* as daily, or almost daily, use of cannabis. Individuals with cannabis dependence are often lethargic, may lack motivation, and may suffer attentional disturbances and memory problems, which may be one of the major problems with young users who may experience impaired psychosocial development. Cannabis abuse is associated with episodic use and maladaptive behavior, possibly leading to cannabis-induced organic mental disorders including *cannabis intoxication*, characterized by such symptoms as impaired judgment and panic attacks, and *cannabis delusional disorder*, depicted by symptoms such as marked anxiety and persecutory delusions (9).

Psychomotor Abilities

Comparable to alcohol, marijuana may adversely affect psychomotor abilities. Although Heishman, Stitzer, and Bigelow (73) reported minimal performance impairment with low doses of marijuana, Hollister (81), summarizing numerous studies regarding the effects of marijuana on psychomotor performance, indicated that if the dose was high enough or the task complex enough, impairment was shown. The impaired judgment associated with cannabis intoxication may underlie the increased risk of motor vehicle accidents and fatalities (142).

Respiratory Diseases

Because marijuana is smoked, it is logical to assume that the health risks to the lungs would be comparable to cigarette smoking, and to some extent they are. Marijuana users typically smoke only 3 to 4 marijuana cigarettes per day—much less than the typical tobacco cigarette smoker—which may minimize health risks. On the other hand, marijuana users also inhale more deeply and retain the smoke in the lungs for a greater period of time and actually deposit more tar in the lungs per cigarette compared to tobacco cigarettes (207). Thus, habitual smoking of 3 to 4 marijuana cigarettes per day is comparable to smoking 20 tobacco cigarettes per day as a risk factor for developing chronic bronchitis and epithelial damage in the central airways (207).

Summary

The effects of marijuana use on health are controversial (125). In a major review Hollister (81) noted field studies in countries such as Jamaica (where marijuana is smoked for years) have failed to detect any major health consequences from chronic heavy use of cannabis, but also noted those studies have many deficiencies. Nevertheless, Hollister (81) stated one is forced to conclude that cannabis is a relatively safe drug as social drugs go, noting also that to date it compares favorably with tobacco and alcohol, if not with caffeine. One should bear in mind, however, the very long time that it took to determine the ill effects on health of these accepted social drugs.

Cocaine

Cocaine is an alkaloid derivative of the leaves of the coca plant, *erythroxylon coca*, which grows extensively in the northern mountains of South America. Its illicit use is attributed to its psychoactive effects; systemically, cocaine stimulates both the central and sympathetic nervous systems, leading to euphoria, mood enhancement, and a decreased sensation of fatigue. Although cocaine once was considered a wonder drug eliciting powerful stimulating effects but having no adverse side effects, such is not the case. Cocaine is strongly addictive and can lead to a variety of health problems, including death (41). In the United States, the National Institute on Drug Abuse considers cocaine the drug of greatest national public health concern (60).

Psychological Disorders

Cocaine has been classified as a highly addictive drug (75). The American Psychiatric Association lists *cocaine dependence* and *cocaine abuse* as psychoactive substance-use disorders, several of the associated psychological and behavioral changes include depression, irritability, and paranoid ideation. Cocaine-induced organic disorders include *cocaine intoxication, delirium,* and *delusional disorder* (9). The initial psychological effects—intense pleasure for about 30 min—are followed by depression, anxiety, or sadness, which then leads to craving for more. Cocaine smoking and intravenous use often progress from infrequent use to cocaine abuse or dependence within only a few weeks or months (9). If we compare the risk reduction objectives for alcohol, marijuana, and cocaine in *Healthy People 2000*, the Public Health Service wants Americans (a) to decrease excess consumption of alcohol, (b) to decrease the regular use of marijuana, but (c) to not even experiment once or twice with cocaine, primarily because cocaine may be so addictive (193).

Cardiovascular and Cerebrovascular Diseases

The adverse effects of cocaine on the cardiovascular system appear to be related to acute bouts of cocaine abuse. Several reviewers (63,105) noted that some of the most serious adverse effects of cocaine use involve the cardiovascular system, with multiple mechanisms of action eliciting potentially life-threatening cardiovascular responses. Cocaine use may exert direct toxic effects on the myocytes or block sodium channels possibly leading to dysrhythmias (105), which may be exemplified by epidemiologic data showing an increased likelihood (RR of 3.4) of heart palpitations with cocaine use (154). Cocaine may also induce myocardial ischemia via coronary vasospasm and increased myocardial oxygen demand (105) in both diseased and nondiseased coronary arteries (52), which may elicit symptoms of myocardial infarction (93,141) and sudden death (41), even in elite athletes (199).

Stroke is another reported complication of cocaine abuse, and although the pathogenesis is uncertain, there are probably a number of factors involved (109), including evidence of peripheral vasospasm (141).

Summary

As noted, cocaine is a very dangerous drug that may be highly addictive and may even be lethal in a single dose. Additionally, its use is significantly associated with other forms of drug abuse, and if used intravenously, is significantly related to human immunodeficiency virus (HIV) seropositivity (146).

Anabolic/Androgenic Steroids (AAS)

Anabolic/androgenic steroids (AAS) represent a class of synthetic drugs designed to mimic the effects of testosterone. AAS are used nonmedically by athletes primarily for their ergogenic potential, but may also be used by nonathletes for psychosocial reasons such as enhanced body image and self-esteem (169).

The ergogenicity of AAS has been the subject of several major reviews (6,47,112,211) and when combined with proper resistance training and diet, reviewers agree that AAS may increase lean body mass. Most reviewers (6,94,112,186,201,202) suggest that AAS may enhance muscular strength development, a judgment supported by a recent review of laboratory studies that included meta-analysis as part of the evaluative criteria (47).

AAS may be potent ergogenics and the Council on Scientific Affairs of the American Medical Association (7) has noted that abuse of AAS for nonmedical purposes is a growing problem with associated health risks. The use of AAS is quite extensive. Approximately 1 million Americans use AAS, including 5% to 7% of high school students, primarily male athletes (210). Nonmedical use is substantially higher in certain athletes such as weight lifters and bodybuilders (28). Because of the potential health risks, one of the risk reduction objectives in *Healthy People 2000* is the reduction of AAS use among high school students (193).

For several reasons there is some controversy relative to the magnitude of the health risks associated with AAS use, including (a) reversibility of most risks upon cessation of AAS use (112); (b) the fact that the most common users are young, healthy, athletic males (205); (c) the nature of the research with humans, which are primarily case studies or retrospective studies with poorly selected samples (112); and (d) limited research into the long-term effects (7). Although the need for more concerted research is recognized, the following discussion highlights some of the major health risks associated with AAS use.

Psychological Disorders

Psychiatric and psychological alterations are major toxicities of AAS (65). Some of the manifestations include increased aggression, hostility, depression (22), drug-induced psychoses (157), and increased tendency to commit violent crimes, including homicide (157). Long-term, high-dose use may lead to dependence (22,90). A recent review concluded that although AAS may have psychological and behavioral effects in some individuals, the effects are variable, and additional research is needed to clarify the association between AAS and psychiatric and psychological changes (13).

Liver Disorders

Friedl (57) noted that 17-alkyl-substituted androgens have certain established health consequences, all involving the liver, possibly due to production of hepatocyte hyperplasia. Patients involved in AAS therapy have exhibited liver impairment resulting in cholestatic hepatitis with jaundice, potentially life-threatening hepatic lesions characterized by blood-filled cysts known as peliosis hepatis, benign hepatomas, and malignant tumors characteristic for hepatocellular carcinoma, as seen in several case studies involving androgen-using athletes (57,112). Friedl (57) noted the reports involving athletes represent symptomatic cases in which abdominal pain necessitated medical attention and subsequent detection, suggesting there may remain a number of undetected cases of tumors because the individual remains unsymptomatic. Although rare, these forms of liver pathology may be fatal (57,112).

Cardiovascular and Cerebrovascular Disorders

One of the most consistent effects of alkylated AAS is an alteration of serum lipids, most notably a decrease in HDL cholesterol, but also increases in total and low-density lipoprotein (LDL) cholesterol. Friedl (57) has indicated this is the single significant adverse effect that has been clearly established for AAS self-administration by athletes, a finding that has been supported in all major reviews (7,57,112). Other risk factors associated with atherosclerosis such as glucose intolerance, insulin resistance, and hypertension have also been associated with AAS use (65,76,186). There are over a half-dozen reported case studies of myocardial infarctions (57,112,118,119) and cerebrovascular accidents (57,106,112) in athletes, primarily weight lifters and bodybuilders using AAS, including two that have resulted in death (118,119). Another case study documents an AAS-related death due to pulmonary embolism (179).

Summary

As indicated previously, most of the information relative to the health risks of AAS has been derived from case studies and therapeutic trials. Despite an increasing number of such reports, a technical review committee of the National Institute of Drug Abuse concluded that definitive data regarding adverse effects of nonmedical use of AAS have yet to be developed (39). Although useful to enhance awareness, such studies are not as powerful as stronger epidemiologic designs to substantiate a strong association between AAS use and life-threatening health conditions. This is the general conclusion of most reviewers, who indicate the need for better controlled research (7,57,112).

Role of Physical Activity in Prevention and Treatment of Drug Misuse and Abuse

It is obvious at this point that drug abuse is an international health problem. Governments spend billions in associated health care costs, and millions of individuals experience personal tragedies and wasted lives, even elite athletes in their prime. Reducing drug abuse is a major worldwide health objective, and officials generally agree that prevention is a key factor (8).

Although many questions remain unanswered concerning the most appropriate approach to prevention of drug abuse, one strategy that may be effective involves social learning techniques such as the development of general coping skills through enhanced personal and social competence. Multiple behavioral techniques may be involved, and the best opportunity currently offered appears to be comprehensive community planning (8). In this regard, physical activity and exercise may be an important component of a comprehensive prevention program, conferring such benefits as improved mood, enhanced self-concept, increased confidence, and reduced symptoms of anxiety and mild-to-moderate depression (128, 187). Unfortunately, the available data supportive of exercise as a therapeutic modality for prevention of drug abuse are somewhat limited.

Association Between Physical Activity and Drug Abuse

The association between levels of physical activity, exercise, or fitness and drug abuse may be negative, neutral, or positive.

In general, smoking status has a negative association with health-related attitudes and behaviors, the higher the level of smoking, the less healthful the attitudes and behaviors (148). Recent studies have shown inverse relationships between smoking status and leisure-time physical activity (108), amount of physical exercise (42,48,95,163,168), and endurance capacity (124). Decreased levels of physical exercise have also been reported for users of smokeless tobacco (48). Regarding marijuana and cocaine, college athletes reported less use compared to a group of nonathletic peers (10).

Although acute alcohol consumption may impair exercise performance and chronic ingestion leading to alcoholism may decrease physical working capacity (25,203), the general relationship between social drinking and exercise or fitness is rather inconsistent (16). In the Tecumseh Health Study, moderate drinkers had higher levels of $\dot{V}O_2$max compared to nondrinkers and heavy drinkers (137), whereas other researchers reported no relationship between alcohol intake and performance in a 12 min run when other variables such as smoking were controlled (124). In collegiate athletic populations there appears to be little difference between athletes and their nonathletic peers relative to alcohol consumption. In one study the percentage of athletes who drank was 3% lower, although approximately 90% in both groups reported drinking (10). In another study athletes consumed greater quantities of alcohol compared to nonathletic controls (145).

The association between certain types of physical activity and anabolic steroid use is generally positive because anabolic steroids are used primarily for their ergogenic potential (28,169,210). The use of smokeless tobacco may also be very prevalent in certain sports (49).

Physical Activity and Exercise for Prevention of Drug Abuse

Primary prevention programs for drug abuse are designed to defer or preclude initiation of drug use, whereas secondary and tertiary prevention programs involve, respectively, counseling of persons in the early stages of abuse, and rehabilitation of the chronic drug abuser (8). Because most drug abuse begins in childhood or adolescence, using exercise for primary prevention should be planned at this life stage. Studies with adolescents have shown that sport participation is inversely related to cigarette use, and participants generally perceive smoking as a health risk (188). However, in this same report, the investigators noted that the sport participants consumed less alcohol, but contrary to their viewpoint on smoking, held the perception that alcohol would not impact on their health (188). Other studies with adolescents suggest that alcohol use may actually be positively associated with physical activity, particularly in younger males. Classifying students as *least*, *moderate*, or *most active*, Faulkner and Slattery (51) reported heavier alcohol consumption in the most active students (males under the age of 16 years) whereas Carr, Kennedy, and Dimick (26) found that male high school athletes consume alcohol significantly more than male nonathletes. No differences were noted between female counterparts in both studies.

Exercise has been included as a component of comprehensive secondary and tertiary treatment programs for substance abuse; however, research data are sparse and deal primarily with alcoholism and smoking cessation. In a 1985 review Taylor, Sallis, and Needle (187) cited only four uncontrolled studies suggestive of a therapeutic effect. However, they noted that although exercise has been employed in substance abuse treatment programs, the importance of exercise per se has not been demonstrated. Research conducted subsequent to their review supports this perspective.

Exercise training may influence smoking cessation. Seventy percent of the male participants in a 16-km race who smoked around the time they began jogging quit smoking as joggers (124); correctional officers engaged in a 6.5-week exercise-training program reported favorable, but modest, changes in smoking consumption (87). In an experimental study comparing a smoking cessation program with and without exercise (control), those who exercised were able to abstain for a longer period of time, with none of the 10 control subjects and 2 of the 7 exercising subjects maintaining abstinence at 12 months. The authors noted that these are preliminary data but supportive of the role of exercise as a component of a behavioral smoking cessation treatment (123). Conversely, compared to two control groups, an exercise program initiated following a standard smoking cessation program coupled with maintenance meetings was no more effective in maintaining abstinence for 18 months, although 34% were still abstainers (167).

Recognizing the methodological problems associated with previous research reviewed by Taylor et al. (187) relative to the role of exercise in treatment of alcoholism, Palmer, Vacc, and Epstein

(152) controlled some of the design problems and found that a 4-week exercise program based on American College of Sports Medicine guidelines elicited significant improvements in state anxiety, trait anxiety, and depression. This suggested that modifying treatment programs to include physical exercise appears worthwhile. Collingwood, Reynolds, Kohl, Smith, and Sloan (35) reported that an 8- to 9-week structured fitness program with adolescents—if it improved performance in a 1-mile run (improvers)—resulted in significantly lower substance use patterns and higher levels of abstinence as compared to nonimprovers. Therefore, physical training may be a useful supplement to intervention programs for adolescent substance abusers. Three months of physical training did reduce anxiety in eight drug and alcohol addicts. Although encouraged to continue with the exercise program following discharge from the treatment program, none did. In an 18-month follow-up, five patients had resumed the addiction. The investigators noted that physical training may be of significance in treatment of addicts; however continued contact appears to be the decisive point (152,174), an important issue that merits additional research (152).

Summary

The role of physical activity and exercise in the prevention of drug abuse is promising, although the data are limited. Most studies have focused on the mental health benefits of exercise such as reduced depression and anxiety, yet exercise may also be useful for physical health reasons. For example, exercise may help to counteract the weight gain associated with smoking cessation, or may help mitigate the fall in HDL-cholesterol levels following reduced alcohol consumption.

Although some research is available relative to these issues, the severity of the problem of drug abuse merits a significant amount of additional research to help clarify the relationship between physical activity, exercise, and the prevention of drug abuse.

References

1. Abelin, T. Epidemiology of alcohol and its sequelae in Switzerland. Ther. Umsch. 47:379-383; 1990.
2. Agurell, S.; Halldin, M.; Lindgren, J.; Ohlsson, A.; Widman, M.; Gillespie, H.; Hollister, L. Pharmacokinetics and metabolism of Δ^1-tetrahydrocannabinol and other cannabinoids with emphasis on man. Pharmacol. Rev. 38:21-43; 1986.
3. Akiba, S.; Hirayama, T. Cigarette smoking and cancer mortality risk in Japanese men and women: Results from reanalysis of the six prefecture cohort study data. Environ. Health Perspect. 87:19-26; 1990.
4. Albers, M. Osteoporosis: A health issue for women. Health Care Women Int. 11:11-19; 1990.
5. Alleyne, B.; Stuart, P.; Copes, R. Alcohol and other drug use in occupational fatalities. J. Occup. Med. 33:496-500; 1991.
6. American College of Sports Medicine. Position stand on the use of anabolic-androgenic steroids in sports. Med. Sci. Sports Exerc. 19:534-539; 1987.
7. American Medical Association. Council on Scientific Affairs. Medical and nonmedical uses of anabolic-androgenic steroids. JAMA. 264:2923-2927; 1990.
8. American Medical Association. Board of Trustees. Drug abuse in the United States. Strategies for prevention. JAMA. 265:2102-2107; 1991.
9. American Psychiatric Association. Diagnostic and statistical manual of mental disorder. 3rd ed. Revised (DSM-III-R). Washington, DC: APA; 1987.
10. Anderson, W.; Albrecht, R.; McKeag, D.; Hough, D.; McGrew, C. A national survey of alcohol and drug use by college athletes. Phys. Sportsmed. 19(2):91-104; 1991.
11. Andrade, R.; Escolar, J.; Valdivielso, P.; Gonzalez-Santos, P. Apolipoprotein distribution in plasma HDL subfractions in alcohol consumers. Drug Alcohol Depend. 26:161-168; 1990.
12. Anthony, H. Reactive changes in the blood of smokers and the development of arterial diseases and COPD, a review: Evidence of associations between changes and subsequent disease with implications for the evaluation of harmful effects of cigarettes, and for susceptibility to the chronic effects of inhaled pollutants. Rev. Environ. Health. 8:25-86; 1989.
13. Bahrke, M.; Yesalis, C.; Wright, J. Psychological and behavioural effects of endogenous testosterone levels and anabolic-androgenic steroids among males. A review. Sports Med. 10:303-337; 1990.
14. Balkau, B.; Eschwege, E.; Ducimetiere, P.; Richard, J.; Warnet, J. The high risk of death by alcohol related diseases in subjects diagnosed as diabetic and impaired glucose tolerant: The Paris Prospective Study after 15 years of follow-up. J. Clin. Epidemiol. 44:465-474; 1991.

15. Benowitz, N. Nicotine and smokeless tobacco. CA. 38:244-247; 1988.
16. Blair, S.; Kohl, H.; Paffenbarger, R.; Clark, D.; Cooper, K.; Gibbons, L. Physical fitness and all-cause mortality. A prospective study of healthy men and women. JAMA. 262:2395-2401; 1989.
17. Blank, S.; Duncan, D.; Meadows, G. Suppression of natural killer cell activity by ethanol consumption and food restriction. Alcohol Clin. Exp. Res. 15:16-22; 1991.
18. Boeing, H.; Frentzel-Beyme, R.; Berger, M.; Berndt, V.; Gores, W.; Korner, M.; Lohmeier, R.; Menarcher, A.; Mannl, H.; Meinhardt, M.; Muller, R.; Ostermeier, H.; Paul, F.; Schwemmle, K.; Wagner, K.; Wahrendorf, J. Case-control study on stomach cancer in Germany. Int. J. Cancer. 47:858-864; 1991.
19. Boffetta, P.; Garfinkel, L. Alcohol drinking and mortality among men enrolled in an American Cancer Society prospective study. Epidemiology. 1:342-348; 1990.
20. Bonaa, K.; Thelle, D. Association between blood pressure and serum lipids in a population. The Tromso study. Circulation. 83:1305-1314; 1991.
21. Boyle, P.; Macfarlane, G.; Maisonneuve, P.; Zheng, T.; Scully, C.; Tedesco, B. Epidemiology of mouth cancer in 1989: A review. J. R. Soc. Med. 83:724-730; 1990.
22. Brower, K.; Blow, F.; Young, J.; Hill, E. Symptoms and correlates of anabolic-androgenic steroid dependence. Br. J. Addict. 86:759-768; 1991.
23. Burke, T.R. The economic impact of alcohol abuse and alcoholism. Public Health Rep. 103:564-568; 1988.
24. Camargo, C. Moderate alcohol consumption and stroke. Stroke. 20:1611-1626; 1989.
25. Campillo, B.; Fouet, P.; Bonnet, J.; Atlan, G. Submaximal oxygen consumption in liver cirrhosis. Evidence of severe functional aerobic impairment. J. Hepatol. 10:163-167; 1990.
26. Carr, C.; Kennedy, S.; Dimick, K. Alcohol use among high school athletes: A comparison of alcohol use and intoxication in male and female high school athletes and non-athletes. J. Alcohol Drug Educ. 36:39-43; 1990.
27. Cassidenti, D.; Vijod, A.; Vijod, M.; Stanczyk, F.; Lobo, R. Short-term effects of smoking on the pharmacokinetic profiles of micronized estradiol in postmenopausal women. Am. J. Obstet. Gynecol. 163:1953-1960; 1990.
28. Catlin, D.; Hatton, C. Use and abuse of anabolic and other drugs for athletic enhancement. Adv. Intern. Med. 36:399-424; 1991.
29. Chambless, L.; Doring, A.; Filipia, K.; Keil, U. Determinants of HDL-cholesterol and the HDL-cholesterol/total cholesterol ratio. Results of the Lubeck blood pressure study. Int. J. Epidemiol. 19:578-585; 1990.
30. Chappard, D.; Plantard, B.; Petitjean, M.; Alexandre, C.; Riffat, G. Alcoholic cirrhosis and osteoporosis in men: A light and scanning electron microscopy study. J. Stud. Alcohol. 52:269-274; 1991.
31. Cheng, S.; Suominen, H.; Rantanen, T.; Parkatti, T.; Heikkinen, E. Bone mineral density and physical activity in 50- 60-year-old women. Bone Miner. 12:123-132; 1991.
32. Christen, A.; McDaniel, R.; McDonald, J. The smokeless tobacco 'time bomb.' Postgrad. Med. 87:69-74; 1990.
33. Chu, S.; Stroup, N.; Wingo, P.; Lee, N.; Peterson, H.; Gwinn, M. Cigarette smoking and the risk of breast cancer. Am. J. Epidemiol. 131:244-253; 1990.
34. Clark, L. Role of electrolytes in the etiology of alcohol-induced hypertension. Magnesium. 8:124-131; 1989.
35. Collingwood, T.; Reynolds, R.; Kohl, H.; Smith, W.; Sloan, S. Physical fitness effects on substance abuse risk factors and use patterns. J. Drug Educ. 21:73-84; 1991.
36. Collins, A. An analysis of the addiction liability of nicotine. Adv. Alcohol Subst. Abuse. 9:83-101; 1990.
37. Combs, A.; Acosta, D. Toxic mechanisms of the heart: A review. Toxicol. Pathol. 18:583-596; 1990.
38. Contaldo, F.; D'Arrigo, E.; Carandente, V.; Cortese, C.; Coltorti, A.; Mancini, M.; Taskinen, M.; Nikkila, E. Short-term effects of moderate alcohol consumption on lipid metabolism and energy balance in normal men. Metabolism. 38:166-171; 1989.
39. Cowart, V.S. NIDA may join in anabolic steroid research. JAMA. 261:1855-1856; 1989.
40. Creath, C.; Cutter, G.; Bradley, D.; Wright, J. Oral leukoplakia and adolescent smokeless tobacco use. Oral Surg. Oral Med. Oral Pathol. 72:35-41; 1991.
41. Cregler, L. Adverse health consequences of cocaine abuse. J. Natl. Med. Assoc. 81:27-38; 1989.
42. Dai, S.; Marti, B.; Rickenbach, M.; Gutzwiller, F. Sports correlate with positive living habits. Results from the population survey of the Swiss MONICA project. Schweiz. Z. Sportmed. 38:71-77; 1990.
43. Dewey, W. Cannabinoid pharmacology. Pharmacol. Rev. 38:151-178; 1986.
44. Diehl, A.; Fuller, J.; Mattock, M.; Salter, A.; el-Gohari, R.; Keen, H. The relationship between

high density lipoprotein subfractions to alcohol consumption, other lifestyle factors, and coronary heart disease. Atherosclerosis. 69: 145-153; 1988.

45. Dryman, A.; Anthony, J. An epidemiologic study of alcohol use as a predictor of psychiatric distress over time. Acta Psychiatr. Scand. 80:315-321; 1989.
46. Earnest, D. NSAID-induced gastric injury: Its pathogenesis and management. Semin. Arthritis Rheum. [Suppl. 2]. 19:6-10; 1990.
47. Elashoff, J.; Jacknow, A.; Shain, S.; Braunstein, G. Effects of anabolic-androgenic steroids on muscular strength. Ann. Intern. Med. 115:387-393; 1991.
48. Eliasson, M.; Lundblad, D.; Hagg, E. Cardiovascular risk factors in young snuff-users and cigarette smokers. J. Intern. Med. 230:17-22; 1991.
49. Ernster, V.; Grady, D.; Greene, J.; Walsh, M.; Robertson, P.; Daniels, T.; Benowitz, N.; Siegel, D.; Gerbert, B.; Hauck, W. Smokeless tobacco use and health effects among baseball players. JAMA. 264:218-224; 1990.
50. Ewertz, M. Smoking and breast cancer risk in Denmark. Cancer Causes Control. 1:31-37; 1990.
51. Faulkner, R.; Slattery, C. The relationship of physical activity to alcohol consumption in youth, 15-16 years of age. Can. J. Public Health. 81:168-169; 1990.
52. Flores, E.; Lange, R.; Cigarroa, R.; Hillis, L. Effect of cocaine on coronary artery dimensions in atherosclerotic coronary artery disease: Enhanced vasoconstriction at sites of significant stenoses. J. Am. Coll. Cardiol. 16:74-79; 1990.
53. Fodor, J.; Chockalingam, A. The Canadian consensus report on non-pharmacological approaches to the management of high blood pressure. Clin. Exp. Hypertens. 12:729-743; 1990.
54. Ford, E.; DeStefano, F. Risk factors for mortality from all causes and from coronary heart disease among persons with diabetes. Findings from the national health and nutrition examination survey I epidemiologic follow-up study. Am. J. Epidemiol. 133:1220-1230; 1991.
55. Forman, D. The etiology of gastric cancer. IARC Sci. Publ. 105:22-32; 1991.
56. Frankel-Conrat, H.; Singer, B. Nucleoside adducts are formed by cooperative reactions of acetaldehyde and alcohols: Possible mechanisms for the role of alcohol in carcinogenesis. Proc. Natl. Acad. Sci. 85:3758-3761; 1988.
57. Friedl, K. Reappraisal of the health risks associated with the use of high doses of oral and injectable androgenic steroids. NIDA Res. Monogr. 102:142-168; 1990.
58. Gao, Y.; Zheng, W.; Gao, R.; Jin, F. Tobacco smoking and its effect on health in China. IARC Sci. Publ. 105:62-67; 1991.
59. Garbe, S.; Garbe, E. Health in the USSR in the era of Perestroika. Cah. Sociol. Demogr. Med. 30:5-45; 1990.
60. Gawin, F. Cocaine abuse and addiction. J. Fam. Pract. 29:193-197; 1989.
61. Ghadirian, P.; Simard, A.; Baillargeon, J. Tobacco, alcohol, and coffee and cancer of the pancreas. A population-based, case-control study in Quebec, Canada. Cancer. 67:2664-2670; 1991.
62. Glantz, S.; Parmley, W. Passive smoking and heart disease. Epidemiology, physiology, and biochemistry. Circulation. 83:1-12; 1991.
63. Goldfrank, L.; Hoffman, R. The cardiovascular effects of cocaine. Ann. Emerg. Med. 20:165-175; 1991.
64. Gorelick, P. The status of alcohol as a risk factor for stroke. Stroke. 20:1607-1610; 1989.
65. Graham, S.; Kennedy, M. Recent developments in the toxicology of anabolic steroids. Drug Saf. 5:458-476; 1990.
66. Groover, J. Alcoholic liver disease. Emerg. Med. Clin. North Am. 8:887-902; 1990.
67. Hamet, P.; Mongeau, E.; Lambert, J.; Bellavance, F.; Daignault-Gelinas, M.; Ledoux, M.; Whissell-Cambiotti, L. Interactions among calcium, sodium, and alcohol intake as determinants of blood pressure. Hypertension. [Suppl. 1]. 17:I150-I154; 1991.
68. Handa, K.; Tanaka, H.; Shindo, M.; Kono, S.; Sasaki, J.; Arakawa, K. Relationship of cigarette smoking to blood pressure and serum lipids. Atherosclerosis. 84:189-193; 1990.
69. Hartung, G.; Foreyt, J.; Reeves, R.; Krock, L.; Patsch, W.; Patsch, J.; Gotto, A. Effect of alcohol dose on plasma lipoprotein subfractions and lipolytic enzyme activity in active and inactive men. Metabolism. 39:81-86; 1990.
70. Hartung, G.; Kohl, H.; Blair, S.; Lawrence, S.; Harris, T. Exercise tolerance and alcohol intake. Blood pressure relation. Hypertension. 16:501-507; 1990.
71. Hays, R.; Stacy, A.; DiMatteo, M. Covariation among health-related behaviors. Addict. Behav. 9:315-318; 1984.
72. Hebert, J.; Kabat, G. Implications for cancer epidemiology of differences in dietary intake associated with alcohol consumption. Nutr. Cancer. 15:107-119; 1991.
73. Heishman, S.J.; Stitzer, M.; Bigelow, G.E. Alcohol and marijuana: Comparative dose effect

profiles in humans. Pharmacol. Biochem. Behav. 31:649-655; 1988.

74. Hellerstedt, W.; Jeffery, R.; Murray, D. The association between alcohol intake and adiposity in the general population. Am. J. Epidemiol. 132:594-611; 1990.
75. Henningfield, J.; Cohen, C.; Slade, J. Is nicotine more addictive than cocaine? Br. J. Addict. 86:565-569; 1991.
76. Hickson, R.; Ball, K.; Falduto, M. Adverse effects of anabolic steroids. Med. Toxicol. Adverse Drug Exp. 4:254-271; 1989.
77. Higgins, M. Risk factors associated with chronic obstructive lung disease. Ann. N.Y. Acad. Sci. 624:7-17; 1991.
78. Hillbom, M.; Kaste, M. Alcohol abuse and brain infarction. Ann. Med. 22:347-352; 1990.
79. Hojnacki, J.; Deschenes, R.; Cluette-Brown, J.; Mulligan, J.; Osmolski, T.; Rencricca, N.; Barboriak, J. Effect of drinking pattern on plasma lipoproteins and body weight. Atherosclerosis. 88:49-59; 1991.
80. Holbrook, T.; Barrett-Connor, E.; Wingard, D. A prospective population-based study of alcohol use and non-insulin-dependent diabetes mellitus. Am. J. Epidemiol. 132:902-909; 1990.
81. Hollister, L. Health effects of cannabis. Pharmacol. Rev. 38:1-20; 1986.
82. Horan, M.; Lenfant, C. Epidemiology of blood pressure and predictors of hypertension. Hypertension. [Suppl. 2]. 15:I20-I24; 1990.
83. Howe, G.; Jain, M.; Burch, J.; Miller, A. Cigarette smoking and cancer of the pancreas: Evidence from a population-based case-control study in Toronto, Canada. Int. J. Cancer. 47:323-328; 1991.
84. Howe, G.; Rohan, T.; Decarli, A.; Iscovich, J.; Kaldor, J.; Katsouyanni, K.; Marubini, E.; Miller, A.; Riboli, E.; Toniolo, P. The association between alcohol and breast cancer risk: Evidence from the combined analysis of six dietary case-control studies. Int. J. Cancer. 47:707-710; 1991.
85. Jackson, R.; Scragg, R.; Beaglehole, R. Alcohol consumption and risk of coronary heart disease. Br. Med. J. 303:211-216; 1991.
86. Jensen, G.; Nyboe, J.; Appleyard, M.; Schnohr, P. Risk factors for acute myocardial infarction in Copenhagen, II: Smoking, alcohol intake, physical activity, obesity, oral contraception, diabetes, lipids, and blood pressure. Eur. Heart J. 12:298-308; 1991.
87. Jette, M.; Sidney, K. The benefits and challenges of a fitness and lifestyle enhancement program for correctional officers. Can. J. Public Health. 82:46-51; 1991.
88. Kannel, W.B. New perspectives on cardiovascular risk factors. Am. Heart J. 114:213-219; 1987.
89. Kaprio, J.; Koskenvuo, M. Twins, smoking and mortality: A 12-year prospective study of smoking-discordant twin pairs. Soc. Sci. Med. 29:1083-1089; 1989.
90. Kashkin, K.; Kleber, H. Hooked on hormones: An anabolic steroid addiction hypothesis. JAMA. 262:3166-3170; 1989.
91. Kaugars, G.; Mehailescu, W.; Gunsolley, J. Smokeless tobacco use and oral epithelial dysplasia. Cancer. 64:1527-1530; 1989.
92. Kaye, S.; Folsom, A.; Prineas, R.; Potter, J.; Gapstur, S. The association of body fat distribution with lifestyle and reproductive factors in a population study of postmenopausal women. Int. J. Obes. 14:583-591; 1990.
93. Keller, K.; Lemberg, L. Myocardial infarction in the young adult. Heart Lung. 20:95-97; 1991.
94. Kleiner, S. Performance-enhancing aids in sport: Health consequences and nutritional alternatives. J. Am. Coll. Nutr. 10:163-176, 1991.
95. Klesges, R.; Eck, L.; Isbell, T.; Fulliton, W.; Hanson, C. Smoking status: Effects on the dietary intake, physical activity, and body fat of adult men. Am. J. Clin. Nutr. 51:784-789; 1990.
96. Kneller, R.; McLaughlin, J.; Bjelke, E.; Schuman, L.; Blot, W.; Wacholder, S.; Gridley, G.; CoChien, H.; Fraumeni, J. A cohort study of stomach cancer in a high-risk American population. Cancer. 68:672-678; 1991.
97. Koo, L.; Ho, J. Worldwide epidemiological patterns of lung cancer in nonsmokers. Int. J. Epidemiol. [Suppl. 1]. 19:S14-S23; 1990.
98. Kornhuber, H.; Backhaus, B.; Kornhuber, A.; Kornhuber, J. The main cause of diabetes (type II): "Normal" alcohol drinking. Versicherungsmedizin. 42:132-142; 1990.
99. Koskinen, P.; Kupari, M. Alcohol consumption of patients with supraventricular tachyarrhythmias other than atrial fibrillation. Alcohol Alcohol. 26:199-206; 1991.
100. Koyama, H.; Suzuki, S.; Satoh, H. Effect of alcohol ingestion on urinary excretion and intraerythrocyte concentrations of sodium and potassium. Tohoku J. Exp. Med. 162:73-78; 1990.
101. Krall, E.; Dawson-Hughes, B. Smoking and bone loss among postmenopausal women. J. Bone Miner. Res. 6:331-338; 1991.
102. Krewski, D.; Wigle, D.; Clayson, D.; Howe, G. Role of epidemiology in health risk management. Recent Results Cancer Res. 120:1-24; 1990.

103. Kupari, M.; Koskinan, P. Time of onset of supraventricular tachyarrhythmia in relation to alcohol consumption. Am. J. Cardiol. 67:718-722; 1991.
104. Lamb, D.; Williams, M. editors. Ergogenics: Enhancement of performance in exercise and sport. Dubuque, IA: Brown and Benchmark; 1991.
105. Laposata, E. Cocaine-induced heart disease: Mechanisms and pathology. J. Thorac. Imaging. 6:68-75; 1991.
106. Laroche, G. Steroid anabolic drugs and arterial complications in an athlete-a case history. Angiology. 41:964-968; 1990.
107. La Vecchia, C.; Boyle, P.; Franceschi, S.; Levi, F.; Maisonneuve, P.; Negri, E.; Lucchini, F.; Smans, M. Smoking and cancer with emphasis on Europe. Eur. J. Cancer. 27:94-104; 1991.
108. Lazarus, N.; Kaplan, G.; Cohen, R.; Leu, D. Smoking and body mass in the natural history of physical activity: Prospective evidence from the Alameda County study, 1965-1974. Am. J. Prev. Med. 5:127-135; 1989.
109. Levine, S.; Brust, J.; Futrell, N.; Ho, K.; Blake, D.; Millikan, C.; Brass, L.; Fayad, P.; Schultz, L.; Selwa, J. Cerebrovascular complications of the use of the "crack" form of alkaloidal cocaine. N. Engl. J. Med. 323:699-704; 1990.
110. Lindholm, J.; Steiniche, T.; Rasmussen, E.; Thamsborg, G.; Nielsen, I.; Brockstedt-Rasmussen, H.; Storm, T.; Hyldstrup, L.; Schou, C. Bone disorder in men with chronic alcoholism: A reversible disease? J. Clin. Endocrinol. Metab. 73:118-124; 1991.
111. Lindqvist, P. Homicides committed by abusers of alcohol and illicit drugs. Br. J. Addict. 86:321-326; 1991.
112. Lombardo, J.; Hickson, R.; Lamb, D. Anabolic/androgenic steroids and growth hormone. In: Lamb, D.R.; Williams, M.H., eds. Ergogenics: Enhancement of performance in exercise and sport. Dubuque, IA: Brown and Benchmark; 1991:249-284.
113. Longnecker, M. A case-control study of alcoholic beverage consumption in relation to risk of cancer of the right colon and rectum in men. Cancer Causes Control. 1:5-14; 1990.
114. Longnecker, M.; Berlin, J.; Orza, M.; Chalmers, T. A meta-analysis of alcohol consumption in relation to risk of breast cancer. JAMA. 260:652-656; 1988.
115. Longnecker, M.; Orza, M.; Adams, M.; Vioque, J.; Chalmers, T. A meta-analysis of alcoholic beverage consumption in relation to risk of colorectal cancer. Cancer Causes Control. 1:59-68; 1990.
116. Lopez, A. Competing causes of death. A review of recent trends in mortality in industrialized countries with special reference to cancer. Ann. N.Y. Acad. Sci. 609:58-76; 1990.
117. Low, B.; Andrews, S. Adolescent suicide. Med. Clin. North Am. 74:1251-1264; 1990.
118. Luke, J.; Farb, A.; Virmani, R.; Sample, R. Sudden cardiac death during exercise in a weight lifter using anabolic androgenic steroids: Pathological and toxicological findings. J. Forensic Sci. 35:1441-1447; 1990.
119. Lyngberg, K. Myocardial infarction and death of a body builder after using anabolic steroids. Ugeskr. Laeger. 153:587-588; 1991.
120. MacMahon, B. Risk factors for cancer of the pancreas. Cancer. 50:2676-2680; 1982.
121. Maier, H.; Dietz, A.; Gewelke, U.; Seitz, H.; Heller, W. Tobacco- and alcohol-associated cancer risk of the upper respiratory and digestive tract. Laryngorhinootologie. 69:505-511; 1990.
122. Marcus, A.; Crane, L.; Shopland, D.; Lynn, W. Use of smokeless tobacco in the United States: Recent estimates from the current population survey. NCI Monogr. 8:17-23; 1989.
123. Marcus, B.; Albrecht, A.; Niaura, R.; Abrams, D.; Thompson, P. Usefulness of physical exercise for maintaining smoking cessation in women. Am. J. Cardiol. 68:406-497; 1991.
124. Marti, B.; Abelin, T.; Minder, C.; Vader, J. Smoking, alcohol consumption, and endurance capacity: An analysis of 6,500 19-year-old conscripts and 4,100 joggers. Prev. Med. 17:79-82; 1988.
125. Martin, B. Cellular effects of cannabinoids. Pharmacol. Rev. 38:45-72; 1986.
126. Mathew, R.; Wilson, W. Substance abuse and cerebral blood flow. Am. J. Psychiatry. 148:292-305; 1991.
127. Mazess, R.; Barden, H. Bone density in premenopausal women: Effects of age, dietary intake, physical activity, smoking, and birth-control pill. Am. J. Clin. Nutr. 53:132-142; 1991.
128. McCalla, S.; Minkoff, H.; Feldman, J.; Delke, I.; Salwin, M.; Valencia, G.; Glass, L. The biologic and social consequences of perinatal cocaine use in an inner-city population: Results of an anonymous cross-sectional study. Am. J. Obstet. Gynecol. 164:625-630; 1991.
129. McGill, H. Smoking and the pathogenesis of atherosclerosis. Adv. Exp. Med. Biol. 273:9-16; 1990.
130. Medina-Mora, M.; Tapia, C.; Rascon, M.; Solache, G.; Otero, B.; Lazcano, F.; Marino, M. Epidemiologic status of drug abuse in Mexico. Bull. Pan Am. Health Organ. 24:1-11; 1990.

131. Mesko, T.; Dunlap, J.; Sutherland, C. Risk factors for breast cancer. Compr. Ther. 16:3-9; 1990.
132. Meyers, H.; Zepeda, S.; Murdock, M. Alcohol and trauma. An endemic syndrome. West. J. Med. 153:149-153; 1990.
133. Miller, G.; Beckles, G.; Maude, G.; Carson, D. Alcohol consumption: Protection against coronary heart disease and risks to health. Int. J. Epidemiol. 19:923-930; 1990.
134. Miller, N. Consequences of alcohol addiction. Kans. Med. 90:339-343; 1989.
135. Misawa, K.; Matsuki, H.; Kasuga, H.; Yokoyama, H.; Hinohara, S. An epidemiological study on the relationships among HDL-cholesterol, smoking and obesity. Nippon Eiseigaku Zasshi. 44:725-732; 1989.
136. Moller, H.; Boyle,P.; Maisonneuve, P.; La Vecchia, C.; Jensen, O. Changing mortality from esophageal cancer in males in Denmark and other European countries, in relation to changing levels of alcohol consumption. Cancer Causes Control. 1:181-188; 1990.
137. Montoye, H.; Gayle, R.; Higgins, M. Smoking habits, alcohol consumption, and maximal oxygen uptake. Med. Sci. Sports Exerc. 12:316-321; 1980.
138. Moore, R.; Levine, D.; Southard, J.; Entwisle, G.; Shapiro, S. Alcohol consumption and blood pressure in the 1982 Maryland hypertension survey. Am. J. Hypertens. 3:1-7; 1990.
139. Moushmoush, B.; Abi-Mansour, P. Alcohol and the heart. The long-term effects of alcohol on the cardiovascular system. Arch. Intern. Med. 151:36-42; 1991.
140. Muscat, J.; Huncharek, M. Firearms and adult, domestic homicides. The role of alcohol and the victim. Am. J. Forensic Med. Pathol. 12:105-110; 1991.
141. Myers, G.; Hansen, T.; Jain, A. Left main coronary artery and femoral artery vasospasm associated with cocaine use. Chest. 100:257-258; 1991.
142. National Institute on Drug Abuse. Marijuana and health. Eighth annual report to the U.S. Congress. DHHS publication no. (ADM) 81-945, 1980. Washington, DC: Public Health Service. U.S. Department of Health and Human Services; 1981. Available from: U.S. Government Printing Office, Washington, DC.
143. National Institute on Drug Abuse. National household survey on drug abuse. Population estimates 1990. DHHS publication no. (ADM) 91-1732, 1990. Washington, DC: Public Health Service. U.S. Department of Health and Human Services. Available from: U.S. Government Printing Office, Washington, DC.
144. National Research Council. Diet and health: Implications for reducing chronic disease risk. Washington, DC: National Academy Press; 1989.
145. Nattiv, A.; Puffer, J. Lifestyles and health risks of collegiate athletes. J. Fam. Pract. 38:585-590; 1991.
146. Nelson, K.; Vlahov, D.; Cohn, S.; Odunmbaku, M.; Lindsay, A.; Anthony, J.; Hook, E. Sexually transmitted diseases in a population of intravenous drug users: Association with seropositivity to the human immunodeficiency virus (HIV). J. Infect. Dis. 164:457-463; 1991.
147. Novello, A. Surgeon General's report on the health benefits of smoking cessation. Public Health Rep. 105:545-548; 1990.
148. Oleckno, W.; Blacconiere, M. A multiple discriminant analysis of smoking status and health-related attitudes and behaviors. Am. J. Prev. Med. 6:323-329; 1990.
149. Olkkonen, S.; Honkanen, R. The role of alcohol in nonfatal bicycle injuries. Accid. Anal. Prev. 22:89-96; 1990.
150. Olsen, G.; Mandel, J.; Gibson, R.; Wattenberg, L.; Schuman, L. A case-control study of pancreatic cancer and cigarettes, alcohol, coffee, and diet. Am. J. Public Health. 79:1016-1019; 1989.
151. Palmer, J.; Rosenberg, L.; Clarke, E.; Stolley, P.; Warshauer, M.; Zauber, A.; Shapiro, S. Breast cancer and cigarette smoking: A hypothesis. Am. J. Epidemiol. 134:1-13; 1991.
152. Palmer, J.; Vacc, N.; Epstein, J. Adult inpatient alcoholics: Physical exercise as a treatment intervention. J. Stud. Alcohol. 49:418-421; 1988.
153. Patel, B.; D'Arville, C.; Iwahashi, M.; Simon, F. Impairment of hepatic insulin receptors during chronic ethanol administration. Am. J. Physiol. 261:6199-6205; 1991.
154. Petronis, K.; Anthony, J. An epidemiologic investigation of marijuana- and cocaine-related palpitations. Drug Alcohol Depend. 23:219-226; 1989.
155. Pettersson, P.; Ellsinger, B.; Sjoberg, C.; Bjorntorp, P. Fat distribution and steroid hormones in women with alcohol abuse. J. Intern. Med. 228:311-316; 1990.
156. Pohorecky, L. Interaction of alcohol and stress at the cardiovascular level. Alcohol. 7:537-546; 1990.
157. Pope, H.; Katz, D. Homicide and near-homicide by anabolic steroid users. J. Clin. Psychiatry. 51:28-31; 1990.
158. Pouilles, J.; Ribot, C.; Tremollieres, F.; Bonneu, M.; Brun, S. Risk factors of vertebral

osteoporosis. Results of a study of 2279 women referred to a menopause clinic. Rev. Rhum. Mal. Osteoartic. 58:169-177; 1991.
159. Preston-Martin, S. Evaluation of the evidence that tobacco-specific nitrosamines (TSNA) cause cancer in humans. Crit. Rev. Toxicol. 21:295-298; 1991.
160. Puig, T.; Marti, B.; Rickenbach, M.; Dai, S.; Casacuberta, C.; Wietlisbach, V.; Gutzwiller, F. Some determinants of body weight, subcutaneous fat, and fat distribution in 25-64 year old Swiss urban men and women. Soz. Praventivmed. 35:193-200; 1990.
161. Regan, T. Alcohol and the cardiovascular system. JAMA. 264:377-381; 1990.
162. Reinke, L.; Rau, J.; McCay, P. Possible roles of free radicals in alcohol tissue damage. Free Radic. Res. Commun. 9:205-211; 1990.
163. Revicki, D.; Sobal, J.; DeForge, B. Smoking status and the practice of other unhealthy behaviors. Fam. Med. 23:361-364; 1991.
164. Riboli, E.; Cornee, J.; Macquart-Moulin, G.; Kaaks, R.; Casagrande, C.; Guyader, M. Cancer and polyps of the colorectum and lifetime consumption of beer and other alcoholic beverages. Am. J. Epidemiol. 134:157-166; 1991.
165. Rimm, E.; Giovannucci, E.; Willett, W.; Colditz, G.; Ascherio, A.; Rosner, B.; Stampfer, M. Prospective study of alcohol consumption and risk of coronary disease in men. Lancet. 338:464-468; 1991.
166. Rothman, K.; Cann, D.; Fried, M. Carcinogenicity of dark liquor. Am. J. Public Health. 79:1516-1520; 1989.
167. Russell, P.; Epstein, L.; Johnston, J.; Block, D.; Blair, E. The effects of physical activity as maintenance for smoking cessation. Addict. Behav. 13:215-218; 1988.
168. Sallis, J.; Hovell, M.; Hofstetter, C.; Faucher, P.; Elder, J.; Blanchard, J.; Caspersen, C.; Powell, K.; Christenson, G. A multivariate study of determinants of vigorous exercise in a community sample. Prev. Med. 18:20-34; 1989.
169. Salva, P.; Bacon, G. Anabolic steroids: Interest among parents and nonathletes. South. Med. J. 84:552-556; 1991.
170. Savolainen, M.; Hannuksela, M.; Seppanen, S.; Kervinen, K.; Kesaniemi, Y. Increased high-density lipoprotein cholesterol concentration in alcoholics is related to low cholesteryl ester transfer protein activity. Eur. J. Clin. Invest. 20:593-599; 1990.
171. Scragg, R.; Stewart, A.; Jackson, R.; Beaglehole, R. Alcohol and exercise in myocardial infarction and sudden coronary death in men and women. Am. J. Epidemiol. 126:77-85; 1987.
172. Seidell, J.; Cigolini, M.; Deslypere, J.; Charzewska, J.; Ellsinger, B.; Cruz, A. Body fat distribution in relation to physical activity and smoking habits of 38-year-old European men. The European fat distribution study. Am. J. Epidemiol. 133:257-265; 1991.
173. Selby, J.; Newman, B.; Quesenberry, C.; Fabsitz, R.; Carmelli, D.; Meaney, F.; Slemenda, C. Genetic and behavioral influences on body fat distribution. Int. J. Obes. 14:593-602; 1990.
174. Sell, E.; Christensen, N. The effect of physical training on physical, mental and social conditions in drug and/or alcohol addicts. Ugeskr. Laeger. 151:2064-2067; 1989.
175. Senay, E. Drug abuse and public health. A global perspective. Drug Saf. [Suppl. 1]. 6:1-65; 1991.
176. Shaper, A. Alcohol and mortality: A review of prospective studies. Br. J. Addict. 85:837-861; 1990.
177. Shaper, A.; Phillips, A.; Pocock, S.; Walker, M.; Macfarlane, P. Risk factors for stroke in middle aged British men. Br. Med. J. 302:1111-1115; 1991.
178. Shopland, D.; Eyre, H.; Pechacek, T. Smoking attributable cancer mortality in 1991: Is lung cancer now the leading cause of death among smokers in the United States? J. Natl. Cancer Inst. 83:1142-1148; 1991.
179. Siekierzynska-Czarnecka, A.; Polowiec, Z.; Kulawinska, M.; Rowinska-Zakrzewska, E. Death caused by pulmonary embolism in a body builder taking anabolic steroids (metanabol). Wiad. Lek. 43:972-975; 1990.
180. Slap, G.; Vorters, D.; Chaudhuri, S.; Centor, R. Risk factors for attempted suicide during adolescence. Pediatrics. 84:762-772; 1989.
181. Slemenda, C.; Hui, S.; Longcope, C.; Johnston, C. Cigarette smoking,obesity, and bone mass. J. Bone Miner. Res. 4:737-741; 1989.
182. Smart, R.; Mann, R. Factors in recent reductions in liver cirrhosis deaths. J. Stud. Alcohol. 52:232-240; 1991.
183. Stampfer, M.; Colditz, G.; Willett, W.; Speizer, F.; Hennekens, C. A prospective study of moderate alcohol consumption and the risk of coronary disease and stroke in women. N. Engl. J. Med. 319:267-273; 1988.
184. Steinberg, D.; Pearson, T.; Kuller, L. Alcohol and atherosclerosis. Ann. Intern. Med. 114: 967-976; 1991.
185. Stemmermann, G.; Nomura, A.; Chyou, P.; Yoshizawa, C. Prospective study of alcohol intake and large bowel cancer. Dig. Dis. Sci. 35:1414-1420; 1990.
186. Strauss, R.; Yesalis, C. Anabolic steroids in the athlete. Annu. Rev. Med. 42:449-457; 1991.

187. Taylor, C.; Sallis, J.; Needle, R. The relation of physical activity and exercise to mental health. Public Health Rep. 100:195-202; 1985.
188. Thorlindsson, T.; Vilhjalmsson, R.; Valgeirsson, G. Sport participation and perceived health status: A study of adolescents. Soc. Sci. Med. 31:551-556; 1990.
189. Tien, A.; Anthony, J. Epidemiological analysis of alcohol and drug use as risk factors for psychotic experiences. J. Nerv. Ment. Dis. 178:473-480; 1990.
190. Troisi, R.; Heinold, J.; Vokonas, P.; Weiss, S. Cigarette smoking, dietary intake, and physical activity: Effects on body fat distribution—the normative aging study. Am. J. Clin. Nutr. 53:1104-1111; 1991.
191. Tuyns, A. Alcohol and cancer. Proc. Nutr. Soc. 49:145-151; 1990.
192. Umbricht-Schneiter, A.; Santora, P.; Moore, R. Alcohol abuse: Comparison of two methods for assessing its prevalence and associated morbidity in hospitalized patients. Am. J. Med. 91:110-118; 1991.
193. United States Department of Health and Human Services. Public Health Service. Healthy people 2000: National health promotion and disease prevention objectives. Washington, DC: U.S. Government Printing Office, 1991.
194. United States Department of Transportation. Drunk driving facts. National Center for Statistics and Analysis. RPO717, 1988, August.
195. Vaillant, G.; Schnurr, P.; Baron, J.; Gerber, P. A prospective study of the effects of cigarette smoking and alcohol abuse on mortality. J. Gen. Intern. Med. 6:299-304; 1991.
196. Vatten, L.; Kvinnsland, S. Cigarette smoking and risk of breast cancer: A prospective study of 24,329 Norwegian women. Eur. J. Cancer. 26:830-833; 1990.
197. Veenstra, J.; Ockhuizen, T.; van de Pol, H.; Wedel, M.; Schaafsma, G. Effects of a moderate dose of alcohol on blood lipids and lipoproteins postprandially and in the fasting state. Alcohol Alcohol. 25:371-377; 1990.
198. Velema, J.; Walker, A.; Gold, E. Alcohol and pancreatic cancer. Insufficient epidemiologic evidence for a causal relationship. Epidemiol. Rev. 8:28-41; 1986.
199. Wadler, G.I.; Hainline, B. Drugs and the athlete. Philadelphia: Davis; 1989.
200. Whitney, S.; Conti, J. Adolescent drug abuse: Problem and prospectus. Med. Law. 9:972-985; 1990.
201. Williams, M. Drugs and athletic performance. Springfield, IL: C.C. Thomas; 1974.
202. Williams, M. Drugs and sport performance. In: Ryan, A.; Allman, F., eds. Sports medicine. New York: Academic Press; 1989:183-210.
203. Williams, M. Alcohol, marijuana, and beta blockers. In: Lamb, D.R.; Williams, M.H., eds. Ergogenics: Enhancement of performance in exercise and sport. Dubuque, IA: Brown and Benchmark; 1991:331-372.
204. Williams, M. Lifetime fitness and wellness: A personal choice. 3rd ed. Dubuque, IA: Brown; [1993].
205. Windsor, R.; Dumitru, D. Anabolic steroid use by athletes. How serious are the health hazards? Postgrad. Med. 84:37-49; 1988.
206. Winn, D. Smokeless tobacco and cancer: The epidemiologic evidence. CA. 38:236-243; 1988.
207. Wu, T.; Tashkin, D.; Djahed, B.; Rose, J. Pulmonary hazards of smoking marijuana as compared to tobacco. N. Engl. J. Med. 318:347-351; 1988.
208. Wynder, E.; Fujita, Y.; Harris, R.; Hirayama, T.; Hiyama, T. Comparative epidemiology of cancer between the United States and Japan. A second look. Cancer. 67:746-763; 1991.
209. Xie, J.; Lesaffre, E.; Kestaloot, H. The relationship between animal fat intake, cigarette smoking, and lung cancer. Cancer Causes Control. 2:79-83; 1991.
210. Yesalis, C.; Anderson, W.; Buckley, W.; Wright, J. Incidence of the nonmedical use of anabolic-androgenic steroids. NIDA Res. Monogr. 102:97-112; 1990.
211. Yesalis, C. Wright, J.; Lombardo, J. Anabolic-androgenic steroids: A synthesis of existing data and recommendations for future research. Clin. Sports Med. 1:109-134; 1989.
212. Zatonski, W.; Becher, H.; Lissowska, J.; Wahrendorf, J. Tobacco, alcohol, and diet in the etiology of laryngeal cancer: A population-based case-control study. Cancer Causes Control. 2:3-10; 1991.

PART VI

Physical Activity and Fitness Across the Life Cycle

Chapter 62

Physical Activity: Relationship to Growth, Maturation, and Physical Fitness

Robert M. Malina

Regular physical activity is generally viewed as having a favorable influence on the growth, biological maturation, and physical fitness of children and youth. Rarick (78, see also 79), for example, suggests that "a certain 'minima' of muscular activity are essential for supporting 'normal growth' and for maintaining the protoplasmic integrity of the tissues" (p. 460). Others suggest a stimulatory or accelerating influence on growth, sexual maturation, and function (19,71). Concern for potentially negative consequences of physical activity in the context of training for sport on growth and maturation, more so for girls than boys, is also apparent. Some (33,37) have concluded that each year of training before menarche delays menarche by about 0.4 to 0.5 years. Others inquire (44), based on a few case studies that appear to be constitutional delay: "What are the mechanisms of slowed growth and delayed or suppressed puberty induced by intensive physical activity?" (p. 3).

Much concern is also expressed for the state of physical fitness and generally low levels of habitual physical activity among contemporary children and youth. The concern is usually framed in the context of adult health issues, primarily cardiovascular fitness and mortality from ischemic heart disease, low back problems, and so on (53) and not relative to the health status of children and youth.

In the context of the preceding, what is the influence of regular physical activity on growth, maturation, and fitness? Can formal training enhance growth and maturation beyond limits set by the genotype? Or, can regular training inhibit growth and delay maturation? Can effects of training be effectively partitioned from other factors associated with sport, such as extremely selective criteria and perhaps dietary restrictions applied in some sports (e.g., ballet and gymnastics)? More appropriate to the consensus conference, can observations and conclusions derived from highly select and specialized samples be extended to the general population of children and youth? Do they cause undue concern among parents and others for the health of children involved in sport? A recent publication of the American Medical Association and the American Dietetic Association (1) asks: "Can adolescents be too active?" and cautions:

> Some fitness programs may be detrimental to adolescents if they mandate prolonged, strenuous exercise and/or very low body fat to maximize their competitive edge. . . . These regimes may delay sexual maturation, decrease bone growth and ultimate height, and cause temporary amenorrhea in females. Excessive activity may also result in a very low body weight, inadequate mineralization of the skeleton, anemia due to red blood cell destruction, and episodic bone fractures. (p. 4)

Given concern for the lack of physical activity and fitness among contemporary populations in developed countries, this caution is hardly applicable to the vast majority of children and youth. A more appropriate issue is how can activity and fitness levels of children and youth be increased. In the context of these questions and concerns, effects of regular physical activity on indicators of growth, maturation, and fitness of children and youth are considered.

Definitions of Relevant Terms

Growth

Growth refers to increase in size, either of the body as a whole or of its parts. Growth is characterized by increases in stature and weight, and changes in physique, body composition, and various systems. Heart volume, lung function, aerobic power, and muscular strength are related to body size and have growth patterns that are generally similar to those for stature and weight (59).

Maturation

Maturation refers to the tempo (rate) and timing of progress toward the mature biological state, and is most often viewed in the context of sexual (secondary sex characteristics), skeletal (skeletal age), and somatic (age at peak height velocity or PHV) maturation. Skeletal maturation spans the growth period, whereas sexual and somatic maturation are limited to adolescence.

Physical Fitness

Physical fitness includes muscular, motor, and cardiorespiratory fitness, as well as body composition and metabolic components (15). The components change with growth and maturation and many follow a pattern of growth similar to that for stature and weight (59). The metabolic component will not be considered.

Physical Activity

Physical activity (15) includes "any body movement produced by the skeletal muscles and resulting in a substantial increase over the resting energy expenditure" (p. 3). The measurement of habitual physical activity and energy expenditure during childhood is a difficult task and needs further attention. Data for large samples of children are derived from questionnaires, interviews, and occasionally diaries, whereas pedometers and heart rate integrators are used less often (47). Estimates of energy expenditure for adequately nourished samples of children with the doubly labeled water method are presently limited but are becoming available (22).

Activity and Training

Physical activity is not the same as regular training. The former refers to the child's level of habitual activity (e.g., hr/week or an activity score). Although some activity occurs in the context of school physical education, a significant percentage of activity occurs outside of school and in organized youth sport programs. However, only a small percentage of children and youth train. *Training* refers to systematic, specialized practice of activities related to a specific sport or sport discipline for most of the year or to specific short-term experimental programs (e.g., 15 weeks of endurance running or resistance training).

Inferences about the influence of regular physical activity and training on growth and maturation are based largely on short-term experimental training studies, comparisons of the growth and maturity characteristics of athletes and nonathletes, and several comparisons of active and inactive children. Longitudinal studies that span childhood and adolescence and that control for physical activity are few. Criteria used to classify children as active or inactive also vary.

Studies of athletes focus primarily on those disciplines characterized by early entry into formal training, especially swimming, gymnastics, and ballet. Elite young athletes are a select group and differ from the general population in size, physique, and maturity status. Differences are apparent as early as 3 to 4 years of age in female gymnasts (75) and 7 years of age in female swimmers (2). Successful young ballet dancers tend to have the thinness and proportional features of elite ballerinas (21). Boys who are successful in sports at relatively young ages tend to be advanced in biological maturity status and are thus, on average, taller and heavier than their chronological age peers. This is especially evident in age group swimming, American football, baseball, and track (48).

Care is thus in order in generalizing from observations on elite young athletes. It cannot be assumed a priori that differences in growth and maturation between young athletes and nonathletes are due to regular training.

Activity and Growth

Stature and Weight

Regular physical activity has no apparent effect on statural growth (49,54). Early data suggest both a stimulatory (9,88) and inhibitory (82) influence of training on statural growth of males. However, subject selection and maturity status were not controlled, and the observed changes were quite small. In contrast to stature, early studies indicate an increase in body weight (9,41), which probably reflects late adolescent growth of muscle mass and the effects of training. Improved nutritional status during the training programs may be a contributing factor (41).

Longitudinal data on active and inactive boys followed from late childhood through adolescence indicate no differences in stature (8,54,62,63). However, data for boys and girls active in sports during childhood and adolescence indicate, on average, taller statures and greater weights from 8 to 18 years of age (56). The growth pattern of the boys is that of early maturers since they are advanced in skeletal age and age at PHV. The pattern of the girls is that of tall, average maturers whose skeletal and chronological ages do not differ and whose ages at PHV and menarche are only slightly later than the reference data.

The growth status of young athletes varies with the sport. Among female gymnasts and swimmers, the former are already shorter than average and the latter are already taller than average prior to gymnastics and swim training, respectively (2,75), which is consistent with cross-sectional data at older ages (54). Parents of gymnasts are also shorter than those of swimmers (75), which would imply a genotypic factor in body size. Elite distance runners 9 to 15 years of age, though somewhat shorter than normally active nonrunners, have similar growth rates (89,90). Young runners of both sexes have the linearity of physique that is characteristic of adult distance runners (90).

The limitations of studies of young athletes in making inferences about training and statural growth are obvious. There is variation among sport disciplines, and sport selection, whether by the athlete, parent, coach, or some combination is a critical factor. The data suggest no influence of physical activity and training on statural growth. In well-nourished children stature is mediated primarily by the genotype. Body weight, on the other hand, may be influenced by regular activity and training, resulting in alterations of body composition.

Body Composition

Regular physical activity and training for sports are associated with a decrease in fatness in both sexes and occasionally with an increase in fat-free mass (FFM) in boys (14,70,72,102). Changes in fatness depend on continued, regular activity (or caloric restriction) for their maintenance, but it is difficult to partition effects of training on FFM from expected age-associated increases during growth.

Longitudinal data on changes in body composition associated with activity are limited. Regularly active boys (6 hr/week sport training) had a larger FFM and less relative fatness than boys with moderate and low levels of physical activity from 11 to 17 years of age (70). The differences in FFM reflect, in part, maturity-associated variation because the active boys were taller and heavier than boys in the other two groups from age 11 to 17 years, experienced earlier PHV (93), and were more advanced in skeletal maturation between age 13 to 16 years (70). Moderately active boys and boys with normal activity did not differ in maturity status; they differed in relative fatness but not in FFM. This would suggest that more intensive training may be needed to induce changes in FFM. Note that increases in FFM with training do not consistently occur in older adolescents and young adults (31).

Young athletes involved in several sports have less relative fatness than nonathletes. Males, both athletes and nonathletes, show a decline in relative fatness during adolescence, but athletes tend to have less relative fatness. Relative fatness does not increase with age during adolescence in female athletes as it does in nonathletes. As a result, the difference between female athletes and nonathletes is greater than the corresponding trend in males (59).

Indicators of physical activity are moderately related to skinfold thickness in 8- to 9-year-old boys and girls; that is, the more active have less subcutaneous fat, and account for about 18% of the variance in fatness (73). Cross-sectional data indicate thinner skinfold thicknesses in active children (84) and young athletes (72,90) than in reference samples. However, boys and girls in upper and lower quartiles of energy expenditure followed from 6 to 12 years of age (86), and active and inactive boys followed from 13 to 18 years of age (8) do not differ from each other in skinfold thicknesses. Boys and girls involved in sports and followed longitudinally from 8 to 18 years of age have skinfold thicknesses that do not differ from local reference data (56).

Although the data are somewhat variable, variation in body composition in conjunction with regular physical activity or inactivity in children and youth is largely associated with fatness and minimal changes in FFM. Changes in FFM are confounded by maturity-associated variation during adolescence, especially in males.

Sex differences in the responsiveness of FFM, fatness, and fat distribution to training during growth merit consideration. Young adult males decline in relative fatness and subcutaneous fat, and increase in FFM after 15 weeks of aerobic training, but young adult females do not (98). The evidence for young adult males also suggests greater reduction in trunk than in extremity skinfold thicknesses after 15 (98) and 20 weeks (25) of aerobic training. In contrast, reduction in subcutaneous fat with aerobic training in young adult females is evenly distributed between extremity and trunk (98).

Males, on average, experience a reduction in extremity and an increase in trunk skinfold thicknesses during adolescence, which results in proportionally greater accumulation of subcutaneous fat on the trunk. Females, on the other hand, accumulate subcutaneous fat on the extremities and trunk at a generally similar rate (58). It would be of interest to learn whether fat accumulation on the trunk is reduced in adolescent males involved in regular training, or whether both extremity and trunk skinfold thicknesses are similarly less in actively training females.

Activity and Biological Maturation

Skeletal age, age at PHV, age at appearance of secondary sex characteristics, and age at menarche are indicators of biological maturity status. They are sufficiently interrelated to suggest a general maturity factor that underlies the timing and tempo of the adolescent growth spurt and sexual maturation. This factor probably discriminates among individuals who are early, average, or late in the timing of adolescent events. On the other hand, there is variation among maturity indicators so that no single system provides a complete description of the timing and tempo of growth and maturation of an individual child during adolescence (11). There also is no consistent relationship between the age at which breast, genital, or pubic hair development begins and the rate of progress from the immature to the mature state. For example, some boys pass from genital Stages 2 (initial enlargement of the genitalia) through 5 (mature state) in about 2 years, whereas others take about 5 years (60).

Somatic Maturity

Age at PHV and magnitude of PHV are not affected by regular activity or training (8,42,54,56, 62,63,93). Corresponding data for girls are limited to a small sample of girls engaged in club sports who show a somewhat later age at PHV than local reference data (56). Estimates of ages at PHV for elite young athletes are not available except for an earlier age at PHV in four elite Japanese distance runners (42).

Skeletal Maturation

Regular activity does not accelerate or delay skeletal maturation of the hand and wrist, the area most often used to assess skeletal age. Longitudinal observations on children regularly training for sports—gymnastics, figure skating, tennis, volleyball, cycling, ice hockey, and rowing—indicate corresponding gains in chronological and skeletal ages over periods of 3 to 4 years (43,69). Further, with athletes classified as having skeletal ages in advance of, on par with, or behind their chronological ages, about 80% remained in the same category after 3 to 4 years of training; those who changed categories did so in no consistent pattern (69). Active and inactive boys do not differ in skeletal age from 13 to 18 years of age (8). Boys active in sports are advanced in skeletal maturation, whereas girls active in sports do not differ from reference data from age 10 to 15 years (56).

Corresponding data for elite young athletes are largely cross-sectional, so that inferences about training effects are not warranted. Girls engaged in ballet, gymnastics, and track tend to have skeletal ages that lag behind chronological age, whereas those involved in swimming tend to have skeletal ages that are somewhat advanced relative to chronological age (20,48,55,103). Boys successful in baseball, track, swimming, cycling, and rowing tend to have, on average, skeletal ages in advance of chronological age (48,55). Cross-sectional data for boys in ice hockey and soccer indicate similar skeletal and chronological ages in late childhood or early adolescent players, but advanced skeletal ages in adolescent participants (17,59).

The process of skeletal maturation of the hand and wrist is thus not affected by regular training. However, as skeletal maturity of the hand and wrist is attained, at about age 16 to 17 years in girls and age 18 to 19 years in boys, the differences between those of contrasting maturity status is reduced and eventually eliminated.

Sexual Maturation

Longitudinal data on the sexual maturation of either girls or boys undergoing regular physical activity or training are limited. Much of the discussion focuses on later mean ages at menarche of athletes compared to the general population with the inference that training delays menarche (46). The data are largely retrospective and do not consider other factors that may influence menarche.

Athletes in a variety of sports attain menarche, on average, later than nonathletes (46,52,59). Standard deviations are generally more than 1 year. Thus, many athletes do in fact attain menarche close to or earlier than the mean for nonathletes, and many nonathletes attain menarche later than athletes. Also, black athletes attain menarche earlier than white athletes (52). Mothers of ballet dancers attain menarche later than nondancer controls (16), and sisters of university swimmers also tend to attain menarche later than average (94). Thus, familial tendency for later maturation in athletes must be considered. There is also a need to complement the retrospective data with status quo estimates (using probit analysis) in larger samples of young athletes.

Based on the correlation of years of training (intensity not specified) before menarche and age at menarche, some (33,37) have concluded that premenarcheal training in swimming, running, and ballet "delays" menarche by about 0.4 to 0.5 year for each year of premenarcheal training. Correlation does not imply causality. Assume, for example, that two girls begin formal training at 7 years of age, one being genotypically an early maturer, attaining menarche at age 11 years, and the other genotypically a late maturer, attaining menarche at age 15 years. The former will have only 4 years while the latter will have 8 years of premenarcheal training. The association of years of premenarcheal training with a later menarche is likely an analytical artifact. Further, computer simulation of quasi-experimental designs used in studies of the association between age at menarche and age at initiation of training before menarche indicates biased estimates of the statistical parameters (95).

If training is related to later menarche, it probably interacts with or is confounded by other factors so that the specific effects of training per se may be difficult to extract. Linearity of physique is associated with later maturation in both sexes (59,97), and some sports select for slenderness (e.g., ballet, distance running, and gymnastics). Dietary practices associated with an emphasis on thinness or an optimal weight for performance in young ballerinas and gymnasts may be additional contributory factors. Significant numbers of ballet dancers have eating problems (18,37), and the diets of (formerly) East German gymnasts were maintained in slight negative energy balance to maintain optimal weights for performance (40). The demands of exercise also compete with those of growth and maturational processes for the available energy.

It is important to emphasize that not all athletes experience late menarche. Late menarche (age 16+ years) and extremely late menarche (age 18+ years) occur in a small percentage of athletes. These athletes would be classified as having *primary amenorrhea* (91). Note, however, that normally 95% and 98% of women have attained menarche by 16 and 18 years of age, respectively (67). The most common cause of primary amenorrhea among athletes is constitutional delay followed by congenital factors (91). In addition to genotype, other factors in the environments of athletes, for example, dietary alteration, weight loss, psychological stress, or overtraining, among others, may be contributory. The etiology of late menarche in some athletes may be multifactorial. The situation is analogous to menstrual dysfunction where several factors in addition to training are involved (52,67,91).

Other factors that may influence menarche are not often considered in studies of athletes. Family size or number of siblings in the family is an example. Girls from larger families tend to attain menarche later than those from smaller families, and the estimated magnitude of the sibling number effect is similar in athletes and nonathletes (52).

Caution is needed in extending observations on samples of select, elite female athletes to the general population. The popular literature often implies a direct relationship between later maturation and training, and this may result in undue concern in parents and perhaps withdrawal of some girls from sport participation.

The relationship between systematic training and sexual maturation of boys has not been considered, although it has been suggested (104) that "boys may be better prepared physically for metabolic demands during the development of reproductive maturity" (p. 370). The underlying neuroendocrine processes are generally similar, and stresses associated with training for sports affect boys as well as girls. With the exception of wrestling, emphasis on extreme weight regulation is not characteristic of sports for boys. In contrast, some literature suggests that the growth and maturation of males may be more susceptible to environmental alteration, whereas that of females may be better buffered against environmental stress (10,96).

Activity and Specific Tissues

The skeleton provides the framework of the body and is its main mineral reservoir, and skeletal muscle is the major work-producing and oxygen-consuming tissue. Adipose tissue represents energy in stored form, and in excessive amounts is a risk factor for several degenerative diseases in adulthood. The three tissues are influenced by regular physical activity.

Skeletal Tissue

Experimental studies of growing animals indicate greater skeletal mineralization, density, and bone mass in response to regular training (45). Studies of human adults indicate similar results—individuals with a history of regular physical activity or training in childhood and youth have an increased bone mass (3,4,45,65). Because specialized training in sports was begun during youth, the results may represent beneficial effects of activity on bone mineralization during growth.

Corresponding data for children and youth are limited. Observations of amateur baseball players suggest increased mineral content of the humerus of the preferred arm (107). Differences between the preferred and nonpreferred humeri increased with age, which suggests a training effect, assuming that older players participated in specialized throwing activity longer than younger players. Physical activity in the preceding year accounted for a small percentage of the variance (6.7%–15.0%) of whole-body and lumbar bone mineral content among adolescent girls age 14 to 18 years (13), and recalled childhood physical activity was positively related to calcaneal bone density in women age 20 to 35 years (61). Although limited, the preceding observations are important because bone mineral established during childhood and youth may be a determinant of adult bone mineral status (4).

In contrast to the positive effect of physical activity on bone mineralization, excessive training associated with altered menstrual function contributes to bone loss in some athletes and increases susceptibility to stress fractures (26,27,105). Restrictive diets are a contributory factor (34). There thus may be a threshold for some adolescents and young adults. Regular physical activity may have a beneficial effect on the integrity of skeletal tissue up to a point. However, when physical activity is excessive, menstrual function may be altered. Dietary deficiencies are an additional factor. Thus, under conditions of altered menstrual function and a deficient diet, physical activity may have a negative influence on skeletal integrity.

Late menarche per se may be a risk factor for stress fractures in professional ballet dancers (105), whereas years of "serious" training prior to menarche are related the incidence of stress fractures in runners (36). However, ages at menarche in university athletes experiencing stress fractures do not differ from athletes in the same sport not experiencing stress fractures. There is also no association between age at onset of specialized training and stress fractures: 7 athletes began specialized training near menarche (within ± 0.5 year), 7 began before menarche, and 15 began after menarche (57). Hence, late menarche by itself may not be a risk factor for stress fractures. Other factors such as dietary restriction, training errors, running surface, and so on, may be involved in a multifactorial etiology.

Muscle Tissue

Data on the effects of training on muscle tissue of growing children, although limited, indicate changes that are generally in the same direction as those observed in young adults (5). Changes are specific to the type of training program. Muscular hypertrophy is associated with high-resistance activities such as weight training in adolescent boys, and may not occur or may occur to a much lesser extent in preadolescent boys and in other forms of training. There is no strong evidence to suggest that fiber-type distribution in youth can be changed as a result of training (30,32,39).

Endurance training is associated with increased succinate dehydrogenase (SDH) and phosphofructokinase (PFK) activities in 11-year-old boys (30). However, 3 months of endurance training in 16-year-old boys resulted only in increased SDH activity, whereas 3 months of sprint training resulted only in increased PFK activity (32). Differences in training protocols may account for the differences observed in 11- and 16-year-old boys. The endurance-trained adolescent boys also showed increased areas of Type I and Type II fibers, but the sprint-trained boys did not. After 6 months of no supervised training, however, SDH and PFK returned to pretraining levels (32). This observation indicates an important feature of training studies: Changes in response to short-term programs are generally not permanent and depend on regular activity for maintenance. Monitoring changes associated with training after a training program ceases would permit a more accurate evaluation of the effects of training. Data for females are lacking. Nevertheless, physical training has the potential to be an important modifying factor of muscle metabolic capacity in growing children.

Adipose Tissue

Information on the effects of regular activity or training on adipose tissue cellularity and metabolism of children is lacking. The decrease in fatness associated with training in adults is attributable solely to a reduction in adipocyte size (12). Trained adults also have increased ability to mobilize and oxidize fat, which is associated with increased lipolysis. Increases in lipolysis also occur in sedentary adults exposed to aerobic training, and the increase in lipolysis is greater in males than in females (24).

Corresponding observations on training and adipose tissue metabolism in children are not presently available. Given the similarity in the response of muscle tissue to training in children and adults, it may be reasonable to assume similar metabolic responses of adipose tissue to training in children and adults. Further, adipose tissue cellularity increases gradually during childhood and then more rapidly with the onset of puberty (59). Possible effects of regular training on adipose cellularity during growth have not been addressed.

Activity and Fitness

Studies of physical activity and fitness take several forms, including those that compare the fitness characteristics of active and inactive children, those that assess the relationship between physical activity and fitness, and those that consider the effects of specific training programs on components of fitness.

Active and Inactive Children

The majority of data are derived from boys. Because studies differ in criteria for activity and performance tasks, results of specific longitudinal studies are summarized. In two studies of Czechoslovakian boys (one study from age 12 to 15 years [43,77] and the other from age 11 to 17 years [92,93]), boys actively training for sports (about 4–6 hr/week) improved more in maximal oxygen uptake (absolute and relative) than boys spending less time in physical activity. In the short-term study, actively training boys also improved more in static strength and heart rate response to standardized work loads than control subjects and dropouts from the programs (43,77).

In the Saskatchewan Growth Study (62,63), inactive boys (ascertained by parental questionnaires, teacher assessments, and sport participation inventory) had lower absolute and relative maximal aerobic power than active boys and those with average levels of physical activity from age 8 to 16 years. Inactive boys also had an adolescent spurt in $\dot{V}O_2max$ that was less than that observed in the normally active and highly active boys. Active boys had a greater relative $\dot{V}O_2max$ before, during, and after the growth spurt than normally active and inactive boys.

Active boys (5+ hr/week in addition to physical education) followed longitudinally from age 13 to 18 years in the Leuven Growth Study of Belgian Boys performed better than inactive boys in pulse recovery after a step test and a flexed arm hang test (8). However, active and inactive boys did not differ in abdominal strength, lower back flexibility, static arm strength, and several motor fitness items.

Active Dutch boys (time spent in physical activity) followed longitudinally from age 13 to 16 years performed better in several components of fitness: maximal aerobic power, 12 min run, flexed arm hang, and shuttle run (100). Only maximal aerobic power and the endurance run were better in active girls from age 13 to 16 years. Active and inactive boys and girls did not differ in abdominal and static arm strength, lower back flexibility, speed of limb movement, and the standing long jump. Also, active and inactive girls did not differ in the flexed arm hang and shuttle run (100).

The evidence indicates higher levels of cardiorespiratory endurance in active boys and girls, although the data for girls are limited. Cross-sectional data also indicate better endurance performance in active children and youth, but generally better levels of motor fitness in more active boys (66,80,84) and girls (66). It is difficult to determine whether differences observed in cross-sectional studies reflect the influence of physical activity or prior selection. It is possible that more skilled individuals are more physically active (106).

Relationship Between Activity and Fitness

Indicators of physical activity (e.g., time per week, global ratings, etc.) are significantly but moderately related to 1.6-km run/walk performance in 8- to 9-year-old children (73); to maximal aerobic power, motor skills, and strength of 12-year-old children (87); and to PWC 170, strength, and motor ability of 17- to 18-year-old boys (106).

Specific Training Programs

Specific training programs are designed around the issue of trainability, that is, How responsive are children at different ages during growth and maturation to a training stimulus? Trainability is related to the concept of readiness or critical periods—time(s) when children are more susceptible to stimulatory effects of training.

Regular instruction and practice of motor skills in physical education result in improved levels of motor fitness (101). Results vary among studies, but emphasize the importance of physical education instruction. Systematic instruction and practice of skills in the context of organized youth sport programs also contribute to the development of motor fitness.

It may be difficult to partition practice and learning effects in motor skill development from those associated with growth and maturation. Motor performance in boys improves more or less linearly with age during middle childhood and continues to improve through adolescence, showing a clear adolescent spurt (7). Among girls, motor performance tends to reach a plateau at about 14 to 15 years of age. A question that merits study is whether the plateau apparent in the motor fitness of adolescent females can be improved by enhanced opportunity, instruction, and practice.

Strength is significantly improved after 14 weeks of hydraulic resistance training in prepubertal boys age 6 to 11 years (81,108) and after 12 weeks of isometric (35) training in prepubertal boys and girls age 7 to 11 years (35). Pubertal boys also gain significantly in strength with resistance training

(76,85). However, prepubertal boys make greater relative gains in strength than pubertal boys. Corresponding data for adolescent girls are not extensive, but indicate increases in both static and functional strength in response to several training programs (68,85). Younger girls (less than age 13.5 years) also tend to make greater relative gains than older girls (68).

Hypertrophy of muscle tissue associated with resistance training is observed in some (35) but not other (108) studies of prepubertal children. The difference may be methodological. The former used ultrasound measurements; the latter used limb circumferences uncorrected for thickness of subcutaneous fat. Nevertheless, strength gain without hypertrophy emphasizes the role of the neuromuscular system in the physiological increase in strength associated with training.

Hypertrophy ordinarily accompanies strength training in pubertal boys. However, the male adolescent growth spurt and sexual maturation are also accompanied by a marked spurt in muscle mass and strength, which occurs on average after PHV (7,59), so it may be difficult to partition training-associated gains from those that accompany the growth spurt and sexual maturation. The female adolescent spurt in muscle mass and strength is about one half of the magnitude of that in boys (7,59). Low levels of androgens probably limit gains in strength and muscle mass in adolescent females (85).

Results of one study (38), which emphasized both muscular strength and endurance, suggest differential responses that depend on age. Younger boys made greater relative gains in maximal strength, whereas older boys made greater relative gains in muscular endurance.

Changes in $\dot{V}O_2$max (ml/min^{-1}/kg^{-1}) in response to endurance training appear to vary with age in children and youth (59). The data (64,74,83) suggest relatively little trainability of maximal aerobic power (less than 5%) in children under 10 years of age. It is not certain whether this is a consequence of low trainability (i.e., a low adaptive potential to aerobic training), initially high levels of physical activity, or inadequacies of training programs. If it can be assumed, for example, that young children are habitually more physically active than adolescents and adults, a more intensive aerobic-training program may be required to induce significant changes in maximal aerobic power. On the other hand, most activities of young children proceed at submaximal rates; therefore maximal aerobic power may not be the appropriate measure. It may be more appropriate to consider changes in submaximal work efficiency in response to training (59).

During puberty, responses of aerobic power to training are clearly apparent. Relative gains may reach about 20%, and there is no sex difference (64,74,83). The variability among studies probably relates to sampling and methodological differences. Training protocols vary and outside activity is difficult to control. When older children and adolescents are rather sedentary at the start of the program, short-term training studies generally yield improvements in maximal aerobic power that are similar to those observed in young adults (59,74). In addition, individual differences in the timing of the adolescent growth spurt may be a source of variation. Maximal oxygen uptake shows a clear adolescent spurt, which parallels growth- and maturity-related changes in heart, blood, and lung volumes (59).

Studies of strength and aerobic training during childhood and adolescence ordinarily do not include a follow-up component, thus persistence of training-related gains cannot be evaluated. Nevertheless, active boys have a greater relative $\dot{V}O_2$max than inactive boys before, during, and after the adolescent spurt (62).

Tracking Fitness and Activity

Tracking of indicators of motor and health-related fitness from childhood through late adolescence is moderate at best (50,51). The interage correlations thus have limited predictive utility. Information on tracking of activity habits or energy expenditure is extremely limited. Interage correlations for physical activity and total energy expenditure reach only .35 for boys and girls from age 6 to 12 years, and the correlation for more intense activity is low (.13) (86).

Tracking of fitness from adolescence into adulthood is also moderate (6). At present, the role of physical activity and fitness during childhood and youth as favorable influences on the health status of adults or as preventive factors in several diseases of adulthood is not yet established (50). Some evidence suggests a relationship between adolescent and adult physical activity. Interage correlations between sport participation scores during adolescence and at age 30 years in males are low, but increase from age 13 to 17 years so that the correlation between activity at age 17 and at age 30 years reaches .39 (99). Other data suggest that males who are more fit during late childhood and adolescence (23) and males and females who are more active during adolescence (28,29,99) are more likely to be active as adults.

Summary

Physical activity is generally viewed as having a favorable influence on the growth, biological maturation, and fitness of children and youth. Inferences about the role of physical activity as a factor affecting growth, maturation, and fitness are based largely on comparisons of active and inactive individuals, children regularly training for specific sports, and short-term experimental studies. Caution is needed in extending observations on samples of athletes, especially select female athletes, to the general population. Longitudinal studies that span childhood and adolescence and that control for physical activity are limited.

Regular physical activity has no effect on statural growth and on indices of biological maturation used in growth studies (skeletal age, age at menarche, age at PHV). In well-nourished children and youth, these variables are primarily regulated by genetic factors. Some discussion focuses on later menarche in female athletes. These data are associational and retrospective, are based on small samples, and do not control for other factors that influence menarche.

Regular physical activity is an important factor in the regulation of body weight. It is often associated with a decrease in fatness in both sexes and occasionally with an increase in FFM, more often in boys. However, it is difficult to partition training effects from expected age- and maturity-associated changes in body composition, particularly during male adolescence. Changes in fatness depend on continued activity (or caloric restriction) for their maintenance. Information on the possible influence of physical activity on fat distribution in children and youth is lacking.

Regular physical activity is associated with greater skeletal mineralization, density, and bone mass. In contrast, training for sports in association with altered menstrual function and perhaps dietary deficiencies can contribute to bone loss in some adolescent athletes and may increase susceptibility to stress fractures.

The effects of regular physical activity on skeletal muscle tissue are specific to the type of training program (e.g., resistance or endurance training). Metabolic responses of muscle to training in growing individuals are similar to those observed in adults, but the magnitude of responses varies.

Information on the influence of regular physical activity on adipose tissue metabolism and cellularity of children is lacking.

Active children generally show better responses to motor, strength, and aerobic power tests than inactive children. Responses to short-term training programs are rather specific to the type of program. Regular instruction and practice of motor skills result in improved motor fitness, whereas strength-training programs result in significant gains in muscular strength and endurance. The trainability of maximal aerobic power in children under 10 years of age is limited. It is not certain whether this observation is the consequence of low trainability, initially high levels of activity, or inadequacies of training programs. During puberty, responses to aerobic training improve considerably.

Tracking (interage correlations) for indicators of fitness from childhood through adolescence and from adolescence into adulthood tend to be moderate. Nevertheless, some evidence indicates that those who are more fit and active during adolescence are more likely to be active as young adults.

References

1. American Medical Association/American Dietetic Association. Targets for adolescent health: Nutrition and physical fitness. Chicago; American Medical Association; 1991.
2. Astrand, P.O.; Engstrom, L.; Eriksson, B.O.; Karlberg, P.; Nylander, I.; Saltin, B.; Thoren, C. Girl swimmers. Acta Paediat. [Suppl.] 147; 1963.
3. Bailey, D.A.; Malina, R.M.; Mirwald, R.L. Physical activity and growth of the child. In: Falkner, F.; Tanner, J.M., eds. Human growth. Vol. 2. Postnatal growth, neurobiology. New York: Plenum Press; 1986:147-170.
4. Bailey, D.A.; McCulloch, R.G. Bone tissue and physical activity. Can. J. Sport Sci. 15:229-239; 1990.
5. Bar-Or, O. Pediatric sports medicine for the practitioner. New York: Springer-Verlag; 1983.
6. Beunen, G.; Lefevre, J.; Claessens, A.L.; Lysens, R.; Maes, H.; Renson, R.; Simons, J.; Vanden Eynde, B.; Vanreusel, B.; Van Den Bossche, C. Age-specific correlation analysis of longitudinal physical fitness levels in men. Eur. J. Appl. Physiol. 64:538-545; 1992.
7. Beunen, G.; Malina, R.M. Growth and physical performance relative to the timing of the adolescent spurt. Exerc. Sport Sci. Rev. 16:503-540; 1988.
8. Beunen, G.P.; Malina, R.M.; Renson, R.; Simons, J.; Ostyn, M.; Lefevre, J. Physical activity and growth, maturation and performance: A longitudinal study. Med. Sci. Sports Exerc. 24:576-585; 1992.

9. Beyer, H.G. The influence of exercise on growth. J. Exp. Med. 1:546-558; 1896.
10. Bielicki, T.; Charzewski, J. Sex differences in the magnitude of statural gain of offspring over parents. Hum. Biol. 49:265-277; 1977.
11. Bielicki, T.; Koniarek, J.; Malina, R.M. Interrelationships among certain measures of growth and maturation rate in boys during adolescence. Ann. Hum. Biol. 11:201-210; 1984.
12. Bjorntorp, P.; Grimby, C.; Sanne, H.; Sjostrom, L.; Tibblin, G.; Wilhelmsen, L. Adipose tissue fat cell size in relation to metabolism in weight-stable, physically active men. Horm. Metab. Res. 4:178-182; 1972.
13. Blimkie, C.J.; Rice, S.; Webber, C.; Martin, J.; Levy, D.; Parker, D. Bone density, physical activity, fitness, anthropometry, gynecologic, endocrine and nutrition status in adolescent girls. In: Coudert, J.; Van Praagh, E., eds. Children and exercise XVI: Pediatric work physiology. Paris: Masson; 1992:201-203.
14. Boileau, R.A.; Lohman, T.G.; Slaughter, M.H. Exercise and body composition of children and youth. Scand. J. Sports Sci. 7:17-27; 1985.
15. Bouchard, C.; Shephard, R.J. Physical activity, fitness and health: The model and key concepts. (Chapter 3 in this volume.)
16. Brooks-Gunn, J.; Warren, M.P. Mother-daughter differences in menarcheal age in adolescent girls attending national dance company schools and non-dancers. Ann. Hum. Biol. 15:35-43; 1988.
17. Cacciari, E.; Mazzanti, L.; Tassinari, D.; Bergamaschi, R.; Magnani, C.; Zappulla, F.; Nanni, G.; Cobianchi, C.; Ghini, T.; Pini, R.; Tani, G. Effects of sport (football) on growth: Auxological, anthropometric and hormonal aspects. Eur. J. Appl. Physiol. 61:149-158; 1990.
18. Calabrese, L.H.; Kirkendall, D.T.; Floyd, M.; Rapoport, S.; Williams, G.W.; Weiker, G.G.; Bergfeld, J.A. Menstrual abnormalities, nutritional patterns, and body composition in female classical ballet dancers. Phys. Sportsmed. 11:86-98; 1983, February.
19. Chen, J.D. Growth, exercise, nutrition and fitness in China. Med. Sports Sci. 31:19-32; 1991.
20. Claessens, A.L.; Malina, R.M.; Lefevre, J.; Beunen, G.; Stijne, V.; Maes, H.; Veer, F.M. Growth and menarcheal status of elite female gymnasts: Participants at the 24th world championship artistic gymnastics, Rotterdam, The Netherlands, 1987. Med. Sci. Sports Exerc. 24:755-763; 1992.
21. Clarkson, P.M.; Freedson, P.S.; Skrinar, M.; Keller, B.; Carney, D. Anthropometric measurements of adolescent and professional classical ballet dancers. J. Sports Med. Phys. Fitness. 29:157-162; 1989.
22. Davies, P.S.W.; Livingstone, M.B.E.; Prentice, A.M.; Coward, W.A.; Jagger, S.E.; Stewart, C.; Strain, J.J.; Whitehead, R.G. Total energy expenditure during childhood and adolescence. Proc. Nutr. Soc. 15:13; 1991.
23. Dennison, B.A.; Straus, J.H.; Mellits, E.D.; Charney, E. Childhood physical fitness tests: Predictor of adult physical activity levels? Pediatrics. 82:324-330; 1988.
24. Despres, J-P.; Bouchard, C.; Savard, R.; Tremblay, A.; Marcotte, M.; Theriault, G. The effect of a 20-week endurance training program on adipose tissue morphology and lipolysis in men and women. Metabolism. 33:235-239; 1984.
25. Despres, J-P.; Bouchard, C.; Tremblay, A.; Savard, R.; Marcotte, M. Effects of aerobic training on fat distribution in male subjects. Med. Sci. Sports Exerc. 17:113-118; 1985.
26. Dhuper, S.; Warren, M.P.; Brooks-Gunn, J.; Fox, R. Effects of hormonal status on bone density in adolescent girls. J. Clin. Endocrinol. Metab. 71:1083-1088; 1990.
27. Drinkwater, B.L.; Nilson, K.; Chestnut, C.H.; Bremner, W.J.; Shainholtz, S.; Southworth, M.B. Bone mineral of amenorrheic and eumenorrheic athletes. N. Engl. J. Med. 311:277-281; 1984.
28. Engstrom, L.-M. The process of socialization into keep-fit activities. Scand. J. Sports Sci. 8:89-97; 1986.
29. Engstrom, L.-M. Exercise adherence in sport for all from youth to adulthood. In: Oja, P.; Telama, R., eds. Sport for all. Amsterdam: Elsevier Science; 1991:473-483.
30. Eriksson, B.O.; Gollnick, P.D.; Saltin, B. The effect of physical training on muscle enzyme activities and fiber composition in 11-year-old boys. Acta Paediatr. Belg. [Suppl.]. 28:245-252; 1974.
31. Forbes, G.B. Body composition in adolescence. In: Falkner, F.; Tanner, J.M., eds. Human growth. Volume 2. Postnatal growth. New York: Plenum Press; 1978:239-272.
32. Fournier, M.; Ricci, J.; Taylor, A.W.; Ferguson, R.J.; Montpetit, R.R.; Chaitman, B.R. Skeletal muscle adaptation in adolescent boys: Sprint and endurance training and detraining. Med. Sci. Sports Exerc. 14:453-456; 1982.
33. Frisch, R.E.; Gotz-Welbergen, A.B.; McArthur, J.W.; Albright, T.; Witschi, J.; Bullen, B.; Birnholz, J.; Reed, R.B.; Hermann, H. Delayed menarche and amenorrhea of college athletes in relation to age of onset of training. JAMA. 246:1559-1563; 1981.

34. Frusztajer, N.T.; Dhuper, S.; Warren, M.P.; Brooks-Gunn, J.; Fox, R.P. Nutrition and the incidence of stress fractures in ballet dancers. Am. J. Clin. Nutr. 51:779-783; 1990.
35. Fukunaga, T.; Funato, K.; Ikegawa, S. The effects of resistance training on muscle area and strength in prepubescent age. Ann. Physiol. Anthropol. 11:357-364; 1992.
36. Grimston, S.K.; Engsberg, J.R.; Kloiber, R.; Hanley, D.A. Menstrual, calcium, and training history: Relationship to bone health in female runners. Clin. Sports Med. 2:119-128; 1990.
37. Hamilton, L.H.; Brooks-Gunn, J.; Warren, M.P.; Hamilton, W.G. The role of selectivity in the pathogenesis of eating problems in ballet dancers. Med. Sci. Sports Exerc. 20:560-565; 1988.
38. Ikai, M. The effects of training on muscular endurance. In: Kato, K., ed. Proceedings of the international congress of sports sciences. Tokyo: University of Tokyo Press; 1966:145-158.
39. Jacobs, I.; Sjodin, B.; Svane, B. Muscle fiber type, cross-sectional area and strength in boys after 4 years endurance training. Med. Sci. Sports Exerc. [Abstract]. 14:123; 1982.
40. Jahreis, G.; Kauf, E.; Frohner, G.; Schmidt, H.E. Influence of intensive exercise on insulin-like growth factor I, thyroid and steroid hormones in female gymnasts. Growth Regul. 1:95-99; 1991.
41. Jokl, E.; Cluver, E.H.; Goedvolk, C.; de Jongh, T.W. Training and efficiency. Johannesburg: South African Institute for Medical Research, Report no. 303; 1941.
42. Kobayashi, K.; Kitamura, K.; Miura, M.; Sodeyama, H.; Murasse, Y.; Miyashita, M.; Matsui, H. Aerobic power as related to body growth and training in Japanese boys: A longitudinal study. J. Appl. Physiol. 44:666-672; 1978.
43. Kotulan, J.; Reznickova, M.; Placheta, Z. Exercise and growth. In: Placheta, Z., ed. Youth and physical activity. Brno, Czechoslovakia: J.E. Purkyne University Medical Faculty; 1980:61-117.
44. Laron, Z.; Klinger, B. Does intensive sport endanger normal growth and development? In: Laron, Z.; Rogol, A.D., eds. Hormones and sport. New York: Raven Press; 1989:1-9.
45. Malina, R.M. The effects of exercise on specific tissues, dimensions and functions during growth. Stud. Phys. Anthropol. 5:21- 52; 1979.
46. Malina, R.M. Menarche in athletes: A synthesis and hypothesis. Ann. Hum. Biol. 10:1-24; 1983.
47. Malina, R.M. Energy expenditure and physical activity during childhood and youth. In: Demirjian, A., ed. Human growth: A multidisciplinary review. London: Taylor and Francis; 1986:215-225.
48. Malina, R.M. Biological maturity status of young athletes. In: Malina, R.M., ed. Young athletes: Biological, psychological and educational perspectives. Champaign, IL: Human Kinetics; 1988:121-140.
49. Malina, R.M. Growth and maturation: Normal variation and effect of training. In: Gisolfi, C.V.; Lamb, D.R., eds. Perspectives in exercise science and sports medicine. Volume 2. Youth, exercise, and sport. Indianapolis: Benchmark Press; 1989:223-265.
50. Malina, R.M. Growth, exercise, fitness, and later health outcomes. In: Bouchard, C.; Shephard, R.J.; Stephens, T.; Sutton, J.R.; McPherson, B.D., eds. Exercise, fitness, and health. Champaign, IL: Human Kinetics; 1990:637-665.
51. Malina, R.M. Tracking of physical fitness and performance during growth. In: Beunen, G.; Ghesquiere, J.; Reybrouck, T.; Claessens, A.L., eds. Children and exercise. Stuttgart: Ferdinand Enke; 1990:1-10.
52. Malina, R.M. Darwinian fitness, physical fitness and activity. In: Mascie-Taylor, C.G.N.; Lasker, G.W., eds. Applications of biological anthropology to human affairs. Cambridge: Cambridge University Press; 1991:143-184.
53. Malina, R.M. Fitness and performance: Adult health and the culture of youth. In: Park, R.J.; Eckert, H.M., eds. New possibilities, new paradigms? (American academy of physical education papers no. 24). Champaign, IL: Human Kinetics; 1991:30-38.
54. Malina, R.M. Effects of physical activity on growth in stature and the adolescent growth spurt. Med. Sci. Sports Exerc.; [Accepted for publication, 1993].
55. Malina, R.M.; Beunen, G.; Wellens, R.; Claessens, A. Skeletal maturity and body size of teenage Belgian track and field athletes. Ann. Hum. Biol. 13:331-339; 1986.
56. Malina, R.M.; Bielicki, T. Growth and maturation of boys and girls active in sport: Longitudinal observations from 8-18 years; [In preparation].
57. Malina, R.M.; Bonci, C.; Ryan, R. Age at menarche and premenarcheal training: Relationship to stress fractures in university athletes; [In preparation].
58. Malina, R.M.; Bouchard, C. Subcutaneous fat distribution during growth. In: Bouchard, C.; Johnston, F.E., eds. Fat distribution during

growth and later health outcomes. New York: Liss; 1988:63-84.

59. Malina, R.M.; Bouchard, C. Growth, maturation, and physical activity. Champaign, IL: Human Kinetics; 1991.
60. Marshall, W.A.; Tanner, J.M. Puberty. In: Falkner, F.; Tanner, J.M., eds. Human growth. Volume 2. Postnatal growth, neurobiology. New York: Plenum Press; 1986:171-209.
61. McCulloch, R.G.; Bailey, D.A.; Houston, C.S.; Dodd, B.L. Effects of physical activity, dietary calcium intake and selected lifestyle factors on bone density in young women. Can. Med. Assoc. J. 142:221-227; 1990.
62. Mirwald, R.L.; Bailey, D.A. Maximal aerobic power. London, Ontario: Sports Dynamics; 1986.
63. Mirwald, R.L.; Bailey, D.A.; Cameron, N.; Rasmussen, R.L. Longitudinal comparison of aerobic power in active and inactive boys 7.0 to 17.0 years. Ann. Hum. Biol. 8:405-414; 1981.
64. Mocellin, R. Jugend und sport (Children and sport). Med. Klin. 70:1443-1457; 1975.
65. Montoye, H.J. Better bones and biodynamics. Res. Q. Exerc. Sport. 58:334-348; 1987.
66. Moravec, R. Vplyv vykonavanych pohybovych aktivit na telesny rozvoj a pohybovu vykonnost 7-18 rocnej mladeze (The influence of performed motor activities on physical development and motor efficiency of 7-18 years old youth). Teor. Praxe Tel. Vych. 37:596-606; 1989.
67. Neinstein, L.S. Menstrual problems in adolescents. Med. Clin. North Am. 74:1181-1203; 1990.
68. Nielsen, B.; Nielsen, K.; Behrendt Hansen, M.; Asmussen, E. Training of "functional muscular strength" in girls 7-19 years old. In: Berg, K.; Eriksson, B.O., eds. Children and exercise IX. Baltimore: University Park Press; 1980: 69-78.
69. Novotny, V. Veranderungen des knochenalters im verlauf einer mehrjahrigen sportlichen belastung. Med. Sport. 21:44-47; 1981.
70. Parizkova, J. Particularities of lean body mass and fat development in growing boys as related to their motor activity. Acta Paediatr. Belg. [Suppl.]. 28:233-242; 1974.
71. Parizkova, J. Functional development and the impact of exercise. In: Berenberg, S.R., ed. Puberty: Biological and psychosocial components. Leiden, Holland: Stenfert Kroese; 1975:198-219.
72. Parizkova, J. Body fat and physical fitness. The Hague, Holland: Martinus Nijhoff; 1977.
73. Pate, R.R.; Dowda, M.; Ross, J.G. Associations between physical activity and physical fitness in American children. Am. J. Dis. Child. 144:1123-1129; 1990.
74. Pate, R.R.; Ward, D.S. Endurance exercise trainability in children and youth. Adv. Sports Med. Fitness. 3:37-55; 1990.
75. Peltenburg, A.L.; Erich, W.B.M.; Zonderland, M.L.; Bernink, M.J.E.; van den Brande, J.L.; Huisveld, I.A. A retrospective growth study of female gymnasts and girl swimmers. Int. J. Sports Med. 5:262-267; 1984.
76. Pfeiffer, R.D.; Francis; R.S. Effects of strength training on muscle development in prepubescent, pubescent, and postpubescent males. Phys. Sportsmed. 14:134-143; 1986.
77. Placheta, Z. Physical fitness development. In: Placheta, Z., ed. Youth and physical activity. Brno, Czechoslovakia: J.E. Purkyne University Medical Faculty; 1980:118-140.
78. Rarick, G.L. Exercise and growth. In: Johnson, W.R., ed. Science and medicine of exercise and sport. New York: Harper and Brothers; 1960:440-465.
79. Rarick, G.L. Exercise and growth. In: Johnson, W.R.; Buskirk, E.R., eds. Science and medicine of exercise and sport. 2nd ed. New York: Harper & Row; 1974:306-321.
80. Renson, R.; Beunen, G.; Ostyn, M.; Simons, J.; Uyttebrouck, J.; Van Gerven, D.; Vanreusel, B. Differentiation of physical fitness in function of sport participation. Hermes [Leuven]. 15:435-444; 1981.
81. Rians, C.B.; Weltman, A.; Cahill, B.R.; Janney, C.A.; Tippett, S.R.; Katch, F.I. Strength training for prepubescent males: Is it safe? Am. J. Sports Med. 15:483-489; 1987.
82. Rowe, F.A. Growth comparisons of athletes and non-athletes. Res. Q. 4:108-116; 1933.
83. Rowland, T.W. Aerobic response to endurance training in prepubescent children: A critical analysis. Med. Sci. Sports Exerc. 17:493-497; 1985.
84. Ruffer, W.A. A study of extreme physical activity groups of young men. Res. Q. 36:183-196; 1965.
85. Sale, D.G. Strength training in children. In: Gisolfi, C.V.; Lamb, D.R., eds. Perspectives in exercise science and sports medicine. Volume 2. Youth, exercise, and sport. Indianapolis: Benchmark Press; 1989:165-216.
86. Saris, W.H.M.; Elvers, J.W.H.; van't Hof, M.A.; Binkhorst, R.A. Changes in physical activity of children aged 6 to 12 years. In: Rutenfranz, J.; Mocellin, R.; Klimt, F., eds. Children and exercise XII. Champaign, IL: Human Kinetics; 1986:121-130.
87. Schmucker, B.; Rigauer, B.; Hinrichs, W.; Trawinski, J. Motor abilities and habitual

physical activity in children. In: Ilmarinen, J.; Valimaki, I., eds. Children and sport. Berlin: Springer-Verlag; 1984:46-52.

88. Schwartz, L.; Britten, E.H.; Thompson, L.R. Studies in physical development and posture. 1. The effect of exercise in the physical condition and development of adolescent boys. Public Health Bull. 179:1-38; 1928.

89. Seefeldt, V.; Haubenstricker, J.; Branta, C.; Evans, S. Physical characteristics of elite young distance runners. In: Brown, E.W.; Branta, C.F., eds. Competitive sports for children and youth. Champaign, IL: Human Kinetics; 1988:247-258.

90. Seefeldt, V.; Haubenstricker, J.; Branta, C.; McKeag, D. Anthropometric assessment of body size and shape of young runners and control subjects. In: Weiss, M.R.; Gould, D., eds. Sport for children and youths. Champaign, IL: Human Kinetics; 1986:247-254.

91. Shangold, M.M. Menstruation. In: Shangold, M.M.; Mirkin, G., eds. Women and exercise: Physiology and sports medicine. Philadelphia: Davis; 1988:129-144.

92. Sprynarova, S. Longitudinal study of the influence of different physical activity programs on functional capacity of the boys from 11 to 18 years. Acta Paediatr. Belg. [Suppl.]. 28:204-213; 1974.

93. Sprynarova, S. The influence of training on physical and functional growth before, during and after puberty. Eur. J. Appl. Physiol. 56:719-724; 1987.

94. Stager, J.M.; Hatler, L.K. Menarche in athletes: The influence of genetics and prepubertal training. Med. Sci. Sports Exerc. 20:369-373; 1988.

95. Stager, J.M.; Wigglesworth, J.K.; Hatler, L.K. Interpreting the relationship between age of menarche and prepubertal training. Med. Sci. Sports Exerc. 22:54-58; 1990.

96. Stinson, S. Sex differences in environmental sensitivity during growth and development. Yearbook Phys. Anthropol. 28:123-147; 1985.

97. Tanner, J.M. Growth at adolescence, 2nd ed. Oxford: Blackwell; 1962.

98. Tremblay, A.; Despres, J.P.; Bouchard, C. Alteration in body fat and fat distribution with exercise. In: Bouchard, C.; Johnston, F.E., eds. Fat distribution during growth and later health outcomes. New York: Liss; 1988:297-312.

99. Vanreusel, B.; Renson, R.; Beunen, G.; Claessens, A.; Lefevre, J.; Lysens, R.; Maes, H.; Simons, J.; Vanden Eynde, B. Adherence to sport from youth to adulthood: A longitudinal study on socialization. In: Proceedings of the international congress on youth, leisure and physical activity. London: E & FN Spon; [In press].

100. Verschuur, R. Daily physical activity: Longitudinal changes during the teenage period. Haarlem, Holland: Uitgeverij de Vrieseborch; 1987.

101. Vogel, P.G. Effects of physical education programs on children. In: Seefeldt, V., ed. Physical activity and well-being. Reston, VA: American Alliance for Health, Physical Education, Recreation and Dance; 1986:455-509.

102. Von Dobeln, W.; Eriksson, B.O. Physical training, maximal oxygen uptake, and dimensions of the oxygen transporting and metabolizing organs in boys 11-13 years of age. Acta Paediatr. Scand. 61:653-660; 1972.

103. Warren, M.P. The effects of exercise on pubertal progression and reproductive function in girls. J. Clin. Endocrinol. Metab. 51:1150-1157; 1980.

104. Warren, M.P. Effects of undernutrition on reproductive function in the human. Endocr. Rev. 4:363-377; 1983.

105. Warren, M.P.; Brooks-Gunn, J.; Hamilton, L.H.; Warren, L.F.; Hamilton, W.G. Scoliosis and fractures in young ballet dancers. N. Engl. J. Med. 314:1348-1353; 1986.

106. Watson, A.W.S.; O'Donovan, D.J. The relationship of level of habitual physical activity to measures of leanness-fatness, physical working capacity, strength, and motor ability in 17 and 18 year old males. Eur. J. Appl. Physiol. 37:93-100; 1977.

107. Watson, R.C. Bone growth and physical activity in young males. In Mazess, R.B., ed. International conference on bones minimal measurement. Washington, DC: Department of Health, Education, and Welfare; 1975:380-386.

108. Weltman, A.; Janney, C.; Rians, C.B.; Strand, K.; Berg, B.; Tippett, S.; Wise, J.; Cahill, B.R.; Katch, F.I. The effects of hydraulic resistance strength training in pre-pubertal males. Med. Sci. Sports Exerc. 18:629-638; 1986.

Chapter 63

Childhood and Adolescent Physical Activity and Fitness and Adult Risk Profile

Oded Bar-Or

Working Definitions

The following are working definitions and clarifications regarding terms used in this review.

Physical activity (PA) is both a physical/physiologic phenomenon and a behavioral one. As agreed at the 1988 International Conference on Exercise, Fitness and Health (19), the physiologic definition of PA is: "Any bodily movement produced by skeletal muscles and resulting in energy expenditure." The units by which such movements are measured are *power* or *work*. A child behaviorist's definition would address also the type of activity; the environment in which the child performs it (e.g., playground, school); the use of toys or apparatus; and the interaction with friends and family members. Even though a quantitative analysis of the behavioral components of PA is not always feasible, these factors have to be considered in order to understand why some children are less active than others.

Risk Factors During Childhood and Adolescence

In adults, *risk factors* have been identified as those physical and behavioral characteristics that are linked to the development of certain chronic diseases. Extensive research has yielded information on the strength of such links in adults. A question remains, however, as to whether the same risk factors can be presumed also for children and adolescents. Factors that have been studied include abnormal lipoprotein profile, obesity, hypertension, low insulin sensitivity, and physical hypoactivity even though future research may prove that, when measured during childhood, some of these factors are not relevant in the prediction of future illness.

Childhood refers to the period until the start of puberty, whereas *adolescence* denotes the period that starts with puberty and ends with adulthood. For brevity's sake, however, childhood will be used in this text to denote in a general sense the years until adulthood, unless the context requires a more precise distinction between childhood and adolescence.

Scope of This Review

Various models have been constructed to suggest possible relationships between children's PA and physical fitness (PF) on the one hand and their health as adults on the other. An example is the model suggested by Blair, Clark, Cureton, and Powell (15), in which PA during childhood may affect adult health via three avenues: (a) directly, (b) through its effect on the child's health, or (c) through its effect on adult PA (which in turn affects adult health). An additional possible link is that PA during childhood determines the child's PF, which in turn, may affect adult health (a) directly, (b) through adult PA and PF, or (c) through the child's health. Such assumptions may be plausible, but they have not yet been tested. Indeed, there is no prospective work that can link health in adult years with a childhood activity pattern with any degree of certainty. The direction taken in this review is therefore to examine the evidence for short-term effects of enhanced PA on the risk profile in childhood.

Several reviews have been published during the last decade on the possible link between PA during childhood and a presumed risk profile (7,8,15,28, 66,71,72,75,83,90,117). These reviews, plus an analysis of recent original studies, served as basis for this chapter.

Adult Health Risk: A Pediatric Issue?

Although the clinical endpoints of diseases such as coronary heart disease (CHD), hypertension (HT), and osteoporosis typically occur in adulthood, there is mounting evidence, particularly for CHD and HT, that these diseases have antecedents already during childhood and adolescence (1,10,11, 70,109,113,127). Likewise, there is a fairly strong relationship between adult obesity and adolescent obesity (e.g., 25,100). It is thus fair to state that indeed these diseases are a legitimate pediatric issue and that their recognition and prevention in early life is of paramount public health importance.

Constraints in Research

Several constraints have impeded research on the effects of physical activity and fitness on children's risk profile.

Assessment of Activity and Body Composition

Methods used to assess PA of adults are not necessarily valid for children. Examples include self-reported activity diaries and recall questionnaires that may be too demanding for young children and often require additional information by parents and teachers (3–5,57). Even though recall questionnaires and activity logs have been constructed in recent years specifically for children, many often-quoted studies have used nonvalidated questionnnaires or activity logs. Motion counters (e.g., LSI, Caltrac) have a much lower validity for preschoolers (56,58) than for adults, probably because young children's body movements during play include muscle groups not usually used by adults. For example, when a motion sensor is attached to the waist or the leg it may not pick up movements of the upper limbs performed during rope climbing. In this regard it is interesting that the validity of the Caltrac for obese children seems higher than for the nonobese (56), possibly because the former may use a less varied repertoire of movements.

Tables constructed for adults that summarize calorie equivalents of various activities may not be valid for children (for reviews see 6,89) because energy requirements per kilogram body weight at any given walking or running speed are higher the younger or smaller the individual (e.g., 2,64,106). Running training in adolescents may induce a decrease in the energy cost of running (27), which further complicates the interpretation of changes induced by a training intervention.

Likewise, assessment of adiposity is often based on techniques, equations, and assumptions made for adults, but not validated for children. Specifically, the density of various lean body tissues (e.g., bone and muscle) changes during growth, as does the water content of the body as a whole (18). As a result, conversion equations from skinfold or body density to percent body fat must change with the age or maturational stage of the subject. Yet, some of the oft-quoted studies on obesity as a pediatric risk factor have used adult-based equations.

Training Effects Versus Growth and Maturation

Several physiologic functions that respond to training also change in conjunction with growth or maturation. Some of the changes are in the same direction (e.g., a decrease in submaximal heart rate or an increase in muscle power and strength), whereas others change in the opposite direction (e.g., maximal oxygen uptake per kilogram in girls, submaximal blood lactate). Likewise, several of the risk factors for CHD change with growth and maturation irrespective of the person's activity level. Examples are an increase in arterial blood pressure (113), a reduction in high-density lipoprotein (HDL) cholesterol during puberty in boys (112), a reduction in insulin sensitivity during puberty (76), and an increase in adiposity during puberty in girls. It is thus difficult to separate changes that are induced by enhanced PA from those that accompany maturation per se, especially if a control group is not matched for biological age.

Tracking

To assess the carryover effect of an intervention from childhood to adulthood, one must first know how each dependent variable would track over years without the intervention. Tracking of physiologic or behavioral characteristics has been used in the context of prediction and stability, that is, the ability to predict subsequent status from earlier measurements and the maintenance of relative rank within a group over time. Its determination requires longitudinal data. Bloom (17) has suggested an interage correlation of .5 or more as an index of stability. Using this index, the stability of health-related fitness and of several risk factors for cardiovascular disease is generally moderate to low (8,54,66,67,78). Most interage correlations over intervals of 5 or more years, especially if they span puberty, are below .5 and thus have limited predictive value. An exception is the 8-year observation—from age 13.5 to 21.5 years—of Amsterdam students (54) for whom some of the interage correlations exceeded .60.

From late adolescence to adulthood, stability is usually better for lipoprotein profile than for fatness. Stability of blood pressure is sometimes higher and sometimes lower than for other risk factors. In the above Amsterdam study, for example, *r* values for blood pressure were considerably lower (.32–.51) than for lipoproteins (.42–.70) and adiposity (.59–.62). Similarly, Palti, Gofin, Adler, Grafstein, and Belmaker (78) found low stability of systolic and diastolic BP (r = .32 and .29, respectively). BP, obesity, and lipoprotein profile track better at the upper quartiles of their distributions, particularly among males, than at lower quartiles.

Attitudes toward physical activity are less stable in 10- to 12-year-old students than in 16- to 18-year-old students (98,104). Involvement in physical activity is quite stable during high school years, but the relationship between attitude and involvement is rather low (98). Given the many factors that affect a person's activity, it would be surprising if the activity pattern were stable from childhood to late adolescence.

Activity Versus Fitness

The role of enhanced PA in the reduction of coronary risk has been demonstrated for adults, even when the effects of PF are partialed out. Similar data are not available for children. Furthermore, it is likely that many children who are more active than their peers represent a group preselected for its higher PF and motor aptitude.

Enhanced Activity as Part of a Multidisciplinary Intervention

For some risk factors, intervention programs that have shown promising and sustained results are multidisciplinary in nature. The best example is the combination of low-calorie diet, enhanced energy expenditure, and behavior modification in the treatment of juvenile obesity. In such interventions it is impossible to tease out the specific effects of enhanced PA.

Short-Term Effects of Activity on Risk Factors

Although cross-sectional studies show that active children have a more favorable coronary risk profile than their sedentary counterparts, there is little evidence (based on longitudinal observations) that in healthy children enhanced PA indeed reduces the risk. One possible explanation is that in the general child population the risk is low and therefore is not likely to drop further with an exercise intervention. Indeed, whatever the changes in coronary risk that can be assigned to the intervention, they seem to affect children who already have a high risk, that is, those with obesity, HT, and dyslipoproteinemia. The following discussion will therefore focus on those who already are at a high percentile of the respective risk factors.

Adiposity

Depending on criteria for obesity, sampling, and methods of assessing adiposity, the prevalence of juvenile obesity in North America has been reported to range from 10% to 25%. Nationwide surveys (45,87) suggest that this prevalence is on the rise. Obesity is thus the most common pediatric chronic illness in North America. Obese children have a greater clustering of other coronary risk factors such as high blood pressure, low insulin sensitivity, and hyperlipoproteinemia than do their leaner counterparts (9,55,103). Without a doubt juvenile obesity poses a major public health challenge.

Activity Pattern in Obese Children

Cross-sectional studies have often (e.g., 22,23, 26,91) but not always (e.g., 96,107,110,124) suggested that nonobese children and adolescents are more physically active than their obese counterparts. One reason for the inconsistency in findings about the relationship between obesity and hypoactivity is the way in which energy expenditure has been reported: Some of the authors who did not find such a relationship have calculated calorie expenditure in absolute terms without correction for body mass or fat-free mass. An example is the report by Waxman and Stunkard (124), who found a lower degree of activity (as assessed by an observer) among obese boys than among their nonobese siblings. These authors reported a higher calorie expenditure among the obese. However, by correcting their values for body mass one would reach an opposite conclusion. In a large sample of U.S. children and adolescents (30) a strong relationship was found between the time spent watching television and the likelihood of obesity.

One approach that will help to decide whether or not hypoactivity is indeed a cause of childhood obesity is to study infants before they are obese and then follow them up longitudinally, also monitoring their food intake and other environmental variables. An attempt in this direction is the study by Berkowitz, Agras, Korner, Kraemer, and Zeanah (12) who monitored the activity (a mattress that served as a capacitance-type transducer to monitor movement) of 1- to 3-day-old babies and then assessed their adiposity (log body mass index) at age 4 to 8 years. The authors found no correlation ($n = 52$) between adiposity of the children and their activity levels as infants. Roberts, Savage, Coward, Chew, and Lucas (85) using doubly labeled water to assess total energy expenditure of nonobese 3-month-old babies, assessed their adiposity (skinfold thickness) at 1 year of age. The total energy expenditure of those who became obese at 1 year was 79% of that found in the infants who remained lean (256 ± 27 kJ vs. 324 ± 22 kJ per kilogram per 24 hr, respectively), strongly suggesting that the lower energy expenditure preceded the development of obesity. More research is needed to further determine the role of hypoactivity compared with other (genetic and environmental) factors in the etiology of juvenile obesity.

Exercise as a Single Intervention

Enhanced PA over several weeks can induce a short-term reduction in body fat of obese children and adolescents (81,82). Sasaki, Shindo, Tanaka, Ando, and Arakawa (93) have reported a sustained decrease in excess body weight of 11-year-old girls and boys over a 2-year, school-based program of 20 min running, 7 days per week. This study is important because of the long duration of the intervention. Its weakness, however, is that the controls were nonobese children, rather than obese children who did not train. Sasaki et al.'s results are contrasted with an earlier prolonged intervention by Moody, Wilmore, Girandola, and Royce (73) in which 15- and 29-month jogging programs resulted in a very mild (2.53% and 3.14%) decrease in percent fat of obese female adolescents. These conflicting findings may be explained by the lower training dose in Moody et al.'s program. Specific effects of training on fat distribution have been shown for young adult males (29), but no data are available for children.

An important question regarding the efficacy of exercise interventions in childhood obesity is whether components of energy expenditure such as basal metabolism or the thermic effect of food would be modified by the intervention. Likewise, would a regimented training program induce changes in the spontaneous activity of the child? In a recent study, Blaak, Westerterp, Bar-Or, Wouters, and Saris (14) administered a 4-week cycling program 5 days per week to 10- to 11-year-old mildly obese Dutch boys. This intervention induced an increase in the total daily metabolic rate, as assessed by doubly labeled water, above and beyond the 10% to 12% increase expected from the program itself. There was no change in the sleeping metabolic rate or in the spontaneous activity (questionnaire and heart rate monitoring). The possibility that obese boys, when given a regimented exercise program, would compensate by decreasing their spontaneous PA has therefore not been confirmed. It is important to find out whether a similar pattern would be obtained for children who are more obese, or for those from other societies.

Exercise in Conjunction With Other Interventions

Programs that include a combination of exercise, low-calorie diet, and behavior modification seem more efficacious than those using only one of the above interventions, particularly if both child and parent undergo behavior modification (21,35, 36,65). Low-calorie diets are the most common treatment for obesity. One problem, particularly with a very low calorie diet (e.g., 2,000–2,500 kJ per 24 hr), is that it may induce a loss of fat-free mass and not only of fat mass. Such loss of fat-free mass can reach 20% to 35% of the total reduction in body mass (13,20). Exercise, on the other hand, may induce an increase in fat-free mass. For obese adults there is evidence that exercise reduces the catabolic effect of a low-calorie diet when both are combined (59,97,128). There is no information on this effect in obese children. Because of the possibly deleterious sequelae of catabolism to growth, this important area merits further research.

Dietary restriction has long been known to reduce the basal metabolic rate. Several studies with adults attempted to find out whether the addition of exercise may counteract the above effect of low-calorie diets. Results so far have been inconclusive, as recently reviewed by Poehlman, Melby, and Goran (84). Again, no studies are available on children regarding this issue.

Arterial Blood Pressure (BP)

Enhanced PA has been shown to induce a short-term reduction in resting systolic and diastolic BP particularly among adults with hypertension (for reviews see 41,99). There is still a controversy, however, as to whether such a reduction would be sustained over a long time (41). In children, as recently reviewed by Lauer, Burns, Mahoney, and Tipton (62), several cross-sectional studies have shown a lower BP in those with high aerobic fitness than in those with lower fitness (38,39,49,51,79 ,108). Such a relationship is evident as early as 5 years of age (46). Immobilized children seem to have higher resting BP than hospitalized, but not immobilized, children (116).

The results of longitudinal intervention studies are less consistent. Among normotensive children and adolescents there seems to be no training-induced reduction in resting BP (34,63). Among adolescents with hypertension some studies (32,47,48) report a decrease in resting BP, but others (61,63) found no effect. In general, obese children and adolescents have a higher BP than the non-obese population, although little attempt (e.g., 126) has been made to separate obesity from large body size per se. In a recent study (86) a combined 20-week exercise, behavior modification, and low-calorie diet regimen induced a similar weight loss, with a greater decrease in BP (and in forearm vascular resistance) of obese adolescents, than did behavior modification and diet alone. Several months after cessation of the training, the BP of hypertensive adolescents returned to pretraining levels (47,48).

In children and adolescents with HT, BP during high-intensity exercise is often higher than in non-hypertensive youth (e.g., 95), athough the increment from rest to maximal exercise is not different between these groups (31). The Task Force on Blood Pressure Control in Children (113) has recommended that, despite the high BP during intense exercise, young patients with mild and moderate HT should not curtail their physical activities. The Task Force further recommends that "in the absence of long-term outcome of weight training on BP and coronary artery disease . . . exercise programs be developed around aerobic forms."

Lipoprotein Profile

Several cross-sectional studies have shown that physically active children or children with higher aerobic fitness have a more favorable lipoprotein profile (or components thereof) than do less active children or those with lower aerobic fitness (33,39,44,74,88,115,118,121). Most of these studies suggest that more active children have lower triglyceride and higher HDL-cholesterol levels. An example is a comparison of 11- to 13-year-old sedentary children and track athletes from Finland (118). Among the girl athletes, serum triglycerides were 0.68 mmol/L, compared with 1.11 mmol/L among the sedentary girls. High-density lipoprotein cholesterol (HDL-C) in these groups were 1.61 mmol/L versus 1.29 mmol/L. The respective values for the boys were 1.67 mmol/L versus 1.32 mmol/L for HDL-C, and 0.73 mmol/L versus 0.98 mmol/L (NS) for triglycerides.

The above studies are quite consistent in suggesting a positive association between a favorable lipid and lipoprotein profile and PA; however, one cannot exclude preselection in these cross-sectional observations. Indeed, several intervention studies have not shown any consistent training effect on serum lipids and lipoproteins (33,37,40,42,43,52,63, 93,94,125). In only one study (37), which followed children who at the start of the program were non-obese and eulipidemic, was there a training-induced decrease in serum triglycerides or total cholesterol. Two studies (37,42) reported an increase in HDL-C and one study (94) found a *decrease* in HDL-C.

The discrepancy between the cross-sectional and the longitudinal findings is puzzling. One possibility is that the active children in the cross-sectional studies represent a preselected group that, genetically or otherwise, has a predisposition to a healthier lipid profile. Another explanation is that the above intervention programs, which lasted no more than 3 months, were too brief to induce biochemical changes in children (whose preintervention lipid and lipoprotein levels are healthier than in adults). The study by Sasaki et al. (93) is a case in point: obese 11-year-old girls and boys underwent a 7-day-per-week activity program for 2 years. Their HDL-C levels increased by 16% (boys) and 19% (girls) after 1 year and remained unchanged in the second year. Triglyceride levels decreased in the girls by 26% at the end of the second year, but not in the boys. The generalizability of Sasaki et al.'s findings is not clear, however, because the program was also accompanied by fat loss, and the study did not include a control group of similarly obese children who did not train.

There are some indications that hyperlipidemic children are more responsive to training than those who are eulipidemic (43,125). Much more research is needed to study this at-risk population.

Bone Mass and Density

One of the determinants of the risk for osteopenia and osteoporosis in advanced age seems to be peak bone mass during young adulthood. Bone mineral content increases markedly during puberty (53,68,105), reaching peak during young adulthood (77). Although heredity is a major determinant of peak bone mass, it is also likely that environmental factors are important. For example, calcium consumption during growth may affect peak bone mass (92). Although there is no definitive evidence regarding the impact of PA during childhood and adolescence on peak bone mass, several (16,60,102,119), but not all (53), recent cross-sectional studies have shown a relationship between bone density or bone mass on the one hand

and habitual activity on the other. Young adults who were active in their youth had a greater bone mineral content than did those who were less active (69,111). To date there are no reports of prospective studies that have assessed the effect of enhanced PA on bone mass of children and adolescents.

Although enhanced PA may induce a higher peak bone mass, there may be a threshold beyond which any additional activity may induce mineral bone loss and susceptibility to stress fractures (e.g., 123). Further research is needed regarding this dose–response pattern and the interaction between mineral bone mass and density on the one hand and PA, body weight, nutritional status (calcium intake in particular), and estrogen activity on the other.

Health Care Delivery: Clinic- Versus School-Based Programs

Assuming that enhanced physical activity during childhood has its merits in the prevention or lessening of adult risk, a question remains as to the best means of delivery of health-related exercise programs. Although assessment of risk can be done adequately in a hospital or a clinic, such an environment is not conducive to, nor cost effective for, the delivery of large-scale exercise programs. Schools, on the other hand, have several advantages insofar as they provide (a) a large pool of children who have a high risk profile or who are candidates for developing such a profile, (b) a pool of at least some of the relevant professionals (health educator, physical educator, dietitian, nurse, behavior counselor), and (c) sport facilities for year-round activities. Moreover, the children are captive participants for 8 to 10 months of the year, and lines of communication with the parents are well established. Most importantly, programs within a school do not carry the clinical stigma that exists in clinics and hospitals and deters many young individuals (e.g., obese adolescents) from participating.

The school environment can thus be conducive to delivering multidisciplinary educational and therapeutic programs (e.g., nutrition education, enhanced exercise classes, and behavior modification for management of obesity). In many schools, the professional best equipped to coordinate such a program is the physical education teacher, who also has experience in health education. Physical education teachers are (or can become) adept in fitness testing and anthropometry, and they are in a position to notice first if a child becomes overweight. One example of a large-scale, school-based program is the Heart Smart project, conducted in Jefferson Parish county, Louisiana. This is a multidisciplinary intervention in which enhanced aerobic activity is one component (24). Although there are no blueprints for optimal school-based programs, there are indications that such programs can be efficacious.

Vogel (120) in an extensive review of school-based intervention programs in the United States, Canada, Western Europe, Australia, and Israel concluded that the programs improved the students' knowledge regarding a healthy lifestyle and their attitudes toward physical activity and health-related fitness, increased their activity levels, and caused a decrease in adiposity. Simons-Morton, Parcel, O'Hara, Blair, and Pate (101), reported that intervention programs in the United States, Canada, and Australia were accompanied by, among others, an increase in aerobic fitness, total heartbeats throughout the day, and more time spent on moderate to vigorous PA. Ward and Bar-Or (122) reviewed 13 school-based programs for juvenile obesity. Most of the interventions induced a mild decrease in adiposity compared with no change in nonparticipant controls. The above findings are related to special school-based projects and do not prove that regular physical education curricula are efficacious in affecting coronary risk. In point of fact, there are indications that some regular physical education programs in the United States are comprised of very little moderate to vigorous PA (80,90,114).

Conclusion

There are no prospective data up to this time that support or reject the hypothesis that childhood physical activity per se affects the risk for chronic disease in adulthood. While cross-sectional studies show differences between active and less active children (and adolescents) in components of coronary risk and in bone mineral mass, there is little evidence that short-term interventions in healthy children modify these components. Even when such an intervention does reduce a risk factor, as in resting blood pressure or in adiposity, the effect is short-lived, reverting to preintervention values soon after the intervention has stopped.

Challenges for Future Research

Methodology

1. What are the *gold standards* to measure energy expenditure of children under free-living conditions and to assess behavioral aspects of children's activity?

2. Using the above gold standards, which other valid tools can assess energy expenditure and behavioral aspects of activity?
3. What are the optimal educational and marketing strategies that might increase leisure-time activity among teenagers?

Activity, Fitness, and Health

4. Which fitness components are health-related during childhood and which are relevant to health in future years?
5. What are the causes for drop in habitual activity during the second decade of life and for the relatively low activity level of teenage females?
6. What is the tracking of activity patterns and its relationship to the tracking of health outcomes from childhood to early adulthood?
7. What is the role of hypoactivity in the etiology of childhood obesity?
8. What factors (hereditary and environmental) determine differences in activity, fitness, and coronary risk among children of different racial, ethnic, and socioeconomic backgrounds?
9. Can a cause-and-effect relationship be confirmed between bone mineral acquisition during growth and physical activity? If so, what is the optimal activity level beyond which bone mineral content diminishes?

Response to Training

10. What are the biological variables that affect interindividual differences in trainability among children?
11. What are the biological and psychosocial factors that affect responsiveness to activity intervention in childhood obesity and other risk factors?
12. What is the optimal multidisciplinary program to promote long-term control of juvenile obesity?
13. What are the effects of regimented training programs on the overall energy expenditure and spontaneous activity of healthy children and those with coronary risk?
14. Does enhanced activity in early years affect health-related attitudes?
15. Can exercise counteract the protein loss induced by very low-calorie diets?

Assuming limited financial resources for research, preference should be given to longitudinal and interventional studies of children who already have adult risk factors for coronary heart disease and those with a family history of premature coronary heart disease.

References

1. Armstrong, N.; Balding, J.; Gentle, P.; Kirby, B. Estimation of coronary risk factors in British schoolchildren: A preliminary report. Br. J. Sports Med. 24:61-66; 1990.
2. Åstrand, P.O. Experimental studies of physical working capacity in relation to sex and age. Copenhagen: Munskgaard; 1952.
3. Baranowski, T. Validity and reliability of self report measures of physical activity: An information-processing perspective. Res. Q. Exerc. Sport. 59:314-327; 1988.
4. Baranowski, T.; Bouchard, C.; Bar-Or, O.; Bricker, T.; Heath, G.; Kimm, S.Y.S.; Malina, R.; Obarzanik, E.; Pate, R.; Strong, W.B.; Truman, B.; Washington, R. Assessment, prevalence, and cardiovascular benefits of physical activity and fitness in youth. Med. Sci. Sports Exerc. 24:S237- S247; 1992.
5. Baranowski, T.; Dworkin, R.J.; Cieslik, C.J.; Hooks, P.; Clearman, D.R.; Ray, L.; Dunn, J.K.; Nader, P.R. Reliability and validity of self report of aerobic activity: Family health project. Res. Q. Exerc. Sport. 55:309-317; 1984.
6. Bar-Or, O. Pediatric sports medicine for the practitioner. New York: Springer-Verlag; 1983.
7. Bar-Or, O. Physical conditioning in children with cardiorespiratory disease. Exerc. Sport Sci. Rev. 13:305-334, 1985.
8. Bar-Or, O.; Malina, R.M. Activity, fitness and health in children and adolescents. In: Cheng, L., ed. Proceedings of the Harvard conference on nutrition and fitness of children and youth; [In press].
9. Becque, M.D.; Katch, V.L.; Rocchini, A.P.; Charles, R.M.; Moorehead, C. Coronary risk incidence of obese adolescents: Reduction by exercise plus diet intervention. Pediatrics. 81:605-612; 1988.
10. Berenson, G.S. Causation of cardiovascular risk factors in children. New York: Raven Press; 1986.
11. Berenson, G.S.; McMahan, C.A.; Voors, A.W., editors. Cardiovascular risk factors in children—the early natural history of atherosclerosis and essential hypertension. New York: Oxford University Press; 1980.
12. Berkowitz, R.I.; Agras, W.S.; Korner, A.F.; Kraemer, H.C.; Zeanah, C.H. Physical activity and adiposity: A longitudinal study from birth to childhood. J. Pediatr. 106:734-738; 1985.
13. Blaak, E.E.; Bar-Or, O.; Westerterp, K.R.; Saris, W.H.M. Effect of VLCD on daily energy expenditure and body composition in obese boys. Int. J. Obes. [Suppl. 2]. 14:86; 1990.

14. Blaak, E.E.; Westerterp, K.R.; Bar-Or, O.; Wouters, L.J.M.; Saris, W.H.M. Total energy expenditure and spontaneous activity in relation to training in obese boys. Am. J. Clin. Nutr. 55:777-782; 1992.
15. Blair, S.N.; Clark, D.B.; Cureton, K.J.; Powell, K.E. Exercise and fitness in childhood: Implications for a lifetime of health. In: Gisolfi, C.V.; Lamb,D.L., eds. Perspectives in exercise science and sports medicine, vol. 2. Youth, exercise and sport. Indianapolis: Benchmark Press; 1989:401-430.
16. Blimkie, C.J.; Rice, S.; Webber, C.; Martin, J.; Levy, D.; Parker, D. Bone density, physical activity, fitness, anthropometry, gynecologic, endocrine and nutrition status in adolescent girls. In: Coudert, J.; Van Praagh, E., eds. Pediatric work physiology. Children and exercise XVI. Paris: Masson; 1992:201-203.
17. Bloom, B.S. Stability and change in human characteristics. New York: Wiley; 1964.
18. Boileau, R.A.; Lohman, T.G.; Slaughter, M.H. Exercise and body composition of children and youth. Scand. J. Sports Sci. 7:17-27; 1985.
19. Bouchard, C.; Shephard, R.J.; Stephens, T.; Sutton, J.R.; McPherson, B.D., editors. Exercise, fitness, and health: A consensus of current knowledge. Champaign, IL: Human Kinetics; 1990.
20. Brown, M.R.; Klish, W.J.; Hollander, J.; Campbell, M.A.; Forbes, G.B. A high protein, low calorie liquid diet in the treatment of very obese adolescents: Long-term effect on lean body mass. Am. J. Clin. Nutr. 38:20-31; 1983.
21. Brownell, K.D.; Kelman, J.H.; Stunkard, A.J. Treatment of obese children with and without their mothers: Change in weight and blood pressure. Pediatrics. 71:515-523; 1983.
22. Bruch, H. Obesity in childhood. IV. Energy expenditure of obese children. Am. J. Dis. Child. 60:1082-1109; 1940.
23. Bullen, B.A.; Reed, R.B.; Mayer, J. Physical activity of obese and non-obese adolescent girls appraised by motion picture sampling. Am. J. Clin. Nutr. 14:211-223; 1964.
24. Butcher, A.H.; Frank, G.C.; Harsha, D.W.; Serpas, D.C.; Little, S.D.; Nicklas, T.A.; Hunter, S.M.; Berenson, G.S. Heart smart: A school health program meeting the 1990 objectives for the nation. Health Educ. Q. 5:17-34; 1988.
25. Charney, E.; Goodman, H.C.; McBride, M.; Lyon, B.; Pratt, R. Childhood antecedents of adult obesity. Do chubby infants become obese adults? New Engl. J. Med. 295:6-9; 1976.
26. Corbin, C.B.; Pletcher, P. Diet and physical activity pattern of obese and nonobese elementary school children. Res. Q. Assoc. Health Phys. Educ. 39:922-928; 1968.
27. Daniels, J.; Oldridge, N. Changes in oxygen consumption of young boys during growth and running training. Med. Sci. Sports. 3:161-165; 1971.
28. Despres, J.P.; Bouchard, C.; Malina, R.M. Physical activity and coronary heart disease risk factors during childhood and adolescence. Exerc. Sport Sci. Rev. 18:243-261; 1990.
29. Despres, J.P.; Bouchard, C.; Tremblay, A.; Savard, R.; Marcotte, M. Effects of aerobic training on fat distribution in male subjects. Med. Sci. Sports Exerc. 17:113-118; 1985.
30. Dietz, W.H.; Gortmaker, S.L. Do we fatten our children at the TV set? Obesity and television viewing in children and adolescents. Pediatrics. 75:807-812; 1985.
31. Dlin, R. Blood pressure response to dynamic exercise in healthy and hypertensive youths. Pediatrician. 13:34-43; 1986.
32. Duncan, J.J.; Farr, J.E.; Upton, S.J.; Hagan, R.D.; Oglesby, M.E.; Blair, S.N. The effects of aerobic exercise on plasma catecholamines and blood pressure in patients with mild essential hypertension. JAMA. 254:2609-2613; 1985.
33. DuRant, R.H.; Linder, C.W.; Harkess, J.W.; Gray, R.G. The relationships between physical activity and serum lipids and lipoproteins in black children and adolescents. J. Adolesc. Health Care. 3:75-81; 1982.
34. Dwyer, T.; Coonan, W.E.; Leitch, D.R.; Hetzel, B.S.; Baghurst, R.A. An investigation of the effects of daily physical activity on the health of primary school students in South Australia. Int. J. Epidemiol. 12:308-313; 1983.
35. Epstein, L. Treatment of childhood obesity. In: Brownell, K.D.; Foreyt, J.P., eds. Handbook of eating disorders. New York: Basic Books; 1986.
36. Epstein, L.H.; Valosky, A.; Wing, R.R.; McCurley, J. Ten-year follow-up of behavioral, family-based treatment for obese children. JAMA. 264:2519-2523; 1990.
37. Fisher, A.G.; Brown, M. The effects of diet and exercise on selected coronary risk factors in children. Med. Sci. Sports Exerc. 14:171; 1982.
38. Fraser, G.E.; Phillips, R.L.; Harris, R. Physical fitness and blood pressure in school children. Circulation. 67:405-412; 1983.
39. Fripp, R.R.; Hodgson, J.L.; Kwiterovich, P.O.; Werner, C.J.; Schuler, H.G.; Whitman, V. Aerobic capacity, obesity, and atherosclerosis risk factors in male adolescents. Pediatrics. 75:813-818; 1985.
40. Gaul, C.A.; Docherty, D.; Wenger, H.A. The effects of aerobic training on blood lipid profiles of young females. Can. J. Sport Sci. 14:112P; 1989.

41. Gilders, R.M.; Dudley, G.A. Endurance exercise training and treatment of hypertension: The controversy. Sports Med. 13:71-77; 1992.
42. Gilliam, T.B.; Burke, M.B. Effects of exercise on serum lipids and lipoproteins in girls, ages 8 to 10 years. Artery. 4:203-213; 1978.
43. Gilliam, T.B.; Freedson, P.S. Effects of a 12-week school physical fitness program on peak VO_2, body composition and blood lipids in 7- to 9-year-old children. Int. J. Sports Med. 1:73-78; 1980.
44. Gilliam, T.B.; Freedson, P.S.; MacConnie, S.E.; Geenen, D.L.; Pels, A.E., III. Comparison of blood lipids, lipoproteins, anthropometric measures and resting and exercise cardiovascular responses in children, 6-7 years old. Prev. Med. 10:754-764; 1981.
45. Gortmaker, S.L.; Dietz, W.H.; Sobol, A.M.; Wehler, C.A. Increasing pediatric obesity in the United States. Am. J. Dis. Child. 141:535-540; 1987.
46. Gutin, B.; Basch, C.; Shea, S.; Contento, I.; DeLozier, M.; Rips, J.; Irigoyen, M.; Zybert, P. Blood pressure, fitness, and fatness in 5- and 6-year-old children. JAMA. 264:1123-1127; 1990.
47. Hagberg, J.M.; Ehsani, A.A.; Goldring, D.; Hernandez, A.; Sinacore, D.R.; Holloszy, J.O. Effect of weight training on blood pressure and hemodynamics in hypertensive adolescents. J. Pediatr. 104:147-151; 1984.
48. Hagberg, J.M.; Goldring, D.; Ehsani, A.A.; Heath, G.W.; Hernandez, A.; Schehchtman, K.; Holloszy, J.O. Effect of exercise training on the blood pressure and hemodynamic features of hypertensive adolescents. Am. J. Cardiol. 52:763-768; 1983.
49. Hansen, H.S.; Hyldebrandt, N.; Froberg, K.; Nielsen, J.R. Blood pressure and fitness in school children. Scand. J. Clin. Lab. Invest. [Suppl.] 192:42-46; 1989.
50. Harshfield, G.A.; Dupaul, L.M.; Alpert, B.S. Aerobic fitness and the diurnal rhythm of blood pressure in adolescents. Hypertension. 15(6):810-814; 1990.
51. Hofman, A.; Walter, H.J.; Connelly, P.A.; Vaughan, R.D. Blood pressure and physical fitness in children. Hypertension. 9:188-191; 1987.
52. Hunt, H.F.; White, J.R. Effects of 10 weeks of vigorous daily exercise on serum lipids and lipoproteins in teenage males. Med. Sci. Sports Exerc. 12:93; 1980.
53. Katzman, D.K.; Bachrach, L.K.; Carter, D.R.; Marcus, R. Clinical and anthropometric correlates of bone mineral acquisition in healthy adolescent girls. J. Clin. Endocrinol. Metab. 73:1332-1339; 1991.
54. Kemper, H.C.G.; Snel, J.; Verschuur, R.; Storm-van Essen, L. Tracking of health and risk indicators of cardiovascular diseases from teenager to adult: Amsterdam growth and health study. Prev. Med. 19:642-655; 1990.
55. Khoury, P.; Morrison, J.A.; Kelly, K.; Mellies, M.; Horvitz, R.; Glueck, C.J. Clustering and interrelationships of coronary heart disease risk factors in schoolchildren, ages 6-19. Am. J. Epidemiol. 112:524-538; 1980.
56. Klesges, L.M.; Klesges, R.C. The assessment of children's physical activity: A comparison of methods. Med. Sci. Sports Exerc. 19:511-517; 1987.
57. Klesges, R.C.; Haddock, C.K.; Eck, L.H. A multimethod approach to the measurement of childhood physical activity and its relationship to blood pressure and body weight. J. Pediatr. 116:888-893; 1990.
58. Klesges, R.C.; Klesges, L.M.; Swenson, A.M.; Pheley, A.M. A validation of two motion sensors in the prediction of child and adult physical activity levels. Am. J. Epidemiol. 122:400-410; 1985.
59. Kreitzman, S.N. Lean body mass, exercise and VLCD. Int. J. Obes. [Suppl. 2]. 13:17-25; 1989.
60. Kröger, H.; Kotaniemi, A.; Vainio, P.; Alhava, E. Bone densitometry of the spine and femur in children by dual-energy x-ray absorptiometry. Bone Miner. 17:75-85; 1992.
61. Laird, W.P.; Fixler, D.E.; Swanbom, C.D. Effect of chronic weight lifting on blood pressure in hypertensive adolescents. Prev. Med. [Abstract]. 8:184; 1979.
62. Lauer, R.M.; Burns, T.L.; Mahoney, L.T.; Tipton, C.M. Blood pressure in children. In: Gisolfi, C.V.; Lamb, D.R., eds. Perspectives in exercise science and sports medicine. Vol. 2 Youth, exercise and sport. Indianapolis: Benchmark Press; 1989:431-459.
63. Linder, C.W.; DuRant, R.H.; Mahoney, O.M. The effect of physical conditioning on serum lipids and lipoproteins in white male adolescents. Med. Sci. Sports Exerc. 15:232-236; 1983.
64. MacDougall, J.D.; Roche, P.D.; Bar-Or, O.; Moroz, J.R. Maximal aerobic capacity of Canadian schoolchildren: Prediction based on age-related oxygen cost of locomotion. Int. J. Sports Med. 4:194-198; 1983.
65. Mahan, L.K. Family-focused behavioral approach to weight control in children. Pediatr. Clin. North Am. 34:983-996; 1987.
66. Malina, R.M. Growth, exercise, fitness, and later outcomes. In: Bouchard, C.; Shephard, R.J.; Stephens, T.; Sutton, J.R.; McPherson,

B.D., eds. Exercise, fitness, and health: A concensus of current knowledge. Champaign, IL: Human Kinetics; 1990:637-653.

67. Malina, R.M. Tracking of physical fitness and performance during growth. In: Beunen, G.; Ghesquiere, J.; Reybrouck, T.; Claessens, A.L., eds. Children and exercise XIV. Band 4, Schriftenreihe der Hamburg-Mannheimer-Stiftung fur Informationsmedizin; 1990:1-10.

68. McCormick, D.P.; Ponder, S.W.; Fawcett, H.D.; Palmer, J.L. Spinal bone mineral density in 335 normal and obese children and adolescents: Evidence for ethnic and sex differences. J. Bone Miner. Res. 6:507-513; 1991.

69. McCulloch, R.G.; Bailey, D.A.; Houston, C.S.; Dodd, B.L. Effects of physical activity, dietary calcium intake and selected lifestyle factors on bone density in young women. Can. Med. Assoc. J. 142:221-227; 1990.

70. McGill, H.C., Jr. Morphologic development of the atherosclerotic plaque. In: Lauer, R.M.; Shekelle, R.R., eds. Childhood prevention of atherosclerosis and hypertension. New York: Raven Press; 1980:41-49.

71. Montoye, H.J. Risk indicators for cardiovascular disease in relation to physical activity in youth. In: Binkhorst, R.; eds. Children and exercise IX. Champaign, IL: Human Kinetics; 1985:3-25.

72. Montoye, H.J. Physical activity, physical fitness, and heart disease risk factors in children. In: Stull, G.A.; Eckert, H.M., eds. Effects of physical activity on children. Champaign, IL: Human Kinetics; 1986:127-152.

73. Moody, D.L.; Wilmore, J.H.; Girandola, R.N.; Royce, J.P. The effects of a jogging program on the body composition of normal and obese high school girls. Med. Sci. Sports. 4:210-213; 1972.

74. Nizankowska-Blaz, T.; Abramowicz, T. Effects of intensive physical training on serum lipids and lipoproteins. Acta Paediatr. Scand. 72:357-359; 1983.

75. Nudel, D.B. Exercise and coronary artery disease risk factors in children. Pediatr. Rev. Commun. 2:207-220; 1988.

76. Orchard, T.J.; Becjer, D.J.; Kuller, L.H.; Wagner, D.K.; LaPorte, R.E.; Drash, A.L. Age and sex variations in glucose tolerance and insulin response: Parallel with cardiovascular risk. J. Chronic Dis. 35:123-132; 1982.

77. Ott, S.M. Editorial: Attainment of peak bone mass. J. Clin. Endocrinol. Metab. 71:1082A-1082C; 1990.

78. Palti, H.; Gofin, R.; Adler, B.; Grafstein, O.; Belmaker, E. Tracking of blood pressure over an eight year period in Jerusalem school children. J. Clin. Epidemiol. 41:731-735; 1988.

79. Panico, S.; Celentano, E.; Krogh, V.; Jossa, F.; Farinaro, E.; Trevisan, M.; Mancini, M. Physical activity and its relationship to blood pressure in school children. J. Chronic Dis. 40:925-930; 1987.

80. Parcel, G.S.; Simons-Morton, B.G.; O'Hara, N.M.; Baranowski, T.; Kolbe, L.J.; Bee, D.E. School promotion of healthful diet and exercise behavior: An integration of organizational change and social learning theory interventions. J. Sch. Health. 57:150-156; 1987.

81. Parizkova, J. Physical training in weight reduction of obese adolescents. Ann. Clin. Res. [Suppl. 34]. 14:63-68; 1982.

82. Parizkova, J.; Vaneckova, M.; Vamberova, M. A study of changes in some functional indicators following reduction of excessive fat in obese children. Physiol. Bohemoslov. 11:351-357; 1962.

83. Pate, R.R.; Blair, S.N. Exercise and the prevention of atherosclerosis: Pediatric implications. In: Strong, W.B., ed. Atherosclerosis: Its pediatric aspects. New York: Grune & Stratton; 1978:251-286.

84. Poehlman, E.T.; Melby, C.L.; Goran, M. The impact of exercise and diet restriction on daily energy expenditure. Sports Med. 11:78-101; 1991.

85. Roberts, S.B.; Savage, J.; Coward, W.A.; Chew, B.; Lucas, A. Energy expenditure and intake in infants born to lean and overweight mothers. N. Engl. J. Med. 318:461-466; 1988.

86. Rocchini, A.P.; Katch, V.; Anderson, J.; Hinderliter, J.; Becque, D.; Martin, M.; Marks, C. Blood pressure in obese adolescents: Effect of weight loss. Pediatrics. 82:16-23; 1988.

87. Ross, J.G.; Pate, R.R.; Lohman, T.G.; Christenson, G.M. Changes in the body composition of children. J. Phys. Educ. Recr. Dance. 58:74-77; 1987.

88. Sady, S.P.; Berg, K.; Smith, J.L.; Savage, M.P.; Thompson, W.H.; Nutter, J. Aerobic fitness and serum high-density lipoprotein cholesterol in young children. Hum. Biol. 56:771-781; 1984.

89. Sallis, J.F.; Buono, M.J.; Fredson, P.S. Bias in estimating caloric expenditure from physical activity in children. Implications for epidemiological studies. Sports Med. 11:203-209; 1991.

90. Sallis, J.F.; McKenzie, T.L. Physical education's role in public health. Res. Q. Exerc. Sport. 62:124-137; 1991.

91. Sallis, J.F.; Patterson, T.L.; Buono, M.J.; Nader, P.R. Relation of cardiovascular fitness and physical activity in cardiovascular disease

risk factors in children and adults. Am. J. Epidemiol. 127:933-941; 1988.

92. Sandler, R.B.; Slemenda, C.W.; LaPorte, R.E.; Cauley, J.A.; Schramm, M.M.; Barresi, M.L.; Kriska, A.M. Postmenopausal bone density and milk consumption in childhood and adolescence. Am. J. Clin. Nutr. 42:270-274; 1985.
93. Sasaki, J.; Shindo, M.; Tanaka, H.; Ando, M.; Arakawa, K. A long-term aerobic exercise program decreases the obesity index and increases the high density lipoprotein cholesterol concentration in obese children. Int. J. Obes. 11:339-345; 1987.
94. Savage, M.P.; Petratis, M.M.; Thomson, W.H.; Berg, K.; Smith, J.L.; Sady, S.P. Exercise training effects on serum lipids of pubescent boys and adult men. Med. Sci. Sports Exerc. 18:197-204; 1986.
95. Schieken, R.M.; Clarke, W.R.; Lauer, R.M. The cardiovascular responses to exercise in children across the blood pressure distribution. The Muscatine study. Hypertension. 5:71-78; 1983.
96. Schoeller, D.A.; Bandini, L.G.; Levitsky, L.L.; Dietz, W.H. Energy requirements of obese children and young adults. Proc. Nutr. Soc. 47:241-246; 1988.
97. Schrub, J.-C.; Wolf, L.-M.; Courtois, H.; Javet, F. Fasting with muscular exercise, changes in weight and nitrogen balance. La Nouvelle Presse Medicale. 22:875-878; 1975.
98. Schutz, R.W.; Smoll, F.L. The (in)stability of attitudes toward physical activity during childhood and adolescence. In: McPherson, B.D., ed. Sport and aging. Champaign, IL: Human Kinetics; 1986:187-197.
99. Seals, D.R.; Hagberg, J.M. The effect of exercise training on human hypertension: A review. Med. Sci. Sports Exerc. 16:207-215; 1984.
100. Seidman, D.S.; Laor, A.; Gale, R.; Stevenson, D.K.; Danon, Y.L. A longitudinal study of birth weight and being overweight in late adolescence. Am. J. Dis. Child. 145:782-785; 1991.
101. Simons-Morton, B.G.; Parcel, G.S.; O'Hara, N.M.; Blair, S.N.; Pate, R.R. Health-related physical fitness in childhood: Status and recommendation. Annual Rev. Public Health. 9:403-425; 1988.
102. Slemenda, C.W.; Miller, J.Z.; Hui, S.L.; Reister, T.K.; Johnston, C.C., Jr. Role of physical activity in the development of skeletal mass in children. J. Bone Miner. Res. 6:1227-1233; 1991.
103. Smoak, C.G.; Burke, G.L.; Webber, L.S.; Harsha, D.W.; Srinivasan, S.R.; Berenson, G.S. Relation of obesity to clustering of cardiovascular disease risk factors in children and young adults. The Bogalusa heart study. Am. J. Epidemiol. 125:364-372; 1987.
104. Smoll, F.L.; Schutz, R.W. Children's attitudes towards physical activity: A longitudinal analysis. J. Sport Psychol. 2:144-154; 1980.
105. Southard, R.N.; Morris, J.D.; Mahan, J.D. Bone mass in healthy children: Measurement with quantitative DXA. Radiology. 179:735-738; 1991.
106. Spurr, G.B.; Barc-Nieto, M.; Reins, J.C.; Ramirez, R. Marginal malnutrition in school-aged Colombian boys: Efficiency of treadmill walking in submaximal exercise. Am. J. Clin. Nutr. 39:452-459; 1984.
107. Stefanik, P.A.; Heald, F.P.; Mayer, J. Caloric intake in relation to energy output of obese and nonobese adolescent boys. Am. J. Clin. Nutr. 7:55-62; 1959.
108. Strazzulo, P.; Cappuccio, P.; Trevisan, M.; De Leo, A.; Krogh,V.; Giorgione, N.; Mancini, M. Leisure time physical activity and blood pressure in schoolchildren. Am. J. Epidemiol. 127:726-733; 1988.
109. Strong, J.P.; McGill, H.C. The pediatric aspects of atherosclerosis. J. Athero. Res. 9:251-265; 1969.
110. Stunkard, A.J.; Pestka, J. The physical activity of obese girls. Am. J. Dis. Child. 103:116-121; 1962.
111. Talmage, R.V.; Anderson, J.B. Bone density loss in women: Effects of childhood activity, exercise, calcium intake and estrogen therapy. Calcium Tissue Res. 36:552; 1984.
112. Tamir, I.; Heiss, G.; Glueck, C.J.; Christensen, B.; Kwiterovich, P.; Rifkind, B.M. Lipid and lipoprotein distribution in white children ages 6-19 yr. The lipid research clinics program prevalence study. J. Chronic Dis. 34:27-39; 1981.
113. Task Force on Blood Pressure Control in Children. Report of the second task force on blood pressure control in children—1987. Pediatrics. 79:1-25; 1987.
114. Taylor, W.C.; Simons-Morton, B.G.; Snider, S.A.; Huang, I.W. Amount of physical activity in physical education classes. Pediatr. Exerc. Sci. 4:185; 1992.
115. Thorland, W.G.; Gilliam, T.B. Comparison of serum lipids between habitually high and low active pre-adolescent males. Med. Sci. Sports Exerc. 13:316-321; 1981.
116. Turner, M.C.; Ruley, E.J.; Buckley, K.M.; Strife, C.F. Blood pressure elevation in children with orthopedic immobilization. J. Pediatr. 95:989-992; 1979.
117. Vaccaro, P.; Mahon, A.D. The effects of exercise on coronary heart disease risk factors in children. Sports Med. 8:139-153; 1989.

118. Valimaki, I.; Hursti, M.L.; Pihlakoski, L.; Viikari, J. Exercise performance and serum lipids in relation to physical activity in school children. Int. J. Sports Med. 1:132-136; 1980.
119. Virvidakis, K.; Georgiou, E.; Korkotsidis, A.; Ntalles, K.; Proukakis, C. Bone mineral content of junior competitive weightlifters. Int. J. Sports Med. 11:244-246; 1990.
120. Vogel, P.G. Effects of physical education programs on children. In: Seefeldt, V., ed. Physical activity and well-being. Reston, VA: American Alliance of Health, Physical Education, Recreation and Dance; 1986:455-509.
121. Wanne, O.; Viikari, J.; Valimaki, I. Physical performance and serum lipids in 14-16-year-old trained, normally active, and inactive children. In: Ilmarinen, J.; Valimaki, I., eds. Children and sport. Berlin: Springer; 1984:241-246.
122. Ward, D.S.; Bar-Or, O. The role of the physician and the physical education teacher in the treatment of obesity at school. Pediatrician. 13:44-51; 1986.
123. Warren, M.P.; Brooks-Gunn, J.; Hamilton, L.H.; Warren, L.F.; Hamilton, W.G. Scoliosis and fractures in young ballet dancers. N. Engl. J. Med. 314:1348-1353; 1986.
124. Waxman, M.; Stunkard, A.J. Caloric intake and expenditure of obese boys. J. Pediatr. 96:187-193; 1980.
125. Widhalm, K.; Maxa, E.; Zyman, H. Effect of diet and exercise upon the cholesterol and triglyceride content of plasma lipoproteins in overweight children. Eur. J. Pediatr. 127:121-126; 1978.
126. Wilson, S.L.; Gaffney, E.A.; Laird, W.P.; Fixler, D.E. Body size, composition, and fitness in adolescents with elevated blood pressures. Hypertension. 7:417-422; 1985.
127. Wynder, E.L. Coronary artery disease prevention: Cholesterol, a pediatric perspective. Prev. Med. 18:323-409; 1989.
128. Zuti, W.B.; Golding, L.A. Comparing diet and exercise as weight reduction tools. Phys. Sportsmed. 4:49-53; 1976.

Chapter 64

Physical Activity, Fitness, and Female Reproductive Morbidity

Anne B. Loucks

Despite high ratings on the traditional components of physiological fitness, many physically active women fail endocrinological tests of reproductive fitness (48,92,144). As in postmenopausal women, hypoestrogenism in amenorrheic physically active women causes rapid skeletal demineralization, predisposing them to stress fractures and osteoporosis (41,55,57,88,96,105,147). There are some indications that bone density increases after menses resume (56,87), but further follow-up indicates that the gain reaches a plateau beneath the normal level (54).

Hypoestrogenism also lowers apolipoprotein levels in amenorrheic athletes (86), potentially increasing their risk of developing coronary artery disease. Meanwhile, the suppressed luteal phase progesterone levels in asymptomatic, regularly menstruating, physically active women may predispose them to breast cancer (47,99,130). Thus, the need arises to distinguish the behavioral etiologies of these reproductive morbidities from unrelated practices in physically active lifestyles and to distinguish the linking neuroendocrine mechanisms from the general neuroendocrine response to physical activity. This new knowledge will reveal whether the reproductive and traditional components of physiological fitness are mutually exclusive in some or all women. (Note, the concept of morbidity is used here in the sense defined by Bouchard and Shephard [25] as "any departure, subjective or objective, from a state of physical or psychological well-being short of death.")

Low body weight and fatness do not account for the occurrence of reproductive morbidities in physically active women (for reviews see 35,90, 128,131), and neither do hyperandrogenism and hyperprolactinemia (51,89). Hence, these hypotheses are not discussed here. This review considers the two hypotheses most actively studied at the present time: exercise stress, mediated by neurotransmitters and hormones of the adrenal axis; and energy availability, mediated by one or more metabolic signals.

The acute release of cortisol and other so-called "stress" hormones during intense and prolonged exercise underlies the hypothesis that activation of the adrenal axis by physical activity disrupts the ovarian axis. In amenorrheic athletes, baseline cortisol levels are, indeed, mildly elevated (51,53,92), and those amenorrheic athletes who spontaneously resumed menses within 6 months after an initial testing did have lower cortisol levels than others who did not resume (53). Paradoxically, baseline adrenocorticotropic hormone (ACTH) levels are normal in amenorrheic athletes (51,92), suggesting that the setpoint for ACTH regulation has been reset, perhaps by increased corticotropin-releasing hormone (CRH) stimulation in the presence of increased cortisol negative feedback. In addition, ACTH and cortisol responses to CRH administration (74,92) and to exercise (51,89) are blunted in amenorrheic athletes, apparently also due to increased cortisol negative feedback. One study failed to detect these characteristics but employed a brief exercise stimulus and sampled blood only briefly after the exercise bout during the confounding midday surge in cortisol levels (73).

The adrenal axis abnormalities in amenorrheic athletes distinguish them from regularly menstruating athletic and sedentary women (51,92). That these abnormalities are also seen in other types of hypothalamic amenorrheic women (16,19,22,26, 65,81,135) raises doubt as to whether "the stress of exercise" is the stimulus causing either hypercortisolism or reproductive morbidity in amenorrheic athletes. Warren's early observations of reproductive morbidities in ballet dancers led her to suggest that the morbidities are due to "energy drain" (146). Later, several investigators reported that women in some sports and performance arts do, in fact, consume much less energy in their diet than would be expected, considering their level of physical activity (55,92,96,103). Indeed, triiodothyronine (T_3) levels are low in amenorrheic athletes (91,96,103), and so, too, is their resting metabolic rate (103). These observations are consistent with the idea that amenorrheic, physically active women may have acclimated to a self-imposed, chronic energy deficiency by reducing their basal metabolic rate (which accounts for most energy utilization) and by avoiding the energy-consuming anabolic processes of the menstrual cycle.

For this review, reports were compiled on the results of true experiments that disrupted reproductive function by three means: (a) exercise training, (b) stress or stress hormones, and (c) energy availability. Articles were obtained through computerized searches of the literature and from the author's personal files. Available information on the influence of stress hormones and energy availability on the reproductive system is reviewed in detail after brief summaries of the responses of the adrenal axis to stress and of the thyroid axis to energy availability. In conclusion, the evidence is evaluated according to criteria for establishing causation in medical and physiological research (50).

Experimental Induction of Reproductive Morbidities by Exercise Training

Historically, few true experiments have investigated the effect of exercise training on reproductive function. Most experiments have utilized animal models, and most of these have used rodents. Three unsatisfactory exercise protocols have been employed in the animal studies: (a) affording animals free access to running wheels, (b) forcing animals to swim or to run on motor-driven wheels or treadmills, and (c) training animals to run for food rewards. The free-exercise method suffers from the inability of the investigator to control the quantity, intensity, or duration of the exercise. The forced-exercise method controls the exercise regimen, but is confounded by psychological distress associated with the forcing technique, commonly electroshock, which is known to have its own influence on the reproductive system. In addition, without intentional control of dietary intake, studies employing either of these methods may be confounded by differences in energy availability. Meanwhile, the confounding of exercise and energy availability is inherent in the rewarded-exercise method.

A recent refinement of the forced-exercise method aims to reduce the level of psychological distress by confining monkeys in a plexiglass cage on top of a treadmill. It is claimed that the monkeys eventually learn to enjoy running, at which time the cage can be removed. The inferential strength of the rewarded-exercise method is improved by including a nonexercising control group with matched food intake.

Most studies have sought effects on reproductive cyclicity, either estrus or menses, or on pubertal development. Inferences about pubertal development in exercising animals have usually been confounded by differences in energy availability, as reflected in an associated delay in growth. Recent studies have examined more rapidly responding outcome variables such as reproductive hormone levels and pulsatility, which permit the influence of energy availability to be more readily distinguished from those of body size and composition. Ovarian function is critically dependent on the frequency with which pulses of luteinizing hormone (LH) are released from the pituitary gland. An introduction to LH pulsatility and its assessment has recently been published (59).

During experiments culminating in his proposed General Adaptation Syndrome, Selye demonstrated that he could induce anestrus, ovarian atrophy, and adrenal hypertrophy in female rats by abruptly imposing prolonged, strenuous exercise training in the form of forced running (129). Since then, an increased prevalence of anestrus has been induced in female rats by forced swimming (4,6) and forced running (42,44), and amenorrhea has been induced in women by voluntary running (15,37). Less strenuous and more gradually progressive exercise protocols have not induced anestrus or amenorrhea (23,29,36,122,129), but have reduced gonadotropin sensitivity to gonadotropin-releasing hormone (GnRH) (29).

Forced swimming delays puberty in female rats (108). An experimental protocol better simulating natural conditions (i.e., increased foraging activity for less food) demonstrates that fat deposition supersedes pubertal development in foraging female mice (109,110). Treadmill running for food rewards can delay puberty for prolonged periods of time until the associated suppression of LH pulsatility is rapidly reversed and the delay is terminated by relaxation of the exercise regimen (94).

The few published studies that have sought acute effects of exercise on LH pulsatility have yielded inconsistent results (49,82,100). The low precision of the statistical techniques for assessing pulsatility from brief blood sampling periods limits the measurability of LH pulsatility in such protocols.

Although early studies were widely interpreted as evidence of the counterregulatory influence of "exercise stress" on the female reproductive system, the "stress of exercise" was routinely confounded with its energy cost in cross-sectional, longitudinal, animal, and human studies of the "activity-stress paradigm." Indeed, cortisol is a glucocorticoid, and blood glucose level is an extremely sensitive regulator of adrenal axis activation by CRH (149). In addition, carbohydrate administration during prolonged exercise has recently been shown to prevent the usual acute rise in cortisol levels in rats (132) and men (136). Thus, the reproductive morbidities observed in physically active women may derive not from exercise stress inherent in physical activity, but rather from a failure to supplement the diet in compensation for the energy expended in physical activity. The following sections summarize the evidence supporting these two hypotheses.

Stress, Mediated by the Adrenal Axis

With its isolation, purification, and characterization as a 41-amino acid peptide in the early 1980s (142), CRH was initially thought to be the major if not the sole means of stimulating the release of ACTH from the pituitary. Subsequent research quickly revealed that ACTH is also released and regulated by catecholamines, gastrin-releasing peptide, vasopressin, somatostatin, glucocorticoids, and several other hormones (for reviews see 3,5).

A recent review of the peripheral and central mechanisms by which stress influences all three levels of the hypothalamic–pituitary–gonadal (HPG) axis has appeared elsewhere (119). For brevity, the authors of that review use the word "stress" "without differentiation" to mean "any stimulus that disturbs the homeostasis of the organism," but they acknowledge that "the effects of stress on reproductive functions and the mechanisms mediating these effects depend on the type, duration, and frequency of the stimulus (45), as well as on the influence of the steroid milieu on adrenergic and opiate components that have an impact on the HPG axis" (119). For example, exercise is known to elevate ACTH much more than a maximal dose of CRH (133). Footshock and immobilization are the means by which the effect of stress on the HPG axis has been most commonly studied.

In castrated male rats, the suppression of LH pulsatility by inescapable intermittent footshock (118) is blocked by the central administration of CRH and opioid antagonists (112,118). The suppression of LH pulsatility by central administration of exogenous CRH (2,106,111,120) is also blocked by central administration of a β-endorphin antagonist (2,112). Thus, the disruption of LH pulsatility by footshock is clearly mediated by a CRH–ß-endorphin pathway. More specifically, CRH has been shown to suppress LH pulsatility by inhibiting the release of GnRH by the hypothalamic pulse generator (63), which is reflected in a reduced frequency of pulse generator neuronal activity that can be blocked by opioid antagonism (150).

The opioid modulation of GnRH release can be either inhibited or facilitated by catecholamine pathways (117). Evidence indicates, however, that the function of opioids is to provide fine control of the GnRH pulse generator's sensitivity to feedback by elevated estrogens and progesterone, and that opioids play little role in the suppression of LH either in prepuberty (except in rodents) or during the nonbreeding season in seasonally breeding species when other powerful inhibitory pathways involving dopamine are predominant (for a review see 69). A variety of other peptides and transmitters have also been shown to modulate GnRH release (64,104).

Chronic peripheral administration of ACTH also suppresses LH pulsatility in rats, sheep, and bulls (78,98,121). Exogenous ACTH reduces GnRH-induced LH release in heifers (97) and rams (62) and inhibits the preovulatory LH surge in cows (134), gilts (12), and female rhesus monkeys (101). In female mice the ACTH-induced delay of puberty is blocked by opioid antagonism (152). In rats ACTH suppression of LH pulsatility occurs only when the adrenals are intact (93,121), but in rhesus monkeys, CRH inhibits LH release via a central mechanism without involvement of the adrenal glands (151).

Corticosteroids antagonize estrogen-dependent changes in pituitary sensitivity to GnRH in rats (7) and they inhibit the LH surge in cows (134), ovulation in gilts (12), and the estradiol-stimulated growth of uterine tissue in rats (116). Corticosteroids appear to have little effect on the ovary in rats, for ovulation continues to be induced by small doses of LH in rats that have received large doses of a corticosteroid agonist (8). However, chronic cortisol administration blocks the normal follicular rise in estrogens, the gonadotropin surge, and the luteal rise in progesterone by direct action at the ovary in rhesus monkeys (68).

ACTH and corticosterone do not affect LH pulsatility in ovariectomized rats, and neither do surgery and leg fracture, yet immobilization does (21). A recent review based primarily on studies of female rats concludes that corticosteroids may either stimulate or inhibit reproduction depending on the length of exposure and the background of estrogen priming (30). With estrogen priming, acute exposure to stress, ACTH, or corticosteroids facilitates gonadotropin secretion and ovulation, whereas chronic exposure without estrogen priming is inhibitory. In male rats the analogous sensitivity of the gonadal axis to suppression by corticosteroid agonist depends on the presence of testosterone (31).

In regularly menstruating women, sustained infusion of CRH into the peripheral circulation during the luteal phase, when sex steroids are elevated, raises cortisol levels and suppresses LH levels (13). The LH effect is selectively reversible by subsequent administration and preventable by prior administration of an opioid antagonist (13).

These studies tend to support the hypothesis that the ovarian axis in physically active women may be inhibited by chronic activation of the adrenal axis. To our knowledge, however, only one study has independently controlled corticosteroid levels during an exercise-training protocol, and that study found the induced disruption of estrous cycles in adrenalectomized female rats to be unaffected by the presence or absence of corticosteroids (44).

Energy Availability, Mediated by a Metabolic Signal

Many observations in field biology indicate that reproductive function in mammals is dependent on energy availability (33). As a result, reproductive function is characteristic of populations in particular environments rather than of species, with different populations of the same species demonstrating seasonal or continuous breeding depending on local environmental conditions. Such observations include studies of several human populations, including desert dwellers (143) and eskimos (58), among whom conception is limited to times of high nutrition. Of special interest in the present context is that the mammalian dependence of reproductive function on energy availability is mediated primarily through the distinctive energy requirements of females. Indeed, ecologists often view the two sexes almost as if they were entirely different species because the nature of the energetic costs of their reproductive efforts varies so greatly (141).

A recent sequence of experiments has focused on how energy availability determines reproductive function in female hamsters. The investigators have induced anestrus in several ways besides food restriction, including administration of pharmacological inhibitors of carbohydrate and fat metabolism (123,124), insulin administration (145), and cold exposure (125). These experiments demonstrate unambiguously that, at least in hamsters, it is the availability of oxidizable metabolic fuels at the level of cellular metabolism—rather than at the level of the blood or the diet—that governs reproductive function. Thus, the metabolic signals linking energy availability to reproductive function may operate at the level of cellular physiology. Notably, the effect is independent of body size and composition (124), and catabolic energy demands at the organismal level such as thermogenesis (125) interfere with energy availability at the cellular level. Clearly, the extrapolation from the energy cost of thermogenesis to the energy cost of physical activity is a short one.

Dietary restriction suppresses LH levels or reduces LH pulse frequency in male and female rats (34,75,76,83), heifers (85), lambs and ewes (61,138), men (40), and women (60). This effect is dependent on the presence of estrogen in female rats (38) and is not accompanied by a rise in cortisol levels in men (40). It is rapidly reversed by refeeding (34), in proportion to the size of the refeed meal in male monkeys (107). Furthermore, starvation-induced reductions in LH, follicle-stimulating hormone (FSH), and testosterone levels and in pituitary LH and FSH messenger ribonucleic acid (mRNA) in male rats are fully reversed by periodic GnRH administration (17).

The effect of energy availability on the reproductive system is a highly active and rapidly advancing area of research. Recent presentations have reported that

- food restriction disrupts the GnRH neuronal system (18),
- prolonged exercise training enhances hypothalamic content of GnRH but suppresses its release (95),
- the retardation of reproductive development due to prolonged exercise is reversed by pulsatile GnRH administration despite a continued lack of body growth (95),
- opioid inhibitors do not reverse hypoglycemia-induced reduction in LH levels (70),
- retardation of the reproductive development due to a growth-restrictive diet is mediated by dopamine (77),
- the effect of food restriction on LH pulsatility results from a metabolic signal rather than psychological stress (126),
- the preovulatory LH surge is attenuated by pharmacological inhibitors of carbohydrate and fat oxidation (52),
- exogenous estrogen priming selectively restores the LH surge without restoring ovulation during retarded follicular development (102,125),
- lack of energy availability disrupts LH pulsatility very rapidly (before an animal is ketotic and while it is still euglycemic) (71),

- the LH disruption occurs at the time when insulin levels fall during a transition from an energy-storing to an energy-mobilizing state (127), and
- amenorrhea induced in monkeys by exercise training can be reversed by increased feeding without a reduction in the exercise regimen (39).

Evidence is conflicting concerning whether food restriction activates the adrenal axis and increases cortisol levels (14,40,60,79), and whether or not opioids mediate the influence of energy availability on reproductive function (38,46,70).

Regardless of the frequent confounding influences of physical activity and dietary intake on the rate of pubertal development, it is clear that reproductive development continues in males under conditions in which it is completely blocked in females (1,66,67,148). The controlling influence of energy availability, rather than body weight or composition, is evident from the initiation of LH pulsatility within a few hours and ovulation within 3 or 4 days after the start of ad libitum feeding in severely growth-restricted female rats, long before significant changes in body size and composition could occur (32).

If the energy expended in physical activity reduces the energy available for reproductive function, then experimental protocols involving prolonged exercise (like those restricting energy and especially carbohydrate intake) should suppress T_3 levels and resting metabolic rate (RMR), which accounts for most energy utilization. For reference, a relatively recent review of animal research on *low-T_3 syndrome,* otherwise known as *euthyroid sick syndrome* or *nonthyroidal disease,* is available elsewhere (139). The literature on the effect of exercise and exercise training on thyroid metabolism has not been reviewed for some time (137). A detailed review on that topic is beyond the scope of this document, so only a few general remarks will be made.

Potentially confounding influences in studies of exercise-training effects on thyroid function include the distinctive energy requirements of males and females, obesity and anorexia as they may have already affected thyroid status, age, and diet. Studies have found T_3 levels to remain unchanged (11,24,27,43) or to decline (28,80,84,114) as a result of exercise training. None of these studies was performed in nonobese young adult women under controlled dietary conditions. One (80) is particularly noteworthy in that T_3 levels rose in exercising mice fed ad libitum but declined in exercising mice pair-fed with sedentary controls eating ad libitum, and declined in exercising mice pair-fed with sedentary controls on a restrictive diet.

One study found RMR to increase during an exercise-training program (113), but dietary intake also increased during that study. Most studies have reported exercise training to have no effect on RMR (9,10,20,72,114,140). None of these studies has been performed in nonobese young adult women under controlled dietary conditions, either.

Implications for Women's Physical Activity, Fitness, and Health

By the diagnostic criteria for causation (50) it must be admitted that no true randomized, prospective, cohort experiments have demonstrated unequivocally that physical activity induces reproductive morbidities in women. Nevertheless, data from unrandomized, prospective experiments strongly indicate that abruptly imposed, prolonged, and intense physical activity can induce reproductive morbidities in at least some women, and the data from females of other mammalian species are consistent with this conclusion. There does appear to be a dose–response gradient in the effect, because more gradually imposed, brief, and less strenuous physical activity has been ineffective at inducing anestrus and amenorrhea. The association of physical activity with reproductive morbidities seems to make epidemiological sense, as the prevalence of amenorrhea is highest in those practicing the most rigorous regimens.

The association does not yet make biological sense, however, in that the specific neuroendocrine mechanism of the morbidities has not been demonstrated. Whether or not the reproductive morbidities seen in physically active women are analogous to those seen under conditions of electroshock and starvation is unclear. They may be caused by the "stress of exercise" or by failure to compensate the diet for the energy expended during exercise, by both, or by neither. To date, these two influences have been confounded in almost all studies of the effects of the "activity-stress paradigm" on reproductive function.

Certain kinds of stresses definitely do activate the adrenal axis and disrupt the reproductive system in vivo, and physical activity definitely activates the adrenal axis under certain circumstances, but a causal link between physical activity, adrenal activation, and the reproductive morbidities observed in women has not been demonstrated. If this linkage is established, it will be important to determine whether women can perform physical activity in such a way that reproductive morbidities can be avoided without sacrificing the benefits of physical activity on the traditional components of physiological fitness.

Strong evidence also indicates that reproductive function in humans as well as in other mammals depends on energy availability and that the reproductive system in females is more susceptible to energy deficiency than that in males. Thus, failure to compensate the diet for energy expended in physical activity may trigger as yet unidentified metabolic signals to suppress reproductive function. Nevertheless, the ability to prevent reproductive morbidities in physically active women by supplementing their diets has yet to be demonstrated, and whether or not women in specific sports can achieve aesthetic and competitive goals while consuming diets that prevent reproductive morbidities is unknown.

In light of the reproductive morbidities in physically active women, the proposed model and key concepts proposed by Bouchard and Shephard (25) concerning the relationships between levels of habitual physical activity, physical and physiological fitness, and health (25) appear to be deficient in three respects. First, the model does not include a reproductive component of health-related fitness, especially as it pertains to the reproductive ability and skeletal integrity of women (25). Consequently, the concept of health-related fitness fails to recognize that an important component of fitness related to health status can be *un*favorably influenced by habitual physical activity (25). In addition, the concept of physical activity does not include the substantial reduction in resting metabolic rate that may occur when a high level of physical activity is performed without a compensatory increase in caloric intake (25). These deficiencies seriously and especially impair understanding of the relationships between levels of habitual physical activity, physical and physiological fitness, and health in women.

References

1. Aguilar, E.; Pinella, L.; Guisado, R.; Gonzalez, D.; Lopez, F. Relation between body weight, growth rate, chronological age, and puberty in male and female rats. Rev. Esp. Fisiol. 40:82-86; 1984.
2. Almeida, O.F.X.; Nikolarakis, K.E.; Herz, A. Evidence for the involvement of endogenous opioids in the inhibition of luteinizing hormone by corticotropin-releasing factor. Endocrinology. 122:1034-1041; 1988.
3. Antoni, F.A. Hypothalamic control of adrenocorticotropin secretion: Advances since the discovery of 41-residue corticotropin-releasing factor. Endocr. Rev. 7:351-378; 1986.
4. Asahina, K.; Kitahara, F.; Yamanaka, M.; Akiba, T. Influences of excessive exercise on the structure and function of rat organs. Jpn. J. Physiol. 9:322-326; 1959.
5. Axelrod, J.; Reisine, T.D. Stress hormones: Their interaction and regulation. Science. 224:452-459; 1984.
6. Axelson, J.F. Forced swimming alters vaginal estrous cycles, body composition, and steroid levels without disrupting lordosis behavior or fertility in rats. Physiol. Behav. 41:471-479; 1987.
7. Baldwin, D.M. The effect of glucocorticoids on estrogen-dependent luteinizing hormone release in the ovariectomized rat and on gonadotropin secretion in the intact female rat. Endocrinology. 105:120-128; 1979.
8. Baldwin, D.M.; Sawyer, C.H. Effects of dexamethasone on LH release and ovulation in the cyclic rat. Endocrinology. 94:1397-1403; 1974.
9. Ballor, D.L. Exercise training elevates RMR during moderate but not severe dietary restriction in obese male rats. J. Appl. Physiol. 70(5):2303-2310; 1991.
10. Ballor, D.L. Effect of dietary restriction and/or exercise on 23-h metabolic rate and body composition in female rats. J. Appl. Physiol. 71(3):801-806; 1991.
11. Balsam, A.; Leppo, L.E. Effect of physical training on the metabolism of thyroid hormones in man. J. Appl. Physiol. 38(2):212-215; 1975.
12. Barb, C.R.; Kraeling, R.R.; Rampacek, G.B.; Fonda, E.S.; Kiser, T.E. Inhibition of ovulation and LH secretion in the gilt after treatment with ACTH or hydrocortisone. J. Reprod. Fertil. 64:85-92; 1982.
13. Barbarino, A.; De Marinis, L.; Tofani, A.; Della Casa, S.; D'Amico, C.; Mancini, A.; Corsello, S.M.; Sciuto, R.; Barini, A. Corticotropin-releasing hormone inhibition of gonadotropin release and the effect of opioid blockade. J. Clin. Endocrinol. Metab. 68:523-528; 1989.
14. Beer, S.F.; Bircham, P.M.M.; Bloom, S.R.; Clark, P.M.; Hales, C.N.; Hughes, C.M.; Jones, C.T.; Marsh, D.R.; Raggatt, P.R.; Findlay, A.L.R. The effect of a 72-h fast on plasma levels of pituitary, adrenal, thyroid, pancreatic and gastrointenstinal hormones in healthy men and women. J. Endocrinol. 120:337-350; 1989.
15. Beitins, I.Z.; McArthur, J.W.; Turnbull, B.A.; Skrinar, G.S.; Bullen, B.A. Exercise induces two types of human luteal dysfunction: Confirmation by urinary free progesterone. J. Clin. Endocrinol. Metab. 72:1350-1358; 1991.

16. Berga, S.L.; Mortola, J.F.; Girton, L.; Suh, B.; Laughlin, G.; Pham, P.; Yen, S.S.C. Neuroendocrine aberrations in women with functional hypothalamic amenorrhea. J. Clin. Endocrinol. Metab. 68:301-308; 1989.
17. Bergendahl, M.; Perheentupa, A.; Huhtaniemi, I. Starvation-induced suppression of pituitary-testicular function in rats is reversed by pulsatile gonadotropin-releasing hormone substitution. Biol. Reprod. 44:413-419; 1991.
18. Berriman, S.J.; Wade, G.N. Food deprivation decreases *c-fos* expression in gonadotropin-releasing hormone (GnRH) neurons in syrian hamsters. Soc. Neurosci. Abstr. [Abstract]. 17:544.5; 1991.
19. Biller, B.M.K.; Federoff, H.J.; Koenig, J.I.; Klibanski, A. Abnormal cortisol secretion and responses to corticotropin-releasing hormone in women with hypothalamic amenorrhea. J. Clin. Endocrinol. Metab. 70:311-317; 1990.
20. Bingham, S.A.; Goldberg, G.R.; Coward, W.A.; Prentice, A.M.; Cummings, J.H. The effect of exercise and improved physical fitness on basal metabolic rate. Br. J. Nutr. 61:155-173; 1989.
21. Blake, C.A. Effects of "stress" on pulsatile luteinizing hormone release in ovariectomized rats. Proc. Soc. Exp. Biol. Med. 148:813-815; 1975.
22. Boesgaard, S.; Hagen, C.; Andersen, A.N.; Djursing, H.; Fenger, M. Cortisol secretion in patients with normoprolactinemic amenorrhea. Acta Endocrinol. (Copenh.). 118:544-550; 1988.
23. Bonen, A. Recreational exercise does not impair menstrual cycles: A prospective study. Int. J. Sports Med. 13:110-120; 1992.
24. Bosello, O.; Ferrari, F.; Tonon, M.; Cigolini, M.; Micciolo, R.; Renoffio, M. Serum thyroid hormone concentration during semi-starvation and physical exercise. Horm. Metab. Res. 13:651-652; 1981.
25. Bouchard, C.; Shephard, R.J. Physical activity, fitness and health: A model and key concepts. (Consensus DOC-017). The 1992 international consensus symposium on physical activity, fitness & health; 1992 May 5-9; Toronto, Canada.
26. Boyar, R.M.; Hellman, L.D.; Roffwarg, H.; Katz, J.; Zumoff, B.; O'Connor, J.; Bradlow, H.L.; Fukushima, D.K. Cortisol secretion and metabolism in anorexia nervosa. N. Engl. J. Med. 296:190-193; 1977.
27. Boyden, T.W.; Pamenter, R.W.; Rotkis, T.C.; Stanforth, P.; Wilmore, J.H. Thyroidal changes associated with endurance training in women. Med. Sci. Sports Exerc. 16:243-246; 1984.
28. Boyden, T.W.; Pamenter, R.W.; Stanforth, R.P.; Rotkis, T.C.; Wilmore, J.H. Evidence for mild thyroidal impairment in women undergoing endurance training. J. Clin. Endocrinol. Metab. 53:53-56; 1982.
29. Boyden, T.W.; Pamenter, R.W.; Stanforth, P.; Rotkis, T.; Wilmore, J.H. Impaired gonadotropin responses to gonadotropin-releasing hormone stimulation in endurance-trained women. Fertil. Steril. 41:359-363; 1984.
30. Brann, D.W.; Mahesh, V.B. Role of corticosteroids in female reproduction FASEB J. 5:2691-2698; 1991.
31. Briski, K.P.; Sylvester, P.W. Acute inhibition of pituitary LH release in the male rat by the glucocorticoid agonist decadron phosphate. Neuroendocrinology. 54:313-320; 1991.
32. Bronson, F.H. Food-restricted, prepubertal female rats: Rapid recovery of luteinizing hormone pulsing with excess food, and full recovery of pubertal development with gonadotropin-releasing hormone. Endocrinology. 118:2483-2487; 1986.
33. Bronson, F.H. Seasonal regulation of reproduction in mammals. In: Knobil, E.; Neill, J.D., eds. The physiology of reproduction, volume 2. New York: Raven Press; 1988:1831-1871.
34. Bronson, F.H.; Heideman, P.D. Short-term hormonal responses to food intake in peripubertal female rats. Am. J. Physiol. (Regulatory Integrative Comp. Physiol. 28) 259:R25-R31; 1990.
35. Bronson, F.H.; Manning, J.M. The energetic regulation of ovulation: A realistic role for body fat. Biol. Reprod. 44:945-950; 1991.
36. Bullen, B.A.; Skrinar, G.S.; Beitins, I.Z.; Carr, D.B.; Reppert, S.M.; Dotson, C.O.; Fencl, M. de M.; Gervino, E.V.; McArthur, J.W. Endurance training effects on plasma hormonal responsiveness and sex hormone excretion. J. Appl. Physiol.: Respir. Environ. Exerc. Physiol. 56: 1453-1463; 1984.
37. Bullen, B.A.; Skrinar, G.S.; Beitins, I.Z.; von Mering, G.; Turnbull, B.A.; McArthur, J.W. Induction of menstrual disorders by strenuous exercise in untrained women. N. Engl. J. Med. 312:1349-1353; 1985.
38. Cagampang, F.R.A.; Maeda, K.-I.; Tsukamura, H.; Ohkura, S.; Ôta, K. Involvement of ovarian steroids and endogenous opioids in the fasting-induced suppression of pulsatile LH release in ovariectomized rats. J. Endocrinol. 129:321-328; 1991.
39. Cameron, J.L.; Nosbisch, C.; Helmreich, D.L.; Parfitt, D.B. Reversal of exercise-induced amenorrhea in female cynomolgus monkeys (Macaca fascicularis) by increasing food in-

take. Proceedings of the Endocrine society 72nd annual meeting; Abstract 1042. 285:1990.
40. Cameron, J.L.; Weltzin, T.E.; McConaha, C.; Helmreich, D.L.; Kaye, W.H. Slowing of pulsatile luteinizing hormone secretion in men after forty-eight hours of fasting. J. Clin. Endocrinol. Metab. 73:35-41; 1991.
41. Cann, C.E.; Martin, M.C.; Genant, H.K.; Jaffe, R.B. Decreased spinal mineral content in amenorrheic women. JAMA. 251:626-629; 1984.
42. Carlberg, K.A.; Fregly, M.J. Disruption of estrous cycles in exercise-trained rats. Proc. Soc. Exp. Biol. Med. 179:21-24; 1985.
43. Caron, P.J.; Sopko, G.; Stolk, J.M.; Jacobs, D.R.; Nisula, B.C. Effect of physical conditioning on measures of thyroid hormone action. Horm. Metab. Res. 18:206-208; 1986.
44. Chatterton, R.T., Jr.; Hartman, A.L.; Lynn, D.E.; Hickson, R.C. Exercise-induced ovarian dysfunction in the rat. Proc. Soc. Exp. Biol. Med. 193:220-224; 1990.
45. Collu, R.; Gibb, W.; Ducharme, J.R. Effects of stress on the gonadal function. J. Endocrinol. Invest. 7:529-537; 1984.
46. Cosgrove, J.R.; Booth, P.J.; Foxcroft, G.R. Opioidergic control of gonadotrophin secretion in the prepubertal gilt during restricted feeding and realimentation. J. Reprod. Fertil. 91:277-284; 1991.
47. Cowan, L.D.; Gordis, L.; Tonascia, J.A.; Jones, G.S. Breast cancer incidence in women with a history of progesterone deficiency. Am. J. Epidemiol. 114:209-217; 1981.
48. Cumming, D.C.; Vickovic, M.M.; Wall, S.R.; Fluker, M.R. Defects in pulsatile LH release in normally menstruating runners. J. Clin. Endocrinol. Metab. 60:810-812; 1985.
49. Cumming, D.C.; Vickovic, M.M.; Wall, S.R.; Fluker, M.R.; Belcastro, A.N. The effect of acute exercise on pulsatile release of luteinizing hormone in women runners. Am. J. Obstet. Gynecol. 153:482-485; 1985.
50. Department of Clinical Epidemiology and Biostatistics, McMaster University Health Sciences Center. How to read clinical journals: IV. To determine etiology or causation. Can. Med. Assoc. J. 124:985-990; 1981.
51. De Souza, M.J.; Maguire, M.S.; Maresh, C.M.; Kraemer, W.J.; Rubin, K.R.; Loucks, A.B. Adrenal activation and the prolactin response to exercise in eumenorrheic and amenorrheic runners. J. Appl. Physiol. 70:2378-2387; 1991.
52. Dickerman, R.W.; Schneider, J.E.; Wade, G.N. Decreased availability of metabolic fuels or food deprivation attenuates the preovulatory LH surge in syrian hamsters. Soc. Neurosci. Abstr. 16:Abstract 168.19; 1990.
53. Ding, J-H.; Sheckter, C.B.; Drinkwater, B.L.; Soules, M.R.; Bremner, W.J. High serum cortisol levels in exercise-associated amenorrhea. Ann. Intern. Med. 108:530-534; 1988.
54. Drinkwater, B.L.; Bruemner, B.; Chesnut, C.H., III. Menstrual history as a determinant of current bone density in young athletes. JAMA. 263:545-548; 1990.
55. Drinkwater, B.L.; Nilson, K.; Chesnut, C.H., III; Bremner, W.J.; Shainholtz, S.; Southworth, M.B. Bone mineral content of amenorrheic and eumenorrheic athletes. N. Engl. J. Med. 311:277-281; 1984.
56. Drinkwater, B.L.; Nilson, K.; Ott, S.; Chesnut, C.H., III. Bone mineral density after resumption of menses in amenorrheic athletes. JAMA. 256:380-382; 1986.
57. Dugowson, C.E.; Drinkwater, B.L.; Clark, J.M. Nontraumatic femur fracture in an oligomenorrheic athlete. Med. Sci. Sports Exerc. 23: 1323-1325; 1991.
58. Ehrenkranz, J.R.L. Seasonal breeding in humans: Birth records of the labrador eskimo. Fertil. Steril. 40:485-489; 1983.
59. Evans, W.S.; Sollenberger, M.J.; Booth, R.A., Jr.; Rogol, A.D.; Urban, R.J.; Carlsen, E.C.; Johnson, M.L.; Veldhuis, J.D. Contemporary aspects of discrete peak-detection algorithms. II. The paradigm of the luteinizing hormone pulse signal in women. Endocr. Rev. 13:81-104; 1992.
60. Fichter, M.M.; Pirke, K.M. Hypothalamic pituitary function in starving healthy subjects. In: Pirke, K.M.; Ploog, D., eds. The psychobiology of anorexia nervosa. Berlin: Springer-Verlag; 1984:124-135.
61. Foster, D.L.; Olster, D.H. Effect of restricted nutrition on puberty in the lamb: Patterns of tonic luteinizing hormone (LH) secretion and competency of the LH surge system. Endocrinology. 116:375-381; 1985.
62. Fuquay, J.W.; Moberg, G.P. Influence of the pituitary-adrenal axis on the induced release of luteinizing hormone in rams. J. Endocrinol. 99:151-155; 1983.
63. Gambacciani, M.; Yen, S.S.C.; Rasmussen, D.D. GnRH release from the mediobasal hypothalamus: *In vitro* inhibition by corticotropin-releasing factor. Neuroendocrinology. 43:533-536; 1986.
64. Gambacciani, M.; Yen, S.S.C.; Rasmussen, D.D. GnRH release from the mediobasal hypothalamus: *In vitro* by oxytocin regulation. Neuroendocrinology. 42:181-183; 1986.

65. Gold, P.W.; Gwirtsman, H.; Avgerinos, P.C.; Nieman, L.K.; Gallucci, W.T.; Kaye, W.; Jimerson, D.; Ebert, M.; Rittmaster, R.; Loriaux, D.L.; Chrousos, G.P. Abnormal hypothalamic-pituitary-adrenal function in anorexia nervosa. N. Engl. J. Med. 314:1335-1342; 1986.
66. Hamilton, G.D.; Bronson, F.H. Food restriction and reproductive development in wild house mice. Biol. Reprod. 32:773-778; 1985.
67. Hamilton, G.D.; Bronson, F.H. Food restriction and reproductive development: Male and female mice and male rats. Am. J. Physiol. (Regulatory Integrative Comp. Physiol. 19) 250:R370-R376; 1986.
68. Hayashi, K.T.; Moberg, G.P. Influence of the hypothalamic-pituitary-adrenal axis on the menstrual cycle and the pituitary responsiveness to estradiol in the female rhesus monkey (Macaca mulatta). Biol. Reprod. 42:260-265; 1990.
69. Haynes, N.B.; Lamming, G.E.; Yang, K-P.; Brooks, A.N.; Finnie, A.D. Endogenous opioid peptides and farm animal reproduction. Oxf. Rev. Reprod. Biol. 11:111-145; 1989.
70. Heisler, L.E.; Reid, R.L.; Van Vugt, D.A. Naloxone infusion does not reverse the hypoglycemia-induced reduction in luteinizing hormone levels observed in chair restrained ovariectomized rhesus monkeys. Soc. Neurosci. Abstr. 17:Abstract 544.6; 1991.
71. Helmreich, D.L.; Parfitt, D.B.; Cameron, J.L. Definition of metabolic states associated with the suppression and restoration of LH secretion caused by fasting and refeeding in rhesus monkeys. Soc. Neurosci. Abstr. 17:Abstract 544.7; 1991.
72. Henson, L.C.; Poole, D.C.; Donahoe, C.P.; Heber, D. Effects of exercise training on resting energy expenditure during caloric restriction. Am. J. Clin. Nutr. 46:893-899; 1987.
73. Hohtari, H.; Elovainio, R.; Salminen, K.; Laatikainen, T. Plasma corticotropin-releasing hormone, corticotropin, and endorphins at rest and during exercise in eumenorrheic and amenorrheic athletes. Fertil. Steril. 50:233-238; 1988.
74. Hohtari, H.; Salminen-Lappalainen, K.; Laatikainen, T. Response of plasma endorphins, corticotropin, cortisol, and luteinizing hormone in the corticotropin-releasing hormone stimulation test in eumenorrheic and amenorrheic athletes. Fertil. Steril. 55:276-280; 1991.
75. Howland, B.E. Gonadotropin levels in female rats subjected to restricted feed intake. J. Reprod. Fertil. 27:467-470; 1971.
76. Howland, B.E. The influence of food restriction and subsequent refeeding on gonadotropin secretion and serum testosterone levels in the male rat. J. Reprod. Fertil. 44:429-436; 1975.
77. I'Anson, H.; Manning, J.M.; Foster, D.L. Dopaminergic inhibition of LH (GnRH) release in the growth restricted hypogonadotropic lamb. Soc. Neurosci. Abstr. 17:Abstract 544.3; 1991.
78. Johnson, B.H.; Welsh, T.H., Jr.; Juniewicz, P.E. Suppression of luteinizing hormone and testosterone secretion in bulls following adrenocorticotropin hormone treatment. Biol. Reprod. 26:305-310; 1982.
79. Kant, G.J.; Anderson, S.M.; Dhillon, G.S.; Mougey, E.H. Neuroendocrine correlates of sustained stress: The activity-stress paradigm. Brain Res. Bull. 20:407-414; 1988.
80. Katzeff, H.L.; Bovbjerg, D.; Mark, D.A. Exercise regulation of triiodothyronine metabolism. Am. J. Physiol. (Endocrinol. Metab. 18) 255:E824-E828; 1988.
81. Kaye, W.H.; Gwirtsman, H.E.; George, D.T.; Ebert, M.H.; Jimerson, D.C.; Tomai, T.P.; Chrousos, G.P.; Gold, P.W. Elevated cerebrospinal fluid levels of immunoreactive corticotropin-releasing hormone in anorexia nervosa: Relation to state of nutrition, adrenal function, and intensity of depression. J. Clin. Endocrinol. Metab. 64:203-208; 1987.
82. Keizer, H.A.; Bonen, A. Exercise-induced changes in gonadotropin secretion patterns. Int. J. Sports Med. 5:206-208; 1984.
83. Kotsuji, F.; Takeshi, A.; Kamitani, N.; Tominaga, T. The synthesis and release of gonadotropins in response to gonadotropin-releasing hormone of the rat anterior pituitary gland during weight reduction. Acta Endocrinol. (Copenh.). 122:628-632; 1990.
84. Krotkiewski, M.; Sjöström, L.; Sullivan, L.; Lundberg, P.-A.; Lindstedt, G.; Wetterqvist, H.; Björntorp, P. The effect of acute and chronic exercise on thyroid hormones in obesity. Acta Med. Scand. 216:269-275; 1984.
85. Kurz, S.G.; Dyer, R.M.; Hu, Y.; Wright, M.D.; Day, M.L. Regulation of luteinizing hormone secretion in prepubertal heifers fed an energy-deficient diet. Biol. Reprod. 43:450-456; 1990.
86. Lamon-Fava, S.; Fisher, E.C.; Nelson, M.E.; Evans, W.J.; Millar, J.S.; Ordovas, J.M.; Schaefer, E.J. Effect of exercise and menstrual cycle status on plasma lipids, low density lipoprotein particle size, and apolipoproteins. J. Clin. Endocrinol. Metab. 68:17-21; 1989.
87. Lindberg, J.S.; Powell, M.R.; Hunt, M.M.; Ducey, D.E.; Wade, C.E. Increased vertebral bone mineral in response to reduced exercise in amenorrheic runners. West. J. Med. 146:39-42; 1987.

88. Linnell, S.L.; Stager, J.M.; Blue, P.W.; Oyster, N.; Robertshaw, D. Bone mineral content and menstrual regularity in female runners. Med. Sci. Sports Exerc. 16:343-348; 1984.
89. Loucks, A.B.; Horvath, S.M. Exercise-induced stress responses of amenorrheic and eumenorrheic runners. J. Clin. Endocrinol. Metab. 59:1109-1120; 1984.
90. Loucks, A.B.; Horvath, S.M. Athletic amenorrhea: A review. Med. Sci. Sports Exerc. 17:56-72; 1985.
91. Loucks, A.B.; Laughlin, G.A.; Mortola, J.F.; Girton, L.; Nelson, J.C.; Yen, S.S.C. Hypothalamic-pituitary-thyroidal function in eumenorrheic and amenorrheic athletes. J. Clin. Endocrinol. Metab. 75:514-518; 1992.
92. Loucks, A.B.; Mortola, J.F.; Girton, L.; Yen, S.S.C. Alterations in the hypothalamic-pituitary-ovarian and hypothalamic-pituitary-adrenal axes in athletic women. J. Clin. Endocrinol. Metab. 68:402-411; 1989.
93. Mann, D.R.; Jackson, G.G.; Blank, M.S. Influence of adrenocorticotropin and adrenalectomy on gonadotropin secretion in immature rats. Neuroendocrinology. 34:20-26; 1982.
94. Manning, J.M.; Bronson, F.H. Effects of prolonged exercise on puberty and luteinizing hormone secretion in female rats. Am. J. Physiol. (Regulatory Integrative Comp. Physiol. 26) 257:R1359-R1364; 1989.
95. Manning, J.M.; Bronson, F.H. Suppression of puberty by prolonged exercise in female rats: Effects on hormone levels, and recovery on reproductive function with gonadotropin-releasing hormone. Soc. Neurosci. Abstr. 16:Abstract 168.20; 1990.
96. Marcus, R.; Cann, C.; Madvig, P.; Minkoff, J.; Goddard, M.; Bayer, M.; Martin, M.; Guadiani, L.; Haskell, W.; Genant, H. Menstrual function and bone mass in elite women distance runner. Ann. Intern. Med. 102:158-163; 1985.
97. Matteri, R.L.; Moberg, G.P. Effect of cortisol or adrenocorticotrophin on release of luteinizing hormone induced by luteinizing hormone releasing hormone in the dairy heifer. J. Endocrinol. 92:141-146; 1982.
98. Matteri, R.L.; Moberg, G.P.; Watson, J.G. Adrenocorticotropin-induced changes in ovine pituitary gonadotropin secretion *in vitro*. Endocrinology. 118:2091-2096; 1986.
99. Mauvais-Jarvis, P.; Sitruk-Ware, R.; Kuttenn, F. Luteal phase defect and breast cancer genesis. Breast Cancer Res. Treat. 2:139-150; 1982.
100. McArthur, J.W.; Gilbert, I.; Henery, R.J.; Quinn, J.; Perry, L.; Cramer, D.; Kirkland, M.; Pedoe, D.S.T.; Rees, L.H.; Besser, G.M.; Turnbull, B.A. The effects of submaximal endurance exercise upon LH pulsatility. Clin. Endocrinol. 32:115-126; 1990.
101. Moberg, G.P.; Watson, J.G.; Hayashi, K.T. Effects of adrenocorticotropin treatment on estrogen, luteinizing hormone and progesterone secretion in the female rhesus monkey. J. Med. Primatol. 11:235-241; 1982.
102. Morin, L.P.; Donham, R.S.; Stetson, M.H. Luteinizing hormone during the estrous cycle of the food deprived hamster. Soc. Neurosci. Abstr. 17:Abstract 544.4; 1991.
103. Myerson, M.; Gutin, B.; Warren, M.P.; May, M.T.; Contento, I.; Lee, M.; Pi-Sunyer, F.X.; Pierson, R.N., Jr.; Brooks-Gunn, J. Resting metabolic rate and energy balance in amenorrheic and eumenorrheic runners. Med. Sci. Sports Exerc. 23:15-22; 1991.
104. Negro-Vilar, A. The median eminence as a model to study presynaptic regulation of neural peptide release. Peptides. 3:305-310; 1982.
105. Nelson, M.E.; Fisher, E.C.; Catsos, P.D.; Meredith, C.N.; Turksoy, R.N.; Evans, W.J. Diet and bone status in amenorrheic runners. Am. J. Clin. Nutr. 43:910-916; 1986.
106. Ono, N.; Lumpkin, M.D.; Samson, W.K.; McDonald, J.K.; McCann, S.M. Intrahypothalamic action of corticotrophin-releasing factor (CRF) to inhibit growth hormone and LH release in the rat. Life Sci. 35:1117-1123; 1984.
107. Parfitt, D.B.; Church, K.R.; Cameron, J.L. Restoration of pulsatile luteinizing hormone secretion after fasting in rhesus monkeys (Macaca mulatta): Dependence on size of the refeed meal. Endocrinology. 129:749-756; 1991.
108. Pellerin-Massicote, J.; Brisson, G.R.; St-Pierre, C.; Rioux, P.; Rajotte, D. Effect of exercise on the onset of puberty, gonadotropins, and ovarian inhibin. J. Appl. Physiol. 63:1165-1173; 1987.
109. Perrigo, G.; Bronson, F.H. Foraging effort, food intake, fat deposition and puberty in female mice. Biol. Reprod. 29:455-463; 1983.
110. Perrigo, G.; Bronson, F.H. Behavioral and physiological responses of female house mice to foraging variation. Physiol. Behav. 34:437-440; 1985.
111. Petraglia, F.; Sutton, S.; Vale, W.; Plotsky, P. Corticotropin-releasing factor decreases plasma luteinizing hormone levels in female rats by inhibiting gonadotropin-releasing hormone release into hypophysial-portal circulation. Endocrinology. 120:1083-1088; 1987.
112. Petraglia, F.; Vale, W.; Rivier, C. Opioids act centrally to modulate stress-induced decrease

in luteinizing hormone in the rat. Endocrinology. 119:2445-2450; 1986.
113. Poehlman, E.T.; Danforth, E., Jr. Endurance training increases metabolic rate and norepinephrine appearance rate in older individuals. Am. J. Physiol. (Endocrinol. Metab. 24) 261:E233-E239; 1991.
114. Poehlman, E.T.; Tremblay, A.; Nadeau, A.; Dussault, J.; Thériault, G.; Bouchard, C. Heredity and changes in hormones and metabolic rates with short-term training. Am. J. Physiol. (Endocrinol. Metab. 13) 250:E711-E717; 1986.
115. Pryor, S.; Bronson, F.H. Relative and combined effects of low temperature, poor diet, and short daylength on the productivity of wild housemice. Biol. Reprod. 25:734-743; 1981.
116. Rabin, D.S.; Johnson, E.O.; Brandon, D.D.; Liapi, C.; Chrousos, G.P. Glucocorticoids inhibit estradiol-mediated uterine growth: Possible role of the uterine estradiol receptor. Biol. Reprod. 42:74-80; 1990.
117. Rasmussen, D.D.; Kennedy, B.P.; Ziegler, M.G.; Nett, T.M. Endogenous opioid inhibition and facilitation of gonadotropin-releasing hormone release from the median eminence *in vitro*: Potential role of catecholamines. Endocrinology. 123:2916-2921; 1988.
118. Rivier, C.; Rivier, J.; Vale, W. Stress-induced inhibition of reproductive functions: Role of endogenous corticotropin-releasing factor. Science. 231:607-609; 1986.
119. Rivier, C.; Rivest, S. Effect of stress on the activity of the hypothalamic-pituitary-gonadal axis: Peripheral and central mechanisms. Biol. Reprod. 45:523-532; 1991.
120. Rivier, C.; Vale, W. Influence of corticotropin-releasing factor on reproductive functions in the rat. Endocrinology. 114:914-921; 1984.
121. Rivier, C.; Vale, W. Effect of the long-term administration of corticotropin-releasing factor on the pituitary-adrenal and pituitary-gonadal axis in the male rat. J. Clin. Invest. 75:689-694; 1985.
122. Rogol, A.D.; Weltman, A.; Weltman, J.Y.; Seip, R.L.; Snead, D.B.; Levine, S.; Haskvitz, E.M.; Thompson, D.L.; Schurrer, R.; Dowling, E.; Walberg-Rankin, J.; Evans, W.S.; Veldhuis, J.D. Durability of the reproductive axis in eumenorrheic women during 1 yr of endurance training. J. Appl. Physiol. 72:1571-1580; 1992.
123. Schneider, J.E.; Wade, G.N. Availability of metabolic fuels controls estrous cyclicity of Syrian hamsters. Science. 244:1326-1328; 1989.
124. Schneider, J.E.; Wade, G.N. Decreased availability of metabolic fuels induces anestrus in golden hamsters. Am. J. Physiol. (Regulatory Integrative Comp. Physiol. 27) 258:R750-R755; 1990.
125. Schneider, J.E.; Wade, G.N. Effects of diet and body fat content on cold-induced anestrus in Syrian hamsters. Am. J. Physiol. (Regulatory Integrative Comp. Physiol. 28) 259:R1198-R1204; 1990.
126. Schreihofer, D.A.; Parfitt, D.B.; Cameron, J.L. Evidence that the suppression of hypothalamic-pituitary-gonadal axis activity during fasting results from a nutritional signal and not the psychological stress of food deprivation. Soc. Neurosci. Abstr. 16:Abstract 168.17; 1990.
127. Schreihofer, D.A.; Parfitt, D.B.; Cameron, J.L. Effects of overfeeding on subsequent fasting-induced suppression of pulsatile LH secretion in male rhesus monkeys (*Macaca mulatta*). Soc. Neurosci. Abstr. 17:Abstract 544.8; 1991.
128. Scott, E.C.; Johnson, F.E. Critical fat, menarche, and the maintenance of menstrual cycles: A critical review. J. Adolesc. Health Care. 2:249-260; 1982.
129. Selye, H. The effect of adaptation to various damaging agents on the female sex organs in the rat. Endocrinology. 25:615-624; 1939.
130. Sherman, B.M.; Korenman, S.G. Inadequate corpus luteum function: A pathophysiological interpretation of human breast cancer epidemiology. Cancer. 33:1306-1312; 1974.
131. Sinning, W.E.; Little, K.D. Body composition and menstrual function in athletes. Sports Med. 4:34-45; 1987.
132. Slentz, C.A.; Davis, J.M.; Settles, D.L.; Russell, R.P.; Settles, S.J. Glucose feedings and exercise in rats: Glycogen use, hormone responses, and performance. J. Appl. Physiol. 69:989-994; 1990.
133. Smoak, B.; Deuster, P.; Rabin, D.; Chrousos, G. Corticotropin-releasing hormone is not the sole factor mediating exercise-induced adrenocorticotropin release in humans. J. Clin. Endocrinol. Metab. 73:302-306; 1991.
134. Stoebel, D.P.; Moberg, G.P. Effect of adrenocorticotropin and cortisol on luteinizing hormone surge and estrous behavior of cows. J. Dairy Sci. 65:1016-1024; 1982.
135. Suh, B.Y.; Liu, J.H.; Berga, S.L.; Quigley, M.E.; Laughlin, G.A.; Yen, S.S. Hypercortisolism in patients with functional hypothalamic-amenorrhea. J. Clin. Endocrinol. Metab. 66: 733-739; 1988.
136. Tabata, I.; Ogita, F.; Miyachi, M.; Shibayama, H. Effect of low blood glucose on plasma CRF, ACTH, and cortisol during prolonged physical exercise. J. Appl. Physiol. 71:1807-1812; 1991.

137. Terjung, R.L.; Winder, W.W. Exercise and thyroid function. Med. Sci. Sports. 7(1):20-26; 1975.
138. Thomas, G.B.; Mercer, J.E.; Karalis, T.; Rao, A.; Cummins, J.T.; Clarke, I.J. Effect of restricted feeding on the concentrations of growth hormone (GH), gonadotropins, and prolactin (PRL) in plasma, and on the amounts of messenger ribonucleic acid for GH, gonadotropin subunits, and PRL in the pituitary glands of adult ovariectomized ewes. Endocrinology. 126:1361-1367; 1990.
139. Tibaldi, J.M.; Surks, M.I. Animal models of nonthyroidal disease. Endocr. Rev. 6:87-102; 1985.
140. Tremblay, A.; Nadeau, A.; Després, J.P.; St-Jean, L.; Thériault, G.; Bouchard, C. Long-term exercise training with constant energy intake. 2: Effect on glucose metabolism and resting energy expenditure. Int. J. Obes. 14:75-84; 1990.
141. Trivers, R.L. Parental investment and sexual selection. In: Campbell, B., ed. Sexual selection and the descent of man. Chicago: Aldine Press; 1972:136-171.
142. Vale, W.; Speiss, J.; Rivier, C.; Rivier, J. Characterization of a 41-residue ovine hypothalamic peptide that stimulates secretion of corticotropin and β-endorphin. Science. 213:1394-1397; 1981.
143. Van der Walt, L.A.; Wilmsen, E.N.; Jenkins, T. Unusual sex hormone patterns among desert-dwelling hunter-gatherers. J. Clin. Endocrinol. Metab. 46:658-663; 1978.
144. Veldhuis, J.D.; Evans, W.S.; Demers, L.M.; Thorner, M.O.; Wakat, D.; Rogol, A.D. Altered neuroendocrine regulation of gonadotropin secretion in women distance runners. J. Clin. Endocrinol. Metab. 61:557-563; 1985.
145. Wade, G.N.; Schneider, J.E.; Friedman, M.I. Insulin-induced anestrus in Syrian hamsters. Am. J. Physiol. (Regulatory Integrative Comp. Physiol. 29) 260:R148-R152; 1991.
146. Warren, M.P. The effects of exercise on pubertal progression and reproductive function in girls. J. Clin. Endocrinol. Metab. 51:1150-1157; 1980.
147. Warren, M.P.; Brooks-Gunn, J.; Hamilton, L.H.; Warren, L.F.; Hamilton, W.G. Scoliosis and fractures in young ballet dancers: Relation to delayed menarche and secondary amenorrhea. N. Engl. J. Med. 314:1348-1353; 1986.
148. Widdowson, E.M.; Mavor, W.O.; McCance, R.A. The effect of undernutrition and rehabilitation on the development of the reproductive organs: Rats. J. Endocrinol. 29:119-126; 1964.
149. Widmaier, E.P.; Plotsky, P.M.; Sutton, S.W.; Vale, W.W. Regulation of corticotropin-releasing factor secretion in vitro by glucose. Am. J. Physiol. (Endocrinol. Metab. 18) 255:E287-E292; 1988.
150. Williams, C.L.; Nishihara, M.; Thalabard, J.C.; Grosser, P.M.; Hotchkiss, J.; Knobil, E. Corticotropin-releasing factor and gonadotropin-releasing hormone pulse generator activity in the rhesus monkey. Neuroendocrinology. 52:133-137; 1990.
151. Xiao, E.; Luckhaus, J.; Niemann, W.; Ferin, M. Acute inhibition of gonadotropin secretion by corticotropin-releasing hormone in the primate: Are the adrenal glands involved? Endocrinology. 124:1632-1637; 1989.
152. Yasukawa, N.; Monder, H.; Michael, S.D.; Christian, J.J. Opiate antagonist counteracts reproductive inhibition by porcine ACTH extract. Life Sci. 22:1381-1390; 1978.

Chapter 65

Physical Activity, Fitness, and Reproductive Health in Women: Clinical Observations

Naama W. Constantini
Michelle P. Warren

Physical activity has a profound effect on the age of menarche, menstrual cyclicity, and the normal function of the postovulatory luteal phase. These problems, which are reversible, appear to have multiple causes and originate in most of the cases from apparent hypothalamic dysfunction and suppression of the gonadotropin-releasing hormone (GnRH) pulse generator. Attempts at understanding the original pathogenesis have been confounded by the inability to control for many of the causal variables, the scarcity of longitudinal studies, and the difficulty of their design. Athletic menstrual dysfunction (MD) can be reproduced by extensive physical training, but full-fledged hypoestrogenic amenorrhea is not produced by strenuous exercise alone in a normal population.

The prolonged hypoestrogenism that occurs with several athletic activities may also have a major impact on the skeleton. Failure to reach peak bone mass, loss of bone, failure of weight-bearing bone to mineralize with stress, and increased fractures, particularly stress fractures, are evolving issues. Estrogen replacement may be indicated under certain circumstances.

Clinical Problems of the Reproductive System in the Female Athlete and Their Prevalence

Delayed Puberty

Delayed Menarche

Menarche, the onset of menstrual cycles that occurs toward the end of puberty, varies greatly from one individual to another and may be influenced by several factors (25,40,64,68) such as

- race,
- socioeconomic status,
- family size,
- nutrition,
- climate,
- altitude,
- disease, and
- physical activity.

Mean age of menarche in the United States is 12.8 years with a standard deviation of 1.2 years (73). *Delayed menarche* is defined as absence of periods at age 14 years (57). The age of menarche for athletic females has been observed to be later than that of nonathletic females and to vary among different modalities of exercise and at different competitive levels (42) (Table 65.1). Women involved in those aerobic sports encouraging thinness such as ballet dancing, long-distance running, and gymnastics tend to have a later age of menarche than other athletes (Table 65.1).

Altered Pubertal Progression

Menarche is only one event in the sequence of puberty. It is not yet clear whether the stages of *thelarche* (breast development) and *pubarche* (development of pubic hair) as defined by Tanner (63), are delayed, too. Physical examination of the athletes should be performed to assess this question; questionnaires (such as those done in most studies) are not sufficient.

One study (64) showed that in 15 ballet dancers menarche and thelarche were markedly delayed, whereas pubarche was not affected. Their bone age was found to be retarded as well. Ballet training during adolescent years appears to prolong the prepubertal state and cause delayed menarche, and periods of rest often lead to a striking catch-up in puberty (64). The peak height velocity (PHV)

…le 65.1 **Age of Menarche in Athletes of Different Sport Activities**

Sport	Study	n	Average age (years)
Control in U.S.	Zacharias et al. (73)	633	12.8
Ballet dancing	Warren and Brooks-Gunn (68)	64[a]	13.3
	Frisch et al. (26)	69	13.7
	Abraham et al. (1)	29	14.8
Running	Dale et al. (17)	90	12.9
	Frisch et al. (24)	17	13.8
Track and field	Malina et al. (41)	66	13.6
Volleyball	Malina et al. (42)	18	14.2
Skating	Warren and Brooks-Gunn (68)	25[b]	13.6
Swimming	Fauno et al. (22)	107	12.6
	Warren and Brooks-Gunn (68)	72[c]	12.9
	Constantini et al. (15)	51[d]	13.8
	Stager and Hatler (59)	140	14.2

[a]25% were premenarcheal. [b]24% were premenarcheal. [c]4% were premenarcheal. [d]26% were premenarcheal.

that immediately precedes menarche is therefore also delayed, so these athletes are taller at menarche as they continue to grow 3 cm to 4 cm each year prior to the growth spurt.

Menstrual Dysfunction

Secondary Amenorrhea and Oligomenorrhea

The prevalence of these problems varies widely (Table 65.2) due to the lack of standard definition for *secondary amenorrhea* and *oligomenorrhea* in numerous reports as well as differences between the population surveyed in terms of age, sport modality, level of activity and performance, training prior to menarche, and other methodological errors.

Definitions used for secondary amenorrhea vary from absence of menstruation for 3, 4, 5, 6, or for up to 12 months, or less than two or three menses per year. Irregularity is sometimes defined by number of menses per year, such as 3 to 6 (52) or 2 to 10 (29), or by the number of days between menses. Clinically, these different definitions may reflect different problems; complete amenorrhea may be hypoestrogenic or euestrogenic, whereas irregular menses, irrespective of frequency, may reflect an euestrogenic-anovulatory state. We suggest the following definitions (57):

- Primary amenorrhea—delay of menarche beyond age 16 years
- Secondary amenorrhea—absence of menstruation for more than 5 or 6 months in women who previously were cyclical
- Eumenorrhea—menstrual cycles that recur consistently at intervals between 21 and 36 days
- Oligomenorrhea—cycle intervals greater than 36 days

In this review we use the term *menstrual irregularities* to include both secondary amenorrhea and oligomenorrhea.

The first few cycles after menarche are usually irregular and anovulatory, but the precise incidence of this phenomenon is not known (31). This interval of irregularity may last from 1 to 3 years and is generally followed by normal cycles (24). Figure 65.1 presents the incidence of menstrual irregularities after menarche in adolescent swimmers compared to age-matched controls: Both the prevalence and the duration of menstrual irregularities are significantly higher in the swimmers. Runners and dancers were also found to have greater incidence of post-menarche irregularities (24,64).

In the general adult population the prevalence of menstrual irregularities is estimated to be from 1.8% to 5% (45,56); whereas surveys of adult athletes show 6% to 79% (Table 65.2). These variations reflect the methodological problems previously mentioned.

Short Luteal Phase and Anovulation

Recent works have suggested that many of the so-called eumenorrheic athletes (i.e., those with

Table 65.2 Surveys of the Prevalence of Menstrual Irregularities in Athletes (Amenorrhea and Oligomenorrhea)

Athletic activity	Study	*n*	% irregularities
General population	Pettersson et al. (45)	1,862	1.8
	Singh (56)	900	5
Ballet dancing	Abraham et al. (1)	29	79
	Frisch et al. (26)	69	58
	Brooks-Gunn et al. (9)	53	59
Running	Feicht et al. (23)	128	6–43
	Dale et al. (17)	90	24
	Shangold and Levine (54)	394	24
	Sanborn et al. (51)	237	26
	Frisch et al. (24)	38	61
	Glass et al. (29)	67	34
Cycling	Sanborn et al. (51)	33	12
Swimming	Sanborn et al. (51)	197	12
	Fauno et al. (22)	110	16

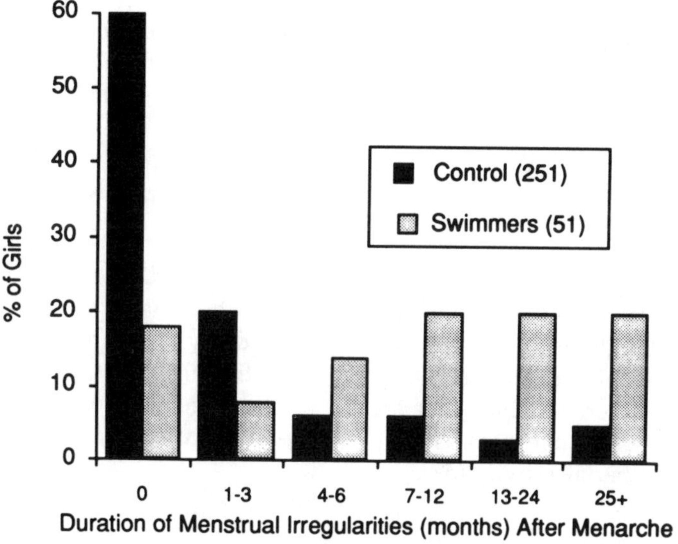

Figure 65.1 The distribution of length of menstrual irregularities in adolescent swimmers compared to controls. Note that 60% of the control group did not suffer any irregularity and only 5% suffered from prolonged MD, whereas 18% of the swimmers had initially normal cycles and 40% had irregularities lasting more than a year.

regular cycles) are actually suffering from hidden menstrual dysfunctions such as *anovulatory cycles* (defined as cycles without basal body temperature [BBT] shifts or progesterone rises) or inadequate luteal phases with or without prolonged follicular phases (8,38,46).

Shangold, Freeman, Thysen, and Gatz (53) found a reduction in the length of the luteal phase and reduced levels of progesterone in a 30-year-old runner, which correlated with her running distance. Bonen, Belcastro, Ling, and Simpson (8) found the same phenomena in 4 regularly menstruating teenage swimmers compared to age-matched controls (4.5 ± 0.6 days in the swimmers vs. 7.8 ± 3.0 days in the control). Loucks, Mortola, Girton, and Yen (38) demonstrated shorter luteal phases and lower urinary excretions of pregnanediol glucuronide in athletes with regular cycles compared to sedentary women. In a prospective study, Bullen et al. (12)

induced disturbed ovarian function in 4 out of 7 subjects after 8 weeks of training.

The exact prevalence of these less obvious forms of menstrual dysfunction is not known, as these athletes consider themselves perfectly regular. Dale, Gerlach, and Wilhite (17) found that only 50% of the runners ovulated during a test month (reflected by a low progesterone level) whereas 83% of the control group did so. Short luteal phase and anovulation might represent a mild form of the athletic reproductive system dysfunction that can lead to amenorrhea under greater stress.

Factors Associated With Athletes' Reproductive System Dysfunction

The factors associated with athletic reproductive system dysfunction can be divided into three major categories: (a) genetic, (b) environmental, and (c) reproductive maturity. It seems that many of these factors work together to influence the reproductive system in female athletes and that the same environmental changes can bring out different pathophysiology depending on the athlete's genetic predisposition.

Genetic Factors

The high correlation that exists in menarcheal age between mothers and daughters in nonathletes seems to be less pronounced in athletes (10,59). In active females there are other variables that are better predictors of menarcheal age such as leanness (9) and intense prepubertal activity (59).

Reproductive Maturity

Amenorrheic athletes have a later age of menarche (4,23,26) and a higher incidence of prior irregularities (52,54) than athletes with regular cycles. These findings suggest that women engaged in athletic activity have an a priori tendency to menstrual dysfunction and that exercise alone is not a causative factor. It has been suggested (40) that the physical characteristics associated with late maturation and amenorrhea attract these girls into athletic activity and to success. Older athletes and those with previous pregnancies have a lower incidence of amenorrhea (4,17,54,58). These are probably not cause-effect relationships but rather signs of hypothalamic–pituitary–gonadal axis maturity.

Environmental Factors

One of the major environmental factors associated with reproductive system dysfunction in women athletes concerns the issue of energy and nutrient balance. Many athletes become highly concerned with their body composition, seeking to alter it by means of strict diets and intense training. This may often lead to eating disorders, negative caloric balance, and changes of weight.

Sport Modality

Differences in the age of menarche and in the prevalence of menstrual irregularities are seen in various sports (Tables 65.1 and 65.2). They are attributed in part to different body sizes and shapes (39), energy expenditures (9), and eating behaviors (5,50). Swimmers, for example, exhibit very little if any dieting behavior because low weight is not required and caloric expenditure is relatively high (5,9,68). By contrast, athletic activities requiring thin bodies, such as ballet dancing, long-distance running, and gymnastics tend to have a much higher prevalence of irregularities and a later age of menarche (9,67), which might be due to their pathological eating behavior and negative energy balance.

Training Prior to Menarche

Many studies have shown that later age of menarche is related to prior training (15,24,26,61), and researchers have concluded that sport participation delays menarche. However, social (40) and genetic (10,59) factors also seem to influence menarcheal age. Randomized prospective cohort studies are necessary to verify the influence of training.

Mental Stress

Mental stress plays an important role in hypothalamic dysfunction, and many athletes are subjected to constant psychological stress during training and competitions. Some studies have suggested that amenorrhea is associated with a greater perceived stress in exercise (52), but this is not a constant finding (3,28,65).

Performance Level

The better performing athletes tend to have later age of menarche (39,61) and higher incidence of menstrual irregularities (52). However, it has been suggested (59) that the higher the competitive level, the more likely inherited traits (including delayed menarche and MD) contribute to an athlete's success.

Pathogenesis of Athletes' Reproductive System Dysfunction

The link between exercise, the associated factors previously mentioned, and MD is not quite clear. It seems that several axes regulated by the hypothalamus and involving the endocrine system are disturbed in athletes with menstrual disorders.

The most frequent hormonal pattern seen in athletes is a *hypothalamic amenorrhea* (see Figure 65.2), with GnRH dysfunction as reflected by altered pulsatility of luteinizing hormone (LH) and follicular-stimulating hormone (FSH), low gonadotrophins, and hypoestrogenism (4,16,33,38). This type of amenorrhea has been described in sports requiring low weight (for better performance or aesthetic appearance) such as long-distance running and ballet dancing. Many of these lean athletes exhibit pathological eating behaviors (9,11,50), and it has been proposed that their very low weight or negative caloric balance may cause these disturbances (19,64). Indeed, this hypothalamic dysfunction is very similar to that found in women suffering from *anorexia nervosa* (17,66,72).

In sports such as swimming and basketball, where low body weight is not required and muscle mass is of great importance, eating disorders are uncommon (5,9,50). The hormone profile in these athletes might therefore be different (33). Elevated levels of LH, inappropriate increase in the LH:FSH ratio, and normal levels of estrogen have been observed in swimmers (8,15). Young swimmers were also found to have higher-than-average levels of androgens (15,62), which can adversely affect the menstrual cycle. Future research should target this type of athlete.

Complications of Athletes' Reproductive System Dysfunction

Infertility

The exact incidence of infertility among athletes is not known, as there are many "regular cycling" women who in fact have a short luteal phase or anovulation. Many athletes are not concerned with their fertility so the incidence of this problem is unknown. To our knowledge, there are no published data on the percentage of women with infertility related to exercise, nor are there studies on the prevalence of infertility among athletes who try to conceive. A 10% incidence of infertility among marathon runners (54) included half who reported infertility prior to running. Naturally, athletes suffering from hypothalamic amenorrhea will have infertility.

Osteoporosis and Skeletal Problems

Osteoporosis and skeletal problems related to osteopenia are surfacing as complications of athletic activity in amenorrheic athletes (6,14,20,34,36,43, 70). Scoliosis has been reported in 24% of ballet dancers (70), much higher than in the nonathletic population (2,7,14). The prevalence of stress fractures among athletes with menstrual irregularities is much higher than among their regularly menstruating counterparts (14,20,34,36,43). Dancers with stress fractures have a higher incidence of and a longer duration of amenorrhea than those without such fractures (70), and runners with menstrual irregularities were found to have not only higher incidence of stress fractures (45% compared to 29% in regular cycling runners) but also more multiple ones (6).

Injuries such as stress fractures and collapse of the femoral head resembling aseptic necrosis may be due to overuse of bone weakened by osteopenia. Osteopenia, particularly of trabecular bone, is common and the rate of bone loss is similar to that associated with menopause, 5% per year (14,20). Exercise, which has been shown to halt or even reverse bone loss in postmenopausal women apparently does not protect the amenorrheic young athlete from a decrease in bone density (69). On the contrary, the compensatory increase in bone density seen in stressed bones is deficient in amenorrheic dancers (see Figure 65.3a,b). In addition, the delayed puberty of these young athletes may interfere with attaining their peak bone mass; bone mass accretion continues into the late 20s, but this process may not progress normally in the absence of estrogen (19,27,69). These findings would be of importance to recreational athletes as well as to those training for competition or preparing for a career, and they would drastically alter our attitude toward the safety of athletic participation.

We have recently shown (27) that aberrant nutrition and nutritional patterns may affect the skeleton even before changes in bone density are noted; dancers with recent stress fractures had a higher prevalence of nutritional aberrations and weight fluctuations when compared to dancers without fractures. Surprisingly there were no differences in bone density measurement between the groups studied, although there was a trend toward lower values in the fracture group. Thus, bone density measurements appear to be a reflection of only one parameter of bone health. Longitudinal studies on these problems are needed.

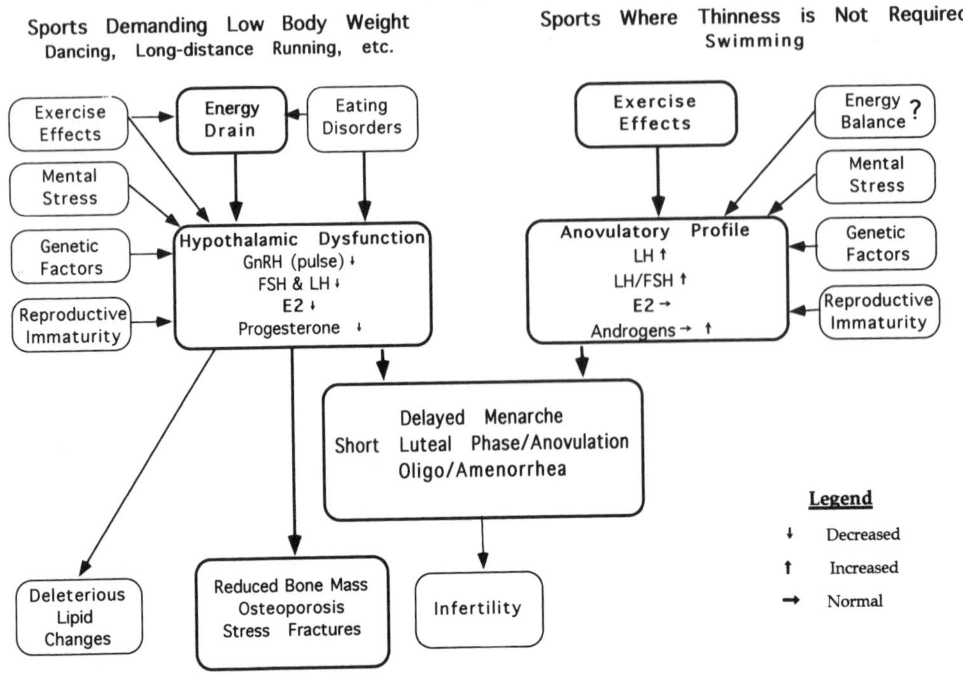

Figure 65.2 This figure schematically illustrates a hypothesis of two different mechanisms leading to athletes' MD: the first (left side) is seen in sports demanding very low weight and results in hypothalamic dysfunction, prolonged periods of hypoestrogenism with the serious consequence of osteoporosis. The second (right side) suggests a different mechanism that might exist in sports that do not require thinness, such as swimming (8, 15).

Other Complications of Menstrual Dysfunction

Metabolic Changes: Lipid and Carbohydrate Metabolism

Risk of Coronary Heart Disease. Exogenous or endogenous changes in estradiol (E2) status can lead to significant alterations in lipid and carbohydrate metabolism (13). E2 normally increases the levels of triglycerides and high-density lipoprotein (HDL) HDL-2 and enhances lipolysis in muscle and adipose tissues. E2 also inhibits gluconeogenesis and glycogenolysis (13).

Habitual physical activity has an important role in the primary prevention of coronary artery disease through the known beneficial effect on plasma lipoproteins (32): High-density lipoprotein (HDL) and apolipoprotein-A-I (apo-A-I) levels increase while low-density lipoprotein (LDL) and apolipoprotein-B (apo-B) levels decrease. Data indicates that these beneficial effects of strenuous exercise (except for apo-B levels) are reversed by exercise-induced hypoestrogenic amenorrhea (32).

Performance. During exercise E2 appears to enhance lipid oxidation and lessen glycogen depletion in liver and skeletal muscle when compared to an estrogen-deficient state (13). The significance of this phenomenon on the performance of hypoestrogenic athletes is not certain.

Endometrial Hyperplasia and Cancer

The risk of endometrial hyperplasia and adenocarcinoma due to a chronic, unopposed estrogen level has been raised (31), but so far has not been reported.

Reduced Basic Metabolic Rate (BMR)

Many female athletes appear to have low energy availability, as their energy (caloric) demands for exercise by far exceed their caloric intake. Some studies have shown lower BMR in amenorrheic compared to eumenorrheic athletes (44), but recent studies (71) have questioned this concept. Hypothalamic suppression in amenorrheic athletes may be an exaggerated adaptation of the body to preserve energy. Other systems might also be affected by saving energy.

Potential Benefits of Delayed Puberty and Menstrual Dysfunction

The changes in the reproductive system in athletes are associated with physical benefits in terms of

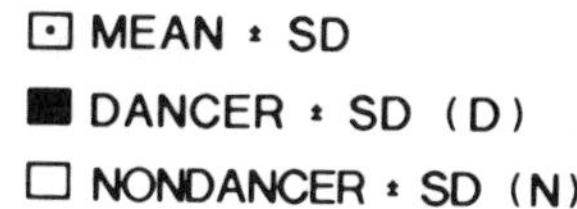

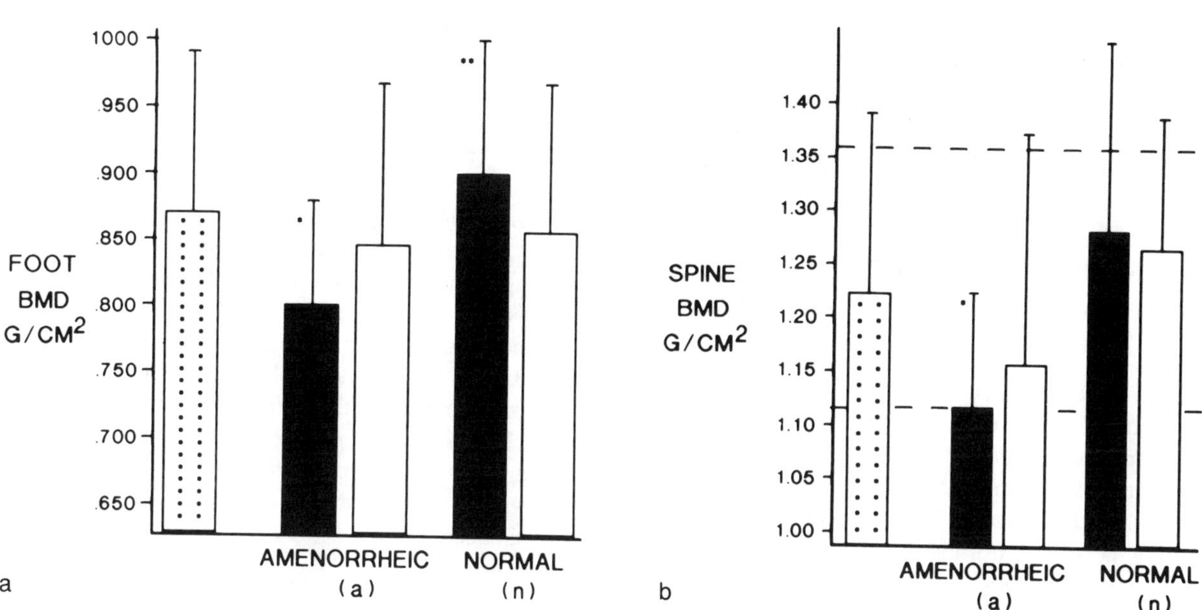

Figure 65.3 Foot (Figure 65.3a) and spine (Figure 65.3b) bone mineral densities in normal and amenorrheic subjects. Groups are divided into dancers and non-dancers. Stippled bar = mean of all values. Two-way ANOVA shows a significant ($p<0.05$) effect of amenorrhea on bone mineral density even when controlling for age, but was eliminated by controlling for weight. Multiple comparisons show that amenorrheic dancers differ from normal dancers even when controlling for age and weight. Normal dancers were higher than both amenorrheic groups when controlling for age.

performance and aesthetic appearance (especially in weight-bearing sports). Late maturing athletes tend to perform better than the early maturing girls (23,39). The later maturing girl is characteristically taller, lighter, and leaner than her early maturing peers (39,68). The greater height is due to later closure of the epiphysis, which is estrogen-dependent (65). Amenorrheic athletes (who were often late maturers) are also lighter and leaner compared with eumenorrheic athletes (29,43,52,54,58). Dancers (64) were observed to have a decreased upper: lower body ratio and a significantly increased arm span when compared to their female siblings or to the normal population.

Androgen levels have consistently been shown to increase in response to acute exercise (37), and in several studies on trained athletes their basal levels were found to be in the upper limits of normal (15,17). These elevated levels may be of great advantage to the exercising athlete as they help build and maintain bone and muscle mass. Exercise might decrease premenstrual syndrome (30,48) and favorably affect menstruation by shortening bleeding duration and reducing flow and cramps (2,17). Another potential benefit of amenorrheic athletes might be their energy efficiency, that is, lowered BMR and thermic responses to food (68). Thus, an effect of training, which appears exaggerated in amenorrheic athletes, may be to decrease caloric need.

Evaluation of Delayed Puberty and Menstrual Dysfunction

The diagnosis of exercise-associated MD (amenorrhea, oligomenorrhea, and infertility) is still one of exclusion, and it is important to first rule out other common causes of amenorrhea. A full history should be taken with special emphases on type of activity and competitive level, energy output, nutrition, eating behavior, changes in weight, and fractures history. Signs and symptoms of androgen excess, galactorrhea, and hot flashes should be looked for. Physical and pelvic examinations and measurement of blood concentrations of prolactin, thyroid function tests, FSH, LH, T, dehydroeplandrosterone-sulfate (DHEA-S), E2, and βHCG should be done. A progestin challenge test might be indicated to induce withdrawal bleeding (Provera, 10 mg for 5 days).

In athletes with hypoestrogenic amenorrhea and other MD with either low estrogen or low progesterone, evaluation of bone density is recommended, as both estrogen and progesterone can affect bone density (49).

Management of Athletes With Reproductive System Dysfunction

When treatment is prescribed, several factors must be considered: (a) the age of the athlete, (b) her diet and caloric balance, (c) the type of sport, (d) the kind of MD and its duration, (e) her estrogen status, and (f) her fertility intentions (i.e., pregnancy, contraception, etc.).

The most rational approach to an athlete's MD is to reduce the amount of exercise or increase the caloric intake (if there is a negative caloric balance). A 10% decrease in exercise (either duration or intensity) or gain of 1 to 2 kg is recommended (21,47). However, the ideal energy balance for an athlete to maintain her menses without losing the artistic and athletic advantages of thinness is not yet known and is probably different from one athlete to another.

Management of the Athlete With Oligomenorrhea or Amenorrhea

After ruling out diseases, explanation and reassurance therapy should be started. Medroxyprogesterone, 10 mg for 5 to 10 days every month will prevent the risk of endometrial hyperplasia and adenocarcinoma. If there is no withdrawal bleeding and if the athlete has low levels of E2, therapy to prevent osteoporosis should be given as discussed later. Oral contraceptives are a reasonable option if contraception is required, and clomiphene if pregnancy is desired.

Management of the Athlete With Short Luteal Phase

It seems that athletes with luteal phase deficiency do not require treatment unless they wish to conceive. Reduction or cessation of exercise will often reverse this condition, but many athletes prefer hormonal treatment over a change in their lifestyle. These include progesterone suppositories, clomiphene citrate, or gonadotropin therapy.

Management of the Athlete With Delayed Puberty

A quandary arises in the premenarcheal patient with delayed menarche. These young athletes should be encouraged to decrease the intensity of their exercise as rest may lead to a catch-up in puberty (64). Improvement of nutritional intake may also be beneficial. Institution of hormonal therapy should be initiated only after discussion with the patient and her parents and if menarche has not occurred by the age of 16 years. This is to encourage an increase in bone mass that does not occur normally in the hypoestrogenic adolescent (69). If growth is not completed, as measured by bone age (closed epiphysial plates), estrogen replacement *should not* be given unless growth cessation is acceptable.

Prevention and Management of Osteoporosis

Hormone Replacement

The main concern about amenorrhea appears to be the serious consequences of osteoporosis, stress fractures, and other skeletal problems due to reduced bone mass. If a decrease in exercise or an increase in weight is not feasible or is rejected by the patient, cyclic estrogen in combination with a progestin should be given in order to prevent the bone demineralization. The doses currently recommended are based on studies on post-menopausal women. Unfortunately, the effect of estrogen replacement on the bones of amenorrheic athletes has not been studied yet. Conjugated estrogens (Premarin or its equivalent) is given in doses of 0.625 mg for 25 days with 10 mg of medroxyprogesterone (Provera) added on days 16 through 25. A week without therapy follows. This dose is thought to prevent further loss of bone mass in an athlete with amenorrhea of recent onset but not to replace bone loss that has already occurred following amenorrhea of longer duration. If periods are desired, the patient may need to take 1.25 to 2.5 mg of Premarin each day.

Side effects are unlikely to occur with these very small doses of estrogen; but they might include headaches, elevated blood pressure, and blood clots. Overstimulation of the endometrium is prevented by Provera therapy. The long-term consequences of low doses of estrogens (given with progesterone) are as yet unknown.

The contraindications to the use of estrogen are: (a) unexplained vaginal bleeding; (b) breast, uterine, or cervical cancer; (c) past history of cerebrovascular accident or deep vein thrombosis; (d) cardiac disease; (e) hypertension; (f) diabetes mellitus; and (g) active hepatic disease.

Calcium Supplementation

The benefits of both exercise and estrogen depend on the adequacy of dietary calcium (18,20). Many athletes consume insufficient amounts of calcium (20) and supplementation should be given. The recommended daily calcium requirement is 1,500 mg to the hypoestrogenic athlete and 1,000 mg to the euestrogenic one (55).

Prognosis of Athletes' Reproductive System Dysfunction

No study has been published that reports the percentage of amenorrheic athletes who display spontaneous reversal, but it seems that most of the abnormalities in the menstrual cycle are reversible with reduction of training or weight gain (46,60). Some athletes will not resume menses, and it seems that in these cases the MD is not solely the result of exercise.

Progression of sexual development and the onset of menarche were observed to occur during times of rest in ballet dancers (64). The long-term effects of delayed puberty on growth and development are yet unknown. It has been suggested that delayed menarche will prevent attaining peak bone mass and will predispose the adolescent athlete to fragile skeleton, vertebral instability, and curvature (19,27,69). The trabecular bone density seems to increase in amenorrheic athletes who resume their menses (21,35), but no one knows yet if the original loss of 5% per year (14,20) can be completely reversed.

Future Research on Athletes' Reproductive System Dysfunction

Future research should address several issues:

1. The growth and development of highly active girls in different sport modalities, including all stages of puberty (thelarche, pubarche, PHV, and menarche). Does delayed puberty in athletes influence peak bone mass, and if it does is it reversible?
2. The prevalence and character of the various types of MD. Are inadequate luteal phase, oligomenorrhea, and secondary amenorrhea one continuity or rather different endpoints of reactions and adaptations to exercise?
3. The importance of nutrition, eating disorders, and negative energy balance in the pathogenesis of MD in exercising women. Both quality and quantity of diet should be assessed and the physiological and endocrine mechanisms associated with it need to be evaluated.
4. The contribution of the other factors (i.e., genetic, training intensity, sport modality, etc.) to the development of MD and the pathophysiology of these disturbances. What is the role (if any) of opiates or other transmitters in the development of reproductive system abnormalities?
5. The different hormonal profiles and mechanisms involved in athletes' MD in different sport modalities.
6. Benefits versus risks of intensive exercise in premenopausal women; immediate and prolonged clinical consequences with special emphasis on the skeleton and the cardiovascular system.
7. Who should be treated with what, and for how long? Does estrogen therapy indeed prevent bone loss in amenorrheic athletes and what is the optimal dose? Should menarche be induced in girls with delayed puberty, and if so at what age?

In summary, reproductive system dysfunction of the female athlete has become a well-recognized entity and a major clinical concern in these premenopausal women. The pathophysiology of this syndrome is not yet understood and the optimal treatment has still to be established.

References

1. Abraham, S.F.; Beumont, P.J.V.; Fraser, I.S.; Llewellyn-Jones, D. Body weight, exercise and menstrual status among ballet dancers in training. Br. J. Obstet. Gynaecol. 89:507-510; 1982.
2. Akella, P.; Warren, M.P.; Jonnavithula, S.; Brooks-Gunn, J. Scoliosis in ballet dancers. Med. Probl. Performing Artists. (Sept.):84-86; 1991.
3. Anderson, J.L. Women's sports and fitness programs at the U.S. Military Academy. Phys. Sportsmed. 7:72-80; 1980.

4. Baker, E.; Mathur, R.S.; Kirk, R.F.; Williamson, H.O. Female runners and secondary amenorrhea: Correlation with age, parity, mileage, and plasma hormonal and sex-hormone-binding globulin concentrations. Fertil. Steril. 36:183-187; 1981.
5. Barr, S.I. Relationship of eating attitudes to anthropometric variables and dietary intakes of female collegiate swimmers. J. Am. Diet. Assoc. 91(8):976-977; 1991.
6. Barrow, G.W.; Saha, S. Menstrual irregularity and stress fractures in collegiate female distance runners. Am. J. Sports Med. 16(3):209-216; 1988.
7. Becker, T.J. Scoliosis in swimmers. Clin. Sports Med. 5:149-158; 1986.
8. Bonen, A.; Belcastro, A.N.; Ling, W.Y.; Simpson, A.A. Profiles of selected hormones during menstrual cycles of teenage athletes. J. Appl. Physiol. 50(3):545-551; 1981.
9. Brooks-Gunn, J.; Burrow, C.; Warren, M.P. Attitudes toward eating and body weight in different groups of female adolescent athletes. Int. J. Eat. Disord. 7(6):749-757; 1988.
10. Brooks-Gunn, J.; Warren, M.P. Mother-daughter differences in menarcheal age in adolescent girls attending national dance company schools and non-dancers. Ann. Hum. Biol. 15(1):35-43; 1988.
11. Brooks-Gunn, J.; Warren, M.P.; Hamilton, L.H. The relationship of eating disorders to amenorrhea in ballet dancers. Med. Sci. Sports Exerc. 19(1):41-44; 1987.
12. Bullen, B.A.; Skrinar, G.S.; Beitins, I.Z.; et al. Endurance training effects on plasma hormonal responsiveness and sex hormone excretion. J. Appl. Physiol. 56(6):1453-1463; 1984.
13. Bunt, J.C. Metabolic actions of estradiol: Significance for acute and chronic exercise responses. Med. Sci. Sports Exerc. 22(3):286-290; 1990.
14. Cann, C.E.; Martin, M.C.; Genant, H.K.; Jaffe, R.B. Decreased spinal mineral content in amenorrheic women. JAMA. 251:626-629; 1984.
15. Constantini, W.N.; Persitz, E.; Warren, M.P. Athletic amenorrhea in swimmers: A different mechanism. Med. Sci. Sports Exerc. 25(5):5141; 1993.
16. Cumming, D.C.; Vickovic, M.M.; Wall, S.R.; Fluker, M.R. Defects in pulsatile LH release in normally menstruating runners. J. Clin. Endocrinol. Metab. 60(4):810-812; 1985.
17. Dale, E.; Gerlach, D.H.; Wilhite, A.L. Menstrual dysfunction in distance runners. Obstet. Gynecol. 54:47-53; 1979.
18. Dalsky, G.P. Effect of exercise on bone: Permissive influence of estrogen and calcium. Med. Sci. Sports Exerc. 22(3):281-285; 1990.
19. Dhuper, S.; Warren, M.P.; Brooks-Gunn, J.; Fox, R.P. Effects of hormonal status on bone density in adolescent girls. J. Clin. Endocrinol. Metab. 71:1038-1088; 1990.
20. Drinkwater, B.L.; Nilson, K.; Chesnut, C.H., III; Bremner, W.J.; Shainholtz, S.; Southworth, M.B. Bone mineral content of amenorrheic and eumenorrheic athletes. N. Engl. J. Med. 311(5):277-281; 1984.
21. Drinkwater, B.L.; Nilson, K.; Ott, S.; Chesnut, C.H., III. Bone mineral density after resumption of menses in amenorrheic athletes. JAMA. 256:380-382; 1986.
22. Fauno, P.; Kalund, S.; Kanstrup, I.L. Menstrual patterns in Danish elite swimmers. Eur. J. Appl. Physiol. 62:36-39; 1991.
23. Feicht, C.B.; Johnson, T.S.; Martin, B.J.; Sparkes, K.E.; Wagner, W.W., Jr. Secondary amenorrhea in athletes. Lancet. 2:1145-1146; 1978.
24. Frisch, R.E.; Gotz-Welbergen, A.V.; McArthur, J.W. Delayed menarche and amenorrhea of college athletes in relation to age of onset of training. JAMA. 246(14):1559-1563; 1981.
25. Frisch, R.E.; Revelle, R. Height and weight at menarche and a hypothesis of menarche. Arch. Dis. Child. 46:695-701; 1971.
26. Frisch, R.E.; Wyshak, G.; Vincent, L. Delayed menarche and amenorrhea in ballet dancers. N. Engl. J. Med. 303:17-19; 1980.
27. Frusztajer, N.T.; Dhuper, S.; Warren, M.P.; Brooks-Gunn, J.; Fox, R.P. Nutrition and the incidence of stress fractures in ballet dancers. Am. J. Clin. Nutr. 51:779-783; 1990.
28. Galle, P.C.; Freeman, M.G.; Galle, G.R.; Huggins, G.R.; Sondheim, S.T. Physiologic and psychologic profiles in a survey of women runners. Med. Sci. Sports Exerc. 39:633-639; 1983.
29. Glass, A.R.; Deuster, P.A.; Kyle, S.B.; Yahiro, J.A.; Vigersky, R.A.; Schoomaker, E.B. Amenorrhea in olympic marathon runners. Fertil. Steril. 48:740-745; 1987.
30. Hale, R.W. Exercise, sports and menstrual dysfunction. Clin. Obstet. Gynecol. 26(3):728-735; 1983.
31. Highet, R. Athletic amenorrhea: An update on aetiology, complications and management. Sports Med. 7:82-108; 1989.
32. Lamon-Fava, S.; Fisher, E.C.; Nelson, M.E.; et al. Effect of exercise and menstrual cycle status on plasma lipids, low density lipoprotein particle size, and apolipoproteins. J. Clin. Endocrinol. Metab. 68:17-21; 1989.
33. Lessing, J.B.; Brenner, S.H.; Weiss, G. Menstrual dysfunction in athletic women. Harefuah. 108(4):193-196; 1985.
34. Lindberg, J.S.; Fears, W.B.; Hunt, M.M.; Powell, M.R.; Boll, D.; Wade, C.E. Exercise-induced

amenorrhea and bone density. Ann. Intern. Med. 101:647-648; 1984.

35. Lindberg, J.S.; Powell, M.R.; Hunt, M.M.; Ducey, D.E.; Wade, C.E. Increased vertebral bone mineral in response to reduced exercise in amenorrheic runners. West. J. Med. 146(1):39-42; 1987.
36. Lloyd, T.; Buchanan, J.R.; Bitzer, S.; Waldman, C.J.; Myers, C.; Ford, B.G. The relationship of diet, athletic activity, menstrual status and bone density among collegiate women. Am. J. Clin. Nutr. 46:681-684; 1987.
37. Loucks, A.B.; Horvath, S.M. Athletic amenorrhea: A review. Med. Sci. Sports Exerc. 17(1):56-72; 1985.
38. Loucks, A.B.; Mortola, J.F.; Girton, L.; Yen, S.S.C. Alterations in the hypothalamic-pituitary-ovarian and the hypothalamic-pituitary-adrenal axes in athletic women. J. Clin. Endocrinol. Metab. 68:402-411; 1989.
39. Malina, R.M. Physical growth and maturity characteristics of young athletes. In: Magill, R.A.; Ash, M.J.; Smoll, F.L., eds. Children in sport: A contemporary anthology. Champaign, IL: Human Kinetics; 1978:79-101.
40. Malina, R.M. Menarche in athletes: A synthesis and hypothesis. Ann. Hum. Biol. 10:1-24; 1983.
41. Malina, R.M.; Harper, A.B.; Avent, H.H.; Campbell, D.E. Age at menarche in athletes and non-athletes. Med. Sci. Sports Exerc. 5(1):11-13; 1973.
42. Malina, R.M.; Spirduso, W.W.; Tate, C.; Baylor, A.M. Age at menarche and selected menstrual characteristics in athletes at different competitive levels and in different sports. Med. Sci. Sports Exerc. 10(3):218-222; 1978.
43. Marcus, R.; Cann, C.; Madvig, P.; et al. Menstrual function and bone mass in elite women distance runners. Ann. Intern. Med. 102:158-163; 1985.
44. Myerson, M.; Gutin, B.; Warren, M.P.; et al. Resting metabolic rate and energy balance in amenorrheic and eumenorrheic runners. Med. Sci. Sports Exerc. 23(1):15-22; 1991.
45. Pettersson, F.; Fries, H.; Nillius, S.J. Epidemiology of secondary amenorrhea: Incidence and prevalence rates. Am. J. Obstet. Gynecol. 7:80-86; 1973.
46. Prior, J.C.; Ho Yuen, B.; Clement, P.; Bowie, L.; Thomas, J. Reversible luteal phase changes and infertility associated with marathon training. Lancet. (July):269-270; 1982.
47. Prior, J.C.; Vigna, Y.M. Gonadal steroids in athletic women: Contraception, complications and performance. Sports Med. 2:287-295; 1985.
48. Prior, J.C.; Vigna, Y.M.; Sciarretta, D.; Alojado, N.; Schulzer, M. Conditioning exercise decreases premenstrual symptoms: A prospective, controlled 6-month trial. Fertil. Steril. 47:402-408; 1987.
49. Prior, J.C.; Vigna, Y.M.; Schechter, M.T.; Burgess, A.E. Spinal bone loss and ovulatory disturbances. N. Engl. J. Med. 323:1221-1227; 1990.
50. Rosen, L.W.; McKeag, D.B.; Hough, D.O.; Curley, V. Pathogenic weight-control behavior in female athletes. Phys. Sportsmed. 14(1):79-86; 1986.
51. Sanborn, C.F.; Martin, B.J.; Wagner, W.W., Jr. Is athletic amenorrhea specific to runners? Am. J. Obstet. Gynecol. 143:859-861; 1982.
52. Schwartz, B.; Cumming, D.C.; Riordan, E.; Selye, M.; Yen, S.S.C.; Rebar, R.W. Exercise-associated amenorrhea: A distinct entity? Am. J. Obstet. Gynecol. 141:662-670; 1981.
53. Shangold, M.M.; Freeman, R.; Thysen, B.; Gatz, M. The relationship between long-distance running, plasma progesterone, and luteal phase length. Fertil. Steril. 31:130-133; 1979.
54. Shangold, M.M.; Levine, H.S. The effect of marathon training upon menstrual function. Am. J. Obstet. Gynecol. 143:862-869; 1982.
55. Shangold, M.M.; Rebar, R.W.; Wentz, A.C.; Schiff, I. Evaluation and management of menstrual dysfunction in athletes. JAMA. 263:1665-1669; 1990.
56. Singh, K.B. Menstrual disorders in college students. Am. J. Obstet. Gynecol. 1210:299-302; 1981.
57. Speroff, L.; Glass, R.H.; Nathan, G.K. Clinical gynecologic endocrinology and infertility. Baltimore: Williams & Wilkins; 1983.
58. Speroff, L.; Redwine, D.B. Exercise and menstrual function. Phys. Sportsmed. 8(5):42-52; 1980.
59. Stager, J.M.; Hatler, L.K. Menarche in athletes: The influence of genetics and prepubertal training. Med. Sci. Sports Exerc. 20(4):369-373; 1988.
60. Stager, J.M.; Ritchie-Flanagan, B.; Robertshaw, D. Reversibility of amenorrhea in athletes. N. Engl. J. Med. 310(1):51-52; 1984.
61. Stager, J.M.; Robertshaw, D.; Meischer, E. Delayed menarche in swimmers in relation to age at onset of training and athletic performance. Med. Sci. Sports Exerc. 16(6):550-555; 1984.
62. Sutton, J.R.; Coleman, M.J.; Casey, J.; Lazarus, L. Androgen response during physical exercise. Br. Med. J. 1:520-522; 1973.
63. Tanner, J.M. Growth and adolescence. Oxford: Blackwell Scientific; 1962.
64. Warren, M.P. The effects of exercise on pubertal progression and reproductive function in girls. J. Clin. Endocrinol. Metab. 51(5):1150-1157; 1980.

65. Warren, M.P. The effects of altered nutritional states, stress and systemic illness on reproduction in women. In: Vaitukaitis, J.L., ed. Clinical reproductive neuroendocrinology. New York: Elsevier Science; 1982:177-206.
66. Warren, M.P. The effects of undernutrition on reproductive function in the human. Endocr. Rev. 4:363-377; 1983.
67. Warren, M.P. Anorexia, bulimia, and exercise-induced amenorrhea: Medical approach. In: Bardin, C.W., ed. Current therapy in endocrinology and metabolism. Philadelphia: B.C. Becker, Inc.; 1991:12-16.
68. Warren, M.P.; Brooks-Gunn, J. Delayed menarche in athletes: The role of low energy intake and eating disorders and their relation to bone density. In: Laron, Z.; Rogol, A.D., eds. Hormones and sport. Vol. 55. New York: Serono Symposia Publications from Raven Press; 1989:41-54.
69. Warren, M.P.; Brooks-Gunn, J.; Fox, R.P.; Lancelot, C.; Newman, D.; Hamilton, W.G. Lack of bone accretion and amenorrhea: Evidence for a relative osteopenia in weight bearing bones. J. Clin. Endocrinol. Metab. 72:847-853; 1991.
70. Warren, M.P.; Brooks-Gunn, J.; Hamilton, L.H.; Warren, L.F.; Hamilton, W.G. Scoliosis and fractures in young ballet dancers: Relation to delayed menarche and secondary amenorrhea. N. Engl. J. Med. 314:1348-1353; 1986.
71. Wilmore, J.H.; Wambsgans, K.C.; Brenner, M.; Broeder, C.E.; et al. Is there energy conservation in amenorrheic compared with eumenorrheic distance runners? J. Appl. Physiol. 72(1):15-22; 1992.
72. Yates, A.; Leehey, K.; Shisslak, C.M. Running an analogue of anorexia? N. Engl. J. Med. 308:251-255; 1983.
73. Zacharias, L.; Rand, W.M.; Wurtman, R.J. A prospective study of sexual development and growth in American girls: The statistics of menarche. Obstet. Gynecol. Surv. 31:325-337; 1976.

Chapter 66

Physical Activity, Fitness, and Health of the Pregnant Mother and Fetus

Marshall W. Carpenter

Both pregnancy and exercise require profound changes in mammalian physiology involving alterations in ventilation, cardiac output, organ perfusion, and mobilization of fuels. Despite increased investigatory interest in maternal exercise, little is known at present about the interaction of pregnancy and maternal exercise. As a result, the impact of physical activity level and fitness on the health of the pregnant mother and fetus is largely unexplored by scientific means. This chapter will explore the current status of knowledge regarding cardiovascular and pulmonary changes associated with normal pregnancy, maternal physiologic response to acute exercise at maximal aerobic capacity and under submaximal conditions, maternal thermoregulation, and changes in maternal endocrine responses to acute exertion. This chapter will also review information on fetoplacental homeostasis during maternal exercise derived from animal and human experimental studies. Information about maternal and fetal effects of maternal training and detraining will be explored as well as the effect of maternal exercise on maternal diabetes during pregnancy. Finally, the chapter will briefly review research questions of interest at the present time.

Maternal Cardiovascular Adaptations to Pregnancy

Plasma Volume

Most maternal cardiovascular adaptations to pregnancy occur in the first third of pregnancy and thereby precede the increased metabolic demands of the conceptus. Plasma volume is measurably increased by 6 to 8 weeks gestation and is increased to 45% above prepregnancy values by 34 weeks gestation (40,57). Red cell volume increases approximately 30%, but its later peak results in a dilutional anemia (57).

Cardiac Function

A preconceptional cohort study has demonstrated a 20% increase in stroke volume and 23% increase in cardiac output by 8 weeks gestational age, estimated by echocardiography (12). This study confirmed earlier studies using both dye dilution techniques and echocardiography with postpartum control values (49,50,67). The increase in cardiac output is much greater than the 13% increase in body mass that typically occurs during human pregnancy, suggesting that changes in cardiac output may be a product of stimuli other than peripheral metabolic demands in pregnancy. Cardiac output appears to increase up to 34% from prepregnancy values (53). Cardiac output later in pregnancy can be altered by maternal position during its measurement and may actually decline in the third trimester (50,65,73,76). Maternal heart rate increases approximately 20 beats per minute through the second trimester over that noted in the postpartum period (73,78).

Echocardiography has demonstrated an increase in ventricular wall thickness and end-diastolic ventricular volume, both of which peak at the end of the second trimester (49,67). These changes are consistent with other studies demonstrating a peak stroke volume at 24 weeks gestation that decreases thereafter until term (73).

Vascular Resistance

The relationship between increased cardiac output, increased blood volume, and decreased peripheral vascular resistance is uncertain. Hormonal effects on castrated nonpregnant animals suggest that the primary event may be a decreased peripheral vascular resistance (53), but this has not been adequately explored in humans. Systemic vascular resistance was measured during recumbency by catheterization studies in pregnant women of varying gestational ages (65). Systemic vascular resistance was at its lowest point in the first trimester.

Venous compliance is also increased during pregnancy, particularly in the lower extremities (8,35).

Respiratory Changes During Pregnancy

Total lung capacity is probably unchanged by pregnancy. Functional residual capacity is reduced by 18% in pregnancy (27). Maximal expiratory flow-volume curves demonstrate that small airway closing volumes are often higher than functional residual capacity, suggesting that pregnancy may predispose to reduced ventilation:perfusion ratios in parts of the lung. Minute ventilation (VE) increases approximately 50% during pregnancy (47). This is due, primarily, to increased tidal volume as respiratory rate remains unchanged. The ventilatory equivalent (the ratio of ventilation to $\dot{V}O_2$) is increased at rest during pregnancy by 17%, resulting in a decrease in arterial partial pressure of carbon dioxide (PCO_2) from 39 to 31 torr (10,70,79). This results in a mild respiratory alkalemia (plasma pH = 7.44). Resting oxygen uptake ($\dot{V}O_2$) increases up to 30% during pregnancy (47,64,79). Half of this increase occurs by 8 weeks gestation, and three quarters of the increase by 15 weeks gestation (20). The increase in resting $\dot{V}O_2$ however, is proportionate to total body mass when compared to postpartum values (16,18).

Maternal Physiologic Response to Acute Exercise at Maximal Aerobic Capacity

Cardiac Output–Oxygen Uptake Relationship

The marked alteration of maternal cardiovascular and respiratory function that characterizes pregnancy has suggested that neuroendocrine physiologic control of cardiorespiratory function may be altered in pregnancy. However, recent observations have confirmed that basic physiologic control mechanisms are conserved during gestation. These questions are best addressed by examination of maternal response to maximal aerobic power output, which is defined by a plateau of $\dot{V}O_2$ ($\dot{V}O_2$max) with increasing work load. Conservation of cardiorespiratory response to exercise during pregnancy is demonstrated in several ways. Cardiac output, in the nonpregnant state, increases linearly with $\dot{V}O_2$ as exercise intensity increases in a 5 to 6:1 ratio, probably maintained by central neural mechanisms (34,52,60). During pregnancy, incremental exercise to $\dot{V}O_2$max, produces a 6.15 ratio compared to a postpartum ratio of 6.18 (70).

Heart Rate at Maximal Oxygen Uptake

Likewise, age-specific heart rate at $\dot{V}O_2$max is probably unchanged by pregnancy (56,70). These studies documented similar mean maximal heart rates of 182 and 174 beats per minute (bpm) with cycle exercise, and the former found 178 bpm during maximal treadmill exercise during pregnancy, all similar to postpartum values. Both studies demonstrated that $\dot{V}O_2$max expressed as either L/min or ml/kg/min did not differ between pregnancy and postpregnancy tests.

Cardiac Function at Maximal Oxygen Uptake

Cardiac output (L/min) at $\dot{V}O_2$max, determined by acetylene rebreathing during cycle exercise, was observed to be increased in pregnancy compared to postpartum values. Stroke volume continued to increase with incremental exercise intensity even at maternal heart rates of more than 140 bpm (70), which is not observed under similar conditions in the nonpregnant state (6,44). It is possible that altered cardiac ventricular compliance not only contributes to increased stroke volume at rest but increases the contribution of stroke volume to cardiac output at extreme levels of exercise intensity. Evidence for this is found in the altered slope of percent $\dot{V}O_2$max versus pulse (69). This change causes Astrand's predictive model based on observations of maximal exertion in nonpregnant individuals to overestimate $\dot{V}O_2$max by 8% in gravidae in mid- to late pregnancy. Stroke volume was higher at $\dot{V}O_2$max during pregnancy compared to the postpartum observations. The increased Q at $\dot{V}O_2$max was associated with a reciprocal decrease in $(a\text{-}\bar{v})O_2$ difference during pregnancy compared to postpartum tests as predicted by the Fick equation $[\dot{V}O_2 = Q \cdot (a\text{-}\bar{v})DO_2]$.

Ventilation at Maximal Oxygen Uptake

Both studies observed an increase of minute ventilation at $\dot{V}O_2$max. This was also found to be increased at rest and at all work loads. The association of ventilation with $\dot{V}O_2$ and $\dot{V}CO_2$ is unaffected by pregnancy. Gestational age did not appear to affect maternal cardiorespiratory response to exertion in either cycle or treadmill exertion at $\dot{V}O_2$max

(56). These investigations (Table 66.1) suggest that neural mechanisms that control ventilatory and cardiac functional response to exertion are not affected by pregnancy.

Maternal Physiologic Response to Acute Exercise at Submaximal Aerobic Capacity

Caloric Requirements of Submaximal Exercise

Although maximal oxygen uptake appears to be unchanged during pregnancy, at least compared to postpartum values, oxygen uptake at rest and the caloric requirement of submaximal exercise appear to be increased in pregnancy. Pregnancy is characterized by an average 13% (12 kg) increase in weight in humans, approximately 4 kg of which is fetus and placenta, 5 kg is amniotic, intra- and extravascular fluid, and the remainder maternal tissue of varying metabolic activity. The effect of maternal weight gain during pregnancy on rest and submaximal exercise caloric costs and efficiency has been uncertain. Oxygen uptake during submaximal cycle ergometry has not been found to be consistently elevated during pregnancy (9,47,51,64,70,75).

One study observed that absolute oxygen consumption (L/min) is 14% higher at rest, 9% higher during weight-supported cycle exercise and 12% higher during weight-bearing treadmill exercise compared to postpartum values at identical power outputs (16). No difference between pregnancy and postpartum values was observed when oxygen uptake was expressed as a function of body weight. Difference between pregnancy and postpartum values was minimized during weight-supported exertion and when weight-bearing exertion during pregnancy was compared to the same external power output postpartum with weight added to equal body weight during pregnancy (Table 66.2) (15). These observations suggest that about 50% of the differences in O_2 uptake are attributable to weight gain, 25% by the increased O_2 uptake at rest, and 25% by pregnancy changes that render exertion during pregnancy less efficient (higher $\dot{V}O_2$ at same external power output or work load).

Exercise Efficiency

The effect of pregnancy on exercise efficiency is controversial. Graded treadmill exercise during the latter half of pregnancy and postpartum have shown that the caloric requirement for fixed work loads increases in pregnancy and decreases postpartum (9) and that this effect disappears when oxygen uptake is expressed per body weight. Others did not find a significant increase in caloric requirement during pregnancy with treadmill exertion but found a drop postpartum (47). Some observers note that $\dot{V}O_2$max and maximal aerobic power appear to be unaffected by pregnancy and that oxygen uptake at rest is increased. They have

Table 66.1 Effect of Pregnancy on Response to Maximal Aerobic Exertion

Variable	Sady et al. (70) Cycle ± SD Antepartum	Sady et al. (70) Cycle ± SD Postpartum	Lotgering et al. (56) (≥ 5 weeks) Cycle ± SEM Antepartum	Lotgering et al. (56) (≥ 5 weeks) Cycle ± SEM Postpartum	Lotgering et al. (56) (≥ 5 weeks) Treadmill ± SEM Antepartum	Lotgering et al. (56) (≥ 5 weeks) Treadmill ± SEM Postpartum
$\dot{V}O_2$						
L/min	1.91 ± 0.32	1.83 ± 0.31	2.16 ± 0.08	2.19 ± 0.07	2.38 ± 0.09	2.39 ± 0.08
ml/(kg · min)	27.3 ± 4.76	28 ± 5.13				
$\dot{V}E$ (L/min)	90.5 ± 13.91	82.1 ± 14.32*	94.6 ± 2.9	89.58 ± 3	99.6 ± 3.3	91.7 ± 2.6*
RER	1.17 ± 0.054	1.22 ± 0.097*				
HR (beats/min)	182 ± 7.8	184 ± 7.1	174 ± 2	178 ± 2*	178 ± 2	183 ± 2*
$\dot{Q}$ (L/min)	16 ± 2.46	13.93 ± 2.08*				
SV (ml/v beat)	88 ± 14.4	76 ± 11.5*				
(a-$\bar{v}$)O_2 difference (ml/100 ml)	11.99 ± 1.69	13.19 ± 1.49*				

Note. L/min = liters per minute; ml/kg/min = milliliters per kilogram per minute; RER = respiratory exchange ratio; HR = heart rate; beats/min = beats per minute; $\dot{Q}$ = cardiac output; SV = stroke volume; $\dot{V}E$ = minute ventilation; (a-$\bar{v}$)O_2 difference = arterial–mixed venous oxygen difference; ml/100 ml = milliliters per 100 milliliters.
*$p < .01$ antepartum vs. postpartum.

Table 66.2 Absolute and Relative $\dot{V}O_2$ During Weight-Bearing and Supported Exercise

Exercise mode	Antepartum	Postpartum	p value
	1/min		
Cycle ergometer	1.04 ± 0.08	0.95 ± 0.09	.014
Treadmill	1.45 ± 0.19	1.27 ± 0.20	.0001
Weighted treadmill		1.36 ± 0.20	.02
	ml/(kg · min)		
Cycle ergometer	14.8 ± 1.5	15.0 ± 2.4	> .05
Treadmill	20.4 ± 1.4	19.8 ± 0.9	> .05
Weighted treadmill		19.2 ± 0.9	.02

Note. Values are means ± SD. Cycle ergometer exercise was at 60 watts; treadmill exercise was at 4.0 km/h, 10% grade. Ante- to postpartum significance levels are reduced to $p = .025$ for treadmill comparisons using Bonferoni's correction of paired t tests. See reference 16.

surmised from this that the same increment of external work per time to reach maximal aerobic power can thereby be accomplished with a reduced increment in $\dot{V}O_2$ and have concluded that exercise efficiency (power/$\dot{V}O_2$) is higher in pregnancy.

Others observed that a certain amount of vertical work on a treadmill required less $\dot{V}O_2$ during pregnancy compared to antenatal values (20) and suggested that this resulted from higher exercise efficiency during pregnancy. However, (a) the effect of work intensity (power) on work-associated oxygen uptake (58), (b) the uncertain effect of pregnancy-related changes in body composition on the metabolic cost at rest and exercise, and (c) the unmeasured effect of pregnancy on the accrual of oxygen debt all leave the potential effect of pregnancy on exercise efficiency uncertain.

Recovery From Exertion

Pregnancy also affects recovery from intense upright exertion. Stroke volume measured 3 min after cessation of exertion was observed to fall 26% from preexercise values compared to an 11% decline between exercise and recovery in the same individuals postpartum (61). The alterations in recovery stroke volume may be secondary to increased venous capacitance in the lower extremities or to obstruction of returning blood flow because of the enlarged uterus. Either or both may result in transiently decreased venous return to the heart and decreased cardiac preload immediately after exercise cessation. It is unknown whether the decrease in stroke volume corresponds to a fall in cardiac output and reduction of uterine perfusion in the recovery period in pregnant women. The possibility of recovery phase deficits in uterine perfusion suggests that exercising pregnant women should be careful to follow a prolonged period of cool-down, decrescendo exercise.

Thermoregulation During Exercise in Pregnancy

Fetal Costs of Maternal Hyperthermia

Hyperthermia can result from prolonged exertion in increased ambient temperatures. Maternal hyperthermia may compromise homeostasis in the conceptus. First, organogenesis may be affected during the first trimester. Core temperature elevations about 40 °C have resulted in increased rates of teratogenesis in animal models (45). Second, maternal exercise-related hyperthermia probably reduces fetal metabolic reserve. The increased maternal core temperature decreases oxygen affinity for maternal and fetal hemoglobin and makes heat exchange between the fetus and its environment less efficient. Both of these changes in fetal environment may increase fetal cardiac output, which is highly heart-rate-dependent, and thereby increase cardiac work and metabolic requirements. To this is added the probable reduction of uterine perfusion resulting from maternal exercise.

Thermogenesis of Maternal Exercise

Accordingly, there has been interest in the thermogenic effects of submaximal exertion on exercising women. Cycle exercise at approximately 60% of maximal aerobic power (15,22,41) and treadmill exercise at approximately the same level of intensity have produced a rise in rectal temperatures of 0.3 °C to 1.0 °C during exertion measured by thermistor probe. The rise in temperature appears to be inversely related to gestational age (22,41). These experiments were performed at temperatures of 19 °C to 21 °C with a relative humidity of 30% to 55%. The duration of exercise was less than 30 min. These data are reassuring with respect to maternal exertion under controlled ambient conditions. Maternal thermoregulatory capacity under conditions of increased ambient heat or humidity have not been examined. In none of these studies was there evidence of fetal asphyxia based on monitoring done either during or after exercise sessions. In these human studies, however, there is inadequate evaluation of fetal homeostasis with respect to changes in maternal temperature. It is possible that modest changes in maternal core temperature during more prolonged periods of exertion may have a demonstrable effect on fetal homeostasis.

Maternal Endocrine Response to Exertion

The endocrinologic response to exercise mediates the alteration of perfusion of nonexercising and exercising vascular beds and the mobilization of fuel. In the nonpregnant state, exercise results in an immediate increase in norepinephrine concentration. Plasma epinephrine concentration is also increased with prolonged and intense exertion. At rest, plasma norepinephrine and epinephrine concentrations appear to be unchanged in pregnancy (7). Exertion appears to produce changes in norepinephrine and epinephrine of similar amplitude in pregnancy as in the nonpregnant state (1,5).

In the nonpregnant state, insulin concentration appears to fall shortly after the onset of vigorous exertion in response to alpha-adrenergic stimulation of the pancreas (37) despite a 15% to 20% rise in plasma glucose. A resulting fourfold rise in glucose production has been measured after 40 min of moderate exertion (36). Maternal insulin response has been tested during mild exertion during pregnancy (3). However, the degree of exertional intensity was probably inadequate to provoke a significant fall in insulin concentration. The effect of pregnancy on exercise-induced rises and concentrations in glucagon, growth hormone, and cortisol has not been tested under the conditions of prolonged and intense exertion required to elicit these responses in nonpregnant individuals.

Fetoplacental Homeostasis During Maternal Exercise

Fetal Gas Exchange in Animal Models During Maternal Exercise

The capacity for marked increases in caloric expenditure during exertion is predicated not only on increased perfusion to exercising muscle but also upon vasoconstriction in nonexercising vascular beds, particularly that of the viscera. Splanchnic perfusion falls linearly with increased oxygen uptake (66). Uterine blood flow is also reduced during moderate to extreme exertion during pregnancy in ungulate models and humans. Sheep exercised at 70% maximum oxygen consumption for 40 min demonstrate a 24% reduction of uterine blood flow at a time when maternal blood volume is decreased by 14% (54). Under these conditions the fetus sustains an 11% fall in partial pressure of oxygen (PO_2). Despite this, however, total uterine oxygen consumption is maintained (55). Another study found that when pregnant ewes were exercised to exhaustion, uterine blood flow fell 28% and fetal arterial PO_2 was reduced 30% without net lactate production or reduction of uterine or umbilical oxygen uptake (19).

These experiments suggested that exercise during human pregnancy might result in significant alterations in fetal environment and could potentially compromise fetal oxygen uptake. These studies also demonstrated, however, that even under conditions of extreme maternal exertion, the sheep fetus was able to maintain metabolic homeostasis during short-term maternal exertion.

Fetal Heart Rate During and After Maternal Exertion in Humans

Concerns about human exercise, however, were raised by observations of fetal bradycardia even with mild to moderate maternal exertion (2,4,42). However all of these observations were made with Doppler detection of fetal heart motion and were therefore subject to maternal movement artifact. The observation that fetal bradycardia would, in some cases, begin immediately after initiation of maternal exertion also suggested that maternal artifact may have been a confounder in these studies (42,63).

Subsequent studies have examined women in mid- and late pregnancy during submaximal and maximal aerobic exertion and monitored fetal heart rate response by direct continuous observation by two-dimensional fetal cardiac imaging during (14) and after these exercise protocols (14,56).

In the first study, 85 submaximal and 79 maximal exercise tests were performed on a cycle ergometer. Only one fetal bradycardia was observed during maternal exertion, and that during a maternal vagal hypotensive episode.

Of the 79 tests of maximal voluntary exertions, 15 were followed by brief fetal bradycardia, all within 4 min of the cessation of maternal exercise. Within 30 min of cessation of maternal exercise, however, fetal heart rate recordings showing physiologic increases of fetal heart rate with fetal movement were documented in all pregnancies. In the second study, 33 women accomplished maximal aerobic exertion at 16 weeks, 25 weeks, and 35 weeks without untoward fetal effects. Women whose maximal exercise was followed by fetal bradycardia demonstrated higher peak oxygen uptake suggesting that physical fitness does not protect against and may even predispose toward post-exertional fetal bradycardia.

Baseline fetal heart rate has been demonstrated to increase following maternal exertion of moderate degree (25). Observation of fetal heart rate during maternal exertion of approximately 60% $\dot{V}O_2$max demonstrates an increase in fetal heart rate after approximately 20 min of maternal exercise. This rise in fetal heart rate response does not seem to be related to changes in maternal core temperature (15).

Effects of Maternal Exercise Training on Maternal and Perinatal Outcome

The epidemiology of workplace environment on maternal health and perinatal outcome occupies a sizable body of literature and will not be addressed here. The complex interaction of maternal aerobic exertion, isometric physical exertion, ambient temperature, humidity, noise, and exposure to chemicals and trauma can be set aside methodologically by examining recreational or laboratory maternal exercise effects on the pregnancy. Likewise, maternal confounders such as social factors, cigarette, alcohol, and drug exposure and prior adverse obstetrical history can be excluded from the prospective trials of maternal exercise.

Maternal Exercise-Training Effects on Aerobic Capacity

The effect of exercise training during pregnancy on aerobic capacity has been investigated in several observational cohort studies and randomized trials of exercise training during pregnancy. Dressendorfer (30) followed a single patient through two pregnancies and was able to demonstrate a 10% increase in extrapolated $\dot{V}O_2$max documented on incremental treadmill testing. This patient maintained her exercise training as per an exercise log. Erkkola (32) examined 62 pregnancies without exercise training and demonstrated a 17% increase in physical work capacity defined, in part, by a work load per heart rate at peak exertional effort.

A second study (33) (presumably on different patients) was a randomized trial of observed, mixed exercise training. At 26 weeks, compared to nonexercised controls, the physical work capacity increased 12% and the work load heart rate ratio had increased 16%. At 38 weeks this increment had further widened to 16% and 20%, respectively, compared to nonexercising controls. This exercise trial extended from the first through the third trimester. A small, late-pregnancy, randomized trial of unobserved swimming exercise training demonstrated a 10% decline in oxygen uptake at a pulse of 146 bpm in controls compared to a 0.7% decline in this variable among exercisers (71).

Collings (26) performed an observational cohort study in late pregnancy and demonstrated a 4% decline in extrapolated $\dot{V}O_2$max on a cycle ergometer among nonexercising women and an 18% increase in this variable among exercising women. Kulpa et al. (48) in a randomized exercise trial extending from the first through the third trimester demonstrated that exercisers had twice the increment in exercise capacity of that observed in controls during pregnancy. This was demonstrated, presumably, by oxygen uptake at a predetermined heart rate on a treadmill. Exercise during this study was documented by log and was not supervised. South-Paul et al. (72) in a randomized trial of supervised cycle exercise in late pregnancy demonstrated a 9% increase in extrapolated $\dot{V}O_2$max determined on a cycle ergometer among exercisers and only a 1% increase in this variable among nonexercising controls.

None of these studies was careful to document the means of randomization, if this took place. Exercise intensity and duration were not quantified in these trials; many of these studies did not supervise the exercise intervention. Pregnancy-related changes in measures of exercise capacity among nonexercising women were quite variable, making it unclear whether pregnancy alone has a negative or a positive effect on exercise capacity. However, chronic exercise stress of moderate intensity appears to consistently produce a measurable cardiorespiratory training effect in either extrapolated $\dot{V}O_2$max or some measure of power or oxygen uptake at a specified heart rate. This can be demonstrated over an exercise trial interval of as little as 10 weeks based on these studies.

Maternal Exercise-Training Effects on Maternal and Perinatal Outcome

Most prospective studies of the effect of maternal exercise training on maternal and perinatal outcome have not been randomized (17,21,23,24,28, 38,48) (Table 66.3). Among nonrandomized observational cohort studies the percent of absolute weight gain found among exercising women was between 76% and 89% of that found among nonexercising women. However, many of these studies were detraining studies where the control group consisted of active trainers who themselves elected to discontinue training during the pregnancy. Some studies did not adequately characterize the level of activity of either group prior to enlistment in the study. Also, these studies generally did not directly observe the level of activity among those who continued exercise training during pregnancy.

None of these studies showed differences in gestational age at delivery and none showed increased incidence of preterm birth among trainers. Most studies showed an increase of birth weight among offspring of nonexercising control subjects ranging between 62 and 623 g above trainers. However, one of these studies showed a birth-weight difference of 151 g that favored the offspring of trainers.

Hall and Kaufmann (38) demonstrated an inverse correlation between exertional frequency during pregnancy and cesarean section rate. However, in this study, the rate of exertional frequency was a matter of self-selection on the part of clients in a for-profit exercise program, and decision making regarding the cesarean section rate was not described. Otherwise, among nonrandomized trials, only one study showed a significant difference in cesarean section rates favoring the training group (21). In this study the cesarean section rate of 6% among 87 trainers contrasted with the cesarean section rate of 30% among 44 control patients. Because the weight differential between the offspring of the two groups is only 407 g, it is unclear why the incidence of secondary arrest in labor was 14% among controls and 2% among exercising subjects, nor is it clear why the cesarean section rate among controls was as high as 30%.

Two randomized trials (17,48) examined pregnancy and labor complications and found no increase in problems among those who exercised. However, the number of subjects in each study (N = 38 and 85) may have been inadequate to demonstrate differences in the frequency of relatively uncommon events. The former study (17) was a randomized trial of sedentary women in contrast with previous studies. All exercise was served in the laboratory and the subjects were sedentary at the time of enlistment in the study. This investigation demonstrated no difference in gestational age or birth weight at delivery and no significant difference in cesarean section rate (Table 66.4).

Uterine activity has been examined with an abdominally applied pressure transducer both during (31) and immediately after (74) maternal exertion. The former study demonstrated that nonrecumbent exercise was associated with increased uterine contractions during exertion. However, the latter demonstrated no evidence of increased uterine activity immediately after cessation of maternal exertion. Because neither these nor other studies have adequately documented intrauterine pressure, the accuracy of transabdominal monitoring in establishing uterine activity has not been validated. Data derived from pregnancies subjected to acute and chronic exercise stress suggest that maternal exertion does not predispose to preterm labor. The effect of maternal exertion on perinatal outcome among patients who are predisposed to preterm labor (e.g., pregnancies complicated by twins, polyhydramnios, or uterine anomalies) has not been examined.

The differences between nonrandomized and randomized exercise studies with respect to pregnancy outcome, namely maternal weight gain, birth weight, labor abnormalities, and cesarean section rates suggest that nonrandomized studies may be biased by subject self-selection of exercise and the generalizability of their findings limited by the effects of chronic athletic training prior to conception. Limited data from randomized protocols suggest that, at least among sedentary women exposed to exertional training during pregnancy, such intervention does not predispose to maternal nutritional deprivation, fetal growth compromise, or preterm labor (17,48).

Exercise and Gestational Diabetes

Gestational Diabetes

Compared to nondiabetic nonpregnant women, nondiabetic pregnant women have higher insulin:glucose ratios during oral glucose tolerance tests suggesting insulin resistance. Also, normal gravida demonstrate decreased glucose uptake during the euglycemic hyperinsulinemic clamp at similar insulin and glucose concentrations compared to nonpregnant controls (68). These authors also demonstrated decreased adipocyte insulin

Table 66.3 Exercise Training Effects on Aerobic Capacity During Pregnancy

Author	Design	Number of pregnancies in such group	Training variable	Response to pregnancy	Response to training
Dressendorfer (30)	Observational cohort; pre- and postpregnancy; exercise log, running	2	Extrapolated $\dot{V}O_2max$, incremental treadmill	—	10% increase
Erkkola (32)	Observational cohort; 1st through 3rd trimester; observed mixed training	62	Physical work capacity, work load/peak heart rate	17% increase	
Erkkola (33)	Randomized trail; 1st through 3rd trimester; observed mixed training	31/31	Physical work capacity, work load/peak heart rate	—	26 weeks vs. controls 12% increase PWC 16% increase WL/HR 38 weeks vs. controls 16% increase PWC 20% increase WL/HR
Sibley et al. (71)	Randomized trial; late pregnancy; unobserved swimming	6/7	$\dot{V}O_2$[ml/(kg · min)] at pulse = 146, treadmill	10.4% decline	0.7% decline
Collings et al. (26)	Observational cohort; late pregnancy; observed mixed training	8/12	Extrapolated $\dot{V}O_2max$, cycle ergometer	4% decline	18% increase
Kulpa et al. (48)	Randomized trial; 1st through 3rd trimester; exercise log, mixed training	47/38	MET at predetermined HR, treadmill	—	~ 100% increase compared to controls
South-Paul et al. (72)	Randomized trial; late pregnancy; observed cycle exercise	7/10	Extrapolated $\dot{V}O_2max$, cycle ergometer	1% increase	95 increase

Note. $\dot{V}O_2max$ = maximal volume of oxygen consumed per minute during exercise; — = not applicable; PWC = physical work capacity; WL/HR = work load per heart rate; ml/(kg · min) = milliliter per kilogram per minute; MET = metabolic equivalent.

Table 66.4 Controlled Trials of Chronic Maternal Exercise Effects on Pregnancy Outcome

Author	Design	Number controls/ exercisers	Maternal weight gain of controls/ exercisers (kg)	Gestational age at delivery (controls/exercisers)	Arrest in labor controls/ exercisers (%)	Fetal body weight differences of controls/exercisers (g)	Fetal distress for controls/exercisers (%)	Percent deliveries by cesarean section
Dale et al. (28)	Observational cohort; continuance of training; unobserved running	11/12	12.9/11.2	—	—	62	—	—
Clapp and Dickstein (24)	Observational cohort, matched; continuance of training; unobserved mixed exercise	29/29	16.0/12.2	280/274 days	—	623	12.5/10.3	12.5/10.3
Hall and Kaufmann (38)	Observational cohort; four exercise frequency levels; observed mixed exercise	393/82/ 309/61	—	40/40/40/40 weeks	—	−151 (lowest–highest)	—	28/23/19/17
Clapp (23)	Observational cohort; continued vs. detraining; unobserved running and aerobics	55/42	16.4/13.5	—	—	310	25/14	30/6
Clapp (21)	Observational cohort; continued vs. detraining; unobserved running and aerobics	44/87	—	281/279 days	14/2	407	—	—
Kulpa et al. (48)	Randomized (?) trial; unknown pretraining state; unobserved mixed exercise	47/38	14.9/13.3	—	—	—	—	—
Carr et al. (17)	Randomized trial; sedentary subjects; observed cycle exercise	20/18	—	40/40 weeks	—	−23	—	10/17

Note. — = no data available.

binding during late pregnancy. Others have demonstrated reduced maximal insulin responsiveness (39) suggesting that postreceptor events in addition to insulin receptor interactions are also influenced by pregnancy.

Gestational diabetes is defined as diminished glucose tolerance demonstrated during an oral glucose tolerance test during pregnancy. This condition is characterized by reduced insulin-mediated glucose uptake during an euglycemic clamp (13) and abnormalities in insulin release during an intravenous glucose tolerance test when patients with gestational diabetes compared to healthy pregnant controls (11). Therefore, women with gestational diabetes have abnormalities in both insulin release and insulin action, which also characterize Type II diabetes (62,77).

Exercise Effects on Insulin Action and Glycemia

Exercise appears to have effects on receptor and postreceptor events. Single bouts of exercise produce increased insulin sensitivity for as long as 48 hr postexertion. Also, insulin responsiveness, the maximal glucose uptake achieved by insulin, is increased by a single bout of exercise (59). In addition, suppressibility of endogenous glucose production by insulin also appears to be increased by a single exercise bout in Type II diabetic men (29). Detraining among nondiabetic men and women results in reduced insulin sensitivity but no change in insulin responsiveness (46).

These latter observations suggest that training may increase insulin receptor number or affinity but not postreceptor events in muscle and fat. Limited information is available regarding the effect of single bouts of exercise or exercise training in gestational diabetes. Jovanovic-Peterson et al. (43) performed a controlled exercise trial for 6 weeks in 19 gestational diabetic subjects, all of whom were given diet therapy. Baseline glycosylated hemoglobin, as well as fasting and 1 hr post-50 g oral glucose challenge values, were the same in both groups. The 6-week exercise trial resulted in significant differences of glycosylated hemoglobin (4.7% in controls vs. 4.2% in trainers), and in significant reductions of fasting glucose values (87.6 mg/dl vs. 70.1 mg/dl, respectively) and 1-hr challenge test results (187.3 mg/dl vs. 105.9 mg/dl, respectively).

What is remarkable about this study is that the exercise intervention consisted of only 20 min of arm crank exercise at maternal heart rates less than 140 bpm three times per week. The authors estimated that exertional intensity never exceeded 50% maximal oxygen uptake. This effect on the fasting glycemia and glycosylated hemoglobin concentrations suggests that exercise intervention of only modest intensity, perhaps not enough to produce cardiorespiratory training effects, may have a salutary effect on gestational diabetes.

Gestational diabetes is associated with a 20% to 30% incidence of fetal macrosomia with an increased risk of birth trauma and neonatal metabolic abnormalities all of which have been associated with the degree of maternal hyperglycemia or obesity. Treatment of gestational diabetes at the present time is logistically difficult and often associated with inadequate surveillance of maternal glycemia. Treatment of this disorder with modest exercise intervention rather than insulin may be logistically easier, less costly, and potentially more acceptable to affected pregnant women. Confirmatory studies of the clinical efficacy of prescribed exercise training in gestational diabetes are presently lacking.

Research Questions

Prioritization of research interests may be predicated on a broad array of assumptions regarding biology, public health, and social issues. Consequently, any list of research priorities is incomplete and subject to revision. The National Heart, Lung, and Blood Institute of the National Institutes of Health sponsored a consensus conference on "Physical Activity and Cardiovascular Health" in August, 1991. Recommendations made during the conference were focused on research design and content.

The design recommendations concerned establishing standards of randomized, controlled trials of exercise intervention when feasible (depending on research hypotheses) and improving standards of description of experimental conditions and quantification of exertional intervention and effects. The recommendation of content for future research included

1. the interaction of exercise stress and pregnancy in normal pregnancy, lactation, and puerperium;
2. the interaction of exercise and pregnancy complicated by maternal and fetal disease;
3. the impact of exercise on pregnancy complicated by chronic maternal cardiovascular or metabolic disease; and
4. the effect of maternal activity, including workplace exertion, on maternal and perinatal outcome.

References

1. Airaksinen, K.E.J.; et al. Effect of pregnancy on autonomic nervous function and heart rate in diabetic and nondiabetic women. Diabetes Care. 10:748-751; 1987.
2. Artal, R.; Paul, R.H.; Romeo, Y.; Wiswell, R. Fetal bradycardia induced by maternal exercise. Lancet. 2:258; 1984.
3. Artal, R.; Platt, L.D.; Sperling, M.; Kammula, R.K.; Jilek, J.; Nakamura, R. Exercise in pregnancy I. Maternal cardiovascular and metabolic responses in normal pregnancy. Am. J. Obstet. Gynecol. 140:123; 1981.
4. Artal, R.; Rutherford, S.; Romem, Y.; Kammula, R.K.; Dorey, F.J.; Wiswell, R.A. Fetal heart rate responses to maternal exercise. Am. J. Obstet. Gynecol. 155:729-733; 1986.
5. Artal, R.; Wiswell, R.; Romeo, Y. Hormonal responses to exercise in diabetic and nondiabetic pregnant patients. Diabetes. [Suppl. 2]. 34:78-80; 1985.
6. Astrand, P.O.; Cuddy, T.E.; Saltin, B.; Stenberg, J. Cardiac output during submaximal and maximal work. J. Appl. Physiol. 19:268; 1964.
7. Barron, W.M.; Mujais, S.K.; Zinaman, M.; Bravo, E.L.; Lindheimer, M.D. Plasma catecholamine responses to physiologic stimuli in normal human pregnancy. Am. J. Obstet. Gynecol. 154:80-84; 1986.
8. Barwin, B.N.; Roddie, I.C. Venous distensibility during pregnancy determined by graded venous congestion. Am. J. Obstet. Gynecol. 125(7):921-923; 1976.
9. Blackburn, M.W.; Calloway, D.H. Basal metabolid rate and work energy expenditure of mature, pregnant women. J. Am. Diet. Assoc. 69:24-28; 1976.
10. Boutourline-Young, H.; Boutourline-Young, E. Alveolar carbon dioxide levels in pregnant parturient and lactating subjects. J. Obstet. Gynaecol. Br. Comm. 63:509-528; 1956.
11. Buchanan, T.; Metzger, B.; Freinkel, N. Impaired B-cell function rather than exaggerated insulin resistance distinguishes gestational diabetes from normal pregnancy. 47th annual meeting. Indianapolis: American Diabetes Association; 1987.
12. Capeless, E.; Clapp, J. Cardiovascular changes during pregnancy. Society of gynecologic investigation scientific program and abstracts 36th annual meeting. 165; 1989.
13. Carpenter, M.; Terry, R.; Carr, S.; Haydon, B.; Dorcas, B.; Thompson, P.; Coustan, D.; Cowett, R. Endogenous glucose production mediates insulin resistance in normal but not gestational diabetic pregnancy. Abstract 41. Society for Gynecologic Investigation Annual Meeting; San Antonio, TX; 1992.
14. Carpenter, M.W.; Sady, S.P.; Hoegsberg, B.; Sady, M.A.; Haydon, B.; Cullinane, E.M.; Coustan, D.R.; Thompson, P.D. Fetal heart rate response to maternal exertion. JAMA. 259:20; 1988.
15. Carpenter, M.W.; et al. Maternal exercise duration and intensity affect fetal heart rate. American College of Sports Medicine annual meeting, Baltimore, MD; 1989.
16. Carpenter, M.W.; Sady, S.P.; Sady, M.A.; Haydon, B.; Coustan, D.R.; Thompson, P.D. Effect of maternal weight gain during pregnancy on exercise performance. J. Appl. Physiol. 68(3): 1173-1176; 1990.
17. Carr, S.R.; Carpenter, M.W.; Terry, R.; Lengle, A.; Haydon, B. Obstetrical outcome in aerobically trained women. Orlando, FL: Society for Perinatal Obstetricians; 1992.
18. Clapp, J.F. Cardiac output and uterine blood flow in the pregnant ewe. Am. J. Obstet. Gynecol. 130:419; 1978.
19. Clapp, J.F. Acute exercise stress in the pregnant ewe. Am. J. Obstet. Gynecol. 136:489; 1980.
20. Clapp, J.F. Oxygen consumption during treadmill exercise before, during and after pregnancy. Abstract 175. Society for gynecologic investigation annual meeting. 1989.
21. Clapp, J.F. The course of labor after endurance exercise during pregnancy. Am. J. Obstet. Gynecol. 163:1799-1804; 1990.
22. Clapp, J.F. The changing thermal response to endurance exercise during pregnancy. Am. J. Obstet. Gynecol. 165:1684; 1991.
23. Clapp, J.F.; Capeless, E.L. Neonatal morphometrics after endurance exercise during pregnancy. Am. J. Obstet. Gynecol. 163:1805-1811; 1990.
24. Clapp, J.F.; Dickstein, S. Endurance exercise and pregnancy outcome. Med. Sci. Sports Exerc. 16(6):556-562; 1984.
25. Collings, C.; Curet, L.B. Fetal heart rate response to maternal exercise. Am. J. Obstet. Gynecol. 151:498-501; 1985.
26. Collings, C.M.S.; Curette, L.B.; Mullin, J.P. Maternal and fetal responses to a maternal aerobic exercise program. Am. J. Obstet. Gynecol. 145:702; 1983.
27. Cugell, D.W.; Frank, N.R.; Gaensler, E.A.; Badger, T.L. Pulmonary function in pregnancy. I. Serial observations in normal women. Am. Rev. Tuberc. 678:568; 1953.
28. Dale, E.; Mullinax, K.M.; Bryan, D. Exercise during pregnancy: Effects on the fetus. Can. J. Appl. Sport Sci. 7:2, 98-103; 1982.

29. Devlin, J.T.; Hirshman, M.; Horton, E.D.; Horton, E.S. Enhanced peripheral and splanchnic insulin sensitivity in NIDDM men after single bout of exercise. Diabetes. 36:434-439; 1987.
30. Dressendorfer, R.H. Physical training during pregnancy and lactation. Phys. Sportsmed. (February): pp. 74-80; 1978.
31. Durak, E.P.; Jovanovic-Peterson, L.; Peterson, C.M. Comparative evaluation of uterine response to exercise on five aerobic machines. Am. J. Obstet. Gynecol. 162:754-756; 1990.
32. Erkkola, R. The physical work capacity of the expectant mother and its effect on pregnancy, labor and the newborn. Int. J. Gynaecol. Obstet. 14:153-159; 1976.
33. Erkkola, R. The influence of physical training during pregnancy on physical work capacity and circulatory parameters. Scand. J. Clin. Lab. Invest. 36:747-754; 1976.
34. Faulkner, J.A.; Heigenhauser, G.F.; Schork, M.A. The cardiac output-oxygen uptake relationship of men during graded bicycle ergometry. Med. Sci. Sports Exerc. 9:148-154; 1977.
35. Fawer, R.; Dettling, A.; Weihs, D.; Welti, H.; Schelling, J.L. Effect of the menstrual cycle, oral contraception and pregnancy on forearm blood flow, venous distensibility and clotting factors. Eur. J. Clin. Pharmacol. 13:251-257; 1978.
36. Felig, P.; Wahren, J. Role of insulin and glucagon in the regulation of hepatic glucose production during exercise. Diabetes. [Suppl. 1]. 28:31-75; 1979.
37. Galbo, H. Hormonal and metabolic adaptation to exercise. New York: GT Verlag, Inc.; 1983.
38. Hall, D.C.; Kaufmann, D.A. Effects of aerobic and strength conditioning on pregnancy outcomes. Am. J. Obstet. Gynecol. 157:1199-1203; 1987.
39. Hjollund, E.; Pedersen, O.; Espersen, T.; Klebe, J.G. Impaired insulin receptor binding and postbinding defects of adipocytes from normal and diabetic pregnant women. Diabetes. 35: 598-603; 1986.
40. Hytten, F.E.; Paintin, D.B. Increase in plasma volume during normal pregnancy. J. Obstet. Gynaecol. Br. Comm. 70:402; 1963.
41. Jones, R.L.; et al. Thermoregulation during aerobic exercise in pregnancy. Obstet. Gynecol. 65:340; 1985.
42. Jovanovic, L.; Kessler, A.; Peterson, C.M. Human maternal and fetal response to graded exercise. J. Appl. Physiol. 58(5):1719-1722; 1985.
43. Jovanovic-Peterson, L.; Durak, E.P.; Peterson, C.M. Randomized trial of diet versus diet plus cardiovascular conditioning on glucose levels in gestational diabetes. Am. J. Obstet. Gynecol. 161:415; 1989.
44. Karpman, V.L. Cardiovascular system and physical exercise, chapter 4: Pumping action of the heart and blood flow in great vessels. Boca Raton, FL: CRC Press; 1987:139-145.
45. Kilhim, L.; Ferm, V.H. Exencephaly in fetal hamsters following exposure to hyperthermia. Teratology. 14:323-326; 1976.
46. King, D.S.; Dalsky, G.P.; Clutter, W.E.; Young, D.A.; Staten, M.A.; Cryer, P.E.; Holloszy, J.O. Effects of exercise and lack of exercise on insulin sensitivity and responsiveness. J. Appl. Physiol. 64(5):1942-1946; 1988.
47. Knuttgen, H.G.; Emerson, K. Physiological response to pregnancy at rest and during exercise. J. Appl. Physiol. 36(5):549-553; 1974.
48. Kulpa, P.J.; White, B.M.; Visscher, R. Aerobic exercise in pregnancy. Am. J. Obstet. Gynecol. 156:1395-1403; 1987.
49. Laiard-Meeter, K.; van de Ley, G.; Bom, T.; Wladimiroff, J.W. Cardiocirculatory adjustments during pregnancy—an echocardiographic study. Clin. Cardiol. 2:328-332; 1979.
50. Lees, M.M.; Taylor, S.H.; Scott, D.B.; Keer, M.G. A study of cardiac output at rest throughout pregnancy. J. Obstet. Gynaecol. Br. Comm. 74:3; 1967.
51. Lehmann, V.; Regnat, K. Untersuchung sur korperlichen belastungsfahigkeit schwangeren frauen. Der einfluss standardisierter arbeit auf herzkreislaufsystem, ventilation, gasaustausch, kohlenhydratstoffwechsel und saure-basen-haushalt. Z Beburtshilfe Perinato. 180:279-289; 1976.
52. Lewis, S.F.; Taylor, W.F.; Graham, R.M.; Pettinger, W.A.; Schutte, E.; Blomqvist, C.G. Cardiovascular responses to exercise as functions of absolute and relative work load. J. Appl. Physiol. 54:1314-1323; 1983.
53. Longo, L.D. Maternal blood volume and cardiac output during pregnancy: A hypothesis of endocrinologic control. Am. J. Physiol. 245:R720-R729; 1983.
54. Lotgering, F.K.; Gilbert, R.D.; Longo, L.D. Exercise responses in pregnant sheep: Oxygen consumption, uterine blood flow, and blood volume. J. Appl. Physiol. 55(3):834-841; 1983.
55. Lotgering, F.K.; Gilbert, R.D.; Longo, L.D. Exercise responses in pregnant sheep: Blood gases, temperatures, and fetal cardiovascular system. J. Appl. Physiol. 55(3):842-850; 1983.
56. Lotgering, F.K.; Van Doorn, M.B.; Struijk, P.C.; Pool, J.; Wallenburg, H.C.S. Maximal aerobic exercise in pregnant women: Heart rate, O_2 consumption, CO_2 production and ventilation. J. Appl. Physiol. 70(3):1016-1023; 1991.

57. Lund, C.J.; Donovan, J.C. Blood volume during pregnancy. Am. J. Obstet. Gynecol. 98(23):393-403; 1967.

58. Margaria, R.; Cerretelli, P.; Aghemo, P.; Sassi, G. Energy cost of running. J. Appl. Physiol. 18:367-370; 1963.

59. Mikines, K.J.; Farrell, P.A.; Sonne, B.; Tronier, B.; Balbo, H. Postexercise dose-response relationship between plasma glucose and insulin secretion. Am. J. Physiol. 63(3):988-999; 1988.

60. Mitchell, J.H.; Schmidt, R.F. Cardiovascular reflex control by afferent fibers from skeletal muscle receptors. In: Shepherd, J.T.; Abboud, F.M., eds. Handbook of physiology. Section 2: The cardiovascular system volume III. Peripheral circulation and organ blood flow, part 2. Bethesda, MD: American Physiological Society; 1983:623-660.

61. Morton, M.J.; Paul, M.S.; Campos, G.R.; Hart, M.V.; Metcalfe, J. Exercise dynamics in late gestation: Effects of physical training. Am. J. Obstet. Gynecol. 152:91-97; 1985.

62. Olefsky, J.M. Lilly lecture 1980. Insulin resistance and insulin action: In vitro perspective. Diabetes. 30(2):148-162; 1981.

63. Paolone, A.M.; Shangold, M.; Paul, D.; Minnitti, J.; Weiner, S. Fetal heart rate measurement during maternal exercise-avoidance of artifact. Med. Sci. Sports Exerc. 19:6; 1987.

64. Pernoll, M.L.; Metcalfe, J.; Schlenker, T.T.; Welch, J.E.; Matsumoto, J.A. Oxygen consumption at rest and during exercise in pregnancy. Respir. Physiol. 25:285; 1975.

65. Rose, D.J.; Bader, M.E.; Bader, R.A.; Braunwald, E. Catheterization studies of cardiac hemodynamics in normal pregnant women with reference to left ventricular work. Am. J. Obstet. Gynecol. 72:2; 1956.

66. Rowell, L.B. Human circulation. Regulation during physical stress. New York: Oxford University Press; 1986.

67. Rubler, S.; Damani, P.M.; Pinto, E.R. Cardiac size and performance during pregnancy estimated with echocardiography. Am. J. Cardiol. 40:534-540; 1977.

68. Ryan, E.D.; O'Sullivan, M.J.; Skyler, J.S. Insulin action during pregnancy: Studies with the euglycemic clamp technique. Diabetes. 34:380-389; 1985.

69. Sady, S.A.; Carpenter, M.W.; Sady, M.A.; Haydon, B.; Hoegsberg, B.; Cullinane, E.M.; Thompson, P.D.; Coustan, D.R. Prediction of $\dot{V}O_2max$ during cycle exercise in pregnant women. J. Appl. Physiol. 65:657-661; 1988.

70. Sady, S.A.; Carpenter, M.W.; Thompson, P.D.; Sady, M.A.; Haydon, B.; Coustan, D.R. Cardiovascular response to cycle exercise during and after pregnancy. J. Appl. Physiol. 66:336-341; 1989.

71. Sibley, L.; Ruhling, R.O.; Cameron-Foster, J.; Christensen, C.; Bolen, B.S. Swimming and physical fitness during pregnancy. J. Nurse Midwifery. 26(6):3-12; 1981.

72. South-Paul, J.E.; Rajagopal, E.R.; Tenholder, M.F. The effect of participation in a regular exercise program upon aerobic capacity during pregnancy. Obstet. Gynecol. 71:175; 1988.

73. Ueland, K.; Novy, M.J.; Peterson, E.N.; Metcalfe, J. Maternal cardiovascular dynamics. Am. J. Obstet. Gynecol. 104:6; 1969.

74. Veille, J.C.; Hohimer, R.A.; Burry, K.; Speroff, L. The effect of exercise on uterine activity in the last eight weeks of pregnancy. Am. J. Obstet. Gynecol. 151:727-730; 1985.

75. Ueland, K.; Novy, M.J.; Metcalfe, J. Cardiorespiratory responses to pregnancy and exercise in normal women and patients with heart disease. Am. J. Obstet. Gynecol. 115:4-10; 1973.

76. Walters, W.A.W.; MacGregor, W.G.; Hills, M. Cardiac output at rest during pregnancy and the puerperium. Clin. Sci. 30:1-11; 1966.

77. Ward, W.K.; Johnson, C.L.W.; Beard, J.C.; Benedetti, T.J.; Halter, J.B.; Porte, D. Insulin resistance and impaired insulin secretion in subjects with histories of gestational diabetes mellitus. Diabetes. 34:861-869; 1985.

78. Wilson, M.; Morganti, A.; Zervoudakis, J.; Letcher, K.L.; Romney, B.M.; et al. Blood pressure, the renin-aldosterone system and sex steroids throughout normal pregnancy. Am. J. Med. 68:97-104; 1980.

79. Wolfe, L.A.; Ohtake, P.J.; Mottola, M.F.; McGrath, M.J. Physiological interactions between pregnancy and aerobic exercise. Exerc. Sport Sci. Rev. 17:295; 1989.

Chapter 67

Exercise, Training, and the Male Reproductive System

David C. Cumming
Garry D. Wheeler

Effects of strenuous physical exercise, particularly endurance training, on the reproductive system have been widely recognized in women; delayed menarche, oligomenorrhea, inadequate luteal phase, and anovulatory cycles occur—although probably less frequently than was originally thought (18). The effects of various forms of physical activity on the hypothalamic–pituitary–gonadal (HPG) axis have also been examined extensively in men. As anticipated, the effects of physical activity on the male reproductive system vary with the intensity and duration of the activity and the fitness of the individual. Relatively short, intense exercise usually increases and more prolonged exercise usually decreases serum testosterone levels. There are similarities in the chronic reproductive effects ofexercise in both sexes. Endurance and other forms of training can induce subclinical inhibition of normal reproductive function, but clinical expression of reproductive dysfunction with exercise is uncommon in men. The long-term, physiological suppressionof the hypothalamic–pituitary–testicular axis in men is probably not of major significance, but it is clear that further investigation in several areas is desirable.

In this chapter, the acute and chronic effects of strenuous physical activity on the HPG axis in men will be reviewed together with an examination of possible mechanisms that may be involved in those changes.

Control of Male Reproductive Function

The testes, under control of gonadotropin-releasing hormone (GnRH) and gonadotropins [luteinizing hormone (LH) and follicle-stimulating hormone (FSH)] manufacture spermatozoa, androgens, and some nonsteroidal substances, notably inhibin. Spermatozoa transmit the genetic material from the male; cytodifferentiation of sperm requires 64 days for completion, a figure that should be remembered in planning any prospective study of the effects of activity on spermatogenesis. Androgens are responsible for the development and maintenance of male secondary sex characteristics; the principal androgen, testosterone, is produced from cholesterol in the smooth endoplasmic reticulum in Leydig cells by pathways similar to those in the ovary and adrenal (Figure 67.1). Inhibin exerts inhibitory feedback on FSH levels.

LH primarily regulates androgenesis; FSH together with a small proportion of the testosterone is responsible for spermatogenesis (Figure 67.2.) Prolactin may also be involved in regulation of testicular sex steroid production through receptors in the adult human testis (83). LH and FSH synthesis and secretion are controlled by GnRH. Pulsatile GnRH is as necessary in men as in women for

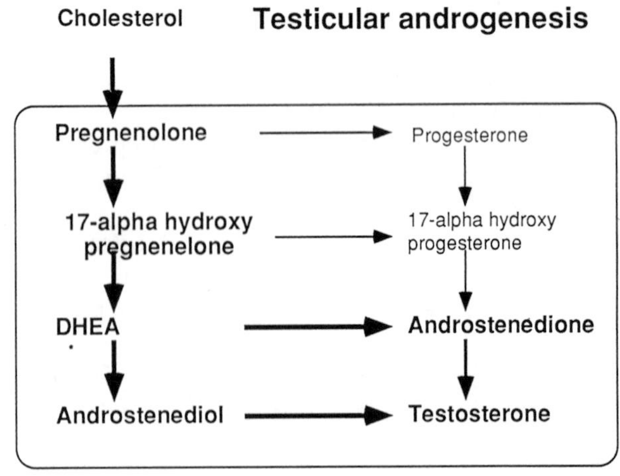

Figure 67.1 Pathways of testicular steroidogenesis.

normal pituitary function (72,73). A circhoral oscillator defines GnRH pulsatile release, which innduces LH pulses at 90- to 110-min intervals. FSH pulsatile release is difficult to demonstrate because of the small pulse amplitude and relatively long half-life of FSH versus LH (respectively, 150 min and 20 min).

The detailed interactions and physiological significance of inputs to the hypothalamic–pituitary unit (Table 67.1) are poorly understood. Sex steroids interact with neuronal elements in the hypothalamus and gonadotropin-secreting cells in the pituitary to affect particularly serum LH levels (negative feedback). The mechanism of testosterone-mediated gonadotropin inhibition at the pituitary level is not known: Possible mechanisms include reduction of gonadotropin receptor number or receptor uncoupling from subsequent biochemical events. Feedback at the hypothalamic level is indirect since steroids modulate the function of other neuronal systems that act on the GnRH-producing neuron without steroids entering the GnRH-secreting cells. Among the neural systems that have been investigated are those producing dopamine, norepinephrine, γ-aminobutyric acid (GABA), and β-endorphin. It is generally thought that dopamine and β-endorphin are inhibitory, whereas noradrenaline and GABA stimulate LH release. A number of other systems are probably involved in GnRH–gonadotropin axis inhibition but their physiological significance is not known. Investigation in the human is primitive, generally relying on the use of single agonists or antagonists to the various systems.

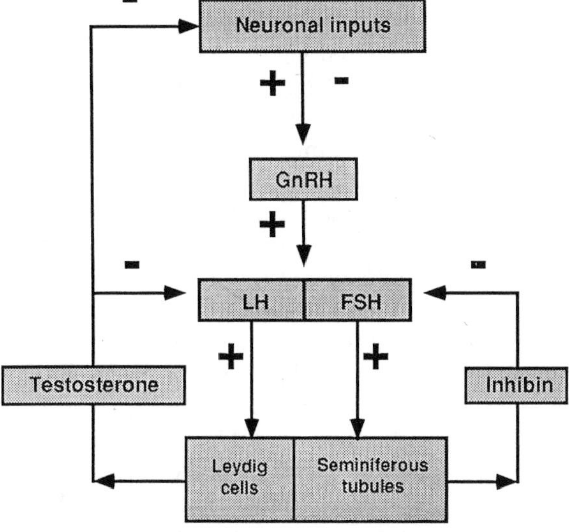

Figure 67.2 Interactions in the regulation of the hypothalamic-pituitary gonadal axis.

Exercise and training can change several factors that modulate the circulating testosterone levels (Table 67.2.). There is a temporal variation in serum testosterone levels and (noted earlier) serum LH levels. Pulsatile testosterone release is difficult to demonstrate and response to an LH pulse does not occur in less than 20 to 30 min (3,10,48,49,63,72,73,81). This is important in examining testosterone responses to short-term, strenuous physical activity.

Testosterone is bound in circulation to a specific, high-affinity plasma protein, sex-hormone-binding globulin (SHBG) and to albumin, which has a large capacity but low affinity. Testosterone is also bound to cortisol-binding globulin but in quantities that have little effect on the response to activity. Substantial changes can occur in serum albumin without significant effects on total testosterone levels. Therefore, measurement of hemoconcentration as the sole indicator of change in testosterone is of little value; to make any valid comment about hemoconcentration, SHBG levels must be measured. A small amount (less than 2%) of testoster-

Table 67.1 Inputs Into the Hypothalamic–Pituitary Unit

Inputs
Brain stem autonomic and reticular structures
Areas of the limbic forebrain (e.g., amygdala and septum)
Photic input from the retina to the suprachiasmatic nuclei
Local neuronal systems
Nonsteroidal factors (e.g., inhibin) from the seminiferous tubules
Sex steroids from the Leydig cells
Other systems including corticotropin-releasing factor, thymus, prolactin, and ependymal tanacytes

Table 67.2 Factors Determining Exercise- or Training-Associated Changes in Serum Testosterone Levels

Factor	
Synthesis/secretion	— gonadotropin-mediated (LH and FSH)
	— other (prolactin, catecholamines)
Testicular blood flow	— catecholaminergic and other controls
Protein binding	— specific, high affinity (SHBG, CBG)
	— nonspecific, low affinity (albumin)
Clearance	— target tissue uptake and metabolism
	— hepatic metabolism

one circulates as the free steroid. Testosterone binding to SHBG reduces its clearance, and it seems likely that the biologically active portion of the hormone is that bound to albumin plus the small unbound fraction (74,97), which together amount to approximately 35% of the total levels. Most (95%) of the 4 to 10 mg of testosterone secreted daily is from direct synthesis in the testes. In males, approximately half of the testosterone produced is cleared through the liver and the remainder is cleared through extrahepatic metabolism by androgen target organs including muscle (7). Modifications of binding or clearance are as significant as changes in synthesis and secretion in determining the effects of physical activity on circulating testosterone.

Acute Exercise and the HPG Axis in Men

Increased serum testosterone levels have been reported during relatively strenuous free and treadmill running, weight training, and ergometer cycling and have ranged from 13% to 185% (e.g., see Figure 67.3) (14,19,31,34,35,45,51,54, 56,58,60,69,84,85,91,98,108). One unexpected exception was the consistent decrease in serum testosterone levels seen in elite swimmers undertaking a tethered swim graded to maximum over approximately 14 min (21). Increased androstenedione and estrogens have also been reported (19,60). There is conflicting evidence about gonadotropin response: LH and FSH levels have been reported as unchanged (14,34,108), increased, (e.g., see Figure 67.4) (19,58,60), or decreased (85). It is difficult to understand the exercise-associated increase in serum testosterone levels because levels increase more quickly than anticipated from any increase in serum LH, which responds inconsistently to short-term intense exercise. Sutton, Coleman, and Casey (91) summarized the difficulty in explaining the effects of short-term, strenuous physical activity on testicular androgens in 1973 and suggested a range of possible mechanisms through which testosterone could increase (Table 67.3).

Nonspecific mechanisms associated with short-term, exercise-induced serum testosterone increases include decreased metabolic clearance rate (MCR) and hemoconcentration through decreased plasma volume. Testosterone is cleared via hepatic and extrahepatic mechanisms. Hepatic blood flow approximates 1,250 L per square meter per day; MCR of testosterone through the liver is approximately half this value. This implies that the 50% reduction in hepatic blood flow that occurs during strenuous exercise (82,99) should have little effect on the MCR of testosterone. However, clearance through the liver depends on protein binding and hepatic blood flow. Binding to SHBG inhibits hepatic testosterone metabolism whereas albumin binding does not (74). Thus the splanchnic extraction of testosterone approximates 50%. The real hepatic reserve may, therefore, be smaller than anticipated from blood flow and clearance rate figures. The metabolic clearance rate of testosterone has been described as reduced during physical activity (16,92). Exercise rates in both studies were moderate and the time course of clearance changes seems to be later than that of testosterone increments reported elsewhere (19,108).

Changes in hemoconcentration were considered important in some (34,54,69,108) but by no means all studies (19,58,59,60,65,67,85,92,98). The assumptions are (a) that the measured components (e.g., hematocrit and hemoglobin) accurately reflect degree of fluid loss, (b) that changes are not influenced by the differential binding of the steroid, and (c) that other physiological changes (e.g., increased temperature) do not affect binding. The association constants of testosterone with SHBG (1.6–1.9 $\cdot$ 10^9 L/mol) and albumin (4 $\cdot$ 10^4 L/mol) are very different (15). Because of the characteristics of testosterone binding, even substantial changes in albumin have little influence on the circulating testosterone levels. Based on the association constants, it can be calculated that if the serum albumin doubled without change in SHBG, the increase in total testosterone would approximate 6%. Although variable hemoconcentration has been reported with different forms of exercise, circulating SHBG, unlike serum protein, changes little with short- or longer term running, and increases in the testosterone:SHBG ratio suggest that hemoconcentration played no significant role (58).

For nonspecific mechanisms to be responsible for the acute, exercise-induced, serum testosterone increase, we would expect all circulating steroids to be affected in the same manner, given that MCR and hemoconcentration do not differentiate among hormones. The temporal patterns of change among the various steroid hormones do not provide this picture (19, see Figure 67.3). The timing of the testosterone increase was distinct from those of androstenedione and dehydroepiandro sterone (DHEA), adrenal androgens whose increments were simultaneous with that of cortisol (19). The clear difference in responses among the hormones

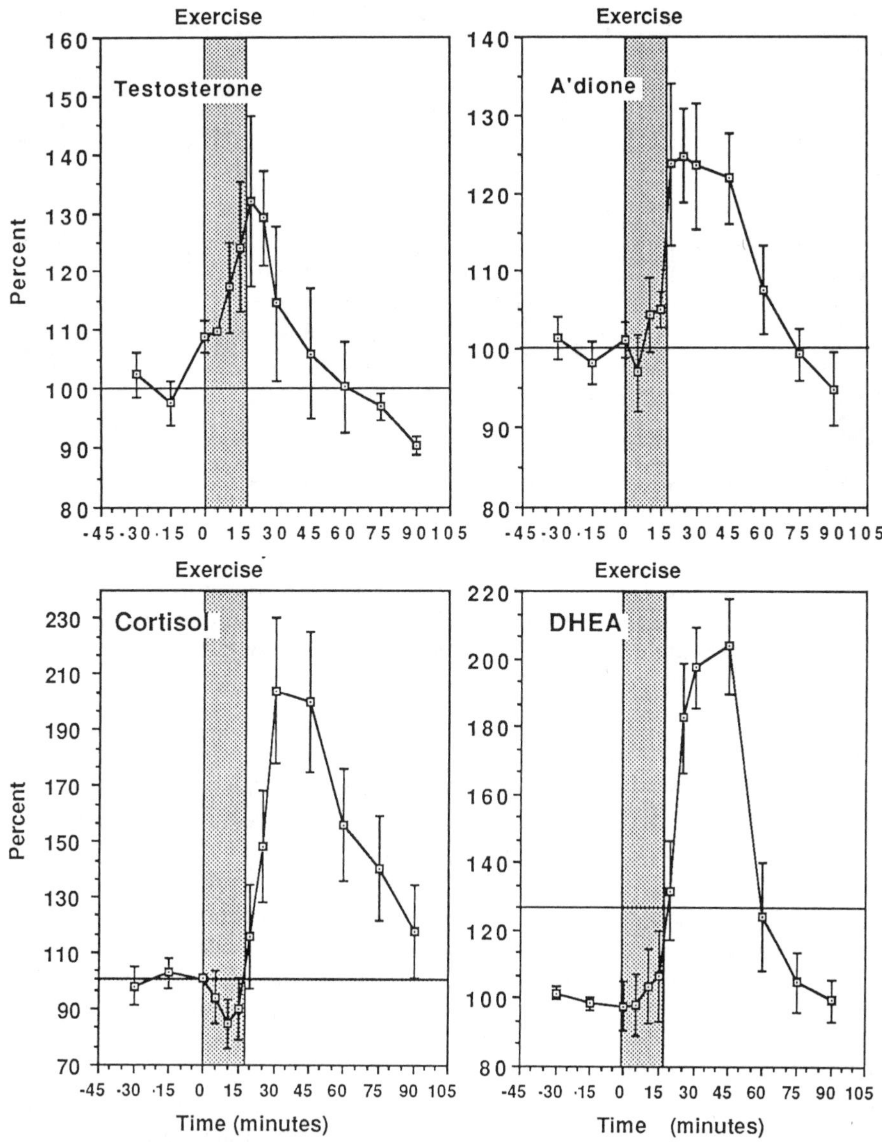

Figure 67.3 Serum testosterone, androstenedione (adione), cortisol and dehydroepiandrosterone (DHEA) prior to during and subsequent to an incremental, maximal intensity Cycle ergometer exercise in five active but untrained males. The values are shown as percent change from a baseline which consisted of the mean of the first two values. (Redrawn from data in reference 19.)

suggests that specific testicular mechanisms are involved.

What mechanism could exist independently from gonadotropin stimulation of testosterone? Dexamethasone suppression did not influence the exercise-induced testosterone response, an expected finding that indicated little adrenal contribution to the increment (90). The involvement of the sympathetic system in testicular testosterone production suggested that a direct neural pathway may stimulate testosterone production during exercise in some species (27,61). Circulating catecholamine levels also increase substantially during exercise (34). β-blockade inhibits testosterone responses to exercise, whereas L-dopa, phentolamine, and clonidine had no effect (45,55). Interestingly β-blockade at doses used in the studies reduces hepatic perfusion (13) and would, therefore, be likely to increase rather than decrease testosterone levels if this impaired hepatic blood flow were the mechanism.

As a consistent increase in testosterone was observed prior to cycle ergometry (19) and testosterone levels were proportional to anticipated work load (108), there is an anticipatory rise in serum testosterone levels that is presumably independent of hepatic perfusion or hemoconcentration. It remains unclear exactly

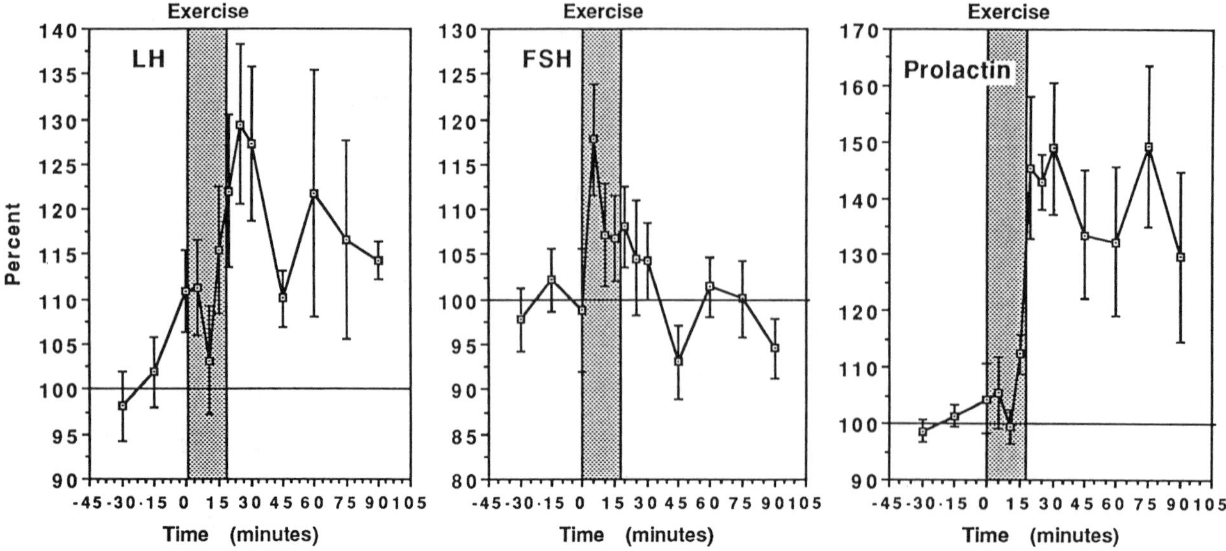

Figure 67.4 Serum LH, FSH and prolactin (Prl) prior to during and subsequent to an incremental, maximal intensity cycle ergometer exercise in five active but untrained males. The values are shown as percent change from a baseline which consisted of the mean of the first two values. (Redrawn from data in reference 19.)

Table 67.3 Possible Mechanisms Involved in the Testosterone Increase That Occurs With Short-Term Exercise

Nonspecific mechanisms
- — decreased metabolic clearance through decreased hepatic perfusion
- — hemoconcentration through decreased plasma volume

Specific mechanisms
- — gonadotropin-mediated increase in production of testosterone

what mechanisms may be operative in increasing serum testosterone levels in any particular exercise protocol and it is possible that the mechanisms responsible early in exercise may differ from those observed subsequently.

The Effects of Prolonged Exercise on the HPG Axis in Men

Prolonged submaximal exercise bouts (i.e., those exceeding 2 hr) may be associated with complex changes in circulating androgens. Responses have been examined under laboratory conditions and during free activity such as marathon and ultramarathon races, as well as cross-country skiing. Several studies have reported an initial testosterone increase with exercise followed by a decline to or below baseline values, (e.g., see Figure 67.5) (11,23,24,41,46,52,62,64,71,85,87,93–95,102). The decrease appears proportional to the preceding work load (52). Serum testosterone levels may fall following short-term, strenuous physical activity (34,60). Physical and psychological stresses such as surgery, myocardial infarction, and simulated warfare training also result in decreased testosterone levels (1,100,101). Several mechanisms may be important in decreased circulating testosterone levels during and following prolonged exercise including suppressed gonadotropin release, or a more direct effect by elevated prolactin, cortisol, or catecholamine levels.

Alterations in β-endorphin have been popularly blamed for acute exercise-associated suppression of the HPG axis in both men and women, although this has been difficult to prove because opiate antagonism does not prevent the exercise-induced decrease in LH observed by some (but by no means all) investigators (28,62,66,85,87,93). Response to GnRH has been reduced (57) and increased (93) following prolonged, exhaustive exercise. Pulsatile LH release did not decrease following 60 and 120 min of treadmill running in men, although the area under the multiple sample curve is decreased after exercise (62,66). The response of testosterone levels to stimulation with human chorionic gonadotropin (HCG) has also been described as reduced (57).

We are therefore again faced with the difficulty in explaining a change in serum testosterone levels that does not appear mediated by alterations in central control. Prolactin responses to intense or prolonged exertion are transient and unlikely to

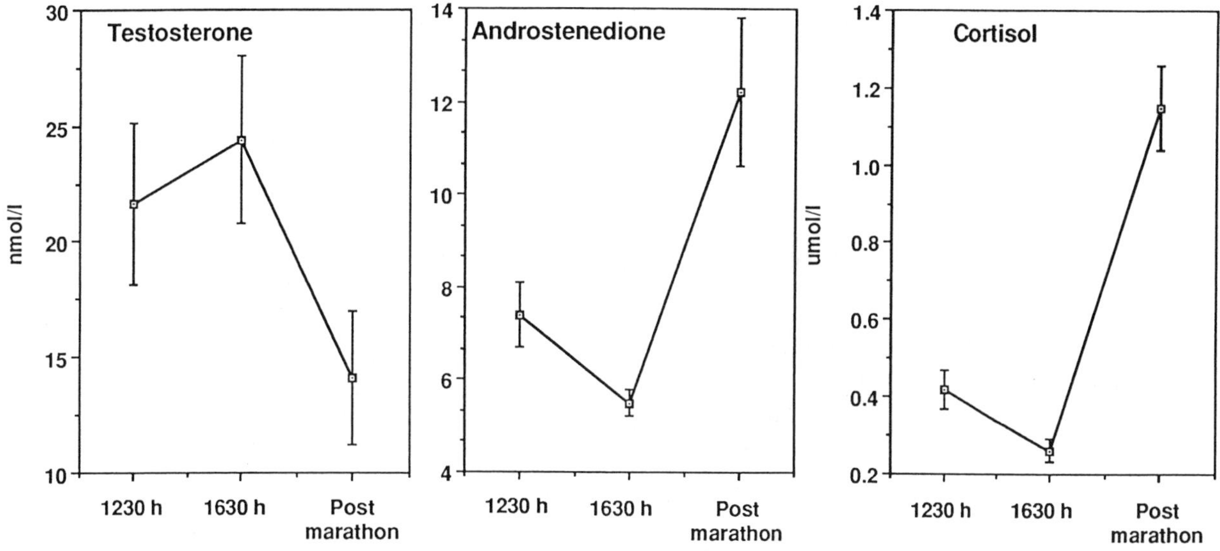

Figure 67.5 Plasma testosterone, androstenedione, and cortisol in eleven subjects prior to and following a noncompetitive run. (Redrawn from data in reference 24.)

influence postexercise testosterone levels. Decreases in serum testosterone followed increments in cortisol levels induced by insulin hypoglycemia or from injection of hydrocortisone hemisuccinate (20). Increases in serum cortisol accompany prolonged or intense exercise and therefore a similar mechanism may be operative (19,24). A decline in serum testosterone levels was observed with an exercise-induced cortisol increment (19). A persistent increase in catecholamines, which may be related to testicular resistance to endogenous gonadotropins, accompanies and follows physical activity (93). The cause for the exercise-associated physiological decline in serum testosterone levels remains unclear. It is possible that the decline results from a subtle interference at either hypothalamic or gonadal levels or because of increased androgen utilization following strenuous exercise for repair of structural and metabolic injury to the tissues.

The Effects of Endurance Training on the HPG Axis in Men

The consistent testosterone decline following prolonged submaximal exercise suggested that there may be a physiological suppression of circulating testosterone associated with chronic involvement in endurance training (e.g., see Figure 67.6). Several cross-sectional and prospective studies have now supported this idea (5,17,33,36,37,39–41, 71,89,96,103–106). Military training including a heavy physical exercise component resulted in an increase in mean plasma testosterone, androstenedione, and luteinizing hormone without change in SHBG levels (77). Prospective studies using relatively light training regimes also produced increased levels of testosterone (47,68,75). Some cross-sectional and prospective studies have reported no change in serum testosterone even with heavy training (6,76).

Symptomatic changes in testicular androgenesis and spermatogenesis are slower and less clearly definable than equivalent changes in the reproductive system of women, in whom the endocrine control of reproduction is both interactive and cyclic. There is some evidence that males with a high level of physical activity may have some impairment of fertility (5). In general there is little evidence of a decline in measures of sperm function even in runners with low physiological androgen levels (Figure 67.7). Mean semen variables in 12 high-mileage runners with serum testosterone levels at least one standard deviation below the mean were almost identical to those in a group of would-be sperm donors. Normal sperm counts are found in runners even with very strenuous training regimes (6,8,9,22). However, in an artificial insemination program donors with a high physical activity profile and low semen volume had significantly lower pregnancy rates than those with moderate activity and low semen volume (8,9). When semen volume was at a more standard level there was no reduction in fertility.

Anecdotal data has also suggested that libido may be impaired in some runners during periods

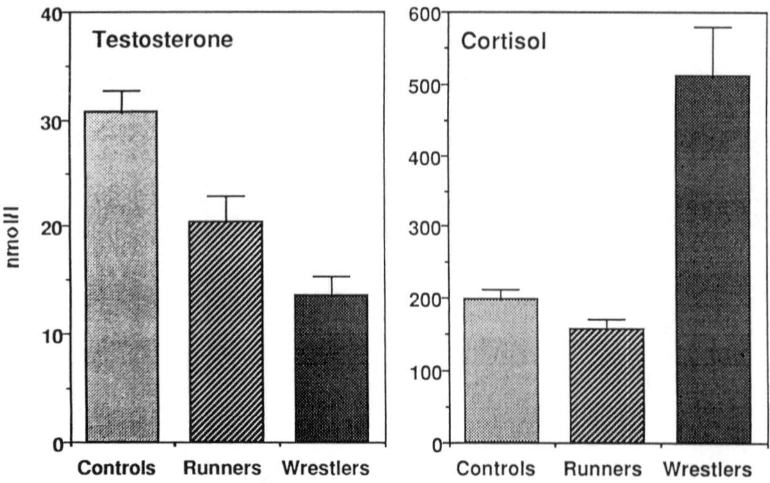

Figure 67.6 Serum testosterone and cortisol levels in controls, runners running at least 65 km per week (from reference 106), and wrestlers at peak season (Wheeler and Cumming, unpublished data).

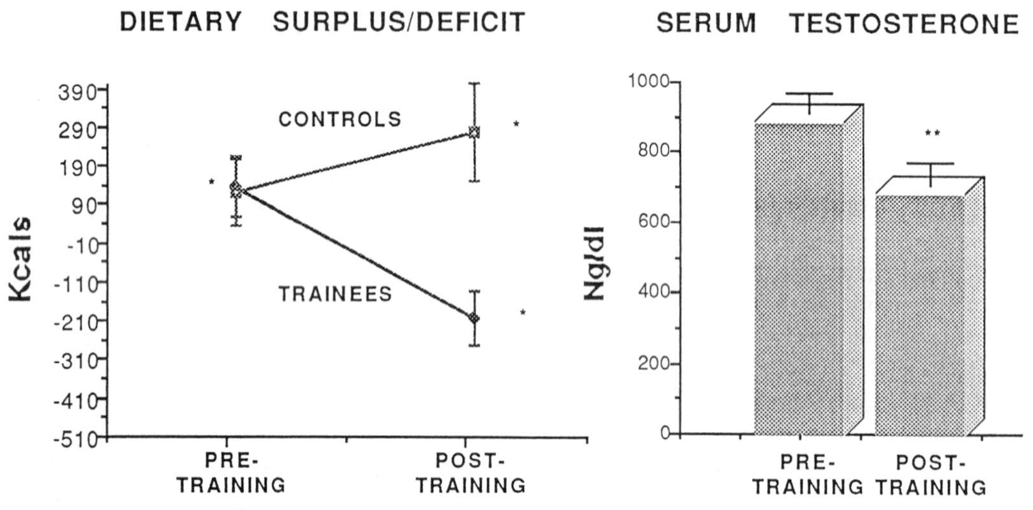

Figure 67.7 Sperm volume, sperm count, motility, progressivity, and percent of normal forms in 12 runners running at least 40 miles per week with testosterone levels greater than 1 standard deviation below the mean and 15 would-be sperm donors (Cumming, unpublished data).

of intense endurance training (106). Reduced testosterone levels may play a role in this but chronic fatigue could also be significant. A large scale study of sexuality in runners was published in *The Runner* (26). Although the scientific validity may be questioned, it is surprising that almost one quarter of the male respondents to the questionnaire would be prepared to give up sex before running and almost half have admitted that they sometimes felt too tired from running to engage in sex. The positive replies to this question increased with increasing mileage. Fitness training in middle-aged men has been reported to increase sexual drive and sexual activity in a group of previously sedentary men (mean age 44 years) (107). So little is known of short- or long-term problems with exercise-induced, symptomatic reproductive change in men that it is impossible at present to provide advice on the management of problems other than to review with the athlete having problems the possibility of decreasing the exercise load.

Androgen-dependent skeletal muscle hypertrophy and androgen synergism with growth hormone is well accepted. The decline in testosterone in rats undergoing endurance training was accompanied by increased excretion of products of muscle catabolism (25). Increased utilization of testosterone may be needed to maintain muscle in chronic exercisers, so basal testosterone or testosterone:cortisol ratios may be important (38). It is possible that one consequence of severe training regimes is a reduction of muscle damage repair because of lowered circulating testosterone levels. Concomitant catabolic effects of high cortisol levels (e.g., in *overtraining syndrome*) and inability of testosterone to prevent muscle catabolism could contribute in this regard. Testosterone and growth hormone also interact in stimulating cardiac muscle hypertrophy (70): It is possible that significant lowering of testosterone levels could influence repair of cardiac muscle.

The number of lower limb injuries, particularly *shin splints* and *stress fractures*, has increased dramatically in the high-mileage runner (88). Shin splints represent the effects of chronic mechanical stress on the bone with possible associated impairment of bone repair mechanisms. Maintenance of bone mass is steroid-dependent: Interaction of bone mass and circulating testosterone levels has been demonstrated in healthy aging men (32). The declining testosterone levels associated with high-mileage runners, particularly in the fourth and fifth decade of their lives, raise the question of implications of the early development of osteoporosis in these men. Exercise in the well-nourished male runners may prevent age-related decreases in bone mineral content, however, a case report has described osteoporotic fractures in a hypogonadal marathoner with *anorexia nervosa* (4,79). Clearly the anorexia is more significant, yet the report raised the question of how much exercise-associated hypogonadism could produce a similar, if less dramatic, effect (78).

The aerobic capacity of runners is dependent on central and peripheral factors. There is a correlation between fitness as judged by maximal oxygen consumption and reductions in exercise-associated decreases in testosterone (77). Testosterone increases synthesis of erythropoietin, which stimulates red cell manufacture: Lowered testosterone levels *could* be related to exercise-associated anemia that has been described in endurance-trained athletes. It is, however, difficult to believe that the physiological reductions in serum testosterone levels generally observed in endurance-trained athletes could affect erythropoiesis.

Physical inactivity, male gender, and elevated blood lipids are among the well-recognized risk factors for atherosclerotic heart disease. Androgens are important in regulating blood lipid levels: The blood levels of high-density lipoprotein cholesterol (HDL-C) in the blood of men are significantly lower than values in women. Because HDL-C has a cardioprotective effect, the risk of atherosclerosis is increased in men. In contrast, endurance training has been associated with lower overall cholesterol, lower low-density lipoprotein cholesterol (LDL-C) and higher HDL-C (29, 43,50,86). This change in pattern may contribute to the beneficial effects of exercise on atherosclerotic heart disease.

It is unclear whether the physiological reductions in androgens could play a significant role in these changes. Androgens may also be important in hepatic and renal function in the brain including effects on aggression and in the immune system. Although there have been concerns over the normal functioning of the immune system in endurance-trained athletes, any effect of lowered but still physiological serum testosterone levels on the immune system and hepatic and renal function remains speculative. Social and other pressures influence aggression, so that any short-term increases or longer term reduction in serum testosterone levels would be unlikely to influence mood and behavior.

The fall in serum testosterone levels must result from decreased production rates, decreased binding, or increased clearance. There is scant evidence of decreased binding (106). No studies have shown long-term increases in hepatic or extrahepatic clearance of testosterone in endurance-trained or other athletes, although basal estradiol clearance is increased in women athletes, presumably through increased hepatic metabolism (53). If testosterone levels fell because of increased hormone utilization by muscle, one might expect a compensatory gonadotropin increase and therefore restoration of normal testicular testosterone production. As demonstrated herein, some authors have suggested that this may happen; however, evidence has suggested a reduction in LH activity that could be responsible for the reductions in total and free testosterone associated with chronic involvement in running. Evidence of altered LH pulsatile release in male runners is conflicting with evidence in support of (62,66) and against it (80,105). LH pulse frequency is not significantly altered in runners with exercise (62,66). GnRH-induced LH response appears to be impaired (62). No evidence has supported increased opioidergic tone as being important in the generation of GnRH–LH suppression in athletes, and the effects of catecholamines have received little attention (28,80). Chronic elevation of serum cortisol levels has been associated with overtraining or a shift in cortisol:testosterone ratios associated with strenuous exercise (2). It is possible but unlikely that such a change could exert a direct effect on testicular testosterone production. Serum prolactin levels are chronically depressed rather than elevated and therefore not likely to be involved in the change in testosterone in highly trained male runners (104).

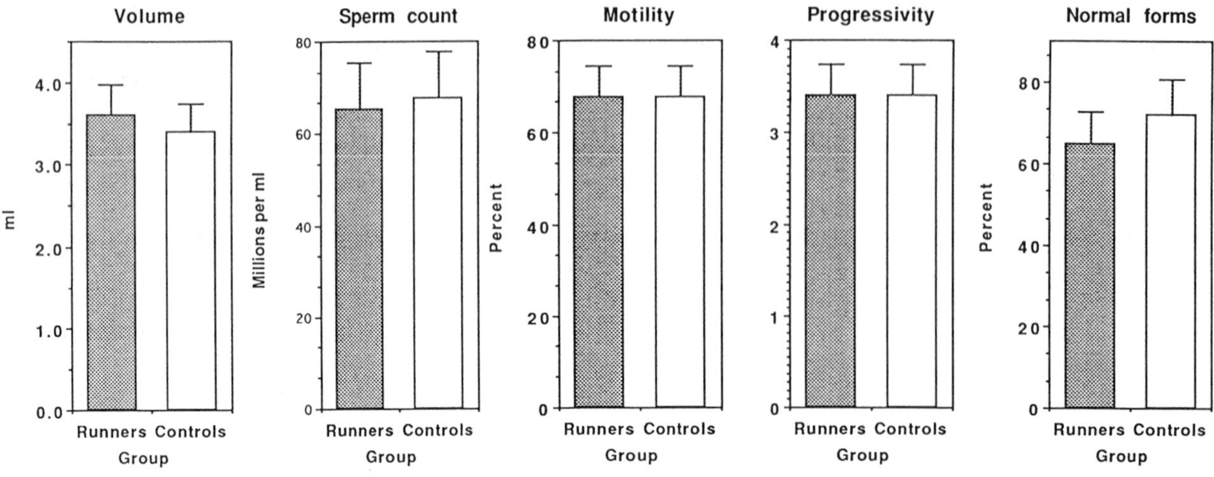

Figure 67.8 Estimated dietary surplus/deficit in control subjects and individuals undergoing 6 months of running training (Wheeler and Cumming, unpublished data).

Suppression of the HPG axis in men is associated with starvation, vegetarian diet, and low-fat, high-fiber diet (42,44,110). An anorectic subgroup with reduced total and free testosterone and a preoccupation with caloric intake and lean body mass was described among a group of 20 high-mileage runners (5). The significant reductions in total and free testosterone in wrestlers during the season were associated with their practices in trying to make weight (89). Within the season, times of dietary and fluid restriction around competition were responsible for further weight loss in wrestlers (103).

The possibility of an association between exercise and anorexia nervosa has been raised (30,105,109), but the reliability of human data has been strongly criticized (12). Although there were significant correlations among total and free testosterone and body weight and body fat in young male wrestlers (89), no correlation was observed between physiological reductions in serum testosterone levels and body fat in cross-sectional studies of runners and controls (89,105,106) and in young wrestlers followed longitudinally. A longitudinal study of sedentary individuals undergoing a 6-month training schedule found that with running the initial dietary surplus was converted to a deficit as the running increased (Figure 67.8), whereas sedentary controls over the same time actually increased their surplus (Wheeler and Cumming, unpublished data). Serum testosterone levels fell by some 30% over the 6 months and a regression analysis indicated that caloric deficit per kilogram of body weight was the most significant predictor of posttraining testosterone levels ($p < .05$).

It seems likely that chronic effects of endurance training on the HPG axis in men result from a mechanism of inhibition that is central and analogous to that described in women, perhaps involving a nutritional–metabolic influence. The possibility of peripheral effects of increased utilization of steroids is worthy of further investigation. It is unlikely that clinical expression of reproductive suppression with training is common in men. Further investigation is essential to provide continuing reassurance that "exercise is good for you," to define the physiological boundaries, and the effects of overstepping them.

References

1. Aakvaag, A.; Sand, T.; Opstad, P.K.; Fonnum, F. Hormonal changes in young men during prolonged physical strain. Eur. J. Appl. Physiol. 39:283-291; 1978.
2. Adlercreutz, H.; Harkonen, M.; Kuopposalmi, K.; Naveri, H.; Huhtaniemi, H.; Tikkanen, H.; Remes, K.; Dessypris, A.; Karvonen, J. Effect of training on plasma anabolic and catabolic steroid hormones and their responses during physical exercise. Int. J. Sports Med. [Suppl.]. 7:27-28; 1986.
3. Alford, F.P.; Baker, H.W.G.; Patel, Y.C.; Rennie, G.C.; Youatt, G.; Berger, H.G.; Hudson, B. Temporal patterns of circulating hormones as assessed by continuous blood sampling. J. Clin. Endocrinol. Metab. 36:108-116; 1973.
4. Aloia, J.F.; Cohn, S.H.; Babu, T.; Abesamic, C.; Kalici, N.; Ellis, K. Skeletal mass and body composition in marathon runners. Metabolism. 27:1793-1796; 1978.
5. Ayers, J.W.T.; Komesu, Y.; Romain, T.; Ansbacher, R.A. Anthropometric, hormonal and

psychologic correlates of semen quality in endurance trained male athletes. Fertil. Steril. 43:917-921; 1985.
6. Bagatell, C.J.; Bremner, W.J. Sperm counts and reproductive hormones in male marathoners and lean controls. Fertil. Steril. 53:688-692; 1990.
7. Baird, D.T.; Horton, R.; Longcope, C.; Tait, J.F. Steroid dynamics under steady state conditions. Recent Prog. Horm. Res. 25:611-624; 1969.
8. Baker, E.R.; Leuker, R.; Stumpf, P.G. Relationship of exercise to semen parameters and fertility success of artificial insemination donors. Fertil. Steril. [Abstract.] 41:107S; 1984.
9. Baker, E.R.; Stevens, C.; Leuker, R. Relationship of exercise to semen parameters and fertility success of artificial insemination donors. J. SC Med. Assoc. 84:580-582; 1988.
10. Baker, H.W.G.; Santen, R.J.; Berger, H.G.; de Kretser, D.M.; Hudson, B.; Peperell, R.J.; Bardin, C.W. Rhythms in the secretion of gonadotropins and gonadal steroids. J. Steroid Biochem. 6:793-801; 1975.
11. Berchtold, P.; Berger, M.; Cuppers, H.J.; Herrmann, J.; Nieschlag, E.; Rudorff, K.; Zimmerman, H.; Kruskemper, H.L. Non-glucoregulatory hormones (T4, T3, rT3, TSH, testosterone) during physical exercise in juvenile-type diabetics. Horm. Metab. Res. 10:269-273; 1978.
12. Blumenthal, J.A.; O'Toole, L.C.; Chang, J.L. Is running an analogue of anorexia nervosa? JAMA. 252:520-523; 1984.
13. Bowdle, T.A.; Freund, P.R.; Slattery, J.T. Propranolol reduces bupivacaine clearance. Anesthesiology. 66:36-38; 1987.
14. Brisson, G.R.; Volle, M.A.; Desharnais, M.; Dion, M.; Tanaka, M. Pituitary-gonadal axis in exercising man. Med. Sci. Sports Exerc. [Abstract]. 9:47; 1977.
15. Burke, C.W.; Anderson, D.C. Sex hormone binding globulin is an estrogen amplifier. Nature. 240:38-40; 1972.
16. Cadoux-Hudson, T.A.; Few, J.D.; Imms, F.J. The effect of exercise on the production and clearance of testosterone in well trained young men. Eur. J. Appl. Physiol. 54:321-325; 1985.
17. Craig, B.W.; Brown, R.; Everhart, J. Effects of progressive resistance training on growth hormone and testosterone levels in young and elderly subjects. Mech. Ageing Dev. 49:159-169; 1989.
18. Cumming, D.C. The reproductive effects of exercise and training. Curr. Probl. Obstet. Gynecol. Fertil. 10:221-285; 1987.
19. Cumming, D.C.; Brunsting, L.A., III.; Strich, G.; Greenberg, L.; Ries, A.L.; Rebar, R.W. Reproductive hormone increases in response to acute exercise in men. Med. Sci. Sports Exerc. 18:369-373; 1986.
20. Cumming, D.C.; Quigley, M.E.; Yen, S.S.C. Acute suppression of circulating testosterone levels by cortisol in man. J. Clin. Endocrinol. Metab. 57:671-673; 1983.
21. Cumming, D.C.; Wall, S.R.; Quinney, H.A.; Belcastro, A.N. Decrease in serum testosterone levels with maximal intensity swimming exercise in trained male and female swimmers. Endocr. Res. 13:31-41; 1987.
22. Cumming, D.C.; Wheeler, G.D.; McColl, E.M. The effects of exercise on reproductive function in men. Sports Med. 7:1-17; 1989.
23. de Lignieres, B.; Plas, J-N.; Commandre, F.; Morville, R.; Viani, J-L.; Plas, F. Secretion testiculaire d'androgenes apres effort physique prolongue chez l'homme. Nouv. Presse. Med. 5:2060-2064; 1976.
24. Dessypris, K.; Adlercreutz, H. Plasma cortisol, testosterone, androstenedione and luteinizing hormone (LH) in a non-competitive marathon run. J. Steroid Biochem. 7:33-37; 1976.
25. Dohm, G.L.; Louis, T.M. Changes in androstenedione, testosterone and protein metabolism as a result of exercise. Proc. Soc. Exp. Biol. Med. 158:622-625; 1978.
26. Editorial. Special survey. Running and sex. The Runner. (May):26-35; 1982.
27. Eik-Nes, K.B. On the relationship between testicular blood flow and secretion of testosterone in anesthetized dogs stimulated with human chorionic gonadotropin. Can. J. Physiol. Pharmacol. 42:671-677; 1964.
28. Elias, A.N.; Fairshter, R.; Pandian, M.R.; Domurat, E.; Kayaleh, R: Beta-endorphin/beta-lipotropin release and gonadotropin secretion after acute exercise in physically conditioned males. Eur. J. Appl. Physiol. 58:522-527; 1989.
29. Enger, S.; Herbjornsen, K.; Erikssen, P., Fretland, A. High density lipoproteins and physical activity: The influence of physical exercise, age and smoking on HDL-cholesterol and the HDL/total cholesterol ratio. Scand. J. Clin. Lab. Invest. 37:251-255; 1977.
30. Epling, W.F.; Pierce, W.D.; Stefan, L. A theory of activity-based anorexia. Int. J. Eat. Disord. 3:27-46; 1983.
31. Fahey, T.D.; Rolph, R.; Moongee, P.; Nagel, J.; Mortara, S. Serum testosterone, body composition, and strength of young adults. Med. Sci. Sports Exerc. 1:31-34; 1976.
32. Foresta, C.; Ruzza, G.; Mioni, R.; Guarneri, G.; Gribaldo, R.; Meneghello, A.; Mastrogiacomo, I. Osteoporosis and decline of gonadal function in the elderly man. Horm. Res. 19:18-22; 1984.
33. Frey, M.A.B.; Doerr, B.M.; Srivastava, L.M.; Glueck, C.J. Exercise training, sex hormones

and lipoprotein relationships in men. J. Appl. Physiol. 54:757-762; 1983.

34. Galbo, H.; Hummer, L.; Petersen, I.B.; Christensen, N.J.; Bie, N. Thyroid and testicular hormone responses to graded and prolonged exercise in man. Eur. J. Appl. Physiol. 36:101-106; 1977.
35. Gawel, M.J.; Park, D.M.; Alaghband-Zadeh, J.; Rose, F.C. Exercise and hormonal secretion. Postgrad. Med. J. 55:373-376; 1979.
36. Hackney, A.C.; Sinning, W.E.; Bruot, B.C. Reproductive hormonal profiles of endurance-trained and untrained males. Med. Sci. Sports Exerc. 2:60-65; 1988.
37. Hackney, A.C.; Sinning, W.E.; Bruot, B.C. Hypothalamic-pituitary-testicular axis function in endurance-trained males. Int. J. Sports Med. 11:98-103; 1990.
38. Hakkinen, K. Neuromuscular and hormonal adaptations during strength and power training. A review. J. Sports Med. Phys. Fitness. 29:9-26; 1989.
39. Hakkinen, K.; Keskinen, K.L.; Alen, M.; Komi, P.V.; Kauhanen, H. Serum hormone concentrations during prolonged training in elite endurance-trained and strength-trained athletes. Eur. J. Appl. Physiol. 59:233-238; 1989.
40. Hakkinen, K.; Pakarinen, A.; Alen, M.; Kauhanen, H.; Komi, P.V. Relationships between training volume, physical performance capacity and serum hormone concentrations during prolonged weight training in elite weight lifters. Int. J. Sports Med. [Suppl.]. 8:61-65; 1987.
41. Hakkinen, K.; Pakarinen, A.; Alen, M.; Kauhanen, H.; Komi, P.V. Neuromuscular and hormonal responses in elite athletes to two successive strength training sessions in one day. Eur. J. Appl. Physiol. 57:133-139; 1988.
42. Hamalainen, E.K.; Adlercreutz, H.; Puska, P.; Pietinen, P. Decrease of serum total and free testosterone during a low-fat, high fibre diet. J. Steroid Biochem. 18:369-370; 1983.
43. Hartung, G.H.; Foreyt, J.P.; Mitchell, R.E.; Vlasek, I.; Gotto, A.M. Relation of diet to high-density-lipoprotein cholesterol in middle aged marathon runners, joggers and inactive men. N. Engl. J. Med. 302:357-361; 1980.
44. Hill, P.; Wynder, E.; Garbacrewski, L.; Garnes, H.; Walker, A.R.P.; Hellman, P. Plasma hormones and lipids in men at different risk for coronary heart disease. Am. J. Clin. Nutr. 33:1010-1018; 1980.
45. Jezova, D.; Vigas, M. Testosterone response to exercise during blockade and stimulation of adrenergic receptors in man. Horm. Res. 15:141-147; 1981.
46. Johansson, C.; Tsai, L.; Hultman, E.; Tegelman, R.; Pousette, A. Restoration of anabolic deficit and muscle glycogen consumption in competitive orienteering. Int. J. Sports Med. 11:204-207; 1990.
47. Johnson, C.C.; Stone, M.H.; Byrd, R.J.; Lopez-s, A. The response of serum lipids and plasma androgens to weight training exercise in sedentary males. J. Sports Med. Phys. Fitness. 23:39-44; 1983.
48. Judd, H.L.; Parker, D.C.; Siler, T.M.; Yen, S.S.C. Elucidation of the nocturnal rise in testosterone in pubertal boys. J. Clin. Endocrinol. Metab. 38:710-713; 1974.
49. Judd, H.L.; Rebar, R.; Vandenberg, G.; Yen, S.S.C. Effect of luteinizing hormone releasing factor on Leydig cell function. J. Clin. Endocrinol. Metab. 38:8-13; 1974.
50. Kantor, M.A.; Cullinane, E.M.; Herbert, P.N.; Thompson, P.D. Acute increase in lipoprotein lipase following prolonged exercise. Metabolism. 33:454-457; 1984.
51. Karvonen, J.; Peltola, E.; Saarela, J.; Nieminen, M.M. Changes in running speed, blood lactic acid concentration and hormone balance during sprint training performed at an altitude of 1860 metres. J. Sports Med. Phys. Fitness. 30:122-126; 1990.
52. Keizer, H.; Janssen, G.M.; Menheere, P.; Kranenburg, G. Changes in basal plasma testosterone, cortisol, and dehydroepiandrosterone sulfate in previously untrained males and females preparing for a marathon. Int. J. Sports Med. [Suppl. 3]. 10:S139-S145; 1989.
53. Keizer, H.A.; Doorfman, J.; Bunnik, G.S.J. Influence of physical exercise on sex hormone metabolism. Med. Sci. Sports Exerc. 48:765-769; 1980.
54. Kindermann, W.; Schnabel, A.; Schmitt, W.M.; Biro, G.; Cassens, J.; Weber, F. Catecholamines, growth hormone, cortisol, insulin and sex hormones in aerobic and anaerobic exercise. Eur. J. Appl. Physiol. 49:389-399; 1982.
55. Kindermann, W.; Schnabel, A.; Schmitt, W.M.; Biro, G.; Hippchen, M. Catecholamine, STH, cortisol, glucagon, insulin und sexualhormone bei korperlicher belastung und beta1-blockade. Klin. Wochenschr. 60:505-512; 1982.
56. Kraemer, W.J.; Marchitelli, L.; Gordon, S.E.; Harman, E.; Dziados, J.E.; Mello, R.; Frykman, P.; McCurry, D.; Fleck, S.J. Hormonal and growth factor responses to heavy resistance exercise protocols. J. Appl. Physiol. 69:1442-1450; 1990.
57. Kujala, U.M.; Alen, M.; Huhtaniemi, I.T. Gonadotrophin-releasing hormone and human chorionic gonadotrophin tests reveal that both hypothalamic and testicular endocrine

functions are suppressed during acute prolonged physical exercise. Clin. Endocrinol. 33:219-225; 1990.

58. Kuopposalmi, K. Plasma testosterone and sex-hormone-binding capacity in physical exercise. Scand. J. Clin. Lab. Invest. 40:411-418; 1980.
59. Kuopposalmi, K.; Naveri, H.; Harkonen, N.; Adlerkreutz, H. Plasma cortisol, a'dione, testosterone and luteinizing hormone in running exercise of various intensities. Scand. J. Clin. Lab. Invest. 40:403-409; 1980.
60. Kuoppasalmi, K.; Naveri, H.; Rehunen, S.; Harkonen, M.; Adlercreutz, H. Effect of strenuous anaerobic running on plasma growth hormone, cortisol, luteinizing hormone, testosterone, androstenedione and estrone and estradiol. J. Steroid Biochem. 7:823-829; 1976.
61. Levin, J.; Lloyd, C.W.; Lobotsky, J.; Friedrich, E.H. The effect of epinephrine on testosterone production. Acta Endocrinol. 55:184-192; 1967.
62. MacConnie, S.E.; Barkan, A.; Lampman, R.M.; Schork, M.A.; Beitins, I.Z. Decreased hypothalamic gonadotropin releasing hormone secretion in male marathon runners. N. Engl. J. Med. 315:411-417; 1986.
63. Marshall, J.C.; Anderson, D.C.; Fraser, T.R.; Marsoulis, P. Human luteinizing hormone in man: Studies of metabolism and biological action. J. Endocrinol. 56:431-439; 1973.
64. Mateev, G.; Djarova, T.; Ilkov, A.; Sachanska, T.; Klissurov, L. Hormonal and cardiorespiratory changes following simulated saturation dives to 4 and 11 ATA. Undersea Biomed. Res. 17:1-11; 1990.
65. Mathur, D.N.; Toriola, A.L.; Dada, O.A. Serum cortisol and testosterone levels in conditioned male distance runners and non-athletes after maximal exercise. J. Sports Med. Phys. Fitness. 26:245-250; 1986.
66. McColl, E.M.; Wheeler, G.D.; Gomes, P.; Bhambhani, Y.; Cumming, D.C. The effects of acute exercise on LH pulsatile release in high mileage male runners. Clin. Endocrinol. 31:617-629; 1989.
67. McConnell, T.R.; Sinning, W.E.; Exercise and temperature effects on human sperm production and testosterone levels. Med. Sci. Sports Exerc. 16:51-55; 1984.
68. Mendoza, S.G.; Carrasco, H.; Zerpa, A.; Briceno, Y.; Rodriguez, F.; Speirs, J.; Glueck, C.J. Effect of physical training on lipids, lipoproteins, apolipoproteins, lipases, and endogenous sex hormones in men with premature myocardial infarction. Metabolism. 40:368-377; 1991.
69. Metivier, G.; Gauthier, R.; de la Chevotriere, J.; Grymala, D. The effect of acute exercise on the serum levels of testosterone and luteinizing (LH) hormone in human male athletes. J. Sports Med. Phys. Fitness. 20:235-237; 1980.
70. Mooradian, A.D.; Morley, J.E.; Korenman, S.G. Biological actions of androgens. Endocr. Rev. 8:1-28; 1987.
71. Morville, R.; Pesquies, P.C.; Guezzenec, C.Y.; Serrurier, B.D.; Guignard, M. Plasma variations in testicular and adrenal androgens during prolonged physical exercise in man. Ann. Endocrinol. 40:501-510; 1979.
72. Naftolin, F.; Judd, H.L.; Yen, S.S.C. Pulsatile patterns of gonadotropins in man: The effect of clomiphene with and without testosterone. J. Clin. Endocrinol. Metab. 36:285-288; 1973.
73. Naftolin, F.; Yen, S.S.C.; Tsai, C.C. Rapid cycling of plasma gonadotropins in normal men as demonstrated by frequent sampling. New Biol. 236:92-93; 1972.
74. Pardridge, W.M. Transport of protein bound hormones into tissues in vivo. Endocr. Rev. 2:103-123; 1981.
75. Peltonen, P.; Marniemi, J.; Hietanen, E.; Vuori, I.; Enholm, C. Changes in serum lipids, lipoproteins and heparin releasable lipolytic enzymes during moderate physical training in man: A longitudinal study. Metabolism. 30:518-526; 1981.
76. Raz, I.; Israeli, A.; Rosenblit, H.; Bar-On. H. Influence of moderate exercise on glucose homeostasis and serum testosterone in young men with low HDL-cholesterol level. Diabetes Res. 19:31-35; 1988.
77. Remes, K.; Kuopposalmi, K.; Adlercreutz, H. Effects of longterm physical training on plasma testosterone, androstenedione, luteinizing hormone, sex hormone binding globulin capacity. Scand. J. Clin. Lab. Invest. 39:743-749; 1979.
78. Riggs, B.L. Exercise, hypogonadism and osteopenia. JAMA. 256:392-393; 1986.
79. Rigotti, N.A.; Neer, R.M.; Jameson, L. Osteopenia and bone fractures in a man with anorexia nervosa and hypogonadism. JAMA. 256:385-388; 1986.
80. Rogol, A.D.; Veldhuis, J.D.; Williams, F.A.; Johnson, M.L. Pulsatile secretion of gonadotropins and prolactin in male marathon runners. Relation to the endogenous opiate system. J. Androl. 5:21-27; 1984.
81. Roth, J.C.; Grumbach, M.M.; Kaplan, S.L. Effect of synthetic luteinizing factor on serum testosterone and gonadotropins in prepubertal, pubertal and adult males. J. Clin. Endocrinol. Metab. 37:680-686; 1973.
82. Rowell, L.B. Human cardiovascular adjustments to exercise and thermal stress. Physiol. Rev. 53:75-159; 1974.
83. Rubin, R.T.; Poland, R.E.; Sobel, I.; Tower, B.B.; Odell, W.D. Effects of prolactin and prolactin plus luteinizing hormone on plasma

testosterone levels in normal adult men. J. Clin. Endocrinol. Metab. 47:447-452; 1978.

84. Sakamoto, K.; Wakabayashi, I.; Yoshimoto, S.; Masui, H.; Katsuno, S. Effects of physical exercise and cold stimulation on serum testosterone level in men. Nippon Eiseigaku Zasshi. 46:635-638; 1991.
85. Schmid, P.; Pusch, P.P.; Wolf, W.W.; Pilger, E.; Pessenhofer, H.; Schwaberger, G.; Pristautz, H.; Purstner, P. Serum FSH, LH and testosterone in humans after physical exercise. Int. J. Sports Med. 3:84-89; 1982.
86. Schriewer, H.; Jung, K.; Gunnewiig, V.; Assmann, G. Serum lipids and lipoproteins during a twenty day run of 1,100 kilometers. Ann. Sports Med. 1:71-74; 1983.
87. Schurmeyer, T.; Jung, K.; Nieschlag, E. The effects of an 1100 kilometer run on testicular adrenal and thyroid hormones. Int. J. Androl. 7:276-282; 1984.
88. Stanish, W. Overuse injuries in athletes: A perspective. Med. Sci. Sports Exerc. 16:1-7; 1984.
89. Strauss, R.H.; Lanese, R.R.; Malarkey, W.B. Weight loss in amateur wrestlers and its effect on testosterone levels. JAMA. 254:3337-3338; 1985.
90. Sutton, J.R.; Coleman, M.J.; Casey, J. Adrenocortical contribution to serum androgens during physical exercise. Med. Sci. Sports Exerc. [Abstract]. 6:72; 1974.
91. Sutton, J.R.; Coleman, M.J.; Casey, J.; Lazarus, L. Androgen responses during physical exercise. Br. Med. J. 1:520-522; 1973.
92. Sutton, J.R.; Coleman, M.J.; Casey, J.H. Testosterone production rate during exercise. In: Landry, F.; Orban, W.A.R., eds. 3rd international symposium on biochemistry of exercise. Miami, FL: Symposium Specialists; 1978:227-234.
93. Tanaka, H.; Cleroux, J.; de Champlain, J.; Ducharme, J.R.; Collu, R.J.: Persistent effects of a marathon run on the pituitary-testicular axis. Endocrinol. Invest. 9:97-101; 1986.
94. Tegelman, R.; Carlstrom, K.; Pousette, A. Hormone levels in male ice hockey players during the night after a 26-hour cup tournament. Andrologia. 22:261-268; 1990.
95. Urhausen, A.; Kinderman, W. Behaviour of testosterone, sex hormone binding globulin (SHBG) and cortisol before and after a triathlon. Int. J. Sports Med. 8:305-308; 1987.
96. Urhausen, A.; Kullmer, T.; Kindermann, W. A 7-week follow-up study of the behaviour of testosterone and cortisol during the competition period in rowers. Eur. J. Appl. Physiol. 56:528-533; 1987.
97. Vermeulen, A.; Verdonck, L.; Van Der Straeten, M.; Orie, N. Capacity of testosterone binding globulin in human plasma and its influence on specific binding of testosterone and its clearance rate. J. Clin. Endocrinol. Metab. 29:1470-1480; 1969.
98. Vogel, R.B.; Books, C.A.; Ketchum, C.; Zauner, C.W.; Murray, F.T. Increase of free and total testosterone during submaximal exercise in normal males. Med. Sci. Sports Exerc. 17:119-123; 1984.
99. Wahren, J.; Felig, P.; Ahlborg, G.; Jorfeldt, l. Glucose metabolism during leg exercise in man. J. Clin. Invest. 50:2715-2725; 1971.
100. Wang, C.; Chan, V.; Tse, T.F.; Yeung, R.T.T. Effect of acute myocardial infarction on pituitary-testicular function. Clin. Endocrinol. 9:249-253; 1978.
101. Wang, C.; Chan, V.; Yeung, R.T.T. Effect of surgical stress on pituitary-testicular function. Clin. Endocrinol. 9:255-256; 1978.
102. Webb, M.L.; Wallace, J.P.; Hamill, C.; Hodgson, J.L.; Mashaly, M.M. Serum testosterone concentration during two hours of moderate intensity treadmill running in trained men and women. Endocr. Res. 10:27-38; 1984.
103. Wheeler, G.D.; McFadyen, S.G.; Symbaluk, D.; Pierce, W.D.; Cumming, D.C. The effects of training on serum testosterone and cortisol levels in wrestlers. Clin. J. Sports Med. 2:257-260; 1992.
104. Wheeler, G.D.; Singh, M.; Pierce, W.D.; Epling, W.F.; Cumming, D.C. Endurance training decreases serum testosterone levels in men without change in LH pulsatile release. J. Clin. Endocrinol. Metab. 72:422-425; 1991.
105. Wheeler, G.D.; Wall, S.R.; Belcastro, A.N.; Conger, P.; Cumming, D.C. Are anorexic tendencies prevalent in the habitual runner? Br. J. Sports Med. 20:77-81; 1986.
106. Wheeler, G.D.; Wall, S.R.; Belcastro, A.N.; Cumming, D.C. Reduced serum testosterone and prolactin levels in male distance runners. JAMA. 252:514-516; 1984.
107. White, J.R.; Case, D.A.; McWhirter, D.; Mattison, A.M. Enhanced sexual behavior in exercising men. Arch. Sex. Behav. 19:193-209; 1990.
108. Wilkerson, J.E.; Horvath, S.M.; Gutin, B. Plasma testosterone during treadmill exercise. J. Appl. Physiol. 49:249-253; 1980.
109. Yates, A.; Leehay, K.; Shisslak, C.M. Running an analogue of anorexia nervosa. N. Engl. J. Med. 308:251-255; 1983.
110. Zubiran, S.; Gomez-Mont, F. Endocrine disturbance in chronic human malnutrition. Vitam. Horm. 11:97-102; 1952.

Chapter 68

Physical Activity, Fitness, Health, and Aging

James M. Hagberg

Demography and Epidemiology of Aging

In industrialized societies the proportion of individuals reaching old age has been increasing and this aging of the population is predicted to continue in the foreseeable future. In 1980, 1 of every 10 Americans was more than 65 years old (11). Only 6 years later, the proportion was 1 of every 8, which represented 29 million people over 65 years old. However, this rapid and dramatic change represents only the tip of the iceberg—by 2020, 1 of every 6 Americans will be over 65 years old, and by 2040 the proportion will be between 1 and every 4 or 5 Americans. Perhaps the most sobering fact is that by 2040 the total American population over 65 years old will be 70 million.

Diseases of the cardiovascular (CV) system cause over half of the deaths in these older Americans (11). Since this proportion increases from age 65 to 85 years, cardiovascular diseases (CVD) will continue to account for an ever-increasing proportion of the deaths of older men and women. High-density lipoprotein (HDL) and low-density lipoprotein (LDL) cholesterol levels, blood pressure (BP), diabetes mellitus, and left ventricular hypertrophy are important CVD risk factors in people over age 65 years (45,59,60). Thus, because these CVD risk factors are present in almost epidemic proportions in older individuals, and because CVD accounts for the large majority of mortality in older populations, it would appear most appropriate to direct intervention strategies at these risk factors in an effort to prevent or forestall the development of CVD in the elderly.

It is also imperative to reduce disability in the elderly, because the extension of life by merely prolonging the period of disability that often precedes death in the elderly is an unacceptable benefit to most. A major cause of disability in the elderly is, once again, CVD, which results in strokes. Another major cause of disability is falls, which result in fractures, other injuries, and a fear of falling that in many cases disables older individuals. Many of the factors that increase the older person's risk of falling are environmental in nature, for example, stairs and clutter (7,71,102). However, various neuromuscular factors have also been shown to increase an older person's risk of falling, including losses of strength, flexibility, and balance (71,102).

Potential Role for Exercise as an Intervention in the Elderly

The proposal that exercise may be beneficial for older persons has been primarily based on the facts that in younger persons it improves nearly all risk factors for CVD and disability, and daily physical activity levels are higher in younger than older persons (21,66). Also underlying this proposal is the fact that many of the age-associated losses in physiological function can be elicited by decreasing physical activity in younger persons. However, until recently only minimal evidence was available to substantiate the beneficial effects of exercise training in older individuals.

To appropriately assess the effects of exercise training on older individuals would require a large, long-term clinical trial. However, no such studies have been done, and they are unlikely to be initiated in these times of fiscal limitations. Two simpler approaches have, however, provided fairly strong evidence substantiating the benefits of exercise training for the elderly. One approach has been to study older well-trained athletes. The second approach involves exercise intervention studies in populations smaller than those required in clinical trials.

Results of Studies in Older Trained Athletes

Cardiovascular Function in Older Athletes

The primary index of maximal CV function in studies of older, as well as younger, athletes is maximal

O_2 consumption ($\dot{V}O_2$max), since it is generally believed to be limited by maximal cardiac output. As in younger individuals, older endurance-trained athletes have $\dot{V}O_2$max values that are markedly higher than those of their sedentary peers (cf. 42,48), with many older athletes having $\dot{V}O_2$max values in $ml \cdot min^{-1} \cdot kg^{-1}$ nearly twice those of their sedentary age-matched peers and higher than those of even the average 20- to 30-yr-old individual. Older resistive-trained individuals, on the other hand, have $\dot{V}O_2$max values comparable to those of their sedentary peers (54).

Few studies have measured cardiovascular function directly in older athletes. Older runners studied by Hagberg et al. (42) had 20% higher maximal cardiac outputs than their sedentary peers. These older athletes' maximal cardiac output was lower than that of training-matched younger runners. However, this difference was due only to the older athletes' lower maximal heart rate, as maximal stroke volume and arteriovenous O_2 difference ([a-$\bar{v}$]O_2 difference) were similar in the two groups. Saltin (86) and Rivera et al. (81) found that older orienteers and runners, respectively, had a lower maximal $\dot{V}O_2$, cardiac output, heart rate, stroke volume, and (a-$\bar{v}$)O_2 difference than younger athletes. However, the older athletes in these studies were undergoing much less training than the younger athletes, which may have resulted in their smaller maximal stroke volume and (a-$\bar{v}$)O_2 difference.

Another important question is if older athletes who continue to train exhibit the same rate of decline in $\dot{V}O_2$max with age as sedentary persons. Early studies indicated that older athletes experienced the same (38,50,57,77,86,99) and in some cases even a greater (76,82) decline in $\dot{V}O_2$max with age than their sedentary peers. However, these early studies were generally confounded by the fact that in most cross-sectional comparisons the older athletes were training much less than their younger counterparts, and in the longitudinal investigations the athletes decreased their training as they aged (82). Heath, Hagberg, Ehsani, and Holloszy (48) first compared young and older endurance athletes matched on the basis of their training. The difference in $\dot{V}O_2$max between these young and older athletes amounted to a 5% decline per decade—a rate of decline in $\dot{V}O_2$max half of that which they and others reported in relatively unscreened, sedentary populations studied cross-sectionally (39,48,50). A subsequent study that matched young and older runners for their training regimens also reported this same reduced rate of decline in $\dot{V}O_2$max (42).

Recently the results of longitudinal studies in older athletes have been published. Pollock, Foster, Knapp, Rod, and Schmidt (76) found that $\dot{V}O_2$max did not decrease in athletes aged 60 years who had maintained a relatively constant training program over the preceding 10 years. In otherwise similar athletes whose training decreased over the 10 years $\dot{V}O_2$max fell by 12.5%. More recently Rogers, Hagberg, Martin, Ehsani, and Holloszy (83) studied only endurance-trained, older (62 ± 2 years) athletes and found that the decline in $\dot{V}O_2$max over 8 years was 5.5% per decade—half that evident in their sedentary men.

Thus, these cross-sectional and longitudinal data generally indicate that the expected rate of decline in $\dot{V}O_2$max with aging can be reduced by roughly one half, not by eliminating the direct effects of aging per se, but by maintaining older individuals' physical activity levels comparable to those of younger persons. The minimal data available indicate that the hemodynamic determinants of $\dot{V}O_2$max, other than maximal heart rate, also change very little with age in studies of older athletes matched to younger athletes on the basis of their training regimens.

Cardiovascular Disease Risk Factors in Older Athletes

Plasma Lipoprotein-Lipids

Older endurance athletes also have markedly better lipoprotein-lipid profiles than their sedentary peers. Seals et al. (89) found that runners with a mean age of 60 years had nearly 50% higher HDL levels than sedentary men of the same age who had the same total cholesterol, LDL, and triglyceride (TG) levels and nearly the same body fat. The older athletes did have lower total cholesterol, LDL, and TG levels than their sedentary peers with a body composition more representative of men this age. These differences in lipoprotein-lipids in older athletes also extend to HDL_2 and HDL_{2b} levels (15,72) and may be due to the decreased hepatic lipase activities evident in these athletes (15). On the other hand, resistive-trained athletes aged 41 to 64 years had worse plasma TG and HDL levels than their sedentary, body-fat-matched peers (54).

Glucose Tolerance and Insulin Sensitivity

Older endurance-trained athletes also have enhanced glucose tolerance and insulin sensitivity compared to their sedentary peers. Runners with a mean age of 60 years studied by Seals et al. (90) had glucose tolerance similar to that of athletes 34 years younger, and 50% better than that of their lean and normal body composition sedentary peers. These older athletes had the same plasma insulin responses to an oral glucose tolerance test (OGTT) as young athletes—responses that were roughly only 1/3 and 1/6 of those of their lean and normal body composition sedentary peers, respectively. These same differences extend to slightly older and somewhat less fit athletes (15). These data are consistent with the conclusion that endurance exercise training has maintained the older athletes' glucose tolerance and insulin sensitivity at levels similar to those of athletes 30 to 40 years younger. On the other hand, resistive-trained athletes 41 to 64 years old studied by Hurley et al. had larger OGTT plasma glucose and insulin responses than their sedentary body-fat-matched peers (54).

In older runners 10 days of inactivity did not change glucose tolerance compared to when they were training, although plasma insulin levels increased by nearly 100% (84). However, in 4 of these older athletes OGTT plasma glucose and insulin responses both deteriorated, and 2 of them had mildly impaired glucose tolerance after only 10 days of inactivity. In the remaining 10 athletes only plasma insulin responses deteriorated with inactivity. These two subgroups of older athletes did not differ in age, body composition, $\dot{V}O_2max$, or training. As a group, these older athletes' glucose and insulin responses after 10 days of inactivity were not different from those of their habitually sedentary peers. These data indicate that these older athletes, who are representative of those studied in St. Louis for the last 10 years (42,48,83,84,89,90), appear to forestall the metabolic effects of aging only when they are training regularly. When they stop training even for a short time they are similar, in terms of glucose and insulin metabolism, to their sedentary peers.

Risk Factors for Falls in Older Athletes

A number of risk factors for falls have been studied in older athletes. Older endurance-trained individuals generally have enhanced reaction times and motor abilities compared to their sedentary peers (28,78,95,101). Sipila, Viitasalo, Era, and Suominen (98) recently found that older endurance-trained athletes aged 70 to 81 years had greater arm and leg muscular strengths than their sedentary peers; thus even endurance activities may attenuate the decline in muscular strength that normally occurs with aging. Pollock et al. (76) found that lean body mass decreased by 4% over 10 years of training in older athletes who were first studied at age 50 years. This loss of lean body mass occurred in these older runners' and walkers' upper bodies, because their arm girths decreased and thigh girths were unchanged. In addition, two of these athletes who did upper body weight training and another who was a cross-country skier did not decrease lean body mass over the 10 years. On the other hand, Rogers et al. (83) found no decrease in lean body mass over 8 years in older runners studied initially at age 54 years. Thus, these data provide some indication that endurance exercise can alter the loss of lean body mass that normally occurs with aging, especially in the specific muscle groups involved in the exercise. However, due to the specificity of training it is doubtful that exercise training involving only the lower limbs could exert a systemic effect and thereby maintain the skeletal muscle mass in the uninvolved muscles of the upper body.

A number of studies have compared bone density in athletes and their sedentary peers, although very few such studies have been done in older male or female athletes (see 100). The data that are available, however, generally indicate that the older athletes have higher bone densities than their sedentary peers (100).

Summary of Studies in Older Athletes

The evidence from older endurance athletes is consistent with the conclusion that endurance exercise training has numerous physiological benefits for older individuals. These benefits include enhanced CV function and a metabolic profile conveying a low CVD risk. It is also clear that older endurance athletes have benefited in terms of their risk factors for falls. On the other hand, CV function appears unaffected and the metabolic CVD risk factors are actually worse in the minimal number of middle-aged to older resistive-trained individuals that have been studied.

Effects of Endurance Exercise Training on Older Men and Women

The training programs older athletes maintain are much more vigorous than those older sedentary men and women would initiate to improve their present and future health status. From a public health point of view a more important question is whether these same adaptations evident in highly trained older athletes can be elicited with less intense exercise training in older sedentary individuals.

CV Adaptations to Endurance Training in Older Men and Women

Early studies found men and women over 60 years of age could not elicit the training-induced increase in $\dot{V}O_2$max evident in younger persons (39). However, a number of studies have now shown that older individuals can, in fact, achieve the same or greater relative increases in $\dot{V}O_2$max as younger populations (75). As evidence of this, men and women aged 60 to 69 years have been shown to elicit 26% to 30% increases in $\dot{V}O_2$max with 6 to 12 months of training (44,61,91). Hagberg et al. also found a 22% increase in $\dot{V}O_2$max in 70- to 79-yr-old men and women with 6 months of training (43).

In the young, training intensity must be greater than 60% to 65% $\dot{V}O_2$max to increase $\dot{V}O_2$max significantly (75). However, Seals, Hagberg, Hurley, Ehsani, and Holloszy (91) elicited a 12% increase in $\dot{V}O_2$max in 60- to 69-yr-old men and women with 6 months of training at 40% of heart rate reserve (HRR). Seals and Reiling also recently reported 9% and 14% increases in $\dot{V}O_2$max in older hypertensives with 6 months of training at 46% HRR and an additional 6 months at 57% HRR, respectively (93). Thus, training at intensities that do not generally increase $\dot{V}O_2$max in younger individuals appears capable of doing so in persons over 60 years of age.

In some cases low-intensity training increased $\dot{V}O_2$max in older individuals as much as higher intensity training; however, these studies have generally used relatively short (8–10 weeks) training programs (8,33). Kohrt et al. (61) also recently reported that training intensity, duration, and frequency in men and women aged 60 to 69 years were not related to the increase in $\dot{V}O_2$max elicited with 9 to 12 months of training; however, by design their ranges of training intensities, frequencies, and durations were minimal. In addition, in older individuals subjected to graded levels of exercise training, moderate to high training intensities increased $\dot{V}O_2$max beyond that elicited with lower intensities (43,91,93). Thus, the available evidence indicates that low-intensity training elicits a small but significant increase in $\dot{V}O_2$max, and that higher intensity training in older individuals is associated with more substantial increases in $\dot{V}O_2$max.

Despite the fact that older individuals can elicit the same training-induced increases in $\dot{V}O_2$max as younger persons, an early study indicated that older men and women increased their $\dot{V}O_2$max with training only by widening their $(a-\bar{v})O_2$ difference while their maximal stroke volume and cardiac output were unchanged (91). However, more recent data using radionuclide techniques show that maximal stroke volume and cardiac output increased in men aged 60 to 69 years in response to 12 months of training that elicited a 23% increase in $\dot{V}O_2$max (27). Their CV adaptations included an increase in left ventricular (LV) end-diastolic volume, indicative of enhanced preload, and a decrease in LV end-systolic volume and an increase in LV ejection fraction—both indicative of increases in contractility. Somewhat similar findings have been reported previously by Schocken, Blumenthal, Port, Hindle, and Coleman (87), although they did not find an increase in LV ejection fraction in response to 12 weeks of training in men and women with an average age of 72 years.

Thus, older individuals appear to elicit the same beneficial training-induced CV adaptations as younger men and women. The next, and perhaps more important, question is whether or not they can also improve their CVD risk factors with exercise training.

CVD Risk Factors and Endurance Exercise Training in Older Persons

Plasma Lipoprotein-Lipids

Plasma HDL and LDL levels are major CVD risk factors in the elderly (59). Plasma TG levels are also a CVD risk factor in the elderly when analyzed on a univariate basis; however, they convey little CVD risk when all other risk factors are taken into account (59). Relatively few studies have assessed the impact of exercise training on lipoprotein-lipids in older men and women. Seals, Hagberg, Hurley, Ehsani, and Holloszy (92) found that 6 months of low-intensity training did not alter plasma lipoprotein-lipids in men and women aged 60 to 69 years. Six additional months of high-intensity training that resulted in small decreases in body weight and body fat in these same subjects increased HDL levels by 14% and decreased TG levels by 21%; total cholesterol and LDL levels did not change (92). Blumenthal et al. reported transient reductions in both total cholesterol and LDL levels that were not sustained with 14 months of training in men and women aged 60 to 83 years (9). However, plasma HDL levels increased by 8% and TG levels decreased by 20% with training in these older men and women who also tended to decrease their body weight with training. Foster, Hume, Byrnes, Dickinson, and Chatfield (33) recently found that total cholesterol and HDL levels did not change with 10 weeks of low- to moderate-intensity training in women aged 67 to 89 years. Their results may be due to the lack of training-induced changes in body weight or composition, or to the short training program, because it appears in younger men and women that training duration must exceed 12 weeks to elicit significant changes in lipoprotein-lipids (104).

Thus, the findings from endurance exercise training studies in older men and women are generally consistent with the increased HDL levels, decreased TG levels, and unchanged total cholesterol and LDL levels found with training in younger populations. However, as with younger individuals, it may be necessary for exercise training to reduce body weight and fat before the improvements in plasma lipoprotein-lipids occur.

Blood Pressure

Hypertension is a major CVD risk factor in the elderly (45,59,60), and it is present in more than 50% of some subsets of older Americans (60). Numerous medications are available to reduce BP and they result in dramatic reductions in mortality and morbidity in individuals with marked BP elevations (60). However, in individuals with mild to moderate elevations in BP, the efficacy of treatment with antihypertensive medications is still under debate (60,62). This has led to a search for nonpharmacological modalities including exercise training as alternative interventions for individuals with mild elevations in BP.

Previously Hagberg (40) concluded that both systolic and diastolic BP are reduced by roughly 10 mmHg with exercise training in essential hypertensives and that the magnitude of the training-induced BP reduction was independent of age. Since then additional studies have continued to support these conclusions. Hagberg, Montain, Martin, and Ehsani (44) found that 9 months of low-intensity training lowered systolic and diastolic BP by 20 and 12 mmHg, respectively, in male and female hypertensives aged 60 to 70 years. In that same study, 9 months of higher intensity training in another group of hypertensives decreased systolic BP by slightly less (8 mmHg) and diastolic BP by the same as the reduction elicited by lower intensity training. In a small group of 70- to 79-yr-old male and female hypertensives, Cononie et al. found that systolic and diastolic BP were reduced by 8 and 9 mmHg, respectively, with 6 months of training (17). Two earlier, less well-controlled studies also reported similar BP reductions in older hypertensives with exercise training (14,29). Seals and Reiling recently reported that 6 months of low-intensity training lowered casual BP in male and female essential hypertensives with an average age of 61 years (93). However, as with a previous study in younger hypertensives (36), these same reductions were not evident when BP was measured using ambulatory BP monitoring.

Thus, endurance exercise training lowers BP in older males and females with essential hypertension to the same degree as in younger hypertensive individuals. It is possible that the ambulatory BP of hypertensives may not as consistently demonstrate the same training-induced reductions in BP as those observed with casually measured BP. The minimal data available in older hypertensives indicate that low-intensity training may be as efficacious in lowering BP as higher intensity training—a finding important from both a safety viewpoint and the potential for applying exercise training to the large number of elderly hypertensives present in industrialized societies.

Glucose Tolerance

A third major CVD risk factor in the elderly is diabetes, which is primarily in the form of non-insulin-dependent diabetes mellitus (NIDDM) in this population. NIDDM develops every year in 6% to 10% of the population over 60 years of age (30). Thus NIDDM in elderly populations is also virtually at epidemic levels. Most studies have assessed the effects of exercise training in subjects with normal glucose metabolism. However, Holloszy, Schultz, Kusnierkiewicz, Hagberg, and Ehsani (52) have studied the effects of 1 year of intensive exercise training in males with CVD that had varying degrees of glucose intolerance. The average age of their men was 56 years; thus, as a whole they cannot be considered elderly, though a number of their patients were over 60 years old. Their three groups (those with NIDDM, with impaired, and with high-normal glucose tolerance) improved their glucose tolerance with training and lost 4 to 5 kg of their initial 85-kg body weight. The improvements were such that in five patients with NIDDM training reduced their OGTT glucose response areas by 60%, and three had normal glucose tolerance after training. In those with impaired glucose tolerance, the training program reduced OGTT glucose response areas by 40%, and all 12 patients had normal glucose tolerance after training. Those with high-normal glucose tolerance also improved their OGTT glucose response areas by 40%.

The only comparable data in older subjects is a trend toward an improvement in glucose tolerance with 6 months of exercise training in men and women 70 to 79 years of age who had high-normal plasma OGTT glucose responses (49). The less dramatic improvement in glucose tolerance in this group may be because they did not lose as much weight as the patients of Holloszy et al. (52) and because their glucose tolerance was only in the high-normal range at the start of the training program (49). Thus, the minimal data that are available are consistent with the possibility that endurance exercise training may improve and potentially normalize glucose tolerance in older individuals who initially have some degree of glucose intolerance.

Insulin Resistance

The pathology underlying NIDDM is resistance to the glucose uptake-stimulating effects of insulin rather than deficient insulin secretion. In fact, most individuals with NIDDM have elevated, not reduced, plasma insulin levels. Early in the course of NIDDM glucose metabolism is maintained close to normal by these elevated plasma insulin levels. However, elevated plasma insulin levels have recently been proposed to have wide-ranging, deleterious effects on the CV system, vascular smooth muscle, sympathetic nervous system, BP, renal function, and lipid metabolism (79). Thus, if insulin resistance and the accompanying hyperinsulinemia that develop with aging could be slowed, a number of negative consequences attributed to aging might also be attenuated.

Numerous studies in young to middle-aged persons demonstrate that exercise training improves insulin sensitivity. It is now also clear that the same beneficial adaptations can be elicited in older men and women. Although, again, their subjects were largely middle-aged, the most striking results are from Holloszy et al., who found 55% to 75% reductions in OGTT insulin response areas in CVD patients (initially diabetic, impaired, or high-normal glucose tolerance) following 1 year of intensive training, which also improved glucose tolerance and resulted in some weight loss (52). Seals et al. (92) have also reported that older men and women (average age 62 years) decreased their OGTT insulin response areas by 23% with 1 year of training that decreased their body weight and body fat but had no effect on their initially normal glucose tolerance. More recently, Kahn et al. (58) studying men with an average age of 69 years and Hersey et al. (49) studying men and women aged 70 to 79 years reported on subjects who underwent 6 months of exercise training and showed similar reductions in OGTT insulin response areas along with decreases in body weight and body fat, but unchanged glucose tolerance. Tonino (103) and Kahn et al. (58) have also found evidence for enhanced insulin sensitivity with exercise training in older individuals using glucose clamp studies and intravenous glucose tolerance tests, respectively.

In younger individuals two mechanisms contribute to the training-induced enhancement of insulin sensitivity. A portion of the improved insulin sensitivity may be more directly a result of the reduction in body mass, primarily body fat, that occurs with exercise training. Another portion of this adaptive response may be a result of the acute effect of exercise rather than a cumulative effect of long-term exercise training (47), and may be a function of the degree of muscle glycogen depletion that results from the exercise (31). Insulin sensitivity is enhanced in both trained and untrained young individuals for up to 24 hr after a single bout of relatively intense exercise, and a portion of the effect dissipates in young, trained individuals with 10 days of inactivity, even though body composition and $\dot{V}O_2max$ are unchanged (47). However, insulin sensitivity in these young athletes after 10 days of inactivity was still greater than that in young, sedentary individuals with somewhat greater body fat stores.

In older subjects this acute insulin sensitivity effect may require more than one bout of exercise, perhaps because of their diminished exercise capacities and, hence, their reduced ability to deplete muscle glycogen during a single exercise session. Rogers et al. found that in middle-aged NIDDM patients a single exercise session had no effect on glucose or insulin metabolism, but that 7 days of exercise, which would result in a cumulative depletion of muscle glycogen stores, improved both OGTT glucose and insulin responses (85). Cononie, Goldberg, Rogus, and Hagberg have also found improved OGTT plasma insulin responses after 7, but not 1, days of exercise in men and women aged 70 to 79 years (16).

In summary, the improvement in insulin sensitivity that occurs with exercise training may be more a function of training-induced changes in body composition in older men and women than in younger individuals. This may be due to the relatively low exercise capacities of older individuals, even after exercise training that increases their $\dot{V}O_2max$. The proposed mechanism underlying this differential response of older men and women, a reduced capacity to deplete muscle glycogen stores, is supported by evidence from (a) endurance-trained older athletes who have high maximal exercise capacities and who have a marked deterioration in insulin sensitivity following 10 days of inactivity that does not result in alterations in their body composition (84), and (b) men and women aged 70 to 79 years who improved their body composition and OGTT plasma insulin responses with training but experienced no deterioration in their insulin responses with 10 days of inactivity following 6 months of training (49).

Obesity

Excess body fat is an independent predictor of CVD risk on a univariate basis, but when considered in a multivariate analysis it conveys minimal independent risk (59). However, because obesity is associated with increased prevalence of dyslipidemia, hypertension, and NIDDM it remains an important factor in an older individual's CVD risk profile even if the relationship is not direct and independent. The obesity that develops with aging is also generally the result of an accumulation of visceral abdominal fat (96,97) which is associated with the greatest CVD risk.

Exercise-training- and dietary-induced weight loss in older, obese men both reduce abdominal fat stores to the greatest degree (25,88). Most exercise-training studies that improved metabolic CVD risk factors in older men and women elicited at least small reductions in body weight and body fat (see preceding), even though their subjects were of relatively normal body weight and fatness. However, in older, obese men exercise training without weight loss apparently has no effect on plasma lipoprotein-lipids, OGTT glucose, or insulin responses (18, 63). These results are similar to those of Segal et al. (94), which indicated that insulin sensitivity was not altered in lean, obese, or diabetic young men with exercise training when body composition was not altered.

Thus it appears, that, as in younger individuals, obesity may overwhelm the ability of exercise training to elicit improvements in metabolic CVD risk factors, and that reductions in body weight and body fatness must accompany exercise training to result in beneficial changes in these metabolic CVD risk factors. From the viewpoint of risk factors for falls, exercise training in older, obese men also did not attenuate the loss in lean body mass that accompanied their weight loss (24).

Effects of Endurance Exercise Training in Older Individuals with CVD

Numerous studies have assessed the effects of exercise training on individuals with CVD (41). However, only recently have Ades and colleagues reported that, in terms of exercise capacity, heart rate, and BP responses, middle-aged and older CVD patients adapt similarly to 12 weeks of exercise training (1,2). These results are consistent with the earlier, generally accepted conclusion that training-induced adaptations in patients with CVD are only peripheral in nature, that is, within skeletal muscle and the autonomic nervous system as opposed to central CV adaptations within the heart (41). In the past 10 years evidence has accumulated that, with a substantially larger training stimulus, middle-aged CVD patients can elicit myocardial adaptations along with the conventional peripheral adaptations (41). Although many subjects in these studies were over 60 years of age, no data have been reported specifically describing the effects of this greater training stimulus on central and peripheral training-induced adaptations in older CVD patients.

Thus, only minimal data are available concerning the effects of exercise training on the physiologic and metabolic variables critical to the future CV health of older CVD patients. The available data are consistent with those from middle-aged CVD patients. However, the possibility has not been investigated that a greater training stimulus than that generally used might elicit improvements in myocardial function similar to those in younger CVD patients.

Risk Factors for Falls and Endurance Exercise Training in the Elderly

In the elderly, in addition to CVD, another main cause of disability and mortality is falling (45). An older person's risk of falling is a complex interaction between environmental and physiological factors; however, prominent risk factors are osteoporosis and neuromuscular factors including strength, flexibility, and balance deficits (7,71,102).

Osteoporosis is thought to be one age-associated, structural deterioration that can be reversed with exercise training in older individuals, specifically postmenopausal women. A number of studies have addressed this proposition, but only recently have they used appropriate study designs and bone density assessment techniques (see 100). Dalsky, Stocke, Ehsani, Slatopolsky, and Birge (23) first demonstrated an actual increase in lumbar bone mineral density in women aged 55 to 70 years with exercise training. Their subjects increased lumbar bone density (measured by dual photon absorptiometry) by 5.2% with 9 months and by 8.4% with 22 months of exercise training. In a subsequent study women aged 60 to 83 years who were at high risk for bone fracture increased the bone mineral density of their radius with 4 months of exercise training that included upper body calisthenics and arm ergometry (10). Previous and subsequent longitudinal studies in young and middle-aged women also generally indicate that exercise training increases bone mineral density (see 100). Thus, it appears that appropriate exercise programs can increase bone mineral density, at least in the lumbar region, in older women; however, no similar data are available for femoral neck bone density—a critical site for hip fractures.

In young and middle-aged persons endurance exercise training does not increase muscular strength. However, men and women aged 70 to 79 years responded to 6 months of endurance exercise training, primarily walk/jogging, with increases in lower limb strength (17). This is not a systemic effect, however, as these individuals did not increase their upper body strength, and men and women aged 60 to 83 years in another study also did not increase their grip strength with 4 months of cycle and arm ergometry and walk/jogging (10).

Dustman et al. (26) found that 4 months of exercise training in 55- to 70-yr-old men and women elicited improvements in simple reaction times and other neurocognitive tasks. However, simple reaction time and its component premotor and motor times were not altered by 6 months of endurance or resistive exercise training in individuals 70 to 79 years of age (74). Thus, although two other studies have shown that short-term exercise training improves reaction time in older persons (26,35), most results indicate that endurance or strength training in older individuals does not improve reaction times (73).

Deficits in balance and flexibility can, however, be improved in older individuals with specifically designed programs. Brown and Holloszy recently found that 3 months of flexibility, balance, gait, and weight-bearing strength exercises increased hip range of motion and eyes-open and -closed, one-legged balance in those with deficits initially (13). Munns also reported that 12 weeks of flexibility exercises in men and women aged 65 to 88 years improved range of motion at six joint sites by an average of 22% (70).

Thus, it appears that endurance exercise training has the capacity to improve bone density and perhaps even muscular strength in older men and women. However, most evidence indicates it is not effective in improving neurocognitive functions that are risk factors for falls. It also appears that to improve balance and flexibility, older individuals require exercise programs that specifically address these risk factors for falls.

Effects of Resistive Training in Older Men and Women

The exercise discussed thus far has been of the cardiovascular type. Another form of exercise available to older individuals is resistive training, which is known to result in markedly different responses and adaptations. However, some resistive-training-induced responses evident in young and middle-aged individuals could be even more important in elderly individuals where deficits in skeletal muscle mass and strength are risk factors for falls (7,71,102).

Some early studies reported that older men did not increase their muscular strength with resistive training (64). However, numerous studies have now shown that both older men and women elicit substantial increases in muscular strength with resistive training (3,4–6,12,13,20,37,67,69). The most dramatic evidence of their adaptive capacities was recently provided by Frontera, Meredith, O'Reilly, Knuttgen, and Evans (34) and Fiatarone et al. (32), who found 107% to 227% increases in leg flexor and extensor muscle strength in men aged 60 to 96 years in response to 8 to 12 weeks of specific leg extension training.

While an increase in muscle strength decreases an older person's risk of falling, an increase in muscle mass would also be of benefit because it (a) would allow for further increases in strength, (b) would reverse the age-associated loss of lean body mass, and (c) could result in other metabolic adaptations (68). However, an early study indicated that the elderly elicited training-induced increases in muscle strength via neurologic adaptations and did not increase skeletal muscle mass, whereas in younger individuals both mechanisms contribute equally to increases in muscular strength (69). More recent studies have shown that older subjects increase the size of their Type II muscle fibers, those that atrophy with age and disuse, with resistive training (5,6,20). Even more recently, Frontera et al. (34) and Fiatarone et al. (32), using computerized tomography, have shown 9% to 12% increases in muscle cross-sectional area as a result of specific single muscle training in men aged 60 to 69 years. However, these studies did not stress enough of the body's muscle mass to elicit an increase in total lean body mass.

Studies that have used total-body muscle-strengthening programs in the elderly have not found corresponding increases in total lean body mass (43,53), although their techniques were probably not sensitive enough to detect potential changes. In one study (43) the estimated total lean body mass did not increase with 26 weeks of total-body resistive training in men and women aged 70 to 79 years; however, specific muscle girths increased indicating that muscular hypertrophy probably did occur. A more recent study in 50- to 70-yr-old men that used magnetic resonance imaging found an 8% increase in midthigh, cross-sectional muscle area and increases in other muscle girths as a result of 16 weeks of total-body resistive training; although, again, lean body mass assessed by underwater weighing did not increase (80). The men in this study also elicited 3.8% and 2% increases in bone mineral density in the femoral neck and the lumbar spine, respectively, as a result of the resistive training (67). Because bone mineral density is known to be related to muscular strength (see 100), these data raise the possibility that resistive training may also have the capacity to increase bone mineral density at critical skeletal sites in older individuals.

Whereas resistive training is most prominently associated with increases in muscular strength and mass, it has also been reported to improve plasma lipoprotein-lipids, OGTT plasma insulin responses, and BP in young to middle-aged individuals (40,53,68). However, most studies have not found improvements in these CVD risk factors with resistive training in young and middle-aged populations (55). A recent study in men and women aged 70 to 79 years found no changes in BP or OGTT plasma glucose or insulin responses as a result of 6 months of resistive training that did not change their estimated lean body mass (17,49). On the other hand, Craig, Everhart, and Brown (19) found a 20% improvement in OGTT plasma insulin responses in men and women aged 60 to 69 years with 12 weeks of resistive training that did increase their lean body mass. Resistive training has been reported to result in only minimal, if any, improvements in CV function in older individuals (19,43,53,56,80).

Summary of the Effects of Exercise Training in Older Men and Women

It is clear that older men and women generally elicit the same beneficial adaptations in response to endurance exercise training as do younger individuals. These adaptations, including improved CV function, body composition, and CVD risk factor profiles, all run counter to those found with aging and decrease the older person's risk for CVD mortality and disability.

Resistive training should be recommended for older individuals primarily to attenuate the losses of muscle strength and mass that occur with aging. Resistive training also holds the potential for improving metabolic CVD risk factors, especially if lean body mass is increased, and for improving bone density; however, additional research is required to document these adaptations in older persons.

Summary and Conclusions

In 1983 Holloszy concluded that much of the positive attention that exercise training had received was based "on emotional reactions and wishful thinking," and that this lack of valid scientific information applied especially well to exercise recommendations for elderly populations (51). A decade of research on the effects of exercise training for older persons has now brought us to the point where exercise training *can* and *should* be recommended for most older individuals. This conclusion is based on these facts: (a) Although definitive evidence documenting the beneficial effects of exercise training on mortality and disability in the elderly is still lacking, it is clear that risk factor profiles for many of the pathologies that limit the quality and quantity of life for older individuals are beneficially affected by exercise training; and (b) No data indicate that exercise training has a deleterious effect on older individuals.

An exercise program for older persons should be multifactorial stressing cardiovascular and strength activities while also including flexibility and balance components similar to physical fitness guidelines proposed by Cureton nearly 50 years ago (22). Thus, specific prescriptions for cardiovascular, strength, flexibility, and balance activities should be included in older individuals' exercise programs to optimize their future health. Although it is clear that exercise training can and should be recommended for most older individuals, more studies are necessary (a) to ascertain that these beneficial training effects are generalizable to all older men and women, (b) to determine the most appropriate training prescriptions to elicit these beneficial adaptations, and (c) to determine if the mechanisms underlying these beneficial responses in the elderly are the same as those in young and middle-aged populations.

References

1. Ades, P.A.; Grunvald, M.H. Cardiopulmonary exercise testing before and after conditioning in older coronary patients. Am. Heart J. 120:585-589; 1990.
2. Ades, P.A.; Hanson, J.S.; Gunther, P.G.S.; Tonino, R.P. Exercise conditioning in the elderly coronary patient. J. Am. Geriatr. Soc. 35:121-124; 1987.
3. Agre, J.C.; Pierce, L.E.; Raab, D.M.; McAdams, M. Light resistance and stretching exercise in elderly women: Effect upon strength. Arch. Phys. Med. Rehabil. 69:273-276; 1988.
4. Aniansson, A.; Grimby, G.; Rundgren, A.; Svanborg, A.; Orlander, J. Physical training in old men. Age Ageing 9:186-187; 1980.
5. Aniansson, A.; Gustafsson, E. Physical training in old men with special reference to quadriceps muscle strength and morphology. Clin. Physiol. 1:73-86; 1981.

6. Aniansson, A.; Ljungberg, P.; Rundgren, A.; Wetterqvist, H. Effect of a training programme for pensioners on condition and muscular strength. Arch. Gerontol. Geriatr. 3:229-241; 1984.
7. Baker, S.B.; Harvey, A.H. Fall injuries in the elderly. Clin. Geriatr. Med. 1:501-508; 1985.
8. Belman, M.J.; Gaesser, G.A. Exercise training below and above the lactate threshold in the elderly. Med. Sci. Sports Exercise. 23:562-568; 1991.
9. Blumenthal, J.A.; Emery, C.F.; Madden, D.J.; Coleman, R.E.; Riddle, M.W.; Cobb, F.R.; Sullivan, M.J.; Higginbotham, M.B. Effects of exercise training on cardiorespiratory function in men and women over 60 years of age. Am. J. Cardiol. 67:633-639; 1991.
10. Blumenthal, J.A.; Emery, C.; Madden, D.; Coleman, R.E.; Riddle, M.W.; McKee, D.C.; Reasoner, J.; Williams, R.S. Cardiovascular and behavioral effects of aerobic exercise training in healthy older men and women. J. Gerontol. 44:M147-M157; 1989.
11. Brock, D.B.; Guralnik, J.M.; Brody, J.A. Demography and epidemiology of aging in the U.S. In: Schneider, E.L.; Rowe, J.W., eds. Handbook of the biology of aging. 3rd ed. San Diego: Academic Press; 1990: 3-23.
12. Brown, A.B.; McCartney, N.; Sale, D.G. Positive adaptations to weight-lifting training in the elderly. J. Appl. Physiol. 69:1725-1733; 1990.
13. Brown, M.; Holloszy, J.O. Effects of a low intensity exercise program on selected physical performance characteristics of 60 to 71 yr olds. Aging. 3:129-139; 1991.
14. Buccola, V.A.; Stone, W.J. Effects of jogging and cycling on physiological and personality variables in aged men. Res. Quart. 46:134-139; 1975.
15. Busby, J.; Goldberg, A.P.; Krauss, R.M.; Hagberg, J.M. Lipoprotein-lipids, lipase activities, and glucose tolerance in older endurance-trained athletes. Atherosclerosis [Submitted].
16. Cononie, C.C.; Goldberg, A.P.; Rogus, E.; Hagberg, J.M. Effects of 7 consecutive days of exercise on plasma insulin in 60-80 yr olds. J. Gerontol. [Submitted].
17. Cononie, C.C.; Graves, J.E.; Pollock, M.L.; Phillips, M.I.; Sumners, C.; Hagberg, J.M. Effect of exercise training on blood pressure in 70-79 yr old men and women. Med. Sci. Sports Exerc. 23:505-511; 1991.
18. Coon, P.J.; Bleecker, E.R.; Drinkwater, D.T.; Meyers, D.A.; Goldberg, A.P. Effects of body composition and exercise capacity on glucose tolerance, insulin, and lipoprotein lipids in healthy older men: A cross-sectional and longitudinal intervention study. Metabolism. 38:1201-1209; 1989.
19. Craig, B.W.; Everhart, J.; Brown, R. Influence of high-resistance training on glucose tolerance in young and elderly subjects. Mech. Ageing Dev. 49:147-157; 1989.
20. Cress, M.E.; Thomas, D.P.; Johnson, J.; Kasch, F.W.; Cassens, R.G.; Smith, E.L.; Agre, J.C. Effect of training on $\dot{V}O_2$max, thigh strength, and muscle morphology in septuagenarian women. Med. Sci. Sports Exerc. 23:752-758; 1991.
21. Cunningham, D.; Montoye, H.; Metzner, H.; Keller, J. Active leisure time activities as related to age among males in a total population. J. Gerontol. 23:551-559; 1968.
22. Cureton, T.K. Physical fitness appraisal and guidance. St. Louis: Mosby; 1947.
23. Dalsky, G.P.; Stocke, K.S.; Ehsani, A.A.; Slatopolsky, E.; Birge, S.J. Weight-bearing exercise training and bone mineral content in postmenopausal women. Ann. Intern. Med. 108:824-828; 1988.
24. Dengel, D.R.; Hagberg, J.M.; Drinkwater, D.T.; Lakatta, L.E.; Goldberg, A.P. Effects of aerobic exercise and weight loss on body composition in older obese men. Metabolism. [Submitted].
25. Dengel, D.R.; Hagberg, J.M.; Lakatta, L.E.; Goldberg, A.P. Effects of aerobic exercise and hypocaloric feeding on fat distribution in older obese men. J. Gerontol. [Submitted].
26. Dustman, R.E.; Ruhling, R.O.; Russell, E.M.; Shearer, D.E.; Bonekat, H.W.; Shigeoka, J.W.; Woods, J.S.; Bradford, D.C. Aerobic exercise training and improved neuropsychological function of older individuals. Neurobiol. Aging. 5:35-42; 1984.
27. Ehsani, A.A.; Ogawa, T.; Miller, T.R.; Spina, R.J.; Jilka, S.M. Exercise training improves left ventricular systolic function in older men. Circulation. 83:96-103; 1991.
28. Elsayed, M.; Ismail, A.H.; Young, R.J. Intellectual differences of adult men related to age and physical fitness before and after an exercise program. J. Gerontol. 35:383-387; 1980.
29. Emes, C.G. The effects of a regular program of light exercise on seniors. Int. J. Sports Med. Phys. Fitness. 19:185-190; 1979.
30. Everhart, J.; Knowler, W.C.; Bennett, P.H. Incidence and risk factors for noninsulin-dependent diabetes. In: Diabetes in America: Diabetes data compiled 1984. NIH publication 85-1468. U.S. Department of Health and Human Services; 1985:IV1-IV35.
31. Fell, R.D.; Terblanche, S.E.; Ivy, J.L.; Young, J.C.; Holloszy, J.O. Effect of muscle glycogen

content on glucose uptake following exercise. J. Appl. Physiol. 52:434-437; 1982.

32. Fiatarone, M.A.; Marks, E.C.; Ryan, N.; Meredith, C.N.; Lipsitz, L.; Evans, W.J. High-intensity strength training in nonagenarians: Effects on skeletal muscle. JAMA. 263:3029-3034; 1990.
33. Foster, V.L.; Hume, G.J.E.; Byrnes, W.C.; Dickinson, A.L.; Chatfield, S.J. Endurance training for elderly women: Moderate versus low intensity. J. Gerontol. 44:M184-M188; 1989.
34. Frontera, W.; Meredith, C.; O'Reilly, K.; Knuttgen, H.; Evans, W. Strength conditioning in older men: Skeletal muscle hypertrophy and improved function. J. Appl. Physiol. 64:1038-1044; 1988.
35. Gibson, D.; Karpovich, P.V.; Gollnick, P.D. Effects of training upon reflex and reaction times. Res. report DA-49-007-MD-889. Washington, DC: Office of the Surgeon General; 1961.
36. Gilders, R.M.; Voiner, C.; Dudley, G.A. Endurance training and blood pressure in normotensive and hypertensive adults. Med. Sci. Sports Exerc. 21:629-636; 1989.
37. Grimby, G. Physical activity and effects of muscle training in the elderly. Ann. Clin. Res. 20:62-66; 1988.
38. Grimby, G.; Saltin, B. Physiological analysis of middle-aged and old athletes. Acta Med. Scand. 179:513-526; 1966.
39. Hagberg, J.M. Effect of training on the decline of $\dot{V}O_2$max with aging. Fed. Proc. 46:1830-1837; 1987.
40. Hagberg, J.M. Exercise, fitness, and hypertension. In: Bouchard, C.; Shephard, R.J.; Stephens, T.; Sutton, J.R.; MacPherson, B.D., eds. Exercise, fitness, and health. Champaign, IL: Human Kinetics; 1988:455-466.
41. Hagberg, J.M. Physiologic adaptations to prolonged high-intensity exercise training in patients with coronary artery disease. Med. Sci. Sports Exerc. 23:661-667; 1991.
42. Hagberg, J.M.; Allen, W.K.; Seals, D.R.; Hurley, B.F.; Ehsani, A.A.; Holloszy, J.O. A hemodynamic comparison of young and older endurance athletes during exercise. J. Appl. Physiol. 58:2041-2046; 1985.
43. Hagberg, J.M.; Graves, J.E.; Limacher, M.; Woods, D.R.; Leggett, S.H.; Cononie, C.; Gruber, J.J.; Pollock, M.L. Cardiovascular responses of 70-79 yr old men and women to exercise training. J. Appl. Physiol. 66:2589-2594; 1989.
44. Hagberg, J.M.; Montain, S.J.; Martin, W.H.; Ehsani, A.A. Effect of exercise training on 60-69 yr old persons with essential hypertension. Am. J. Cardiol. 64:348-353; 1989.
45. Harris, T.; Cook, E.F.; Kannel, W.; Schatzkin, A.; Goldman, L. Blood pressure experience and risk of cardiovascular disease in the elderly. Hypertension. 7:118-124; 1985.
46. Haupt, B.J.; Graves, E. Detailed diagnoses and surgical procedures for patients discharged from short-stay hospitals: United States, 1979. DHHS pub. #(PHS) 82-1274. Washington, DC: U.S. Department of Health and Human Services; 1982.
47. Heath, G.W.; Gavin, J.R., III; Hinderliter, J.M.; Hagberg, J.M.; Bloomfield, S.A.; Holloszy, J.O. Effects of exercise and lack of exercise on glucose tolerance and insulin sensitivity. J. Appl. Physiol. 55:512-517; 1983.
48. Heath, G.W.; Hagberg, J.M.; Ehsani, A.A.; Holloszy, J.O. A physiological comparison of young and older endurance athletes. J. Appl. Physiol. 51:634-640; 1981.
49. Hersey, W.C.; Graves, J.E.; Pollock, M.L.; Gingerich, R.; Heath, G.W.; Spierto, F.; McCole, S.D.; Hagberg, J.M. Endurance exercise training improves body composition and plasma insulin responses in 70-79 yr old men and women. Metabolism [Submitted].
50. Hodgson, J.L.; Buskirk, E.R. Physical fitness and age, with emphasis on cardiovascular function in the elderly. J. Am. Geriatr. Soc. 25:385-392; 1977.
51. Holloszy, J.O. Exercise, health, and aging: A need for more information. Med. Sci. Sports Exerc. 15:1-5; 1983.
52. Holloszy, J.O.; Schultz, J.; Kusnierkiewicz, J.; Hagberg, J.M.; Ehsani, A.A. Effects of exercise on glucose tolerance and insulin resistance. Acta Med. Scand. [Suppl.]. 711:55-65; 1986.
53. Hurley, B.F.; Hagberg, J.M.; Goldberg, A.P.; Seals, D.R.; Ehsani, A.A.; Brennan, R.E.; Holloszy, J.O. Resistive training can reduce coronary risk factors without altering $\dot{V}O_2$max or percent body fat. Med. Sci. Sports Exerc. 20:150-154; 1988.
54. Hurley, B.F.; Hagberg, J.M.; Seals, D.R.; Ehsani, A.A.; Goldberg, A.; Holloszy, J.O. Glucose tolerance and lipoprotein-lipids in middle-aged powerlifters. Clin. Physiol. 7:11-19; 1987.
55. Hurley, B.F.; Kokkinos, P.F. Effects of weight training on CAD risk factors. Sports Med. 4:231-238; 1987.
56. Hurley, B.F.; Seals, D.R.; Ehsani, A.A.; Cartier, L.-J.; Dalsky, G.P.; Hagberg, J.M.; Holloszy, J.O. Effects of high-intensity strength training on cardiovascular function. Med. Sci. Sports Exerc. 16:483-488; 1984.
57. Irving, J.B.; Kusumi, F.; Bruce, R.A. Longitudinal variations in maximal oxygen consumption in healthy men. Clin. Cardiol. 3:134-136; 1980.

58. Kahn, S.E.; Larson, V.G.; Beard, J.; Cain, K.; Schwartz, R.S.; Veith, R.C.; Stratton, J.R.; Cerqueira, M.D.; Abrass, I.B. Effects of exercise on insulin action, glucose tolerance, and insulin secretion in aging. Am. J. Physiol. 258:E937-E943; 1990.
59. Kannel, W.B.; Gordon, T. Evaluation of cardiovascular risk in the elderly: The Framingham study. Bull. NY. Acad. Med. 54:573-591; 1978.
60. Kaplan, N.M. Clinical hypertension. 5th ed. Baltimore: Williams & Wilkins; 1990.
61. Kohrt, W.M.; Malley, M.; Coggan, A.; Spina, R.; Ogawa, T.; Ehsani, A.A.; Bourey, R.E.; Martin, W.H., III; Holloszy, J.O. Effects of gender, age, and fitness level on response of $\dot{V}O_2$max to training in 60-71 yr olds. J. Appl. Physiol. 71:2004-2011; 1991.
62. Kuller, L.H.; Hulley, S.B.; Cohen, J.D.; Neaton, J. Unexpected effects of treating hypertension in men with ECG abnormalities: A critical analysis. Circulation. 73:114-123; 1986.
63. Lampman, R.M.; Schteingart, D.E. Moderate and extreme obesity. In: Franklin, B.A.; Gordon, S.; Timmis, G.C., eds. Exercise in modern medicine. Baltimore: Williams & Wilkins; 1898:156-174.
64. Larsson, L. Physical training effects on muscle morphology in sedentary males at different ages. Med. Sci. Sports Exerc. 14:203-206; 1982.
65. Makrides, L.; Heigenhauser, G.J.F.; Jones, N.L. High-intensity endurance training in 20-30 and 60-70 yr old healthy men. J. Appl. Physiol. 69:1792-1798; 1990.
66. McGandy, R.B.; Barrows, C.H.; Spanias, A.; Meredith, A.; Stone, J.L.; Norris, A.H. Nutrient intakes and energy expenditure in men of different ages. J. Gerontol. 21:581-587; 1966.
67. Menkes, A.; Mazel, S.; Redmond, R.; Koffler, K.; Libanati, C.; Zizic, T.; Hagberg, J.M.; Pratley, R.E.; Hurley, B.F. Strength training increases regional bone mineral density in middle-aged and older men. J. Appl. Physiol. [Submitted].
68. Miller, W.J.; Sherman, W.M.; Ivy, J.L. Effect of strength training on glucose tolerance and post-glucose insulin response. Med. Sci. Sports Exerc. 16:539-543; 1984.
69. Moritani, T.; DeVries, H.A. Potential for gross muscle hypertrophy in older men. J. Gerontol. 35:672-682; 1980.
70. Munns, K. Effects of exercise on the range of joint motion in elderly subjects. In: Smith, E.L.; Serfass, R.C., eds. Exercise and aging. Hillside, NJ: Enslow Publishers; 1981:167-178.
71. Nevitt, M.C.; Cumming, S.R.; Kidd, S.; Black, D. Risk factors for recurrent nonsyncopal falls: A prospective study. JAMA. 261:2663-2668; 1989.
72. Northcote, R.J.; Canning, G.C.; Todd, I.C.; Ballantyne, D. Lipoprotein profiles of elite veteran endurance athletes. Am. J. Cardiol. 61:934-935; 1988.
73. Ostrow, A.C. Physical activity and the older adult: Psychological perspectives. Princeton, NJ: Princeton Book Co.; 1984:78.
74. Panton, L.; Graves, J.E.; Pollock, M.L.; Hagberg, J.M.; Chen, W. Effect of aerobic and resistance training on fractionated reaction time and speed of movement. J. Gerontol. 45:M26-M31; 1990.
75. Pollock, M.L. The quantification of endurance training programs. Exerc. Sport Sci. Rev. 1:155-188; 1973.
76. Pollock, M.L.; Foster, C.; Knapp, D.; Rod, J.L.; Schmidt, D.H. Effect of age and training on aerobic capacity and body composition of master athletes. J. Appl. Physiol. 62:625-631; 1987.
77. Pollock, M.L.; Miller, H.S.; Wilmore, J.H. Physiological characteristics of champion American track athletes 40 to 75 yrs of age. J. Gerontol. 29:645-649; 1974.
78. Powell, R.R.; Pohndorf, R.H. Comparison of adult exercisers and nonexercisers on fluid intelligence and selected physiological variables. Res. Q. Exerc. Sport. 42:70-77; 1971.
79. Reaven, G.M. The role of insulin resistance in human disease. Diabetes. 37:1595-1607; 1988.
80. Redmond, R.; Menkes, A.; Koffler, K.; Hagberg, J.M.; Goldberg, A.P.; Hurley, B.F. Effects of strength training on muscle size and injury in older men. J. Appl. Physiol. [Submitted].
81. Rivera, A.M.; Pels, A.E.; Sady, S.P.; Sady, M.A.; Cullinane, E.M.; Thompson, P.D. Physiological factors associated with the lower maximal oxygen consumption of masters runners. J. Appl. Physiol. 66:949-954; 1989.
82. Robinson, S.; Dill, D.B.; Robinson, R.D.; Tzankoff, S.P.; Wagner, P.D. Physiological aging of champion runners. J. Appl. Physiol. 41:46-51; 1976.
83. Rogers, M.A.; Hagberg, J.M.; Martin, W.H., III; Ehsani, A.A.; Holloszy, J.O. Decline in $\dot{V}O_2$max with aging in master athletes and sedentary men. J. Appl. Physiol. 68:2195-2199; 1990.
84. Rogers, M.A.; King, D.S.; Hagberg, J.M.; Ehsani, A.A.; Holloszy, J.O. Effect of 10 days of physical inactivity on glucose tolerance in master athletes. J. Appl. Physiol. 68:1833-1837; 1990.
85. Rogers, M.A.; Yamamoto, C.; King, D.S.; Hagberg, J.M.; Ehsani, A.A.; Holloszy, J.O. Improvement in glucose tolerance after 1 wk

of exercise in patients with mild NIDDM. Diabetes Care. 11:613-618; 1988.

86. Saltin, B. The aging endurance athlete. In: Sutton, J.R.; Brock, R.M., eds. Sports medicine for the mature athlete. Indianapolis: Benchmark Press; 1986:59-80.
87. Schocken, D.D.; Blumenthal, J.A.; Port, S.; Hindle, P.; Coleman, R.E. Physical conditioning and left ventricular performance in the elderly: Assessment by radionuclide angiocardiography. Am. J. Cardiol. 52:359-364; 1983.
88. Schwartz, W.P.; Shuman, V.; Larson, K.C.; Cain, G.W.; Fellingham, J.C.; Beard, S.E.; Kahn, J.R.; Stratton, M.D.; Abrass, I.B. The effect of intensive endurance exercise training on body fat distribution in young and older men. Metabolism. 40:545-551; 1991.
89. Seals, D.R.; Allen, W.K.; Hurley, B.F.; Dalsky, G.P.; Ehsani, A.A.; Hagberg, J.M. Elevated high-density lipoprotein cholesterol levels in older endurance athletes. Am. J. Cardiol. 54:390-393; 1984.
90. Seals, D.R.; Hagberg, J.M.; Allen, W.K.; Hurley, B.F.; Dalsky, G.P.; Ehsani, A.A.; Holloszy, J.O. Glucose tolerance in young and older athletes and sedentary men. J. Appl. Physiol. 56:1521-1525; 1984.
91. Seals, D.R.; Hagberg, J.M.; Hurley, B.F.; Ehsani, A.A.; Holloszy, J.O. Endurance exercise training in older men and women. I. Cardiovascular response to exercise. J. Appl. Physiol. 57:1024-1029; 1984.
92. Seals, D.R.; Hagberg, J.M.; Hurley, B.F.; Ehsani, A.A.; Holloszy, J.O. Effects of endurance training on glucose tolerance and plasma lipid levels in older men and women. JAMA. 252:645-649; 1984.
93. Seals, D.R.; Reiling, M.J. Effect of regular exercise on 24-hr arterial blood pressure in older hypertensive humans. Hypertension. 18:583-592; 1991.
94. Segal, K.R.; Edano, A.; Abalos, A.; Albu, J.; Blando, L.; Tomas, M.; Pi-Sunyer, F.X. Effect of exercise training on insulin sensitivity and glucose metabolism in lean, obese, and diabetic men. J. Appl. Physiol. 71:2402-2411; 1991.
95. Sherwood, D.E.; Seider, D.J. Cardiorespiratory health, reaction time, and aging. Med. Sci. Sports. 11:186-189; 1979.
96. Shimokata, H.; Andres, R.; Coon, P.J.; Elahi, D.; Muller, D.C.; Tobin, J.D. Studies in the distribution of body fat. II. Longitudinal effects of change in weight. Int. J. Obes. 13:455-464; 1988.
97. Shimokata, H.; Tobin, J.D.; Muller, D.C.; Elahi, D.; Coon, P.J.; Andres, R. Studies in the distribution of body fat. I. Effects of age, sex, and obesity. J. Gerontol. 44:M66-73; 1989.
98. Sipila, S.; Viitasalo, J.; Era, P.; Suominen, H. Muscle strength in male athletes aged 70-81 yrs and a population sample. Eur. J. Appl. Physiol. 63:399-403; 1991.
99. Skinner, J.S. Age and performance. In: Keul, J.; ed. Limiting factors of physical performance. W. Germany: Thieme Publishers; 1973:271-282.
100. Snow-Harter, C.; Marcus, R. Exercise, bone mineral density, and osteoporosis. In: Holloszy, J.O., ed. Exercise and sport science reviews (vol. 19). Baltimore: Williams & Wilkins; 1991:351-388.
101. Spirduso, W.W.; Clifford, P. Replication of age and physical activity effects on reaction and movement times. J. Gerontol. 33:26-30; 1978.
102. Tinetti, M.E.; Speechley, M.; Ginter, S.F. Risk factors for falls among elderly persons living in the community. N. Engl. J. Med. 319:1701-1707; 1988.
103. Tonino, R.P. Effect of physical training on the insulin resistance of aging. Am. J. Physiol. 256:E352-E356; 1989.
104. Wood, P.D.; Stefanick, M.L. Exercise, fitness, and atherosclerosis. In: Bouchard, C.; Shephard, R.J.; Stephens, T.; Sutton, J.R.; MacPherson, B.D., eds. Exercise, fitness, and health. Champaign, IL: Human Kinetics; 1988:409-423.

PART VII

Risks of Activity Versus Inactivity

Chapter 69

Risks of Exercising: Musculoskeletal Injuries

Russell R. Pate
Caroline A. Macera

An extensive body of knowledge now links regular participation in exercise to higher levels of physical fitness and to reduced risk of developing chronic diseases such as coronary heart disease, hypertension, and diabetes. It is well established that chronic participation in vigorous forms of exercise can produce or maintain higher levels of cardiorespiratory fitness (1) and muscular strength (17,93). Also, vigorous, habitual exercise has been shown to cause improvements in chronic disease risk factors such as blood lipid profiles (94), blood pressure (14), body composition, and glucose metabolism. In addition, the results of recent epidemiological studies suggest that moderate amounts of physical activity are associated with very substantial reductions in risk of chronic disease morbidity and all-cause mortality (4,6,24, 43,59,60,61,66). Such findings have prompted public health authorities to endorse regular, moderate-to-vigorous exercise as an important component of a healthy lifestyle.

Although the health benefits of regular exercise are very significant, it has long been recognized that these benefits do not come without cost. As participation in exercise became more prevalent during the 1970s and 1980s it became evident that exercise can produce negative health outcomes in at least some participants. It is now known that exercise, if used improperly, can aggravate some existing disease states (77). Among healthy persons, who constitute most of the population, one of the greatest of the perceived costs of regular exercise is risk of musculoskeletal injuries. Such injuries increase the burden on the health care system, can be financially and emotionally costly to the participant, and may be a deterrent to continued participation in exercise.

Studies of patient groups treated in hospital emergency rooms and physician's offices have clearly indicated that a great many persons experience musculoskeletal injury while engaged in organized and individual exercise and sporting activities. However, because such studies do not allow observation of rates of injury in specified populations, they fail to provide information concerning the incidence of and risk factors for musculoskeletal injuries during exercise participation. Such information is needed to fully evaluate the cost:benefit ratio associated with being a regular exerciser. Accordingly, this paper is intended to review the existing epidemiological literature concerning the incidence of and risk factors for musculoskeletal injury during participation in exercise. A secondary purpose is to indicate important directions for future research on these issues.

Delimitations

As noted, the health benefits of exercise are now widely accepted by public health authorities. As a result, public health initiatives designed to increase exercise participation in the population have become increasingly common. A prime example is *Healthy People 2000* (21), a document produced by the U.S. Public Health Service that includes over 200 health objectives that are designed to guide the activities of health agencies during the 1990s. Included in *Healthy People 2000* are 12 objectives that deal specifically with increasing exercise participation. We believe that public health promotional efforts, like those embodied in *Healthy People 2000*, constitute the most cost-effective and feasible approach to increasing the prevalence of appropriate exercise behavior in society at large. Accordingly, we have organized this chapter in a manner that we think is consistent with the "public health approach" to exercise promotion.

In addition, we have opted to focus principally on musculoskeletal injuries as observed in groups of adults. Although the incidence of sports- and activity-related injuries appears to be high among youth and deserves full attention, this report is limited to adults because (a) the evidence linking regular exercise to better health is most clear for adults; and (b) the types of activities, rates of participation, and types of injury differ between youth and adults.

The second major delimitation is that primary attention will be given to injuries associated with the forms of exercise that are most prevalent in the adult population. There are, of course, a very large number of activities that are engaged in by some adults. However, as will be discussed, most North Americans who are physically active report participating in one or more of a relatively small number of particularly popular activities. It is our assumption that, if the percentage of active adults is appreciably increased through public health initiatives, most of this increased activity would probably come in the forms of exercise that are now most prevalent. Consequently, it seems most important that the injury risks associated with these activities be understood.

Prevalent Modes of Exercise

Over the past decade several population surveys of exercise behavior have been conducted in the United States and Canada. As noted in a review by Stephens, Jacobs, and White (80), there is considerable consistency across the various surveys in the relative rankings of specific modes of leisure-time physical activity. Stephens et al. (80) reported that the most popular activities in order of decreasing prevalence are walking, swimming, calisthenics, bicycling, jogging, bowling, and softball.

The most recent national survey in the United States for which results are available is the Behavioral Risk Factor Surveillance System (BRFSS) conducted in 1989 by 40 state health departments in cooperation with the U.S. Centers for Disease Control. BRFSS is a telephone survey that includes the question: "During the past month, did you participate in any physical activities or exercises such as running, calisthenics, golf, gardening, or walking for exercise?" (92). Approximately two thirds (67.7%) of the 67,293 respondents answered that question in the affirmative. Those answering "yes" were asked to indicate the specific activities (up to two) in which they had participated for the most time during the preceding month.

Table 69.1 lists the specific activities that were reported by more than 1% of the respondents as either the primary or secondary form of activity used during the previous month. The listing of activities in Table 69.1 is, in general, consistent with the earlier conclusions of Stephens. Walking, jogging, swimming, and cycling—all activities that are considered aerobic conditioning exercises—were found to be quite popular. In addition, gardening, aerobic dance, weight lifting, and golf were reported by sizable numbers of respondents. Based on these BRFSS data and the earlier report of Stephens et al. (80), the following specific exercise activities will be addressed in this paper: walking, running/jogging, swimming, softball, aerobic dance/calisthenics, cycling, and tennis/racket sports. Also, leisure activities with recreational vehicles were included because these activities may involve unique risks of injury.

Clinical Studies

Our knowledge of the incidence of and risk factors for musculoskeletal injuries associated with exercise is limited. Nonetheless, it does seem certain that a great many persons do experience injury as a result of participation in exercise and sport. This general conclusion is supported by the collective results of several types of investigations that appear in the literature. Of these, the most common is the clinical study in which the records of patients passing through a clinical practice are surveyed to determine the percentage of patients whose injuries were associated with exercise or sports. Also, these studies can provide information concerning the most common types of injuries and can describe the clinical course of the various types of injured patients. Examples of these clinical studies from various countries are provided in the reference list (12,27,48,51,53,57,62,79).

These studies all demonstrate that considerable numbers of patients go to clinics for treatment of musculoskeletal injuries associated with exercise. However, from an epidemiological standpoint, these clinical studies are severely limited because they cannot provide information on the prevalence or incidence of exercise-related injury in a population. The limitations of "nondenominator" studies have been discussed in detail (66). Briefly, without knowing the size of the population from which the clinical cases were drawn we learn little about the public health impact of a series of cases.

Communitywide Studies

Much better information concerning the incidence or prevalence of activity-related injury can be provided by studies in which entire communities are observed. In recent years a small number of these studies have been completed, most of them in

Table 69.1 Most Prevalent Forms of Leisure-Time Physical Activity in American Adults in 1989*

Activity	Number of respondents	% of all respondents N = 67,293	% of active respondents N = 45,607
Walking	23,642	35.1	51.8
Gardening	4,726	7.0	10.4
Running/jogging	4,464	6.6	9.8
Aerobic dance	4,400	6.5	9.6
Bicycling	2,617	3.9	5.7
Weight lifting	2,604	3.9	5.7
Golf	2,252	3.4	4.9
Swimming laps	2,173	3.3	4.8
Basketball	1,558	2.3	3.4
Home exercise	1,516	2.3	3.3
Calisthenics	1,504	2.2	3.3
Stationary cycling	1,304	1.9	2.9
Softball	1,041	1.6	2.3
Racquet sports	1,025	1.5	2.2
Nothing	21,686	32.2	—

Note. — = not applicable. *Determined by the Behavioral Risk Factor Surveillance System (BRFSS).

Scandinavia. For example, Sandelin, Sartavirta, Lattila, Vuolle, and Sarna (73), observing the population of greater Helsinki, Finland, in 1980, reported 670 ± 1,232 sports injuries per 10,000 persons, and this corresponded to approximately 14% of all injuries. De Loes and colleagues (10,11) studied a rural municipality in Sweden and found that 17% of all injuries were activity-related. In contrast with the study of Sandelin et al., de Loes reported a considerably lower rate of injury (150 per 10,000), probably because a more restrictive definition of injury was applied.

Another approach to studying the epidemiology of activity-related injuries has been to observe the incidence of specific types of injuries and to quantify the percentage of those injuries associated with sports or exercise. Studying ankle fractures in Rochester, Minnesota, Daly, Fitzgerald, Melton, and Ilstrip (9) reported an overall incidence rate of 187 per 100,000 person-years. Thirty-six percent of these fractures were associated with sport participation. Hede, Jensen, Blyme, and Sonne-Holm (23) found that 38% of openly operated meniscal lesions in the knee followed sport-related injuries. So the unavoidable conclusion must be that large numbers of injuries do arise from participation in exercise.

Activity-Specific Injury Risks

As mentioned, a major purpose of this chapter is to summarize and evaluate the existing research on injury risks associated with participation in those specific forms of exercise that are currently most prevalent among adults in North America. An overriding goal is to provide information that might aid in performing a cost–benefit analysis for each activity. Our knowledge of injury risks varies widely across the different activities. This discussion begins with running/jogging, the fitness activity for which our knowledge of injury risk is by far the most extensive.

Running/Jogging

In 1989 about 7% of adults in the U.S. reported running or jogging as their primary or secondary leisure-time activity (Table 69.1). Population-based studies of runners have consistently reported annual rates of musculoskeletal injuries that range from 35% (36) to 65% (45). This variation in injury rates may be due to the diversity of populations studied and the different definitions of injury applied among the studies. Most injuries occur to the lower extremities, especially the knee, foot, and ankle. The most frequently reported types of musculoskeletal injuries are sprains, strains, stress fractures, and various overuse injuries (e.g., patellar or achilles tendinitis).

Many factors that may influence risk of injury in runners have been identified and summarized by Powell, Kohl, Casperson, and Blair (65). These factors are usually divided into two general categories: (a) personal characteristics of the runner, such as gender, age, running experience, previous injury, body composition, and psychological factors; and (b) training characteristics, such as weekly mileage, frequency, speed, racing activity, warm-up, time of run, and running surface. In general, personal factors are not amenable to modification while training aspects are within the control of the runner.

Among population-based studies of recreational and elite runners in which the type, duration, and intensity of running activities were under control of the runner, the injury rate was similar for men and women (31,46,47,49,88). Contrary to expectation, rates of injury among runners did not increase with increasing age (46,47,50,87). Studies of marathon runners have also reported a lower rate of injuries among older runners (over age 40 years) compared to younger runners and a lower injury rate among those who had previously competed in a marathon (55). In addition, Kretsch et al. (40) found that older marathon participants (over age 40 years) report fewer race day symptoms than younger runners.

These results are consistent with the notion that those who have a propensity to running injuries may choose other types of physical activity. Furthermore, older runners may have had more running experience, thus enabling them to avoid overuse injuries. Alternatively, older runners may exhibit musculoskeletal adaptation to running, thus explaining the lower injury rate. Yet, one study found that while the injury rate actually decreased among older runners, the amount of time lost due to injuries increased, suggesting an age-related slowing of recuperative ability (50). So, whereas age may not be a determining factor for predicting injuries, the injuries sustained due to running may require more time to heal than those occurring among younger individuals.

Some studies found that inexperienced runners are at increased risk of injury during a 1-year follow-up (47,50). The lower injury rate among more seasoned runners (similar to the lower injury rate among older runners) may be due to the self-selection of injury-prone individuals into other types of physical activities. The lower injury rate among more experienced runners could also be due to a musculoskeletal adaptive process that would actually result in a decrease in injury rate as the years of training increase, even if weekly mileage was high. This idea is supported by a finding that non-elite marathon runners had lower injury rates than expected given their training mileage (26).

Almost every relevant epidemiologic study has identified the report of a previous injury as a risk factor for future injuries (28,36,47,50,87). In marathon studies those who required treatment during and immediately after the marathon were more likely to have had an injury before the race (40). In earlier studies this effect was not adjusted for other running characteristics such as running mileage, and it was not clear whether a previous injury represented additional risk for future injuries after controlling for distance. However, several studies have been published that found a previous injury to be a significant predictor of injury during follow-up even after controlling for distance (47, 50,87). It is not clear whether this finding suggests (a) incomplete healing of the original injury, (b) a personal propensity or susceptibility for reinjury, or (c) an uncorrected biomechanical problem.

The effect of high or low weight or percent body fat has been examined from several perspectives. Pollock et al. (64) found that among those beginning a running program, those with a high percentage of body fat had more injuries. However, in this study as in studies of habitual runners, there were very few obese individuals. Some studies found no clear effect of body composition on injury rates (36,47), whereas other studies reported a U-shaped relationship such that both the lightest group and the heaviest group were at increased risk for injuries (50). The population studies do not support any particular risk of injury associated with heavy body weight (or high percent body fat). However, it was very difficult to sort out this factor because many people start running to lose weight, and those who have been running for a while are usually lean.

A review of the sports medicine literature suggested that several personality traits are associated with an increased risk of injury (34), but very few carefully controlled studies have examined these issues among habitual runners. In a small, 1-year follow-up of 40 runners, Type A behavior, but not running mileage, was associated with an increase in running injuries, particularly multiple injuries (15). Although one could postulate that certain psychological problems with attendant attention deficits or motor control problems could place afflicted runners at increased risk of injuries, this has yet to be demonstrated.

Studies in different populations with different definitions of injury have consistently reported an increase in injuries with an increase in distance run, with risk increasing after about 33 km/week (20 miles/week) (7,28,36,47,50,64,72,87). This factor remained a strong predictor of injury even after adjusting for other running-related practices. Lysholm and Wiklander (45) also found a positive association between the injury rate during any given month and the training distance covered during the previous month among marathon runners. However, Bovens et al. (7) found no relationship between injuries in a given week and the distance covered in the previous week.

At present, there is no definitive data on the effect of abrupt increases in training practices on injury risk. However, some studies found that the injury rate per unit of exposure time (i.e., 1,000 training hours) actually decreased with longer training distances (7). Lysholm and Wiklander (45) found a lower injury rate per unit of exposure for long-distance runners but not for sprinters and middle-distance runners. However, even if the injury rate per unit exposure decreases, the absolute number of injuries will increase with increasing mileage.

If weekly mileage is a determining factor for injuries, a related question is whether the risk of injury is lower if the same total weekly mileage is run over many days instead of a few days per week (29). Compared to less than 3 days of running, some investigators found that any increase in the number of days run resulted in an increase in injury rate; however, this effect did not persist after controlling for total mileage (47,87). This finding suggests that cumulative mileage was more indicative of injury than the lack of rest between runs as suggested by the clinical data (29). Marti (49) examined this issue by observing a subgroup of runners who had similar weekly mileage, but ran this mileage in two, three, or four training sessions per week. Marti found no significant differences in the injury rate among the groups. The speed at which a runner runs was not an important factor after adjusting for total mileage (47,50,87).

It has been reported that previous participation in a marathon, when considered alone, is a significant predictor of injury for both men and women during 1 year of follow-up (47). However, after adjusting for other indicators of running activity such as training mileage the increased injury risk associated with marathon participation was no longer evident. Another study shows that during a marathon those with previous marathon experience have a lower percentage of muscle or joint problems than those without previous marathon experience (55). So, although marathon participation suggested high injury rates during training and perhaps during the race itself (52), the injury rates for runners during subsequent recreational running was apparently more dependent on training mileage than past marathon participation.

Another dimension to racing activity was whether runners classified themselves as competitive or as recreational. Walter, Hart, McIntosh, and Sutton (87) reported that competitive runners were at almost twice the risk of injury as recreational runners during a 1-year follow-up. However, this finding was no longer significant after adjusting for weekly mileage and previous injury, suggesting that competitive runners were also more likely to be high mileage runners and to have reported previous injuries.

Although clinical studies suggest that hard running surfaces or running in the morning are associated with an increased risk of injuries (29), population studies have not found such differences, especially after controlling for weekly mileage (47,50,87). Similarly, studies that examined the timing of the first run of the day found that the injury rates do not differ among those who run primarily early in the morning and those who run at other times (5,47).

Although stretching is often recommended as a safety measure for preventing injuries (29), no population-based study of runners found that this practice reduced the injury rate. Several studies showed no difference in injury rates between those who stretch and those who do not stretch before running (36,47). In an uncontrolled analysis, Jacobs and Berson (28) reported a higher injury rate among runners who reported stretching regularly compared to those who did not. Without controlling for previous injury or running mileage, this result was difficult to interpret. Walter et al. (87) found that the risk of injury was higher among those who stretched irregularly compared to those who always or never stretched. However, after controlling for weekly mileage and previous injury, this effect was no longer significant.

The differences in the findings of the various studies are not surprising because the characteristics of stretching are rarely fully investigated as to type and duration. It may well be that certain stretching practices are effective in preventing injuries whereas others are not. This issue needs further investigation.

Walking

Walking has been consistently reported as the most prevalent form of exercise among adults in North America. The 1989 BRFSS indicated that 35% of all respondents (and 52% of those reporting some activity) participated in walking for exercise. Walking is generally seen as an activity that involves low risk of musculoskeletal injury. This impression may be correct, but it has not been confirmed by scientific investigation. Indeed, we were unable to find a single published epidemiologic study of injuries in habitual walkers.

Data reported by Sandelin et al. (73) on activity-related injuries in greater Helsinki, Finland, seem to indicate that the injury rate for walking is lower than for many other activities. In that study walking was found to be the most popular activity, practiced by 75% of the sample surveyed. However, walking did not appear in the list of activities that was associated with a sizable percentage of the observed injuries. This implies that the injury risk associated with walking was low.

Calisthenics/Aerobic Dance

Although the BRFSS data indicate that 2.2% of American adults in 1989 reported engaging in calisthenics as a primary or secondary activity, the actual participation rate is probably much higher as this activity may precede or follow participation in a number of other activities. Although much has been written about avoidance of improper calisthenic exercises, we are aware of no epidemiologic studies of injury risk with this form of activity.

Aerobic dance includes a variety of exercise programs that vary in intensity. The common features include rhythmic movements set to music. BRFSS data indicate that 6.5% of American adults participate in this activity, but this percentage is much higher among women. Cross-sectional and prospective studies on injuries among aerobic dance participants have yielded surprisingly consistent results. The overall percent who report injuries is about 49%–45% among students and 75% among instructors (16,68,69). Almost half of the women currently in a program report having had a previous injury (69); 23% of these injuries required a visit to a physician. Although the injury rate for this activity is high, very few of these injuries result in long-term curtailment of activity. Garrick, Gillien, and Whiteside (16) report that 80% of the injuries only affected the participant during the aerobics class. The most common site of injury is the shin, consistently accounting for over 20% of the injuries for both instructors and students.

The only risk factor that has been consistently identified among the studies on aerobic dance was frequency of dance class participation. Those participating more than four times per week had a higher injury rate than those participating less than four times per week (16,68). However, the rate of injury per hour of aerobics decreased as the number of hours of participation increased, a trend that is similar to that noted herein with running. Other risk factors identified in cross-sectional studies include type of footwear and floor type (68). In the Garrick et al. (16) prospective study prior orthopedic problems and lack of exposure to other fitness endeavors were associated with higher injury percentages.

Bicycling

BRFSS data indicate that about 3.9% of American adults participate in bicycling as their primary or secondary activity. Stationary cycling is reported by 1.9% of BRFSS respondents. Many clinical series have described a range of injuries seen by medical personnel. Most of these reports have focused on head trauma (20,71,82). The studies that included noninjured as well as injured cyclists found annual injury rates that ranged from 4.6% (35) to about 13% (41). However, most of the injuries reported were minor and required only self-treatment or no treatment at all.

Studies of bicycle-touring participants (42,90) have also found low rates of musculoskeletal problems during the tour. In a study of urban cyclists, Sgaglione, Suljaga-Petchell, and Frankel (75) found increased cycling mileage and length of cycling time were associated with increased accidents. The difficulty in comparing injury rates and risk factors among the various studies is that the study population varies by type of cycling (recreation, transportation, and sport), and the equipment and riding environment associated with each type of cycling may vary substantially.

The most common type of injury requiring hospitalization is head trauma (20). A case-control study of head trauma among bicyclists demonstrated the effectiveness of safety helmets in reducing the severity of head trauma (82). Other studies have similarly concluded that safety helmets are effective in preventing severe injury and even death (71). Although there is general agreement on the efficacy of helmets in preventing or reducing head trauma, not all riders use helmets. One study found that those who used helmets were also likely to use seat belts, be married, have a high educational level, and believe that they are susceptible to injury (89).

The use of a helmet may effectively prevent or reduce the consequences of head trauma, however, there is some evidence that the characteristics of the helmet itself may lead to neck pain. In his study of cyclists on an 8-day tour Weiss (90) found that 20% reported significant neck and shoulder pain. Although the risk factors for this pain could not be identified from the study, the cyclists attributed the pain to road vibration and to neck hyperextension due to bicycling helmets that obscured the upper field of vision.

Racquet Sports

BRFSS data indicate that 1.5% of American adults participate in racquet sports (tennis, squash, and racquetball) as their primary or secondary activity. The information on injuries associated with these sports comes primarily from clinic populations (2).

Very few population-based studies have been conducted for these sports and most of these studies involve competitive or organized groups.

A prospective study of 1,327 competitive squash players found an injury rate of 6.5% during the season (8). Most squash injuries involved the head and upper extremities, and resulted in loss of playing time (3,8). Among the risk factors identified are age (over age 40 years), novice skill level, and increased playing time.

A prospective study of tennis elbow among 500 tennis players found a 2-month incidence of 9.1% and a 2-month prevalence of 14.1% (19). The risk factors for tennis elbow included older age and increased playing time (19). While the major injury among tennis players is tennis elbow, this was not the case for badminton players (25). In this study, the annual injury rate was 9% for men and 14% for women; but the predominant injuries were cramps and blisters.

Swimming

The 1989 BRFSS data (Table 69.1) indicate that 3% to 4% of American adults participate in swimming as a primary or secondary exercise activity. Sports medicine practitioners recognize that shoulder pain, medial knee pain, and pain in the dorsum of the foot are common musculoskeletal problems in swimmers (32). Unfortunately there are few epidemiologic studies of injuries in swimmers. Our search of the literature failed to identify a single study in which the subjects were adults who participated in swimming as a fitness or health enhancement activity.

Younger, competitive swimmers have been studied. Vizsolyi et al. (86) surveyed 391 competitive teenage swimmers and found that 73% of breaststroke specialists and 48% of nonbreaststrokers reported a history of medial knee pain (i.e., *breaststroker's knee*). Older athletes, those who trained more frequently, and those who reported more years of competitive swimming were more likely to report a history of knee pain. Rather similar findings were reported by Rovere and Nichols (70), who studied 36 teenage and young adult swimmers who specialized in the breaststroke.

Use of All-Terrain and Recreational Vehicles

All-terrain vehicle (ATV) and recreational vehicle (RV) use is not typically viewed as a mode of exercise, even though it is a popular leisure-time activity in many parts of North America. Clinical evidence indicates rising morbidity and mortality rates as a result of ATV use (18,38,63). Smith and Middaugh (78) investigated injury and mortality associated with use of three-wheeled ATVs in Alaska over 2 years. Injury, hospitalization, and mortality rates were 6.61, 5.8, and 0.36 per 1,000 ATV sales per year. Significantly different death rates have been reported for ATV and motorcycle use (85). Most prevalent injuries are lower extremity fractures or dislocations. Risk factors associated with ATV or RV injury are

- younger age,
- lack of helmet use,
- alcohol consumption,
- weekend use,
- driver inattention and inexperience,
- recklessness, and
- the season from July to September.

Legislative regulation of ATVs and RVs under consideration in many states may curtail these rising injury and mortality rates.

Softball

In 1989 approximately 1.6% of American adults reported participation in softball. The existing literature includes two prospective studies of softball injuries. One of these studies compared rates of sliding injuries with stationary versus breakaway bases (30). Markedly lower injury rates were observed with breakaway bases (0.3 vs. 7.2 injuries per 100 games). In a 1-year study of softball injuries among United States Army personnel in Hawaii, 83 participants from 288 softball teams (number of individual players was not reported) were referred for treatment in an orthopedic clinic (91). Over 40% of these injuries were associated with sliding.

Summary and Recommendations for Future Research

Previous reviews of the epidemiologic literature on exercise-related musculoskeletal injuries have concluded with great consistency that the existing knowledge base is quite limited (37,39,76). In the years that have intervened since the publication of those previous reviews the relevant epidemiologic literature has expanded considerably. Nonetheless, we must conclude that our knowledge of the epidemiology of exercise-related injuries is still very limited and that many of the deficiencies noted by previous reviewers still exist.

In recent years considerable attention has been focused on the study of injury risk in runners; as a result we now have a much improved understanding of the incidence of and risk factors for injury in habitual runners. These recent findings are reviewed herein; they support the conclusion that injury risk in runners is considerable (35%–65% per year), and that risk is positively related to level of exposure to the activity (e.g., miles run per week) and to previous injury. Some evidence indicates that so-called training errors may increase injury risk. However, most previous studies have not used the methodologies that would test this hypothesis in a definitive manner. Prospective studies are needed that carefully and concurrently monitor both training behavior and injury experience in a sizable cohort of runners.

Unfortunately our knowledge of injury risk with other highly prevalent forms of exercise continues to be very limited. Particularly deficient is our knowledge of injury risk with walking and gardening. According to BRFSS data these are the two most frequently reported modes of activity in American adults and our search of the epidemiologic literature revealed no large-scale studies of injury risk with participation in either of them. As both walking and gardening are already highly prevalent, involve moderate intensity, and are readily accessible to large segments of the adult population, these activities are likely to play important roles in future community-based physical activity promotion programs. The common perception is that walking and gardening carry minimal risk of musculoskeletal injury. The validity of this perception should be directly addressed in future studies. Likewise we need to know more about the injury risks associated with other common forms of exercise. Activities such as weight lifting, aerobic dance, and cycling have become increasingly popular in recent years, yet relatively little is known about the risk factors for injury among participants in these activities.

As noted by previous reviewers, future studies of exercise-related injuries should employ appropriate epidemiologic methods. The concerns raised previously by Koplan, Siscovick, and Goldbaum (37) and Walter, Sutton, McIntosh, and Connolly (88) are still applicable. Future studies of exercise-related injuries should

1. provide carefully developed and precisely presented definitions of "injury,"
2. include denominator data so that injury cases can be related to an at-risk population,
3. make every effort to minimize selection bias,
4. monitor injury experience, activity behavior, and other potential behavioral risk factors concurrently, and
5. employ prospective research designs.

In our view an overriding goal of future studies of exercise-related injuries should be to provide information that can guide future efforts to promote public health through increased physical activity. Accordingly, we consider it important that future studies quantify exposure to the various forms of exercise in such a manner as to facilitate comparisons across activities and performance of risk–benefit analyses. Acceptable approaches include expression of exercise participation as hours of activity per week or estimated kilocalories of energy expended per week. With a knowledge of the relationship between level of exposure to specific forms of exercise and injury risk it should be possible to identify those activities that optimize the long-term health benefits while minimizing the costs.

Acknowledgment

The authors express their appreciation to Mr. J. David Branch for his assistance with the preparation of this paper.

References

1. American College of Sports Medicine. ACSM position stand: The recommended quantity and quality of exercise for developing and maintaining cardiorespiratory and muscular fitness in healthy adults. Med. Sci. Sports Exerc. 22(2):265-274; 1990.
2. Barrell, G.V.; Cooper, P.J.; Elkington, A.R.; MacFadyen, J.M.; Powell, R.G.; Tormey, P. Squash ball to eye ball: The likelihood of squash players incurring an eye injury. Br. Med. J. 283:893-895; 1981.
3. Berson, B.L.; Rolnick, A.M.; Ramos, C.G.; Thornton, J. An epidemiologic study of squash injuries. Am. J. Sports Med. 9(2):103-106; 1981.
4. Blair, S.N.; Goodyear, N.N.; Gibbons, L.W.; Cooper, K.H. Physical fitness and incidence of hypertension in healthy normotensive men and women. JAMA. 252:487-490; 1984.
5. Blair, S.N.; Kohl, H.W.; Goodyear, N.N. Rates and risks for running and exercise injuries: Studies in three populations. Res. Q. Exerc. Sports. 58(3):221-228; 1987.
6. Blair, S.N.; Kohl, H.W.; Paffenbarger, R.S.; Clark, D.G.; Cooper, K.H.; Gibbons, L.W. Physical fitness and all-cause mortality: A prospective study of healthy men and women. JAMA. 262(17):2395-2401; 1989.

7. Bovens, A.M.; Janssen, G.M.E.; Vermeer, H.G.W.; Hoeberigs, J.H.; Janssen, M.P.E.; Verstappen, F.T.J. Occurrence of running injuries in adults following a supervised training program. Int. J. Sports Med. 10:S186-S190; 1989.
8. Clemett, R.S.; Fairhurst, S.M. Head injuries from squash: A propective study. N.Z. Med. J. 92:1-3; 1980.
9. Daly, P.J.; Fitzgerald, R.H.; Melton, L.J.; Ilstrip, D.M. Epidemiology of ankle fractures in Rochester, Minnesota. Acta Orthop. Scand. 58:539-544; 1987.
10. de Loes, M. Medical treatment and costs of sports-related injuries in a total population. Int. J. Sports Med. 11(1):66-71; 1990.
11. de Loes, M.; Goldie, I. Incidence rate of injuries during sport activity and physical exercise in a rural Swedish municipality: Incidence rates in 17 sports. Int. J. Sports Med. 9(6):461-467; 1988.
12. Deveraeux, M.D.; Lachmann, S.M. Athletes attending a sports injury clinic—a review. Br. J. Sports Med. 17(4):137-142; 1983.
13. Dowling, P.A. Prospective study of injuries in United States Ski Association freestyle skiing—1976-77 to 1979-80. Am. J. Sports Med. 10(5):268-275; 1982.
14. Duncan, J.J.; Farr, J.E.; Upton, S.J.; Hagan, R.D.; Oglesby, M.E.; Blair, S.N. The effects of aerobic exercise on plasma catecholamines and blood pressure in patients with mild essential hypertension. JAMA. 254:2609-2613; 1985.
15. Fields, K.B.; DeLaney, M.; Hinkle, J.S. A prospective study of type A behavior and running injuries. J. Fam. Pract. 30:425-429; 1990.
16. Garrick, J.G.; Gillien, D.M.; Whiteside, P. The epidemiology of aerobic dance injuries. Am. J. Sports Med. 14(1):67-72; 1986.
17. Gettman, L.R.; Ayres, J.J.; Pollock, M.L.; Jackson, A. The effect of circuit weight training on strength, cardiorespiratory function, and body composition of adult men. Med. Sci. Sports. 10(3):171-176; 1978.
18. Greene, M.A.; Metzler, M.H. Trauma associated with three and four-wheeled all-terrain vehicles. J. Trauma. 28(3):391-394; 1988.
19. Gruchow, H.W.; Pelletier, D. An epidemiologic study of tennis elbow. Am. J. Sports Med. 7(4):234-238; 1979.
20. Guichon, D.M.P.; Myles, S.T. Bicycle injuries: One year sample in Calgary. J. Trauma. 15(6):504-506; 1975.
21. Healthy people 2000. National health promotion and disease prevention objectives. DHHS publication no. (PHS) 91-50212. Washington, DC: U.S. Department of Health and Human Services. Public Health Service; 1990. Available from: U.S. Government Printing Office, Washington, DC.
22. Heath, G.W.; Kendrick, J.S. Outrunning the risks: A behavioral risk profile of runners. Am. J. Prev. Med. 5(6):347-352; 1989.
23. Hede A.; Jensen, D.B.; Blyme, P.; Sonne-Holm, S. Epidemiology of meniscal lesions in the knee. Acta Orthop. Scand. 61(5):435-437; 1990.
24. Helmick, S.P.; Ragland, D.R.; Leung, R.W.; Paffenbarger, R.S. Physical activity and reduced occurrence of non-insulin-dependent diabetes mellitus. N. Engl. J. Med. 325:147-152; 1991.
25. Hensley, L.D.; Paup, D.C. A survey of badminton injuries. Br. J. Sports Med. 13:156-160; 1979.
26. Holmich, P.; Christensen, S.W.; Darre, E.; Jahnsen, F.; Hartvig, T. Non-elite marathon runners: Health, training and injuries. Br. J. Sports Med. 23(3):177-178; 1989.
27. Jackson, D.S.; Furman, W.K.; Berson, B.L. Patterns of injuries in college athletes: A retrospective study of injuries sustained in intercollegiate athletics in two colleges over a two-year period. Mt. Sinai J. Med. 47(4):423-426; 1980.
28. Jacobs, S.J.; Berson, B.L. Injuries to runners: A study of entrants to a 10,000 meter race. Am. J. Sports Med. 14:151-155; 1986.
29. James, S.L.; Bates, B.T.; Osternig, L.R. Injuries to runners. Am. J. Sports Med. 6(2):40-50; 1978.
30. Janda, D.H.; Wojtys, E.M.; Hankin, F.M.; Benedict, M.E. Softball sliding injuries: A prospective study comparing standard and modifed bases. JAMA. 259:1848-1850; 1988.
31. Johansson, C. Injuries in elite orienteers. Am. J. Sports Med. 14(5):410-415; 1986.
32. Johnson, J.E.; Sim, F.H.; Scott, S.G. Musculoskeletal injuries in competitive swimmers. Mayo Clin. Proc. 62:289-304; 1987.
33. Kannus, P.; Jarvinen, M. Incidence of knee injuries and the need for further care. A one year prospective follow-up study. J. Sports Med. 29:321-325; 1989.
34. Kelly, M.J. Psychological risk factors and sports injuries. J. Sports Med. Phys. Fitness. 30:202-221; 1990.
35. Kiburz, D.; Jacobs, R.; Reckling, F.; Mason, J. Bicycle accidents and injuries among adult cyclists. Am. J. Sports Med. 14(5):416-419; 1986.
36. Koplan, J.P.; Powell, K.E.; Sikes, R.K.; Shirley, R.W.; Campbell, C.C. An epidemiologic study of the benefits and risks of running. JAMA. 248(23):3118-3121; 1982.
37. Koplan, J.P.; Siscovick, D.S.; Goldbaum, G.M. The risks of exercise: A public view of injuries and hazards. Public Health Rep. 100(2):189-194; 1985.
38. Krane, B.D.; Ricci, M.A.; Sweeney, W.B.; Deshmukh, N. All-terrain vehicle injuries. A review

at a rural level II trauma center. Am. Surg. 54(8):471-474; 1988.

39. Kraus, J.F.; Conroy, C. Mortality and morbidity from injuries in sports and recreation. Annu. Rev. Public Health. 5:163-192; 1984.
40. Kretsch, A.; Gragan, R.; Duras, P.; Allen, F.; Sumner, J.; Gillam, I. 1980 Melbourne marathon study. Med. J. Aust. 141:809-814; 1984.
41. Kruse, D.L.; McBeath, A.A. Bicycle accidents and injuries. Am. J. Sports Med. 8(5):342-344; 1980.
42. Kulund, D.N.; Brubaker, C.E. Injuries in the bikecentennial tour. Phys. Sportsmed. 6(6):74-78; 1978.
43. Leon, A.S.; Connett, J.; Jacobs, D.R.; Rauramaa, R. Leisure-time physical activity levels and risk of coronary heart disease and death. JAMA. 258(17):2388-2395; 1987.
44. Lloyd, T.; Triantafyllou, S.J.; Baker, E.R.; Houts, P.S.; Whiteside, J.A.; Kalenak, A.; Stumpf, P.G. Women athletes with menstrual irregularity have increased musculo-skeletal injuries. Med. Sci. Sports Exerc. 18(4):374-379; 1986.
45. Lysholm, J.; Wiklander, J. Injuries in runners. Am. J. Sports Med. 15(2):168-171; 1987.
46. Macera, C.A.; Pate, R.R.; Davis, D.R.; Jackson, K.L.; Woods, J. Postrace morbidity among runners. Am. J. Prev. Med. 7:194-198; 1991.
47. Macera, C.A.; Pate, R.R.; Powell, K.E.; Jackson, K.L.; Kendrick, J.S.; Craven, T.E. Predicting lower-extremity injuries among habitual runners. Arch. Intern. Med. 149:2565-2568; 1989.
48. Maehlum, S.; Daljord, O.A. Acute sports injuries in Oslo: A one year study. Br. J. Sports Med. 18(3):181-185; 1984.
49. Marti, B. Benefits and risks of running among women: An epidemiologic study. Int. J. Sports Med. 9(2):92-98; 1988.
50. Marti, B.; Vader, J.P.; Minder, C.E.; Abelin, T. On the epidemiology of running injuries. The 1984 Bern Grand-Prix study. Am. J. Sports Med. 16(3):285-294; 1988.
51. Matheson, G.O.; MacIntyre, J.G.; Taunton, J.E.; Clement, D.B.; Lloyd-Smith, R. Musculoskeletal injuries associated with physical activity in older adults. Med. Sci. Sports Exerc. 21(4):379-385; 1989.
52. Maughan, R.J.; Miller, J.D.B. Incidence of training-related injuries among marathon runners. Br. J. Sports Med. 17(3):162-165; 1983.
53. McKenna, S.; Borman, B.; Findlay, J.; de Boer Student, M. Sports injuries in New Zealand. N.Z. Med. J. 99:899-901; 1986.
54. McMaster, W.C.; Walter, M. Injuries in soccer. Am. J. Sports Med. 6(6):354-357; 1978.
55. Nicholl, J.P.; Williams, B.T. Injuries sustained by runners during a popular marathon. Br. J. Sports Med. 17(1):10-15; 1983.
56. Nielsen, A.B.; Yde, J. Epidemiology and traumatology of injuries in soccer. Am. J. Sports Med. 17(6):803-807; 1989.
57. Orava, S.; Hulkko, A.; Jormakka, E. Exertion injuries in female athletes. Br. J. Sports Med. 15(4):229-233; 1981.
58. O'Toole, M.L.; Hiller, D.B.; Smith, R.A.; Sisk, T.D. Overuse injuries in ultraendurance triathletes. Am. J. Sports Med. 17(4):514-518; 1989.
59. Paffenbarger, R.S.; Hale, W.E. Work activity and coronary heart mortality. N. Engl. J. Med. 292:545-550; 1975.
60. Paffenbarger, R.S.; Hyde, R.T.; Wing, A.L.; Hsieh, C. Physical activity, all-cause mortality, and longevity of college alumni. N. Engl. J. Med. 314:605-613; 1986.
61. Paffenbarger, R.S.; Wing, A.L.; Hyde, R.T.; Jung, D.L. Physical activity and incidence of hypertension in college men. Am. J. Epidemiol. 116:245-257; 1983.
62. Pelletier, R.L.; Anderson, G.; Stark, R.M. Profile of sports/leisure injuries treated at emergency rooms of urban hospitals. Can. J. Sport Sci. 16(1):99-102; 1991.
63. Percy, E.C.; Duffey, J.P. All-terrain vehicle injuries. A sport out of control. West. J. Med. 150(3):296-299; 1989.
64. Pollock, M.L.; Gettman, L.R.; Milesis, C.A.; Bah, M.D.; Durstine, L.; Johnson, R.B. Effects of frequency and duration of training on attrition and incidence of injury. Med. Sci. Sports. 9(1):31-36; 1977.
65. Powell, K.E.; Kohl, H.W.; Casperson, C.J.; Blair, S.N. An epidemiological perspective on the causes of running injuries. Phys. Sportsmed. 14(6):100-114; 1986.
66. Powell, K.E.; Thompson, P.D.; Casperson, C.J.; Kendrick, J.S. Physical activity and the incidence of coronary heart disease. Annu. Rev. Public Health. 8:253-287; 1987.
67. Raskin, R.J.; Rebecca, G.S. Posttraumatic sports-related musculo-skeletal abnormalities: Prevalence in a normal population. Am. J. Sports Med. 11(5):336-339; 1983.
68. Richie, D.H.; Kelso, S.F.; Bellucci, P.A. Aerobic dance injuries: A retrospective study of instructors and participants. Phys. Sportsmed. 13(2):130-140; 1985.
69. Rothenberger, L.A.; Chang, J.I.; Cable, T.A. Prevalence and types of injuries in aerobic dancers. Am. J. Sports Med. 16(4):403-407; 1988.
70. Rovere, G.D.; Nichols, A.W. Frequency, associated factors, and treatment of breaststroker's knee in competitive swimmers. Am. J. Sports Med. 13(2):99-104; 1985.
71. Sacks, J.J.; Holmgreen, P.; Smith, S.M.; Sosin, D.M. Bicycle-associated head injuries and

deaths in the United States from 1984 through 1988. JAMA. 266:3016-3018; 1991.

72. Samet, J.M.; Chick, T.W.; Howard, C.A. Running-related morbidity: A community survey. Ann. Sports Med. 1(1):30-34; 1982.
73. Sandelin, J.; Santavirta, S.; Lattila, R.; Vuolle, P.; Sarna, S. Sports injuries in a large urban population: Occurrence and epidemiological aspects. Int. J. Sports Med. 9(1):61-66; 1988.
74. Sedgwick, A.W.; Smith, D.S.; Davies, M.J. Musculo-skeletal status of men and women who entered a fitness programme. Med. J. Aust. 148:385-391; 1988.
75. Sgaglione, N.A.; Suljaga-Petchell, K.; Frankel, V.H. Bicycle-related accidents and injuries in a population of urban cyclists. Bull. Hosp. J. Dis. Orthop. Inst. 42(1)80-91; 1982.
76. Siscovick, D.S. Risks of exercising: Sudden cardiac death and injuries. In: Bouchard, C.; Shephard, R.J.; Stephens, T.; Sutton, J.R.; McPherson, B.D., eds. Exercise, fitness, and health. Champaign, IL: Human Kinetics; 1990:707-713.
77. Siscovick, D.S.; Weiss, N.S.; Fletcher, R.H.; Lasky, T. The incidence of cardiac arrest during vigorous exercise. N. Engl. J. Med. 311:874-877; 1984.
78. Smith, S.M.; Middaugh, J.P. Injuries associated with three-wheeled, all-terrain vehicles, Alaska, 1983 and 1984. JAMA. 255(18):2454-2458; 1986.
79. Sonne-Holm, S.; Sorensen, C.H. Risk factors with acute sports injuries. Br. J. Sports Med. 14:22-24; 1980.
80. Stephens, T.; Jacobs, D.R.; White, C.C. A descriptive epidemiology of leisure time physical activity. Public Health Rep. 100(2):147-157; 1985.
81. Tator, C.H.; Edmonds, V.E. Sports and recreation are a rising cause of spinal cord injury. Phys. Sportsmed. 14(5):157-167; 1986.
82. Thompson, R.S.; Rivara, F.P.; Thompson, D.C. A case-control study of the effectiveness of bicycle safety helmets. N. Engl. J. Med. 320(21): 1361-1367; 1989.
83. Tsai, S.P.; Bernacki, E.J.; Baun, W.B. Injury prevalence and associated costs among participants of an employee fitness program. Prev. Med. 17:475-482; 1988.
84. Valliant, P.M. Personality and injury in competitive runners. Percept. Mot. Skills. 53:251-253; 1981.
85. Vasilakis, A.; Vargish, T.; Apelgren, K.N.; Moran, W.H. All terrain vehicles (ATVs). A recreational gamble. Am. Surg. 55(3):142-144; 1989.
86. Vizsolyi, P.; Taunton, J.; Robertson, G.; Filsinger, L.; Shannon, H.S.; Whittingham, D.; Gleave, M. Breaststroker's knee. An analysis of epidemiological and biochemical factors. Am. J. Sports Med. 15(1):63-71; 1987.
87. Walter, S.D.; Hart, L.E.; McIntosh, J.M.; Sutton, J.R. The Ontario cohort study of running-related injuries. Arch. Intern. Med. 149:2561-2564; 1989.
88. Walter, S.D.; Sutton, J.R.; McIntosh, J.M.; Connolly, C. The etiology of sports injuries: A review of methodologies. Sports Med. 2:47-58; 1985.
89. Wasserman, R.C.; Waller, J.A.; Monty, M.J.; Emery, A.B.; Robinson, D.R. Bicyclists, helmets and head injuries: A rider-based study of helmet use and effectiveness. Am. J. Public Health. 78(9):1220-1221; 1988.
90. Weiss, B.D. Nontraumatic injuries in amateur long distance bicyclists. Am. J. Sports Med. 13(3):187-192; 1985.
91. Wheeler, B.R. Slow-pitch softball injuries. Am. J. Sports Med. 12(3):237-240; 1984.
92. White, C.C.; Powell, K.E.; Hogelin, G.C.; Gentry, E.M.; Forman, M.R. The behavioral risk factor surveys: IV. The descriptive epidemiology of exercise. Am. J. Prev. Med. 3:304-310; 1987.
93. Wilmore, J.H.; Parr, R.B.; Girandola, R.N.; Ward, P.; Vodak, P.A.; Barstow, T.J.; Pipes, T.V.; Romero, G.T.; Leslie, P. Physiological alterations consequent to circuit weight training. Med. Sci. Sports. 10(2):79-84; 1978.
94. Wood, P.D.; Haskell, W.L.; Blair, S.N.; Williams, P.T.; Krauss, R.M.; Lindgren, F.T.; Albers, J.J.; Ho, P.H.; Farguhar, J.W. Increased exercise level and plasma lipoprotein concentrations: A one-year, randomized, controlled study in sedentary, middle-aged men. Metabolism. 32(1):31-39; 1983.

Chapter 70

Risks of Exercising: Cardiovascular Including Sudden Cardiac Death

Paul D. Thompson
Mary C. Fahrenbach

The cardiovascular complications of vigorous physical activity include cerebrovascular accidents, symptomatic cardiac arrhythmias, aortic dissection, myocardial infarction, and sudden cardiac death (50). There is a paucity of data on the incidence of nonfatal cardiovascular complications during exercise. Collection of such cases in the general population is difficult, and the imprecise onset of some acute coronary syndromes obscures their relationship to exercise. Consequently this presentation will focus on exercise-related sudden cardiac death, a topic previously reviewed for this conference by Dr. David Siscovick (45), a prominent researcher in this field. We will summarize our present understanding of this problem and identify areas of potential future investigation. In addition, we will discuss recent reports of transient cardiac dysfunction after prolonged exertion and address new studies that question the value of vigorous exercise training in patients with severe cardiac disease.

The Pathology of Exercise-Related Deaths

The prevalence of occult atherosclerotic coronary artery disease (CAD) in the United States has been estimated from autopsies of traumatic deaths and from coronary angiography in patients with valvular heart disease to be approximately 5% of the adult population (7). This prevalence far exceeds that for other potentially fatal cardiac conditions. It is not surprising, therefore, that CAD is the predominant cause of sudden death in the general population and in individuals over age 30 years who die during physical activity.

Pathology in Children and Young Adults Dying During Exercise

A variety of other cardiac abnormalities are associated with exercise-related deaths in individuals under age 30 years. These include

- hypertrophic cardiomyopathy;
- congenital coronary artery anomalies including abnormal origin of and course of a coronary artery, hypoplastic coronaries, and myocardial bridging;
- aortic stenosis;
- aortic dissection often associated with Marfan's syndrome;
- myocarditis;
- idiopathic dilated cardiomyopathy;
- mitral valve prolapse;
- idiopathic cardiac hypertrophy; and
- infiltrating cardiomyopathies such as amyloidosis (56,59).

Right ventricular dysplasia has also been associated with sudden cardiac death (SCD) during exercise (8). Most collected series of exercise-related deaths include some cases with no pathologically defined cause of death. These cases may represent undiagnosed conduction system abnormalities such as ventricular preexcitation (12), more subtle conduction system pathology (1), or even exercise-induced coronary spasm (60).

Coronary Artery Pathology in Adults Dying During Exercise

Ventricular fibrillation (VF) is the immediate cause of most sudden cardiac deaths. VF occurs in hearts made electrically unstable by an acute myocardial infarction (MI), potentially transient ischemia, or a prior MI with reduced left ventricular function (6). Evidence of an acute coronary lesion is common in SCD victims. A recent MI or a fresh coronary artery thrombus was found at autopsy in 30% to 66% of SCD cases (13,43). Careful coronary artery examination demonstrated coronary plaque disruption in 64% of the victims (13). A concomitant coronary thrombus was present in 42% of those with plaque rupture, whereas a thrombus alone was found in 23%. Less than half (41%) of the victims had evidence of an acute MI, possibly because they did not survive long enough for pathological changes to appear (13). Advanced CAD without an acute coronary lesion was found in only 12% of SCDs (13).

There are few autopsy series that have searched for acute coronary lesions in adult victims of exercise-related SCD. We found evidence of an acute coronary thrombus or intramural hemorrhage in 7 of 13 (54%) men who died during or immediately after jogging (53). Only 2 (15%) had evidence of an acute MI. Two others had old MIs, and advanced CAD alone was present in the remaining 4 men. Caution must be exercised in accepting these results. Cases were collected from different medical examiners' records and autopsies were not performed by a standardized protocol. Nevertheless, these results suggest that roughly half of exercise-related SCD victims sustain an acute coronary event, whereas an equal number are likely to have died from exercise-induced ischemia. Supporting the role of myocardial ischemia is the observation that new Q waves or enzymatic evidence of an acute MI appear in less than 30% of patients resuscitated from an exercise-related cardiac arrest (6).

Mechanisms of Exercise-Related Sudden Death

Conventional wisdom suggests that ischemia is induced during exercise by increased myocardial oxygen demand secondary to increases in heart rate and systolic blood pressure (51). Exercise can also reduce myocardial oxygen supply by provoking coronary spasm (60). Such inappropriate vasoconstriction occurs where coronary endothelial vasodilatory capacity is impaired by atherosclerosis (24). Coronary spasm may also lead to thrombus formation by restricting normal blood flow (21). Consequently, spasm may contribute to both exercise-induced ischemia and coronary thrombosis.

Alternatively, exercise may induce thrombosis directly or by plaque disruption. Chan, Davies, and Chambers (5) reported a 34-year-old man whose symptoms of an anterior wall MI began 30 min after he completed a 42-km footrace in 3 hr, 15 min. Coronary arteriography 5 hr later demonstrated occlusion of the left anterior descending (LAD) coronary artery and nonocclusive clot in the right coronary artery (see Figure 70.1). The patient was treated with streptokinase into the LAD without effect, but had entirely normal coronaries when studied 10 days later. The presence of probable thrombi in two coronary arteries argues against simultaneous plaque disruption in this patient.

Others (2), however, have identified evidence of plaque disruption in victims of exercise-related

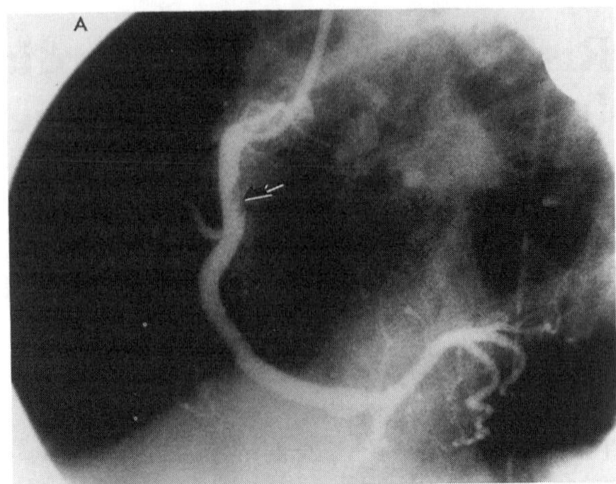

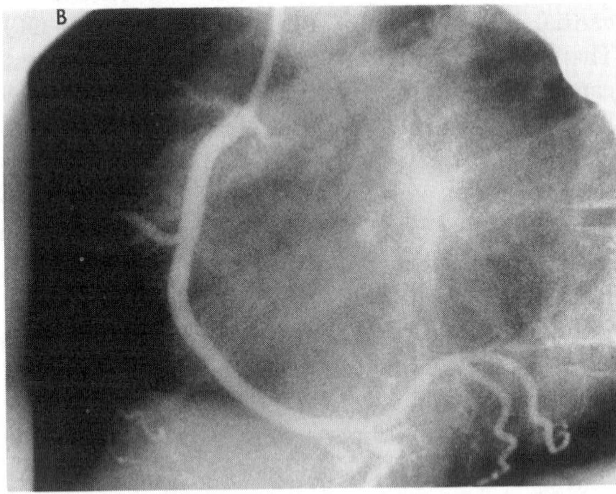

Figure 70.1 (A) Right coronary angiogram in the left anterior oblique view in a 35-year-old man who developed chest pain 30 min after completing a 42-km footrace (5). The angiogram was obtained 5 hr after the onset of symptoms. There is a nonocclusive filling defect at the arrow consistent with a coronary thrombus. (B) Repeat angiography 10 days later shows resolution of the defect. Reprinted with permission of the American College of Cardiology (Journal of the American College of Cardiology, 6[6], 1322-1325, 1984).

SCDs and suggested that the increased heart rate and vessel wall stress during exercise initiate the vascular injury. The thrombus in this situation results from the endothelial disruption. On the other hand, exercise may simply enlarge an existing intimal tear. Angioplasty reduces coronary artery stenosis in part by initiating a controlled dissection. Reports of acute coronary occlusions during stress testing performed after a recent angioplasty suggest that exercise can amplify existing coronary disruptions, ultimately producing thrombotic coronary occlusion (9,37).

All of the above mechanisms—exercise-induced ischemia, exercise-induced spasm, primary coronary thrombosis, and thrombosis due to plaque disruption initiated or exacerbated by exercise—probably contribute to some exercise deaths. Nevertheless, the available autopsy data (53) suggest that ischemia secondary to advanced, stable CAD and thrombosis secondary to endothelial disruption account for most exercise-related SCDs in adults.

The Incidence of Exercise-Related Sudden Cardiac Death

Methodological Concerns in Determining the Incidence of Exercise Deaths

The incidence of death during physical activity has been estimated using a variety of populations including Finnish cross-country skiers (57,58); British (30), American (40), Finnish (28), and Israeli (11) military personnel; participants in fitness facilities (22); and the general young (42) and adult (47,52) population. Unfortunately, methodological considerations limit the comparability and generalizability of most of these studies. The definition of an exercise-related event varies, and some studies include cases that occurred up to 24 hr after (28,30) exertion. Presentation of incidence figures also varies and major assumptions are frequently required to calculate annual death rates from the data provided.

Because CAD is the predominant cause of exercise deaths, incidence figures vary widely depending on the prevalence of CAD in the study population. Low incidence rates in military personnel, for example, reflect their younger age, a lower prevalence of CAD, and the use of screening examinations to eliminate potentially fatal cardiac malformations such as aortic stenosis, hypertrophic cardiomyopathy, and Marfan's syndrome. Even among military personnel, however, the incidence of exercise deaths may vary with the population studied. Phillips et al. examined deaths in Air Force recruits during 6 weeks of basic training (40). Seventeen of 19 sudden cardiac deaths occurred during physical activity. Myocarditis was found at autopsy in four (21%) of these deaths. This incidence of myocarditis is much higher than reported in other studies of military personnel and may reflect a higher prevalence of viral infections from barracks living or myocarditis from recent vaccinations. Both barracks living and vaccinations are common among new recruits, but not as frequent in more senior personnel.

Exercise Deaths in the General Population

Two studies have examined the incidence of exercise SCD in unselected adult populations. The incidence of death during jogging for men in the state of Rhode Island aged 30 to 65 years has been estimated as 1 death per 7,620 joggers (13 deaths per 100,000 joggers) per year (52). Half of the victims had known CAD. If these men are eliminated and no other joggers had diagnosed CAD, the yearly incidence could be estimated as only 1 death per 15,240 asymptomatic joggers (7 deaths per 100,000 joggers). Nevertheless, the hourly death rate during jogging (1 death per 396,000 jogging hr) is 7 times greater than that during less vigorous activities.

There are several limits to this study's design (52). The prevalence of joggers was based on self-report obtained by a random digit telephone survey. Self-report may overestimate the number of joggers and underestimate the rate of jogging deaths. On the other hand, the study design may have overestimated the risks of exercise. Telephone calls were placed between 5:00 and 8:00 p.m. The first person over age 15 years to answer the phone was interviewed. If joggers were running during this time period, the prevalence of joggers would have been underestimated and their death rate overestimated.

Despite these potential problems, similar rates for cardiac arrest during vigorous exercise have been reported for previously healthy men 25 to 75 years old in Seattle, Washington (47). The incidence of exertion-related cardiac arrests was only 1 per 18,000 men (6 cardiac arrests per 100,000 men) annually, however the hourly rate again was higher than that during other activities.

The agreement in the exercise "death" rate among previously healthy men between these two studies is reassuring, but both results must be taken as estimates. Only 10 exercise deaths in the Rhode Island study and 9 in the Seattle, Washington, study were used to calculate the incidence figures. Consequently, slight variation in the number of cases would have a large impact on the final estimate.

There are no published incidence figures for exercise-related SCD in women and few female deaths are included in most series. This probably reflects the delayed development of CAD in women and lower rates of physical activity among postmenopausal women in our society.

We also know of no good incidence figures for exercise-related deaths in young subjects. Much of the data that is available was obtained for military personnel and cannot be applied to the general population for the reasons previously delineated. We estimated the annual cardiovascular death rate during exercise for Rhode Island men under age 30 years as approximately 0.36 deaths per 100,000 men (42). The denominator for this estimate was all Rhode Island men of this age, however, and was not restricted to young men who exercise. Consequently, this figure underestimates the risk of exercise for young men.

Cardiac Event Rates in Patients With Known Coronary Artery Disease

Studies on the risk of cardiac rehabilitation provide insight into the incidence of nonfatal cardiac events among patients with known CAD. Two studies have surveyed a large enough sample of programs to provide reliable information. In the mid-1970s Haskell compiled questionnaire data from 30 rehabilitation centers (25). There was 1 cardiac arrest, myocardial infarction, and death every 33,000, 233,000, and 116,000 patient-hours of participation, respectively. Van Camp and Peterson surveyed 167 rehabilitation programs in 1985 (54). These authors reported 1 cardiac arrest, MI, and death every 112,000, 294,000, and 784,000 patient-hours of participation, respectively. The lower exercise event rates in the later study may be due to improved patient selection and supervision as well as to better treatment of underlying CAD.

Both studies suggest that cardiac arrest is more frequent than myocardial infarction in this patient group. This conclusion may not be applicable to the general population, however. Most patients in rehabilitation programs have sustained prior myocardial damage, and the risk of ventricular fibrillation increases with the degree of myocardial dysfunction (6). These studies also demonstrate that prompt treatment of cardiac arrest contributes to the low mortality in cardiac rehabilitation programs.

The Relative Risks of Exercise

Despite low absolute incidence figures, the occurrence of cardiac complications during exercise remains a significant problem. Both the Rhode Island and Seattle, Washington, studies (47,52) as well as others (19,58) conclude that exercise acutely increases the risk of SCD. In Helsinki, Finland, 3.7% of SCDs (within 1 hr of onset of symptoms), 6.3% of delayed cardiac deaths, and 6.8% of nonfatal cardiac events occurred during physical activity (43). These figures underestimate the percentage of exercise events, because unwitnessed deaths such as those during sleep were not included in the denominator. Furthermore, an additional 9% of SCDs occurred immediately after snow shoveling, sport, or other exceptional physical activity so that physical activity contributed to approximately 14% of all SCDs (43). Similar figures are available from the general population of Seattle where approximately 11% of cardiac arrests are associated with physical or emotional stress (6). Surprisingly, given the increase in CAD with age, the relative risk of exercise compared to rest is actually greater in young compared to older adult men (47,52). This is largely because the incidence of cardiac deaths at rest is so low in the young men (45).

An important question is whether someone who has had an exercise-related event would have encountered a similar fate in the near future if they had not exercised. Vuori, Makarainen, and Jaaskelainen (58) noted that instantaneous deaths were more frequent with concurrent physical activity. This raises the possibility that the myocardial demands of exercise increase the fatality rate of any coronary events that happen during exertion. Indirect support for the concept that physical stress only hastens a potential event comes from a study of the February 1978 Rhode Island blizzard (17). On the day of this storm, the death rate from ischemic heart disease nearly doubled compared to the February average for the previous 5 years. The death rate remained elevated for several days, but then decreased below the usual February average so that the overall death rate in February 1978 was similar to that for the preceding 5 years (Figure 70.2). This suggests that the physical and emotional stress of the storm only hastened the inevitable. Nevertheless, given the therapeutic tools available for managing CAD, the onus falls on clinicians to identify and treat those patients with the potential for exercise-related events before they occur.

Preventing Exercise-Related Cardiac Complications

Cardiovascular testing has often been recommended to identify individuals at risk for exercise-related cardiac events. Unfortunately, there are problems with this approach. The rarity of exercise deaths limits the yield of any screening procedures. Also, cardiovascular testing in active individuals may not be predictive of future cardiac events. Cardiac abnormalities in athletes are often variants of normal conditions (16), and normal exercise tests in active adults are not necessarily reassuring because exercise-related CAD deaths may be due to an abrupt change in a coronary lesion due to plaque rupture of thrombus. Such previously noncritical stenoses are unlikely to have been detected by prior exercise testing. Finally, the costs of complex screening strategies present a formidable economic burden.

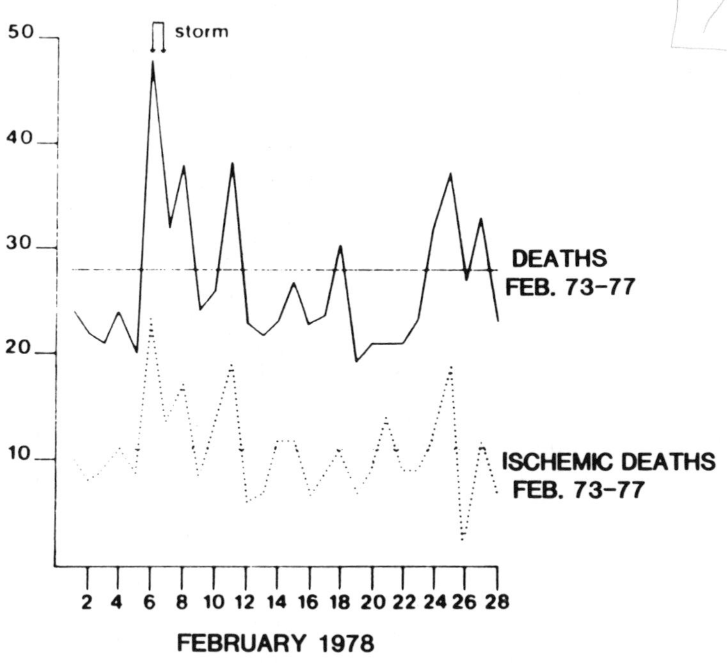

Figure 70.2 Daily total and ischemic heart disease deaths in Rhode Island, USA in February 1978 (17). The horizontal lines indicate the average February death rates for the prior 5 Februaries. The arrows indicate the storm that deposited 52 in. of snow in 24 hr on the state. *Note*. From "Blizzard Morbidity and Mortality: Rhode Island, 1978," by G. Faich and R. Rose, *American Journal of Public Health*, 69(10) 1050-1052, 1979. Copyright 1979 by the American Public Health Association. Reproduced with permission of the American Public Health Association.

Two studies have demonstrated the low yield of screening examinations for college-age athletes. Lewis et al. (29) obtained two-dimensional echocardiograms on 265 college athletes. Ventricular septal thickness was above normal in 13% of the men and markedly enlarged in 3 of these athletes. The ratio of the septum to posterior left ventricular wall was normal in all cases, however, so that no athlete was diagnosed as having hypertrophic cardiomyopathy.

Maron, Bodison, Wesley, Tucker, and Green (32) screened 501 college athletes and selected 90 for additional testing because of abnormalities in their personal or family medical history, physical examination, or resting electrocardiogram. Three athletes had thickening of the ventricular septum, but none had classic findings of hypertrophic cardiomyopathy or was prohibited from competition. These studies demonstrate that important cardiac abnormalities among young athletes are rare and that the cardiac adaptations to physical activity can produce abnormalities that obscure the separation of healthy from pathological conditions in this population.

Similar problems plague the use of routine exercise stress testing in active adults. False-positive ST-segment changes are more common in physically active individuals, possibly because cardiac enlargement alters the repolarization pattern of the myocardium (48). Also, in an asymptomatic population of middle-aged men, the largest number of sudden deaths occurs among the men with a normal ST-segment response, whereas an ischemic response predicts nonfatal events (34). Epstein and Maron (15) have estimated that if 10,000 asymptomatic men undergo screening exercise electrocardiography, only 1 sudden death would occur among men with positive tests, but that 4 deaths would occur in men with normal electrocardiographic results. Such analyses question the wisdom of routine exercise testing to prevent exercise cardiac complications in asymptomatic populations.

An alternative approach is to limit exercise testing to populations at high risk for CAD and consequently at high risk for exercise-related cardiac complications. The Lipid Research Clinics Primary Prevention Trial was a double-blind, clinical trial comparing the effect of cholestyramine versus placebo in the prevention of CAD in hyperlipidemic men. All 3,617 male participants underwent baseline and yearly submaximal exercise testing to 90% of their age-predicted maximal heart rate (46). Sixty-two men (1.7%) experienced an exercise-related cardiac event, but only 11 had a previously positive exercise test. The authors concluded that such testing could not be recommended for screening active individuals even in a high-risk population.

Radionuclide techniques would improve the sensitivity and specificity of exercise testing. Nevertheless, such procedures still have a high rate of false-positive results in an asymptomatic population, have a substantial cost, and would not detect noncritical coronary lesions that progress rapidly by plaque rupture or thrombosis during exertion.

Despite the limitations of routine, extensive screening procedures, we do recommend that active individuals undergo baseline and periodic examinations by a physician familiar with the individual's medical history. Such examinations should seek symptoms of exercise intolerance and exclude cardiac abnormalities that increase the risk of exercise complications including aortic stenosis, Marfan's syndrome, and hypertrophic cardiomyopathy (16). We also suggest that these encounters be used to inform active individuals of the nature of prodromal cardiac symptoms and their need for prompt attention. Up to 50% of exercise-related SCD victims in one series (53) reported new symptoms to relatives but continued their exercise regimens. Unfortunately, such symptoms are nonspecific, and angina pectoris appears to be more frequent in cardiac event survivors than in SCD (43).

Research Questions on the Cardiovascular Risks of Exercise

Can the Risk:Benefit Ratio for Exercise Be Improved?

No discussion of the cardiovascular risks of physical activity should be interpreted as an indictment of exercise. Epidemiologic and clinical studies provide compelling evidence that physical inactivity is an important risk factor for CAD (41). Similarly, meta-analysis of cardiac rehabilitation studies suggests that this activity decreases postinfarction mortality by 21% (38)—a reduction comparable to the only other widely acknowledged, beneficial intervention, beta-adrenergic blockade (33). Nevertheless, exercise does increase the risk of cardiac complications for some patient groups, such as those with unstable angina, Marfan's syndrome, and hypertrophic cardiomyopathy. Are there other patient groups for whom the risks outweigh the benefits? Is there a quantity or quality of exercise that produces comparable benefits with less risk? The following section will address these issues.

Do the Risks of Vigorous Exercise Outweigh the Benefits?

Epidemiological studies examining the relationship of physical activity to CAD have classified individuals largely on the basis of their occupational or recreational activity histories. Those studies, including several gradations of activity among the more active group, have generally demonstrated decreasing rates of CAD with increasing levels of physical activity (41). For example, in Seattle, Washington, the incidence of cardiac arrest decreased progressively with increased time spent in activities requiring more than 5 kcal per minute (47). Nevertheless, it is unlikely that many subjects in these occupational and recreational studies performed the extreme levels of physical activity practiced by some middle-aged competitive athletes. Would similar benefits be demonstrated for exercise at high levels of exertion or would the risks outweigh the benefits?

Anecdotal reports of death during vigorous activity abound. Are these aberrations or a warning that extreme exertion carries significant risk? Cobb and Weaver estimated that the risk of SCD for CAD patients is increased 164-fold during exercise stress testing (6). The incidence of first MI among Harvard alumni decreases with increasing levels of physical activity up to an estimated expenditure of 2,999 kcal per week (39). Above this level, however, there is a slight increase in MI incidence (Figure 70.3). This increase may be due to subject misclassification because of reporting errors on the exercise history form (Ralph Paffenbarger, personal communication). Multiple regression analysis of the data eliminates this trend and also suggests that vigorous sports are more beneficial than milder activities (Figure 70.4). Nevertheless, it is probable that the risk of exercise increases with its intensity; and it is possible that the greatest risk reduction with exercise occurs with modest increases in activity (3). At present, sufficient information is not available to conclude definitively that the benefits of intense or extreme exertion are worth the risk.

Are the Effects of Exercise-Induced Myocardial Ischemia Good or Bad?

In 1802 William Heberden (26) reported that one of his patients was "nearly cured" of his angina pectoris by the "task of sawing wood for half an hour every day" (p. 224). Modern studies have also documented the ability of exercise training to delay the onset of pain and to improve exercise tolerance in patients with angina pectoris (51). Many patients do not develop symptoms with exercise-induced ischemia, and even in symptomatic patients ischemia often appears before discomfort. Such ischemia has not been considered deleterious and could even serve as a stimulus for

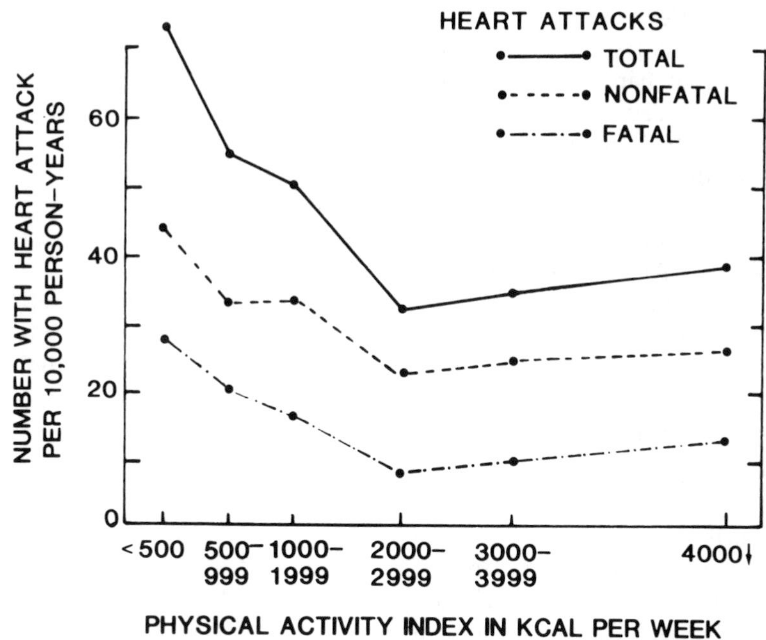

Figure 70.3 Age-adjusted first heart attack rates by estimated physical activity in a 6- to 10-year follow-up of Harvard male alumni. See reference 39. Reproduced with permission of the *American Journal of Epidemiology*.

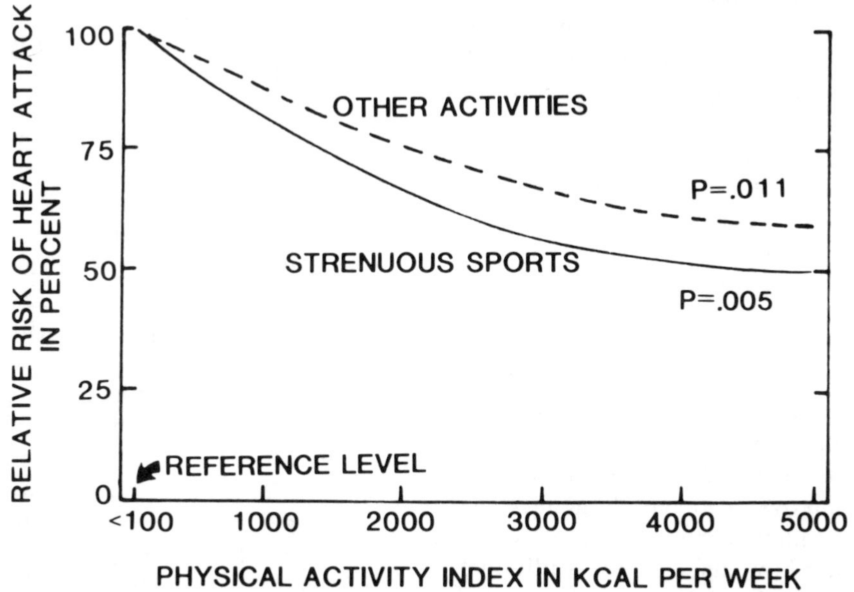

Figure 70.4 Relative risk of first heart attack by estimated physical activity for strenuous sports and other activities in Harvard alumni. Relative risk is adjusted for age, follow-up interval, and alternate type of physical activity. See reference 39. Reproduced with permission of the *American Journal of Epidemiology*.

coronary collateral development. Recent animal studies documenting myocardial dysfunction after even brief (less than 20 min) coronary occlusion, however, have challenged this view (4). Such dysfunction can be produced in exercising dogs with coronary stenoses, and the severity of dysfunction increases with both the intensity of exercise and the duration of occlusion (27). Some experts (4,14) suggest that repeated episodes of ischemia have a cumulative effect and can ultimately produce myocardial necrosis such as the minor myocardial fibrotic foci often found in CAD victims (20).

Patients with severe CAD and exercise-induced ischemia can develop left ventricular dysfunction after only a symptom-limited exercise test (18). In this study, the peak rate of left ventricular filling was decreased for 48 hr after exercise in 15 CAD patients, but had returned to baseline 7 days after exertion (18). On the other hand, some animals subjected to repetitive coronary occlusions appear to develop a tolerance to the ischemia (20). These provocative studies do not detract from the conclusion that patients with CAD develop better effort tolerance with exercise training. They remind us, however, that subsets of CAD exist and that the long-term effects of repetitive exercise-induced ischemia in man is not known.

What Is the Significance of Exercise-Induced Myocardial Dysfunction?

A discussion of the cardiovascular risks of physical activity would be incomplete without noting recent observations in endurance athletes of transient myocardial dysfunction following prolonged exercise. Various authors have noted reductions in systolic (10,36,44,55) and diastolic (35) performance after such prolonged exertion as the Ironman Triathlon (10), a treadmill run to exhaustion (44), and a 24-hr footrace (36). These conclusions are derived from echo/Doppler parameters that may not accurately reflect cardiac function during the changes in fluid volume and heart rate that accompany such events. Nevertheless, animal studies also document reductions in isometric tension development and shortening velocity (31) as well as decreased myocardial glycogen content (23) in myocardial samples from exercise-exhausted rats.

The significance of these studies to clinical medicine is unclear. It is a clinical impression that patients with heart failure do not tolerate successive days of unaccustomed physical activity. Also, it is possibly significant that 12% (2/16) of patients with left ventricular dysfunction undergoing exercise training discontinued their participation because of increasing heart failure (49). Additional studies are needed on the effects of exercise training in patients with heart failure. Documentation of the long-term effects of extreme athletic activity on myocardial function would also be reassuring, although there is no evidence that such activity has persistent deleterious effects.

Summary

Exercise transiently increases the risk of SCD in people with underlying heart disease, however the absolute incidence of exercise-related SCD in the general population is low. There is little data available on the incidence of nonfatal cardiac complications. Clinical strategies to reduce the incidence of exercise SCD are limited by the rarity of such events and the low sensitivity and specificity of available tests. Information is needed on the amount and type of exercise that would improve cardiovascular health in the general population with the least increment in risk. In addition, questions remain on the long-term risk and benefits of exercise in patients with exercise-induced ischemia and with resting myocardial dysfunction.

References

1. Bharati, S.; Lev, M. Congenital abnormalities of the conduction system in sudden death in young adults. JACC. 8:1096-1104; 1986.
2. Black, A.; Black, M.M.; Gensini, G. Exertion and acute coronary artery injury. Angiology. 26:759-783; 1975.
3. Blair, S.N.; Kohl, H.W., III; Paffenbarger, R.S., Jr.; Clark, D.G.; Cooper, K.H.; Gibbons, L.W. Physical fitness and all-cause mortality. JAMA. 262:2395-2401; 1989.
4. Braunwald, E.; Kloner, R.A. The stunned myocardium: Prolonged, postischemic ventricular dysfunction. Circulation. 66:1146-1149; 1982.
5. Chan, K.L.; Davies, R.A.; Chambers, R.J. Coronary thrombosis and subsequent lysis after a marathon. JACC. 4:1322-1325; 1984.
6. Cobb, L.A.; Weaver, W.D. Exercise: A risk for sudden death in patients with coronary heart disease. J. Am. Coll. Cardiol. 7:215-219; 1986.
7. Cohn, P.F. Asymptomatic coronary artery disease. Mod. Concepts Cardiovasc. Dis. 50:55-60; 1981.
8. Corrado, D.; Thiene, G.; Nava, A.; Rossi, L.; Pennelli, N. Sudden death in young competitive athletes: Clinicopathologic correlations in 22 cases. Am. J. Med. 89:588-596; 1990.
9. Dash, H. Delayed coronary occlusion after successful percutaneous transluminal coronary angioplasty: Association with exercise testing. Am. J. Cardiol. 52:1143-1144; 1982.
10. Douglas, P.S.; O'Toole, M.L.; Hiller, W.D.B.; Hackney, K.; Reichek, N. Cardiac fatigue after prolonged exercise. Circulation. 76:1206-1213; 1987.
11. Drory, Y.; Kramer, M.R.; Lev, B. Exertional sudden death in soldiers. Med. Sci. Sports Exerc. 23:147-151; 1991.
12. Duvernoy, W.F.C. Sudden death in Wolff-Parkinson-White syndrome. Am. J. Cardiol. 39:472; 1977.

13. El Fawal, M.A.; Berg, G.A.; Wheatley, D.J.; Harland, W.A. Sudden coronary death in Glasgow: Nature and frequency of acute coronary lesions. Br. Heart J. 57:329-335; 1987.
14. Ellestad, M.H. Is exercise harmful in ischemic heart disease? Am. J. Noninv. Cardiol. 1:15-17; 1987.
15. Epstein, S.E.; Maron, B.J. Sudden death and the competitive athlete: Perspectives on preparticipation screening studies. J. Am. Coll. Cardiol. 7:220-230; 1986.
16. Fahrenbach, M.C.; Thompson, P.D. The preparticipation sports examination: Cardiovascular considerations for screening. Cardiol. Clin. 10:319-333; 1992.
17. Faich, G.; Rose, R. Blizzard morbidity and mortality: Rhode Island, 1978. Am. J. Public Health. 69:1050-1052; 1979.
18. Fragasso, G.; Benti, R.; Sciammarella, M.; Rossetti, E.; Savi, A.; Gerundini, P.; Chierchia, S.L. Symptom-limited exercise testing causes sustained diastolic dysfunction in patients with coronary disease and low effort tolerance. JACC. 17:1251-1255; 1991.
19. French, A.J.; Dock, W. Fatal coronary arteriosclerosis in young soldiers. JAMA. 124:1233-1237; 1944.
20. Geft, I.L.; Fishbein, M.C.; Ninomiya, K.; Hashida, J.; Chaux, E.; Yano, J.; Y-Rit, J.; Genov, T.; Shell, W.; Ganz, W. Intermittent brief periods of ischemia have a cumulative effect and may cause myocardial necrosis. Circulation. 66:1150-1153; 1982.
21. Gertz, S.D.; Uretsky, G.; Wajnberg, R.S.; Navot, N.; Gotsman, M.S. Endothelial cell damage and thrombus formation after partial arterial constriction: Relevance to the role of coronary artery spasm in the pathogenesis of myocardial infarction. Circulation. 63:476-486; 1981.
22. Gibbons, L.W.; Cooper, K.H.; Meyer, B.M.; Ellison, R.C. The acute cardiac risk of strenuous exercise. JAMA. 244:1799-1801; 1980.
23. Goldfarb, A.H.; Kendrick, Z.V. Effect of an exercise run to exhaustion on cAMP in the rat heart. J. Appl. Physiol. 51:1539-1542; 1981.
24. Gordon, J.B.; Ganz, P.; Nabel, E.G.; Fish, R.D.; Zebede, J.; Mudge, G.H.; Alexander, R.W.; Selwyn, A.P. Atherosclerosis influences the vasomotor response of epicardial coronary arteries to exercise. J. Clin. Invest. 83:1946-1952; 1989.
25. Haskell, W.L. Cardiovascular complications during exercise training of cardiac patients. Circulation. 57:920-924; 1978.
26. Heberden, W. Commentary on the history and cure of diseases. In: Willius, F.A.; Keys, T.E., eds. Cardiac classics. St. Louis: Mosby; 1941:224.
27. Homans, D.C.; Laxson, D.D.; Sublett, E.; Pavek, T.; Crampton, M. Effect of exercise intensity and duration on regional function during and after exercise-induced ischemia. Circulation. 83:2029-2037; 1991.
28. Koskenvuo, K. Sudden deaths among Finnish conscripts. Br. Med. J. 2:1413-1415; 1976.
29. Lewis, J.F.; Maron, B.J.; Diggs, J.A.; Spencer, J.E.; Mehrotra, P.P.; Curry, C.L. Preparticipation echocardiographic screening for cardiovascular disease in a large, predominantly black population of collegiate athletes. Am. J. Cardiol. 64:1029-1033; 1989.
30. Lynch, P. Soldiers, sport, and sudden death. Lancet. 1:1235-1237; 1980.
31. Maher, J.T.; Goodman, A.L.; Francesconi, R.; Bowers, W.D.; Hartley, L.H.; Angelakos, E.T. Responses of rat myocardium to exhaustive exercise. Am. J. Physiol. 222:207-212; 1972.
32. Maron, B.J.; Bodison, S.A.; Wesley, Y.E.; Tucker, E.; Green, K.J. Results of screening a large group of intercollegiate athletes for cardiovascular disease. J. Am. Coll. Cardiol. 10:1214-1221; 1987.
33. May, G.S.; Eberlein, K.A.; Furberg, C.D.; Passamani, E.R.; Demets, D.L. Secondary prevention after myocardial infarction: A review of long-term trials. Prog. Cardiovasc. Dis. 24:331-352; 1982.
34. McHenry, P.L.; O'Donnell, J.; Morris, S.N.; Jordan, J.J. The abnormal exercise electrocardiogram in apparently healthy men: A predictor of angina pectoris as an initial coronary event during long-term follow-up. Circulation. 70:547-551; 1984.
35. Niemela, K.; Palatsi, I.; Ikaheimo, M.; Airaksinen, J.; Takkunen, J. Impaired left ventricular diastolic function in athletes after utterly strenuous prolonged exercise. Int. J. Sports Med. 8:61-65; 1987.
36. Niemela, K.O.; Palatsi, I.J.; Ikaheimo, M.J.; Takkunen, J.T.; Vuori, J.J. Evidence of impaired left ventricular performance after an uninterrupted competitive 24 hour run. Circulation. 70:350-356; 1984.
37. Nygaard, T.W.; Beller, G.A.; Mentzer, R.M.; Gibson, R.S.; Moeller, C.M.; Burwell, L.R. Acute coronary occlusion with exercise testing after initially successful coronary angioplasty for acute myocardial infarction. Am. J. Cardiol. 57:687-688; 1986.
38. Oldridge, N.B.; Guyait, G.H.; Fischer, M.E.; Rimm, A.A. Cardiac rehabilitation after myocardial infarction: Combined experience of randomized clinical trials. JAMA. 260:945-950; 1988.
39. Paffenbarger, R.S.; Wing, A.L.; Hyde, R.T. Physical activity as an index of heart attack

risk in college alumni. Am. J. Epidemiol. 108:161-175; 1978.

40. Phillips, M.; Robinowitz, M.; Higgins, J.R.; Boran, K.J.; Reed, T.; Virmani, R. Sudden cardiac death in Air Force recruits. JAMA. 256:2696-2699; 1986.
41. Powell, K.E.; Thompson, P.D.; Caspersen, C.J.; Kendrick, J.S. Physical activity and the incidence of coronary heart disease. In: Breslow, L.; Fielding, J.E.; Lave, L.B., eds. Annual review of public health. Palo Alto, CA: Annual Reviews, Inc.; 1987:253-287.
42. Ragosta, M.; Crabtree, J.; Sturner, W.Q.; Thompson, P.D. Death during recreational exercise in the state of Rhode Island. Med. Sci. Sports Exerc. 16:339-342; 1984.
43. Romo, M. Factors related to sudden death in acute ischaemic heart disease. Acta Med. Scand. [Suppl.]. 547:1-92; 1972.
44. Seals, D.R.; Rogers, M.A.; Hagberg, J.M.; Yamamoto, C.; Cryer, P.E.; Ehsani, A.A. Left ventricular dysfunction after prolonged strenuous exercise in healthy subjects. Am. J. Cardiol. 61:875-879; 1988.
45. Siscovick, D.S. Risks of exercising: Sudden cardiac death and injuries. In: Bouchard, C.; Shephard, R.J.; Stephens, T.; Sutton, J.R.; McPherson, B.D., eds. Exercise, fitness, and health. Champaign, IL: Human Kinetics; 1990:707-713.
46. Siscovick, D.S.; Ekelund, L.G.; Johnson, J.L.; Truong, Y.; Adler, A. Sensitivity of exercise electrocardiography for acute cardiac events during moderate and strenuous physical activity. Arch. Intern. Med. 151:325-330; 1991.
47. Siscovick, D.S.; Weiss, N.S.; Fletcher, R.H.; Lasky, T. The incidence of primary cardiac arrest during vigorous exercise. N. Engl. J. Med. 311:874-877; 1984.
48. Spirito, P.; Maron, B.J.; Bonow, R.O.; Epstein, S.E. Prevalence and significance of an abnormal S-T segment response to exercise in a young athletic population. Am. J. Cardiol. 51:1663-1666; 1983.
49. Sullivan, M.J.; Higginbotham, M.B.; Cobb, F.R. Exercise training in patients with severe left ventricular dysfunction. Circulation. 78:506-515; 1988.
50. Thompson, P.D. Cardiovascular hazards of physical activity. In: Terjung, R.L., ed. Exercise and sports sciences reviews. Philadelphia: The Franklin Institute Press; 1982:208-235.
51. Thompson, P.D. The benefits and risks of exercise training in patients with chronic coronary artery disease. JAMA. 259:1537-1540; 1988.
52. Thompson, P.D.; Funk, E.J.; Carleton, R.A.; Sturner, W.Q. Incidence of death during jogging in Rhode Island from 1975 through 1980. JAMA. 247:2535-2538; 1982.
53. Thompson, P.D.; Stern, M.P.; Williams, P.; Duncan, K.; Haskell, W.L.; Wood, P.D. Death during jogging or running. JAMA. 242:1265-1267; 1979.
54. Van Camp, S.P.; Peterson, R.A. Cardiovascular complications of outpatient cardiac rehabilitation programs. JAMA. 256:1160-1163; 1986.
55. Vanoverschelde, J-L.J.; Younis, L.T.; Melin, J.A.; Vanbutsele, R.; Leclercq, B.; Robert, A.R.; Cosyns, J.R.; Detry, J-M.R. Prolonged exercise induces left ventricular dysfunction in healthy subjects. J. Appl. Physiol. 70:1356-1363; 1991.
56. Virmani, R.; Robinowitz, M.; McAllister H.A., Jr. Exercise and the heart. Pathol. Annu. 20:431-462; 1985.
57. Vuori, I. The cardiovascular risks of physical activity. Acta Med. Scand. [Suppl.]. 711:205-214; 1984.
58. Vuori, I.; Makarainen, M.; Jaaskelainen, A. Sudden death and physical activity. Cardiology. 63:287-304; 1978.
59. Waller, B.F. Exercise-related sudden death in young (age $\leq$ 30 years) and old (age > 30 years) conditioned subjects. In: Wenger, N.K., ed. Cardiovascular clinics: Exercise and the heart. Philadelphia: Davis; 1985:9-73.
60. Yasue, H.; Omote, S.; Takizawa, A.; Nagao, M.; Miwa, K.; Tanaka, S. Circadian variation of exercise capacity in patients with prinzmetal's variant angina: Role of exercise-induced coronary arterial spasm. Circulation. 59:938-947; 1979.

PART VIII

Dose–Response Issues from Two Perspectives

Chapter 71

Dose–Response Issues From a Biological Perspective

William L. Haskell

Any physical activity that requires sustained or repeated movement of a relatively large skeletal muscle mass activates many of the body's systems to support the process of muscle contraction. During and following this muscle contraction, local biochemical factors, along with activation of the central nervous system, stimulate the increased activity of various hormones and enzymes that help regulate key metabolic functions; and there are major shifts in cardiorespiratory performance. If the activity is of sufficient intensity and duration, the renal, hepatic, gastrointestinal, and immune systems become involved. Also, physical activity exerts physical forces on the bones, muscles, and connective tissue as a result of muscle contraction or in response to gravity. The improvement in function or health status produced by performing repeated bouts of physical activity results from (a) the body's immediate response to the exercise, (b) the adaptations that occur over time in the body's attempt to increase its capacity or efficiency to respond to the exercise stimulus (*training response*), or (c) some combination of these acute and more chronic responses.

This chapter presents an overview of some of the major issues or concepts that need to be considered in attempting to determine how much of what type of physical activity is required to achieve specific health-related outcomes. Its focus is on the biological responses to physical activity that may be the basis for the inverse association between physical activity and clinical manifestations of various diseases. For many of the clinical outcomes of interest to this consensus conference, very few experimental studies have been conducted that systematically address the issue of dose–response. In many cases, for both clinical and biological outcomes, physical activity dose has been inferred from observational studies. In most experimental (training) studies, a single dose of exercise has been prescribed and a dose–response relationship defined by analyzing the variation in response in relation to adherence by program participants. Both of these approaches can provide some insight into dose–response, but they lack the scientific rigor required to accurately define the dose–response relationship for a wide variety of biological and clinical outcomes. Of major concern in both instances is the problem of self-selection bias. A detailed review of the dose–response relationship between physical activity and many of the health-related biological outcomes of interest has been left to the authors assigned to review the relationship between physical activity or physical fitness and the specific diseases or pathological conditions for this consensus conference. The primary focus of this chapter is a presentation of some of the major conceptual and applied issues that need consideration in developing dose–response guidelines for exercise-induced, health-related outcomes.

Physical Activity, Physical Fitness, and Health

Traditionally it has been promulgated that physical activity improves health by means of an increase in physical fitness: That is, regular exercise leads to an increase in fitness (especially cardiorespiratory fitness), and by achieving fitness, health is improved. If this is the process, then for physical activity to improve health there first needs to be a significant improvement in cardiorespiratory fitness, and the degree of improvement in health status is closely tied to the magnitude of this improvement in fitness. It is becoming more and more apparent that the relationship is not so simple for such diseases as coronary heart disease or adult-onset diabetes. Indeed, other relationships between physical activity, fitness, and health possibly exist (Figure 71.1): (a) Physical activity may improve fitness and health simultaneously but separately, (b) activity may improve fitness but not a specific health outcome, or (c) physical activity

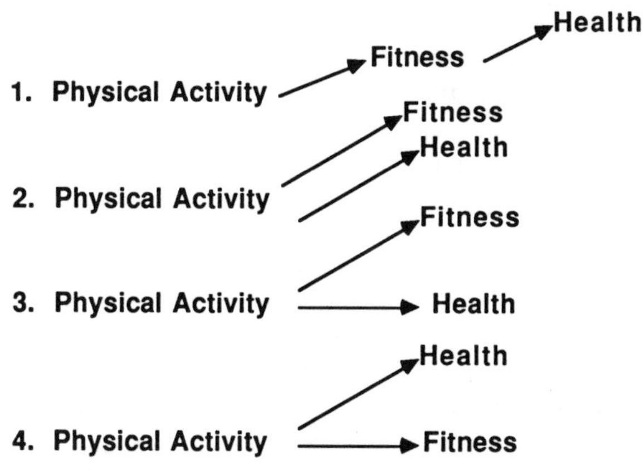

Figure 71.1 Possible causal relationships among Physical activity, physical fitness, and health. From "Physical Activity and Health: The Need to Define the Required Stimulus," by William Haskell, The American Journal of Cardiology, 55:4D-9D, 1984. Reprinted by permission.

may improve some aspects of health but not significantly improve traditional or accepted measures of fitness.

Due to the specificity of exercise (adaptations occur only in those systems or tissues that are activated by the exercise), it is likely that all of the physical activity–fitness–health relationships depicted in Figure 71.1 exist when considering the wide variety of health-related outcomes ascribed to physical activity and enhanced fitness. Some health outcomes may occur as a result of an increase in cardiorespiratory fitness while others may occur only if the metabolic capacity of the skeletal muscle is enhanced. At the same time, as a result of the same exercise stimulus, biological responses may occur that have a positive effect on long-term health outcomes, but do not influence performance capacity (fitness).

Issues Regarding Dose–Response

The *dose* aspect of the dose–response relationship incorporates various characteristics of physical activity including type (dynamic vs. static, arms vs. legs, amount of muscle mass used, etc.), intensity (absolute or relative to capacity), duration of session, frequency of sessions, number of sessions, and length of time over which sessions are performed (days, months, or years). The *response* component is what happens as a result of the activity and may be expressed as the biological, psychological, physical, performance, or health consequences of the activity. Some responses are relatively easy to measure accurately and reliably, such as body weight or number of kilograms that can be lifted, whereas other responses, such as changes in the rate of progression of coronary atherosclerosis or enhancement of a clinically useful immune response are currently very difficult.

The Need for a Revision in Terminology

Over the past several decades in the attempt to better define the health benefits of physical activity, a variety of new terms or revisions of existing words have occurred. It has been proposed that the term *physical activity* be used for body movement that is not specifically performed to improve physical working capacity or health-related fitness, which is designated as *exercise* (3). Also, *health-related fitness* has been introduced to differentiate health outcomes from improvement in physical working capacity (*physical fitness*). Physical fitness has frequently meant the capacity to perform endurance exercise, therefore it has nearly become synonymous with cardiorespiratory capacity and maximal oxygen uptake, ignoring the other components of physical fitness (muscle strength and power, speed, flexibility, agility, and balance).

Given the complexity of the biological responses to all forms of physical activity and the need to be able to accurately describe the specific responses to exercise, further refinement of the dose–response lexicon is needed. Instead of using the label *physical fitness*, the specific performance parameter of interest should be used, such as endurance capacity, maximal oxygen uptake, muscle strength, muscle endurance, and so forth. *Health-related fitness* should mean an improvement in performance that contributes to health (but infrequently used as such). Rather, specific biological or psychological parameters should be defined; for example, improved lipoprotein profile, enhanced glucose disposal, increased cardiopulmonary efficiency, and so on. It is apparent that some biological changes in response to physical activity that enhance various parameters of performance also contribute to improved health status. When these changes are used to describe health outcomes, it would clarify their meaning if the term *fitness* was not applied; improvement in oxygen transport capacity or efficiency should not be labeled as an improvement in *cardiorespiratory fitness*, neither should a change in lipoprotein or carbohydrate metabolism be labeled a change in *metabolic fitness*. Continuation of the application of *fitness* to the biological changes produced by physical activity would likely lead to such terms as *neurohormonal fitness* or *immune fitness* and produce more confusion than clarification.

Dose for Performance Versus Health

It is important that the parameters of the dose–response relationship for health-related outcomes not be confined to just those typically considered when evaluating the dose–response for improving athletic or physical performance. For example, the volume of activity per day (rather than that for a specific training session), or the volume of activity per day above a specific intensity threshold may need to be considered. The nature of the exercise dose may be very different for selected biologic changes required for improved health status compared to that required for improved performance. In fact, the maximal or supramaximal exercise intensity used by some athletes to enhance physical performance for athletic competition may even have some detrimental health outcomes.

Interaction Between Dose–Response and Personal Characteristics

A variety of personal characteristics may influence the dose–response relationship for any specific biological outcome, and the nature of the interaction between physical activity dose and these personal characteristics probably varies from one biological response to another. These characteristics would include at least age, gender, clinical status, nutritional status, use of medications, smoking status, and baseline physical activity and fitness levels. Superimposed on all of these characteristics is the interindividual response variation due to heredity (2). One example of an environmental factor altering the dose–response relationship is the influence of cigarette smoking on the increase in plasma high-density lipoprotein cholesterol (HDL-C) usually produced by endurance training. Several studies have shown that continuation of smoking during training blunts the increase in HDL-C (4,25). It is speculated that smoking interacts with the exercise effect on HDL-C by reducing the activity of lipoprotein lipase (17).

Individual Variability of Dose–Response

For many of the favorable biological responses attributed to physical activity, very little is known about their response to a specific dose of activity. Data are available that describe reasonably well the type, intensity, and amount of activity that improve maximal oxygen uptake of a group (1), and an adequate prescription probably can be constructed for other health-related outcomes such as adiposity or improvement in insulin resistance. However, even for these responses, very little is known about why there is substantial variation in the response to the same dose of physical activity among individuals who appear to be relatively homogeneous regarding key characteristics.

For example, Dionne et al. (6) reported the individual changes in maximal oxygen uptake of sedentary men aged 24 to 29 years to a highly standardized endurance-training program (12 weeks, 3 times per week, 20 min per session at onset of blood lactic acid [OBLA]). Among the 29 men training at Arizona State University, the increase in maximal oxygen uptake ranged from 0.07 to 0.96 L per minute, a 14-fold difference (Figure 71.2). Interindividual variations in the responses of other biological variables to exercise have been reported (2,20), but so far little attention has been given to this important issue in the discussion of the exercise prescription. Why such variations exist is not well understood and requires substantial investigation.

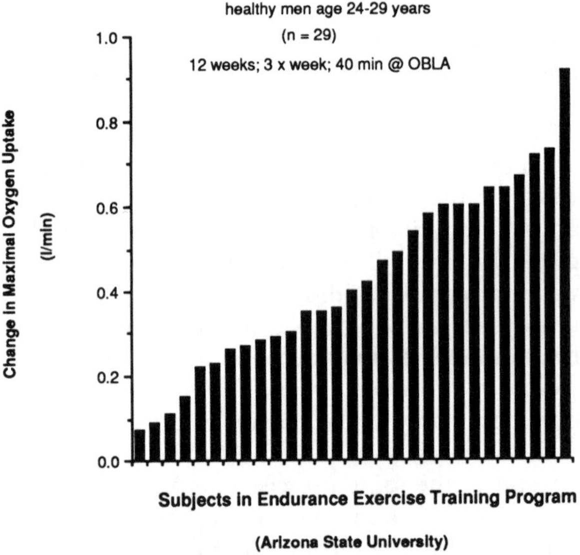

Figure 71.2 Interindividual variation in the changes in maximal oxygen uptake in response to a standardized endurance-training program.

Absolute Versus Relative Intensity

For many of the specific biological changes produced by physical activity, it has not been determined if the intensity component of the dose is more related to absolute intensity (e.g., a set rate of energy expenditure, a specific resistance in kilograms, etc.) or to intensity relative to a person's capacity (e.g., percent of aerobic capacity, percent voluntary maximal contraction, etc.). For example, for weight loss the response is more closely related to absolute intensity (e.g., number of calories per minute) rather than to percent of capacity, whereas the increase in aerobic capacity is more related to relative intensity (e.g., percent $\dot{V}O_2max$ or maximal heart rate) than absolute intensity.

Some investigators and coaches have attempted to develop training regimens where intensity is based on the lactate or anaerobic threshold. Substantial controversy still exists regarding this concept; however, it brings into focus a potentially important issue regarding exercise intensity and specificity of the response. If the response is dependent on a substantial increase in sympathetic nervous system drive, then the exercise probably needs to be at or above the anaerobic threshold, as the increase in plasma catecholamine concentration appears to be increased significantly only above 60% of aerobic capacity.

On the other hand, if the response does not require substantial activation of the sympathetic system, then lower intensity exercise may be an adequate stimulus. Also, there is increasing evidence that lower intensity endurance-type exercise is more effective in lowering systemic arterial blood pressure in borderline or moderate hypertensive patients than higher intensity activity (18,26). It could be that sustained stimulation of the sympathetic nervous system during higher intensity activity may negate some of the beneficial effects of exercise on resting blood pressure produced by other mechanisms.

Specificity of the Response

In order to accurately define the required dose, the specific measure of interest has to be identified due to the specificity of the exercise effect. Substantial data exist demonstrating that the dose–response relationship varies widely for different outcomes. For example, the stimulus for changes in fat and carbohydrate metabolism are most likely to be responsive to increases in metabolic rate or total energy expenditure above some threshold, whereas changes in bone density are likely due primarily to the stress placed on bone by vigorous muscular contraction or the force of gravity. The recent report by Duncan, Gordon, and Scott (7) demonstrates that although intensity may be key in increasing aerobic capacity, volume of exercise may be more important for increasing HDL-C.

Mechanisms of Action

To understand why a specific dose of exercise is needed to produce a specific health-related effect, it is necessary to have some idea of the nature of the mechanism of action (12). For example, if the desired effect is a reduction in systemic arterial blood pressure, then to understand why a certain dose of exercise is required it would be useful to know how this decrease in blood pressure is achieved. Is the lower blood pressure due to a decrease in cardiac output or a decrease in peripheral vascular resistance and what biological changes lead to a reduction in each of these? Independent of its effect on adiposity, some data indicate that exercise could impact blood pressure control through a variety of mechanisms, including its effects on the sympathetic nervous system, insulin sensitivity, electrolyte balance, neural and baroreflex mechanisms, and changes in vascular structure (24,26).

Not understanding a mechanism of action could lead to a major misunderstanding regarding the required dose of exercise for a specific health-related benefit. For example, it has generally been implied or stated by many authors of scientific manuscripts reporting exercise-training studies that if the physical activity regimen improved $\dot{V}O_2max$, then the activity would likely contribute to the prevention of coronary heart disease. If no improvement in $\dot{V}O_2max$ was observed then it was assumed the activity lacked health benefits. It is generally accepted that the major factors involved in the increase in $\dot{V}O_2max$ with endurance training are hemodynamic or related to enhanced oxygen transport by the cardiorespiratory system (23). However, these hemodynamic factors seem unlikely to be responsible for the primary preventive effect that exercise appears to provide against coronary artery disease. It is much more likely that various metabolic changes produced by regular exercise influence the process of atherosclerosis. Thus, even though hemodynamic and metabolic changes may occur with the exercise dose that improves $\dot{V}O_2max$, these metabolic changes may be responsive to a much different dose (e.g., lower intensity) than that required for hemodynamic changes.

Acute Response Versus Training Response

The traditional approach to the physical activity dose–response issue has been to consider that the dose of activity must produce a *training response* to be of benefit. A training response is a temporary or extended change in structure or function that results from performing repeated bouts of exercise and is usually considered to be independent of the effects produced by a single bout of exercise. However, there is increasing evidence that some of the major health-related biological changes produced by physical activity may be due more to acute biological responses during and for some time following each bout of activity than to a training response or an interaction between these two types of responses. An example of an *acute response* is that a 45-min bout of stationary cycling at 70% of $\dot{V}O_2max$ by older men and women with moderate hypertension significantly decreases systolic blood pressure for at least 3 hr postexercise (11).

Also, it has been demonstrated that in hypertriglyceridemic men, fasting plasma triglyceride concentration the morning after a 45-min bout of exercise at approximately 75% of aerobic capacity is lower than when such exercise is not performed (19). Over a 5-day period, if exercise is performed every day, triglyceride concentration decreases further the following day. Thus, this acute response is augmented by repeated bouts of exercise. This effect occurs even if the increased caloric expenditure is compensated for by increased caloric intake (10), and is likely due to an increase in lipoprotein lipase activity in response to the exercise (17). This could be called an *augmented acute response* in that repeated bouts of exercise during the week produce a greater effect than a single bout; however, there is no further decrease even after weeks of exercise training on a regular basis.

In Figure 71.3 four different exercise response profiles to the same dose of exercise are depicted. Response A represents an acute response in which the benefit occurs after one or several bouts of exercise and does not improve any further with continued exercise. Response B shows a *rapid response* in which more benefit is derived early with a relative plateauing of the response after a few weeks of training (22). Response C shows a nearly linear training response throughout the entire 12 weeks, and Response D depicts a *delayed response* that only occurs after a number of weeks of training.

The concept of an interaction between acute and chronic effects of exercise on health-related biological changes is depicted in Figure 71.4. It is likely

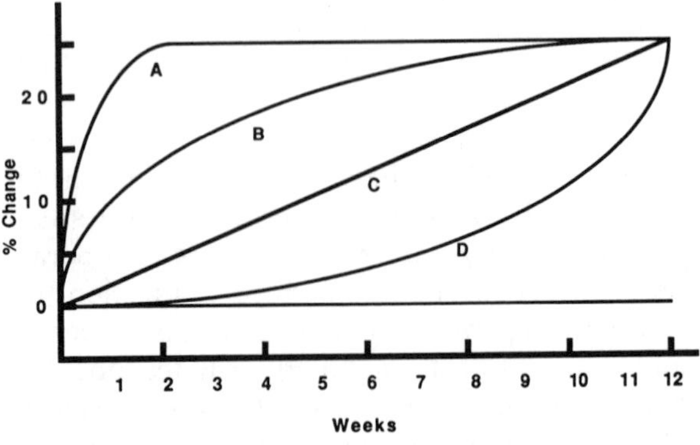

Figure 71.3 Various biological response profiles in response to frequent bouts of physical activity.

that as a person's physical working capacity increases and the absolute intensity of exercise performed during an exercise session is increased (relative intensity stays the same), the acute responses to various physiological or biochemical reactions will be enhanced. This would be true for any benefit directly tied to the magnitude of energy expended during the exercise session. An example of such a benefit might be the enhanced insulin-mediated glucose uptake observed in response to a single bout of exercise by highly trained endurance athletes (14). If such changes prove to provide significant clinical benefits, then major changes may need to be made in exercise program guidelines designed to promote specific aspects of health.

Dose–Response for Disease Prevention Versus Disease Treatment

When the effects of exercise training are evaluated for a specific health-related outcome, most often its significance is considered in the context of a treatment modality. For example, a comprehensive review of the literature on blood-pressure-lowering effects of endurance exercise training indicates that in normotensive persons the decrease in both systolic and diastolic blood pressure is approximately 3 mmHg, a 6-mmHg decrease in borderline hypertensive patients, and a 7- to 9-mmHg decrease in hypertensive patients (8). When this level of blood pressure reduction is compared to the greater reductions achieved by the use of antihypertensive medications (compounded by the difficulty in getting many patients to increase their activity), the frequent reaction by medical personnel is to dismiss the use of exercise as a primary means of blood pressure control. However, this magnitude of blood pressure reduction or the prevention of the age-related rise in pressure observed in many Western societies would have a powerful effect on decreasing the prevalence of hypertension in the population.

A relatively small downward shift of the distribution of blood pressure in the population significantly reduces the prevalence of hypertension. For example, in Figure 71.5 are data relating the prevalence of hypertension and mean blood pressure levels to leisure-time physical activity status among women 60 to 89 years of age living in Ranch Bernardo, California (21). The blood pressures are adjusted for age. The average mean blood pressure for women who were moderately active (133/74 mmHg) is lower than that observed in women reporting no regular leisure-time activity (142/77 mmHg). Associated with this relatively small difference in blood pressure is an approximate 50%

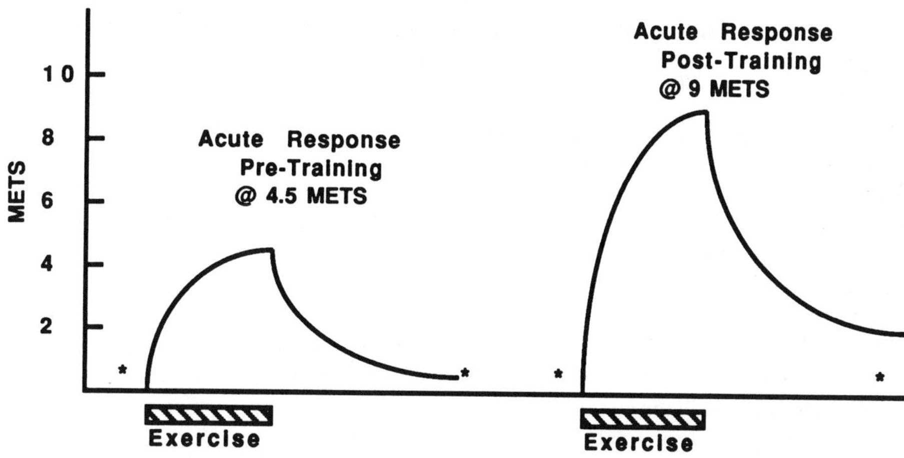

Figure 71.4 Interaction between acute and chronic effects of exercise to produce favorable biological changes.

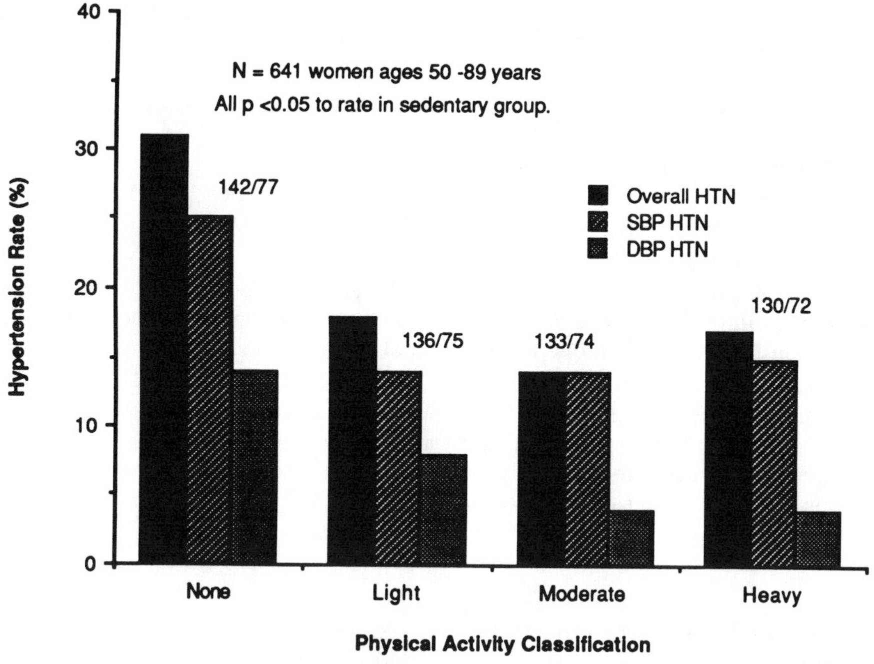

Figure 71.5 Relationship between habitual physical activity and the prevalence of hypertension (HTN) in older women.

reduction in the prevalence of hypertension. Thus, it is important to consider this population effect of the exercise response when considering the potential health benefit of the various biological outcomes from exercise.

Such a benefit on the risk of coronary heart disease mortality in the population might be observed from relatively small increases in HDL-C. It appears that a 1 mg/dl-higher HDL-C is associated with an approximate 3.5% lower risk of coronary heart disease mortality (9). If exercise increases HDL-C by even 4 mg/dl in the population (which by most standards would be considered a relatively small change), it might reduce CHD mortality by as much as 14%.

Multiple Biological Changes Contributing to a Single Clinical Benefit

It is important to realize that some of the clinical benefits of physical activity, that is the reduction in the frequency or severity of clinical manifestation of the disease, may not be due to one but several or numerous biological changes and that each of these changes may have a different dose–response relationship. For example, the reduction in coronary heart disease mortality associated with a more physically active lifestyle is likely due to the effects of increased activity on a number of different biological mechanisms (Table 71.1). In some cases, the increase in activity may reduce the

Table 71.1 Biological Mechanisms by Which Exercise May Contribute to the Primary or Secondary Prevention of Coronary Heart Disease*

Maintain or increase myocardial oxygen supply
- Delay progression of coronary atherosclerosis (possible)
  - Improve lipoprotein profile (increase HDL-C:LDL-C ratio) (probable)
  - Improve carbohydrate metabolism (increase insulin sensitivity) (probable)
  - Decrease platelet aggregation and increase fibrinolysis (probable)
  - Decrease adiposity (usually)
- Increase coronary collateral vascularization (unlikely)
- Increase epicardial artery diameter (possible)
- Increase coronary blood flow (myocardial perfusion) or distribution (possible)

Decrease myocardial work and oxygen demand
- Decrease heart rate at rest and during submaximal exercise (usually)
- Decrease systolic and mean systemic arterial pressure during submaximal exercise (usually) and at rest (possible)
- Decrease cardiac output during submaximal exercise (probable)
- Decrease circulating plasma catecholamine levels (decrease sympathetic tone) at rest (probable) and during submaximal exercise (usually)

Increase myocardial function
- Increase stroke volume at rest and during submaximal and maximal exercise (likely)
- Increase ejection fraction at rest and during exercise (likely)
- Increase intrinsic myocardial contractility (possible)
- Increase myocardial function resulting from decreased "afterload" (probable)
- Increase myocardial hypertrophy (probable), but this may not reduce CHD risk

Increase electrical stability of myocardium
- Decrease regional ischemia at rest or during submaximal exercise (possible)
- Decrease catecholamines in myocardium at rest (possible) and during submaximal exercise (probable)
- Increase ventricular fibrillation threshold due to reduction of cyclic AMP (possible)

Note. * = Expression of likelihood that effect will occur for an individual participating in endurance-type training program for 16 weeks or longer at 65% to 80% of functional capacity for 25 min or longer per session (300 kcal) for 3 or more sessions per week ranges from unlikely, possible, likely, probable, to usually. HDL-C = high-density lipoprotein cholesterol: LDL-C = low-density lipoprotein cholesterol: CHD = coronary heart disease; AMP = adenosine monophosphate.

rate of atherosclerosis or alter platelet aggregation, blood clotting, or fibrinolysis. In other cases it may reduce myocardial work, increase electrical stability, or alter vascular remodeling (13). If this occurs, then the clinical benefit of physical activity is the result of the combined changes of each of these biological changes.

This concept is depicted in Figure 71.6 for selected biological changes produced by physical activity thought to reduce the risk of coronary heart disease. At various points along the dose–response curve for coronary heart disease the magnitude of the benefit contributed by each of the biological responses will vary, some contributing more at the lower level of the dose scale with others only contributing at a much higher dose. This figure is a schematic representation of this concept because available data are inadequate to establish a data-based relationship between such biological and clinical outcomes.

Not only does it appear that exercise produces multiple positive biological changes that may reduce the risk of CAD, but exercise's minimum side effects make it an even more attractive intervention. For example, many of the medications used to treat hypertension produce detrimental side effects on lipid or glucose metabolism (increase in triglycerides, decrease in HDL-C, decreased glucose tolerance), whereas exercise tends to have a positive effect. These benefits are especially noticeable when exercise is added to a low-fat, calorie-restricted diet.

Optimal Versus Adequate Versus Minimal Dose

Currently we know a substantial amount about what the *adequate* dose of exercise is to achieve many health-related biological or physical changes, but we still know very little about the *optimal* or *minimal* dose of exercise for such effects. For exercise prescriptions or guidelines to be scientifically sound and produce the desired effects,

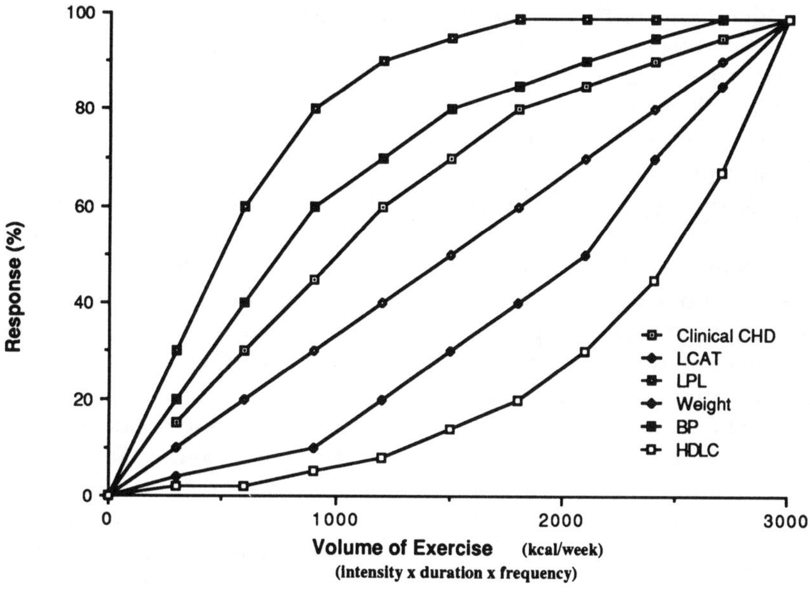

Figure 71.6 Dose–response relationships between volume of exercise, biological responses, and coronary heart disease. Total CVD = total cardiovascular disease, BP = blood pressure, HDL-C = high-density lipoprotein cholesterol.

it is important to develop the data required to understand what the optimal dose of exercise is to achieve a desired outcome. This optimal dose would maximize benefit and minimize risk and cost. What the minimal dose is for a specific benefit is what much of the general public would like to know (not how much do I have to do, but how little can I get away with). Although information on the minimal or optimal dose of exercise required to achieve many health-related biological and physical changes is incomplete, it is still adequate for use in the design and implementation of specific exercise program recommendations directed at improving health-related outcomes.

Discussion

The exact exercise stimulus required for producing a change in any of the health-related biological factors other than for possibly $\dot{V}O_2$max and body weight is not known. It is only by trial and error research that the dose–response relationship can be established. For example, we do not know the relative role that changes in intensity, duration, or volume of exercise play in producing beneficial clinical changes. It may be that for some benefits intensity is not critical, and for others only volume of exercise influences the response. On the other hand, if beneficial changes are related to the amount of fat metabolism that occurs during exercise, then lower intensity exercise will be of greater value. But, if the changes are related to the magnitude of sympathetic drive stimulated by the exercise, then time spent at a higher intensity of exercise would be most effective.

It generally appears that for most health-related biological changes there is a dose relationship throughout nearly the full range of exercise. Yet in some cases there may be an upper threshold where greater intensity or volume may actually be less beneficial than a lower dose. Several studies suggest this may be the case for blood pressure (15,18).

Because the risk of orthopedic and cardiac injury and the acceptability of a specific exercise regimen by many persons is closely linked to exercise intensity, establishing dose–response data for intensity and specific health benefits is a high priority. In middle-aged and older men and women some data demonstrate that moderate intensity (40%–60% of aerobic capacity) exercise provides significant health-related benefits at low risk and good adherence. The trade-off of longer exercise duration or more frequent sessions at lower intensity for higher intensity shorter exercise sessions needs further evaluation (16). Also, the health benefits of multiple short bouts of exercise per day versus a single longer bout needs to be investigated further (5). A brief, but more frequent stimulus, especially for some functions like platelet aggregation or fibrinolysis, might be more effective than a longer bout every other day or two.

The greatest health benefits from exercise appear to occur when very sedentary persons begin a regular program of moderate-intensity endurance-type exercise. Further increases in intensity or amount of exercise produce further benefits in some, but not all, biological responses. The primary stimulus for many of these changes is a sustained, repeated increase in metabolic rate; any way this can be achieved during physical activity is of benefit.

Standard exercise recommendations based on the stimulus required to produce a significant increase in aerobic capacity have been incorporated as part of the usual exercise prescription for health (aerobic activity at moderate intensity for 30 min or 4 kcal/kg body weight, 3 times or more per week). Although such a prescription is probably *adequate*, it may not be *optimal* or *minimal*, and selected health benefits will require more specificity.

Major Research Questions on the Biological Aspects of Dose–Response

1. For various key biological changes associated with major health outcomes, determine the optimal dose of physical activity required for a significant improvement. Define the dose in terms of the type, intensity, duration, and frequency of exercise and the time course of the response (acute vs. chronic).
2. Determine the magnitude of the interindividual variation in the dose–response relationship for the major health-related biological outcomes produced by exercise. Identify the components of the variation due to heredity and those due to various environmental factors.
3. Evaluate the acute effects of physical activity on major biological outcomes that have potential health benefits. Consider a wide variety of physical activity profiles, including low-intensity exercise performed for hours at a time as well as short bouts repeated frequently throughout the day.
4. Begin to determine the optimal dose–response for the prevention of various pathological conditions as well as their treatment. For example, the dose–response characteristics of exercise for the prevention of the age-related increase in arterial blood pressure may be different than that for the lowering of already elevated blood pressure.
5. Develop a program of research to investigate the interaction of the dose of physical activity and other personal characteristics, such as various dietary components, on major health-related outcomes.

References

1. American College of Sports Medicine. The recommended quality and quantity of exercise for developing and maintaining fitness in healthy adults. Med. Sci. Sports Exerc. 22:265-274; 1990.
2. Bouchard, C. Discussion: Heredity, fitness, and Health. In: Bouchard, C.; Shephard, R.J.; Stephens, T.; Sutton, J.R.; McPherson, B.D., eds. Exercise, fitness, and health. Champaign, IL: Human Kinetics; 1988:147-153.
3. Caspersen, C.J.; Powell, K.E.; Christenson, G.M. Physical activity, exercise and physical fitness: Definitions and distributions for health-related research. Public Health Rep. 100:126-134; 1985.
4. Cowan, G.O. Influences of exercise on high density lipoproteins. Am. J. Cardiol. 52:13B-16B; 1983.
5. DeBusk, R.F.; Hakansson, U.; Sheehan, M.; Haskell, W.L. Training effects of long versus short bouts of exercise. Am. J. Cardiol. 65:1010-1013; 1990.
6. Dionne, F.T.; Turcotte, L.; Thibault, C.; Bonlay, M.R.; Skinner, J.S.; Bouchard, C. Mitochondrial DNA sequence polymorphism, VO_2max and response to endurance training. Med. Sci. Sports Exerc. 23:177-185; 1991.
7. Duncan, J.J.; Gordon, N.F.; Scott, C.B. Women walking for health and fitness. JAMA. 66:3295-3299; 1991.
8. Fagard, R.H.; Tipton, C.M. Physical activity, fitness, and hypertension. In Physical activity, fitness and health, Champaign, IL: Human Kinetics; 1994. (Chapter 43 of this volume.)
9. Gordon, D.J.; Probstfield, J.L.; Garrison, R.J.; Neaton, J.D.; Castelli, W.L.; Knoke, J.D.; Jacobs, D.R.; Bangdlwala, S.; Tyroler, H.A. High-density lipoprotein cholesterol and cardiovascular disease. Four prospective American studies. Circulation. 79:8-15; 1989.
10. Gyntelberg, F.; Brennan, R.; Holloszy, J.; Schonfeld, G.; Rennie, M.; Weidman, S. Plasma triglyceride lowering by exercise despite increased food intake in patients with Type IV hyperlipoproteinemia. Am. J. Clin. Nutr. 30:716-720; 1977.
11. Hagberg, J.M.; Montain, S.J.; Martin, W.H. Blood pressure and hemodynamic responses after exercise in older hypertensives. J. Appl. Physiol. 63:270-276; 1987.
12. Haskell, W.L. Physical activity and health: The need to define the required stimulus. Am. J. Cardiol. 55:4D-9D; 1984.

13. Haskell, W.L. Mechanisms by which physical activity may enhance the clinical status of cardiac patients. In: Pollock, M.; Schmidt, D., eds. Heart disease and rehabilitation. New York: Wiley; 1986:303-324.
14. Heath, G.W.; Gavin, J.R.; Hinderlith, J.M.; Hagberg, J.M.; Bloomfield, S.A.; Holloszy, J.O. Effects of exercise and lack of exercise on glucose tolerance and insulin sensitivity. J. Appl. Physiol. 55:512-517; 1983.
15. Jennings, G.; Nelson, L.; Nestel, P.; Esler, M.; Korner, P.; Burton, D.; Bazelmans, J. The effects of changes in physical activity on major cardiovascular risk factors, hemodynamics, sympathetic function, and glucose utilization in man: A controlled study of four levels of activity. Circulation. 73:30-40; 1986.
16. King, A.C.; Haskell, W.L.; Taylor, C.B.; Kraemer, H.C.; DeBusk, R.F. Group- vs. home-based exercise training in healthy older men and women: A community-based clinical trial. JAMA. 266:1535-1542; 1991.
17. Lithell, H.; Hellsing, K.; Lundqvist, G.; Malmberg, P. Lipoprotein lipase activity of human skeletal muscle and adipose tissue after intense physical exercise. Acta Physiol. Scand. 105:312-315; 1979.
18. Nelson, L.; Jennings, G.L.; Elser, M.D.; Kover, P.I. Effects of changing levels of physical activity on blood pressure and haemodynamics in essential hypertension. Lancet. 8505:473-476; 1986.
19. Oscai, L.B.; Patterson, J.A.; Bogard, D.L.; Beck, R.J.; Rothermel, B.L. Normalization of serum triglycerides and lipoprotein electrophoretic patterns by exercise. Am. J. Cardiol. 30:775-780; 1972.
20. Poehlman, E.T.; Tramblay, A.; Nadeau, A.; Dussault, J.; Theriault, G.; Bouchard, C. Heredity and changes in body composition and adipose tissue metabolism after short-term exercise training. Eur. J. Appl. Physiol. 250:E711-E717; 1987.
21. Reaven, P.D.; Barrett-Conner, E.; Edelstein, S. Relation between leisure-time physical activity and blood pressure in older women. Circulation. 83:559-565; 1991.
22. Rogers, M.A.; Yamamoto, C.; King, D.S.; Hagberg, J.M.; Ehsan, A.A.; Holloszy, J.O. Improvement in glucose tolerance after 1 week of exercise in patients with mild NIDDM. Diabetes Care. 11:613-618; 1986.
23. Saltin, B. Cardiovascular and pulmonary adaptations to physical activity. In: Bouchard, C.; Shephard, R.J.; Stephens, T.; Sutton, J.R.; McPherson, B.D., eds. Exercise, fitness, and health. Champaign, IL: Human Kinetics; 1988:187-203.
24. Seals, D.R.; Hagberg, J.M. The effect of exercise training on human hypertension: A review. Med. Sci. Sports Exerc. 16:207-215; 1984.
25. Stanford, B.A.; Matter, S.; Fell, R.; Sady, S.; Cresanta, M.; Papanek, P. Cigarette smoking, physical activity and alcohol consumption: Relationship to blood lipids and lipoproteins in postmenopausal females. Metabolism. 33:585-590; 1984.
26. Tipton, C.M. Exercise and hypertension: A review. In: Holloszy, J.O., ed. Exercise and sport sciences reviews. Baltimore: Williams & Wilkins; 1991:447-505.

Chapter 72

Dose–Response Issues From a Psychosocial Perspective

W. Jack Rejeski

There is a growing body of literature supporting the popular belief that exercise interventions have positive effects on various psychosocial outcomes. For example, quantitative reviews of the literature have shown that aerobic exercise is effective in countering both depression (31) and anxiety (33). Ewart, Taylor, Reese, and Debusk (15) found that even single bouts of treadmill testing could be effective in increasing cardiac patients' confidence toward walking and stair climbing, whereas confidence toward dissimilar tasks (sexual intercourse and weight lifting) were strongest after the implications of treadmill data had been explained by a physician and nurse. Yet other investigators have reported that aerobic exercise may decrease the self-report of daily hassles (8) and dampen physiological reactivity to acute stress (9). Despite these developments, however, a question that has both practical as well as theoretical significance is whether these reported effects are mediated by the dose of activity. In other words, is there an optimal treatment intervention? Is more necessarily better? Are there points at which we see diminishing returns?

With the general goal of examining dose–response issues from a psychosocial perspective, the content of this chapter has two specific objectives: (a) to clarify the meaning and implications of the phrase "dose–response issues from a psychosocial perspective," and (b) to provide a review of the existing dose–response literature.

Dose of Activity From a Psychosocial Perspective: Meaning and Implications

I suspect that the scientific interest in dose–response relationships with exercise can be traced to the extensive literature on this topic in drug therapy. Yet it is good to recognize that the concept of dose–response curves for behavior and for exercise in particular is both reductionistic and complex. The concept is reductionistic because it espouses a stimulus–response paradigm, one that ignores cognitive and emotional input by the perceiver. Although biological cues (the stimulus) play an important role in determining the affective and behavioral outcomes of exercise, it is critical to remember that people respond as "active" rather than "passive" agents; that is, they are involved in interpreting a given dose of activity and making decisions on their response. This point has been very clear in my own research on perceived exertion (34) as well as work by Morgan and others (26). For example, in one study (39) we had males run for 20 min at 85% of their $\dot{V}O_2$max on two different occasions, once when subjects thought they were running for 20 min and another when they believed they would be running for 30 min. Exertional ratings for minutes 3 through 16 were statistically lower on the day subjects believed they would have to run for 30 min, suggesting that they adopted a different mental set for the more demanding trial in order to cope with the larger dose of exercise.

Along with the need to conceptualize the exerciser as an "active agent" is the task of delineating the stimulus. The concept of *dose* encompasses several well-known dimensions of an exercise prescription; that is, type of activity, frequency, intensity, duration, and even length of training. Investigators also have the choice of examining acute bouts of exercise or the chronic effects of training. In this sense, dose of activity is central to any consensus statement that is made about exercise.

Finally, it is important to reflect on the various responses in question. Figure 72.1 provides a broad overview of typical outcomes that are relevant to such an inquiry. This organizational structure yields several key points. First, a psychosocial perspective encompasses measures related to affect or emotion, cognition, perception, biological functioning, and overt behavior. Also, there is no clear

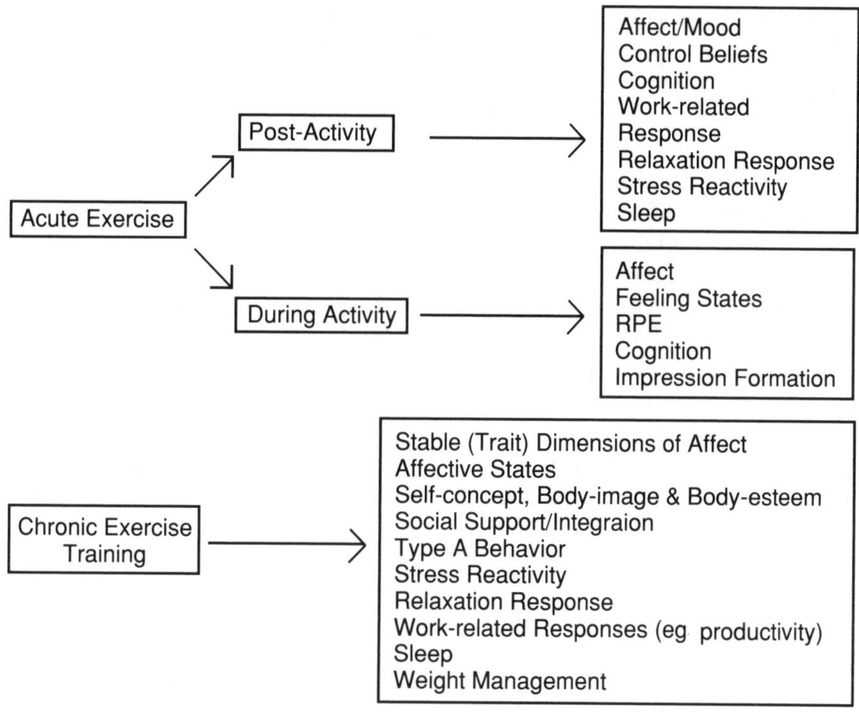

Figure 72.1 Psychosocial-related outcomes of exercise.

separation of biological, psychological, and social processes, a view that is consistent with the biopsychosocial model in medicine first proposed by Engle in 1977 (13).

Second, although much of the attention in the literature on acute exercise has focused on post-exercise responses, it is extremely important to consider outcomes that take place during activity itself. Why do some people thrive on levels of activity that others find aversive? What is the impact of task aversion on long-term compliance? An additional consideration with in-task responses is how observers interpret the exerciser's behavior (37). Although this is a sharp departure from traditional research, observers' perceptions of the demands that accompany a given dose of exercise have relevance to how people reinforce those who engage in such behavior. These perceptions also have implications for constructs such as efficacy beliefs, attitudes, intentions, and subjective norms.

Third, the breadth of potential responses depicted in Figure 72.1 argues strongly against ever identifying a single mechanism of action for dose–response relationships. The fact that there is not a single cause common to all outcomes should not come as a great surprise. The early work of Kenyon (19) demonstrated that people have diverse motives for engaging in physical activity. Moreover, the dynamics of why exercise may enhance cognition differ greatly from the social goals of impression management (21) or the challenge of or threat to physical recovery from coronary heart disease (38). In other words, the response itself is an important contributing factor to our understanding of dose–response relationships.

And fourth, there is no reason to believe that any single response can be predicted from a given dose of activity. This point may be most obvious in the area of impression management. Although exercise is an important means of controlling aspects of one's social self (18,44), there is considerable variability in desired exercise images people choose or are forced to project. For some, being labeled "an exerciser" may be sufficient, a feat that can be achieved with minimal effort. On the other hand, there are those who seek the social comparative rewards of having a more muscular body or sleek-looking appearance than other men or women. Quite logically, in this latter instance the desired psychosocial and physical outcomes are dependent on a far more demanding dose of activity.

Areas for Consideration

Obviously it is beyond the scope of any single chapter to elaborate on every endpoint identified in Figure 72.1. Furthermore, there are very few experiments pertinent to this organizational structure where varying doses of activity have been systematically manipulated. Although it is possible to examine dose–response effects by contrasting training variables (e.g., low- vs. high-intensity exercise) from different publications, such an approach has inherent liabilities via method variance and lack of correspondence in operation of terms. In view of these limitations I have chosen to focus the remainder of my discussion on content areas where published research has provided specific data that is relevant to developing a psychosocial perspective on dose–response relationships. With the exception of quantitative reviews, very little attention is given to cross-study comparisons. This approach led to the identification of two broad areas: (a) postexercise affect, and (b) psychophysiological function and weight control.

Posttask Affect

The first topic for consideration is existing evidence that posttask affect may be moderated by the dose of an activity. Rather than treating individual responses (e.g., depression or anxiety) separately, I have elected to group studies under three broad themes: (a) improved affect, (b) baseline mood states, and (c) the potential negative effects of overload.

Improved Affect

There are four studies that have attempted to evaluate whether a particular dose of activity is instrumental to enhanced affect. Two of these investigations have dealt with chronic exercise training. Utilizing a randomized control group design, Moses, Steptoe, Matthews, and Edwards (30) recently contrasted *moderate aerobic exercise* (20 min at 60% HRmax, three times per week for 10 weeks) with what they termed *high-intensity work* (30 min at 60%–70% HRmax, 3 times per week for 10 weeks) and two distinct control groups. In a relatively unfit population (see Table 72.1), it was the moderate-exercise group that experienced reductions in tension and confusion. The mood states for the high-intensity group did not differ from trends seen in attention- or wait-list-control conditions. In addition, at a 3-month follow-up, those subjects that had participated in the moderate exercise therapy reported fewer coping deficits than any other group. There were no effects observed for depression or other subscales of a modified Profile of Mood States (POMS). One further point worth mentioning is that, as expected, it was the high-intensity group that made the greatest gains in physical work capacity.

Berger and Owen (2) elected to study dose by using intact groups whose activities were characterized as providing a naturalistic environment for studying varying physical demands: swimming, body conditioning, fencing, yoga, and lecture classes. Over a 14-week period, chronic training in any of the four modes of activity produced no changes in affective functioning. This study, however, had several serious flaws including (a) the use of single intact classes, (b) confounds within treatments (e.g., yoga offers far more than simply low-level activity), and (c) treatment leaders' awareness of the experimental hypothesis (i.e., on an a priori basis the authors hypothesized that the chronic training would not alter mood profiles).

As far as acute exercise is concerned, Farrell, Gustafson, Morgan, and Pert (16) studying a group of highly trained runners found reductions in postexercise tension or anxiety after demanding as compared to relatively light physical work. The exact opposite conclusion was reached by Berger and Owen (2) following pre- to postchanges in POMS scores collected during a single bout of exercise; however, as indicated previously, the internal validity of this study is highly suspect. One other dose–response study in the area of acute exercise is a paper by Roy and Steptoe (42). The purpose of this research was to examine the effects of varying the intensity of exercise on psychological responses to subsequent psychosocial threat. As shown in Table 72.1, subjects participated in one of three different treatment conditions with increasing physical demand. After completing their respective exercise bouts, subjects engaged in a problem-solving task were given two brief periods of recovery and completed posttask self-rating scales for positive and negative affect. None of the groups stood out as having a unique pattern in mood upon recovery from psychosocial threat. Regrettably, however, no data were available on pretask apprehension after subjects had been introduced to the stressor.

The Moderating Role of Baseline Mood

A frequently discussed position in research on affective function is conceptually similar to the law of initial values in psychophysiology. The argument is that if subjects' preintervention profiles are within normal limits then the window for change is significantly reduced, a situation that will minimize group differences and yield poor statistical power. Surprisingly, data from meta-analyses on

Table 72.1 Improved Affect

Study	n, gender, M age (years), fitness (ml · kg^{-1} · min^{-1})	Design	Measures	Major findings
Berger & Owen (2)	170, both, ~22, none reported	Intact classes: swimming, body conditioning, fencing, yoga, and two lecture controls; assessed both acute and chronic effects	POMS	Yoga, the low-intensity work, improved mood more than other group
Farrell et al. (16)	7, male, 27.4, 61.1	Within subjects; 80-min run at 40% and 60% $\dot{V}O_2max$, plus 40 min-run at 80% $\dot{V}O_2max$	POMS	Tension reduced only after runs at 60% and 80% $\dot{V}O_2max$
Moses et al. (30)	75, both, 18 to 60, ~34	Randomized between subjects, 10 weeks; 20 min at 60% HRmax, 30 min at 60% to 75% HRmax, light exercise, and wait-list control; 3-month follow-up	Modified POMS and coping scale	20-min group had greater change in tension and confusion when compared to other groups; they also had better coping skills at 3-month follow-up
Roy & Steptoe (in press)	30, male, 21.3, ~44.1	Randomized between subjects, 3 groups; control, 20 min at 25 W, and 20 min at 100 W; subjects rested and were then stressed after each treatment	Single items: relaxation, exhaustion, worry, and happiness	The groups did not differ in affect following the stressor; subjects' tension increased following the 100-W condition

Note. n = number in sample; M = mean; ml · kg^{-1} · min^{-1} = milliliters per kilogram per minute; POMS = Profile of Mood States; $\dot{V}O_2max$ = maximal volume of oxygen consumed per minute during exercise; HRmax = maximal heart rate; W = watts.

anxiety and depression (31,33) do not support a moderating influence for baseline levels of affective functioning. Yet, North, McCullagh, and Vu Tran (31) did find that the largest effect size (ES) for depression occurred in a group whose purpose for exercise was medical rehabilitation. Parenthetically, depression is common in such groups and the origin is frequently reactive rather than endogenous.

There are three studies in the dose–response literature that warrant consideration in evaluating the possible effects of baseline values on changes in affect. These include the work by (a) Lennox, Bedell, and Stone (22); (b) Blumenthal, Emery, and Rejeski (3); and (c) Sexton, Maere, and Dahl (43). Neither study (a) nor (b), both randomized group designs, found differences in various parameters of affective functioning following roughly 3 months of training with either a low or moderate program of exercise (see Table 72.2). Interestingly, the mean pretest scores in these studies approximated the 50th T-score from published norms. These results may seem at odds with the previously discussed data by Moses et al. (30), however, this investigation employed a modified version of the POMS that lacks published normative data. Thus, it is impossible to ascertain the pretreatment status of their subjects.

Despite poor experimental control, a study by Sexton and his colleagues (43) is pertinent to the potential role that pretreatment affective dysfunction may play in evaluating the efficacy of exercise in the arena of mental health. Specifically, these authors piggybacked multimodal psychotherapy and two different intensities of exercise (low and moderate) in the treatment of psychiatric patients with documented anxiety or depressive symptomology. After the completion of an 8-week treatment, both groups manifested improvement in psychological functioning even though the high-intensity group experienced greater gains in estimated $\dot{V}O_2max$. Most important was the finding that the high-intensity exercise had a much higher dropout rate than the low-intensity program.

Negative Effects of Overload

In addition to the potential compliance problems associated with more demanding exercise regimens is the concern that high-intensity programs may actually foster negative affective states (Table 72.3). For example, in the realm of collegiate swimming, Morgan and his colleagues (27,28) have published descriptive data that suggest that overtraining leads to staleness, a condition that is marked by elevation in depression and anxiety as well as a decrease in vigor. Whereas an experiment published in 1987 (27, Experiment 3) documented the negative effects of overtraining across a 6-month period, later work (28) suggested that even short-term exposure (about 1 week) to demanding physical work can create elevations in negative affect that covary with signs of physiological stress.

In the realm of exercise prescriptions that are more typical of preventive and rehabilitative medicine is the recent work of Steptoe and his associates. In one study Steptoe and Cox (46) studied women who completed four separate 8-min trials of exercise. Subjects rode a cycle ergometer at both 25 W and 100 W; both with and without music as a form of distraction. Immediately following the 100-W conditions subjects reported increased tension or anxiety, whereas after completing the 25-W trials there were noticeable increases in vigor and exhilaration. Although this finding has been replicated on two different occasions (42,45), its clinical significance is far from obvious. For example, elevation in tension or anxiety immediately postexercise may be a false positive; that is to say, increased sympathetic nervous system activity that occurs with exercise may create elevated tension that shares little in common with the tension accompanying psychological distress (36). Additionally, there is evidence from Steptoe's own laboratory that the negative effects of demanding aerobic exercise on tension or anxiety are relatively short-lived (42).

The only other research that has specifically examined the potential negative effects of more traditional doses of exercise therapy are two experiments published in the early 1970s by Morgan, Roberts, and Feinerman (29, see Table 72.3). At this time in the history of exercise psychology, one hypothesis was that the accumulation of lactic acid, which increases in direct proportion to exercise intensity, might trigger undesirable psychological change (e.g., elevated anxiety). In the first experiment, university professors engaged in progressive exercise tests with one of four different endpoints: a target heart rate (HR) of 150 beats per minute (bpm), 160 bpm, 170 bpm, or 180 bpm. Contrary to theoretical predictions, there were no group differences in posttask depression. The second experiment involved college males and females. Neither anxiety nor depression (assessed immediately following exercise) was differentially affected by varying the intensity of exercise, that is, 17 min bouts at about 118 bpm or about 135 bpm.

In closing this section, I would like to comment on one other paper in the exercise literature that is relevant to future research directions. Cameron and Hudson (7) performed a questionnaire study in an attempt to discover whether certain groups

Table 72.2 Moderating Role of Baseline Mood

Study	*n*, gender, *M* age (years), fitness	Design	Measures	Major findings
Blumenthal et al. (3)	70, male, 54, 22.59 $ml \cdot kg^{-1} \cdot min^{-1}$	Randomized between subjects design with cardiac patients, 2 groups, 12 weeks; 30 to 40 min at > 40% HRR or > 70% HRR	SCL-90, CDC-D, STAI	Neither group changed as a function of exercise; subjects' affect was normal prior to beginning of study
Lennox et al. (22)	47, both, ~45, ~10 min on Bruce test	Randomized between subjects design, 3 groups, 13 weeks; 30-min stimulus phase at 70% to 80% HRmax; light weights and volleyball, wait-list control	MAACL and DACL given 7 days prior to and following exercise	No differences; normal mood scores at pretest
Sexton et al. (43)	52, both, ~37, ~30	Psychiatric patients given therapy and randomized to either walk (comfortable pace) or jog program (70% HRmax); treatment lasted 8 weeks with 6-month follow-up	STAI, SCL-90, BDI	Joggers made greater gains in aerobic fitness although both groups had improved affect; higher dropout in jogging condition

Note. n = number in sample; M = mean; $ml \cdot kg^{-1} \cdot min^{-1}$ = milliliters per kilogram per minute; HRR = heart rate reserve; SCL-90 = symptom checklist-90; CDC-D = Centers for Disease Control-Depression Scale; STAI = state/trait anxiety inventory; HRmax = maximal heart rate; MAACL = multiple affect adjective checklist; DACL = depression adjective checklist; BDI = Beck depression inventory.

Table 72.3 Negative Effects of Overload

Study	*n*, gender, *M* age (years), fitness	Design	Measures	Major findings
Cameron & Hudson (7)	82, both, 34.4, none reported	Questionnaire study; subjects with anxiety disorders and healthy subjects were asked to recall the anxiety felt with five different levels of exercise.	6-point unipolar anxiety measure	13 of 66 (20%) reported that exercise increased anxiety in a dose-dependent manner
Morgan et al. (29, Exp. 1)	120, males, faculty, none reported	Randomized posttest-only group between subjects; four conditions: progressive exercise up to 150, 160, 170, or 180 bpm	DACL, 5-min postexercise	No differences between groups
Morgan et al. (29, Exp. 2)	36, both, students, none reported	Randomized posttest-only group between subjects; three conditions, 17 min: 3.5 mph, 0% grade (HR = ~118) or 3.5 mph, 5% grade (HR = ~135), and control	IPAT anxiety and DACL given immediately after	No differences between groups
Morgan et al. (27)	15 to 130, both, college competitive swimmers	Reported on seven retrospective studies; subjects given POMS at various points in season; natural increase in training across a 6-month period. Used a general university control in one analysis to rule out effects of academics.	POMS	Total mood disturbance highest when training was most severe; recovered with taper; depression and anxiety was up and vigor was down; not caused by academics
Morgan et al. (28)	12, male, college competitive swimmers	Subjects swam an average of 9,000 m/day for 10 days at 94% of $\dot{V}O_2max$ after season was complete.	POMS daily well-being	By Day 5, TMD was up; those subjects with stressed physiology also had higher TMDs
Steptoe & Cox (46)	32, female, 18 to 23, 2.99 $L \cdot min^{-1}$ (fit) 2.24 $L \cdot min^{-1}$ (unfit)	Subjects completed single session of 4 trials: 100 W and 25 W both with and without music.	Modified POMS right after trials	100 W yielded more tension and anxiety; 25 W produced more vigor and exhilaration

Note. *n* = number in sample; *M* = mean; bpm = beats per minute; min = minute; mph = miles per hour; HR = heart rate; DACL = depression adjective checklist; POMS = Profile of Mood States; m = meters; $\dot{V}O_2max$ = maximal volume of oxygen consumed per minute during exercise; TMD = total mood disturbance; $L \cdot min^{-1}$ = liters per minute; W = watts.

of individuals may be psychologically sensitive to physiological changes that occur with exercise. These investigators simply asked subjects whether they had ever experienced anxiety in conjunction with exercise of varying intensities. Thirteen of 66 patients with documented anxiety disorders reported exercise-induced anxiety that was dose-dependent, a trend that was most pronounced for individuals prone to panic attacks. Despite the crude experimental approach taken in this research, the issue of exercise sensitivity is an important one given the frequency with which exercise is prescribed for the treatment of both anxiety and depression. Parenthetically, our clinical exercise laboratory at Wake Forest University has conducted well over 1,000 graded exercise tests on patients with documented cardiovascular disease. To my knowledge, we have never had a patient experience an acute episode of anxiety following testing, even though some of these individuals have documented anxiety disorders.

Summary

Perhaps the most useful outcome from reviewing the extant literature on dose–response effects for exercise on affective functioning is that it reveals an important void in the developing field of exercise psychology. Of those studies involving chronic exercise, the most significant contribution to date is the work by Moses et al. (30). The notion that lower levels of aerobic exercise may have greater psychosocial payoffs than more traditional prescriptions (i.e., 30 min at 70% $\dot{V}O_2max$, three times per week) cannot be ignored from a clinical perspective. In fact, the research by Sexton et al. (43) suggests that there may be negative effects from more demanding exercise regimens in that they may lead to higher dropout rates.

Recent meta-analyses of the anxiety (33) and depression (31) research are mixed when it comes to any conclusions concerning dose–response relationships; however, it may be that dose–response effects do not generalize across different outcomes. For example, the data of Petruzzello, Landers, Hatfield, Kubitz, and Salazar (33) suggest that intensity of exercise does not have a differential impact on reductions seen in state or trait anxiety, whereas North et al. (31) concluded that there was insufficient data for any analysis of how exercise intensity might influence depression. Although I do not question the value of the meta-analytic approach taken by Petruzzello et al. (33), even the authors recognize that it is not an easy task to classify existing studies as to exercise intensity (personal communication with S. Petruzzello, January 1991). There is a great deal of method variance in its calculation, and few published studies provide adequate manipulation checks on target HR ranges.

On the subject of duration, neither quantitative review found that the length of individual exercise sessions influences effect sizes (ES). It is important to note, however, that the lowest category considered in the anxiety analysis (33) ranged from 0 to 20 min. Close examination of the studies in this category reveals that 20 min was the modal treatment manipulation. Thus, it is difficult to say what the impact might be of very brief exercise bouts (e.g., 10 min). Furthermore, from the North et al. (31) review it is not clear how the authors tested for the moderating influence of exercise duration on depression.

One area where the meta-analyses on anxiety and depression do seem to agree is the importance of the length of training. The ESs for both trait anxiety and depression are largest when programs exceed about 4 months (see Figures 72.2 and 72.3).

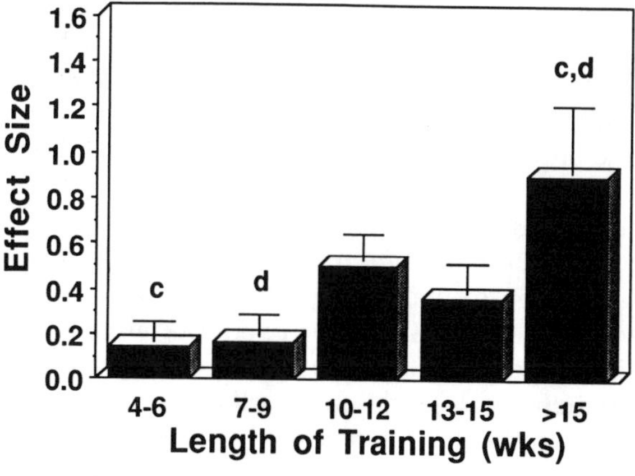

Figure 72.2 The effects of length of training on anxiety. Adapted from Petruzzello et al. (33).

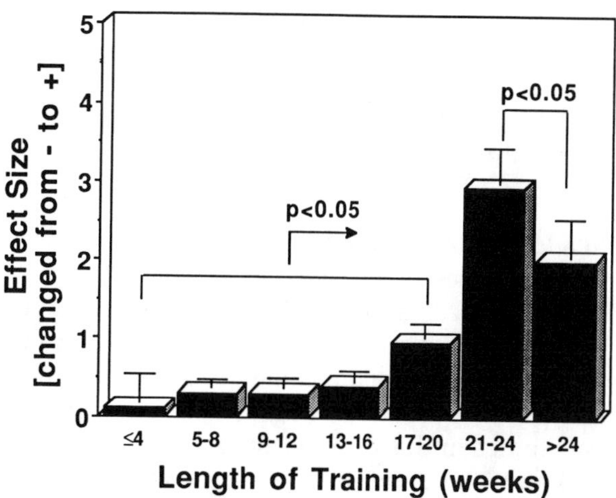

Figure 72.3 The effects of length of training on depression. Adapted from North et al. (31).

Yet there is little question that acute bouts of exercise can be effective in reducing state anxiety and, to the surprise of some (11), produce ESs for depression that are significant (ES = −0.31), albeit about half the magnitude found with chronic training (ES = −0.59).

Finally, I could not locate a single study that addressed the potential role of varying doses of exercise on self-esteem or more specific forms such as body esteem. There is, however, a very intriguing unpublished report by Rodin (40) at Yale University. In this study, Rodin randomly assigned unfit subjects (i.e., individuals who were not involved in any systematic exercise for at least 2 years), to four, 12-week treatment conditions: (a) exercise, (b) exercise with efficacy feedback, (c) language training, and (d) language training with efficacy feedback. The efficacy manipulation involved repeated information that "what they were doing was something difficult, something that they should feel proud about, and something that few others could do quite as well" (p. 12). The results were quite striking in that either exercise or the language treatment when combined with the high-efficacy manipulation caused greater changes in self-esteem, mood, reductions in stress or anxiety, and improved performance on cognitive tasks than the conditions lacking such feedback. However, there was a trend on some measures for the feedback to be more effective with exercise than the language treatment, suggesting that exercise provides an ideal climate for psychosocial interventions. Although these data must be regarded as preliminary, they do offer further support to my position that the affect-related outcomes of a particular dose of activity are dependent, in part, on the exerciser as an active agent. What people believe they are doing or have done is extremely important in determining dose–response relationships from a psychosocial perspective.

Physiological Outcomes and Weight Control

In addition to the potential moderating effect that varying doses of physical activity have on self-reported affect, several investigators have examined the influence of intensity or duration of training on physiological outcomes, and a single study has been published on weight control. The principal studies in this area are summarized in Tables 72.4 and 72.5 under two headings: (a) the effects of varying doses of acute exercise on electromyographic activity (EMG), central nervous system (CNS) activity (Hoffman reflex), and psychosocial stress reactivity, or (b) the effects of varying doses of chronic exercise on psychosocial stress reactivity and weight loss.

EMG and CNS Function

There are only two dose–response investigations that I could locate on EMG or CNS function; both elected to manipulate the intensity of exercise while maintaining a constant duration (either 15 or 20 min; see Table 72.4). As part of an EMG study conducted in 1972 deVries and Adams (10) had subjects walk for 15 min at an intensity of either 100 bpm or 120 bpm. These conditions were contrasted with drug therapy and an attention control group to determine whether the intensity of exercise was a determining factor in postexercise EMG. The results of this research demonstrated that exercise at 100 bpm was more effective in lowering EMG than an attention control rest period. Although the EMG data following exercise at 120 bpm did not differ from the control group when evaluated at the established experiment error rate, these data were statistically significant at the $p < .10$ level. Parenthetically, deVries and Adams's study did not provide a strong test of dose effects because of the similarity between the two treatment groups.

In 1983 Bulbulian and Darabos (6) published an investigation that examined the effects of two diverse exercise intensities (40% or 75% $\dot{V}O_2$max) on an index of CNS function—the Hoffman reflex. As shown in Figure 72.4, the largest change (reduction) in the postexercise Hmax:Mmax ratio occurred following the 75% $\dot{V}O_2$max condition, whereas the smallest change was reported for the control condition; the 40% $\dot{V}O_2$max condition produced a response that was intermediate. If one

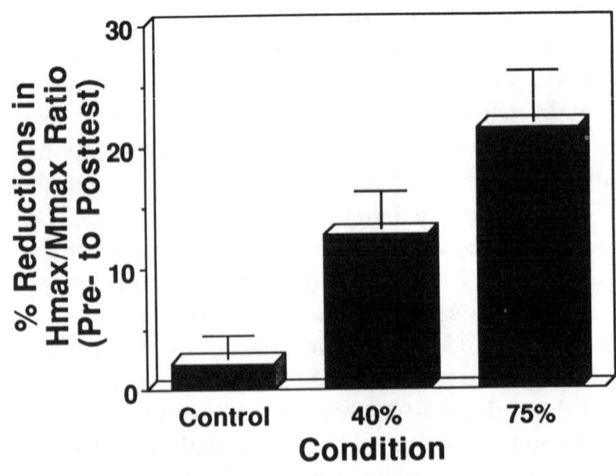

Figure 72.4 The effects of different doses of acute exercise on the Hoffman Reflex. Adapted from Bulbulian and Darabos (6).

Table 72.4 Effects of Dose of Acute Exercise on EMG, CNS Activity, and Psychosocial Stress Reactivity

Study	*n*, gender, *M* age (years), fitness (ml · kg^{-1} · min^{-1})	Design	Measures	Major findings
Bulbulian & Darabos (6)	10, both, 28.7, 55.8	Within subjects, three 20-min conditions: no exercise, 40% $\dot{V}O_2$max, and 75% $\dot{V}O_2$max	Hoffman reflex	10 min after treatments the Hoffman reflex lowest after 75% bout
deVries & Adams (10)	10, both, 62.6, none reported	Within subjects, five conditions: meprobamate, placebo, 15-min walk at 100 bpm and 120 bpm, and 15-min reading control	EMG 30 min, 1 hr, 1 1/2 hr after treatments	Walking at 100 bpm led to lower EMG than control; 120-bpm trial reached $p < .1$ level.
McGowan et al. (25)	12, male, 21 to 29, 47.04	Within subjects: attention control, 15 min at 40%, 55%, and 70% $\dot{V}O_2$max; 15-min rest followed by mental stressor	EMG, HR; mood assessed after stressor	No differences between groups on any of the measures
Rejeski et al. (36)	12, male, 30, 58.8	Within subjects, three conditions: attention control, 30 min at 50% $\dot{V}O_2$max, and 60 min at 80% $\dot{V}O_2$max; 30-min rest followed by mental stressor	BP, HR; POMS given after acute stressor	Lowest reactivity in MAP following heavy trial; highest reactivity in control condition; light exercise intermediate
Roy & Steptoe (in press)	30, male, 21.3, ~44	Between subjects, 3 conditions: 20 min at 25 W, 20 min at 100 W, and attention control; 20-min rest followed by mental stressor	BP, HR, RR, SCL, baroreflex	HR was blunted in a work-dependent fashion.

Note. EMG = electromyography; CNS = central nervous system; *n* = number in sample; *M* = mean; ml · kg^{-1} · min^{-1} = milliliters per kilogram per minute; min = minute; $\dot{V}O_2$max = maximal volume of oxygen consumed per minute during exercise; bpm = beats per minute; *p* = probability; HR = heart rate; BP = blood pressure; POMS = Profile of Mood States; MAP = mean arterial pressure; W = watts; RR = respiratory rate; SCL = skin conductance level.

accepts that the Hoffman reflex is an index of muscular tension or stress, then the implication in these data is that the therapeutic benefits of relatively brief exercise (20 min) are dependent on a fairly demanding exercise stimulus.

Acute Exercise and Stress Reactivity

The second group of investigations has examined the effects of acute exercise on psychophysiological stress reactivity. The earliest study in this category conducted by McGowan, Robertson, and Epstein (25) exercised subjects at 40%, 55%, and 75% $\dot{V}O_2$max for 15 min and included an attention control group. These manipulations were followed by a brief period of rest and exposure to a mental challenge. When contrasted with the control condition, there was no evidence from the physiological data (EMG or HR) or an assessment of mood states taken during a recovery period following the stressor that any of the exercise bouts blunted reactivity to acute stress. As recognized by the authors, however, the use of HR as an index of cardiovascular reactivity following acute exercise does have several limitations.

Recently, in my own laboratory (35) we had trained cyclists participate in three counterbalanced treatment conditions: (a) an attention control, (b) exercise at 50% $\dot{V}O_2$max for 30 min, and (c) exercise at 80% $\dot{V}O_2$max for 60 min. These manipulations were followed by 30 min of rest and participation in a brief bout of mental stress. As seen in Figure 72.5, there were clear dose–response effects for mean arterial pressure during psychosocial threat that are similar to the resting Hoffman reflex data reported by Bulbulian and Darabos (6). These results have since been replicated and extended in a group of less fit individuals (42). In this latter study, Roy and Steptoe manipulated intensity while holding duration constant at 20 min (see Table 72.4). Ebbesen, Prkachin, and Mills (12) recently failed to support a dose–response effect between varying levels of acute exercise and stress-induced elevation in blood pressure; however, their data may be influenced by a ceiling effect in that the lowest level of exercise was 84% of maximal heart rate for 1 hr.

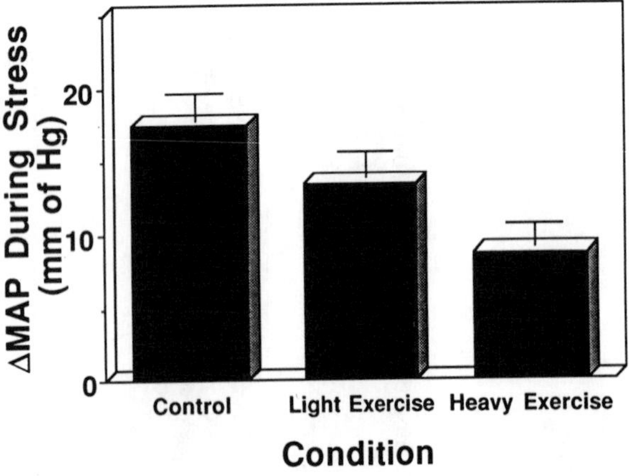

Figure 72.5 The effects of different doses of acute exercise on blood pressure. Adapted from Rejeski et al. (36).

Chronic Exercise

There are three studies involving chronic exercise that have addressed very different questions regarding how exercise dosage might influence psychosocial outcomes. The first, conducted by Steptoe, Moses, Matthews, and Edwards (47), examined the effects that two levels of exercise training have on various psychosocial outcomes during mental stress (see Table 72.5). After 10 weeks of training, neither moderate- nor high-intensity exercise regimens altered physiological responses to acute stress reactivity when contrasted with an attention control condition. However, in cross-sectional comparisons on pretest data, level of physical conditioning did moderate stress reactivity. Thus, either these cross-sectional comparisons reflect genetic influence or else duration of training is a key variable for consideration in future research.

The second study involves the stress-buffering capacity of exercise on self-reported illness in female children. In a 9-month prospective study, Brown and Siegel (5) found an interaction between amount of exercise and levels of stress on illness reporting. Specifically, exercise only reduced illness reporting in children who were under high stress; children under low stress reported a low incidence of illness irrespective of their level of activity. Unfortunately, the measurement of exercise in this study was crude in that children listed the total time in hours per week spent in various fitness or sport-related activities. Despite this limitation an additional analysis of interest is one in which the authors partitioned the data by anaerobic or aerobic activities. Both groups of tasks yielded the same stress-buffering potential against self-reported illness. This is interesting in light of a recent randomized trial on depression in psychiatric patients (23). In this study anaerobic work (weight training) without change in estimated $\dot{V}O_2$max lowered depression to the same degree as an aerobic program where estimated $\dot{V}O_2$max was increased.

The final study in this grouping involves the complex role that dose of activity may play in

Table 72.5 Effects of Dose of Chronic Training on Psychosocial Stress Reactivity and Weight Loss

Study	*n*, gender, *M* age (years), fitness	Design	Measures	Major findings
Brown & Siegel (5)	364, female, 7 to 11, varied	9-month prospective study; pretest data on exercise and stress; posttest assessment of exercise, stress, and self-reported illness	Self-reported illness	Exercise has stress-buffering potential on self-reported illness that appears dose-related.
Epstein et al. (14)	42, both, 8 to 12, ~32% overweight	Crossed dietary restrictions with either programmed aerobic exercise or unstructured, discontinuous fitness and sport activities; intervention lasted for 8 weeks, followed for 17 months	Weight, BMI	Equivalent weight and BMI changes at 8 weeks in lifestyle and aerobic groups; lifestyle better at follow-ups
Steptoe et al. (47)	75, both, 18 to 60, 40.2 $ml \cdot kg^{-1} \cdot min^{-1}$ (fit), 29.1 $ml \cdot kg^{-1} \cdot min^{-1}$ (unfit)	Randomized between subjects design, 10 weeks: 30 min 70% to 75% HRmax, 20 min at 60% to 65% HRmax, attention control or wait-list control	BP, HR, RR, SCL, O_2	No effects on reactivity to problem-solving task

Note. n = number in sample; M = mean; BMI = body mass index; $ml \cdot kg^{-1} \cdot min^{-1}$ = milliliters per kilogram per minute; HRmax = maximal heart rate; BP = blood pressure; HR = heart rate; RR = respiratory rate; SCL = skin conductance level; O_2 = oxygen.

weight management—an important health behavior (14). In this study obese children were randomly assigned to either programmed aerobic exercise or a self-selected multiactivity intervention that was characterized by low-intensity, discontinuous bouts of physical activity. The common ingredient to both treatments was that children were required to achieve equivalent daily caloric expenditures. Despite greater initial aerobic gains made by the programmed group, Figure 72.6 illustrates that after 8 weeks of treatment the two

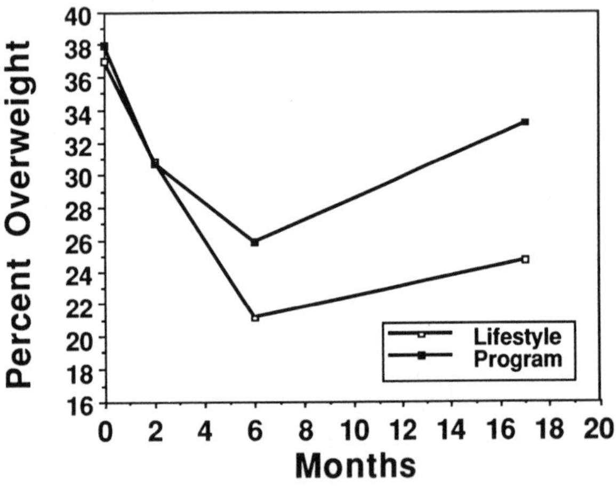

Figure 72.6 Long-term effects of physical activity on weight loss. Adapted from Epstein et al. (14).

groups made nearly identical reductions in weight. More important, after several months of follow-up testing, compliance to the exercise therapy was better in the less structured and lower intensity treatment protocol. In fact, at 17 months those in the structured aerobic exercise had regained most of the weight lost in the initial 8-week period.

Summary

Although it is premature to reach any definitive conclusions regarding the effects of varying doses of acute or chronic exercise on physiological outcomes or weight management, there are several results from the previously reviewed literature that deserve emphasis. First, the Bulbulian and Darabos (6) research argues for the position that exercise performed at high intensity has a more dramatic effect on resting CNS function than low-intensity exercise. In a recent meta-analysis, however, Petruzzello et al. (33) concluded that physiological indexes of anxiety do not appear to be moderated by the intensity of work. This contradiction might lead one to question whether the finding by Bulbulian and Darabos (6) was due to a Type I error. Conversely, the conclusion reached in the meta-analysis by Petruzzello et al. (33) must be viewed in light of several limitations: (a) The ES for exercise intensity with the physiological indexes of anxiety represents a composite of 10 different measures, (b) the blood pressure data did not include the rather extensive literature on exercise hypotension following acute exercise, and (c) it is important to underscore that the quantitative analysis of exercise intensity involved contrasting data from different experiments.

Second, the role that intensity of acute exercise has on cardiovascular responses to subsequent psychosocial stress is compelling in light of the link between acute stress reactivity and various cardiovascular disorders (20), however, there is no support for the external validity of these findings. More important, the work by Brown and Siegel (5) as well as Epstein et al. (14) provides support for the position that dose–response relationships depend on the outcome and population under consideration. This point is reinforced by a study that we conducted several years ago, a joint venture of the cardiac rehabilitation programs at Duke University and Wake Forest University. In that study (4) cardiac rehabilitation patients were randomly assigned to either light (less than 40% symptom-limited $\dot{V}O_2max$) or heavy (greater than 70% symptom-limited $\dot{V}O_2max$) exercise. After 3 months of training, both groups made equivalent gains in symptom-limited $\dot{V}O_2max$ and there was no evidence that intensity of exercise had a differential effect on various psychosocial outcomes (3).

Finally, although the research described in Tables 72.4 and 72.5 did not manipulate duration of training, the meta-analysis performed by Petruzzello et al. (33) did conclude that exercise below 20 min in duration produced a larger ES (ES = 0.78) than studies where the duration was 31 to 40 min (ES = 0.31) or more than 41 min (ES = 0.28). I think we should be cautious in interpreting this result for two reasons. First, as expected, reactivity data from our own laboratory (35) as well as Steptoe's (42) has shown increases in post-exercise HR following more demanding work, yet greater decreases in blood pressure as exercise intensity increases. Thus, it is inappropriate to aggregate physiological measures in examining dose–response effects. And second, there is a more basic issue of the psychological meaning that we should ascribe to physiological data that are collected in conjunction with acute exercise. Conceivably, mild elevation in sympathetic nervous system activity 10 to 20 min postexercise may occur in conjunction with positive affective states (36). In other words, following acute bouts of exercise, there can be considerable ambiguity regarding the psychological meaning of somatic states, a point that again emphasizes the importance of characterizing the subject as an active agent.

Concluding Comments

Although I realize that we have to be cautious in reaching any definitive conclusions regarding the relationships between various doses of exercise and the responses identified in Figure 72.1, there are several conceptually based propositions that emerge from this review. These have implications for future research, the scientific objectives of this conference, and issues in clinical exercise settings. First, the stimulus properties inherent to the concept *dose of exercise* are enormously complex. From an objective viewpoint, there are different types of activities with varied physiologic demands, numerous permutations of intensity, duration, and frequency, as well as effects from acute versus chronic training. Moreover, when people exercise they are doing far more than simply moving physically. As numerous studies suggest (14,34,40), the social environment provided with exercise training (e.g., enjoyment, peer support, or interactions with exercise leaders) may be as important to psychosocial outcomes as the activity itself. This variance, a critical aspect of defining the dose of any physical activity, must be taken seriously in future programs of research; unless of course we adhere to the principle of Cartesian dualism and choose to ignore the external validity of our data.

Second, future research must acknowledge (a) the broad range of responses that deserve consideration, (b) individual differences, and (c) the inevitable existence of complex biopsychosocial interactions. If we accept these points, then it follows that no single dose of activity will ever have universal appeal for every desired program objective (3,30). As Epstein's (14) data indicate, there are instances in which discontinuous, free-living, multiactivity programs are likely to produce maximum yield, particularly when the objective is long-range maintenance of an effect.

On the other hand, there are those cases in which people are likely to benefit from more focused, demanding, continuous activity (35,42). This position is certainly consistent with other psychological literature that has recognized the importance of individual need states and the merits of studying behavior at a specific rather than general unit of analysis (41). It also has strong implications for the methods employed in exercise prescription. For example, in the context of behavioral medicine, it makes little sense to focus on an optimal aerobic training stimulus when the physical dysfunction people experience is related to activities of daily living that are tied to inadequacies in balance, flexibility, or strength.

Third, this chapter has emphasized that the social psychology of the individual organism is critical to an understanding of dose–response relationships. Certainly Morgan's 1985 review (26) dealing with psychogenic factors and exercise metabolism is supportive of this position as is my own research on ratings of perceived exertion (RPE) (34). In fact Hardy, Hall, and Presholdt (17) have published a very interesting paper on RPE that serves to underscore the potential role played by social influence. In Experiment 1 subjects exercised either with or without a coactor. At the same relative work load (i.e., 50% $\dot{V}O_2$max), subjects reported lower RPEs when exercising in the presence of another performer as compared to the alone condition. Furthermore in Experiment 2, subjects exercised in the presence of a coactor who either gave low-intensity or high-intensity nonverbal cues of exertion. The lowest RPEs were reported in the low-intensity condition. Clearly social cognition is relevant to the definition that exercisers give to any dose of activity. Moreover, these definitions may differ from that of the investigator or health care provider.

Finally, there has been far too much emphasis placed on the role of changes in maximal aerobic power as the key exercise manipulation for chronic dose–response studies of psychosocial outcomes (23,40). In fact, although genetic influences can serve as powerful determinants of fitness- and health-related behavior, I believe it is misguided to theorize that explanations for psychosocial outcomes will ultimately be reduced to some physiological system (e.g., cardiac-related cortical activity) or neurochemical activity (see Peele [32]). Rather, the particular biological input to improved psychosocial functioning varies with the response or the individual exerciser. Hence, there is no primacy intended for variables in a biopsychosocial model of health and fitness; rather, a key assumption is the notion of reciprocal determinism (1).

References

1. Bandura, A. Self-efficacy mechanisms in physiological activation and health-promoting behavior. In: Madden, J., ed. Neurobiology of learning, emotion, and affect. New York: Raven Press; 1991:229-269.
2. Berger, B.G.; Owen, D.R. Stress reduction and mood enhancement in four exercise modes: Swimming, body conditioning, hatha yoga,

and fencing. Res. Q. Exerc. Sport. 59:148-159; 1988.

3. Blumenthal, J.A.; Emery, C.F.; Rejeski, W.J. The effects of exercise training on psychosocial functioning after myocardial infarction. J. Cardiopul. Rehabil. 8:183-193; 1988.
4. Blumenthal, J.A.; Rejeski, W.J.; Walsh-Riddle, M.; Emery, C.F.; Miller, H.; Roark, S.; Ribisl, P.M.; Morris, P.B.; Brubaker, P.; Williams, R.S. Comparison of high- and low-intensity exercise training after acute myocardial infarction. Am. J. Cardiol. 61:26-30; 1988.
5. Brown, J.D.; Siegel, J.M. Exercise as a buffer of life stress: A prospective study of adolescent health. Health Psychol. 7:341-353; 1988.
6. Bulbulian, R.; Darabos, B.L. Motor neuron excitability: The Hoffman reflex following exercise of low and high intensity. Med. Sci. Sports Exerc. 18:697-702; 1986.
7. Cameron, O.G.; Hudson, C.J. Influence of exercise on anxiety level in patients with anxiety disorders. Psychosomatics. 27:720-723; 1986.
8. Cramer, S.R.; Nieman, D.C.; Lee, J.W. The effects of moderate exercise training on psychological well-being and mood state in women. J. Psychosom. Res. 35:437-449; 1991.
9. Crews, D.J.; Landers, D.M. A meta-analytic review of aerobic fitness and reactivity to psychosocial stressors. Med. Sci. Sports Exerc. 19:S114-S120; 1987.
10. deVries, H.A.; Adams, G.M. Electromyographic comparison of single doses of exercise and meprobamate as to effects on muscular relaxation. Am. J. Phys. Med. 51:130-141; 1972.
11. Dunn, A.L.; Dishman, R.K. In: Holloszy, J.O., ed. Exercise and sport sciences reviews. Baltimore: Williams & Wilkins; 1991:41-98.
12. Ebbesen, B.L.; Prkachin, K.M.; Mills, D.E. Effects of acute exercise on cardiovascular reactivity. J. Behav. Med.; [In press].
13. Engel, G.L. The need for a new medical model: A challenge for biomedicine. Science. 196:129-136; 1980.
14. Epstein, L.H.; Wing, R.R.; Koeske, R.; Ossip, D.; Beck, S. A comparison of lifestyle change and programmed aerobic exercise on weight and fitness changes in children. Behav. Ther. 13:651-665; 1982.
15. Ewart, C.K.; Taylor, C.B.; Reese, L.B.; Debusk, R.F. Effects of early postmyocardial infarction exercise testing on self-perception and subsequent physical activity. Am. J. Cardiol. 51:1076-1080; 1983.
16. Farrell, P.A.; Gustafson, A.B.; Morgan, W.P.; Pert, C.B. Enkephalins, catecholamines, and psychological mood alterations: Effects of prolonged exercise. Med. Sci. Sports Exerc. 19:347-353; 1987.
17. Hardy, C.J.; Hall, E.G.; Presholdt, P.H. The mediational role of social influence in the perception of exertion. J. Sport Psychol. 8:88-104; 1986.
18. Hart, E.A.; Leary, M.R.; Rejeski, W.J. The measurement of social physique anxiety. J. Sport Exerc. Psychol. 11:94-104; 1989.
19. Kenyon, G.S. A conceptual model for characterizing physical activity. Res. Q. 39:96-105; 1966.
20. Krantz, D.S.; Manuck, S.B. Acute psychophysiologic reactivity and risk of cardiovascular disease. Psychol. Bull. 96:435-464; 1984.
21. Leary, M.R.; Kowalski, R.M. Impression management: A literature review and two-component model. Psychol. Bull. 107:34-47; 1990.
22. Lennox, S.S.; Bedell, J.R.; Stone, A.A. The effect of exercise on normal mood. J. Psychosom. Med. 34:629-636; 1990.
23. Martinsen, E.W.; Hoffart, A.; Solberg, O. Comparing aerobic with nonaerobic forms of exercise in the treatment of clinical depression: A randomized trial. Compr. Psychiatry. 30:324-331; 1989.
24. McAuley, E.; Courneya, K.S.; Lettunich, J. Effects of acute and long-term exercise on self-efficacy responses in sedentary middle-aged males and females. Gerontologist. 31:534-542; 1991.
25. McGowan, C.R.; Robertson, R.J.; Epstein, L.H. The effect of bicycle ergometer exercise at varying intensities on the heart rate, EMG and mood state responses to a mental arithmetic stressor. Res. Q. Exerc. Sport. 56:131-137; 1985.
26. Morgan, W.P. Psychogenic factors and exercise metabolism: A review. Med. Sci. Sports Exerc. 17:309-316; 1985.
27. Morgan, W.P.; Brown, D.R.; Raglin, J.S.; O'Connor, P.J.; Ellickson, K.A. Psychological monitoring of overtraining and staleness. Br. J. Sports Med. 21:107-114; 1987.
28. Morgan, W.P.; Costill, D.L.; Flynn, M.G.; Raglin, J.S.; O'Connor, P.J. Mood disturbance following increased training in swimmers. Med. Sci. Sports Exerc. 20:408-414; 1988.
29. Morgan, W.P.; Roberts, J.A.; Feinerman, A.D. Psychologic effect of acute physical activity. Arch. Phys. Med. Rehabil. 52:422-425; 1971.
30. Moses, J.; Steptoe, A.; Matthews, A.; Edwards, S. The effects of exercise training on mental well-being in the normal population: A controlled trial. J. Psychosom. Res. 33:47-61; 1989.
31. North, T.C.; McCullagh, P.; Vu Tran, Z. Effect of exercise on depression. In: Pandolf, K.B., ed. Exercise and sport sciences reviews. Baltimore: Williams & Wilkins; 1990:379-415.

32. Peele, S. Can biochemistry eliminate addiction, mental illness, and pain. Am. Psychol. 36:807-817; 1981.
33. Petruzzello, S.J.; Landers, D.M.; Hatfield, B.D.; Kubitz, K.A.; Salazar, W. A meta-analysis on the anxiety-reducing effects of acute and chronic exercise. Sports Med. 11:143-182; 1991.
34. Rejeski, W.J. Perceived exertion: An active or passive process? J. Sport Exerc. Psychol. 7:371-378; 1985.
35. Rejeski, W.J.; Gregg, E.; Thompson, A.; Berry, M. The effects of varying doses of acute aerobic exercise on psychophysiological stress responses in highly trained cyclists. J. Sport Exerc. Psychol. 13:188-199; 1991.
36. Rejeski, W.J.; Hardy, C.J.; Shaw, J. Psychometric confounds of assessing state anxiety in conjunction with acute bouts of vigorous exercise. J. Sport Exerc. Psychol. 13:65-74; 1991.
37. Rejeski, W.J.; Lowe, C.A. Nonverbal expression of causally relevant information. Per. Soc. Psychol. Bull. 6:436-440; 1980.
38. Rejeski, W.J.; Morley, D.; Sotile, W. Cardiac rehabilitation: A conceptual framework for psychological assessment. J. Cardiopulm. Rehabil. 5:172-180; 1985.
39. Rejeski, W.J.; Ribisl, P.M. Expected task duration and perceived effort: An attributional analysis. J. Sport Exerc. Psychol. 2:227-236; 1980.
40. Rodin, J. The psychological effects of exercise. New Haven, CT: Yale University; 1988. Unpublished manuscript.
41. Rotter, J.B.; Chance, J.E.; Phares, E.J. Applications of a social learning theory of personality. New York: Holt, Rinehart & Winston; 1972.
42. Roy, M.; Steptoe, A. The inhibition of cardiovascular responses to mental stress following aerobic exercise. Psychophysiology; [In press].
43. Sexton, H.; Maere, A.; Dahl, N.H. Exercise intensity and reduction in neurotic symptoms. Acta Psychiatr. Scand. 80:231-235; 1989.
44. Silberstein, L.R.; Mishkind, M.E.; Striegel-Moore, R.H.; Timko, C.; Rodin, J. Men and their bodies: A comparison of homosexual and heterosexual men. Psychosom. Med. 51:337-346; 1989.
45. Steptoe, A.; Bolton, J. The short-term influence of high and low physical exercise on mood. Psychol. Health. 2:91-106; 1988.
46. Steptoe, A.; Cox, S. Acute effects of aerobic exercise on mood. Health Psychol. 7:329-340; 1988.
47. Steptoe, A.; Moses, J.; Matthews, A.; Edwards, S. Aerobic fitness, physical activity, and psychophysiological reactions to mental stress. Psychophysiology. 27:264-274; 1990.